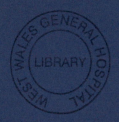

PEDIATRIC
Ophthalmology
and Strabismus

PEDIATRIC
Ophthalmology
and Strabismus

THIRD EDITION

Edited by

David Taylor FRCS FRCP FRCOphth DSc(Med)
Professor of Pediatric Ophthalmology, Institute of Child Health and
Consultant Ophthalmologist, Great Ormond Street Hospital for Children
London, UK

and

Creig S Hoyt MD
The Theresa and Wayne Caygill Professor and Chairman of the
Department of Ophthalmology; Director of the Beckman Vision Center,
University of California San Francisco, California, USA

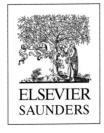

ELSEVIER
SAUNDERS

Edinburgh   London   New York   Oxford   Philadelphia   St Louis   Sydney   Toronto   2005

SAUNDERS
An imprint of Elsevier Limited

First edition 1990
Second edition 1997
Third edition 2005
    Reprinted 2005

ISBN 0 7020 2708 1

British Library Cataloguing in Publication Data
A catalogue record for this book is available from the British Library

Library of Congress Cataloguing in Publication Data
A catalogue record for this book is available from the Library of Congress

Notice
Medical knowledge is constantly changing. Standard safety precautions must be followed, but as new research and clinical experience broaden our knowledge, changes in treatment and drug therapy may become necessary r appropriate. Readers are advised to check the most current product information provided by the manufacturer of each drug to be administered to verify the recommended dose, the method and duration of administration, and contraindications. It is the responsibility of the practitioner, relying on experience and knowledge of the patient, to determine dosages and the best treatment for each individual patient. Neither the Publisher nor the editors assume any liability for any injury and/or damage to persons or property arising from this publication.
The Publisher

ELSEVIER   your source for books,
            journals and multimedia
            in the health sciences
www.elsevierhealth.com

Working together to grow
libraries in developing countries

www.elsevier.com | www.bookaid.org | www.sabre.org

ELSEVIER   BOOK AID   Sabre Foundation
            International

Commissioning Editor: Paul Fam
Project Development Manager: Shuet-Kei Cheung
Project Manager: Jess Thompson
Illustration Manager: Mick Ruddy
Design Manager: Jayne Jones
Illustrator: Martin Woodward

Printed in China
Last digit is the print number : 9 8 7 6 5 4 3 2

The
publisher's
policy is to use
**paper manufactured
from sustainable forests**

CONTENTS

v

CONTENTS

Section 5: Selected Topics in Pediatric Ophthalmology

Section 6: Eye Movements and Strabismus

CONTENTS

Section 7: Appendix – Problems

vii

FOREWORD

This unique book presents a whole panorama of present pediatric ophthalmology and strabismus.

Based on Taylor's *Pediatric Ophthalmology*, the text has been extensively updated, enriched, and revised with an additional section on Strabismus. With a large variety of clarifying illustrations and a selected bibliography, this masterpiece is an invaluable source of knowledge and reference for libraries and ophthalmic offices worldwide.

We ophthalmologists thank the authors for their vital contribution to this specialty.

Alberto O Ciancia MD
2004

Eight years have elapsed since the second edition of *Pediatric Ophthalmology* was published. During this period there has been an exponential outpouring of clinical discoveries and innovative research, making mandatory the compilation of a new edition, which we now welcome. Creig Hoyt, a major contributor to the two previous editions has joined David Taylor as co-editor of this new edition, in which 108 authors contribute 122 separate pediatric ophthalmology topics, 25 of which are new. Most of the original chapters have been entirely rewritten.

A major part of pediatric ophthalmology involves the management of strabismus. This section has therefore, been expanded from 5 to 18 chapters. It now includes all the recent findings of neuroscience that address the issue of amblyopia and strabismus and places them in clinical perspective. There is also new knowledge about extraocular rectus muscle pulleys and the scientific basis of strabismus.

Both editors are known for their clinical acumen, their insistence on remaining current clinically and for expanding research arenas. Nevertheless, their dedication to their patients is paramount. Their approach is reflected in their choice of author and subject matter. Several chapters focus on addressing the patients' needs, attending to the patient as a whole, and communicating sensitively to parents and child.

The current edition is the combined work of gifted, investigative, dedicated clinicians and perceptive, enlightened and energetic editors. The acquisition of new medical knowledge accelerates at a pace defying total comprehension. One can only salute the multiple authors who have crystallized such an enormous amount of material in their quality works collected in this text. Readers will appreciate their efforts and patients will be grateful for their continued commitment.

This edition, now entitled *Pediatric Ophthalmology and Strabismus*, will be, and deserves to be, an invaluable resource for those practising pediatric ophthalmology, for those in training, and for those having anything to do with eye care in children.

Professor Anthony Murray MD
2004

The third edition of *Pediatric Ophthalmology and Strabismus* comprises the right volume arriving at the right time. This multi-authored text is written by the most knowledgeable specialists of our time. It has been seven years since the second edition and it is astonishing how much new information has accumulated over these years. Molecular genetics has moved the watershed area between genetic taxonomy and clinical denomination in ophthalmology in the direction of genetics, and understanding genetics in ophthalmology and embryology is now a must for clinicians. These subjects are explained for the beginner as well as the advanced reader, and all references have been completely updated. Several chapters discuss ethics in clinical ophthalmology underlining the importance of empathy in counseling families and treating the whole child, not only the disorder. The discussion on education of the visually impaired child is central to the present wave of de-institutionalization and mainstreaming. It is the task of the pediatric ophthalmologist to explain to the teacher, the difference between the (mainly) ophthalmic causes of visual impairment, cerebral visual impairment, and delayed visual maturation; the present edition will be of great help in this endeavor.

The most common disorder in pediatric ophthalmology is strabismus; treatment or prevention of amblyopia accounts for the major clinical workload. Eye movement disorders are therefore broadly covered, again with due regard to both the experienced reader and the novice.

It is fascinating to read the clinical sections, look at the pictures, tables, and graphic illustrations which all have superb educational merit. The illustrator, Martin Woodward is commended for his contributions.

Mette Warburg DMSci MD
2004

PREFACE

We have been exceptionally fortunate to have the best list of contributors to this book that we could have imagined. We drafted the outline, invited the 110 best authors we could think of, matching them carefully to the chapters needing to be written. We asked them to help produce the best book on pediatric ophthalmology and strabismus; we wanted chapters that related to each other, were clinically comprehensive and at a very high academic and practical level whilst being a 'masterpiece of compression'. All but one accepted the challenge and they completed their contribution on time and to a standard that we had only dreamed of. Our very sincere thanks go to each and every one of them: they have made this book. We have had the enjoyment of conceptualising, collating, editing, illustrating and realising the project. Enjoyment is the right word, we have enjoyed each other's company, enjoyed the association with the contributors, the clanging of ideas with each other, the learning of how much we did not know about a subject we thought we were pretty cool about, but above all we look forward to the final production of this book and, hopefully getting it into the hands of those who will use it to benefit children.

We could not have picked a better publisher to help us. We were a little nervous that we would be a tiny cog in the giant Elsevier wheel and would have all of the disadvantages and none of the advantages stemming from that. Paul Fam and his team at Elsevier, especially Shuet-Kei Cheung, Helen Sofio and Jess Thompson saw to it that our fears were unfounded and they made it an enjoyable experience for both of us and the authors: many thanks to them.

We believe that the illustrations are a vital part of the whole, not just a way of distracting a reader who happens to have a short attention span! Many of the illustrations have been supplied by the editors but were taken by the Medical Illustration department at Great Ormond Street Hospital who deserve our thanks for their skills unfailingly delivered with efficiency and good humour. Martin Woodward has done a fantastic job in producing lively and informative artwork. Occasionally, we may have not acknowledged the source of photographs accurately (unintentionally, in the second edition, none of Rob Morris' excellent photographs were attributed to him!), if this has been done again, apologies to the offended!

This book will not make anyone into a brilliant pediatric ophthalmologist—but we hope that it will be part of the process by which many professionals become expert in helping children with eye and vision problems. So what is it that makes a good pediatric ophthalmologist, optometrist or orthoptist? If we understand that process, it has come more through the mistakes that we have both made over our years as doctors. Having a long list of mistakes to ones name (often well-hidden!) is what is called experience. Everyone makes mistakes: mistakes are a powerful way of learning and by learning from the mistakes of others we can help prevent their repetition- we hope that this book will distil the experience of the authors into a brew that will help create great pediatric ophthalmologists!

Good doctors are not born but made. They are made by three processes: Learning, Understanding and Compassion.

Learning has to be life-long. Learning has little to do with the CME programmes, working time directives, curriculae, examinations, or revalidation so beloved of Colleges, Academies and doctors' trade organisations or guilds. These artefacts are by-products of our profession's inability to adequately train good doctors in sufficient numbers and to stimulate them to continue their training without a heavy stick and a large golden carrot. What we hope is that this book, like the first two editions, will be used in the clinic to help answer questions sparked by the problems confronting individual patients. By extracting scraps of the knowledge in the chapters so generously contributed by the authors on the problems posed by patients and by learning further from other sources, a lasting, unforgettable and enjoyable framework of knowledge can be built up. Teaching is a small part of learning and it is two way: the teacher learns as much as the taught. Real learning stems from a need to find out more, to challenge the accepted, to question the unquestionable.

Understanding starts with learning; it is an intellectual ability to project oneself into the position of the patient and family and from it springs wisdom- an ability to judge rightly and to make decisions and recommendations based on that judgement. Understanding is based on an ability to project oneself into the situation of the patient, to learn what they want and need and it is the starting point for a professional to go about improving their lot from that standpoint. Sure, understanding is based on learning and can be helped by a knowledge of technology etc. but it cannot be based on the technology alone- how many shallow, ill-judged decisions do we know that were based on readings from machines alone?

Compassion is a quality that is born of nature but is nurtured by training in the right environment. Unlike in the world of our own teachers, it is now OK to wear compassion with pride: it is a way of showing patients that we really care and by which they can know that we are acting for their interests above all others.

A 'successful' doctor usually has a combination of a variety of attributes- an extensive reference list with publications in high impact-factor journals, a large practise, a long list of lectures given (preferably overseas), membership of at least a few influential committees, presidency of this or that. These criteria will not, hopefully, be the life aim of a pediatric ophthalmologist; there are a number of colleagues who do not have prestigious hospital appointments, have minimal publications, and are not members of powerful committees, yet their opinion is continually sought by their peers and patients who beat a path to their door. These colleagues, who are often successful in at least one of the meanings of the word, have learned the art of blending learning, understanding and compassion. There is no qualification, no roster, no letters after the name just the unspoken acknowledgement by patients and colleagues.

We have suggested that you cannot get learning, understanding and compassion from a book or for that matter from the Internet, electronic media or elsewhere. So where is the fount? There is only one way- in the clinic, at the 'bedside', or in the operating theatre. It is by listening to patients; by listening to other professionals (senior and junior) in several disciplines and combining it with learning from other sources, and by apprenticeship that a good pediatric ophthalmologist can be made: hopefully helped by this book!

We would have achieved little without the help of Debbie and Anna who have been supportive and positively critical and who are a refuge for us from a hectic professional life. Strength in diversity!

David Taylor
Creig S Hoyt
London and San Francisco
August 2004

LIST OF CONTRIBUTORS

Gillian G W Adams BSc MB ChB FRCS (Ed) FRCOphth
Consultant Ophthalmic Surgeon
Department of Strabismus and Pediatrics
Moorfields Eye Hospital
London, UK

Daniel L Adams PhD
Assistant Professor
Koret Vision Center
Department of Ophthalmology
University of California San Francisco
San Francisco, USA

John R Ainsworth BMBS BMedSc FRCOphth FRCSEd
Paediatric Ophthalmologist
Eye Department
Birmingham Children's Hospital
Steelhouse Lane
Birmingham, UK

Luis Amaya MD
Consultant Ophthalmic Surgeon
Eye Ear and Mouth Unit
Maidstone District General Hospital
Maidstone
Kent, UK

Abudulaziz H Awad MD
Senior Academic Consultant
Pediatric Ophthalmology Division
King Khaled Eye Specialist Hospital
Riyadh, Saudi Arabia

Haroon R Awan MB ChB MMed Ophth
Country Representative
Sight Savers International
Islamabad, Pakistan

Katharine Barr MBBS
Medical Student
University College London
London, UK

Robert B Bhisitkul MD PhD
Associate Professor of Clinical
 Ophthalmology
Department of Ophthalmology
University of California San Francisco
San Francisco, USA

Valérie Biousse MD
Associate Professor of Ophthalmology
 and Neurology
Cyrus H. Stone Professor of
 Ophthalmology
Neuro-Ophthalmology Unit
Emory University
Atlanta, USA

Graeme C M Black MA MB BCh DPhil FRCOphth
Consultant Ophthalmologist
Department of Clinical Genetics
Central Manchester and Manchester
 Children's
University Hospital NHS Trust
Manchester, UK

John A Bradbury FRCS FRCOphth MBChB
Consultant Ophthalmologist
Department of Ophthalmology
Bradford Royal Infirmary
Bradford, UK

Michael C Brodsky MD
Professor of Ophthalmology and
 Pediatrics
Arkansas Children's Hospital
Little Rock
Arkansas, USA

Donal Brosnahan FRCS FRCOphth
Ophthalmic Surgeon
Our Lady's Hospital for Sick Children
Crumlin
Dublin, Eire

J Raymond Buncic MD FRCSC
Professor of Ophthalmology, University
 of Toronto
Department of Ophthalmology
Hospital for Sick Children
Toronto, Ontario, Canada

Susan M Carden MBBS FRANZCO FRACS
Senior Lecturer, University of Melbourne
Department of Ophthalmology
Royal Children's Hospital
Bentleigh, Victoria, Australia

Ingele Casteels MD PhD
Consultant Ophthalmologist, and
 Assistant Professor
Department of Ophthalmology
University Hospitals Leuven
Leuven, Belguim

Helen S L Chan MBBS FRCP (C) FAAP
Professor of Pediatrics
University of Toronto
Toronto, Ontario, Canada

Wilma Chang MD
Research Assistant
Department of Ophthalmology and
 Visual Sciences
British Columbia Childrens Hospital
Vancouver, British Columbia, Canada

Michael P Clarke FRCOphth
Reader in Ophthalmology
Department of Ophthalmology
Royal Victoria Infirmary
Newcastle Upon Tyne, UK

Maureen Cleary MB ChB MD
Consultant Metabolic Medicine
Metabolic Office
Great Ormond Street Hospital
London, UK

J Richard O Collin MA MB Bchir FRCS FRCOphth
Consultant Surgeon
Adnexal Service
Moorfields Eye Hospital,
 and Honorary Consultant Ophthalmic
 Surgeon
Great Ormond Street Hospital for
 Children
London, UK

John K G Dart MA DM FRCS FRCOphth
Consultant Ophthalmologist
Corneal and External Disease Service
Moorfields Eye Hospital
London, UK

Susan H Day MD
Chair and Program Director
California Pacific Medical Center
San Francisco, California, USA

Luis Carlos F de Sa MD
Consultant in Ophthalmology
Instituto Da Crianca-HC
Sao Paulo Eye Center
University of Sao Paulo
Sao Paulo, Brazil

Philippe Demaerel MD PhD
Consultant Neuroradiologist
Department of Radiology
University Hospitals K.U. Leuven
Leuven, Belgium

Joseph L Demer MD PhD
Professor of Ophthalmology and
    Neurology
Jules Stein Eye Institute
The University of California Los Angeles
Los Angeles, California, USA

Hélène Dollfus MD PhD
Professor of Medical Genetics
Hôpitaux Universitaires de Strasbourg
Hôpital de Hautepierre
Strasbourg, France

Sean P Donahue MD PhD
Associate Professor of Ophthalmology,
    Neurology and Pediatrics
Vanderbilt University School of Medicine
Nashville, Tennesse, USA

Clive Edelsten MRCP FRCOphth
Consultant Ophthalmologist
Department of Rheumatology
Great Ormond Street Hospital for
    Children
London, UK

**John S Elston MBBS BSc MD FRCS
FRCOphth**
Consultant Ophthalmologist
Oxford Eye Hospital
Radcliffe Infirmary
Oxford, UK

Vasudha Erraguntla MBBS DO
Pediatric Ophthalmologist
Saskatoon City Hospital
Saskatoon, Canada

**Alistair R Fielder FRCS FRCP
FRCOphth**
Professor of Ophthalmology
Department of Visual Neuroscience
Imperial College
Charing Cross Hospital
London, UK

Peter J Francis FRCOphth PhD
Consultant Ophthalmologist and Senior
    Lecturer
Eye Department
St Thomas Hospital
London, UK

Douglas R Fredrick MD
Associate Professor of Clinical
    Ophthalmology
Department of Ophthalmology
University of California San Francisco
San Francisco, California, USA

Anne B Fulton MD
Associate Professor of Ophthalmology
    Harvard Medical School; and Senior
    Associate in Ophthalmology
Department of Ophthalmology
The Children's Hospital
Boston, Massachusetts, USA

Brenda L Gallie MD FRCS(C)
Professor
University of Toronto
University Health Network
Princess Margaret Hospital
Cancer Information Division
Toronto, Ontario, Canada

Siobhan Garbutt BSc PhD
Postdoctoral Fellow
Department of Physiology
University of California San Francisco
San Francisco, California, USA

**Clare E Gilbert MB ChB FRCOphth MD
MSc**
Senior Lecturer
International Centre for Eye Health
Department of Infectious Tropical
    Diseases
London School of Hygiene and Tropical
    Medicine
London, UK

William V Good MD
Senior Scientist
The Smith-Kettlewell Eye Research
    Institute
San Francisco, USA

**John R Grigg MBBS FRANZCO
FRACS**
Consultant Ophthalmologist
Sydney Eye Hospital and The Children's
    Hospital at Westmead; and Senior
    Lecturer
University of Sydney
New South Wales, Australia

Yoshikazu Hatsukawa MD
Director, Eye Department
Osaka Medical Center and Research
    Institute for Maternal and Child Health
Osaka, Japan

**Hugo W A Henderson BA MBBS
FRCOphth**
Oculoplastic Fellow
Adnexal Service
Moorfields Eye Hospital
London, UK

Elise Héon MD FRCS
Professor and Ophthalmologist-in-chief
Department of Ophthalmology and
    Vision Research
Hospital for Sick Children
Toronto, Ontario, Canada

**Richard W Hertle MD FAAO FACS
FAAP**
Chief of Pediatric Ophthalmology
Director of the Laboratory of Visual and
    Ocular Motor Physiology
Children's Hospital of Pittsburgh;
Visiting Professor
Department of Ophthalmology
Pittsburgh Eye and Ear Institute
University of Pittsburgh School of
    Medicine
The University of Pittsburgh Medical
    Center
Pittsburgh, USA

Peter Hodgkins BSc FRCS FRCOphth
Consultant Ophthalmologist
Southampton Eye Unit
Southampton, UK

Graham E Holder BSc MSc PhD
Director of Electrophysiology
Department of Electrophysiology
Moorfields Eye Hospital
London, UK

David A Hollander MD MBA
Fellow, Cornea and External Disease
Jules Stein Eye Institute
Los Angeles, California, USA

Gerd Holmström MD PhD
Associate Professor
Department of Ophthalmology
University Hospital
Uppsala, Sweden

Creig S Hoyt MD
The Theresa and Wayne Caygill
Professor and Chairman of the
   Department of Ophthalmology;
Director of the Beckman Vision Center
University of California San Francisco
   California, USA

David G Hunter MD PhD
Ophthalmologist-in-chief
Harvard Medical School
Children's Hospital Boston
Boston, Massachusetts, USA

**Robyn V Jamieson MBBS PhD FRACP
PhD**
Consultant Clinical Geneticist
Department of Clinical Genetics
The Children's Hospital at Westmead
Sydney, Australia

Arthur Jampolsky MD
Founder
Smith-Kettlewell Eye Research Institute
San Francisco, California, USA

James E Jan MD FRCP(C)
Pediatric Neurologist
Department of Pediatrics
University of British Columbia
Vancouver, British Columbia, Canada

Hanne Jensen MD PhD
Consultant Ophthalmologist National
   Eye Clinic for the Visually Impaired
Hellerup, Denmark

**Peng Tee Khaw PhD FRCP FRCS
FRCOphth FIBiol FRCPath FMedSci**
Professor of Glaucoma and Ocular
   Healing
Glaucoma Unit and Ocular Repair and
   Regeneration Biology Unit
London, UK

Stephen P Kraft MD FRCSC
Professor of Ophthalmology
The Hospital for Sick Children
University of Toronto
Toronto, Ontario, Canada

Burton J Kushner MD
John W and Helen Doolittle Professor of
   Ophthalmology
Department of Ophthalmology and
   Visual Sciences
University of Wisconsin
Madison, USA

Pamela J Kutschke CO
Chief Orthoptist
Department of Ophthalmology
University of Iowa Hospitals and Clinics
Iowa City, USA

Scott R Lambert MD
Professor of Ophthalmology and
   Pediatrics
Emery Eye Center
Atlanta, USA

David Laws MB BCh FRCOphth
Consultant in Ophthalmology
Ophthalmology Department
Singleton Eye Hospital
Swansea, Wales

John P Lee FRCS FRCP FRCOphth
Consultant Ophthalmic Surgeon
Director, Strabismus and Pediatric
   Services
Moorfields Eye Hospital
London, UK

R John Leigh MD
Professor of Neurology
Department of Neurology and Veteran
   Affairs Medical Center and University
   Hospitals
Cleveland, Ohio, USA

Alki Liasis PhD
Senior Clinical Scientist
The Tony Kriss Visual Electrophysiology
   Unit
Eye Department
Great Ormond Street Hospital for
   Children
London, UK

Ian C Lloyd FRCS FRCOphth
Consultant Pediatric Ophthalmologist
The Royal Eye Hospital
Manchester, UK

Christopher J Lyons MB FRCS FRCSC
Associate Professor
University of British Columbia,
Department of Ophthalmology
British Columbia Children's Hospital
Vancouver, British Columbia, Canada

**Caroline J MacEwen MB ChB MD
FRCS FRCOphth FFSEM**
Consultant Ophthalmologist
Department of Ophthalmology
Ninewells Hospital
Dundee, UK

Nancy C Mansfield MD
Assistant Professor of Clinical
   Ophthalmology
Keck School of Medicine
University of Southern California
California, USA

**Frank J Martin MBBS (Syd.)
FRCOphth FRACS FRANZCO**
Associate Professor
University of Sydney
Sydney, Australia

D Luisa Mayer PhD
Assistant Professor of Ophthalmology
Harvard Medical School, and Clinical
   Associate of Ophthalmology
Department of Ophthalmology
The Children's Hospital
Boston, USA

**Michel Michaelides MD BSc MBBS
MRCOphth**
Clinical Research Fellow
Department of Molecular Genetics
Institute of Ophthalmology
University College London; and
   Specialist Registrar in Ophthalmology
Moorfields Eye Hospital
London, UK

Neil R Miller MD
Frank B Walsh Professor
Department of Ophthalmology and
   Neurology
Wilmer Eye Institute
Baltimore, Maryland, USA

Hans Ulrik Møller PhD
Consultant Ophthalmologist
Department of Ophthalmology
Viborg Hospital
Viborg, Denmark

Anthony T Moore MA FRCS FRCOphth
Duke-Elder Professor of Ophthalmology
Moorfields Eye Hospital
London, UK

**Andrew A M Morris BM BCh PhD
FRCPCH**
Consultant in Pediatric Metabolic Medicine
Willink Unit
Royal Manchester Children's Hospital
Manchester, UK

**Robert Morris MRCP FRCS
FRCPOphth**
Consultant Ophthalmic Surgeon
Southampton Eye Unit
Southampton General Hospital
Southampton, UK

A Linn Murphree MD
Director
The Retinoblastoma Centre
Children's Hospital of Los Angeles
Los Angeles, California, USA

Nancy J Newman MD
Professor of Ophthalmology and
    Neurology
Leo Delle Jolley Professor of
    Ophthalmology
Emory University
Atlanta, USA

Ken K Nischal FRCOphth
Consultant Ophthalmic Surgeon
Department of Ophthalmology
Great Ormond Street Hospital for
    Children
London, UK

Maria Papadopoulos MBBS FRACO
Consultant Ophthalmic Surgeon
Glaucoma Unit
Moorfields Eye Hospital
London, UK

Cameron F Parsa MD
Assistant Professor
The Wilmer Eye Institute
Johns Hopkins University School of
    Medicine
Baltimore, Maryland, USA

**Anthony G Quinn MB ChB DCH
FRANZCO FRCOphth**
Consultant Ophthalmologist
West of England Eye Unit
Royal Devon and Exeter Hospital
Exeter, UK

Graham E Quinn MD MSCE
Professor of Ophthalmology
Pediatric Ophthalmology
The Childrens Hospital of Philadelphia
Philadelphia, Pennsylvania, USA

**Jugnoo S Rahi MBBS FRCOphth
MRCPCH Msc PhD**
Clinical Senior Lecturer in Ophthalmic
Epidemiology and Honorary
Consultant Opthalmologist
Centre for Paediatric Epidemiology and
    Biostatistics
Institute of Child Health
Great Ormond Street Hospital
London, UK

Michael X Repka MD
Professor of Ophthalmology and
    Pediatrics
John Hopkins Hospital
Baltimore, Maryland, USA

Jack Rootman MD FRCSC
Professor of Ophthalmology and
    Pathology
Department of Ophthalmology and
    Visual Sciences
University of British Columbia
Vancouver, British Columibia, Canada

Arthur L Rosenbaum MD
Chief, Division of Pediatric
    Ophthalmology,
Vice-chairman
Department of Ophthalmology
Jules Stein Institute
University of California Los Angeles
Los Angeles, California,USA

**Isabelle M Russell-Eggitt MA DO
FRCS FRCOphth**
Consultant Pediatric Ophthalmologist
Great Ormond Street Hospital for
    Children
London, UK

**Alison Salt MBBS MSc DCH FRCPCH
FRACP**
Consultant Pediatrician (Neurodisability)
Neurodisability Service
The Wolfson Center
Great Ormond Street Childrens Hospital;
and Moorfields Eye Hospital
London, UK

David A Sami MD
Pediatric Ophthalmologist
Department of Pediatric Ophthalmology
Children's Hospital
Boston, Massachusetts, USA

Alvina Pauline D L Santiago MD
Clinical Associate Professor
University of the Philippines College of
    Medicine
Department of Ophthalmology
Philippines General Hospital
Quezon City, Philippines

Seang-Mei Saw MBBS MPH PhD
Associate Professor
Department of Community, Occupational
    and Family Medicine
National University Singapore
Singapore, Republic of Singapore

William E Scott MD
Professor of Medicine
Department of Ophthalmology
University of Iowa Hospital
Iowa City, USA

Janet H Silver OBE DSc MPhil FBCO
Formerly Principal Optometrist
Optometry Department
Moorfields Eye Hospital
London, UK

**Martin P Snead MA MD FRCS
FRCOphth**
Consultant Ophthalmic Surgeon
Vitreoretinal Service
Addenbrookes Hospital
Cambridge, UK

Danilo S Soriano MD
Consultant in Ophthalmology
Children's Hospital
Department of Pediatrics
University of Sao Paolo
Sao Paulo, Brazil

Jane Sowden MA PhD
Senior Lecturer in Developmental Biology
Developmental Biology Unit
Institute of Child Health
University College London
London, UK

**Lynne Speedwell BSc MSc (Health
Psy) FCOptom DCLP FAAO**
Head of Optometry
Department of Ophthalmology
Great Ormond Street Childrens Hospital
London, UK

Angela Tank
Secretary to David Taylor
Great Ormond Street Hospital
London, UK

**David Taylor FRCS FRCP FRCOphth
DSc(Med)**
Professor of Pediatric Ophthalmology
Institute of Child Health and Consultant
    Ophthalmologist
Great Ormond Street Hospital for
    Children
London, UK

Dorothy Thompson PhD
Consultant Clinical Scientist
The Tony Kriss Visual Electrophysiology
    Unit Eye Department
Great Ormond Street Hospital for
    Children
London, UK

Christine Timms DBO (T)
Orthoptist
Orthoptic Department
Great Ormond Street Hospital
London, UK

Lawrence Tychsen MD
Professor of Opthalmology and Visual
    Sciences
Pediatrics, Anatomy and Neurobiology
St Louis Childrens Hospital
St Louis, USA

Jimmy M Uddin MA FRCOphth
Consultant Ophthalmic Surgeon
Orbital Service, Adnexal Service
Moorfields Eye Hospital
London, UK

Alain Verloes MD PhD
Head
Clinical Genetics Unit
Hôpital Robert Debre
Paris, France

Anthony J Vivian FRCS FRCOphth
Consultant Ophthalmologist
Addenbrooks Hospital
Cambridge and West Sussex Hospital
    NHS Trust
Eye Treatment Centre
Bury St Edmunds, UK

**David Webb MD FRCP FRCPath
MRCPH**
Consultant Haematologist
Great Ormond Street Children's Hospital
London, UK

Mark Wilkins MA MD FRCOphth
Fellow in Corneal and External Diseases
Moorfields Eye Hospital
London, UK

Mark G Wood MD
Assistant Professor
Health Sciences Center
University of New Mexico
Alberquerque, USA

CHAPTER

1 Epidemiology of Visual Impairment and Blindness in Childhood

Jugnoo S Rahi and Clare E Gilbert

The aims of this chapter are, firstly, to familiarize the reader with important issues in the interpretation of epidemiological studies of childhood visual impairment and, secondly, to synthesize currently available data to provide a global picture regarding the frequency, causes, and prevention of visual impairment and blindness in childhood. For more information about the epidemiology of individual disorders, please refer to their respective chapters, as well as the further reading list and references at end of this chapter.

WHAT IS EPIDEMIOLOGY?

Literally, this science comprises "studies upon people."[1] Ophthalmic epidemiology has both its *origins* and its *applications* in clinical and public health ophthalmology. Its aims are:

- to shed light on the causes and natural history of ophthalmic disorders;
- to enhance the accuracy and efficiency of diagnosis;
- to improve the effectiveness of treatment and preventive strategies; and
- to provide quantitative information for planning of services.

EPIDEMIOLOGICAL REASONING

This is based on the following principles:

- the occurrence of disease is not random, but rather a balance between *causal* and *protective* factors;
- disease causation, modification, and prevention are studied by systematic investigation of *populations*, defined by place and time, to gain a more complete overview than can be achieved by studying individuals; and
- the inference that an association between a risk factor and a disease is *causal* requires, firstly, the explicit exclusion of chance, bias, or confounding as alternative explanations for the observed association and, secondly, evidence of a con-

sistent, strong, and biologically plausible association, in correct temporal sequence, and preferably exhibiting a dose–response relationship.

FRAMING THE QUESTION

Decisions in clinical practice or service provision are ideally based on "three-part questions" that incorporate the *reference population* (e.g., children under 2 years with infantile esotropia), *the risk factor or intervention* (e.g., prematurity or strabismus surgery), and the *outcomes* (e.g., parent-reported improvement in cosmesis and objective improvement in alignment and stereopsis). The focus of the question–be it frequency, causes, or treatment/ prevention of disease–determines the study design required to address it: for example, a *descriptive* study (e.g., cross-sectional prevalence study) or an *analytical* study (either *observational*, e.g., case–control or cohort studies, or *interventional*, e.g., randomized controlled trials).

WHO IS A VISUALLY IMPAIRED CHILD?

The answers given by the affected child, her parents, her teacher, her social worker, her rehabilitation specialist, her pediatrician, and her ophthalmologist will be equally valid but may differ substantially. However, comparisons within and between countries, and over time, of the frequency, causes, and treatment/ prevention of visual impairment require a standard definition. Thus the WHO's taxonomy (Table 1.1) has been adopted for epidemiological research, despite the recognized difficulties of measuring visual acuity in very young children and those unable to cooperate with formal testing. Thus the need remains for a better system of classification that is applicable to children of different ages and that may allow consideration of other visual parameters such as near acuity, visual fields, binocularity, and contrast sensitivity.

Table 1.1 World Health Organization classification of levels of visual impairment

Level of visual impairment	Category of vision	Visual acuity in better eye with optical correction
Slight, if acuity less than 6/7.5 or LogMAR 0.2	Normal vision	6/18 or better (LogMAR 0.4 or better)
Visual impairment (VI)	Low vision	Worse than 6/18 up to 6/60 (LogMAR 0.5 to 1.0)
Severe visual impairment (SVI)	Low vision	Worse than 6/60 up to 3/60 (logMAR 1.1 to 1.3)
Blind (BL)	Blindness	Worse than 3/60 (worse than logMAR 1.3) to no light perception *or* visual field ≤ 10 degrees around central fixation

Note: Adapted with permission from World Health Organisation (WHO). International Statistical Classification of Diseases and Health Related Problems. 10th Revision. Geneva, World Health Organisation, 1992.

Equally, the importance of both *measures of functional vision* and *measures of vision-related quality of life* is increasingly recognized. The former assess the child's ability to perform tasks of daily living that depend on vision, such as the ability to navigate independently. The latter elicit the child's and/or parent's view of the gap, caused by the visually impairing disorder and its therapy, between the child's expectations and actual experiences in terms of his/her physical, emotional/psychological, cognitive, and social functioning.[2,3] This interest is timely with a major revision underway of the International Classification of Impairment, Disability and Handicap, to incorporate important recent shifts in the conceptual frameworks underpinning understanding of the disability.[4]

MEASURING THE FREQUENCY AND BURDEN OF CHILDHOOD VISUAL IMPAIRMENT AND BLINDNESS

The analogy of running a bath (or filling a water trough) serves to illustrate different measures of frequency and burden of disease.

The speed with which water runs in to the bath equates with *incidence*–i.e., the *rate* of new occurrence of disease *in a given population* over a *specified time period*: for example in the UK the annual incidence of congenital cataract is 2.5 per 10,000 children aged one year or less.[5]

The degree to which the bath is full at a particular moment (a balance between how fast water is running into the bath and how much is running out through the plug or overflow) equates to the prevalence of disease–i.e., the *proportion* of a *given population* that has disease at a particular *point in time*. This in turn reflects both the incidence of the disease and its duration–i.e., new cases of disease added to the pool while others are "lost" from it through death, cure, or migration. For example currently in the UK the prevalence in childhood of amblyopia with an acuity of worse than 6/12 (LogMAR 0.3) is 1%.[6] Finally, the comparison of how a bath is valued more broadly, versus a shower or versus staying unwashed, might be seen to equate with measures of utility such as disability-adjusted life years (DALYs) or quality-adjusted life years (QALYs).[4] These incorporate both morbidity and mortality into a single measure to be used to compare different states of health within and between countries in order to identify economic and other priorities in health-care provision: for example throughout the world, blindness is categorized in the penultimate class of increasingly severe disability.[7]

These indices provide complementary information. Incidence is useful in identifying and monitoring secular trends, such as the emergence or disappearance of risk factors, in provision of services and in planning research, for example estimating likely recruitment time in clinical trials. Prevalence provides a measure of the size of the problem in a community at a given time, and thus is helpful in allocating resources and can be used to evaluate services, if changes in prevalence can be attributed solely to changes in outcome or duration of disease as a result of treatment rather than changes in underlying incidence.

"COSTS" OF CHILDHOOD VISUAL IMPAIRMENT

Visual impairment in childhood impacts on the child's development, education, and care given by families and professionals, and shapes the adult she becomes, influencing profoundly her

employment and social prospects and opportunities throughout life.[8–10] Thus although the prevalence and incidence of visual impairment are considerably lower in childhood than in adult life in all regions of the world, the relative burden, when considered in terms of years of life lived with visual impairment ("person-years of visual impairment") is considerable. Personal and social costs are important but difficult to measure. There has been a greater focus on the economic costs of childhood visual impairment, measured in terms of loss of economic productivity. This is considerable, amounting to about a quarter of costs of adult blindness in some countries[11–13]; for example, a recent annual estimate of the cumulative loss of gross national product attributable to childhood visual impairment was US$22 billion.[12–13]

SPECIFIC ISSUES IN THE EPIDEMIOLOGICAL STUDY OF VISUAL IMPAIRMENT AND BLINDNESS IN CHILDHOOD

Case definition–A standard definition applicable to all children remains problematic, as discussed above.

Rarity–That visual impairment and blindness in childhood is uncommon poses significant methodological challenges in trying to achieve sufficiently large and representative populations of affected children to allow unbiased and meaningful study.

Complex, multidisciplinary management–For a complete picture, information must be sought from the different professionals involved in the care of visually impaired or blind children, which, in the case of the many children with additional nonophthalmic impairments or chronic disorders, adds even further layers of complexity.

Long-term outcomes important–In pediatric ophthalmology, as in all pediatric disciplines, developmental issues must be accounted for, and thus assessment of meaningful outcomes, such as final visual function or educational placement, requires long-term follow-up in epidemiological studies.

Ethics–There is increasing emphasis on issues of proxy consent (by parents) and children's autonomy regarding treatment decisions, which may impact on participation in ophthalmic epidemiological research.

POTENTIAL SOURCES OF INFORMATION ON FREQUENCY AND CAUSES OF VISUAL IMPAIRMENT

Theoretically, there are a number of sources to turn to for epidemiological information about childhood visual impairment or blindness, but in reality only a few are available in most countries. This explains the incomplete picture of visual impairment that currently exists.

1. *Population-based prevalence studies*–Although the ideal source for robust information, studies of whole populations of children identifying those with visual impairment, such as the British national birth cohort studies,[14,15] are uncommon, as they need to be very large (e.g., a study of 100,000 children would be required in an industrialized country to identify 100 to 200 children with visual impairment or blindness), and thus are costly and difficult to do.

2. *Population-based incidence studies*–Even greater difficulties exist in conducting incidence studies, explaining the greater paucity of incidence data.

3. *Special needs/disability registers, surveys, and surveillance*–Specific studies and/or surveillance systems[16] or registers of childhood disability can provide information about visual impairment, but it is important to recognize the potential for bias as certain visually impaired children may be over-represented in these sources, for example those with multiple impairment.

4. *Surveys of schools for the visually impaired*–In developing countries studies of children enrolled in special education have provided some useful information on causes but the inherent bias in such sources–that many blind children, particularly those with additional nonophthalmic impairments, may not have access to special education–needs to be taken into account in their interpretation.

5. *Visual impairment registers*–These exist in many industrialized countries but if registration is voluntary and is also not a prerequisite for accessing special educational or social services, then registers may be incomplete as well as biased, reflecting differences in both parental preferences and professionals' practices regarding registration of eligible children.[17]

6. *Visual impairment teams*–Increasingly children in industrialized settings are evaluated by multidisciplinary teams, and if these serve geographically defined populations then useful information about visual impairment can be derived.

7. *Disorder-specific ophthalmic surveillance schemes*–Research on uncommon ophthalmic conditions in children can be undertaken using a range of specific population-based surveillance schemes, for example those for congenital anomalies (e.g., for study of anophthalmia or microphthalmia) or adverse drug reactions (e.g., for study of visual loss with vigabatrin) although underascertainment in such work is recognized. A recently established national active surveillance scheme comprising all senior ophthalmologists in the United Kingdom (the British Ophthalmological Surveillance Unit[18]) has facilitated the study of uncommon ophthalmic disorders, including the first population-based study incidence study of severe visual impairment and blindness in childhood.[19] This provides an important new model for ophthalmic epidemiological research.

8. *Community-based rehabilitation programs*–In many developing countries rehabilitation of blind and visually impaired children and adults within their community is being adopted. Where information about the size of the catchment population is available it is possible to derive estimates of prevalence through such programmes.[20]

9. *Surveillance using key informants*–In many developing countries, it may be possible to identify key community and religious leaders, health-care workers, and others who know their communities well and thus can identify children believed to have visual impairment and/or ocular abnormalities, and if such information can be combined with the size of the population at risk, then estimates of prevalence and causes can be derived.[21]

Irrespective of the sources, there is always potential for underascertainment, which is especially problematic in research on rare ophthalmic disorders, when a sufficiently large and representative sample must be achieved to enable meaningful and unbiased analysis. Therefore it is important to use multiple sources, wherever possible, to gain a more complete picture of childhood visual impairment.

VISUAL IMPAIRMENT IN THE BROADER CONTEXT OF CHILDHOOD DISABILITY

Multiple impairments

In industrialized countries, *at least* half of all severely visually impaired and blind children have, in addition, motor, sensory, or learning impairments and/or chronic systemic disorders, which confer further disadvantage in terms of development, education, and independence.[19,22] Currently, in developing countries the available evidence suggests that this proportion is lower than that in industrialized settings. This reflects differences in the relative importance of etiological factors (e.g., vitamin A deficiency and ophthalmia neonatorum, which result in purely ocular disease) as well as differences in survival with blinding conditions associated with systemic diseases with high rates of multiple impairment (e.g., prematurity, congenital rubella syndrome, or cortical blindness following cerebral malaria, meningitis, or cerebral tumors).[21]

Thus it can be argued that for research on etiology and interventions, as well as for provision of services, one should think of *two* populations: children with isolated visual impairment versus those with visual impairment in the context of other impairments or systemic diseases.

Mortality

It is estimated that in developing countries, where the major cause of blindness remains corneal scarring due to vitamin A deficiency,[23,24] about half of all children who become blind each year die within a few years of onset of blindness.[23,24] The available prevalence data suggest that there is an association between prevalence of blindness in children and under-5 mortality rates (U5MR) for a country, enabling this readily available indicator to be used as a proxy for blindness rates in children. In industrialized countries with very low U5MRs the prevalence of blindness is approximately 3–5 per 10,000 children whereas in countries with U5MRs of >250/1,000 live births the prevalence of blindness is likely to be nearer 12–15 per 10,000 children.

Recent data from the United Kingdom indicating 10% mortality among children in the year following diagnosis of severe visual impairment or blindness[19] are consistent with previous reports in Sweden[25] and the USA[26] of increased mortality in children with visual impairment, when compared with the total child population.

It is important to recognize that as prevalence studies of older visually impaired children exclude those who died earlier in childhood, they may provide both an underestimate of true frequency and a biased picture regarding causes.

Groups at high risk of visual impairment

It is increasingly important to both research and resource allocation to consider visual impairment against the backdrop of broader secular trends in childhood disability. In particular there is now good evidence that certain children are at increased risk of serious visual loss: those of low birthweight,[27,28] those from socio-economically deprived families,[19] and in industrialized countries, those from ethnic minorities.[19] These issues are discussed below in relation to secular trends.

FREQUENCY OF CHILDHOOD VISUAL IMPAIRMENT AND BLINDNESS

Prevalence

The estimated prevalence of childhood blindness (BL) in different regions of the world, together with the absolute number of affected children, is shown in Table 1.2.[23,24]

Of the 1.4 million blind (BL) children in the world the overwhelming majority live in the least affluent regions of the world–where both the prevalence of visual impairment and the size of the population at risk (children) are greatest. Currently, as an approximate guide for estimating the total number of blind children in a country at a given time, it can be assumed that there are about 60 blind children per million total (adult and child) population in industrialized countries, whereas there are about 600 per million total population in the poorest developing countries.

The prevalence of visual impairment (VI) and severe visual impairment (SVI) are not known for many regions of the world. However, in general, blindness accounts for about one-third or less of all visual impairment. Thus in industrialized countries, the prevalence of VI, SVI, and BL combined is about 10 to 22 per 10,000 children aged <16 years while in some developing countries it may be as high as 30 to 40 per 10,000.[29]

Incidence

Estimates of the incidence of childhood visual impairment are available for only a few countries. Using pooled data from the Scandinavian visual impairment registers the overall annual incidence of VI, SVI, and BL combined was reported to be 0.8 per 10,000 individuals <19 years old in 1993.[30] More recently, from a population-based study in the United Kingdom, the annual age group-specific incidence was reported to be highest in the first year of life at 4.0 per 10,000, with the cumulative incidence (life-time risk) increasing to 5.3 per 10,000 by 5 years old, and further to 5.9 per 10,000 by 16 years old.[19]

"CAUSES" OF VISUAL IMPAIRMENT

Taxonomy

Understanding of the relative importance of different causes of visual impairment, including comparisons between countries and within countries over time, has been enhanced by the introduction of a dual taxonomy in which, for each child, the "anatomical sites" affected are assigned together with etiological factors categorized according to the timing of their action.[31] This taxonomy was proposed and used initially in work in developing countries but has recently been extended for use in research in industrialized countries[19] and is shown in Table 1.3.

Data from a variety of sources, collected or reclassified or using this classification system, are presented in Tables 1.4 and 1.5. Most of the data from developing countries have been obtained from examining children in schools for the blind, while that from industrialized countries come mainly from registers of the blind.

Using the same taxonomy, estimates of the relative contributions of different causes to the global picture are presented in Tables 1.6 and 1.7.

Variations by region and over time

The pattern of causes of visual impairment and blindness in children in a given country at a particular time reflects the prevailing balance between the determinants of individual ophthalmic disorders (biological, environmental, and social) and the strategies and resources available for their prevention or treatment. This at least partly explains the considerable regional variations in the relative importance of different disorders (Tables 1.4 and 1.5), although it is important to remember that direct comparison of data from different sources in this way is not necessarily entirely valid.

Equally, the changing balance between risk factors and treatment/prevention that accompanies economic and social development explains the major trends over time within countries. For example, ophthalmia neonatorum has disappeared, while cerebral visual impairment and retinopathy of prematurity

Table 1.2 Estimated prevalence and magnitude of childhood blindness (BL) by region[35]

Region (World Bank)	Total number of children (millions)	Prevalence of blindness (BL) per 1000 children aged 0–15 years	Estimates of number blind (BL) children	% Blind children worldwide
Former socialist economies (FSE)	78	0.51	40,000	2.9
Established market economies (EME) e.g., Scandinavia, Republic of Ireland[36,37]	170	0.30	50,000	3.6
Latin America and Caribbean (LAC) e.g., Chile[38]	170	0.62	100,000	7.1
Middle East Crescent (MEC) e.g., Morocco[39]	240	0.80	190,000	13.6
China[40]	340	0.50	210,000	15.0
India[20,41]	350	0.80	270,000	19.3
Other Asia and islands (OAI) e.g., Bangladesh, Nepal, Mongolia[21,42,43]	260	0.83	220,000	15.6
Sub-Saharan Africa (SSA) e.g., Malawi, Gambia, Nigeria, Benin, Cameroon[44–48]	260	1.24	320,000	22.9
Total:	1868	0.75	1,400,000	100

With permission from WHO/IAPB. Preventing blindness in children. Report of a WHO/IAPB Scientific Meeting WHO/PBL/00.77. Geneva, World Health Organisation (WHO) 2000.

Table 1.3 Classification of the causes of childhood visual impairment or blindness, according to the anatomical site(s) affected, and the etiological factors by their timing of action

Anatomical site(s) affected	Etiological factor(s) by timing of action
Whole globe and anterior segment Microphthalmia/anophthalmia Anterior segment dysgenesis Coloboma-multiple sites Others **Glaucoma** Primary Secondary **Cornea** Sclerocornea Keratomalacia Other corneal scar **Lens** Cataract Aphakia Subluxed **Uvea** Anidiria Uveitis Coloboma—single site **Retina** Retinopathy of prematurity Retinal and macular dystrophies Oculo-cutaneous albinism Retinitis/neuroretinitis Retinal detachment Retinoblastoma Other **Optic nerve** Hypoplasia Atrophy (primary or secondary) Neuritis/neuropathy Others **Cerebral/visual pathways** Neuro-degenerative disorders Hypoxic/ischemic encephalopathy Nonaccidental injury Infection Structural abnormalities Tumor Other **Other** Idiopathic nystagmus High refractive error	**Prenatal** Hereditary —Autosomal recessive, autosomal dominant, X-linked —Chromosomal Hypoxia/ischaemia Infection Prenatal drug Others Presumed prenatal but factor unknown **Perinatal + Neonatal** Hypoxia/ischemia Infection Non-accidental injury Others Presumed peri/neonatal but factor unknown **Childhood** Tumor Nutritional Infection Hydrocephalus/Increased cranial pressure Hypoxia /ischemia Non-accidental injury Accidental injury Specific systemic disorders Presumed childhood but factor unknown **Undetermined timing of insult and factors unknown**

Note: Modified with permission from Gilbert C, Foster A, Negrel A-D, Thylefors B, et al. Childhood blindness: a new form for recording causes of visual loss in children. Bull World Health Organ 1993; 71: 485–489.

Table 1.4 Regional variation in the causes of blindness in children—anatomical sites affected

Anatomical site affected	Wealthiest EME (% total)	FSE (% total)	LAC (% total)	MEC (% total)	China (% total)	India (% total)	OAI (% total)	Poorest SSA (% total)
Globe/anterior segment	10	12	12	14	26	25	21	9
Glaucoma	1	3	8	5	9	3	6	6
Cornea	1	2	8	8	4	27	21	36
Lens	8	11	7	20	19	11	19	9
Uvea	2	5	2	4	1	5	3	5
Retina	25	44	47	38	25	22	21	20
Optic nerve	25	15	12	8	14	6	7	10
Cerebral/visual pathways and other	28	8	4	3	2	1	2	5
Total:	100	100	100	100	100	100	100	100

Table 1.5 Regional variation in the causes of blindness in children — etiological factors according to timing of action

| | Region | | | | | | | |
| Timing of action | Wealthiest → | | | | | | | → Poorest |
	EME (% total)	FSE (% total)	LAC (% total)	MEC (% total)	China (% total)	India (% total)	OAI (% total)	SSA (% total)
Prenatal (definite)								
1. Hereditary	45	18	22	53	31	26	27	20
2. Other intrauterine factors	7	6	8	2	0	2	3	3
Perinatal (definite)	24	28	28	1	2	2	9	6
Childhood (definite)	10	5	10	7	14	28	14	34
Unknown[a]	14	43	32	37	53	42	47	37
Total:	100	100	100	100	100	100	100	100

[a]Available data used for this table require classification as "unknown" of those disorders with *presumed* other "timing of action," e.g., congenital anomalies presumed to be of prenatal origin.

Table 1.6 Major causes of blindness in children, and estimates of numbers affected by anatomical site

Anatomical site	Number affected	% total	Main disorders worldwide
Retina	381,000	27	Hereditary dystrophies, retinopathy of prematurity
Cornea	231,000	16	Scarring due to vitamin A deficiency, measles, ophthalmia neonatorum, use of harmful traditional eye remedies
Whole globe	230,000	16	Microphthalmos, anophthalmos, coloboma
Lens	170,000	13	Cataract
Optic nerve	167,000	12	Atrophy, hypoplasia and coloboma
Cerebral/visual pathways and other	103,000	7	Cerebral visual impairment, refractive errors
Glaucoma	68,000	5	
Uvea	50,000	4	Coloboma, uveitis
Total	1,400,000	100	

Table 1.7 Major causes of blindness in children, and estimates of numbers affected by etiological category

Category	Number affected	% total
Prenatal (definite)		
1. Hereditary	423,000	30
2. Intrauterine	50,000	4
Childhood (definite)	260,000	19
Perinatal (definite)	151,000	11
Unknown[a]	516,000	36
Total	1,400,000	100

[a]Available data used for this table require classification as "unknown" of those disorders with *presumed* other "timing of action," e.g., congenital anomalies presumed to be of prenatal origin.

Importantly, the current picture of childhood visual disability in industrialized countries can, inevitably, be expected to be replicated in those countries currently in economic transition.[19]

Other sources of variations in pattern of "causes"

It is essential to remember that the *relative* importance of different disorders will also vary by the level of visual impairment studied. For example, albinism, congenital cataract, and retinopathy of prematurity are all likely to be relatively more important if children with all levels of visual impairment (VI, SVI, or BL) are included, whereas cerebral visual impairment is likely to be relatively more important if only those with blindness are studied.

Furthermore, patterns may differ according to whether prevalent cases or incident cases are studied, since survival is an important issue. For example, studies of secondary school-age children with long-standing visual loss (prevalent cases) may exclude those children with severe acute vitamin A deficiency-related corneal disease, those of extremely low birthweight, or those with severe systemic diseases, all associated with death in early childhood.

have emerged, and the inherited retinal dystrophies have gained ground as the major causes of visual impairment in children in the industrialized world during the past century.[32,33] By contrast, congenital cataract remains an important cause of severe visual loss in many developing countries despite the marked recent improvement in visual outcomes evident in industrialized nations where early detection occurs and specialist management is available.

PREVENTION OF VISUAL IMPAIRMENT AND BLINDNESS IN CHILDHOOD

Children are a priority in "Vision 2020",[23,24] the global initiative against avoidable visual impairment led by the World Health Organization and the International Agency for Prevention of Blindness. As the causes of visual loss vary considerably, country-specific programs are being developed and implemented, based on the specific priorities for prevention, treatment, and rehabilitation. All programs combine disease control strategies with human resource, technological, and infrastructure development. In many countries these programs will interface with existing broader governmental initiatives to improve the health of children or improve services for children with disability.

Strategies to prevent visual impairment or blindness can be categorized as follows:

Primary prevention–to prevent the occurrence of ophthalmic disease.

Examples include rubella immunization programs, which prevent congenital rubella infection-associated cataract and retinopathy; vitamin A supplementation, and measles immunization to prevent corneal scarring; avoidance of known ocular teratogens in pregnancy through public antenatal and general public health education campaigns; and preconceptional genetic counseling of families with known genetic eye disease.

Secondary prevention–to prevent established ophthalmic disease from causing serious visual loss.

This would include both screening and surveillance examinations to ensure early detection and prompt referral of children with suspected ophthalmic disease, such as cataract. Equally it incorporates prompt and specialist treatment by pediatric ophthalmic professionals of specific disorders such as retinopathy of prematurity, cataract, and glaucoma.

Tertiary prevention–to maximize residual visual function and prevent disadvantage due to established visual impairment.

In the main, this incorporates major activities relating to assessing and meeting special educational needs; providing low vision aids; mobility training, and other rehabilitation programs; and providing social support and services to families of affected children. It also includes specific ophthalmic treatment aimed at restoring useful residual sight in advanced disease, such as optical iridectomy for corneal scarring.

ROLE OF OPHTHALMIC PROFESSIONALS IN PREVENTION OF CHILDHOOD VISUAL IMPAIRMENT

Ophthalmic professionals have a key role to play in the effective implementation of primary, secondary, and tertiary preventive strategies through their ability to:

- provide specialist pediatric ophthalmic care, combining medical, surgical, and optical management of specific disorders;
- educate/train nonophthalmic colleagues, such as pediatricians, family doctors, or community eye workers, to ensure effective implementation of screening or surveillance programs aimed at early detection and prompt referral of children suspected of having specific eye diseases (e.g., congenital cataract) as well as those at high risk for visual impairment (e.g., preterm infants, those with major neuro-developmental disorders, or those with a family history of blinding eye disease);
- contribute to multidisciplinary visual impairment teams, ideally combining medical, educational, and social service professionals, to ensure comprehensive and coordinated care of all visually impaired children and their families;
- contribute to specific assessments of special educational needs and certification of eligibility for special services, in particular, notification to visual impairment registers, where these exist;
- contribute to monitoring visual impairment in the geographically defined population they serve; and
- to participate in/undertake epidemiological research that strengthens the evidence base for practice and policy.

SELECTED FURTHER READING

1. Gilbert C, Rahi J, Quinn G. Visual impairment and blindness in children. In: Johnson G, Minassian D, Weale R, West S, editors. The epidemiology of eye disease. 2nd ed. London: Arnold; 2003.
2. Sackett DL, Haynes RB, Guyatt GH, Tugwell P. Clinical epidemiology. 2nd ed. Boston: Little Brown; 1991.
3. Rothman KJ, Greenland S, editors. Modern epidemiology. 2nd ed. Philadelphia: Lippincott-Raven; 1998.

REFERENCES

1. Last JM. A Dictionary of Epidemiology. Oxford: Oxford University Press; 1988.
2. World Health Organisation (WHO). Measurement of quality of life in children. Geneva: Division of Mental Health, WHO; 1993.
3. Eiser C, Morse R. Quality of life measures in chronic diseases of childhood. Health Technol Assess 2001; 5: 1-157.
4. Barbotte E, Guillemin F, Chau N, Lorhandicap Group. Prevalence of impairments, disabilities, handicaps and quality of life in the general population: a review of recent literature. Bull World Health Organ 2001; 79: 1047–55.
5. Rahi JS, Dezateux C, British Congenital Cataract Interest Group. Measuring and interpreting the incidence of congenital ocular anomalies: lessons from a national study of congenital cataract in the UK. Invest Ophthalmol Vis Sci 2001; 42: 1444–8.
6. Williams C, Harrard RA, Harvey I, Sparrow JM; ALSPAC Study Team. Screening for amblyopia in preschool children: results of a population-based randomised controlled trial. Avon Longitudinal Study of Pregnancy and Childhood. Ophthalmic Epidemiol 2001; 8: 279–95.

7. Murray CJ, Lopez AD. Regional patterns of disability-free life expectancy and disability-adjusted life expectancy: Global Burden of Disease Study. Lancet 1997; 349: 1347–52.
8. Jan JE, Freeman RD. Who is a visually impaired child? Dev Med Child Neurol 1998; 40: 65–7.
9. Jan JE, Freeman RD, Scott EP. The family of the visually impaired child. In: Jan JE, Freeman RD, Scott EP, editors. Visual Impairment in Children and Adolescents. 1st ed. New York: Grune Stratton; 1977; p. 159–86.
10. Nixon HL. Mainstreaming and the American Dream. Sociological Perspectives on Coping with Blind and Visually Impaired Children. New York, American Foundation for the Blind; 1991.
11. Smith AF, Smith JG. The economic burden of global blindness: a price too high! Br J Ophthalmol 1996; 80: 276–7.
12. Shamanna BR, Dandona L, Rao GN. Economic burden of blindness in India. Indian J Ophthalmol 1998; 46: 169–72.
13. Frick KD, Foster A. The magnitude and cost of global blindness: an increasing problem that can be alleviated. Am J Ophthalmol 2003; 135: 471–6.
14. Tibbenham AD, Peckham CS, Gardiner PA. Vision screening in children tested at 7, 11, and 16 years. Br Med J 1978; 1: 1312–4.

15. Stewart-Brown S, Haslum MN. Partial sight and blindness in children of the 1970 birth cohort at 10 years of age. J Epidemiol Community Health 1988; 42: 17–23.

16. Mervis CA, Yeargin-Allsopp M, Winter S, Boyle C. Aetiology of childhood vision impairment, metropolitan Atlanta, 1991–1993. Paediatr Perinat Epidemiol 2000; 14: 70–7.

17. Evans J. Causes of blindness and partial sight in England and Wales 1990–91. Studies on Medical and Population Subjects No 57. London: HMSO; 1995.

18. Foot B, Stanford M, Rahi J, Thompson J. The British Ophthalmological Surveillance Unit: an evaluation of the first three years. Eye 2003; 17: 9–15.

19. Rahi JS, Cable N, on behalf of the British Childhood Visual Impairment Study Group (BCVISG). Severe visual impairment and blindness in children in the UK. The Lancet, 2003; 362: 1359–65.

20. Dandona L, Williams JD, Williams BC, Rao GN. Population based assessment of childhood blindness in Southern India. Arch Ophthalmol 1998; 116: 545–6.

21. Bulgan T, Gilbert CE. Prevalence and causes of severe visual impairment and blindness in children in Mongolia. Ophthalmic Epidemiology 2001; 9: 1–11.

22. Rahi JS, Dezateux C. Epidemiology of visual impairment. In: David TJ, editor. Recent Advances in Paediatrics 19. London: Churchill Livingstone; 2001: 97–114.

23. Gilbert CE, Foster A. Blindness in children: control priorities and research opportunities. Br J Ophthalmol 2001; 85: 1025–7.

24. Gilbert CE, Foster A. Childhood blindness in the context of VISION 2020–The right to sight. Bull World Health Organ 2001; 79: 227–32.

25. Blohme J, Tornqvist K. Visually imparied Swedish children. The 1980 cohort study–aspects on mortality. Acta Ophthalmol Scand 2000; 78: 560–5.

26. Boyle CA, Decoufle P, Holmgreen P. Contribution of developmental disabilities to childhood mortality in the United States: a multiple-cause-of-death analysis. Paediatr Perinat Epidemiol 1994; 8: 411–22.

27. Crofts B, King B, Johnson A. The contribution of low birthweight to severe vision loss in a geographically defined population. Br J Ophthalmol 1998; 82: 9–13.

28. Hack M, Flannery D, Schluchter M, et al. Outcomes in young adulthood for very-low-birthweight infants. N Engl J Med 2002; 346: 149–57.

29. Gilbert CE, Anderton L, Dandona L, Foster A. Prevalence of visual impairment in children: a review of available data. Ophthalmic Epidemiol 1999; 6: 73–82.

30. Rosenberg T, Flage T, Hansen E, et al. Incidence of registered visual impairment in the Nordic child population. Br J Ophthalmol 1996; 80: 49–53.

31. Gilbert C, Foster A, Negrel A-D, Thylefors B. Childhood blindness: a new form for recording causes of visual loss in children. Bull World Health Organ 1993; 71: 485–9.

32. Jay B. Causes of blindness in schoolchildren. Br Med J 1987; 294: 1183–4.

33. Fraser GR, Friedmann AI. The Causes of Blindness in Childhood. 1st ed. Baltimore: Johns Hopkins Press; 1967.

34. World Health Organization (WHO). International statistical classification of diseases and health related problems. 10th revision. Geneva: World Health Organisation; 1992.

35. WHO/IAPB. Preventing blindness in children. Report of a WHO/IAPB scientific meeting. WHO/PBL/00.77. Geneva: World Health Organization (WHO); 2000.

36. Riise R, Flage T, Hansen E, et al. Visual impairment in Nordic children. I. Nordic registers and prevalence data. Acta Ophthalmol 1992; 70: 145–54.

37. Goggin M, O'Keefe M. Childhood blindness in the Republic of Ireland: a national survey. Br J Ophthalmol 1991; 75: 425–9.

38. Maul E, Barroso S, Munoz SR, et al. Refractive error study in children: results from La Florida, Chile. Am J Ophthalmol 2000; 129: 445–54.

39. World Health Organization (WHO). Prevalence and causes of blindness and low vision, Morocco. Wkly Epidem. Rec 1994; 69: 129–36.

40. Zhao J, Pan X, Sui R, et al. Refractive error study in children: results from Shungi District, China. Am J Ophthalmol 2000; 129: 427–35.

41. Sil AK, Basu S, Acharya N. Prevalence of chldhood blindness in Orissa. Available at http://aios.org/Contents/Data/Community/13.pdf; 2003.

42. Cohen N, Rahman H, Sprague J, et al. Prevalence and determinants of nutritional blindness in Bangladeshi children. World Health Stat Q 1995; 38: 317–30.

43. Pokharel GP, Negrel A-D, Munoz SR, Ellwein LB. Refractive error study in children: results from Mechi Zone, Nepal. Am J Ophthalmol 2000; 129: 436–44.

44. Tielsch JM, West KP Jr, Katz J, et al. Prevalence and severity of xerophthalmia in southern Malawi. Am J Epidemiol 1986; 124: 561–8.

45. Faal H, Minassian D, Sowa S, Foster A. National survey of blindness and low vision in The Gambia: results. Br J Ophthalmol 1989; 73: 82–7.

46. Abiose A, Murdoch I, Babalola O, et al. Distribution and aetiology of blindness and visual impairment in mesoendemic onchocercal communities, Kaduna State, Nigeria. Kaduna Collaboration for Research on Onchocerciasis. Br J Ophthalmol 1994; 78: 8–13. [Published erratum Br J Ophthalmol 1995 Feb; 79: 197.]

47. World Health Organisation (WHO). Prevalence and causes of blindness and low vision, Benin. Wkly Epidem.Rec 1991; 66: 337–44.

48. Wilson MR, Mansour M, Ross Degnan D, et al. Prevalence and causes of low vision and blindness in the extreme North Province of Cameroon, West Africa. Ophthalmic Epidemiol 1996; 3: 23–33.

CHAPTER 2 Normal and Abnormal Visual Development

Daniel L Adams

THE DEVELOPING VISUAL PATHWAYS

Human vision requires precise collaboration of diverse structures. From the eye to the cerebral cortex, the components mature in parallel, each influencing the development of the whole.

Some developmental processes follow an innate plan that is programmed using molecular cues forming "hard-wired" neural circuits. Others are controlled by the neuronal activity within the system itself that arises spontaneously, or from visual stimulation. Thus, the anatomical configuration of the visual system is sculpted by both nature and nurture.

In a developing individual, visual experience adjusts the neural structures such that they best represent the world they are exposed to. Combined with the innate, "hard-wired," plan, this produces an efficient visual system because only elements that function appropriately are maintained: "use it or lose it."

Reliance on visual experience makes the system vulnerable: a fault during development may be detrimental. With anomalous visual experience, the system develops abnormally. Thus, the processes that normally generate an efficient visual system can also cause abnormal development.

An example is monocular deprivation. Here, a problem that obscures vision in one eye, like a congenital cataract, disrupts the development of "down stream structures" generating a permanent visual loss that persists after removal of the cataract.

The interdependent elements of the visual system must all develop appropriately. A fault at any point from eye to brain can have effects on the whole system. The normal development of each component will be discussed individually.

The eye

The eyes differentiate early from the neural plate. They first appear as the optic pits by the fifth week of gestation, and then extend from the neural tube to form the optic vesicles. These spherical pouches invaginate to form the optic cups, attached to the prosencephalon by stalks that become the optic nerves. Further differentiation of the optic cup gives rise to each of the components of the eye. The lens and cornea arise from the surface ectoderm; the retina, pigment epithelia, and optic nerve from neural ectoderm; and the vasculature and sclera from paraxial mesoderm. By three months gestation, each of the major anatomical structures is in place.

At birth, the axial length of the human eye is about 17 mm (about 74% of adult), and increasing by about 0.16 mm/week.[1] The eye grows nonuniformly; most of its increase in volume is from posterior segment growth. The neonatal corneal surface area is 3/4, and the scleral surface area 1/3 of the emmetropic adult's.[2] The lens continues to grow after birth, increasing in diameter more than in thickness, resulting in a less spherical and more disk-like adult shape. By 13 years of age, the eye has reached an average axial length of 23 mm, its developmental endpoint.[3]

The retina

The fovea develops before the peripheral retina,[4-6] yet it is immature at birth.[7,8] It first appears as a bump formed by ganglion cells. Over about the next 25 weeks, foveal ganglion cells and inner nuclear layer cells migrate peripherally, creating the familiar foveal depression at about 15 months.[8,9]

Among the many specializations that endow the primate fovea with supreme vision is its peak density of photoreceptors. At birth, the density of foveal photoreceptor cells is a tiny fraction of the adult's. Peripheral photoreceptor cells migrate toward the fovea from before birth to at least 45 months (longer than the centripetal migration of ganglion cells). As the cones pack together there is a reduction in their diameter; their short, squat inner segments elongate, and the rudimentary stumps of outer segments lengthen into the long, thin appendages of the adult (Fig. 2.1). Since ganglion cells and photoreceptors migrate in opposite directions, extended connecting processes form between the cone pedicles and their cell bodies. Reaching radially as far as 0.4 mm, these specialized axons form the Henle fiber layer, which surrounds the fovea by 2.5 mm in the adult.[10]

The human fovea remains immature, even at six to eight months postpartum. Cell morphology and cell density take 15 months to approach maturity, and it may be four years before the retina is largely adult-like.[11] This time course is consistent with some aspects of visual development measured experimentally.

The retina contains seven principal cell types, each with its own circuitry, organized into layers. The different cell types derive from progenitor cells in the inner layer of the optic cup. A progenitor cell can generate different retinal cell types, right up to its final division, raising the following question "What influences the fate of retinal progenitor cells?" The type of cell a progenitor may become follows a temporal order during development that is preserved between species.[12-14] Ganglion cells develop first, followed in overlapping phases by horizontal cells, cones, amacrine cells, rods, bipolar cells, and Müller cells (Fig. 2.2).[15] The acquisition and loss of ability to differentiate into particular cell types suggests that the progenitor cells' extrinsic factors serially bias them to a particular fate. However, in vitro experiments have not confirmed this. Environmental factors can change the proportions of different cell types generated at a particular stage, but they cannot induce the production of cell types inappropriate for that stage.[16,17] Thus, progenitor cells pass through a number of states during which they are only competent at producing a subset of cell types, and the proportions of cell types that they produce at each stage is

9

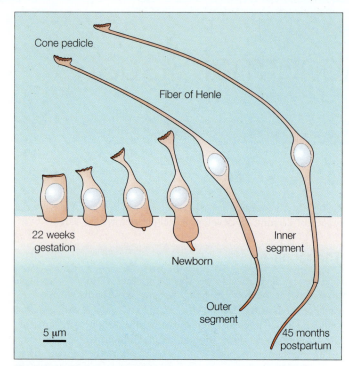

Fig. 2.1 A schematic drawing showing the stages of development of a human foveal cone (left to right) at 22, 24 to 26, and 34 to 36 weeks gestation, newborn, and 15 and 45 months postpartum. The inner segment is present before birth, while the outer segment develops mainly postnatally, being little more than a stump at birth. The cone pedicle and the fiber of Henle are present before birth. All four structures undergo extreme postnatal thinning and elongation. Adapted from Hendrickson AE, Yaodelis C. The morphological development of the human forea. Ophthalmology 1984; 91: 603–12, with permission from the American Academy of Ophthalmology.

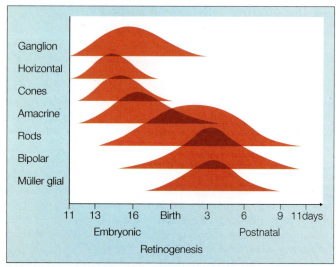

Fig. 2.2 Retinal neurogenesis proceeds in a characteristic sequence. Ganglion cells and horizontal cells differentiate first, followed in overlapping phases by cones, amacrine cells, rods, bipolar cells, and Müller glial cells. Curves represent the relative proportions of cells differentiating at each stage, not their absolute numbers. The time scale refers to mouse development. Adapted from Marquart T, Gruss P. Generating neuronal diversity in the retina: one for nearly all. Trends Neurosci 2002; 25: 32–8. © 2002 with permission from Elsevier.

controlled by environmental factors.[18] This is the "competence model" of retinal development.[19]

Once differentiated, retinal neurons must migrate to their adult positions before they form synapses, and to generate the laminar structure of the retina. This occurs in two stages:

Stage one brings cells imprecisely into bands at roughly the appropriate depths and is moderated by the attractive/repulsive adhesion properties of the cells. Mutations in genes encoding adhesion molecules or integrins disrupt retinal lamination at this stage.[20–22]

Stage two more precisely organizes cells into uniform mosaics, distributed tangentially, and with precise laminar distribution. In the rat, at birth the horizontal cells have migrated to within a ~50-μm-deep sheet, but by day six, they form a regularly spaced monolayer.[23,24] The mechanisms of the second stage may work by maintaining constant distances between cells, perhaps by minimizing dendritic overlap. If one cell is removed from, or cells are added to a developing retinal layer, the others shuffle over to regularize the mozaic.[25]

The chiasm

In primates, ganglion cell axons enter the optic stalk at about six weeks gestation. When they reach the optic chiasm they either cross or remain ipsilateral. Their decision is influenced by (among other factors[26]) adhesion molecules and pathway markers,[27] differential gene expression[28,29] and chiasmal template neurons.[30,31] These mechanisms guide axons using attractive and repulsive molecules.[32] One such family of molecules is the "slits." These are thought to govern where the chiasm forms by defining a restricting corridor. Disrupting slit expression produces a large, more anterior, secondary chiasm and prevents retinal ganglion cell (RGC) axons from finding their way into the appropriate optic tract.[33]

The zinc finger transcription factor, Zic2, is expressed in ipsilaterally projecting RGCs during their growth from the ventrotemporal retina to the chiasm.[34] Zic2 regulates RGC axon repulsion by cues at the chiasmal midline. The proportion of RGC axons that cross is related to the size of the animal's binocular visual field. Retinal Zic2 levels correlate with the animal's degree of binocular vision, suggesting that Zic2 is an evolutionarily conserved determinant of ipsilateral projection.

In primates, the RGCs in nasal and temporal retina are directed to the contralateral and ipsilateral hemispheres respectively, except for a 5° wedge along the vertical meridian (with the overlap increasing with vertical distance from the fovea) where ganglion cells project to either hemisphere.[35] The normal decussation pattern is disrupted in albinos[36] (see Chapter 45) and rarely in otherwise normal primates[37].

Myelination of the optic nerve begins only after all RGC axons have reached the geniculate body (fifth month in humans) and continues into early childhood in a brain-to-eye direction, stopping at the lamina cribrosa.[38] Occasionally, it proceeds into the retina, where it appears as white streaks in the nerve fiber layer.[39] Such errant myelination is normally benign, but rarely it can be associated with a visual deficit.[40,41]

Retinogeniculate projections

About 90% of primate RGCs project to the lateral geniculate body (LGB); the remainder go mostly to the pretectum and the superior colliculus.[42] The LGB contains six principal layers specified by their eye of input and by their cell type (Fig. 2.3). Four of the principal layers (two for each eye) are made up of small, parvocellular (P) cells, and two (one for each eye) contain large, magnocellular (M) cells. Tiny koniocellular (K) cells constitute a third class that occupy the leaflets between the six principal layers.[43]

The layers of the LGB are present at birth. Their development exemplifies the interaction between activity-dependent and hard-wired mechanisms in the formation of the visual pathways. In the

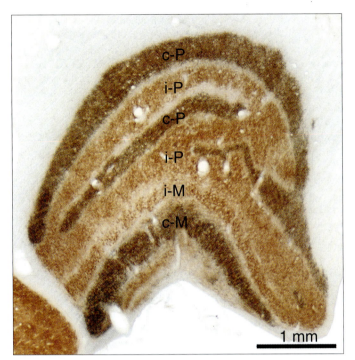

Fig. 2.3 Macaque LGN stained with cytochrome oxidase following injection of a radioactive tracer ([³H] proline) into the right (contralateral) eye. Layers containing the tracer appear dark. The six principal layers are monocular in macaque (and human) and follows the sequence: contra-ipsi-ipsi-contra-ipsi-contra. Layers 1 and 2 are magnocellular, and layers 3–6 are parvocellular. Koniocellular layers are situated between the six principal layers. M, magnocellular; P, parvocellular; c, contralateral; i, ipsilateral.

human, optic tract fibers begin to reach the LGB by about the 11th week. Initially, left and right eye afferents are intermingled over the prospective left and right eye layers.[44] Between weeks 14 and 30, a time corresponding to the formation of eye-specific layers in the geniculate body, the population of RGC axons reduces from 3.5 million to about 1 million.[45,46] Perhaps the purpose of this cell loss is to generate eye-specific layers by eliminating inappropriately connected axons: "selective elimination."[45]

Selective trimming of axon terminal arbors also segregates binocular inputs to the LGB. In the cat, axons innervating the LGB grow promiscuous side-branches that contact cells in both left and right eye columns. By birth, the side-branches contacting the inappropriate layer for their eye are withdrawn, leaving a precise segregation of inputs.[46,47] However, selective elimination of whole retinal afferents (rather than single branches) can account for the segregation of binocular afferents in the primate LGB.[48]

In contrast to the laminar segregation by eye, development of the M and P layers of the LGB does not employ selective elimination of afferent cells. RGCs become M and P types soon after their final mitosis.[49] The P-type retinal afferents reach the geniculate first and innervate the medial segment that will later develop into the four P layers. The M-type retinal afferents arrive later and innervate the lateral segment that will become the two layers of the M division. Thus, retinal afferents innervate their appropriate presumptive M or P divisions exclusively, suggesting selective targeting rather than corrective selective elimination.[50] Thus, the segregation of the geniculate into magnocellular and parvocellular layers is less dependent on visual experience than its segregation by eye.

Geniculocortical connections

Most geniculate cells project to layer 4 of the striate cortex, where inputs from the two eyes differentially activate single cells–"ocular dominance."[51] As an electrode is advanced parallel to the cortical layers, the ocular dominance of cells alternates between the left and right eyes. Small lesions of single (monocular) layers of the LGB cause degeneration of terminals in layer 4 of the striate cortex in a stripy pattern.[52] These 300- to 400-μm-wide stripes of left- and right-eye inputs form a mosaic of discreet columns. The complete pattern of ocular dominance columns can be visualized by radioactive tracer injection into one eye.[53] The tracer is taken up by RGCs and transported to layer 4 of the striate cortex (Fig 2.4).

Formation of the ocular dominance column pattern cannot be dependent on visual experience because (at least in the macaque) it is adult-like at birth.[54,55] However, this does not necessarily mean that it forms independently of neuronal activity. It has long been held that the geniculocortical afferents are initially intermingled and are segregated into ocular dominance columns under the influence of retinal activity.[56–58] Thus, pharmacological blockage of retinal activity abolishes column formation in the cat.[57] The spontaneous waves of neuronal activity that roll across each retina in utero could play a role in column segregation by generating firing patterns in the RGCs that are spatially correlated within, but not between, each eye.[59] This suggests that cells with synchronous activity are segregated into a single ocular dominance column, i.e., cells that "fire together, wire together."[60] However, ferrets binocularly enucleated before their geniculo-cortical afferents arrived at the striate cortex form normal ocular dominance columns.[61] Thus, retinal activity cannot be a prerequisite for columnar segregation in this species. The formation of the ocular dominance column pattern may rely on intrinsic signals, e.g., molecular cues on thalamic axons, on cortical cells, or on both.[62]

Extrastriate cortical areas

Cells in the striate cortex project to multiple extrastriate visual areas, forming an interconnected hierarchy reaching into the

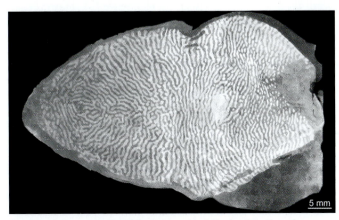

Fig. 2.4 Macaque monkey left striate cortex following injection of a radioactive tracer ([³H] proline) into the left eye. The tracer appears bright. The tissue has been dissected from the rest of the brain, unfolded, and flattened to show the entire striate cortex. The mosaic of ocular dominance columns is visible because the tracer was transported to only those columns belonging to the injected eye. The bright oval to the right of the center is the representation of the blind spot—a monocular region of the visual field.

parietal and temporal lobes. Many regions in this network are defined as single visual areas by their retinotopic organization, cell selectivity, and/or unique pattern of connections with other regions.[63] It is thought that different areas process different visual modalities, e.g., motion, color, and form.[64]

The development of extrastriate cortical areas has been investigated by the early removal of cortical tissue, before any inputs have arrived at the neocortex.[65] If cortical areas form in predetermined regions, subsequent mapping of visual areas in these animals in adulthood would show a reduced number of areas. However, it shows a full compliment of cortical areas, squeezed onto a reduced area of cortex. Thus, the primitive neocortex is an unspecialized substrate whose subdivision into areas occurs in unison.

NORMAL VISUAL DEVELOPMENT

To study visual development, it is important to know about the vision of the newborn. Newborn humans can see. They prefer to look at faces.[66,67] They can even discriminate between mouth opening and tongue protrusion, and rapidly imitate either.[68] They initially fixate simple high-contrast patterns (like their mother's hairline), and are later attracted to more subtle features (like their mother's eyes).

Measurement techniques

Since infants are unable to report what they see, adult vision measurement techniques must be adapted and other indicators of "seeing" used.[69,70] The three most commonly used techniques will be described:

Preferential looking (PL)
Given a choice of looking at a striped grating or a uniform field, an infant will prefer to fix the grating.[71-73] A hidden observer guesses which of two stimuli contains a grating based on the infant's fixation behaviour.[74] As less visible gratings are presented, the observer makes more incorrect inferences. The visual threshold is defined by the grating stimulus that generates only 75% correct inferences from the observer. Also known as "forced choice preferential looking" (FPL), this technique has been successfully used to assess infant visual development.[74-76] However, its reliability is dependent on many trials and it is difficult to hold the infant's attention for the necessary time.[77]

Visually evoked potentials (VEP)
The VEP technique measures electrical activity directly from the scalp using surface electrodes.[78,79] Visual stimulation produces a stereotypical wave of electrical activity, whose amplitude and timing can be measured. Repeated responses are recorded and averaged to improve signal-to-noise ratio. A "transient" VEP is recorded in response to a single event, e.g., a flashed stimulus,[80] and a "steady-state" VEP is a continuous standing wave pattern produced by a rapidly repeating stimulus.[81]

The raw VEP signal must be analyzed to estimate visual acuity. A simple method is to compile a set of transient VEPs using a single high-contrast stimulus, and measure the Snellen acuity in an emmetropic adult with various degrees of optical blur. The infant's acuity can then be estimated by comparing their VEP to the blurred adult set. The acuity of the infant is presumed to be equal to the acuity of the adult whose vision was blurred such that their VEP signals were most similar.[80,82] This method relies on the unlikely assumption that infant and adult VEPs are equivalent.

An alternative method is to present finer and finer grating stimuli until a transient VEP is no longer measurable above noise,[83] or to extrapolate to zero response amplitude, using either the transient[84] or the steady-state VEP.[85] Extrapolation to zero is used because the VEP signal is inherently noisy, making it more difficult to define the exact point where a small signal disappears.

Optokinetic nystagmus (OKN)
A stimulus generates wide-field, drifting OKN that can be used to estimate infant visual acuity because it is only generated by resolvable stimuli and it is easily observed. The earliest investigation used a stimulus attached to a metronome wand;[86] later experiments employed scrolls of paper, printed with gratings and streamed over the infant's visual field by a hand crank.[73,87] Eye movements were observed or measured with electro-oculograms.[88]

Visual acuity

Visual acuity ("grating acuity," "resolution acuity") is a measure of the finest feature detectable by an observer. It can be described as the visual angle subtended by a single stripe element (minutes per stripe), or more formally as its reciprocal (cycles per degree), i.e., the threshold spatial frequency of a 100% contrast square-wave grating.[89] In normal adults, resolution acuity is equal to about 1 min/stripe, or 30 cycles/degree. By setting this value to be equivalent to the standard Snellen acuity of 20/20, it is possible to roughly convert between the two scales.

In classic studies using optokinetic nystagmus, 93 of 100 infants aged 80 minutes to 5 days responded to a 0.56 cycles/degree grating moving at 8.5°/sec, but none responded to a 0.19 cycles/ degree grating moving at the same speed.[87] Using a greater range of grating sizes, a "large percentage" of another 100 newborns responded to a 0.25 cycles/degree grating.[90] Thus, nearly all the infants tested had at least 20/400, and some 20/300, Snellen equivalent vision. Others have found lower values for newborn acuity,[91] but this range is consistent with most investigations of zero- to three-week-old infant acuity, using OKN[73,88] and PL.[75]

Natural variation, nonstandardized testing techniques, different viewing distances, and illuminations produce differences in measured acuity between studies. To overcome this, the standardized Teller Acuity Card system was devised.[92,93] Using these cards, 140 infants showed a mean acuity at one week of 0.9 (± ~0.5 SD) cycles/degree.[94] This data, along with other measures of the development of acuity using PL, is shown in Fig. 2.5.

A comparison of PL with VEP data shows that the VEP technique gives acuity values about 1 to 2 octaves better than PL measures at all ages (an octave is a doubling of acuity). This could be due to the stationary stimuli used in PL studies, whereas VEP studies use temporally modulated gratings that may produce a lower acuity threshold. If checkerboard stimuli are used in VEP studies, the amplitude of the signal shows a peak at a particular check size. If the location of this peak is used instead of the VEP amplitude, the two acuity measures agree.[95] When visual acuity is assessed using VEPs and FPL in the same infants, VEP signals could be detected for spatial patterns that were below threshold for behavioral measures. This could be due to the signal averaging used in the VEP technique.[96] It seems that the increased signal-to-noise ratio generated by averaging in VEP studies is of benefit to the experimenter but not the visual system! If VEP latency is used instead of amplitude, comparable scores can be generated with the two techniques.

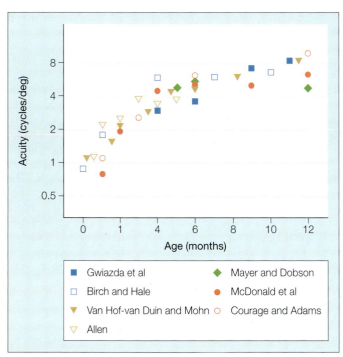

Fig. 2.5 Representative examples of data showing the development of binocular grating acuity in normal infants tested with the PL procedure.[70,94,241–245] With permission from Dobson.[240]

Contrast sensitivity

A more complete evaluation of the spatial performance of the visual system can be gained by measuring many contrast thresholds over a range of spatial frequency. This produces a graph of threshold contrast versus spatial frequency–"contrast sensitivity function."[97,98] The conventionally measured grating acuity is then represented by the abscissa of the x axis (100% contrast). The adult curve has a peak value at 3–5 cycles/degree and a decline in sensitivity at both lower and higher spatial frequencies.

Overall contrast sensitivity of the infant is about 10 times higher than the adult but infants are relatively more sensitive in the low-frequency region. This reduced "low-frequency cut" was demonstrated in a PL study of infants from age 5 to 12 weeks.[99] The low-frequency cut was smallest in the 5-week group, and more pronounced by 12 weeks.

The absence of a low-frequency cut in the 5-week group, and its relatively smaller size in the older groups, suggests that the undeveloped visual pathway might be relatively well suited to transmit coarse features that do not require the high-resolution components of the retina, or it could be central in origin. Inhibitory cortical connections may tune cortical cells to higher spatial frequencies[100,101] and perhaps these are underdeveloped in infants. It could also be artifactual, due to the reduced number of cycles visible in low-frequency stimuli,[102–104] or perhaps infants just prefer to fixate lower spatial frequencies. The effect has been verified by further PL investigations (Fig. 2.6) but the origins of changes in the contrast sensitivity function over the first 3 months of infancy would have to be determined with other techniques.

The maturation of contrast sensitivity has been studied in the infant using the steady-state "sweep VEP,"[105–107] where the spatial frequency of the stimulus is swept over a range of values during recording, while holding contrast constant. These findings substantiated the main PL findings and narrowed the search for

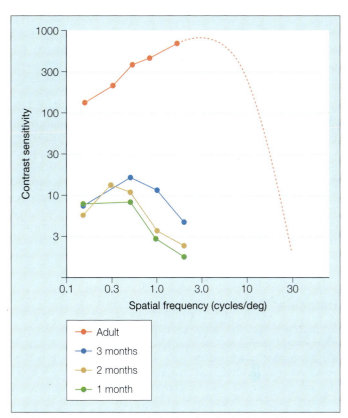

Fig. 2.6 Average contrast sensitivity functions for 1-, 2-, and 3-month-olds and an adult obtained using an FLP procedure. The solid line represents data obtained with the infant apparatus; the dashed portion represents typical high-frequency data for an adult under similar conditions. Data from Banks and Salapatek.[76]

anatomical correlates. The absence of low-frequency attenuation in young infants was reproduced, and its time course clarified. Up to 9 weeks of age, the contrast sensitivity function shows an increase in sensitivity at all spatial frequencies. Thence, sensitivity increases are restricted to the higher frequency domain, indicating an improvement in spatial resolution, rather than sensitivity per se. Thus, the development of low-spatial-frequency vision follows a time-course shorter than that of high spatial frequencies. Given that high spatial frequencies are detected by the fovea, which develops more slowly than the periphery,[7] it is likely that the slow increase in high-spatial-frequency sensitivity is a result of the prolonged development of the fovea. Likewise, since low-spatial-frequency sensitivity is unaffected by exclusion of the fovea,[108] it follows that the early relative sensitivity to low spatial frequencies is due to the relatively advanced maturation of peripheral retina.

Operant training of infant monkeys, shows that the macaque visual system is very similar to the human's, but that it develops much faster.[109] Infant humans and monkeys show the same depression of sensitivity compared to adults. The higher relative sensitivity to low spatial frequencies of human infants is also apparent, as is the differential developmental time-course for low and high spatial frequencies.[110] Young monkeys' foveal contrast sensitivity is similar to the near periphery but develops to a greater degree during maturation.[111] Thus, the developmental time-courses of high- and low-spatial-frequency sensitivity match those of the fovea and peripheral retina, respectively.

To compare the development of grating acuity and contrast sensitivity in the central and peripheral visual field of the human infant, sweep VEPs were measured in infants ranging from 10 to 39 weeks of age.[112] By testing the central and peripheral fields simultaneously, each at a different temporal frequency, it was found that peripheral acuity reached adult values by 26 weeks while central acuity did not reach asymptosy up to 33 weeks. The human infant's fixation sensitivity was better than its peripheral vision at all ages. However, this could be due to the infant using an eccentric fixation strategy, rather like the one an adult might use to view a distant star at night.

Photoreceptor development is probably not the only limiter of maturation of contrast sensitivity.[113] Optical influences are modest because the neonatal media are clear, and accommodation does not affect acuity much over distances between 30 and 150 cm.[114] To gauge any influence the LGB and striate cortex may have on contrast sensitivity is not straightforward because they receive signals already filtered by the immature retina.

Binocular vision

Primates and carnivores perceive depth from their binocular view of the world: stereopsis. For stereopsis to develop, eye movements must point both foveas at the same location in 3-D space and the eyes must move conjugately to maintain binocular fusion. When the images from the eyes are continuously fused, disparities are analyzed by cortical cells for the calculation of depth. Stereopsis is robust: stereograms can still be perceived when one eye's image is blurred.[115,116]

Stereopsis is the result of a neuronal calculation, so it requires specialized stimuli to isolate it from other visual cues. Clinically, stereopsis is often tested with the Titmus test. The patient wears polarized spectacles with the plane of polarization at right angles for each eye. Test images consist of superimposed stereo-pairs, presented differently to each eye by a polarized filter layer. One example is of a large housefly, which stands out from the page to an observer with stereopsis. Others are circles and animal pictures at different depth planes. While these tests are adequate for assessing the presence or absence of stereopsis in children, random dot stereograms[117] are superior because they contain a form that can *only* be seen with stereopsis. Viewed monocularly or by the stereoblind, a random dot stereogram appears as a flat field of noise. When viewed stereoscopically, pictures appear in front of, or behind the plane of the page.

By about two months of age, some infants, tested with random dot stereograms, apparently discriminated disparity when tested with PL and a habituation recovery test.[118] Computers made dynamic random dot stereograms more amenable. Using FPL, infants were presented with a square stimulus, defined by stereo alone, that drifted to the right or left. The hidden observer guessed the direction of the stimulus by the infant's behavior and eye movements.[119] No significant difference from chance was measured in the observer's direction guesses for infants up to 3.5 months of age, and even later (up to 6 months) in a longitudinal experiment.[120]

Random dot stereograms are suited for use with VEPs because they are perceived only if stereopsis is present. Any modulation of the VEP signal at the same frequency as the stimulus is indicative of stereopsis. Random dot stimuli that oscillate in depth (stereograms) or that counterphase in one eye (correlograms) evoke large potentials, enabling reliable determination of stereopsis in infants.[121–123] Stereo stimuli evoked responses in infants at 8 to 20 weeks.[124,125]

Stereoacuity improves until about 24 months, when it approaches adult levels;[126,127] some improvement is from increased interocular distance but most is due to development of the central visual pathways. Disparity-tuned binocular neurons have been found in the striate cortex in both the cat and monkey.[128,129] Although these cells signal the disparity of stimuli, their responses do not necessarily correlate with depth perception.[130,131] Cells in the monkey striate cortex can be tuned to disparity by the sixth postnatal day,[132] several weeks before the onset of stereopsis. Furthermore, infant monkeys have an adult proportion of disparity-tuned cells and their ocular dominance histograms are adult-like.[133] The development of stereopsis is not due simply to a proportional increase in the numbers of disparity-tuned cells in the striate cortex, but to a refinement of their spatial response properties and overall responsiveness. The onset of stereopsis may correlate with the refinement of extrastriate visual connections and increasing populations of disparity-tuned cells in higher visual areas.

Orientation selectivity

Cells activated selectively by bars or gratings presented over a small range of orientations are implicated in form vision.[134] Recordings from striate cortex cells of newborn kittens showed that no neurons were adult-like in their responses to oriented contours.[135] Orientation-selective cells have been found in visually inexperienced macaque striate cortex at three weeks.[136] Even at this early stage, the cells are organized into adult-like columns that are in register with ocular dominance columns.[137]

The relationship between orientation selectivity development and visual experience has been investigated by raising animals in an artificial environment that exposed them to a restricted range of contour orientations: "stripe rearing."[138,139] Stripe-reared cats were first shown to have a larger than normal proportion of cells tuned to the orientation they were exposed to most. Despite the dramatic changes in the distributions of orientation preference of cortical cells, only modest specific behavioral deficits could be measured, incommensurate with the magnitude of the physiological effects.[140] This inconsistency led others to re-examine the phenomenon. At first, no effect was found;[141] later, a small effect was described.[142] The inconsistencies among stripe rearing experiments were probably due to different techniques and sampling methods. The overall effect, though probably real, is certainly not as striking as it was first described.

Motion perception

Motion information is crucial to many visual and motor functions, for example, the encoding of depth through parallax, estimating trajectories, segmenting figures from backgrounds, and controlling posture and eye movements.[143] OKN studies show that motion vision develops early in humans.[144] However, OKN is a crude and reflexive measure of motion sensitivity that does not require fine direction discrimination.

The ability to discriminate opposite directions of motion develops at about 10 to 13 weeks.[145,146] VEP studies show it within the first two months of life.[147,148] Finer discriminations of motion direction have been tested using FPL where infants were presented with windows of dots moving in a different direction to the background dots.[148] The angle between target and background directions was reduced until preferential looking by the infant was no longer detectable. By the age of 12 weeks, infants made quite fine discriminations, on the order of 20°, and by 18 weeks they were down to ~15°. These values are still far from those of adults, who have no trouble making discriminations of less than 1°.

Neural motion perception is thought to result from the activity of direction-selective cells. These are found in layer IVB of the striate cortex,[150] and in many extrastriate cortical areas, most notably V5 (MT).[151] Electrical microstimulation of V5 cells in the monkey has shown that their activity correlates directly with the perception of motion direction and can affect the animal's direction discrimination.[152] Little is known about the development of direction selectivity in area V5. However, single-cell recordings in the striate cortex of 1-week-old monkeys have shown that direction selectivity is absent or very broad. The tuning width was 45°–90° by 2 weeks of age, narrowing to an adult-like 30° by 4 to 8 weeks.[153] Thus, the time-course of direction selectivity in monkey striate cortex approximately matches that of the psychophysical measurement of direction discrimination in the human infant, counting the four-times slower maturation of the human visual system.[109]

Color vision

Early studies suggested that very young infants are able to discriminate different colors.[154] However, most natural-colored stimuli also differ in their real and perceived brightness. To test color vision exclusively it is necessary to use colors of the same perceived brightness that can be discriminated by their wavelength composition alone (isoluminant colors). Different individuals can have different isoluminance points, so to eliminate individual variability, isoluminance points must be measured in every experimental subject. In early studies, adult isoluminance points were used,[155] introducing a luminance confound.[156] FPL techniques for measuring isoluminance points in infants were soon developed.[157,158] FPL-derived isoluminance points are unlikely to be perfectly accurate, so residual luminance artifacts were camouflaged either by testing over small ranges of luminance differences from trial to trial or by dividing the stimuli into a number of tiles and randomly "jittering" luminance.

With the luminance confound removed, the infants' chromatic discrimination can be tested, with FPL, using patterned (preferred) stimuli, commonly two isoluminant color checks or gratings, versus uniform (nonpreferred) intermediate color stimuli. Thus it was shown that 8-week-old infants can distinguish a red and isoluminant gray square-wave grating from a uniform luminance matched stimulus.[158] Female infants were used to reduce the probability of a color-blind infant being tested. A few 4-week-olds, some 8-week-olds, and all 12-week-olds demonstrated color vision.[159–161] Sensitivities to different wavelengths may develop at different times, making infants functionally deuteranopic for a developmental period.[160] However, a wide range of normal variation exists in development of spectral sensitivities.[161,162]

Luminance and chromatic sensitivity are both dependent on the same photoreceptors: red and green cones.[163] If the time-course of changes in contrast sensitivity are the same for luminance and chromatic stimuli, it suggests that their neural correlate lies with the photoreceptors' development,[164] but if their time-course is different, separate (post-receptor) mechanisms may be responsible for each.[165] To differentiate, it is necessary to measure chromatic contrast sensitivity in infants over a range of ages. Using VEPs, it was found that chromatic and luminance contrast sensitivity functions at all ages were well described by curves of a common shape, with developmental changes confined to upward shifts in

sensitivity and rightward shifts in spatial scale.[166–169] Thus, their poorer color discriminative ability (like their poorer luminance contrast sensitivity) is likely due to the smaller percentage of photons caught by their immature photoreceptors.[164]

ABNORMAL VISUAL DEVELOPMENT: AMBLYOPIA

Definition

"Amblyopia" is from the Greek *amblyos*, blunt, and *opia*, vision. Albrecht von Graefe is said to have defined amblyopia as the condition in which the observer saw nothing and the patient very little. This definition remains valid because it emphasizes an important feature of amblyopia–that looking into the eye reveals nothing about the disease itself. Eye examination does reveal factors that cause amblyopia, like cataract, strabismus, and anisometropia. A more formal definition of amblyopia is visual impairment without apparent organic pathology.

Critical periods

The term "critical period" was first used by Konrad Lorenz in his studies of imprinting in birds. It was adopted by Hubel and Wiesel to refer to the time when deprivation changes the ocular dominance of cells in the striate cortex.[170] It falls between 4 and 6 weeks in the cat,[171] when closure of one eye for 3 days or more leads to a visual cortex dominated by cells that respond to the open eye alone. Some susceptibility to deprivation persists until about 9 months.[172] Since Lorenz coined the term, it has taken on a more general use. A critical period can be defined for any function as the time when, if deprived of normal stimulation or unused, the function's development will be permanently disrupted. Visual critical periods begin after the initiation of visual stimulation (eye-opening in cats, birth in primates) and last between weeks and years, depending on the species and visual faculty in question.

Critical periods have been defined for strabismus,[173] for the development of direction selectivity in cat striate cortex,[173] and for orientation selectivity.[175] Neurons with more complex response properties have critical periods that end later than those with earlier-processed properties, like ocular dominance. This is exemplified within the striate cortex, where the critical period is over in layer IV (the input layer) before the other layers.[176]

Critical periods can be inferred by monocular deprivation after various delays. Early monocular deprivation is catastrophic to the visual system because it affects many critical periods. In the monkey, monocular deprivation before 3 months affects absolute light sensitivity, between 3 and 6 months sensitivity to wavelength and brightness, up to 18 months high-spatial-frequency vision, and up to 24 months binocular vision.[177] Human critical periods are less well defined, and can be deduced by studying children with amblyopia following unilateral cataract surgery.[178] By comparing children in whom the age of cataract onset and correction of vision are known, the human critical period for visual acuity loss appears to be much longer than that in cats and monkeys. Weeks of deprivation between 6 and 18 months, and months of deprivation up to age 8 produce permanent visual deficits. Early correction is therefore imperative for visual recovery following deprivation.

Amblyopia may recover in adult humans following loss of the nonamblyopic eye. This can occur well beyond the critical period, when no amount of monocular occlusion would result in the induction of amblyopia. However, improvements have been measured following visual loss of the good eye in teenagers and adults[179] and a 65-year-old.[180] One year after the loss of their good eye, 20% of 254 amblyopes aged 11 years or older had some improvement in their amblyopic eye,[181] and half improved by two or more Snellen lines. At least in a minority of patients, it appears that neural plasticity can occur past the critical period.

Factors other than neural plasticity could also account for the apparent improvement in visual acuity. Fixation may become more stable and accommodation accuracy may improve in an amblyopic eye once the individual is forced to use it alone. Adult recovery from amblyopia may help us understand the factors that normally act to restrain plasticity beyond the critical period but children should remain the focus of detection and treatment.[181]

Causes

Amblyopia is caused by abnormal visual experience: mostly by strabismus, anisometropia, monocular form deprivation, or a combination of these. Defining the cause in any particular patient is not always straightforward because anisometropia and strabismus can arise as a consequence of amblyopia,[182] making it difficult to distinguish cause and effect unless a patient is examined early enough. The three most recognized causes are strabismus, anisometropia, and monocular form deprivation.

Strabismus

Strabismus is a misalignment of the optic axes resulting from motor or sensory deficits.[183] The optic axes may be crossed (esotropic), diverged (exotropic), or vertically misaligned (hyper/hypotropic). Humans are often born with a slight exodeviation, thought to represent the anatomic positions of the divergent orbits.[182] During the first six months, binocular fusion emerges, and a normal infant attains orthotropic vision.[183] One to 2% of infants do not develop binocular fusion and acquire strabismus.[181] Esotropia is the most common form of childhood strabismus and is often associated with hyperopia. Infants are born hyperopic but generally attain emmetropia, though some remain hyperopic until 2–3 years or more.[186] Some of these infants accommodate to correct their blurred vision. Normally, accommodation is reflexively accompanied by a tendency to converge but in hyperopia this reflex can cause the eyes to cross, preventing binocular fusion and resulting in infantile esotropia.

Strabismics rarely complain of double vision because they suppress perception from the deviated eye. Some are able to alternate fixation and suppression between their eyes, and they rarely develop amblyopia. Strabismics who fix constantly with one eye and suppress its deviated fellow are most at risk of developing amblyopia. In adult monkeys made exotropic surgically, the metabolic activity of one or other set of ocular dominance columns was found to be locally depressed.[187] The retinotopic locations of these depressed columns corresponded to the locations of suppression scotomas in human exotropes. Thus, strabismic suppression reduces the activity of cells in the striate cortex. The neural mechanism of suppression may be similar to that of normal binocular rivalry.[188]

Anisometropia

Anisometropia is an interocular difference in refractive power, often the result of a difference in size or shape of the globes. An inequality of greater than 2 diopters is potentially amblyogenic if it persists until the age of 3 or longer.[183,189] In humans, about one-third of cases of anisometropia are accompanied by strabismus. Blurred vision in one eye can sometimes lead to inaccurate

binocular fusion, resulting in a small angle strabismus, but any confounding effects of the strabismus are difficult to isolate.

Anisometropic amblyopia has been produced in primates by daily uniocular administration of the cycloplegic, atropine, from birth to eight months.[188] This provides a realistic model of the effects of anisometropic amblyopia without the confounding factors that exist in humans.[191–193]

Astigmatism occurs when one or more of the refracting surfaces of the eye contain a cylindrical component, resulting in refractive power that varies at different meridians. Astigmatism is common (30 to 70%) in the first two years of life.[194–197] Early astigmatism may not have any detrimental affect on visual development but, if persistent, it is a risk factor for amblyopia.[198]

Astigmatism may be responsible for a form of amblyopia that is orientation specific–"meridional" amblyopia,[199] where subpopulations of cortical cells are selectively affected according to their visual response properties. In humans, the angle and magnitude of meridional amblyopia correlate well with that of astigmatism.[200] Adult monkeys, raised with fixed orientation cylindrical lenses to imitate binocular astigmatism, have shown orientation-specific acuity deficits when tested without the lenses.[190,201]

Monocular form deprivation

It is not the lack of light that causes amblyopia, but the lack of a sharp image. Monocular blur (anisometropia) is a form of monocular form deprivation in an eye with clear optics. Form deprivation can also be caused by light scattering from imperfections in the optical components of the eye. Cataracts are a common cause. Surgery for early cataracts is urgent because, at the peak of the critical period, as little as 2 weeks of deprivation can initiate amblyopia. However, the operated, aphakic eye is far from normal: accommodation is abolished, so focus is fixed at a single distance and anisometropia occurs at some fixation distances. Aggressive patching following cataract surgery may enable some recovery of vision, but it rarely prevents amblyopia entirely.[202–205]

Suturing the lids of one eye of neonatal cats causes profound amblyopia reliably but nonspecifically, because it blocks all modalities of vision. Monkeys raised with one of three different strengths of diffuser spectacle lenses in front of one eye and a clear zero-powered lens in front of the fellow eye were found, in adulthood, to have a close correspondence between the magnitude of the amblyopia and the reduction in retinal image contrast produced by the diffuser lenses.[206] Thus, the depth of non-strabismic amblyopia is strongly influenced by the degree of retinal image degradation early in life.

Classification

Patients are usually classified as strabismic or anisometropic amblyopes based on the symptoms at the time of study. A fundamental distinction exists between strabismic and other forms of amblyopia. Anisometropic and deprivation amblyopias are caused by an optical degradation of one retinal image, but in strabismic amblyopia both retinal images are initially perfect.

It has been proposed that there are distinct patterns of visual deficits in strabismic and anisometropic amblyopes.[207–212] Recently, 427 amblyopes between the ages of 8 and 40 were classified by ocular deviation, surgical history, refractive errors, eccentric fixation and deprivation history, and compared with 68 controls.[213] Measures of acuity, contrast sensitivity, and binocular and stereo vision were undertaken. Three patterns of visual loss corresponding roughly to traditional classifications based on the associated condition were found: strabismics, anisometropes, and strabismic anisometropes. Deprivational amblyopes had functional deficits distinguishable from anisometropes (Fig. 2.7). Thus, two developmental anomalies could account for the patterns of visual loss in amblyopia: poor image formation in one eye (anisometropes) and a loss of binocular function (strabismics). A combination of these factors produces the third, worst affected group (strabismic amblyopes).

Visual deficits

Clinically, amblyopia is characterized by a significant reduction of Snellen visual acuity that does not correct with refraction. However, Snellen acuity is a general measure of visual function. If more specific characteristics of vision are examined, a more precise picture of amblyopia can be gained. Comparing grating acuity, Vernier acuity, and Snellen acuity in strabismic and anisometropic amblyopes shows that grating acuity is more reduced in anisometropic than strabismic amblyopia.[214-218] Conversely, contrast sensitivity is more elevated in strabismic amblyopes than those with preserved binocular vision (including controls) but reduced below normal in anisometropic amblyopes.[213]

Interference effects, characteristics of normal spatial vision, manifest as a reduced discrimination of closely spaced stimuli, e.g., orientation,[219] stereoacuity,[220] and Vernier acuity.[219] Spatial interference, or "crowding," is elevated in amblyopic eyes,[221,222] so amblyopes' poor performance at Snellen charts organized in rows may be improved by using single optotypes.[221,223] Visual measures adversely affected by crowding all rely on hyperacuity; i.e., they are limited by cortical processing rather than the spatial resolution of foveal cones.[224,225] Since amblyopia is thought to be a cortical deficit, diminished hyperacuity and the increased effects of visual crowding are typical in amblyopic individuals.

The acuity and sensitivity deficits in amblyopia could be the result of changes in striate cortex,[226-228] but other deficits are less easily accounted for by "early" visual processing. If strabismic amblyopes are asked to count highly visible features in briefly presented stimuli, they systematically undercount. This suggests a limit to the amount of information to which the amblyopic visual system can attend.[229] Cueing the observer to the relevant part of the display improved performance in amblyopes and normals alike, suggesting that the amblyopic deficit was not the result of reduced spatial attention. It is unlikely that this "high-level" visual processing occurs in striate cortex. The deficits probably reflect unreliable signals reaching higher visual areas.

Anatomical correlates

The balance of left- and right-eye cells in the cat striate cortex can be tilted in favor of one or the other eye by manipulating early visual experience. Immediately after newborn kittens open their eyes, a few weeks of monocular eye-lid closure results in a paucity of cortical cells responding to the closed eye.[230,231] This regime produced monocular deprivation similar to a congenital cataract in humans. In macaques, the changes are accompanied by a change in the relative widths of the ocular dominance columns.[232,233] The normal pattern of ocular dominance columns, roughly equal in width, is remodeled so that the columns belonging to the sutured eye shrink and the space is taken by the expanded columns of the nondeprived eye (Fig. 2.8).

This anatomical evidence of postnatal remodeling of ocular dominance columns in monocular deprivation suggests that amblyopia could be caused by a lack of striate cortex devoted to the deprived eye. However, other forms of amblyopia are not accompanied by differential column shrinkage. The ocular dominance columns of a human strabismic and an anisometropic amblyope were shown to have the same width for both eyes,[234,235] and a naturally occurring anisometropic amblyopic macaque also had normal and equal width ocular dominance columns.[236] Thus, column shrinkage does not necessarily have a causal relationship to amblyopia. Nevertheless, column shrinkage without amblyopia has never been described.

An fMRI study showed a biased share of cortical territory in favor of the nonamblyopic eye in strabismic, anisometropic, and strabismic-anisometropic amblyopes whose visual deficit developed during infancy, but no effect if the deficit developed after two years of age.[237] This finding contradicts the histological

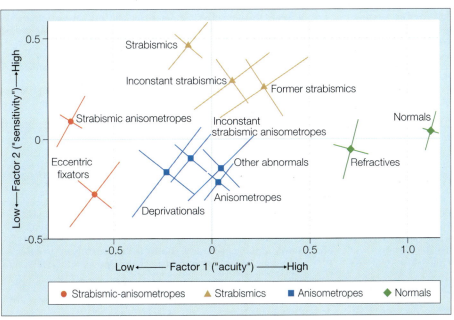

Fig. 2.7 Eleven clinically defined categories of amblyopia in the study of McKee et al.[211] The mean position of each is plotted against "acuity" and "sensitivity," calculated from a number of tests. The normal, strabismic, and anisometropic observers fall into different regions of the two-factor space. The strabismic amblyopes appear to represent a mixture of the strabismic and anisometropic categories. Error bars represent 1 SEM along the principal axes of each category's elliptical distribution. From McKee SP, Levi DM, Movshon JA. The pattern of visual deficits in amblyopia. Journal of Vision 2003; 3: 380–405.

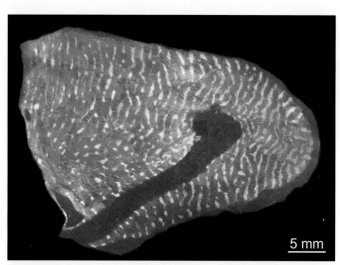

Fig. 2.8 The ocular dominance column pattern of a macaque, following early monocular eye-lid suture to simulate congenital cataract. The columns belonging to the deprived eye (bright) appear shrunken and reduced to small islands, while those of the unaffected eye (dark) have expanded their territory.

studies in humans and animals. Perhaps the humans and animals studied histologically had late-onset amblyopia, occurring after remodeling of the columns was possible. The resolution of fMRI is limited to about 0.5 mm, about the width of a single ocular dominance column, making it difficult to resolve columns, let alone measure the subtle changes that they may undergo in amblyopia. The spatial resolution of histological tissue is not limited.

Anatomical tracer injections have shown that neurons in the striate cortex of strabismics have abnormal wiring. At birth, intralaminar horizontal connections exist between neighboring ocular dominance columns. This pattern of horizontal fibers normally persists into adulthood,[238] but if strabismus is induced during the critical period, there is a change in the horizontal network: projections between left- and right-eye columns are reduced, leaving only fibers that connect cells activated by the same eye.[239]

Amblyopia is caused by anatomical and functional changes in the brain. So far they have only been observed in the striate cortex, but it is unlikely that this is the only region altered; it is merely the best studied. Further investigations of the anatomical wiring and physiological properties of neurons in amblyopic and normal animals and humans may tell us more about the mechanisms that cause amblyopia. One hopes that such knowledge will facilitate new approaches for the treatment and prevention of this disease.

REFERENCES

1. Fledelius HC, Christensen AC. Reappraisal of the human ocular growth curve in fetal life, infancy, and early childhood. Br J Ophthalmol 1996; 80: 918–21.

2. Swan KC, Wilkins JH. Extraocular muscle surgery in early infancy–anatomical factors. J Pediatr Ophthalmol Strabismus 1984; 21: 44–9.

3. Sorsby A, Leary GA. A longitudinal study of refraction and its components during growth. Spec Rec Ser Med Res Counc (GB) 1969; 309: 1–41.

4. Rapaport DH, Stone J. The site of commencement of maturation in mammalian retina: observations in the cat. Brain Res 1982; 281: 273–9.

5. Okada M, Erickson A, Hendrickson A. Light and electron microscopic analysis of synaptic development in Macaca monkey retina as detected by immunocytochemical labeling for the synaptic vesicle protein, SV2. J Comp Neurol 1994; 339: 535–58.

6. La Vail MM, Rapaport DH, Rakic P. Cytogenesis in the monkey retina. J Comp Neurol 1991; 309: 86–114.

7. Abramov I, Gordon J, Hendrickson A, et al. The retina of the newborn human infant. Science 1982; 217: 265–7.

8. Yuodelis C, Hendrickson A. A qualitative and quantitative analysis of the human fovea during development. Vision Res 1986; 26: 847–55.

9. Hendrickson A, Drucker D. The development of parafoveal and mid-peripheral human retina. Behav Brain Res 1992; 49: 21–31.

10. Sjöstrand J, Popovic Z, Conradi N, Marshall J. Morphometric study of the displacement of retinal ganglion cells subserving cones within the human fovea. Graefes Arch Clin Exp Ophthalmol 1999; 237: 1014–23.

11. Hendrickson AE, Yuodelis C. The morphological development of the human fovea. Ophthalmology 1984; 91: 603–12.

12. Carter-Dawson LD, LaVail MM. Rods and cones in the mouse retina. II. Autoradiographic analysis of cell generation using tritiated thymidine. J Comp Neurol 1979; 188: 263–72.

13. Young RW. Cell differentiation in the retina of the mouse. Anat Rec 1985; 212: 199–205.

14. Stiemke MM, Hollyfield JG. Cell birthdays in *Xenopus laevis* retina. Differentiation 1995; 58: 189–93.

15. Livesey FJ, Cepko CL. Vertebrate neural cell-fate determination: lessons from the retina. Nat Rev Neurosci 2001; 2: 109–18.

16. Belliveau MJ, Cepko CL. Extrinsic and intrinsic factors control the genesis of amacrine and cone cells in the rat retina. Development 1999; 126: 555–66.

17. Belliveau MJ, Young TL, Cepko CL. Late retinal progenitor cells show intrinsic limitations in the production of cell types and the kinetics of opsin synthesis. J Neurosci 2000; 20: 2247–54.

18. Cepko CL, Austin CP, Yang X, et al. Cell fate determination in the vertebrate retina. Proc Natl Acad Sci USA 1996; 93: 589–95.

19. Marquardt T, Gruss P. Generating neuronal diversity in the retina: one for nearly all. Trends Neurosci 2002; 25: 32–8.

20. Tomasiewicz H, Ono K, Yee D, et al. Genetic deletion of a neural cell adhesion molecule variant (N-CAM-180) produces distinct defects in the central nervous system. Neuron 1993; 11: 1163–74.

21. Steinberg MS, Takeichi M. Experimental specification of cell sorting, tissue spreading, and specific spatial patterning by quantitative differences in cadherin expression. Proc Natl Acad Sci USA 1994; 91: 206–9.

22. Georges-Labouesse E, Mark M, Messaddeq N, Gansmuller A. Essential role of alpha 6 integrins in cortical and retinal lamination. Curr Biol 1998; 8: 983–6.

23. Scheibe R, Schnitzer J, Rohrenbeck J, et al. Development of A-type (axonless) horizontal cells in the rabbit retina. J Comp Neurol 1995; 354: 438–58.

24. Reese BE, Necessary BD, Tam PP, et al. Clonal expansion and cell dispersion in the developing mouse retina. Eur J Neurosci 1999; 11: 2965–78.

25. Galli-Resta L. Putting neurons in the right places: local interactions in the genesis of retinal architecture. Trends Neurosci 2002; 25: 638–43.

26. Jeffery G. Architecture of the optic chiasm and the mechanisms that sculpt its development. Physiol Rev 2001; 81: 1393–414.

27. Stoeckli ET, Landmesser LT. Axon guidance at choice points. Curr Opin Neurobiol 1998; 8: 73–9.

28. Torres M, Gomez-Pardo E, Gruss P. Pax2 contributes to inner ear patterning and optic nerve trajectory. Development 1996; 122: 3381–91.

29. Trousse F, Marti E, Gruss P, et al. Control of retinal ganglion cell axon growth: a new role for Sonic hedgehog. Development 2001; 128: 3927–36.

30. Sretavan DW, Reichardt LF. Time-lapse video analysis of retinal

ganglion cell axon pathfinding at the mammalian optic chiasm: growth cone guidance using intrinsic chiasm cues. Neuron 1993; 10: 761–77.

31. Sretavan DW, Pure E, Siegel MW, Reichardt LF. Disruption of retinal axon ingrowth by ablation of embryonic mouse optic chiasm neurons. Science 1995; 269: 98–101.

32. Oster SF, Sretavan DW. Connecting the eye to the brain: the molecular basis of ganglion cell axon guidance. Br J Ophthalmol 2003; 87: 639–45.

33. Plump AS, Erskine L, Sabatier C, et al. Slit1 and Slit2 cooperate to prevent premature midline crossing of retinal axons in the mouse visual system. Neuron 2002; 33: 219–32.

34. Herrera E, Brown L, Aruga J, et al. Zic2 Patterns binocular vision by specifying the uncrossed retinal projection. Cell 2003; 114: 545–57.

35. Fukuda Y, Sawai H, Watanabe M, et al. Nasotemporal overlap of crossed and uncrossed retinal ganglion cell projections in the Japanese monkey (Macaca fuscata). J Neurosci 1989; 9: 2353–73.

36. Guillery RW. Visual pathways in albinos. Sci Am 1974; 230: 44–54.

37. Sincich LC, Horton JC. An albino-like decussation error in the optic chiasm revealed by anomalous ocular dominance columns. Vis Neurosci 2003; 19: 541–5.

38. Magoon EH, Robb RM. Development of myelin in human optic nerve and tract. A light and electron microscopic study. Arch Ophthalmol 1981; 99: 655–9.

39. Ali BH, Logani S, Kozlov KL, et al. Progression of retinal nerve fiber myelination in childhood. Am J Ophthalmol 1994; 118: 515–7.

40. Rosen B, Barry C, Constable IJ. Progression of myelinated retinal nerve fibers. Am J Ophthalmol 1999; 127: 471–3.

41. Jean-Louis G, Katz BJ, Digre KB, et al. Acquired and progressive retinal nerve fiber layer myelination in an adolescent. Am J Ophthalmol 2000; 130: 361–2.

42. Schiller PH, Malpeli JG. Properties and tectal projections of monkey retinal ganglion cells. J Neurophysiol 1977; 40: 428–45.

43. Hendry SH, Reid RC. The koniocellular pathway in primate vision. Annu Rev Neurosci 2000; 23: 127–53.

44. Rakic P. Prenatal genesis of connections subserving ocular dominance in the rhesus monkey. Nature 1976; 261: 467–71.

45. Rakic P, Riley KP. Overproduction and elimination of retinal axons in the fetal rhesus monkey. Science 1983; 219: 1441–4.

46. Provis JM. Patterns of cell death in the ganglion cell layer of the human fetal retina. J Comp Neurol 1987; 259: 237–46.

47. Sretavan DW, Shatz CJ. Prenatal development of individual retinogeniculate axons during the period of segregation. Nature 1984; 308: 845–8.

48. Sretavan DW, Shatz CJ. Prenatal development of retinal ganglion cell axons: segregation into eye-specific layers within the cat's lateral geniculate nucleus. J Neurosci 1986; 6: 234–51.

49. Snider CJ, Dehay C, Berland M, et al. Prenatal development of retinogeniculate axons in the macaque monkey during segregation of binocular inputs. J Neurosci 1998; 19: 220–8.

50. Erkman L, McEvilly RJ, Luo L, et al. Role of transcription factors Brn-3.1 and Brn-3.2 in auditory and visual system development. Nature 1996; 381: 603–6.

51. Meissirel C, Wikler KC, Chalupa LM, Rakic P. Early divergence of magnocellular and parvocellular functional subsystems in the embryonic primate visual system. Proc Natl Acad Sci USA 1997; 94: 5900–5.

52. Hubel DH, Wiesel TN. Receptive fields and functional architecture of monkey striate cortex. J Physiol (London) 1968; 195: 215–43.

53. Hubel DH, Wiesel TN. Anatomical demonstration of columns in the monkey striate cortex. Nature 1969; 221: 747–50.

54. Wiesel TN, Hubel DH, Lam DM. Autoradiographic demonstration of ocular-dominance columns in the monkey striate cortex by means of transneuronal transport. Brain Res 1974; 79: 273–9.

55. Horton JC, Hocking DR. An adult-like pattern of ocular dominance columns in striate cortex of newborn monkeys prior to visual experience. J Neurosci 1996; 16: 1791–807.

56. LeVay S, Stryker MP, Shatz CJ. Ocular dominance columns and their development in layer IV of the cat's visual cortex: a quantitative study. J Comp Neurol 1978; 179: 223–44.

57. Stryker MP, Harris WA. Binocular impulse blockade prevents the formation of ocular dominance columns in cat visual cortex. J Neurosci 1986; 6: 2117–33.

58. Katz LC, Shatz CJ. Synaptic activity and the construction of cortical circuits. Science 1996; 274: 1133–8.

59. Wong RO, Meister M, Shatz CJ. Transient period of correlated bursting activity during development of the mammalian retina. Neuron 1993; 11: 923–38.

60. Stellwagen D, Shatz CJ. An instructive role for retinal waves in the development of retinogeniculate connectivity. Neuron 2002; 33: 357–67.

61. Crowley JC, Katz LC. Development of ocular dominance columns in the absence of retinal input. Nat Neurosci 1999; 2: 1125–30.

62. Sengpiel F, Kind PC. The role of activity in development of the visual system. Curr Biol 2002; 12: R818–26.

63. van Essen DC. Organization of visual areas in macaque and human cerebral cortex. In: Werner JS, Chalupa LM, editors. Visual Neurosciences. Cambridge, MA: MIT Press; 2003: 507–21.

64. Zeki S. A vision of the brain. Oxford: Blackwell, 1993.

65. Huffman KJ, Molnar Z, van Dellen A, et al. Formation of cortical fields on a reduced cortical sheet. J Neurosci 1999; 19: 9939–52.

66. Valenza E, Simion F, Cassia VM, Umilta C. Face preference at birth. J Exp Psychol Hum Percept Perform 1996; 22: 892–903.

67. Turati C, Simion F, Milani I, Umilta C. Newborns' preference for faces: what is crucial? Dev Psychol 2002; 38: 875–82.

68. Salapatek P, Cohen LB. Handbook of Infant Perception. Orlando: Academic Press; 1987.

69. Dobson V, Teller DY. Visual acuity in human infants: a review and comparison of behavioral and electrophysiological studies. Vision Res 1978; 18: 1469–83.

70. Mayer DL, Dobson V. Visual acuity development in infants and young children, as assessed by operant preferential looking. Vision Res 1982; 22: 1141–51.

71. Berlyne DE. The influence of the albedo and complexity of stimuli on visual fixation in the human infant. Br J Psychol 1958; 49: 315–8.

72. Fantz RL. Pattern vision in young infants. Psychological Record 1958; 8: 43–7.

73. Fantz RL, Ordy JM, Udelf MS. Maturation of pattern vision in infants during the first six months. J Comp Physiol Psychol 1962; 55: 907–17.

74. Teller DY, Morse R, Borton R, Regal D. Visual acuity for vertical and diagonal gratings in human infants. Vision Res 1974; 14: 1433–9.

75. Atkinson J, Braddick O, Braddick F. Acuity and contrast sensitivity of infant vision. Nature 1974; 247: 403–4.

76. Banks MS, Salapatek P. Acuity and contrast sensitivity in 1-, 2-, and 3-month-old human infants. Invest Ophthalmol Vis Sci 1978; 17: 361–5.

77. Atkinson J, Braddick O, Pimm-Smith E. "Preferential looking" for monocular and binocular acuity testing of infants. Br J Ophthalmol 1982; 66: 264–8.

78. Tyler CW, Apkarian P, Levi DM, Nakayama K. Rapid assessment of visual function: an electronic sweep technique for the pattern visual evoked potential. Invest Ophthalmol Vis Sci 1979; 18: 703–13.

79. Norcia AM, Tyler CW. Spatial frequency sweep VEP: visual acuity during the first year of life. Vision Res 1985; 25: 1399–408.

80. Harter MR, Suitt CD. Visually-evoked cortical responses and pattern vision in the infant: a longitudinal study. Psychonomic Science 1970; 18: 235–7.

81. Regan D. Evoked Potentials in Psychology, Sensory Physiology and Clinical Medicine. New York: Wiley-Interscience; 1972.

82. Harter MR, White CT. Evoked cortical responses to checkerboard patterns: effect of check-size as a function of visual acuity. Electroencephalogr Clin Neurophysiol 1970; 28: 48–54.

83. Marg E, Freeman DN, Peltzman P, Goldstein PJ. Visual acuity development in human infants: evoked potential measurements. Invest Ophthalmol 1976; 15: 150–3.

84. Harter MR, Deaton FK, Odom JV. Maturation of evoked potentials and visual preference in 6–45-day-old infants: effects of check size, visual acuity, and refractive error. Electroencephalogr Clin Neurophysiol 1977; 42: 595–607.

85. Harris L, Atkinson J, Braddick O. Visual contrast sensitivity of a 6-month-old infant measured by the evoked potential. Nature 1976; 264: 570–1.

86. Schwarting DB. Testing infants' vision. Am J Ophthalmol 1954; 38: 714–5.

87. Gorman J, Cogan DG, Gellis SS. An apparatus for grading the visual acuity on the basis of optokinetic nystagmus. Pediatrics 1957; 19: 1088–92.

88. Dayton GO, Jones MH, Aiu P, et al. Developmental study of coordinated eye movements in the human infant. I. Visual activity in the newborn infant: a study based on induced optokinetic nystagmus recorded by electro-oculography. Arch Ophthalmol 1964; 71: 865–70.

89. Riggs LA. Visual acuity. In: Graham CH, editor. Vision and Visual Perception. New York: Wiley; 1965: p. 321–49.

90. Gorman JJ, Cogan DG, Gellis SS. A device for testing visual acuity in infants. Sight Sav Rev 1959; 29: 80–4.

91. Miranda SB. Visual abilities and pattern preferences of premature infants and full-term neonates. J Exp Child Psychol 1970; 10: 189–205.

92. McDonald MA, Dobson V, Sebris SL, et al. The acuity card procedure: a rapid test of infant acuity. Invest Ophthalmol Vis Sci 1985; 26: 1158–62.

93. Teller DY, McDonald MA, Preston K, et al. Assessment of visual acuity in infants and children: the acuity card procedure. Dev Med Child Neurol 1986; 28: 779–89.

94. Courage ML, Adams RJ. Visual acuity assessment from birth to three years using the acuity card procedure: cross-sectional and longitudinal samples. Optom Vis Sci 1990; 67: 713–8.

95. Sokol S. Measurement of infant visual acuity from pattern reversal evoked potentials. Vision Res 1978; 18: 33–9.

96. Sokol S, Moskowitz A. Comparison of pattern VEPs and preferential-looking behavior in 3-month-old infants. Invest Ophthalmol Vis Sci 1985; 26: 359–65.

97. Schade OH. Optical and photoelectric analog of the eye. J Opt Soc Am 1956; 46: 721–39.

98. Campbell FW, Robson JG. Application of Fourier analysis to the visibility of gratings. J Physiol 1968; 197: 551–66.

99. Atkinson J, Braddick O, Moar K. Development of contrast sensitivity over the first 3 months of life in the human infant. Vision Res 1977; 17: 1037–44.

100. Kelly DH. Spatial frequency selectivity in the retina. Vision Res 1975; 15: 665–72.

101. Eschweiler GW, Rauschecker JP. Temporal integration in visual cortex of cats with surgically induced strabismus. Eur J Neurosci 1993; 5: 1501–9.

102. Hoekstra J, van der Goot DP, van den Brink G, Bilsen FA. The influence of the number of cycles upon the visual contrast threshold for spatial sine wave patterns. Vision Res 1974; 14: 365–8.

103. Savoy RL, McCann JJ. Visibility of low-spatial-frequency sine-wave targets: Dependence on number of cycles. J Opt Soc Am 1975; 65: 343–50.

104. Banks MS, Salapatek P. Contrast sensitivity function of the infant visual system. Vision Res 1976; 16: 867–9.

105. Norcia AM, Tyler CW, Allen D. Electrophysiological assessment of contrast sensitivity in human infants. Am J Optom Physiol Opt 1986; 63: 12–5.

106. Norcia AM, Tyler CW, Hamer RD. High visual contrast sensitivity in the young human infant. Invest Ophthalmol Vis Sci 1988; 29: 44–9.

107. Norcia AM, Tyler CW, Hamer RD. Development of contrast sensitivity in the human infant. Vision Res 1990; 30: 1475–86.

108. Campbell FW, Maffei L. Electrophysiological evidence for the existence of orientation and size detectors in the human visual system. J Physiol 1970; 207: 635–52.

109. Teller DY, Regal DM, Videen TO, Pulos PE. Development of visual acuity in infant monkeys (Macaca nemestrina) during the early postnatal weeks. Vision Res 1978; 18: 561–6.

110. Boothe RG, Williams RA, Kiorpes L, Teller DY. Development of contrast sensitivity in infant Macaca nemestrina monkeys. Science 1980; 208: 1290–2.

111. Kiorpes L, Kiper DC. Development of contrast sensitivity across the visual field in macaque monkeys (Macaca nemestrina). Vision Res 1996; 36: 239–47.

112. Allen D, Tyler CW, Norcia AM. Development of grating acuity and contrast sensitivity in the central and peripheral visual field of the human infant. Vision Res 1996; 36: 1945–53.

113. Kiorpes L, Movshon JA. Peripheral and central factors limiting the development of contrast sensitivity in macaque monkeys. Vision Res 1998; 38: 61–70.

114. Salapatek P, Bechtold AG, Bushnell EW. Infant visual acuity as a function of viewing distance. Child Dev 1976; 47: 860–3.

115. Julesz B. Foundations of Cyclopean Perception. Chicago: Univ. of Chicago Press; 1971.

116. Tomac S, Birdal E. Effects of anisometropia on binocularity. J Pediatr Ophthalmol Strabismus 2001; 38: 27–33.

117. Julesz B. Binocular depth perception of computer generated patterns. Bell Systems Technical Journal 1960; 39: 1125–62.

118. Atkinson J, Braddick O. Stereoscopic discrimination in infants. Perception 1976; 5: 29–38.

119. Fox R, Aslin RN, Shea SL, Dumais ST. Stereopsis in human infants. Science 1980; 207: 323–4.

120. Shea SL, Fox R, Aslin RN, Dumais ST. Assessment of stereopsis in human infants. Invest Ophth Vis Sci 1980; 19: 1400–4.

121. Julesz B, Kropfl W, Petrig B. Large evoked potentials to dynamic random-dot correlograms and stereograms permit quick determination of stereopsis. Proc Natl Acad Sci USA 1980; 77: 2348–51.

122. Braddick O, Atkinson J, Julesz B, et al. Cortical binocularity in infants. Nature 1980; 288: 363–5.

123. Petrig B, Julesz B, Kropfl W, et al. Development of stereopsis and cortical binocularity in human infants: Electrophysiological evidence. Science 1981; 213: 1402–5.

124. Braddick O, Wattam-Bell J, Day J, Atkinson J. The onset of binocular function in human infants. Hum Neurobiol 1983; 2: 65–9.

125. Birch EE. Stereopsis in children and its developmental relation to visual acuity. In: Simons K, editor. Early Visual Development, Normal and Abnormal. New York: Oxford University Press; 1993: 224–36.

126. Birch E, Petrig B. FPL and VEP measures of fusion, stereopsis and stereoacuity in normal infants. Vision Res 1996; 36: 1321–7.

127. Ciner EB, Schanel-Klitsch E, Herzberg C. Stereoacuity development: 6 months to 5 years. A new tool for testing and screening. Optom Vis Sci 1996; 73: 43–8.

128. Pettigrew JD, Nikara T, Bishop PO. Binocular interaction on single units in cat striate cortex: simultaneous stimulation by single moving slit with receptive fields in correspondence. Exp Brain Res 1968; 6: 391–410.

129. Poggio GF, Fischer B. Binocular interaction and depth sensitivity in striate and prestriate cortex of behaving rhesus monkey. J Neurophysiol 1977; 40: 1392–405.

130. Cumming BG, Parker AJ. Responses of primary visual cortical neurons to binocular disparity without depth perception. Nature 1997; 389: 280–3.

131. Cumming BG, Parker AJ. Binocular neurons in V1 of awake monkeys are selective for absolute, not relative, disparity. J Neurosci 1999; 19: 5602–18.

132. Chino YM, Smith EL 3rd, Hatta S, Cheng H. Postnatal development of binocular disparity sensitivity in neurons of the primate visual cortex. J Neurosci 1997; 17: 296–307.

133. O'Dell C, Boothe RG. The development of stereoacuity in infant rhesus monkeys. Vision Res 1997; 37: 2675–84.

134. Hubel DH, Wiesel TN. Receptive fields of single neurones in the cat's striate cortex. J Physiol (London) 1959; 148: 574–91.

135. Barlow HB, Pettigrew JD. Lack of specificity of neurones in the visual cortex of young kittens. J Physiol 1971;218:98–101.

136. Wiesel TN, Hubel DH. Ordered arrangement of orientation columns in monkeys lacking visual experience. J Comp Neurol 1974; 158: 307–18.

137. Blasdel G, Obermayer K, Kiorpes L. Organization of ocular dominance and orientation columns in the striate cortex of neonatal macaque monkeys. Vis Neurosci 1995; 12: 589–603.

138. Blakemore C, Cooper GF. Development of the brain depends on the visual environment. Nature 1970; 228: 477–8.

139. Hirsch HV. Visual perception in cats after environmental surgery. Exp Brain Res 1972; 15: 405–23.

140. Blasdel GG, Mitchell DE, Muir DW, Pettigrew JD. A physiological and behavioural study in cats of the effect of early visual experience with contours of a single orientation. J Physiol (London) 1977; 265: 615–36.

141. Stryker MP, Sherk H. Modification of cortical orientation selectivity in the cat by restricted visual experience: a re-examination. Science 1975; 190: 904–6.

142. Stryker MP, Sherk H, Leventhal AG, Hirsch HV. Physiological consequences for the cat's visual cortex of effectively restricting

early visual experience with oriented contours. J Neurophysiol 1978; 41: 896–909.

143. Nakayama K. Biological image motion processing: a review. Vision Res 1985; 25: 625–60.

144. Kremenitzer JP, Vaughan HG Jr, Kurtzberg D, Dowling K. Smooth-pursuit eye movements in the newborn infant. Child Dev 1979; 50: 442–8.

145. Wattam-Bell J. Visual motion processing in one-month-old infants: preferential looking experiments. Vision Res 1996; 36: 1671–7.

146. Wattam-Bell J. Visual motion processing in one-month-old infants: habituation experiments. Vision Res 1996; 36: 1679–85.

147. Wattam-Bell J. Development of motion-specific cortical responses in infancy. Vision Res 1991; 31: 287–97.

148. Hamer RD, Norcia AM. The development of motion sensitivity during the first year of life. Vision Res 1994; 34: 2387–402.

149. Banton T, Dobkins K, Bertenthal BI. Infant direction discrimination thresholds. Vision Res 2001; 41: 1049–56.

150. Hawken MJ, Parker AJ, Lund JS. Laminar organization and contrast selectivity of direction selective cells in the striate cortex of the Old-World monkey. J Neurosci 1988; 8: 3541–8.

151. Zeki SM. Functional organization of a visual area in the posterior bank of the superior temporal sulcus of the rhesus monkey. J Physiol (London) 1974; 236: 549–73.

152. Salzman CD, Britten KH, Newsome WT. Cortical micro-stimulation influences perceptual judgements of motion direction. Nature 1990; 346: 174–7.

153. Hatta S, Kumagami T, Qian J, et al. Nasotemporal directional bias of V1 neurons in young infant monkeys. Invest Ophthalmol Vis Sci 1998; 39: 2259–67.

154. Chase WP. Color Vision in Infants. J Exp Psychol 1937; 20: 203–22.

155. Fagan JF 3rd. Infant color perception. Science 1974; 183: 973–5.

156. Wooten BR. Letter: infant hue discrimination? Science 1975; 187: 275–7.

157. Bornstein MH. Qualities of color vision in infancy. J Exp Child Psychol 1975; 19: 401–19.

158. Peeples DR, Teller DY. Color vision and brightness discrimination in two-month-old human infants. Science 1975; 189: 1102–3.

159. Brown AM. Development of visual sensitivity to light and color vision in human infants: a critical review. Vision Res 1990; 30: 1159–88.

160. Teller DY, Peeples DR, Sekel M. Discrimination of chromatic from white light by two-month-old human infants. Vision Res 1978; 18: 41–8.

161. Hamer RD, Alexander KR, Teller DY. Rayleigh discriminations in young human infants. Vision Res 1982; 22: 575–7.

162. Packer O, Hartmann EE, Teller DY. Infant color vision: the effect of test field size on Rayleigh discriminations. Vision Res 1984; 24: 1247–60.

163. Boynton RM. Human color vision, special limited. Washington, DC: Optical Society of America; 1992.

164. Banks MS, Bennett PJ. Optical and photoreceptor immaturities limit the spatial and chromatic vision of human neonates. J Opt Soc Am A 1988; 5: 2059–79.

165. Morrone MC, Speed HD, Burr DC. Development of visual inhibitory interactions in kittens. Vis Neurosci 1991; 7: 321–34.

166. Movshon JA, Kiorpes L. Analysis of the development of spatial contrast sensitivity in monkey and human infants. J Opt Soc Am A 1988; 5: 2166–72.

167. Morrone MC, Burr DC, Fiorentini A. Development of infant contrast sensitivity to chromatic stimuli. Vision Res 1993; 33: 2535–52.

168. Morrone MC, Fiorentini A, Burr DC. Development of the temporal properties of visual evoked potentials to luminance and colour contrast in infants. Vision Res 1996; 36: 3141–55.

169. Kelly JP, Borchert K, Teller DY. The development of chromatic and achromatic contrast sensitivity in infancy as tested with the sweep VEP. Vision Res 1997; 37: 2057–72.

170. Wiesel TN, Hubel DH. Single cell responses in striate cortex of kittens deprived of vision in one eye. J Neurophysiol 1963; 26: 1003–17.

171. Hubel DH, Wiesel TN. The period of susceptibility to the physiological effects of unilateral eye closure in kittens. J Physiol (London) 1970; 206: 419–36.

172. Daw NW, Fox K, Sato H, Czepita D. Critical period for monocular deprivation in the cat visual cortex. J Neurophysiol 1992; 67: 197–202.

173. Levitt FB, van Sluyters RC. The sensitive period for strabismus in the kitten. Brain Res 1982; 255: 323–7.

174. Daw NW, Wyatt HJ. Kittens reared in a unidirectional environment: evidence for a critical period. J Physiol 1976; 257: 155–70.

175. Kim DS, Bonhoeffer T. Reverse occlusion leads to a precise restoration of orientation preference maps in visual cortex. Nature 1994; 370: 370–2. (Published erratum appears in Nature 1994 Nov 10; 372(6502): 196.)

176. Shatz CJ, Stryker MP. Ocular dominance in layer IV of the cat's visual cortex and the effects of monocular deprivation. J Physiol (London) 1978; 281: 267–83.

177. Harwerth RS, Smith EL, 3rd, Duncan GC, et al. Multiple sensitive periods in the development of the primate visual system. Science 1986; 232: 235–8.

178. Vaegan, Taylor D. Critical period for deprivation amblyopia in children. Trans Ophthalmol Soc UK 1979; 99: 432–9.

179. Vereecken EP, Brabant P. Prognosis for vision in amblyopia after the loss of the good eye. Arch Ophthalmol 1984; 102: 220–4.

180. Tierney DW. Vision recovery in amblyopia after contralateral subretinal hemorrhage. J Am Optom Assoc 1989; 60: 281–3.

181. Rahi JS, Logan S, Borja MC, et al. Prediction of improved vision in the amblyopic eye after visual loss in the non-amblyopic eye. Lancet 2002; 360: 621–2.

182. Lepard CW. Comparative changes in the error of refraction between fixing and amblyopic eyes during growth and development. Am J Ophthalmol 1975; 80: 485–90.

183. von Noorden GK, Campos EC. Binocular Vision and Ocular Motility: Theory and Management of Strabismus, 6th ed. St. Louis, MO: Mosby; 2002.

184. Archer SM, Sondhi N, Helveston EM. Strabismus in infancy. Ophthalmology 1989; 96: 133–7.

185. Sondhi N, Archer SM, Helveston EM. Development of normal ocular alignment. J Pediatr Ophthalmol Strabismus 1988; 25: 210–1.

186. Gwiazda J, Thorn F. Development of refraction and strabismus. Curr Opin Ophthalmol 1999; 10: 293–9.

187. Horton JC, Hocking DR, Adams DL. Metabolic mapping of suppression scotomas in striate cortex of macaques with experimental strabismus. J Neurosci 1999; 19: 7111–29.

188. Blake R, Logothetis NK. Visual competition. Nat Rev Neurosci 2002; 3: 13–21.

189. Abrahamsson M, Fabian G, Sjostrand J. A longitudinal study of a population based sample of astigmatic children. II. The changeability of anisometropia. Acta Ophthalmol (Copenhagen) 1990; 68: 435–40.

190. Boothe RG, Teller DY. Meridional variations in acuity and CSFs in monkeys (Macaca nemestrina) reared with externally applied astigmatism. Vision Res 1982; 22: 801–10.

191. Hendrickson AE, Movshon JA, Eggers HM, et al. Effects of early unilateral blur on the macaque's visual system. II. Anatomical observations. J Neurosci 1987; 7: 1327–39.

192. Kiorpes L, Boothe RG, Hendrickson AE, et al. Effects of early unilateral blur on the Macaque's visual system. 1. Behavioral observations. J Neurosci 1987; 7: 1318–26.

193. Movshon JA, Eggers HM, Gizzi MS, et al. Effects of early unilateral blur on the macaque's visual system. III. Physiological observations. J Neurosci 1987; 7: 1340–51.

194. Atkinson J, Braddick O, French J. Infant astigmatism: its disappearance with age. Vision Res 1980; 20: 891–3.

195. Gwiazda J, Scheiman M, Mohindra I, Held R. Astigmatism in children: changes in axis and amount from birth to six years. Invest Ophthalmol Vis Sci 1984; 25: 88–92.

196. Saunders KJ. Early refractive development in humans. Surv Ophthalmol 1995; 40: 207–16.

197. Ehrlich DL, Braddick OJ, Atkinson J, et al. Infant emmetropization: longitudinal changes in refraction components from nine to twenty months of age. Optom Vis Sci 1997; 74: 822–43.

198. Dobson V, Miller JM, Harvey EM, Sherrill DL. Amblyopia in astigmatic preschool children. Vision Res 2003; 43: 1081–90.

199. Freeman RD, Mitchell DE, Millodot M. A neural effect of partial visual deprivation in humans. Science 1972; 175: 1384–6.

200. Mitchell DE, Freeman RD, Millodot M, Haegerstrom G. Meridional amblyopia: evidence for modification of the human visual system by early visual experience. Vis Res 1973; 13: 535–58.

201. Harweth RS, Smith EL 3rd, Boltz RL. Meridional amblyopia in monkeys. Exp Brain Res 1980; 39: 351–6.

202. Jacobson SG, Mohindra I, Held R. Development of visual acuity in infants with congenital cataracts. Br J Ophthalmol 1981; 65: 727–35.

203. Birch EE, Stager DR, Wright WW. Grating acuity development after early surgery for congenital unilateral cataract. Arch Ophthalmol 1986; 104: 1783–7.

204. Drummond GT, Scott WE, Keech RV. Management of monocular congenital cataracts. Arch Ophthalmol 1989; 107: 45–51.

205. Taylor D, Wright KW, Amaya L, et al. Should we aggressively treat unilateral congenital cataracts? Br J Ophthalmol 2001; 85: 1120–6.

206. Smith EL 3rd, Hung LF, Harwerth RS. The degree of image degradation and the depth of amblyopia. Invest Ophthalmol Vis Sci 2000; 41: 3775–81.

207. von Noorden GK. Classification of amblyopia. Am J Ophthalmol 1967; 63: 238–44.

208. Schapero M. Amblyopia. 1st ed. Philadelphia: Chilton; 1971.

209. Bradley A, Freeman RD. Is reduced Vernier acuity in amblyopia due to position, contrast or fixation deficits? Vision Res 1985; 25: 55–66.

210. Levi DM, Klein SA. Vernier acuity, crowding and amblyopia. Vision Res 1985; 25: 979–91.

211. Hess RF, Holliday IE. The spatial localization deficit in amblyopia. Vision Res 1992; 32: 1319–39.

212. Birch EE, Swanson WH. Hyperacuity deficits in anisometropic and strabismic amblyopes with known ages of onset. Vision Res 2000; 40: 1035–40.

213. McKee SP, Levi DM, Movshon JA. The pattern of visual deficits in amblyopia. J Vision 2003; 3: 380–405.

214. Levi DM, Klein S. Hyperacuity and amblyopia. Nature 1982; 298: 268–70.

215. Levi DM, Klein S. Differences in Vernier discrimination for grating between strabismic and anisometropic amblyopes. Invest Ophthalmol Vis Sci 1982; 23: 398–407.

216. Levi DM, Klein SA, Yap YL. Positional uncertainty in peripheral and amblyopic vision. Vision Res 1987; 27: 581–97.

217. Levi DM, Klein SA, Wang H. Amblyopic and peripheral Vernier acuity: a test-pedestal approach. Vision Res 1994; 34: 3265–92.

218. Levi DM, Klein SA, Wang H. Discrimination of position and contrast in amblyopic and peripheral vision. Vision Res 1994; 34: 3293–313.

219. Westheimer G, Hauske G. Temporal and spatial interference with Vernier acuity. Vision Res 1975; 15: 1137–41.

220. Butler TW, Westheimer G. Interference with stereoscopic acuity: Spatial, temporal, and disparity tuning. Vision Res 1978; 18: 1387–92.

221. Flom MC, Weymouth FW, Kahnemann D. Visual resolution and contour integration. J Ophthalmol Soc Am 1963; 53: 1026–32.

222. Hess RF, Jacobs RJ. A preliminary report of acuity and contour interactions across the amblyope's visual field. Vision Res 1979; 19: 1403–8.

223. Flom MC, Bedell HE, Allen J. Contour integration and visual resolution: Contralateral effects. Science 1963; 142: 979–80.

224. Barlow HB. The Ferrier Lecture, 1980. Critical limiting factors in the design of the eye and visual cortex. Proc R Soc Lond B Biol Sci 1981; 212: 1–34.

225. Westheimer G. Visual hyperacuity. Prog Sensory Physiol 1981; 1: 1–30.

226. Wiesel TN. Postnatal development of the visual cortex and the influence of environment. Nature 1982; 299: 583–91.

227. Smith EL 3rd, Chino YM, Ni J, et al. Residual binocular interactions in the striate cortex of monkeys reared with abnormal binocular vision. J Neurophysiol 1997; 78: 1353–62.

228. Kiorpes L, Kiper DC, O'Keefe LP, et al. Neuronal correlates of amblyopia in the visual cortex of macaque monkeys with experimental strabismus and anisometropia. J Neurosci 1998; 18: 6411–24.

229. Sharma V, Levi DM, Klein SA. Undercounting features and missing features: evidence for a high-level deficit in strabismic amblyopia. Nat Neurosci 2000; 3: 496–501.

230. Wiesel TN, Hubel DH. Comparison of the effects of unilateral and bilateral eye closure on cortical unit responses in kittens. J Neurophysiol 1965; 28: 1029–40.

231. Wiesel TN, Hubel DH. Extent of recovery from the effects of visual deprivation in kittens. J Neurophysiol 1965; 28: 1060–72.

232. Hubel DH, Wiesel TN, LeVay S. Plasticity of ocular dominance columns in monkey striate cortex. Philos Trans R Soc Lond B Biol Sci 1977; 278: 377–409.

233. LeVay S, Wiesel TN, Hubel DH. The development of ocular dominance columns in normal and visually deprived monkeys. J Comp Neurol 1980; 191: 1–51.

234. Horton JC, Stryker MP. Amblyopia induced by anisometropia without shrinkage of ocular dominance columns in human striate cortex. Proc Natl Acad Sci USA 1993; 90: 5494–8.

235. Horton JC, Hocking DR. Pattern of ocular dominance columns in human striate cortex in strabismic amblyopia. Vis Neurosci 1996; 13: 787–95.

236. Horton JC, Hocking DR, Kiorpes L. Pattern of ocular dominance columns and cytochrome oxidase activity in a macaque monkey with naturally occurring anisometropic amblyopia. Vis Neurosci 1997; 14: 681–9.

237. Goodyear BG, Nicolle DA, Menon RS. High resolution fMRI of ocular dominance columns within the visual cortex of human amblyopes. Strabismus 2002; 10: 129–36.

238. Löwel S, Singer W. Experience dependent plasticity of intracortical connections. In: Fahle M, Poggio T, editors. Perceptual Learning. Cambridge, MA: MIT Press; 2002: 3–18.

239. Löwel S, Engelmann R. Neuroanatomical and neurophysiological consequences of strabismus: changes in the structural and functional organization of the primary visual cortex in cats with alternating fixation and strabismic amblyopia. Strabismus 2002; 10:95–105.

240. Dobson V. Visual acuity testing by preferential looking techniques. In: Isenberg SJ, editor. The eye in infancy. St. Louis, MO: Mosby; 1994. 131–56.

241. Gwiazda J, Brill S, Mohindra I, Held R. Infant visual acuity and its meridional variation. Vision Res 1978; 18: 1557–64.

242. Allen JL. The development of visual acuity in human infants during the early postnatal weeks. Seattle: University of Washington; 1979.

243. Van Hof-Van Duin J, Mohn G. Monocular and binocular optokinetic nystagmus in humans with defective stereopsis. Invest Ophthalmol Vis Sci 1986; 27: 574–83.

244. Birch EE, Hale LA. Criteria for monocular acuity deficit in infancy and early childhood. Invest Ophthalmol Vis Sci 1988; 29: 636–43.

245. McDonald M, Ankrum C, Preston K et al. Monocular and binocular acuity estimation in 18- to 36-month-olds: acuity card results. Am J Optom Physiol Opt 1986; 63: 181–6.

CHAPTER

3 Delayed Visual Maturation

Creig S Hoyt

When a baby is referred because the parents are worried about its vision, the cause is usually evident to the ophthalmologist on the first examination. At the very least there is usually a strong suspicion about the site of the problem in the visual or neurological system. In some babies, no apparent cause can be found; their vision just seems worse for their chronological age than it should be, and their estimated or measured visual function is worse than expected. In many of these infants, however, vision improves over time, without specific treatment.

This phenomenon has been recognized for many years. Illingworth[1] first introduced the term "delayed visual maturation" to describe it. He described two children who had been visually unresponsive as infants, but at 6 months of age began to be attentive to visual stimuli. It is noteworthy that one child was considerably late in walking. In all other regards, however, Illingworth's first two patients were not developmentally delayed, except with regard to their visual function.

It should be noted that although Illingworth introduced the term, similar cases had previously been described using other terms. J. Beauvieux[2] and M. Beauvieux[3] noted the anomalous appearance of optic discs in infants whom they referred to as having "temporary visual inattention." With time the discs appeared to assume a normal adult appearance, and the visual function improved. Believing this problem to be due to a defect in the myelination of the optic nerve, the authors coined the term "pseudo-atrophie optique dysgenesie myelinique." M. Beauvieux, however, appreciated that the situation could be more complex, and might be compounded by neurodevelopmental or ocular anomalies that might influence eventual visual outcome.[3] He considered that there were two distinct categories of affected infants. In the first, delayed visual maturation is an isolated anomaly, with rapid and complete recovery within 4–6 months. In the second, because of associated problems such as strabismus, high refractive errors, or mental retardation, visual improvement is slower and less complete.

CLINICAL PRESENTATION

Most parents and many doctors do not expect the newborn baby to see well, so it is only when the child is not fixing and following by 2–4 months of age that they are referred by the parents themselves, or their advisors, to the ophthalmologist or pediatrician. The diagnosis of delayed visual maturation is really done retrospectively, and by exclusion of visual system disease as far as that is possible. It is essential for the diagnosis that the vision should improve with time, but since delayed visual maturation may co-exist with ocular or systemic disease, the eventual vision is not necessarily normal. It is noteworthy that the patient who presents with delayed visual maturation in its isolated form is the

child with no apparent fixation and following reflexes, and no strabismus. The patient thus appears distinctly different than the infant who presents with poor visual function associated with a bilateral anterior visual pathway disorder in which nystagmus is to be expected and in whom pupillary abnormalities may be present. Delayed visual maturation must be distinguished from those infants who present with poor visual function as a result of visual cortex or associated neurovisual pathway pathology. These patients too may present with poor visual fixation and no nystagmus.

CLASSIFICATION

Uemura et al. present a classification of delayed visual maturation that includes three categories.[4] This classification was prompted by the observation that many infants with apparent visual maturation delay were found subsequently to have other significant neurodevelopmental or visual problems. In their original classification, Uemera et al. suggested that type I should include patients who exhibit visual maturation delay with no other anomalies; type II should include infants with visual maturation delay who are mentally retarded or who have a seizure disorder; and type III should include children with a primary visual abnormality and a superimposed visual maturation delay.[4] These authors recognized that the simplistic notion that these children simply had a temporary delay in achieving normal visual milestones was often incorrect.

VISUAL FUNCTION TESTING IN ISOLATED DELAYED VISUAL MATURATION

In these babies general and neurological development is normal, and the only problem is that the baby appears to see less well than expected for his or her age.[1] They have normal ocular examination and no systemic abnormalities.

Thus far, there is a consensus among ophthalmologists that the electroretinogram (ERG) is entirely normal for the adjusted age of the child studied. It should be noted that these ERG studies have been standard flash nonfocal studies. No attempt to date to study these infants with a focal stimulus or foveal-type ERG has been made.

In contrast to the consensus among ERG studies, visually evoked potentials (VEPs) of these patients have produced variable and conflicting results. Mellor and Fielder reported that flash VEPs had delayed latencies as well as reduced amplitudes in four children with delayed visual maturation.[5] All of these children were reported to have normal VEPs when tested after achieving apparent normal visual behavior. Harel et al. described three infants with delayed visual maturation who had flash VEPs with delayed latencies that became normal by 1 year of age.[6] Fielder and Mayer reported a large series of children with delayed visual maturation in which 78% had flash VEPs with prolonged latencies, abnormal wave forms, and decreased amplitudes.[7] The nonspecific stimulus nature of flash VEPs and the multiple recording artifacts that have been noted in infant studies using these techniques suggest that flash VEP studies are probably not specific enough in their stimulus to be useful in evaluating this group of children.

Pattern VEPs have also been reported in these children. Hoyt et al. reported a series of eight children with delayed visual maturation in which seven had pattern onset/offset VEPs with decreased amplitudes and delayed latencies.[8] The authors unfortunately did not report whether these patients were age-matched with normal visually attentive children. Lambert et al. reported the VEP results on nine children with a diagnosis of delayed visual maturation.[9] They reported that there were no abnormalities of amplitude, waveform, or latency in these children as compared to an age-matched population. This study, unfortunately, because of the unreliability and small amplitude of smaller check sizes in very young infants, utilized a stimulus of 100-minute check size as the standard stimulus: this test of visual function and acuity is relatively coarse. Weiss and co-workers reported normal pattern visually evoked potentials in three infants with delayed visual maturation, although they chose to call it "visual inattention."[10]

Tresidder et al. studied 26 infants with delayed visual maturation using a modified forced choice preferential looking apparatus.[11] All infants regardless of the group type showed significant reduction in visual acuity on the initial examination. Visual improvement commenced, variably depending on the type of delayed visual maturation. In sharp contrast, Weiss and co-workers studied 14 infants with delayed visual maturation and no other developmental problems.[10] Visual acuity estimates with Teller Acuity Cards were reported to be normal for age. It is not clear what accounts for the markedly different findings of these two studies.[10,11]

CLINICAL COURSE AND OUTCOME

Group I: isolated delayed visual maturation

Clinically, the profile of the patient in group I is usually relatively constant. Most patients in this group present by 3–4 months of age, and it is very unusual for improvement to be prolonged beyond 6 months. Quite frequently, the short delay during the referral process is enough to allow for considerable improvement so that the diagnosis in these cases can only be made retrospectively by the history.

Because the measurement of visual function in small children is difficult, and indeed the VEP and forced choice preferential looking studies to date conflict in these children, the determination of whether normal vision has been achieved in these infants is largely subjective. However, the eventual outcome should not only be normal for vision but for intellectual and other development.

Several studies have emphasized that children with apparent isolated delayed visual maturation frequently had delays in other spheres of general development upon follow-up examination. Cole et al. reported that several children with delayed visual maturation were slow in learning to speak.[12] Hoyt et al. noted general delays in the motor development of seven of eight children identified with delayed visual maturation.[8] Lambert et

al. in a study of nine children noted that four of the children were delayed by 3–5 months in achieving other developmental milestones such as sitting and walking compared with their unaffected siblings.[9] One additional child was hypotonic with marked developmental delay. They concluded that delayed visual maturation may be only one manifestation of global developmental delay in some infants.

Recent studies have emphasized that seizures, especially infantile spasms or focal partial-complex seizures, may become apparent in infants thought to have isolated visual maturation delay.[13,14] This has been attributed to interference with the cortically related visual attention mechanisms by the seizure acuity.[10,13] A recent report suggests an association of visual maturation delay and auditory neuropathy/dyssynchrony.[15] Auditory neuropathy/dyssynchrony is a temporary hearing impairment with normal cochlear function (as measured by otoacoustic emissions) but absent of severely impaired brainstem auditory evoked potentials.[15]

Group II: delayed visual maturation with systemic disease or mental retardation

Babies who are very premature, who have severe intercurrent illness early in their life, may present with delay in visual development, but this usually improves in the same way as in group I patients, with residual defects only related to their illness. Most patients in this group have severe mental retardation. It is most frequently seen in children who have infantile spasms, or other seizure disorders in relationship to severe birth asphyxia, hypoglycemia, hypocalcemia, tuberous sclerosis, Aicardi syndrome, and so on. In most cases, these are diagnostic clues to the underlying cause and the neurophysiological studies are more frequently normal, especially the electroencephalogram (EEG). Vision appears to improve with the control of seizures in these children. Children with other causes of mental retardation without seizures, such as hydrocephalus or brain malformations, may also exhibit delayed visual maturation often to a lesser degree. The vision is variable and may be stimulated or excited by sound as well as visual stimulation.

In the group in whom structural central nervous system pathology is associated with delayed visual maturation the long-term prognosis is less good. There are often residual visual defects, or problems with visual perception, or hand–eye coordination and the recovery of vision takes considerably longer. This is dramatically demonstrated in the study of Tresidder et al. in which they showed that visual improvement commenced as follows: group I, 7–24 weeks; group II, 22–78 weeks; and group III, 13–28 weeks.[11]

Group III: delayed visual maturation with ocular disease

Children with early onset ocular disease associated with nystagmus may have vision that is much worse than would be expected from the primary disease alone. It is a reasonable hypothesis that these children have a form of delayed visual maturation in addition to their organic defect. This is frequently seen in children with albinism, but may also be seen in children with bilateral cataracts, optic nerve hypoplasia, and so on. Children in this group improve to their final level more slowly, and less fully than in group I, but faster and more completely than group II (see the previous section). Infrequent reports of infants with transient nystagmus and delayed visual maturation add confusion to this group distinction.[16]

DIFFERENTIAL DIAGNOSES

The main differential diagnoses for the baby with poor vision, with no apparent nystagmus and no gross ocular or systemic disorder, are delayed visual maturation versus cortical vision impairment. In most cases the child with significant cortical visual impairment either will have a history of significant perinatal hypoxia or other precipitant causes of this disorder or will present with other associated neurological signs. Occasionally, however, only a magnetic resonance image or computed tomographic scan will be able to discern between these two disorders.[10] New functional brain-imaging techniques using near-infrared optical topography may provide insights into the neural substrates involved in delayed visual maturation.[17]

INVESTIGATION AND MANAGEMENT

Delayed visual maturation is an area where the ophthalmologist and pediatrician or pediatric neurologist must work well together.[18] If the child with suspected delayed visual maturation is developmentally normal, and associated eye or systemic disease has been ruled out by joint consultation, and noninvasive neurophysiological studies are normal or not markedly abnormal, then no further investigations are needed and a good outcome can be expected. These children probably need to be followed rather more carefully than the average patient by their developmental clinician or their general practitioner after their improvement has been observed by the ophthalmologist.

Where the child has eye disease or systemic problems, these should be investigated and managed as appropriate.

REFERENCES

1. Illingworth RS. Delayed visual maturation. Arch Dis Child 1961; 36: 407–9.
2. Beauvieux J. La pseudo-atrophie optique des nouveau-nes. Ann Oculist 1926;163: 881–921.
3. Beauvieux M. La cecite apparente chez le nouveau-ne la pseudo-atrophie grise du nerf optique. Arch Ophthalmol (Paris) 1947; 7: 241–9.
4. Uemera Y, Agucci Y, Katsumi O. Visual development delay. Ophthal Paediatr Genet 1981; 1: 4–11.
5. Mellor DH, Fielder AR. Dissociated visual development: electro-diagnostic studies in infants who are slow to see. Dev Med Child Neurol 1980; 22: 327–35.
6. Harel S, Holtzman M, Feinsod M. Delayed visual maturation. Arch Dis Child 1983; 58: 298–9.
7. Fielder AR, Mayer DL. Delayed visual maturation. Semin Ophthalmol 1991; 5: 182–93.
8. Hoyt CS, Jastrzebski G, Marg E. Delayed visual maturation. Br J Ophthalmol 1983; 63: 127–30.
9. Lambert SR, Kriss A, Taylor D. Delayed visual maturation. Ophthalmology 1989; 96: 524–9.
10. Weiss AH, Kelly JP, Phillips JO. The infant who is visually unresponsive on a cortical basis. Ophthalmology 2001; 108: 2076–87.
11. Tresidder J, Fielder AR, Nicholson J. Delayed visual maturation: ophthalmic and neurodevelopmental aspects. Dev Med Child Neurol 1990; 32: 872–81.
12. Cole GF, Hungerford J, Jones RD. Delayed visual maturation. Arch Dis Child 1984; 59: 107–10.
13. Guzzetta F, Frisone MF, Ricci D et al. Development of visual attention in West syndrome. Epilepsia 2002; 43: 757–63.
14. Shalar E, Hwang PA. Prolonged epileptic blindness in an infant associated with cortical dysplasia. Dev Med Child Neurol 2001; 44: 792.
15. Aldosari M, Mabic A, Husain AM. Delayed visual maturation associated with auditory neuropathy/dyssynchrony. J Child Neurol 2003; 18: 358–61.
16. Bianchi PE, Salati R, Cavallini A, Fazzi E. Transient nystagmus in delayed visual maturation. Dev Med Child Neurol 1998; 40: 263–5.
17. Taga G, Asakawa K, Maki A et al. Brain imaging in awake infants by near-infrared optical topography. Proc Natl Acad Sci USA 2003; 100: 10,722–7.
18. Fielder AR, Russell-Eggitt IR, Dodd KL, Mellor DH. Delayed visual maturation. Trans Ophthalmol Soc UK 1988; 104: 653–61.

CHAPTER
4

Pre- and Postnatal Growth of the Eye, Adnexa, Visual System and Emmetropization

Douglas R Fredrick

The eye is one of the first organs recognizable during embryogenesis. Its normal development depends upon the orderly differentiation and migration of endoderm, mesoderm, neural and surface ectoderm, and neural crest tissue. Knowledge of the timing of ocular organogenesis is vital to understanding diagnosis and treatment of children with congenital ocular anomalies. Ocular anomalies are commonly associated with other structural anomalies, and their recognition can help in the diagnosis of infants with syndromes. Molecular mechanisms controlling ocular growth have led to new classifications of ocular anomalies.

At birth, development is incomplete: concerted postnatal growth, development, and organization of the eye and the whole visual pathway to the cortex is important for the normal development of vision.

Table 4.1 Newborn vs. adult ocular parameters

	Newborn	Adult
Axial length	16.8 mm	23.0 mm
Mean K	55 D	43 D
Optic nerve length	24 mm	30 mm
Corneal diameter	10.0 mm	10.6 mm vertical by 11.7 mm horizontal
Corneal thickness	581 µm	510 µm
Parsplana length	0.5–1.05 mm	3.5–4 mm
Orbital volume	7 cc	30 cc

EMBRYONIC DEVELOPMENT

In the first three weeks of embryonic development, the two main processes that occur are the differentiation of cell type into endoderm, mesoderm, and ectoderm and the organization of these tissues into a tube-like notochord/neural tube structure (see Table 5.1).[1] At day 22 an optic groove forms within the lumen of the forebrain. Over the next three days, the neural tube closes at its caudal and cephalic ends. At day 25 the optic groove has formed in the optic vesicles, which evaginate toward the surface ectoderm, initiating the lens placode. The optic vesicle then begins to invaginate, forming a double-layered optic cup lined by the two layers of the neuroectoderm that form the layers of the retina. The invaginating optic vesicle cradles the lens placode, which develops into the lens vesicle, separating from the surface ectoderm from which it originated. The optic cup is connected to the forebrain by the optic stalk with the embryonic fissure on the ventral surface. The hyaloid artery develops from the internal carotid artery and lies within the embryonic fissure and extends to the optic vesicle. At 6 weeks, the embryonic fissure closes proximally to distally with failure of closure leading to colobomas.

At 7 weeks, the eye has an optic nerve, two-layer retina, and primary lens vesicle. It is surrounded by mesenchyme and neural crest cells, which differentiate into sclera, choroid, iris, cornea, and vitreous between 7 and 15 weeks of age.[2] As the eye develops, neural crest mesenchyme surrounds the craniofacial complex; it migrates from different origins to different ultimate locations (e.g., frontonasal complex versus maxillary processes). Neural crest cells are also important for anterior segment structures of the eye, hence the association of ocular anomalies with craniofacial syndromes.

At birth, normal newborns have the following ocular parameters: axial length 16.8 mm, corneal steepness 55 diopters, and lens power 34 diopters[3] (Table 4.1).

Errors of differentiation, induction, and cell migration early in embryogenesis lead to congenital anomalies of the eye as a whole with more significant anomalies resulting from earlier errors. Conditions such as anophthalmos, microphthalmos with cyst, colobomatous microphthalmos, and teratoma originate prior to 8 weeks. Anomalies occurring between 7 and 15 weeks can cause microphthalmos, anterior segment dysgenesis, persistent hyperplastic primary vitreous, congenital cataract, congenital glaucoma, and lid, muscle, and orbit anomalies.[4]

ORBIT DEVELOPMENT AND ANOMALIES

The face is formed by two embryonic structures:
1. The midline facial structures, the nose and the upper lip, develop from the frontonasal processes; and
2. The lateral aspect of the face develops from the branchial arches.

The orbit first forms during the fifth week. The first branchial process differentiates into the maxillary and mandibular processes, which become the lateral and inferior bones of the orbit. The frontonasal tissue, derived from the forebrain, develops into the nasal and superior bones of the orbit. Between these processes, at 6 weeks, a column of epithelial cells that develops into the nasolacrimal system is interposed between maxillary and frontal tissue. At 6 weeks, the upper eyelid fold develops from the frontonasal process and the lower eyelid develops from the maxillary process.

As the extraocular muscles develop as a cone between 6 and 8 weeks, they grow from anterior to posterior to insert into the developing sphenoid bone. At 8 weeks the upper and lower lid folds completely cover the developing eye and fuse. The outer layer of the lid fold becomes surface ectoderm and skin, the inner layer conjunctiva. The lacrimal gland arises from conjunctiva and neural crest cells in the third month. The extraocular muscles become attached to the sclera anteriorly into the orbital bone and dura mater posteriorly. Ossification of the orbital bone begins in the third month of life, and the angle between the orbital axes becomes reduced as the maxilla develops. In the fifth month, the eyelids separate as the meibomian glands begin to secrete.[5] The extraocular muscles now show myelinated axons. Adipose tissue appears within the orbit and ossification progresses with the annulus of Zinn first identified at 7 months. At birth, bones of the orbit are ossified but separated. The nasolacrimal system becomes patent at term. The volume of the orbit increases and the angle of the orbital axes decreases from 160° at 5 weeks to 65° at birth.

Postnatal growth of the eye is dependent upon normal postnatal growth of the globe. At birth, the orbital volume is 7 cm^3, and as the globe grows rapidly, the orbital volume reaches adult size, 30 cm^3 by the age of 4.[6] Anomalies of the globe formation and development lead to failure of orbital enlargement, making prosthetic fitting more difficult in children with severe microphthalmos and anophthalmos.

MOLECULAR CONTROL OF FACIAL DEVELOPMENT

There is genetic conservation of the molecular control of embryogenesis, the processes that guide the development of the three primordial layers and their subsequent differentiation and control of signal transduction. These gene clusters are divided into groups with different functions:

1. Transcription factors act as on/off switches that control other genes. These include the homeobox (*HOX*) and paired box (*PAX*) genes. Homeobox genes are present in all cells and they encode for a protein that activates or suppresses other gene transcription, and thus these gene products. Abnormal expression leads to abnormal embryogenesis, and *HOX* genes are especially important in human facial development. *PAX* genes, first found in fruit flies, consist of a specific domain of 128 base pairs. Nine different *PAX* genes on different chromosomes important in ocular development have been identified.
2. Signaling molecules, which are important in facial and orbital development, are protein or peptide growth factors that induce neighboring cells in embryogenesis. Examples include transforming growth factor-β (TGF-β), fibroblast growth factors (FGF-1 to FGF-9), and hedgehog proteins.[7] They help guide cell differentiation, motility, apoptosis, and organization.[8]
3. Cell surface receptors are essential to proper and normal embryogenesis: they receive guiding information from gene products. Mutations in the receptors can cause as much dysfunction and maldevelopment as abnormalities in gene expression or peptide formation.

ANOMALIES OF THE ORBITAL EMBRYOGENESIS

Craniosynostosis syndromes

Children with craniosynostosis syndromes, such as Crouzon, Pfeiffer, Apert, or Saethre-Chotzen syndrome, commonly have ocular malformations secondary to abnormal orbital development. These include exophthalmos, strabismus, corneal exposure, spontaneous globe subluxation, and optic neuropathy due to optic nerve compression or intracranial hypertension. They are secondary to abnormalities of fibroblast growth factor receptors (Table 4.2).

Table 4.2 Known genetic markers of specific congenital ocular anomalies

Anomalies/syndrome	Genetic marker
Crouzon/Apert	FGFR2
Treacher Collins	TCOF1
Waardenberg	PAX 3
Microphthalmos	PAX 6
Peters	PAX 6, PITX 3, CYP1B1
Aniridia	PAX 6, WT
Cataract	PAX 6, Bmp 4, 7
Stickler syndrome	COL2A1, COL11A, COL11A2
Alagille syndrome	JAG 1
Oculocutaneous OCA I	TYR
Oculocutaneous Albinism Type 2	OCA 2
Ataxia – Telangiectasia	ATM
Marfan syndrome	FBN 1

Mandibular facial dysostosis (Treacher Collins syndrome) is an autosomal dominant syndrome with ocular manifestations of lower eyelid colobomas, downslanting palpebral fissures, and, occasionally, cataract and cleft palate. A gene *TCOF1* and its product TREACL have been implicated as they may cause abnormal formation of the branchial arches.

Orbital dermoids

When surface ectoderm becomes entrapped in developing orbital mesenchyme at the age of 4 to 6 weeks, subsequent differentiation of these tissues can lead to dermoids. These dermoids most commonly occur at the junction of the frontal and temporal bones, but may be intraorbital. In Goldenhar syndrome, corneal–scleral dermoids are associated with coloboma of eyelid, preauricular skin tags, Duane syndrome, auricular abnormalities, and cardiovascular and vertebral anomalies.

Waardenburg syndrome is an autosomal dominant disorder of sensorineural hearing loss, hypertelorism, heterochromia irides, and white forelock. There are four variations of this syndrome, some due to *PAX3* mutations. In some forms, there is limb involvement with gene clusters interacting abnormally due to the *PAX3* mutation.

MOLECULAR CONTROL OF OCULAR DEVELOPMENT

When embryogenesis and optic vesicle development fails early in development (age 3–6 weeks), abnormalities of the whole eye result. Anophthalmos or complete absence of ocular development is rare: it results from complete failure of optic vesicle formation. Microphthalmos results from abnormal development of the eye in the first trimester. The earlier the malformation, the more severely affected the eye, with microphthalmos with cyst more severe than colobomatous microphthalmos or microphthalmos without coloboma.

When the optic vesicles are completely fused (cyclopia), this is associated with significant lethal neurologic and systemic abnormalities. When the optic vesicles fail to close, colobomatous microphthalmos results, with cystic components often larger than the malformed eye.[9] Smaller localized failure of closure will lead to coloboma of part of the globe (optic nerve, chorioretina, iris, or lens).

PAX6

PAX6, found on the chromosome 11p13, encodes for transcription factors essential for normal ocular and central nervous system development. It is highly conserved. *PAX6* interacts with other cell cycle proteins and regulates proliferation of cells in many ocular tissues including developing retina, which may account for the afoveate retina in aniridia (see Chapter 4.1). Abnormalities of *PAX6* have been found in patients with aniridia, Peters anomaly, ectopia pupillae, and microphthalmos.

PAX6 in mice is involved in normal ganglion cell development, guiding anterior cellular projections to the superior colliculus and lateral geniculate nucleus and is also important in establishing the nasotemporal axis of the retina.[10–17]

ABNORMALITIES OF EYELID DEVELOPMENT

Cryptophthalmos occurs when the globe is covered with skin due to abnormal eyelid development and separation.[18] It may be associated with limb and other anomalies and Fraser syndrome (see Chapter 24).

Failure of the lid structures to develop normally leads to areas of absent lid tissue or eyelid colobomas. When the upper lid is involved, there is often a notch at the medial and middle third of the lid. These are not associated with other ocular or systemic problems. Lower lid colobomas are usually at the middle/lateral junction and are more frequently associated with syndromes such as Treacher Collins or Goldenhar.

DEVELOPMENT OF THE CORNEA
(see Chapter 28)

The structure and cellular composition of the cornea is complete by 7 months, and at birth, the cornea is 10 mm in diameter with a steep curvature averaging 55 diopters. The central cornea is thicker in newborns than in adults, measuring 580 μm, and postnatally, there is continued loss of cellularity of the corneal epithelium with 45% loss in cell density in the first year of life.[19]

ANOMALIES OF THE CORNEA (see Chapter 28)

The presence of corneolenticular adhesion places the child at higher risk for vitreoretinal and systemic abnormalities (a condition known as Peters Plus). Genetic abnormalities that have been described in these patients with multisystem involvement include mutations in *PAX6, PITX2, PITX3,* and *CYP1B1*.[20,21]

DEVELOPMENT OF THE LENS

Primitive lens cells are formed when the optic vesicles contact the surface ectoderm at 27 days to form the lens plate. Invagination of the optic cup in the fifth week is accompanied by evolution of the lens plate to the lens pit then a lens vesicle. The epithelium lining the lens vesicle is arranged with the apices turned inward so that the basement membrane they secrete

forms the lens capsule. The developing lens receives vascular support from the hyaloid artery, which extends from the optic nerve to the posterior lens where it forms the tunica vasculosa lentis. At 7 weeks, the neural crest cells have covered the anterior surface of the lens, separating it from the cornea. Vessels form from the trabecular structures, giving rise to the anterior tunica vasculosa lentis. Lens fiber development is active in the eighth week, and anterior epithelial cells at the equator divide and are pushed posteriorly, which in turn displaces the primary fibers anteriorly. This equatorial division and displacement leads to the creation of the lens sutures, an upright Y-suture anterior and an inverted Y-suture posterior. At 3 months, sutures are found only in the fetal nucleus, not in the embryonal nucleus. In the fourth and sixth month, the lens crystallins change in composition from α-fetal-crystallins to β-crystallins. Between 7 and 9 months, the tunica vasculosa lentis and hyaloid vessels regress.

MOLECULAR CONTROL OF LENS DEVELOPMENT

Normal polarity of the lens fiber development is essential for the formation of optically clear structure. Abnormal polarity may lead to the development of cataracts. A family of genes called bone morphogenic protein (*Bmp4, Bmp7*) genes have been described in a mouse model as being essential to normal lens development.[22–26] *PAX6* is an important mediator in this process. The loss of lens fiber cellular organelles and nuclei with maintenance of cell membrane and crystalline integrity is essential to crystalline lens clarity. To remain optically clear, the secondary lens fibers undergo an apoptotic process in which nuclei shrink and mitochondria degenerate while plasma membrane survives. Disturbance in this cellular ballet may lead to congenital cataracts.

IRIS AND TRABECULAR MESHWORK DEVELOPMENT

Iris stroma and trabecular meshwork structures first appear as neural crest cells migrating into the anterior segment at 7 weeks. In the third month, the anterior rim of the optic cup differentiates as it nears the lens. The external pigmented layer of the neuroectoderm develops folds that will become ciliary processes. Anterior to these folds, iris epithelium develops. The anterior chamber angle begins to form, covered by endothelial cells of neural crest origin. The major arteriolar circle forms at 4 months, when zonules form and distinct trabecular meshwork cells can be seen. At month 5, gaps appear within the trabecular structures and distinct pigmented cells are formed.[27] The pupillary membrane covering the pupil begins to atrophy at the end of 6 months, leaving a clear central visual axis. Macrophages line the surface of the iris and are crucial to normal trabecular development.[28] At 7 months, the iris sphincter and dilator muscle develop and become functional by 32 weeks of age. Iris pigmentation continues after birth for at least 6 months, with pale irides getting darker. Physiologic anisocoria can be seen in 21% of children.[29] The trabecular meshwork continues to show remodeling in the first year of life, and delayed maturation of angle structure may be responsible for some cases of congenital glaucoma.

MOLECULAR CONTROL OF TRABECULAR DEVELOPMENT

PAX6, PITX2, and *FOXC1* are involved in forms of anterior segment dysgenesis; they are widely distributed in developing embryonic tissues, when ocular organogenesis is at its most critical stage.[30–32] They are discussed in Chapter 28.

RETINA DEVELOPMENT

As the optic vesicle contacts the surface ectoderm, induction of the lens plate also induces development of the retina and invagination of the vesicle to form the optic cup. The bilayer nature of the retina is established early, as the inner invaginating neuroepithelium becomes the sensory retina and the external pigmented noninvaginating epithelium becomes the retinal pigment epithelium. By 5 weeks, the inner sensory retinal layer of the cup is apposed against the outer RPE layer of the optic cup. The hyaloid artery extends from the nerve to the developing lens. The primary vitreous has formed and lined the developing retina and posterior lens surface. At the sixth week, the embryonic fissure begins to close by apoptosis, starting in the center of the fissure and moving simultaneously anteriorly and posteriorly. The RPE is a single layer of cuboidal epithelium whereas the cells of the sensory retina replicate and grow thicker. The sensory retina secretes secondary vitreous, which displaces primary vitreous. At 7 weeks, the sensory retina differentiates and cells migrate toward the optic nerve. At week 8, the RPE cells extend to the optic nerve to form the lamina cribrosa. The inner layers of the sensory retina develop into ganglion cells and nerve fiber layers and other cells form Müller cells. Clumps of glial cells form Bergmeister's papilla over the developing optic disc. The sclera and choriocapillaris develop from posterior mesenchyme, and the ophthalmic artery develops. Differentiation progresses in the sensory retina with the posterior retina developing before the peripheral retina, and the inner retinal layers prior to the outer (photoreceptor) layers. Bipolar and horizontal cells develop and migrate inward toward the photoreceptors. By 4 months, the inner layers of the sensory retina have been formed with the photoreceptor layer, inner nuclear, inner plexiform, and ganglion cell layer. The photoreceptors begin to develop and retinal vascularization takes place starting posteriorly and moving peripherally, a process that continues until 8 months. The cones differentiate in the sixth month followed by the rods, which differentiate in the seventh month. Macular differentiation starts in the eighth month and continues postnatally. The ganglion, amacrine, bipolar, horizontal, and Müller cells move away from the fovea, while the photoreceptors move toward the fovea.[33] It is worth noting that while lamination appears highly specific, ectopic functioning photoreceptors can be found in the ganglion cell layer at birth; bipolar cells can be found in the ganglion cell layer in adult rats. The significance of these cells in the wrong location is uncertain.

Postnatally the cones elongate and become narrower, leading to increased foveal cone density, which increases until it reaches its adult configuration by 45 months of age.

MOLECULAR CONTROL OF RETINAL DEVELOPMENT

Whereas genetic control of mechanisms for human ocular, corneal, and iris development has clearly been shown, the identified molecular products controlling retinal development are limited to other mammal species such as mice and rats. There are multiple protein modulators being investigated that control proper differentiation and lamination in developing murine models. Some of these include homeodomain interacting protein kinase 2 (*HIPK2*), sonic hedgehog gene (*SHH*), and distal-less homeobox genes (*Dlx1, Dlx2*) as well as *PAX6.*[34,35] A protein Tubedown-1 (Tbdn-1) has been found to be operative in the regulation of vitreal vasculature, and elucidation of these pathways may be useful in the treatment and control of the neovascular conditions such as diabetic retinopathy or retinopathy of prematurity.[36,37]

DEVELOPMENT OF THE OPTIC NERVE

The optic nerve develops in three phases. In the first phase the embryonal fissure within the optic stalk begins to close at week five, with complete closure by week seven. The optic stalk is the connection between the optic vesicle and forebrain, which serve as the scaffold on which the optic nerve will develop. In the second stage of development, ganglion cells and glial cells from the developing retina begin to penetrate the disc and enter the stalk at 8 weeks of age. By 12 weeks of age there are 1.9 million axons in the developing nerve, with the number of axons peaking at 3.7 million by 17 weeks. The third stage of development occurs between the fourth and eighth month when the numbers of axons begins to decrease and the numbers of glial cells increases. Simultaneously there is an increase in the collagen content of the optic nerve. By eight months the number of axons has decreased to 1.1 million. Myelination begins in the sixth month, starting at the chiasm and moving anteriorly but stopping at the disc. Occasionally, myelination of the axons in the retina occurs, leading to a myelinated nerve fiber layer.

VISUAL CORTEX DEVELOPMENT

Development of the cortical visual centers has been investigated using Macaque monkeys. The lateral geniculate nucleus (LGN) can first be identified at an age that corresponds to 8 to 11 weeks in a human gestational age with ganglion cells reaching the LGN at 10 weeks gestational age. The lamination that characterizes the LGN develops between 22 and 25 weeks gestational age.[38] Concurrently, as the LGN is developing, cells that will form the striate cortex are developing between 10 to 25 weeks. Initially, inputs from the LGN are intermingled with innervation from the LGN, taking place at 26 weeks gestational age. Formation of ocular dominance columns takes place between 26 weeks and term, and a significant amount of cortical visual development continues postnatally. Just as the foveal development is incomplete at birth, so is the lateral geniculate nucleus as well as striate cortex. Synaptic connections in the striate cortex develop to reach a maximum degree of interconnection 8 months postnatally with further refinement that occurs over several years. This refinement of organization is dependent upon a clear retinal image being focused upon the eye transmitted through the optic nerve and received by the developing striate cortex. There is a critical period of cortical development during which any impediment of formed vision leads to permanent abnormal cortical development.[39]

The molecular mechanisms responsible for guidance of developing axons from the retina into the optic nerve to the chiasm and striate cortex have been elucidated in mouse models. These guidance molecules called netrins provide chemotactic and biochemical signals to developing axons. Knockout mice models that show abnormal ganglion cell development with significant optic nerve hypoplasia in mice in which these guidance molecules have been disrupted have been developed.[40]

POSTNATAL GROWTH AND EMMETROPIZATION (see Chapter 6)

At birth, the eye is rarely emmetropic. The optical refractive determinants of the eye–corneal curvature, lens power and location, and axial length–can be quite variable so that the refractive error of the newborn eye ranges from between –2.0 and +4.0 diopters.[41] Within two years, this variability of refractive decreases and the mean value shifts so that the eye becomes closer to emmetropia. This process is called emmetropization, and within populations, it is possible to predict shifts in refractive error so that most infants are born hyperopic and become near emmetropic by 6 to 8 years of age.[42] As the cornea flattens, it loses refractive power, which is balanced by increasing axial length. Whether this balance is guided by genetically encoded mechanisms or whether eye growth is affected by environmental influences has been debated for centuries, and most likely both nature and nurture affect the way the eye develops.

Support for the assertion that eye growth is genetically regulated comes from studies of heritability and prevalence studies. Studies of identical and fraternal twins enable epidemiologists to ascribe a predictability coefficient to inherited traits.[43] Such studies have shown a strong hereditary component determining whether a child will become hyperopic or myopic. Studies of children followed longitudinally for the development of refractive errors have shown that parental history of myopia is one of the strongest predictors that the child will become myopic.[44] Prevalence studies done in different countries examining the prevalence of myopia and hyperopia show the prevalence of myopia varies between 7 and 70% depending on the age, occupation, and educational status of those studied.

The notion that use of the eyes can affect the eventual refractive status has been proposed for centuries. In the 19th century, the association between occupations requiring extensive nearwork and high myopia was established in the European and Asian literature. It has only been in the past three decades that controlled studies to examine the effect of visual input on the developing eye have been designed and conducted. Most myopia research is limited by difficulties with study design, such as measurement of prevalence, rather than the longitudinally conducted studies measuring incidence of myopia, and controlling for factors such as amount of reading, ambient lighting conditions, font size, and nutritional and parental factors have been a problem.[45] When studies of intervention to prevent myopia have

been conducted, these studies have been limited by significant study design problems, such as lack of randomization, lack of control, and lack of long-term follow-up. In the past decade there have been well-conducted studies that have followed school-aged children longitudinally to measure the effect of reading and nearwork on the development of myopia.[46] These studies have shown that there is a strong correlation between the amount of nearwork performed and education attainment level in children who are more likely to become myopic. Such myopia is axial in nature with the eye growing longer and not due to change in cornea curvature, lens power, or position.

Animal models of myopia have been accidentally discovered, then further refined to investigate the effect of visual input on the developing eye: the avian models (chick), primate models (Macaque monkeys), marmosets, or tree shrews.[47,48] All these models have shown that when the eye is deprived from receiving a formed visual image early in life, such eyes develop axial myopia. This form deprivation myopia occurs in a dose-dependent fashion. In the avian model, it can be reversed with restoration of normal retinal imaging or with restoration of a nondefocused visual image. Both axial myopia and axial hyperopia can be induced with defocusing spectacles or contact lenses placed in front of the eye of the visually immature monkey or chicken. In the avian model, this optical defocus leads to biochemical changes that lead to changes in the sclera and choroid of the animals, leading to axial myopia. This seems to be a locally mediated process as hemiretinal formed deprivation leads to hemiretinal axial elongation. Use of these animal models may help identify the relationship between visual input and subsequent biochemical processes that lead to structural changes in the developing eye.

Just as the striate cortex requires a clear visual image in order to develop normally postnatally, ocular growth and development also require formed clear visual image to grow properly. By compiling the epidemiologic data investigating the visual habits of developing children and analyzing that data in the context of animal models of formed deprivation myopia, new theories as to postnatal ocular growth regulations have been developed. It is believed that retinal blur, whether due to form deprivation or abnormal early visual experience in the developing eye, leads to alterations in emmetropization, which, when coupled with a genetic predisposition to myopia, leads to increased axial length in developing children.

Historically, attempts to modulate the visual habits of developing children through the use of contact lenses, bifocals, or pharmacologic agents such as antimuscarinics have shown a limited effect on ocular growth. Antimuscarinics (atropine and more selective agents) are being investigated to see whether the progression of myopia may be slowed, if not prevented, by modulation of mechanisms that may affect both the visual input to the eye and on the developing retina, sclera, and choroid.

REFERENCES

1. Barishak YR. Embryology of the eye and its adnexae. In: Straub W, editor. Developments in Ophthalmology. Basel: Karger; 1992. (vol. 24.)
2. Langman J. Medical Embryology. Baltimore/London: Williams & Wilkins; 1981.
3. Gordon RA, Donzis PB. Refractive development of the human eye. Arch Ophthalmol 1985; 103: 785–9.
4. Levin AV. Congenital eye anomalies. Pediatr Clin North Am 2003; 50: 55–76.
5. Mohamed YH, Gong H, Amemiya T. Role of apoptosis in eyelid

development. Exp Eye Res 2003; 76: 115–23.
6. Dilmen G, Koktener A, Turhan NO, et al. Growth of fetal lens and orbit. Int J Gynaecol Obstet 2002; 76: 267–71.
7. Li C, Guo H, Xu X, et al. Fibroblast growth factor receptor 2 (Fgfr2) plays an important role in eyelid and skin formation and patterning. Dev Dyn 2001; 222: 471–83.
8. Adler R, Belecky-Adams TL. The role of bone morphogenetic proteins in the differentiation of the ventral optic cup. Development 2002; 129: 3161–71.
9. Khairallah M, Messaoud R, Zaouali S, et al. Posterior segment changes associated with posterior microphthalmos. Ophthalmology 2002; 109: 569–74.

10. Saleem RA, Walter MA. The complexities of ocular genetics. Clin Genet 2002; 61: 79–88.

11. Chan CC, Datiles M, Kaiser-Kupfer MI, et al. Congenital iridocorneal malformation in Rieger syndrome. Arch Ophthalmol 2003; 121: 582–3.

12. Graf MH, Jungherr A. Congenital mydriasis, failure of accommodation, and patent ductus ateriosus. Arch Ophthalmol 2002; 120: 509–10.

13. Collinson JM, Quinn JC, Hill RE, et al. The roles of Pax6 in the cornea, retina, and olfactory epithelium of the developing mouse embryo. Dev Biol 2003; 255: 303–12.

14. Li CM, Yan RT, Wang SZ. Chick homeobox gene cbx and its role in retinal development. Mech Dev 2002; 116: 85–94.

15. van Heyningen V, Williamson K. PAX6 in sensory development. Hum Mol Genet 2002; 11: 1161–7.

16. Baumer N, Marquardt T, Stoykova A, et al. Pax6 is required for establishing naso-temporal and dorsal characteristics of the optic vesicle. Development 2002; 129: 4535–45.

17. Simpson T, Price D. Pax6: a pleiotropic player in development. Bioessays 2002; 24: 1041–51.

18. Wolfram-Gabel R, Sick H. Microvascularization of the mucocutaneous junction of the eyelid in fetuses and in neonates. Surg Radiol Anat 2002; 24: 97–101.

19. Riley NC, Lwigale PY, Conrad GW. Specificity of corneal nerve positions during embryogenesis. Mol Vis 2001; 7: 297–304.

20. Pierantoni G, Bulfone A, Pentimalli F, et al. The homeodomain-interacting protein kinase 2 gene is expressed late in embryogenesis and preferentially in retina, muscle, and neural tissue. Biochem Biophys Res Commun 2002; 290: 942–7.

21. Walter MA. PITs and FOXes in ocular genetics. Invest Ophthalmol Vis Sci 2003; 44: 1402–5.

22. Veromann S. Theoretical considerations regarding the study "Alpha-B Crystallin Gene (CRYAB) Mutation Causes Dominant Congenital Posterior Polar Cataract in Humans." Am J Hum Genet 2002; 71: 684–5.

23. Bagchi M, Katar M, Maisel H. Heat shock proteins of adult and embryonic human ocular lenses. J Cell Biochem 2002; 84: 278–84.

24. White TW. Unique and redundant connexin contributions to lens development. Science 2002; 295: 319–20.

25. Sanders EJ, Parker E. The role of mitochondria, cytochrome c and caspase-9 in embryonic lens fibre cell denucleation. J Anat 2002; 201: 121–35.

26. Faber SC, Robinson ML, Makarenkova HP, et al. Bmp signaling is required for development of primary lens fiber cells. Development 2002; 129: 3727–37.

27. McMenamin PG. Human fetal iridocorneal angle: a light and electron microscopic study. Br J Ophthalmol 1989; 73: 871–9.

28. McMenamin PG, Loeffler KU. Cells resembling intraventricular macrophages present in subretinal space in human fetal eyes. Anat Rec 1990; 227: 245–53.

29. Roarty JD, Keltner JL. Normal pupil size and anisocoria in new born infants. Arch Ophthalmol 1990; 108: 94–5.

30. Lines M, Kozlowski K, Walter M. Molecular genetics of Axenfeld-Rieger malformations. Hum Mol Genet 2002; 11: 1177–84.

31. Espana EM, Raju VK, Tseng SC. Focal limbal stem cell deficiency corresponding to an iris coloboma. Br J Ophthalmol 2002; 86: 1451–2.

32. Ramaesh T, Collinson J, Ramaesh K, et al. Corneal abnormalities in (Pax6(+/−) small eye) mice mimic human aniridia-related keratopathy. Invest Ophthalmol Vis Sci 2003; 44: 1871–8.

33. McGuire DE, Weinreb RN, Goldbaum MH. Foveal hypoplasia demonstrated in vivo with optical coherence tomography. Am J Ophthalmol 2003; 135: 112–4.

34. Wang Y, Dakubo G, Howley P, et al. Development of normal retinal organization depends on Sonic hedgehog signaling from ganglion cells. Nat Neurosci 2002; 5831–2.

35. de Melo J, Qui X, Du G, et al. Dlx1, Dlx2, Pax6, Brn3b, and Chx10 Homeobox gene expression defines the retinal ganglion and inner nuclear layers of the developing and adult mouse retina. J Comp Neurol 2003; 461: 187–204.

36. Wagner KD, Wagner N, Vidal VP, et al. The Wilms' tumor gene Wt1 is required for normal development of the retina. EMBO J 2002; 21: 1398–405.

37. Paradis H, Liu C, Saika S, et al. Tubedown-1 in remodeling of the developing vitreal vasculature in vivo and regulation of capillary outgrowth in vitro. Dev Biol 2002; 249: 140–55.

38. Horton JC. The central visual pathways. In: Hart WM, editor. Adler's Physiology of the Eye. 9th ed. St. Louis: Mosby; 1992: 728–72.

39. Hubel H, Wiesel TN, LeVay S. Plasticity of ocular dominance columns in monkey striate cortex. Phil Trans R Soc London 1977; B278: 377.

40. Oster SF, Stretavan DW. Connecting the eye to the brain: the molecular basis of ganglion cell axon guidance. Br J Ophthalmol 2003; 87: 639–45.

41. Brown EV. Net average yearly changes in refraction of atropinized eye from birth to beyond middle life. Arch Ophthalmol 1938; 19: 719–34.

42. Fulton AB, Dobson V, Salem D, et al. Cycloplegic refractions in infants and young children. Am J Ophthalmol 1980; 90: 239–47.

43. Hammond CJ, Snieder H, Gilbert CE, et al. Genes and environment in refractive error: the twin eye study. Invet Ophthalmol Vis Sci 2001; 42: 1232–6.

44. Zadnik K, Sataranio WA, Mutti DO, et al. The effect parental history of myopia on children's eye size. JAMA 1994; 271: 1323–32.

45. Saw SM, Katz J, Schein OD, et al. Epidemiology of myopia. Epidemiol Rev 1996; 18: 175–87.

46. Tay MT, Au Eong KG, Ng CY, et al. Myopia and educational attainment in 421,116 Singaporean males. Ann Acad Med Singapore 1992; 21: 785–91.

47. Raviola E, Wiesel TN. An animal model of myopia. N Engl J Med 1985; 312: 1609–15.

48. Wallman J, Turkel J, Trachtman J. Extreme myopia produced by modest change in early visual experience. Science 1978; 201: 1249–51.

CHAPTER

5 Milestones and Normative Data

Hans Ulrik Møller

At birth the eye looks nearly the same size as in the adult because the corneal diameter is only 1.7 mm smaller; but its volume increases almost threefold up to maturity and its weight doubles, the average for the full-term newborn eye being, respectively, 3.25 cm^3 and 3.40 g. The weight increases nearly 40% by the middle of the second year and nearly 70% by the fifth year.

Many changes occur with maturation: normative data are needed for clinical observations during childhood. Much of the data is old, as the art of anthropometry is unfashionable, but still useful.

EMBRYOLOGY

The development and growth of an embryo and its eyes is a continuous process; however, there is variability in the rate of growth of the different ocular tissues. The cells that will become the iris are visible as migrated neural crest cells in the seventh week, but they remain dormant until the ciliary muscles are formed in the third month.

Unlike man, Mother Nature does not look at an embryo in stages, weeks of gestation, or trimesters; however, the development of the parts of the eyes are meticulously sequenced: understanding the milestones of embryogenesis may help understand teratogenic syndromes (Fig. 5.1, Table 5.1).

The developing eye comprises:
(i) Neuroectoderm (e.g., the optic sulcus, which later becomes the optic vesicle early in the fourth week);
(ii) Surface ectoderm (e.g., the first sign of the lens on day 32);
(iii) Migrated neural crest cells, which are the stem cells of, among other things, the anterior chamber during the seventh week; and
(iv) Mesodermal embryonic layer, which contributes only the vascular endothelial cells and extraocular muscles, which are visible in the fourth week.

Barishak[1] published an extensive chronology of eye development.

INTERCANTHAL DISTANCE AND PALPEBRA

The distance between the inner canthi and the outer canthi and the size and shape of the palpebral fissure are important in diagnosing conditions such as craniofacial malformations and fetal alcohol syndrome.

Palpebral fissure changes in early childhood have recently been studied by analyzing digital imaging:[2] during the first 3 months of life the upper eyelid is at its lowest position compared to the center of the pupil, later raising to its maximum between the age of 3 to 6 months, and then declining linearly until adulthood. The lower eyelid is close to the pupil center at birth, dropping linearly

until the age of 18 months when its position stabilizes. A single lower eyelid crease was the common finding at birth, a double crease at the age of 36 months. Figure 5.2 shows the linear relationship between gestational age and orbital margin horizontal (OMH) as well as vertical (OMV) diameters in the unborn child.[3] Figure 5.3 illustrates the linear relationship between gestational age and conjunctival fornix horizontal (CFH) as well as vertical (CFV) diameters.[3]

The palpebral fissures are 15±2 mm at 32 weeks of gestation, 17±2 mm at birth, 24±3 mm at 2 years of age, and 27±3 mm at the age of 14.[4,5] Interracial differences may exist: the palpebral fissure is longer in black Americans, with a mean of 30 mm at the age of 3 years.[6]

Inner canthal distance and outer orbital distance are 16 and 59 mm, respectively, in premature infants; 20±4 and 69±8 mm in newborn babies; 26±6 and 88±10 mm at the age of 3; and 31±5 and 111±12 mm at the age of 14 (Fig. 5.4).[7]

A universal approach is the canthus index (CI):

$$\text{Canthus Index} = \frac{\text{inner canthus distance} \times 100}{\text{outer canthus distance}}\%.$$

Normals, unrelated to age, lie between 28.4 and 38%.[8] The canthus index of over 1,000 children between 6 and 18 years old was determined as follows[9]:

	Boys	Girls
6 years	38.2% (SD 2.1%)	38.3% (SD 1.8%)
16 years	37.1% (SD 2.6%)	36.6% (SD 1.9%)

TEAR SECRETION

Any nurse on the ROP ward round knows that tearing is not a problem with the youngest premature babies. In preterm babies (30–37 weeks after conception) mean basal tear (with topical anesthesia) secretion is 6.2 (±4.5 SD) mm and at term 9.2 (±4.3) mm tested with a Schirmer tear test strip. Mean reflex tear secretion is 7.4 (±4.8) mm in preterm and 13.2 (±6.5) mm in term infants.[10]

CORNEA

The young premature cornea lacks luster and clarity, making some diagnoses difficult. The shallow anterior chambers, miotic pupils, and bluish irides are features of prematurity.

The corneal diameter in infants at 25–37 weeks post-conceptional age increases by 0.5 mm every 15 days from 6.2 to 9.0 mm (Fig. 5.5).[11,12]

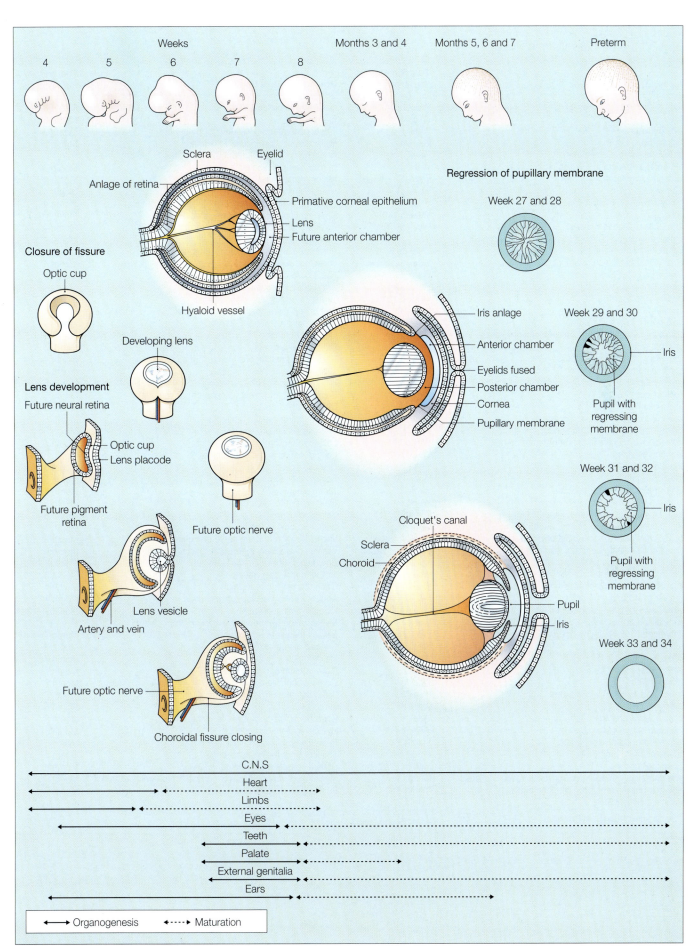

Fig. 5.1 Milestones in ophthalmoembryology.

Table 5.1 Chronological embryology

Development of the eye	The age of the embryo	Development of the eye	The age of the embryo
Optic sulcus, optic primordium	Week 3	Vortex veins pierce sclera	Month 3
Optic cup	Week 4	Eyelids fuse	Month 3
Lens placode	Week 4	Tarsal plate merges with levator palpebrae	Month 3
Retinal disc	Week 4	Extraocular muscles fuse with sclera	Month 3
Embryonic fissure (coloboma)	Week 4	Angle between orbits reduced to 72° due to growth of maxillary processes	Month 3
Primordia, extraocular muscles	Week 4		
Lens pit invaginates	Week 5	Major retinal constituents present	Month 4
Lens vesicle	Week 5	Haller–Zinn arterial circle	Month 4
Primary vitreous, hyaloid vasculature	Week 5	Incipient retinal vascularization	Month 4
Optic stalk	Week 5	Physiological cupping of optic disc	Month 4
Structures of face and orbit	Week 5	Anlage of pars plana	Month 4
Angle between orbits reduced to 160° due to growth of maxillary processes	Week 5	Arterial circle of iris	Month 4
		Pupillary membrane replaces anterior tunica vasculosa lentis	Month 4
Incipient differentiation of retinal pigment epithelium	Week 6	Hyaloid vascular system regresses	Month 4
Primordium of sensory retina	Week 6	Secondary vitreous well developed	Month 4
Secondary vitreous fibrils	Week 6	Tertiary vitreous develops	Month 4
Primary lens fibers	Week 6	Sclera well developed	Month 4
First eyelid folds	Week 6	Descemet's membrane	Month 4
Closure of embryonic fissure	Week 6	Canal of Schlemm	Month 4
Retinal pigment epithelium, one-cell-thick layer of cuboidal cells	Week 6	Palpebral ligaments	Month 4
First fibrils of secondary vitreous	Week 6	Lanugo and sebaceous glands in the caruncle	Month 4
Primitive corneal epithelium	Week 6	First uncrossed chiasm fibers	Month 4
First myofibrils of extraocular muscles	Week 6	Differentiation of photoreceptors	Month 5
Muscles cone visible	Week 6	Rapid growth of retinal vasculature	Month 5
Ciliary ganglion visible	Week 6	Differentiation of cornea	Month 5
Superior anlage of nasolacrimal duct	Week 6	Corneal nerves reach the epithelium	Month 5
Inferior anlage of nasolacrimal duct	Week 6	Adipose tissue in the orbit	Month 5
Proliferation and differentiation of future cornea	Week 6	Loss of ganglion cells in the retina	Month 5
Sensory retina	Week 7	Loss of axons in the optic nerve	Month 5
Choroidal vasculature	Week 7	Cloquet's canal	Month 5
Anterior segment	Week 7	Bowman's membrane	Month 5
Anterior tunica vasculosa lentis	Week 7	Tenon's capsule	Month 5
Embryonic fissure completely closed	Week 7	Eyelids start to separate	Month 5
Neural crest cells for corneal endothelium	Week 7	Scleral spur	Month 5
Neural crest cells for trabecular endothelium	Week 7	Dilator muscle of the iris	Month 6
Neural crest cells for corneal stroma	Week 7	Vascularization of optic nerve completed	Month 6
Neural crest cells to be future iris stroma	Week 7	Vessels of pupillary membrane start to atrophy	Month 6
Anterior chamber between corneal endothelium and lamina irido pupillaris	Week 7	Bowman's membrane well defined	Month 6
Sclera visible	Week 7	Nasolacrimal duct patent	Month 6
Circular eyelid fold	Week 7	Central fovea starts to thin	Month 7
Angle between orbits reduced to 120° due to growth of maxillary processes	Week 7	Adult size of avascular zone of fovea	Month 7
		Fibrous lamina cribosa	Month 7
Maturation of retinal pigment epithelium	Week 8	Myelinization of optic nerve appears from chiasm toward the eye	Month 7
Retinal ganglion cells	Week 8	Circular muscle of ciliary body	Month 7
Axons in optic stalk	Week 8	Iris completes its pigmentation	Month 7
Bergmeister papilla formed	Week 8	Pigmentation of choroid	Month 7
Lacrimal gland	Week 8	Corneal epithelium 4–5 layers	Month 7
Optic nerve has 2,670,000 axons	Week 8	Lens diameter 5 mm	Month 7
Rudimentary chiasm	Week 8	Iris sphincter	Month 8
Hyaloid vascular system fully formed	Week 8	Chamber angle completes formation	Month 8
Y-shaped suture of the lens	Week 8	Hyaloid system disappears	Month 8
Bergmeister papilla disappears	Month 3	Retinal vessels reach nasal ora serrata	Month 8
Anlage of ciliary processes	Month 3	The length of the muscles cone 25 mm	Month 8
Iris epithelium	Month 3	Retinal vessels reach the periphery	Month 9
Lens completely surrounded by tunica vasculosa lentis	Month 3	Myelination of optic nerve is completed to lamina cribosa	Month 9
Lens comprises embryonal and fetal nucleus	Month 3	Pupillary membrane disappears	Month 9
Corneal collagen fibrils	Month 3		

The table is mainly based on Barishak.[1]

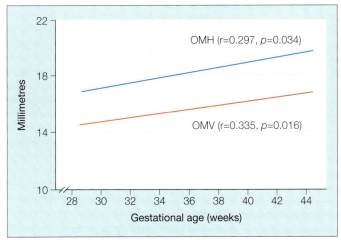

Fig. 5.2 Interocular distance. Linear regression relationship and standard error of the estimate between orbital margin horizontal (OMH) and vertical (OMV) diameters and gestational age. Correlation coefficients with *p* values are indicated. Data from Isenberg et al.[3] With permission from American Academy of Ophthalmology.

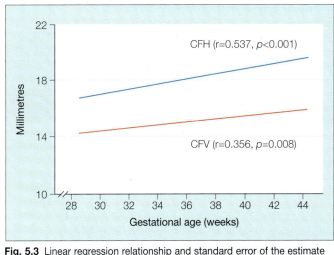

Fig. 5.3 Linear regression relationship and standard error of the estimate between conjunctival fornix horizontal (CFH) and vertical (CFV) diameters and gestational age. Correlation coefficients with *p* values are indicated. Data from Isenberg et al.[3] Redrawn with permission from the publisher.

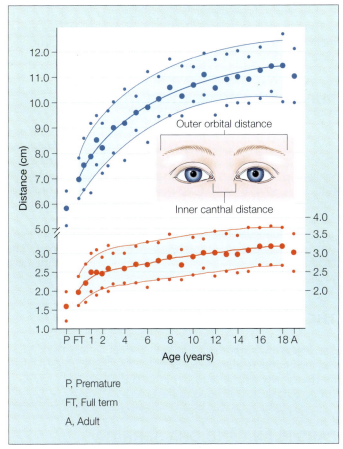

Fig. 5.4 Graphs of inner canthal and outer orbital distances. The large points represent the mean value for each age group, the smaller points represent 2 SD from the mean. The heavy line approximates the 50th percentile, while the shaded area roughly encompasses the range from the third to the 97th percentile. Data from Laestadius et al.[7] With permission from Elsevier.

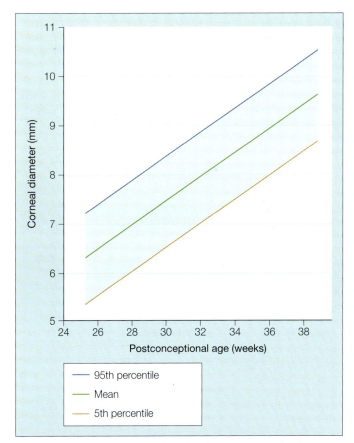

Fig. 5.5 Mean corneal diameter plotted against postconceptional age. From Tucker SM, Enzenauer RW, Levin AV, et al. Corneal diameter, axial length, and intraocular pressure in premature infants. Ophthalmology 1992; 99: 1296–300. With permission from American Academy of Ophthalmology.[11]

At birth the horizontal and vertical diameters of the cornea for full-term boys are 9.8±0.33 mm and 10.4±0.35 mm and for girls 10.1±0.33 mm and 10.7±0.29 mm.[13] The last 2 mm of growth in corneal diameter, i.e., approximately 20%, takes place in early infancy and then more slowly in early childhood. An adult value of 11.7 mm is reached at 7 years.

Corneal refraction in premature infants is 53.1±1.5 diopters, in the neonate 48.4±1.7 diopters, at 1 month 45.9±2.3 diopters, and at 36 months 42.9±1.3 diopters.[14]

Central corneal thickness

Abnormal thickness of the central cornea is a possible source of error in tonometry. Central corneal thickness (CCT) in full-term babies is significantly higher, 0.54 mm, than that of children of more than 2 years of age, who have adult readings of 0.52 mm. CCTs measured with optical pachymetry, corneal curvature are given for premature and full-term babies in Table 5.2.[15]

CCT measured by ultrasonic pachymetry in 13 babies with gestational ages below 33 weeks gives a mean of 0.656 mm (SD ±0.103 mm) 5 days postnatally, and 0.566 (SD ±0.064) at the age of 110 days–a decrease of 12%.[16]

In 74 full-term neonates,[17] also with ultrasonography, CCT is 0.573±0.052 mm (range 0.450–0.691 mm). They have a peripheral corneal thickness of 0.650±0.062 mm (range 0.520–0.830 mm). Table 5.3 shows the decrease in thickness during the first few days of life.

Another study[18] confirms these data and the decrease from the values of day 1 by ultrasonic pachymetry in full-term newborns. They also studied the peripheral corneal thickness: superior corneal thickness was 0.696±0.055 mm, which is significantly thinner than the inferior corneal thickness (0.744±0.062 mm) and the nasal corneal thickness (0.742±0.058 mm), as well as the temporal corneal thickness (0.748±0.055 mm). The peripheral measurement was taken setting the 1.5-mm probe tip

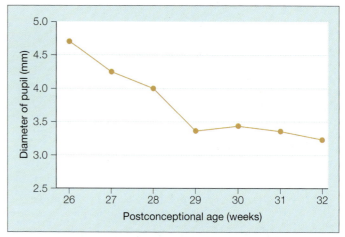

Fig. 5.6 The diameter of the pupil in relative darkness in preterm neonates.[19] With permission from Isenberg et al.[19]

at a tangent to the limbus, i.e., 0.75 mm from the limbus. Adult values are reached at about 3 years of age.

The keratocyte density is around 60,000 cells per cubic millimeter in infancy with a decline of 0.3% per year through life.

The endothelial cell count is more than 10,000 cells per square millimeter at 12 weeks of gestation, 50% of this at birth, and around 4,000 cells per square millimeter in childhood.

PUPIL SIZE AND REACTION TO LIGHT

The pupil, in relative darkness, has a mean diameter of 4.7 mm at 26 weeks of postconceptional age compared to a corneal diameter of 7 mm. The pupils subsequently become progressively smaller reaching 3.4 mm at 29 weeks. There is no reaction to light until a mean of 30.6 weeks (±1 week) postconceptional age.[19] Figure 5.6 shows the change of pupil diameter in relative darkness (<10 ft-c) in preterm neonates.

Using a photographic technique on 88 babies the mean pupil size is 3.8 mm (SD±0.8 mm) in the newborn period. The incidence of anisocoria of less than 1 mm is 21%; no difference was greater than 1 mm.[20]

THE CRYSTALLINE LENS

The lens grows throughout life; information on lens thickness is included in the section "Axial Length." The lens capsule doubles its thickness from birth to old age. The young lens capsule is strong and elastic compared to the elderly.

PARS PLANA AND ORA SERRATA

Morphological and topographic anatomical studies of 15 fetuses at autopsy (age range 24–40 postmenstrual weeks) have shown the average pars plana to be 1.17 mm in width: that is, approximately one-third of that in the adult eye.[21]

The mean value of the distance between the sclerocorneal limbus and the ora serrata is 3.22 mm nasally and 3.33 mm temporally, respectively (Table 5.4). Since there is little growth of the eye between the 30th and 40th weeks of intrauterine life, these values are close to the neonate's.

Table 5.2 Central corneal thickness (CCT) and curvature (R) in newborns and children

Age group	No.	CCT (mm ± SEM)	R (mm ± SEM)
Premature newborns	6	0.545 ± 0.014	6.35 ± 0.09
Mature newborns	19	0.541 ± 0.006	7.11 ± 0.07
Children 2–4 years	10	0.520 ± 0.007	7.73 ± 0.09
Children 5–9 years	15	0.520 ± 0.005	7.81 ± 0.09
Children 10–14 years	11	0.520 ± 0.007	8.01 ± 0.05
Adults (own group and data from literature)		~0.52	~7.8

Ehlers N, Sørensen T, Bramsen T, et al. Central corneal thickness in newborns and children. Acta Ophthalmol (Copenh) 1976; 54: 285–90. With permission from Blackwell Publishing Ltd.

Table 5.3 Central and peripheral corneal thickness (mm) in newborn babies

Corneal thickness	Age (hours)		
	0–24	24–48	48–72
Central	0.58	0.56	0.54
Peripheral	0.63	0.63	0.61

Portellinha W, Belfort R Jr. Central and peripheral corneal thickness in newborns. Acta Ophthalmol (Copenh) 1991; 69: 247–50. With permission from Blackwell Publishing Ltd.

Table 5.4 Values (mm) of the distance from sclerocorneal limbus to the ora serrata in the nasal, temporal, superior, and inferior meridians (mean ± SD)[21]

Nasal meridian	Temporal meridian	Superior meridian	Inferior meridian
3.22	3.33	3.23	3.27
0.30	0.35	0.36	0.37

Bonomo PP. Pars plana and ora serrata anatomotopographic study of fetal eyes. Acta Ophthalmol (Copenh) 1989; 67: 145–50. With permission from Blackwell Publishing Ltd.

Similar figures were obtained from the examination of 76 paraffin-embedded normal eyes from 1-week to 6-year-old children.[22]

Seventy-six percent of the development of the ciliary body has probably been achieved by the age of 24 months. The pars plana, which occupies 75% of the total length of the ciliary body, follows a similar course.

It is estimated that the external distance from the limbus to the ora serrata is approximately 0.3–0.4 mm more than the corresponding dimension of the ciliary body in the specimens used.

OPTIC DISC PARAMETERS

Although one might wish for an objective measurement for optic nerve hypoplasia, this diagnosis is still a subjective one, because it is not only size that is important. The optic disc dimensions of 66 children of low refraction error aged 2–10 years has been analyzed by fundus photography (Table 5.5a).[23] The vertical disc diameter, the disc area, and the cup-to-disc ratio are significantly larger in black than in white children.

The optic disc dimensions (excluding the meninges) studied at autopsy[24] may produce slightly different results due to fixation shrinkage. Considering this shrinkage (an average of 13%) the measurements correlate well with the photographic study (Tables

Table 5.5a Optic disc parameters in 66 volunteers[23]

No. of volunteers	Race	Sex	Age	Cycloplegic refraction	Vertical disc diameter (mm)	Horizontal disc diameter (mm)	Cup-to-disc ratio	Area (mm²)	Neuroretinal rim area (mm²)
16	Black	Female	7.0	+0.8	2.11	1.84	0.32	3.05	2.57
			2.5	1.4	0.21	0.17	0.21	0.54	0.50
14	Black	Male	7.0	+0.5	2.13	1.85	0.40	3.11	2.46
			2.4	0.7	0.19	0.19	0.20	0.56	0.58
18	White	Female	5.2	+1.0	1.88	1.73	0.10	2.57	2.52
			2.4	1.1	0.20	0.17	0.11	0.49	0.48
18	White	Male	6.1	+0.7	1.94	1.79	0.20	2.74	2.54
			2.2	0.7	0.22	0.22	0.18	0.59	0.58

Values are expressed as means; SDs are listed under the means.
With permission from Mansour.[23] © 1992 Slack Inc.

Table 5.5b Mean vertical and horizontal diameters and area of the optic disc for each age group

Age	No. of subjects	Mean diameter (mm) (SD) Vertical	Mean diameter (mm) (SD) Horizontal	Mean area (mm²) (SD)
< 40 weeks gestation	20	1.10 (0.21)	0.93 (0.15)	0.82 (0.26)
Term to 6 months	13	1.37 (0.21)	1.13 (0.19)	1.25 (0.40)
6 months to 2 years	12	1.57 (0.15)	1.40 (0.17)	1.73 (0.32)
2–10 years	17	1.64 (0.20)	1.43 (0.19)	1.87 (0.44)
> 10 years	31	1.73 (0.23)	1.59 (0.21)	2.19 (0.54)

From Rimmer et al, with permission.[24]

Table 5.5c Mean vertical and horizontal diameters and area of the optic nerve for each age group

Age	No. of subjects	Mean diameter (mm) (SD) Vertical	Mean diameter (mm) (SD) Horizontal	Mean area (mm²) (SD)
< 40 weeks gestation	20	1.96 (0.36)	1.79 (0.43)	2.85 (1.16)
Term to 6 months	13	2.38 (0.22)	2.23 (0.30)	4.22 (0.87)
6 months to 2 years	12	2.70 (0.33)	2.55 (0.32)	5.47 (1.26)
2–10 years	17	2.84 (0.39)	2.64 (0.27)	5.95 (1.26)
> 10 years	30	3.06 (0.39)	2.85 (0.32)	6.95 (1.62)

From Rimmer et al, with permission.[24]

5.5b, 5.5c). Approximately 50% of the growth of the optic disc and nerve occurs by 20 weeks of gestation and 75% by birth. Ninety-five percent of the growth of the optic disc and nerve occurs before the age of 1 year.

Newer methods, such as optical coherence tomography, will give more accurate measurements in the clinic.

AXIAL LENGTH

In week 9 of fetal life the eye has a sagittal diameter of 1 mm, rapidly increasing to a mean of 5.1 mm by the age of 12 weeks.[25]

The total axial length of the premature eye was studied in premature babies of 25–37 weeks postconceptional age with A-scan ultrasound;[11] it increases linearly from 12.6 to 16.2 mm.

A later study[26] suggested a second-order exponential function; the measurements given in Table 5.6.

Ultrasound measurements of the newborn eye[27] are as follows:
1. Average anterior chamber depth (including the cornea) 2.6 mm, ranging from 2.4 to 2.9 mm.
2. Average lens thickness 3.6 mm, ranging from 3.4 to 3.9 mm.
3. Average vitreous length 10.4 mm, ranging from 8.9 to 11.2 mm.
4. The total length of the newborn eye is 16.6 mm, ranging from 15.3 to 17.6 mm.

The postnatal longitudinal growth of the emmetropic eye can be divided into three growth periods.[28]
1. A rapid postnatal phase with an increase in length of 3.7–3.8 mm during the first 18 months.
2. A slower phase from the second to the fifth year of life with an increase in length of 1.1–1.2 mm.
3. A slow juvenile phase, which lasts until the age of 13 years with an increase of 1.3–1.4 mm.

Longitudinal growth is minimal after this age.

See Table 5.7 and Fig. 5.7.[28]

EXTRAOCULAR MUSCLES AND SCLERA

Most of the enlargement of the eye is in the first 6 months of extrauterine life. All diameters increase. The anterior, visible part

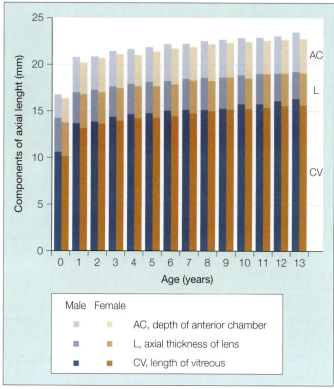

Fig. 5.7 The relationships between the different components of the eye during the growth period. An ultrasound oculometric study. AC, depth of anterior chamber; L, axial thickness of lens; CV, length of vitreous. From Larsen JS. The sagittal growth of the eye. I–IV. Acta Ophthalmol (Copenh) 1971; 49: 239–62, 427–40, 441–53, 873–86. With permission from Blackwell Publishing Ltd.[28]

Table 5.6 Numerical parameters of ocular axial length, and axial growth rate from fetal age 20 weeks to the age of 3 years

Age (weeks)[a]	Axial length (mm)	Growth rate (mm/week)
20	10.08	0.66
30	14.74	0.32
40 (term)	17.02	0.16
50	18.24	0.092
60	18.97	0.059
70	19.48	0.044
80	19.87	0.035
90 (about 1 year)	20.19	0.030
100	20.47	0.026
120	20.93	0.021
140 (about 2 years)	21.31	0.017
170	21.75	0.013
200 (about 3 years)	22.07	0.009

[a]<40 weeks = fetal; >40 weeks = post-term.
From Fledelius and Christensen.[26]

Table 5.7 Axial length in male series

Length of axis (mm)	Days	Months		Years													
	1–5	6	9	1–2	2–3	3–4	4–5	5–6	6–7	7–8	8–9	9–10	10–11	11–12	12–13	13–14
No. of eyes	86	2	4	36	118	110	100	64	64	70	100	80	56	52	56	24
Mean	16.78	18.21	19.05	20.61	20.79	21.27	21.68	21.85	21.97	22.09	22.33	22.43	22.50	22.70	22.97	23.15
SD	0.51	–	–	0.47	0.61	0.55	0.58	0.59	0.71	0.62	0.51	0.47	0.47	0.82	0.71	0.38
SE	0.055	–	–	0.078	0.056	0.052	0.058	0.074	0.089	0.074	0.051	0.053	0.063	0.114	0.095	0.078

SD, standard deviation; SE, standard error.
Larsen JS. The sagittal growth of the eye. I–IV. Acta Ophthalmol (Copenh) 1971; 49: 239–62, 427–40, 441–53, 873–86. With permission from Blackwell Publishing Ltd.

Table 5.8a Breadth of rectus muscle insertions (mm)

Age	No. of specimens	Superior	Medial	Inferior	Lateral
Neonatal	10	7.5	7.6	6.8	6.9
2-3 months	4	7.3	6.8	6.7	7.0
6 months	4	8.9	9.0	8.3	8.4
9 months	4	8.8	8.7	8.3	8.2
20 months	2	10.2	8.9	9.3	7.8
Adult	5	10.8	10.5	9.8	9.2

With permission from Swan and Wilkins.[29] © 1984 Slack Inc.

Table 5.8b Millimeters from clear cornea to rectus muscle insertions

Age	No. of specimens	Superior		Medial		Inferior		Lateral	
		Nasal end	Temporal end	Sup. end	Inf. end	Nasal end	Temporal end	Sup. end	Inf. end
Neonatal	10	6.1	7.6	4.7	5.3	6.0	6.6	6.4	5.8
2 months	3	5.5	5.8	5.2	6.0	5.2	6.2	7.8	5.8
3 months	3	6.9	7.5	5.1	5.8	6.6	7.5	7.5	7.0
6 months	4	7.4	8.3	5.8	6.6	7.2	9.0	7.2	7.1
9 months	4	7.2	9.3	6.2	6.9	7.7	8.8	7.5	7.1
20 months	2	7.1	8.7	7.3	7.6	8.5	9.3	8.5	8.5
Adult	5	7.4	10.0	7.8	7.7	8.0	9.2	8.4	8.5

With permission from Swan and Wilkins.[29] © 1984 Slack Inc.

Table 5.8c Distance in millimeters of oblique muscle insertions from clear cornea and optic nerve

Age	No. of specimens	Superior oblique				Inferior oblique			
		To cornea		To optic nerve		To cornea		To optic nerve	
		Ant. edge	Post. edge	Ant. edge	Post. edge	Ant. edge	Post. edge	Ant. edge	Post. edge
Neonatal	8	9.0	11.6	10.6	5.6	10.2	14.8	8.6	2.2
2–3 months	4	10.3	12.8	10.3	5.6	12.1	16.2	8.2	2.3
6–9 months	8	12.3	14.2	12.0	6.4	13.9	18.0	10.8	3.2
20 months	2	14.2	15.3	12.2	7.8	15.5	19.3	11.7	4.6
Adult	3	14.7	17.7	14.6	8.3	16.2	20.5	14.2	6.6

With permission from Swan and Wilkins.[29] © 1984 Slack Inc.

of the eye in infants, the cornea and the iris, have about 80% of their adult dimensions at birth. The posterior segment increases more. In squint surgery in the very young child the anatomical dimensions make it more difficult to predict outcomes (Tables 5.8a, 5.8b, and 5.8c).

The thickness of the sclera in 6-, 9-, and 20-month specimens is 0.45 mm, similar to that in adult eyes.[29]

VISUAL ACUITY

Most parents appreciate that their newborn baby sees. The neonate stops moving and breathes slowly and regularly when seeing. The image that the brain receives is probably an unfocused, crude outline to which the infant may not accommodate, and it may be mediated via the extrageniculostriate system.

Postnatal maturation of the visual pathways plays an important role in visual development. At birth, the macula is immature; vision at birth may be extramacular. The fovea reaches histological maturity as late as between 15 and 45 months of age, and myelination of the optic nerve is not finished until about the age of 2 years.

"The period between 1 and 3 months is a period of radical changes in visual capabilities and behavior. A rapid rise in acuity, the appearance of the low-frequency cut in contrast sensitivity, the emergence of smooth pursuit eye movements and of symmetrical optokinetic nystagmus, and possibly the establishment of functional binocular vision all occur roughly together."[30]

Lid closure is seen on illumination with a bright light in babies of 25 weeks gestation. The pupillary reflex to light is seen from

Table 5.9 Visual acuity according to different methods, given as Snellen equivalents

Technique	Newborn	2 months	4 months	6 months	1 year
Optokinetic nystagmus	20/400	20/400	20/200		20/60
Preferential looking (one study)	20/400	20/200	20/200	20/150	20/50
Preferential looking (other study)	20/800 to 20/1600	20/1200	20/400	20/300	20/100
Visual evoked potential	20/100 to 20/200	20/80	20/80	20/20 to 20/40	20/40
Information pooled from different sources.					

week 29 to 31. On presenting a red woolen ball at a distance of approximately 17 cm there is evidence that discriminative visual function and tracking eye movements are present by 31–33 weeks gestational age.[31]

The acuity of the newborn infant is close to 6/240, and at 7 weeks of age the infant has eye-to-face contact. Visual acuity rapidly increases to 6/180–6/90 at 2–3 months. At 6 months visual acuity is between 6/18 and 6/9. The assessment of visual acuity, however, depends on the testing method used; here visual acuities are given as Snellen equivalents, which may be a daring interpretation. Table 5.9 summarizes pooled information of visual development, indicating the difficulties in examining infant vision.

Full accommodative ability is not established until 3–4 months of age. Yet is does not appear to be a major limiting factor on reported acuity values.

Stereoacuity tested by means of a two-choice preference procedure could first be demonstrated by the age of 16 weeks. By the age of 21 weeks infants have a stereoacuity of 1 minute of arc or better.[32]

It is difficult to know at what age adult acuity is normally attained; it is likely that it is approached asymptotically over a number of years.

VISUAL FIELD

The visual field of the infant depends on the distance at which the target is presented, whether static or kinetic fields are investigated, how interesting the targets are, and whether a fixation target is present. Between 2 and 4 months the child

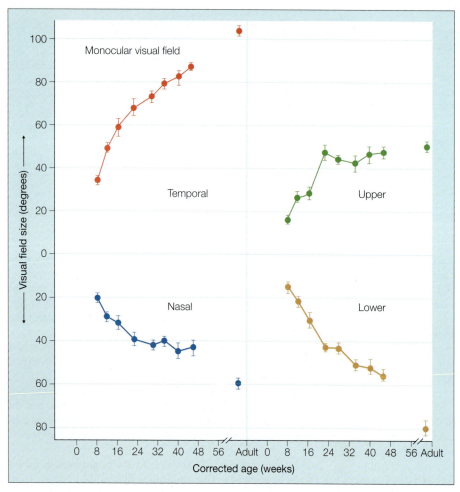

Fig. 5.8 Development of monocular visual field. The horizontal (left) and vertical (right) meridians. Error bars indicate 2 SEM. Redrawn from Mohn and van Hof-van Duin.[33]

Table 5.10 Mean extent of visual field in degrees (±SEM) in each meridian for five age groups

Age group	ST	IT	IN	SN
Right eye				
4 years	59.2 (2.1)	84.7 (1.6)	51.4 (2.4)	47.8 (1.8)
5 years	63.4 (2.4)	88.1 (1.9)	52.4 (2.6)	51.7 (1.6)
7 years	66.8 (1.5)	86.0 (2.0)	53.6 (2.0)	58.4 (1.3)
10 years	66.9 (2.3)	86.7 (1.7)	57.9 (1.9)	60.2 (1.3)
Adult	72.6 (2.7)	94.9 (1.4)	54.0 (1.7)	60.2 (2.1)
Left eye				
4 years	66.1 (2.6)	83.8 (2.5)	59.2 (2.9)	49.1 (1.7)
5 years	66.7 (2.8)	83.0 (2.3)	54.8 (2.3)	52.4 (1.9)
7 years	73.7 (1.4)	89.4 (1.7)	51.9 (1.5)	55.9 (1.3)
10 years	71.8 (2.5)	86.7 (1.8)	52.9 (2.1)	55.8 (2.5)
Adult	70.7 (2.5)	93.4 (1.7)	52.4 (2.0)	57.7 (2.1)

S, superior; I, inferior; T, temporal; N, nasal.
With permission from Wilson et al.[84] © 1991 Slack Inc.

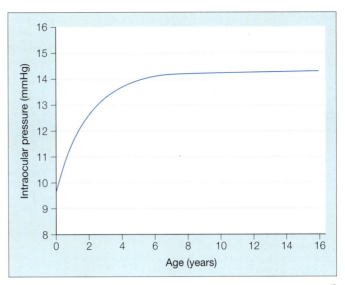

Fig. 5.9 Intraocular pressure by age group. Redrawn from Pensiero et al.[40] © 1992 Slack Inc.

seems to develop the controlled ability to switch attention to a new object.

The binocular visual field of the infant shows little development between birth and 7 weeks. From 2 months there is a rapid expansion of field size until 6–8 months of age. The increase in size of the visual field then continues at a slower rate up to the age of 12 months (Fig. 5.8).

An asymmetry of 13° or more should be considered pathological. The fields were investigated by means of kinetic perimetry using an arc perimeter. Two white balls of 6° diameter served as fixation and peripheral targets.[33] In a similar way[34] normative data were produced for 4- to 12-year-old children (Table 5.10).

REFRACTION OF THE EYE, CORNEAL CURVATURE, AND ASTIGMATISM

Slataper[35] carried out and published the impressive feat of refractions of 35,000 eyes of all ages, but even this was not the end of the story on refractive errors and development. The spectrum of refractive errors is large but the need for normative data when examining any everyday patient is not essential.

There is a large variability among the reported results but most authorities agree that neonatal refractions are distributed in a bell-shaped curve around +2 diopters. Later there is a shift toward emmetropia.

The normative range for astigmatism is as difficult to quantify as refraction. One study of noncycloplegic refractions of 1000 children aged 0–6 years revealed a minus cylinder against-the-rule before the age of 4.5 years, and a minus cylinder with-the-rule after that age.[36]

The smaller eyes of the premature and full-term babies have a more curved cornea of 6.35 mm in contrast to the adult measurement of approximately 7.8 mm (Table 5.2).[15] Keratometer readings were 47.59 diopters (SD ±2.10; range 44.08–50.75 diopters) in the newly born, 45.56 diopters (SD ±2.70; 40.13–52.75 diopters) in the 12- to 18-month age group, and stabilization of the cornea at the age of 54 months with an average of 42.69 diopters (SD ±1.89; range 40.50–47.50 diopters).[37]

INTRAOCULAR PRESSURE

There is no agreed normal range for intraocular pressure in children. An awake measurement of intraocular pressure in children is difficult and a general anesthetic is often required. The anesthetic agents used and the depth of anesthesia may affect the outcome of the measurements.

Most studies show the intraocular pressure is lower in children than in adults. Babies who were 3–11 weeks premature had a mean intraocular pressure value of 18 mmHg (SD ±2.3 mmHg; range 13–24 mmHg) with a Perkins tonometer on healthy, topically anesthetized, relaxed babies under optimal conditions.[38] The face of the tonometer applanator measured 6 mm in diameter and the mean corneal diameter was 8 mm (SD ±0.5 mm). Conflicting results with a hand-held Tonopen applanation tonometer were a mean of 10.3 mmHg (SD ±3.5 mmHg) in 70 premature babies aged 25–37 weeks.[11] Lower values of 11.4±2.4 mmHg using a Perkins tonometer have been published on topically anesthetized full-term neonates.[39]

The intraocular pressure in 460 subjects aged 0–16 years was found, with a noncontact Keeler Pulsair tonometer, to be 9.5±2.3 mmHg in the neonates, rapidly increasing to 14 mmHg at the age of 5 years (Fig. 5.9).[40] Up to 6 months of age these infants were lying down, up to 3 years they were held in their mother's lap, and older children were sitting.

The usefulness of the Keeler Pulsair was confirmed in a study of 53 children aged 6 months to 9 years. Averaged Pulsair readings agreed well with Perkins applanation tonometry values under general anesthesia.[41]

Among the drugs and procedures known to affect intraocular pressure under general anesthesia are ketamine, suxamethonium, laryngoscopy, and intubation. Large amounts of some anesthetic agents, such as halothane, reduce intraocular pressure. Dear et al.[42] found that the mean intraocular pressure among 60 infants was 12 mmHg in normal eyes and 22 mmHg in glaucoma after induction on spontaneous ventilation using nitrous oxide and halothane or isoflurane. Using atracurium and controlled ventilation there was a slight increase in intraocular pressure. Dear et al. recommended measuring the intraocular pressure just after induction, before intubation. This finding was confirmed with constant readings over time in children of different ages after exposure to different concentrations of halothane for 10 minutes before intubation.[43]

REFERENCES

1. Barishak YR. Embryology of the eye and its adnexae. 2nd ed. Basel: Karger; 2001.
2. Paiva RS, Minaire-Filho AM, Cruz AA. Palpebral fissure changes in early childhood. J Pediatr Ophthalmol Strabismus 2001; 38: 219–23.
3. Isenberg SJ, McCarty JW, Rich R. Growth of the conjunctival fornix and orbital margin in term and preterm infants. Ophthalmology 1987; 94: 1276–80.
4. Jones KL, Hanson JW, Smith DW. Palpebral fissure size in newborn infants. J Pediatr 1978; 92: 787.
5. Thomas IT, Gaitantzis YA, Frias JL. Palpebral fissure length from 29 weeks gestation to 14 years. J Pediatr 1987; 111: 267–8.
6. Iosub S, Fuchs M, Bingol N, Stone RK, Gromisch DS, Wasserman E. Palpebral fissure length in black and Hispanic children: correlation with head circumference. Pediatrics 1985; 75: 318–20.
7. Laestadius ND, Aase JM, Smith DW. Normal inner canthal and outer orbital dimensions. J Pediatr 1969; 74: 465–8.
8. Leiber B. Hypertelorismus. Mülheim/Ruhr: HU-Verlag PAIS; 1992. 11: 281–5.
9. Farkas LG, Munro IR. Orbital width index. In: Farkas LG, Munro IR, editors. Anthropometric facial proportions in medicine. Springfield, IL: CC Thomas; 1987. p. 208.
10. Isenberg SJ, Apt L, McCarty JA, Cooper LL, Lim L, Del Signore M. Development of tearing in preterm and term neonates. Arch Ophthalmol 1998; 116: 773–6.
11. Tucker SM, Enzenauer RW, Levin AV, Morin JD, Hellmann J. Corneal diameter, axial length, and intraocular pressure in premature infants. Ophthalmology 1992; 99: 1296–300.
12. al-Umran KU, Pandolfi MF. Corneal diameter in premature infants. Br J Ophthalmol 1992; 76: 292–3.
13. Sorsby A, Sheridan M. The eye at birth: measurement of the principal diameters in forty-eight cadavers. J Anat 1960; 94: 192–5.
14. Weale RA. A biography of the eye. London: HK Lewis; 1982.
15. Ehlers N, Sørensen T, Bramsen T, Poulsen EH. Central corneal thickness in newborns and children. Acta Ophthalmol (Copenh) 1976; 54: 285–90.
16. Autzen T, Bjørnstrøm L. Central corneal thickness in premature babies. Acta Ophthalmol (Copenhagen) 1991; 69: 251–2.
17. Portellinha W, Belfort R Jr. Central and peripheral corneal thickness in newborns. Acta Ophthalmol (Copenhagen) 1991; 69: 247–50.
18. Remon L, Cristobal JA, Castillo J, Palomar T, Palomar A, Perez J. Central and peripheral corneal thickness in full-term newborns by ultrasonic pachymetry. Invest Ophthalmol Vis Sci 1992; 33: 3080–3.
19. Isenberg SJ, Molarte A, Vazquez M. The fixed and dilated pupils of premature neonates. Am J Ophthalmol 1990; 110: 168–71.
20. Roarty JD, Keltner JL. Normal pupil size and anisocoria in newborn infants. Arch Ophthalmol 1990; 108: 94–5.
21. Bonomo PP. Pars plana and ora serrata anatomotopographic study of fetal eyes. Acta Ophthalmol (Copenhagen) 1989; 67: 145–50.
22. Aiello AL, Tran VT, Rao NA. Postnatal development of the ciliary body and pars plana. A morphometric study in childhood. Arch Ophthalmol 1992; 110: 802–5.
23. Mansour AM. Racial variation of the optic disc parameters in children. Ophthalmic Surg 1992; 33: 469–71.
24. Rimmer S, Keating C, Chou T, Farb MD, Christenson PD, Foos RY, et al. Growth of the human optic disc and nerve during gestation, childhood, and early adulthood. Am J Ophthalmol 1993; 116: 748–53.
25. Harayama K, Amemiya T, Nishimura H. Development of the eyeball during fetal life. J Pediatr Ophthalmol Strabismus 1981; 18: 37–40.
26. Fledelius HC, Christensen AC. Reappraisal of the human ocular growth curve in fetal life, infancy and early childhood. Br J Ophthalmol 1996; 80: 918–21.
27. Blomdahl S. Ultrasonic measurements of the eye in the newborn infant. Acta Ophthalmol (Copenhagen) 1979; 57: 1048–56.
28. Larsen JS. The sagittal growth of the eye. I–IV. Acta Ophthalmol (Copenhagen) 1971; 49: 239–62, 427–40, 441–53, 873–86.
29. Swan KC, Wilkins JH. Extraocular muscle surgery in early infancy–anatomical factors. J Pediatr Ophthalmol Strabismus 1984; 21: 44–9.
30. Atkinson J, Braddick O. The development of visual function. In: Davis JA, Dobbing J, editors. Scientific foundation of pediatrics. 2nd ed. London: Heinemann; 1981. p. 865–77.
31. Dubowitz LM, Dubowitz V, Morante A, Verghote M. Visual function in the preterm and full-term newborn infant. Dev Med Child Neurol 1980; 22: 465–75.
32. Held R, Birch E, Gwiazda J. Stereoacuity of human infants. Proc Natl Acad Sci USA 1980; 77: 5572–4.
33. Mohn G, van Hof-van Duin J. Development of the binocular and monocular visual fields of human infants during the first year of life. Clin Visual Sci 1986; 1: 51–64, as well as personal communication 1994.
34. Wilson M, Quinn G, Dobson V, Breton M. Normative values for visual fields in 4- to 12-year-old children using kinetic perimetry. J Pediatr Ophthalmol Strabismus 1991; 28: 151–4.
35. Slataper FJ. Age norms of refraction and vision. Arch Ophthalmol 1950; 43: 466–81.
36. Gwiazda J, Scheiman M, Mohindra I, Held R. Astigmatism in children: changes of axis and amount from birth to 6 years. Invest Ophthalmol Vis Sci 1984; 25: 88–92.
37. Asbell PA, Chiang B, Somers ME, Morgan KS. Keratometry in children. CLAO J 1990; 16: 99–102.
38. Musarella MA, Morin JD. Anterior segment and intraocular pressure measurements of the unanesthetized premature infant. Metab Pediatr Syst Ophthalmol 1982; 8: 53–60.
39. Radtke ND, Cohan BE. Intraocular pressure measurement in the newborn. Am J Ophthalmol 1974; 78: 501–4.
40. Pensiero S, Da Pozzo S, Perissutti P, Cavallini GM, Guerra R. Normal intraocular pressure in children. J Pediatr Ophthalmol Strabismus 1992; 29: 79–84.
41. Evans K, Wishart PK. Intraocular pressure measurement in children using the Keeler Pulsair tonometer. Ophthalmic Physiol Opt 1992; 12: 287–90.
42. Dear G de L, Hammerton M, Hatch DJ, Taylor D. Anaesthesia and intra-ocular pressure in young children. Anaesthesia 1987; 42: 259–65.
43. Watcha MF, Chu FC, Stevens JL, Forestner JE. Effects of halothane on intraocular pressure in anesthetized children. Anesth Analg 1990; 71: 181–4.

Refraction and Refractive Errors: Theory and Practice

CHAPTER **6**

Seang-Mei Saw

INTRODUCTION

To see clearly, the eye must focus the image accurately on the retina.

Emmetropization is the process by which the refractive power of the anterior segment of the eye reduces its power proportionately as the axial length increases. Both active and passive factors combine and refractive error is guided initially toward emmetropia, a balance of the refractive power of the eye and its ocular dimensions. Myopia is a refractive condition in which the emmetropization mechanism is disrupted and the image is focused anterior to the retina: the refractive power is relatively large compared with the length of the eyeball (Fig. 6.1). Children with myopia see near objects clearly, while distant ones are blurred.

ANIMAL MODELS OF MYOPIA

Raviola and Wiesel reported the disruption of ocular growth and development of myopia in infant macaque monkeys with fused eyelids.[1] In recent years, models of form deprivation myopia have been developed in a wide variety of animal species, including chicks, tree shrews, guinea pigs, and adult monkeys. Degradation of near visual images result in retinal signaling mechanisms via neurochemical modulation, the alteration of choroid growth, promotion of remodeling of the sclera, and ultimately the alteration of final eye size and shape. The translation and application of findings from animal experiments to the myopia model in humans is still questionable as there are fundamental differences in the biology and anatomy of humans and animals.

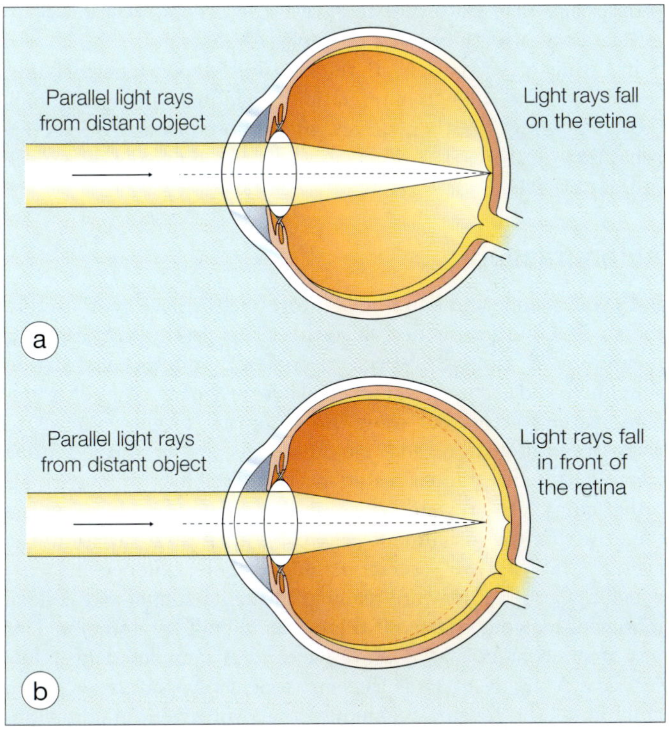

DEFINITION OF MYOPIA

Refractive error is frequently quantified as spherical equivalent (SE) (sphere + half negative cylinder) in diopters (D) on a continuous scale. For each diopter of refractive error, a child may not be able to read the next smaller line on the visual acuity (VA) chart. The distribution of refractive error is narrower than a normal distribution with a peak at emmetropia (Fig. 6.2).

The definitions of myopia involve the imposition of arbitrary cutoffs on this continuous distribution and to date there is no universal definition of myopia. Categorization of refraction measurements limits the comparisons of studies using different criteria, forces the dichotomization of a physiologic continuum, and does not take into account axial length elongation. Distinct criteria, however, facilitate the clinical diagnosis of myopia and guide the choice of interventions and refractive surgical procedures. Commonly used and accepted definitions of myopia include SE of at least –0.5, –0.75, and –1.0 D. Other classifications of myopia include an SE of at least –3.0 D to denote moderate or even high myopia, while high myopia has been defined in several ways: as an SE of at least –6.0, –8.0, and –10.0 D. Health economics often lie behind the choice of one or another definition.

Fig. 6.1 Convergence of light rays in myopic and emmetropic eyes.

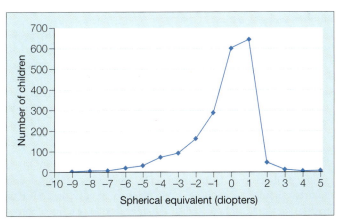

Fig. 6.2 Distribution of refraction (SE) in 1,979 Singapore children aged 7 to 9 years in the SCORM (Singapore Cohort Study of the Risk Factors for Myopia) study.

43

ASSESSMENT OF MYOPIA

Cycloplegic eyedrops

Pseudomyopia may be recorded as there may be habitual accommodation in children or young adults. There is wide individual variation in the extent of excessive accommodation and any bias cannot be corrected by mathematical formulas. Cycloplegic agents are used to inhibit accommodation in children to obtain the "true" manifest refraction often masked by accommodation when viewing a distant target in subjective refraction and auto-refraction procedures. Common agents used include cyclopentolate, tropicamide, and atropine. An ideal cycloplegic agent reveals the full amount of hyperopia, the onset should be rapid, the duration short, the drop should not sting, and there should be few serious adverse effects.[2] There is no perfect cycloplegic agent. Historically, the efficacy of a cycloplegic agent is measured by residual accommodation.

Cyclopentolate is one of the most commonly used cycloplegic agents in clinical practice. Two to three drops of 1% cyclopentolate (0.5% in infants) are administered into each eye five minutes apart, after the instillation of local anesthesia. Cyclopentolate is maximal in 60 min: it provides in 1 hour cycloplegia comparable to 3 days of atropine. The cycloplegic effect lasts for up to 48 hours. The children may complain of transient stinging, "blurred vision," and photophobia; allergic reactions seldom occur. Known rare central nervous system side effects include cerebellar dysfunction, disorientation and hallucinations. Cardiopulmonary side effects are also rare.

Tropicamide (1%) has been used in clinical practice more recently and has a rapid onset of cycloplegia (maximum cycloplegia in 30 min), shorter duration of action, and recovery from mydriasis occurs within 2 to 6 hours. There is a lower incidence of local side effects (primary local effect is transient stinging) compared with cyclopentolate and no psychogenic adverse events. Two to three drops of 1% tropicamide are administered at 5-min intervals and refractions performed after 30 min. In a comparative study of 20 children aged 6 to 12 years, the residual accommodation was 0.47 D greater with tropicamide than with cyclopentolate.[2] Tropicamide has been touted as the latest effective cycloplegic agent because of its high margin of safety. Although there is poorer cycloplegia, the degree of difference to cyclopentolate is marginal.

Although atropine provides the greatest amount of cycloplegia, the onset of cycloplegia requires several hours, and the recovery period may last longer than 2 weeks. Atropine sulfate (0.5 or 1%) is administered twice a day for three days. There are a large number of local and systemic side effects such as dry mouth, flushing of the face, allergic reactions, irritability, tachycardia, and hallucinations. A 10mg dose of atropine is potentially lethal.

Homatropine 2% is not as potent as atropine, and there is also a prolonged mydriatic effect, albeit shorter than atropine. The side effect profile is similar to atropine and is generally not recommended as a cycloplegic agent, but has been useful in penalization (see Chapter 78) because its action of around two days is in between atropine and cyclopentolate and it does not sting.

It is advisable to use shorter-acting agents such as cyclopentolate and tropicamide for refraction. Parents and children should be counseled and warned about the transient mydriatic effects and possibilities of any adverse reactions before cycloplegic drugs are administered. The effects of photophobia may be addressed by wearing wrap-around sunglasses or hats.

Subjective refraction

Subjective refraction is a procedure that determines by subjective means the combination of spherical and cylindrical lenses necessary to place the far point of each of the patient's eyes at infinity. Subjective refraction may be the "gold standard" for refraction in adults but is more difficult to perform in young children. Accommodation may be relaxed by fogging or the use of cycloplegic drugs. The starting point for subjective refraction may be lenses based on an autorefractor or retinoscopy reading. Refinement of the sphere is done by applying an overcorrection with a +2-D lens that should reduce the VA to 0.1 (6/60 or 20/200). If VA is better than this, then more plus lenses are required. Thereafter, the power of the lens is reduced at intervals of 0.25 D by subtracting plus or adding minus, until the best possible vision is obtained. The end-point used in subjective refraction is the "maximum plus lens power (sphere) for best VA."

In children as young as 3 to 4 years, it may be difficult to perform subjective refraction because the child is unable to say whether the new lens is better or worse than the former. The repeatability of subjective refraction was higher (coefficients of repeatability 0.61, 0.22, and 0.49 in the vertical, torsional, and horizontal meridians, respectively), compared with the repeatability of autorefraction measured using the Nikon NRK-8000 and the Nidek AR-1000.[3]

Retinoscopy

Static retinoscopy may be performed if a child fixates at an object at a distance to relax accommodation. Inaccurate retinoscopic findings may be due to incorrect working distances, failure of the patient to fixate on a distant target, or failure to locate the principal meridians. Relaxation of accommodation in static retinoscopy may be achieved by distance fixation or the use of cycloplegic drugs. Retinoscopy may also be performed dynamically when the child fixates on an object at some closer distance, and dynamic retinoscopy may be useful to investigate accommodation or to evaluate the effectiveness of cycloplegic agents.

In a study of 100 patients in the Houston Myopia Control study, retinoscopy and subjective refraction SE findings differed by only 0.01 D,[4] while another survey of retinoscopy and subjective refraction measures of 1,078 eyes of all ages showed a difference of 0.3 to 0.4 D.[5]

Autorefraction

Both stand-alone and hand-held autorefractors have been used to measure a child's refraction since the 1970s. In the past 30 years, measurement time has been decreased, optical construction simplified, and accuracy improved. There are many types of stand-alone autorefractors but most use automatic fogging systems to relax accommodation, and measurements are performed using infrared light. The child is seated in a comfortable position with his or her chin on the rest and the child is instructed to fixate on the target within the instrument (Fig. 6.3). In an ideal situation, the average of at least five accurate readings (sphere, cylinder, and axis) is taken. Corneal curvature readings in the horizontal and vertical meridians may be obtained if there is an in-built keratometer. This test is noncontact and noninvasive, and is completed in a few seconds. A disadvantage is that instrument myopia may occur in children as the fogging techniques that work well on adults are less effective in children. It is also almost impossible to perform

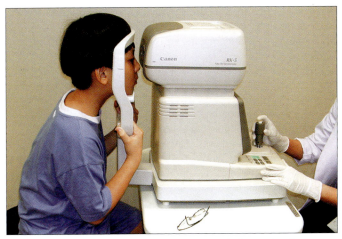

Fig. 6.3 Child's refraction measured using a stand-alone autorefractor.

autorefraction measurements in infants. Children may feel that the fixation target is very close to their eyes. The 95% limits of agreement for five SE readings determined by autorefraction were ±0.31 D, and the 95% limits of agreement in comparison with subjective refraction were ±0.61 D in 12 adults.[6]

The hand-held autorefractor is a portable, small instrument that is useful for the measurement of myopia in rural health settings (Fig. 6.4). In a validation study of the handheld autorefractor in 67 Singapore adults, the Spearman correlation coefficient of the handheld autorefractor versus the stand-alone autorefractor was 0.97, while the coefficient for the handheld autorefractor and subjective refraction was 0.96.

Biometry

Myopia is determined by changes in the following ocular components:
1. Axial length;
2. Vitreous chamber depth;
3. Lens thickness;
4. Anterior chamber depth; and
5. Corneal curvature.

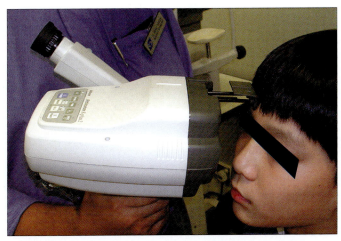

Fig. 6.4 Child's refraction measured using a handheld autorefractor.

A myopic eye has an increased axial length, deeper vitreous and anterior chambers, thinner lens, and steeper cornea for a given axial length (higher axial length/corneal curvature radius ratio (AL/CR)). In other words, the image is focused anterior to the retina in a myopic eye because the axial length is too long or the cornea is too steep. Biometry parameters may be measured using the contact A-scan or noncontact optical coherence tomography (OCT) biometry machines.

A-scan biometry

Biometry parameters including axial length, vitreous chamber depth, lens thickness, and anterior chamber depth may be measured in children using A-scan ultrasound biometry (see Chapter 12).

Optical biometry

Optical biometry is a noncontact biometry machine that uses optical coherence tomography, an optical measurement method. This technique is patient-friendly with no risk of corneal abrasions or infections. The child is asked to sit comfortably and instructed to place his chin on a rest and fixate the instrument target (Fig. 6.5). An average of at least two readings should be taken. A current disadvantage is that vitreous chamber depth is not measured directly and vitreous chamber elongation is nearly always present in myopic eyes. The Spearman correlation coefficient for

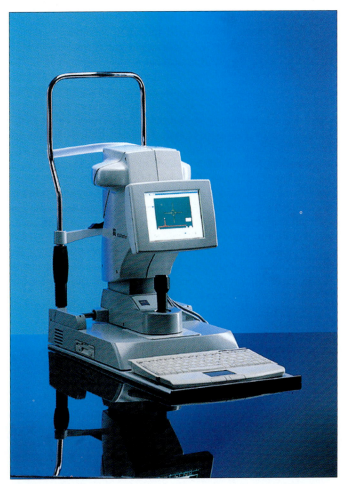

Fig. 6.5 Optical components measured using the noninvasive optical coherence tomography (OCT).

optical biometry versus A-scan biometry axial length measures was 0.96 in 178 children aged 9 to 11 years.[7] The coefficient for the test–retest values were higher for the optical biometry ($r = 1.00$) compared with the A-scan biometry machine ($r = 0.95$).

RECOMMENDATIONS FOR DETERMINING REFRACTIVE ERROR

Cycloplegic drugs should be used in conjunction with retinoscopy, subjective refraction, or autorefraction in measuring refractive error in children and teenagers. Accurate determinations of refractive error in children and most teenagers require the inhibition of excessive accommodation by cycloplegia. If the child is not cooperative during the refraction test, the parent could help to calm the child and the test may be repeated several times. Autorefraction is an ideal method of refractive error measurement in young children because the procedure is fast, noninvasive, and easy to perform, and it does not require the child to follow complex instructions. Retinoscopy is an accurate method for assessing refractive error, and subjective refraction procedures may be too difficult for very young children.

SCREENING FOR REFRACTIVE ERRORS
(see also Chapter 8)

Population-based vision screening to detect refractive errors in children is recommended in populations where myopia is perceived as a major public health problem. The Snellen or logMAR distance VA charts may be used for vision screening to detect habitual VA (defined as VA wearing current correction, if any) worse than 6/12 (logMAR equivalent = 0.3) in either eye. The logMAR letter chart, a logarithmic progression chart with letter-by-letter acuity measurements, has several advantages: the letters used are a given size, there are an identical number of letters on each line, and the letter size changes between rows are set at 0.1 log units. In the Singapore Cohort Study of the Risk Factors for Myopia (SCORM) of children aged 9 to 11 years, the sensitivity and specificity of logMAR VA charts in the prediction of myopia (SE at least –0.5 D) were 91.7 and 91.0%, respectively.[8] If a child has difficulty reading letters, the tumbling "E" or LEA symbols charts may be used instead. Population-wide vision screening can be conducted in schools by nurses or other trained staff on an annual basis. Any child with VA worse than LogMAR 0.3 in either eye should be referred to the optometrist or ophthalmologist for eye examination, including cycloplegic refraction. Screening may be part of a multipronged approach to facilitate the diagnosis of undetected or undercorrected myopia in children.

SOCIOECONOMIC IMPACT OF MYOPIA

Significant myopia is a life-long burden with recurrent costs of spectacles, contact lenses, contact lens solutions, and optometry visits. The economic costs of myopia to individuals and society are substantial.[9] Myopia has repercussions for occupational groups with special visual needs such as air force pilots and combat officers.

Although most myopes live a normal and fulfilling life, the economic, social, and psychological impact of less than optimal vision despite the best optical correction may be significant. For some, being myopic may affect emotional well being, self-esteem, family relationships, and job productivity–impairments

of quality of life are similar to patients with keratoconus. Adults with potentially blinding ocular complications such as retinal detachment or glaucoma may need surgery, medications, and lifelong medical care.

Patient-perceived quality of life utility measures have been reported recently. In a study of 699 myopic teenagers aged 15 to 18 years in Singapore, Saw et al. asked teenagers the number of years he or she was willing to give up in return for perfect vision restored by a new hypothetical technology.[10] The computed time trade-off utility value was 0.93 (0 denotes poor ocular health where the individual would trade off all remaining years of life for a myopia cure and 1.0 indicates perfect health where the individual would not trade any years of remaining life for a hypothetical cure for myopia).

PREVALENCE OF MYOPIA

Caution should be exercised when comparing rates in different surveys as the nature of the study population, definitions of myopia, instruments used to measure myopia, and the use of cycloplegia may differ. Ideally, all prevalence surveys of myopia should be population-based with appropriate sampling strategies, different definitions of myopia presented, and "standard" autorefraction and subjective refraction techniques employed. Small shifts in the cutoff for myopia from SE at least –0.5 D to SE at least –0.75 D may decrease the prevalence rate of myopia by 10%. Prevalence rates of myopia may be highest in urban Asian areas (38.7% in adults 40 to 79 years) and lower in other parts of the world, including the United States (22.7% in adults 40 years and older in East Baltimore), Barbados (21.9% in adults 40 to 84 years in the Barbados Eye Study), and Australia (15% in adults 49 to 97 years old in the Blue Mountains).[11–14]

The Refractive Error Study in Children (RESC) is a joint comparative study of the prevalence rates of refractive errors in countries including China, Chile, Nepal, and India (Fig. 6.6).[15–19] A unique feature of this multicenter study is that the study methodology, definitions, and sampling strategies are identical.

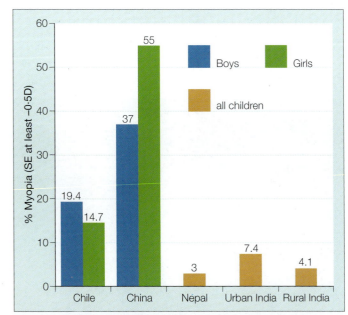

Fig. 6.6 Prevalence rates of myopia (SE at least –0.5 D) in the RESC (Refractive Error Study in Children).

Children aged 5 to 15 years were randomly sampled in clusters in population-based prevalence surveys. Myopia was defined as SE at least –0.5 D and cycloplegic refraction measured using the streak retinoscope and handheld autorefractor. The refractive error rates were highest in rural China (55.0% in 15-year-old females) and lowest in rural Nepal (< 3%). Singapore and Taiwan report one of the highest rates of myopia in children. In one of the largest prevalence surveys, the rate of myopia (SE at least –0.25 D) was 12% in 6 year olds and 84% in 16- to 18-year-old Taiwanese school children (n=11,178).[20] The SCORM study reported myopia rates of 27.8% in 7 year olds, 34.3% in 8 year olds, and 43.9% in 9 year olds.[21] Generally speaking, the reported rates of myopia are higher in Chinese- than in European-derived populations.

The "epidemic" of myopia and high myopia in urban Asian (predominantly Chinese) cities is a recent population-specific phenomenon known as the "cohort effect." The cohort effect occurs when, for example, individuals in their 20s are subject to environmental influences such as reading, which individuals in their 20s 40 years ago were not subjected to. The best explanation for the cohort effect is that the educational demands have risen and both schoolchildren and adults spend excessive time on near-work activities in urban Asian populations. Some researchers assert that the rates of high and pathologic myopia may increase over time, leading to higher rates of myopia-related blindness.

There are little data from longitudinal myopia studies, and although information from repeated cross-sectional data in Asian countries such as Singapore is easily acquired, limited conclusions may be inferred from these data. It is difficult to directly compare data over time as there may be differences in the definitions of myopia, sampling strategies, and profile of populations studied. From cross-sectional data, decreases in myopia rates in adults in their 60s compared with 40s may be a part of the natural aging process, rather than because there are increased rates of myopia in the younger population. There are similar assertions of cohort changes in the Eskimo- and European-derived populations.

AGE OF ONSET, CESSATION, AND PROGRESSION RATES OF MYOPIA

Most infants are born hyperopic and become less hyperopic as they grow older with refraction tending toward emmetropization by age 7 to 9 years.[22] During the first two years of life, the enlarging globe is associated with flattening of the cornea to achieve emmetropia. Asian children are more likely to be born less hyperopic or even emmetropic and a significant proportion may tend toward myopia later in life. It is not completely clear why some children remain hyperopic since birth, some emmetropize, while others become myopic.

Early lifestyle factors in childhood such as an altered visual experience may exert the greatest influence on the development of myopia. An undiagnosed young myopic child may ignore distant objects or express greater difficulty reading from the classroom blackboard. An older myopic child may describe blurred distance vision and express a need for spectacles. The average age of onset of myopia is 10 to 16 years in Caucasian children and 10 years in Asian children, though there may be wide variations.

In teenagers, the refractive distribution curve develops a skew toward the minus direction. The average rate of progression of myopia is –0.3 to –0.5 D per year in Caucasian children[23] and –0.5 to –0.6 D per year in Asian children (Fig. 6.7). Progression is most rapid during the first few years after the initiation of myopia but subsequently plateaus in the later years. It is widely believed that

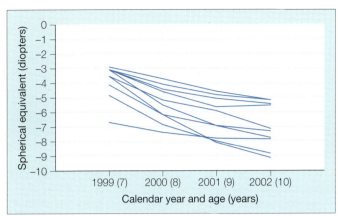

Fig. 6.7 Three-year myopia progression rates of children aged 7 years (n=10) in the SCORM study (Singapore Cohort Study of the Risk Factors for Myopia).

myopia stops during teen-ages (average age of 14 to 18 years) when puberty ceases. Myopia stops progressing earlier in females than in males, possibly following trends of earlier cessation of general body growth in females. An interesting question is how do we predict the final degree of myopia of each child? Children with an earlier age of onset of myopia, more rapid myopia progression, and a parental history of myopia, and who spend excessive cumulative time reading may be more likely to develop high myopia. If children who may develop pathologic myopia in adult life can be accurately identified, effective and safe treatments (if identified in the future) may be targeted at this high-risk group.

RISK FACTORS

The nature versus nurture question for myopia has been hotly debated by researchers for centuries. The exact environmental risk factors or genes involved, as well as the relative importance of genes and environment, are still largely unknown. In populations with a genetic susceptibility to myopia, the effects of environmental influences may be even more pronounced, leading to excessively high rates of myopia. This phenomenon is called gene–environment interaction.

Environmental risk factors

As early as 1885, Fuchs noted that prolonged work requiring close vision may induce myopia, and he defined optimal requirements for the selection of light, design of desks, and appropriate distances while writing. The hypothesis that near work is a major risk factor for myopia is supported by several observations:

1. The risks of myopia are higher in microscopists and visual display terminal workers who spend long hours on visually demanding near work.
2. The rates of myopia have risen rapidly over the past few decades in Asia, whereas the gene pool has not changed: this rise is attributed to increasingly competitive schooling systems.
3. The association of the onset of myopia (average age of onset 7 to 10 years) with schooling suggests that prolonged reading may increase the risks of myopia.
4. Myopia is more common in school-going Eskimo children than in their parents who are mostly illiterate.
5. There is a cohort effect and there are increases in the myopia rates of children born in later cohorts. This could be attributed

to the introduction of compulsory schooling and the increasingly intensive education system over the past few decades as in some Asian countries.

Animal experiments suggest that abnormal visual experience may disrupt postnatal eye growth. The eyes compensate for the hyperopic blur during reading by growing toward myopia in normal eye growth feedback control mechanisms.[24] Disruption of normal feedback mechanisms of the retina may involve neurochemical modulators such as dopamine, growth factors, and muscarinic antagonists, resulting in retina, choroid, and scleral growth modulation.

Epidemiologic data from 1,005 children in the SCORM study shows that the multivariate adjusted odds ratio (OR) of higher myopia (SE at least –3.0 D) for children aged 7 to 9 years who read more than 2 books per week was 3.05 (95% confidence interval (CI) 1.80, 5.18).[25]

In the Orinda Longitudinal Study of 366 eight grade children in 1991 to 1996, the multivariate OR was 1.02 (95% CI 1.008, 1.032) for each diopter-hour per week of near work.[26] Diopter-hour was defined as 3 × (hours spent reading) + 2 × (hours spent playing video games or computer games) + 1 × (hours spent watching television).[26] There are few data on the effects of near-work parameters such as lighting while reading, posture, reading in a moving vehicle, and distance of eye from the book on myopia.

The duration of the light–dark cycle may affect eye growth and myopia development in chicks: constant light produces shallowing of the anterior chamber, vitreous enlargement, and hyperopic refractive error. Several studies have investigated whether light exposure in children may be related to refractive error development and the onset of myopia. In a study of 479 children aged 2 to 16 years in a tertiary Philadelphia hospital, children who slept with the lights at night before aged 2 years had higher risks of myopia in a dose-dependent fashion; but 2 other population-based studies conducted in children in the United States did not show any associations between night lighting and myopia.[27–29] In third-year law students in the United States, decreased exposure to daily darkness was strongly associated with myopia progression. Data suggest that interactions of light with dark and disruptions of the light–dark cycle may influence eye growth and refractive error development. The lack of consistency of the results across all studies precluded a cause–effect relationship, and it is still not possible to conclude from the available evidence that there is a link between night lighting and refractive error development.

Another hypothesis is that myopic children may have higher academic abilities or may perhaps be more intelligent. In a survey of 157,748 Israeli male military recruits aged 17 to 19 years, the rate of myopia was lower in recruits with low intelligence quotient (IQ) (8%) than in recruits with high IQ (27.3%).[30] The rates of myopia were higher in children in the high-ability class (13%) than in those in the low-ability class (7%) in 707 schoolchildren aged 11 to 13 years in New Zealand.[31] These studies may be confounded by an increase in reading activity among those with higher IQ or those who perform better in school. In a study of 1,816 offspring of families 12 to 33 years in Hawaii, there was more negative refraction with higher grades and vocabulary scores, even adjusting for near work.[32] Myopes may have higher IQs and overall academic achievement independent of the greater amount of time spent reading. The relationship between reading, IQ scores, and overall academic ability as well as biometry and refraction parameters is complex and future studies with comprehensive measurements are needed.

Myopia is primarily axial: myopes have longer eyeballs. If overall body growth is proportionate to eye growth, myopes may be taller too. A survey of 106,926 males in Israel aged 17 to 19 years found that the weight and height of myopes were similar to that of nonmyopes.[33] Teasdale and colleagues report the data from 7,950 Danish draftees, and myopic draftees were found to be 0.8 cm taller than emmetropic recruits.[34] In the SCORM study of 1,449 Chinese school children, children who were taller had longer axial lengths, deeper vitreous chambers, flatter corneas, and refractions that tend toward myopia.[35] Indeed, height may be a unique heritable trait in myopic children, or one could argue that an apparent association may be seen because taller children may have higher socioeconomic status, or just be better nourished.

Hereditary factors

Similar high rates of myopia in Chinese, despite different environmental lifestyles in various countries such as China, Singapore, or Taiwan, underscore the importance of genetic factors. Syndromes associated with myopia, such as Ehlers–Danlos syndrome (autosomal dominant), Marfan syndrome (autosomal dominant), and Fabry disease (sex-linked), account for only a small proportion of myopia worldwide. There is, however, substantial evidence that hereditary factors are important but myopia may be multifactorial in origin.

In epidemiologic studies, children with one of two myopic parents have a two- to fourfold higher risk of developing myopia than children with no myopic parents.[36] Parental history of myopia may denote hereditary susceptibility or shared environmental factors among family members with common reading habits. Twin studies in the United Kingdom (226 monozygotic twins and 280 dizygotic twins aged 49 to 79 years) and Taiwan (90 monozygotic and 36 dizygotic twins) have shown that the concordance rate for myopia is higher in monozygotic than dizygotic twins and the estimates of heritability are as high as 90%.[37,38] It is unlikely that myopia is a single gene disease but more likely to be multifactorial in origin.

Several genetic loci for high myopia (18p11.31, 12q 21–23, 7q36) have been identified in family linkage studies of autosomal dominant high myopia. Further work is being performed with several genome-wide scans conducted worldwide. An allelic association between the trabecular meshwork-induced glucocorticoid response (TIGR/myocilin) gene and severe myopia was found in 104 Chinese families.

A Hong Kong DNA sequencing study of 71 adult high myopes (SE at least –6.0 D) and 105 controls identified 6 significantly different single-nucleotide polymorphisms (SNPs) and their interactions in transforming growth β-induced factor (TGIF); thus TGIF may be a possible candidate gene for high myopia.[39]

Individuals with the myopia gene/s may have increased susceptibility to environmental influences. Population-specific phenomenon such as the "epidemic" of myopia in Asia may be a culmination of genetic susceptibility and a competitive educational system. A study of 361 Taiwanese twins found that monozygotic twins with concordant reading habits had myopia concordance rates of 92.4% compared with 79.1% in monozygotic twins with discordant reading habits.[40] This suggests that additive gene–environment interaction (a different effect of environment on persons with different genotypes) may be present, although the index for hereditary factors was zygosity and not parental myopia.

In the SCORM study, reading interacted with parental myopia to increase the risks of higher myopia (SE at least –3.0 D).[41] In contrast, no gene–environment interaction was found in

Caucasian children in the Orinda Longitudinal Study.[26] Studies of myopic twins reared together and apart may help us further understand the mechanism of gene–environment interaction.

EDUCATION OF THE PUBLIC, PARENTS, AND HEALTH-CARE PROFESSIONALS

Structured myopia prevention programs have been implemented in several urban Asian cities where there is increased public concern. Strategies for the implementation of myopia prevention programs have been formulated, myopia research planned in an integrated fashion, and clinical practice guidelines on the role of treatment modalities for myopia progression developed. Possible modifiable risk factors such as breaks while reading have been identified and public education of potential beneficial behavioral changes instituted via school-wide education campaigns, public forums, health fairs, nation-wide mass media, and community-based eye screening programs. These programs, however, have been limited by the paucity of definite evidence for primary preventive strategies, sparse data on the exact genetic markers for myopia, and the lack of a safe and effective treatment to retard the progression of myopia.

INTERVENTIONS TO RETARD MYOPIA PROGRESSION

The safety and efficacy of therapeutic modalities such as optical corrective devices and pharmacological interventions to retard the progression of myopia have been reported in randomized clinical trials, controlled clinical trials, and case series. Most interventions have been evaluated in myopic children and the end-points of interest include the retardation of the progression of myopia and changes in biometry parameters such as axial length.

Eyedrops

Atropine is a nonselective antimuscarinic agent that may retard axial length elongation and prevent form-deprivation myopia by blocking accommodation. It has been used on myopic children to slow progression. Recent evidence from randomized clinical trials conducted in Taiwan assert that a range of concentrations of atropine (0.1, 0.25, 0.5, and 1%) were useful in delaying the progression of myopia in children, though the differences in effects of the atropine and the control group were small and the number of dropouts high.[42,43]

In a double-masked randomized clinical trial of the effect of 1% atropine eyedrops or placebo artificial tears once nightly in one eye of 331 Singapore children aged 6 to 12 years with myopia of –1 to –6 D, the myopia progression and axial elongation rates were significantly retarded in the atropine group compared with the single-lens vision group.[44] The interim one-year analysis of the Atropine in the Treatment of Myopia (ATOM) study found that atropine was generally well tolerated and that the margin of safety was high. A range of local side effects were found, however, in other prior studies including photophobia, blurred vision, allergic blepharitis, mydriasis, and restrictions with outdoor activity. It is advisable to wear photochromatic lenses to block ultraviolet light and multifocal lenses to assist with accommodation. The long-term effects of chronic pupil dilatation and possible risks of ultraviolet light-induced cataract and retinal toxicity are not well understood. The psychological effects of this forced regimen and prolonged

compliance in children need to be tested. The data suggest that the effects of atropine may be reversed once the drug is stopped. However, the regular use of atropine over long periods has not been well assessed. Currently, routine administration of atropine eyedrops to retard myopia progression is not recommended because of possible unwarranted side effects and difficulties with compliance. In children at high risk of developing pathologic myopia in adulthood, atropine eyedrops may be considered but appropriate counseling of parents is needed.

Further studies of the effects of bilateral atropine administration, low concentrations of atropine, and reversal of effects after termination of atropine should be conducted.

The search for safer and more appropriate pharmacological interventions continues, as there are uncertainties associated with the use of atropine. A promising new drug is pirenzepine, a relatively selective M1 and M4 muscarinic receptor antagonist. In two separate Phase II randomized, controlled trials in the United States and Asia, the effects of 2% pirenzepine ophthalmic gel twice a day and 2% pirenzepine gel once at night compared with a placebo have been evaluated in children aged 6 to 12 years.[45] The mean differences in myopia progression after 1 year were 0.26 and 0.37 D, respectively. Pirenzepine significantly decreased the progression of myopia and there were minimal mydriatic and accommodative adverse effects. Further large randomized clinical trials are needed to confirm the effectiveness and high safety profile of pirenzepine before clinical recommendations may be made. Antimuscarinic drugs may have the greatest potential for the desired magnitude of effect (slowing of myopia progression).

Undercorrection

Undercorrection is a time-honored but unproven way of attempting to slow the progression of myopia by prescribing spectacles that are the least strong that the child can manage day-to-day life with. If the detection of optical defocus is defective in undercorrected eyes, there may be a growth response toward hyperopia and perhaps myopia progression may be slowed. This hypothesis was tested in a randomized, single-masked trial of 106 children aged 9 to 14 years in Malaysia: children were randomly allocated to lens undercorrection of 0.75 D or full correction.[46] Contrary to expectations, the undercorrected group had significantly higher rates of progression of myopia, implying that myopic defocus may speed up myopia development. This interesting finding must be substantiated.

Bifocal and multifocal lenses

Increased retinal defocus is one of the causative factors for myopia in animals and high accommodative lag is found in humans with myopia. Bifocals may reduce the accommodative demand and retinal defocus in myopic children. No significant slowing of myopia progression was found in randomized clinical trials evaluating bifocals with additions of +1 to +2 D in Finland, Denmark, the United States, and Hong Kong.[47-50] In a randomized clinical trial of bifocals with +1.50 D additions in 75 esophoric children, there was a barely significant decrease in myopia progression and axial elongation in the bifocal compared with the placebo group.[49]

Although there are no serious adverse effects associated with the wearing of bifocals, there may be problems with compliance as the child may not use the lower segment for reading. Progressive addition multifocal lenses may allow clear vision in all directions and may be more cosmetically acceptable. A large multicenter randomized 3-year clinical trial (Correction of Myopia Evaluation Trial (COMET)) of 469 children aged 6 to 11 years with myopia between –1.25 and –4.50 D from four clinical centers in the United States evaluated the effects of progressive addition lenses with a +2.00-D addition compared with children wearing single-vision lenses.[51] The use of progressive addition lenses significantly slowed myopia progression–this effect was greatest in the first year and the results hold promise, although the difference was not clinically significant. If proven to be effective in future trials, bifocals may be an ideal treatment of progression of myopia because they are safe and compliance is good.

Contact lenses

Contact lenses may increase the quality and size of retinal images and flatten the cornea. Soft contact lenses were not found to be effective in a randomized clinical trial of 175 children in the United States.[52] Soft contact lens wearers have higher risks of infective keratitis and allergic conjunctivitis. Newer rigid gas permeable lenses have increased oxygen permeability and may permanently flatten the cornea.

A randomized clinical trial evaluated the effects of rigid gas permeable contact lenses in children aged 6 to 12 years with low to moderate myopia, and no evidence was found that rigid contact lenses reduce myopia progression.[53] Children reported difficulties in learning to wear contact lenses, adherence to contact lens wear hygiene protocols, and the daily wear of contact lenses over extended periods.

Because of the lack of data to support their efficacy and the associated side effects, this author does not advocate the use of contact lenses as treatments for myopia progression.

Others

A wide variety of other devices for myopia retardation have been evaluated primarily in small noncontrolled trials. Examples of other interventions include:

1. Biofeedback visual training with repeated visual acuity chart testing;
2. Orthokeratology with successive fittings of progressively flatter contact lenses to flatten the cornea;
3. Ocular hypotensive eyedrops (i.e., timolol) that decrease intraocular pressure and vitreous chamber volume; and
4. Facial "Qi Qong" eye exercises to relax ocular muscles.

There is no convincing evidence that any of these effectively reduce myopia progression and they are currently not recommended in myopic children.

CORRECTION OF MYOPIA

The main aim of treatment of myopia with spectacle or contact lenses is to attain optimal vision. Children with poor vision report headaches, experience difficulty reading words on the classroom blackboard, or have falling school grades. Other benefits are the enhancement of binocular vision, reduction of asthenopic symptoms, and risk of strabismus. Early indications for correction include a spherical equivalent of at least –0.5 D with uncorrected VA worse than 6/12. As the average rate of progression of myopia is approximately –0.5 D per year in children, a myopic child should visit his or her optometrist or ophthalmologist once a year. These general guidelines for optometrists and ophthalmologists could be tailored according to the individual child's needs.

Full correction of myopia is common practice but many ophthalmologists undercorrect to prescribe a strong enough lens to allow all day-to-day activities and do not advocate regular review, just reviews when the child notices that the spectacles are inadequate for their needs. This is based on the likelihood that a full correction causes more accommodation drive for near work, which is liable to cause increased myopia. Neither full correction nor undercorrection is proven to be the optimal way.

PATHOLOGICAL OCULAR COMPLICATIONS ASSOCIATED WITH HIGH MYOPIA

Myopia appears to be a benign condition, but high myopia may lead to excessive elongation of the eyeball with degenerative changes in the sclera, choroid, and retinal pigment epithelium and compromised vision. Myopia associated with progressive blinding pathology has been referred to as "malignant myopia," "degenerative myopia," and "pathologic myopia." The prevalence rates of high myopia (defined as SE at least –6.0 D) vary from 5 to 15%, and the rates of pathologic myopia are estimated to be around 1 to 3% in the general population. Pathologic myopia is a leading cause of blindness in many countries, including Japan.

The evidence for pathological complications of myopia or excessive axial elongation is largely from case series of adults with ocular pathology, with little solid evidence from well-conducted cohort and case–control studies. There are little data on the pathologic complications of myopia in children. Table 6.1 shows the evidence for cataract, glaucoma, chorioretinal, and optic disc abnormalities as complications of myopia in adults from cohort, case–control, and cross-sectional studies. Myopia may lead to damage of rod outer segments and increased production of cataractogenic lipid peroxidation by-products. Often, it is not known whether myopia is the result of increased refractive power of the cataractous lens or cataract is the cause of myopia.

Cohort studies allow the delineation of the temporal sequence of events and the incident risks of cataract in myopes compared with nonmyopes. Several cohort studies have shown that myopes, especially high myopes, have higher incident risks of posterior subcapsular, nuclear, and cortical cataracts.[54,55] In the Blue Mountains Eye Study of 2,334 adults aged 49 years and older, the OR of posterior subcapsular and nuclear cataracts were 4.4 (95% CI 1.7, 11.5) and 3.3 (95% CI 1.5, 7.4), respectively.[54] In the Barbados Eye Study of 2,609 adults aged 40 to 84 years, the multivariate adjusted relative risk of incident nuclear cataract was 2.8 (95% CI 2.0, 4.0).[55]

Myopic patients may have increased retinal nerve fiber layer defects, deformability of the lamina cribrosa, and greater susceptibility to glaucomatous optic disc changes. Prior cross-sectional studies have shown that low, moderate, and high myopes have higher risks of glaucoma.[56,57] In the Beaver Dam Eye Study of 4,670 adults aged 43 to 86 years of age, the age- and gender-adjusted ORs of prevalent primary open-angle glaucoma for myopic patients (SE at least –1.0 D) was 1.6 (95% CI 1.1, 2.3).[57] Glaucoma patients with myopia are more likely to have severe glaucomatous visual field defects and optic disc changes (Fig. 6.8). In a survey of 321 children in a tertiary hospital, the mean intraocular pressure of myopic eyes (17.8 mmHg) was higher than that of nonmyopic eyes (17.1 mmHg) ($p<0.01$).

In myopes with excessive axial elongation, mechanical stretching and thinning of the choroid and retinal pigment epithelium may lead to vascular and degenerative changes. The

Table 6.1 Summary of published data on cataract, glaucoma, chorioretinal abnormalities, and optic disc abnormalities as possible complications of myopia

Country	Study population (n)	Results
		Cataract
Australia[54]	Population-based cohort study Blue Mountains Eye Study 49 years and older (n=2,334) (FU=5 years)	Multivariate-adjusted OR of *incident* posterior subcapsular cataract were 4.4 (95% confidence interval (CI) 1.7, 11.5) for those with moderate myopia (SE at least −3.5 D), 0.5 (95% CI 0.2, 2.0) for cortical cataract, and 3.3 (95% CI 1.5, 7.4) for nuclear cataract for those with high myopia (SE at least −6.0 D)
Barbados[55]	Population-based cohort study Barbados Eye Study 40 to 84 years (n=2,609) (FU=4 years)	Multivariate-adjusted relative risk (RR) of *incident* cataract for myopia (SE at least −0.5 D) was 2.8 (95% CI 2.0, 4.0) for nuclear cataract
		Glaucoma
Australia[56]	Population-based cross-sectional study Blue Mountains Eye Study 49 years and older (n=3,654)	Multivariate-adjusted OR of *prevalent* OAG was 3.3 (95% CI 1.7, 6.4) for moderate to high myopia (SE at least −3.0 D) and 2.3 (95% CI 1.3, 4.1) for patients with low myopia (SE < −3.0 D and ≥ −1.0 D)
USA[57]	Population-based cross-sectional study Beaver Dam Eye Study 43 to 86 years (n=4,670)	The age- and gender-adjusted ORs of *prevalent* POAG for myopia (SE at least −1.0D) was 1.6 (95% CI 1.1, 2.3)
		Chorioretinal abnormalities
USA[58,59]	Cross-sectional study Eye clinic patients with myopia (1,437 eyes) Or with hyperopia or emmetropia (n=100)	% of chorioretinal atrophy was 0% if AL < 24.5 mm and 23% if AL ≥ 24.5 mm % with Fuch's spot was 0% if < 26.5 mm and 5.2% if ≥ 26.5 mm % with lacquer cracks was 0% if < 26.5 mm and 4.3% if ≥ 26.5 mm % white without pressure increased from 0% at 20 to 21 mm to 54% at 33 mm % lattice degeneration increased with AL ($p<0.01$)
USA[60]	Case–control study Cases of idiopathic rhegmatogenous retinal detachments and age–sex–race–clinic matched controls (free of retinal disease) from five eye centers, high myopia (SE at least −8 D) excluded (n=1,391)	The multivariate OR of retinal detachment for myopes (SE at least −1 D) was 7.8 (95% CI 5.0, 12.3)
		Optic disc abnormalities
Netherlands[61]	Population-based cross-sectional study Rotterdam study 55 years and older (n=5,114)	The disc area increased by 0.033 mm^2 (95% CI 0.027, 0.038), the neural rim area by 0.029 mm^2 (95% CI 0.025, 0.034), and the prevalence of parapapillary atrophy (zone alpha by 0.4% (95% CI 0.03%, 0.8%), and zone beta by 1.3% (95% CI 0.57, 1.9%)) for each diopter increase toward myopia
Australia[62]	Population-based cross-sectional study 49 years or older in the Blue Mountains, West Sydney (n=3,583)	In eyes with tilted discs (77 eyes), 66.2% were myopic (SE at least −1.0 D), but in eyes without tilted discs (7,089 eyes), 11.3% were myopic ($p<0.001$).

common characteristics of pathologic myopia are fundus changes with or without posterior staphyloma, with varying degrees of visual deterioration. Chorioretinal atrophy, lacquer cracks (multiple whitish-yellow stripes), Fuchs spots (black spots caused by hyperplasia of retinal pigment epithelial cells), and white without pressure are more common in myopic eyes and eyes with elongated axial lengths.[58,59] Myopes may also have higher risks of peripapillary atrophy (Fig. 6.9). This may be accompanied by degeneration of the peripheral retina with lattice degeneration, breaks, tears, and retinal detachment. In the Eye Disease Case–Control Study of idiopathic rhegmatogenous retinal detachments and age–sex–race–clinic matched controls

from five eye centers, the multivariate OR of retinal detachment for myopes was 7.8 (95% CI 5.0, 12.3).[60] The majority of degenerative chorioretinal changes may cause visual loss, but not all lesions are treatable. Nevertheless high myopes should be regularly screened for chorioretinal abnormalities such as retinal breaks that are asymptomatic yet treatable.

Myopia-associated optic disc abnormalities include optic disc tilt, increased disc or neural rim area, larger long:short axis ratio, and rotated discs (Fig. 6.10).[61,62] In the Blue Mountains Eye Study of adults 49 years and older in Australia, 66.2% of eyes with tilted discs were myopic, but only 11.3% of eyes without tilted discs were myopic.[62] As optic disc abnormalities are relatively innocuous

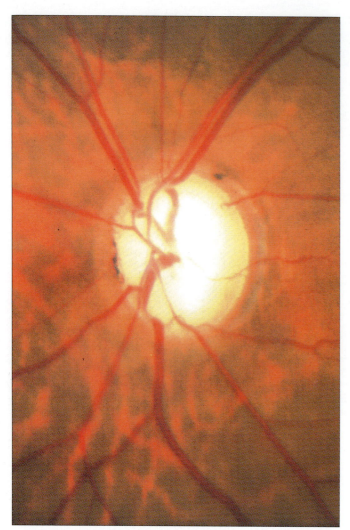

Fig. 6.8 Glaucomatous disc with marked cupping.

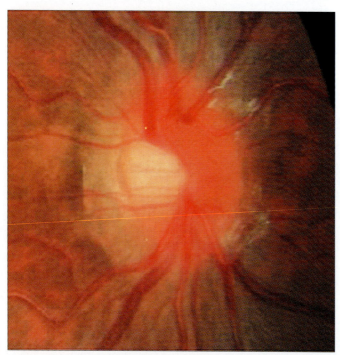

Fig. 6.9 Optic disc with peripapillary atrophy in a myopic child.

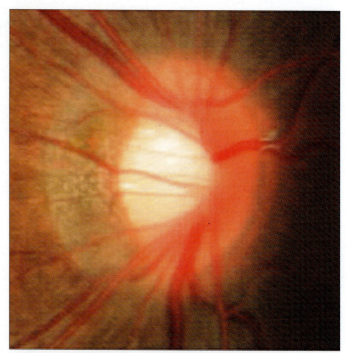

Fig. 6.10 Tilted optic disc in a myopic child: major retinal vessels emerging from the disc are straightened temporally and nasal vessels emerge from main vessel trunks, which are not visible.

and do not threaten vision, regular screening of myopes for these abnormalities is not justified. However, the diagnosis of glaucoma in myopes may be more complex because of the inherent optic disc changes in a myopic eye.

To date, there is no evidence that age-related macular degeneration (AMD) is a complication of myopia. In a study of 3,684 adults aged 43 to 84 years in the Beaver Dam Eye Study, the age-adjusted relative risks of early and late AMD for myopes were 1.0 (95% CI 0.7, 1.3) and 0.5 (95% CI 0.2, 1.5), respectively.[63] The multivariate OR of any AMD for moderate to high myopes in 3,654 adults aged 49 years and older in the Blue Mountains Eye Study was 0.7 (95% CI 0.4, 1.3).[64]

Decreases in vision may be easily correctable optically, but ocular pathologic outcomes and excessive axial elongation may not be prevented. How can the development of pathologic myopia and associated visual loss be prevented? First, children at high risk of developing pathologic myopia in adulthood need to be identified. Children with faster rates of progression of myopia, or an earlier age of onset of myopia, may be at higher risk. Second, the search continues for effective and safe treatments that slow the progression of myopia and prevent the development of pathologic myopia.

ASTIGMATISM

Clinical features of astigmatism

Optical asymmetries in the anterior segment may result in uneven focus and astigmatism. These asymmetries may involve pupillary position, or corneal (cornea astigmatism) or lenticular curvature (lenticular astigmatism). The axis may be "with the rule" (+ axis at 90°), oblique, or "against the rule." Astigmatism is a less well-studied phenomenon than spherical errors but is important because the visual blur associated with uncorrected astigmatism may lead to uncoordinated eye growth and the later development of myopia. Additionally, the risk of amblyopia is higher in children who are astigmatic between 6 and 24 months and rises with increasing astigmatism. The minimum level of astigmatism associated with increased risks of amblyopia is uncertain.

An often-cited observation is that astigmatism is more prevalent in infancy and childhood than in adulthood. The cylinder error at birth diminishes during the first few years of life. Against-the-rule astigmatism is more common in infancy and decreases with age, while with-the-rule astigmatism is more common in later childhood. The axis changes may be contributed by increases in eyelid pressure with age and greater flattening of the cornea in the horizontal meridian. Adults with astigmatism often have amblyopia, which may be a result of habitual blurring since childhood. In a study of 1,000 children aged 0 to 6 years (97% white) in the United States, significant reductions in the amount of astigmatism between 6 months and 4 to 6 years were reported.[65] There are equal proportions of with-the-rule and against-the-rule astigmatism in children 0 to 35 months, and a higher rate of against-the-rule astigmatism before 4.5 years, but a higher rate of with-the-rule astigmatism after that. There was a relatively low rate of oblique axis astigmatism. Another interesting observation is that the incidence rate of astigmatism between 0 and 6 years is almost negligible and a child who does not have astigmatism in infancy is unlikely to develop astigmatism up to age 6 years. Abrahamsson et al. noted in a study in Sweden of 299 astigmatic infants aged 1 to 4 years that infants with with-the-rule or oblique astigmatism may have higher risks of increasing astigmatism and spherical equivalent with age.[66]

A hypothesis that links astigmatism to myopia is that early cylindrical blur may contribute retinal signals that disrupt normal eye growth control mechanisms. Another argument is that astigmatism is just another aberration that occurs in the process of axial myopia development. The rate of combined astigmatism and myopia was 9.8% in Singapore children aged 7 to 9 years and myopia was significantly associated with astigmatism.[67] Gwiazda et al. noted that infants with against-the-rule astigmatism had earlier onset of myopia than infants with with-the-rule or no astigmatism.[68]

Prevalence rates of astigmatism

Comparisons of the prevalence rates of astigmatism across studies are hampered by different definitions and classifications.

Cylinder is a continuous variable with a skewed distribution curve (Fig. 6.11) and any proposed cut-off is at best arbitrary. Common accepted definitions of astigmatism include cylinder of at least –0.50 D, to cylinder of at least –1.00 D. In population-based prevalence surveys in adults, the rates of astigmatism are 37% (cylinder at least –0.75 D) in Australian adults (Blue Mountains Eye Survey) aged 49 to 97 years and 37.8% (cylinder at least –0.5 D) in Singapore Chinese (Tanjong Pagar Eye Survey) aged 40 years and above.[11,14] The prevalence rates of astigmatism vary from 5.2% in children aged 12 to 13 years in Sweden, and 19.2% in children aged 7 to 9 years (cylinder at least –0.5 D) in Singapore.[67,69] In adults, age-related increases in astigmatism were found in the Baltimore Eye Survey and Blue Mountains Study.[12,14] Along with the reported high rates of myopia in recent years, there may be concomitant rises in astigmatism, because of the link between myopia and astigmatism.

The causation of astigmatism is rather obscure and hereditary factors may play a role. High rates of astigmatism have been found in children with retinitis pigmentosa, albinism, and ptosis. Segregation analysis studies reveal a possible single-major locus inheritance for astigmatism; while twin studies have shown higher astigmatism concordance rates in monozygotic twins than in dizygotic twins. A study of 226 monozygotic and 280 dizygotic twins pairs aged 49 to 79 years demonstrated that dominant genetic effects accounted for 47 to 49% and additive genetic factors for 1 to 4% of the variance in total astigmatism. As for corneal astigmatism, dominant genetic factors accounted for 42 to 61% and additive genetic factors 4 to 8% of the total variance.[37] Genome wide-scans have been conducted to identify candidate genes: none have yet been localized.

Little is known about environmental risk factors or gene–environment interaction in the genesis of astigmatism.

Treatment of astigmatism

Vision may be compromised if astigmatism is uncorrected. Vision screening in schools is widespread. Prescription of spectacles should be considered for children who have significant astigmatism (at least 1.5 D) or correctable vision loss. Older children may feel the benefit of the correction of lesser degrees of astigmatism, but it is rarely necessary to prescribe for less than 0.5 D. Significant astigmatism is treated as early in life as possible to prevent amblyopia. The optimal age to start depends on the cooperation of

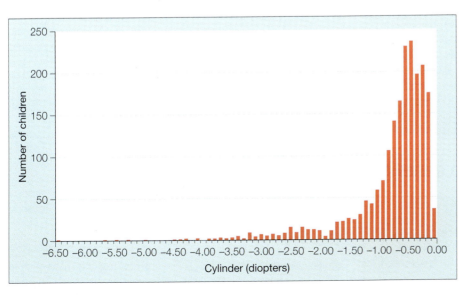

Fig. 6.11 Distribution of cylinder in 1,979 Singapore children aged 7 to 9 years in the SCORM (Singapore Cohort Study of the Risk Factors for Myopia) study.

the child, the severity of the astigmatism, and visual impairment. Infants with astigmatism and no indication for refractive correction may be observed and the refraction repeated.

HYPEROPIA (HYPERMETROPIA)

Clinical features of hyperopia

Hyperopia occurs mostly if the eye is shorter, the cornea is flatter, or the lens power is weaker than usual: it may be overcome by accommodation if the power of accommodation is adequate. Most hyperopic eyes have a shorter axial length with shallower vitreous and anterior chambers. An older patient may present with headaches, blurring of vision, difficulty reading, or the habitual act of holding the book near. If accommodation is inadequate, blurring of vision at distance may also occur. Most children with hyperopia present because of an associated strabismus or amblyopia.

On ophthalmoscopic examination, eyes with high degrees of hyperopia may have a shot-silk retina and optic disc drusen (see Chapter 59). The visual axis may cut the cornea at a considerable distance inside the optic axis, resulting in a pseudo-divergent squint.

Prevalence rates of hyperopia

Hyperopia has received less attention than myopia for several reasons:
1. The rates of hyperopia do not appear to be increasing.
2. It is not perceived as a significant public health problem.
3. Neonates are often born hyperopic and regress with age.
4. Hyperopia is easily correctable by convex spectacle lenses.
5. It is only occasionally linked with any potentially blinding disease.
6. There is no "pathologic hyperopia."

However, hyperopes have significantly increased risks of strabismus and amblyopia.

Hyperopia rates across countries should be compared with caution because there may be differences in the refraction measures and definitions of hyperopia. In the Baltimore Eye Survey of adults aged 40 years or older, the rates of hyperopia (defined as at least +0.5 D) range from 11.8% in blacks aged 40 to 49 years to 68.1% in whites 80 years or older.[12] The hyperopia rates were higher in older adults (possibly an age-related increase), were higher in white than in black men, and declined with higher levels of education. In the Blue Mountains Eye Study conducted in Australia of 3,654 adults aged 49 to 97 years, the prevalence rate of hyperopia (SE at least +0.5 D) was 57.0%.[14] Similar age-related increases in hyperopia were associated with age-related decreases in myopia. In contrast, lower rates of hyperopia (28.4%) (defined as SE at least +0.5 D) were observed in Singapore Chinese aged 40 to 79 years.[11] The multicenter RESC study uses a uniform definition (hyperopia defined as SE at least +2 D) and identical study methodology in different countries (Fig. 6.12). The prevalence rates of hyperopia range from less than 3% in Nepal to 7.7% in urban India.[15–19] A consistent observation is that the hyperopia rates in children decrease with age.

SYNDROME ASSOCIATIONS AND GENETICS OF HYPEROPIA

A variety of associations have been described with hyperopia, including autosomal dominant nanophthalmos, Franceschetti syndrome, Leber Amaurosis and other retinal dystrophies, and autosomal dominant syndrome with congenital stapes ankylosis and broad thumbs.

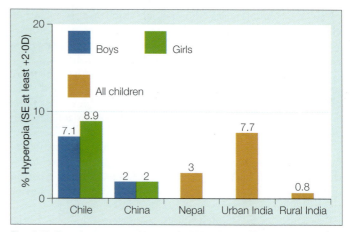

Fig. 6.12 Prevalence rates of hyperopia (SE at least +2.0 D) in the RESC (Refractive Error Study in Children). Repeat key on Fig 6.6 on p. 4.

Hyperopia may be at least partially hereditary. In a study of 226 monozygotic and 280 dizygotic twins aged 49 to 79 years in the United Kingdom, both additive genetic and environmental factors explained the continuous spectrum of myopia/hyperopia and the estimate of heritability was 89% for hyperopia as a dichotomous binary trait.[37] In Finland, the proportion of total variance attributable to additive genetic effects for hyperopia was 0.91 in 600 twin pairs aged 30 to 31 years.[70] The mode of inheritance for hyperopia is most likely to be similar to myopia: hyperopia is not a product of a single gene and is multifactorial in origin. The exact genetic loci are still not known and genome-wide scans to identify relevant loci are ongoing.

Treatment of hyperopia

There is no consensus on the level of hyperopia that warrants correction with spectacles or contact lenses.
1. If there is strabismus or amblyopia associated with the hyperopia, spectacle correction is mandatory.
2. In a preverbal child without strabismus, with hyperopia of over +3.0-D full spectacle correction, even if there is no evidence of visual problems, some authorities suggest the use of spectacles to prevent amblyopia and strabismus. However, there is conflicting evidence as to whether spectacle correction reduces the risk of amblyopia and strabismus, and it is probably safe to wait, carefully observing the young child, until formal vision testing can be done and the natural history of the condition can be observed. In young children who have higher hyperopia, say over +5.0-D spectacle correction, the indications for prescription increase proportionately because the risk of amblyopia increases.
3. In an older child, if the best corrected VA is worse than 0.2 to 0.3 LogMAR (depending on age, the younger the child, the less the need to prescribe) and the degree of hyperopia is more than + 3.0-D full correction, spectacles may be prescribed. Often, vision is good at even higher levels of hyperopia, and the child may not need to wear lenses.
4. Recently, there has been considerable interest in the surgical correction of hyperopia: this is not advocated in children.

ANISOMETROPIA

Anisometropia occurs when there is an interocular difference in refractive state of the right and left eyes. The difference in SE in

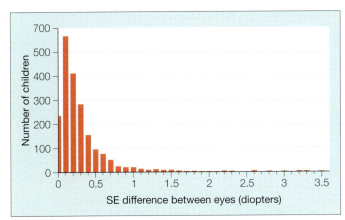

Fig. 6.13 Distribution of the difference in spherical equivalent (SE) in the eyes of 1,979 Singapore children in the SCORM (Singapore Cohort Study of the Risk Factors for Myopia) study.

the right and left eyes is a continuous variable with a skewed distribution (Fig. 6.13). Commonly accepted definitions of anisometropia include SE differences of +0.5, +1.0, and +2.0 D between the right and left eyes. Clinically, anisometropia may be classified as:

Spherical myopic anisometropia;
Spherical hyperopic anisometropia;
Cylindrical myopic anisometropia; and
Cylindrical hyperopic anisometropia.

Complications and adverse effects of all types of anisometropia include spectacle intolerance, defects in binocularity, and amblyopia. The degree of anisometropia is strongly correlated with the severity of amblyopia and reduction in binocular function; hyperopic anisometropia is more likely compared with myopic anisometropia.

The prevalence rate of anisometropia (SE difference of at least +1.0 D) in 3,654 residents aged 49 to 97 years in the Blue Mountains Eye Study was 14.1%.[14] In the Tanjong Pagar survey of 1,232 adults aged 40 to 79 years, the age-adjusted prevalence rate of anisometropia (SE difference of at least +1.0 D) was 15.9%.[11] In adults, rates of anisometropia increase with refractive error or cylinder, but there were no significant gender differences. Myopic eyes were more likely to be anisometropic compared with hyperopic eyes. The prevalence rate of anisometropia (SE at least +1.0 D) was 3.8% in Singapore Chinese aged 7 to 9 years, and 14.4% in Singapore male military conscripts aged 16 to 25 years.[71] In the SCORM study, the severity of anisometropia correlated with the axial length differences between eyes.

A study of data from several countries showed that the increase in the prevalence rate of nonamblyopic anisometropia was 1% for every 7 years in adults ($p < 0.001$), possibly accounted for by an age-related decrease in binocular vision.[72] In a follow-up study of 238 schoolchildren aged 9 to 11 years in Finland over a 3-year period, anisometropia increased in 27%, decreased in 6%, and remained unchanged in 67% of the population.[73] Little is known about the predisposing factors for anisometropia and whether this condition may be hereditary in nature.

It is important to monitor anisometropia and to detect amblyopia by reviewing the child at intervals determined by the severity of the anisometropia and the risk of amblyopia: the younger the child and the greater the anisometropia, the more frequent the reviews.

Anisometropia is a common cause of amblyopia. The mean age of presentation of anisometropic amblyopia is higher than that of strabismic amblyopia. Children with VA worse than LogMAR 0.2 or anisometropia with SE difference of at least 1.0 D will need optical correction. Optimal optical correction with spectacle lenses may ensure good binocular vision; this is especially important in early infancy. More than 3.0 D of anisometropia may be ideally treated with contact lenses to reduce aniseikonia, especially in older children. Some young children can tolerate large amounts of aniseikonia and can develop binocular vision with spectacles.

REFERENCES

1. Raviola E, Wiesel TN. An animal model of myopia. N Engl J Med 1985; 312: 1609–15.
2. Mutti DO, Zadnik K, Egashira S et al. The effect of cycloplegia on measurement of the ocular components. Invest Ophthalmol Vis Sci 1994; 35: 515–27.
3. Elliott M, Simpson T, Richter D, Fonn D. Repeatability and accuracy of automated refraction: a comparison of the Nikon NRK-8000, the Nidek AR-1000, and subjective refraction. Optom Vis Sci 1997; 74: 434–8.
4. Grosvenor T, Perrigin DM, Perrigin J. Three-way comparison of retinoscopy, subjective, and Dioptron Nova refractive findings. Am J Optom Physiol Opt 1985; 62: 63–5.
5. Millodot M, O'Leary D. The discrepancy between retinoscopic and subjective measurements: effect of age. Am J Optom Physiol Opt 1978; 55: 309–16.
6. Rosenfield M, Chiu NN. Repeatability of subjective and objective refraction. Optom Vis Sci 1995; 72: 577–9.
7. Carkeet A, Saw SM, Gazzard G, et al. Measurements of children's axial lengths made with ocular coherence biometry are more repeatable than those made with A-scan ultrasound [Abstract 3613]. 2003 Annual Meeting Abstract and Program Planner accessed at http://www.arvo.org. Association for Research in Vision and Ophthalmology. 5–9 May 2003, Florida.
8. Tong L, Saw SM, Tan D et al. Sensitivity and specificity of visual acuity screening for refractive errors in school children. Optom Vis Sci. 2002; 79: 650–7.
9. Javitt JC, Chiang YP. The socioeconomic aspects of laser refractive surgery. Arch Ophthalmol 1994; 112: 1526–30.
10. Saw SM, Gazzard G, Au-Eong KG, Koh D. Utility values and myopia in teenage school students. Br J Ophthalmol 2003; 87: 341–5.
11. Wong TY, Foster PJ, Hee J et al. Prevalence and risk factors for refractive errors in adult Chinese in Singapore. Invest Ophthalmol Vis Sci 2000; 41: 2486–94.
12. Katz J, Tielsch JM, Sommer A. Prevalence and risk factors for refractive errors in an adult inner city population. Invest Ophthalmol Vis Sci 1997; 38: 334–40.
13. Wu SY, Nemesure B, Leske MC. Refractive errors in a black adult population: The Barbados Eye Study. Invest Ophthalmol Vis Sci 1999; 40: 2179–84.
14. Attebo K, Ivers RQ, Mitchell P. Refractive errors in an older population: the Blue Mountains Eye Study. Ophthalmology 1999; 106: 1066–72.
15. Zhao J, Pan X, Sui R et al. Refractive Error Study in Children: results from Shunyi District, China. Am J Ophthalmol 2000; 129: 427–35.
16. Maul E, Barroso S, Munoz SR et al. Refractive Error Study in Children: results from La Florida, Chile. Am J Ophthalmol 2000; 129: 445–54.
17. Pokharel GP, Negrel AD, Munoz SR, Ellwein LB. Refractive Error Study in Children: results from Mechi Zone, Nepal. Am J Ophthalmol 2000; 129: 436–44.
18. Dandona R, Dandona L, Srinivas M et al. Refractive error in children in a rural population in India. Invest Ophthalmol Vis Sci 2002; 43: 615–22.
19. Murthy GV, Gupta SK, Ellwein LB et al. Refractive error in children in an urban population in New Delhi. Invest Ophthalmol Vis Sci 2002; 43: 623–31.
20. Lin LL, Shih YF, Tsai CB et al. Epidemiologic study of ocular refraction among schoolchildren in Taiwan in 1995. Optom Vis Sci 1999; 76: 275–81.

21. Chua WH, Saw SM, Wu HM, et al. Refractive errors in schoolchildren: the Singapore Myopia Cohort Study. Proceedings of the VIII International Conference on Myopia; 2000 July 7–9, Boston, MA.

22. Saunders KJ. Early refractive development in humans. Surv Ophthalmol 1995; 40: 207–16.

23. Goss DA. Variables related to the rate of childhood myopia progression. Optom Vis Sci 1990; 67: 631–6.

24. Wallman J, McFadden S. Monkey eyes grow into focus. Nat Med 1995; 1: 737–739.

25. Saw SM, Chua WH, Hong CY et al. Nearwork in early onset myopia. Invest Ophthalmol Vis Sci 2002; 43: 332–9.

26. Mutti DO, Mitchell GL, Moeschberger ML et al. Parental myopia, near work, school achievement, and children's refractive error. Invest Ophthalmol Vis Sci 2002; 43: 3633–40.

27. Quinn GE, Shin CH, Maguire MG, Stone RA. Myopia and ambient lighting at night. Nature 1999; 399: 113–4.

28. Zadnik K, Jones LA, Irvin BC et al. Myopia and ambient night-time lighting. CLEERE Study Group. Nature 2000; 404: 143–4.

29. Gwiazda J, Ong E, Held R, Thorn F. Myopia and ambient night-time lighting. Nature 2000; 404: 144.

30. Rosner M, Belkin M. Intelligence, education, and myopia in males. Arch Ophthalmol 1987; 105: 1508–11.

31. Grosvenor T. Refractive state, intelligence test scores, and academic ability. Am J Optom Arch Am Acad Optom 1970; (47): 355–61.

32. Ashton GC. Nearwork, school achievement and myopia. J Biosc Sci 1985; 17: 223–33.

33. Rosner M, Laor A, Belkin M. Myopia and stature: findings in a population of 106,926 males. Eur J Ophthalmol 1995; 5: 1–6.

34. Teasdale TW, Goldschmidt E. Myopia and its relationship to education, intelligence and height. Preliminary results from an on-going study of Danish draftees. Acta Ophthalmol Suppl 1988; 185: 41–3.

35. Saw SM, Chua WH, Hong CY et al. Height and its relationship to refraction and biometry parameters in Singapore Chinese children. Invest Ophthalmol Vis Sci 2002; 43: 1408–13.

36. Mutti DO, Zadnik K. The utility of three predictors of childhood myopia: a Bayesian analysis. Vision Res 1995; 35: 1345–52.

37. Hammond CJ, Snieder H, Gilbert CE, Spector TD. Genes and environment in refractive error: The Twin Eye Study. Invest Ophthalmol Vis Sci. 2001; 42: 1232–6.

38. Lin LL, Chen CJ. Twin study on myopia. Acta Genet Med Gemellol. (Roma)1987; 36: 535–40.

39. Lam DS, Lee WS, Leung YF et al. TGFβ-induced factor: a candidate gene for high myopia. Invest Ophthalmol Vis Sci 2003; 44: 1012–5.

40. Chen CJ, Cohen BH, Diamond EL. Genetic and environmental effects on the development of myopia in Chinese twin studies. Ophthalmic Paediatr Genet 1985; 6: 353–9.

41. Saw SM, Hong CY, Chia KS et al. Nearwork and myopia in young children. Lancet 2001; 357: 90.

42. Shih YF, Chen CH, Chou AC et al. Effects of different concentrations of atropine on controlling myopia in myopic children. J Ocul Pharmacol Ther 1999; 15: 85–90.

43. Yen MY, Liu JH, Kao SC, Shiao CH. Comparison of the effect of atropine and cyclopentolate on myopia. Ann Ophthalmol 1989; 21: 180–2.

44. Chua WH, Balakrishnan V, Tan DTH, et al. Efficacy results from the Atropine in the Treatment of Myopia (ATOM) Study [Abstract 3119]. 2003 Annual Meeting Abstract and Program Planner accessed at http://www.arvo.org. Association for Research in Vision and Ophthalmology. 5–9 May 2003, Florida.

45. Tan DTH, Lam D, Chua WH, et al. Pirenzepine Ophthalmic Gel (PIR): safety and efficacy for pediatric myopia in one-year study in Asia [Abstract 801]. 2003 Annual Meeting Abstract and Program Planner accessed at http://www.arvo.org. Association for Research in Vision and Ophthalmology. 5–9 May 2003, Florida.

46. Chung K, Mohidin N, O'Leary DJ. Undercorrection of myopia enhances rather than inhibits myopia progression. Vision Res 2002; 42: 2555–9.

47. Parssinen O, Hemminki E, Klemetti A. Effect of spectacle use and accommodation on myopic progression: final results of a three-year randomised clinical trial among schoolchildren. Br J Ophthalmol 1989; 73: 547–51.

48. Jensen H. Myopia progression in young school children. A prospective study of myopia progression and the effect of a trial with bifocal lenses and beta blocker eye drops. Acta Ophthalmol Suppl 1991; 200: 1–79.

49. Fulk GW, Cyert LA, Parker DE. A randomized trial of the effect of single-vision vs. bifocal lenses on myopia progression in children with esophoria. Optom Vis Sci 2000; 77: 395–401.

50. Edwards MH, Li RW, Lam CS et al. The Hong Kong progressive lens myopia control study: study design and main findings. Invest Ophthalmol Vis Sci 2002; 43: 2852–8.

51. Gwiazda J, Hyman L, Hussein M et al. A randomized clinical trial of progressive addition lenses versus single vision lenses on the progression of myopia in children. Invest Ophthalmol Vis Sci 2003; 44: 1492–1500.

52. Horner DG, Soni PS, Salmon TO, Swartz TS. Myopia progression in adolescent wearers of soft contact lenses and spectacles. Optom Vis Sci 1999; 76: 474–9.

53. Katz J, Schein OD, Levy B et al. A randomized trial of rigid gas permeable contact lenses to reduce progression of children's myopia. Am J Ophthalmol 2003; 136: 82–90.

54. Younan C, Mitchell P, Cumming RG et al. Myopia and incident cataract and cataract surgery: the Blue Mountains Eye Study. Invest Ophthalmol Vis Sci 2002; 43: 3625–32.

55. Leske MC, Wu SY, Nemesure B, Hennis A; Barbados Eye Studies Group. Risk factors for incident nuclear opacities. Ophthalmology 2002; 109: 1303–8.

56. Mitchell P, Hourihan F, Sandbach J, Wang JJ. The relationship between glaucoma and myopia: the Blue Mountains Eye Study. Ophthalmology 1999; 106: 2010–5.

57. Wong TY, Klein BE et al. Refractive errors, intraocular pressure, and glaucoma in a white population. Ophthalmology 2003; 110: 211–7.

58. Curtin BJ, Karlin DB. Axial length measurements and fundus changes of the myopic eye. I. The posterior fundus. Trans Am Ophthalmol Soc 1970; 68: 312–34.

59. Karlin DB, Curtin BJ. Peripheral chorioretinal lesions and axial length of the myopic eye. Am J Ophthalmol 1976; 81: 625–35.

60. Risk factors for idiopathic rhegmatogenous retinal detachment. The Eye Disease Case–Control Study Group. Am J Epidemiol 1993; 137: 749–57.

61. Ramrattan RS, Wolfs RC, Jonas JB et al. Determinants of optic disc characteristics in a general population: The Rotterdam Study. Ophthalmology 1999; 106: 1588–96.

62. Vongphanit J, Mitchell P, Wang JJ. Population prevalence of titled optic disks and the relationship of this sign to refractive error. Am J Ophthalmol 2002; 133: 679–85.

63. Wong TY, Klein R, Klein BE, Tomany SC. Refractive errors and 10-year incidence of age-related maculopathy. Invest Ophthalmol Vis Sci 2002; 43: 2869–73.

64. Wang JJ, Mitchell P, Smith W. Refractive error and age-related maculopathy: the Blue Mountains Eye Study. Invest Ophthalmol Vis Sci 1998; 39: 2167–71.

65. Gwiazda J, Scheiman M, Mohindra I, Held R. Astigmatism in children: changes in axis and amount from birth to six years. Invest Ophthalmol Vis Sci 1984; 25: 88–92.

66. Abrahamsson M, Fabian G, Sjostrand J. Changes in astigmatism between the ages of 1 and 4 years: a longitudinal study. Br J Ophthalmol 1988; 72: 145–9.

67. Tong L, Saw SM, Carkeet A et al. Prevalence rates and epidemiological risk factors for astigmatism in Singapore school children. Optom Vis Sci 2002; 79: 606–13.

68. Gwiazda J, Bauer J, Thorn F, Held R. Meridional amblyopia does result from astigmatism in early childhood. Clin Vis Sci 1993; 8: 337–44.

69. Villareal MG, Ohlsson J, Abrahamsson M et al. Myopiasation: the refractive tendency in teenagers. Prevalence of myopia among teenagers in Sweden. Acta Ophthalmol Scand 2000; 78: 177–81.

70. Teikari JM, Kaprio J, Koskenvuo M, O'Donnell J. Heritability of defects of far vision in young adults–a twin study. Scand J Soc Med 1992; 20: 73–8.

71. Wu HM, Seet B, Yap EP et al. Does education explain ethnic differences in myopia prevalence? A population-based study of young adult males in Singapore. Optom Vis Sci 2001; 78: 234–9.

72. Weale RA. On the age-related prevalence of anisometropia. Ophthalmic Res 2002; 34: 389–92.

73. Parssinen O. Anisometropia and changes in anisometropia in school myopia. Optom Vis Sci 1990; 67: 256–9.

CHAPTER 7 Refractive Surgery in Children

Luis Amaya

INTRODUCTION

Refractive surgery is an accepted procedure for millions of adults annually. Many children want to get rid of their glasses and contact lenses and ophthalmologists need to determine the safety and benefit of these procedures. Refractive surgery in children is controversial and experimental. It is not a matter of whether the procedures can be carried out technically, but whether it is the best way to correct refractive errors in a way that will benefit them best throughout their lives.

DEVELOPMENT OF REFRACTIVE SURGERY

Sato, in the 1930s, used multiple posterior corneal incisions; these corneas decompensated. Radial keratotomy became common during the 1980s with different algorithms developed using partial thickness radial incisions. In the long term it caused unstable corneas with refractive shifts, corneal erosions, edema, and decompensation.

In photorefractive keratectomy (PRK), the cornea is remodeled with the excimer laser after removing the epithelium. Recovery is long and painful.

In laser in situ keratomileusis (LASIK) the corneal epithelium is intact, providing rapid recovery and reducing pain. Automated microkeratomes have produced more predictable, regular flaps and even surfaces.

REFRACTION CHANGES IN CHILDHOOD

The developing eye poses a challenge and refraction must be unchanged for at least two years before surgery. In the first years of life, there are large changes in refraction, and emmetropization continues throughout development (see Chapter 4).

Refractive errors usually occur in the first two decades. Hyperopia is present very early, and if it is higher than the accommodative amplitude, amblyopia may result. Simple myopia develops later and usually progresses until the teen-ages. Astigmatism is often present at birth, but it often resolves during the first year: it may then remain stable.

INDICATIONS FOR REFRACTIVE SURGERY IN CHILDREN

Monocular amblyopia in older children

Many older anisometropic children refuse to wear any optical correction. Although the best-corrected visual acuity can be good without correction, it can also be poor. Refractive surgery can provide improvement of the amblyopia even without postoperative patching therapy.[1–5]

Amblyopia can improve later in life.[6] With the refractive error corrected, occlusion even at a later age can give some improvement. Refractive surgery for amblyopia in young children is experimental.

Anisometropia

Significant anisometropia is associated with amblyopia,[7] especially in anisohypermetropia.[8] Children with high anisometropia often refuse optical correction and patching; it is common to see older children, treated vigorously for years, with significant residual amblyopia.[9] Refractive surgery may improve the vision and make occlusion easier. Amblyopia from mild anisometropia can be treated with optical correction without patching.[10] Refractive surgery can equalize the refractive error and improve the visual prognosis of anisometropic children even without patching but the long-term effect on growing eyes is unknown. Anisomyopia may have a better refractive and visual prognosis as its treatment is more predictable than hyperopia.

Refractive surgery for anisometropia should be offered only as a last option, and parents must be informed of the uncertain long-term outcome and complications.

Bilateral refractive amblyopia intolerant to other optical devices

Bilateral high refractive errors may induce bilateral amblyopia, but can usually be treated by optical correction alone. Parents may request refractive surgery because their children are discriminated against and bullied.

This is not an indication for refractive surgery because of the future unpredictable changes in refraction, and these children and their parents need only firm and detailed reassurance.

Special activity requirements for good uncorrected vision

Occasionally, refractive surgery may be suggested for children with craniofacial or other deformities that make the fitting of glasses difficult, or some activities (i.e., sport) may be difficult with spectacles. Refractive surgery should not be considered for these reasons.

Stable myopia

As myopia in children progresses, it may stabilize in the teens, but in some cases it progresses into adulthood. Surgical outcome is unpredictable, and the behavior of myopia after refractive surgery in childhood is uncertain. Refractive surgery is not indicated for the vast majority of young myopes.

Hypermetropia

Laser correction of hypermetropia is less predictable, and only mild refractive errors have reasonable results. The refractive error must be stable for at least two years, so most young hypermetropes are excluded. Children should wear glasses or contact lenses until eye growth is completed.

PRK for hypermetropic children can cause recurrence and corneal haze,[2,11] and it may induce astigmatism so it is not indicated for children. There are a few reports on LASIK for hypermetropia in older children: they can be undercorrected since they tolerate some hypermetropia.[12]

Accommodative esotropia

Accommodative strabismus has been treated by refractive surgery,[13,14] but not all patients have a reduction of the esodeviation,[15] some require strabismus surgery, and some lost visual acuity. Refractive surgery for the full hypermetropic defect may result in later myopia. Hypermetropia is less predictably treated and undercorrections are planned, which leaves these children with an accommodative component requiring optical correction. LASIK could be an option in older children with long-standing stable mild hypermetropia, accommodative esotropia with stereopsis. Prospective studies are needed.

EXCIMER LASER SURGERY

PRK

In PRK, laser ablation of the surface of the cornea is produced after removing the epithelium. Recovery time is long and painful. Use of postoperative steroids may continue for 3 months. However, it may be safer than LASIK.

PRK has been used in older children with amblyopia and myopic anisometropia in whom other treatment was unsuccessful,[2,5,11] resulting in reduction of the refractive error, improvement of visual acuity, and low rates of haze. The procedures were done with or without[2] sedation or under general anesthesia using the center of the pupil as the optical zone.[1,11] PRK for myopia in children[1,2,5,11] showed reduction of the refractive error and improvement of vision.

LASIK

LASIK provides quicker rehabilitation, less pain, and less haze since Bowman's membrane is left intact: it provides more predictable and stable results. With a high precision, automated microkeratome, a hinged corneal flap is created. The excimer laser removes tissue from the central exposed cornea, modifying its curvature: the flap is repositioned and rapidly re-adheres.

Preoperative assessment

After full consent, the clinician must judge whether the procedure can be done under local or general anesthesia. Children over 8 years are often willing to cooperate with topical anesthesia. An ophthalmic assessment is required, including best-uncorrected and -corrected visual acuity, cycloplegic refraction, and best subjective visual acuity. Slit lamp and dilated fundus examination are mandatory. Corneal topography (Figs. 7.1 and 7.2) with pachymetry are necessary for the assessment, and subclinical keratoconus, corneal distortions, or very thin corneas can be identified using adult nomograms.

Surgical technique: LASIK

The procedure is performed as a day case: sedation is not used and one eye only is operated on in children. Several topical anesthetic drops are instilled. Strips of adhesive tape are placed at the superior lid edges to keep the eyelashes away from the operating field, and the fellow eye is covered. A lid speculum is placed but when the palpebral fissure is too narrow to allow placement of the suction ring the surgeon or the assistant holds the lids open and places the ring without the speculum. The suction ring is placed and activated; special care must be taken that the cornea is firmly held to provide optimal flap formation. The microkeratome is placed on the ring and moved across the cornea to create the flap. The incision is made so that an adequate hinge is left. The flap is lifted and the exposed stroma is dried. The patient is asked to look at the red light, and the laser is activated. After ablation, the stroma is washed and the flap repositioned. Under general anesthesia, the ring is kept in place without suction while the laser is activated, to keep the eye stable and centered.

COMPLICATIONS

PRK

With PRK in children, corneal haze occurs in up to 40%.[1,2,11] Prolonged use of topical steroids may be required with a risk of steroid-induced glaucoma and regression,[2,11] and induced astigmatism may occur.

When there is a kappa angle, the ablation may not be centered if the surgery is performed under general anesthesia or sedation as active fixation is necessary to guarantee centration.

PRK gives a risk of infection that has not been an issue in the published series involving children. Some recommend topical antibiotics.

LASIK

Although LASIK provides more predictable and stable results, complications can be more severe than those with PRK. Microkeratome malfunction or defective blades can produce irregular corneal cuts: sometimes the procedure must be aborted, and inadequate calibration can cause corneal perforation. The prolonged use of a suction ring increases the intraocular pressure, which can cause optic disc damage or retinal artery occlusion. The corneal flap can be displaced or lost. In patients with cyclotorsion that require astigmatic correction under general anesthesia, inaccurate meridional correction can be avoided by preoperative assessment and using conjunctival vessels as markers.

Displacement, disturbance, loss, folding, or wrinkling[16] of the corneal flap in the postoperative period is frequent in children. The younger the child is, the more likely corneal haze will occur.[17] Deposits under the flap have been reported.[4]

Long-term complications include fluctuating vision, increased sensitivity to light, glare, and haloes, and cataract formation. There can be flap complications such as corneal ulcer formation, corneal epithelial healing defects, dry eye, corneal vascularization, and epithelial cell growth beneath the flap. This may require further corrective surgery or corneal transplant. Corneal ectasia can occur after LASIK, and herpes virus infection may be reactivated.

Phakic intraocular lenses

Phakic intraocular lenses have been implanted in adults for the correction of refractive errors; the long-term complications are not well documented, and implantation in children is not recommended.

THE FUTURE

Only long-term, multicenter, randomized prospective studies will show whether PRK and LASIK are safe and long-term treatments for refractive errors in children. We hope that, by better understanding growth and emmetropization and those factors that result in refractive errors and by manipulating them to create eyes with normal vision, refractive surgery will not be needed.

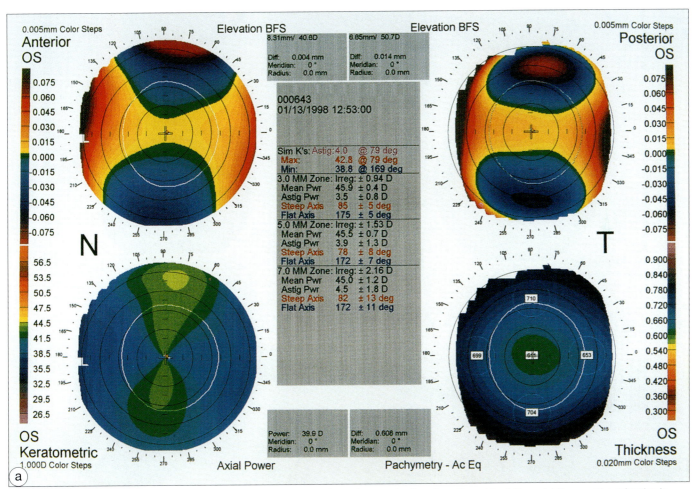

Fig. 7.1 Corneal topography of a nine-year-old boy with anisometropia due to hypermetropic astigmatism of the left eye. (a) Preoperative refraction is +4.00 –2.00 × 180. Uncorrected vision is 20/200. Anterior and posterior surfaces of the cornea illustrate moderate astigmatism (superior right and left, respectively). Keratometric readings (inferior left) and central pachymetry of 0.611 mm (inferior right).

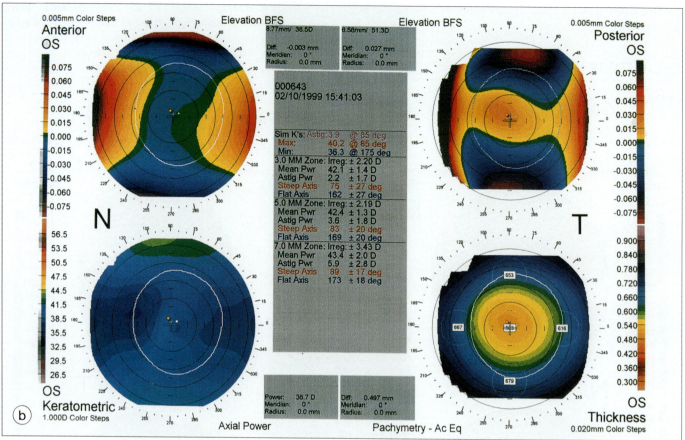

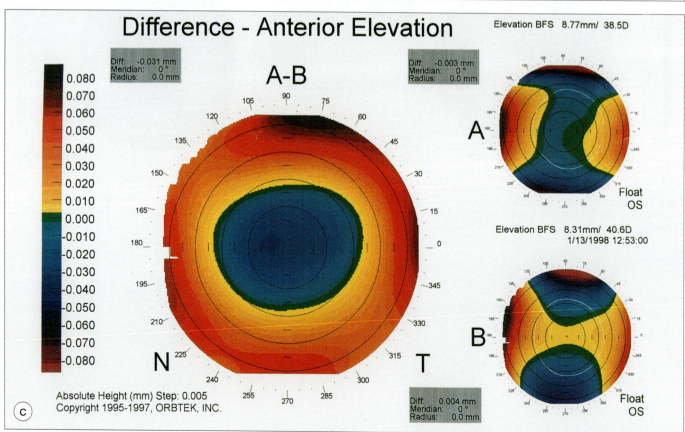

Fig. 7.1 (*Cont'd*) Corneal topography of a nine-year-old boy with anisometropia due to hypermetropic astigmatism of the left eye. (b) One-week postoperative topography. Refraction is +1.00 −1.25 × 180, with an uncorrected vision of 20/40. Central anterior surface is less steep, and keratometry shows significant reduction of astigmatism. Pachymetry at the center is 0.500 mm. (c) Computer composition after superimposing preoperative and postoperative anterior corneal surfaces.

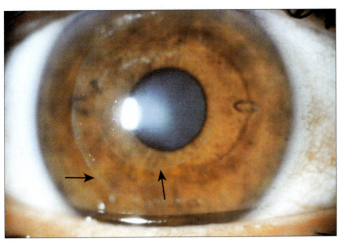

Fig. 7.2 Same boy two days after LASIK surgery. Internal corneal ring (right arrow) corresponds to laser ablation, and external ring to corneal keratectomy (left arrow).

REFERENCES

1. Alio JL, Artola A, Claramonte P, et al. Photorefractive keratectomy for pediatric myopic anismoetropia. J Cataract Refract Surg 1998; 24: 327–30.
2. Nano HD Jr, Muzzin S, Irigaray LF. Excimer laser photorefractive keratectomy in pediatric patients. J Cataract Refract Surg 1997; 23: 736–9.
3. Ibrahim O. Laser in-situ keratomileusis for hyperopia and hyperopic astigmatism. J Refract Surg 1998; 14: S179–82.
4. Rashad KM. Laser in situ keratomileusis for myopic anisometropia in children. J Refract Surg 1999; 15: 429–35.
5. Singh D. Photorefractive keratectomy in pediatric patients. J Cataract Refract Surg 1995; 21: 630–3.
6. El Mallah MK, Chakravarthy U, Hart PM. Amblyopia: Is visual loss permanent? Br J Ophthalmol 2000; 84: 952–6.
7. Abrahamsson M, Sjostrand J. Natural history of infantile anisometropia. Br J Ophthalmol 1996; 80: 860–3.
8. Weakley DR Jr. The association between nonstrabismic anisometropia, amblyopia and subnormal binocularity. Ophthalmology 2001; 108: 163–171.
9. Gregson R. Why are we so bad at treating amblyopia? Eye 2002; 16: 461–2.
10. Flynn JT, Schiffman J, Feuer W, Corona A. The therapy of amblyopia: an analysis of the results of amblyopia therapy utilizing the pooled data of published studies. Trans Am Ophthalmol Soc 1998; 96: 431–50.
11. Astle WF, Huang PT, Ells AL, et al. Photorefractive keratectomy in children. J Cataract Refract Surg 2002; 28: 932–41.
12. Davidorf JM. Pediatric refractive surgery. J Cataract Refract Surg 2000; 26: 1567–8.
13. Maldonado-Bas A, Hoyos J. Strabismus: accommodative component treated by Lasik. Rev Bras Oftalmol 1998; 57: 757–60.
14. Goodman D. Strabismus: accommodative component treated by LASIK. Surv Ophthalmol 1999; 44: 183–4.
15. Stidham DB, Borissova O, Borissov V, Prager TC. Effect of hyperopic laser in situ keratomileusis on ocular alignment and stereopsis in patients with accommodative esotropia. Ophthalmology 2002; 109: 1148–53.
16. Nassaralla BR, Nassaralla JJ Jr. Laser in situ keratomileusis in children 8 to 15 years old. J Refract Surg 2001; 17: 519–24.
17. Agarwal A, Agarwal A, Agarwal T, et al. Results of pediatric laser in situ keratomileusis. J Cataract Refract Surg 2000; 26: 684–9.

CHAPTER

8 Screening

Sean P Donahue

INTRODUCTION

Children are not simply little adults. Although they may have similar problems, such as refractive error and cataract, the management of these conditions, and the importance of early detection, is critically different. The most significant difference between children and adults, with respect to the visual system, is the presence of a time window, called the critical period. The critical period is a window during a child's development in which synaptic connections are established permanently. After the critical period, treatment is much less likely to be effective in restoring vision. Although the length of the critical period varies individually and depending on the type of pathology, identification and treatment during the critical period are critical to successful visual development and avoidance of amblyopia.

For the purposes of screening, the development of a child's vision can be separated into four overlapping age ranges. Each age range has pathology that needs to be identified and treated during that age period in order for successful visual development to occur. These age periods, and their associated pathology, are listed in Table 8.1. What follows is a brief discussion of these periods and screening that, in ideal circumstances, should occur during these periods to detect and treat these problems. The key issues are highlighted for each age group.

GUIDELINES FOR SCREENING

The World Health Organization has studied screening programs for disease as part of a public health program, and has established guidelines for the development of a successful screening program. These guidelines are listed in Table 8.2. As a general rule, the guidelines demand that the condition being screened for is a relatively common problem that is also a public health concern, and for which successful detection and treatment exist. Although these guidelines were designed to encompass all types of screening for different diseases (both ocular and nonocular),

Table 8.2 World Health Organization guidelines for screening

1) The condition sought should be an important health problem.
2) There should be an accepted treatment for patients with recognized disease.
3) Facilities for diagnosis and treatment should be available.
4) There should be a suitable latent or early symptomatic stage.
5) There should be a suitable test or examination.
6) The test should be acceptable to the population.
7) The natural history of the condition, including development from latent to declared disease, should be adequately understood.
8) There should be an agreed policy on whom to treat as patients.
9) The cost of case finding, including diagnosis and treatment of patients diagnosed, should be economically balanced in relation to expenditures on medical care as a whole.
10) Case finding should be a continuous process and not a "once-for-all" project

most of the guidelines remain applicable to screening for common visual problems in children, such as those listed in Table 8.1. The conditions listed in Table 8.1 generally fit these guidelines, although for some (amblyogenic factors), the natural history remains somewhat unknown.

SCREENING PREMATURE INFANTS

Prematurity is a significant cause of blindness (Chapter 51). The multicenter, prospective CRYO-ROP study demonstrated the effectiveness of treatment.[1] Laser photocoagulation is now used and is probably as effective as cryotherapy,[2,3] although no large, multicentered prospective studies have compared the two. The American Academy of Pediatrics has recently revised its guidelines for which children should be screened (Table 8.3).[4] Screening should be done using pupillary dilation and scleral depression, by an ophthalmologist using indirect ophthalmoscopy, beginning at 31–33 weeks of age or 4–6 weeks post-natal age,

Table 8.1 Age ranges and visual pathology to be detected in children

Preterm	Perinatal/ infantile period	Preschool period	Elementary school age
Retinopathy of prematurity	Congenital cataract Glaucoma Anterior segment disorders	Amblyogenic factors Strabismus Anisometropia High refractive error	Refractive error

Table 8.3 Revised screening guidelines for retinopathy of prematurity[4]

1) Infants with birth weight < 1500 gm or gestational age < 28 weeks.
2) Selected infants birth weights 1500-2000 gm with unstable clinical course.
3) Examination by experienced, knowledgeable ophthalmologist using indirect ophthalmoscopy and pupillary dilation.
4) First examination between 4 and 6 weeks postnatal age or 31 and 33 weeks gestational age, whichever is later.
5) Follow-up examination at regular intervals, depending on clinical findings.

whichever is later. Children should continue to undergo screening until 45 weeks postmenstrual age or progression of retinal vascularization into Zone III without previous Zone II ROP or full vascularization occurs.[5]

Recent studies evaluating new technology such as telemedicine show promise. Wide-angle cameras, such as the Retcam, can be used by nurses and other less-trained personnel, but currently cannot visualize the entire ridge reliably enough to assess vascularity.[6] Screening for plus disease may eventually play a role in ROP screening,[7] but because of the very high risk of missing treatable disease, the sensitivity of any such screening program must come close to 100% in order to allow its use.

SCREENING FULL-TERM NEONATES

The eyes of the full-term child should be assessed for the presence of congenital cataract. Untreated complete bilateral congenital cataracts cause nystagmus within three to four months, after which development of good vision is unlikely, despite clearing of the visual axis and correcting the aphakia. For unilateral congenital cataract, 17 weeks is the latest time when a cataract can be removed, occlusion instituted, and 20/20 vision still regained.[8] Thus, detection during the nursery examination or at the six-week examination is vital.

Detection of congenital cataracts is typically performed by red reflex testing by the pediatrician in the newborn nursery and repeated at the 2- and 6-week outpatient examinations. Current recommendations have been made both by the Children's Subgroup of the National Screening Committee of the United Kingdom (http://www.nsc.nhs.uk) and by the American Academy of Pediatrics,[9] and both recommend red reflex screening by primary care doctors within the first two months of postnatal life.

The use of pupillary dilation for the detection of congenital cataracts is controversial. Bills have been introduced into the legislature in several of the states in the United States, requiring pupillary dilation by primary care doctors, with hopes of detecting both congenital cataract and retinoblastoma. However, the extreme rarity of sporadic retinoblastoma (in the absence of family history), the absence of large sporadic tumors in most children under one year of age (when such screening exams are most likely to occur) and the unknown sensitivity of red reflex testing by pediatricians through dilated pupils to detect retinoblastoma in very young children make such a legal mandate extremely controversial.

PRESCHOOL VISION SCREENING

During preschool age (up to age six years), the most common visual conditions are strabismus, asymmetric refractive error (anisometropia), and high bilateral symmetric refractive error such as high hyperopia, all of which can cause amblyopia. Since most preschool children use a working distance of less than one meter, myopic refractive errors in the range of 2 D (diopters) or less are essentially irrelevant, as is mild symmetric regular meridional astigmatism. The prevalence of high myopia and high levels of astigmatism of this population is probably much less than 1%. High hypermetropic refractive errors, however, represent a potential problem. Studies by Atkinson have suggested that the risk of strabismus or amblyopia in children whose refractive error exceeds +3.50 D is 13 times the risk in the general population,[10] and that spectacle correction reduces the risk of strabismus substantially. Despite these issues, the techniques for detecting uncorrected hypermetropia have not

been well described. Furthermore, the relationship between high hyperopia, accommodation, and the prevention of the development of accommodative strabismus is not well understood.

Amblyopia is a significant public health problem. Amblyopia typically affects 3–5% of the population. Detection during the preschool years is critical for successful treatment. Traditional vision screening is the standard method for detecting amblyopia.[11] Many types of traditional screening programs using LEA symbols, Allen cards, Sheriden Gardiner cards, HOTV letters, and Teller acuity cards exist for children who are too young to read Snellen letters. Testing personnel include trained lay personnel, school nurses, pediatricians, pediatric nurses, and, in the United Kingdom, orthoptists. Tests for alignment (cover tests and light reflex tests) and stereopsis (Randot, Titmus, or Lang cards) are variably added to testing protocols. The result, unfortunately, has been a morass of guidelines and mandates.[12] None of these tests has had adequate validation in the primary care physician's office.[13] In addition, compliance with published vision screening guidelines by pediatricians is less than complete.[14]

In 1998, Stewart-Brown and Snowdon presented their results from a review of the existing literature of preschool vision screening.[15] Their review revealed deficits in our knowledge of how amblyopic patients report their specific visual disabilities. In addition, they found no studies where a control group with no treatment was compared to amblyopia treatment, and therefore they concluded that the natural history of amblyopia was unknown. Thus, despite previous retrospective studies demonstrating that orthoptic screening can efficiently identify amblyopic children and that amblyopia treatment improves visual acuity, the report of Stewart-Brown and Snowdon concluded that "screening is not effective ... because there is no evidence that treatment is either effective nor necessary."[15]

The report by Stewart-Brown and Snowdon created a firestorm of controversy both in the United Kingdom and in the United States, but resulted in several better-performed studies demonstrating how preschool vision screening can detect amblyopia, and how successful amblyopia treatment is. Some of these studies are detailed below.

Kvarnstrom et al. reported their results from a Swedish visual screening program of 3,126 children.[16] They found that screening and subsequent diagnosis and treatment have reduced the prevalence of amblyopia at various levels of acuity. Specifically, their program reduced the prevalence of significant amblyopia (visual acuity < 0.3 (approximately 20/60)) from 2 to 0.2%. In addition, 47% of amblyopic children achieved visual acuity better than 20/30 with treatment.

The success of early screening for amblyogenic risk factors was also demonstrated in Haifa, Israel.[17] Eibschitz et al. compared the prevalence and severity of amblyopia in two populations of eight-year-old children in elementary school. One population was screened at infancy, while the second group had no screening performed. The prevalence of amblyopia in the screened group was 1.0% compared to 2.6% in the unscreened group, and the prevalence of amblyopia with acuity of 20/60 or less was 0.1% in the screened population compared to 1.7% in the nonscreened population.

The ALSPAC study team has provided similar results from intensive screening compared to only orthoptic screening alone.[18] The intensive screening group had a prevalence of amblyopia of only 0.6% at age 7.5 years compared to 1.8% following a single orthoptic screening at 37 months. The results of these three large-scale prospective public health studies conclusively demonstrate that amblyopia screening and subsequent treatment significantly decreases the prevalence of amblyopia.

Another concern raised by Stewart-Brown and Snowdon was that the natural history of untreated amblyopia was unknown; that is, some amblyopia would get better without treatment.[15] Simons and Preslan evaluated this hypothesis in 18 children aged 4–6 years who had been screened for amblyopia, and who did not comply with prescribed treatment.[19] They were screened again one year later. One child of the 18, who wore glasses sporadically, showed some improvement in the amblyopic eye. Otherwise, no child showed any improvement: 7 of the 17 (41%) showed a deterioration of acuity, and 3 who had no amblyopia developed it during the year as a result of noncompliance with treatment. This study demonstrates that including any untreated control group in a study of amblyopia would be unethical. A theoretical bias would be that these children were not compliant because they (or their parents) knew they would not improve; however, the demographics of inner city Baltimore, where the study was performed, are such that other factors, primarily social, were much more likely to contribute to the noncompliance.

Perhaps the greatest risk of not treating amblyopia lies in the potential for a loss of vision in the healthy eye later on in life. A Finnish study[20] demonstrated a higher risk of vision loss in the healthy eye of amblyopic individuals than in healthy two-eyed individuals. In 1997, a national surveillance program was performed in the United Kingdom to identify adults with unilateral amblyopia who had newly acquired vision loss in the healthy eye, resulting in acuity of 20/40 or less and precluding driving.[21] These investigators found the projected lifetime risk of vision loss for an amblyopic individual was at least 1.2% (confidence intervals from 1.1 to 1.4%), and that 65% of the 102 people who lost vision in their healthy eye were unable to continue paid employment. The result of these two studies should conclusively demonstrate to critics of visual screening that amblyopia is a significant visual disability.

The cost effectiveness of amblyopia screening has also been clearly demonstrated. Konig and Barry performed an economic evaluation of orthoptic screening in German kindergartens.[22] They evaluated several different screening methodologies, and found binocular visual acuity screening with rescreening of inconclusive results to have favorable cost effectiveness compared to other types of vision screening, with an average cost per detected case of amblyopia of approximately 878 euros. Membreno et al. recently performed an economic evaluation of the cost effectiveness of amblyopia treatment.[23] They demonstrated that amblyopia treatment has a cost per quality-adjusted life year gained of approximately $2,281. This compares favorably to all other ophthalmic interventions for all conditions, with the exception of screening and treatment for retinopathy of prematurity ($678–$1,801/QALY).[24] Membreno et al. also calculated that loss of vision in fellow eyes of amblyopic individuals causes a decrease in the yearly US gross domestic product (GDP) of $7.4 billion, and that amblyopia screening and treatment would return $22 to the GDP for every dollar spent.

Traditional vision screening has several recognized difficulties. These include the lack of cooperation of young children with objective literate targets, the time taken for pediatricians and primary care doctors to screen such children with these techniques, and the lack of insurance reimbursement for vision screening. However, recent new technology and the desire to detect abnormalities before they cause amblyopia has led to the development of new instruments for preschool vision screening such as photoscreening and automated retinoscopy. Several types of photoscreening are currently being marketed, each having various levels of validation. In each photoscreening system, a

picture is taken of the eyes using a flash. The picture is later interpreted to evaluate ocular alignment and the presence of a refractive error. A referral is then made on the basis of suspected levels of refractive error and alignment abnormalities. Although all photoscreening techniques have had some type of validation, it is difficult to compare all the new technologies, since there is no universal agreement on what magnitude refractive error should be detected. In an attempt to reconcile this problem, the vision screening committee of the American Association of Pediatric Ophthalmology and Strabismus has recently reported vision screening guidelines for which amblyogenic factors are considered significant enough to be detected (Table 8.4).[25]

Two large photoscreening programs have been described in the United States. The Alaska Blind Discovery Project utilizes the MTI photoscreener in urban and rural communities in Southern Alaska.[26] Screenings are performed by lay personnel, and interpreted by a pediatric ophthalmologist. During the first three years of the program, over 4,000 screenings were performed on 3,930 children. Positive predictive value has improved from 77 to over 90% for amblyogenic factors.

A larger program has been carried out in Tennessee, USA.[27] This program also utilizes volunteer screeners, the MTI photoscreener, and a central reading center. Over 100,000 children have been screened during the first six years of the program, with a referral rate of slightly greater than 4%, a screenability rate of 96%, and a positive predictive value of 75%.

In addition to the MTI photoscreener, other photoscreening devices are in various levels of development, validation, and use. Space does not permit a discussion of each of them, as this is a rapidly changing field. Further research and development will eventually lead to digital cameras with visual image capturing systems, and an automated image analysis system, to detect pathology rapidly so that an immediate referral can be made. This, commensurate with a mandate for reimbursement for preschool vision screening, will further drive the development of new technology at least in the United States. A statement supporting the use of photoscreening for preschool vision screening has recently been released by the American Academy of Pediatrics.[28]

Automated retinoscopy is also a new technique for vision screening in preschool children. Cordonnier and Kallay have used the handheld Retinomax autorefractor to detect refractive errors in 1,218 children in Brussels, Belgium.[29] Automated refraction cannot detect strabismus, but has a positive predictive value to detect refractive error that ranges from 19 to 69% and a sensitivity of 37–87%.

Comprehensive eye examinations, mandated by the legislature of an individual state, have also been proposed as a method for

---

Table 8.4 Amblyogenic factors to be detected by screening

1) Anisometropia (spherical or cylindrical) > 1.5 D
2) Any manifest strabismus
3) Hyperopia > 3.50 D in any meridian
4) Myopia magnitude > 3.00 D in any meridian
5) Any media opacity > 1 mm in size
6) Astigmatism > 1.5 D at 90° or 180°, > 1.0 in oblique axis (more than 10° eccentric to 90° or 180°)
7) Ptosis ≤ 1 mm margin-reflex distance[a]
8) Visual acuity: per AAP (age-appropriate standards)[31]

[a]Margin-reflex distance is the distance from the corneal light reflex to the upper lid margin, and is a standard objective measurement of ptosis.
With permission from Donahue et al.[25]

vision examinations in the United States, mostly supported by the optometry lobby. In addition to the lack of mandate for what refractive conditions should be detected, what should be required in an examination (cycloplegia or not), and how these conditions should be treated, the manpower issues required to personally examine five million new children in the United States each year are not taken into account with such bills.

Such concerns are evident from an analysis of a recent paper describing the results of a mandated vision screening law introduced in Kentucky.[30] A survey was carried out of optometrists who performed eye examinations on three- to six-year-olds during the years 2000 to 2001 as part of the Kentucky law. They found that spectacles were prescribed for 14% of children, including 11% of three-year-olds. This is particularly bothersome, because no studies have provided data that 11% of otherwise healthy three-year-old children require spectacles, no data were provided on what level refractive error was necessary before spectacles were prescribed, and cycloplegic refraction was not necessarily performed in these children.

SCREENING SCHOOL AGE CHILDREN

Once children reach school age, amblyopia is typically not an issue. The most prevalent ocular pathology in school-aged children is refractive error. Screening for refractive error in school-aged children is typically done within the school system or in the pediatrician's office, or both, with traditional tests of Snellen acuity.[31] The sensitivity and specificity of these screening techniques has never been well described, but nevertheless they are time-honored. It is not until middle elementary years that most children develop myopia and require spectacle correction for it, as most children's visual demands do not require clear distance acuity up until the late elementary years. At that time, traditional vision screening of young elementary children, and relying upon subjective symptoms of blurred distance acuity for older children, is sufficient for identifying individuals with a need for spectacle correction. It should be noted that, in contrast to preschool children, lack of treatment of refractive error in older children will not cause permanent afferent visual system pathology (amblyopia).

REFERENCES

1. Multicenter trial of cryotherapy for retinopathy of prematurity. Preliminary results. Cryotherapy for retinopathy of prematurity cooperative group. Arch Ophthalmol 1988;106:471–9.
2. Paysse EA, Lindsey JL, Coats DK, et al. Therapeutic outcomes of cryotherapy versus transpupillary diode laser photocoagulation for threshold retinopathy of prematurity. J AAPOS 1999; 3: 234–40.
3. White JE, Repka MX. Randomized comparison of diode laser photocoagulation versus cryotherapy for threshold retinopathy of prematurity: 3-year outcome. J Pediatr Ophthalmol Strabismus 1997; 34: 83–7.
4. Screening examination of premature infants for retinopathy of prematurity. Section on Ophthalmology. American Academy of Pediatrics. Pediatrics 2001; 108: 809–11.
5. Reynolds JD, Dobson V, Quinn GE, et al. Evidence-based screening criteria for retinopathy of prematurity: Natural history data from the CRYO-ROP and LIGHT-ROP studies. Arch Ophthalmol 2002; 120: 1470–6.
6. Roth DB, Morales D, Feuer WJ, et al. Screening for retinopathy of prematurity employing the Retcam 120: sensitivity and specificity. Arch Ophthalmol 2001; 119: 268–72.
7. Saunders RA, Bluestein EC, Sinatra RB, et al. The predictive value of posterior pole vessels in retinopathy of prematurity. J Pediatr Ophthalmol Strabismus 1995; 32: 82–5.
8. Cheng KP, Hiles DA, Biglan AW, Pettapiece MC. Visual results after early surgical treatment of unilateral congenital cataracts. Ophthalmology 1991; 98: 903–10.
9. Red Reflex Examination in Infants. Section on Ophthalmology. American Academy of Pediatrics. Pediatrics 2002; 109: 980–1.
10. Atkinson J, Braddick O, Robier B, et al. Two infant vision screening programmes: prediction and prevention of strabismus and amblyopia from photo- and videorefractive screening. Eye 1996; 10: 189–98.
11. Hartmann EE, Dobson V, Hainline L, et al. Preschool vision screening: Summary of a task force report. Ophthalmology 2001; 108: 479–86.
12. Ciner EB, Dobson V, Schmidt PP, et al. A survey of vision screening policy of preschool children in the United States. Surv Ophthalmol 1999; 43: 445–57.
13. Kemper AR, Margolis PA, Downs SM, Bordley WC. A systematic review of vision screening tests for the detection of amblyopia. Pediatrics 1999; 104: 1220–22.
14. Wall TC, Marsh-Tootle W, Evans HH, et al. Compliance with vision-screening guidelines among a national sample of pediatricians. Ambul Pediatr 2002; 2: 449–55.
15. Stewart-Brown SL, Snowdon SK. Evidence-based dilemmas in pre-school vision screening. Arch Dis Child 1998; 78: 406–7.
16. Kvarnstrom G, Jakobsson P, Lennerstrand G. Visual screening of Swedish children: an ophthalmological evaluation. Acta Ophthalmol Scand 2001; 79: 240–4.
17. Eibschitz-Tsimhoni M, Friedman T, Naor J, et al. Early screening for amblyogenic risk factors lowers the prevalence and severity of amblyopia. J AAPOS 2000; 4: 194–9.
18. Williams C, Northstone K, Harrad RA, et al. ALSPAC Study Team. Amblyopia treatment outcomes after screening before or at age 3 years: Follow-up from randomized trial. BMJ 2002; 324: 1549.
19. Simons K, Preslan M. Natural history of amblyopia untreated owing to lack of compliance. Br J Ophthalmol 1999; 83: 582–7.
20. Tommila V, Tarkkanen A. Incidence of loss of vision in the healthy eye in amblyopia. Br J Ophthalmol 1981; 65: 575–7.
21. Rahi JS, Logan S, Timms C, et al. Risk, causes, and outcomes of visual impairment after loss of vision in the non-amblyopic eye: a population-based study. Lancet 2002; 360: 597–602.
22. Konig HH, Barry JC. Economic evaluation of different methods of screening for amblyopia in kindergarten. Pediatrics 2002; 109: e59.
23. Membreno JH, Brown MM, Brown GC, et al. A cost-utility analysis of therapy for amblyopia. Ophthalmology 2002; 109: 2265–71.
24. Brown GC, Brown MM, Sharma S, et al. Cost-effectiveness of treatment for threshold retinopathy of prematurity. Pediatrics 1999; 104: e47.
25. Donahue SP, Arnold RW, Ruben JB. Preschool vision screening: what should we be detecting and how should we report it? Uniform guidelines for reporting results from studies of preschool vision screening. J AAPOS 2003; 7: 314–316.
26. Arnold RW, Gionet EG, Jastrzebski AI, et al. The Alaska Blind Child Discovery project: rationale, methods and results of 4,000 screenings. Alaska Med 2000; 42: 58–72.
27. Donahue SP, Johnson TM, Leonard-Martin TC. Screening for amblyogenic factors using a volunteer lay network and the MTI photoscreener. Initial results from 15,000 preschool children in a statewide effort. Ophthalmology 2000; 107: 1637–44.
28. Committee on Practice and Ambulatory Medicine and Section on Ophthalmology; American Academy of Pediatrics. Use of photo-screening for children's vision screening. Pediatrics 2002; 109: 524–5.
29. Cordonnier M, Kallay O. Non-cycloplegic screening for refractive errors in children with the hand-held autorefractor Retinomax: Final results and comparison with non-cycloplegic photoscreening. Strabismus 2001; 9: 59–70.
30. Zaba JN, Johnson RA, Reynolds WT. Vision examinations for all children entering public school—the new Kentucky law. Optometry 2003; 74: 149–58.
31. American Academy of Pediatrics Committee on Practice and Ambulatory Medicine and Section on Ophthalmology. American Association of Certified Orthoptists. American Association for Pediatric Ophthalmology and Strabismus. American Academy of Ophthalmology. Policy Statement: Eye examination in infants, children and young adults by pediatricians. Pediatrics 2003; 111: 902–7.

History, Examination, and Further Investigation

CHAPTER **9**

Susan H Day and David A Sami

ACCESS AND COMMUNICATION

Timely diagnosis and treatment is essential in pediatric ophthalmology: early recognition of media opacities in infants is critical; ocular tumors need early diagnosis for successful treatment. Service needs must be balanced so that lengthy waiting times for symptomatic children, and especially infants, and those with predisposing conditions are avoided. Office personnel should involve the ophthalmologist if there are any doubts about the urgency of the appointment.

Parents should be advised to bring along baby pictures of the child. Old photos documenting abnormal head posture or unequal red reflex can guide diagnosis and management decisions.

GETTING THE HISTORY

Babies are often referred to the ophthalmologist to answer a seemingly simple question: Does this child see? And if so, how well?

A significant part of a child's motor and social development is vision dependent. Thus, developmental delay may be rooted in poor vision. Conversely, a child with poor growth and development may have abnormalities of the optic nerve and the visual pathways as part of an underlying syndrome (e.g., septo-optic-dysplasia). Perhaps the simplest and most open-ended question to pose is "Are you, or your doctor concerned about any aspect of your child's health and development?" Such a question might elicit a response that, for instance, the child has had a special hearing test, alerting the clinician to possible associated conditions such as retinitis pigmentosa and Waardenburg and Alport syndromes.

Exposure to toxic or infectious agents during pregnancy, in particular toxoplasmosis, rubella, cytomegalovirus, herpes (ToRCH), may be associated with ocular abnormalities. If a congenital infection is suspected, assessment of HIV risk factors is important (see Chapter 23). Confirming appropriate maternal immunizations is also relevant. Any history of fever or rash during pregnancy should be sought. Any history of prematurity and hospitalization should be noted. A review of medications, in particular anticonvulsants, during pregnancy or while breast-feeding should be made. These questions must be carefully phrased, as parents may blame themselves unnecessarily for a congenital defect.

Parents are perceptive of the baby's vision in an intuitive fashion. Beyond intuitive ideas of how good the vision is, they should be questioned about habits directly related to vision or behavior that implies poor sight. The physician must be cautious in considering behavior as vision generated whenever the stimulus also makes a noise. A baby with poor eyesight may stare at bright lights, have flickering eyelid movements, and develop nystagmus noticeable to the parent. Such infants may exhibit eye poking (see Fig. 52.6) or hand waving in front of their eyes. Parents often report that the child does not smile or seems disinterested in his/her environment, and may sit with the chin tucked. Eye contact and mimicking of facial expressions are a profound component of the emotional bond between parent and child in the first months of life.

In older children play habits become important. Normal children often like to be close to an object of interest, such as the TV screen or comic book–presumably due to:

1. Their desire to be immersed in the activity on the screen; and
2. Their ability to accommodate more fully and maintain focus at a shorter viewing distance.

"Near behavior" becomes concerning when the child sits so close that an entire view is not possible without moving the head. A child with poor vision may hold toys within 2–5.5 cm (1–2 inches) of one or both eyes, inspecting the toy in a way that maximizes his or her vision.

Children who are born with poor vision are not likely to tell you that their vision is poor. Children who acquire poor vision will usually only volunteer that they are unable to see well if the visual loss is bilateral. Unilateral visual loss, either acute or chronic, is usually not noticed by a young child unless or until the other eye becomes involved.

Apparent visual difficulty may be present in very specific circumstances, such as in dim or bright illumination. In the former case, the child may become very irritated when the night-light is turned off or has inordinate difficulty in finding his or her way around in dimly-lit situations. Conversely, children with poor photopic vision may hate going outside, insist on protection from the sun, and may prefer to play in more dimly lit areas of an otherwise well-lit room (see Chapters 52 and 53).

An older child should be included in the discussion; valuable information is offered, and rapport is established, which leads to better cooperation during the examination.

APPROACH TO THE EXAM

The doctor's image portrayed when the child is initially seen must be carefully considered. Many pediatric ophthalmologists prefer not to wear a traditional white laboratory coat. Talking directly to the older child (rather than to the parents) initially also focuses the attention appropriately on the patient.

The clinical examination starts with observation of the child as the history is being taken. Is the child interested in his surroundings, does he notice small objects around him? Take note of the child's coordination and his physical habitus (abnormalities of ears, ocular adnexa and eyelids, facial asymmetry, etc.). Make note of any abnormal head posture. Causes of abnormal head position include strabismus, nystagmus with null-point, refractive error (usually astigmatism or myopia), homonymous hemianopia, and torticollis caused by muscular, skeletal, or neurologic deficit.

Retinoscopy and refraction

The retinoscope is an important tool of the pediatric ophthalmologist. Sitting at eye level and examining without touching help to allay the fears of an anxious child. With a few sweeps much information can be gathered regarding amblyogenic factors (media opacities, high refractive error, astigmatism, and anisometropia). Once the child is at ease a lens can be introduced in front of each eye (minimal or no touching required) to get a more accurate measure of refractive error (see Chapter 6).

Slit-lamp examination

Age is never a contraindication to slit-lamp examination.

For infants, the parent may be asked to support the baby in a prone position, with the palm steadying the chin. The parent is instructed to rest the baby's forehead against the slit-lamp headrest (Fig. 9.1). Young children may be supported in their parent's lap, or alternatively can reach the chinrest by placing knees on the exam chair. It may help to have an older sibling or parent demonstrate first to ease apprehension of the child. Older children often manage well by standing at the slit lamp.

Slit-lamp examination is indispensable in evaluation of corneal abnormalities, congenital glaucoma, anterior segment dysgenesis, and iris abnormalities (e.g., transillumination defects in albinism and Lisch nodules in neurofibromatosis), and in children at risk for uveitis (e.g., juvenile rheumatoid arthritis).

Funduscopy

Indirect ophthalmoscopy with a 28-diopter lens followed by closer inspection with a direct ophthalmoscope permits a good balance of "macro and micro" views. Subtle abnormalities of the optic nerve and nerve fiber layer may be missed by indirect examination, especially when a 28-diopter lens is the only one used.

Children over 6 months old can have their pupils dilated with either cyclopentolate 1% or tropicamide 1%, one drop instilled into the conjunctival sac. Infants with dark irides may be difficult to dilate: Tropicamide may be more effective than cyclopentolate. Phenylephrine 2.5% may be used as well. For infants, especially under 6 months, cyclopentolate 0.5% should be used.

Phenylephrine 10% should not be used in children as it may precipitate life-threatening cardiovascular consequences. (See Chapter 6.)

Fundus examination in an uncooperative child can be very challenging. Some children will tolerate the red free light more easily. Suggest that by looking in the eyes you can guess what the child had for breakfast, or describe parts of an animal in the fundus, asking the child to help identify it. Sometimes it helps to demonstrate on parents, to show that it is not painful. If all else fails, note "difficult exam" or "inadequate view" and schedule a second visit.

Examination under sedation (EUS) and examination under anesthesia (EUA)

In children with potential vision-threatening disease (e.g., congenital glaucoma) who cannot cooperate with the examination, an oral form of sedation such as chloral hydrate may be considered (50 mg/kg). Oral sedation usually permits checking of intraocular pressure, and use of a speculum. When tissue manipulation is necessary, oral sedation will likely be insufficient, and a general anesthetic will have to be administered (EUA). Diagnostic intraocular pressure measurements should be made prior to tracheal intubation. The risks of sedation and general anesthesia are similar.

Ultrasound and neuroimaging

High-resolution ultrasound is important for evaluation of anterior segment dysgenesis and preoperative planning. A B-scan

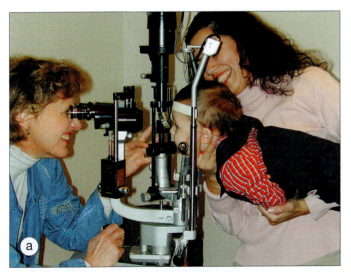
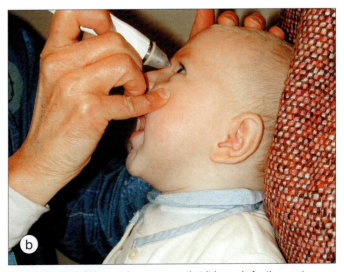

Fig. 9.1 (a) Method for examining infants at the slit lamp. First, the ophthalmologist sets up the slit-lamp microscope so that it is ready for the most important task (i.e., looking for transillumination using a coaxial beam). While the parent (or clinic assistant) holds the baby with the left arm under his tummy, she places his head on the white strap, continually encouraging him. (b) Tono-Pen tonometry. After instillation of an anesthetic drop, the tonometer, with a disposable sheath over the contact point, is briefly touched on the cornea and a digital readout of the intraocular pressure is obtained. (Photo by Dr Hung Pham.)

ultrasound should be performed when media opacities preclude examination of the posterior pole. Ultrasound can often be performed without sedation. Ultrasound should not be performed if a ruptured globe is suspected (see Chapter 12).

Neuroimaging in children often implies the need for a general anesthetic, and the risks associated with it. Magnetic resonance imaging is generally preferred for evaluation of orbital soft tissue disease and demyelinating disease. Computed tomography is typically used in the setting of trauma and for detection of calcific changes associated with retinoblastoma (see Chapter 13).

Examination of the premature baby

This is usually done in a neonatal care unit. The pupils of a premature baby may be difficult to dilate. A combination drop, such as Cyclomydril (cyclopentolate 0.2%, phenylephrine 0.1%), repeated once after 5–10 minutes generally works well. Systemic effects of eye drops may be significant in premature babies.

The major concern is often about retinopathy of prematurity. This should not detract attention from other ocular abnormalities such as anterior segment dysgenesis, congenital glaucoma, and optic nerve defects (see Chapter 51).

The list of equipment needed includes retinoscope (to assess clarity of media and refractive symmetry–slight vitreous haze may be normal in the premature infant), hand-held slit lamp, indirect ophthalmoscope with 20- or 30-diopter lens, scleral depressor or cotton tipped applicator, pediatric size speculum, and portable tonometer (Fig. 9.1b).

ASSESSING THE VISION OF INFANTS

Fixation assessment and CSM notation

Accurate quantification of visual acuity in an infant is difficult.

A popular method for assessment and notation is the CSM method:

Assessment

1. With both eyes uncovered, observations are made for a manifest deviation, alternation of fixation, or abnormal movements (unsteady fixation, nystagmus, or searching eye movements).
2. One eye is covered for about 3 seconds, the fixation behavior of the uncovered eye is observed, and then the covered eye is uncovered.
3. The other eye is then covered for about 3 seconds, the fixation behavior of the uncovered eye is observed, and then the covered eye is uncovered.

Notation

"C" for *central* or foveal fixation is assessed by the corneal light reflex when the other eye is covered;

"S" for *steady* fixation of a still target or one that is moved slightly with the other eye covered. If the left eye is covered and the right eye takes up central fixation steadily, the notation used is "Steady" (S).

"M" for *maintained* fixation is the ability of the child to maintain fixation with the same eye when the other is *un*covered. The position should be maintained at least through the next blink.

"C" and "S" are monocular tests, while "M" is essentially binocular.

For example, a child with right esotropia, right amblyopia, and eccentric fixation without latent or other nystagmus and a normal left eye will likely show uncentral (UC) but steady (S) fixation

with the right eye, but will switch fixation from the right to the preferred left eye once the occluder is removed from the left eye (unmaintained, or UM). This is noted as "Right eye: UC, S, UM. Left eye: CSM." If there is very poor fixation and latent or other nystagmus the right eye will be unsteady (US).

"CSM vision" does not necessarily imply normal visual acuity for age, as it may not detect bilateral visual disability. In cases of unequal visual loss, pronounced objection to the occlusion of one eye as opposed to the other may be an important clue.

Testing babies with very poor vision

In infants with very poor vision, testing the vestibulo-ocular reflex may be useful. The mother may be asked to support the infant with his head resting on her shoulder and to spin around several times. In a normal infant on cessation of spinning there are normally a few beats of nystagmus before the child regains fixation. If vision is very poor or in the presence of severe cerebellar disease there will be prolonged "after-nystagmus."

In the most severe cases the question may be whether the baby can see light at all. Assessing blink response to a bright flash may be useful in this situation. The threat response in the first months of life is generally not reliable.

PUPIL INSPECTION

Abnormalities of the pupillary response to light are generally attributable to diseases of the anterior visual pathway (anterior to chiasm). Media opacities such as cataracts and vitreous hemorrhage generally do not produce a relative afferent pupillary defect (RAPD). *Relative* is the key term here: a child with one blind eye will have equally sized pupils, but unequal reaction to light. It is best to use a bright source of light in a dark room. There are reports of RAPD in amblyopia.[1] The finding is generally subtle. Any difference in pupil size >1 mm (anisocoria) should be noted and investigated. (See Chapter 67 for discussion of pupil abnormalities.)

Pupil reactivity to light is generally absent prior to 29 weeks gestation, and should be detectable by 32 weeks.[2,3]

Older children are prone to accommodate on the light source. Remind the child to look at a distant target and be vigilant for ocular convergence, which can tip off the examiner to accommodation.

Inevitably, parents are curious about the color of their child's eyes. The evolution of iris pigmentation tends to be complete by 9–12 months; in many circumstances, eye color can be predicted much earlier on the basis of the color of the parents' eyes as well as the relative degree of pigmentation of the neonate's eyes. Conditions that result in lightening of the eyes with age are rare; thus, it is fairly safe to provide this information to parents.

ESTIMATING ACUITY IN THE PREVERBAL CHILD

Standard methods of visual acuity testing can rarely be used before the age of 3 years. Near acuity tests, especially with picture optotypes, can often be performed at a young age and should be attempted in cooperative 18- to 24-month-old children.

There are three basic methods for estimating visual acuity in the preverbal or impaired child: optokinetic nystagmus (OKN), preferential looking (PL), and visually evoked potentials (VEP).

Optokinetic nystagmus (OKN)

Although of historic interest, OKN testing is now rarely used in clinical practice.

OKN technique was modified to measure vision in infants, with acuity measured as the finest grating on a rotating drum that elicited a visible nystagmus response.[4] Electroculography was used to increase the sensitivity of detection.[5]

Pitfalls of OKN testing include:

1. The absence of an OKN response to a moving stripe may represent nothing more than a lack of interest or attention; and
2. Equating detection of visual stripes (a task of *resolution* acuity and processing of movement) with a recognition (e.g., Snellen chart) acuity may not be valid.[6]

Preferential looking (PL)

Infants demonstrate a greater tendency to look at a patterned stimulus than a homogeneous field. This assumption has been extended to regard grating or interference patterns too fine to be resolved as similar in arousing interest to a homogenous field. Normal values for development of "acuity" in the first year of life were estimated by identifying spatial stripe frequencies that were fixated longer than a homogeneous field by 75% of infants at a given age.[7] The statistical reliability of this approach was improved by developing a "two-alternative, forced choice, preferential looking test."[8] In this modification the observer is masked to the positions of the striped and homogeneous field, forcing him to predict if the striped stimulus is on the right or left by judging the child's fixation behavior. Thus, it is the observer who is forced to make a choice, not the infant! Often multiple trials are required to arrive at stable acuity thresholds (Fig. 9.2).

Acuity cards were developed in an attempt to make PL more applicable to a busy clinic setting.[9] The cards are large rectangles with grating patterns on each end. One grating is above the resolution limit and the other has variable spatial frequencies. In this paradigm the examiner is not masked to the location of the gratings (Fig. 9.3). Judging preferential left or right gaze in children with horizontal nystagmus can be difficult. Holding the cards vertically may permit more accurate assessment.

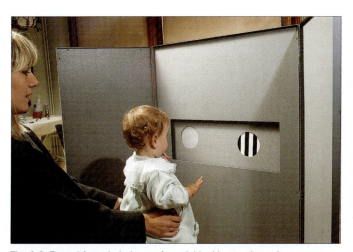

Fig. 9.2 Formal forced-choice preferential looking testing using a screen to hide the examiner. The child is sat on the parent's lap and the examiner shows the series of cards (in this case Keeler cards) while observing the child's responses through the peephole between the test cards.

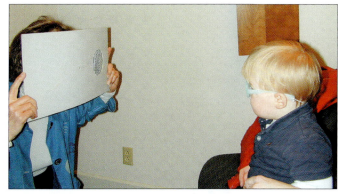

Fig. 9.3 Acuity card technique. To minimize distraction of the child, the examiner "hides" behind the acuity card and observes the child's behavior through a small peephole in the center of the card. Using, in this case Teller cards, the child is presented with two targets on a homogeneous background, one of which matches the background, the other of which contains gratings. If the infant responds by turning the eyes or the head toward the striped target as they are simultaneously presented, then this response is interpreted as an ability of the child to see the target. The child is then presented with progressively smaller gratings until the examiner believes the grating targets are no longer eliciting a response different from the homogeneous targets. Photo by Dr Hung Pham.

PL grating acuity is a resolution, and not a recognition (e.g., Snellen chart), task. In amblyopic children (especially strabismic amblyopia) resolution acuity is characteristically better than recognition acuity. This is also true for children with foveal abnormalities.[10]

Visually evoked potentials (see Chapter 11)

Failure to fixate preferentially on a grating pattern does not automatically imply that a child cannot resolve the pattern. This is particularly relevant for children with motor developmental disabilities, ocular motor apraxia, and cortical visual impairment (CVI); VEPs may then be particularly useful for assessing visual function.[11]

The VEP may be thought of as a transient electroencephalogram (EEG) from which background cerebral "noise" is subtracted to give information regarding surface occipital lobe electrical activity. In general, two types of stimuli, the unpatterned and the patterned, can evoke visual cortical potentials. The quantification of infant vision is limited to patterned stimuli, which in general are bar, checkerboard, or sinusoidal gratings.[12] Correction of any significant refractive errors prior to testing is essential.[13]

Pattern reversal VEP technique (Fig. 9.4) has suggested maturation of 20/20 equivalent grating resolution between the ages of 6 and 12 months. The swept VEP technique, which relies upon extrapolation of the VEP signal generated by a "sweeping" of grating size from large to small in 10 seconds, also suggests this tempo of infant vision development.[14-16] In general VEP acuity thresholds overestimate OKN and PL "acuities" (Table 9.1). This discrepancy may be pronounced in children with developmental delay.[6]

Important features of the VEP waveform are the amplitude of the first positive wave and the implicit time (time between stimulus presentation and peak of the first positive wave). As the grating pattern becomes finer, the peak amplitude decreases and the implicit time increases. The finest grating that elicits a waveform detectibly different from a blank (luminance-matched) screen is the threshold "acuity."

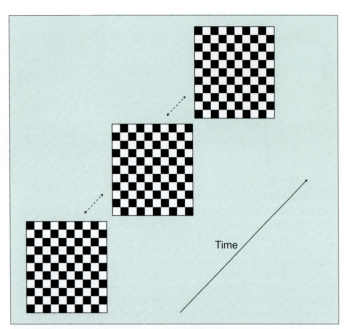

Fig. 9.4 Schematic for pattern-reversal VEP paradigm. The pattern in each square (which can be altered in size) reverses with time. (See Chapter 11.)

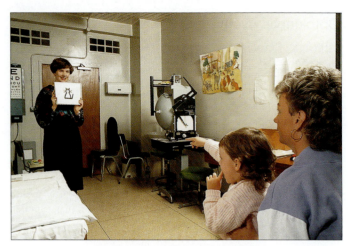

Fig. 9.5 The Kay picture test. The test card is held by the examiner and the child is encouraged to identify the figure being shown or to match it on a card held by the parent. Single, Snellen-equivalent figures and crowded and uncrowded logMAR cards are available. They have cultural limitation due to their being recognition tests.

Table 9.1 Comparison of Visual Acuity development* in the 1st year of life as measured by Optokinetic nystagmus (OKN), Preferential Looking (PL), and Visually evoked potentials (VEP).

	Age 1–2 mo	Age 6–8 mo	Age 10–12 mo	Age at "20/20 acuity"
Modality	Acuity	Acuity	Acuity	
OKN	20/400	20/100	20/60	24–30 mo
PL	20/400	20/100	20/50	18–24 mo
VEP	20/100	20/25	20/20	6–12 mo

*Extrapolation of resolution acuity to recognition acuity may not be valid in all children.

Extrapolating resolution acuity to recognition (e.g., Snellen) acuity may not be valid. The VEP threshold acuity is perhaps best interpreted as an acuity potential, since it does not give information regarding higher order cortical visual processing.

OPTOTYPE TESTING

Optotype testing of visual acuity is usually not possible until 2–3 years of age. An optotype is a symbol that when correctly identified at a given distance (i.e., a particular subtended angle) permits quantification of acuity. Although some children are able to recognize a few letters by the age of 4 years, the complexities of Snellen visual acuity testing may make it unreliable before the age of 6–8 years. Failure to see a line on the chart must raise the question as to whether the child knows what the letter is.

With children, the E game has limitations. First, a child's coordination and left–right discrimination may present apparently inaccurate answers. Some examiners will therefore ignore any miss when left is confused with right. Second, the test is inherently repetitive, and the child's attention span may fall short of the examiner's needs.

Picture optotype testing (e.g., Allen figures, Kay picture test) may be most appropriate for the 2- to 5-year-old age group (Fig. 9.5). One adaptation of optotype testing is the matching technique (e.g., HOTV chart, Sheridan-Gardner single-optotype matching test) (Fig. 9.6). This permits a child to identify an optotype even if he/she does not know its name.

"Poor acuity" may be as much a reflection of visual ability as the child's attention span or lack of interest in the test. The examination must be more of a game than a test, with reinforcement and reward for positive responses. Control of parental coaching must be maintained. Several tries at different times may be necessary. Extraneous competition for the child's attention by active siblings, ringing telephones, or unnecessary movement must be kept at a bare minimum.

Snellen or M units vs logMAR

Although logMAR (log minimum angle of resolution) visual acuity charts (e.g., EDTRS chart) have become the standard for visual acuity testing in clinical research, many clinicians continue to use Snellen acuities in daily practice.

LogMAR visual acuity charts have inherent advantages over traditional Snellen acuity charts.[17,18] These include:

1. Reduced test–retest variability of acuity measurement across the acuity range: with logMAR charts, one can establish a minimum "significant" change regardless of the underlying acuity. As there are equal number of letters in each line, missing 2 letters is just as significant in the 20/40 line as it is on the 20/80 line. This is in contrast to traditional Snellen charts where the number of letters per line increases as the visual acuity line improves. The nongeometric progression of letter sizes in a Snellen chart also adds to difficulty in determining "significant change."

2. From a research standpoint, the nongeometric progression of the Snellen fraction complicates parametric statistical analysis as compared to a log scale.

3. Snellen acuity data may be converted to logMAR by taking a base 10 log of the reciprocal of the Snellen acuity fraction. For example a Snellen acuity of 20/30 = 6/9; 9/6=1.5; $\log^{1.5}$ = 0.18 logMAR.

4. Lack of a systematic approach to letter legibility and "crowding" (see below) in Snellen charts as compared to logMAR charts.

In an effort to promote use of logMAR visual acuity charts investigators have developed more compact logMAR charts for

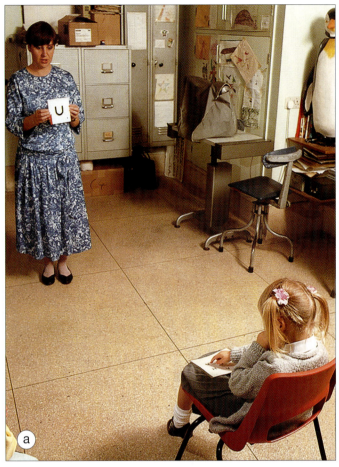

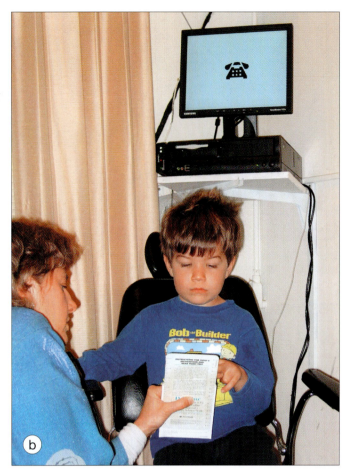

Fig. 9.6 Acuity testing. (a) Sheridan-Gardner single-optotype matching test. Matching optotypes, such as the Sheridan-Gardner single-optotype matching test shown here, cannot be used with children as young as those who can use the picture optotypes but they are nearer to Snellen acuity because recognition is less important. Single-letter tests tend to overestimate acuities in amblyopes. (b) Testing near vision with age-appropriate reading material is an important assessment especially when considering the child's educational needs.

routine clinical use.[19] Still, some clinicians feel that a visual acuity fraction (M units or Snellen acuity) with testing distance in the numerator and letter size in the denominator is more intuitive.

Crowding

Some normal children and even adults achieve better visual acuity results when tested with a single optotype than a line of letters (Fig. 9.6a). This effect is particularly pronounced in amblyopia.[20]

The phenomenon of crowding is more problematic with traditional Snellen charts in which the spacing between letters is not uniform. This phenomenon is less pronounced with logMAR charts.[21]

TESTING COLOR VISION

In a busy clinical setting, color vision testing is practical when it is quick to perform and is simple for the child to understand. This probably accounts for the popularity of the following.

Pseudoisochromatic plates

Ishihara plates (Fig. 9.7a) screen for moderate-to-severe congenital red–green deficiency, but do not test blue–yellow

deficits. Blue–yellow defects may be a feature of acquired diseases such as optic neuritis, retinitis pigmentosa, chorioretinitis, and diabetic retinopathy. It is estimated that 8% of boys have a red–green deficit. Use of the Ishihara plates to test for an acquired deficit (e.g., as the sequelae of optic neuritis) in this subgroup is inappropriate.[22]

City University color vision test

The City University color vision test (Fig. 9.7b) is adaptable to testing children, since the response does not depend on pattern recognition but rather on the identification of individual dots. The child must identify which of four different-colored spots is nearer the same color as the spot around which they are grouped.

Other tests

One can also keep a group of different-colored socks and ask the child to pick out the two which match. Color naming may be useful but should be interpreted with caution because many young children with normal color vision are rather poor at naming colors.

More detailed testing with an anomaloscope, Farnsworth Munsell, or its more simple derivative, the D15 test, can more accurately quantify a color vision defect in an older child.

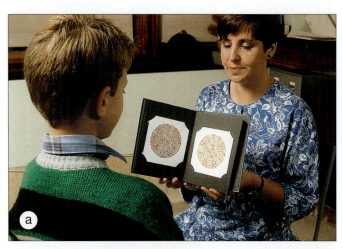
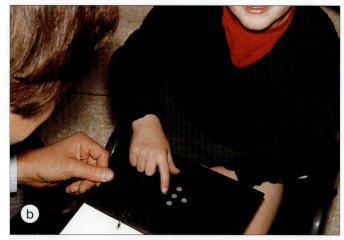

Fig. 9.7 Color vision testing. (a) The commonly used Ishihara test detects red–green defects only. (b) The City University color test. The child must identify which of four colored spots is nearer in color to the central spot.

TESTING CONTRAST SENSITIVITY

Contrast sensitivity may not reach adult levels until age 8 years. One of the problems with contrast testing in children is that age-matched norms have not been well established. Contrast sensitivity testing may be useful in detecting previous optic neuritis in the absence of other signs. From a low-vision perspective contrast sensitivity has been shown to be an important predictor of reading speed, which may have important implications for school-aged children.[23] Examples of contrast sensitivity tests include the Pelli-Robson chart and "Mr. Happy."[24]

ASSESSING VISUAL FIELDS

Although formal assessment of visual fields (e.g., Goldmann, Humphrey) in young children is difficult, confrontation techniques can give the examiner a good idea of significant field defects. The examiner faces the patient and attracts the child's attention centrally; then a toy or light is introduced silently from the periphery. A child with normal fields will make a quick head or eye movement in the direction of the stimulus (Fig. 9.8). Keep in mind that a "boring stimulus" could give the false impression of a field defect. Finger counting or detection of "which finger is wiggling" may be used for older, cooperative children (Fig. 9.9). When in doubt visually evoked response testing may reveal a hemianopic defect. Older children when instructed appropriately can perform reliable Goldmann perimetry (Fig. 9.10).

STRABISMUS

Strabismus is a common referral diagnosis in children. One must constantly keep in mind the interplay between strabismus and amblyopia. In general, the oculomotor examination gives information about the function of cranial nerves III, IV, and VI, as well as the supranuclear control of eye movements (see Chapters 73–90).

Assessing the corneal light reflex

In infancy, assessment of the corneal light reflex (Hirschberg) is the simplest estimate of ocular alignment. One must keep in mind the tendency for children to have a nasal displacement of the corneal light reflex or "positive angle kappa."

Hirschberg

A point source of light is used to assess symmetry of the corneal reflex. The normal corneal reflex is just nasal to the center of the cornea. A small tropia may be easily missed by this method. Grossly, 1-mm decentration of the corneal light reflex corresponds to 15 prism diopters of deviation (or 7°). Assuming a 4-mm pupil, a light reflex at the papillary border would be 2 mm or 30 prism diopters from the center. A light reflex in the mid-iris region is estimated to be 4 mm or 60 prism diopters from the center. Esotropia displaces the reflex temporal and exotropia displaces the reflex nasal (Fig. 9.11). The light source should be in the same line as the examiner's eye. The child should fix not on the light source but preferably on a small, accommodative target, such as a small picture. With this type of stimulus, an accommodative component of the strabismus can more easily be elicited.

Krimsky

A prism is used to center the corneal reflex. This technique is useful for estimating deviation of a nonfixing eye.

Cover–uncover and cross-cover testing

Cover–uncover and cross-cover testing are used to confirm strabismus (Fig. 9.12). These tests may be difficult to perform, since control of fixation is mandatory and often children tend to refixate randomly. When available it is best to use a clear plastic occluder, which is less threatening than a black plastic occluder and allows the observer to monitor the occluded eye. The clear plastic blurs vision enough to permit accurate measurement.

If the child is cooperative and has relatively good vision in both eyes, the cover test is probably the most accurate method for measuring strabismus. The test does not depend on corneal light reflection. Cover–uncover testing permits the examiner to distinguish the type (phoria versus tropia) and the direction (eso, exo, hyper, hypo) of the strabismus. Cross-cover (or alternate-cover) testing is performed by placing the occluder in front of one eye and then quickly moving it to the other eye before fusion can be regained. This may reveal a greater amount of deviation than was apparent with cover–uncover testing. Progressive prism

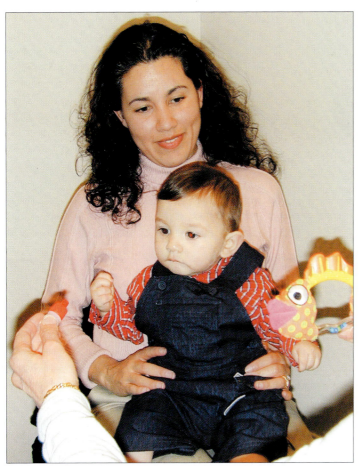
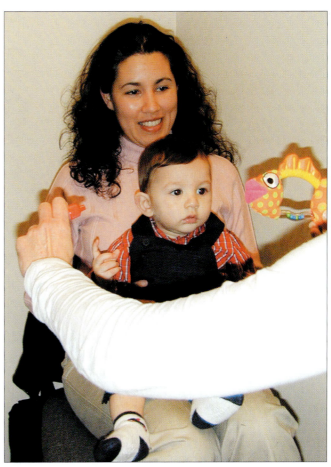

Fig. 9.8 Assessing the visual field of infants. The tester attracts the baby's attention to a toy (right) while bringing in an object, in this case a dropper bottle, silently from the child's right side to see whether the child's attention is drawn to it–which in this case (left) it is! Although seemingly crude, if defects are detected by these methods, they are likely to be functionally significant in the future. (Photo by Dr Hung Pham.)

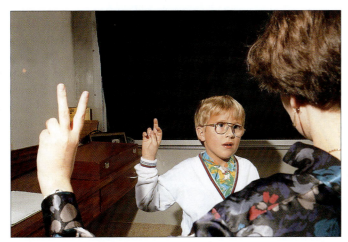

Fig. 9.9 Demonstration of finger counting technique to assess visual fields in older children. While the tester watches the fixation, the child tells her when the tester's fingers are wiggling or may watch or count the fingers if able to do so.

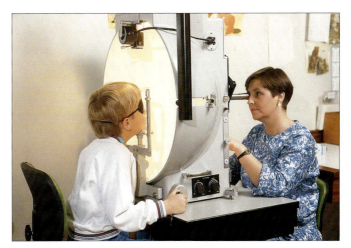

Fig. 9.10 Goldmann perimetry. Older children, with good attention, can be tested on more sophisticated devices such as the Goldmann field analyzer or various forms of automated field analyzer. (See Chapter 10.)

power is placed in front of the deviating eye until a refixation shift is no longer seen. Some children (in particular Asians) have prominent epicanthal folds. This may give a misleading impression of esotropia (pseudostrabismus), particularly when the folds are asymmetric. The symmetry of corneal light reflexes and cover testing should be normal.

A 4-diopter base-out prism

A 4-diopter base-out prism[25] may be used to uncover small angles of strabismus that may not be detected on cover testing. The prism is introduced over one eye while the child is fixing on a distant target. The response is a refixation movement. The test is

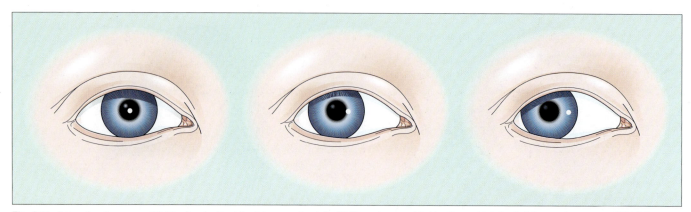

Fig. 9.11 Assessing the corneal light reflex by the Hirschberg method. (Left) Normal corneal light reflex, which is slightly nasal to center. (Middle) Approximately 30-prism-diopter exotropia. (Right) Approximately 60-prism-diopter exotropia.

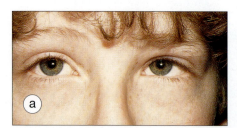
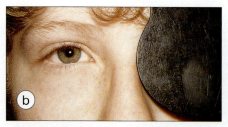
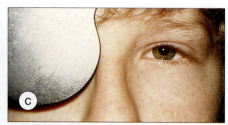

Fig. 9.12 Demonstration of cover test. (a) Note asymmetrical corneal light reflex, suggesting left esotropia. (b) No fixation shift of the right eye when the left eye is covered. (c) Left fixation movement (as evidenced by the light reflex in photograph, although the cover test does not depend on the corneal light reflection for measurement of strabismus) when right eye is covered. This test requires strict control of fixation.

then repeated with the prism held over the fellow eye. If there is a difference between the two eyes a refixation movement is made with the prism over the dominant eye only.

FUSION

Fusion has been artificially divided into stereopsis, sensory fusion, and motor fusion.

Stereopsis

Stereopsis, which mostly applies to near tasks, is a function of retinal disparity, and implies at least reasonably good visual acuity in both eyes. The absence of stereopsis though does not necessarily imply poor visual acuity.[26] Stereopsis is a function of retinal image disparity between the two eyes. It is not synonymous with "depth perception," which contains monocular clues (such as parallax and perspective).

In clinical practice, the Titmus fly and Randot stereopsis test remains the most commonly used form of assessment. A child wearing polarized lenses is asked to point to apparently elevated figures (Fig. 9.13). A stereo acuity of 60 seconds or better virtually proves bifoveal fusion.[27] The less-refined targets may be seen using monocular clues. Other tests use red–green goggles to create disparate images. The Lang and Frisby tests do not require any special glasses. The Lang test also has, on one of the plates, a figure that can be seen by children without binocular vision. The development of stereopsis appears to be most impressive between 3 and 7 months of age.[28]

Sensory fusion

Sensory fusion infers that corresponding retinal points are present in each eye that project to similar areas of the cortical visual map. When fusion is not present, then the abnormal binocular sensory states of diplopia, confusion, or suppression may be present.

Children with strabismus often develop a suppression scotoma of the nondominant eye to avoid diplopia. The size of the scotoma is thought to correlate with the severity of strabismus, amblyopia, and stereopsis. A child with stereo acuity for only the "fly" on the Titmus test will likely have a scotoma larger than that of a child with 100 seconds of stereo acuity. The Worth four-dot test may be used to grossly assess the size of this scotoma. The test is performed at distance and near. The child is instructed to wear a pair of glasses that contain a red filter over one eye and a green filter over the other. A white, a red, and two green circles of light are presented and the child is asked to name the number and color of the lights. When fusion is present, four circles are seen, with the white target changing colors due to retinal rivalry. When diplopia is present, five circles are seen. Suppression results in the child seeing two or three lights, depending on which eye is suppressed. The test subtends 1.25° of the central visual field at 6 m, and 6° at $\frac{1}{3}$ m[27]. The examiner should walk toward the patient with the flash-light until 4 lights are seen. This should give the clinician an idea of the size of the suppression scotoma (Fig. 9.14).

Another way to elicit a suppression scotoma is with Bagolini striated lenses. A point source of light is used and the child is asked to draw the lines in the air just as he sees them. Children with bifoveal fusion see a complete X. If central suppression is present, it will appear as a break in the line corresponding to the suppressing eye. If there is total suppression only one arm of the X will be seen (Fig. 9.15).

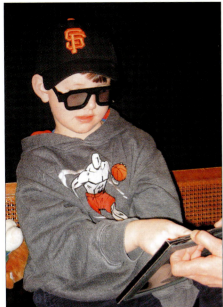
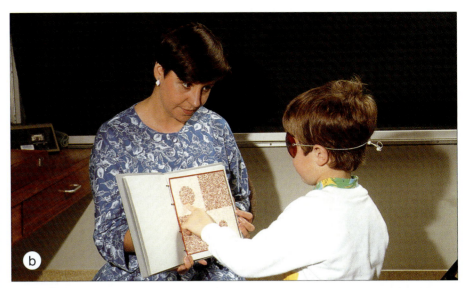
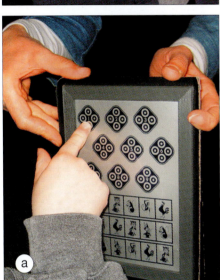
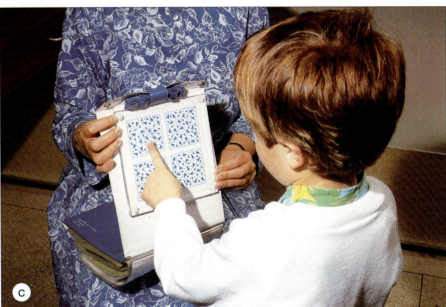

Fig. 9.13 Stereopsis testing. (a) The Titmus stereoacuity test requires the use of Polaroid glasses with the plane of polarization at right angles to each other in the spectacles. The child identifies which circle in 9 groups of four circles is standing forward from the others. Three rows of animal figures can be used for younger children. (Photo by Dr Hung Pham.) (b) Other stereoacuity tests use a red–green system for creating the disparity between the eyes, which allows the child to see shapes on the test card. This child is viewing the demonstration plate. (c) The Frisby test does not require glasses; instead the figures in a central panel of one of the test squares are printed on the other side of the Perspex sheets so that the child can only see it if he or she has binocular depth perception. In this picture this is demonstrated by the flashgun's shadow cast by the test figure to which the child points. The thickness of the Perspex varies; the thicker plates give greater disparity and therefore are easier to see.

Motor fusion

Motor fusion refers to vergence movements. Fusional vergences measure the ability of a child to converge or diverge behind a changing prism to maintain retinal correspondence. An example is the 4-prism-diopter base-out test.

Retinal correspondence

Retinal correspondence refers to the point-to-point coupling of retinal receptor fields with cortical visual maps. With early-onset strabismus, the normal retinal receptor fields may be reordered as a possible adaptation to improve binocularity (anomalous retinal correspondence). In this setting fusional vergences are typically poor.

Screening
SUMMARY

The taking of the history is the beginning of a good eye examination in infants and children. A detailed history of vision behavior may give the ophthalmologist an accurate refinement of where to look for pathology. The mood set by taking a history helps to establish rapport with the child, which makes examination more fun for the child and more rewarding for the doctor.

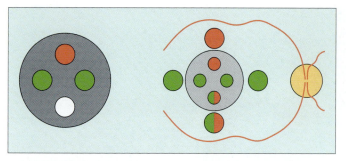

Assessment of visual function includes visual acuity, ocular alignment, visual fields, color vision, and afferent pupillary function. Whenever there is any question of possible vision-threatening disease the ophthalmologist must be persistent in performing an adequate examination and using sedation or even a general anesthetic if necessary. The pediatric ophthalmic exam can become engaging and fun when the physician develops the skills necessary to be playful with children while completing a detailed exam.

Fig. 9.14 Worth four-dot test. A flashlight with a screen containing 4 small circles of light (one white, one red, and two green, left of picture) is presented to the child who is wearing a green lens over one eye and a red lens over the other. When normal fusion is present, 4 lights are seen: 1 red, 2 green, and one that changes or flickers (the white light) due to retinal rivalry. What would the lights look like to a child with a right small-angle esotropia (i.e., right central suppression scotoma) who is wearing a green lens over the right eye and a red lens over the left eye? At distance the green lights fall within suppression scotoma of the right eye, and 2 red lights are reported. As the target is brought closer, the 4 circles will subtend a greater visual angle and are seen outside the suppression scotoma. What if the same child was wearing the red lens over the right eye and the green lens over the left eye? At distance the red light falls within the suppression scotoma and 3 green lights are reported.

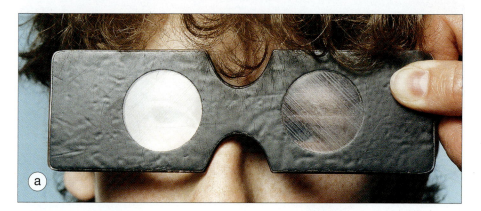

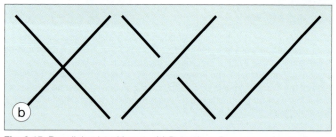

Fig. 9.15 Bagolini striated lenses. (a) Detection of a suppression scotoma with Bagolini striated lenses. Note that the striations in the right and left eye are perpendicular to each other. A point source of light is used and the child is asked to draw the lines in the air just as he sees them. (b) Children with bifoveal fusion see a complete X. If central suppression is present, it will appear as a break in the line corresponding to the suppressing eye. If there is total suppression only one arm of the X will be seen (see text).

REFERENCES

1. Greenwald MJ, Folk ER. Afferent papillary defects in amblyopia. J Pediatr Ophthalmol Strabismus 1983; 20: 63–7.
2. Robinson A, Fielder AR. Pupillary diameter and reaction to light in preterm neonates. Arch Dis Child 1990; 65: 35–8.
3. Isenberg SJ, Dang Y, Jotterand V. The pupils of term and preterm infants. Am J Ophthalmol 1989; 108: 75–9.
4. Gorman JJ, Cogan DG, Gellis SS. An apparatus for grading the visual acuity of infants on the basis of opticokinetic nystagmus. Pediatrics 1957; 19: 1088–92.
5. Dayton GO, Jones MH, Aiu P, et al. Developmental study of coordinated eye movements in the human infant. I. Visual acuity in the newborn human: a study based on induced optokinetic nystagmus recorded by electrooculography. Arch Ophthalmol 1964; 71: 865–70.
6. Lamkin JC. Can this baby see? Estimation of visual acuity in the preverbal child. Int Ophth Clinics 1992; 32: 1–23.
7. Frantz RL. Pattern vision in young infants. Psychol Rec 1958; 8: 43–7.
8. Teller DY, Morse R, Borton R, et al. Visual acuity for vertical and diagonal gratings in human infants. Vision Res 1974; 14: 1433–9.
9. Teller DT, McDonald MA, Preston K, et al. Assessment of visual acuity in infants and children: the acuity card procedure. Dev Med Child Neurol 1986; 28: 779–89.
10. Mayer DL, Fulton AB, Roder D. Grating and recognition acuities of pediatric patients. Ophthalmology 1984; 91: 947–53.
11. Good WV. Development of a quantitative method to measure vision in children with chronic cortical visual impairment. Trans Am Ophth Soc 2001; 99: 253–69.
12. Sokol S. Visually evoked potentials: theory, techniques and clinical applications. Surv Ophthalmol 1976; 21: 18–44.
13. Millodot M, Riggs LA. Refraction determined electrophysiologically: responses to alternation of visual contours. Arch Ophthalmol 1970; 84: 272–8.
14. Marg E, Freeman DN, Peltzman P, et al. Visual acuity development in human infants: evoked potential measurements. Invest Ophthalmol Vis Sci 1976; 15: 150.
15. Sokol S, Dobson V. Pattern reversal visually evoked potentials in infants. Invest Ophthalmol Vis Sci 1976; 15: 58–62.
16. Norcia A, Tyler C. Spatial frequency sweep VEP: visual acuity during the first year of life. Vision Res 1985; 25: 1399–408.
17. Sloan LL. Needs for precise measures of visual acuity. Arch Ophthalmol 1980; 98: 286–90.
18. Rosser DA, Laidlaw DAH, Murdoch IE. The development of a "reduced logMAR" visual acuity chart of use in routine clinical practice. Br J Ophthalmol 2001; 85: 432–6.
19. Laidlaw DAH, Abbot A, Rosser DA. Development of a clinically feasible logMAR alternative to the Snellen chart: performance of the "compact reduced logMAR" visual acuity chart in amblyopic children. Br J Ophthalmol 2003; 87: 1232–4.
20. Morad Y, Werker E, Pinhas N. Visual acuity tests using chart, line and single optotye in healthy and amblyopic children. J AAPOS 1999; 3: 94–7.
21. Stuart J, Burian H. A study of separation difficulty: its relationship to visual acuity in normal and amblyopic eyes. Am J Ophthalmol 1962; 53: 471–7.
22. Kon CH, De Alwis D. A new colour vision test for clinical use. Eye 1996; 10: 65–74.
23. Leat SJ, Woodhouse JM. Reading performance with low vision aids: relationship with contrast sensitivity. Ophthal Physiol Optics 1993; 13: 9–16.
24. Leat SJ, Shute RH, Westall CA. Assessing Children's Vision. Contrast Sensitivity. London: Butterworth-Heinemann; 1999: 194–215.
25. Jampolsky A. The prism test for strabismus screening. J Pediatr Ophthalmol Strabismus 1964; 1: 30–3.
26. Donzis P, Rapazzo J, Burde R, et al. Effect of binocular variations of Snellen's visual acuity on Titmus stereoacuity. Arch. Ophthalmol 1983; 101: 930–2.
27. Moody EA. Ophthalmic examination of infants and children. In: Harley RD, editor. Pediatric Ophthalmology. 2nd ed. Philadelphia: Saunders; 1983: 108–33.
28. Teller D, Movshon A. Visual development. Vision Res 1986; 26: 1483–521.

CHAPTER
10 Visual Fields

D Luisa Mayer and Anne B Fulton

INTRODUCTION

Visual fields are tested in children, as in adults, to diagnose disease and monitor visual deficits. The impact of visual field loss on a child's daily life, mobility, and education cannot be overstated. Visual fields inform parents, teachers, and therapists regarding habilitation and education of infants and children.

Risk of visual field loss instigates referrals for perimetry in children, particularly those with retinal or neurological diseases, about which the perimetrist must have special knowledge. Every patient must be approached with a testable hypothesis about the visual fields.

This chapter will describe confrontation methods for infants and young and handicapped children, and Goldmann kinetic perimetry for preschool children. Automated static perimetry is appropriate for testing some older children. Goldmann visual fields of common defects in children are presented and discussed.

PROCEDURES

Children are not small adults and do not behave like adults. Even a sick child has a playful streak. The perimetrist must be creative and engaging to obtain cooperation and sustain attention. The chance of successful testing is improved if the test is a "game" and if there are positive reinforcements throughout the test.

CONFRONTATION TESTING

Confrontation testing is used to assess visual fields in patients who cannot participate in Goldmann perimetry. A preliminary confrontation test may guide strategies for perimetry. Confrontation methods afford efficient detection of large visual field cuts. Hemianopsia and quadrantanopsia can be appreciated. However, confrontation results are not quantitative. Small changes in visual fields cannot be appreciated reliably by confrontation testing. Descriptions of confrontation testing in adults are found in Harrington and Drake's[1] and Walsh's books.[2]

Essential elements of the confrontation test for young children are an interesting central stimulus, dynamic peripheral stimulus presentation, and observation of orienting eye and head movements to the peripheral stimulus.

To conduct the test:
1. Attract the child's gaze to a small toy or your face; smiles and gentle noises are attractive.
2. Present a small object on a slender stick peripherally in each quadrant.
3. Observe the child's orienting response toward the peripheral stimulus.

The confrontation "game" incorporates reinforcement for the child's orienting response. Reinforcement reduces boredom. Toddlers and handicapped children love games (Fig. 10.1a). For infants under 6 months and older infants with low vision, the examiner's face is a good central fixation target and a small translucent toy on a bright penlight, presented in dim room light, is a good peripheral stimulus.

Typically 12 or fewer trials are possible in an infant, and often the infant must be tested with binocular viewing. However, the child may not orient to the peripheral stimulus if the central stimulus is *too* interesting.[3,4]

SPECIAL PERIMETERS

Special perimeters and methods[5-7] provide an advantage over confrontation testing. Better control of stimulus presentation and monitoring of the child's fixation and responses are possible. These simple instruments were developed to study visual fields in normal infants. Objective and quantitative visual fields have been obtained using sound psychophysical methods in normals[5,6,8] and patients.[4,6,8-10]

Special perimeters used in the authors' clinics (Figs. 10.1b, 10.1c) evaluate children who cannot use the Goldmann perimeter due to age or disability. Static stimulus presentation is used,[11] and the fixation and orienting responses are monitored with a video camera.

GOLDMANN KINETIC PERIMETRY

Goldmann kinetic perimetry is the method of choice in cooperative children (see Table 10.1). Experience and familiarity with the Goldmann instrument are essential; its use is superbly illustrated in Anderson's textbook,[12] and visual field defects are likewise detailed in Harrington and Drake's[1] and Walsh's[2] manuals.

The Goldmann perimeter is designed for adults: small children need accommodations (Fig. 10.1d). The child must be comfortable and the head well positioned. Older children with physical disabilities are often testable in their wheelchairs.

Preparation for testing

Before testing, the examiner shows the child and parent what the child needs to do. Children perform well if the test is cast as a computer game. For example, the authors tell the child, "You are going to shoot the light (star, spaceship) with the buzzer."
1. Teach the child to give a quick response with the buzzer.

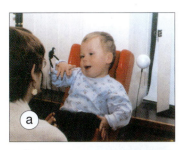

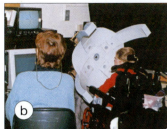

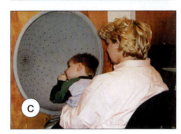

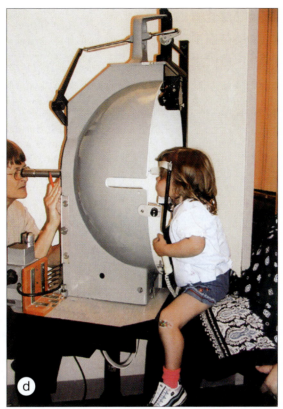

Fig. 10.1 Testing visual fields in young patients.
(a) Confrontation testing. The "Count," a small Dracula figure with wiggly legs and arms, is the central stimulus. The peripheral stimulus, a white Styrofoam sphere on a thin, black wand, is presented at an extreme eccentricity and moved centrally. When the child orients to the white ball, it is time to play and reinforce the orienting response. The Count attacks the white ball and "eats" it, accompanied by the examiner's commentary. The white ball is presented several times in each quadrant. This 21-month-old child had delayed myelination, hypotonia, and visual inattention, despite near normal grating acuity. He responded to the white sphere in all quadrants.
(b) Testing using an arc perimeter with lights embedded on four oblique meridia. A 6-year-old child with spastic quadraparesis and markedly reduced grating acuity is seated in his wheelchair. His seeing field was limited to the left superior quadrant.
(c) Testing with a hemispheric perimeter that has small lights embedded on 24 meridia. A 32-month-old child with neonatal hypoxic ischemic encephalopathy is seated on his parent's lap. He has a dense, inferior altitudinal hemianopic field defect, but normal grating acuity for age.
(d) Goldmann perimetry. A young child seated at the Goldmann perimeter on an adult's lap. Extra padding under the chin positioned her properly. In her left hand, she held the buzzer. The examiner (left side of photograph) monitored fixation through the telescope and presented the stimuli. At 4 years, her blind spots were enlarged due to chronic papilledema; her peripheral fields were full.

Table 10.1 The advantages of Goldmann perimetry in children

1) The child's fixation and responses can be monitored directly.
2) The examiner can communicate efficiently with the child, and reinforce fixation and responses.
3) Strategies for plotting visual fields are more flexible.

2. Open the shutter and project the V-4e target near the center of the bowl.
3. Demonstrate that the light in the bowl goes off the instant the buzzer sounds. (Be sure to close the shutter after the child presses the buzzer!)
4. Point to the black spot in the center of the bowl, and tell the child that you will be watching him through that spot. "Keep your eye on the black spot. The pilot sends the spaceship only when you look at the black spot."

Testing

Communicate frequently with the child. Encourage and reinforce good fixation. The orienting eye movement (OEM) to the per-ipheral target is the response that is monitored. OEMs are natural in young children and, in our experience, are not suppressed until age 8 to 10; then we can rely confidently on the buzzer for the response. The young child must be trained to respond when the light is seen: "Shoot the light with the buzzer!"

Because of reliance on OEMs in a young child, the target light must move from nonseeing to seeing areas of the field. In a child with good fixation, kinetic scanning from seeing to nonseeing areas ("Tap the buzzer when the light hides!") may be used to plot scotomas. Static stimuli work well but are time-intensive.

Because reaction time is delayed, even for OEMs in young children and older children with developmental disabilities, the speed of the kinetic scan must be slower than that in adults. We use 2° to 3° per second. If the scan is too fast, the field will be spuriously constricted; too slow invites loss of fixation and false positives.

A young child's participation is seldom sustained for more than 15 to 20 min. Usually 25 to 75 trials are possible (100s in an adult). Either the trials are divided between eyes or a decision is made as to whether a binocular test will yield informative results. Binocular testing is most useful in children with brain lesions.

Strategies for plotting Goldmann visual fields

In young children, one starts with a large, bright target, such as the V-4e or III-4e. By age 5 or 6 years, children can often be tested with the I-4e in addition to the III-4e. We usually start the test with the larger target. In very cooperative children dimmer targets can be used for relative or subtle field defects. The blind spot cannot be plotted accurately until fixation is held well, usually at age 5–6.

Knowledge of the patient's disease guides stimulus presentation. The strategy for mapping the irregular field defects in retinal diseases differs from that in a patient with a brain lesion. Beside the usual cautions,[2,12] start the kinetic scan from unexpected peripheral locations. This is critical in children with congenital homonymous defects because they have learned to scan anticipatorily into their nonseeing field.

AUTOMATED STATIC PERIMETRY

In general clinical practice, automated static perimetry is increasingly preferred over Goldmann kinetic perimetry, because the tests are sensitive to ocular diseases. In the authors' experience, only normal children aged 8 to 10 years are capable of the vigilant, rapid responses and good fixation required. For older children requiring evaluation of glaucoma fields and other optic nerve disorders, automated perimetry has much to recommend it. Instructions must be carefully stated, and the examiner must remain throughout the test to monitor fixation. The test is stopped to reinstruct the patient if false positives or false negatives increase or if there is a high rate of fixation losses, when repeat testing or other perimetry methods are necessary.

INTERPRETATION OF GOLDMANN VISUAL FIELDS

Clinical validity depends on cautious interpretation of Goldmann visual fields in young patients. Comparison to visual fields obtained in healthy children is desirable. Figure 10.2a shows visual fields from a 4-year-old with a brain tumor. Field sizes for the V-4e and III-4e targets are within the ranges reported in 10-year-old normal children.[13] Vigabitrin therapy may cause irreversible constriction (Fig. 10.2b).

For visual field size in 4- and 5-year-olds, the coefficient of variation is twice that in adults for the same Goldmann targets[14], and abnormal visual fields are more variable than normal ones.[15] This is important when evaluating serial visual fields, although visual field defects may be remarkably stable in young children, as shown in Fig. 10.2b.

Visual field defects

The validity of Goldmann perimetry is supported by the congruent visual field defects found with circumscribed retinal lesions (Fig. 10.3a). Other retinal diseases encountered in pediatric practice include retinal degenerations. Irregular field defects are found and are progressive (Fig. 10.3b).

Chiasmal lesions give rise to bitemporal field defects. The defect depends on the position of the lesion and associated abnormalities (Figs. 10.4a, 10.4b). Variable bitemporal defects are common in chiasmal optic gliomas (Fig. 10.4c). Visual field testing in young patients with treatable tumours is increasingly important as management improves and treatment is offered to more patients. Serial visual fields, paired with MRI scans, contribute to treatment decisions in these patients (see Chapters 33, 34, and 62).

Postchiasmal lesions are often asymmetric even if bilateral, giving rise to quadrantanopsia or hemianopsia contralateral to the more severely involved side (Fig. 10.5a). Field defects due to bilateral postchiasmal lesions are unusual; however, the authors have seen young patients with bilateral, inferior altitudinal field defects.

Perinatally acquired damage to periventricular white matter,[16] periventricular leukomalacia (PVL), occurs in areas that correspond to the optic radiations. Inferior field defects are predicted in lesions affecting the superior optic radiations. Dense, inferior altitudinal hemianopic visual field defects (Fig. 10.5b) are found with PVL.[17,18] Other clinically similar PVL patients show milder, relative inferior field defects. Also, inferior field defects occur in children with neonatal hypoxic ischemic encephalopathy, hemorrhagic strokes, and hypoglycemic brain injury.

To map visual field defects such as shown in Fig. 10.5b, exploration of the horizontal meridian is needed. Move the peripheral target from below upward, perpendicular to the horizon, systematically covering a full range of nasal and temporal eccentricities. Beware of the patient's anticipatory scanning downward, particularly for the less eccentric stimuli.

SUMMARY

Visual fields can be assessed in infants and young children, including those with developmental disabilities. Confrontation methods and Goldmann kinetic perimetry are most often used. Procedures must accommodate the physical and behavioral attributes of the child. Major field defects are detectable in infancy. Relative visual field defects are detected when the child is capable of good fixation and tolerates increased testing time. Sometimes, it takes two tries to get a reliable visual field in a young child. Visual field data bear on diagnosis and treatment. Visual field defects in children impact social and object regard, the development of gross and fine motor skills, spatial orientation and mobility, visual scanning, and other visually mediated activities.

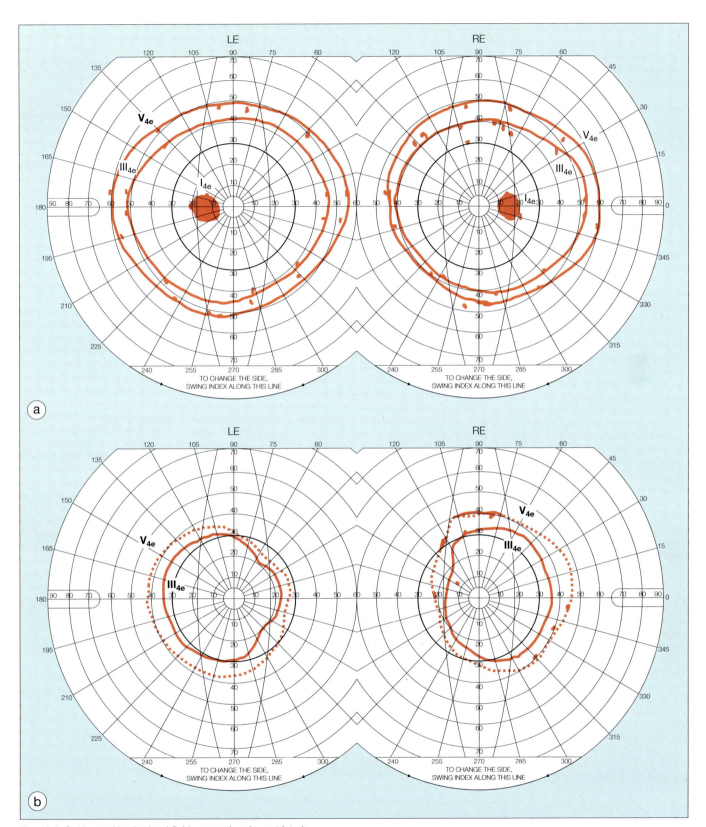

Fig. 10.2 Goldmann kinetic visual fields, normal and constricted.
(a) Monocular visual fields in a 4-year-old child prior to neurosurgery for a recurrent brain tumor. The peripheral fields, plotted with V-4e and III-4e targets, are within the normal limits for 10 year olds (see text). The blind spots, plotted with the I-4e target, appear normal. To obtain these fields, a total of 70 stimulus trials, 35 for each eye, were used.
(b) Monocular visual fields in a 4-year-old child on Vigabatrin monotherapy for epilepsy. The fields are constricted, each eye. This child's mother noted that he bumped into furniture and was very cautious moving in unfamiliar settings. The fields had not improved one year later.

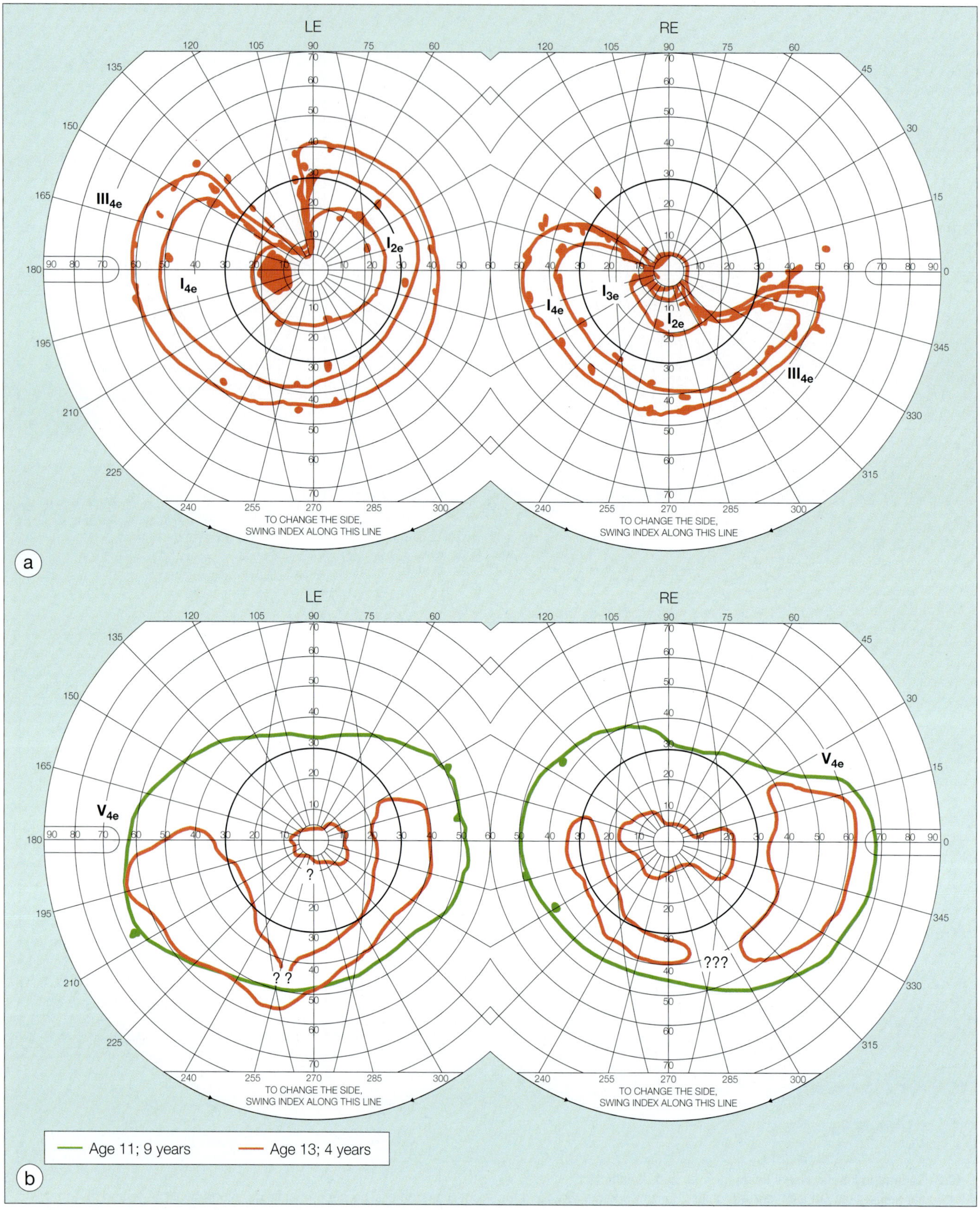

Fig. 10.3 Goldmann visual fields in children with lesions of the retina.

(a) Visual fields in a 6 year old with bilateral chorioretinal colobomas. The upper temporal field cut, left eye, corresponded exactly to an inferior nasal coloboma. The large defect in the superior visual field, right eye, corresponded to an extensive inferior chorioretinal coloboma that involved the optic nerve head. The foveas were spared and letter acuity was 20/25 in each eye. In baseball games, the child could catch grounders but missed pop flies.

(b) Visual fields in a child with retinal degeneration associated with Bardet Biedl syndrome. The V-4e fields at age 11 years (green lines) were within limits for healthy 10 year olds. Two years later, ring scotomas with central and peripheral islands of seeing field (red lines) were documented. In the classroom and unfamiliar surroundings, orientation and mobility were impaired.

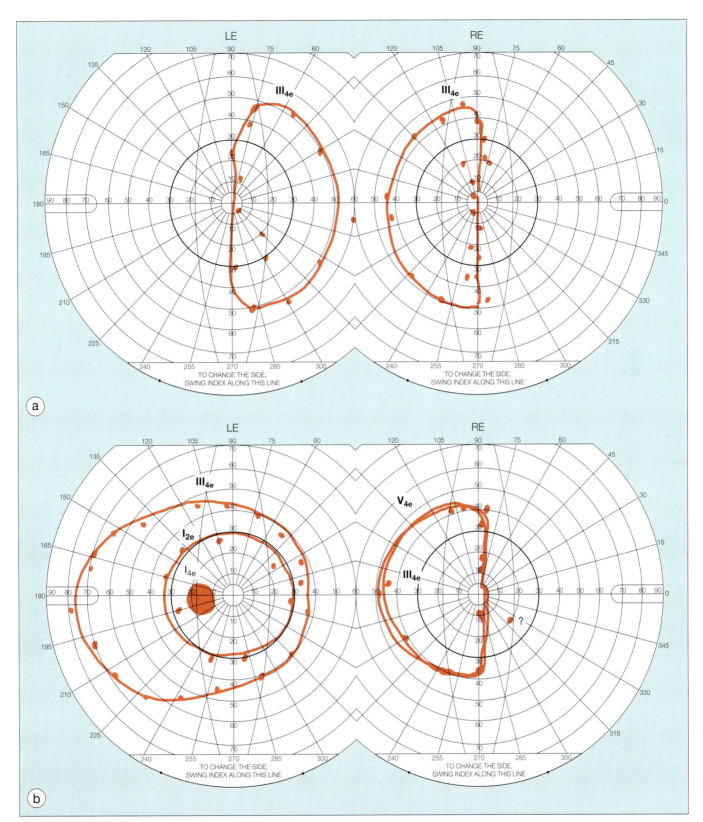

Fig. 10.4 Goldmann visual fields in children with tumors affecting the chiasm.
(a) Bitemporal hemianopsia was documented in a 4 year old with a craniopharyngioma. Despite acuities of 20/20 and 20/50, variable strabismus and "sliding fields" impaired her performance of fine motor tasks, scanning of visual arrays, and mobility. The hemianopic defects were stable over many years.
(b) Temporal field loss in the right eye and full fields in the left eye were shown in a 5 year old, who was status post-resection of the pituitary adenoma, aspiration of suprasellar cysts, and radiation therapy.

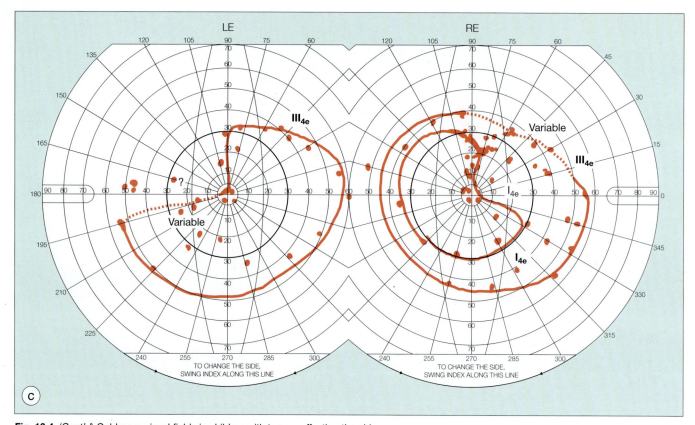

Fig. 10.4 (*Cont'd*) Goldmann visual fields in children with tumors affecting the chiasm.
(c) A superior bitemporal quadrantic field defect was found in a 4 year old after partial resection and chemotherapy for a low-grade astrocytoma of the chiasm.

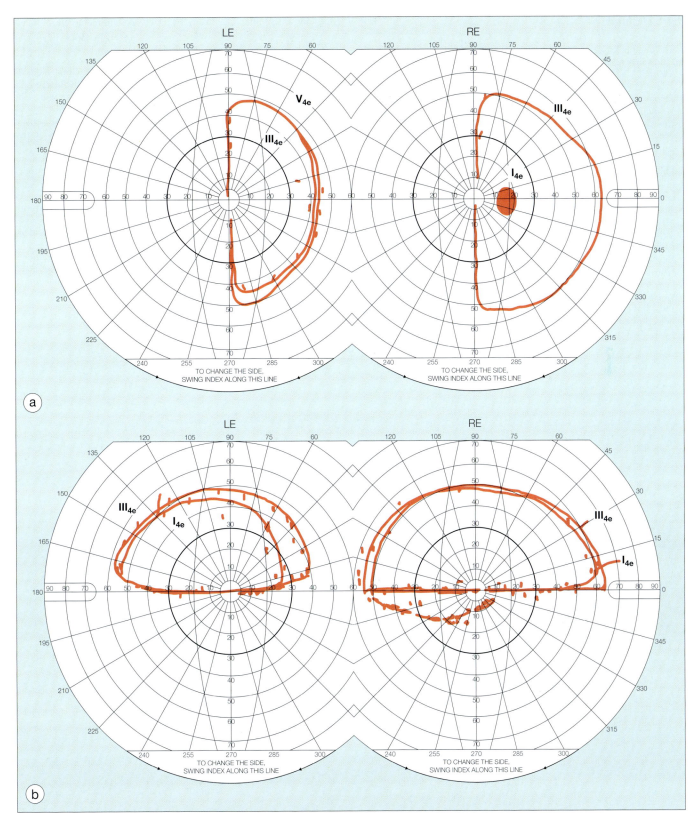

Fig. 10.5 Goldmann visual fields in children with postchiasmal lesions.
(a) A left homonymous hemianopsia is consistent with right porencephaly in a 4 year old. The porencephaly was thought to be secondary to prenatal hemorrhage; there was also evidence of damage to the left hemisphere. There was a left hemiparesis and a seizure disorder. His picture acuities were good in each eye. This child neglected his left field when performing fine motor tasks and other vision-mediated activities.
(b) Bilateral, inferior altitudinal hemianopic field defect was shown in a 5 year old with spastic diplegia. Birth was at 32 weeks gestation and CT images were consistent with periventricular leukomalacia. Parents and teachers reported difficulties in numerous activities requiring attention to the lower visual fields.

REFERENCES

1. Harrington DO, Drake MV. The Visual Fields. Text and Atlas of Clinical Perimetry. 6th ed. St. Louis: Mosby; 1990.
2. Walsh TJ. Visual Fields. Examination and Interpretation. 2nd ed. San Francisco: American Academy of Ophthalmology; 1996.
3. Harvey EM, Dobson V, Narter DB. The influence of a central stimulus on visual field measurements in children from 3.5 to 30 months of age. Optom Vis Sci 1997; 74: 768–74.
4. Mayer DL, Fulton AB. Development of the human visual field. In: Simons K, editor. Early Visual Development. Normal and Abnormal. New York: Oxford University Press; 1993. p. 117–29.
5. Dobson V, Brown AM, Harvey EM, Narter DB. Visual field extent in children 3.5–30 months of age tested with a double-arc LED perimeter. Vision Res 1998; 38: 2743–60.
6. Mayer DL, Fulton AB, Cummings MF. Visual fields of infants assessed with a new perimetric technique. Invest Ophthalmol Vis Sci 1988; 29: 452–9.
7. Mohn G, van Hof-van Duin J. Development of the binocular and monocular visual fields of human infants during the first year of life. Clin Vision Sci 1986; 1: 51–4.
8. Cummings MF, van Hof-van Duin J, Mayer DL, et al. Visual fields of young children. Behav Brain Res 1988; 29: 7–16.
9. Luna B, Dobson V, Scher MS, Guthrie RD. Grating acuity and visual field development in infants following perinatal asphyxia. Dev Med Child Neurol 1995; 37: 330–44.
10. Quinn GE, Miller DL, Evans JA, et al. Measurement of Goldmann visual fields in older children who received cryotherapy as infants for threshold retinopathy of prematurity. Arch Ophthalmol 1996; 114: 425–8.
11. Mayer DL, Fulton AB. Efficient method to screen visual fields of pediatric patients. Invest Ophthalmol Vis Sci 1989; 30(Suppl): 242.
12. Anderson DR. Perimetry With and Without Automation. 2nd edition. St. Louis: Mosby; 1987.
13. Myers VS, Gidlewski N, Quinn GE, et al. Distance and near visual acuity, contrast sensitivity, and visual fields of 10-year-old children. Arch Ophthalmol 1999; 117: 94–9.
14. Goldberg MC, Palafox G, Mayer DL. Maturation of Goldmann kinetic visual fields. Invest Ophthalmol Vis Sci 1992; 33(Suppl): 713.
15. Ross DF, Fishman GA, Gilbert LD, Anderson RJ. Variability of visual field measurements in normal subjects and patients with retinitis pigmentosa. Arch Ophthalmol 1984; 102: 1004–10.
16. Volpe JJ. Neurology of the Newborn. 3rd ed. Philadelphia: Saunders; 1995.
17. Brodsky MC. Periventricular leukomalacia: an intracranial cause of pseudoglaucomatous cupping. Arch Ophthalmol 2001; 119: 626–7.
18. Jacobson LK, Dutton GN. Periventricular leukomalacia: an important cause of visual and ocular motility dysfunction in children. Surv Ophthalmol 2000; 45: 1–13.

CHAPTER 11 Pediatric Visual Electrodiagnosis

Dorothy Thompson and Alki Liasis

INTRODUCTION

Visual electrodiagnostic tests (EDTs) encompass a range of investigations that record bioelectrical activity in response to ocular stimulation. These investigations provide objective and noninvasive measures of the functional integrity of the visual pathway, from retina to cortex, with millisecond resolution. EDTs are well suited for pediatric assessment, as although they require a degree of cooperation, they do not require any participation, in contrast to behavioral tests. Clinically EDTs include the electrooculogram (EOG) and the electroretinogram (ERG), which assess the function of the retinal pigment epithelium (RPE) and retina, and the visual evoked potential (VEP), which assesses the postretinal pathway to the visual cortex.

A range of stimuli is used to elicit ERGs and VEPs, including transient flashes of different intensities, durations, temporal rates, colors, patterns, and multifocal mosaics. Commercial flash stimulators include hand-held strobes and Ganzfelds. Hand-held strobes are advantageous in pediatric testing as they can be manipulated to follow an alert, but restless, child. Ganzfelds are available as static domes with chin rests, or smaller hand-held LED versions, which are held close to the eye and have the advantage of uniformly scattering light over the retina. Patterned stimuli are typically computer generated and presented on television screens, computer monitors, or back projection systems. These patterns contain equal numbers of black-and-white elements (usually checks, more rarely gratings) that either counterphase (reverse from black to white) or appear from a background of uniform gray field of equal mean luminance (pattern onset); thus there is no overall change in mean retinal luminance and light scatter within the eye is minimized. The spatial distribution of the pattern can be scaled for eccentricity, used in multifocal testing, with smaller elements in the center and larger elements at the periphery of the field. This accounts for the change in receptive field sizes across the retina and cortex in an attempt to achieve a topographically proportional recording.

International standards and recommendations for carrying out visual EDTs have been published in an attempt to introduce a global consistency of recording methodology, stimulation, and interpretation of findings, which would enable meaningful comparison of data across laboratories (e.g., ISCEV, the International Society for Clinical Electrophysiology of Vision, available at http://www.iscev.org, or International Federation of Clinical Neurophysiology at http://www.ifcn.info). However, there remain many technical and physiological factors that can mimic pathological changes in the EDTs results, especially in pediatric recording. These are potentially misleading during analysis and must be interpreted with care.

EVOKED POTENTIALS

Technical aspects of averaging, filtering, and display of data

The ERG and VEPs recorded with skin electrodes are of small amplitude compared to the EEG and are extracted using an averaging technique. Signal averaging relies on the evoked activity having a constant, or known, relationship in time to the presentation of the stimulus, while the background activity is random. The process of averaging reduces random noise relative to the signal (signal/noise ratio) and is proportional to n, where n is the number of responses. Noise can be defined as any activity not related to the stimulus, which can be both physiological (e.g., muscle activity) and environmental (e.g., main interference). During the process of averaging the continuous EEG is epoched or portioned into known time intervals before and after each stimulus. A computer sums the waveforms from each of the individual blocks and then divides the summed waveform by the total number of EEG epochs.

A filter bandwidth used during signal acquisition determines the frequency content of the recorded ERG/VEP. The filters usually consist of high- and low-pass filters. The high-frequency filter settings are determined by the analogue-to-digital sampling frequency. Different filter bandwidths are selected for different recording situations. In our department we record flash ERGs employing a bandpass of 0.3–1000 Hz, but manipulation of the filter settings enables investigation of specific activity. For example, although high-frequency oscillatory potentials (OPs) can be observed on the ascending limb of the ERG "b-wave" when a bandpass of 0.3–1000 Hz is used, they are more routinely analyzed using a bandpass of 100–1000 Hz. This filtering removes lower frequency ERG components of the a- and b-waves. In comparison an EOG recording contains both high- and low-frequency information and requires a very wide bandpass. Advice about the calibration of visual EDT equipment is found on the ISCEV website.

Evoked potentials are displayed as measures of voltage (in microvolts) against time (in milliseconds). These waveforms have characteristic morphologies made up of positive and negative peaks. These can be quantified by latency, relative to the onset of stimulus (or implicit time to peak), and size (amplitude), relative to the previous peak or an estimated baseline. The waveform may also be defined qualitatively in terms of its definition or shape compared to normal findings. Nomenclature used to define the various components is usually based on the polarity and latency of the component; for example, p100 of the pattern reversal VEP refers to the positive component that peaks 100 ms after the pattern reverses.

THE ELECTROOCULOGRAM (EOG)

A standing potential arises across the eye because of a difference in ionic activity at the apical end of the RPE cells, where they abut the photoreceptors, compared to their basal ends. The ionic changes are a consequence of the phagocytosis of outer segment discs, and transport of retinal binding proteins in the synthesis of the inter-receptor matrix. The standing potential measures around 6 mV with positivity at the cornea. During a saccade a large potential difference can be detected across electrodes placed on the medial and lateral canthi: the electrode closest to the cornea becomes positive relative to the electrode furthest from the cornea. The EOG is displayed as a voltage/time plot that allows eye movements, including nystagmus, to be graphically characterized.

Prolonged light adaptation causes changes in the ionic activity in the RPE. This is reflected as fluctuations in the amplitude of the EOG, and can be used to assess the functional integrity of the RPE interaction with the photoreceptors. The increase in the EOG amplitude in the light (light rise) is compared to the decrease in amplitude in darkness (dark trough) as a ratio, the Arden index[1] (Fig. 11.1). To acquire an Arden index a patient needs to cooperate sufficiently to make reproducible saccades between 2 LEDs every 2 minutes during a period of 10–15 minutes of dark adaptation followed by 10–15 minutes light adaptation. In normal subjects the dark trough and light rise each occur approximately 8 minutes under either lighting condition. In many laboratories, Arden ratios greater than 1.8 are considered normal. In our experience children around 5 years and upward are capable of completing the investigation with enough encouragement. The EOG is most often used to investigate maculopathies in the pediatric clinic. For example in Best disease the EOG is often markedly subnormal early on while ERG is wholly normal. EOG recordings can be achieved in young infants by a swinging chair to utilize the vestibular-ocular reflex to trigger saccades of 30°, in dark and light.[2]

THE ELECTRORETINOGRAM (ERG)

Rod and cone function, as well as and inner and outer retinal function, can be differentiated by changing wavelength, intensity, and duration of a flash stimuli under different states of dark and light adaptation. The recorded ERG waveform is an algebraic summation of retinal potentials from all retinal areas, which have different polarity, latency, and amplitude. The bright flash ERG has 4 major components labeled alphabetically the a-, b-, c-, and d- waves with oscillatory potentials appearing as a series of wavelets between the a- and b- waves. The d-wave is associated with decreases in light under photopic conditions, but is best seen in response to prolonged on–off flashes. Response to short duration stimuli results in a superimposition of the b- and d-waves.[3]

The a-wave

The a-wave is the first major negative component related to the hyperpolarization of the retinal photoreceptors in response to incident light. It's amplitude increases with intensity (Fig. 11.2a). Changes in the slope of the a-wave have been quantitatively related to the G-protein-triggered photo-transduction amplification cascade, and differential effects on amplification and maximum a-wave amplitude have been described in RP and cone dystrophy.[4–7]

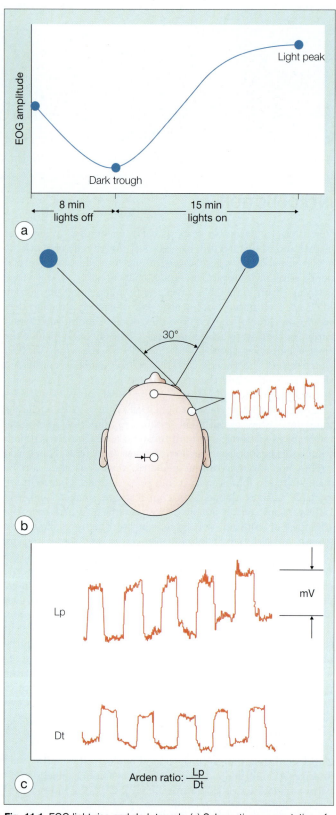

Fig. 11.1 EOG light rise and dark trough. (a) Schematic representation of changes in EOG amplitude over time under photopic and scotopic conditions. (b) The dipole movement as a 30° saccade is made. (c) EOG waveforms recorded during the "dark trough" and "light peak." The ratio of the amplitudes gives the Arden index.

The b-wave

The light-activated photoreceptors activate "on" center, depolarizing bipolar cells, whose activity is thought to be limited in a push-pull model by hyperpolarizing cells.[8] Consequent increases in extracellular potassium ions at the postreceptoral outer plexiform layer are transported through, and depolarize, Muller cells. This spread of ionic current through the depth of the retina produces the corneal positive b-wave. The implicit time of the b-wave can be a measure of receptor sensitivity and will decrease as more cones are stimulated.

The amplitude of the b-wave changes as a function of stimulus intensity (Fig. 11.2a), and mathematically can be described by a Naka-Rushton function. This is a derivation of a Michaelis-Menton equation, which describes a saturating nonlinearity function; however, the derived parameters will vary according to the technique of curve fitting used, and needs to be interpreted with care in clinical circumstances,[9]

$$V/V_{max} = Int/Int + K,$$

where V = trough-to-peak amplitude of the b-wave, V_{max} = maximum value of trough-to-peak amplitude, Int = flash intensity in trolland-second, K = semisaturation value, i.e., when Int $=K$, V is $V_{max}/2$.

The c-wave

The initial movement of ions depletes the amount of potassium ions between the receptor outer segments and the RPE. The net result of this ionic imbalance is recorded as a slow positive wave (c-wave), identifiable, though not invariably, after the b-wave.[3]

Oscillatory potentials

Oscillatory potentials (OPs) represent radial currents through the retina, which are probably generated at the bipolar/amacrine/interplexiform cell layer. Early OPs appear to be associated with rod function and "on" pathways, and the later ones with the cone system and "off" pathway.[10] The OPs are most easily recorded under mesopic conditions to widely spaced 20s flashes. Oscillatory potentials are commonly employed to investigate retinal vascular disturbances in diabetes or in distinguishing subtypes of night blindness.

ERG methodology

Flash ERG international standards

The ISCEV standards define a standard flash as 1.5–3.0 photopic cd/m^2 at the surface of the Ganzfeld bowl with a maximum duration of 5 ms. They recommend that for ERG recordings a contact lens electrode with speculum, pupillary dilation, full field Ganzfeld stimulation, and at least 20 minutes dark adaptation are used. They advocate five standard responses (Fig. 11.3):

Following at least 20 minutes of dark adaptation:

1. Rod response dark-adapted eye by dim white flash;
2. Maximal mixed rod–cone ERG dark-adapted eye and standard flash; and
3. Oscillatory potentials recorded to standard flashes of a dark-adapted eye.

Following at least 10 minutes of light adaptation:

4. A cone response from light-adapted eye to a standard flash; and
5. Cone-mediated 30-Hz flicker of a standard flash.

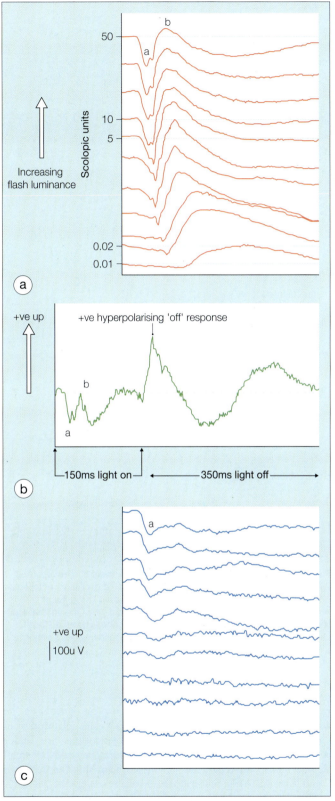

Fig. 11.2 ERG intensity series (a) changes in the ERG waveform as flash luminance increases: recorded with a DTL fiber electrode after the eye is dilated and dark adapted for 20 minutes. A-wave and b-wave amplitudes increase as flash luminance increases and the time to peak of each decreases. 5–10 cd.s.m^2 scotopic units (1.8–3.6 photopic units) is equivalent to the ISCEV standard flash. (b) The ERGs elicited to the onset and offset of a prolonged light flash. (c) The response from a patient with X-L complete CSNB in whom the a-wave develops, but the b-wave does not. This results in giving a "negative" ERG morphology.

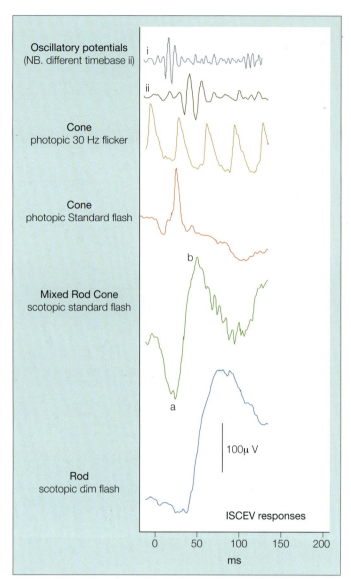

Oscillatory potentials
(NB. different timebase ii)

Cone
photopic 30 Hz flicker

Cone
photopic Standard flash

Mixed Rod Cone
scotopic standard flash

Rod
scotopic dim flash

100μ V

ISCEV responses

ms

Fig. 11.3 Examples of 5 ISCEV responses to Ganzfeld flashes recorded with DTL electrode. The top trace shows the filtered oscillatory potentials on an usual timebase (i), and expanded timebase (ii). These traces illustrate the change in waveform shape that occur when the adaptation level and flash luminance preferential stimulate cones and rods. These Ganzfeld ERGs are summated across the whole retina, whilst a pattern ERG is a localized retinal response.

ISCEV standards recommend that topical anesthesia be administered prior to the use of contact lens electrodes in children. Although the ISCEV recommendations are under review, they currently indicate that restraint be used for small infants, and sedation induced on noncompliant children (between 2 and 6 years). When following these recommendations, the ERG findings must be interpreted with the knowledge that anesthesia can affect the rod ERG b-wave.

The ISCEV standards board acknowledges that achieving a full-standardized protocol may not be possible in all infants and that abbreviated protocols may be used. Abbreviating the period of dark adaptation will introduce further variability in the rod b-wave.

The morphology and amplitude of the ERG varies according to the preponderance of contributing cell to the response. Cone-mediated responses are shorter in component latency than broader longer latency responses evoked by rods. ERGs elicited by stimulation rates above 20/s reflect cone photoreceptor activity, as rods are unable to respond to activation at these stimulation rates. At these higher stimulation rates the responses merge and appear sinusoidal. There is also a postreceptoral contribution to the flicker response.[11]

Recording electrodes

The amplitude of a recorded ERG component is related to the type of recording electrode used, and it is important for laboratories to standardize on the types of electrodes they use. For example in comparison to a Burian Allen contact lens electrode we found the dark-adapted ERG amplitude to be reduced to 56% with gold foil electrodes, to 46% with DTL fiber electrodes, and to 12% with skin electrodes.[12] In some countries especially in Europe disposable electrodes like the DTL fiber and adhesive AgCl skin electrodes are preferred to the reusable Burian Allen contact lens and gold foil electrodes because of the risks of cross-contamination from multiuse electrodes.

In our experience of skin electrodes, disposable adhesive AgCl electrodes are best positioned below the eye, within 1 cm of the lower eyelid margin. If the eyes are deviated, the electrode should be positioned as close as possible to the cornea (e.g., lateral placement in strabismus or superior placement if the eyes are rolled up). Similarly if the midface is flat and eyes protuberant, as in some craniofacial conditions, a slightly temporal electrode position is better if the child is able to direct their gaze laterally toward the electrode.

We routinely perform ERGs on infants and young children using disposable skin electrodes and natural pupils under both darkened and photopic conditions. Colored filters and different intensity lights are used to bias the contribution from rods (dim blue flash (475 nm) in the dark) and cones (brighter red flash (625 nm) or flashes under photopic conditions). In older children who are able to tolerate DTL fiber electrodes, we will record pattern ERG (PERGs) and ISCEV standard flash ERGs in addition to skin ERG recordings. A recent study has demonstrated that ERGs recorded with skin electrodes in response to ISCEV standard stimulation differ only in scale from those recorded with contact lens or gold foil electrodes. Across electrodes there were no statistical differences in the ranges of interindividual amplitudes.[13]

"On and off" contributions to the flash ERG

The ERGs described above are in response to abrupt, transient changes in stimuli. By using prolonged flash stimuli (light on for usually 150 ms or longer), the retinal activity in response to stimulus onset (on responses) and offset (off responses) can be distinguished (Fig. 11.2b). Separating the "on" and "off" responses is of interest when the flash ERG b-wave is abnormal, for example, in some forms of congenital stationary night-blindness (CSNB).[14]

Negative ERGs

Normally the bright flash mixed rod–cone ERG b-wave is 1.5 to 2 times the size of the a-wave. If the a-wave amplitude is preserved, but the b-wave amplitude is markedly attenuated, or not detectable, then the ERG is said to have a "negative" morphology (Fig. 11.2c). This morphology indicates a relative dysfunction of the inner retinal layers, with preservation of receptor activity. There are three main ways in which this can occur:

1. *An interruption of transmission to, and by, the on-bipolar system*: e.g., X-L complete CSNB mutations in nyctalopin associated with disrupted bipolar connection development and on-bipolar pathway dysfunction[15] and incomplete CSNB associated with mutations in a retina-specific calcium channel alpha 1 subunit (CACNA1F) affecting both on and off pathways.[16]

2. *Via mechanical compromise of the inner retinal layers*: e.g., X-L retinoschisis often shows interocular asymmetries in ERGs and VEPs while CSNB tend to be bilaterally symmetric;[17] or an affect to the circulation of the inner retina (central retinal vein or artery occlusion).

3. *An interruption of ionic transmission through the Muller cell current and ERG generation*: e.g., a negative ERG in patients with Duchenne muscular dystrophy is not associated with a functional deficit or altered dark adaptation because only ERG generation is affected rather than actual signal transmission through the bipolar ganglion cell connections.[18,19]

The negative ERG has been associated with the various following conditions:

- Early RP in a subset of RP patients;[20]
- Bull's eye maculopathy;[21]
- Cone dystrophies;[22]
- Melanoma-associated retinopathy–MAR IgG circulating antibodies;[23] and
- Infantile and juvenile neuronal ceroid lipofuscinosis NCL.[24]

All childhood-onset forms of NCL are associated with retinal degeneration and visual failure, but infantile and juvenile forms of NCL are distinguished by negative ERGs early on. In the early stages of the late infantile form the cone b-wave is severely attenuated and markedly increased in latency. Rod responses are mildly abnormal, but more preserved than in infantile or juvenile NCL. The "flash VEP" is reported to be markedly enlarged (12 to 20 times larger than normal), even though the ERG is usually not detectable.[25] This response may not be a true occipital VEP as each flash elicits what appears to be a "sharp" wave with morphology and distribution different to a normal VEP.[24] The high-amplitude spike activity probably represents cortical disinhibition and is analogous to the giant somatosensory evoked potentials that can be observed during finger tapping of these patients.[25]

Focal, pattern, and multifocal ERGs

The flash ERG is a net summation of activity from widespread retinal areas that can mask dysfunction of a localized retinal lesion. To stimulate focal retinal areas the stimulation must be localized and intraocular light scatter minimized. This can be achieved either by bleaching the surrounding retina to reduce the effectiveness of any scattered light–a procedure described as the focal ERG–or more effectively by using patterns with equal numbers of black and white elements localized to the macular and paramacular areas–a procedure known as the pattern ERG (PERG).

PERGs to pattern reversing checks are biphasic with positivity at 50 ms and a negativity at 95 ms, termed p50 and n95, respectively. Clinically and parametrically it has been shown that the p50 represents distal retina and localized macula function while the n95 characterizes more proximal retinal and reflects ganglion cell function.[26] PERGs are most often used to investigate suspected early maculopathy. These responses are on the order of 0.5–8 μV and require signal averaging. They are typically recorded with corneal electrodes that do not impede the eye's optics, e.g., gold foil and DTL fiber electrodes. A check

size of 0.8° presented in a field size of 16° is suggested. In our experience PERGs of half size can be detected with skin electrodes to reversals of 6/s or less. Steady fixation is important and the level of cooperation required to record a PERG may not be achieved in children less than 5–6 years old.

The multifocal ERG technique, (mfERGs) allows local ERG responses to be recorded simultaneously from many regions of the retina.[27] A pattern array of elements, typically hexagons scaled in size according to retinal eccentricity, is modulated in luminance according to an M-sequence. This is a pseudorandom algorithm that guarantees that no stimulus sequence is repeated during an examination. Each element changes luminance according to the pseudorandom sequence, but starts the sequence at a different place to every other element. Response generated by a particular element in this way is uncorrelated with every other element if the "lag," the difference in starting point of the sequence, is greater than the duration of the response. At any one time on average half of the hexagons are black and the other half white. The stimulation rate is quite high, resulting in a flickering appearance of the screen with a relatively stable mean luminance. Responses that are the result of retinal activity associated with a particular area unaffected by stimulation of other areas are termed first-order components while second-order components represent temporal interactions between flashes and short lags relative to the duration of the response. This technique is also very sensitive to fixation instabilities and its application in children is to date largely untried.

THE VISUAL EVOKED POTENTIAL (VEP)

The VEP recorded from electrodes placed on the occipital scalp reflects activity on cortical gyri. The retinotopic map at the occipital lobe determines that the VEP is dominated by activity from the central 5°, predominantly lower field. This macula predominance means that pattern VEPs in children can be used as an index of macula pathway function. If the pattern VEP is diminished, a retinal macula problem should be excluded as a cause of the dysfunction. This can be done using a PERG and fundal imaging. To flash stimulation the retino-geniculo afferent volley causes depolarization in lamina 4c of the striate cortex (area V_1).[28,29] Pattern reversal stimulation activates the same cortical areas as diffuse flash stimulation. In macaque at least, additional supra- and infragranular layers of striate cortex are activated. Other specialized visual areas are also activated, in particular the V_4 complex, which is also involved in generating later components of the flash VEP.[29] Monocular stimulation with a transoccipital array of electrodes, and where possible half-field stimulation, can discriminate optic nerve, chiasmal, and hemisphere anomalies.

Pattern reversal VEPs

Pattern reversal VEPs to full-field stimulation usually have a triphasic waveform with a major positive component around 100 ms (called p100) (Fig. 11.4). Pattern reversal stimulation is used most widely in clinical assessment as its waveform is maintained across the lifespan and half-field abnormalities are more reliably detected with this stimulus mode. The shape of the pattern reversal VEP becomes bifid (like a "W") in dominant optic atrophy when the central scotoma reduces the macula component and concomitantly enhances paramacular components n105 and

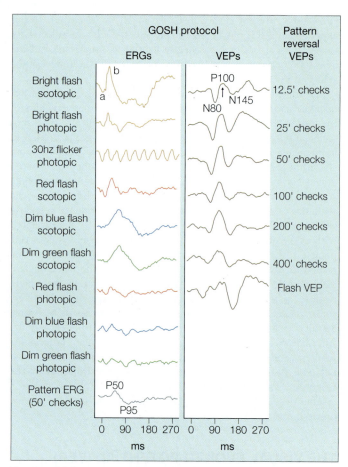

Fig. 11.4 GOSH response array. These responses illustrate the combined skin ERG and VEP averaged recording. The stimulus intensity and wavelength are used to bias the predominantly contributing receptors from rods to cones. The pattern reversal VEP is characterized by its main positive component p100 and the preceding negativity n80. The n80 shows greater prominence to smaller checksizes. The flash VEP has a more complex waveform. NB: the display gains are illustrative.

p135. Half-field stimulation will confirm this mechanism is responsible for the full-field bifid morphology.

Pattern onset VEPs

Pattern onset VEPs are elicited by the abrupt appearance of a pattern usually lasting between 100 and 300 ms. This VEP is characterized by three components with spatially separate generator sources: CI, a positivity around 90ms; CII, negativity at about 110 ms; and CIII, a prominent positivity at around 180–200 ms.[30,31] The negative CII, and probably CIII, has an extrastriate origin and the positive CI a striate cortical origin. Others, however, using dipole localization models suggest CI originates in Brodman area 18 and CII in an area beyond this.[31] In children the most prominent response is the initial positive CI, which is mostly dependent upon contrast and luminance. The "contour" pattern-specific CII emerges only in later childhood; these changes in waveform can confuse the clinical interpretation with age. A VEP is also elicited to pattern-offset, and its waveform properties have a close affinity to the pattern reversal VEP (although component latencies are around 10 ms later than PVEPs).[33]

Electrode placement

AgCl i.e. silver, silver chloride electrodes are used in standard positions over the scalp (international 10:20 system of electrode placement).[34] The largest amplitude is found over the midline 3 cm above the inion. In order to distinguish chiasmal and hemisphere dysfunction it is essential to have a minimum of 3 electrodes over the occipital scalp and record monocular responses. These are distributed equally on either side of the midline, either 4 cm from the midline or half way between the midline and mastoid, if this is smaller in babies. Multichannel recording is especially important in pediatric practice when perimetry or imaging studies are not practical.

Paradoxical lateralization and transoccipital asymmetry

In addition to amplitude, latency, and waveform, the transoccipital distribution of VEP components plays a vital role in VEP analysis, as it can distinguish hemisphere from chiasmal dysfunction. The symmetry of distribution is analyzed by comparing the size and polarity of lateral channel activity from the right and left sides of the head. An uncrossed asymmetry is the term given when the same transoccipital distribution is noted irrespective of which eye is tested, indicating hemisphere dysfunction. In comparison a crossed asymmetry occurs when the transoccipital VEP distribution changes according to which eye is stimulated. The pattern of crossed asymmetry suggests a chiasmal problem, e.g., albinism, achiasmia, or chiasmal compression. A difference of R and L lateral channel responses for each eye can be used to show mirror asymmetry. Other methods for qualitatively scoring the peak of potential distribution across an electrode array or statistically cross-correlating difference potentials have been recently compared.[35]

Half-field stimulation can be used in cooperative children with steady fixation to preferentially stimulate one hemisphere and to distinguish the contribution of paramacular and macula areas to the full-field response. The distribution of the pattern reversal VEP to half-field stimulation shows "paradoxical" lateralization (Fig. 11.5). When a wide lateral half-field is used (extending more than 6° from fixation), the pattern reversal VEP p100 component is largest over the occipital hemisphere *ipsilateral* to the field of stimulation. This distribution arises because the cortical fibers within the contralateral hemisphere corresponding to the stimulated field are orientated in the direction of the ipsilateral hemisphere. This results in a dipole whose activity is recorded over the ipsilateral hemisphere.[36] The ipsilateral n80-p100-n145 complex represents macular pathway activity predominantly, whereas the p75-n105-p150 recorded over the contralateral site reflects mainly paramacular activation of the visual field. For visual half-field lateralization a common reference (e.g., placed on a midfrontal site) is preferable for distinguishing between zones of activity and inactivity.[37]

Steady-state VEPs and sweep VEPs

When the stimulation frequency increases so that responses begin to merge and become sinusoidal recording, conditions are described as steady state. Steady-state techniques are used in sweep VEPs, where many different pattern sizes or contrast levels are swept through rapidly[38,39] (Fig. 11.6). The response is analyzed with Fourier techniques into amplitude and phase. These have been used clinically to assess acuity and contrast

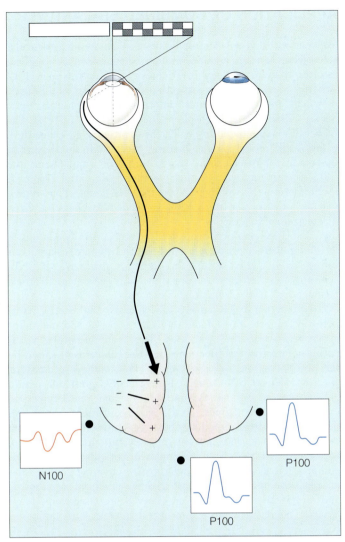

Fig. 11.5 Paradoxical lateralization of pattern VEPs to half-field stimulation. The afferent volley activates cortical generators with dipole-type properties. Electrodes over the midline and hemisphere ipsilateral to the stimulated half-field to pick up p100 activity produced by the visual cortex of the activated contralateral hemisphere.

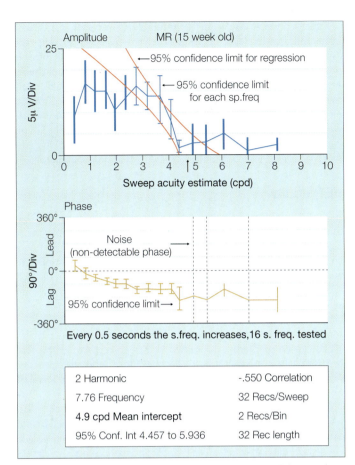

2 Harmonic	-.550 Correlation
7.76 Frequency	32 Recs/Sweep
4.9 cpd Mean intercept	2 Recs/Bin
95% Conf. Int 4.457 to 5.936	32 Rec length

Fig. 11.6 Sweep VEP. Rapid stimulation rates are used to elicit a quasi-sinusoidal VEP characterized by its amplitude and phase. A range of spatial frequencies is presented. There is a trend for VEP amplitude to decrease with increasing spatial frequency. A regression to the baseline or noise level is computed to give an acuity estimate.

sensitivity quickly,[40] but there is a loss of waveform component information that can be very important especially on the first visual EDT assessment. For this reason we prefer transient recording for routine clinical practice.

Adaptations for VEP recording in children

VEPs are changed by the level of alertness, and cannot be done under sedation or anesthesia. VEPs from sleepy young infants can become broader, smaller, and later. Occasionally the recording can become swamped by large-amplitude, slow EEG "sleep" activity, enhancing of VEP components. In some cases high-amplitude, sharp wave transients associated with seizure or epileptiform activity can confound the VEP to such an extent that a VEP cannot be identified in the average. This occurs if the activity is random, but not rejected by the on-line rejection criteria, or becomes time locked to the stimulus.

In our lab, alert babies, infants and children sit on a parent's lap and may need considerable distraction to encourage fixation and to reduce "wriggling" muscle artifacts. A large pattern screen is

important. The ability to switch from cartoons/musical videos to pattern stimulation is useful as it maintains continuity of distraction. It is preferable to use noisy toys dangled in the upper part of the TV to promote central to lower visual field stimulation, which is more likely to be retinotopically represented in the full-field VEP. Close-circuit TV is used to monitor fixation. It is an advantage to be able to pause or interrupt data averaging if a child's fixation wanders and to resume immediately their attention is regained. This facility will enhance the quality and reliability of the recording. Repeated runs are necessary to confirm response reproducibility. We recommend using a series of different checksizes to look for response consistency and subtle variations in amplitude and latency that will give an indication of vision and refractive error. Spectacles should be worn, but this is not always possible; therefore it is important to present an adequate range of checksizes that can withstand moderate refractive error. We use checksizes ranging from 400′ to 6.25′ presented in a 28° field, but start recording with a medium checksize, 50′. This can withstand 8-D spherical blur and hence larger astigmatic blur. If patterns with small element sizes are defocused, PVEP latency increases and the macular response is attenuated in proportion to the degree of refractive error present. Changes in pupil size or eyelid ptosis will also deleteriously affect pattern reversal VEPs. Slow stimulation rates are appropriate for infants less than 8 weeks of age.

Pattern onset stimulation is preferable to reversal in cases of nystagmus or unstable fixation. Pattern onset is valuable for assessing acuity in the older child, particularly if nystagmus is present, and is also useful for identifying abnormal pathway projection in older children with albinism.[41] It is also more difficult to actively defocus pattern onset stimuli. Flash stimulation is more effective in younger children with albinism.[42] In our laboratory, we perform both pattern reversal and onset/offset stimulation on patients with nystagmus, as the tests can be done rapidly, and more complete and complementary information is obtained.

VEP acuity

In normal children an acuity estimate can be made from the size of responses elicited by patterns of decreasing element size.[43] The smallest pattern size to give a response above noise level, or an extrapolation to zero amplitude on a graph of amplitude versus spatial frequency, can be used to estimate threshold VEP acuity.[40,44] Although VEPs show some correlation with behavioral acuity it would be unrealistic to rely upon such a direct correlation in a clinical population as the anatomical substrate differs for each measure. For example, in optic atrophy the pattern VEPs can be markedly attenuated and degraded, yet if the few remaining functioning fibers sample close enough together recognition acuity can be surprisingly good given the level of optic disc pallor.

Estimates of acuity development are higher with VEP techniques in the first 12–18 months of life. After this behavioral estimates exceed VEP acuity.[40,45] In our lab we consider that a good sized pattern reversal VEP to 50' or smaller checks suggests good vision levels, to 100'–200' moderate, and to 400' poor vision levels, while if a flash VEP is detected, but no pattern VEP is recorded, this suggests vision is rudimentary only. PVEPs are a useful benchmark for serial monitoring and are particularly useful for interocular comparisons.[46]

MATURATION OF EVOKED POTENTIALS

Maturation of visual electrophysiological responses is rapid in the first 7 months. VEP latencies decrease reflecting myelination of the visual pathway and increase synaptic organization, and ERGs become larger as the effectiveness of retinal elements increases.[47,48] It is useful to record to a slower repetition rate particularly in the first 6–8 weeks of life, e.g., 1 Hz, and to increase the time window from 300 to 500 ms so that the main positive VEP response sits in the middle of the time window. There can be great individual variability in VEPs in the first days following birth,[49] and attempts have been made to fit logistic curves to help labs who do not have young norms.[50] The spatial tuning of the pattern VEP tends to be low pass in the early weeks, becoming more bandpass by 6 months. The pattern-specific, negative, CII of the pattern onset VEP is immature in infancy and the morphology of the pattern onset VEP becomes more complex in later childhood.

Changes continue throughout life, and each laboratory should establish their own normative data as there can be surprisingly large variability across laboratories even using international standards. It is worth emphasizing that uncomplicated delayed visual maturation, DVM, is a behavioral delay in visual responsiveness, and in contrast the ERG and VEP findings show normal maturation for age. In particular there is *no* concomitant delay in VEP latency.[51]

APPLICATION OF COMBINED ERG AND VEP

We believe that visual electrophysiology in children has particular value when tests are combined rather being individually applied, as often there may be few overt clues to explain the poor visual behavior of an infant. Used together the ERG and VEP provide pertinent and complementary information about retina, optic nerve, chiasmal, and hemisphere function (Fig. 11.7).[52,53] The flash ERG is summated from all areas of retina while the pattern reversal VEP reflects macula pathway function. In the absence of overt signs of maculopathy the pattern VEP supplements the ERG assessment by indicating whether the central region of localized retina is working. When there is doubt about retinal macula integrity a pattern ERG is needed to check localized macula retinal function.

A flash ERG can be diagnostically important in conditions in which fundi are likely to be normal, yet the infant does not fix or follow well. This occurs in Leber's amaurosis, CSNB, achromatopsia, progressive cone dystrophy, early stage RP, toxic retinopathy[54] (see Chapters 52–54).

Used together an ERG and VEP can assess the anterior visual pathway from receptors, inner retina, optic nerve, and chiasm for a sensory reason for nystagmus. They can investigate visual pathway integrity and function when the fundus is obscured by media opacity, e.g., cataract and PHPV, corneal opacity, or anterior segment dysgenesis.[55] They can distinguish the nature and extent of retinal dysfunction, macula involvement in coloboma, maculopathies, ROP, and detachment. They can determine the level of pathway dysfunction discriminating optic nerve, chiasmal, and postchiasmal dysfunction. They have application assessing the visual impact of optic nerve hypoplasia, compression, demyelination, neuropathy, chiasmal compression or mal-development (chiasmal glioma, albinism, achiasmia), and unilateral hemisphere or generalized conditions (e.g., hypoxia, neurodegenerative disorders, hydrocephalus, and raised ICP).

SUMMARY

Visual EDTs are noninvasive and objective. They can be adapted for children to provide sensitive information if normative data and an awareness of potential pitfalls are taken into consideration. A combined ERG and VEP assessment can localize dysfunction in the visual pathway and will be able to provide a qualitative estimate of vision. For these reasons visual EDTs can provide complementary and supplementary information in many diverse clinical presentations; ranging from an infant who does not fix and follow and has unusual eye movements, through to amblyopia not responding to patching, investigation of headaches, and assessment of children who cannot communicate enough for behavioral assessments.

It is very important that the prognostic significance of visual EDT results is weighed in the light of all clinical data and with an awareness of maturational changes. Visual EDTs assess the "visual hardware," but do not tell us about the "software." Although they can suggest the quality of pattern vision the retino-geniculostriate pathway may support, in their current form EDTs cannot tell us how well a child will be able to use the visual data that reach the cortex.

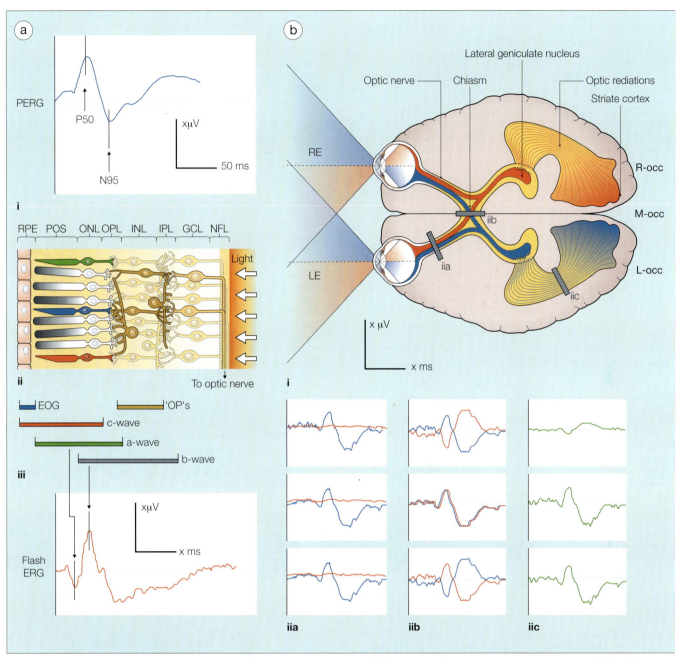

Fig. 11.7 Composite pathway: generators of the ERG and topography of the VEP. (a) Generators of the electroretinogram and pattern ERG. (i) Schematic of the pattern ERG. (ii) Schematic of neuronal architecture of the retina. RPE = retinal pigment epithelial, POS = photoreceptor outer segments, ONL = outer nuclear layer, OPL = outer plexiform layer, INL = inner nuclear layer, IPL = inner plexiform layer, GCL = ganglion cell layer, NFL = nerve fiber layer. Blue, red, and green cells illustrate blue, red, and green cones. Grey cells represent rod photocells. Orange = horizontal cells, light blue = bipolar and amacrine cells, yellow = ganglion cells. (iii) Schematic of a flash ERG. Colored bars indicate approximate source within the retina of the EOG and ERG components. (b) Visually evoked potentials. (i) Schematic of visual pathways from LE and RE. Blue pathways represent right half-field and red the left half-field. Grey bars superimposed on the pathways represent a lesion at the level of the (iia) optic nerve, (iib) chiasm, and (iic) optic radiations and cortex. (Pathway diagram provided by Richard Tibbetts). (ii) Schematic VEP waveforms recorded from the right (R-occ) and left (L-occ) lateral and mid-occipital (M-occ) channels. The blue and red waveforms represent left and right eye stimulation, respectively. The VEPs (iia), (iib), and (iic) are a result of the lesions marked in (Bi).

REFERENCES

1. Arden G, Barrada A, Kelsey JH. New clinical test of retinal function based on the standing potential of the eye. J Physiol 1962; 46: 449–67.

2. Fulton AB, Hartmann EE, Hansen RM. Electrophysiological testing techniques for children. Doc Ophthalmol 1989; 71: 341–54.

3. Granit R. Sensory Mechanisms of the Retina. London: Oxford University Press; 1947.

4. Pugh E, Lamb T. Phototransduction in vertebrate rods and cones: molecular mechanisms of amplification, recovery and light adaptation. In: Stavenga DG, de Grip WJ, Pugh, EN Jr, editors. Handbook of Biological Physics. Amsterdam: Elsevier; 2000: 183–254. (Vol. 3, Chapter 5.)

5. Breton ME, Schueller AW, Lamb TD, et al. Analysis of ERG a-wave amplification and kinetics in terms of the G-protein cascade of phototransduction. Invest Ophthalmol Vis Sci 1994 ;35: 295–309.

6. Breton ME, Quinn GE, Schueller AW. Development of electroretinogram and rod phototransduction response in human infants. Invest Ophthalmol Vis Sci 1995; 36: 1588–602.

7. Tzekov RT, Locke KG, Hood DC, et al. Cone and rod phototransduction parameters in retinitis pigmentosa patients. Invest Ophthalmol Vis Sci 2003; 44: 3993–4000.

8. Sieving PA, Murayama K, Naarendorp F. Push-pull model of the primate photopic electroretinogram: a role for hyperpolarizing neurons in shaping the b-wave. Vis Neurosci 1994; 11: 519–32.

9. Evans LS, Peachey NS, Marchese AL. Comparison of three methods of estimating the parameters of the Naka-Rushton equation. Doc Ophthalmol 1993; 84: 19–30.

10. Wachtmeister L. Oscillatory potentials in the retina: what do they reveal? Prog Ret Eye Res 1998; 17: 485–521

11. Kondo M, Sieving PA. Primate photopic sine-wave flicker ERG: vector modelling and component origins using glutamate analogs. Invest Ophthalmol Vis Sci 2001; 42: 305–12.

12. Esakowitz L, Kriss A, Shawkat F. A comparison of flash electroretinograms recorded from Burian Allen, JET, C-Glide, gold foil, DTL, and skin electrodes. Eye 1993; 7: 169–71.

13. Bradshaw K, Fulton A, Hansen R, et al. Full field skin ERGs are comparable, after scaling, with corneal ERGs in normal adults and children. Abstr BRISCEV meeting 2003.

14. Sieving PA. Photopic ON- and OFF-pathway abnormalities in retinal dystrophies. Trans Am Ophthalmol Soc 1993; 91: 701–73.

15. Bech-Hansen NT, Naylor MJ, Maybaum TA, et al. Mutations in NYX, encoding the leucine-rich proteoglycan nyctalopin, cause X-linked complete congenital stationary night blindness. Nat Genet 2000; 26: 319–23.

16. Boycott KM, Maybaum TA, Naylor MJ, et al. A summary of 20 CACNA1F mutations identified in 36 families with incomplete X-linked congenital stationary night blindness, and characterization of splice variants. Hum Genet 2001; 108: 91–7.

17. Bradshaw K, George N, Moore A, et al. Mutations of the XLRS1 gene causing abnormalities of photoreceptor as well as inner retinal responses of the ERG. Doc Ophthalmol 1999; 98: 153–73.

18. Jensen H, Warburg M, Sjo O, et al. Duchenne muscular dystrophy: negative electroretinograms and normal dark adaptation. Reappraisal of assignment of X linked incomplete congenital stationary night blindness. J Med Genet 1995; 32: 348–51.

19. Fitzgerald K, Cibis G, Giambrone S, et al. Retinal signal transmission in Duchenne muscular dystrophy: evidence for dysfunction in the photoreceptor depolarising bipolar cell pathway. J Clin Invest 1994; 93: 2425–30.

20. Cicedyian A, Jacobsen S. Negative electroretinograms in retinitis pigmentosa. Invest Ophthalmol Vis Sci 1993; 34: 3253–63.

21. Miyake Y, Shiroyama N, Horiguchi M, et al. Bull's eye maculopathy and negative electroretinograms. Retina 1989; 9: 210–5.

22. Kellner U, Foerster MH. Cone dystrophies with negative photopic electroretinogram. Br J Ophthalmol 1993; 77: 404–9.

23. Lei B, Bush RA, Milam AH, et al. Human melanoma-associated retinopathy (MAR) antibodies alter the retinal ON-response of the monkey ERG in vivo. Invest Ophthalmol Vis Sci 2000;41:262–6.

24. Weleber R. The dystrophic retina in multisystem disorders: the electroretinogram in neuronal ceroid lipofuscinoses. Eye 1998; 12: 580–90.

25. Williams RE, Boyd S, Lake BD. Ultrastructural and electrophysiological correlation of the genotypes of NCL. Mol Genet Metab 1999; 66: 398–400.

26. Holder G. Pattern electroretinography (PERG) and an integrated approach to visual pathway diagnosis. In: Fishman GA, Birch D, Holder GE, et al., editors. Electrophysiologic Testing in Disorders of the Retina, Optic Nerve, and Visual Pathway. 2nd ed. Ophthalmology monograph 2. San Francisco: Foundation of the American Academy of Ophthalmology; 2001: 197–235.

27. Multifocal electroretinography: Special issue. The multifocal technique: topographic ERG and VEP responses. Doc Ophthalmol 2001; 100: 49–251.

28. Schroeder CE, Tenke CE, Givre SJ, et al. Striate cortical contribution to the surface recorded pattern reversal VEP in the alert monkey. Vision Res 1991;31:1143–57. (Erratum in: Vision Res 1991; 31(11): 1.)

29. Givre SJ, Schroeder CE, Arezzo JC. Contribution of extra striate area V4 to the surface recorded flash VEP in the awake macaque. Vision Res 1994; 34: 415–28.

30. Jeffreys DA, Axford JG. Source localisations of pattern-specific components of human visual evoked potentials l. Component of striate cortical origin. Exp Brain Res 1972; 6: 1–21.

31. Jeffreys DA, Axford JG. Source localisations of pattern-specific components of human visual evoked potentials ll. Component of extra-striate cortical origin. Exp Brain Res 1972 6: 22–40.

32. Ossenblok P, Spekreijse H. The extra-striate generators of the EP to checkerboard onset. A source localisation approach. Electroenceph Clin Neurophysiol 1991; 80: 181–93.

33. Shawkat FS, Kriss A. A study of the effects of contrast change on pattern VEPs, and the transition between onset, reversal and offset modes of stimulation. Doc Ophthalmol 2000; 101: 73–89.

34. Jasper HH. Report of the committee on methods of clinical examination in electroencephalography. Electroenceph Clin Neurophys 1958; 10: 370.

35. Soong F, Levin AV, Westall CA. Comparison of techniques for detecting visually evoked potential asymmetry in albinism. J AAPOS 2000; 4: 302–10.

36. Barrett G, Blumhardt L, Halliday A, et al. A paradox in the lateralization of the visual evoked response. Nature 1976; 261: 253–5.

37. Halliday A. Evoked Potentials in Clinical Testing. 2nd ed. Edinburgh: Churchill Livingstone; 1993.

38. Tyler CW, Apkarian P, Levi DM, et al. Rapid assessment of visual function: an electronic sweep technique for the pattern visual evoked potential. Invest Ophthalmol Vis Sci 1979; 18: 703–13.

39. Norcia A, Tyler C, Hamer R, et al. Measurement of spatial contrast sensitivity with the swept contrast VEP. Vision-Res 1989; 29; 627–37.

40. Allen D, Tyler C, Norcia A. Development of grating acuity and contrast sensitivity in the central and peripheral visual field of the human infant. Vision Res 1996; 36: 1945–53.

41. Apkarian P. Electrodiagnosis in paediatric ophthalmogenetics. Int J Psychophysiol 1994; 16: 229–43.

42. Kriss A, Russell-Eggitt IM, Harris CM, et al. Aspects of albinism. Ophthalmic Paediatr Genet 1992; 13: 89–100.

43. Sokol S. Measurement of infant visual acuity from pattern reversal evoked potentials. Vision Res 1978; 18: 33–9.

44. Marg E, Freeman DN, Peltzman P, et al. Visual acuity development in human infants: evoked potential measurements. Invest Ophthalmol Vis Sci 1976; 15: 150–3.

45. Orel-Bixler D, Norcia A. Differential growth for steady state pattern reversal and transient onset offset VEPs. Clin Vis Sci 1987; 2: 1–10.

46. Liasis A, Thompson DA, Hayward R, et al. Sustained raised intracranial pressure implicated only by pattern reversal visual evoked potentials after cranial vault expansion surgery. Pediatr Neurosurg 2003; 39: 75–80.

47. Fulton AB; Hansen RM. Electroretinography: application to clinical studies of infants. J Pediatr Ophthalmol Strabismus 1985; 22: 251–5.

48. Nusinowitz S, Birch DG, Birch EE. Rod photoresponses in 6-week and 4-month-old human infants. Vision Res 1998; 38: 627–35.

49. Kraemer M, Abrahamsson M, Sjostrum A. The neonatal development of the light flash visual evoked potential. Doc Ophthalmol 1999; 99: 21–39.

50. McCulloch DL, Orbach H, Skarf B. Maturation of the pattern reversal VEP in human infants: a theoretical framework. Vision Res 1999; 39: 3673–80.

51. Lambert SR, Kriss A, Taylor D. Delayed visual maturation; a longitudinal clinical and electrophysiological assessment. Ophthalmology 1989; 96: 534–29.

52. Kriss A, Russell-Eggitt IM. Electrophysiological assessment of visual pathway function in infants. Eye 1992; 6: 145–53.

53. Lambert SR; Kriss A; Taylor D. Detection of isolated occipital lobe anomalies during early childhood. Dev Med Child Neurol 1990; 32: 451–5.

54. Lambert SR, Taylor D, Kriss A. The infant with nystagmus, normal appearing fundi but an abnormal ERG. Surv Ophthalmol 1989; 34: 176–86.

55. Kriss A, Thompson D, Lloyd I, et al. Pattern VEP findings in young children treated for unilateral congenital cataract. In: Cottlier E, editor. Congenital Cataracts. Austin: RG Landes; 1994: 79.

CHAPTER
12 Diagnostic Ultrasound

Ken K Nischal

INTRODUCTION

Ocular ultrasound is a useful tool in the pediatric ophthalmologist's armamentarium. Improved technology has made reliable ultrasonography readily accessible.

Essentially a piezoelectric crystal is housed in a transducer and stimulated with electric current. This causes the crystal to vibrate, emitting ultrasonic waves. These are reflected back from the target being scanned or absorbed by the target at variable rates. These returning waves stimulate the piezoelectric crystal, which then creates a current. This is converted to a grayscale display to give an ultrasound scan picture in real time. In order for the same piezoelectric crystal to emit ultrasound waves and then absorb returning waves, the electric stimulation of the crystal is rapidly switched on and off.

INSTRUMENTATION

The transducer is most often housed in a case: the ultrasound probe. Transducers may be vector or linear.
1. Vector transducers oscillate back and forth, producing an image in the form of an arc (Fig. 12.1).

2. Linear transducers are aligned in several tightly packed rows and produce an image in the form of a rectangle (Fig. 12.2).

There are various transducers that can be used but the same ocular probes used in adults can be used for children. Examination of the globe is best done using 7- to 10-MHz transducers whereas the orbit is best examined with 5-MHz probes. Linear

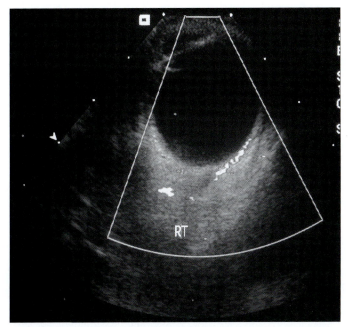

Fig. 12.1 Vector transducers oscillate back and forth producing an image in the form of an arc. This scan shows Doppler imaging also with increased flow in the choroid (see Fig. 12.6).

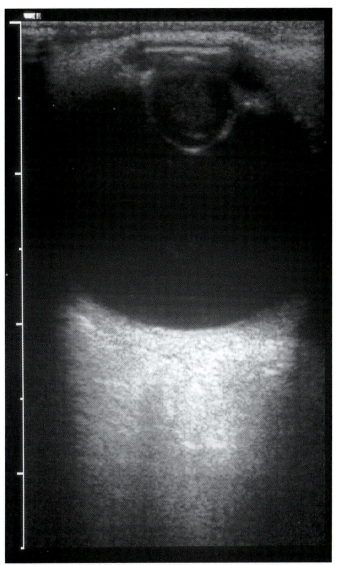

Fig. 12.2 Linear transducers are aligned in several tightly packed rows and produce an image in the form of a rectangle. The scan shows an intumescent lens in a child.

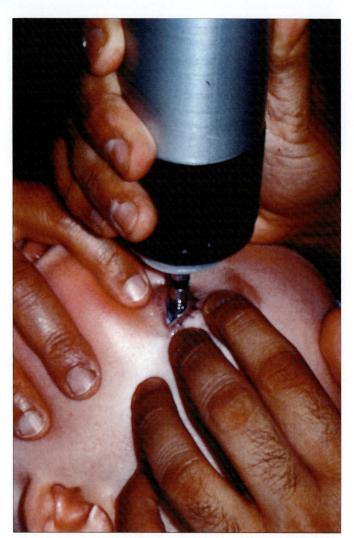

Fig. 12.3 UBM examinations need to be performed with the eyelids open and with a coupling agent between the cornea (front of the eye) and the transducer head.

transducers give much more information of the globe, and vector transducers are useful for orbital examination.

Fifty-megahertz transducers, which allow visualization of the first 5 mm of the eye to microscopic levels of distinction, are available. The most commonly available machine is the ultrasound biomicroscope (UBM), which requires the examination to be performed with the eyelids open and with a coupling agent between the cornea and the transducer head (Fig. 12.3). It usually is performed in children during an examination under anesthetic. All other transducers (5–10 MHz) are performed through the closed lids with coupling agent between the skin and the transducer head. To aid orientation the probe has a marker at one point on its circumference, which corresponds to a point on the display screen.

ROUTINE OF EXAMINATION

A complete but quick examination in children demands a routine. Although sedation with 50 to 100 mg/kg of chloral hydrate has

been used[1] to allow thorough examination, ultrasound is usually performed in children without anesthesia or sedation.[2] Babies can often be examined during feeding.

A simple routine of examination is to scan the eye in the vertical plane (i.e., with the marker on the transducer head pointing to the brow of the patient) and then in the horizontal plane (with the marker on the transducer head nearest the nose). In each plane of examination the optic nerve should be seen and then areas either side of the optic nerve. This results in scans of the superior and inferior areas of the globe and orbit (if scanning in horizontal plane) and scans of the nasal and temporal globe and orbit (if scanning in the vertical plane), together with scans of the optic nerve in both horizontal and vertical planes. This results in a protocol of static scans.

If ever a body organ was designed for dynamic USS the eye is it. By holding the probe still and getting the child to move its eyes or waiting for the child to move them spontaneously dynamic USS will be achieved. In any child who is not unusually myopic, the vitreous should not move during dynamic scanning. If it is seen to move then it is worth commenting upon. Furthermore in retinal detachment, dynamic USS will help confirm the diagnosis in those cases where the ocular media are obscured, e.g., after a hemorrhage into the vitreous after trauma.

High-frequency ultrasound is usually performed with the child under anesthetic, given the close proximity of the transducer to the child's eye, but in infants it may be performed with the child awake.[3] Scans are taken either axially through the pupil or at various clock hours positions either radial or parallel to the limbus (Figs. 12.4 and 12.5).

TYPES OF ULTRASOUND AVAILABLE FOR DIAGNOSTIC USE

There are two main types of ultrasound display:
1. *A-scan* is a single ultrasound wave used to measure the axial length and/or the corneal thickness.
2. *B-scan* is a 2-dimensional grayscale display that is a composite of many ultrasound waves (Fig. 12.6). The frequency of the transducer determines which part of the globe/orbit is examined. Low-frequency transducers (2–5 MHz) allow orbital examination while high-frequency ultrasound (30–50 MHz) allows high-definition imaging of the anterior segment but only to a depth of 5 mm (Figs. 12.4 and 12.5). The addition of Doppler facility allows evaluation of flow superimposed on a B-scan display (Figs. 12.6 and 12.7). Three-dimensional B-scan is also available and can be used for volume measurements.

Axial length measurements are critical for biometry, which has become increasingly important with the increased popularity of intraocular lens implantation in children. Biometry will not be discussed in this chapter.

ULTRASOUND AND THE EYELIDS

It is unusual to need ultrasound evaluation of lesions of the eyelids. Vascular anomalies of the eyelid occasionally need to be confirmed as such with Doppler ultrasound (Fig. 12.7). High-frequency ultrasound evaluation of skin lesions of the eyelid has not proved to be valuable. The eyelids are examined using a coupling agent (usually methylcellulose) with the eyes closed.

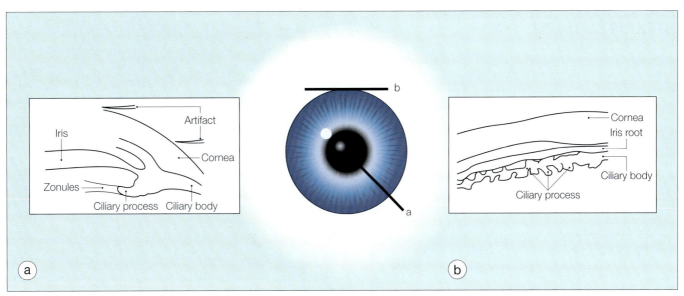

Fig. 12.4 Scans are taken either axially through the pupil or at various clock hours positions either radial or parallel to the limbus.

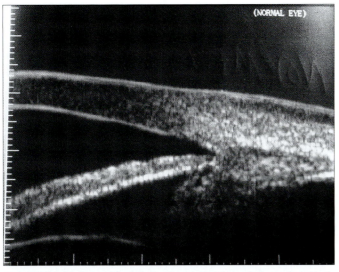

Fig. 12.5 UBM allows high-definition imaging of the anterior segment but only to a depth of 5 mm. Here the ciliary sulcus, ciliary body and processes, angle, iris, and corneoscleral junction are seen.

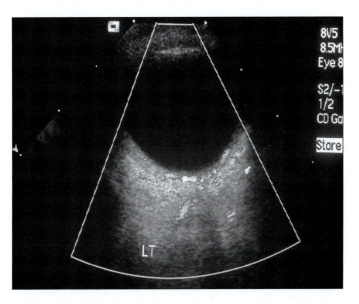

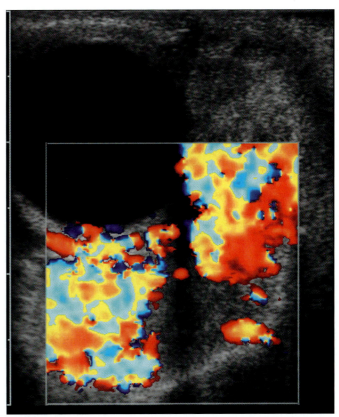

Fig. 12.7 Doppler ultrasound of periorbital hemangioma demonstrating flow in the orbit.

Fig. 12.6 The addition of a Doppler facility allows evaluation of flow superimposed on a B-scan display. This is a child with choroidal hemangioma. Choroidal hemangiomas are best assessed by measuring the retinochoroid-scleral thickness and may further be evaluated by using Doppler ultrasound to demonstrate increased blood flow.

ULTRASOUND OF THE CORNEA AND ANTERIOR SEGMENT

Pachymetry is the measurement of the corneal thickness using an A-scan. Pachymetry is useful in the evaluation of intraocular pressure (IOP) in any child with suspected glaucoma because the thickness of the cornea is proportional to the applanation tonometry-measured IOP. Therefore in cases such as mega-locornea the intraocular pressure may be determined to be artificially lower than it actually is.

The UBM has a 50-MHz transducer suspended on a mechanical arm, which allows relatively easy maneuverability. It provides a B-scan-type display and can also be used for pachymetry. It is very useful for the evaluation of congenital corneal opacification.[4] It allows microscopic evaluation of the cornea, allowing detection of corneal dystrophies such as congenital hereditary endothelial dystrophy (CHED) or posterior polymorphous dystrophy (PPD). In CHED, the cornea is thickened and there is increased echogenicity within the stroma with irregularities in the endothelial layer. In PPD there is an increased echogenicity at Descemet's layer and the endothelium. Peters anomaly can be diagnosed by the finding of a posterior stromal defect with absence of Descemet's membrane and the adjacent endothelium (Fig. 12.8).

Edema is hypoechogenic[4] while scarring is hyperechogenic. Scarring of the cornea sometimes needs to be assessed to decide whether a lamellar keratoplasty or penetrating keratoplasty is more appropriate.

A value of high-frequency ultrasound is its ability to improve surgical planning. In cases of corneal opacification, it allows evaluation of the anterior segment. Keratolenticular, iridolenticular, and iridocorneal adhesions can all be detected prior to surgery (Fig. 12.9).

UBM also allows visualization of the ciliary body, and this has been utilized to aid cycloablation[5,6] and to minimize side-effects of treatment.

UBM is also useful for the assessment of children and adults with cystinosis in whom a plateau-iris-type peripheral iris has been reported[7] and is due to swelling of the ciliary body secondary to cystine crystal deposition.

If a high-frequency ultrasound machine is not available some information can be gained about the anterior segment by using an ordinary probe (7–10 MHz) by using a water bath to scan through. Filling a rubber glove with water most easily does this. Coupling agent is placed on the closed eyelids and the water-filled glove placed on the eyelids. The probe with coupling agent is placed on the glove and scanning commenced. It takes a while

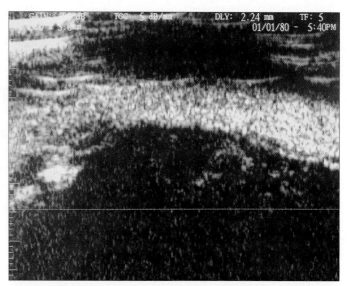

Fig. 12.9 Ultrasound of sclerocornea showing posterior corneal defect with complete disorganization of the anterior chamber.

to appreciate the ocular structures but the globe is displaced to one side of the display screen but details of the anterior segment become more apparent. It is not as efficient or as accurate as high-frequency ultrasound but it is better than nothing.

ULTRASOUND OF THE GLOBE

Globe ultrasound is best performed using a 7- to 10-MHz transducer. A linear transducer allows more information to be viewed from the front of the globe than that using a vector probe; however, vector probes are generally more readily available in dedicated marketed ocular ultrasound machines. Ultrasound is essential for a full evaluation in those conditions causing leukocoria (cataract, retinoblastoma, Coats disease, retinal detachment, toxocariasis), hazy media (vitreous hemorrhage, vitreitis), ocular tumors (retinoblastoma, medulloepithelioma), and structural anomalies (severe microphthalmos/anophthalmos, coloboma).

Leukocoria

Cataract

When there is a limited view of the fundus due to cataract, it is essential to establish that the posterior segment appears normal on ultrasound examination. In particular it is important to exclude or confirm the diagnosis of *persistent hyperplastic primary vitreous* (PHPV) and *posterior lenticonus*. Usually there are clinical indicators of the diagnosis such as microphthalmos, and vascular posterior plaque on lens with a relatively clear anterior lens. There is usually a retrolental band,[8] which may be thick or thin, with evidence of increased posterior capsular echogenicity.[9] Doppler ultrasound is very useful for illustrating blood flow in this persistent hyaloid artery structure (Fig. 12.10) and can indicate the possibility of intraocular bleeding at the tine of any proposed lensectomy. Occasionally secondary retinal detachment with or without gross disorganization of the posterior pole may be seen.[10]

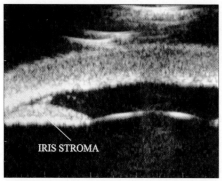

Fig. 12.8 Peters anomaly can be diagnosed by the finding of a posterior stromal defect with absence of Descemet's membrane and the adjacent endothelium.

IRIS STROMA

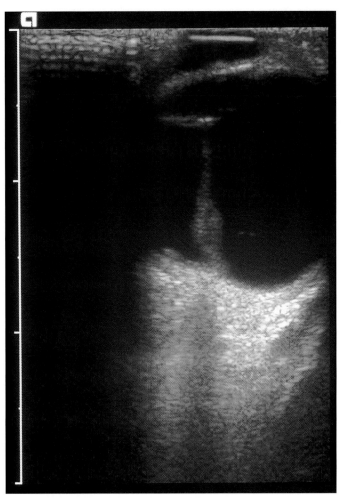

Fig. 12.10 Ultrasound of an eye with PHPV showing a large hyaloid remnant extending from the optic disc to the posterior surface of the lens.

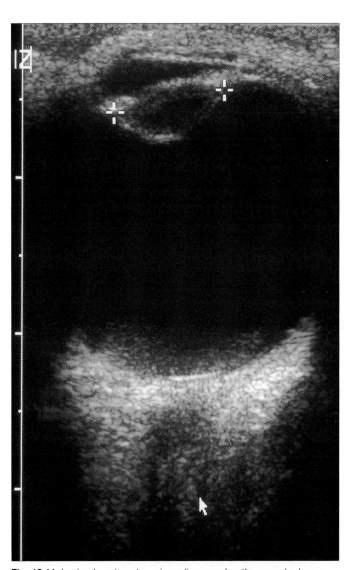

Fig. 12.11 In simple cataracts, using a linear probe, the capsular bag can be measured between two cursors. This is important if implantation is considered, as it will determine whether an implant is possible and, if so, what diameter implant can be used.

High-frequency ultrasound has been used to evaluate cases of PHPV[11] and has demonstrated a double linear echo thought to represent an unusual thickening of the anterior hyaloid face attaching to the peripheral anterior retina.

In simple cataracts, the capsular bag can be measured with a linear probe. This is important if implantation is being considered; as it will determine what diameter implant can be used (Fig. 12.11).

In posterior lenticonus, the posterior lens defect and extrusion of lens cortex posteriorly can be detected preoperatively (Fig. 12.12).

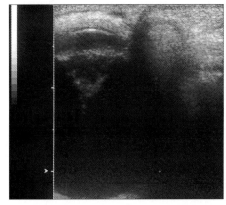

Fig. 12.12 A case of posterior lenticonus: a cone-shaped structure (representing extruding lens material) can be seen extending posteriorly from the posterior lens surface.

Retinal detachment

This may be tractional (most commonly seen in stages IV and V retinopathy of prematurity), exudative, or rhegmatogenous.

Tractional retinal detachment may be total or partial. Total retinal detachment has a typical appearance with a funnel-shaped echogenicity, the mouth of the funnel showing increased linear echogenicity (Fig. 12.13a). Partial retinal detachment behaves in a rigid fashion on dynamic scanning. There is usually no obvious mobile posterior hyaloid face seen in children in cases of tractional retinal detachments.

Exudative detachments can be difficult to diagnose but may show a shallow detachment of the retina, which tends to follow the contour of the posterior wall of the globe. Often the

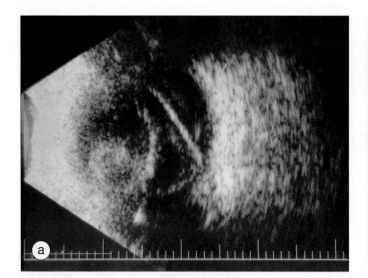

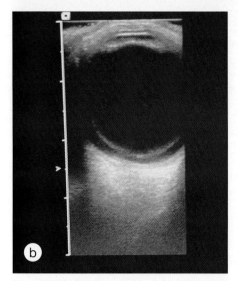

Fig. 12.13 (a) Total retinal detachment has a typical appearance with a funnel-shaped echogenicity. (b) A serous detachment in a child with a nonspecific systemic vasculitis. The detachment receded with systemic steroids.

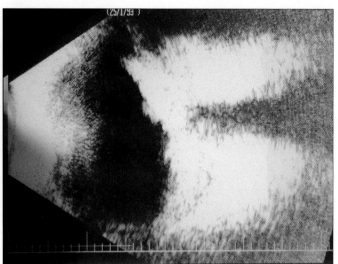

Fig. 12.14 The scan demonstrates folds of retinochoroidal layers together with thickening of the sclera in a child with scleritis associated with Wegener granulomatosis.

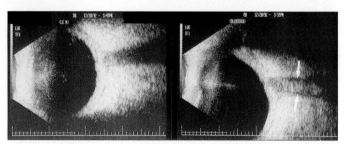

Fig. 12.15 Posterior scleritis may also be suspected if there is fluid seen in Tenon's space.

subretinal space has areas of slightly raised echogenicity.[9] It is almost impossible to demonstrate the "shifting fluid" sign using ultrasound usually because of lack of cooperation from the child. If the exudative retinal detachment is due to posterior scleritis,[12] ultrasound may demonstrate folds of retinochoroidal layers together with thickening of the sclera (Fig. 12.13b). Posterior scleritis may also be suspected if there is fluid seen in Tenon's space (Figs. 12.14 and 12.15). Subhyaloid hemorrhages can be differentiated by finding the retina intact with the echogenicity corresponding to the hemorrhage behind the posterior hyaloid face (Fig. 12.16a). In choroidal hemorrhage (as after trabeculectomy for glaucoma in the presence of a choroidal hemangioma) the retina is anterior to the main area of echogenicity associated with the hemorrhage (Fig. 12.16b).

Rhegmatogenous retinal detachments are rare in children but if seen, the possibility of Stickler syndrome should be considered. To make a diagnosis of a rhegmatogenous detachment, a reflection of a fluid posterior hyaloid face must be seen anterior to the putative retinal detachment (Fig. 12.16c). This is important to recognize because sometimes if there has been some vitreous

hemorrhage the posterior hyaloid face may become coated with blood, detach, and then be mistaken for a detached retina due to an increased echogenicity.

Retinoblastoma (See Chapter 50)

Although CT scan is used to check for extension of the tumor and to confirm the diagnosis, an ultrasound scan helps make the diagnosis. The main differential diagnosis of retinoblastoma is Coats disease, end-stage retinopathy of prematurity, and toxocariasis.

Two-dimensional B-scan USS shows a dome-shaped lesion(s) with or without a retinal detachment, depending on whether the tumor is endophytic or exophytic. To confirm the presence of the almost pathognomonic calcification, the gain is reduced to a minimum; if the original area of high echogenicity remains hyperechogenic then this is likely to be calcification. In tumors that are calcified there is attenuation of USS posterior to the tumor, resulting in an orbital shadow. Calcium may be diffuse or localized within a retinoblastoma.[9,13] If the tumor is necrotic then sometimes there is little or no increased reflectivity. These latter cases can be difficult to distinguish from Coats disease where there is subretinal exudate causing retinal detachment.

Three-dimensional ultrasound may detect growth and response of treatment of retinoblastoma.[14] It allows volume measurements of tumors and allows an appreciation of the size of the base of the tumor rather than merely tumor height. Few machines are available for 3-D ocular ultrasound but all rely on the patient being steady for a number of seconds while data are acquired. For

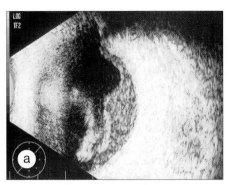 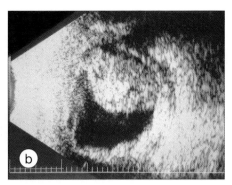 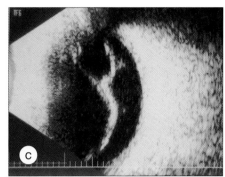

Fig. 12.16 (a) Ultrasound of a subhyaloid hemorrhage. The posterior hyaloid face is coated with blood but there is no detachment. (b) A choroidal hemorrhage/expansion after trabeculectomy in a child with choroidal hemangioma. (c) To make a diagnosis of a rhegmatogenous detachment, a reflection of a fluid posterior hyaloid face must be seen anterior to the putative retinal detachment.

this reason examinations are usually best done in younger children under anesthetic or sedation.

Coats disease

The signs seen on USS in Coats disease depend on the extent of the abnormality. At an early stage where there are vascular anomalies with hard exudates only, USS is often unremarkable. USS is more useful in patients who present later with retinal detachments and leukocoria. These retinal detachments are due to subretinal exudates, which usually contain cholesterol crystals.[9,15] USS examination often reveals tiny low-echogenic opacities, which may be due to the cholesterol crystals or to blood.[10,16] In some long-standing cases calcification may occur but this is more plaque-like, whereas that seen in retinoblastoma is more granular and diffuse on B-scan.[9,10] Otherwise the echogenicity is much less in cases of Coats disease than in those of retinoblastoma. Masses with heterogeneous echoes may be seen in Coats disease, and these are usually due to massive subretinal fibrosis.

Toxocariasis

See the section Vitreitis.

Hazy media

Vitreous hemorrhage

Spontaneous vitreous hemorrhage is very rare in children.[17] Ultrasound can help make the diagnosis, however. Causes include PHPV, choroidal hemangioma, and sickle cell disease.[18]

USS reveals multiple hyperechogenic opacities throughout the vitreous, which are very mobile. The opacities vary in size but in general are very small. If there is blood in the subhyaloid space this tends to be more echogenic, and the posterior hyaloid face becomes coated with blood, resulting in a bright echo from the hyaloid face itself.

Choroidal hemangiomas are best assessed by measuring the retinochoroid-scleral thickness and may further be evaluated by using Doppler ultrasound to demonstrate increased blood flow (Fig. 12.6). In cases of vitreous hemorrhage due to retinal neovascularization as may be seen in sickle cell proliferative retinopathy, there is a stalk-like hyperechogenic lesion attaching the posterior hyaloid face to the retinal surface usually peripherally. In sickle cell disease there may also be subretinal hemorrhage.

In cases of trauma-related vitreous hemorrhage USS is very important to exclude a retinal detachment or posterior perforation. In such circumstances MRI has become more popular as its availability has improved.

Vitreitis

Inflammation within the vitreous is seen as an increased echogenicity of a very fine granular nature (Fig. 12.17). The echogenicity is much less intense than that seen in vitreous hemorrhage. There may be an associated lesion in the periphery or posterior pole such as a granuloma, which may be seen in toxocariasis. This condition may present with a granuloma or as a chronic endophthalmitis. The granuloma shows a reduced echogenicity and may be associated with a tractional retinal detachment or a membrane.[19] High-frequency ultrasound has been used to evaluate cases of toxocariasis where there is a peripheral granuloma.[20] Intermediate uveitis may be suspected if there is an increased echogenicity at the pars plana area with signs of a vitreitis on USS.

Ocular tumors

Retinoblastoma

See the same-titled section under Leukocoria.

Medulloepithelioma

This arises from the medullary epithelium of the ciliary body in children. Ultrasound, especially high-frequency ultrasound, shows a solid mass arising from the ciliary body region, which may or may be associated with iris cysts or localized areas of high echoes due to the presence of cartilage.[9]

Structural anomalies

Colobomas

Usually ultrasound is not needed to make the diagnosis of a coloboma of the retinochoroid or optic disc. When the media are not clear, it is important to recognize a coloboma, especially in microphthalmic eyes with cataract, given the association of microphthalmos with coloboma.

Ultrasound shows a distinct defect of the optic nerve head, which may extend into the adjacent retinochoroid (Fig. 12.18). This defect may reveal single strands extending across the defect, and some authors have described a double-walled lining posteriorly.[21] Occasionally a clear connection between the optic nerve sheath and the defect can be seen.

Anophthalmos and severe microphthalmos

Ultrasound helps differentiate between anophthalmos and severe microphthalmos (Fig. 12.19). USS is performed through the closed lids, and in any case of microphthalmos orbital ultrasound

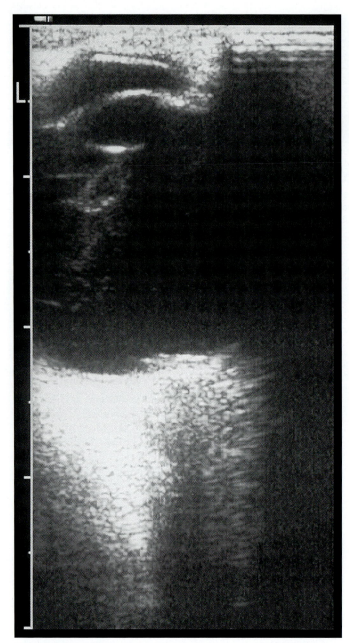

Fig. 12.17 Inflammation within the vitreous is seen as an increased echogenicity of a very fine granular nature.

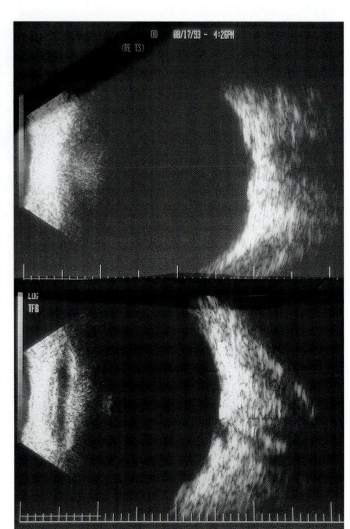

Fig. 12.18 Ultrasound shows a distinct defect of the optic nerve head, which may extend into the adjacent (inferior) retinochoroid; this suggests a coloboma.

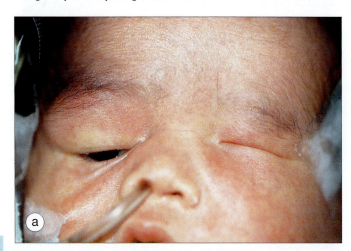

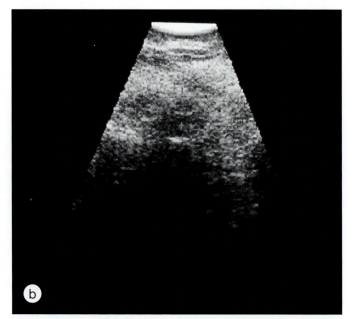

Fig. 12.19 (a) A baby with extreme microphthalmos or anophthalmos of the left eye. (b) Ultrasound shows a very small globe, helping to differentiate between anophthalmos and severe microphthalmos.

can reveal the presence of an orbital cyst. This is seen as a round, almost completely anechoic lesion posterior or adjacent to the microphthalmic eye.[22]

Miscellaneous

Angle recession and supraciliary cleft
High-frequency ultrasound is very useful in making the diagnosis of a supraciliary cleft. There is a separation of the ciliary body from the overlying sclera. Septa can be seen in the supraciliary space.

Optic disc drusen
Optic disc drusen are buried in children and are an important cause of pseudopapilledema. Although by definition they are calcified hyaline bodies in very young children there may be minimal calcification. The diagnosis should be made on USS with a very low gain, showing increased reflectivity deep in the optic nerve head and not just superficially. In young children, to allow maximal detection of reflected ultrasound waves, the probe should be angled so as to avoid the lens. The human lens absorbs ultrasound, and in a patient with early/mildly calcified drusen the reflected waves may be absorbed by the lens and not detected (Fig. 12.20a).

Retinal astrocytoma
These show calcification, which again increases with age. In obviously calcified lesions there is a hyperechoic lesion on the retina with a corresponding orbital shadow (Figs. 12.20b, 12.20c). Novice ultrasonographers can mistake this for the optic nerve.

Optic disc cupping
Some authors describe the use of B-scan ultrasound to evaluate optic disc cupping. Although this is useful in those cases where the media are unclear to help establish the diagnosis of glaucoma, it is not as useful as A-scan measurement of the axial length of the eye for serial evaluation of glaucoma treatment.

ULTRASOUND AND THE ORBIT

Ultrasound of the orbit is best performed using lower frequency vector transducers.

Doppler ultrasound has also been shown to be useful in these cases. The main use of ultrasound of the orbit in the pediatric population is in cases of acquired proptosis. Most commonly this is seen unilaterally with vascular anomalies, neoplasms, and orbital pseudotumor. Cases of thyroid eye disease can be seen in children but ultrasound in these cases is much less useful than MRI to assess the size of the extraocular muscles.

Vascular anomalies

Capillary hemangioma
Both A- and B-scan findings of capillary hemangiomas are characterized by variable internal reflectivity. Areas of low reflectivity correspond to solid hypercellular regions of endothelial proliferation; areas of moderate reflectivity to ectatic vascular channels; and areas of high reflectivity to fibrous septae separating tumor lobules.[23] The resulting scan is one of tightly packed small hypoechoic channels, which show fast flow on Doppler examination (Fig. 12.7).

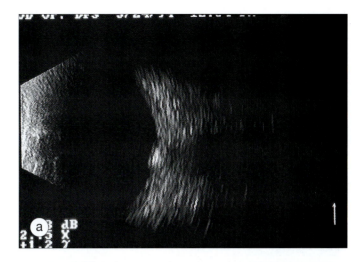

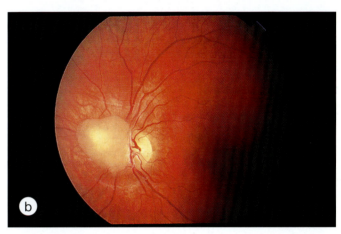

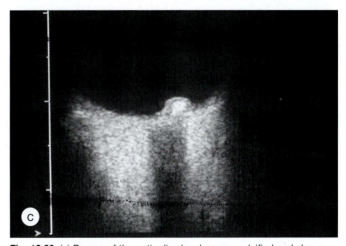

Fig. 12.20 (a) Drusen of the optic disc has become calcified and shows high reflectivity. (b) A hamartoma at the optic disc. (c) Same case as in Fig. 12.20(b). The ultrasound shows central calcification: the size of the lesion can be monitored by ultrasound.

Lymphangioma
These have much larger hypoechoic areas and Doppler ultrasound shows little or no flow through them. Ultimately CT scan or MRI is needed to help evaluate the condition more fully. Capillary hemangiomas show much smaller hypoechoic areas with fast flow on Doppler scanning.

Neoplasms

The main neoplasm that needs excluding is rhabdomyosarcoma. The proptosis here is usually nonaxial but this may be the case in a deep vascular anomaly also. Rhabdomyosarcomas show much more of a homogeneous ultrasound picture with blood flow that usually is less diffusely displayed than that seen in a capillary hemangioma. However, very vascular rhabdomyosarcoma scan be seen and therefore MRI or CT scan should be considered in cases where the diagnosis is unclear.

Orbital pseudotumor

This is part of the spectrum of disease that includes orbital myositis. Contiguous inflammation from orbital pseudotumor may lead to posterior scleritis, fluid in the extraocular muscle sheaths, and fluid in the optic nerve sheath, all of which results in a much better definition of all these structures than normal. The orbital pseudotumor itself may cause indentation of the globe, and in itself is a homogeneously echoic lesion, the posterior edge of which is usually poorly defined.

Miscellaneous

Doppler ultrasound has become increasingly useful in the evaluation of the superior orbital vein. In cases where it is enlarged or has developed fast flow, arteriovenous malformations must be suspected.

REFERENCES

1. Enriquez G, Gil-Gibernau JJ, Garriga V, et al. Sonography of the eye in children: imaging findings. Am J Roentgenol 1995; 165: 935–9.
2. Panarello SM, Priolo E, Vittone P. Pediatric ultrasound: a personal experience during the period 1991–1994. Ophthalmologica 1998; 212(s): 115–7.
3. Kiryu J, Park M, Kobayashi H, et al. Ultrasound biomicroscopy of the anterior segment of the eyes of infants. J Pediatr Ophthalmol Strabismus 1998; 35: 320–2.
4. Nischal KK, Naor J, Jay V, et al. Clinicopathologic correlation of congenital corneal opacification using ultrasound biomicroscopy. Br J Ophthalmol 2002; 86: 62–9.
5. Choong YF, Kouri A, Nischal KK. High frequency ultrasound guided cyclophotocoagulation in pediatric glaucoma. Poster AAPOS March 2003 (unpublished data).
6. Pavlin CJ, Macken P, Trope GE, et al. Ultrasound biomicroscopic imaging of the effects of YAG laser cycloablation in postmortem eyes and living patients. Ophthalmology 1995; 102: 334–41.
7. Mungan N, Nischal KK, MacKeen L, et al. Ultrasound biomicroscopy of the eye in cystinosis. Arch Ophthalmol 2000; 118: 1329–33.
8. Haik BG, Zimmer-Galler I, Smith ME. Ultrasound in the evaluation of leukocoria. J Diagnost Med Sonogr 1989; 3: 116.
9. Byrne SF, Green RL. Ultrasound of the Eye and Orbit. St.Louis: Mosby Yearbook; 1992.
10. Long G, Stringer DA, Nadel HR, et al. B mode ultrasonography–spectrum of paediatric ocular disease. Eur J Radiol 1998; 26: 132–47.
11. MacKeen L, Nischal KK, Lam WC, et al. High-frequency ultrasonography findings in persistent hyperplastic primary vitreous. J AAPOS 2000; 4: 217–24.
12. Woon WH, Stanford MR, Graham EM. Severe idiopathic posterior scleritis in children. Eye 1995; 9: 570–4.
13. Roth DB, Scott IU, Murray TG, et al. Echography of retinoblastoma: histopathologic correlation and serial evaluation after globe-conserving radiotherapy or chemotherapy. J Pediatr Ophthalmol Strabismus 2001; 38: 136–43.
14. Finger PT, Khoobehi A, Ponce-Contreras MR, et al. Three dimensional ultrasound of retinoblastoma: initial experience. Br J Ophthalmol 2002; 86: 1136–8.
15. Shields JA, Shields CL, Honavar SG, et al. Clinical variations and complications of Coats disease in 150 cases: the 2000 Sanford Gifford Memorial Lecture. Am J Ophthalmol 2001; 131: 561–71.
16. Smirpniotopoulos JG, Bargalo N, Mafee MF. Differential diagnosis of leukocoria: radiologic pathologic correlation. Radiographics 1994; 14: 1059–79.
17. Nischal KK, James JN, McAllister J. The use of dynamic ultrasound B-scan to detect retinal tears in spontaneous vitreous haemorrhage. Eye 1995; 9: 502–6.
18. Onder F, Cossar CB, Gultan E, et al. Vitreous hemorrhage from the persistent hyaloid artery. J AAPOS 2000; 4: 190–1.
19. Schneider C, Arnaud B, Schmitt-Bernard CF. [Ocular toxocariasis. Value of local immunodiagnosis.] J Fr Ophtalmol 2000; 23: 1016–9.
20. Tran VT, LeHoang P, Herbort CP. Value of high-frequency ultrasound biomicroscopy in uveitis. Eye 2001; 15: 23–30.
21. Singh J, Ghose S. Isolated coloboma of the optic nerve head: an echographic evaluation. Ann Ophthalmol 1987; 19: 184–6.
22. Fledelius HC. Ultrasonic evaluation of microphthalmos and coloboma. A discussion of 3 cases, with emphasis on microphthalmos with orbital cyst. Acta Ophthalmol Scand Suppl 1996; (219): 23–6.
23. Basta LL, Anderson LS, Acers TE. Regression of orbital hemangioma detected by echography. Arch Ophthalmol 1977; 95: 1383–6.

CHAPTER 13 Neuroimaging of the Visual Pathway in Children

Philippe Demaerel

INTRODUCTION

The contribution of neuroradiological examination to the diagnosis of visual disorders in children has significantly changed with the advent of magnetic resonance (MR) imaging.

Computed tomography (CT) is still an excellent technique for imaging the eye and orbit but the irradiation of the soft tissues should be particularly considered.

The main advantage of MR imaging is the absence of ionizing radiation. MR imaging is superior to CT because of its better soft tissue contrast and multiplanar capability; it is the modality of choice for imaging the visual pathway. CT remains the modality of choice for visualizing the bones, for demonstrating calcification, and for depicting foreign bodies in the orbits and brain.

The applications of both techniques and the different approach in adults and children will be discussed. Ultrasound is discussed in Chapter 12. Catheter angiography is rarely required in children with visual disturbances and will therefore not be discussed in this chapter.

ANATOMICAL CONSIDERATIONS REGARDING CT AND MR IMAGING

The bony orbital structures are best seen on CT. The orbital portion of the optic nerve can be adequately visualized with both techniques but the optic nerve can more easily be differentiated from its surrounding sheath on MR imaging (Fig. 13.1).

For the globe, MR has some distinct advantages. On CT, the lens and the ciliary bodies can be seen separating the anterior chamber from the vitreous. In addition, MR imaging can differentiate the lens capsule, and the macula can be identified in most cases (Fig. 13.2). The sclera can usually be differentiated from the choroid, ciliary body, and iris. Using high-resolution MR imaging with dedicated surface coils, it is possible to define the septum orbitale in most patients[1]: treatment differs depending on whether orbital cellulitis is pre- or postseptal.

CT and MR imaging are comparable in demonstrating the extraocular muscles and the lacrimal gland.

MR is preferable for imaging the intracranial portion of the optic nerve and the chiasm and for a detailed analysis of the posterior

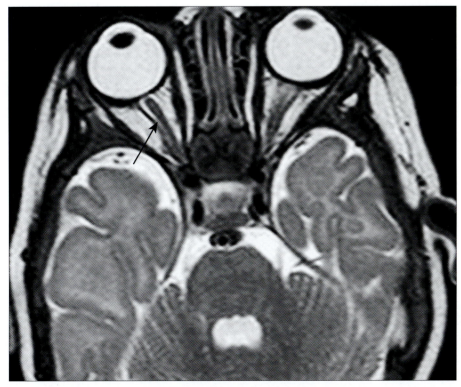

Fig. 13.1 Axial T2-weighted images. Normal appearance of the right optic nerve (arrow).

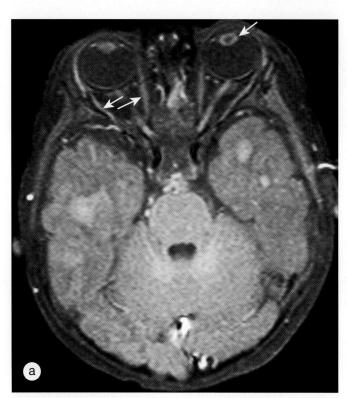
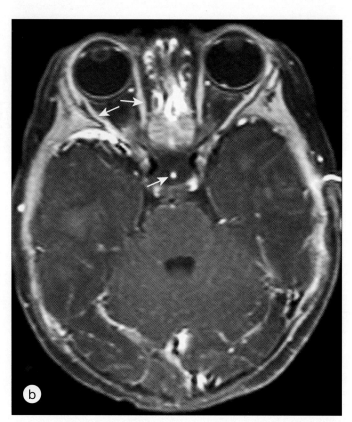

Fig. 13.2 Axial T1-weighted images with fat saturation (a) before and (b) after intravenous contrast administration. Note the differentiation between the lens and the lens capsule (a, arrows). Note the normal enhancement of structures such as the extraocular muscles, the vascular structures, the choroid and the pituitary stalk (b, arrows).

visual pathway. With high-resolution MR images it may be possible to identify the lateral geniculate nucleus and the fibers of the optic radiation.

TECHNICAL CONSIDERATIONS

CT has made significant progress in the past decade. Many radiology departments offer the spiral or helical technique. A chosen volume is exposed to continuous radiation. The newest generation multislice CT scanners allows a fast and high-resolution imaging of any part of the body.

The author performs CT in the axial plane using 120 kV and 120 mA. In spiral mode, a slice thickness of 1.5 mm with a pitch of 2.3 is used. The pitch is the longitudinal distance the patient travels per tube rotation divided by the nominal slice width. Thereafter, 1.5-mm slices are reformatted in a plane parallel to the optic nerve (almost parallel to the canthomeatal line) and perpendicular to this imaging plane. Small lesions can clearly be identified. Direct coronal imaging, which is difficult to obtain in children, is rarely necessary thanks to the excellent quality of the reformatted spiral CT images. For imaging of the orbital tissues, window width/level values of 350/80 Hounsfield units are recommended. For bone assessment, high-resolution bone scale images should be obtained using window width/level values of 2500/500 Hounsfield units.

CT is associated with several limitations: the radiation exposure, the potential risk of iodinated contrast agents, and the beam-hardening (caused by the bone adjacent to the soft tissues) and dental amalgam artifacts. The main disadvantage is the radiation

dose to the lens.[2,3] The dose depends on slice thickness and number of slices. On the author's multislice spiral scan an examination of the orbit results in approximately 8 mSv to the lens in a child and 13 mSv in an adult. This is far below the dose that can cause cataracts (500 mSv/year during 5 years). It is also useful to know that the natural background radiation per year is approximately 2.5 mSv.

The author advocates the use of a contrast agent in most patients except for the assessment of developmental abnormalities, in suspected ischemia, following trauma, and (much less frequent in children) in thyroid eye disease.

Iodinated contrast agents may improve the detection of a lesion or its characterization. Contrast media distribute both into the blood plasma and into the interstitial fluid compartment of the organs. Normal neuronal structures do not enhance because of the blood–brain barrier, which consists of tight junctions between the cells of blood vessels. It is important to realize that anatomical structures without a blood–brain barrier, such as the meninges, vascular structures, the pituitary stalk, the pineal gland, the cavernous sinuses, the uvea, and the extraocular muscles, will normally enhance (Fig. 13.2). Anything that disrupts the blood–brain barrier will also enhance.

Adverse reactions to contrast administration have been reported in up to 3% of patients. Usually mild, severe adverse reactions occur in approximately 1:40,000, but can be more frequent in elderly patients.[4] Because of renal toxicity, patients with impaired renal function should not be given an iodinated contrast agent.

The advantages of MR imaging include the absence of ionizing radiation, direct multiplanar imaging, and the availability of safe MR-specific contrast agents. MR imaging is based on the interaction between a high-field magnet and hydrogen nuclei in the body, which have magnetic properties themselves and are abundantly present in all tissues, resulting in high-quality images. Nowadays, the resolution from head coils is sufficient in most patients; special surface coils are usually unnecessary.

The mechanism of action of a MR contrast agent is analogous to that of iodinated contrast agents in CT. Contrast media may improve lesion detection and/or lesion characterization. MR contrast agents are gadolinium chelates, which are safe products compared with the iodinated contrast media. Gadolinium is a paramagnetic metal used clinically. The metal is always encapsulated by a chelate, and both substances protect each other from having toxic effects. Fasting before the injection of a MR contrast agent, which is required for iodinated contrast agents, is not necessary. Severe adverse reactions are rare at 1:350,000.[5] Mild and moderate reactions are much less frequent than with iodinated contrast media in CT.

Tumours, infectious diseases, and cranial nerve palsy are typical indications for the administration of a contrast agent (Fig. 13.3).

The disadvantages of MR imaging compared with CT include the high installation and running cost. Most MR scanners are closed systems in a claustrophobic, noisy, narrow tube and almost all children below 5 years need sedation or general anesthesia (Fig. 13.4).[6,7] Many children do not require sedation for CT because of the rapidity of the examination. Multislice brain or orbital spiral CT can be achieved within one minute. Occasionally simple immobilization may be sufficient.

Various drugs are available when sedation is required. Oral chloral hydrate has been one of the safest drugs for children. Intramuscular or intravenous administration of pentobarbital (Nembutal) has also proved to be popular. At the author's institution the anesthesiologists induce with Sevofluorane and use a laryngeal mask and the child breaths spontaneously. Following the induction, propofol (Diprivan) is started. Due to its rapid degradation by the liver, the child can easily be aroused after the examination upon terminating the infusion. The monitoring of children under the continuous supervision of the anesthesiologist must be performed using nonferromagnetic MR-compatible equipment. MR imaging of the brain and orbits takes approximately 25 min.

Finally, one should be extremely careful with ferromagnetic materials. These should not be exposed to the strong magnetic field. Ventricular shunts will cause so-called susceptibility artifacts but can safely be examined. Shunts with transcutaneous magnetically adjustable valves, however, need to be checked radiologically after the MR examination and may need readjustment.

WHEN TO RECOMMEND CT OR MR IMAGING

As far as the eyeball itself is concerned, the role of CT is limited to those patients where ultrasound is technically difficult or when the sonographic observations are difficult to interpret.

Indications for CT include leukocoria, trauma, and proptosis of the eyeball. The detection of calcification in a child younger than 3 years of age is highly suggestive of retinoblastoma, although a minority of retinoblastomas present without calcification (Fig. 13.5).

CT is preferable for the detection of calcification (e.g., retinoblastoma, drusen) and for assessing the interface between bone and air, both of which appear black on MR imaging. Fractures are best seen on CT (Fig. 13.6). Several craniofacial anomalies affect vision with an abnormal shape or size of the orbits (Fig. 13.7). These include several types of craniosynostoses, fibrous dysplasia, and osteopetrosis.[8] The author prefers CT in the early assessment of suspected hemorrhage and brain edema

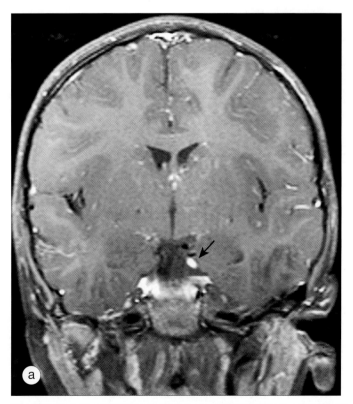
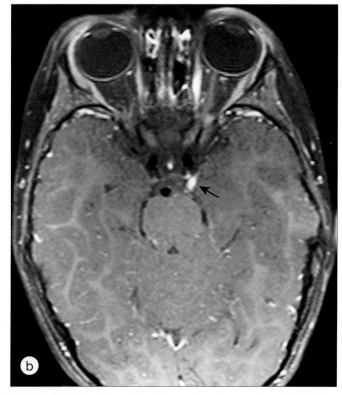

Fig. 13.3 Coronal and axial contrast-enhanced T1-weighted images with fat saturation in a patient with neuritis of the oculomotor nerve (a and b, arrow).

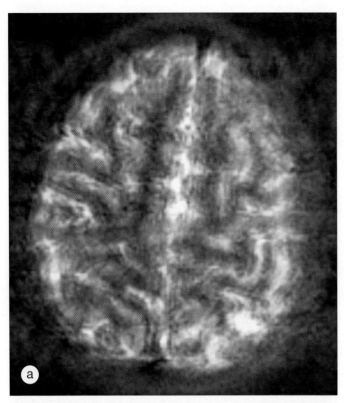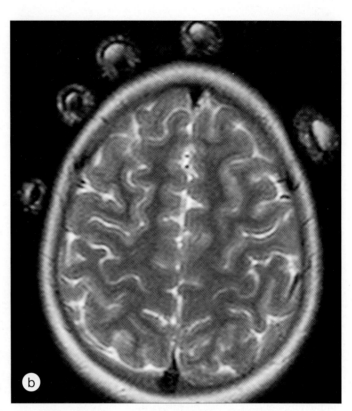

Fig. 13.4 Axial T2-weighted images. (a) Some form of sedation is necessary in most children under five years of age to avoid motion artifacts. (b) Although holding the head is certainly not routine, it was successful in this patient. Note the images of the parent's fingers on the childs skull.

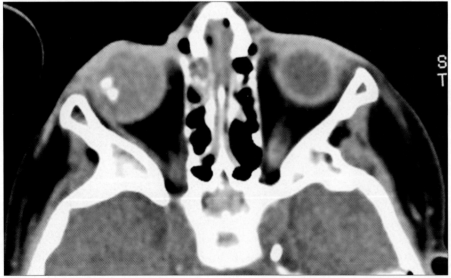

Fig. 13.5 Axial unenhanced CT in a patient with a partly calcified retinoblastoma of the right eye.

(Fig. 13.8). CT is also excellent for assessing preseptal cellulitis and the assessment of possible abscess formation and/or postseptal extension (Fig. 13.9). Clinical distinction between preseptal cellulitis without or with postseptal extension is difficult in the young child. CT is mandatory because more aggressive therapy is required when postseptal.

When an intraocular or intraorbital foreign body is suspected, CT is indicated to detect glass or metal.[9,10] If such materials are excluded, MR imaging may be useful to depict plastic (polyethylene or polystyrene) or wood fragments, but only after a metallic foreign body has been excluded.[11,12]

For the majority of patients, MR imaging is preferred over CT (Table 13.1).[13]

The imaging strategy in pediatric MR imaging of the brain and orbits has undergone significant changes.[14] Most MR examinations still use T1- and T2-weighted images. The T2-weighted images are best for detection of pathology. We use a T2-weighted double-echo short-time inversion recovery sequence, which offers an excellent differentiation between gray and white matter (Fig. 13.10). T1-weighted images are better for delineating the anatomical structures and are also necessary as pre-contrast sequence. It is important to know that fat will appear bright on

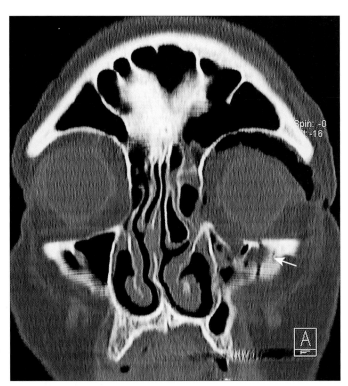

Fig. 13.6 Coronal CT at bone window setting demonstrates the fracture of the left orbital floor (white arrow to the fracture).

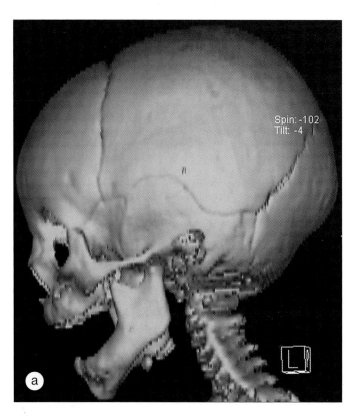

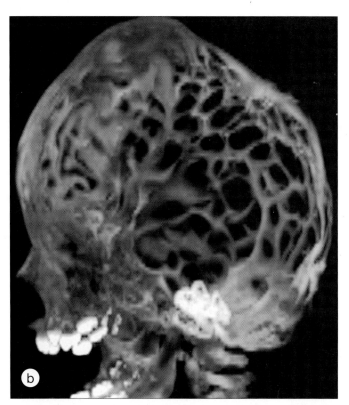

Fig. 13.7 Three-dimensional CT (a) in a healthy child and (b) in a patient with Pfeiffer syndrome, showing the "beaten metal" appearance caused by raised intracranial pressure leading to abnormally modeled skull bones.

T1 and dark on T2, while cerebrospinal fluid will appear bright on T2 and dark on T1. The administration of a contrast agent, usually gadopentetate dimeglumine, will enhance most pathological conditions. Enhancing structures appear bright on T1-weighted images.

The slice thickness of most sequences is at least 3 mm but one can obtain a three-dimensional gradient-echo T1-weighted volumetric sequence that offers between 124 and 160 1-mm slices, which can then be reformatted in any plane with an identical slice thickness. This is particularly useful for assessing congenital pathology of the optic nerve. More recently, a three-dimensional T2-weighted sequence has become available.

Several sequences have been developed to improve the visualization of pathology. A fluid-attenuated inversion recovery (FLAIR) sequence produces heavily T2-weighted images while simultaneously suppressing the signal from cerebrospinal fluid. The technique has been used in many pathological conditions and proved particularly useful for documenting periventricular leukomalacia secondary to a perinatal anoxic-ischemic insult in prematurely born infants.[15] A T2-weighted gradient-echo sequence is mandatory whenever axonal shearing injuries (Fig. 13.11) are suspected or hemosiderin deposition sought. This technique is strongly recommended in the assessment of accidental and nonaccidental cranial injury.

Because of the bright appearance of fat on T1-weighted images, the author uses so-called fat-suppressed T1-weighted images for imaging the orbit. This allows easy identification of abnormalities because the normal, high signal of the orbital fat is suppressed.

MR imaging can also be used to visualize the arteries and veins. The technique is based on an enhancement of the signal of flowing blood, without injection of a contrast agent, and a simultaneous suppression of the background tissues (Fig. 13.12). The sequences and the parameters are different for arterial and venous flow.

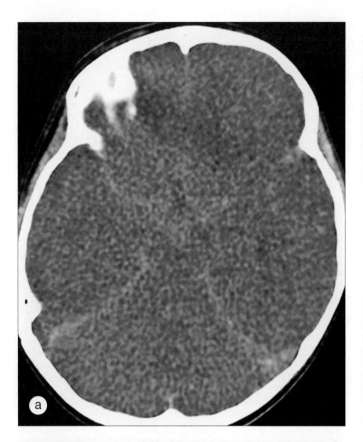

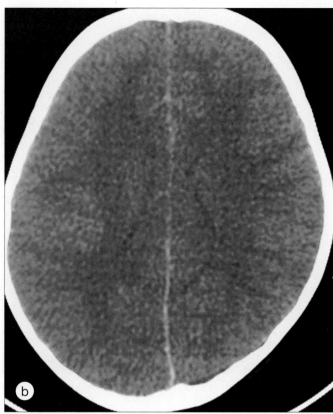

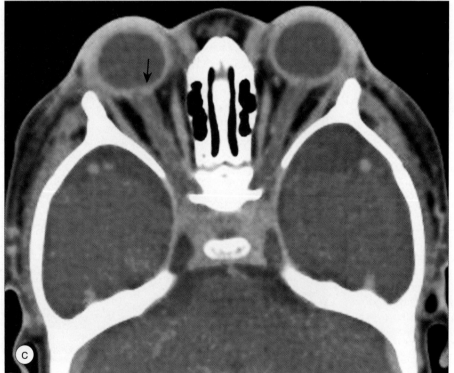

Fig. 13.8 Axial unenhanced CT in a child with massive brain edema. (a) The sulci are not visible (effaced). (b) The ventricles are narrowed and the basal cisterns are obliterated. (c) There is elevation of the optic disc, indicating severely raised intracranial pressure (arrow).

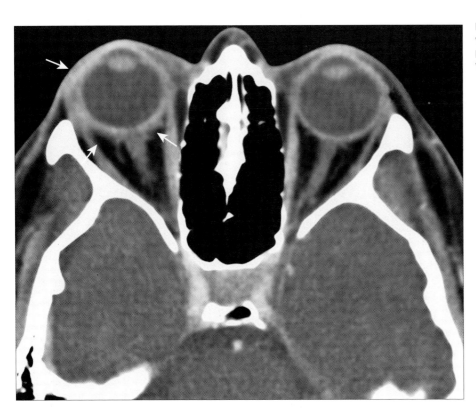

Fig. 13.9 Axial contrast-enhanced CT in a child with preseptal cellulitis showing as a thickening of preseptal and periocular tissue (arrows) compared with the unaffected eye.

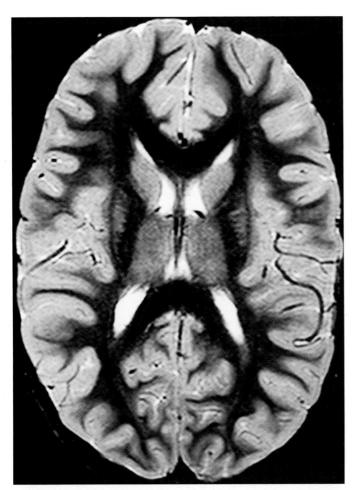

Fig. 13.10 Axial T2-weighted MR image using the double-echo short tau inversion recovery sequence to obtain an optimal differentiation between the gray and the white matter for the assessment of myelination.

Recent ischaemia is best seen on diffusion-weighted images. This technique detects restricted diffusion at a microscopical level, as a result of cell death.

MR imaging is recommended for imaging the optic chiasm and the posterior visual pathway (Fig. 13.13). Typical examples that illustrate the superiority of MR imaging include inflammatory (e.g., Lyme disease) and demyelinating diseases (e.g., Devic disease, multiple sclerosis), congenital abnormalities, phakomatoses (e.g., von Hippel–Lindau disease, tuberous sclerosis, Sturge Weber syndrome, neurofibromatosis), and hypoxic-ischemic encephalopathy and periventricular leukomalacia.[16,17] Perinatal visual loss is an important research and medicolegal topic.[15,18]

Using MR imaging, cortical damage could be differentiated from subcortical parenchymal damage.[19] The ophthalmological dysfunction associated with these injuries was different. Whereas horizontal conjugate gaze deviation and exotropia were more common in cortical injury, tonic downgaze, esotropia, and optic nerve hypoplasia were more frequent when there was a predominant white matter injury.

In children with neurofibromatosis, MR is an important part of the diagnostic work-up (Fig. 13.13). When progressive disease is diagnosed in children with a visual pathway glioma or when there is loss of visual function, chemotherapy may be indicated. At the author's institution, MR imaging is used for the follow-up at 2, 5, and 9 months during chemotherapy and every 3 to 6 months after the treatment.[15] Visual pathway gliomas can spontaneously regress.[20]

Septo-optic dysplasia consists of an absence or hypoplasia of the septum pellucidum and hypoplasia of the anterior visual pathway (Fig. 13.14). MR imaging may support the clinical observations and a further classification may be possible. Five different types have been distinguished, each with different associations and prognosis.[21]

MR imaging of the brain stem, cerebellum, pituitary gland, and cranial nerves is far superior to CT, partly due to the multiplanar imaging capability. The cerebellum, brain stem, pituitary gland,

Table 13.1 Indications for CT and MR imaging in pediatric ophthalmology

Suspected abnormality	Initial imaging modality	Additional imaging modality
Retinoblastoma	CT	MR to assess spread along optic nerve and subarachnoid tumour dissemination
PHPV, Coats, ROP	CT	
Craniofacial anomalies	CT	
Ocular/orbital trauma	CT	
(Non)accidental cranial trauma	CT	MR if CT remains normal or doubtful and for late follow-up
Optic nerve head drusen	CT	
Capillary hemangioma	CT	
Lymphangioma	CT	MR to confirm the diagnosis by showing the septations and cysts with fluid–fluid blood levels
Orbital varices	CT (incl. Valsalva)	
Plexiform neurofibroma	MR	
Visual pathway glioma	MR	
Dermoid/epidermoid	CT	
Rhabdomyosarcoma	CT	MR to better delineate the full extent of involvement
Phacomatoses	MR	CT to demonstrate calcification
Preseptal/orbital cellulitis	CT	
Optic nerve hypoplasia, septo-optic dysplasia	MR	
Cerebellar, brain stem, and pituitary gland pathology	MR	
Microphthalmos, anophthalmos	MR	
Disorders of extraocular motility	MR	
Metabolic disorders	MR	
Cranial nerve palsies	MR	
Periventricular leukomalacia in premature born children	Ultrasound usually done in neonatal unit	MR for definition

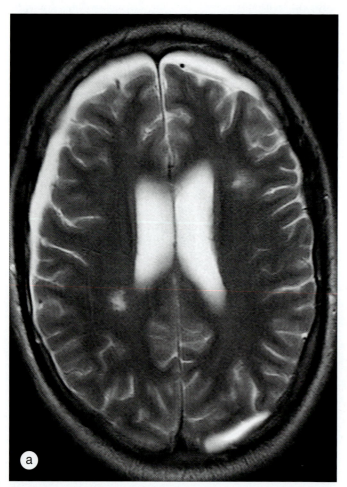 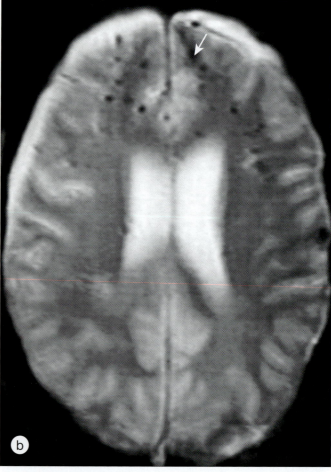

Fig. 13.11 (a) Axial T2-weighted and (b) axial T2*-weighted gradient-echo images. Apart from the subdural collection in both frontal regions and in the left occipital lobe, the post-traumatic axonal shearing injuries are much better seen on the gradient-echo image (b), arrow.

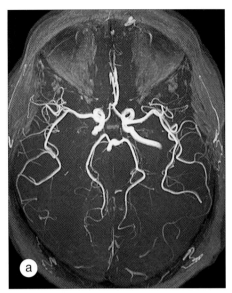
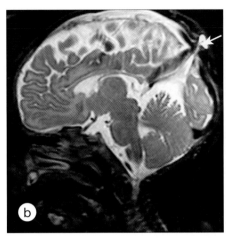
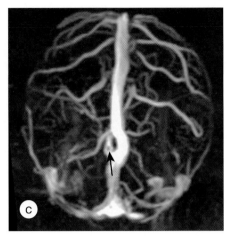

Fig. 13.12 MR angiogram. (a) Three dimensional "time-of-flight," maximum intensity projection, (b) sagittal T2-weighted image, and (c) 2D phase contrast venous MR angiogram. Note the clear visualization of large- and middle-sized arteries without administrating a contrast agent (a) in a child with a parietal encephalocele; the venous MR angiogram (c) shows the splitting (arrow) of the superior sagittal sinus by the encephalocele.

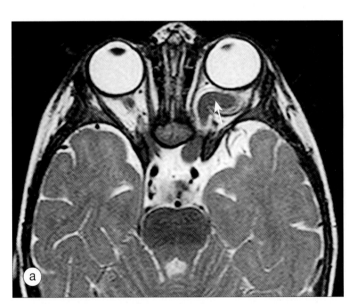
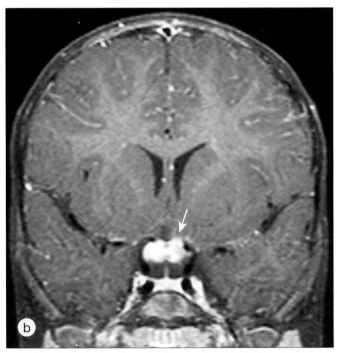

Fig. 13.13 (a) Axial T2-weighted in a child with NF1 and a left optic nerve glioma: note the "kink" in the enlarged optic nerve (arrow), which extends through the optic foramen. Note that proptosis is not apparent on the scan because the orbit has gradually enlarged coronally. (b) Coronal contrast-enhanced T1-weighted MR images showing enlarged and enhanced chiasm (arrow).

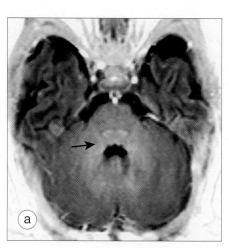

Fig. 13.14 Axial T2-weighted image in a child with septo-optic dysplasia and an absence of the septum pellucidum, which gives the appearance of an undivided anterior ventricle (arrow).

and optic chiasm are imaged in the coronal and sagittal planes. In children with congenital ocular motor apraxia, cerebellar abnormalities were found in 63% of them. Most of these patients had inferior vermian dysplasia.[22]

The assessment of the myelination is an advantage of MR imaging. T1- and T2-weighted images are necessary. The progress of myelination will be better seen on T1-weighted images during the first 6 months of life while thereafter T2-weighted images are needed (Figs 13.15 and 13.16). The other set of images is necessary to assess structural changes. Myelinated fiber tracts return a high signal on T1-weighted images and a low signal on T2-weighted images.

Changes with age on MRI images of young children are substantial, especially in the first year of life. At birth, myelin should be present in the dorsal brain stem, in the ventrolateral region of the thalamus, in the central part of the centrum semiovale, and in the dorsal limb of the internal capsule[14] (Fig. 13.15). At approximately three months of age, the optic radiation should be myelinated (Fig. 13.16). The splenium and the genu of the internal capsule are myelinated at 5 and 7 months, respectively (Fig. 13.16). The different rate of myelination on T1- and T2-weighted images remains a matter of debate. It has been suggested that the interaction with water of cholesterol and galactocerebrosides on the surface of the myelin membrane is responsible for the increase in signal on T1-weighted images. The decreasing signal on T2-weighted images correlates with the maturation and tightening of the myelin sheath around the axon. The signal decrease corresponds to a decrease in axonal and extracellular water.

The myelination progresses in the caudocranial and postero-anterior directions and from the periventricular region toward the subcortical region.

A child is considered fully myelinated between 15 and 18 months of age.

Functional MR imaging has been used to investigate the relationship between the progressive myelination of the visual pathway and the cortical function.[23] Using a photic stimulation, Yamada et al. found a rapid inversion of response, which is related to rapid synapse formation and brain maturation.

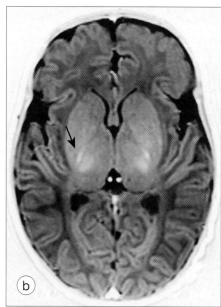

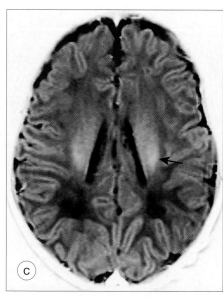

Fig. 13.15 Axial true inversion recovery T1-weighted images in a 6 week old with normal myelination. Myelination can be seen in the dorsal brain stem (a, arrow), in the ventrolateral region of the thalamus (b, arrow), and in the central part of the centrum semiovale (c, arrow).

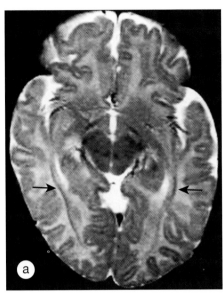
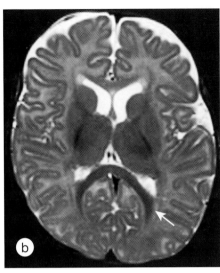
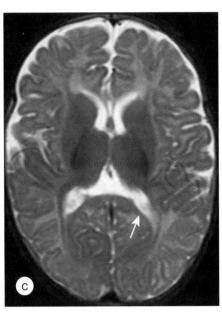

Fig. 13.16 Axial T2-weighted MR images. (a) The normal myelination of the optic radiation at 3 months of age, (b) normal myelination of the splenium of the corpus callosum (arrow), and (c) delayed myelination of the splenium of the corpus callosum in a 5 month-old girl (arrow). Note that on T2 images the myelin is dark.

REFERENCES

1. Hoffmann KT, Hosten N, Lemke AJ, et al. Septum orbitale: high-resolution MR in orbital anatomy. Am J Neuroradiol 1998; 19: 91–4.
2. Dixon AD, Dendy Ph. Spiral CT: how much does radiation dose matter? Lancet 1998; 352: 1082–3.
3. Czechowski J, Janeczek J, Kelly G, Johansen J. Radiation dose to the lens in sequential and spiral CT of the facial bones and sinuses. Eur Radiol 2001; 11: 711–3.
4. Cohan RH, Dunnick NR. Intravascular contrast media: adverse reactions. Am J Roentgenol 1987; 149: 665–70.
5. Tishler S, Hoffman JC Jr. Anaphylactoid reactions to IV gadopentetate dimeglumine. Am J Neuroradiol 1990; 11: 1167–9.
6. Cauldwell CB, Fisher DM. Sedating pediatric patients: Is propofol a panacea? Radiology 1993; 186: 9–10.
7. Bloomfield EL, Masaryk TJ, Caplin A, et al. Intravenous sedation for MR imaging of the brain and spine in children: pentobarbital versus propofol. Radiology 1993; 186: 93–7.
8. Denis D, Genitori L, Conrath J, et al. Ocular findings in children operated on for plagiocephaly and trigonocephaly. Childs Nerv Syst 1996; 12: 683–9.
9. Gor DM, Kirsch CF, Leen J, et al. Radiologic differentiation of intraocular glass: evaluation of imaging techniques, glass types, size, and effect of intraocular hemorrhage. Am J Roentgenol 2001; 177: 1199–203.
10. Finkelstein M, Legmann A, Rubin PA. Projectile metallic foreign bodies in the orbit: a retrospective study of epidemiologic factors, management, and outcomes. Ophthalmology 1997; 104: 96–103.
11. Weinacht S, Zaunbauer W, Gottlob I. Optic atrophy induced by an intraorbital wooden foreign body: the role of CT and MRI. J Peditr Ophthalmol Strabismus 1998; 35: 179–81.
12. Ho VT, McGuckin JF Jr, Smergel EM. Intraorbital wooden foreign body: CT and MR appearance. Am J Neuroradiol 1996; 17: 134–6.
13. Newton TH, Bilaniuk LT. Radiology of the Eye and Orbit. New York: Raven Press; 1990. (Modern neuroradiology; vol 4.)
14. Barkovich AJ. Pediatric Neuroimaging. 3rd edition. Baltimore: Lippincott Williams & Wilkins; 2000.
15. Casteels I, Demaerel P, Spileers W, et al. Cortical visual impairment following perinatal hypoxia: clinicoradiologic correlation using magnetic resonance imaging. J Pediatr Ophthalmol Strabismus 1997; 34: 297–305.
16. Demaerel P, de Ruyter N, Casteels I, et al. Visual pathway glioma in children treated with chemotherapy. Eur J Paediatr Neurol 2002; 6: 207–12.
17. Sorkin JA, Davis PC, Meacham LR, et al. Optic nerve hypoplasia: Absence of posterior pituitary bright signal on magnetic resonance imaging correlates with diabetes insipidus. Am J Ophthalmol 1996; 122: 717–23.
18. Uggetti C, Egitto MG, Fazzi.E, et al. Cerebral visual impairment in periventricular leukomalacia: MR correlation. Am J Neuroradiol 1996; 17: 979–85.
19. Brodsky MC, Fray KJ, Glasier CM. Perinatal cortical and subcortical visual loss: mechanisms of injury and associated ophthalmologic signs. Ophthalmology 2002; 109: 85–94.
20. Perilongo G, Moras P, Carollo C, et al. Spontaneous partial regression of low-grade glioma in children with neurofibromatosis-1: a real possibility. J Child Neurol 1999; 14: 352–6.
21. Brodsky MC, Glasier CM. Optic nerve hypoplasia: Clinical significance of associated central nervous system abnormalities on magnetic resonance imaging. Arch Ophthalmol 1993; 111: 66–74.
22. Sargent MA, Poskitt KJ, Jan JE. Congenital ocular motor apraxia: Imaging findings. Am J Neuroradiol 1997; 18: 1915–22.
23. Yamada H, Sadato N, Konishi Y, et al. A milestone for normal development of the infantile brain detected by functional MRI. Neurology 2000; 55: 218–23.

CHAPTER 14 Genetics, Ophthalmology, and Genetic Testing

Graeme C M Black

Studies suggest that, in developed countries, between a third and a half of the diagnoses underlying childhood blind or partial-sighted registration are genetic, a figure likely to be an underestimate.[1,2] In many developing countries, where visual disability is significantly more common, genetic conditions also represent an important group contributing to childhood blindness.[3] Although many common conditions have a substantial inherited contribution, many of the "genetic" conditions referred to in this context are monogenic, or Mendelian, conditions. Although most of these are rare, many of the issues regarding diagnosis and counseling apply to the group as a whole. It is therefore possible to consider a common approach to many aspects of their clinical management.

GENETIC COUNSELING

Genetic counseling should provide the necessary information for patients and their families to understand the condition that affects them as well as its implications for, for example, future reproductive decision-making. Thus the focus is on passing information back to families, which must be based on a complete family history and an accurate diagnosis. The construction of a full and accurate, three-generation pedigree underpins genetic counseling (see Figs. 14.1–14.3). It is important to be clear about certain "sensitive" issues such as consanguinity (see discussion on recessive inheritance in New Mutations) as well as stillbirths/abortions and infant deaths. This is seldom achieved within the normal time constraints of a busy outpatient consultation and referral for either genetic counseling or the opinion of a clinical geneticist may be sought either separately or in a joint ophthalmic genetic clinic.

In many cases, the ocular abnormalities will represent one facet of a multisystemic condition, and such a referral represents an important opportunity to secure the diagnosis. Whether or not a condition is genetic, this represents an opportunity to help an affected individual or his/her family to understand the underlying cause and its implications for the future and for the wider family and the reproductive risks. The aim is to give sufficient time for answering questions and for passing on sufficient information that an individual may be able to make his own, informed choices and decisions.

MENDELIAN INHERITANCE

Recently, the major focus of attention has been on understanding genes implicated in single-gene, or Mendelian, disorders. The majority follow one of three inheritance patterns—autosomal dominant, autosomal recessive, or X-linked. Many such conditions are highly variable (heterogeneous) both within and between families. The extent of this variability can be highly disease-specific and is often a major consideration when counseling families.

Autosomal dominant inheritance

Conditions inherited in an autosomal dominant fashion may affect any part of the eye. Examples include some forms of anterior segment dysgenesis (Rieger syndrome, iridogoniodysgenesis), corneal dystrophy (granular, Meesmann), congenital cataract (autosomal dominant congenital cataract, ADCC), vitreoretinopathy (Stickler syndrome), and retinal dystrophy (forms of retinitis pigmentosa, Best syndrome). These conditions are carried on the autosomes (chromosomes 1–22) and an affected individual carries one normal and one defective copy or allele of the gene in question.

In the majority of cases, individuals who have inherited an autosomal dominant condition will have a strong family history including one or other parent. The full family history, such as shown in Fig. 14.1, then illustrates a two- or multigenerational condition in which there may be evidence of male-to-male transmission. In such cases the family will often (although not always) have a clear understanding about the likely impact for future affected individuals. Individuals with such a condition have a

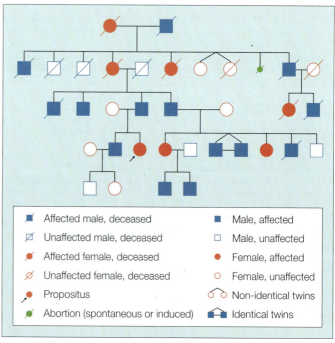

Fig. 14.1 Pedigree construction illustrating autosomal dominant inheritance.

Legend:
- Affected male, deceased
- Unaffected male, deceased
- Affected female, deceased
- Unaffected female, deceased
- Propositus
- Abortion (spontaneous or induced)
- Male, affected
- Male, unaffected
- Female, affected
- Female, unaffected
- Non-identical twins
- Identical twins

50% chance of passing the faulty gene on to each of their off-spring, with the risks being identical for both males and females.

There may be significant phenotypic variability between affected individuals representing in either variable *penetrance* or *expressivity* of a mutant gene:

PENETRANCE

For many genetic conditions, in particular those of autosomal dominant inheritance, the chance of gene carriers developing symptoms is not 100%–that is, the mutation shows *reduced penetrance*. For certain conditions (e.g., certain forms of autosomal dominant retinitis pigmentosa, inherited coloboma, and cataract), gene carriers may not manifest signs of the conditions but have an identical risk of passing the condition on to their off-spring as those who do manifest symptoms. This is one of the most important reasons for examining the parents of a child with, for example, coloboma or anterior segment dysgenesis.

EXPRESSIVITY

Within a family, all individuals affected by a single gene disorder carry the same genetic fault or mutation within that gene. However, the manifestations of that condition may vary widely. In this case the condition (or more properly the mutant allele) is said to demonstrate *variable expressivity*. Examples include Marfan syndrome, neurofibromatosis type 1, and oculocutaneous albinism whose ocular and extraocular manifestations may show a wide range within families even amongst individuals in whom the mutant allele has phenotypic manifestations (i.e., amongst those in whom the mutation is penetrant). The reasons for this are poorly understood although environment, genetic background, and chance developmental events are all likely to contribute. Importantly, where a condition varies widely within a family, the degree of severity in one individual, which has a huge influence upon their decision making, is often of little or no significance in predicting the severity of outcome for his or her siblings or offspring.

NEW MUTATIONS

In some cases a condition that is clearly autosomal dominant and is also highly penetrant will be inherited without a family history in either parents. For example this is seen in a number of cases of aniridia or retinoblastoma, where it is assumed that this results from a new mutation that has occurred in the process of copying one or other parent's DNA. In such cases the recurrence risks for future siblings of the affected individual are much lower than 50%. This risk figure will not be zero and may be hard to calculate as there is a risk of *gonadal mosaicism*–that is, that one parent carries the mutation in a proportion of his/her sperm or eggs and can therefore pass the condition to other children.

In such cases where, for a autosomal dominant condition, there is no family history the exact nature of the mutation may be difficult to predict. For example, cases of sporadic aniridia may result from a deletion of the short arm of chromosome 11, which can remove other, neighboring genes at the same time. This is seen in patients with WAGR syndrome in whom a deletion results in *W*ilms tumor, *a*niridia, *g*enitourinary abnormalities, and intellectual *r*etardation. This is termed a *co-deletion* or *contiguous gene syndrome*. It is for this reason that patients with sporadic

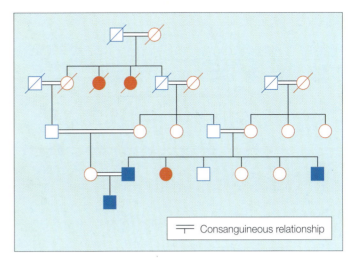

Fig. 14.2 Pedigree construction illustrating autosomal recessive inheritance in the presence of consanguinity.

aniridia require either renal ultrasound screening or molecular evidence that the Wilms tumor gene, *WT1*, is unaffected by the new mutation (see discussion on Fig. 14.5).

Autosomal recessive inheritance

Conditions inherited in an autosomal recessive fashion include forms of oculocutaneous albinism, congenital cataract (autosomal recessive congenital cataract, ARCC), and retinal dystrophy (forms of Leber congenital amaurosis, achromatopsia). These conditions also result from defects in genes that lie on the autosomes. In this case an affected individual carries two defective copies of a single gene that have, in the majority of cases, been inherited from either parent. As parents carry one normal and one faulty copy of the gene in question they are termed *carriers* of the condition.

Most individuals who have inherited a recessive condition have no history of the condition in previous generations. This is not always the case as there may be more than two partnerships in which both father and mother are carriers of the same faulty gene. Situations where it is more likely that both parents are carriers–for example, consanguinity–increase the risks of a recessive condition (see Fig. 14.2). Counseling for recessive conditions in all circumstances should be nonjudgmental and should aim to pass over information while seeking to minimize the feelings of guilt and responsibility that may accompany such knowledge.

Where both partners are carriers of a recessive gene they have a 1/4 risk of each child being affected by the same condition. Unaffected children have a 2/3 risk of being carriers. Thus for Stargardt disease, which may have a disease frequency of 1 in 10,000 and which has a carrier frequency of around 1 in 50, the risks to the offspring of affected individual and their children is low (~1 and 0.65%, respectively).

X-linked inheritance

Amongst the monogenic disorders that result from defects in genes that lie on the X-chromosome are developmental disorders of the anterior (e.g., megalocornea, Nance-Horan syndrome) and posterior segments (e.g., Norrie disease) and retinal dystrophies (retinitis pigmentosa, cone dystrophy, congenital stationary night

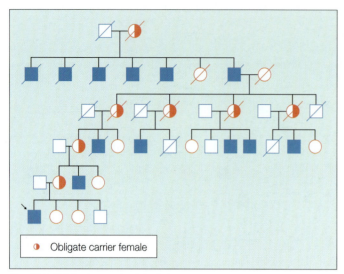

● Obligate carrier female

Fig. 14.3 X-linked recessive inheritance.

blindness, choroideremia, and retinoschisis). In addition, a number of well-recognized X-linked multisystemic syndromes, such as Lowe oculocerebrorenal syndrome, are associated with major ocular complications that may manifest during childhood.

Classically it is assumed that X-linked conditions affect only males–that is, that they are inherited in an X-linked recessive pattern (see Fig. 14.3). This is the case in X-linked retinoschisis, X-linked ocular albinism (XLOA), and Norrie disease. Since females carry two X chromosomes and one is inactivated in each somatic cell there is sufficient expression of the normal allele to preclude deleterious manifestations of the disorder. There may be clinical signs of carrier status (such as the "mud-splattered" fundus appearances of XLOA carrier females) that are helpful diagnostically. In this case, the recognition of an X-linked condition (and hence the guidelines for counseling) depends upon recognizing the presence of affected males, often in multiple generations who are all related through the female line (i.e., the affected gene has never been passed from father to son). Affected males may pass the faulty gene on only to their daughters, who are thus obligate gene carriers. Obligate gene carriers have a 50:50 chance of passing the faulty gene to their children of whom only the males will (in general) show signs of the condition in question.

Manifestations of X-linked conditions in females

For a small number of conditions, mutations in X-linked conditions have manifestations in both females and males–termed X-linked dominant inheritance. In certain cases, such as incontinentia pigmenti, these mutations are lethal in males and here the disorder is seen only in females. However, even amongst classical X-linked recessive disorders some carrier females may show signs or symptoms. Skewing of X-inactivation that causes preferential expression of the mutant allele in sufficient cells can thus result in manifestations of the condition. This has rarely been described in Norrie disease and choroideremia.

For certain X-linked conditions disease manifestation in carriers is more common. This may make the recognition of an X-linked pedigree–and subsequent counseling–tricky. This is the case with some XLRP families where a majority of females manifest symptoms of night blindness at some stage, usually from middle life onward. In almost all cases this will be considerably later than their affected male relatives, which is an important

guide to the presence of an X-linked condition. Although the severity of such manifestations, which may be neither trivial nor visually insignificant, may be influenced by X-inactivation, it is likely that they represent a predictable manifestation of the carrier state. This must be taken into account when counseling family members in order that the simplistic and falsely optimistic notion that "X-linked conditions do not affect females" is not inappropriately perpetuated.

MITOCHONDRIAL, OR MATERNAL, INHERITANCE

Mitochondria are cellular organelles found within the cytoplasm. They contain their own small circular genome (16–17,000 base pairs of DNA), which is distinct from the nuclear genome. Mitochondrial DNA (mtDNA) encodes a small number of genes, including important components of the electron-transport chain, whose genetic code is also different from that used for nuclear genes. MtDNA gene mutations include Leber hereditary optic neuropathy (LHON, Chapter 60) and Kearnes-Sayre syndrome (KSS, Chapter 65).

Mitochondria are inherited exclusively from the ovum; thus, a mtDNA mutation can only be passed on from mother to child, i.e., *maternally inherited*. LHON is the best known of the ophthalmic genetic conditions that are maternally inherited, but it is important to remember that it is also not typical of the group because, unlike other such conditions, it shows a male bias (around 80–90% of affected individuals in the UK are male).

Mitochondrial conditions can be highly variable. In many cases where individuals carry mtDNA mutations in all of their cells, as is seen for most patients with LHON, the basis for this variability is poorly understood. For example, it is not known why only a minority of LHON mutation carriers (even males) will manifest symptoms. However, amongst many patients with mitochondrial myopathies such as KSS, only a proportion of their mitochondria carry mtDNA mutations while others remain normal, a state termed heteroplasmy. Since each cell has many mitochondria, where heteroplasmy occurs this can contribute to phenotypic variability, since the ratio of mutant to normal mtDNA may vary between the cells or tissues of a single individual. Most importantly, the level of heteroplasmy can also vary between different individuals of the same family.

Maternal inheritance is apparently clearcut; yet the disorders caused by mtDNA mutations are highly variable in their penetrance and expression, transforming the processes of mutation detection and prognosis estimation into complex issues and making counseling challenging.

HETEROGENEITY AMONGST SINGLE-GENE DISORDERS

Molecular analysis of an increasing number of inherited ocular conditions has demonstrated that similar or identical clinical disorders may be caused by mutations in one of several genes (see Table 14.1). For example, retinitis pigmentosa is not one but a large number of genetically distinct, but in many cases clinically indistinguishable, conditions. The observation that defects in a large number of the genes may cause identical phenotypic manifestations is termed *locus heterogeneity*. This has implications for diagnosis, counseling, and genetic testing of such conditions. It is also commonly recognized that different defects within one gene may cause a wide range of different clinical entities (see Table

Table 14.1 Examples of locus heterogeneity amongst inherited ophthalmic conditions

Condition	Inheritance pattern	Locus	Gene	Chromosomal location
Zonular pulverulent cataract	Autosomal dominant	CZP1	GJA8	1q21–q25
		CZP1	CRYGC	2q33–q35
		CZP3	GJA3	13q11
Coppock-like cataract	Autosomal dominant	CZP3	CRYBB2	22q11.2
		CCL	CRYGC	2q33–q35
Posterior polar cataract	Autosomal dominant	CTPP		1pter–p36.1
		CPP3	CRYGC	20p12–q12
Retinitis pigmentosa	Autosomal dominant	RP18	CRYGC	1q13–q23
		RP4	RHO	3q21–q24
		RP7	RDS/peripherin	6p21.2–cen
		RP9	RDS/peripherin	7p13–p15
		RP10	RDS/peripherin	7q31.3
		RP1	RP1	8q11–q13
		RP27	NRL	14q11.2
		RP13	NRL	17p13.3
		RP17	NRL	17q22
		RP11	NRL	19q13.4
Oculocutaneous albinism	Autosomal recessive	OCA1	TYR	11q14–q21
		OCA2	P gene	15q11.2–q12
		OCA3	TRP1	9p23
Retinitis pigmentosa	X-linked	RP23	TRP1	Xp22
		RP3	RPGR	Xp21.1
		RP2	RP2	Xp11.3
		RP24	RP2	Xq26–q27

Table 14.2 Examples of allelic heterogeneity amongst inherited ophthalmic conditions

Chromosomal location	Gene	Condition	Inheritance
5q31	BIGH3	Reis-Bucklers dystrophy	AD
		Thiel-Behnke dystrophy	AD
		Granular dystrophy	AD
		Avellino dystrophy	AD
		Lattice dystrophy (type I)	AD
Xp11	NDP	Norrie disease	XL
		Familial exudative vitreoretinopathy	XL
6p21.1-cen	RDS/peripherin	ADRP	AD
		Pattern/butterfly macular dystrophy	AD
		Central areolar choroidal dystrophy	AD
3q21–q24	Rhodopsin	ADRP	AD
		ARRP	AR
		Congenital stationary night blindness	AD
		Sectoral RP	AD

AD, autosomal dominant; AR, autosomal recessive; XL, X-linked.

14.2). This is termed *allelic heterogeneity* and results from differential effects of distinct mutations within the same gene. One of the factors determining clinical outcome is the position and effect of a mutation on the encoded protein.

Genetic testing

Many genes responsible for inherited ophthalmic conditions have been identified. Where available, genetic testing can provide valuable information regarding diagnosis, prognosis, and reproductive risks. Sadly, such developments are not easily translated into routinely available genetic tests. This technological delay can result in difficulties meeting the expectations of patients or

clinical needs. Although there are few "rules" for molecular testing, the following guidelines may help.

Karyotype analysis

In the molecular era it is somewhat unfashionable to think in terms of whole chromosomes. However, it should not be forgotten that chromosome rearrangements such as deletions and translocations have been the starting point for the identification of many of the genes such as *PAX6* (aniridia), *PITX2* (Rieger syndrome), and *FOXC2* (iridogoniodysgenesis) that underlie inherited ocular disease.[4–9] Therefore, detailed karyotype analysis will be considered by geneticists to exclude a chromosomal rearrangement. This may include the analysis of individuals who have multiple congenital abnormalities (see Fig. 14.4).

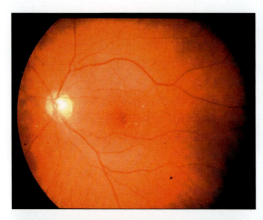

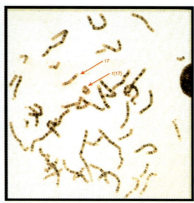

Fig. 14.4 Cytogenetically visible arrangements. In this patient karyotype analysis was undertaken to seek an explanation for an unusual constellation of abnormalities including bilateral flecked retinas (left), learning difficulties, short stature, and severe epilepsy. In this case a ring chromosome 17 is present in which the ends (telomeres) of the chromosome are lost and the chromosome forms a ring (right). The rearrangement is rare but is a recognized differential diagnosis of flecked retina. Neither parent carried the rearrangement.

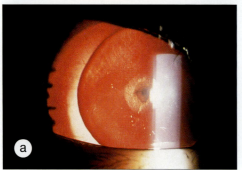

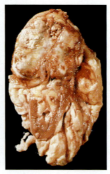

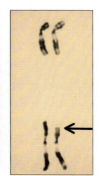

Fig. 14.5 Aniridia may occasionally be sporadic. WAGR syndrome caused by cytogenetically visible 11p deletion. A young child presented with delay, genitourinary abnormalities, and aniridia. There was no family history of aniridia. He was found to have a Wilms tumor in the superior pole of kidney. Karyotype analysis reveals a 11p deletion (arrow), which encompasses the PAX6 (aniridia) and the WT1 genes (Wilms tumor). (a) Aniridia, showing the lack of the iris revealing the edge of the lens, and an anterior polar cataract (common in PAX6 mutations). The ciliary processes are visible on the left. (b) Microdeletion syndrome of chromosome causing aniridia/Wilms tumor. Patients 1 and 2 are born with sporadic aniridia. Chromosome analysis is normal. FISH analysis shows two signals in patient 2 but not in patient 1. This indicates that patient 1 is at high risk of Wilms tumor.

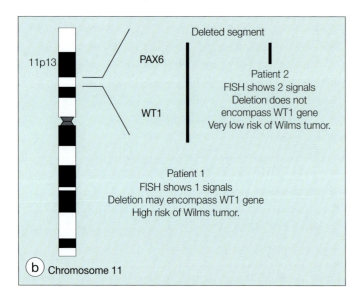

Fluorescence in situ hybridization (FISH).

Karyotype analysis may also be indicated for patients with a condition that is usually monogenic but is associated with an unusual constellation of features, as is the case with patients with WAGR syndrome (Fig. 14.5a). However, routine chromosome analysis can only identify large chromosomal rearrangements, whereas smaller alterations may be beyond the resolution of conventional microscopy. Unlike the example illustrated in Fig. 14.5a, a deletion cannot always be detected microscopically. In circumstances where the gene underlying a monogenic disorder has been identified and where a nonetheless chromosomal rearrangement is suspected, fluorescence *in situ* hybridization (FISH)–a molecular cytogenetic technique–can be used to enable identification of cytogenetically invisible (submicroscopic) chromosome rearrangements (see Fig. 14.5b).

FISH is also valuable for confirming the diagnosis of recognizable submicroscopic deletion dysmorphism syndromes; in some cases these may be associated with ophthalmic abnormalities including deletions of chromosome 4p (Wolf-Hirschhorn syndrome: coloboma/strabismus) and 22q11 deletion syndrome (DiGeorge syndrome: microphthalmia/coloboma).[10–12] Submicroscopic deletions are suspected in those with multiple congenital abnormalities (in particular in those with developmental delay), which are sporadic and present in those with normal karyotypes.

Genetic testing for mutations underlying monogenic disorders

In the past, molecular genetic analysis relied on limited information since the number of known gene mutations causing disease was limited. In some cases testing therefore relied upon indirect methods such as linkage studies. This is seldom the case now and the majority of analyses aim to test for mutations in known genes. The methods utilized are beyond the scope of this text but ultimately rely upon the identification of a sequence variation that alters the expression or function of a gene or protein and is shown to be pathogenic or disease-causing (Fig. 14.6).

Where genetic testing is appropriate this will usually be performed on a peripheral blood sample from an affected family member who is therefore certain to carry a familial mutation. Testing of an unaffected relative is only helpful to exclude the

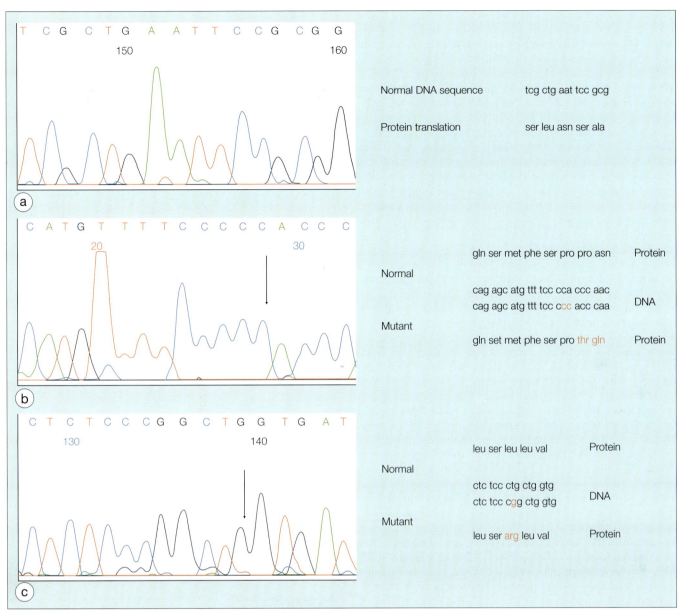

Fig. 14.6 DNA sequencing and mutation identification. (a) An electropherogram from direct DNA sequencing. Shown are a series of peaks corresponding to consecutive bases in a DNA sequence. The green corresponds to adenine, red to thymidine, blue to cytosine, and black to guanine. (b) Frameshift mutation causing Rieger syndrome. Shown is a sequence of *PITX2* in patient with Rieger syndrome, an autosomal dominant condition. The arrowed base is an insertion of a single C residue. When translated, the triplet code is now out of frame by 1 base pair. This totally alters the translated protein's amino acid sequence and leads to a premature stop codon later in the protein that results in Rieger syndrome. (c) Missense mutation causing Norrie disease. Shown is the sequence of the *NDP* gene in a patient with Norrie syndrome, an X-linked condition. The sequence is of genomic DNA and shows abnormal sequences as the male patient only has a single mutant X chromosome. The arrowed base is changed from T to G. When translated, the triplet codon is changed from CTG (leucine) to CGG (arginine). This single amino acid alteration is not seen in the normal population and results in Norrie disease.

presence of a genetic change and should generally be performed after a mutation has been identified in the family.

For the majority of genes that underlie Mendelian disorders, the identification of pathogenic mutation is labor-intensive and time-consuming and requires a detailed analysis of the whole gene. In some cases there is a strong relationship between phenotype and genotype. This exists amongst certain monogenic macular dystrophies where the majority of cases of Sorsby dystrophy and Doyne Honeycomb dystrophy (Malattia Leventinese) result from single-point mutations in the *TIMP3* and *EFEMP1* genes, respectively.[13,14] The same is true for the stromal corneal dystrophies linked to chromosome 5q31 and

caused by mutations in the *BIGH3* gene, where the range of mutations causing granular, lattice type I, and Bowman's layer (Thiel-Behnke and Reis-Buckler) dystrophies is very limited.[15] In these circumstances, the molecular identification of this point mutation is straightforward (although the identification of a laboratory willing to do it might be less so).

However, in the majority of cases where mutation identification is attempted, the task is not simple. Usually, where a mutation is suspected, the whole gene must be screened. In the case of *ABCA4*, which is mutated in Stargardt disease, and encompasses 51 exons and 6,000–7,000 base pairs of DNA, this is an enormous task beyond the scope of most diagnostic laboratories.[16] Furthermore the pick-up rate, amongst those known to harbor mutations in *ABCA4*, is considerably less than 100%.[17] This means that a negative result is of limited value as it neither excludes a mutation in the *ABCA4* gene nor in any other. Finally, for many molecules, there is a significant degree of *normal* variation seen in both the gene and, importantly, its encoded protein. The task of defining whether a variation, altering a single amino acid, is pathogenic is onerous and, in the absence of a functional protein assay, may even be impossible.

Therefore, the process of mutation screening can take several months. In conditions where mutation of a number of genes can cause an identical phenotype (retinitis pigmentosa is the most obvious example), there is no way to choose one from a number of genes: this may make testing impractical in a clinical setting using current techniques.

The ethics of genetic testing

Genetic testing–in most cases–is undertaken by means of a peripheral blood sample sent, with ease, for DNA extraction, followed by the required molecular analysis. For the clinician it is therefore little different from a full blood count. As always, appearances can be deceptive; this is a complex area for which a clinician needs to be prepared. It is all too easy to act without thought and end up facing a complicated situation that could have been avoided, even to the extent of discovering signs suggesting false paternity. There are no hard and fast rules. Indeed, one may be forgiven for thinking that there are no rules! Although much has been written on ethics and genetic testing, presymptomatic testing, and carrier diagnosis for a wide spectrum of conditions such as Huntington disease and early-onset cancer syndromes, little has been said about their application to ophthalmology. In such circumstances, it is perhaps wise to seek advice and, at the very least, to use the experience of clinical genetics colleagues in guiding practice.

Clinical examination

The examination of asymptomatic relatives may be as effective as–and far quicker than–a "genetic test." This may be invaluable when examining parents for evidence of an unsuspected disc coloboma, but there are circumstances where such an examination should be avoided, or at the very least may need to be discussed with the patient. Therefore, examining the children of a concerned parent with an autosomal dominant retinal dystrophy, or with Sorsby fundus dystrophy may be a generous and simple act, *but* does the child (or young adult) know *why you are examining him?* And would he (or she) give consent if they knew the potential consequences of such a simple action? Do they want to know that they could go blind in the future? Do they realize that this may have consequences for their future insurability?

Testing is easily done, of course, but impossible to undo.

Presymptomatic or predictive testing

Clinical examination of an asymptomatic individual–who may not even be "the patient"–may result in his or her being given a genetic diagnosis. This is exactly the same as performing a presymptomatic genetic test, a circumstance for which an individual would ordinarily be given considerable preparation. For example, when those with a family history of Huntingdon disease consider a genetic test it would usually take three full counseling sessions of 45 minutes before a blood test would be considered.[18]

This would allow the clinician to explain not only the nature of the condition but also the pros *and cons* of testing at that particular time. A significant number of those beginning such an exercise decline the test before completing the process.

In the case of Huntington disease, counseling and testing is generally undertaken for adults who are capable of understanding the process to which they are being subjected. This situation would be analogous to that encountered by an adult individual whose first-degree relatives have Sorsby fundus dystrophy and who is concerned to know his/her risks of developing similar problems. It is important to ensure that the implications of such testing are fully thought through and that the patient is aware of the full implications of such testing. It may be that this is best achieved outside of a busy ophthalmic outpatient clinic and by those most comfortable with the processes involved.

Genetic testing of children

Testing of children for later-onset conditions is also an area into which a clinician may be pushed, in particular by parents and guardians who are understandably concerned for their children's well being. In all cases where a condition is untreatable and where there are no obvious clinical advantages of knowing whether an individual is a gene carrier, the motivation behind testing must be clear. Where the advantages of "knowing" lie simply in satisfying a parent's understandable curiosity, it may be appropriate to delay testing until the child is of an age to understand the reasoning behind testing, or even to consent to it him/herself.[19]

Carrier testing (e.g., for X-linked conditions)

Genetic testing of female carriers of X-linked conditions, or of nonmanifesting gene carriers, is another area that needs careful consideration. In the case of X-linked ocular albinism, for example, this may not have implications for a woman's personal health. However, the timing of such testing and the reproductive implications (e.g., prenatal diagnosis, presymptomatic testing of children) need to be judged and to have been discussed prior to testing. Again it is often helpful to involve clinicians, such as clinical geneticists, who are familiar and comfortable with such processes.

Prenatal diagnosis

The number of ocular conditions for which genetic testing is now available increases year upon year. This means that where a test is available to a family it is now possible to test those at risk of developing the condition, born or unborn. Clinical geneticists therefore oversee the process of prenatal diagnosis for a large number of patients who cover a wide range of conditions.

The impact of prenatal diagnosis upon ophthalmic genetics can only increase as testing becomes more widely available on a service (as opposed to research) basis. For a prenatal test to be possible in the timeframe required during early pregnancy it is usually necessary for a mutation to have already been found in an affected individual in the family. This implies that a family will have had some form of genetic "work-up" in the past. Genetic testing–and prenatal diagnosis in particular–is a subject that rouses strong emotions amongst both patients and professionals alike. Whether an individual opts for testing during pregnancy is a time-consuming and complex process that needs to be approached sensitively, without judgment, and in a nondirective manner by those who have experience of such situations.

REFERENCES

1. Rahi JS, Cable N. British Childhood Visual Impairment Study Group. Severe visual impairment and blindness in children in the UK. Lancet 2003; 362: 1359–65.
2. Alagaratnam J, Sharma TK, Lim CS, et al. A survey of visual impairment in children attending the Royal Blind School, Edinburgh using the WHO childhood visual impairment database. Eye 2002; 16: 557–61.
3. Dandona R, Dandona L. Childhood blindness in India: a population based perspective. Br J Ophthalmol 2003 Mar; 87: 263–5.
4. Andersen SR, Geertinger P, Larsen HW, et al. Aniridia, cataract and gonadoblastoma in a mentally retarded girl with deletion of chromosome II. A clinicopathological case report. Ophthalmologica 1977; 176: 171–7.
5. Francke U, Holmes LB, Atkins L, et al. Aniridia-Wilms' tumor association: evidence for specific deletion of 11p13. Cytogenet Cell Genet 1979; 24: 185–92.
6. Makita Y, Masuno M, Imaizumi K, et al. Rieger syndrome with de novo reciprocal translocation t(1;4) (q23.1;q25). Am J Med Genet 1995; 22: 57: 19–21.
7. Schinzel A, Brecevic L, Dutly F, et al. Multiple congenital anomalies including the Rieger eye malformation in a boy with interstitial deletion of (4) (q25→q27) secondary to a balanced insertion in his normal father: evidence for haplotype insufficiency causing the Rieger malformation. J Med Genet 1997; 34: 1012–4.
8. Lehmann OJ, Ebenezer ND, Ekong R, et al. Ocular developmental abnormalities and glaucoma associated with interstitial 6p25 duplications and deletions. Invest Ophthalmol Vis Sci 2002; 43: 1843–9.
9. Nishimura DY, Swiderski RE, Alward WL, et al. The forkhead transcription factor gene FKHL7 is responsible for glaucoma phenotypes which map to 6p25. Nat Genet 1998; 19: 140–7.
10. Mayer UM, Bialasiewicz AA. Ocular findings in a 4 p- deletion syndrome (Wolf-Hirschhorn). Ophthalmic Paediatr Genet 1989; 10: 69–72.
11. Wieczorek D, Krause M, Majewski F, et al. Effect of the size of the deletion and clinical manifestation in Wolf-Hirschhorn syndrome: analysis of 13 patients with a de novo deletion. Eur J Hum Genet 2000; 8: 519–26.
12. Morrison DA, FitzPatrick DR, Fleck BW. Iris coloboma and a microdeletion of chromosome 22: del(22)(q11.22). Br J Ophthalmol 2002; 86: 1316.
13. Wijesuriya SD, Evans K, Jay MR, et al. Sorsby's fundus dystrophy in the British Isles: demonstration of a striking founder effect by microsatellite-generated haplotypes. Genome Res 1996; 6: 92–101.
14. Stone EM, Lotery AJ, Munier FL, et al. A single EFEMP1 mutation associated with both Malattia Leventinese and Doyne honeycomb retinal dystrophy. Nat Genet 1999; 22: 199–202.
15. Munier FL, Frueh BE, Othenin-Girard P, et al. BIGH3 mutation spectrum in corneal dystrophies. Invest Ophthalmol Vis Sci 2002; 43: 949–54.
16. Webster AR, Heon E, Lotery AJ, et al. An analysis of allelic variation in the ABCA4 gene. Invest Ophthalmol Vis Sci 2001; 42: 1179–89.
17. Briggs CE, Rucinski D, Rosenfeld PJ, et al. Mutations in ABCR (ABCA4) in patients with Stargardt macular degeneration or cone-rod degeneration. Invest Ophthalmol Vis Sci 2001; 42: 2229–36.
18. Craufurd D, Tyler A. Predictive testing for Huntington's disease: protocol of the UK Huntington's prediction consortium. J Med Genet 1992; 29: 915–8.
19. Craufurd D, Donnai D, Kerzin-Storrar L, et al. Testing of children for "adult" genetic diseases. Lancet 1990; 335: 1406.

CHAPTER 15 The Visually Impaired Child and Family

James E Jan

WHO IS A VISUALLY IMPAIRED CHILD?

The concept of visual impairment has gradually changed:[1] the emphasis has shifted from acuity, field size, and legal blindness to a more functional definition, which includes ocular and brain conditions with acuity loss, eye movement disorders, and visual inattentiveness, which prevent the effective use of vision. In industrial nations, the majority of visually impaired children now have congenital rather than acquired visual loss, total blindness has become less common, and most have additional developmental disabilities. The prevalence of ocular visual disorders has dropped, while the neurological causes of visual loss have significantly increased. In Western countries, recent medical advances, especially in pre- and perinatal care, have resulted in increased survival rates of critically ill infants who previously would have died of severe neurological deficits. Although the definition of "visual impairment" has expanded, severe visual loss is still infrequent.

CONVEYING THE DIAGNOSIS

Generally, children with visual impairment are first referred to ophthalmologists, who play a critical role in their diagnosis and management and shoulder the burden of making the final diagnosis.

Introducing the parents to the fact that their child has visual impairment is a hard task. It is difficult to describe their devastation after such news. The manner in which the parents are told can positively or adversely affect them and their children for years to come. How doctors present their medical findings and related issues is influenced by their own attitudes about blindness, especially when there is no treatment. Thus, it is crucial for all physicians to examine their own feelings and then convey the diagnosis truthfully, in lay terms, with compassion, patience, and optimism but without giving unrealistic hopes for visual recovery and allow time for questions. Doctors should not be hesitant to show their own feelings to avoid the complaint that "the doctor did not care."

Often the parents are so anxious during the initial office visit that they can remember little afterward; therefore more than one appointment may be necessary. It is important that both parents should be present. Second medical opinions are extremely beneficial, even when the diagnosis appears to be certain. Most affected children appear to be severely or totally blind in early infancy; yet the majority will develop useful vision. Therefore the diagnosis of total blindness should be avoided, unless it is absolutely certain. Refer the child *as soon as possible* to a pediatric clinic specializing in the habilitation of visually impaired children, or, when such does not exist, to a pediatrician familiar with neurodevelopmental issues. When surgical procedures are planned, early referral may be overlooked, to the detriment of the family and the child.

PARENTS

The parents have a realistic basis for their emotional difficulties following the diagnosis because they will have to deal with the heavy physical and emotional demands, for years to come. After they have been informed that, instead of being perfect, their baby has a visual impairment and perhaps neurodevelopmental disabilities, they experience a series of intense feelings such as shock, denial, grief, guilt, despair, and anger. It is clear that *how* this emotional crisis is handled by the parents and by the professionals will profoundly affect the life of the child. It is not unusual for the parents to cry repeatedly in the doctor's office, which in fact is a good sign. It is more worrisome when they show little or no emotion, because they are not moving through the various emotional stages. Most mothers have guilt feelings: that they did something wrong during the pregnancy that could have caused the problems. Even when they do not mention their guilt, it needs to be strongly stated that it is not their fault.

Much can be done to help the parents during this critical period. Doctors can offer practical and easily understood information on the type of visual disorder and disability. Most parents have access to the Internet, but they often obtain incorrect information. The parents will need repeated explanations on how the impaired sight affects their child's development. Experienced professionals realize that raising a visually impaired child is an enormous burden on the family. In the process of successful habilitation, professionals, no matter how dedicated and well-trained, cannot replace the parents who will carry out the major portion of the work. Therefore, when a therapeutic team is created around the child, the parents must be active participants.

Parents often need help to deal with the attitudes of their extended families, also with the prejudices of the public and sometimes with complex cultural issues. Both mother and father must be involved in the process of habilitation and the needs of the siblings should not be neglected. Feeling sorry for, or over-protection, are extremely damaging to a visually impaired child. Parents' group discussions are helpful, not only for educational purposes, but for dealing with the social and cultural issues facing each family.

EARLY INTERVENTION

The most vulnerable period for the parents is after the diagnosis of the visual disorder. Their concern over vision overshadows everything, underlining the important role of the ophthalmologists.

Intervention services should be introduced at this time, which begins by giving realistic information to the parents.

The habilitation (or rehabilitation) of visually impaired children is based on the fact that their physical, emotional, and intellectual growth responds to skilled, early intervention.[2] The professionals assigned to the family as vision consultants or counselors must first develop a trusting relationship with the parents and subsequently keep them advised on developmental issues. It is critical that they should be well trained and are supported by a larger diagnostic multidisciplinary team. Without understanding the children's abilities and weaknesses, it is difficult to advise the family and may even be harmful, if incorrect information is given.

DEVELOPMENT

Motor development

Much has been written about motor development, the rate of which depends on the severity and type of visual disorder, on the presence of additional neurological disabilities, and to a large extent, on the opportunities to acquire skills. Thus, children who are raised in a rich, stimulating environment provided by loving, informed parents, who are supported by professionals, develop faster than when they are understimulated. Even bright, intelligent infants with severe visual loss reared under ideal circumstances have delays in some of their motor skills. Crawling may not begin until around the first birthday and independent walking until 18 months or two years of age. In contrast, unsupported sitting and standing may be age-appropriate. Understimulated congenitally blind infants frequently develop generalized hypotonia with poor posture, delayed motor skills, and poor coordination, and tend to walk with an insecure, wide-based gait, with their feet everted.[3] When intervention services are not introduced during the first two years of life these neurological problems become permanent.

Blind infants are usually quiet and passive and require encouragement to be mobile. They may not acquire skills through accidental learning, as do the sighted. To the severely visually impaired, motor tasks such as sitting, pushing, pulling, jumping, early aspects of orientation and mobility, even chewing must be taught. Partially sighted children usually learn to move about quite normally and cannot be distinguished from the sighted, unless they are required to carry out balance activities, such as standing on one foot.

The development of visual motor skills, arrangement of objects in space, and constructive play are also affected. Children must have enrichment of their visual environment in an appropriate preschool setting, to be able to best progress. Teachers should be aware that young, visually impaired children often avoid activities such as construction toys, puzzles, and drawing, because they find these difficult. When trying to use their partial sight, they will often adopt head tilts or head turns, which are aimed at improving vision and controlling nystagmus. These and other postural adaptations should not be discouraged.

Conceptual development

The effect of visual impairment is also noticeable in cognition. Vision is an integrative sense, because it enables the perception of the entire image without losing the concept of it as a whole. Severe visual loss forces the observer to fragmented processing of information, as only a part of the object can be seen or felt at one time. The image must be built up out of components, and the relationships to other objects are frequently lost.

The attention span of young visually impaired children is usually shorter for meaningful exploration than that of the sighted. Self-initiated exploration is also reduced because they are frequently not aware of their surroundings. They are not as ready to investigate, so they may become overly passive and understimulated if experiences are not brought to them. Therefore, when they are assessed about their knowledge of their environment, delays are frequent. This does not necessarily indicate a lack of cognitive ability, but more likely insufficient opportunity to acquire the skills and information that would be expected in a sighted child of similar age. Deliberate intervention, making experiences available, and encouraging them to use their vision is essential.

Language development

For visually impaired infants to learn from their hearing, structuring of the environment is required by minimizing background noises especially from radio or TV, and they need encouragement to listen to meaningful sounds. They learn to recognize voices and anticipate events through sound, smell, and touch. Blind infants may not turn their heads or show the expected motor responses to auditory clues as do the sighted, and as a result, they are occasionally misdiagnosed as being deaf.

A common misconception is that blindness does not interfere with the acquisition of language.[4] In the absence of the full range of sensory information, the language concepts, as well as words and phrases retained from overheard conversations, tend to become based on auditory memory rather than on direct experience. When this happens, the language skills become more self-oriented, and word meanings will be limited. Children with these types of language difficulties are sometimes able to use quite sophisticated sentences, without actually being completely clear of the meaning. Appropriate intervention services should minimize this major problem. For the majority of children who are free from neurological disabilities, articulation is not a problem.

Social and emotional development

Most visually impaired infants have markedly poor vision during their first few months of life, which then improves with maturation. Thus, the parents miss the rewarding experiences of mutual gaze and smiling, an important part of the bonding process. Although these infants do smile and respond to voices and touch, these responses are subtle, making them appear indifferent to others and giving rise to the risk that they may be left alone and understimulated. The early intervention specialist must interpret the infant's signals to the parents and encourage them to keep their babies nearby and talk to them often in order to develop a strong relationship.

It becomes difficult for older children in peer groups to gauge their effect on others, because they may not be able to read body language. Some of their peers may move quickly in and out of their visual range and they may not be able to see who is available for play. This can lead to a sense of isolation and somewhat egocentric behavior, which persists longer than in sighted children. Because visually impaired children need more structure and predictability in their environments they are often more resistant to change, while their behavior may appear rigid.

THE DISABLED VISUALLY IMPAIRED CHILD

Neurodevelopmental disabilities are associated with a number of ocular disorders and seen in almost all children with cortical visual impairment.[5] Today, the majority of visually impaired children have additional disabilities, which make the habilitation considerably more complex.[6] For intervention specialists, it is no longer satisfactory to have experience only with visual disorders, because the various neurodevelopmental disabilities interact with each other and affect the child and their use of residual vision. The increase in the associated disabilities has facilitated the emergence of teamwork between a variety of professionals.

Cognition

Cognition is frequently affected in visually impaired children. The diagnosis of intellectual deficit is difficult and should be made only by psychologists; otherwise, the abilities could be over- or underestimated. Children with severe visual loss are capable of memorizing words and phrases, but without much first-hand experience, they may have little understanding of their meanings. Therefore, the psychologist must separate understimulation from intellectual deficit, making the interpretation of the test results important.

Cerebral palsy

Cerebral palsy is more detrimental for visually impaired children than for the sighted. It can result in loss of mobility, it affects touch, and it prevents the child from gaining first-hand experience while the frequently associated eye movement disorders may interfere with the use of residual vision.

Epilepsy

Epileptic disorders are more common among the visually impaired than in the general population. One time it was incorrectly assumed that the loss of vision itself can predispose to seizures, but it is now realized that the higher prevalence of epilepsy is due to neurological damage. Seizure disorders, such as infantile spasms, may result in cortical visual impairment, which is generally temporary and disappears with successful treatment. If possible, sedative anticonvulsant drugs should be avoided because sedation seriously interferes with learning.

Chronic sleep disorders

Sleep difficulties are common in visually impaired children and need to be appropriately diagnosed and treated early. Furthermore, when they do not sleep, the rest of the family does not sleep either. Sleep-deprived children may be so exhausted that they do not respond to various therapies or fail in the educational system. Chronic sleep deprivation permanently affects the motor and intellectual development. Untreated sleep disturbance of multidisabled visually impaired children is a common reason for their parents to relinquish their care, as they are unable to cope.

Deaf–blind children

The deaf–blind should not be viewed as visually impaired with hearing loss, or hearing impaired with visual loss, because their management is unique. See Chapter P15.

TEAMWORK

The interaction of visual loss and the various disabilities on the development is complex, and the multidisciplinary approach may be the most efficient way to deal with visually impaired children, in both the diagnostic and management processes.[7] These teams include ophthalmologists, pediatricians, and other physicians with a variety of training, nurses, a psychologist, speech-language pathologist, audiologist, physiotherapist, and orientation and mobility specialist, among others. Because genetic causes are so frequent, the involvement of the geneticist is required in most instances. These large, highly specialized, and expensive teams can only exist in major medical centers but close cooperation between the various professionals dealing with the visually impaired is now a necessity everywhere. It is felt that, in some circumstances, the single practitioner model no longer works efficiently, but in some cultures and economies it is, if anything at all, the only help available.

Team evaluation and management has many advantages. Since severe visual impairment is an infrequent disability, over time team members will develop considerable experience. Each professional is informed of the opinions of the others by conferences and/or reports. Thus, the care of visually impaired children becomes high quality and well coordinated, rather than fragmented.

Team members have specific roles. They are required to advocate for the blind, educate the community, and participate in publications and research. They also need to continually educate the parents, who must be active participants in the team. Therefore, the parents should receive all reports related to their children. Although this may be threatening to some professionals, when the parents feel that they are team members, they are much more cooperative and effective in the management of their children.

BLIND MANNERISMS

Many children with severe visual impairment exhibit one or more types of self-stimulating behaviors, which are also called "blind mannerisms." Some of these involve the visual system, while others manifest in motor activities. Blind mannerisms result from disordered physiological mechanisms; therefore when they occur, they need to be carefully analyzed and then appropriately managed. They should not be confused with autism or Tourette syndrome.

The stereotyped behaviors, which involve the visual system, include eye rubbing, pressing, poking, gazing compulsively at light, staring at hands, flicking fingers in front of the eyes against a light source, pulling on eyelids, tapping or hitting their globes, and repeatedly blinking or rolling the eyes. Rubbing, pressing, and poking the eyes are grouped together under the term "oculodigital phenomena" but they are different. Eye rubbing is observed in normal or disabled children, who are sleepy or tired. Eye pressing occurs in children who have severe bilateral, but usually not total congenital visual loss. Most commonly, eye pressers have retinopathies, but they can have other lesions, but optic atrophy, optic nerve hypoplasia, and cortical visual impairment are unusual.

The cause of eye pressing is unknown: it may be that it stimulates the brain for which functioning retinal ganglion cells appear to be a prerequisite. This type of primitive stimulation occurs when the child's vision is so impaired that he cannot give rise to well-formed, sustained images. This mannerism is seen when the child is bored or anxious or during various activities such as listening to music. It tends to be prolonged, but it is not painful. Due to chronic eye pressing, the orbits may eventually become enlarged, distorted, with an unsightly appearance. The parents must continually keep the children's hands busy and remove them from their eyes during the first years of life, when eye pressing is most intense. Later, the urge to eye press diminishes, and the management is easier.

Eye poking is deliberate and harmful. Most of these children exhibit their own repertoire of several self-injurious behaviors. Usually, eye poking causes pain and it is not unusual for them to scream afterward. Eye poking occurs in severely multidisabled or emotionally disturbed children, who are not necessarily visually impaired. It can cause corneal scarring, infection, retinal detachment, intraocular bleeding, and cataracts and may lead to blindness. The treatment is difficult.

Light gazing, a compulsive need to stare into lights, is one of the many clinical signs of cortical visual impairment. Visually impaired children who flicker their fingers in front of their eyes against a light source are also light gazers. The urge to light gaze can be mild or so severe that occasionally the child stares into the sun, risking the development of solar retinopathy.

There are a number of self-stimulating behaviors characterized by repetitive motor activities, such as rocking, head rolling, body swaying, twitching, tapping, and hand flapping. These blind mannerisms occur mostly in immobile, understimulated children with neurodevelopmental disabilities and marked visual impairment. These stereotyped behaviors diminish or even entirely disappear when there is exposure to appropriate physical activity. It is assumed that this primitive neurological self-stimulation is caused by inadequate movement input.

PROMOTION OF VISION DEVELOPMENT

Vision, which is a complex sense, is much more than acuity. Children require constant experience to develop their visual skills. While, in the absence of disabilities, this developmental process is more or less spontaneous, infants with impaired vision must be steadily encouraged to use their sight. Visual interaction with the environment can be reduced by severe acuity or field loss, defective eye movements, marked developmental delay, sedative medications for the treatment of epilepsy, or even ill health. Although visual learning continues throughout life, the rate of acquisition of visual skills is greatest during infancy. The development and structuring of the visual brain is influenced by visual input.[8] Therefore, in this critical early period, the visual environment for young children must be rich, meaningful, and increasingly complex; otherwise, there is a loss of opportunity to fully develop their visual sense. Appropriate encouragement to use vision can significantly improve visual potentials;[9] therefore, programs for promoting visual development are widespread. The process should be started after the diagnosis, whether it is an ocular or brain disorder. However, professionals working with visually impaired infants must first test and understand their visual abilities. It is important to avoid repetitive visual stimuli, like flashing lights, and to make interactions to be increasingly meaningful in order to make them a learning experience. The facilitation of visual development could be carried out by all members of the family, throughout the day when the infant is alert. For parents to be involved in the visual and neuro-developmental habilitation of their infants is extremely rewarding.

The majority of children with significant congenital visual loss appear to have little or no vision during early infancy; yet most develop useful sight later. There are two reasons for this. First, certain visual parameters, such as acuity, fields, eye movements, accommodation, perception, and cognitive factors rapidly improve after birth. Second, the vision of these infants may be so severely reduced by the combination of physiologic, ocular, or neurologic factors that they cannot use their vision spontaneously and experience delayed visual development. Because the maturation of the brain and visual system is stimulus-dependent, techniques that encourage these infants to use their sight are critical.

BEHAVIORAL PROBLEMS

Professionals not familiar with visually impaired children may draw the wrong conclusions from their mannerisms, speech, posture, facial expressions, and psychological test results. Therefore, there is a significant risk for these children to be misdiagnosed as emotionally disturbed or unintelligent. Yet most studies still agree that behavioral disorders are more common among the visually impaired than the sighted, especially when there are additional disabilities.

The assessment of behavioral deviations is a complex process; it cannot be done quickly, without knowledge of the past history and family dynamics, and it often requires multiple persons and settings.[10] The cause is often simple, but when more complex, the treatment needs to be directed to the family. Again, it is critical that the psychologist or psychiatrist be familiar with visual impairment and be part of a larger diagnostic team.

EDUCATION

Visual disorders can have a major impact on the education of students: normally learning requires a well-functioning visual system. The education of the blind has evolved into a highly specialized and respected field. After the parents, the educators are the most important in the lives of visually impaired children. The teachers who plan the curricula and teach the students require special training and working experience. The dedication, time commitment, skills, and healthy attitudes of the teachers are a prerequisite for the later success of visually impaired students in adult life.

In addition to the usual subjects adopted for the visually impaired curriculum planning includes concept formation, orientation and mobility, daily living techniques, nonvisual communication in reading, writing, speaking, and listening, the use of recently developed technical aids, physical and sex education, and the arts. To succeed, the educators need to understand the ocular or neurological visual disorders, the cognitive abilities, and the health issues facing their students. This requires good parent–teacher relationships and access to vital information from ophthalmologists. The distance acuity determines where the students should sit in the classroom and how much blackboard work is required of them. Those with homonymous hemianopia must be seated so that their functioning visual field is directed toward the teacher and the class. Children with severe peripheral field loss but intact macular vision function better if they are further away from the blackboard, rather than close to it. Students with photosensitivity (as in aniridia and albinism) must not be placed next to a window where the glare is most intense. Appropriate lighting, individually adjusted, is critically important. Impaired accommodation, abnormal contrast sensitivity or color perception, and eye movement disorders can all adversely affect learning. It is helpful for the educators to understand the reasons for the head turn and the head shaking associated with nystagmus. When the visual disorder is progressive, as in retinitis pigmentosa, the rate of deterioration determines the timely introduction of Braille and assistive devices. Also, the uses of visual aids are much more effective when the educators are involved in the instructions.

Since so many visually impaired children have complex neuro-developmental disabilities, educators require information about cognitive deficits, anticonvulsant medications, what to do when a student has an epileptic seizure in the classroom, and how to care for a visually impaired student who has cerebral palsy. Educators for the visually impaired often accompany students to appointments with ophthalmologists and other physicians, and it is helpful when they receive copies of the medical reports. Not only the ophthalmologist but also the educators should be participants in the team that provides care to each visually impaired child.

The education of children with cortical visual impairment and ocular visual loss differs.[11] With pure ocular disorders, the transmission of signals from the eyes to the brain may be reduced, but the process of analysis is sound. Thus, visual enrichment and training to scan more efficiently are useful. For children with cortical visual impairment, this approach does not work: visual input must be controlled, to avoid "overloading." Visual images should be simple in form and presented in isolation. In their training, teachers for the visually impaired should be exposed to the management of neurological visual disorders that are increasingly common.

Until recently, severely visually impaired students were educated in segregated schools. Due to changes in social attitudes in many regions of the world, they have been "integrated" into classrooms, resulting in benefits and disadvantages.[12] Full integration often tends to be detrimental to the multidisabled visually impaired, who best learn in a carefully controlled classroom.

ASSISTIVE TECHNOLOGY

The technological revolution has had a markedly beneficial effect on the visually impaired. Assistive or adoptive technology has dramatically improved the way they are educated or trained and increased their employment opportunities. When assistive technology is offered, the visual and intellectual abilities are evaluated, costs and social issues considered, devices are selected, adjusted, and maintained, the school and home environments are often modified, the students, parents, and educators are instructed how to use them, while the services are coordinated with other therapies. Assistive technology is a basic tool, like pencil and paper for sighted students, and as they grow this is a continuous process. It can enhance, not replace, basic skills.

There are a great number of devices listed on the Web. These range from magnification programs for computer screens, Windows-based tutorials, Braille translation of software, portable note takers, Braille writing equipment, scanners, and specialized programs to simulate the human voice, to a variety of video magnifiers or closed-circuit televisions.

It is beneficial to introduce these services, even before school age, so that young, visually impaired children may have a chance to learn how to scribble, draw, or color: early referrals are important. Professionals who provide assistive technology should also be members of the team that offers services to that child. Low vision clinics, operated by ophthalmologists or optometrists, do not work well in isolation, and they should be familiar with assistive technology or work with professionals who are.

ORIENTATION AND MOBILITY

Orientation is the understanding of one's location, while mobility is movement from one area to another. Orientation and mobility (O&M) teaches concepts and skills to children with visual impairment and how to travel safely and efficiently in different environments. O&M specialists need to known about visual disorders, the cognitive abilities, the understanding of concepts, the extent of their early environmental exposure, the interaction of additional neurodevelopmental disabilities, and motivational and emotional issues, and they must be members of a team supporting the child. It is founded on the acquisition of skills in early childhood, when basic sensory awareness of the environment is formed: it is much more than just cane training!

O&M cannot be taught by words or by miniature models, but only in the real world and by direct experience. Although it begins in infancy, formal instructions are often started in preschool years. The most common methods of mobility are sighted guides, cane, alternative mobility devices, guide dogs, and electronic travel aids.

SEX EDUCATION

Children who are severely visually impaired may have distorted concepts about sexuality because it is through sight that sexual behaviors are mainly learnt. This ignorance is partly attributed to social taboos on touching, and parents are often embarrassed to discuss issues that sighted children may discover for themselves.

Sex education must start early and needs to embrace not just anatomy or reproduction, but correct vocabulary, feelings, function, courting, human sexual relationships, family values, and principles of marriage. Children and their parents require counseling, because of the complexity of human sexuality, as it relates to blindness. It should be part of the habilitation process, which emphasizes the importance of proper training for professionals who carry out the intervention.

THE JOB MARKET

Although the severely visually impaired are capable of performing a great variety of jobs, and many blind individuals achieve remarkable careers, according to census figures only one in four are employed, and their mean monthly earnings are significantly lower than those of nondisabled individuals. They require support from agencies and extra education and training, often beyond the high school level, and need to be knowledgeable with assistive devices. When they have additional neurological disabilities, their employment records are worse.

In view of these obstacles, families must prepare their children for adult employment early in life, nurturing their abilities with a positive but realistic attitude. The preparation continues until, and beyond, employment in adulthood. In this prolonged process, the role of parents, teachers, vocational counselors, and agencies for the visually impaired is critical.

SUGGESTED BIBLIOGRAPHY FOR PARENTS

A great variety of educational material exists for parents. Service providers tend to have their favorite resources. Most are listed on the Internet.

Holbrook MC, editor. Children with Visual Impairment: a Parents' Guide. Bethesda, MD: Woodbine House; 1996.

Pogrund RL, Fazzi DL, editors. Early Focus: Working with Young Children Who are Blind or Visually Impaired and their Families. 2nd ed. New York: AFB Press; 2002.

Rayner S, Drouillard R. Get a Wiggle On: a Guide for Helping Visually Impaired Children Grow. Mason, MI: Ingham Intermediate School District; 1975.

Sonsken P, Stiff B. Show Me What My Friends Can See. A Developmental Guide for Parents of Babies with Severely Impaired Sight and their Professional Advisors. London: Institute of Child Health; 1991.

REFERENCES

1. Jan JE, Freeman RD. Who is a Visually Impaired child? Dev Med Child Neurol 1998; 40: 65–7.
2. Shonkoff JP, Hauser-Cram P. Early intervention for disabled infants and their families: a quantitative analysis. Pediatrics 1987; 80: 650–8.
3. Jan JE, Robinson GC, Scott E, Kinnis C. Hypotonia in the blind child. Dev Med Child Neurol 1975; 17: 35–40.
4. Kekelis LS, Andersen ES. Family communication styles and language development. J Visual Impair Blindness 1984; 78: 54–65.
5. Mervis CA, Boyle CA, Yeargin-Allsopp M. Prevalence and selected characteristics of childhood visual impairment. Dev Med Child Neurol 2002; 44: 538–42.
6. Sonsken PM, Dale N. Visual impairment in infancy: impact on neurodevelopmental and neurobiological processes. Dev Med Child Neurol 2002; 44: 782–91.
7. Langley MB. ISAVE: individualized, systematic assessment of visual efficiency. For the developmentally young and individuals with multihandicapping conditions. Louisville, KY: American Printing House for the Blind; 1998. (vols. 1 & 2.)
8. Blakemore C. Sensitive and vulnerable periods in the development of the visual system. Ciba Found Symp 1991; 156: 129–47.
9. Sonsken PM, Petrie A, Drew KJ. Promotion of visual development of severely visually impaired babies: evaluation of a developmentally based programme. Dev Med Child Neurol 1991; 33: 320–35.
10. Freeman RD, Goetz E, Richards DP et al. Blind children's early emotional development: do we know enough to help? Child Care Health Dev 1989; 15: 3–28.
11. Groenveld M, Jan JE, Leader P. Observations on the habilitation of children with cortical visual impairment. J Visual Impair Blindness 1990; 84: 11–15.
12. Hatlen PH, Curry SA. In support of specialized programs for blind and visually impaired children: the impact of vision loss on learning. J Visual Impair Blindness 1987; 81: 7–13.

CHAPTER 16 Helping a Family with a Visually Impaired Child

Nancy C Mansfield and A Linn Murphree

The diagnosis of visual impairment in a child has an enormous emotional impact. It is shattering to parents, siblings, grandparents, and extended family, and to the community in which they live. The following discussion is based on the authors' clinical training and experience working with families of blind and visually impaired children for the past 27 years.

LIFE WITHOUT A SAFETY NET

We often refer to the life of a family given the diagnosis of visual disability in a child as a life "without a safety net"; this is because when a couple learns that they are going to have a baby, they have expectations of their life after the birth of the baby. Although these expectations are individual, some are universal. They expect that their child will face only "normal" challenges: broken bones, ear tubes for recurrent infections, or removal of the tonsils or adenoids. Most families expect colic or a period of adjustment to life with a new baby. Most have fears about being able to provide all that a baby requires. They expect that their child will be free from unreasonable harm and to be able to live out their dreams and hopes for their children.

This "safety net" is, in reality, a form of denial. As we watch the amazing Cirque du Soleil performers, we are horrified if they appear to lose their balance, because we know that they will not survive a fall, because they perform without a safety net.

This "safety net for life" keeps our children and us safe as well. We expect that nothing terribly "bad" will happen to our family. Bad things happen to other people, people on TV shows. The reality of having such a belief is one of life's most important fantasies. This form of denial (as none of us are ever really safe from harm) enables us to function each day.

What happens to a family when this "safety net" is taken away by a diagnosis of blindness or other disability in the baby? When a family first learns that their child probably does not see well, they are devastated. Confusion, shock, helplessness, fear, depression, and profound sadness overwhelm everyone involved. The news affects mothers and fathers, brothers and sisters, the extended family, friends, co-workers, and even the community in which they live. The research of grief specialists[1-4] confirms this.

Ramifications for daily living

What are the ramifications in terms of daily living once a family learns that their baby has a serious diagnosis? The family no longer feels the same safety that they had before the diagnosis. After the diagnosis, every cough is pneumonia; every headache a brain tumor; everyday activities are fraught with dangers. Living with a child with special needs is a chronic problem because it is never finished and it poses life-long challenges to the family as well as the children.

It is normal for parents to experience extreme anxiety. Many have symptoms of post-traumatic stress disorder. Depression and anxiety become normal: at the same time the couple must go on, make crucial decisions, and raise their children. Families have feelings of denial, anger, and guilt. They suffer a tremendous loss, not only the loss of their dreams, but also a loss of the baby they expected to bring home from the hospital. A mourning period is usually associated with this loss, and parental reactions are compared to the feelings associated with a death in the family.

Ophthalmologists often have expectations that families should "accept the situation" especially if no treatment is available, and after they have given what they perceive to be a rational and logical explanation for the visual impairment. In fact, just the opposite is true. Parents should not be expected to accept what is, to them, "unacceptable." Their not being willing to "accept the situation" by expressing anger, resistance, or aggressive questioning does not make them "bad" or "difficult" parents–just "normal" ones.

With the news, families experience a loss of control over their lives: professionals take over and the family find themselves in a world they are not prepared to handle. Even the most resourceful have difficulty navigating a hospital, even more the overwhelming challenges of a neonatal intensive care unit. The number of people that a family encounters is staggering. Nothing is certain and every nuance, every gesture of the professional staff takes on significance for the family. "Is something wrong with the baby they are not telling me?" "What does 'that' mean?" "I don't want to sound stupid, but what did she just say? Will the baby survive today, tonight, forever?" "Will the baby have a normal life?" These are all questions families ask themselves during their stay in the hospital and beyond.

Stress on the marriage

A special needs baby puts enormous stress on a marriage. In the USA, the divorce rate among couples with a disabled child approaches 80% compared with just over 50% in families without a disabled child. Men and women handle stress and grief differently, communication becomes strained, and often couples feel estranged and isolated from their partner. Mothers say, "he doesn't care, he never even cries." In Western culture, men handle their feelings differently to their wives. Women often interpret this as a loss of love or unwillingness on the part of their husband or partner to participate in the required daily decision-making.

Learning to cope

How do families survive the stress of having a disabled child? Couples survive by first understanding that they do not have to "accept" the "unacceptable." Instead, they learn to cope. Learning to cope requires support, understanding, and nonjudgmental help on the part of professionals, extended family members, and friends. Counseling is critical to the "coping process" as no one is prepared to deal with the associated stress of a disabled baby or child. With counseling help for the individual parents, the couple, and eventually the entire family including the children, families learn to live one day at a time. Eventually they return to the previous family lifestyle with the modifications required following the loss of life's "safety net." Parents and children can learn to accommodate to the visual and/or hearing loss of their child, but rarely without regular, experienced, and supportive help from an empathetic counselor or therapist.

THE IMPACT OF VISUAL IMPAIRMENT ON CHILD DEVELOPMENT

Development of a visually impaired child is different from what is expected.[1,5,6] Vision is one of the major stimuli to the timing of developmental milestones in a sighted child. The milestones still happen in the absence of vision but "out-of-kilter." Late milestones may trigger anxiety, which can be mitigated if the ophthalmologist discusses with the parents their altered timing.

For the first years of life, vision is the primary stimulus that encourages sighted infants to interact with the world. The desire to peer over the crib's edge is what challenges a normally developing baby to push up; this is critical as the baby's neck muscles become stronger and leads to pushing up to all fours, crawling, sitting, etc. Because development is a sequence of mastering one situation to the challenge of the next, infants with a visual problem start with an impediment.

Children without good vision like to be on their backs with as much of the surface of the crib touching their bodies. This provides them with a sense of security and certainty about their surroundings. With no visual stimulus, they feel insecure and resist being placed on their stomachs, which is extremely important as it encourages infants to raise their heads up to see. Without this encouragement, being placed on their stomach is one thing visually impaired babies usually resist. They cry and may get upset in this position. Consequently, parents are often not willing to place the baby in this position and offer other forms of stimulation to encourage the baby to raise his or her head. The act of raising the head is critical in the development of the neck muscles, which must be strong enough for the baby to push up from the floor or surface of the crib.

When a sighted infant sees a parent or family member approach the crib, he or she usually expresses happiness and excitement by movement of the arms and legs and making noises. The nonsighted child becomes still to hear the approaching parent better: this stillness may be misinterpreted as disinterest and, unless warned of this, some parents of visually impaired children rarely pick them up.

All developmental milestones are delayed in blind babies. These babies often do not sit up at the appropriate age because the world is no more interesting to them sitting up than lying down. They feel less secure seated than on their backs, and they do not feel any need to master this important skill. For sighted babies, the seated position is preferred as their view of everything is increased. A very young sighted baby stands on the parent's lap to enhance their view: not so for a child with poor vision.

Visually impaired children do not acquire motor skills naturally like their sighted counterparts. They do not reach out and grasp objects because there are no objects to see. They do not crawl after a toy because they cannot see it. Blind children are slow to develop a sense of balance because of low muscle tone and they cannot orient themselves as do their sighted peers.

Sounds are more difficult to trace to people or objects. Ordinary household machines such as the vacuum cleaner, washing machine, and lawnmower may frighten blind children, as they have less awareness of them. Each sound must be systematically introduced and explained while allowing the child to touch the object so that they are not so startled or frightened. This taxes all members in the household as most do not think about the ordinary noises that are around us and may be quite loud.

Early emotional and social development is often delayed because blind children cannot see their parents and have no way of knowing when they are present or absent, far or near. The development of a sense of self or "I" is driven by vision. Since we address children by name, blind babies often do not know who they are in relation to others because they cannot see themselves, which slows their self-identity. Since they do not have the eye contact that sighted children rely on, blind babies cannot "read" facial expressions or body language such as smiles of approval or frowns of reproach. Instead they rely on tone, clarity, and directness of the person addressing them to get the same information as their sighted counterpart. Their body language is often "off" as they cannot imitate others. Imitation accounts for a lot of what a baby learns in the first year; much of it is visual and must be made up for in other ways by the visually impaired baby.

Language development is difficult. Firstly, pronouns develop relatively late for blind babies, as it is difficult to discriminate between "you," "me," and "I" when you cannot see. Reciprocity or the understanding of taking turns when we speak is also a challenge for visually impaired children. Thus, most blind babies begin their use of language by using "echolalia" (repeating words or phrases) to make their needs known. This is acceptable as a first step, but must be worked on with the parents so that the child moves to the next step, which is appropriate use of the phrases acquired from the use of "echolalia."

Words like "up" and "down" have little meaning to a child who cannot see what direction an adult is referring to. A child who recognizes his father's face can easily learn to match the face with the word "daddy," but this does not happen in the same way or at the same time with a blind baby.

Walking independently is another example of a seemingly simple behavior that automatically happens between certain ages. This is true for sighted children, but not for the visually impaired child. In addition to the motor skills required to walk, children use imitation to master this skill. They are motivated to get to a toy, other child, or parent faster by walking than by crawling or rolling. Blind children must be stimulated to take those first steps and rewarded with hugs and kisses. They must feel secure that someone will be there to catch them if they fall and they must, by feeling their environment, learn what is around them and whether it is safe to proceed. This takes time and patience. A blind child may begin walking at age two or more, compared with fourteen months in sighted children.

An airplane journey takes one hour; in a car, the same trip takes seven hours: this concept of space and its relation to the world is difficult to master without vision. Sighted children quickly learn that objects are permanent and continue to exist whether they can be seen or not. For blind children objects seem to appear and disappear without any permanence or consistency. This affects much of daily life: the ability to navigate one's bedroom, house, block, or another's house, the ability to walk down the street, etc.

Language takes on a new meaning. Often blind children are very literal in their interpretation of everyday expressions of time and space. "I am going to catch the bus," for example, can be confusing to a blind child unless each developmental step that comes before the understanding of this concept is mastered.

Piaget taught that object permanence is a crucial step in child development; this is especially so for a blind child, as trust and understanding of the world rely on the understanding and application of this milestone. Sighted children learn early that the family dog is the same dog whether he is sleeping indoors or is outdoors playing. This concept of object permanence or consistency is a challenge to even the most resourceful and bright blind child.

Daily living activities are challenging for visually impaired children; it takes time to teach them how to dress and undress, where clothes are kept, how to identify what garment goes with another, and whether something is on inside out or not. Buttoning a shirt, learning how to zipper, putting on jeans in time for school, and tying shoes are all very difficult tasks for visually impaired children and put pressure on the whole family. Grooming skills, so important in later childhood, are difficult to master. Hair combing, hair washing, nail trimming, and make-up application are all difficult and require patience by the parent.

THE NEEDS OF THE FAMILY OF A VISUALLY-IMPAIRED CHILD

The family of a newly diagnosed visually impaired child needs a great deal of support, understanding, and *nonjudgmental* help.[5] Interventions from professionals are critical. These include at various times:
1. Counseling;
2. Parent organizations;
3. Special education;
4. Physical therapy; and
5. Language specialists.

Some guidelines that may be of help to pediatric ophthalmologists in making referrals are listed in Table 16.1. Access to the Internet opens a host of resources for those to whom it is

---

Table 16.1 Key resources and referrals for the family of a visually impaired child

Worldwide
See Chapter P32

USA
1. The local school district office or State Department of Education (even if the visually impaired child is an infant)
2. Internet sites
   a. National Organization for Rare Diseases, Inc. (NORD): http://www.rarediseases.org
      This site is where to start searching for a specific disease.
   b. Rare Genetic Diseases/Family Village: http://www.familyvillage.wisc.edu/lib_gene.htm
      This is a site for genetic diseases; it has many links to specific organizations.
   c. National Institutes of Health Office of Rare Diseases: http://rarediseases.info.nih.gov
   d. Institute for Families: http://www.instituteforfamilies.org
   e. Retinoblastoma International: http://www.retinoblastoma.net

---

available. A good place to start is the National Organization for Rare Diseases (http://www.nord.org).

In the United States, one of the first places parents should contact is the office of the local school board or the local office of the State Department of Education. Most states have assigned the local schools the task of providing appropriate intervention and assistance for children, including newborns, with visual abnormalities. The contents of Table 16.1 may be freely reproduced and distributed to families with children newly diagnosed with visual impairment.

The Hadley School for the Blind is a resource that provides distance learning (correspondence courses) free of charge to any family member of a visually impaired child. Their Web site is http://www.Hadley-school.org/Web_Site/1aa_about_hadley.asp.

Understanding that the world of the blind child, even if he or she is very intelligent, is starkly different from that of the sighted child helps the ophthalmologist to provide direction and resources for their families. An understanding and concerned physician can have a profound and positive impact on the life of the family with a visually impaired child.

REFERENCES

1. Halliday C. The Visually Impaired Child: Growth, Learning, Development–Infancy to School Age. Louisville, KY: American Printing House for the Blind; 1971.
2. Fraiberg SH, Fraiberg L. Insights for the Blind: Comparative Studies of Blind and Sighted Infants. New York: Basic Books; 1977.
3. Fraiberg SH. The Magic Years: Understanding and Handling the Problems of Early Childhood. New York: Scribner's & Sons; 1965.
4. Moses K. The Impact of Childhood Disability. Ways Magazine, Spring 1987.
5. Brazelton TB. Toddlers and Parents: a Declaration of Independence. New York: Dell; 1974.
6. Sonksen PM, Stiff B. Show Me What My Friends Can See: a Guide for Parents and Professionals. London: Wolfson Centre; 1997.

CHAPTER 17   The Low Vision Clinic

Janet H Silver and Elizabeth Gould

BACKGROUND

For a definition and the epidemiology of visual handicap, see Chapter 1.

DEVICES

Low vision aids (LVAs) fall into the following groups:
   Simple hand- and stand-magnifiers;
   Telescopes: face mounted and hand held; and
   Electronic magnifiers (see Further Reading).
   The calculation of magnification is complex, particularly for hand and stand magnifiers. Magnification (M) was derived from

$$(1)$$
$$M = f/4,$$

where f = the back vertex power in diopters. However, an argument can be made for

$$(2)$$
$$M = f/4 + 1.$$

Thus a +20 lens is labeled as 5× using Formula (1) and 6× using Formula (2). Furthermore, if the lens is closer to the object than its focal length, its effective magnification is reduced and an accommodative effort or spectacle correction is required.

Spectacle magnifiers too may be labeled by either method (commonly, $f/4$) but a 5×-labeled lens (i.e., 20 D) has different effects, depending on the refractive error of the user:

1. An uncorrected –12.00-diopter myope will have a total optical system of (+12.00 + 20.00 =) +32 diopters; material must be placed (100/32 =) 3.3 cm from the eye. The magnification (using $f/4$) will be 8×.
2. A +12.00 aphakic using the same spectacle magnifier produces only 2× (+20.00 – 12.00 = +8.00), for use at (100/8 =) 12.5 cm.

Here all simple magnifiers are described by their effective power in diopters to the nearest diopter.

Spectacle-mounted LVAs present a larger image at the retina: electronic and some stand and dome magnifiers usually produce a large image that can be scanned. Other strategies are enlargement, large print, contrast, extra illumination, and simply moving closer. For children, sitting near the blackboard or TV or enlarging material is often preferable

Several organizations (Keeler (UK), Designs for Vision (USA), and Zeiss (Germany)) produce complete kits, usually with prescribing instructions. Combined Optical Industries produce the most comprehensive range of magnifiers. It is preferable to assemble a basic prescribing kit appropriate to the circumstances and enlarge it as experience and needs develop. A "starter kit"

might include hand, stand, and spectacle magnifiers; a series of hand-held and face-mounted telescopes; and a CCTV.

The practitioner must understand the relationship between lens power, focal length, and image size. If a normal reading distance is 25 cm, when print is moved to 12.5 cm the angle subtended is twice as large – and in the emmetropic eye +8.00 is required to focus that image, but a –12.00 myope will need –4.00, +12.00 aphakic +20.00. The retinal image size will be similar. We will state the reciprocal of the near point (the distance from the eye or the back vertex of a spectacle magnifier (in centimeters) to the plane of the reading chart) when magnification is quoted.

Telescopic lenses are calculated differently. Distant vision telescopes are afocal, and may incorporate a prescription, or are focusable. For near, plus lenses are incorporated into the objective or added as caps; magnification then is normally calculated on angle subtended as previously described.

EQUIPMENT AND TEST MATERIALS

Some additions to standard equipment are required if the practitioner is seeing children. For older children, items such as a map and dictionary are useful. New patients should bring with them examples of what they can and cannot manage. A distinction is made between a congenital and an acquired visual impairment. In the former, the child "does not know what he is missing." If a selection of common problem materials is available in the waiting area the child may request help. Although such material does not measure vision, the expression on a child's face when he identifies correctly a photograph or inspects an insect gives as good an indication of the potential use of an LVA as does a conventional acuity chart.

Visual acuity is important in establishing the magnification needed. Snellen charts are constructed on the basis of the elements of the 6-m line subtending one minute of arc at the retina of the viewer; the whole figure subtends 5°. However, crowding and confusion elements are lost at low acuity levels. Charts with multiple characters at each level like Sonksen-Silver charts are more appropriate in the low vision clinic. Charts using symbols are often culturally specific and older children can read letter charts. Children of 3 years will normally match reliably. Picture and symbol tests such as Lea, Cardiff, and Kay plates have merits, and eye clinics are adopting LogMAR charts. With acuity of less than about 6/24 (20/60) we prefer to use a reduced distance: 3/18 is almost identical to 6/36 (20/120) but more comfortable for the child.

The "N series" of reading charts uses standard printer's typefaces and sizes, are sensibly constructed, and are widely available. Where such charts are not readily available, alternatives can be produced with a computer using standard "N" fonts. There is an arithmetic relationship between the different sizes, and the correlation between Snellen and these cards is well understood. Maclure charts devised specifically for children check the near vision rather than the reading ability.

Other information such as visual fields; color vision; contrast sensitivity, ultrasound, and electrophysiology is helpful. Refraction is crucial to low vision assessment. Using a cycloplegic is necessary at a separate visit or as confirmation at the end, since accommodation provides significant magnification. Each child is refracted personally as it builds cooperation and rapport and gives information about the media. A refractionist can gain the cooperation of most 3-year-olds for long enough to give an accurate retinoscopy. If the mother, or other fixation target, is at 2 m, an allowance of one-half diopter can be made for accommodation. We do not use a trial frame for small children, but prefer to hold the lenses in front of the eye, or even work over present glasses if their power is reliable. With lower acuities, small cylinders can safely be ignored, but oblique astigmatism of ±1.00 or more should be corrected.

Subjective refraction is not usually possible, but small errors matter little. When the child has nystagmus both eyes should always be kept uncovered with the eye not under consideration being fogged; +2.00 after the allowance for working distance fogs to about 6/60 (20/200).

Occlusion is necessary if there is a large strabismus: if the dominant eye is covered, the squinting eye will fix the target, enabling accurate retinoscopy.

Where there is no retinoscopy reflex we must depend on subjective responses: depending on the level of cooperation, we may start with the chart at 1 m and perhaps ±3.00 extending the distance and making the necessary adjustments as indicated by the improving acuity. A surprising number of children come to the low vision clinic uncorrected, and while +3.00 may not make much improvement for distance or near acuity in the clinic, it will be significant for extended reading or when incorporated into spectacles. A special correction for aphakes may be needed for intermediate tasks such as using computers. Preverbal aphakes may be overcorrected by about 2.00 to 3.00 diopters (see Chapter 47).

LOW VISION ASSESSMENT

The life, difficulties, interests, needs, and ambitions of the child are paramount and can best be clarified by getting to know him and his family at the first contact. This is an enabling situation, with the ultimate target of giving the child the means to cope with normal materials in a normal environment, both in his school life and later. The greatest difficulty may be reading the blackboard or small print: it is important to know the distance at which any material is to be viewed. There may be an interest in making models, reading comics, or other visually demanding activities. Many children become bored quickly, so prioritized shortcuts may be needed.

After noncycloplegic refraction and the optimum levels of magnification have been determined, the different methods of achieving this are demonstrated. The alternatives need to be discussed fully with the child and parents, showing the benefits and limitations of the device. Where the difficulty is with occasional small print, a small portable magnifier is often best (Figs. 17.1 and 17.2), but if standard textbooks or library books present difficulties a face-mounted appliance must be considered (Figs. 17.3–17.5). CCTV has great advantages in that the child

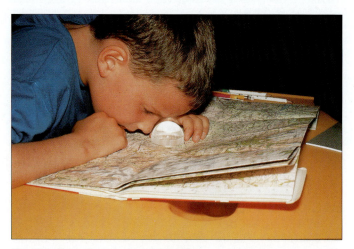

Fig. 17.1 Alexander using dome magnifier.

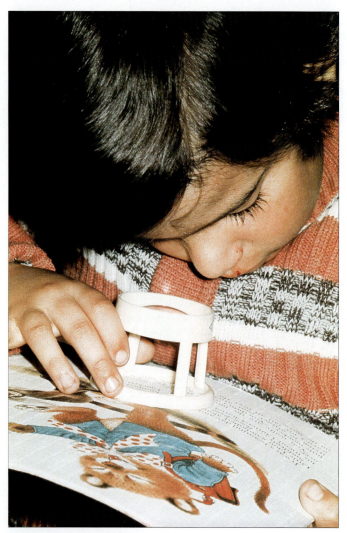

Fig. 17.2 Daniel using stand magnifier.

can use as much magnification as the task requires. CCTV is well accepted, and in combination with a laptop computer it extends the range of materials available.

When demonstrating the benefits of a hand-held telescope with the black/whiteboard, its potential use for outings, theater trips, spectator sports, bus numbers, etc. should be mentioned.

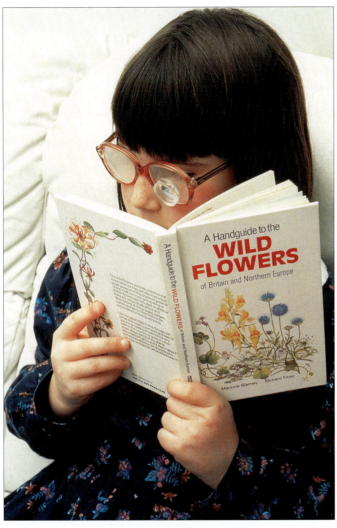

Fig. 17.3 Anna reading with bifocal spectacle magnifier.

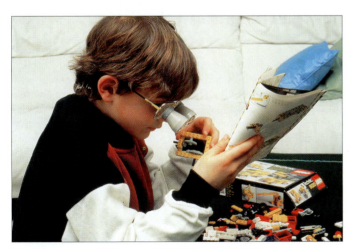

Fig. 17.4 James with his near vision telescopic spectacle.

In bilateral disorders such as albinism or macular dystrophies, if the level of vision is similar in both eyes, there are advantages in keeping patients binocular, as the field is better and it is more comfortable.

Reading music is difficult. Before finding a solution, the instrument played, the optimum distance from the music, and the

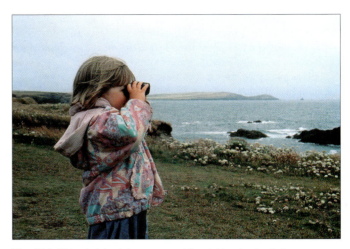

Fig. 17.5 Distant vision telescope used for sightseeing by Sally.

closest practical distance need to be known. Telescopic appliances usually give the required range but their restricted field of view and their appearance may limit success. Although enlarged music is cumbersome it is often the only practical solution.

Children are best seen first at about age 3. Some children are uncooperative, have not yet developed sufficient hand–eye coordination, or are uninterested at that age, but they become familiar with the informal and relaxed environment and build a relationship with the practitioner. The assessment can as easily be carried out on the floor or outdoors as in the standard, often frightening, consulting room chair. White coats went out with the Ark! Some bricks, crayons, or a simple tray jigsaw, for example, will keep most young children occupied.

If a child is being taxed either visually or intellectually he may become uncooperative or restless but the low vision assessment can be made to seem like play. He may become absorbed in a new "toy" (the magnifier) that is presented to him although it is often difficult to decide which one is preferred.

In the final discussion with the parents, they should understand the potential of magnification for their child, so that at school his magnifiers will help with nursery-type material. With even very small children it is important to try to determine adequate levels of magnification required for various tasks. A child may have a large low-powered magnifier for pictures, and a high-powered device for detail.

Before the clinician prescribes a low vision aid, the child must understand its potential use and, in the case of the younger child, that he must be able to both manipulate it and understand its use. Many young children place a stand magnifier over an object, look through it, and then remove the magnifier to check whether the object is really there; however, if they learn to use a magnifier early, it becomes part of their personal equipment and is used without conscious thought.

At the end of the assessment an aid may be loaned from stock, with full instructions on its use and care. Face-mounted prescription devices must be dispensed by an optician competent in this specialized area.

Reassurance that low vision aids cannot damage a child's vision nor exacerbate the disease is needed.

TRAINING

Learning how to use low vision aids is important, so encouragement or supervised training is desirable if a child is to use the devices competently. Such training is expensive and may be avoidable if the aid matches the current interests and dexterity of the child. If the tasks performed with the device are important he rapidly becomes adept. Parents and teachers can provide encouragement. Written instructions can be useful.

Children with low vision who have been educated in schools for the blind may have been taught to acquire information by nonvisual means only, and may even sight-read Braille! Some are unfamiliar with alpha-numeric script, in which case a low vision aid may be introduced for photographs and other graphic material first and print later.

FOLLOW-UP VISITS

Children may benefit from regular clinic attendance: their requirements change with new activities as dexterity and skills improve. We ask that materials for the next school year be brought to the clinic so that everything is accessible. If outgrown, damaged, or mislaid, appliances may need replacing. Parents or children worried about damage to a loaned appliance can be reassured that it can still be used or replaced.

Initial follow-up visits may be at about six months, but sooner if a complex appliance has been prescribed, if the vision is changing, or for a very young child. Subsequent visits can be annual for the child who is happy with his devices and where no problems are anticipated. Parents need to be able to contact the practitioner in the event of difficulties.

The procedure at follow-up is the same: the parents and child explore the value and limitations of existing loaned appliances. When and where are they used? With older children, are they used both at school and at home? Has the full potential of the appliance been appreciated, e.g., is the telescope that is used for blackboard work or outings also used when supporting the football team?

Does a younger child use the appliance spontaneously or only at an adult's instigation? This may happen when the aid is kept by the teacher or parent to prevent loss or damage. Any problems with new tasks need to be discussed; once the value of magnification has been demonstrated, a series of previously unrecognized visual difficulties can become apparent to child, parent, or teacher.

Finally, if the provision of an appliance had been deferred, the situation needs to be reevaluated. The deferment may have been because the child was not ready for a face-mounted appliance for cosmetic reasons, but after using a hand magnifier, the advantages of the previously rejected appliance become apparent. A reason for deferring the provision of appliances is that supplying a child (especially a young child) with too many new gadgets simultaneously may result in the rejection of all of them. The prudent practitioner solves the most pressing (usually school-related) problems but reassures the child that next time help may be available for important hobbies like painting small objects or building models.

Most children go through a period when all devices (sometimes including the practitioner!) are rejected. The reasons are cosmetic or pressure to conform. We have a relaxed attitude to this, suggesting that the device can be useful at home, and the situation will be reviewed later. The phase is usually brief.

LIGHT SENSITIVITY

Children with retinal dystrophies, albinism, aniridia, or other conditions can get increased comfort if a dark lens is put on as they leave the house and removed as they return. Many patients prefer to wear a red or brown lens. The spectacle lens needs side-shielding to prevent the back of the lens acting as a mirror and for extra protection. Lenses that cut out UV and short-wavelength visible light are preferable, usually with a 25% light transmission (it can be made darker or bleached). Since a standard CR39 lens cuts off completely at 350 nm, this with a red or brown tint is an economic and practical solution. Since most glare comes from above, and most environments have low-contrast materials at floor level, a graduated tint, quite dark at the top and fading quickly to nil at the midline, is often helpful, as is a hat with an adjustable brim.

STARTING A SERVICE

We have worked mainly in a dedicated eye hospital clinic in an industrialized country: such clinics do not exist everywhere so it may be more appropriate to start with a limited service, increasing hardware and scope as expertise and demand increases. Locally produced devices should be used, augmented by the more expensive imported equipment where necessary.

FURTHER INFORMATION

A list of low vision aids available within the UK (and many available in other countries) can be found at http://www.tiresias.org. It is intended for professionals working with visually disabled people. There is also information on nonvisual devices; the site has data on nearly 2000 devices, including supplier, current price, and date of last update. The TechDis Accessibility Database (http://www.niad.sussex.ac.uk) contains a useful listing of electronic devices.

In 2000, *The Lighthouse Handbook on Vision Impairment and Vision Rehabilitation* in two volumes was published.

CHAPTER
18

Ocular Manifestations of Intrauterine Infections

Scott R Lambert

While most maternal infections during pregnancy do not affect the developing fetus, there are several notable exceptions, including the TORCH infections (i.e., toxoplasmosis, syphilis, rubella, cytomegalovirus (CMV), and herpes simplex), varicella, and lymphocytic choriomeningitis virus. Neonates may be infected either by hematogenous spread or by an ascending infection from the maternal genitourinary tract, or during the delivery process. Primary rubella and varicella infections impart life-long immunity, virtually eliminating any risk of an intrauterine infection during subsequent pregnancies, while other infections such as CMV and toxoplasmosis may recur.[1,2] Maternal syphilis infection may result in significant intrauterine disease, regardless of whether it is a primary, secondary, or latent infection.

Intrauterine infections may injure the fetus by disturbing embryogenesis, damaging vital organs, or as an ongoing infection extending into postnatal life. Rubella infections primarily damage the fetus by interfering with embryogenesis and as a consequence rarely result in serious malformations after the first trimester. Varicella and CMV infections damage the fetus by causing necrosis of vital organs and may result in severe abnormalities even if contracted during the second and, rarely, the third trimesters of gestation. Intrauterine syphilis continues to damage neonates postnatally as an ongoing infection.

Intrauterine infections are difficult to distinguish on clinical grounds alone. Laboratory confirmation may sometimes be obtained by culturing the responsible pathogen; cultures from neonates with intrauterine CMV, rubella, and herpes simplex infections are frequently positive. Other infections, such as varicella and toxoplasmosis, are difficult to culture after intrauterine infections and usually require serological confirmation of the diagnosis. An elevated titer of immunoglobulin M (IgM) antibodies in a neonate suggests an intrauterine infection since maternal IgM antibodies are too large to cross the blood–placental barrier. An elevated titer of IgG antibodies is less specific since maternal IgG antibodies cross the blood–placental barrier; however, a higher IgG antibody titer in a neonate than in the mother is suggestive of an intrauterine infection.

RUBELLA

In 1941, congenital cataracts occurred in 78 children following a rubella epidemic in Australia. Most had white central opacities with a clear peripheral zone. In 68 instances, the mothers had had symptomatic rubella infections while pregnant with the affected children. In addition, many of these children had microphthalmos, growth retardation, and congenital heart defects. The congenital rubella syndrome has since been expanded to include sensorineural hearing loss, mental retardation, hepatosplenomegaly, thrombocytopenic purpura, microcephaly, osteopathy, lymphadenopathy, diabetes, abnormal dermatoglyphics, a retinal pigmentary

disturbance, glaucoma, and keratitis.[3,4] Computed tomography (CT) may show low-density areas and flecks of calcification of the white matter, and calcification in the basal ganglia.

The prevalence of these abnormalities correlates closely with the gestational stage during which the rubella infection occurs. Intrauterine infections during the first 3 months of pregnancy result in a 50% incidence of the rubella embryopathy, whereas infections after the fourth gestational month rarely result in the full rubella syndrome.

Cataracts are present in 20–30% of children with the congenital rubella syndrome.[5] They are bilateral 75% of the time and conform closely to Gregg's original description. The rubella virus has been cultured from the cataractous lenses of children with the congenital rubella syndrome up to 4 years of age and is probably responsible for the intense inflammatory response that may occur after cataract surgery.[6]

The most common ocular abnormality of the congenital rubella syndrome is a pigmentary retinopathy (Fig. 18.1). It is usually bilateral and is present in 40% of affected patients. The retinopathy is characterized by mottled pigmentary changes throughout the fundi, which are most marked in the posterior pole. Although progression of the pigmentary changes may occur, the vision typically remains 6/12 or better.[7] Rarely subretinal neovascularization may occur with a precipitous fall in the visual acuity. The electro-oculogram and electroretinogram are usually normal, indicating that the function of the retinal pigment epithelium and retina are not affected by the pigment mottling.[8] A disturbance of iris pigmentation is also common (Fig. 18.2) and may be associated with glaucoma.

The corneas of infants with the rubella syndrome may be hazy (Fig. 18.3), secondary either to a keratitis (Fig. 18.4) or less commonly to an elevation of the intraocular pressure. The keratitis typically clears in weeks or a few months. Glaucoma is found most frequently in eyes with iris hypoplasia and microphthalmos. It occurs in approximately 10% of children with the congenital rubella syndrome.[9] Severe anterior segment damage may result from the combination of keratitis, glaucoma, and cataract. There are now sixty-year follow-up data on some of Gregg's original cohort. It is noteworthy that 41% of these now have negative rubella titers. The data also suggest that HLA-A1 and HLA-B8 may be risk factors for developing the rubella embryopathy syndrome.[10]

The development of an attenuated rubella virus vaccine and its subsequent widespread usage beginning in 1969 has dramatically decreased the incidence of the congenital rubella syndrome in the developed world.[11] Whereas 30,000 children were estimated to have been born with the congenital rubella syndrome during the rubella epidemic of 1964 in the USA, the condition is now rare there. However, rubella continues to be an important cause of congenital cataracts in developing countries where vaccination

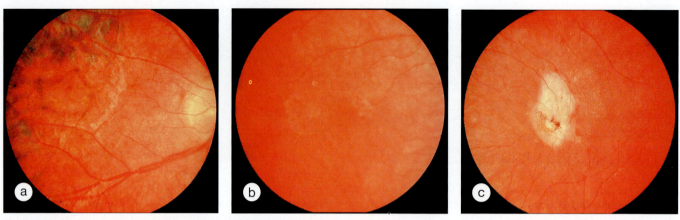

Fig. 18.1 Congenital rubella retinopathy. (a) There are diffuse retinal pigment epithelial changes most marked at the posterior pole. The acuity is 6/12. (b) Subtle RPE changes in rubella retinopathy. (c) Macular neovascular membrane.

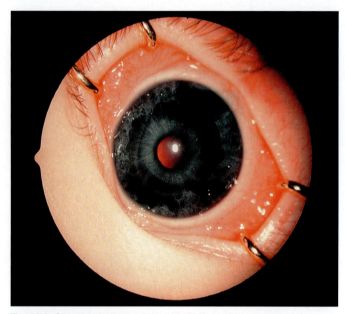

Fig. 18.2 Congenital rubella with mottled iris atrophy.

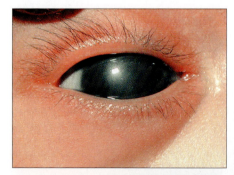

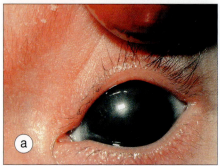

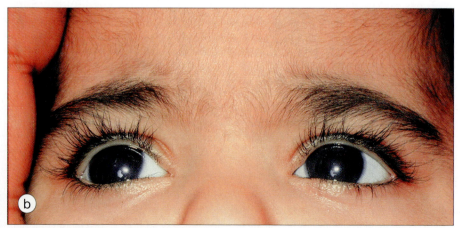

Fig. 18.3 (a) Neonate with congenital rubella with hazy large appearing corneas. The intraocular pressure was normal. (b) Same patient aged 3 years. The intraocular pressure has not been raised at any of the subsequent examinations. The corneas had cleared by 3 months of age.

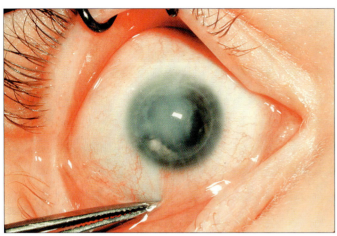

Fig. 18.4 Congenital rubella with microphthalmos, cataract, iris damage, glaucoma, and corneal scarring: it had had a corneal graft and had navigation vision.

against the rubella virus is not routinely followed.[12] Moreover, even with improved surgical techniques for managing rubella cataracts the visual outcomes remain discouragingly poor.[13]

The rubella vaccine is a live attenuated vaccine but has no effect on the developing fetus. Analysis of the wild virus and the live attenuated vaccine virus suggest that there is a variable region in the gene coding for nonstructural protein NSP-1 that may be the molecular basis of rubella embryopathy.[14] There is no compelling evidence that the rubella vaccine is a contributing factor in the development of autism.[15]

TOXOPLASMOSIS

Intrauterine toxoplasmosis was first recognized as a cause of chorioretinitis and intracranial calcification in 1939.[16] Chorioretinitis is the most frequently recognized feature of the congenital toxoplasmosis syndrome (Fig. 18.5). Other common findings include intracranial calcification, seizures, hydrocephalus, microcephaly, hepatosplenomegaly, jaundice, anemia, and fever. In the USA, it has been estimated to have an incidence ranging from 1 in 1000 live births to 1 in 10,000 live births.[17] Only 10–15% of the offspring of women who become infected with toxoplasmosis during the first trimester demonstrate serological evidence of intrauterine disease. However, these children typically have the most severe manifestations of the syndrome. Rare cases of congenital toxoplasmosis where the mother was infected years before the pregnancy but maintained persistent IgG antibodies have been reported.[18] A higher percentage of fetuses infected during the later stages of gestation are seropositive for toxoplasmosis, but usually have minimal if any abnormalities.[19] However, it is now recognized that some of these infants who are apparently normal on initial examination develop chorioretinitis, blindness, hydrocephalus, mental retardation, and deafness later in childhood.[20] The importance of the placenta in transmitting the infection to the fetus is evident from studies of monozygotic and dizygotic twins.[21]

Toxoplasmosis is acquired from eating undercooked meat or exposure to cat feces. Marked regional differences occur in the prevalence of seropositivity to toxoplasmosis presumably due to differing dietary and living customs. For example, 54% of pregnant women in France are seropositive to toxoplasmosis[22] versus only 30% of the U.S. population.[23] Women of childbearing years emigrating from an area of low immunity to a region of high immunity are at the greatest risk of contracting toxoplasmosis.

Ocular manifestations of congenital toxoplasmosis include chorioretinitis (Fig. 18.5), microphthalmos, cataracts, panuveitis, and optic atrophy. The chorioretinal scarring is usually heavily pigmented and associated with areas of chorioretinal atrophy. A large prospective study demonstrated a 30% incidence of chorioretinal scarring in infants with congenital toxoplasmosis;[24] in severe disease, it may approach 100%.[25] The chorioretinal scarring is usually bilateral and frequently involves the macula. Chorioretinitis is progressive with the incidence increasing in one study from 11% at 1 year of age to 23% by 7 years of age.[26]

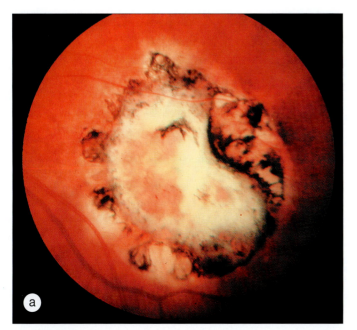

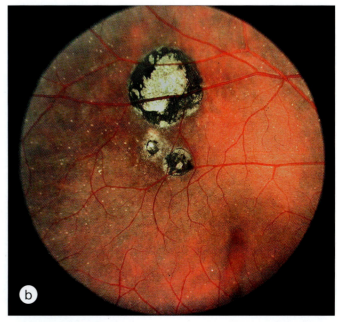

Fig. 18.5 (a) Raised congenital toxoplasmosis macular scar. (b) Paramacular congenital toxoplasmosis scar.

Toxoplasmosis acquired after birth only rarely results in chorioretinitis. Recently vasoproliferative tumors of the sensory retina have been identified to occur on the edge of presumed congenital toxoplasmosis chorioretinal scars.[27]

It is recommended that all neonates with serological evidence of an intrauterine toxoplasmosis infection, whether or not they have signs of active infection, be treated with a 1-year course of pyrimethamine and sulfadiazine with the concurrent administration of folic acid to reduce the hemotoxicity of pyrimethamine.[28] A reduction in the incidence of adverse neurological sequelae has been reported in children treated with this drug regimen; however, 80% of these children still developed chorioretinitis. Similarly, prenatal treatment has not been shown to alter the incidence of chorioretinitis.[29]

Women seronegative to toxoplasmosis should not eat undercooked meat and should minimize their exposure to cats during pregnancy. Fruits and vegetables, which might be contaminated with toxoplasmosis oocytes, should be washed carefully before being eaten. If a pregnant woman is found to have a primary toxoplasmosis infection, treatment with spiramycin may mitigate the severity of the disease in her offspring.

CYTOMEGALOVIRUS

A congenital CMV infection is the most common intrauterine infection occurring in 1% of all newborns in the United States; however, only 10% of children with congenital CMV are symptomatic as newborns.[30] Intrauterine CMV infections damage the fetus as a consequence of tissue necrosis, although recent evidence from a mouse model suggests that mesenchymal cells may be specifically targeted and may lead to disruption of organogenesis.[31] Infections early in gestation are probably more embryopathic, although it is often difficult to determine the gestational age at which the infection occurred. Abnormalities associated with congenital CMV infections include jaundice, hepatosplenomegaly, microcephaly, sensorineural hearing ion, psychomotor retardation, cerebral calcifications (Fig. 18.6), malformations of cortical development, a petechial rash, keratitis (Fig. 18.7), optic atrophy, and chorioretinitis. Recent evidence suggests that congenital cytomegalovirus infection may be a significant cause of maldevelopment in otherwise unaffected children.[32]

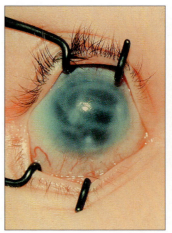
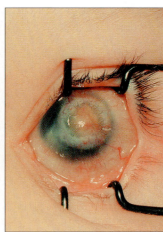

Fig. 18.7 Congenital CMV with bilateral keratopathy and glaucoma.

Ocular manifestations of congenital CMV are not common, but include chorioretinitis, microphthalmos, cataracts, keratitis (Fig. 18.7), and optic atrophy.[33] Congenital CMV infections result in chorioretinal scarring in 6% of infants after a primary maternal CMV infection and 2% of infants after a recurrent maternal CMV infection.[34] Congenital CMV chorioretinal scars are usually less heavily pigmented than those associated with congenital toxoplasmosis.

The diagnosis of congenital CMV should be suspected in neonates with hepatosplenomegaly, jaundice, petechiae or thrombocytopenia, cerebral calcification, chorioretinitis, and microcephaly. The diagnosis should be confirmed by viral isolation since these findings occur in association with many other congenital infections. The virus can usually be cultured from the urine and saliva for many months after birth. Culturing CMV from an infant during the first 3 weeks of life is usually proof of a congenital infection. Most maternal CMV infections are believed to be acquired from younger children in a family or a daycare setting rather than from casual contacts in the community.[35] Postnatal therapy with ganciclovir may reduce the severity of sensorineural hearing loss but it has only a minimal effect on neurodevelopmental outcomes. Ganciclovir has not been shown to alter the time to resolution of CMV retinitis in infants with congenital CMV.[36]

HERPES SIMPLEX

Herpes simplex infections most commonly occur in neonates delivered to mothers with active genital herpes simplex infections. This may be related to infection with herpes simplex virus HSV-1 primarily manifesting as a labialis or HSV-2 causing a vulvovaginitis.[37] The risk of neonates becoming infected is much higher after primary genital herpes infection than from recurrent infections. Although most infants are infected during parturition, a small percentage are infected secondary to an infection ascending into the uterus after premature rupture of the amniotic membranes or postnatal inoculation. The herpes simplex HSV-2 is responsible for most neonatal infections.

Neonatal herpes simplex infections are often first detected as a cutaneous vesicular eruption. In 50% of infants, this then progresses to a systemic infection. Systemic involvement may result in hepatitis, pneumonia, disseminated intravascular coagulation, or encephalitis. Seventy percent of neonates with

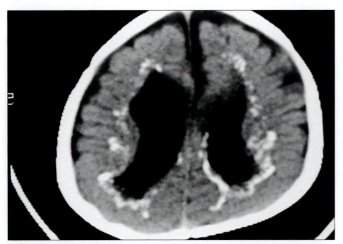

Fig. 18.6 Congenital CMV infection with periventricular calcification, hydrocephalus, and cerebral atrophy shown on this CT scan.

disseminated infections have involvement of both the viscera and the central nervous system.

Ocular involvement most commonly consists of blepharo-conjunctivitis with vesicles on the eyelids or a keratitis with epithelial dendrites. Chorioretinitis with an accompanying vitritis and optic atrophy may also occur, particularly in infants with central nervous system involvement. The chorioretinitis typically involves the peripheral retina and results in well-circumscribed hyperpigmented scars. A recrudescence of the herpes virus in these scars later in life can result in acute retinal necrosis.[38] On rare occasions a fulminant retinitis that involves the entire retina may develop during infancy. Cataracts may also form secondary to the accompanying uveitis. In addition, cortical visual impairment is a common sequela after herpes simplex encephalitis. Rarely, hematogenous transplacental spread of the virus rather than infection within the birth canal occurs. This has been associated with persistence of fetal vasculature in the affected infant.[39]

A disseminated neonatal herpes simplex infection is associated with a high mortality rate. In addition, a high percentage of children surviving herpes simplex encephalitis are neurologically handicapped. Because of the risk of dissemination, all neonates less than 1 month of age with a herpes simplex infection, even if it is initially limited to cutaneous or ocular involvement, should be treated with systemic acyclovir. Herpetic keratitis should be treated with either acyclovir ointment or trifluorothymidine solution topically. Herpes simplex blepharoconjunctivitis should also be treated with topical antiviral therapy as prophylaxis against the development of keratitis.

The diagnosis of a herpes simplex infection should be considered in infants with progressive icterus, fever, hepatosplenomegaly, and cutaneous vesicular lesions. The isolation of herpes simplex virus from fresh vesicles or from corneal scrapings confirms the diagnosis.

SYPHILIS

Congenital syphilis only occurs in fetuses exposed to *Treponema pallidum* after the 16th gestational week. Virtually all of the offspring of women with primary syphilis acquired after the 16th gestational week have congenital syphilis, whereas the incidence decreases to 90% with secondary syphilis and 30% with latent syphilis. Syphilis infections acquired at an earlier gestational age frequently result in fetal death.

Congenital syphilis is associated with early manifestations occurring during infancy secondary to an active infection or late manifestations occurring later in childhood secondary to ongoing inflammation or a hypersensitivity reaction. Early manifestations include skeletal abnormalities, rhinitis, a maculopapular rash, fissures around the lips, nares, and anus, hepatosplenomegaly, anemia, and uveitis. Late manifestations include sensorineural hearing loss, bone changes, dental abnormalities, and interstitial keratitis. The finding of interstitial keratitis, deafness, and malformed incisors is known as Hutchinson's triad.

Ocular manifestations of congenital syphilis include chorio-retinitis, interstitial keratitis, anterior uveitis, iridoschisis, and optic atrophy. Interstitial keratitis occurs in 10–40% of children with untreated congenital syphilis.[40] It most commonly occurs in individuals of 5–20 years of age. It is characterized by either sectorial or diffuse corneal edema infiltrated by interstitial vessels. Visual loss occurs secondary to corneal scarring and residual ghost vessels. It is bilateral in 80% of affected children and usually accompanied by an iridocyclitis and iris atrophy. It occurs secondary to a hypersensitivity reaction and responds to topical

corticosteroids. The chorioretinitis occurring with congenital syphilis most commonly results in peripheral areas of pigment mottling, but in severe cases may result in extensive pigmentary changes resembling retinitis pigmentosa. This form of syphilitic chorioretinitis is sometimes referred to as pseudoretinitis pigmentosa.

Congenital syphilis predominantly occurs in the offspring of young, unmarried women with poor antenatal care. Improved antenatal care, community surveillance of known cases of syphilis, and follow-up after treatment could prevent many cases of congenital syphilis.[41,42]

The diagnosis of congenital syphilis may be difficult to establish in neonates since few have symptoms of the disease and serological tests may initially be negative. A quantitative rapid plasma reagin (RPR) or venereal disease reference laboratory (VDRL) result higher in an infant than in the mother is highly suggestive of congenital disease. Occasionally dark-field microscopy or a direct fluorescent antibody test of a scraping from a fresh lesion will reveal *T. pallidum*, which is very sensitive to penicillin. A 10-day course of intravenous penicillin is usually adequate to treat congenital syphilis; however, a more protracted course of treatment is occasionally necessary. Serologies should be repeated after a course of penicillin to ensure that the treatment was adequate.

VARICELLA

In 1947, a child was reported with multiple birth defects following an intrauterine varicella infection.[43] The abnormalities included a hypotrophic limb, low birth weight for gestational age, seizures, cortical atrophy, and cicatricial skin lesions. Subsequent reports have confirmed these findings and expanded the congenital varicella syndrome to include chorioretinitis, cataracts, microphthalmos, Horner syndrome, and neuropathic bladder. Unlike the rubella syndrome, which occurs almost exclusively after first trimester infections, the congenital varicella syndrome frequently occurs after second, and even third, trimester infections. Several pro-spective studies have shown that the risk of the varicella embryopathy developing after a maternal varicella infection during the first trimester is 0.4–2%.[44] In some instances, the congenital varicella syndrome may be overlooked since the clinical findings may be subtle and nonspecific. Attempts to culture the varicella virus from congenitally infected neonates have been unsuccessful.

Chorioretinitis (Fig. 18.8) is the most common ocular mani-festation of the syndrome. It closely resembles toxoplasmosis chorioretinitis with either single or multiple deeply pigmented chorioretinal scars and atrophy.[45] It may be unilateral or bilateral. In some instances the chorioretinal scarring may be so severe as to result in tractional retinal detachments.

Mature cataracts in microphthalmic eyes (Fig. 18.9) may also occur with the congenital varicella syndrome. The associated chorioretinal disease often limits the visual potential of these eyes even if the cataracts are extracted.

A unilateral Horner syndrome also occasionally occurs with the congenital varicella syndrome (Fig. 18.10).

Varicella infections usually occur during childhood and confer life-long immunity. However, 5–16% of women of childbearing years are seronegative to varicella.[46] An estimated 0.7 cases of primary varicella infections occur per 1,000 pregnancies. Severe infection during pregnancy has led to pneumonitis and even death.

Although the risks to the fetus of acquiring the congenital varicella syndrome are small, because the associated malformations may be so severe it has been recommended that pregnant women

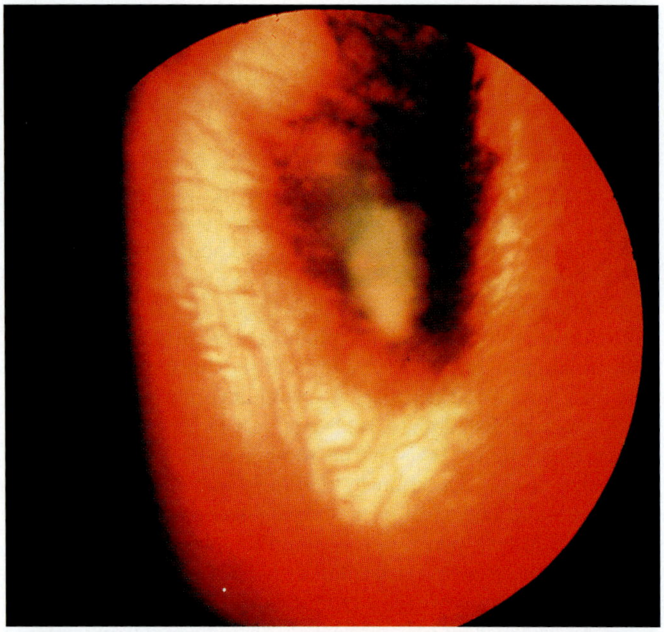

Fig. 18.8 Chorioretinal scar in a child with congenital varicella syndrome.

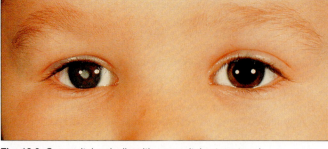

Fig. 18.9 Congenital varicella with congenital cataract and microphthalmos.

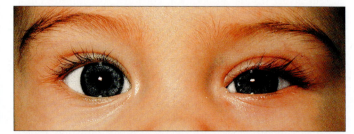

Fig. 18.10 Congenital varicella with Horner syndrome in the left eye.

exposed to varicella who are seronegative should promptly receive an injection of Zoster immunoglobulin. Although this does not prevent an infection from developing, it may attenuate the severity of the infection.[47]

LYMPHOCYTIC CHORIOMENINGITIS VIRUS

Lymphocytic choriomeningitis virus (LCMV) was first recognized as an intrauterine infection in 1955. The most common manifestations of this intrauterine infection include hydrocephalus, periventricular calcification, microcephaly, and chorioretinitis.[48] Humans are believed to acquire the infection from exposure to the urine, feces, or saliva of LCMV-infected feral mice or hamsters. In some locales, up to 10% of feral mice are infected with LCMV.

Ocular manifestations of a congenital LCMV infection include chorioretinitis and optic atrophy.[49] The chorioretinitis is most commonly present in the periphery, but it can also occur in the macula. LCMV chorioretinal scars can be indistinguishable from those of congenital toxoplasmosis.[50]

The diagnosis of a congenital LCMV infection can be established through serological testing of the mother and infant. Since antibodies to LCMV are uncommon in the general population (0.3–5%), seropositivity in the mother and infant are highly suggestive of the disease. Although ribavirin has been shown to be effective in the management of other arenavirus infections, its efficacy with congenital LCMV has not been established. No vaccine exists to prevent LCMV infections. Women can reduce their risk of contracting LCMV during pregnancy by minimizing their exposure to rodents. Up to 40% of women with infants with intrauterine-acquired LCMV infections have had a known exposure to rodents during their pregnancy.

REFERENCES

1. Embil JA, Ozene RL, Haldone EV. Congenital CMV infection in two siblings from consecutive pregnancies. J Pediatr 1970; 77: 417–21.
2. Stagno S, Pass RF, Cloud G, et al. Primary cytomegalovirus infection in pregnancy: incidence, transmission to foetus, and clinical outcome. J Am Med Assoc 1986; 256: 1904–8.
3. Alfano JE. Ocular aspects of the maternal rubella syndrome. Trans Am Acad Ophthalmol Otolaryng 1966; 70: 235–66
4. Wolff SM. The ocular manifestations of congenital rubella. Trans Am Ophthalmol Soc 1972; 70: 577–614.
5. Givens KT, Lee DA, Jones T, Ilstrup DM. Congenital rubella syndrome: ophthalmic manifestations and associated systemic disorders. Br J Ophthalmol 1993; 77: 358–63.
6. Cotlier E, Fox J, Smith M. Rubella virus in the cataractous lens of congenital rubella syndrome. Am J Ophthalmol 1966; 62: 233–6.
7. Collis WJ, Cohen DN. Rubella retinopathy. A progressive disorder. Arch Ophthalmol 1970; 84: 33–5.
8. Krill AE. The retinal disease of rubella. Arch Ophthalmol 1967; 77: 445–9.
9. Sears ML. Congenital glaucoma in neonatal rubella. Br J Ophthalmol 1967; 51: 744–8.
10. Forrest JM, Turnbull FM, Sholler GF, et al. Gregg's congenital rubella patients sixty years later. Med J Austral 2002; 177: 664–7.
11. Krugman S, editor. International conference on rubella immunization. Am J Dis Child 1969; 118: 1–410.
12. Eckstein M, Vijayalakshmi P, Killeder M, et al. Etiology of childhood cataract in South India. Br J Ophthalmol 1996; 80: 628–32.
13. Vijayalakshmi P, Srivastava KK, Poornima B. Visual outcome of cataract surgery in children with congenital rubella syndrome. J AAPOS 2003; 7: 91–5.
14. Hofmann J, Renz M, Meyer S, et al. Phylogenetic analysis of rubella virus including new genotype I isolates. Virus Res 2003; 96: 123–8.
15. Miller E. Measles-mumps-rubella vaccine and the development of autism. Seminar Pediatr Infect Dis 2003; 14: 199–206.
16. Wolf A, Cowen D, Paige BH. Toxoplasmosis encephalomyelitis. III. A new case of granulomatous encephalomyelitis due to a protozoan. Am J Pathol 1939; 15: 657–94.
17. Remington JS, Desmonts G. Toxoplasmosis. In: Remington JS, Klein JO, editors. Infectious Diseases of the Fetus and Newborn Infants. 3rd ed. Philadelphia: WB Saunders; 1990: 89–195.

18. Silveira C, Ferreira R, Muccioli C, et al. Toxoplasmosis transmitted to a newborn from the mother infected twenty years earlier. Am J Ophthalmol 2003; 136: 370–1.

19. Desmonts G, Couvreur J. Congenital toxoplasmosis: a prospective study of 378 pregnancies. N Engl J Med 1974; 290(2): 1110–16.

20. Koppe JG, Loewer-Sieger DH, Roever-Bonnet H. Results of 20-year follow-up of congenital toxoplasmosis. Lancet 1986; 1: 254–6.

21. Peyron F, Ateba AB, Wallon M, et al. Congenital toxoplasmosis in twins. Pediatr Infect Dis 2003; 22: 695–701.

22. Ancelle T, Goulet V, Tirard-Fleury V, et al. La toxoplasmose chez la femme enceinte en France en 1995. Résultats d'une enquête nationale périnatale. Bulletin Epidemiologique Hebdomadaire 1996; 51: 227–9.

23. Grant A. Varicella infection and toxoplasmosis in pregnancy. J Perinatal Neonatal Nursing 1996; 10: 17–29.

24. Guerina NG, Hsu HW, Meissner HC, et al. Neonatal serologic screening and early treatment for congenital *Toxoplasma gondii* infection. N Engl J Med 1994; 330: 1858–63.

25. Meenken C, Assies J, van Nieuwenhuizen O, et al. Long-term ocular and neurological involvement in severe congenital toxoplasmosis. Br J Ophthalmol 1995; 79: 581–4.

26. Gras L, Gilbert RE, Ades AE, Dunn DT. Effect of prenatal treatment on the risk of intracranial and ocular lesions in children with congenital toxoplasmosis. Int J Epidemiol 2001; 30: 1309–13.

27. Lafaut BA, Meire FM, Leys AM, et al. Vasoproliferative retinal tumors associated with chorioretinal scars in presumed congenital toxoplasmosis. Graefes Arch Clin Exp Ophthalmol 1999; 237: 1033–8.

28. McAuley J, Boyer KM, Patel D, et al. Early and longitudinal evaluations of treated infants and children and untreated historical patients with congenital toxoplasmosis: the Chicago Collaborative Treatment Trial. Clin Infect Dis 1994; 18: 38–72.

29. Brézin AP, Thulliez P, Couvreur J, et al. Ophthalmic outcomes after prenatal and postnatal treatment of congenital toxoplasmosis. Am J Ophthalmol 2003; 135: 779–84.

30. Fowler KB, Stagno S, Pass RF. Maternal immunity and prevention of congenital cytomegalovirus infection. JAMA 2003; 289: 1008–11.

31. Tsutsui Y, Kashiwai A, Kawamura N, Kadota C. Microphthalmia and cerebral atrophy induced in mouse embryos by infection with murine cytomegalovirus in midgestation. Am J Pathol 1993; 143: 804–13.

32. Zucca C, Binda S, Borgatti R, et al. Retrospective diagnosis of congenital cytomegalovirus infection and cortical maldevelopment. Neurology 2003; 61: 710–2.

33. Coats DK, Demmler GJ, Paysse EA, et al. and the Congenital CMV Longitudinal Study Group. Ophthalmologic findings in children with congenital cytomegalovirus infection. J AAPOS 2000; 4: 110–16.

34. Fowler KB, Stagno S, Pass RF, et al. The outcome of congenital cytomegalovirus infection in relation to maternal antibody status. N Engl J Med 1992; 326: 663–7.

35. Pass RF, Little A, Stagno S, et al. Young children as a probable source of maternal and congenital cytomegalovirus infection. N Engl J Med 1987; 316: 1366–70.

36. Noffke AS, Mets MB. Spontaneous resolution of cytomegalovirus retinitis in an infant with congenital cytomegalovirus infection. Retina 2001; 21: 541–2.

37. Riley LE. Herpes simplex virus. Semin Perinatol 1998; 22: 284–92.

38. Thompson WS, Culbertson WW, Smiddy WE, et al. Acute retinal necrosis caused by reactivation of herpes simplex virus type 2. Am J Ophthalmol 1994; 118: 205–11.

39. Corey RP, Flynn JT. Maternal intrauterine herpes simplex virus infection leading to persistent fetal vasculature. Arch Ophthalmol 2000; 118: 837–40.

40. Ruusuvaara P, Setala K, Kivela T. Syphilitic interstitial keratitis with bilateral funnel-shaped iridiocorneal adhesions. Eur J Ophthalmol 1996; 6: 6–10.

41. Carey JC. Congenital syphilis in the twenty first century. Curr Womens Health Rep 2003; 3: 299–302.

42. Tikhonova L, Salakhov E, Southwick K. Congenital syphilis in the Russian Federation. Sex Transm Infect 2003; 79: 106–10.

43. Laforet EG, Lynch CL. Multiple congenital defects following maternal varicella. Report of a case. N Engl J Med 1947; 236: 534–7.

44. Harger JH, Ernest JM, Thurnau GR, et al. Frequency of congenital varicilla syndrome in a prospective cohort of 347 pregnant women. Obstet Gynecol 2002; 100: 260–5.

45. Lambert SR, Taylor D, Kriss A, et al. Ocular manifestations of the congenital varicella syndrome. Arch Ophthalmol 1989; 107: 52–6.

46. Gershon AA, Raker R, Steinberg S, et al. Antibody to varicella zoster virus in parturient women and their offspring during the first year of life. Pediatrics 1976; 58: 692–6.

47. McIntosh D, Isaacs D. Varicella zoster virus infection in pregnancy. Arch Dis Child 1993; 68: 1–20.

48. Barton LL, Mets MB. Congenital lymphocytic choriomeningitis virus infection: decade of rediscovery. Clin Infect Dis 2001; 33: 370–4.

49. Mets MB, Barton LL, Khan AS, Ksiazek TG. Lymphocytic chorio-meningitis virus: an underdiagnosed cause of congenital chorioretinitis. Am J Ophthalmol 2000; 130: 209–15.

50. Brézin AP, Thulliez P, Cisneros B, et al. Lymphocytic choriomeningitis virus chorioretinitis mimicking ocular toxoplasmosis in two otherwise normal children. Am J Ophthalmol 2000; 130: 245–7.

CHAPTER
19

Conjunctivitis of the Newborn (Ophthalmia Neonatorum)

Scott R Lambert

Conjunctivitis of the newborn is the term used by the World Health Organization to describe conjunctivitis during the neonatal period. Previously it was referred to as ophthalmia neonatorum. It was originally described in 1750 and is one of the most common infections occurring during the first month of life. Its incidence has been reported to be as high as 7–19% of all newborns.[1,2] See also Chapters P2 and P3.

The period of time after birth until the onset of neonatal conjunctivitis is quite variable and may be helpful in suggesting the causative agent. Conjunctivitis during the first few days of life commonly occurs as a toxic effect of topically administered silver nitrate at the time of birth. Gonococcal conjunctivitis usually develops 1 to 3 days after birth, chlamydial conjunctivitis 5 to 25 days after birth. Prophylactic treatment with erythromycin may prolong the interval until chlamydial conjunctivitis is detected. Chlamydial conjunctivitis was not detected in infants who had received erythromycin prophylaxis until 9–45 days after birth, whereas infants who received silver nitrate prophylaxis presented with chlamydial conjunctivitis 6–26 days after birth.[3] Conjunctivitis caused by other bacterial pathogens may occur at any time during the first month of life.

The pathogens for neonatal conjunctivitis vary geographically due to differences in the prevalence of maternal infections and the use of prophylactic antibiotics or silver nitrate. In a large hospital in Nairobi, Kenya where 6% of all pregnant women had cervical gonococcal cervicitis, 3% of all newborns had gonococcal conjunctivitis.[4] In contrast, gonococcal conjunctivitis is rare in neonates in the USA, with prevalences as low as 0.4%.

LABORATORY STUDIES

Because of the difficulty in distinguishing between the various types of neonatal conjunctivitis by clinical characteristics alone, laboratory studies are paramount in establishing the correct diagnosis and selecting the best treatment. A Gram stain should be performed on a conjunctival scraping from the palpebral conjunctiva of all infants with conjunctivitis. If Gram-negative diplococci are present in polymorphonuclear leucocytes, the child should be treated for presumed gonococcal conjunctivitis. The identification of Gram-negative coccobacilli on a Gram stain of the conjunctiva correlated with the isolation of *Haemophilus* species but Gram-positive cocci did not correlate with positive cultures of *Staphylococcus aureus*, enterococci, or *Streptococcus pneumoniae*.[5] White blood cells are also more frequent on the Gram stain of infants with conjunctivitis than on that of controls.

McCoy cell culture has been the standard for diagnosing *Chlamydia* conjunctivitis in the past. Although the specificity of this technique is 100%, the sensitivity varies between 65 and 85%, and several days are needed before the culture results are available. Polymerase chain reaction (PCR) analysis achieves a comparable specificity, with a higher sensitivity. Talley et al.[6] compared PCR tests with McCoy cell cultures and found that only two of seven (28%) patients with positive PCR had positive McCoy cell cultures, suggesting a much higher sensitivity for PCR analysis. They also emphasized the fact that the diagnosis could be established more quickly with the PCR analysis, which allowed earlier treatment.

A Giemsa stain may be helpful in identifying intracytoplasmic inclusion bodies in infants with chlamydial conjunctivitis. Unlike adults with chlamydial conjunctivitis, intracytoplasmic inclusion bodies may be seen in 60–80% of all infants with chlamydial conjunctivitis.

GONOCOCCAL CONJUNCTIVITIS

Gonococcal conjunctivitis in newborns is common in developing countries. However, because of its propensity to produce a severe keratitis, a gonococcal infection should be excluded in all children with neonatal conjunctivitis by Gram staining and culturing a conjunctival scraping. *Neisseria gonorrhoeae* isolates are resistant to penicillin in many urban areas in the USA and many other parts of the world (50–60% in certain areas of Africa). For this reason, infants with gonococcal conjunctivitis should be treated with a third-generation cephalosporin for 7 days in areas where penicillinase-producing strains of *N. gonorrhoeae* are endemic (1% or more of isolates). Irrigation of the eyes with saline at least hourly until the accompanying ocular discharge is eliminated is also recommended. Newborn infants whose mothers are known to have a gonococcal infection at the time of delivery should receive a single dose of ceftriaxone (25–50 mg/kg) soon after birth, in addition to ocular prophylaxis. A concurrent infection with *Chlamydia trachomatis* should be considered in neonates who do not respond.

CHLAMYDIAL CONJUNCTIVITIS

Chlamydia trachomatis is one of the most commonly isolated pathogens in infants with neonatal conjunctivitis in industrialized countries, with a prevalence of three to four per 1000 live births. It usually begins in one eye but often becomes bilateral (Fig. 19.1). Because chlamydial conjunctivitis may also be associated with a neonatal pneumonitis, it is important that the correct diagnosis be promptly established.[7] The pneumonitis generally develops during the first 6 weeks of life and is associated with a nasal discharge, cough, and tachypnea. The recommended treatment for infants with chlamydial conjunctivitis is a 14-day course of oral erythromycin syrup (50 mg/kg per day) in four divided

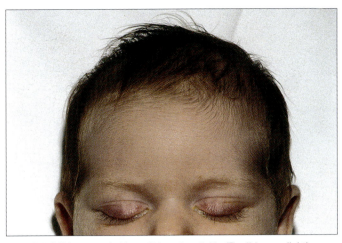

Fig. 19.1 Mild neonatal chlamydial conjunctivitis. The lids are slightly swollen and there is a discharge.

doses.[8] Oral erythromycin not only treats chlamydial pneumonitis and eradicates nasopharyngeal carriage of *Chlamydia*, but it is also more effective than topical erythromycin in preventing a relapse of chlamydial conjunctivitis. However, chlamydial conjunctivitis may recur even after a course of oral erythromycin, possibly due to poor compliance with antibiotic therapy, an inadequate dose of antibiotics, or a reinfection. A second course of oral erythromycin should be given when a recurrence occurs. Adjuvant therapy with topical erythromycin or tetracycline may also be beneficial. In addition, parents of infected children should be treated with oral tetracycline or erythromycin for 2 weeks. If possible, pregnant women with chlamydial cervicitis should be treated before delivery of their child with oral erythromycin. Untreated chlamydial conjunctivitis usually resolves spontaneously after 8–12 months but may result in the formation of a micropannus and scarring of the tarsal conjunctiva. In addition, children with untreated chlamydial conjunctivitis are at increased risk of developing a pneumonitis or otitis.[9]

NONGONOCOCCAL, NONCHLAMYDIAL CONJUNCTIVITIS

The most common pathogen isolated from neonates with conjunctivitis in most studies is *S. aureus*.[2,10] Other Gram-positive organisms including *Staphylococcus epidermidis*, *Streptococcus viridans*, and *S. pneumoniae* can also frequently be cultured from newborns with conjunctivitis. Gram-negative organisms such as enterococcus, *Escherichia coli*, *Serratia* spp., and *Pseudomonas* spp. account for a smaller percentage of cases.[11] Conjunctival cultures are negative in up to 25% of children with neonatal conjunctivitis. Broad-spectrum antibiotics should be administered to infants with severe conjunctivitis until culture results have identified the pathogen and its antibiotic sensitivity. Infants with mild to moderate conjunctivitis may be treated with lid hygiene alone until a microbe has been isolated. Lid hygiene alone may be sufficient for infants with negative conjunctival cultures.

CONGENITAL DACRYOSTENOSIS

A congenital nasolacrimal duct obstruction (see Chapter 31) is also frequently associated with neonatal conjunctivitis. Dacryostenosis should be suspected in children with unilateral conjunctivitis and epiphora who have a reflux of mucopurulent material from the lacrimal puncta after massaging the lacrimal sac. Dacryocystitis in infants with congenital dacryostenosis is usually caused by *Haemophilus* spp. and *S. pneumoniae*.[5] Congenital dacryostenosis should be treated initially with topical antibiotics and massaging of the lacrimal sac to increase the hydrostatic pressure in the lacrimal sac.[12] If the dacryostenosis fails to resolve spontaneously by 6–12 months of age, the nasolacrimal system should be probed. A dacryocystocele is an enlargement of the lacrimal sac secondary to a distal and proximal obstruction of the nasolacrimal system. Although mucinous material may be expressed from the lacrimal sac by massaging a dacryocystocele, the lacrimal sac rapidly fills again, presumably due to the ball-valve effect of the proximal obstruction.

VIRAL CONJUNCTIVITIS

Viral conjunctivitis occurs infrequently in neonates. Herpes simplex conjunctivitis can develop in neonates exposed to a maternal herpes infection at the time of birth. Vesicles may be present on the eyelids or on other parts of the body. Herpetic keratitis may also develop. The diagnosis can be confirmed by culturing the fluid in a vesicle. Neonates with a suspected herpes simplex infection should be treated with systemic acyclovir to reduce the risk of a disseminated infection developing.

PROPHYLAXIS

Crédé[13] introduced 2% silver nitrate as a prophylactic treatment for conjunctivitis in newborns in Leipzig in 1881. The widespread use of silver nitrate prophylaxis was subsequently associated with a dramatic decline in the incidence of gonococcal conjunctivitis in newborns throughout Europe and the USA. Topical erythromycin and tetracycline are also now used for ocular prophylaxis in newborns. All are considered to be quite effective in preventing gonococcal conjunctivitis,[14] but less effective as a prophylactic treatment for chlamydial conjunctivitis. Bell et al.[15] randomized 630 infants to silver nitrate, erythromycin, or no prophylaxis. Mild conjunctivitis developed in 17% of the infants. Although the incidence of conjunctivitis was slightly lower in the children receiving silver nitrate and erythromycin prophylaxis, the effect was modest and the conjunctivitis was caused in most cases by microorganisms of low virulence that were believed to be acquired postnatally. These findings suggest that most cases of neonatal conjunctivitis are caused by postnatally acquired pathogens. This helps to explain why the incidence of conjunctivitis in newborns is similar between infants born by caesarean section and those by vaginal delivery.

Povidone-iodine is less costly than silver nitrate or erythromycin and is equally efficacious as a prophylaxis for neonatal conjunctivitis.[16]

REFERENCES

1. Pierce JM, Ward ME, Seal DV. Ophthalmia neonatorum in the 1980s: incidence, aetiology and treatment. Br J Ophthalmol 1982; 66: 728–31.
2. Dannevig L, Straume B, Melby K. Ophthalmia neonatorum in northern Norway II. Microbiology with emphasis on Chlamydia trachomatis. Acta Ophthalmol 1992; 70: 19–25.
3. Bell TA, Sandstrom KI, Gravett MG, et al. Comparison of ophthalmic silver nitrate solution and erythromycin ointment for prevention of natally acquired Chlamydia trachomatis. Sex Trans Dis 1987; 14: 195–200.
4. Laga M, Naamara W, Brunham RC, et al. Single-dose therapy of gonococcal ophthalmia neonatorum with ceftriaxone. N Engl J Med 1986; 315: 1382–5.
5. Sandstrom KI, Bell TA, Chandler JW, et al. Microbial causes of neonatal conjunctivitis. J Pediatr 1984; 5: 706–11.
6. Talley AR, Garcia-Ferrer KF, Laycock KA, et al. Comparative diagnosis of neonatal chlamydial conjunctivitis by polymerase chain reaction and McCoy cell culture. Am J Ophthalmol 1994; 117: 50–7.
7. Harrison HR, Phil D, English MG, et al. Chlamydia trachomatis infant pneumonitis. Comparison with matched controls and other infant pneumonitis. N Engl J Med 1978; 298: 702–8.
8. Peter G. Red Book: Report of the Committee on Infectious Diseases. 20th ed. Elk Grove, IL: American Academy of Pediatrics; 1991.
9. Beem MO, Saxon EM. Respiratory tract colonization and a distinctive pneumonia syndrome in infants with Chlamydia trachomatis. N Engl J Med 1977; 296: 306–10.
10. Zanoni D, Isenberg SJ, Apt L. A comparison of silver nitrate with erythromycin for prophylaxis against ophthalmia neonatorum. Clin Pediatr 1992; 31: 295–8.
11. Sandstrom I. Treatment of neonatal conjunctivitis. Arch Ophthalmol 1987; 105: 925–8.
12. Crigler LW. The treatment of congenital dacrocystitis. JAMA 1923; 81: 23–4.
13. Crede CSF. Reports from the obstetrical clinic in Leipzig: prevention of eye inflammation in the newborn. Arch Gynaekol 1881; 17: 50–3.
14. Laga M, Plummer FA, Piot P, et al. Prophylaxis of gonococcal and chlamydial ophthalmia neonatorum. N Engl J Med 1988; 318: 653–7.
15. Bell TA, Grayson JT, Krohn MA, et al. Randomized trial of silver nitrate, erythromycin, and no eye prophylaxis for the prevention of conjunctivitis among newborns not at risk for gonococcal ophthalmitis. Pediatrics 1993; 92: 755–60.
16. Isenberg SJ, Apt L, Wood M. A controlled trial of Povidone-iodine as prophylaxis against ophthalmia neonatorum. N Engl J Med 1995; 2: 562–6.

CHAPTER
20 Preseptal and Orbital Cellulitis

Jimmy M Uddin

The initial diagnosis of infective preseptal and orbital cellulitis is clinical. The primary goal is to prevent rapid deterioration and serious sequelae such as visual loss, cavernous sinus thrombosis, cerebral abscess, osteomyelitis, and septicemia. It must be managed promptly with appropriate antibiotics and medical support within a multidisciplinary team consisting of pediatricians, ophthalmologists, ENT surgeons, nurses, and others. Regular evaluation is required, looking for progression of signs or deterioration of the clinical picture. Neuroimaging is necessary to determine the extent of the disease.

DEFINITION

Preseptal cellulitis is a descriptive, clinical, term applying to patients who present with signs of inflammation confined largely to the eyelids, these being redness, swelling, and pain. However, orbital cellulitis may present as preseptal cellulitis due to contiguous spread from the orbit or sinuses to preseptal tissues with few or subtle orbital signs. The presence of decreased or painful eye movements or proptosis, signs of optic neuropathy, or radiological evidence of orbital inflammation or collections signifies orbital cellulitis.

ANATOMY

The orbital septum marks the anterior extent of the orbit. It is firmly adherent at the orbital rim with the orbital periosteum (periorbita) as the arcus marginalis, and it extends to the upper and lower tarsal plates. *Preseptal* cellulitis occurs when the infection is anterior to the orbital septum, confined to the eyelids. The orbital septum acts as a physical barrier to lesions spreading posteriorly to the orbit (the postseptal space). *Orbital* cellulitis involves infection of the postseptal space and usually results from adjacent infected sinuses, commonly the ethmoids. Many vessels and nerves pierce the thin lamina papyracea between the ethmoid sinuses and the orbit: infection can easily spread through these and other naturally occurring perforations, to lift off the loosely attached periosteum within the anterior orbit, resulting in a subperiosteal abscess. An orbital abscess results from breach of the periosteum by infection or seeding into the orbit. Extension of infection from the ethmoids into the brain may result in meningitis and cerebral abscesses.

The drainage of the eyelids, sinuses, and orbits are largely by the orbital venous system, which empty into the cavernous sinus via the superior and inferior orbital veins. Since this system is devoid of valves, infection may spread in both preseptal and orbital cellulitis, leading to the serious sight- and life-threatening complication of cavernous sinus thrombosis.

CLASSIFICATION

Infective orbital cellulitis and its complications can be classified into five types:
1. Preseptal cellulitis;
2. Orbital cellulitis;
3. Subperiosteal abscess;
4. Orbital abscess; and
5. Cavernous sinus thrombosis.[1]

These types are not mutually exclusive and do not necessarily progress in that order. Uzcategui et al.[2] have updated this with additional computed tomography (CT) findings (Table 20.1).

Table 20.1 Classification of orbital cellulitis		
Stage	**Signs and symptoms**	**CT findings**
Preseptal cellulitis	Eyelid swelling, occasional fever	If performed, sinusitis may be present
Orbital cellulitis	Proptosis, decreased painful eye movements, chemosis	Sinusitis, mild soft tissue changes in the orbit
Subperiosteal abscess	Signs of orbital cellulitis, systemic involvement	Subperiosteal abscess, globe displacement, soft tissue changes in the orbit
Orbital abscess	Signs of orbital cellulitis, systemic involvement, ophthalmoplegia, visual loss	Orbital collection of pus with marked soft tissue changes of the fat and muscles
Intracranial complication	Signs of orbital or rarely preseptal cellulitis, marked proptosis, cranial nerve palsies (III, IV, V, VI)	Intracranial changes: cavernous sinus thrombosis, extradural abscess, meningitis, and osteomyelitis

Modified from Uzcategui N, Warman R, Smith A, et al. Clinical practice guidelines for the management of orbital cellulitis. J Pediatr Ophthalmol Strabismus 1998; 35: 73–9. © 1998 Slack Inc.

PRESEPTAL CELLULITIS

Preseptal cellulitis is about five times more common than orbital cellulitis, especially in children under the age of 5 years,[3] and is often secondary to lid and cutaneous infections–styes, impetigo, erysipelas, herpes simplex, varicella (Fig. 20.1)–or dacryocystitis. It is also associated with upper respiratory tract infections or uncomplicated sinusitis (Fig. 20.2) as well as secondary to lid trauma (Fig. 20.3).

Infective preseptal cellulitis must be distinguished from other causes of lid edema associated with adenoviral keratoconjunctivitis, atopic conjunctivitis, or, rarely, Kawasaki disease. Thirteen out of 80 (16%) children referred to a children's hospital with preseptal cellulitis were subsequently found to have adenoviral keratoconjunctivitis. The most common physical finding was an easily visible whitish membrane on the palpebral conjunctiva. These children either were culture positive for adenovirus, had corneal signs associated with adenovirus, or had a clear exposure to a person with adenovirus. These children were younger than 2 years and may have been more difficult to examine than older children. Also, older children with adenovirus infections tend to have less eyelid swelling while corneal findings predominate. Correct diagnosis can reduce unnecessary and prolonged hospitalization and treatment.[4] Preseptal progressed to orbital cellulitis in a case despite antibiotic treatment and without CT evidence of sinus disease; when a swinging pyrexia, cervical lymphadenopathy, macular rash, and swollen, dry lips developed, the diagnosis of Kawasaki disease was confirmed.[5] Treatment with intravenous gamma globulin and aspirin reduces potentially severe morbidity in this condition.

CLINICAL ASSESSMENT

History

Children with preseptal cellulitis associated with an upper respiratory tract infection or sinusitis present in the winter months with preceding nasal discharge, cough, fever, localized tenderness, and general malaise, followed typically by unilateral eyelid swelling. Bilateral involvement is rare. Otherwise, there is history of a localized lid infection or trauma with swelling spreading from an identifiable point.

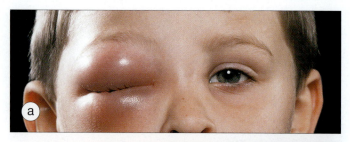
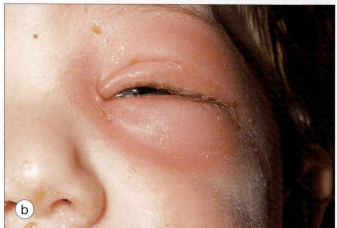

Fig. 20.2 (a) Preseptal cellulitis associated with sinusitis in an otherwise healthy child. (b) Preseptal cellulitis due to *Haemophilus influenzae* in a 6-month-old infant.

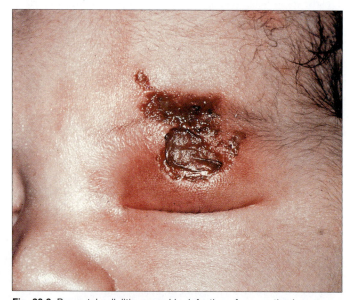

Fig. 20.3 Preseptal cellulitis caused by infection of a necrotic ulcer caused by a forceps injury (Dr S. Day's patient).

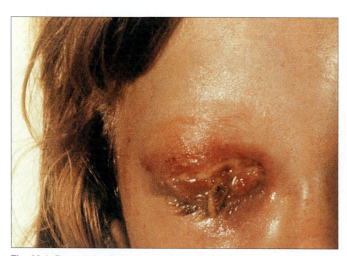

Fig. 20.1 Preseptal cellulitis caused by spread from a stye in a patient with leukemia.

Examination

The child may be generally unwell and febrile. The cellulitis may range from a mild localized involvement, with or without an abscess, to generalized tense upper and lower lid edema spreading to the cheek and brow, which may preclude examination of the eye. Localized causes such as styes, trauma, and dacryocystitis should be evident. There will be an absence of proptosis and optic nerve function, and extraocular movements will be normal.

It can be difficult to differentiate with certainty between preseptal and orbital cellulitis, especially in young children who may be more difficult to examine or when signs of orbital involvement are subtle. Therefore, the diagnosis may change from preseptal to orbital cellulitis if orbital signs become more obvious clinically or by imaging.[6]

The clinical picture may vary with the organism involved. In staphylococcal infections there is a purulent discharge, while Haemophilus infection leads to a nonpurulent cellulitis with a characteristic bluish-purple discoloration of the eyelid with irritability, raised temperature, and otitis media. In streptococcal infection there is usually a sharply demarcated red area of induration,[7] heat, and marked tenderness. Preseptal cellulitis may be complicated by meningitis, particularly if the infection is due to *Haemophilus influenzae* type B.[8]

MANAGEMENT

In children who develop preseptal cellulitis following an upper respiratory tract infection, cultures should be taken from the nose, throat, conjunctiva, and any accessible aspirates of the periorbital edema.

Children with mild to moderate preseptal cellulitis can be managed in the same way as uncomplicated sinusitis on an outpatient basis with oral broad spectrum antibiotics or as an inpatient with intravenous antibiotics if more severe (Table 20.2).[9,10]

In young children, management is best undertaken by a pediatrician in consultation with an ophthalmologist. An ENT surgeon and infectious diseases specialist may also be required.

Surgical treatment is seldom necessary.

Sinus X-rays may be difficult to interpret in children under 2 years due to the lack of development of the sinuses and are generally unhelpful. Lumbar puncture may be required to rule out meningitis, particularly if the infecting organism is thought to be *H. influenzae*. A CT scan (Fig. 20.4) to exclude orbital involvement is indicated when marked lid swelling prevents an adequate examination of the globe.[11]

Children with a local cause for the periorbital edema, such as dacryocystitis, need specific treatment for the underlying condition and rarely need further investigation.

Lid trauma may result in suppurative cellulitis, when the causative agent is usually *Staphylococcus aureus* or a beta-hemolytic *Streptococcus*. It is usually sufficient to culture the wound discharge as there is rarely any bacteremia, and blood cultures are usually negative.[12] Parenteral antibiotics are administered and tetanus prophylaxis is provided, if appropriate. If the skin has been penetrated by organic material or following animal bites, penicillin G should be added to cover anaerobic organisms. However, rarely beta-hemolytic *Streptococcus* may cause necrotizing fasciitis, which is characterized by a rapidly progressive tense and shiny cellulitis, with excessive edema and poorly demarcated borders with a violaceous skin discoloration. Frank necrosis develops and streptococcal toxic shock syndrome is common (Fig. 20.5). Treatment is with immediate hospitalization with a multi-

Table 20.2 Initial antibiotic treatment of preseptal and orbital cellulitis	
Preseptal cellulitis	*Associated with trauma/suppurative* Oxacillin or nafcillin 150–200 mg/kg per day in divided doses (P.O. or I.V.) *Associated with upper respiratory tract infection* Cefuroxime 100–150 mg/kg per day *or* amoxicillin-clavulanate (augmentin) or ampicillin 50–100 mg/kg per day *and* chloramphenicol 75–100 mg/kg per day (I.V. in divided doses)
Orbital cellulitis	Ceftazidime 100–150 mg/kg per day *or* cefotaxime 100–150 mg/kg per day *or* ceftriaxone 100–150 mg/kg per day (I.V. in divided doses) and oxacillin or nafcillin 150–200 mg/kg per day (in divided doses) Vancomycin should be considered in resistant cases. Clindamycin should be added in necrotizing fasciitis.

Note: The exact dose will vary with age and severity of infection.

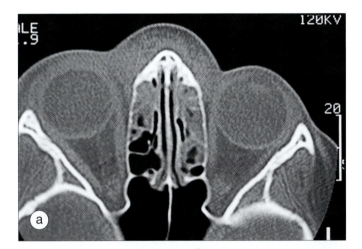

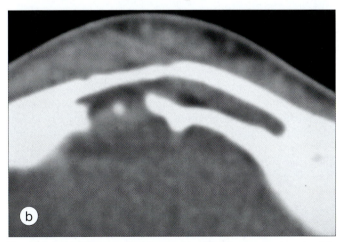

Fig. 20.4 (a, b) CT scans of a 13-year-old child with an anomalous frontal sinus. The initial cellulitis responded to low doses of antibiotics, which were then stopped. One month later she developed osteomyelitis, meningitis, and frontal lobe edema.

disciplinary team implementing resuscitation and medical support with immediate high-dose intravenous antibiotics including a penicillin or third-generation cephalosporin and clindamycin. Surgical debridement should be considered if there is not a clear response to medical treatment.[13,14]

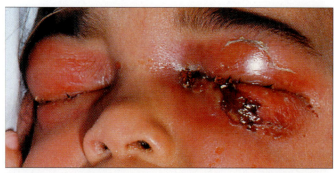

Fig. 20.5 Beta-hemolytic *Streptococcus* may cause necrotizing fasciitis. (Courtesy of Mr G. Rose)

ORBITAL CELLULITIS

Etiology

Orbital cellulitis is more frequent in children over 5 years (average age 7 years), and in over 90% is secondary to sinusitis,[15,12] especially of the ethmoid. It is more common in cold weather when the frequency of sinusitis increases. Other less common causes are penetrating orbital trauma, especially when there is a retained foreign body, dental infections,[16] extraocular muscle and retinal surgery,[17] and hematogenous spread during a systemic infectious illness.

Orbital cellulitis is always serious and potentially sight- and life-threatening, giving rise to a variety of systemic and ocular complications (Table 20.3). In the preantibiotic era one-fifth of patients died from septic intracranial complications, and one-third of the survivors had visual loss in the affected eye.[18] This poor outlook has been dramatically altered by the introduction of effective antibiotics and changing spectrum of causative organisms, but prompt diagnosis and vigorous treatment are still essential.

History

The usual presentation is with a painful red eye and increasing lid edema in a child who has had a recent upper respiratory tract infection. The child is usually miserable, pyrexial, and unwell.

Examination

There is conjunctival chemosis and injection and signs of orbital dysfunction, including proptosis, reduced and painful extraocular movements, and optic nerve dysfunction (Fig. 20.6). Orbital cellulitis is constrained by the septum at the arcus marginalis; thus, the preseptal soft tissue signs may be less dramatic than those in preseptal cellulitis.

Table 20.3 Complications of orbital cellulitis

Optic neuritis
Optic atrophy
Exposure keratitis
Central retinal artery occlusion[19]
Retinal and choroidal ischemia[20]
Subperiosteal and orbital abscess[23, 24]
Cavernous sinus thrombosis[39]
Meningitis[12]
Brain abscess
Septicemia[22]

There may be involvement of cranial nerves III, IV, and VI, especially with superior orbital fissure and cavernous sinus involvement. Visual loss when it occurs is usually due to an associated optic neuritis but may also be caused by exposure keratitis or even a retinal vascular occlusion (Fig. 20.7).[19–21]

The acute, sometimes explosive, onset of pain, fever, and systemic illness helps to differentiate orbital cellulitis from most other causes of inflammatory proptosis (Fig. 20.8, Table 20.4).

Management

Children with orbital cellulitis should be admitted under the care of pediatricians, ophthalmologists, ENT surgeons, and the infectious disease team. Blood cultures, nasal, throat, and conjunctival microbiology swabs may also be taken. These are often negative, but a positive result is helpful in planning antibiotic treatment if there is failure of initial therapy. This should not delay immediate and appropriate intravenous antibiotics and fluid resuscitation where necessary.

The initial treatment of orbital cellulitis in infants should be with high-dose intravenous third-generation cephalosporin such as cefotaxime, ceftazidime, or ceftriaxone combined with a penicillinase-resistant penicillin (Table 20.2). In older children sinusitis is frequently caused by mixed aerobic and anaerobic organisms so clindamycin may be substituted for penicillinase-resistant penicillin. An alternative regimen is the combination of

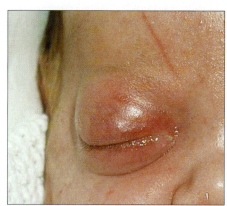

Fig. 20.6 Orbital cellulitis: proptosis, preseptal erythema, and fever suggest the diagnosis.

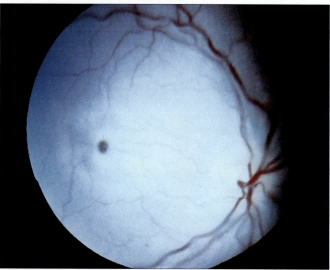

Fig. 20.7 Central retinal artery occlusion in orbital cellulitis (Dr S. Day's patient).

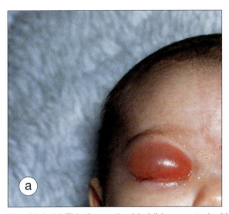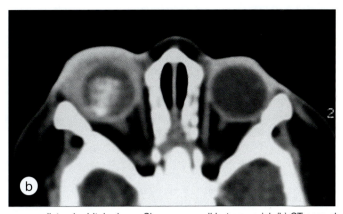

Fig. 20.8 (a) This 9-month-old child presented with a severe unilateral orbital edema. She was unwell but apyrexial. (b) CT scan shows bilateral retinoblastoma; large and calcified on the right, small on the left. She was treated with systemic steroids, which abolished the orbital edema, the right eye was enucleated, and the left was given local treatment. She is alive and well 7 years later with a left visual acuity of 6/5.

Table 20.4 The differential diagnosis of inflammatory proptosis	
Infection	Orbital cellulitis or cavernous sinus thrombosis
Idiopathic and specific inflammation	Orbital idiopathic inflammation, myositis, sarcoidosis, and Wegener granulomatosis
Neoplasia	Leukemia, Burkitt lymphoma, rhabdomyosarcoma, ruptured retinoblastoma, metastatic carcinoma, histiocytosis X (Letterer–Siwe variety), dermoid cyst (rupture and inflammation), and ethmoid osteoma
Trauma	Traumatic hematoma, orbital emphysema, retained foreign body
Systemic conditions	Sickle cell disease (bone infarction)
Endocrine dysfunction	Dysthyroid exophthalmos (very rare)

Modified from Jain and Rubin.[24]

penicillinase-resistant penicillin with chloramphenicol. The initial regime may be modified in the light of later culture results. Nasal decongestants such as ephedrine may be helpful in promoting intranasal drainage of infected sinuses. The child should be monitored closely for deterioration of ocular and systemic signs and management modified.

Plain X-rays may confirm sinus disease but are generally considered to be unhelpful. In the absence of any local cause for the orbital cellulitis a careful search should be made for any septic focus elsewhere in the body. If there are signs of meningism, lumbar puncture is indicated. As in preseptal cellulitis close liaison between pediatrician, ENT surgeon, and ophthalmologist is required for optimal treatment.

Investigations

Computed tomography is the investigation of choice and will define the extent of sinus disease, subperiosteal and orbital abscess, or intracranial involvement. Although a CT scan may detect subperiosteal and orbital abscesses not apparent clinically or on plain films,[11,21] the management of mild and moderate orbital cellulitis without optic nerve compromise or intracranial complications is initially medical. Imaging may be unnecessary unless there is a poor response to intravenous antibiotics, increasing systemic signs, progression of orbital signs, or expectant surgical management. Orbital ultrasound may also detect orbital abscess but is less reliable.[21,22]

MICROBIOLOGY OF PRESEPTAL AND ORBITAL CELLULITIS

Historically, the most commonly feared pathogen implicated in both preseptal and orbital cellulitis, as well as sinusitis, was *H. influenzae* type B (Hib). Vaccination against Hib was widely available from 1990. In a study of cases of preseptal and orbital cellulitis from 1980 to 1989 compared with cases from 1990 to 1998, 315 patients, 297 of which were preseptal and 18 were orbital cellulitis, were identified. Before 1990 12% were found positively to be Hib-related cellulitis and after 1990, 3.5%. The overall rate of cellulitis also declined by 60% in the 1990s.[3] The dramatic decline of culture-positive infection may also be due to higher threshold for admission (managed care), improved general child health, and earlier and more aggressive outpatient use of antibiotics (e.g., oral cephalosporins).

In younger children, the most common pathogens after the decline in Hib infections are *S. aureus* and *Staphylococcus epidermidis*; *Streptococcus pneumoniae*, *pyogenes*, and *sanguinis*; and *Moraxella catarrhalis*.[3,6] This mirrors the microbiology of sinusitis. Older children have bacteriologically more complex sinus infections and therefore orbital cellulitis.[23] Polymicrobial infections and anaerobic infections are more common. Anaerobic organisms include *Peptostreptococcus*, *Veillonella*, *Bacteroides*, *Fusobacterium*, and *Eubacterium*. Other Gram-negative organisms such as *Pseudomonas*, *Klebsiella*, atypical mycobacteria, *Mycobacterium tuberculosis*, and *Eikenella corrodens* have also been isolated from orbital infections.[24]

Fungal infections are rare but should be excluded when orbital cellulitis occurs in an immunosuppressed or diabetic child.[25] Gram-negative organisms, Gram-positive bacteria, and fungi are also more prevalent in these patients. Those with cystic fibrosis are more likely to be infected with *Pseudomonas aeruginosa* or *S. aureus*.

Blood cultures are more likely to be positive with Hib infections and rarely positive with other infections. Tissue cultures can be positive in over 50% but results are of dubious significance unless from a pointing abscess or collection drained at surgery.[26,27]

SUBPERIOSTEAL AND ORBITAL ABSCESS

The incidence of subperiosteal and orbital abscess complicating orbital cellulitis was probably about 10%,[28] but is now declining. Most have sinus infection. In subperiosteal abscess, a purulent infection within a sinus, usually the ethmoids, breaks through the thin orbital bony wall (lamina papyracea) and lies beneath the loosely adherent periosteum, which is easily lifted off the bone, giving a convex "lens" type of appearance on CT scanning. An orbital abscess occurs either when a subperiosteal abscess breaches the periorbita or when a collection of pus forms within the orbit.

The usual causative organism is *Staphylococcus* but *Streptococcus*, *H. influenzae*, and anaerobic organisms may also be responsible. Unless there is nonaxial proptosis or a palpable fluctuant swelling at the orbital rim, it is difficult to distinguish orbital abscess from uncomplicated orbital cellulitis clinically. It should be suspected whenever there is marked systemic toxicity and severe orbital signs, or when orbital cellulitis is slow to respond to adequate doses of intravenous antibiotics. The presence of subperiosteal abscess may be indicated by lateral displacement of the globe away from the infected sinus, impaired adduction, and resilience on retropulsion.[29]

All studies have recommend hospitalization for intravenous antibiotic therapy (Table 20.2) and repeated eye examinations to evaluate progression of infection or involvement of the optic nerve.

CT scanning (Fig. 20.9) at presentation is not always necessary, especially if there is mild orbital cellulitis with clear findings of sinusitis and without optic nerve compromise or intracranial signs.

A CT scan is indicated if the presentation is unusual, severe, or in an older child or there are optic nerve or intracranial signs. Also, if the child does not respond to treatment, it would be advisable to image the sinuses, orbits, and intracranial compartment with a CT scan (Fig. 20.10). A contrast-enhanced scan gives additional information in differentiating an abscess, which is amenable to drainage, from a phlegmon (purulent tissue inflammation), which is not. Serial orbital ultrasound has been used to follow the course of the abscess after treatment.

An orbital abscess should be drained but the management of subperiosteal abscess is more controversial[6] because they may resolve with medical treatment.[6,23,30] In a review of 37 patients with subperiosteal abscess secondary to sinusitis it was noted that resolution occurred in 83% of patients under 9 years of age who were treated medically or who had negative cultures on drainage.[31] In contrast only 25% of those aged between 9 and 14 years cleared without drainage or had negative cultures on drainage. The remaining group, aged 15 years and over, were refractory to medical therapy alone.

Nine children (2 months to 4 years) with subperiosteal abscesses were managed with a third-generation cephalosporin and vancomycin in the first 24 to 36 hours; only one required surgical drainage, this case being culture-negative. This supports an initial medical management approach for most patients with subperiosteal or orbital abscesses resulting in orbital cellulitis.[6]

Garcia and Harris[23] advocate a nonsurgical management of subperiosteal abscess with the presence of four criteria:

1. Age less than 9 years;
2. No visual compromise;
3. Medial abscess of modest size; and
4. No intracranial or frontal sinus involvement.

In their prospective study of 29 patients fulfilling the above criteria, 27 (93%) were managed successfully exclusively medically. Only 2 patients had surgical intervention with successful outcomes.[23]

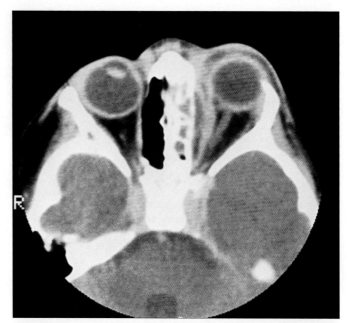

Fig. 20.9 CT scan showing left ethmoidal sinusitis and subperiosteal abscess.

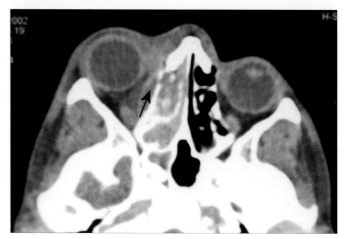

Fig. 20.10 Subperiosteal abscess in a child with orbital cellulitis secondary to ethmoid sinusitis: note the dome-shaped abscess contained by periosteum (arrow).

Thus it would seem reasonable to initially treat medically if vision is normal, the subperiosteal abscess is of moderate size, in the absence of intracranial extension, and the child is under 9 years of age.[32]

OSTEOMYELITIS OF THE SUPERIOR MAXILLA

This rare condition, which usually presents in the first few months of life with fever, general malaise, and marked periorbital edema, may be confused with orbital cellulitis or subperiosteal abscess.[32] There may be conjunctival chemosis, mild proptosis, and early central abscess formation in the superior maxilla with pointing at the inner or outer canthus. The diagnosis should be suspected if there is pus in the nostril and edema of the alveolus and palate on the affected side. A fistula may be present in the area of the first deciduous molar.

S. aureus is the usual infecting organism but the mode of infection is uncertain; it may result from hematogenous spread to the dental sac of the first deciduous molar, which has a rich blood supply, or may develop secondary to mastitis in the mother.

Treatment is with high-dose intravenous antibiotics chosen on the basis of culture and sensitivity and surgical drainage of the abscess preferably via the nose.[32]

CAVERNOUS SINUS THROMBOSIS

Since the introduction of antibiotics this dreaded complication of orbital cellulitis has become rare. In the preantibiotic era the mortality rate was almost 100%.[33] In its early stages cavernous sinus thrombosis may be difficult to distinguish clinically from orbital cellulitis. In the former there is more severe pain and a marked systemic illness, proptosis develops rapidly, and there may be third, fourth, and sixth cranial nerve palsies compared with the purely mechanical limitation seen in orbital cellulitis.

Hyperalgesia in the distribution of the fifth cranial nerve is common. The presence of retinal venous dilatation and optic disc swelling, especially if bilateral, is very suggestive of cavernous sinus thrombosis. In the later stages, bilateral involvement in cavernous sinus thrombosis makes the clinical distinction from orbital cellulitis easier.

Diagnosis can be confirmed by performing CT or MRI scan. Cavernous sinus thrombosis is most frequently associated with *S. aureus* infection.[34]

Management is best undertaken by a pediatric neurologist or neurosurgeon and involves treatment with high-dose intravenous antibiotics, anticoagulants, and systemic steroids in selected cases.

FUNGAL ORBITAL CELLULITIS

Fungal orbital cellulitis is rare in childhood but may cause orbital infection in children who are acidotic, diabetic, or immunosuppressed.

ORBITAL MUCORMYCOSIS

Orbital fungal infection should be suspected in any diabetic or immunosuppressed[25] child or one with gastroenteritis and metabolic acidosis[35] who develops a rapidly progressive orbital cellulitis, especially if accompanied by necrosis of the skin or nasal mucosa.

Fungal orbital cellulitis has been described in otherwise healthy children.[36,37] Untreated, it is rapidly fatal.

Colonization of the sinuses by spores followed by direct or hematogenous spread to the orbit occurs, which is heralded by periorbital pain, marked lid edema, conjunctival chemosis, and proptosis. Later spread to the orbital apex results in third, fourth, and sixth cranial nerve palsies and optic neuropathy. Central retinal artery occlusion may occur. CT scanning normally shows ethmoid or maxillary sinusitis. Zygomycetes have a tendency to invade arteries, causing thrombosis and subsequent ischemic necrosis; involvement of the facial arteries causes gangrene of the nose, palate, and facial tissues. Once spread to the cavernous sinus and intracranial vessels has occurred, the prognosis is very poor.

To confirm the diagnosis, scrapings from infected tissues should be cultured and Gram and Giemsa stained. Larger tissue biopsies should be fixed in 10% formalin and processed for histological examination. These fungi have an affinity for hematoxylin and are therefore easily recognized in hematoxylin and eosin sections.

The management of this condition consists of specific antifungal therapy/correction of the underlying metabolic or immunological abnormality and surgical debridement of necrotic tissues. The specific treatment of choice is amphotericin B, which should be given intravenously and may also be used locally to irrigate infected sinuses.[38] It is nephrotoxic so renal function should be carefully monitored.

REFERENCES

1. Chandler JR, Langenbrunner DJ, Stevens ER. The pathogenesis of orbital complications of acute sinusitis. Laryngoscope 1970; 80: 1414–28.
2. Uzcategui N, Warman R, Smith A, Howard CW. Clinical practice guidelines for the management of orbital cellulitis. J Pediatr Ophthalmol Strabismus 1998; 35: 73–9
3. Ambati BK, Ambati J, Azar N, et al. Periorbital and orbital cellulitis before and after the advent of *Haemophilus influenzae* type B vaccination. Ophthalmology 2000; 107: 1450–3.
4. Ruttum MS, Ogawa G. Adenovirus conjunctivitis mimics preseptal and orbital cellulitis in young children. Pediatr Infect Dis J 1996; 15: 266–7.
5. Sheard RM, Pandey KR, Barnes ND, Vivian AJ. Kawasaki disease presenting as orbital cellulitis. J Pediatr Ophthalmol Strabismus 2000; 37: 123–5.
6. Starkey CR, Steele RW. Medical management of orbital cellulitis. Pediatr Infect Dis J 2001; 20: 1002–5.
7. Jones DB. Discussion on paper by Weiss, et al. Bacterial periorbital cellulitis and orbital cellulitis in childhood. Ophthalmology 1983; 90: 201–3.
8. Ciarallo LR, Rowe PC. Lumbar puncture in children with periorbital and orbital cellulitis. J Pediatr 1993; 122: 355–9.

9. Durand M. Intravenous antibiotics in sinusitis. Otolaryngol Head Neck Surg 1999; 7: 7.
10. Healy GB. Comment on: "Chandler, et al. The pathogenesis of orbital complications in acute sinusitis. Laryngoscope 1970; 80: 1414–28." Laryngoscope 1997; 107: 441–6.
11. Goldberg F, Berne AS, Oski FA. Differentiation of orbital cellulitis from preseptal cellulitis by computed tomography. Paediatrics 1978; 62: 1000–5.
12. Weiss A, Friendly D, Eglin K, et al. Bacterial periorbital and orbital cellulitis in childhood. Ophthalmology 1983; 90: 195–203.
13. Rose GE, Howard DJ, Watts MR. Periorbital necrotising fasciitis. Eye 1991; 5: 736–40.
14. Stevens DL. Streptococcal toxic shock syndrome associated with necrotizing fasciitis. Annu Rev Med 2000; 51: 271–88.
15. Watters E, Wallar PH, Hiles DA, Michaels RH. Acute orbital cellulitis. Arch Ophthalmol 1976; 94: 785–8.
16. Flood TP, Braude LS, Jampol LM, Herzog S. Computed tomography in the management of orbital infections associated with dental disease. Br J Ophthalmol 1982; 66: 269–74.
17. von Noorden GK. Orbital cellulitis following extraocular muscle surgery. Am J Ophthalmol 1972; 74: 627–9.
18. Duke-Elder S. Acute orbital inflammations. In: Duke-Elder S, editor. The Ocular Adnexa. London: Henry Kimpton; 1952: 5427–48. (System of Ophthalmology, Vol. 5.)

19. Jarrett WH, Gutman FA. Ocular complications of infection in the paranasal sinuses. Arch Ophthalmol 1969; 81: 683–8.

20. Sherry T. Acute infarction of the choroid and retina. Br J Ophthalmol 1973; 57: 133–7.

21. Schramm VL, Myers EN, Kennerdell J. Orbital complications of acute sinusitis. Evaluation, management and outcome. Otolaryngology 1978; 86: 221–30.

22. Krohel GB, Krauss HR, Christensen RE, Minckler D. Orbital abscess. Arch Ophthalmol 1980; 98: 274–6.

23. Garcia GH, Harris GJ. Criteria for nonsurgical management of subperiosteal abscess of the orbit. Ophthalmology 2000; 107: 1454–1458

24. Jain A, Rubin PA. Orbital cellulitis in children. Int Ophthalmol Clin 2001 Fall; 41: 71–86.

25. Schwartz JN, Donnelly EH, Klintworth GK. Ocular and orbital phycomycosis. Surv Ophthalmol 1977; 22: 3–28.

26. Donahue SP, Schwartz G. Preseptal and orbital cellulitis in childhood. A changing microbiologic spectrum. Ophthalmology 1998; 105: 1902–5.

27. Ferguson MP, McNab AA. Current treatment and outcome in orbital cellulitis. Aust N Z J Ophthalmol 1999; 27: 375–9.

28. Hornblass A, Herschorn BJ, Stern K, Grimes C. Orbital abscess. Surv Ophthalmol 1984; 29: 169–78.

29. Harris GJ. Subperiosteal abscess of the orbit. Arch Ophthalmol 1983; 101: 751–7.

30. Rubin SE, Zito J. Orbital sub-periosteal abscess responding to medical therapy. J Pediatr Ophthalmol Strabismus 1994; 31: 325–6.

31. Harris GJ. Subperiosteal abscess of the orbit. Ophthalmology 1994; 101: 585–95.

32. Cavenagh F. Osteomyelitis of the superior maxilla in infants. Br Med J I960; 1: 468–72.

33. Grove WE. Septic and aseptic types of thrombosis of the cavernous sinus. Arch Otolaryngol 1936; 24: 29–50.

34. Southwick FS, Richardson EP, Swartz MN. Septic thrombosis of the dural sinuses. Medicine 1986; 65: 82–106.

35. Hale LM. Orbito-cerebral phycomycosis. Arch Ophthalmol 1971; 86: 39–43.

36. Blodi FC, Hannah FT, Wadsworth JA. Lethal orbitocerebral phycomycosis in otherwise healthy children. Am J Ophthalmol 1969; 67: 698–705.

37. Whitehurst FO, Listen TE. Orbital aspergillosis: Report of a case in a child. J Pediatr Ophthalmol Strabismus 1981; 18: 50–4.

38. Lee EJ, Lee MY, Hung YC, Wang LC. Orbital rhinocerebral mucormycosis associated with diabetic ketoacidosis: report of survival of a 10-year-old boy. J Formos Med Assoc 1998; 97: 720–3.

39. Clune JP. Septic thrombosis within the cavernous sinus. Am J Ophthalmol 1963; 56: 33–9.

CHAPTER 21 Endophthalmitis

Donal Brosnahan

Infectious endophthalmitis occurs when bacteria, fungi, parasites, or viruses enter the eye following a breach of the outer wall of the eye (exogenous endophthalmitis) or when organisms enter the eye from a source elsewhere in the body (endogenous endophthalmitis). Exogenous endophthalmitis most frequently arises following surgical intervention but may be a consequence of traumatic injury to the eye. Endogenous endophthalmitis usually results from hematogenous spread of infection from a distant focus. Exogenous endophthalmitis may be subclassified into acute and chronic. The classification of endophthalmitis is of importance as each type has a characteristic clinical setting, differing spectrum of microorganisms, and varying visual prognosis.

EXOGENOUS BACTERIAL ENDOPHTHALMITIS

Exogenous endophthalmitis in adults occurs most frequently following intraocular surgery (70–90%). The most commonly performed intraocular procedure in adults is cataract extraction, which has a reported incidence of postoperative endophthalmitis of 0.1–0.38%.[1] The incidence of endophthalmitis in children undergoing cataract extraction (Fig. 21.1) is unknown. Wheeler et al. surveyed 350 pediatric ophthalmologists and reported an incidence of 0.07% in children undergoing surgery for congenital cataracts and glaucoma.[2] The authors identified upper respiratory infection and nasolacrimal duct obstruction as possible risk factors. Good et al. reported an incidence of 0.45% in a retrospective review of 651 cases of cataract extraction in children.[3]

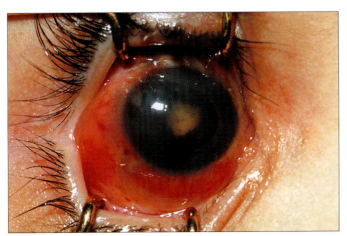

Fig. 21.1 Bacterial endophthalmitis following infant cataract surgery and intraocular lens implantation.

In adults the incidence of endophthalmitis is higher in patients undergoing intracapsular cataract extraction and surgery complicated by rupture of the posterior capsule.[4] Surgery for congenital cataract usually involves breach of the posterior capsule whether by lensectomy or primary capsulotomy following lens aspiration, and one might expect an incidence of postoperative endophthalmitis similar to that following intracapsular extraction, capsular rupture, and anterior vitrectomy. Endophthalmitis may develop following the removal of sutures postoperatively when pathogens may enter the eye along suture tracts. Neuteboom and de Vries-Knoppert reported endophthalmitis following Nd:YAG laser capsulotomy.[5]

Trauma is a significant cause of endophthalmitis in children. Endophthalmitis following penetrating injury accounts for approximately 20% of most large reported series. The incidence of endophthalmitis after penetrating injury ranges from 4 to 20% and is particularly high when injury occurs in a rural setting.[6] As many as 85% of patients in the Endophthalmitis Vitrectomy Study (EVS) achieved final visual acuity of 20/400 or better while only 22–42% achieved this level of acuity following post-traumatic endophthalmitis.[7,8]

Poor visual outcome may result from a delay in diagnosis as signs of inflammation may be attributed to the injury itself. There may be a delay in wound closure and also a retained intraocular foreign body, which may adversely affect outcome. The final visual acuity will also be affected by trauma to ocular structures. Infection often results from virulent organisms, with higher rates of Gram-negative infection with species such as *Bacillus* spp.

Antimetabolites such as 5-fluorouracil and mitomycin C are often used to augment filtration surgery for glaucoma in children and increase success rates. The use of mitomycin is associated with significant morbidity with one study showing 23% incidence of infection or bleb leak after 5 years.[9] Morad et al. reported 3 cases of endophthalmitis in 60 eyes following use of an Ahmed drainage device for pediatric glaucoma, where two eyes became phthisical.[10] Infection was related to tube exposure in two cases. The incidence of endophthalmitis following glaucoma surgery in adults is similar to that found with cataract surgery. Al-Hazami et al. reported an incidence of 0.4% in 254 eyes of children undergoing filtration surgery with mitomycin C.[11] The onset of endophthalmitis is frequently delayed, occurring months or years after surgery.

Infection associated with filtration surgery is often sub-classified clinically into blebitis, which is defined as mucopurulent material in and around the bleb associated with anterior segment activity but without hypopyon. If a hypopyon is present or there is evidence of vitreous activity a diagnosis of bleb-associated endophthalmitis may be made. There is strong evidence of increased risk of post-trabeculectomy endophthalmitis in patients who have diabetes mellitus, an episode of blebitis, and also an

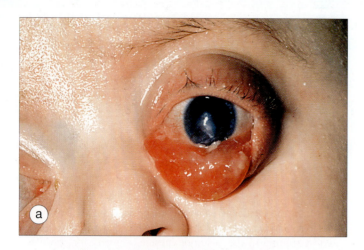

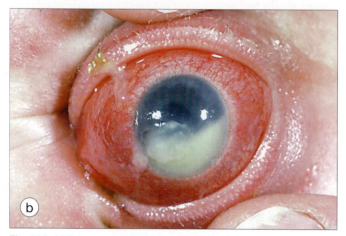

Fig. 21.2 (a) Exposure keratitis with conjunctival chemosis in a child with subluxation of the globe caused by shallow orbits in Crouzon disease. (b) Same patient with endophthalmitis and hypopyon following exposure keratitis.

association with the use of antimetabolites such as 5-fluorouracil and mitomycin C.[12,13]

Endophthalmitis following strabismus surgery is rare with a reported incidence of 1:3,500 to 1:185,000.[14] Recchia et al. reported endophthalmitis in 6 patients after pediatric strabismus surgery. It has not been proven that scleral perforation is a prerequisite for the development of endophthalmitis. Needles and sutures are frequently contaminated despite the use of preoperative povidone-iodine. Carothers et al. noted 19% of needles and 25% of sutures were culture positive in a prospective study of patients undergoing strabismus surgery.[15] Endophthalmitis has been reported in the absence of scleral perforation, presumably due to intrascleral inoculation from contaminated needles or sutures or possibly due to endogenous spread.

Exogenous endophthalmitis may also arise secondary to suppurative keratitis (Fig. 21.2) associated with exposure or trauma.

CLINICAL PRESENTATION

The clinical presentation of bacterial endophthalmitis depends on the route of infection and the virulence of the organism. Acute postoperative endophthalmitis typically presents 1–3 days after surgery with pain and decreased vision. There is often associated lid swelling, conjunctival injection, corneal edema, and chemosis.

Intraocular findings include uveitis, hypopyon, vitreous cells, and occasionally sheathing of blood vessels.

Infection with less virulent organisms may result in chronic or late onset endophthalmitis, which may run a more indolent course with exacerbations and remissions. Intraocular inflammation is less severe though hypopyon and vitreous activity may be present. The presence of creamy white plaques on the posterior capsule is suggestive of *Propionibacterium acnes* infection. In endophthalmitis following penetrating injury there may be a persistent severe uveitis and vitreous haze often with infiltration of the wound edges. Retinal periphlebitis may be an early sign of bacterial endophthalmitis in those cases where fundus examination is possible. Endophthalmitis should always be suspected after intraocular surgery or traumatic perforation whenever the degree of inflammation is greater than expected. If there is concern, serial and frequent examinations should be performed.

The main differential diagnoses are from fungal endophthalmitis and severe uveitis. Rarely retinoblastoma or metastatic tumour may present with uveitis and hypopyon.

PATHOGENIC ORGANISMS

The Endophthalmitis Vitrectomy Study (EVS) prospectively studied 420 cases of infectious endophthalmitis presenting within 6 weeks of cataract extraction or secondary intraocular lens implantation.[16] Positive culture was obtained from 69.3% of intraocular specimens. Gram-positive bacteria were isolated in 94.2% of cases and Gram-negative bacteria in 6.5% of isolates. *Staphylococcus epidermidis*, which forms part of the normal skin flora, was by far the most common Gram-positive isolate (70%), followed by *Staphylococcus aureus* (9.9%), *Streptococcus* species (2.2%), and *P. acnes*. *Proteus* and *Pseudomonas* were the most commonly identified Gram-negative organisms. *Haemophilus influenzae* has also been identified in other series.[17] Weinstein et al.'s study of children with endophthalmitis reported similar results with 75% of culture-positive cases being caused by Gram-positive organisms.[18] *S. epidermidis*, *Streptococcus pneumoniae*, and *S. aureus* have been identified as the most frequent infecting agents in children following cataract extraction.

When endophthalmitis is related to glaucoma surgery the spectrum of organisms differs in that *Streptococcus* species predominate. *Haemophilus influenzae* is also isolated more frequently than *S. epidermidis*. This difference may reflect the fact that endophthalmitis is often of late onset, with invasion of organisms through thin-walled or leaking blebs. There is also an increased risk of late endophthalmitis associated with inferiorly placed filtration blebs.[19] In a case–control study Jampel et al. found increased incidence of endophthalmitis associated with full-thickness filtration procedures, inferior-placed blebs, bleb leakage, and the use of mitomycin.[13] If endophthalmitis develops in the early postoperative period *S. epidermidis* is more frequently cultured.

S. pneumoniae, *S. aureus*, *H. influenzae*, and *S. epidermidis* have been isolated in cases of endophthalmitis associated with strabismus surgery. The number of reported cases is small, though it appears that infection with more virulent organisms is more frequent than that following cataract surgery. Visual prognosis is poor as a consequence of delayed diagnosis and the virulence of the infecting organisms.

In adults with endophthalmitis associated with trauma, *S. epidermidis* and *Bacillus* spp. are the pathogens most frequently identified. In a review of post-traumatic endophthalmitis in children *Streptococcus* species were isolated in 25.9%, *Staphylococcus* in 18.5%, and *Bacillus* spp. in 22% of cases, respectively.

BACTERIOLOGICAL INVESTIGATION

Culture specimens from aqueous, vitreous, and any other obviously infected site should always be obtained before starting therapy. Children with suspected endophthalmitis will require examination under anesthesia to facilitate thorough examination and collection of specimens for culture. The microbiologist should be informed to ensure that appropriate culture media are available in the operating room and to perform immediate Gram and Giemsa stains.

Aqueous and vitreous specimens are plated out on blood agar, chocolate agar, and thioglycolate broth and incubated at 37°C for bacterial isolation; further specimens are incubated at 25°C on Sabouraud's medium and blood agar for fungal growth. In addition, specimens should be placed on glass slides for Gram and Giemsa stains. Culture for up to 2 weeks is required to allow growth of anaerobes such as *P. acnes*, which may be sequestered in folds of the posterior capsule. If *P. acnes* is clinically suspected, removal of capsular remnants for culture may be helpful in confirming the diagnosis.

Polymerase chain reaction (PCR) is a highly sensitive and specific test, which can be employed to identify bacteria, fungi, and viruses from ocular samples. PCR allows rapid identification of microorganisms, which in turn results in early diagnosis and appropriate antibiotic therapy. This technique is particularly helpful in culture-negative cases where a preponderance of Gram-negative organisms have been identified using PCR. Although PCR testing is not routinely performed, its role continues to expand.

Aqueous samples may be obtained by a paracentesis; vitreous specimens should be obtained by use of a mechanical suction cutting device. Where a three-port vitrectomy is planned, specimens should be obtained before the infusion is turned on to avoid dilution of the specimen. Approximately 0.2 ml is removed for culture and staining. In infants the pars plana is poorly developed and therefore sclerotomies should be anteriorly placed. If lensectomy and anterior vitrectomy have been performed, specimens may be obtained via an anterior approach. Once all specimens have been obtained, intravitreal antibiotics may be given. In cases of penetrating injury any foreign body retrieved should be sent for culture.

TREATMENT

Treatment of endophthalmitis has been greatly influenced by the EVS of eyes with endophthalmitis post cataract surgery.[16]
1. Immediate vitrectomy is not indicated if the visual acuity is better than light perception.
2. If visual acuity is light perception only then there is a significant benefit from vitrectomy.
3. There is no additional therapeutic benefit from the use of systemic antibiotics.

It has not been established whether EVS findings can be applied to endophthalmitis in children, to bleb-associated infection, or to traumatic endophthalmitis. In light of the higher incidence of more pathogenic organisms in traumatic and bleb-related endophthalmitis it is reasonable to undertake early

vitrectomy. Treatment regimens need to take into account the clinical setting and the likely infecting organisms. Furthermore it may not be possible to establish the level of vision in infants.

If vision is better than light perception, vitreous sampling should be followed by intravitreal antibiotic injection. If vitrectomy is not performed, then a single-port vitreous sampling ("tap") may be performed. Vitreous sampling will create a space in the vitreous cavity into which antibiotics may be injected. If vision is perception of light, then a three-port vitrectomy is performed. Vitrectomy in these patients is often difficult due to the presence of corneal edema and media opacity. Vitrectomy in infants is particularly hazardous due to the poorly developed pars plana. In infants it may be necessary to perform lensectomy to gain access to the vitreous cavity (Table 21.1).

At the time of administration of intravitreal antibiotics, the type of organism is usually unknown, and therefore the antibiotics chosen should provide broad-spectrum cover. Intravitreal vancomycin (see Table 21.2) provides good cover for Gram-positive organisms. Cephalosporins such as ceftazidime are effective against Gram-negative bacteria. Aminoglycosides such as gentamicin and amikacin are also effective against Gram-negative organisms. Aminoglycosides, particularly gentamicin, have been shown to be toxic to the retina when given intravitreally. If indicated, intravitreal injection can be repeated after 48 hours.

The role of intravenous antibiotics is controversial, as the EVS did not find any additional benefit with their use; yet they are commonly used. Ocular penetration of vancomycin and ceftazidime following intravenous administration is good, gentamicin and amikacin less so. Subconjunctival antibiotics are not commonly used in children. Topical antibiotics may also be used to supplement intravitreal injection (vancomycin 50 mg/ml and

Table 21.1 Vitrectomy in endophthalmitis

Advantages of vitrectomy	Disadvantages of vitrectomy
Removal of organisms and toxins	Technically difficult in small eye
Removal of loculated infection	Media opacities increase risk of complication
Removal of inflammatory cells Better antibiotic distribution	Lensectomy may be required

Table 21.2 Initial antibiotic treatment of bacterial endophthalmitis

Intravitreal antibiotics
Vancomycin 1 mg in 0.1 ml of normal saline
and amikacin 0.4 mg in 0.1 ml of normal saline
or ceftazidime 2.25 mg in 0.1 ml of normal saline

Systemic antibiotics
Vancomycin 44 mg/kg per day
and ceftazidime 100–150 mg/kg per day
or ciprofloxacin 5–10 mg/kg per day

Topical antibiotics
Vancomycin 50 mg/ml hourly
ceftazidime 50 mg/ml hourly
or gentamicin 14 mg/ml hourly

Note: Therapy should be reviewed when culture results are available. Dosages may need to be adjusted for children less than 1 year of age.

ceftazidime 50 mg/ml or gentamicin 14 mg/ml). Antibiotic therapy should be reviewed in the light of clinical response and culture results. Inflammation is controlled with steroids applied topically, subconjunctivally, and systemically (1 mg/kg). Intravitreal steroids have been shown to have a beneficial effect.[20]

PREVENTION

In postoperative infection the patient is the most common source of infection; children with extraocular infection such as blepharitis or conjunctivitis or with impaired nasolacrimal drainage should have surgery deferred until these conditions are remedied. Surgery should also be deferred in the presence of upper respiratory tract infection.

Preoperative application of topical povidone-iodine 5% solution to the conjunctival sac has been shown to decrease bacterial counts and probably reduces the incidence of endophthalmitis; however, it must be applied five minutes before surgery. In cases of penetrating injury, povidone-iodine should not be applied. There may be a beneficial effect from administering intravitreal antibiotics after repair of penetrating injuries where there is a known higher rate of endophthalmitis. Although used, antibiotics in irrigating solutions during cataract surgery have not been shown to decrease the incidence of endophthalmitis. Many surgeons inject antibiotics subconjunctivally when performing intraocular surgery although its effectiveness in reducing endophthalmitis is unproven.

ENDOGENOUS BACTERIAL ENDOPHTHALMITIS

Metastatic endophthalmitis results from hematogenous spread from a distant focus of infection such as meningitis (Fig. 21.3), bacterial endocarditis, abdominal sepsis, skin infection, and otitis media. Endogenous bacterial endophthalmitis represents 2–8% of all endophthalmitis and is bilateral in 14–50% of cases.[21]

The patient may present with symptoms and signs similar to those seen in postoperative infection though the clinical setting is quite different. Presentation is often to a pediatrician because of systemic symptoms or the child may be under the care of the pediatrician for treatment of a predisposing condition such as meningitis or endocarditis. Diabetes mellitus and gastrointestinal infection are also significant risk factors. Initially symptoms may be mild and diagnosis is often delayed. Red eye in a patient with

sepsis should prompt full ophthalmological examination. The differential diagnosis includes conjunctivitis, uveitis, and orbital cellulitis. The presence of significant vitreous inflammation and posterior segment changes such as vasculitis and localized choroidal or retinal infiltration suggests an infective etiology.

Endogenous endophthalmitis is most commonly due to Gram-positive organisms such as *S. aureus* and *Streptococcus* species. Wong et al. found a preponderance of Gram-negative species in an Asian population.[22] *H. influenzae* and *Neisseria meningitidis* remain important causes in children though the incidence could be expected to decrease in populations with immunization programs.

Metastatic endophthalmitis should be managed in the same way as postoperative infection. When aqueous and vitreous samples have been taken, intravitreal antibiotics to cover Gram-negative and gram-positive organisms are given. If the child is too ill to undergo anesthesia, therapy may be guided by blood culture results, which may be positive in up to 72% of cases.[23] There may be a role for vitrectomy in this condition, which is often caused by highly pathogenic bacteria and frequently has a very poor visual outcome. The patient's underlying medical condition influences whether systemic steroids are appropriate. Patients presenting with endophthalmitis need evaluation by a pediatrician or infectious disease specialist.

EXOGENOUS FUNGAL ENDOPHTHALMITIS

Fungal endophthalmitis may rarely complicate penetrating trauma in children, especially if there is a retained wooden foreign body. Symptoms and signs of infection may develop weeks or months after the injury, following which there is slow progression with uveitis, vitritis, and later hypopyon and vitreous abscess. In suspected fungal endophthalmitis aqueous and vitreous samples are taken as for bacterial endophthalmitis. Giemsa stain will often show fungal hyphae and allow prompt diagnosis. If fungal infection is confirmed, amphotericin B is injected intravitreally. Vitrectomy should be considered if there is significant vitreous involvement.

ENDOGENOUS FUNGAL ENDOPHTHALMITIS

Candida albicans is the organism most commonly identified in endogenous fungal endophthalmitis although *Aspergillus*

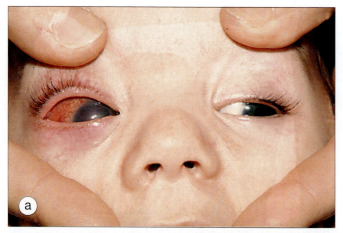
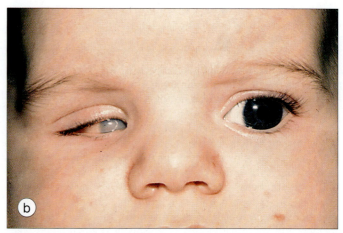

Fig. 21.3 (a) Metastatic meningococcal endophthalmitis leading to (b) phthisis bulbi.

Table 21.3 Risk factors for endogenous endophthalmitis in children

Endocarditis
Meningococcal infection
Prematurity
Intravenous feeding
Immunosuppression
Broad-spectrum antibiotics

fumigatus, Histoplasma capsulatum, Coccidioides immitis, Blastomycosis dermatidis, Cryptococcus neoformans, and *Sporotrichum schenckii* have all been implicated. Endophthalmitis is usually associated with *Candida* septicemia; risk factors include immunosuppression, intravenous feeding, and prematurity.[24] Systemic candidiasis may occur in up to 4% of premature babies and is associated with indwelling catheters and use of broad-spectrum antibiotics (Table 21.3). The prevalence of *Candida* endophthalmitis has been estimated to be 28–45% in patients with *Candida* septicemia although postmortem studies have shown histopathological evidence of intraocular infection in 85% of cases. Donahue et al. in a large prospective study detected *Candida* chorioretinitis in 9.3% of patients with positive blood cultures, yet found no cases of endophthalmitis.[25] These findings were attributed to stricter diagnostic criteria and a possible effect of earlier systemic treatment.

The presence of a red eye in a child with any of the known risk factors should prompt dilated fundus examination. The typical appearance of intraocular *Candida* infection is chorioretinitis with a predilection for posterior pole involvement. The creamy white chorioretinal lesions enlarge and extend into the vitreous to form "puff balls" (Fig. 21.4), which, when multiple, have a "string of pearls" appearance. The degree of vitreous inflammation is variable. The anterior segments may be involved to a varying degree and secondary cataract has been reported. *Aspergillus* endophthalmitis is typically more severe with large confluent areas of chorioretinitis.

If fungemia is suspected, blood and urine samples are obtained to identify the organism. If the diagnosis is in doubt, vitreous sampling as for bacterial endophthalmitis is essential to identify the organism and determine sensitivity. Giemsa stain and Sabouraud's

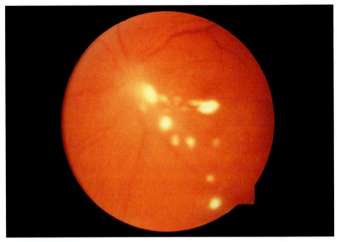

Fig. 21.4 Endogenous *Candida* endophthalmitis in an immunosuppressed child. Note characteristic "string of pearls" appearance of vitreous infiltrates.

media are used to identify and culture fungi. PCR has also been successfully used to rapidly identify fungi in intraocular samples.

If the chorioretinal lesions are small and there is mild vitreous involvement, systemic treatment with amphotericin B or fluconazole is used. Ocular penetration of amphotericin B is limited although there are reports of successful outcome with systemic treatment alone. Although amphotericin B with or without flucytosine has been the treatment of choice there may be significant renal and hepatic toxicity. If culture and sensitivity indicate that the fungus is sensitive to fluconazole it can be substituted for amphotericin B. Fluconazole has better ocular penetration and has fewer systemic side effects; however, resistance is a common problem. The role of newer antifungal agents such as voriconazole and caspofungin in fungal endophthalmitis has yet to be evaluated.

When there is significant vitreous involvement, then intravitreal amphotericin (5 μg in 0.1 ml of normal saline) is given and vitrectomy should be considered. As with all forms of endogenous endophthalmitis the involvement of a pediatrician or infectious diseases specialist is essential.

REFERENCES

1. Desai P, Minassenian DC, Reidy A. National cataract survey 1997–8: a report of the results of the clinical outcomes. Br J Ophthalmol 1999; 83: 1336–40.
2. Wheeler DT, Stager DR, Weakley DR. Endophthalmitis following pediatric intraocular surgery for congenital cataract and congenital glaucoma. J Pediatr Ophthalmol Strabismus 1992; 29: 139–41.
3. Good WV, Hing S, Irvine AR, et al. Postoperative endophthalmitis in children following cataract surgery. J Pediatr Ophthalmol Strabismus 1990; 27: 283–5.
4. Norregaard JC, Thoning H, Bernth-Petersen P, et al. Risk of endophthalmitis after cataract extraction: results from the International Cataract Surgery Outcomes Study. Br J Ophthalmol 1997; 81: 102–6.
5. Neuteboom GH, de Vries-Knoppert WA. Endophthalmitis after Nd:YAG laser capsulotomy. Doc Ophthalmol 1988; 70: 175–8.
6. Verbraeken H, Rysselaere M. Post-traumatic endophthalmitis. Eur J Ophthalmol 1994; 4: 1–5.
7. Endophthalmitis Vitrectomy Study Group. Results of the Endophthalmitis Vitrectomy Study. Arch Ophthalmol 1995; 113: 1479–96.
8. Sternberg P Jr, Martin DF. Management of endophthalmitis in the post-endophthalmitis vitrectomy study era Arch Ophthalmol 2001; 119: 754–5.
9. DeBry PW, Perkins TW, Heatley G, et al. Incidence of late onset bleb related complications following trabeculectomy with mitomycin. Arch Ophthalmol 2002; 120: 297–300.
10. Morad Y, Donaldson CE, Kim YM, et al. The Ahmed drainage implant in the treatment of pediatric glaucoma. Am J Ophthalmol 2003; 135: 821–9.
11. Al–Hazmi A, Zwaan J, Awad A, et al. Effectiveness and complications of mitomycin C use during pediatric glaucoma surgery. Ophthalmology 1998; 105: 1915–20.
12. Lehmann OJ, Bunce C, Matheson MM, et al. Risk factors for the development of post-trabeculectomy endophthalmitis. Br J Ophthalmol 2000; 84: 1349–53.
13. Jampel HD, Quigley HA, Kerrigan-Baumrind LA, et al. Glaucoma Surgical Outcomes Study Group. Risk factors for late-onset infection following glaucoma filtration surgery. Arch Ophthalmol 2001; 119: 1001–8.
14. Recchia FM, Baumal CR, Sivalingam A, et al. Endophthalmitis after pediatric strabismus surgery. Arch Ophthalmol 2000; 118: 939–44.

15. Carothers TS, Coats DK, McCreery KM, et al. Quantification of incidental needle and suture contamination during strabismus surgery. Binoc Vis Strabismus 2003; 18: 75–9.

16. Han DP, Wisniewski SR, Wilson LA, et al. Spectrum and susceptibilities of microbiologic isolates in the Endophthalmitis Vitrectomy Study. Arch Ophthalmol 1996; 122: 1–17.

17. Doft BH. The Endophthalmitis Vitrectomy Study. Arch Ophthalmol 1991; 109: 487–8.

18. Weinstein GS, Mondino BJ, Weinberg RJ, Biglan AW. Endophthalmitis in a pediatric population. Ann Ophthalmol 1979; 11: 935–43.

19. Caronia RM, Liebmann JM, Friedman R, et al. Trabeculectomy at the inferior limbus. Arch Ophthalmol 1996; 114: 387–91.

20. Meredith TA, Aguilar HE, Miller MJ, et al. Comparative treatment of experimental *Staphylococcus epidermidis* endophthalmitis. Arch Ophthalmol 1990; 108; 857–60.

21. Okada AA, Johnson RP, Liles WC, et al. Endogenous bacterial endophthalmitis: Report of a ten year retrospective study. Ophthalmology 1994; 101: 832–8.

22. Wong JS, Chan TK, Lee HM, Chee SP. Endogenous bacterial endophthalmitis: An East Asia experience and a reappraisal of a severe ocular affliction. Ophthalmology 2000; 107: 1483–91.

23. Baley JE, Annable WL, Kliegmann RM. Candida endophthalmitis in the premature infant. J Pediatr 1981; 98: 458–61.

24. Edwards JE, Foos RY, Montgomerie JZ, Guze LB. Ocular manifestations of Candida septicemia. Review of 76 cases of hematogenous Candida endophthalmitis. Medicine 1974; 53: 47–75.

25. Donahue SP, Greven CM, Zuravleff JJ, et al. Intraocular candidiasis in patients with candidemia. Clinical implications derived from a prospective study. Ophthalmology 1994; 101: 1302–9.

CHAPTER
22

External Eye Disease and the Oculocutaneous Disorders

John K G Dart and Mark Wilkins

INTRODUCTION

External eye disease includes a spectrum of disorders from the most common to the very rare. This chapter, whilst comprehensive, is not all-inclusive and is focused on common problems as well those rare disorders that present major management problems.

BLEPHARITIS

Chronic blepharitis is a leading cause of external disease in all age groups although patterns of disease differ in children and adults. The term is used to describe a group of disorders in which the lid margin is usually involved although not always inflamed. The disease is poorly understood with no consensus about classification, usually based on McCulley's modification of Thygeson's for adult disease,[1] few unifying pathological concepts and heterogeneous clinical features which may or may not include:

- Conjunctivitis.
- Keratitis (the latter is typically, but not always, associated with lid margin disease).
- Dermatological associations.

Blepharitis in children differs from adult disease in that seborrheic blepharitis, meibomitis and meibomian seborrhea are uncommon; dermatological associations are less frequent; and the corneal component is probably more common than in adults with different clinical features. Dividing the disease into anterior and posterior lid margin, depending on whether the signs occur anterior or posterior to the grey line, simplifies the classification and treatment which differs for anterior and posterior lid margin disease. Different types of blepharitis may co-exist in the same patient. Table 22.1 outlines a classification for pediatric chronic blepharitis and summarizes the symptoms and signs.

Pathogenesis

The pathogenesis of chronic blepharitis is poorly understood. In staphylococcal blepharitis disease is associated with *Staphylococcus aureus* and *S. epidermidis* colonization, and sometimes frank infection, of the lid margins. Colonization by *S. aureus* is often transient and the numbers of either organism may be no greater than in normal controls. Although folliculitis, styes and lid margin

Table 22.1 Classification and clinical features of blepharitis in children

Anterior lid margin Staphylococcal blepharitis			Posterior lid margin Meibomian dysfunction and meibomitis[1]	
Associated skin disease Atopic eczema Impetigo Ectodermal dysplasia			Acne rosacea[1] Ectodermal dysplasia	
Main features **Symptoms** Redness Watering Pain Photophobia Discharge Rubbing			Usually none	
Signs[2] **Lids** Unilateral/patchy lid margin involvement Folliculitis Styes	**Conjunctiva[3]** Hyperemia Mixed follicular and papillary hyperplasia Bulbar conjunctival phlyctenule	**Cornea[3]** Marginal infiltrates Coarse subepithelial punctate KERATITIS Epithelial punctate keratitis Punctate erosions Sectional vascularization Circumcorneal vascularization Corneal phlyctenule Chalazia	Chalazia Inspissated secretions expression difficult Irregular lid margins	
[1]Rare in children. [2]Often largely unilateral. [3]May occasionally occur without clinically apparent lid disease.				

ulcers may be due to infection by *S. aureus* the persistence of lid inflammation after treatment, and the development of sterile marginal ulcers and phlyctenules, are not explained by infection alone. The superficial keratopathy can be simulated in animals by exposure to bacteria free culture filtrates of staphylococci. The importance of cell-mediated immunity in the pathogenesis of the disease was shown by experimental studies in rabbits immunized with either whole *S. aureus*, or with cell wall ribitol-teichoic acid; both ulcerative keratitis, phlyctenules and marginal corneal ulcers developed after secondary challenge providing evidence for the hypothesis that these changes were due to the development of hypersensitivity to both viable and killed organisms. These findings could not be reproduced for *S. epidermidis*. Our understanding of the causes of these blinding complications of chronic blepharitis is based on these experiments. However the evidence for a similar pathogenesis in humans is minimal and the role of a hypersensitivity response is assumed rather than supported by data.[2–6]

Posterior lid margin disease has been attributed to three factors; keratinization of the meibomian ductules, the effect of bacterial lipases on the meibum at the lid margin and primary abnormalities in the production of meibum by individuals with meibomian gland disease.[7] Chalazion is a sterile granuloma that probably results from a tissue response to lipid extruded from blocked meibomian glands

Anterior blepharitis is predominantly staphylococcal in children and may involve the lid margin alone or occur with a conjunctivitis (blepharoconjunctivitis) or keratoconjunctivitis (blepharokeratoconjunctivitis). Discomfort and inflammation of the lid margins occurs in the presence of styes or folliculitis. Fibrinous scales are seen along the lid margin; where they are centered on a lash they are termed collarettes (Fig. 22.1). In mild cases children may present with chronically uncomfortable red eyes. The blepharitis may be very asymmetrical, so that children present with a unilateral red eye. The symptoms are more severe in patients with an associated keratoconjunctivitis (Table 22.1). Photophobia can be severe in these cases, is often noticed by the parents, and may be bad enough to limit activity. The signs of lid disease as well as of keratoconjunctivitis are often asymmetrical although asymptomatic eyes usually show some clinical signs. Mild disease activity, without symptoms, results in inferior tarsal conjunctivitis and inferior punctate keratopathy.

In advanced disease the conjunctivitis, usually mixed follicular and papillary, extends from the lower to the upper tarsal conjunctiva (Fig. 22.2), there may be a limbitis and conjunctival phlyctenules (Fig. 22.3). The corneal disease results in an intense inferior punctate keratopathy, with peripheral corneal scarring and vascularization at the site of phlyctenules, and inferior marginal ulceration (Fig. 22.4). Vision may be affected, sometimes severely, by extension of marginal infiltrative keratitis with sectoral vascularization (Fig. 22.5), by central phlyctenules (Fig. 22.6) or by subepithelial punctate opacities (Fig. 22.7). Rarely acute corneal perforations occur at the site of corneal phlyctens. All these aspects of the disease are thought to be due to a cell-mediated immune response to staphylococcal antigen.

Posterior blepharitis arises from meibomian gland dysfunction. Apart from the development of unsightly chalazia, and the short-term discomfort sometimes associated with the development of these, this condition is usually asymptomatic in children.

Dermatological associations with blepharitis are less common in children than in adults, rosacea is rare in children.[8,9] However ectodermal dysplasia is associated with both anterior and posterior lid margin disease and treatment of blepharitis will improve comfort and the ocular surface in patients with this.

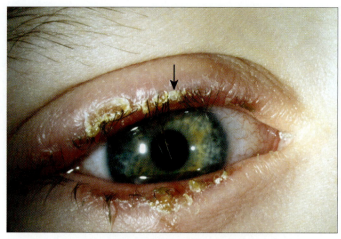

Fig. 22.1 Anterior staphylococcal blepharitis with fibrinous exudates on the anterior lid margin. The arrow indicates a collarette. (Courtesy of Mala Viswalingham.)

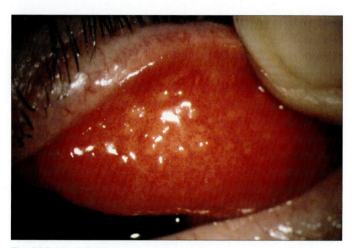

Fig. 22.2 Mixed follicular and papillary blepharoconjunctivitis. The larger pale elevations are follicles surrounded by small hyperemic papillae. (Courtesy of Mala Viswalingham.)

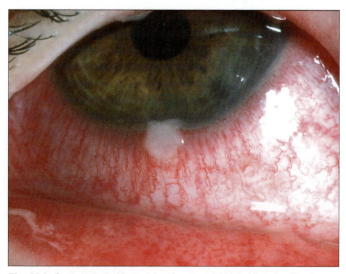

Fig. 22.3 Conjunctival phlyctenule. (Courtesy of Mala Viswalingham.)

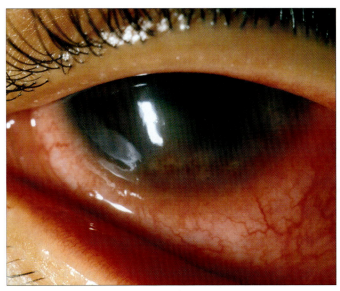

Fig. 22.4 Intense peripheral corneal vascularization and infiltrate in blepharokeratoconjunctivitis. (Courtesy of Mala Viswalingham.)

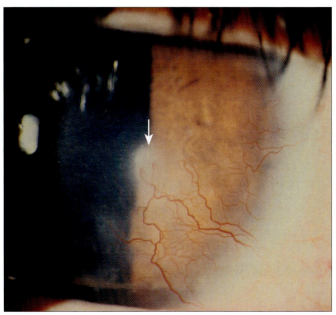

Fig. 22.5 Sectoral vascularization and scarring in blepharokeratoconjunctivitis with a new infiltrate at the apex of the lesion (see arrow). (Courtesy of Mala Viswalingham.)

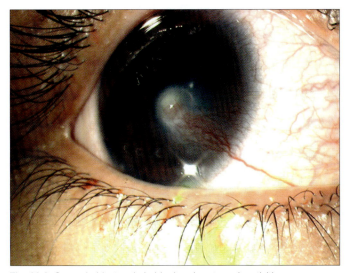

Fig. 22.6 Corneal phlyctenule in blepharokeratoconjunctivitis.

Treatment of chronic blepharitis and chalazion

The rationale for treatment is based on our imperfect understanding of the causes of the disease and is outlined in Table 22.2. The management strategy for anterior lid margin disease is to treat any acute episode of infection and then to reduce the population of bacteria on the lid margin, by simple lid hygiene and short courses of topical antibiotic, and to manage the presumed hypersensitivity response with topical steroids. Fortunately these management strategies are usually effective.[1,2] Parents and physicians often express concern about the long-term use of topical steroid that is necessary to control both the corneal components of this disease and to maintain comfort. Because central corneal scarring (Fig. 22.8) is so difficult to correct, compared to the steroid cataract that might potentially result, the use of long-term topical steroid can be justified in severe disease providing steroid glaucoma is detected. Blepharitis is uncommon before 3 years of age and most children will co-operate with tonometry. Four monthly examinations under anesthesia for tonometry are rarely needed.

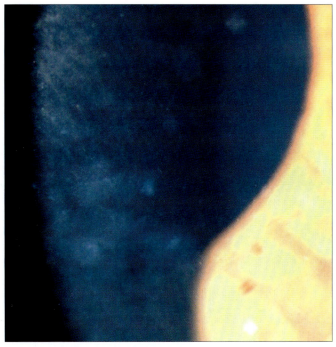

Fig. 22.7 Subepithelial punctate opacities in blepharokeratoconjunctivitis.

Chalazion is the most common problem resulting from posterior lid margin disease. Sixty percent of chalazia will resolve in 6 months and the remainder resolve spontaneously given longer. Treatment of individual chalazia, by incision and curettage, is justifiable for large lesions that affect vision by altering corneal astigmatism or when children want a cosmetic procedure. Prophylactic treatment, outlined in Table 22.2, is worthwhile for those children with frequent recurrences and is aimed at normalizing the meibomian secretions and preventing the accumulation of secretions in the gland lead to the development of chalazia.

Table 22.2 The treatment of chronic blepharitis

Aims of treatment for anterior lid margin disease	Therapeutic guidelines
Treat infection	Staphylococcal and mixed staph/seborrheic groups
	Topical antibiotics: chloramphenicol ointment (or fucithalmic), 4× daily to lid margins
	Oral oxytetracycline or erythromycin (as Erymax), 250 mg bd for 10 days
Clean lid margins	"Lid scrubs": 1–2× daily with cotton wool bud dampened in boiled water to remove debris or with proprietary lid cleaning pads[1]
Lid hyperemia and exudate	Topical Oc chloramphenicol and hydrocortisone 0.5–1% to lid margins 2–4× daily for 1 month
For associated conjunctivitis (papillary or mixed follicular and papillary)	
Reduce inflammation	G FML 0.1% 4× daily for 1 week, progressively reducing to ×1 daily over a further 4 weeks
For keratitis	
Coarse punctate keratitis and/or marginal keratitis and/or phlyctenular keratoconjunctivitis	G FML 0.1% 4× daily for 1 week, progressively reducing to ×1 daily over a further 4 weeks[2]
Corneal thinning and perforation	Exclude and treat any concomitant microbial keratitis and establish disease control by methods summarized above, apply tissue glue to perforations. Carry out tectonic keratoplasty, if necessary, once the inflammation is controlled
Aims of treatment for posterior lid margin disease	**Therapeutic guidelines**
Mechanically unblock meibomian glands	Apply hot compresses for 5 minutes to liquefy meibomian secretions, followed by massage[1] of tarsal plate with cotton wool bud (or finger), to express lipid from glands, 1–2× daily
Alter meibomian secretions	Oral erythromycin 125–250 mg bd or, in children over 12 years, oxytetracycline 250 mg bd or doxycycline 100 mg od[2]

[1]Lid scrubs , lid massage and low dose systemic antibiotics take about 4–6 weeks to start to work.
[2]More prolonged courses of steroid or more potent steroids may be needed under specialist ophthalmological supervision.

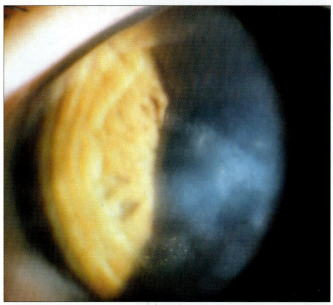

Fig. 22.8 Central cornea scaring following the resolution of blepharokeratoconjunctivitis after several years of active disease. (Courtesy of Mala Viswalingham.)

Table 22.3: Classification of other causes of chronic blepharitis in children by pathogenesis

Cause	Example
Fungal	*Candida*
Parasitic	*Phthirus pubis* (pubic louse) and pediculosis (head and body lice)
Protozoal	Leishmania
Autoimmune	Systemic lupus

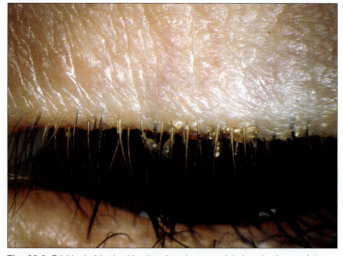

Fig. 22.9 Pthiriasis blepharitis showing the eggs (nits) at the base of the lashes.

Other causes of chronic blepharitis

The remaining causes of chronic blepharitis are all uncommon and often misdiagnosed as one of the types of chronic blepharitis described in Table 22.1. Their pathogenesis is clear. They should always be considered when therapy for staphylococcal blepharitis fails; some of the causes are outlined in Table 22.3. One of the commonest of these is lash infestation by lice (Fig. 22.9). Pubic lice (*Pthirus pubis*) are a more frequent inhabitant of lashes than head and body lice (*Pthirus palpebrarum*). Treatment is directed at the nonocular infestation and its causes, sexually transmitted diseases and child abuse must be considered in the case of *Pthirus pubis*, and pediatricians involved. Local ocular treatment is by physical removal of the eggs (nits) and lice at the slit lamp followed by use of liquid paraffin eye ointment on the lid margin

Table 22.4 Acute blepharitis	
Acute anterior lid margin	Folliculitis (infected lash follicles) External hordeoleum (stye) Angular (at lateral canthus) Impetigo Pustular (herpes)
Acute posterior lid margin	Chalazion Internal hordeoleum

twice daily for 10 days to suffocate the adult and hatching lice. Pilocarpine ointment is also directly toxic to adult lice. Physostigmine and mercury containing ophthalmic ointments, said to be effective against both lice and eggs, are no longer available in the UK. The insecticides for use on body hair are toxic to the eye and direct application to the lashes should be avoided.

Acute blepharitis

Acute blepharitis is a well-defined group of conditions, which may overlap with chronic blepharitis, these are summarized in Table 22.4.

Phlyctenular keratoconjunctivitis is characterized by inflammatory conjunctival and corneal nodules, may occur in settings other than that of chronic anterior lid margin blepharitis. Phlyctenules represent a cell-mediated response to antigens, usually staphylococcal, but may occur with tuberculosis, and infection with protozoa (leishmania), parasitic worms and local chlamydial and candida infection. Children developing phlyctenules, in areas where tuberculosis is common, should be screened for tuberculosis, when the signs of chronic staphylococcal blepharitis are absent. Corneal phlyctenules can lead to perforation of the cornea, as well as to loss of vision due to scarring, when intensive topical steroid therapy, with antibiotics if an epithelial defect is present, are needed. Systemic antibiotics, as recommended for the management of the other manifestations of blepharitis in Table 22.2, appear to reduce the frequency and severity of relapses.[10]

CONJUNCTIVITIS

Conjunctivitis in the neonatal period, ophthalmia neonatorum, is described in Chapter 19. In older children a working diagnosis of the causes of conjunctivitis can be reached using the algorithm in Fig. 22.10 which bases the working diagnosis on the length of history and the predominant clinical signs.

Acute bacterial conjunctivitis

Acute bacterial conjunctivitis is a common disorder in young children. It is bilateral, mucopurulent, with papillary conjunctivitis. *H. influenzae* and *S. pneumoniae* and *Moraxella* are common causes.[11,12] Transmission is by hand or by spread from the nasopharynx. Molecular analysis has shown that in a child with conjunctivitis the strain of *H. influenzae* isolated from the conjunctiva matches the strain from the nasopharynx[13] and the middle ear.[14] As many as one quarter of children with conjunctivitis may also have an otitis media which may be asymptomatic.[14,15] Cultures are unnecessary in patients with signs of bacterial conjunctivitis. Bacterial conjunctivitis can usually be differentiated

from viral conjunctivitis by the absence of the following signs that are often present in viral conjunctivitis:

- Systemic symptoms of an upper respiratory tract infection.
- Preauricular lymphadenopathy.
- A mixed follicular and papillary conjunctivitis.
- A diffuse punctate keratopathy within 3 days of the onset.
- A watery discharge. Some patients with viral conjunctivitis will go on to develop a mucopurulent discharge.

Hyperpurulent bacterial conjunctivitis

Hyperpurulent bacterial conjunctivitis is an important disease because of its morbidity. It is severe with rapid onset of lid swelling, excessive discharge, tenderness, conjunctival swelling and preauricular lymphadenopathy. The most common organisms involved are *N. gonorrhea* and *N. meningitidis*, although staphylococci, streptococci and *Pseudomonas* sp. also cause this. *N. gonorrhea* is usually sexually acquired beyond the neonatal period. It can cause microbial keratitis and rapid progression to corneal perforation. *N. meningitidis* (Fig. 22.11) can also cause keratitis but is associated with systemic meningococcal disease.

Membranous bacterial conjunctivitis

Membranous bacterial conjunctivitis in which the conjunctival epithelium necroses and sloughs, resulting in a membrane firmly adherent to the underlying substantia propria that separates with bleeding, is caused by *C. diphtheriae* and *S. pyogenes*. There may be associated corneal infiltrates, epithelial sloughing or frank microbial keratitis. There may be a bacteriemia or systemic disease. Conjunctival scarring with symblepharon, entropion, trichiasis and tear deficiency follow. The differential is from pseudomembranous conjunctivitis, in which the inflammation is less severe causing thick conjunctival exudates without epithelial necrosis which may be caused by:

- *Neisseria* sp. as a complication of hyperpurulent conjunctivitis.
- A severe acute conjunctivitis caused by *Haemophilus influenzae*, *S. pyogenes*, *S. aureus*.
- *Candida*.
- Adenovirus and herpes simplex virus.

Stevens–Johnson syndrome and ligneous conjunctivitis produce a similar appearance but in a completely different clinical setting (see below).

Diagnosis
Diagnosis is clinical for acute conjunctivitis. Investigations are only necessary for persistent acute conjunctivitis when nonbacterial causes should be included in the differential. For hyperpurulent and membranous conjunctivitis urgent Gram stain, and cultures, are required to exclude infection with *Neisseria* sp. and confirm the diagnosis. Viral cultures should be included.

Treatment
Acute bacterial conjunctivitis is usually a self-limiting condition, but topical therapy has been shown to produce a more rapid clinical resolution, and a higher eradication rate of bacteria.[16] No single topical preparation covers all possible pathogens.

Topical treatment
Frequency is 6–8× daily with drops, or 4× daily with ointments, for 2 or 3 days until the symptoms are controlled after which treatment frequency can be halved for another 3 days. Treatment choices are:
- Broad spectrum single agents–chloramphenicol.

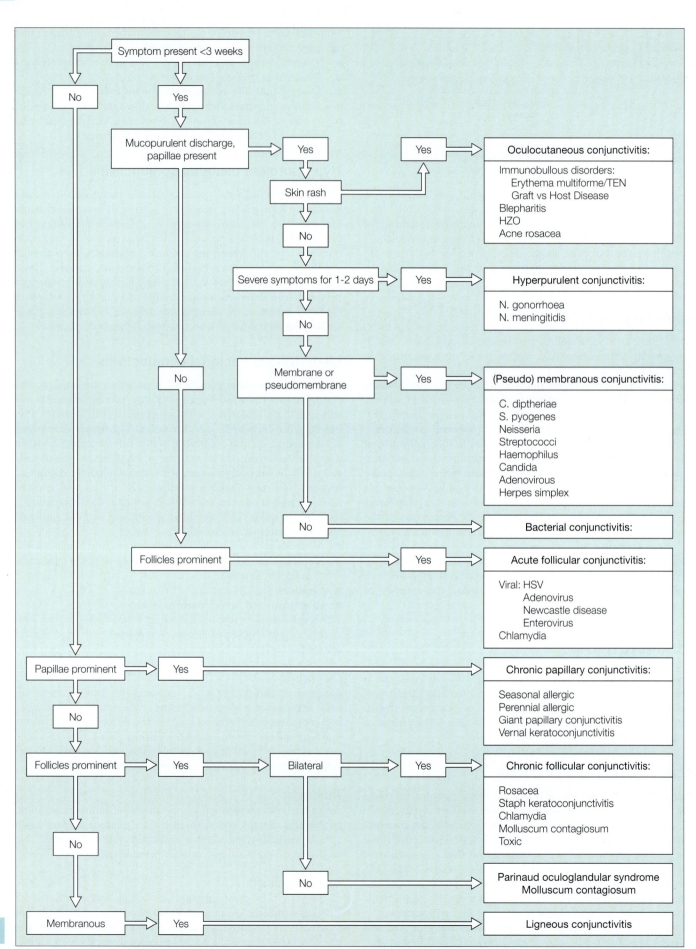

Fig. 22.10 Algorithm for the differential diagnosis of conjunctivitis.

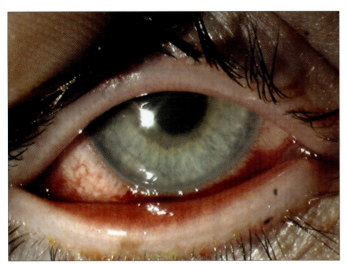

Fig. 22.11 Hyperacute *N. meningitides* conjunctivitis with a central corneal epithelial erosion. (Courtesy of Seema Verma.)

- Broad-spectrum combinations–polymyxin B sulfate with trimethoprim, polymyxin B sulfate with bacitracin zinc, gramicidin with neomycin sulfate and polymyxin B sulfate.
- Gram-positive infections–trimethoprim and polymyxin B sulfate.
- Gram-negative infections–gentamicin, tobramycin.

Quinolones (i.e. ciprofloxacin and ofloxacin) are effective broad spectrum agents to which streptococci are relatively resistant. However acquired resistance to both Gram-positive and Gram-negative organisms is becoming a problem and their broad spectrum ophthalmic use should be restricted to their use in keratitis.

Systemic treatment

This is necessary for patients with hyperpurulent or membranous conjunctivitis and immunosuppressed patients. These should be admitted for observation until the diagnosis and management have been confirmed, and for observation, as both systemic and acute corneal complications can develop rapidly. Hyperpurulent conjunctivitis suspected to be due to gonococcus requires a single intramuscular injection of ceftriaxone (50 mg/kg). For suspected *N. meningitidis*, and other suspected bacterial causes of membranous conjunctivitis, penicillin G intramuscularly, or by infusion, is given 4× daily.[17] Adjunctive topical therapy is not needed, unless the cornea is involved, when any keratitis should be treated with broad spectrum therapy (see below) until the microbiological diagnosis has been established. For *Haemophilus influenzae* conjunctivitis, with otitis media, oral amoxicillin, cefuroxime or cefixime is indicated.[18]

Acute follicular conjunctivitis

An acute follicular conjunctivitis, usually a mixed follicular and papillary reaction, is the typical conjunctival response to infection by viral or chlamydial organisms. Adenovirus, herpes virus and chlamydia account for the majority of cases in which a causative organism can be identified. Newcastle disease virus and enteroviruses also cause keratoconjunctivitis.

Adenovirus causes a range of infections of mucosal surfaces. Some of these only affect the conjunctiva and others cause respiratory infection and genital infection which may or may not

be associated with keratoconjunctivitis. These disease syndromes are caused by different adenovirus serotypes, although there is some overlap; for example adenovirus type 8 is almost exclusively associated with epidemic keratoconjunctivitis whereas type 11 may cause upper respiratory tract infection, acute follicular conjunctivitis, pharyngoconjunctival fever (PCF), epidemic keratoconjunctivitis (EKC) and venereal disease.

The three syndromes affecting the eyes are acute follicular conjunctivitis, pharyngoconjunctival fever and epidemic keratoconjunctivitis.[19]

Acute follicular conjunctivitis is a mild disease most often caused by serotypes 1–11 and 19, is common in children, and is often associated with an acute upper respiratory tract infection. It requires no treatment and there are no sequelae.

Pharyngoconjunctival fever is commonly caused by serotypes 3,4 and 7 and is a more severe disease which is often heralded by a high fever, pharyngitis, acute follicular conjunctivitis (Fig. 22.12) and sometimes malaise vomiting and diarrhea, particularly in children. There may be petechial conjunctival hemorrhages with the follicular conjunctivitis, a punctate keratopathy is usual (Fig. 22.13), but the later development of subepithelial infiltrates, as in EKC, is infrequent. The disease usually resolves fully, without treatment, within 2 weeks.

Epidemic keratoconjunctivitis, most often caused by serotypes 8, 19 and 37 generally causes a conjunctivitis with a variable

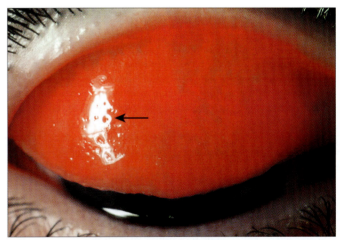

Fig. 22.12 Acute follicular adenovirus conjunctivitis within 24 hours of onset. The small follicles can be seen in the specular reflex (arrow) surrounded by infiltrated and hyperemic conjunctiva.

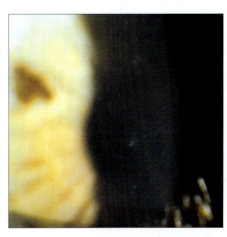

Fig. 22.13 Epithelial infiltrates from the same case as Fig. 22.12.

preauricular and submandibular lymphadenopathy. There may less often be an associated upper respiratory tract infection, urethritis and cervicitis. The symptoms and signs are usually of rapid onset and predominantly unilateral. This syndrome is often epidemic and transmitted by contact with:

- Infected hands.
- Infected towels.
- Contaminated ophthalmic instruments.
- Infected eye drops.
- Droplet infection from patients with an associated upper respiratory tract infection.
- Contaminated surfaces where the virus is now known to survive for prolonged periods.

The presenting features are severe discomfort, photophobia, conjunctival edema, and small subconjunctival hemorrhages. Pseudomembranes can develop on the tarsal conjunctiva, usually after 7 days. A marked punctate keratitis is often present in the first few days; this is followed after 3–5 days by a focal epithelial keratitis. These corneal changes are then followed after 2 weeks by the development of subepithelial infiltrates. By week 3 the epithelial changes subside, leaving the subepithelial infiltrates which may persist for weeks, months or years.

Treatment

No treatment is required for mild cases. A short course of broad spectrum topical antibiotics may be given at the onset when the differential diagnosis is hyperacute bacterial conjunctivitis. These are unnecessary once a typical viral keratitis has developed. Topical steroids potentiate viral replication within the first two weeks of infections when they should be avoided unless early pseudomembrane formation is severe. After 2 weeks viral cultures are negative and topical steroid, dexamethasone 0.1% for severe disease or fluorometholone, for milder disease, is very effective in treating both pseudomembranes and symptomatic keratitis. The use of topical steroids in the treatment of adenovirus keratoconjunctivitis remains controversial and untested by clinical trials. Early use (within 1–2 weeks) of topical steroids may increase the viral load and exacerbate the late keratopathy whereas late use (after 2 weeks) may result in prolonging the recovery from the keratopathy even though virus can seldom be recovered at this stage. Topical steroids will result in rapid resolution of symptoms and signs of the disease and our recommendation is to use these to control symptoms that are causing significant patient morbidity, after discussing the option not to treat with the family.

Prevention

Prevention is important as this is a highly infectious disease. Children should be kept off school for 2 weeks if the index of suspicion of EKC is high. Good personal hygiene, with the use of separate face towels, is essential to avoid spread. Patients attending our hospital, with acute conjunctivitis, are seen promptly in a separate area where they cannot mix with other patients or contaminate surfaces unnecessarily.

Herpes simplex

Herpes simplex conjunctivitis or blepharoconjunctivitis (Fig. 22.14) is common in children developing the primary infection although these disorders may also represent recurrent disease following asymptomatic primary infection. The conjunctivitis is often unilateral, follicular and associated with preauricular lymphadenopathy. After 1 week, vesicles can develop on the conjunctiva

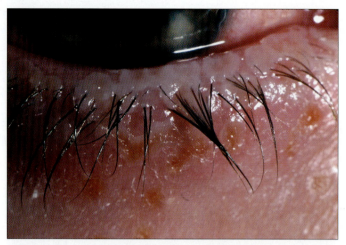

Fig. 22.14 Herpes simplex virus blepharoconjunctivitis showing focal skin lesions and unruptured vesicles at the lid margin. (Courtesy of Mala Viswalingham.)

or lids. A keratitis may develop at the same time. When it does it ranges from diffuse punctate to dendriform. Corneal stromal involvement may occur with the first clinical manifestation of the disease (although this is not necessarily the primary infection) although it usually occurs with recurrences. Atopes, and the immunocompromised, often present with bilateral herpes conjunctivitis or keratitis. Treatment of conjunctivitis or blepharoconjunctivitis is with acyclovir ointment five times a day for 1 week, or if topical acyclovir is unavailable, vidarabine or trifluorothymidine. Oral acyclovir is also effective. The management of HSV keratitis is discussed below.

Chlamydia

Chlamydial conjunctivitis from C. *trachomatis* serotypes D–K is sexually acquired outside of the neonatal period. It presents with a follicular and papillary conjunctivitis with mucopurulent discharge and preauricular lymphadenopathy. Initially there is acute conjunctival inflammation and infiltrate with follicles becoming prominent, particularly in the lower tarsal and bulbar conjunctiva. The cornea can show a superficial punctate keratitis followed by subepithelial opacities and peripheral vessels in chronic disease. Diagnosis is by conjunctival smears and culture. Treatment is with a single dose of azithromycin or a 2 week course of erythromycin. Children need further investigation for other sexually transmitted diseases, and assessment as to whether they are the victims of sexual abuse.

Chronic follicular conjunctivitis

The normal conjunctiva in children may have prominent clear conjunctival follicles in the fornices extending into the tarsal conjunctiva which can be distinguished from the diseased conjunctiva by the absence of an associated conjunctival infiltrate obscuring the tarsal conjunctival vessels (Fig. 22.15). Most patients with a chronic follicular conjunctivitis have a mixed papillary and follicular reaction. Blepharoconjunctivitis is probably the commonest cause of this and has already been discussed. Acute chlamydial disease, discussed above, will become chronic and persist for months, if untreated, and should always be considered as a cause of chronic follicular disease with the other rare chlamydial infections (endemic trachoma, feline pneumonitis,

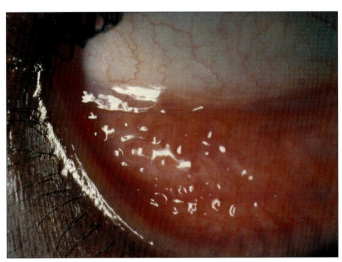

Fig. 22.15 Conjunctival folliculosis.

psittacosis and lymphogranuloma venereum). Moraxella conjunctivitis and chronic canaliculitis, caused by *Actinomyces* sp. are also rare causes of a chronic mixed papillary and follicular conjunctivitis. Other common causes are described below. Toxic conjunctivitis may cause a predominantly papillary or mixed papillary and follicular conjunctivitis and is discussed in the section on papillary conjunctivitis.

Molluscum contagiosum

Molluscum contagiosum is a frequently missed cause of a chronic relapsing follicular conjunctivitis (Fig. 22.16). It is usually, but not always unilateral, and with Parinaud's oculoglandular syndrome should be considered as a cause of unilateral follicular conjunctivitis. The molluscum lesions may be very small and are usually in the lash line, they can also mimic a sebaceous cyst. Treatment is by curettage of the lesion; histopathology of the curetting will confirm the diagnosis. Symptoms usually subside rapidly without treatment after the removal of the molluscum; a 2 week course of topical steroid can be given, but its use deferred, unless symptoms persist.

Parinaud oculoglandular syndrome

Parinaud's oculoglandular syndrome is a rare condition causing a unilateral granulomatous conjunctivitis which in children may also be follicular. This syndrome is usually a rare manifestation of

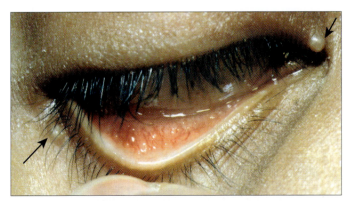

Fig. 22.16 Molluscum contagiosum showing molluscum skin lesions (arrows) and the associated inferior tarsal follicular conjunctivitis. Reproduced with permission from Bruns T, Breathnach S, et al. The Skin and Eyes. In: Rook's Textbook of Dermatology: 7th edition. London: Blackwell Publishing Ltd; 2004.

cat-scratch disease, caused by *Bartonella henselae* and *Afipia felis*, when inoculation of the organisms is directly into the conjunctiva rather than by the skin trauma which is the usual route. This results in conjunctivitis and regional lymphadenopathy which generally resolve spontaneously after some weeks. The diagnosis can be confirmed by serology at a national reference center. Treatment with oral doxycycline or erythromycin or ciprofloxacin has been reportedly effective. Other causes of Parinaud oculoglandular syndrome include tularemia, sporotrichosis, tuberculosis and syphilis amongst other rare associations.

Ophthalmia nodosa

Caterpillar or other insect hairs, both barbed and unbarbed, can cause a prolonged inflammatory conjunctivitis; keratitis, iridocyclitis and even endophthalmitis have been recorded.

Chronic papillary conjunctivitis

Chronic papillary conjunctivitis occurs in all patients with moderate or severe allergic eye disease. Seasonal and perennial allergic conjunctivitis, vernal keratoconjunctivitis and giant papillary conjunctivitis all occur in children and are discussed here.[20] A chronic papillary reaction also occurs in some patients with toxic keratoconjunctivitis, and keratoconjunctivitis artefacta which are discussed below.

Seasonal and perennial allergic conjunctivitis (SAC and PAC)

Seasonal allergic conjunctivitis, also known as hay fever conjunctivitis, is a type I hypersensitivity response to a seasonal allergen such as grass or tree pollen. In individuals with PAC there is usually a response to the seasonal allergens that precipitate SAC but, in addition, there is a clinically significant type 1 response to allergens that are present year round, or which may increase in the winter, such as house dust mite and animal dander. Both conditions are usually bilateral and symmetrical resulting in itching, tearing, photophobia, and the production of sticky white and stringy mucous discharge. The conjunctiva is hyperemic, although relatively pale conjunctival edema, which rapidly resolves, may be present during acute exacerbations. Conjunctival papillae are uncommon in SAC, probably because of the short duration of each episode, whereas in PAC a chronic papillary reaction (Fig. 22.17) is a normal finding. The cornea is usually unaffected. It is now recognized that together with the classic type I hypersensitivity reaction resulting in IgE mediated mast cell degranulation, there is a late-phase reaction with recruitment of TH2 cells by cytokines released from mast cells.[21]

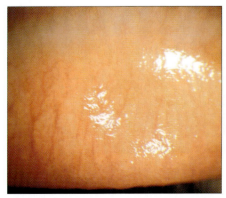

Fig. 22.17 Upper tarsal conjunctival infiltrate. Note the hazy view of the tarsal blood vessels due to the thickened conjunctiva, and the very small papillae in the specular reflex (compare with the larger size of follicles in Figs 22.2, 22.12, 22.15 and 22.16).

Vernal keratoconjunctivitis

Vernal keratoconjunctivitis (VKC) is an uncommon childhood condition that resolves in 90% by adulthood. It usually presents between the ages of 3 and 5. It is a perennial condition with seasonal exacerbations, classically in the spring, hence the name "vernal". It is more common in boys, in patients with a personal or family history of atopy, and in children in warm, dry climates.

VKC presents with bilateral itch, tearing, foreign body sensation and photophobia. Associated with this is the production of a dense mucus discharge. The intense photophobia and discomfort may result in behavioral problems.

Clinical signs and pathogenesis in VKC

Understanding the pathogenesis is important to the rational management of the disease. The conjunctival signs may predominate in the tarsal conjunctiva, when the disease is known as palpebral VKC (Fig. 22.18), or the limbus, when it is known as limbal VKC (Fig. 22.19) although a mixed picture sometimes occurs. In palpebral VKC the florid conjunctival infiltrate leads to the development of compound ("giant") papillae on the upper tarsal conjunctiva. This results in thickening of the upper lid and a ptosis. In limbal VKC papillae develop along the limbus; during

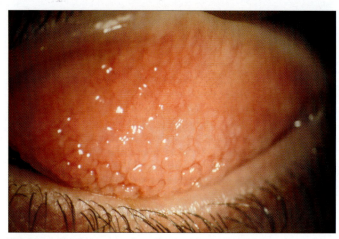

Fig. 22.18 Giant (compound) papillae in palpebral vernal keratoconjunctivitis.

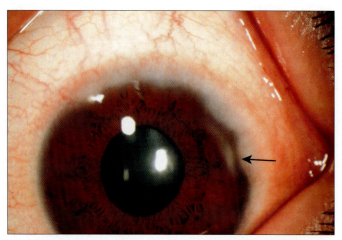

Fig. 22.19 Pale limbal papillae in limbal vernal. The arrow identifies an arcus (pseudogerontoxon) that sometimes develops after severe inflammation in limbal vernal.

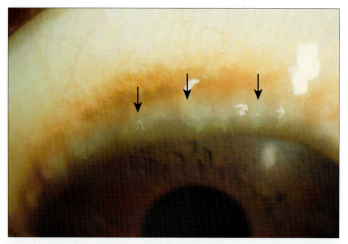

Fig. 22.20 Trantas dots in limbal VKC. These are very small pale dots at the apices of the papillae (see arrows).

exacerbations white pinhead size Horner–Trantas dots, composed of eosinophilic debris, are seen at the apices of the limbal papillae and occasionally elsewhere on the conjunctiva (Fig. 22.20). In severe cases the papillae coalesce to form a thickened gelatinous ring which may extend into the cornea.

The difference in severity between VKC and SAC/PAC is due to the cellular response seen in the conjunctiva. Like SAC and PAC, VKC involves a type I and type IV hypersensitivity response. However in VKC the type IV response triggers the recruitment of large numbers of T helper cells which in turn leads to increased numbers of eosinophils, basophils, macrophages, mast cells, and fibroblasts.[22] Release of inflammatory mediators by these cells results in severe corneal complications.[23]

The corneal component of the disease may affect vision severely and is usually worst in palpebral disease; Figure 22.21 illustrates a simplified pathogenesis of vernal plaque. During reactivation of disease (Fig. 22.21a) the most frequent corneal sign is a diffuse punctate epitheliopathy, affecting the upper half of the cornea, where it is in contact with the upper tarsus (Fig. 22.21b), although this may extend to involve the whole cornea. In more severe exacerbations mucous adheres to the punctate erosions and this may progress to the development of confluent punctate corneal erosions and the development of a macroerosion (Fig. 22.21c). Macroerosions may resolve without corneal signs but, within a day or two of progressive disease, mature into a raised corneal plaque (Fig. 22.21d) (vernal plaque or shield ulcer) consisting of mucous and eosinophilic debris adherent to Bowman's layer. Plaques leave ring scars that affect vision (Fig. 22.21e). Plaques usually occur in the superior half of the cornea, where the corneal epithelium is in direct contact with the tarsal conjunctiva, but these will involve the visual axis in severe disease. Plaque results from release of inflammatory mediators by eosinophils and mast cells in the papillae rather than from mechanical abrasion by the papillae. Because of these corneal changes VKC is a sight threatening process that requires prompt and appropriate treatment.

Giant (contact lens associated) papillary conjunctivitis is a conjunctival foreign body response, typically in children wearing ocular prostheses or contact lenses, and less often to exposed sutures or exposed scleral buckles. Symptoms are of itch, irritation and mucous production. Where a contact lens triggers the conjunctivitis they also complain of blurred vision and reduced wear time. On examination giant (>0.3 mm) papillae are seen on the upper tarsal conjunctiva. Although a type I and type IV

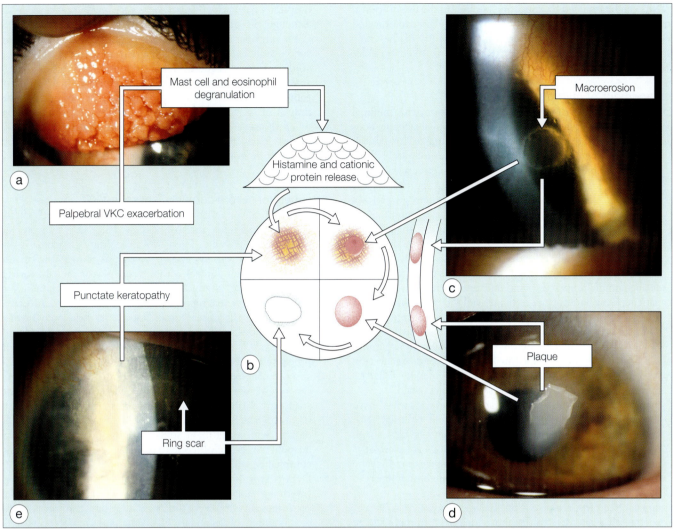

Fig. 22.21 The pathogenesis of vernal plaque. (a) The tarsal conjunctiva becomes inflamed with increased mucous production due to mast cell degranulation and histamine release. Eosinophil degranulation releases cationic proteins that are epitheliotoxic resulting in (b) associated corneal punctate keratopathy with adherent mucous. (c) If the inflammation continues a confluent area of epithelium breaks down to form a macroerosion. (d) Epithelial and eosinophilic debris are deposited on Bowman's membrane in the base of the macroerosion to form a vernal plaque. (e) Whether this is removed with lamellar dissection or epithelializes a ring scar results. The diagram illustrates the corneal staining pattern with Rose Bengal. Figures (a) and (d) reproduced with permission from Bruns T, Breathnach S, et al. The Skin and Eyes. In: Rook's Textbook of Dermatology: 7th edition. London: Blackwell Publishing Ltd; 2004.

hypersensitivity response is again responsible the lower level of eosinophilic infiltration probably explains why the cornea is rarely involved.

Diagnosis

These clinical features, with a personal or family history of atopy, are sufficient to confirm the diagnosis for most cases. Laboratory investigations are only needed in patients not responding to therapy or who require topical (or systemic) steroid therapy for relief of symptoms when the diagnosis is uncertain. Conjunctival cytology for eosinophils and mast cells is difficult to carry out well and requires an experienced pathologist for interpretation. It is usually positive in acute exacerbations of VKC and in about 50% of patients with SAC and PAC. Serum IgE and skin prick tests, although often requested by parents, have no value as the results do not indicate the antigens precipitating the eye disease. Identification of a potential allergen rarely causes a change in therapy, providing that appropriate environmental controls, including restricting the movement of pets around the house,

have been implemented. Upper tarsal conjunctival biopsy is the gold standard for confirmation of the disease but is often negative in patients treated with topical steroids; it should be carried out after a 2 week washout of topical steroids and is only necessary to confirm a very uncertain clinical diagnosis. Tear IgE is locally produced in the eye and elevated in most patients with atopic eye diseases but false positives occur in patients with atopic dermatitis having very high serum IgE due to conjunctival transudation. However an easily performed office test for tear IgE is now available (*Lacrytest* from Adiatec SA, France) and a positive result will confirm the diagnosis in all except the highly atopic.

Treatment

Treatment involves the use of a combination of drugs including mast cell stabilizers, topical and systemic antihistamines, non-steroidal anti-inflammatory drops, steroids and cyclosporine. Guidelines for the use of all these drugs are given below. Exacerbations of VKC may occur very rapidly and demand prompt access to the clinic.

Visits can be reduced by educating families in the use of topical steroids, so that changes in both the potency preparation and frequency of use can be introduced independently of the clinic with reporting of this at routine attendances to maintain side-effect monitoring.

Management of mild disease

Management of mild disease (conjunctival disease with minimal corneal involvement as in seasonal and perennial allergic conjunctivitis (SAC and PAC), giant papillary conjunctivitis (GPC) and mild vernal keratoconjunctivitis (VKC) is as follows.

- Mast cell stabilizers are very safe and quite effective; topical cromones (sodium cromoglycate 2–4%, or the newer nedocromil, lodoxamide) are first line treatment given 1–4× daily depending on symptoms. The newer cromones have been more effective in trials of SAC[24,25] and are the authors' first choice. Patients need to be told that they can take 1–2 weeks to be fully effective.

- Olopatadine has both mast cell stabilizing activity and antihistaminic properties[26] and may be a useful alternative for patients using both topical cromones and topical antihistamines.

- Topical antihistamines are effective for relief of symptoms in SAC and PAC but, in our experience, have little effect in GPC or VKC. The potent new topical antihistamines (levocabastine or emedastine) or a second generation systemic antihistamine (such as loratadine) may be added to the use of the mast cell stabilizers already described.

- Nonsteroidal anti-inflammatory drugs: several trials have shown that oral aspirin has been helpful in children with vernal keratoconjunctivitis, however they must be old enough to meet the recommendations for its use. Topical ketorolac is unhelpful in severe disease in our experience but may be useful as an alternative or adjunctive to mast cell stabilizers in SAC and PAC.

- Topical steroids are used to manage disease that is not adequately responsive to the above measures. In more severe disease both mast cell stabilizers and antihistamines may not be tolerated until the inflammation is brought under control with high-dose topical steroids when these steroid sparing drugs can be reintroduced and the steroid tailed off. Steroids complement the action of the mast cell stabilizers and antihistamines and their use is minimized by adding the steroid to the nonsteroidal drugs that have been found helpful for milder disease in any individual patient. A "safe" steroid with a lower (1%) risk of precipitating glaucoma (fluorometholone or rimexolone), used 1–4× daily as required, is adequate for the management of exacerbations in mild disease.

- Additional treatment for GPC includes replacing scratched rigid contact lenses or prostheses, optimizing their fit to reduce conjunctival trauma, and the use of a rigorous hygiene regimen with a microsphere cleaner and protein removing tablets 1–3× weekly. Topical steroids can be used freely in blind eyes with prostheses. Steroids are usually only necessary in CL users who have atopic eye disease with keratoconus; intraocular pressure measurement is less precise in keratoconus and discs and fields need careful monitoring to prevent steroid side-effects when steroids are used for prolonged periods.

- Topical cyclosporine is not yet available commercially, although a preparation designed for use in dry eye (Restasis Allergan USA) was licensed in the USA in 2003 and is expected to be available in Europe soon. It has shown promise in trials for atopic keratoconjunctivitis and may be effective in VKC. Trials of cyclosporine 2% in oil (available from some hospital pharmacies) have been very encouraging in VKC although the oil-based products are poorly tolerated.[27] The 0.2% veterinary ointment (Optimmune, Schering) has been successfully used by the authors. Adverse effects, apart from stinging, are infrequent and introduction of the drug as a steroid sparing agent, for patients requiring high doses of topical steroids, has allowed reduction or complete withdrawal of steroids in many cases. It is used by the authors when the severity of the corneal disease demands prolonged use of strong topical steroids. Topical cyclosporine is most successfully tolerated if introduced during remissions and used 2–3× daily.

Treatment of severe corneal disease in VKC

- Substitute dexamethasone 0.1% or prednisolone forte 1% for the "safe" steroids and use 2–12× daily. Use unpreserved drops where possible. These will precipitate glaucoma in 1% of patients, as well as cataract, so that as soon as the disease is brought under control with a frequency of 2× daily switch back to a "safe" steroid. Very high treatment frequency is needed to treat macroerosion. Drops may be more effective if applied to the upper fornix. Upon the development of a macroerosion some practitioners will reduce the steroid because of concern about corneal melting; however this will precipitate the development of plaque and melting, in the absence of infection, probably never occurs. Bacterial keratitis can rarely supervene and a short course of intensive broad spectrum antibiotics given if it is suspected. Steroid ointment, such as Betnesol, may be useful at night and during the day, to reduce treatment application frequency. Admission to hospital may be helpful due to the change of environment and compliance with a complicated regimen.

- Depot steroid injections given into the upper fornix (methylprednisolone acetate 40 mg) can be very effective for control of severe disease although their safety in terms of the development of secondary glaucoma and cataractogenesis is uncertain.

- Systemic immunosuppression may be needed in severe exacerbations of disease, a 3–4 week course of systemic steroids starting at a dose of 1 mg/kg can bring the disease under control while topical therapy is introduced. Patients with a previous history of labial or ocular herpes should be put on oral prophylaxis with acyclovir 400 mg bd or 200 mg bd if under 2 years old; topical prophylaxis is unnecessary and may complicate the clinical signs in patients with a complex keratoconjunctivitis. For a small number of patients systemic cyclosporine (Neoral, Novartis) starting at 5 mg/kg can be very helpful.

- Vernal plaque is managed by control of the underlying conjunctival disease that has precipitated plaque formation. If plaques are left as persistent epithelial defects they will vascularize or become infected. If the plaque does not epithelialize spontaneously this can be achieved rapidly by a superficial keratectomy with a scleral pocket knife. It is essential to have good disease control before carrying this out to avoid a rapid recurrence.

Oculocutaneous conjunctivitis

Several of the immunobullous disorders result in conjunctivitis (oculocutaneous conjunctivitis) which can in turn cause blinding corneal disease. Of these disorders pemphigus vulgaris, bullous and cicatricial pemphigoid, epidermolysis bullosa, linear IgA disease, dermatitis herpetiformis and lichen planus rarely cause disease in children and will not be discussed further here. Of the remaining conditions erythema multiforme minor causes a self-limiting papillary conjunctivitis with relatively minor involvement of the skin and mucosa. However Stevens–Johnson syndrome (also known as erythema multiforme major), toxic epidermal necrolysis (TEN), a more severe form of STS, and graft-versus-host disease (GVHD) may all cause severe and very similar ocular disease with the same treatment options and these will be discussed here.

Immunobullous disorders

Stevens–Johnson syndrome and toxic epidermal necrolysis cause malaise and a prodrome followed by the development of skin lesions (Fig. 22.22). The typical lesions are target in appearance and can progress to a papular rash. Blisters and bullae are extensive in severe SJS and TEN. Mucosal lesions are common especially the lips and buccal mucosa. However any mucosal surface in the body can be affected. In severe cases the mortality rate varies from 5% in SJS to 25% in SJS/TEN. In Germany a national reporting system identified an incidence of 1.8 per million affecting all ages. It is more common in patients with human immunodeficiency virus (HIV). Typically the disease has been precipitated by infections, such as herpes simplex virus, influenza and mycoplasma, and drugs. Drugs that have been implicated in a case–control study are both antibiotics (co-trimoxazole, sulfonamides, aminopenicillins, quinolones and cephalosporins) and drugs used for the therapy of chronic diseases (carbamazepine, phenobarbital, phenytoin, valproic acid, oxicam-NSAIDs and allopurinol). Cell-mediated immunity has been implicated in the skin reactions and circulating autoantibodies producing an allergic vasculitis secondary to deposition of immune complexes in blood vessel walls.

The ocular complications of SJS and TEN are identical and around 70% of patients admitted for treatment of these diseases will develop eye disease.[28] It is the eye disease which leads to the most profound long-term morbidity in many of these patients. In addition, the eye disease, unlike the lesions affecting the remaining mucosal surfaces, may progress years after the acute episode

has resolved. The ocular disease is more common in affected children.

Acute ocular complications usually occur concurrently with the skin disease but may sometimes precede it by several days. The conjunctivitis varies from a papillary reaction with watery discharge to a membranous conjunctivitis with sloughing of the conjunctival epithelium (Fig. 22.23). Corneal epithelial defects are common and may progress to corneal ulceration with or without bacterial superinfection.[29] The morbidity of the disease may be due to the acute corneal complications but is more usually due to the results of the conjunctival scarring (Fig. 22.24).

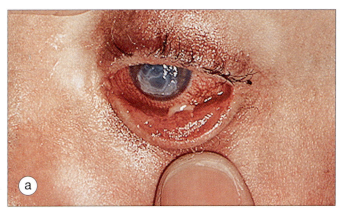

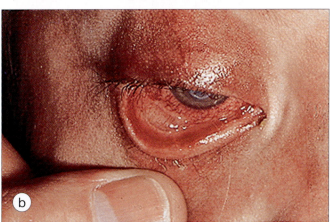

Fig. 22.23 Conjunctival inflammation and necrosis in acute Stevens–Johnson syndrome. There is an associated keratitis (a) and a full thickness loss of conjunctival epithelium (b).

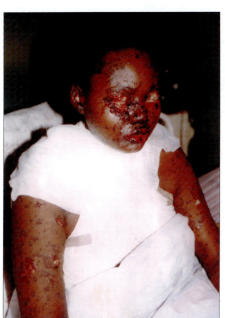

Fig. 22.22 Skin and lid lesions in acute Stevens–Johnson syndrome. The corneas of this patient are shown 15 years later in Fig. 22.26.

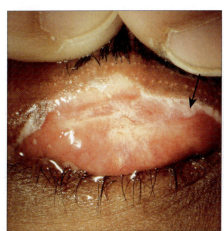

Fig. 22.24 Late upper tarsal scarring in Stevens–Johnson syndrome. Shows marginal keratinization (arrow) and typical linear scarring in the marginal sulcus and sheet scarring in the central tarsus.

Table 22.5 Ocular effects of SJS and TEN

Ocular effects	Resulting symptoms and signs
Loss of goblet cells Loss of accessory lacrimal glands Scarring of meibomian gland orifices	Disrupted tear film leading to poor vision and punctate keratopathy
Metaplasia of meibomian gland epithelium with development of metaplastic lashes	Trichiasis secondary to metaplastic lashes
Conjunctival scarring and obliteration of lacrimal gland ductules	Very dry eye with secondary conjunctival and corneal squamous metaplasia
Keratinization due to squamous metaplasia	Exacerbates drying and discomfort
Conjunctival scarring with fornix shortening and symblepharon formation	May cause lagophthalmos
Retroplacement of meibomian gland orifices	Disrupts tear film
Entropion of upper and lower lids with trichiasis of both metaplastic and normal lashes Lid shortening Corneal epithelial failure secondary to limbal inflammation	Severe ocular surface damage

Chronic ocular complications are numerous. The severe conjunctival inflammation leads to the following sequence of events (summarized in Table 22.5):

- Loss of goblet cells and the accessory conjunctival lacrimal glands as well as disruption of the meibomian gland orifices leading to meibomian gland dysfunction (MGD).
- This results in a disrupted tear film and, in mildly affected cases, may be the principal problem causing chronic discomfort, photophobia and slightly reduced vision because of a combination of the disrupted tear film and a punctate keratopathy secondary to this.
- In more severely affected cases the conjunctival inflammation leads to cicatrization of the lacrimal ductules resulting in a severely dry eye (Fig. 22.25) accompanied by squamous metaplasia and keratinization of both the conjunctival and corneal components of the ocular surface resulting in severe discomfort and loss of vision.
- In addition the meibomian gland ductal epithelium undergoes metaplasia resulting in the development of fine metaplastic lashes.
- The conjunctival shortening leads both to entropion, resulting in ocular surface abrasion by normal, as well as any metaplastic lashes, and may also cause lid shortening leading to reduced eye closure (lagophthalmos) which is easily overlooked.

- Lash abrasion and trichiasis leads to the development of corneal epithelial defects which, as a result of the poor tear film, may develop into persistent corneal epithelial defects.
- Persistent epithelial defect predisposes to corneal stromal melts and perforation often precipitated by infection.
- The severe inflammation may also lead to ocular surface failure, not only as a result of squamous metaplasia, but also by loss of corneal epithelial progenitor cells (stem cells) (Fig. 22.26).
- Chronic or acute episodes of conjunctival inflammation may persist after the systemic disease has resolved or recur months or years later (recurrent SJS). These recurrences do not occur in nonocular tissues and their pathogenesis is obscure.[31,32]

Graft-versus-host-disease (GVAD). Ocular complications are common in patients with graft-versus-host disease resulting from involvement of both the conjunctiva and of the lacrimal gland.[32–34] In acute GVHD conjunctivitis ranges from hyperemia, through chemosis, to a pseudomembranous conjunctivitis with or without corneal epithelial sloughing. Severe conjunctival involvement is a marker for the severity of acute GVHD and was found to occur in 12% of patients in one study who had a 90% mortality. In chronic GVHD the same study found conjunctival involvement in 11% of patients for whom it was also associated with disease severity. Some of these patients develop a severe scarring response like that of cicatricial pemphigoid. Lacrimal gland involvement occurs in about 50% of patients with chronic GVHD who develop a Sjögren-type picture of dry eyes. The pathogenesis of the conjunctival disease has been examined in a few cases and appears similar to the findings in the skin.

Management of the ocular component of the immunobullous disorders

In the acute phase the management of these conditions is supportive and empirical. Glass rodding and the use of conformers to maintain the conjunctival fornices are probably no substitute for daily conjunctival hygiene by an ophthalmologist, with local anesthetic, to remove inflammatory debris and break down any conjunctival adhesions. Lubricant ointment may be used to prevent exposure keratitis in intensive care. Bacterial superinfection must be treated promptly. Topical steroids may be useful for severe conjunctival inflammation but should be used cautiously when there is a corneal epithelial defect.

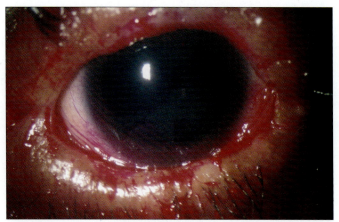

Fig. 22.25 Very dry eye in late Stevens–Johnson syndrome. Shows fornix shortening, diffuse corneal punctate stain with Rose Bengal, and anterior corneal stromal scarring resulting from the initial keratitis.

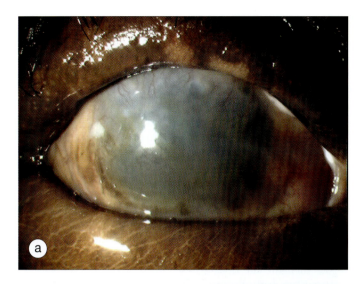

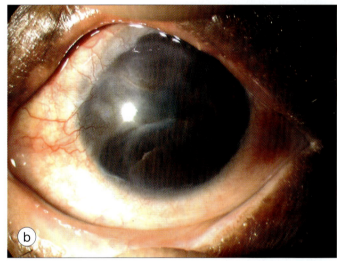

Fig. 22.26 The corneas 15 years after the acute episode of Stevens–Johnson syndrome shown in Fig. 22.22. The right cornea (a) has complete surface failure and is covered by a fibrovascular membrane. The left cornea (b) has partial corneal failure and residual nasal corneal scarring is left after a partial surface reconstruction. The vision is 20/40 with a rigid contact lens.

In the chronic phase the treatment aims are the *management of the ocular surface disease, the elimination or minimalization of treatment toxicity* and, in the minority of these patients who have recurrent inflammation or progressive cicatrization, suppression of inflammation with *immunosuppressive therapy.* Successful management demands identification of the components of the disorder due to surface disease, treatment toxicity, and inflammation related to activity of the underlying disease as well as the early detection and treatment of secondary corneal infection. ALL of these must be managed for successful control of this group of diseases.

Management of the ocular surface disease[35]

- *Trichiasis*: epilate in the short term, use electrolysis or laser for odd lashes, cryotherapy for misdirected lashes and surgery for entropion (inferior retractor plication for lower lid and anterior lamellar reposition for upper lid).
- *Blepharitis*: use oral tetracyclines and institute a lid hygiene regimen.

- *Dry eye and filaments*: use nonpreserved lubricants, the mucolytic gutt. acetylcysteine 5–10% and punctal occlusion to conserve tears (once any blepharitis has been controlled).
- *Keratinization*: topical retinoic acid 0.05% is effective in about 30% of patients but only available in specialized centers.
- *Persistent corneal epithelial defect*: exclude infection, treat ingrowing lashes, use nonpreserved lubricants, therapeutic lenses (silicone hydrogel, limbal fit rigid corneal or scleral lenses in dry eyes) and, if these measures are unsuccessful, close the eye with a botulinus toxin protective ptosis or temporary tarsorrhaphy. Autologous serum drops can be very effective if these measures fail.
- *Corneal perforation*: temporize with therapeutic contact lenses and/or corneal glue followed by keratoplasty only if absolutely necessary as the outcome of keratoplasty is usually very poor.

Eliminating or minimizing treatment toxicity

Treatment toxicity results principally from the preservative benzalkonium chloride (BZK), a component of most reusable bottles of eye drop preparations, and also from glaucoma medications and the aminoglycoside antibiotics. The effects of topical treatment toxicity cannot be distinguished from those of the ocular surface disease. After the withdrawal of toxic topical therapy the mean recovery period is 2 weeks but may extend to 3 months. Management of this component requires that the use of:

- Unnecessary topical treatment is avoided.
- Unpreserved drops are used as far as possible.
- Alternatives to aminoglycoside antibiotics, which are very toxic, are prescribed.

Immunosuppressive therapy

- For mild hyperemia and edema low-dose topical steroid may be helpful.
- For moderate and severe disease unresponsive to topical therapy (hyperemia, intense conjunctival infiltration with or without progressive conjunctival scarring and shortening) systemic immunosuppressive therapy can produce good symptomatic relief and control of disease. Azathioprine and cyclosporine can be used separately or combined for the management of severe disease. A short course of high-dose oral prednisolone (1 mg/kg) can be used to start therapy, with one of these drugs, for the management of severe exacerbations of inflammation. Dapsone may be useful but, because of the potential for causing SJS, is usually avoided for this disease. The use of this drug regimen in GVHD must be coordinated with the hematologists managing the bone marrow transplant as mild GVHD may be beneficial; most, but not all, patients with GVHD causing severe conjunctivitis are already on systemic immunosuppressive therapy. However the ophthalmologist may need to liaise over the level of control that is necessary to prevent the development of blinding complications.

Toxic conjunctivitis and keratoconjunctivitis

Toxic conjunctival and corneal reactions to topical medication are common in adults but rare in children, probably because chronic conjunctival disease is less common and because self medication is less common.[6] However in children with chronic disease such as glaucoma, allergic conjunctivitis and recurrent herpes simplex virus ocular disease toxicity should be considered as a cause of both chronic follicular and papillary reactions.

Toxic follicular reactions, with or without inflammation, may be associated with pseudodendritic or geographic ulcers and punctal stenosis. Offending drugs include atropine, miotics, epinephrine and antivirals. Nonprogressive scarring may also occur (pseudotrachoma), but is rare, and is probably the consequence of prolonged or severe toxic follicular conjunctivitis thought to be the result of the mitogenic effect of these drugs. A toxic papillary response is most commonly the result of exposure to benzalkonium chloride which is the most widely used preservative for topical medications.

Conjunctivitis artefacta

Conjunctivitis artefacta (see Chapters 70 and 71) is usually either as a result of the abuse of topical preparations or from mechanical trauma and may be seen in teenage children.[6] The topical anesthetics and the more toxic antivirals (idoxuridine and trifluorothymidine) are amongst the more commonly abused drops. However it is often almost impossible to be certain of the diagnosis which must always therefore be a diagnosis of exclusion. A frank discussion with the child and parents of the possibility that this may be the diagnosis, and to explore the existence of any potential precipitating social and emotional factors, whilst continuing to offer full conservative therapy for the resulting pathology (conjunctival and corneal inflammation and/or ulceration) is usually helpful as may be the involvement of a pediatrician to whom the uncertainty of the diagnosis must be made clear. It is important to remember that mucous fishing syndrome, as a response to chronic cause of conjunctivitis such as atopic conjunctivitis and congenital or acquired corneal anesthesia, particularly in very young children, has been mistaken for keratoconjunctivitis artefacta, as has molluscum contagiosum, and should be considered in the differential diagnosis of such patients.

Ligneous conjunctivitis

Ligneous conjunctivitis is a rare cause of membranous conjunctivitis. Although it occurs in all age groups it usually affects infants and young children with a preponderance in females. The clinical appearance is characteristic and once seen unlikely to be misdiagnosed (Fig. 22.27). Typically the disease involves the upper tarsal conjunctiva although the bulbar and lower tarsal conjunctiva may be involved. Some chronic cases may differ in having very little coagulum over an elevated tissue mass.

The disease may be preceded by a febrile illness and can be generalized with the development of lesions at extraocular mucosal sites including the upper respiratory tract, middle ear, and cervix. There is also an association with hydrocephalus. In addition conjunctival trauma, typically surgery (ptosis, strabismus,

chalazion, and cataract) may precipitate ocular disease and surgical excision, without appropriate ancillary treatment, is accompanied by accelerated recurrence so that clinical recognition of the condition before excision biopsy is important. The condition may be unilateral or bilateral and there may be a family history.

Recent studies have utilized functional assays of plasminogen to show reduced activity in affected patients and genetic studies have demonstrated associated mutations in the plasminogen gene. A plasminogen deficient mouse model develops a similar disease.[36] These findings have lead to the treatment of one severely affected case, with intravenous plasminogen concentrate,[37] and three further cases treated by local excision followed by topical plasminogen concentrate with good results.[38] Before the demonstration of the role of plasminogen deficiency a success rate of 75% (17 patients) was shown for excision biopsy with meticulous hemostasis, and immediate hourly application of topical heparin and steroid, continued until the conjunctival inflammation had subsided.[39] This treatment is still appropriate when plasminogen concentrate is unobtainable; currently the situation in the UK. The other topical treatments that have been proposed, including sodium cromoglycate, topical cyclosporine and topical steroids have been disappointing.

Until both larger trials of treatment with topical plasminogen have been done, and plasminogen concentrate becomes widely available, conservative therapy should be considered in patients whose lesions do not threaten vision by virtue of their size or corneal involvement, and who have no significant discomfort. Lesions may resolve spontaneously and cause minimal problems for long periods.

KERATITIS

Corneal infection is rare in the normal eye because of the protective effects of a normal blink, normal tear volume and stability, normal tear constituents including antimicrobials, normal corneal sensation and an intact corneal epithelium. The cornea is at risk of infection when any of these are compromised.

Microbial keratitis[40]

Epidemiology

A series of studies of microbial keratitis in children (Fig. 22.28), without a viral etiology, have found that the main risk factors for infection are trauma, ocular disease (severe vernal keratoconjunctivitis, trichiasis, congenital corneal anesthesia, orbital tumor, tear insufficiency, and exposure), systemic

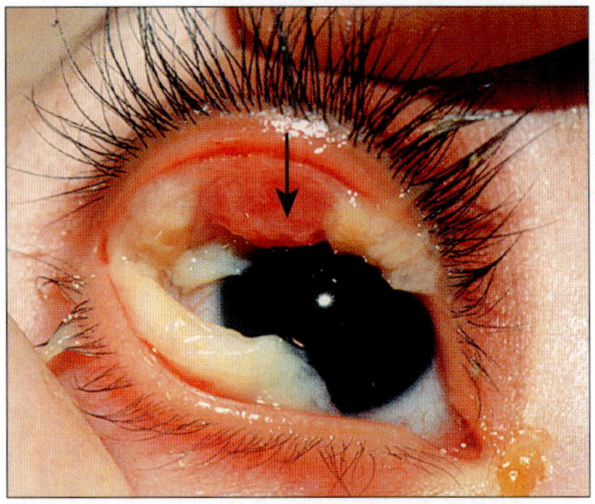

Fig. 22.27 Ligneous conjunctivitis showing typical membranes. The central area of thickened hyperemic conjunctiva on the upper tarsus (arrow) is the appearance that is sometimes seen in chronic cases which may no longer have membranes.

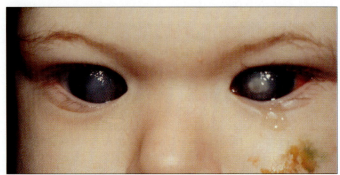

Fig. 22.28 Buphthalmic child with a left bacterial keratitis.

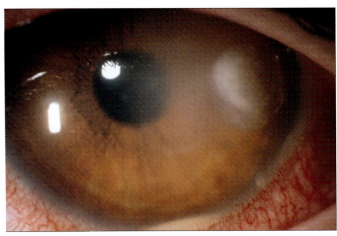

Fig. 22.29 Pseudomonas keratitis in a child using soft contact lenses to correct myopia.

disease (systemic immunodeficiency, Stevens–Johnson syndrome vitamin A deficiency and measles), and prior ocular surgery.[41–45] The relative contribution of these risk factors varies with age, gender, and geographical location. In children up to 3 years of age systemic illness and congenital external ocular disease are the main risk factors.[42,44] Contact lens wear is an important cause of microbial keratitis in studies from the developed world[42,44] but not in those from the developing one[43,45] (Fig. 22.29). Boys have a higher rate of microbial keratitis than girls, possibly because they experience higher rates of ocular trauma.[41] Although the organisms responsible vary, all centers report high rates of staphylococcal, streptococcal and pseudomonal infection. Fungi are the cause of infection in 10–18% overall and are much more common in subtropical and tropical environments. Polymicrobial infections are also common.

Clinically microbial keratitis is distinguished from sterile keratitis by a larger size, the location and the degree of pain and inflammation as described in Table 22.6. One of the most important characteristics of sterile lesions is their proximity to the limbal vascular arcades, thought to be due to their immune etiology, and the presence of the higher concentrations of the complement fixing antibody in the perilimbal cornea.[46]

Investigation

Children who may have sterile lesions can be treated expectantly without investigation. However most cases of acute onset microbial keratitis, in adults, are due to contact lens wear or previous surface disease and respond to appropriate broad spectrum therapy without the need for diagnostic tests. However corneal cultures provide material for microbiological diagnosis whilst removing necrotic tissue and enhancing antibiotic penetration as well as providing local epidemiological data and direct therapy in patients who develop progressive keratitis. For these reasons culture is ideal for all cases and mandatory for the following:

- Where the clinical diagnosis of bacterial disease is uncertain.
- When the underlying cause is not apparent.
- In patients who are locally or systemically immunosuppressed and who may develop infected corneal ulcers without an infiltrate.

Endophthalmitis does not follow bacterial keratitis without corneal perforation (unlike fungal keratitis) so that anterior chamber and vitreous taps are not indicated when perforation is absent. Corneal culture materials should be available in the emergency room and include, as a minimum, a slide for microscopy and Gram staining, and blood agar plates. In temperate regions, most corneal isolates, including fungi, will grow on these media. Specialised media are required to culture *Acanthamoeba* and to optimise the growth of fungi. Ocular specimens should be inoculated directly onto the media avoiding the use of transport and storage media. In our center the readily available 21-gauge hypodermic needle is preferred to the use of a platinum spatula for taking specimens. Samples are taken as small biopsies from the edges of the lesion. In children an examination under anesthesia is often required both for a full examination and to permit these diagnostic tests.

Sixty percent of severely infected and 25% of smaller lesions are culture positive using the conventional diagnostic techniques described above. Growth of most pathogens can be expected after 48 hours. Cultures of fungi and *Acanthamoeba* spp. may take up to 10 days to grow, after which several more days may pass before *in vitro* sensitivity test results are available. Whilst cultures should be incubated for a minimum of 14 days before being reported as culture negative.

The initial examination

This should include assessment of the following indices for comparison with later examinations:

- Degree of pain, indicating disease activity.
- Dimensions of the lesion, recording the maximum length and width of the epithelial defect and infiltrate, using the variable slit beam.
- Estimate of maximal stromal thinning expressed as a percentage of normal corneal thickness.
- Height of any hypopyon.

Table 22.6 Distinguishing characteristics of microbial and sterile keratitis		
	Presumed microbial	**Presumed sterile**
Definition	High probability that replicating bacteria are the principal factor in the pathogenesis. As a result microbial investigations may assist in the management	High probability that replicating bacteria are *not* involved in the pathogenesis. Consequently microbial investigations will be irrelevant to the management. Laboratory investigations are not available to confirm the diagnosis
Clinical criteria	Central lesions Lesions >1 mm Epithelial defect Severe, progressive pain Severe corneal suppuration Uveitis	Peripheral lesions Lesions <1 mm in diameter, *or* >1 mm diameter within the limbal zone Intact epithelium (early) or late epithelial defect Mild, nonprogressive pain Mild corneal suppuration No uveitis

- Intensity of the anterior chamber reaction including presence of fibrin (a contracting clot heralds resolution), cells and flare.
- Include a full assessment of ocular surface integrity with special consideration of factors such as lid function, the tear film and corneal sensation.

Treatment

Treatment can be simplified by separating it into a sterilization phase and a healing phase. It is important to remember that sterilization usually precedes both epithelial healing and the resolution of inflammatory signs, both of which may be delayed by preservative related toxicity, or prolonged topical treatment.

Choice of initial antibiotics

This should depend on local epidemiological knowledge regarding both the common corneal pathogens and their antimicrobial susceptibilities. In temperate climates bacterial isolates account for over 90% of the infections whereas in tropical climates up to 50% may be fungal (usually identifiable by the results from the smears). Polymicrobial infection occurs in about 10% of cases.

For most centers the choice of topical antibiotics, for bacterial keratitis, is outlined in Table 22.7 and consists of either a combination of a commercially unavailable fortified aminoglycoside, or a commercially available quinolone, combined with a fortified cephalosporin or fluoroquinolone monotherapy. Adult studies have shown that fluoroquinolone monotherapy is comparable to an aminoglycoside/cephalosporin combination[47-49] but resistance is an increasing problem in some parts of the USA and India although not in the UK. However fluoroquinolones may not adequately treat streptococcal keratitis, an important cause of microbial keratitis in children, and it is prudent to use a combination of a quinolone with fortified cephalosporin for pediatric cases.

Sterilization phase

See algorithm in Fig. 22.30a. Hourly administration of topical antibiotic therapy for five days leaves a wide margin of safety for most bacterial infections, and compares well with gradual reduction of high dose antibiotic treatment.

Older children may not need to be admitted, but where good compliance is unlikely, or overnight treatment is necessary, as in severe infections (axial lesions, lesions 6 mm or more in diameter, >50% stromal thinning), then admission is preferable if the family cannot comply with this rigorous treatment regimen. A systemic antibiotic is only indicated where the ulcer is close to the limbus to prevent scleral spread, if there is associated hyper-purulent conjunctivitis (see above),in the immunocompromised child or if a corneal perforation is present.

Adjunctive therapy at this stage may include cycloplegics, analgesics, and hypotensive agents for secondary glaucoma. A broad spectrum subconjunctival injection can be given at the end of an examination under anesthesia but is painful and does not enhance the effect of intensive topical therapy.

Daily review can be confusing as the inflammatory reaction may be enhanced by endotoxin release. Review at 48 hours allows detection of rapidly progressive cases and assessment of any culture results. Definite progression at this stage (increased stromal thinning, or a clear expansion of the ulcer) is unusual, and implies that patients are insensitive to, or not complying with, antimicrobial therapy. Rapid early progression can be treated by admitting the patients to ensure compliance and reviewing the microbiology results. Unless these indicate resist-

---

Table 22.7 Choice of topical antibiotics for bacterial keratitis

Organism	Preferred antimicrobial[a,b]	Alternative antimicrobials[a,b]
Bacteria		
Staphylococcus	Quinolone[c]	Cefuroxime 50 mg/ml + aminoglycoside[d] 15 mg/ml
Streptococcus	Cefuroxime 5% (50 mg/ml) + quinolone	Penicillin G 5000 international units/ml
Pseudomonas	Quinolone	Ceftazidime 50 mg/ml + aminoglycoside 15 mg/ml
Enterobacter	Quinolone	Ceftazidime 50 mg/ml + aminoglycoside 15 mg/ml
Moraxella	Quinolone	Aminoglycoside 15 mg/ml
Mycobacteria	Ciprofloxacin 0.3% (3 mg/ml)	Amikacin 50 mg/ml
Fungi	Econazole 1% (10 mg/ml)	Amphotericin 0.15–0.3% (1.5–3 mg/ml) Miconazole 1% Chlorhexidine 0.02%[e] Natamycin 5%
Amoeba	PHMB 0.02%	Hexamidine 0.1% Chlorhexidine 0.02% Propamidine 0.1%

[a]These are broad recommendations that must be tailored to regional data on the prevalence of different microbes and their antimicrobial susceptibility. In particular the choice of quinolone monotherapy must be guided by local epidemiological information. Commercially available quinolones in the UK are ofloxacin and ciprofloxacin to which there is little resistance; in parts of the USA and India resistance to these quinolones is high, new generation quinolones (moxifloxacin and gaitfloxacin) may be appropriate substitutes, or alternative combination therapy with a cephalosporin and aminoglycoside should be used.

[b]With the exception of the quinolones, natamycin, and propamidine all the antimicrobials for topical use in keratitis must be manufactured by a hospital pharmacy or extemporaneously. In the UK all of these are available from Moorfields Eye Hospital Pharmacy (162 City Road, London EC1V 2PD). If there is no hospital pharmacy prepared to manufacture these drugs then the aminoglycosides (gentamicin and tobramycin) can be made up by fortifying the commercially available topical 0.3% preparations with an intravenous preparation. The cephalosporins and penicillin are made up from intravenous preparations, to the required concentration (the manufacturers advice on the stability of the intravenous preparation should be used to determine the period of use).

[c]Antimicrobial concentrations given in percentages can be converted to mg/ml by multiplying the percentage by a factor of 10, i.e. 0.3% = 3 mg/ml.

[d]Gentamicin or tobramycin (the latter is preferred by some authors as less toxic and more active against *P. aeruginosa*).

[e]More effective than natamycin in a recent trial (Rahman MR, Johnson GJ, Husain R, et al. Randomized trial of 0.2% chlorhexidine gluconate and 2.5% natamycin for fungal keratitis in Bangladesh. Br J Ophthalmol 1998;82(8):919–925).

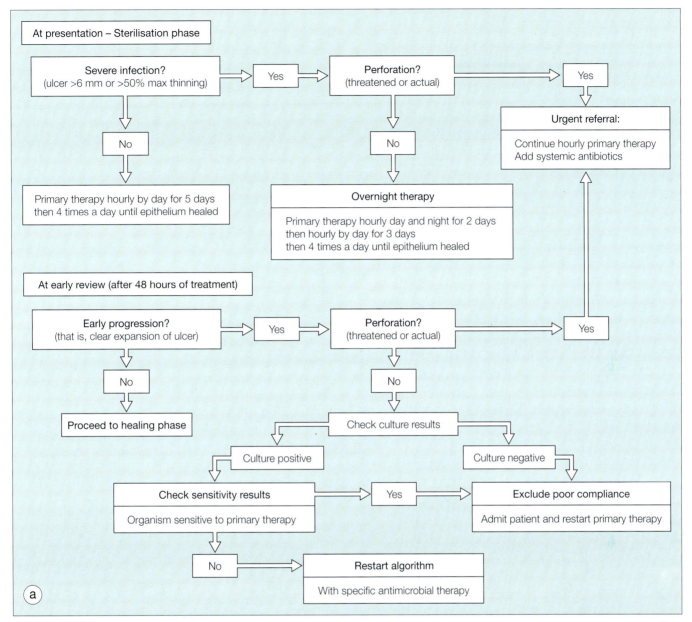

Fig. 22.30 (a) Management of microbial keratitis at presentation, and at the 48 hour review, for the sterilization phase of microbial keratitis therapy. The bold arrows indicate the route followed by the majority of cases. Reproduced with permission from Allan BD, Dart J. Strategies for the management of microbial keratitis. British Journal of Ophthalmology 1995; 777–786.

ance to the primary therapy, a change to an alternative therapy is not indicated. The initial broad spectrum antibiotic therapy is continued hourly day and night for two days, followed by a further three days of hourly treatment during the day. Further progression after this point is an indication for specialist referral.

Even with early recognition and appropriate management, surgery rates are high in children, ranging from 6–28%.[41–45] Threatened or actual perforation indicate urgent referral as emergency penetrating keratoplasties in these circumstances carry a poor prognosis for vision, are difficult to perform well, and can often be avoided even after perforation. Later treatment such as tectonic grafts, debridement, conjunctival flap and penetrating keratoplasty may have their place but the visual prognosis is often poor due to the scarring from the disease and amblyopia in younger children.

Review at one week (see algorithm in Fig. 22.30b) is necessary to determine whether the disease is progressive, or resolving.

Clear evidence of poor compliance or, in culture positive cases, resistance to the choice of antibiotic are indications for re-entering the sterilization phase using appropriate specific therapy. Deteriorating or static cases should be referred for the management of progressive microbial keratitis, whereas cases in which resolution is partial, may safely enter the second phase of treatment directed at encouraging healing.

Healing phase

See Fig. 22.30b. Healing is commonly retarded by persisting inflammation, treatment toxicity or untreated underlying ocular surface disease. Antibiotic treatment can be reduced to prophylactic levels, usually four times a day, at this stage to avoid toxicity, and unpreserved medication used wherever possible. Ocular surface disease (dry eyes, exposure, entropion, and blepharitis) must be treated.

181

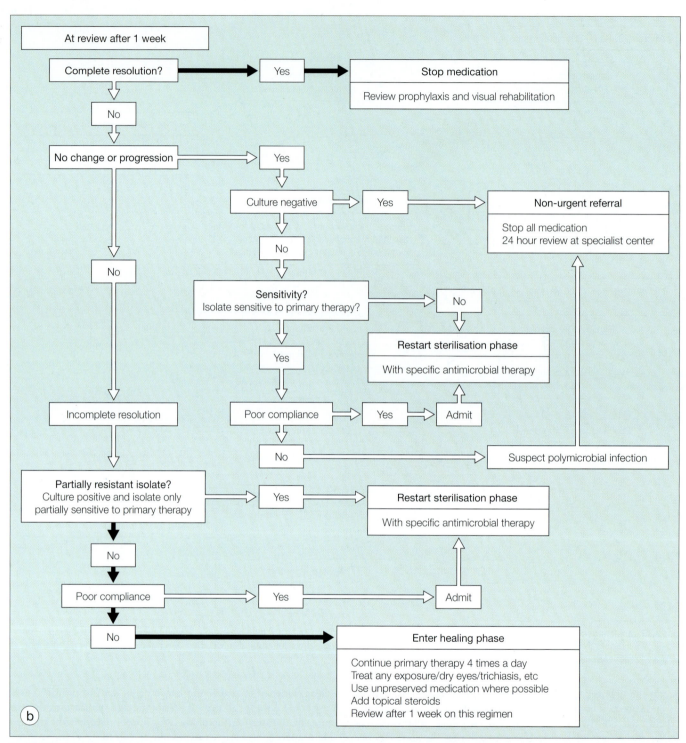

Fig. 22.30 (b) Strategies for managing patients with microbial keratitis at review after one week of therapy. Most cases follow the route shown by the bold arrows. For fungal and amoebic keratitis a prolonged treatment phase is needed to eliminate persistent organisms.

Use of topical corticosteroids

Complete resolution of anterior chamber and corneal inflammatory signs is normal in microbial keratitis without steroid treatment. Corticosteroids enhance microbial growth in fungal or herpes simplex infection (but not in bacterial infection treated with effective antibiotics) and their use is unwise unless the diagnosis of bacterial keratitis has been confirmed beyond reasonable doubt. To date, there have been no prospective randomized controlled trials evaluating the role of corticosteroids as adjunctive therapy in the management of microbial keratitis.[50] Our practice is to introduce topical steroids to dampen a severe inflammatory response in patients whose ulcers are not healing during the second, healing phase, of treatment. Bacterial keratitis is a major risk factor for corneal graft rejection and failure in corneal graft recipients in whom frequent dose topical corticosteroid therapy should be introduced at the outset to protect against a rejection episode.

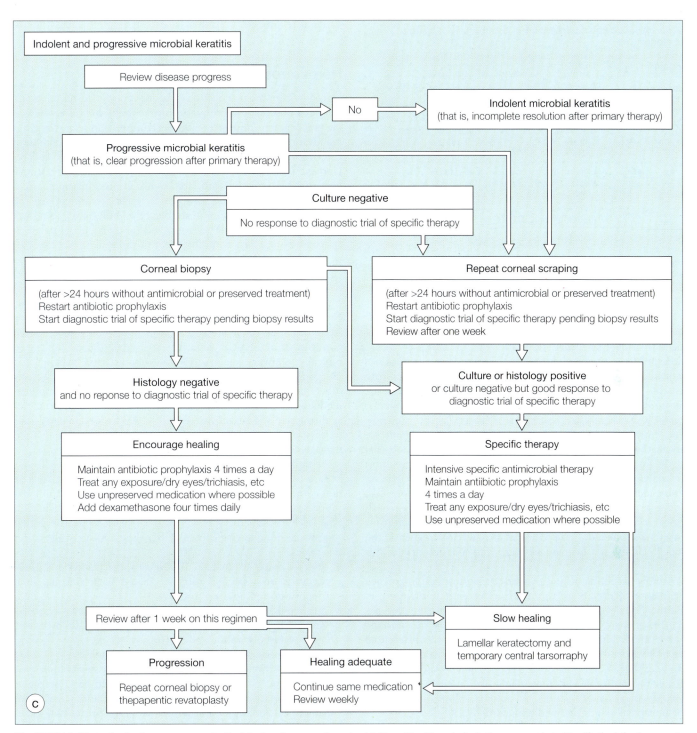

Fig. 22.30 (c) Strategies for the management of indolent and progressive microbial keratitis. The priority in these cases is to identify the infecting agent and institute appropriate specific antimicrobial therapy wherever possible.

Progressive and indolent keratitis

See Fig. 22.30c. Keratitis may actively progress or persist because of a failure of adequate re-epithelialization (indolent microbial keratitis). Progressive microbial keratitis after 5 days of intensive broad spectrum topical antibiotic treatment is an indication for specialist management and reculture, including specialist media (Table 22.8) or corneal biopsy. Prior to biopsy or reculture antibiotic treatment, and the use of any preserved adjunctive medication, should be stopped for 24 hours. When a biopsy is performed half should be sent for histology while the other half is cultured (Table 22.8). Fastidious or slow growing organisms can take 3 weeks to culture; the microbiology service must be informed of the differential diagnosis when receiving the inoculated media. A trial of therapy directed at the organism most likely to be causing the infection on clinical and epidemiological grounds, can be started while awaiting the pathology results.

Failure to heal may require a lamellar keratectomy, to debride necrotic tissue and obtain further specimens for pathology or a

Table 22.8: Organisms involved in progressive microbial keratitis

Organism	Histology	Culture
Acanthamoeba	Calcofluor white Immunofluorescence	Non-nutrient agar seeded with *E. coli*
Fungi	Gram Calcofluor white Giemsa PAS	Sabouraud's agar Brain–heart infusion
Herpes simplex	Electron microscopy Immunohistochemistry and/or molecular techniques (both often unreliable)	Cell culture
Mycobacteria Anaerobes Nocardia Microsporidia	Ziehl–Neelsen Gram Ziehl–Neelsen Modified trichrome	Lowenstein–Jensen Thioglycolate Muller–Hinton

therapeutic keratoplasty. Fungal and amoebic cases require prolonged treatment to ensure sterilization.

Microbial keratitis in children is uncommon, but when it does occur recent surveys have suggested that 10–18% of culture positive cases are due to fungi.[41–45] This probably reflects the predisposing factors in children, namely trauma, systemic illness, ocular disease. *Candida*, *Fusarium* and *Aspergillus* spp. are common. Fungal keratitis is characterized by a white stromal infiltrate with feathery borders, satellite lesions, hypopyon and endothelial plaque formation but may be clinically indistinguishable from bacterial disease. Treatment is region specific and is dependent on local epidemiological data and clinical practice. In London, UK, econazole 1% is the topical treatment of choice, with amphotericin B 0.15–0.3% being used when *Candida albicans* keratitis is suspected. In the USA natamycin 5% is frequently the drug of choice for filamentary fungi and amphotericin B for candida.

With the exception of fungal keratitis the causes of progressive keratitis in Table 22.8 are very rare, or currently unreported, in children. However *Acanthamoeba keratitis*, for example, has occurred in two children under the age of 10 in the authors' practice and failure to include these rare causes in the differential diagnosis will lead to missed or delayed therapeutic opportunities.

In unexplained and progressive keratoconjunctivitis, biotinidase deficiency, a treatable condition, should be considered: affected children may have seizures, hypotonia, alopecia, pinpoint maculopapular skin rashes and optic atrophy.

Herpes simplex virus keratitis

Corneal infection by herpes simplex virus (HSV) produces dendritic, geographic and disciform lesions. Disciform keratitis appears as a grey vascularized stromal opacity with corneal anesthesia and a uveitis; it has been described following neonatal herpes simplex infection.[51] Disciform keratitis also occurs rarely with the Epstein–Barr and varicella-zoster infection. Varicella, mumps and cytomegalovirus also cause a stromal keratitis. Dendrites are more common than geographic or disciform lesions in chronic HSV cases and carry a better visual prognosis.[52] Purely epithelial disease is treated using a topical antiviral such as acyclovir five times a day. Systemic acyclovir can be used for epithelial disease in children, where application of a topical

antiviral is difficult.[53] Stromal disease is treated using systemic acyclovir with topical steroids.

Herpes zoster ophthalmicus

Herpes zoster, the reactivation of latent varicella-zoster infection, has been described in immunocompetent children, even following vaccination. However immunosuppression can trigger a reactivation. Where the reactivation involves the distribution of the trigeminal nerve it is known as herpes zoster ophthalmicus. Corneal involvement can manifest as a dendritic or stromal keratitis, this can be associated with uveitis, glaucoma, progressive outer retinal necrosis and scleritis. Treatment for the corneal disease is with topical steroids. Systemic antivirals reduce the severity of the ocular disease, and postherpetic neuralgia, if started within 3 days from the onset of the rash.

Interstitial keratitis

Interstitial keratitis (IK) is nonulcerative inflammation of the corneal stroma.[54] It may be diffuse, sectoral, peripheral, focal (nummular) and may affect any layer. Commonly encountered patterns of interstitial keratitis are subepithelial infiltrates, typically following adenovirus keratoconjunctivitis, marginal and phlyctenular keratitis (discussed above). However there are many other clinical phenotypes, including both infectious and immune-mediated causes, for which the history and findings are often not as distinctive and diagnostic tests few. This brief summary aims to give some guidelines to recognition of these and their management.

Of these other causes most are thought to be the result of a hypersensitivity response to antigens, or antigen bearing cells, in the corneal stroma for which treatment is topical immunosuppression with steroids. This is generally very effective. This type of hypersensitivity response is thought to be the pathogenesis of the following causes of IK, although the evidence for this varies:

- Herpes zoster stromal keratitis–either a focal anterior stromal keratitis or a late keratitis associated with scarring, lipid deposition and lipid keratopathy.
- Epstein–Barr and mumps virus–usually focal stromal keratitis.
- Congenital syphilis–acute corneal swelling followed by intense vascularization and scarring.
- Tuberculosis–phlyctenular or similar to syphilis.
- Leprosy–stromal infiltration followed by vascularization.
- Lyme disease–focal nummular opacities. In early stages of Lyme disease around 10% of affected children have conjunctivitis and VII and other cranial nerve palsies may occur later.

Other rarer causes, also thought to be due to a hypersensitivity phenomenon are nummular in appearance and include Dimmer nummular keratitis, and the keratitis associated with brucellosis. Recognition of this group of disorders is often easy, providing the association with stromal keratitis is recalled, because of their association with systemic disease. However they must always be differentiated from herpes simplex stromal keratitis for which antiviral therapy is required; if in doubt about the diagnosis treatment should include oral aciclovir.

Another group of causes of IK are due to the interaction of live organisms in the corneal stroma with the host immune response. This group includes the most common cause of stromal keratitis, herpes simplex virus (HSV) discussed above. Others include some cases of lepromatous keratitis and onchocerciasis. The importance of understanding the pathogenesis in this group of causes is that treatment requires both antimicrobial therapy as well as topical immunosuppression.

A further group of diseases are those due to infection, in which the host immune response is absent. Infectious crystalline keratopathy is associated with the chronic use of topical steroid therapy, often following graft surgery, and has a typical crystalline appearance at the edge of the lesion. Microsporidial stromal keratitis is very slowly progressive and may have little or no associated inflammation. Both of these causes require corneal biopsy for diagnosis.

Lastly Cogan syndrome is a systemic vasculitis associated with focal anterior stromal and subepithelial infiltrates, or posterior stromal coarse granular infiltrates. A few cases may also have inflammation involving other ocular tissues including the conjunctiva, episclera, uvea and retinal vessels. The importance of recognizing this condition is the association with deafness and vestibular symptoms, which may either precede or follow the onset of the ocular signs, and which require urgent treatment with high doses of oral immunosuppressives to prevent rapid progression. The disease is associated with a systemic vasculitis.

This extensive list of disorders causing IK is not however exhaustive, but shows the diagnostic dilemmas posed by the development of nonulcerative stromal inflammation and opacification.

LARYNGO-ONYCHOCUTANEOUS SYNDROME (LOGIC OR SHABBIR SYNDROME)

This devastating condition which comprises skin, laryngeal and ocular mucous membrane sloughing and granulation tissue in Punjabi Muslim children is autosomal recessively inherited. In the first year of life relentlessly progressive (Fig. 22.31) conjunctival, laryngeal, nailbed, oral and esophageal granulomas appear that are resistant to all forms of treatment. The gene lies on chromosome 18q11.2, a region which includes the laminin alpha3 gene (*LAMA3*), in which loss-of-expression mutations cause the lethal skin disorder junctional epidermolysis bullosa.

EPISCLERITIS

Episcleritis occurs in self-limiting attacks lasting up to a month and recurring after an interval of some months. The eye becomes red in a circumscribed area deep to the conjunctiva (Fig. 22.32) which may be swollen ("nodular") and irritable. No cause is found in children but in adults there is a definite association with gout. Treatment with a short course of topical steroids usually shortens the attack and oral nonsteroidal anti-inflammatory agents may help. For scleritis, see Chapter 44.

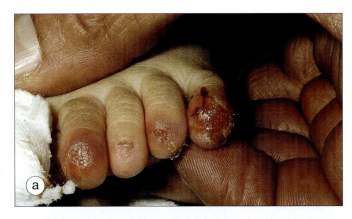

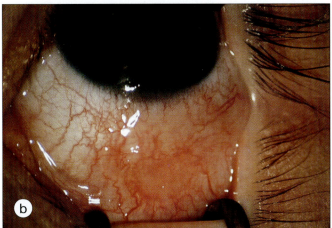

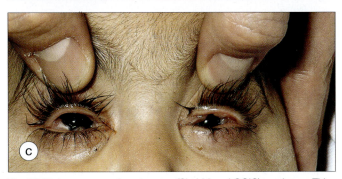

Fig. 22.31 Laryngo-onychocutaneous (Shabbir or LOGIC) syndrome. This syndrome comprises laryngeal, nailbed (a), oral and esophageal lesions. In (b) a conjunctival granuloma with a necrotic slough can be seen, and in (c) there is bilateral conjunctival and nasal mucosal and skin involvement.

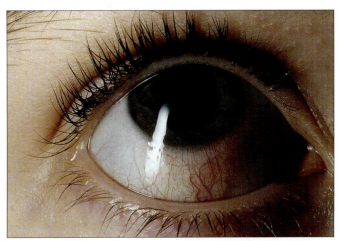

Fig. 22.32 Episcleritis.

REFERENCES

1. McCulley JP, Dougherty JM, Deneau DG. Classification of chronic blepharitis. Ophthalmology 1982; 89: 1173–80.

2. Mondino BJ, Kowalski R, Ratajczak HV, et al. Rabbit model of phlyctenulosis and catarrhal infiltrates. Arch Ophthalmol 1981; 99: 891–5.

3. Mondino BJ, Dethlefs B. Occurrence of phlyctenules after immunization with ribitol teichoic acid of Staphylococcus aureus. Arch Ophthalmol 1984; 102: 461–3.

4. Mondino BJ, Brawman-Mintzer O, Adamu SA. Corneal antibody levels to ribitol teichoic acid in rabbits immunized with staphylococcal antigens using various routes. Invest Ophthalmol Vis Sci 1987; 28: 1553–8.

5. Mondino BJ, Caster AI, Dethlefs B. A rabbit model of staphylococcal blepharitis. Arch Ophthalmol 1987; 105: 409–12.

6. Dart J. Corneal toxicity: the epithelium and stroma in iatrogenic and factitious disease. Eye 2003; 17: 886–92.

7. McCulley JP, Sciallis GF. Meibomian keratoconjunctivitis. Am J Ophthalmol 1977; 84: 788–93.

8. Erzurum SA, Feder RS, Greenwald MJ. Acne rosacea with keratitis in childhood. Arch Ophthalmol 1993; 111: 228–30.

9. Jenkins MS, Brown SI, Lempert SL, et al. Ocular rosacea. Metab Pediatr Syst Ophthalmol 1982; 6: 189–95.

10. Culbertson WW, Huang AJ, Mandelbaum SH, et al. Effective treatment of phlyctenular keratoconjunctivitis with oral tetracycline. Ophthalmology 1993; 100: 1358–66.

11. Gigliotti F, Williams WT, Hayden FG, et al. Etiology of acute conjunctivitis in children. J Pediatr 1981; 98: 531–6.

12. Weiss A, Brinser JH, Nazar-Stewart V. Acute conjunctivitis in childhood. J Pediatr 1993; 122: 10–14.

13. Trottier S, Stenberg K, Von Rosen IA, et al. Haemophilus influenzae causing conjunctivitis in day-care children. Pediatr Infect Dis J 1991; 10: 578–84.

14. Bodor FF, Marchant CD, Shurin PA, et al. Bacterial etiology of conjunctivitis-otitis media syndrome. Pediatrics 1985; 76: 26–8.

15. Bodor FF. Conjunctivitis-otitis syndrome. Pediatrics 1982; 69: 695–8.

16. Gigliotti F, Hendley JO, Morgan J, et al. Efficacy of topical antibiotic therapy in acute conjunctivitis in children. J Pediatr 1984; 104: 623–6.

17. Barquet N, Gasser I, Domingo P, et al. Primary meningococcal conjunctivitis: report of 21 patients and review. Rev Infect Dis 1990; 12: 838–47.

18. Bodor FF. Systemic antibiotics for treatment of the conjunctivitis-otitis media syndrome. Pediatr Infect Dis J 1989; 8: 287–90.

19. Gordon YJ, Aoki K, Kinchington PR. Adenovirus keratoconjunctivitis. In: Pepose JS, Holland GN, Wilhelmus KR, editors. Ocular Infection and Immunity. St Louis: Mosby, 1995: 877–94.

20. Hannouche D, Hoang-Xuan T. Allergic conjunctivitis. Inflammatory Diseases of the Conjunctiva. Stuttgart: Thieme, 2001: 53–70.

21. Trocme SD, Sra KK. Spectrum of ocular allergy. Curr Opin Allergy Clin Immunol 2002; 2: 423–7.

22. Abu El-Asrar AM, Struyf S, Van Damme J, et al. Role of chemokines in vernal keratoconjunctivitis. Int Ophthalmol Clin 2003; 43: 33–9.

23. Abu El-Asrar AM, Van Aelst I, Al-Mansouri S, et al. Gelatinase B in vernal keratoconjunctivitis. Arch Ophthalmol 2001; 119: 1505–11.

24. Caldwell DR, Verin P, Hartwich-Young R, et al. Efficacy and safety of lodoxamide 0.1% vs cromolyn sodium 4% in patients with vernal keratoconjunctivitis. Am J Ophthalmol 1992; 113: 632–7.

25. Verin PH, Dicker ID, Mortemousque B. Nedocromil sodium eye drops are more effective than sodium cromoglycate eye drops for the long-term management of vernal keratoconjunctivitis. Clin Exp Allergy 1999; 29: 529–36.

26. Sharif NA, Xu SX, Miller ST, et al. Characterization of the ocular antiallergic and antihistaminic effects of olopatadine (AL-4943A), a novel drug for treating ocular allergic diseases. J Pharmacol Exp Ther 1996; 278: 1252–61.

27. Gupta V, Sahu PK. Topical cyclosporin A in the management of vernal keratoconjunctivitis. Eye 2001; 15: 39–41.

28. Pleyer U, Häberle H, Baatz H, et al. Acute manifestations of oculo-muco-cutaneous disorders: erythema multiforme major, Steven-Johnson syndrome, and toxic epidermal necrolysis. In: Pleyer U, Hartmann C, Sterry W, editors. Oculodermal Diseases. Buren: Æolus Press, 1997: 169–92.

29. Arstikaitis MJ. Ocular aftermath of Stevens-Johnson syndrome. Arch Ophthalmol 1973; 90: 376–9.

30. Chan LS, Soong HK, Foster CS, et al. Ocular cicatricial pemphigoid occurring as a sequela of Stevens-Johnson syndrome. JAMA 1991; 266: 1543–6.

31. Foster CS, Fong LP, Azar D, et al. Episodic conjunctival inflammation after Stevens-Johnson syndrome. Ophthalmology 1988; 95: 453–62.

32. Jabs DA, Hirst LW, Green WR, et al. The eye in bone marrow transplantation. II. Histopathology. Arch Ophthalmol 1983; 101: 585–90.

33. Jabs DA, Wingard J, Green WR, et al. The eye in bone marrow transplantation. III. Conjunctival graft-vs-host disease. Arch Ophthalmol 1989; 107: 1343–8.

34. Hirst LW, Jabs DA, Tutschka PJ, et al. The eye in bone marrow transplantation. I. Clinical study. Arch Ophthalmol 1983; 101: 580–4.

35. Elder MJ, Bernauer W, Dart JK. The management of ocular surface disease. Dev Ophthalmol 1997; 28: 219–27.

36. Schuster V, Seregard S. Ligneous conjunctivitis. Surv Ophthalmol 2003; 48: 369–88.

37. Schott D, Dempfle CE, Beck P, et al. Therapy with a purified plasminogen concentrate in an infant with ligneous conjunctivitis and homozygous plasminogen deficiency. N Engl J Med 1998; 339: 1679–86.

38. Watts P, Suresh P, Mezer E, et al. Effective treatment of ligneous conjunctivitis with topical plasminogen. Am J Ophthalmol 2002; 133: 451–5.

39. De Cock R, Ficker LA, Dart JG, et al. Topical heparin in the treatment of ligneous conjunctivitis. Ophthalmology 1995; 102: 1654–9.

40. Allan BD, Dart JK. Strategies for the management of microbial keratitis. Br J Ophthalmol 1995; 79: 777–86.

41. Clinch TE, Palmon FE, Robinson MJ, et al. Microbial keratitis in children. Am J Ophthalmol 1994; 117: 65–71.

42. Cruz OA, Sabir SM, Capo H, et al. Microbial keratitis in childhood. Ophthalmology 1993; 100: 192–6.

43. Kunimoto DY, Sharma S, Reddy MK, et al. Microbial keratitis in children. Ophthalmology 1998; 105: 252–7.

44. Ormerod LD, Murphree AL, Gomez DS, et al. Microbial keratitis in children. Ophthalmology 1986; 93: 449–55.

45. Vajpayee RB, Ray M, Panda A, et al. Risk factors for pediatric presumed microbial keratitis: a case-control study. Cornea 1999; 18: 565–9.

46. Bates AK, Morris RJ, Stapleton F, et al. 'Sterile' corneal infiltrates in contact lens wearers. Eye 1989; 3: 803–10.

47. Ofloxacin monotherapy for the primary treatment of microbial keratitis: a double-masked, randomized, controlled trial with conventional dual therapy. The Ofloxacin Study Group. Ophthalmology 1997; 104: 1902–9.

48. Hyndiuk RA, Eiferman RA, Caldwell DR, et al. Comparison of ciprofloxacin ophthalmic solution 0.3% to fortified tobramycin-cefazolin in treating bacterial corneal ulcers. Ciprofloxacin Bacterial Keratitis Study Group. Ophthalmology 1996; 103: 1854–62.

49. O'Brien TP, Maguire MG, Fink NE, et al. Efficacy of ofloxacin vs cefazolin and tobramycin in the therapy for bacterial keratitis. Report from the Bacterial Keratitis Study Research Group. Arch Ophthalmol 1995; 113: 1257–65.

50. Wilhelmus KR. Indecision about corticosteroids for bacterial keratitis: an evidence-based update. Ophthalmology 2002; 109: 835–42.

51. Hammond CJ, Harden AF. Progressive corneal vascularisation as a previously unreported complication of neonatal herpes simplex infection. Br J Ophthalmol 1994; 78: 654–6.

52. Beigi B, Algawi K, Foley-Nolan A, et al. Herpes simplex keratitis in children. Br J Ophthalmol 1994; 78: 458–60.

53. Schwartz GS, Holland EJ. Oral acyclovir for the management of herpes simplex virus keratitis in children. Ophthalmology 2000; 107: 278–82.

54. Wilhelmus KR, Liesang TJ. Interstitial keratitis. Ophthalmology Clinics of North America 1994; 7.

55. McLean WH, Irvine AD, Hamill KJ, et al. An unusual N-terminal deletion of the laminin α-3a isoform leads to the chronic granulation tissue disorder laryngo-onycho-cutaneous syndrome. Hum Mol Genet. 2004;13: 365.

Systemic Infections and the Eye: AIDS

CHAPTER **23**

Luis Carlos F de Sa and Danilo S Soriano

HIV infection and AIDS have had a profound clinical impact on children all over the world. Through June 1998 an estimated 30.6 million people were infected, with 1.1 million children younger than the age of 15 years (UNAIDS report on the Global HIV/AIDS Epidemic). In developing nations, children account for more than 10% of people with HIV/AIDS infection,[1] and 23% (2.7 million) of AIDS-related deaths have occurred in children younger than 15 years, while in the United States HIV-infected children younger than 13 years represent only 1% of all AIDS cases.[2]

TRANSMISSION

Approximately 80% of the children with HIV/AIDS infection are younger than 5 years and result of vertical transmission from mother to child. Perinatal transmission of HIV infection, during the immediate peripartum period, represents more than 90% of newly reported pediatric AIDS cases.[3] The transmission rate for perinatally acquired HIV infection can be reduced substantially with the employment of antiretroviral therapy (antepartum, peripartum, and postpartum delivery of zidovudine).[4] Breast-feeding has been implicated as a postnatal mode of mother-to-child HIV infection, but the decision to breast-feed should be based on the status of the mother's serology, risk factors (drug users, sexual partners of known HIV-positive), and availability of good oral food substitutes and safe water supply for reconstituting dried milk. Pediatric HIV transmission has also been attributed to blood and blood products and to sexual abuse in young children and infants.

ETIOLOGY AND PATHOGENESIS

HIV belongs to the family of retroviruses described almost 50 years ago. HIV-1 and -2 are the two species identified: HIV-1 is the more prevalent and almost uniformly associated with AIDS cases.[5] This RNA virus infects cell membranes utilizing an integral enzyme, reverse transcriptase, which is carried in its core and which becomes integrated into the host-cell genome. Genetic mapping of HIV has identified several genes common to other retroviruses, including *gag*, *pol*, and *env*, used in the process of replication. Five other HIV genes–*tat*, *rev*, *vif*, *nef*, and *vpr*–also help in the process of HIV activation and replication, and newer therapy trials have targeted these genes.

Leukopenia, lymphopenia, and decreased CD4 T-lymphocyte cells with an expanded CD8 population resulting in an inverted CD4/CD8 ratio are common findings in adult HIV infection.[5] With the involvement of CD4 cells, interleukin-2 (IL-2) production is decreased, which weakens the immune amplification system. In addition to T-lymphocyte dysfunction,

B-lymphocyte, natural killer, and cytotoxic T-cells, as well as monocytes and macrophages, are also affected in HIV infection. The human fetus and neonate are more susceptible to the effects of HIV infection because of the immaturity of the immune system, which may account for the rapid expression and fatality of early infection.

Classification of pediatric HIV infection is composed of four clinical categories (N, A, B, C), according to disease severity,[6] with N being asymptomatic, A mildly symptomatic, B moderately symptomatic, and C severely symptomatic. Category C accounts for children with AIDS-specific characteristics: wasting, opportunistic infections, encephalopathy, and malignancies (excluding lymphoid interstitial pneumonitis/pulmonary lymphoid hyperplasia). Clinical category B represents children with specific HIV-related illness including single episodes of bacteremia, lymphoid interstitial pneumonitis/pulmonary lymphoid hyperplasia, anemia, thrombocytopenia, and leiomyosarcomas but excluding diseases of category C. Clinical category A includes children with two or more specific HIV illnesses like lymphadenopathy, hepatomegaly, splenomegaly, sinusitis, otitis, dermatitis, and parotiditis but excludes children of category B or C.

DIAGNOSIS

HIV infection screening in many countries has been a part of routine prenatal care of pregnant women since antiretroviral therapy for HIV-positive pregnant women became available, especially in industrialized countries.

Prenatal diagnosis in the fetus, including sampling of chorionic villus and amniotic fluid, is associated with a higher risk for the fetus, including bleeding and contamination. Noninvasive techniques like fetal ultrasonography provide unspecific and not very predictive information.

The diagnosis of HIV infection in a child born from a seropositive mother may be problematic because of the possibility of passive transfer of maternal antibodies. However, with measurements of viral RNA and DNA copy numbers as well as culture techniques and PCR assay, the diagnosis of HIV infection in infants has improved considerably, although any positive test should be repeated for confirmation. PCR assay should not be performed on cord blood because of the risk of maternal blood contamination.

In children older than 18 months serologic tests for specific antibodies (against the envelope proteins, core proteins, and enzyme bands) are used to establish the diagnosis of HIV infection, especially when culture and PCR are unavailable. Most common enzyme immunoassay tests measure IgG antibodies to HIV, and since these antibodies are passively transferred, most children will therefore be tested positive at birth, although only

Table 23.1 Guidelines for diagnosis of HIV infection in children younger than 13 years of age

A. Child less than 18 months of age, HIV seropositive or born to an HIV-infected mother

AND

■ Positive viral detection assays on two separate specimens (excluding cord blood) from one or more of the HIV tests:
HIV culture
HIV polymerase chain reaction
HIV antigen (P24)

OR

■ Meets criteria for AIDS diagnosis on the 1987 AIDS surveillance case definition.

B. Child more than 18 months of age, born to an HIV-infected mother, or any child infected by blood/blood products, or other known modes of infection, who:

■ Is HIV seropositive on two positive viral detection assays, enzyme immunoassay and confirmatory test:
Western blot
Immunofluorescence assay

OR

■ Meets any of the criteria in A.

Adapted from Center for Disease Control and Prevention.[6]

a minority will be infected. These IgG antibodies will disappear between 6 and 12 months of age in 75% of infants, although persistence of maternal antibodies will be detected in up to 2% until 18 months of age. In children older than 13 years, serologic tests for specific antibodies, PCR assays, and culture are currently used methods for diagnosis of HIV infection. Table 23.1 outlines the current guidelines for diagnosis of HIV infection in children younger than 13 years of age.

CLINICAL MANIFESTATIONS

HIV infection in infants and children differs from that in adults. Common clinical features include growth delay, failure to thrive, lymphadenopathy, malaise, fever, loss of energy, respiratory tract infections, diarrhea, chronic and recurrent sinusitis/otitis, and mucocutaneous candidiasis. Although toxoplasmosis, cryptococcal infection, and malignancies are uncommon in children, lymphocytic interstitial pneumonitis and serious bacterial infections are almost exclusively restricted to pediatric HIV infection.

HIV causes a depression of cellular immunity that will predispose patients to develop opportunistic infections due to agents including bacteria (tuberculosis, syphilis), virus (CMV, herpes zoster, herpes simplex), and protozoal (toxoplasmosis, *Pneumocystis carinii*). In many patients, ocular involvement is part of systemic involvement but the infection may be asymptomatic, which in turn makes diagnosis a more difficult problem. Multiple infections in AIDS patients are also frequent, and despite serology status and knowledge of systemic infection, diagnosis of a specific infection site like the eye can be problematic.

OCULAR MANIFESTATIONS

The ocular manifestations of AIDS have been described in adults including (a) noninfectious microangiopathy with cotton-wool spots associated or not with hemorrhages; (b) opportunistic infections affecting the retina like cytomegalovirus (CMV), herpes zoster, syphilis, toxoplasmosis, *Candida albicans*, and atypical mycobacterial retinitis; (c) conjunctival, eyelid, and/or orbital involvement including malignancies such as Kaposi sarcoma and lymphoma; and (d) neuro-ophthalmic lesions.[7]

The incidence of ocular complications is lower in children than in adults with AIDS.[8–11] Young children rarely complain of visual loss, and advanced involvement may occur unless screening protocols are started at young ages. As the child grows, reaching their teens, they behave like adults, reporting when visual loss occurs, but the incidence of ocular disease also increases, reaching similar proportions to adults.

Ocular manifestations in children with HIV infection may be classified as opportunistic infections (CMV, herpes zoster, toxoplasmosis, etc.) and noninfectious manifestations.

CMV retinitis

CMV retinitis is the most common ocular infection in children with AIDS. It may occur in up to 5.4% of children with AIDS, while in the adult population the incidence may vary from 12 to 32%.[9–11] When the CD4 count falls below 100 the incidence increases to 16%, lower than the 50% in adult population with a similar CD4 count.[9]

CMV retinitis is usually painless and not associated with external inflammatory signs. As children often do not complain of visual loss, it is common for them to present with advanced retinitis, bilateral involvement, and visual acuity less than 20/200. Typically CMV retinitis is easily recognized with white granular retinal opacification associated with exudates and hemorrhages (Figs. 23.1a, 23.1b). The retinitis may start in an area of prior cotton-wool spot (Fig. 23.2) and generally spreads along the vascular arcades or the optic nerve. An abrupt transition between the normal retina and the necrotic area is common (Fig. 23.3). Large atrophic holes may appear in the necrotic area, which may lead to retinal detachment. The anterior chamber and vitreous are minimally affected, although patients on highly active antiretroviral therapy (HAART) may present with greater inflammatory signs.

Treatment should be started soon after the diagnosis, and the most commonly used antivirotics are ganciclovir, foscarnet, and cidofovir. The agents are all virostatic, and once therapy is initiated treatment must be continued generally for the life of the patient. Some patients on HAART may stop their specific anti-CMV therapy, depending on their CD4 counts, but the efficacy and safety of this treatment are still unknown. Treatment includes a 2- to 3-week induction dose followed by long-term maintenance therapy. Intravenous ganciclovir is initially given at doses of 5 mg/kg/day b.i.d. and followed by 5–6 mg/kg given on daily basis for at least 5 days a week. Oral ganciclovir can also be used, avoiding catheter complications. Toxicity of ganciclovir is related particularly to bone marrow depression with severe neutropenia in 10–25% of patients. Foscarnet is given every 8 hours, 60 mg/kg followed by 90–120 mg/kg/day. Foscarnet may cause renal dysfunction in up to 30% of patients. Both drugs can be associated in order to decrease side effects and to improve control of the retinitis. Cidofovir was approved by the FDA in 1996, and it can be used for treatment and prophylaxis of CMV retinitis.

In the unusual cases where CMV infection is restricted to the eye, local therapy with intravitreal injection may be used in adults, but is not feasible for children. Ganciclovir intraocular implants are an alternative local treatment, but may require additional oral or intravenous therapy.

Reactivation is a problem, and it may occur at some point in many patients while on maintenance therapy because of viral resistance and/or declining host immunity.

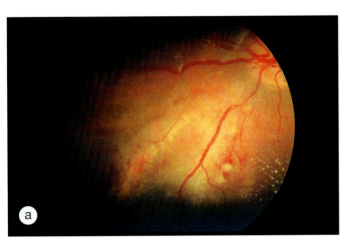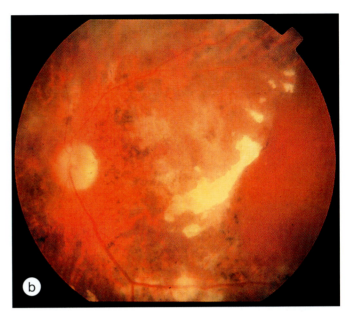

Fig. 23.1 (a, b) A 14-year-old boy with CMV retinitis in his right eye with white granular retinal opacification associated with exudates and vitreous opacities.

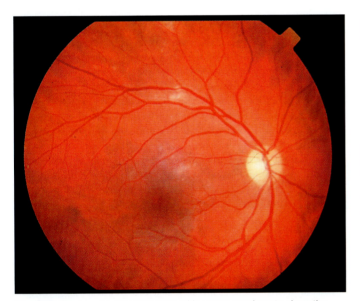

Fig. 23.2 Same patient 5 years later, with cotton-wool spots along the temporal superior vascular arcades and close to the fovea.

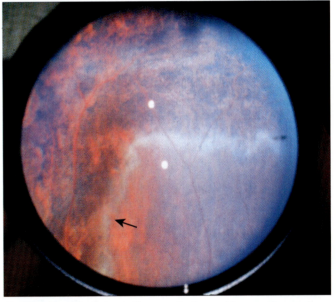

Fig. 23.3 Transition between the normal retina and the necrotic area in a 3-year-old girl with cicatricial CMV retinitis.

TOXOPLASMOSIS

Ocular toxoplasmosis is the second most common ocular infection in children with AIDS, after CMV retinitis, with an incidence ranging between 0.4 and 2.5%.[10] In children, ocular lesions are frequently the result of congenital or intrauterine infection, although reactivation may occur as in adults. It may also occur in the absence of previous ocular infection, and association with central nervous system involvement is frequently found in over 40% of patients.[9] Vitreous involvement with inflammation, which turns the vitreous hazy, is much more common than in CMV infection.

Treatment should include sulfadiazine 100 mg/kg/day four times daily associated with pyrimethamine 1 mg/kg/day and leucovorin 0.5 mg/kg/day, three times a week. Sulfadiazine 50 mg/kg/day four times daily on three days a week is used for maintenance therapy although pyrimethamine may also be used for prophylaxis.

Other intraocular manifestations

Several other infections have been described in children with AIDS,[8-11] including syphilis, *P. carinii*, and herpes. Syphilis is frequently associated with optic neuritis. *P. carinii* generally produces choroiditis, and it is associated with disseminated systemic infection. Herpes simplex and herpes zoster may cause retinitis but are rarely found in children. Herpes zoster may mimic CMV retinitis, and it can also present with a special appearance described as progressive outer retinal necrosis ("PORN"), with rapid progression. Treatment with acyclovir, ganciclovir, and foscarnet has been used with moderate success.

Children treated with dideoxyinosine (DDI) may present with retinal and retinal pigment epithelial atrophy, which have been associated with ocular toxicity.[12] These lesions are usually bilateral and located in the mid/far periphery. Clofazimine used for treatment of atypical mycobacteria may also cause macular pigmentary changes, producing a bull's eye appearance.[13]

Noninfectious manifestations include cotton-wool spot, retinal and/or arterial occlusions, and retinal hemorrhages. Cotton-wool spot is one of the most common manifestations of HIV infection in adults. It results from microvascular infarct of the nerve fiber layer, with secondary retinal edema (Fig. 23.2). It is rarely seen in children younger than 8 years of age, and it usually improves in 4–6 weeks.

Neuro-ophthalmic and orbital manifestations[9,10]

Optic neuropathy is one of the most common neuro-ophthalmic findings in children with HIV infection, and it can be caused by viral, bacterial, and fungal infections. Among the fungi *Cryptococcus neoformans* is the most common, and it is frequently associated with cryptococcus meningitis, requiring I.V. amphotericin-B therapy. Since children do not complain of visual loss it is important to distinguish optic neuropathy from papilledema caused by raised intracranial pressure. CNS toxoplasmosis is one of the most common causes of disc swelling.

Paretic strabismus and diplopia may also occur in children infected with HIV, and they may result from CNS or orbital or cranial nerve involvement.

A work-up for neuro-ophthalmic involvement may require brain and orbital imaging, blood sampling, and lumbar puncture.

Orbital lesions may present with proptosis, visual loss, and diplopia due to restrictive or paretic strabismus. Malignancies including lymphoma and Kaposi sarcoma, infections caused by bacterial, parasitic, and fungal infections, and an inflammatory disease like orbital pseudotumor are the main causes of orbital involvement.[10]

Molluscum contagiosum[14] (Fig. 23.4) and verrucae of the eyelids are cutaneous manifestations found in children with HIV infection. Although benign in immunocompetent patients, molluscum has been described as more confluent and more disseminated in patients with HIV infection. Follicular conjunctivitis and even corneal involvement may be associated with eyelid molluscum. Treatment includes surgical excision, cryotherapy, and chemical cautery but recurrence is common.

External and anterior chamber disease

Dry eyes with or without a dry mouth occurs in 2–56% of children with HIV infection.[10] This Sjögren-like syndrome may be asymptomatic or associated with conjunctival injection and

red eyes. Treatment includes artificial tears/ointment for ocular lubrication and, in more severe cases, punctal occlusion.

Conjunctival and corneal involvement, particularly ulcerative keratitis, may rarely occur in children with AIDS.

Anterior uveitis rarely occurs in patients with HIV infection, and it may be idiopathic or associated with intraocular infection or autoimmune inflammation or related to medications. Drug-induced anterior uveitis has been associated with cidofovir, rifabutin, and oligonucleotides.[10] Clinical presentation may vary from cells and flare in the anterior chamber to severe inflammation with hypotony and hypopyon.

GENERAL TREATMENT

Prenatal care should include improved nutrition, prompt treatment of acute infections, and avoidance of drugs and other related substances to prevent premature birth and low birth weight. General care of the newborn is the same for children born to seronegative mothers, but should include special considerations regarding immunizations, administration of immunoglobulin, prophylaxis of *Pneumocystis carinii* pneumonia with TMP/SMX, and attention to developmental milestones and nutritional status.

In the past few years, with the use of HAART, the prognosis for the HIV-infected child has improved considerably. It is clear that early therapy with a combination of agents provides the best way to preserve immune function, decreasing the chance of disease progression. Usually the combination therapy includes a protease inhibitor (nelfinavir, ritonavir, or indinavir; the latter is not yet approved for pediatric use) and two dideoxynucleoside reverse transcriptase inhibitors (zidovudine, didanosine, lamivudine, stavudine, zalcitabine). Alternative regimens may include other drugs like non-nucleoside reverse transcriptase inhibitors but since standards of care are still evolving, long-term tolerance and efficacy are unknown.

Clinical course and prevention

In the past few years a major decrease in mortality and morbidity in HIV-infected children was observed due to the use of more effective treatment and prophylaxis of infections and complications. Children with HIV infection generally present a more accelerated course than adults but the disease may vary according to the time of infection. In infants infected perinatally, about one-third become symptomatic in the first two years and the others in the next year, except for a minority group that remain asymptomatic up to 8 years of age.[1] When an infant is infected by blood transfusion the disease tends to have a prolonged asymptomatic period.

High virus copy number, early manifestation of symptoms (opportunistic infections, hepatosplenomegaly, encephalopathy), and the birth of a child to a mother with low CD4 counts and a high virus load are factors associated with a more accelerated course.

Education and prevention of further infections are the main targets for controlling HIV infection. Regarding pediatric AIDS, it is crucial to identify seropositive pregnant women because intervention in this group of patients is essential for preventing infant contamination. Pregnant women should receive antiretroviral therapy (zidovudine) early in pregnancy as well as during labor, which significantly decreases the transmission rate. Cesarean

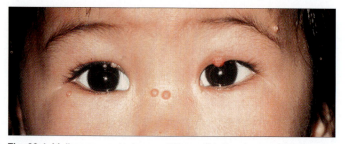

Fig. 23.4 Molluscum contagiosum of the eyelids in a 4-year-old girl.

section may also decrease dramatically the transmission rate when compared to vaginal delivery. However, in developing countries the use of antiretroviral therapy, cesarean section, and avoidance of breast-feeding are often not feasible and new strategies should be developed.

Visual loss is a significant cause of morbidity in children with HIV infection. Regularly scheduled ophthalmic examination should be performed in these patients, in order to avoid blindness. The frequency of examination depends mainly on age, CD4 counts, and general health of the child.

REFERENCES

1. Mueller BU, Pizo PA. Acquired immunodeficiency syndrome in the infant. In: Remington JS, Klein KO, editors. Infectious Diseases of the Fetus and Newborn Infant. 5th ed. Philadelphia: Saunders; 2001: 447–75. (vol. 1.)
2. Centers for Disease Control and Prevention. U.S. HIV and AIDS cases reported through December 1997. HIV/AIDS Surveillance report: year-end edition. MMWR Morb Mortal Wkly Rep 1997; 9: 1–44
3. Rogers MF, Caldwell MB, Gwinn ML, Simonds RJ. Epidemiology of pediatric human immunodeficiency virus infection in the United States. Acta Paediatr Suppl 1994; 400: 5–7.
4. Connor EM, Sperling RS, Gelber R, et al. Reduction of maternal–infant transmission of human immunodeficiency virus type 1 with zidovudine treatment: Pediatric AIDS Clinical Trials Group Protocol 076 Study Group. N Eng J Med 1994; 331: 1173–80.
5. Hanson C, Shearer T. AIDS and other acquired immunodeficiency diseases. In: Feigin RD, Cherry JD, editors. Textbook of Pediatric Infectious Diseases. 4th ed. Philadelphia: Saunders; 1998: 954–79. (vol. 1.)
6. Center for Disease Control and Prevention. 1994 revised classification system for human immunodeficiency virus infection in children less than 13 years of age. MMWR Morb Mortal Wkly Rep 1994; 43: 1–17.
7. Jabs DA. Ocular manifestations of HIV infection. Trans Am Ophthalmol Soc 1995; 93: 623–83.
8. Dennehy PJ, Warman R, Flynn JT, et al. Ocular manifestations in pediatric patients with acquired immunodeficiency syndrome. Arch Ophthalmol 1989; 107: 978–82.
9. Smet MD, Nussenblatt RB. Ocular manifestations of HIV in the pediatric population. In: Pizo PA, Wilfert CM, editors. Pediatric AIDS. The challenge of HIV infection in infants, children, and adolescents. 2nd ed. Baltimore: Williams & Wilkins; 1994: 457–66.
10. Whitcup SM, Robinson MR. Ocular manifestations of HIV in the pediatric population. In: Pizo PA, Wilfert CM, editors. Pediatric AIDS. The challenge of HIV infection in infants, children, and adolescents. 3rd ed. Philadelphia: Lippincott Williams & Wilkins; 1998: 309–21.
11. Livingston PG, Kerr NC, Sullivan JL. Ocular disease in children with vertically acquired human immunodeficiency virus infection. J AAPOS 1998; 2: 177–81.
12. Whitcup SM, Dastgheib K, Nussenblatt RB, et al. A clinicopathologic report of the retinal lesions associated with didanosine. Arch Ophthalmol 1994; 112: 1594–8.
13. Craythorn JM, Swartz M, Creel DJ. Clofazimine-induced bull's-eye retinopathy. Retina 1986; 6: 50–2.
14. Pelaez CA, Gurbindo MD, Cortés C, Munoz-Fernandez MA. Molluscum contagiosum involving the upper eyelids in a child infected with HIV-1. Pediatric AIDS HIV Infect 1996; 7: 43–6.

CHAPTER 24 Disorders of the Eye as a Whole

Jane Sowden and David Taylor

INFLUENCE OF THE EYE ON THE DEVELOPMENT OF THE ORBIT

Although the absence of a developing eye in itself does not affect the initial development of a bony orbit,[1] the growth of the orbit is highly influenced by the presence or absence of an eye. At birth, the normal eye occupies a higher percentage of the orbital volume; growth of the orbital volume increases dramatically during the first year of life.

How does absence of an eye, either congenitally or surgically at an early age, influence the growth of the orbit? Although orbital volume cannot be assessed with plain X-rays, the horizontal and vertical measurement of the orbital rim can be taken easily: these parameters are reduced in adults who had anophthalmos or had the eye removed within the first year of life. In humans, cats, and rabbits this retardation of orbital growth is approximately halved when an orbital implant is used, and the severity of the overall reduction in volume diminishes if the insult occurs at a later date. Orbital growth appears to be complete by the age of 15 years, so that subsequent enucleation will not result in any clinically appreciable size difference.[2]

Determination of the influence of an eye on orbital volume cannot be detected radiologically, but measurements of skulls have shown a 60% reduction in volume.

Orbital growth may be secondarily influenced by radiotherapy. This consideration, as well as intracranial radiotherapeutic effects, becomes important clinically in the management of children with retinoblastoma, rhabdomyosarcoma, and other radiosensitive neoplasms involving the orbit.

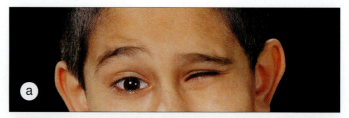
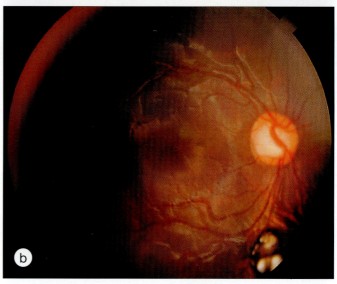

Fig. 24.1 (a) Left clinical anophthalmos with no perception of light. (b) The right eye had 0.0 LogMAR acuity. There is a small coloboma inferior to the optic disc. The mother had a clinically insignificant coloboma.

ANOPHTHALMOS AND MICROPHTHALMOS

Anophthalmos and microphthalmos are rare, occurring in around 10–19 per 100,000 live births.[3–5] They are often associated with other abnormalities but there is no uniting causation, and clustering of cases (which might suggest an environmental cause) probably does not occur.[3,6]

Anophthalmos

Anophthalmos is the term used when the eye is nonexistent (Fig. 24.1), or more commonly when a tiny cystic remnant of the eye is present, the term "clinical anophthalmos" may be used, which emphasizes that there is a spectrum: anophthalmos merges with microphthalmos.

Variable secondary abnormalities of the orbit occur and orbital growth is always retarded to some extent. Extraocular muscles may be absent, and the optic foramen size is often decreased. The conjunctival sac may be small.

Anophthalmos represents either a complete failure of budding of the optic vesicle or early arrest of its development. To differentiate between anophthalmos and extreme microphthalmos, the examiner can touch the lids to feel for any movements representing rudimentary extraocular muscle function. Neuroimaging or ultrasound may demonstrate some buried residual soft tissue mass in cases of extreme microphthalmos, but histological sectioning alone can clarify the presence of neural ectoderm-derived cells or microphthalmos, or their absence in true anophthalmos. Functional assessment using electrophysiology may demonstrate rudimentary, but useful, function in cases thought to be anophthalmic on clinical examination. Unilateral anophthalmos is often associated with anomalies of the other eye.[7]

Many underlying causes for anophthalmos have been proposed: these merge almost imperceptibly with the causes of microphthalmos (see next section). Bilaterality and severity imply an early teratogenic event.[8]

The ophthalmologist's management of clinical anophthalmos is twofold:

1. To stimulate growth of the adnexal structures and orbit. Orbital expansion can be achieved by the use of serially larger prostheses, and hydrophilic or inflatable expanders.[9–11]
2. Support for the parents of such a child is essential: the impact of blindness is bad enough but when the cause is anophthalmos it seems worse. When bilateral, blindness is inevitable and networking with the appropriate agencies will provide support. A search for possible causes may help ease guilt. Genetic counseling will help the parents understand the risks of future children being involved. When unilateral, emphasis must be placed on the integrity of the fellow eye if this is the case and on the relatively normal life that can be expected in a monocular child. Safety glasses may be considered at an early age to protect the good eye.

Microphthalmos

The net volume of a microphthalmic eye is reduced. Often, clinical suspicion is created on the basis of cornea size. Although microphthalmos is usually associated with a small cornea, there may be microphthalmos with a normal cornea[12] and microcornea without microphthalmos.[13] Ultrasonographic determination of an axial length less than 21 mm in an adult or 19 mm in a 1-year-old child substantiates a diagnosis of microphthalmos.[14] This represents 2 SD below normal.

Bilateral microphthalmos is a relatively rare condition,[15] but it accounted for approximately 10% of blind children in one study.[16]

The defect of vision depends on whether it is bilateral and on the severity of the microphthalmos, specifically the horizontal corneal diameter and the presence of cataract and coloboma.[17]

Microphthalmos may be designated as simple (without other ocular disease) or complex (associated with cataract, retinal or vitreous disease, or more complex malformations).[14,18] It can be further divided into colobomatous (Fig. 24.2) and non-colobomatous categories[12,19] on the basis of associated uveal abnormalities. The association between eye growth and closure of the fetal fissure is linked and important since closure of the cleft is completed early in development.[20]

Microphthalmos probably represents a nonspecific growth failure in response to a very wide variety of prenatal insults. Many causal associations of microphthalmos have been suggested, and possible causes must be kept in mind while considering the child's overall health. Bateman[12] and others have carefully identified and classified microphthalmos according to heredity, environmental causes, chromosomal aberration, and unknown causes that have additional systemic abnormalities.[21]

Isolated microphthalmos
Idiopathic microphthalmos
Some eyes that are otherwise healthy may be below 2 SD in size. Vision is variably affected, depending on the degree to which the eye is microphthalmic. There may be no obvious inheritance pattern, but care is needed in genetic counseling because of the possibility of new mutations and recessive inheritance.

Inherited isolated microphthalmos
Many cases are sporadic.[22,23]

1. Autosomal dominant.[24] Some families (Fig. 24.3) have shown a dominant gene for coloboma with variable expression with extreme microphthalmos at one end of the spectrum and

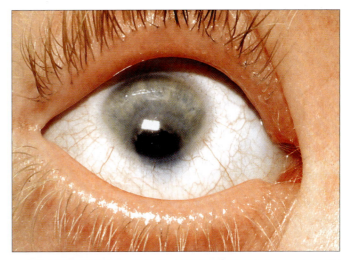

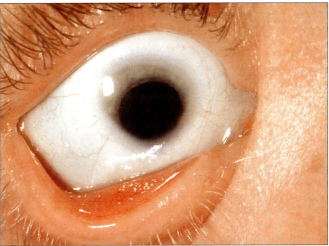

Fig. 24.2 Colobomatous microphthalmos. Both eyes are generally small with an inferior coloboma in the fundus. Although vision was limited to an acuity of 2/60 in each eye, the patient had a useful field and navigated without problems.

coloboma, sometimes quite trivial colobomatous defects, at the other.
2. Autosomal recessive.[25] The high rate of consanguinity in one study suggests an autosomal recessive inheritance in some cases.[26]
3. X-linked recessive, some with mental retardation.[27]

Microphthalmos with ocular and systemic disease
Other eye abnormalities and systemic diseases are frequent in babies presenting because of microphthalmos: there are 231 syndromes associated with microphthalmos in the GENEEYE database.[28] Accordingly, patients with microphthalmos must be examined with a view to excluding associated disease.

Microphthalmos with ocular abnormalities
Microphthalmos is a nonspecific response to a wide variety of influences; therefore it occurs with many severe eye diseases, including the following:

1. Anterior segment malformations, i.e., Peters anomaly, Rieger anomaly, and so on[29] (Chapter 28).
2. Cataract (see Chapter 47): one family with a translocation defect t(2;16), the breakpoint at 16p13.3.[30] Many congenital

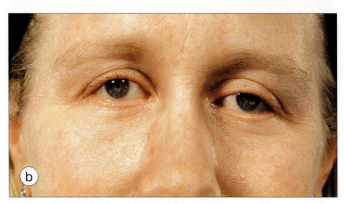

Fig. 24.3 (a) Bilateral marked noncolobomatous microphthalmos.
(b) Mother of the child in (a) showing bilateral noncolobomatous microphthalmos.

cataracts occur in microphthalmic eyes and some specific syndromes.

3. Persistent hyperplastic vitreous (see Chapter 47).[31] Traboulsi and Parks[32] described this in the autosomal dominant oculodentodigital syndrome.
4. Retinal diseases: microphthalmos may be secondary to severe, widespread intraocular disease:
   - Retinopathy of prematurity (see Chapter 51);
   - Retinal dysplasia (see Chapter 41);
   - Retinal folds;[33] and
   - Retinal degeneration and glaucoma.
5. Aniridia. A three-generation family with aniridia, anophthalmos, and microcephaly.[34]
6. Coloboma (see Chapter 59). Coloboma is the most common association of microphthalmos[35,36] and is found in many of the microphthalmos syndromes to be discussed in the following.

Gene mutations associated with anophthalmos and microphthalmos

PAX6

Gene mutations are rare as a cause of microphthalmos,[4,37] but a family in which both parents who had PAX6-related cataracts and aniridia had a child with total anophthalmos, microcephaly, agenesis of the corpus callosum, and choanal atresia was described.[38]

SOX2

A submicroscopic deletion containing SOX2 was identified at the 3q breakpoint in a child with t(3;11)(q26.3;p11.2) associated with bilateral anophthalmos. Subsequent SOX2 mutation analysis identified de novo truncating mutations of SOX2 in 4 of 35 (11%) individuals with anophthalmos.

PAX2 and SHH (sonic hedgehog)

Mutations in PAX2 are found in cases of the renal-coloboma syndrome (ocular colobomas, vesicoureteral reflux (VUR), and kidney anomalies).[39] Upstream expression of sonic hedgehog (SHH) controls PAX2. A deletion in the SHH gene was identified in a three-generation family with iris and uveoretinal colobomas and co-segregated with the phenotype.[40]

CHX10

Human CHX10 is expressed in progenitor cells of the developing neuroretina and in the inner nuclear layer of the mature retina. A human microphthalmia locus was mapped on chromosome 14q24.3, CHX10 cloned at this locus, and CHX10 mutations were identified in nonsyndromic autosomal recessive microphthalmia, cataracts, and severe abnormalities of the iris.[41]

Microphthalmos with systemic disease

1. The Temple-al Gazali syndrome (Fig. 24.4). X-linked dominant *m*icrophthalmia with *l*inear *s*kin defects (MLS) syndrome or the *m*icrophthalmos, *d*ermal *a*plasia, and *s*clerocornea (MIDAS) syndrome is the result of a deletion of Xp22.2-pter;[42,43] patients have linear, irregular areas of skin aplasia especially of the head and neck, microphthalmos with variable sclerocornea, and sometimes normal intelligence.[44–46] They are female or at least have two X chromosomes;[21,47] it is lethal in males.
2. Chromosomal syndromes. Chromosomal disorders are often associated with colobomatous microphthalmos,[22,23,30] often with mental retardation.[48]
3. Mental retardation. Many patients with microphthalmos-associated syndromes are mentally retarded.[27,48,49]
4. Macrosomia/cleft palate.[50]
5. Facial defects:
   - Fryns "anophthalmos plus" syndrome: microphthalmos, facial clefts, and choanal atresia;[51–53]
   - The branchio-oculofacial syndrome: broad nose with large lateral pillars, branchial sinuses, and orbital cysts;[54,55]
   - Fronto-facio-nasal dysplasia[56] (Fig. 24.5);
   - Cerebro-oculo-nasal syndrome: anophthalmia/microphthalmia, abnormal nares, and central nervous system anomalies;[57] and
   - Unilateral hamartomatous proboscis with ipsilateral microphthalmos, choanal atresia, and mildly hypoplastic left nose.[58]

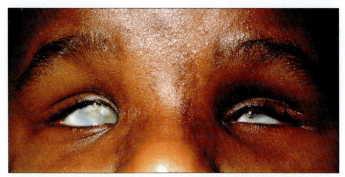

Fig. 24.4 *M*icrophthalmos, *d*ermal *a*plasia, and *s*clerocornea (MIDAS or Temple-al-Gazali) syndrome showing extreme microphthalmos and characteristic skin lesions.

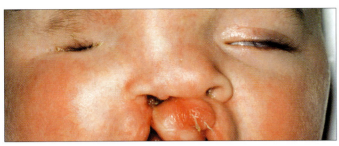

Fig. 24.5 Right clinical anophthalmos, left microphthalmos in a child with bilateral cleft lip and palate associated with fronto-facio-nasal dysplasia.

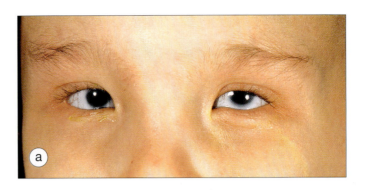

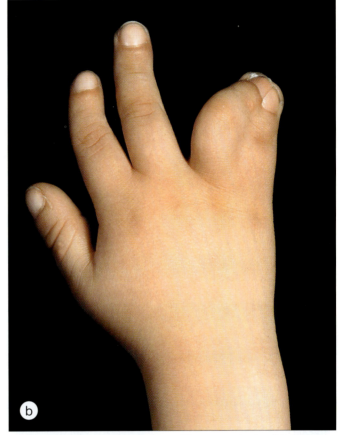

Fig. 24.6 (a) Bilateral microphthalmos, thin nose, and epicanthic folds in a patient with the oculo-dento-digital syndrome. (b) Cutaneous syndactyly of fingers and camptodactyly in the oculo-dento-digital syndrome.

6. Delleman syndrome. Skin tags, punched-out lesions of the skin on ears and elsewhere, mental retardation, hydrocephalus, brain malformations, and orbital dermoid cysts.[59,60]
7. Ectodermal dysplasia.[61]
8. Blepharophimosis, ptosis, epicanthus inversus. Fujita et al.[62] described a boy with a chromosomal deletion (3)(q12 q32).
9. X-linked microcephaly, urogenital anomalies.[63]
10. Growth retardation, microcephaly, brachycephaly, oligophrenia syndrome (GOMBO syndrome).[64]
11. The oculodentodigital syndrome.[32,65] Digital anomalies (Fig. 24.6): bilateral cutaneous syndactyly of fingers and camptodactyly. Facial and ocular anomalies: microphthalmos-epicanthal folds, small midface, thin nose with hypoplastic alae nasi and small nares. Dental anomalies: partial dental agenesis and enamel hypoplasia. Glaucoma.[66,67]
12. Fetal infections: Rubella, varicella, influenza, toxoplasmosis, and parvovirus infections.[68,69]
13. Fetal toxins: vitamin A (and retinoic acid in mice[70]), alcohol, warfarin, LSD,[71] thalidomide, hyperthermia,[72] carbamazepine.[73] The fungicide benomyl is now not thought to be a cause of microphthalmos.[3,74]
14. Microphthalmos with syndactyly, oligodactyly, and other limb defects and mental retardation: "Waardenburg recessive anophthalmia syndrome."[75]
15. Cross syndrome. This autosomal recessive syndrome associates microphthalmos with corneal opacities and albinism and severe mental retardation.[76]
16. The Lenz microphthalmia syndrome:[36,77] microphthalmia with mental retardation, malformed ears, skeletal anomalies; it is inherited in an X-linked recessive pattern and is probably genetically heterogeneous.[78]
17. The "micro" syndrome: microphakia, microphthalmos, characteristic lens opacity, atonic pupils, cortical visual impairment, microcephaly, developmental delay by 6 months of age, and microgenitalia in males. Autosomal recessive.[79]

The ophthalmologist faced with a new patient with microphthalmos must address several questions:
1. What is the level of vision?
2. What is the refractive error? If it is asymmetrical, is amblyopia present?
3. Are any colobomas present?
4. Is there evidence of glaucoma?
5. Is there evidence of congenital infection, chromosomal abnormality, or environmental factors?
6. Is there a risk of involvement in future children?
7. Are there life-threatening associations (such as cardiac defect) or factors that may alter parental expectations of the child (such as mental retardation or deafness)?

Ophthalmic intervention *per se* is limited to prescribing glasses to offset amblyogenic refractive errors, arranging for assessment of low vision, helping the ocularist in management and fitting of cosmetic shells or contact lenses in nonseeing eyes, and diagnosing and treating glaucoma and cataracts. Microphthalmic eyes with corneal opacities may rarely be successfully treated by corneal grafting.

Microphthalmos with orbital cyst
This form of microphthalmos can present with progressive swelling from birth (Fig. 24.7): it is sometimes known as a congenital cystic eye.[80] The eye often cannot be seen, and the uninitiated ophthalmologist may initially fear a neoplasm. This condition is a colobomatous microphthalmos where cyst formation occurs on the course of the optic nerve, often with free communication with the eye.[81,82] Presentation may be as an orbital mass distending the lids and hiding the eye or as proptosis

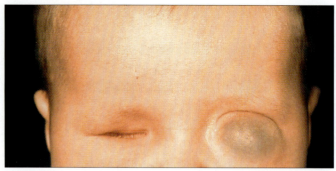

Fig. 24.7 Right clinical anophthalmos and left microphthalmos with cyst. The baby had presented at birth with a clinically anophthalmic right eye and extreme colobomatous microphthalmos in the left eye. A blue swelling was initially thought to be vascular but it transilluminated and was found to be a cyst associated with microphthalmos.

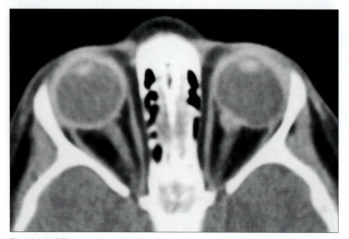

Fig. 24.8 CT scan of a girl with unilateral small cyst (shows as a protuberance adjacent to the optic nerve where it joins the eye) in a colobomatous eye with temporal scleral ectasia.

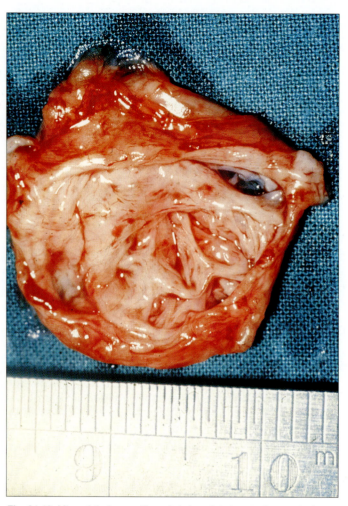

Fig. 24.10 Microphthalmos with cyst: trabeculated cyst after surgical removal.

in which a microphthalmic eye is visible. Ultrasonography and CT or MRI scanning[83] aid in its diagnosis. Although management is initially conservative, especially for small cysts (Fig. 24.8), large cysts may be managed either with repeated aspiration[83,84] (Fig. 24.9) or by surgical removal[85] (Fig. 24.10). If the cyst is not growing too rapidly, the cyst may be left in place until some orbital growth is achieved. Because of the communication of the cyst with the eye (Fig. 24.11), the removal of the cyst may necessarily deflate the microphthalmic eye, which may need to be removed.

Cryptophthalmos

The cryptophthalmos syndrome[86] describes the concurrence of microphthalmos with a varying degree of skin covering the eyeball and lids being variably attached to the cornea.

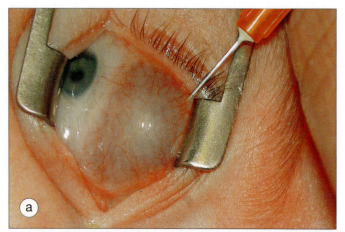

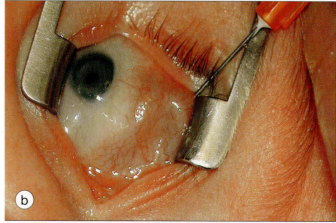

Fig. 24.9 (a) A unilateral coloboma with cyst in an infant. The mother had bilateral chorioretinal colobomas not affecting vision. The cyst is about to be aspirated under topical anesthesia. (b) After aspiration, the cyst collapses. Some cases need repeated aspirations and may eventually require surgical removal.

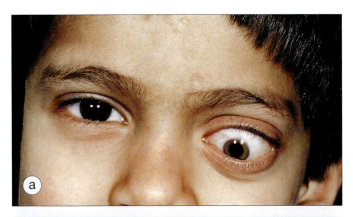

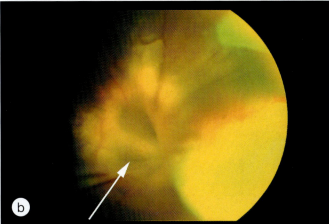

Fig. 24.11 (a) Microphthalmos with cyst. The left eye was small and proptosed by an expanding cyst that had free communication with the eye so that the eye would collapse if the cyst was aspirated. (b) Fundus photograph of the left eye of the child in (a) showing (arrow) the colobomatous defect in communication with the cyst. See also Fig. 40.8.

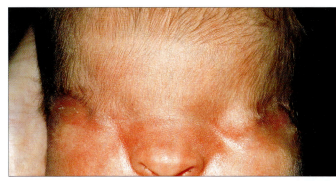

Fig. 24.12 Complete cryptophthalmos. Note the characteristic abnormality of the hair extending to the brow and the abnormality of the nose.

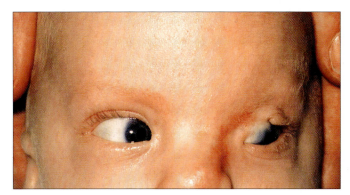

Fig. 24.13 Partial cryptophthalmos of the left eye. The eye is small and the cornea is opaque. There is a colobomatous upper lid and a characteristic "lick" of hair from the temple to the brow with a unilateral nose abnormality.

The locus of FS1 is at chromosome 4q21, although it is genetically heterogeneous. Mutation analysis identified five frameshift mutations in *FRAS1*, which encodes one member of a family of novel proteins related to an extracellular matrix (ECM).[87] The composition of the extracellular space underlying epithelia could account for the Fraser syndrome manifestations in humans.[88] Francois[89] described three subgroups:

1. Complete cryptophthalmos (Fig. 24.12). The lids are replaced by a layer of skin without lashes or glands, and the skin is fused with the microphthalmic eye without a conjunctival sac. Normal electrophysiological responses have been recorded in this form of cryptophthalmos.[90]
2. Incomplete cryptophthalmos (Fig. 24.13). The lids are colobomatous (often medially) or rudimentary and there is a small conjunctival sac. The exposed cornea is often opaque.
3. Abortive form. In this form the upper lid is partly fused with the upper cornea and conjunctiva and may be colobomatous.[86] The globe is often small.

The systemic associations include nose deformities, cleft lip and palate, syndactyly, abnormal genitalia, renal agenesis, mental retardation, and many others.[86,91,92] Prenatal diagnosis can be made by ultrasound.[93] Surgical treatment is often unsatisfactory and mainly indicated to protect an eye at risk from further deterioration of corneal clarity (see also Chapter 26). Multiple procedures may be required, even for the incomplete form.[94]

Nanophthalmos

Nanophthalmos (Fig. 24.14) is a rare disease characterized by a small eye, high hypermetropia, a weak but thick sclera with abnormal collagen,[95] a tendency to angle closure glaucoma in young patients,[96] and uveal effusion. There is an increased fibronectin level in nanophthalmic sclera and cells.[97] Fibronectin is a glycoprotein involved with cellular adhesion and healing.

Any surgery, but especially intraocular surgery and even laser trabeculoplasty,[98–101] may be complicated by severe uveal effusion and should be avoided where possible. Vortex vein decompression may reduce the incidence of uveal effusion.[98] Some cases may be autosomal recessive. A consanguineous family had seven affected offspring, with a pigmentary retinopathy, cystic macular degeneration, high hypermetropia, nanophthalmos, and angle closure glaucoma.[102]

Cyclopia and synophthalmos

Complete (cyclopic) or partial (synophthalmos) fusion of the two eyes is a very rare birth defect. The brain also fails to develop two hemispheres, and the orbit has gross deformities.[103–105] The defects are rarely compatible with life.

These conditions result from inadequate embryonic neural tissue anteriorly, with subsequent maldevelopment of midline mesodermal structures. The brain is almost always malformed; the telencephalon fails to divide, and a large dorsal cyst develops. Midline structures such as the corpus callosum, septum

197

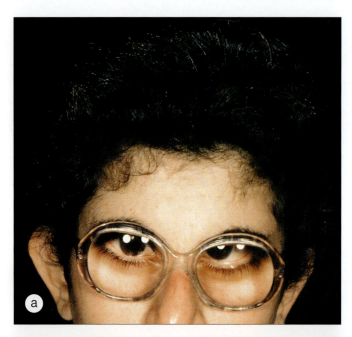

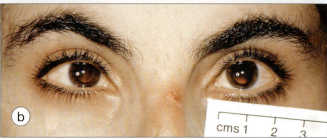

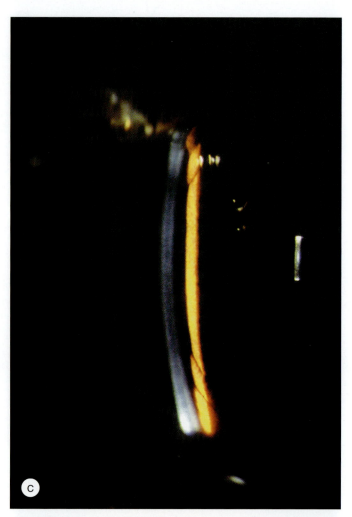

Fig. 24.14 (a) Nanophthalmos showing the high hypermetropia. The phakic correction was +10.0 right, +11.0 left. (b) Nanophthalmos showing small eyes and abnormal red reflex with coaxial illumination. (c) Nanophthalmos showing the shallow anterior chamber. The eyes are prone to angle closure glaucoma. (d) Nanophthalmos showing the crowded optic disc and prominent yellow foveal pigment with a fold between the fovea and the macula. Nanophthalmic eyes are very prone to choroidal effusions in response to intraocular surgery.

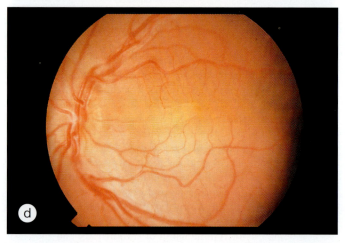

pellucidum, and olfactory lobes are often not present and anomalies may extend to the mesencephalic region with thalamic abnormalities.

The orbits are markedly affected as a consequence of the abnormal development of midline mesodermal structures. The normal nasal cavity is replaced by the "pseudo-orbit,"[106] and the bones show multiple malformations, especially in midline structures. The defects additionally involve the skull, with absence of the sella turcica and clinoids.

The eyes are more commonly partly fused than completely fused. One optic nerve is present, and no chiasm is recognizable. Structures are best developed laterally, such as the muscles innervated by cranial nerves IV and VI in comparison to those innervated by cranial nerve III. Other intraocular abnormalities such as persistent hyperplastic primary vitreous, cataract, coloboma, and microcornea may exist.[107]

Chromosomal aberrations are commonly present.[108] Familial occurrences and association with consanguineous marriages have also been noted.[109]

Other etiological considerations include maternal health[110] and toxic factors. Evidence for this is based on a high incidence in animals who grazed on an alkaloid-containing substance. The importance of cyclopia and synophthalmos is primarily one of academic embryological interest; the overwhelming systemic abnormalities place management of this condition in the hands of perinatologists and geneticists.

Diplophthalmos
A unilateral double eye with ipsilateral temporoparietal porencephaly, supernumerary teeth, and cervical cyst was reported in one case.[111]

REFERENCES

1. Mann I. Developmental Abnormalities of the Eye. Cambridge: Cambridge University Press; 1937.
2. Hintschich C, Zonneveld F, Baldeschi L, et al. Bony orbital development after early enucleation in humans. Br J Ophthalmol 2001; 85: 205–8.
3. Dolk H, Busby A, Armstrong BG, et al. Geographical variation in anophthalmia and microphthalmia in England, 1988–94. BMJ 1998; 317: 905–9.
4. Morrison D, FitzPatrick D, Hanson I, et al. National study of microphthalmia, anophthalmia, and coloboma (MAC) in Scotland: investigation of genetic aetiology. J Med Genet 2002; 39: 16–22.
5. Busby A, Dolk H, Collin R, et al. Compiling a national register of babies born with anophthalmia microphthalmia in England 1988–1994. Arch. Dis. Child (Fetal Neonatal Edition) 1998; 79: 168–73.
6. Cuzick J. Clustering of anophthalmia and microphthalmia is not supported by the data. BMJ 1998; 317: 910.
7. O'Keefe M, Webb M, Pashby RC, et al. Clinical anophthalmos. Br J Ophthalmol 1987; 71: 635–8.
8. Guyer DR, Green WR. Bilateral extreme microphthalmos. Ophthal Pediatr Genet 1984; 4: 81–90.
9. Tucker SM, Sapp N, Collin R. Orbital expansion of the congenitally anophthalmic socket. Br J Ophthalmol 1995; 79: 667–71.
10. Gossman MD, Mohay J, Roberts DM. Expansion of the human microphthalmic orbit. Ophthalmology 1999; 106: 2005–9.
11. Wiese KG, Vogel M, Guthoff R, et al. Treatment of congenital anophthalmos with self-inflating polymer expanders: a new method. J Craniomaxillofac Surg 1999; 27: 72–6.
12. Bateman JB. Microphthalmos. Int Ophthalmol Clin 1984; 24: 87–107.
13. Judisch GF, Martin-Casals A, Hanson JW, et al. Oculodentodigital dysplasia. Four new reports and a literature review. Arch Ophthalmol 1979; 97: 878–84.
14. Weiss AH, Kousseff BG, Ross EA, et al. Complex microphthalmos. Arch Ophthalmol 1989; 107: 1619–24.
15. Heinonen OP, Shapiro S, Slone D. Birth defects and drugs in pregnancy. Massachusetts: Publishing Sciences Group; 1977.
16. Fujiki K, Nakajima A, Yasuda N, et al. Genetic analysis of microphthalmos. Ophthal Paediatr Genet 1989; 1: 139–49.
17. Elder MJ. Aetiology of severe visual impairment and blindness in microphthalmos. Br J Ophthalmol 1994; 78: 332–4.
18. Weiss AH, Kousseff BG, Ross EA, et al. Simple microphthalmos. Arch Ophthalmol 1985; 107: 1625–30.
19. Warburg M. Classification of microphthalmos and coloboma. J Med Genet 1993; 30: 664–9.
20. Mann I. The Development of the Human Eye. London: British Medical Association; 1964.
21. Lindsay EA, Gutto A, Ferrero GB, et al. Microphthalmia with linear skin defects (MLS) syndrome. Am J Med Genet 1994; 49: 229–34.
22. Warburg M. Genetics of microphthalmos. Int Ophthalmol 1981; 4: 45–65.
23. Warburg M. Diagnostic precision in microphthalmos and coloboma of heterogenous origin. Ophthal Paediatr Genet 1981; 1: 37–42.
24. Russel-Eggitt I, Fielder A, Levene M. Microphthalmos in a family. Ophthal Paediatr Genet 1985; 6: 121–8.
25. Kohn G, Shawwa EL, Rayyes E. Isolated "clinical anophthalmia" in an extremely affected Arab kindred. Clin Genet 1988; 33: 321–4.
26. Hornby SJ, Dandona L, Foster A, et al. Clinical findings, consanguinity, and pedigrees in children with anophthalmos in southern India. Dev Med Child Neurol 2001; 43: 392–8.
27. Graham CA, Redmond RM, Nevin L. X-linked clinical anophthalmos: localisation of the gene to Xq27-Xq28. Ophthal Paediatr Genet 1991; 12: 43–8.
28. Baraitser M, Winter R, Russel-Eggitt I, et al. GENEEYE. 2003. Bushey: London Medical Databases Ltd. Available at http://www.lmdatabases.com.
29. De Paepe A, Leroy J, Nuytinck L, et al. Osteoporosis-pseudoglioma syndrome. Am J Med Genet 1993; 45: 30–7.
30. Yokoyama Y, Narahara K, Tsuji K, et al. Autosomal dominant congenital cataract and cataract associated with a familial translocation +(2;16). Hum Genet 1992; 90: 177–8.
31. Haddad R, Font RL, Resser F. Persistent hyperplastic primary vitreous: a clinicopathological study of 62 cases and review of the literature. Surv Ophthalmol 1978; 23: 123–43.
32. Traboulsi EI, Parks MM. Glaucoma in oculo-dento-osseous dysplasia. Am J Ophthalmol 1990; 109: 310–3.
33. Young ID, Fielder AR, Simpson K. Microcephaly, microphthalmos, and retinal folds: report of a family. J Med Genet 1987; 24: 172–4.
34. Edwards J, Lampert R, Hammer M, et al. Ocular defects and dysmorphic features in three generations. J Clin Dysmorphol 1984; 2: 8–12.
35. Pagon RA, Graham JM, Zonana J, et al. Coloboma, congenital heart disease, and choanal atresia with multiple anomalies: CHARGE association. J Pediatr 1981; 99: 223–7.
36. Traboulsi EI, Lenz W, Gonzales-Ramas M, et al. The Lenz microphthalmia syndrome. Am J Ophthalmol 1988; 105: 40–5.
37. Hanson IM. PAX6 and congenital eye malformations. Pediatr Res 2003; 54: 1–6.
38. Glaser T, Jepeal L, Edwards J, et al. PAX6 gene dosage effect in a family with congenital cataracts, aniridia, anophthalmia, and central nervous system defects. Nature Genet 1994; 7: 463–71.
39. Cunliffe HE, McNoe LA, Ward TA, et. al. The prevalence of PAX2 mutations in patients with isolated colobomas or colobomas associated with urogenital anomalies. J Med Genet 1998; 35: 806–12.
40. Schimmenti LA, de la Cruz J, Lewis RA, et al. Novel mutation in sonic hedgehog in non-syndromic colobomatous microphthalmia. Am J Med Genet 2003; 116A: 215–21.
41. Percin EF, Ploder LA, Yu JJ, et al. Human microphthalmia associated with mutations in the retinal homeobox gene CHX10. Nat Genet 2000; 25: 397–401.
42. Enright F, Campbell P, Stallings RL, et al. Xp22.3 microdeletion in a 19-year-old girl with clinical features of MLS syndrome. Pediatr Dermatol 2003; 20: 153–7.
43. Prakash SK, Cormier TA, McCall AE, et al. Loss of holo-cytochrome c-type synthetase causes the male lethality of X-linked dominant microphthalmia with linear skin defects (MLS) syndrome. Hum Mol Genet 2002; 11: 3237–48.
44. Al Gazali LI, Mueller RF, Caine A, et al. Two 46,XX,t(X;Y) females with linear skin defects and congenital microphthalmia: a new syndrome of Xp22.3. J Med Genet 1990; 27: 59–63.
45. McLeod SD, Sugar J, Elejalde BR, et al. Gazali-Temple syndrome. Arch Ophthalmol 1994; 112: 851–2.
46. Temple IK, Hurst JA, Hing S, et al. De novo deletion of Xp22.2pter in a female with linear skin lesions of the face and neck, microphthalmia and anterior chamber eye anomalies. J Med Genet 1990; 27: 56–8.
47. Stratton RF, Walter CA, Paulgar BR, et. al. Second 46,XX male with MLS syndrome. Am J Med Genet 1998; 76: 37–41.
48. Warburg M, Friedrich U. Coloboma and microphthalmos in chromosomal aberrations. Chromosomal aberrations and neural crest cell developmental field. Ophthal Paediatr Genet 1987; 8: 105–18.
49. Wilkes G, Stephenson R. Microphthalmia, microcornea and mental retardation: an autosomal recessive disorder. Proc Or Genet Center 1983; 2: 14–9.
50. Teebi AS, al Saleh QA, Hassoon MM, et al. Macrosomia microphthalmia with or without cleft palate and early infant death: a new autosomal recessive syndrome. Clin Genet 1989; 36: 174–7.
51. Warburg M, Jensen H, Prause JU, et. al. Anophthalmia-microphthalmia-oblique clefting syndrome: confirmation of the Fryns anophthalmia syndrome. Am J Med Genet 1997; 73: 36–40.
52. Wiltshire E, Moore M, Casey T, et al. Fryns "Anophthalmia-Plus" syndrome associated with developmental regression. Clin Dysmorphol 2003; 12: 41–3.
53. Fryns JP, Legius E, Moerman P, et al. Apparently new "anophthalmia-plus" syndrome in sibs. Am J Med Genet 1995; 58: 113–4.

54. Fielding DW, Fryer AL. Recurrence of orbital cysts in the brancio-oculo facial syndrome. J Med Genet 1992; 29: 430–1.

55. McCool M, Weaver DD. Brancio-oculo-facial syndrome: broadening the spectrum. Am J Med Genet 1994; 49: 414–21.

56. Reardon W, Winter RM, Taylor D, et al. Frontofacionasal dysplasia: a new case and review of the phenotype. Clin Dysmorph 1994; 3: 70–9.

57. Ercal D, Say B. Cerebro-oculo-nasal syndrome: another case and review of the literature. Clin Dysmorphol 1998; 7: 139–41.

58. Guerrero JM, Cogen MS, Kelly DR, et al. Proboscis lateralis. Arch Ophthalmol 2001; 119: 1071–4.

59. De Cock R, Merizian A. Delleman syndrome: a case report and review. Br J Ophthalmol 1992; 76: 115–6.

60. Tambe KA, Ambekar SV, Bafna PN. Delleman (oculocerebro-cutaneous) syndrome: few variations in a classical case. Eur J Paediatr Neurol 2003; 7: 77–80.

61. Wallis CE, Beighton P. Ectodermal dysplasia with blindness in sibs on the island of Rodrigues. J Med Genet 1992; 29: 323–5.

62. Fujita H, Meng J, Kawamura M, et al. Boy with a chromosome deletion(3)(q12q23) and blepharophimosis syndrome. Am J Med Genet 1992; 44: 434–6.

63. Siber M. X-linked recessive microcephaly microphthalmia with corneal opacities, spastic quadriplegia, hypospadius and cryptorchidism. Clin Genet 1984; 26: 453–6.

64. Verloes A, Delfortrie J, Lambott C. GOMBO syndrome of growth retardation, ocular abnormalities, microcephaly, brachydactyly and digephrenia: a possible "new" recessively inherited syndrome. Am J Med Genet 1989; 32: 13–8.

65. Ioan DM, Dumitriu L, Belengeariu V, et al. The oculo-dento-digital syndrome: male-to-male transmission and variable expression in a family. Genet Couns 1997; 8: 87–90.

66. Braun M, Seitz B, Naumann GO. Juvenile open angle glaucoma with microcornea in oculo-dento-digital dysplasia (Meyer-Schwickerath-Weyers syndrome). Klin Monatsbl Augenheilkd 1996; 208: 262–3.

67. Widder RA, Engels B, Severin M, et al. A case of angle-closure glaucoma, cataract, nanophthalmos and spherophakia in oculo-dento-digital syndrome. Graefes Arch Clin Exp Ophthalmol 2003; 241: 161–3.

68. Burton PA, Caul EO. Fetal cell tropism of human parvovirus B19. Lancet 1988; ii: 767.

69. Hartwig NG, Vermeij-Keers C, Van Elsacker-Niele AM, et al. Embryonic malformations in a case of intrauterine Parvovirus B19 infection. Teratology 1989; 39: 295–302.

70. Ozeki H, Shirai S. Developmental eye abnormalities in mouse fetuses induced by retinoic acid. Jpn J Ophthalmol 1998; 42: 162–7.

71. Bogdanoff B, Rorke LB, Yanoff M, et al. Brain and eye abnormalities: possible sequelae to prenatal use of multiple drugs including LSD. Am J Dis Child 1972; 123: 145–8.

72. Milunksy A, Ulcickas M, Rothman AJ, et al. Maternal heat exposure and neural tube defects. JAMA 1992; 268: 882–5.

73. Sutcliffe AG, Jones RB, Woodruff G. Eye malformations associated with treatment with carbamazepine during pregnancy. Ophthalmic Genet 1998; 19: 59–62.

74. Willshaw HE. How dangerous a world is it? Br J Ophthalmol 1998; 82: 6–7.

75. Tekin M, Tutar E, Arsan S, et al. Ophthalmo-acromelic syndrome: report and review. Am J Med Genet 2000; 90: 150–4.

76. Lerone M, Persagno A, Taccone A, et al. Oculocerebral syndrome with hypopigmentation. Clin Genet 1992; 41: 87–9.

77. Forrester S, Kovach MJ, Reynolds NM, et al. Manifestations in four males with and an obligate carrier of the Lenz microphthalmia syndrome. Am J Med Genet 2001; 98: 92–100.

78. Ng D, Hadley DW, Tifft CJ, et al. Genetic heterogeneity of syndromic X-linked recessive microphthalmia-anophthalmia: is Lenz microphthalmia a single disorder? Am J Med Genet 2002; 110: 308–14.

79. Ainsworth JR, Morton JE, Good P, et al. Micro syndrome in Muslim Pakistan children. Ophthalmology 2001; 108: 491–7.

80. Hayashi N, Repka MX, Ueno H, et al. Congenital cystic eye: report of two cases and review of the literature. Surv Ophthalmol 1999; 44: 173–9.

81. Leatherbarrow B, Kwartz J, Noble J. Microphthalmos with cyst in monozygous twins. J Pediatr Ophthalmol Strabismus 1990; 27: 294–8.

82. Pasquale LR, Romayananda N, Kubacki J, et al. Congenital cystic eye with multiple ocular and intracranial anomalies. Arch Ophthalmol 1991; 109: 985–7.

83. Weiss A, Martinez C, Greenwald M. Microphthalmos with cyst: clinical presentations and computed tomographic findings. J Pediatr Ophthalmol Strabismus 1985; 22: 6–12.

84. Raynor M, Hodgkins P. Microphthalmos with cyst: preservation of the eye by repeated aspiration. J Pediatr Ophthalmol Strabismus 2001; 38: 245–6.

85. McLean CJ, Ragge NK, Jones RB, et al. The management of orbital cysts associated with congenital microphthalmos and anophthalmos. Br J Ophthalmol 2003; 87: 860–3.

86. Walton WT, Enzenauer RW, Cornell FM. Abortive cryptophthalmos: a case report and a review of cryptophthalmos. J Pediatr Ophthalmol Strabismus 1990; 27: 129–33.

87. McGregor L, Makela V, Darling SM, et al. Fraser syndrome and mouse blebbed phenotype caused by mutations in FRAS1/Fras1 encoding a putative extracellular matrix protein. Nat Genet 2003; 34: 203–8.

88. Vrontou S, Petrou P, Meyer BI, et al. Fras1 deficiency results in cryptophthalmos, renal agenesis and blebbed phenotype in mice. Nat Genet 2003; 34: 209–14.

89. Francois J. Syndrome malformatif avec cryptophtalmie. Acta Genet Med Gemellol (Roma) 1969; 18: 18–50.

90. Hing S, Wison-Holt N, Kriss A, et al. Complete cryptophthalmos: case report with normal flash VEP and ERG. J Pediatr Ophthalmol Strabismus 1990; 27: 133–6.

91. Brazier DJ, Hardman-Lea SJ, Collin JR. Cryptophthalmos: surgical treatment of the congenital symblepharon variant. Br J Ophthalmol 1986; 70: 391–5.

92. Thomas IT, Frias JL, Felix V, et al. Isolated and syndromic cryptophthalmos. Am J Med Genet 1986; 25: 85–98.

93. Rousseau T, Laurent N, Thauvin-Robinet, et al. Prenatal diagnosis and intrafamilial clinical heterogeneity of Fraser syndrome. Prenat Diagn 2002; 22: 692–6.

94. Dibben K, Rabinowitz YS, Shorr N, et al. Surgical correction of incomplete cryptophthalmos in Fraser syndrome. Am J Ophthalmol 1997; 124: 107–9.

95. Stewart DH, Streeten BW, Brockhurst RJ, et al. Abnormal scleral collagen in nanophthalmos: an ultrastructural study. Arch Ophthalmol 1991; 109: 1017–9.

96. Ritch R, Chang BM, Liebmann JM. Angle closure in younger patients. Ophthalmology 2003; 110: 1880–9.

97. Yue BY, Kurosawa A, Duvall J, et al. Nanophthalmic sclera. Fibronectin studies. Ophthalmology 1988; 95: 56–60.

98. Brockhurst RJ. Cataract surgery in nanophthalmic eyes. Arch Ophthalmol 1990; 108: 965–7.

99. Good WV, Stern WH. Recurrent nanophthalmic uveal effusion syndrome following laser trabeculoplasty. Am J Ophthalmol 1988; 106: 234–5.

100. Jin JC, Anderson DR. Laser and unsutured sclerotomy in nanophthalmos. Am J Ophthalmol 1990; 109: 575–81.

101. Villada JR, Osman AA, Alio JL. Cataract surgery in the nanophthalmic eye. J Cataract Refract Surg 2001; 27: 968.

102. MacKay CJ, Shek MS, Carr RE, et al. Retinal degeneration with nanophthalmos, cystic macular degeneration, and angle closure glaucoma. A new recessive syndrome. Arch Ophthalmol 1987; 105: 366–71.

103. Roessler E, Muenke M. Midline and laterality defects: left and right meet in the middle. Bioessays 2001; 23: 888–900.

104. Sezgin I, Sungu S, Bekar E, et al. Cyclopia-astomia-agnathia-holoprosencephaly association: a case report. Clin. Dysmorphol 2002; 11: 225–6.

105. Situ D, Reifel CW, Smith R, et. al. Investigation of a cyclopic, human, term fetus by use of magnetic resonance imaging (MRI). J Anat 2002; 200: 431–8.

106. Duke Elder S. Anomalies in the size of the eye. Normal and abnormal development. London: Kimpton; 1964: 429–51, 488–90. (System of Ophthalmology, Vol III, Part 2.)

107. Spencer WH. Abnormalities of scleral thickness and congenital anomalies. In Spencer WH, editor. Ophthalmic Pathology. An Atlas and Textbook. Philadelphia: Saunders, 1985: 394–5.
108. Kuchle M, Kraus J, Rummelt C, et al. Synophthalmia and holoprosencephaly in chromosome 18p deletion defect. Arch Ophthalmol 1991; 109: 136–8.
109. Howard RO. Chromosomal abnormalities associated with cyclopia and synophthalmia. Trans Am Ophthalmol Soc 1977; 75: 505–38.
110. Stabile M, Bianco A, Iannuzzi S, et al. A case of suspected keratogenic holoprosencephaly. J Med Genet 1985; 22: 147–9.
111. Stefani FH, Hausmann N, Lund OE. Unilateral diplophthalmos. Am J Ophthalmol 1991; 112: 581–6.

CHAPTER 25

Developmental Anomalies of the Lids

Hélène Dollfus and Alain Verloes

Developmental anomalies of the eyelids can be isolated or syndromic conditions. Their clinical and syndromic evaluations are closely linked to dysmorphology: the study of abnormal human development. The examination of a patient with developmental anomalies includes the examination of the eye, lids, and orbital region as well as the other parts of the face and the body.

Four categories of developmental anomalies, also applicable to eyelids, have been described:

1. A *malformation sequence* is a single morphogenetic defect;
2. A *deformation* results from mechanical constraints on a normal embryo;
3. A *disruption sequence* results from the destruction of a normal structure; and
4. A *dysplasia* is when the primary defect lies in the differentiation and organization of a tissue.[1]

When identified, the etiology of congenital anomalies can vary: *in utero* exposure to exogenous teratogens (i.e., alcohol) or to an obstetrical hazard (i.e., amniotic bands), chromosomal anomalies (i.e., trisomy, monosomy, or structural rearrangement as deletion, duplication, or translocation), or a defect in the genes implicated in development.[2]

NORMAL DEVELOPMENT AND ANATOMY OF THE EYELIDS

Embryology of the eyelids

Development of the eyelids is characterized by three main stages in all mammals:

1. initial development;
2. fusion; and
3. final reopening.

Initial development

During the first month of embryonic development, the optic vesicle is covered by a thin layer of surface ectoderm. During the second month, active cellular proliferation of the adjacent mesoderm results in the formation of a circular fold of mesoderm lined on both sides by ectoderm. This fold constitutes the rudiments of the eyelid, which gradually elongates over the eye. The mesodermal portion of the upper lid arises from the frontal nasal process, the lower lid from the maxillary process. The covering layer of ectoderm becomes skin on the outside and the conjunctiva on the inside. Tarsal plate, connective, and muscular tissues of the eyelids are derived from the mesodermal core.

Fusion

Fusion of the eyelids by an epithelial seal begins at the two extremities at 8 weeks and is soon complete, covering the corneal epithelium. The eyelids remain adherent to each other until the end of the fifth to the seventh month.

Final reopening

Separation begins from the nasal side, and is usually completed during the sixth or seventh month of development. Very rarely, this process is incomplete at birth in a full-term infant (Fig. 25.1).[3]

The specialized structures in the lids develop between 8 weeks and 7 months, and by term the lid is fully developed with functioning muscles, lashes, and meibomian glands.

MORPHOLOGY AND ANATOMY OF THE EYELIDS

The eyelids have several characteristic horizontal and vertical folds.

The most conspicuous is a well-demarcated horizontal skin crease 3–4 mm above the upper lid margin, which flattens out on depression and becomes deeply recessed when the upper lid is elevated. It divides each lid into an orbital and tarsal portion. The *orbital portion* lies between the margin of the orbit and the crease, and the *tarsal portion* lies in direct relationship to the globe. A tarsal plate composed of dense connective tissue is found in both the upper and lower eyelids. The upper lid tarsal plate has a marginal length of 29 mm and is 10–12 mm wide. The lower lid tarsal plate is about 4 mm wide.

The *palpebral fissure*–the opening between the upper and lower lids–is the entrance into the conjunctival sac bounded by the margins of the eyelids. This aperture forms an asymmetrical ellipse that undergoes complex changes during infancy.[4] After birth, the upper lid has its lowest position with the lower eyelid margin close to the pupil center. Between ages 3 and 6 months, the position of the upper lid reaches its maximum and then declines linearly. The distance between the pupil center and the lower eyelid margin increases linearly until age 18 months and stabilizes.[4] By adulthood, the upper eyelid covers the upper 1–2 mm of the cornea while the lower lid lies slightly below its inferior margin.[5] Normally, palpebral fissures have a slight outer-upward inclination as the outer canthus is positioned 1 or 2 mm higher then the inner canthus. The normal orientation of the eyelids varies depending on ethnic origin. Palpebral fissure length increases during normal development.[6]

Epicanthus *palpebralis* (or epicanthal fold) is defined as a vertical cutaneous fold arising from the nasal root and directed toward the internal part of the upper lids (Fig. 25.2). It can be subdivided into the areas where they occur such as preseptal, pretarsal, or orbital. Sometimes the fold may cover the inner canthus. It is a normal finding in fetuses of all races and commonly found in young children who have a flat nasal bridge.

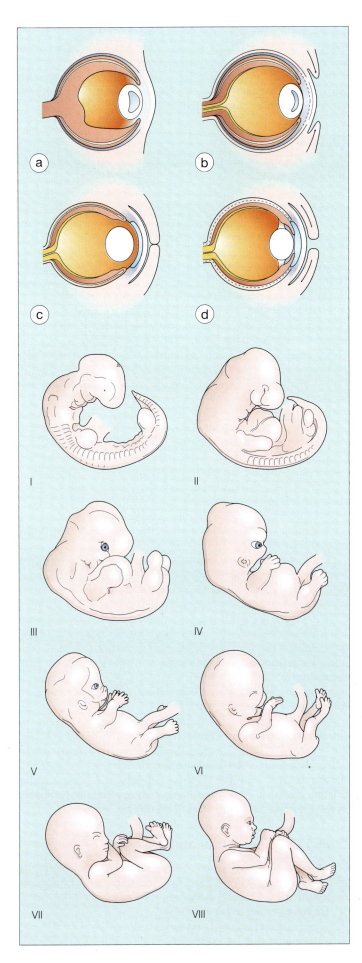

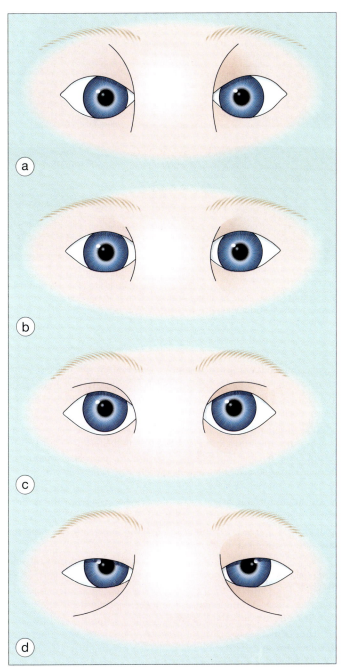

Fig. 25.2 Epicanthus. (a) Superciliaris; (b) palpebralis (most frequent); (c) tarsalis ("Asian epicanthus"); (d) inversus (blepharophimosis–ptosis–epicanthus inversus syndrome).

Fig. 25.1 Development of the eyelids. Schematic representation of the eyelids (a–d) and of the development of the embryo and the fetus (after 2 months). Main stages of the development of the eyelids (a–d). (a) Before 6 weeks: optic vesicle covered with surface ectoderm. (b) Between 6 and 8 weeks: superior and inferior folds elongated over the eye. (c) Soon after 8 weeks of development: fusion of the superior and inferior folds of the eyelids until the seventh month. (d) From the seventh month to birth; the eyelids are open. (I–VIII) Main stages of development of a human being with regard to eyelid development. (I) Embryo aged 31–35 days (no eyelids). (II) Embryo aged 6 weeks (the eyelids start to appear). ((III) Embryo aged 7 weeks. (IV and V) Embryo during the 8th week. (VI) Embryo aged 9 weeks (the eyelids have started to fuse). (VII) Fetus aged 4 months (eyelids are fused). (VIII) Fetus close to birth (eyelid can open).

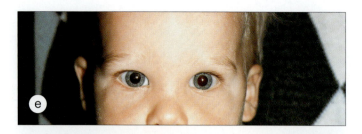

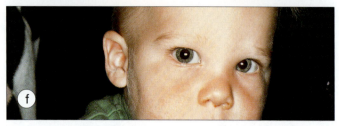

Fig. 25.2 Epicanthus. *(Cont'd)* (e) Epicanthus in the straight-ahead position. This child can be seen to have a broad base to his nose and mild epicanthus. In the straight-ahead position his eyes appear straight. (f) On looking right the adducting eye appears to be convergent, giving rise to a pseudosquint.

Epicanthus palpebralis is present as a normal morphologic feature in many populations, mostly in Asians. As opposed to epicanthus palpebralis, epicanthus *inversus* is defined as a dermal fold arising from the lower lid and diminishing toward the upper lid (see blepharophimosis).

The principle muscle involved in opening the upper lid and in maintaining normal lid position is the *levator palpebrae superioris*. Müller's muscle and the frontalis muscle play accessory roles.

The levator palpebrae superioris arises as a short tendon blended with the underlying origin of the superior rectus from the undersurface of the lesser wing of the sphenoid bone. The levator palpebrae superioris is innervated by branches from the superior division of the oculomotor nerve.

Müller's muscle is composed of a thin band of smooth muscle fibers about 10 mm in width that arise on the inferior surface of the levator palpebrae superioris. It courses anteriorly, directly between the levator aponeurosis and the conjunctiva of the upper eyelid to insert into the superior margin of the tarsus. Branches of the ocular sympathetic pathway innervate the fibers of Müller's muscle. The eyelid is indirectly elevated by attachment of the frontalis muscle into the superior orbital portions of the *orbicularis oculi muscle*. The frontalis muscle is innervated by the temporal branch of the facial nerve.

CLINICAL EVALUATION OF THE EYELIDS

In dysmorphology, the clinical assessment of craniofacial features, including eyelid malformations, is based on the overall subjective qualitative clinical evaluation but also on objective quantitative measurements. Qualitative anomalies are relatively easy to define as present or absent compared to an "ideal" human phenotype. The frequency of a feature in the general population defined as a "variant" (present in more than 1% of human beings) must be distinguished from an "anomaly." A number of anomalies useful in dysmorphology are quantitative. This means that an objective definition of an abnormal phenotype requires the knowledge of the normal variation of the trait (usually defined as ±2 SD (standard deviation) for any measurement) in a population of a given ethnic background or at a given age (see Chapter 5). Some anomalies are subjective e.g. "a coarse face."

In clinical practice, morphological measurements can be easily performed with transparent ruler measurements. The measurements are usually compared to a normal database.[5]

Clinical landmarks

Many anomalies of the lids are related to or correlated with an abnormal orbital structure. Hypertelorism and hypotelorism, for instance, refers to anomalies of the skull, but they influence critically the appearance of the eyelids. The normal distance between the orbits varies during embryogenesis and after birth in accordance with the general craniofacial development.

The embryonic separation of the globes, defined by the angle between the optic nerves at the chiasm of the fetus, progresses from a widely divergent 180° angle between the ocular axes in the first weeks of development to an angle of 70° at birth and 68° in adulthood[7,8] (Fig. 25.3a). The interorbital distance, defined as the shortest distance between the inner walls of the orbits, increases with age[9] (Fig. 25.3b). The most accurate interorbital measurements are the bony interorbital distances from X-rays (Waters incidence (half-axial projection) or from posteroanterior cephalograms) or computed tomograms used usually for pre-surgical evaluation.[10]

In clinical practice, evaluation of the interocular distances is based on the measurement of the following lid-based landmarks that can be easily compared to normal values:[11–15]

Interpupillary distance;
Inner intercanthal distance;
Outer intercanthal distances; and
Horizontal palpebral length.

An approximate "rule of thumb" estimation of normality is to consider that the inner intercanthal distance is equivalent to the palpebral length (Fig. 25.4).

Different quantitative methods have been used for children and for adults with tables presenting the evolution of the interocular distances according to age (see Chapter 5). The routine clinical method for assessing interocular distance is based on a biometric study that includes measurements of the inner intercanthal distance, the outer intercanthal distance, and the interpupillary distance in Caucasians from birth to 14 years. The normal intercanthal distance is 20 ± 2 mm (1 SD) at birth increasing to 26 ± 1.5 mm by 2 years of age. The normal interpupillary distance is 39 ± 3 mm at birth increasing to 48 ± 2 mm by 2 years of age.[4]

Ethnic variations of orbital features are important as the distances may vary considerably from the published data. For example a study comparing newborns from England and Africa showed that the Caucasian and the African newborns had the same inner canthal distance, whereas the outer canthal distance and palpebral fissure length were significantly smaller in the Caucasian newborn than in the African newborn.[16]

Eyelid developmental anomalies

Developmental anomalies of the eyelids include variable eyelid malformations sometimes important in dysmorphology diagnosis. Systematic clinical eyelid evaluation is based on:
1. Distances between the eyelids;
2. General morphology of the eyelids;
3. Palpebral fissures and slanting;

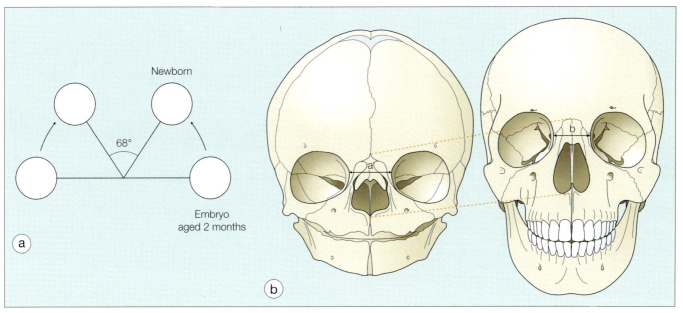

Fig. 25.3 Evolution of the ocular axis and the inner interorbital wall during development of a human face. (a) Ocular axis from 180° for an 8-week-old embryo to 68° for a newborn (adapted from Zimmermann et al.[8]). (b) Evolution of the bony orbit: a face from newborn compared to an adult.

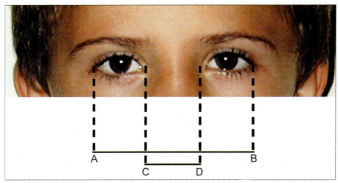

Fig. 25.4 Normal interocular distances. "The rule of the thumb" in a five-year-old child: inner intercanthal distance is equivalent to palpebral length (AB = BC = CD).

4. Position of the eyelids; and
5. Evaluation of the eyebrows and eyelashes.

ABNORMAL DISTANCES BETWEEN THE EYELIDS AND ORBITS

Conditions with abnormal distances between the eyelid landmarks are defined in Table 25.1 and schematically presented in Fig. 25.5.

Hypotelorism

Hypotelorism can be the result of a skull malformation or failure in brain development. Hypotelorism occurs in more than 60 syndromes (Fig. 25.6). For instance, in trigonocephaly, a craniosynostosis caused by premature closure of the metopic sutures results in a triangular skull with a prominent frontal protuberance and hypotelorism.[17]

Holoprosencephaly is a rare major malformation of the brain frequently associated with craniofacial anomalies.[18,19] Holoprosencephaly results from an abnormal cleavage and morphogenesis of the embryonic forebrain during the third week, with alobar or semilobar development of the telencephalon associated with missing or incomplete development of the midline structures of the face. Severity of midfacial anomalies correlates usually, but not universally, with the severity of the underlying brain malformation.[20,21] The related craniofacial anomalies constitute a spectrum extending from a single median orbit with more or less fused eye globes (cyclopia) with an overhanging proboscis to milder facial abnormality consisting of a single maxillary incisor with hypotelorism (Table 25.1). Holoprosencephaly may be due to environmental/maternal factors (such as maternal diabetes), chromosomal abnormalities (trisomy 13, 18q deletion), or single gene defects[22] (Table 25.2).

Hypertelorism

Hypertelorism occurs in more then 550 disorders (Fig. 25.7, Fig. 25.8). Three pathogenic mechanisms have been suggested:[9]
1. The early ossification of the lesser wings of the sphenoid, fixing the orbits in fetal position;
2. The failure of development of the nasal capsule, allowing the primitive brain vesicle to protrude into the space normally occupied by the capsule, resulting in morphokinetic arrest in the position of the eyes as in frontal encephalocele;[23] and
3. A disturbance in the development of the skull base as in craniosynostosis syndromes (as in Crouzon or Apert syndrome) or in midfacial malformations such as frontonasal dysplasia.

The widow's peak (low median implantation on the scalp hair on the forehead) is a consequence of ocular hypertelorism as the two fields of hair-suppression are further apart than usual with the fields failing to overlap sufficiently high on the forehead.

Table 25.1 Conditions with abnormal spacing of the orbits and eyelids

Condition	Definition	Comments
Hypertelorism	Increased distance of the inner and outer intercanthal distances	1. Not only the increased inner intercanthal distance (a common mistake) 2. Exclude erroneous hypertelorism (misleading adjacent structures) in cases of: Flat nasal bridge Epicanthic folds Exotropia Widely spaced eyebrows Narrow palpebral fissures Isolated dystopia canthorum
Hypotelorism	Reduced distance between the medial walls of the orbits with reduced inner and outer intercanthal distances	Exclude illusory hypotelorism in cases of: Esotropia Closely spaced eyebrows
Telecanthus	Increased distance between the inner canthi *Primary telecanthus*: increased distance between the inner canthi (normally spaced outer canthi and normal interpupillary measurement) *Secondary telecanthus*: increased inner canthi distance (associated with ocular hypertelorism)	Often mistaken as hypertelorism
Dystopia canthorum	Lateral displacement of the inner canthi (telecanthus) together with lateral displacement of the lacrimal puncta	Clinical tip: an imaginary vertical line passing through the lacrimal punctum cuts the cornea

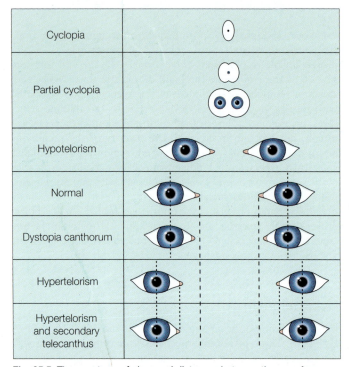

Fig. 25.5 The spectrum of abnormal distances between the eyes from cyclopia to hypertelorism.

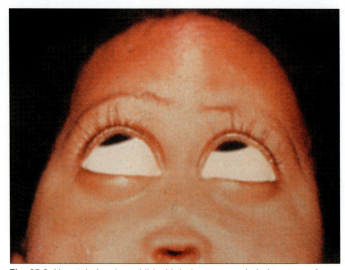

Fig. 25.6 Hypotelorism in a child with holoprosencephaly (courtesy of Dr Sylvie Odent).

Telecanthus and dystopia canthorum

Telecanthus, wide set eyes, is a common feature in syndromes, whereas dystopia canthorum is a specific feature of Waardenburg syndrome (WS) type 1[24] (Fig. 25.9). This condition is an autosomal dominant syndrome with variable expressivity, characterized by dystopia canthorum with a broad nasal root, often poliosis and a white forelock, heterochromia irides, and various degrees of sensorineural hearing loss.[25] WS type 2 differs from WS type 1 by the absence of dystopia canthorum (type 3 is a variant of type 1 with limb anomalies, whereas type 4 is associated with Hirschsprung disease).[26]

MAJOR MALFORMATIONS OF EYELID

Ablepharon

Ablepharon is defined as the absence of lids. It has been reported in several settings. In the Neu–Laxova syndrome, ablepharon is associated with intrauterine growth retardation, syndactyly, swollen "collodion" skin, microcephaly, and severe developmental brain defects.[27]

In the autosomal recessive ablepharon-macrostomia syndrome, patients have congenitally absent or rudimentary eyelids,[28] a hypoplastic nose, ambiguous genitalia, an absent zygoma, and macrostomia with possible familial recurrence[29] (Fig. 25.10).

Table 25.2 Gene identification in syndromes with developmental eyelid anomalies cited in this chapter (updated June 2003)

Name of syndrome	Type of eyelid anomaly	Gene identification (reference)	Extra ocular manifestation
Holoprosencephaly	Cyclopia or more or less severe hypotelorism	SHH (sonic-hedgehog)[94] SIX3 (since oculis homeobox 3)[95] TGIF (TG interacting factor)[96] ZIC2 (zinc finger protein of cerebellum)[97]	Malformation of the brain induces secondary craniofacial anomaly
Apert syndrome	Hypertelorism Protrusion of the eyes Asymmetry of orbits Strabismus	FGFR2 (Fibroblast growth factor receptor 2)[98]	Severe craniosynostosis Major syndactyly
Crouzon syndrome	Hypertelorism Protrusion of the eyes Asymmetry of orbits	FGFR2-FGFR3 (Fibroblast growth factor receptor 2 and 3)[99]	Craniostenosis Severe to moderate
Coffin Lowry syndrome	Hypertelorism Down-slanting palpebral fissures	RPS6KA3 (Ribosomal protein S6 kinase)[100]	X-linked mental retardation syndrome
Waardenburg syndrome	Telecanthus Dystopia canthorum (distinguishes WS1 and WS2)	PAX3 (Paired-box 3) (WS type 1)[101] MITF (Microphthalmia associated transcription factor) (WS type 2)[102]	Iris heterochromia Variable deafness White forelock
Fraser syndrome	Cryptophthalmos	FRAS1 (extracellular matrix protein)[103]	Renal agenesis or hypoplasia, laryngal stenosis, syndactyly
Hay Wells—EEC3	Sparse eyebrows and eyelashes	P63 protein[104,105]	Ectrodactyly-ectodermal dysplasia-clefting syndrome
Treacher–Collins syndrome	Down-slanting palpebral fissures Occasional colobomas of eyelids	TCOF1 (Treacher–Collins Franceschetti gene 1)[106]	First branchial arch syndrome
Cohen syndrome	Wavy eyelid	COH1 (Cohen syndrome gene 1)[107]	Microcephaly, mental retardation, intermittent neutropenia, retinal dystrophy
BPES type I and type II	Blepharophimosis Ptosis Epicanthus inversus	FOXL2 (Forkhead box C 2)[108,109]	Genotype–phenotype correlations for BPES type I and BPES type II for female infertility
Saethre–Chotzen syndrome	Ptosis	TWIST (Rarely FGFR2 and FGFR3)[110,111]	Variable craniosynostosis Minor limb and ear anomalies
Noonan syndrome	Ptosis	PTPN11[112]	Webbing of the neck, pectus excavatum, pulmonic stenosis, cryptorchidism
Rubinstein–Taybi syndrome	Heavy high-arched eyebrows Down-slanting palpebral fissures Ptosis	CBP (CRE-binding protein)[113]	Broad thumbs and toes, characteristic facies, mental retardation
Alopecia universalis (AD)	Absent eyebrows and eyelashes	HR (human homolog of mouse hairless gene)[114]	Absent hair on all the body
Ectodermal dysplasia anhydrotic (EDA) (XL)	Absent or sparse eyebrows and eyelashes	Ectodysplasin A gene[115]	Abnormal sweating and dentition
Lymphedema-distichiasis syndrome	Distichiasis Ptosis	FOXC2[116,117]	Lymphedema

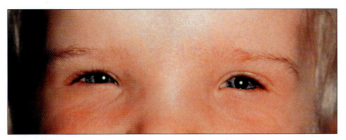

Fig. 25.7 Hypertelorism in Optiz syndrome (esophageal abnormalities, hypospadias, and other midline defects). Image courtesy of Clinique ophthalmologique des Hôpitaux Universitaires de Strasbourg.

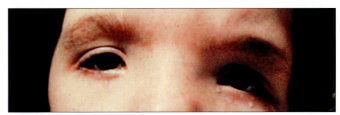

Fig. 25.8 Hypertelorism in Coffin–Lowry syndrome (a mental retardation syndrome).

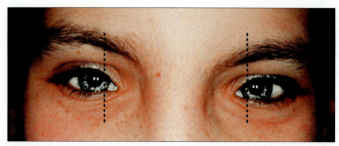

Fig. 25.9 Telecanthus and dystopia canthorum. A teenager with Waardenburg syndrome. Note that an imaginary vertical line at the level of the puncta cuts the cornea.

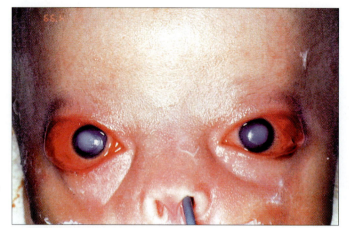

Fig. 25.10 Bilateral ablepharon. Ablepharon macrostomia syndrome. Image courtesy of Dr AA Cruz.

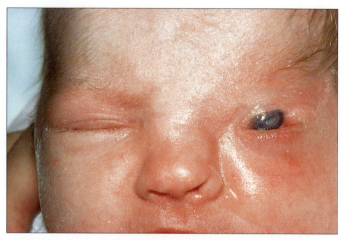

Fig. 25.11 Cryptophthalmos. Unilateral partial abortive cryptophthalmos (symblepharon): the upper lid is fused to the eye.

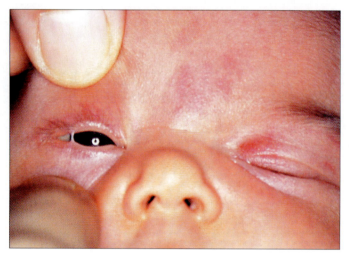

Fig. 25.12 Ankyloblepharon. Image courtesy of Dr AA Cruz.

Cryptophthalmos (see Chapter 24)

Cryptophthalmos is a rare malformation in which there is a failure of development of the eyelid folds with continuity of the skin from the forehead to the cheek.[30,31]

In complete cryptophthalmos, the epithelium that is normally differentiated into cornea and conjunctiva becomes part of the skin that passes continuously from the forehead to the cheek. The eyebrow is usually absent and the globe microphthalmic.

In the incomplete form, a rudimentary lid and conjunctival sac is present.

Abortive cryptophthalmos presents with a normal lower lid and an absent or abnormal upper lid, the forehead skin passing directly to and fusing with the superior cornea (Fig. 25.11).

Cryptophthalmos may be an isolated finding or present as part of Fraser syndrome.[30] Fraser syndrome, a rare autosomal recessive syndrome, combines cryptophthalmos, hypoplasia of the genitalia, laryngeal stenosis, and renal hypoplasia or agenesis.

Ankyloblepharon

Ankyloblepharon is a partial or complete adhesion of the ciliary edges of the superior and inferior eyelids. *Ankyloblepharon filiforme ad natum* is usually a sporadic isolated malformation in which the upper and lower lids are joined by tags (easily cured by a rapid simple surgical procedure)[32] (Fig. 25.12). Ankyloblepharon may be inherited as an autosomal dominant trait, and may occur in association with ectodermal defects and cleft lip and/or palate in Hay–Wells syndrome,[33] an allelic variant of the ectodactyly–ectodermal dysplasia–cleft lip palate (EEC) syndrome

(see Chapter 31). Ankyloblepharon has been also reported in trisomy 18.[34]

Clefting or notching of the eyelids ("coloboma")

Notches or clefts of the eyelid have been described as eyelid colobomas although there is no embryological relation with the eyeball colobomatous anomalies due to malclosure of the embryological fissure. The shape is usually triangular with the base at the lid margin, and the size may vary from a discrete notch to a major defect with the threat of exposure keratopathy requiring surgical procedures.[35]

Eyelid colobomas may be found in all areas of the eyelids but are most common in the nasal half of the upper lid. More than one lid may be involved in the same patient, or there may be multiple colobomas in the same lid.

The eye itself may be normal or show abnormalities such as corneal opacities, and iris and retinal colobomas extending to microphthalmos and anophthalmos. There may be associated bands limiting ocular motility, and strabismus is common.[36] The causes of eyelid colobomas remain uncertain. For some authors they are equivalent to facial clefts, but intrauterine factors may play a major role.[37] Amniotic bands may cause mechanical

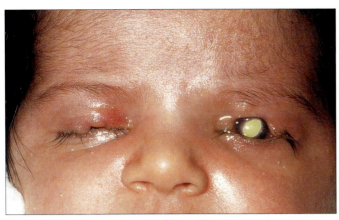

Fig. 25.13 Coloboma of the eyelid. Bilateral lid colobomas in a patient with Goldenhar syndrome. Since birth this child has corneal exposure on the left from a large lid coloboma that has given rise to drying of the cornea, corneal ulceration, and ultimately scarring.

disruptive clefting of the eyelids in the amniotic deformity adhesions mutilations (ADAM) syndrome.[38]

Coloboma of the upper lid can occur in the oculo-auriculo-vertebral dysplasia syndrome (Goldenhar syndrome) (Fig. 25.13). Coloboma of the lower lid is a common feature of the autosomal dominant Treacher–Collins syndrome.[39,40]

ABNORMAL PALPEBRAL FISSURES

Palpebral fissure orientation

Abnormal orientation, or slanting, of the palpebral fissures are described as "up-slanting" when the outer canthus is positioned higher than usual or as "down-slanting" when the outer canthus is lower than usual.

In trisomy 21, up-slanting of the palpebral fissures, though not specific, is the most common ocular and facial feature[41,42] (Fig. 25.14).

Hypoplastic malar bones often result in down-slanting palpebral fissures. It is a characteristic finding in first or second branchial arch malformations such as the Treacher–Collins syndrome characterized by a narrow face with hypoplasia of supraorbital rims, zygomas, and hypoplastic ear (Fig. 25.15).

The palpebral fissure may have a "wave shape" in the Cohen syndrome defined by a specific facial gestalt, developmental delay, and retinal degeneration[43] (Fig. 25.16).

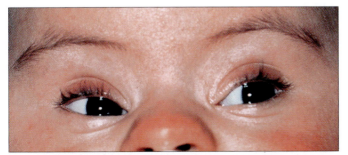

Fig. 25.14 Up-slanting palpebral fissures in a child with trisomy 21. Image courtesy of Clinique ophthalmologique des Hôpitaux Universitaires de Strasbourg.

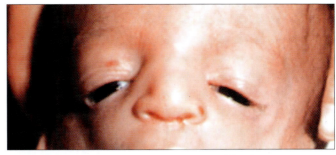

Fig. 25.15 Down slanting palpebral fissures in a child with Treacher–Collins syndrome.

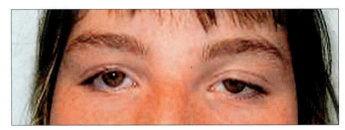

Fig. 25.16 "Wavy palpebral" fissures in Cohen syndrome (associated with retinal dystrophy). Image courtesy of Dr Y Alembik.

Long palpebral fissures

The palpebral fissure length may be increased with an enlargement of the palpebral aperture.

Euryblepharon is a condition of generalized enlargement of the palpebral aperture, usually greatest in the lateral aspect.[44] There is localized outward and downward displacement of the lateral canthus, with a downward displacement of the lower lid. This may superficially mimic the appearance of congenital ectropion (the whole length eversion of the lower lid defines congenital ectropion). It may occur as an isolated anomaly, may be inherited as an autosomal dominant trait, or may be associated with trisomy 21[45] or with craniofacial dysostosis.

Euryblepharon is characteristic of the Kabuki syndrome, defined by postnatal growth retardation, mental retardation, and a facial gestalt reminiscent of the makeup of the actors of a traditional Japanese theatre[46,47] (Fig. 25.17).

Short palpebral fissures

A moderate reduction of the palpebral length may be the consequence of excessive curvature of the palpebral rim ("almond-shaped fissures") and can be found in trisomy 21.

Blepharophimosis is a malformation defined by a considerable reduction in the horizontal dimensions of the palpebral fissure. Blepharophimosis can be isolated or part of various syndromes and should not be confused with ptosis (which has normal horizontal distance of fissures).[48]

The fetal alcohol syndrome (due to alcohol consumption during pregnancy) associates growth retardation, microcephaly, and cognitive impairment. It is one of the most common causes of blepharophimosis.[49]

The blepharophimosis–ptosis–epicanthus inversus syndrome (BPES) is an autosomal dominant condition defined by the presence of marked blepharophimosis, ptosis associated with hypoplasia of the tarsal plates, and epicanthus inversus (Fig. 25.18).

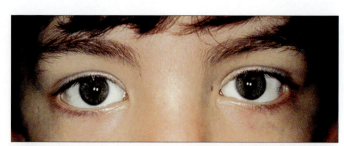

Fig. 25.17 Euryblepharon in Kabuki syndrome.

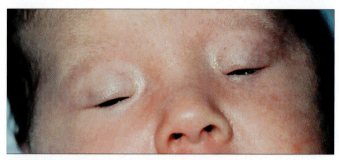

Fig. 25.18 Blepharophimosis–ptosis–epicanthus inversus syndrome (BPES) in a 2-month-old child.

Two clinical types of BPES have been defined:[50]
1. BPES I is characterized by transmission through males only and menstrual irregularity and infertility due to ovarian failure in the affected females.
2. BPES type II does not have the associated infertility[50] and transmission is through both sexes.

Early milestones may be thought to be delayed because of suspicions of hypotonia and backward head tilt.

Ohdo syndrome is a usually sporadic syndrome defined by blepharophimosis, ptosis, dental hypoplasia, partial deafness, and mental retardation.[51]

Ptosis and/or blepharophimosis are also observed in chromosomal syndromes. Blepharophimosis with ptosis is, for instance, a hallmark of chromosome 3p deletion.[52]

ABNORMAL POSITION OF THE EYELIDS

Ectropion

Congenital ectropion refers to an outward rotation of the eyelid margin present at birth. It may occur in the upper or lower lids, rarely as an isolated anomaly. Associations of congenital or acquired ectropion include the blepharophimosis syndrome, trisomy 21,[53] mandibulofacial or other facial dysostoses, skin disorders, i.e., lamellar ichthyosis[54] or congenital cutis laxa microphthalmos, buphthalmos, and orbital cysts.

Congenital skin disorders may lead to congenital ectropion as, for instance, in congenital cutis laxa with looseness of the lid or the harlequin ichthyotic babies with cicatricial ectropion (Fig. 25.19). Therapy may be initially conservative using lubrication. Surgical intervention is indicated for exposure keratitis or cosmesis.

Eversion

Congenital eversion of the lids is an acute ectropion. It can occur intermittently in neonates when the child cries. It is caused by spasm of the orbicularis muscle and usually corrects itself spontaneously. If it becomes established the conjunctiva becomes chemotic and may obscure the globe. This condition, which has been reported in association with trisomy 21, black babies, and difficult deliveries, should be treated initially by pressure patching or repositioning of the lids and taping and in second intention with surgery[55] (Fig. 25.20).

Epitarsus

Primary epitarsus is an apron-like fold of conjunctiva attached to the inner surface of the upper lid. It occurs secondary to conjunctivitis and amniotic bands or as a congenital anomaly.[56]

Epiblepharon

Epiblepharon is a condition characterized by the presence of a horizontal fold of skin across either the upper or lower eyelid, which forces the lashes against the cornea. There is a familial tendency. It occurs more frequently in chubby-cheeked and in Asian infants.[57] Epiblepharon usually corrects itself within the

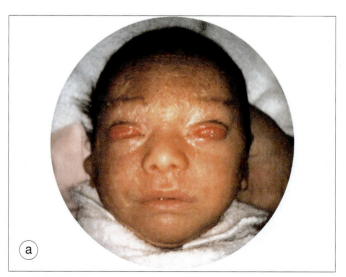

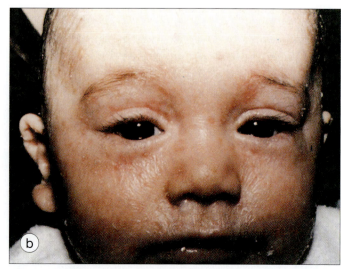

Fig. 25.19 Ectropion. (a) Bilateral ectropion in a patient with severe congenital ichthyosis. (b) Same patient after bilateral lid suture (Dr Geoffrey Hipwell's patient).

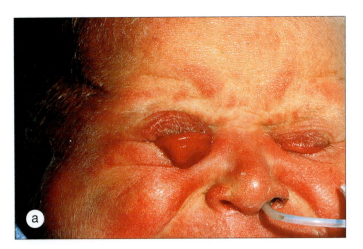

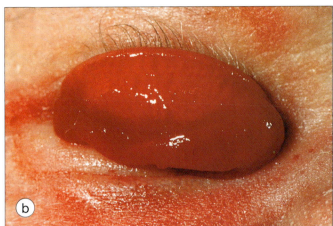

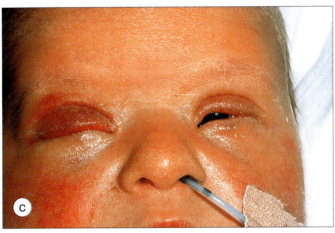

Fig. 25.20 Lid eversion. (a) This neonate with Down syndrome developed lid eversion when crying that rapidly became permanently present. The birth history was unremarkable. (b) The lid eversion was maintained by the very marked chemosis. (c) After taping the lids for 4 days the swelling resolved, leaving bruising, indicating that hemorrhaging may play a causative role.

first 2 years of life as a result of differential growth of the facial bones; occasionally surgery to remove a strip of skin and fat from the lid margin is necessary. It is seldom associated with keratitis (Fig. 25.21).

Entropion

Congenital entropion refers to turning inward of the lid margin, with associated malposition of the tarsal plate. It usually involves the lower lid, although involvement of the upper lid has been documented. Congenital entropion must be distinguished from epiblepharon, where a skinfold causes a secondary turning of the lower lid eyelashes. Entropion may be secondary to microphthalmos and enophthalmos, resulting from lack of support of the posterior border of the eyelid.

The etiology of primary congenital entropion is controversial: hypertrophy of the marginal portion of the orbicularis muscle and disinsertion of the lower lid retractors have been considered responsible factors by various authors.[58–60]

Protection of the cornea is paramount. Congenital entropion, as opposed to congenital epiblepharon, requires prompt surgical intervention to prevent corneal scarring and infection[61] (Fig. 25.22). Surgical procedures are usually directed toward myocutaneous resection and plication or reattachment of the lower lid retractors to the inferior tarsal border. A trial of simpler treatment may be worthwhile.

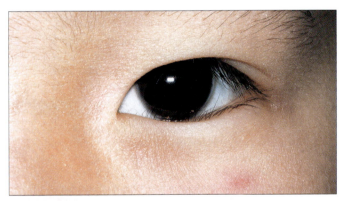

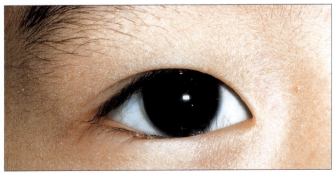

Fig. 25.21 Epiblepharon. In this child the lower lid lashes have turned in from birth, but the cornea has remained undamaged. Spontaneous improvement usually occurs.

211

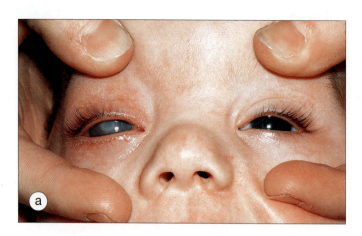

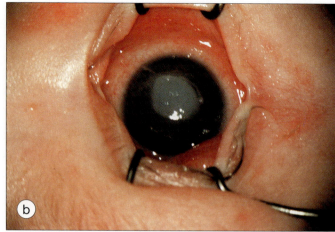

Fig. 25.22 Congenital entropion. (a) Shortly after birth this child's eye was found to be swollen. During examination under anesthetic right upper lid entropion was found. (b) A corneal abrasion caused by the entropion.

Lid retraction in infancy

Occasionally infants may present with a history of one or both eyelids appearing to be retracted. Upper lid retraction is considered to exist when the resting position of the lid is above the superior limbus. For lower lid retraction the affected lower lid rests below the inferior limbus. There is often significant asymmetry between the two sides. There are several conditions that can give rise to this appearance:

1. Physiological, in the newborn.
2. Congenital idiopathic lid retraction.[62] There are patients in whom one eyelid, usually the upper, is retracted. Several anatomical variants may be responsible for this, such as an increase in the number and size of the levator muscle fibers and a thickened or shortened levator aponeurosis or orbital septum. No definite etiology has been established.
3. A false appearance of lid retraction may be given by ipsilateral proptosis or contralateral ptosis when the child is trying to elevate the ptotic lid, and with inferior rectus fibrosis, double elevator palsy, Brown syndrome, or orbital pathology, which restrict upward movement of the eye.
4. Bilateral lid elevation with an upgaze palsy is the classic "setting sun" sign in hydrocephalus of any cause and also in dorsal midbrain disease.
5. Lid retraction, unilateral or bilateral, may occur with the Marcus Gunn jaw-winking phenomenon. Sometimes there is no ptosis–the lid just elevates.
6. Neonatal Graves disease.[63]
7. A sequel to third nerve palsy with aberrant regeneration.[64]
8. Myasthenic patients may have transient lid retraction, a "twitch," after looking down for a period.
9. Lid lag is a defective relaxation of the lids that occurs in hyperthyroidism, myopathic disease, a congenitally short levator tendon,[65] or occasionally myasthenia gravis.
10. Seventh nerve palsy.
11. Levator fibrosis.[66]
12. Vertical nystagmus.

Treatment necessarily depends upon the etiology. For primary congenital eyelid retraction, initial management should consist of observation and lubrication. Indications for surgical intervention include corneal exposure and cosmesis.

PTOSIS

Ptosis is usually classified as congenital or acquired but many conditions, such as third nerve palsies and Horner syndrome, may be either. The essential differentiation is between a simple congenital dystrophy or dysgenesis of the levator muscle and other causes of ptosis. If the levator is dystrophic, it will not relax properly and there will be some lid lag on downgaze; whereas if the levator muscle is not dystrophic, the ptotic eyelid will remain ptotic in all positions of gaze.

The following classification emphasizes this differentiation and covers most of the causes of ptosis.

Classification

Congenital ptosis

Simple congenital ptosis is by far the most common type of ptosis in childhood (Figs. 25.23–25.26). It is due to a dystrophy or dysgenesis of the levator palpebrae superioris muscle. Lid lag on downgaze and the extent of the skin crease are also usually related to the levator function. In view of the close embryological development of the levator and superior rectus muscles, it is not surprising that a ptosis may be associated with a superior rectus weakness. There is no well-defined pattern of heredity, and it is not known why an isolated unilateral dystrophy of the levator muscle should be relatively common.

Aponeurotic defects may occur anywhere in the aponeurosis. They are associated with good levator function and no lid lag on downgaze. The most common sites are at the origin or insertion of the aponeurosis. If a defect occurs at the origin and the terminal aponeurosis is normal, the child will have a ptosis with good levator function and a normal skin crease. If the defect occurs at the insertion of the aponeurosis, as commonly occurs with trauma, the ptosis will be associated with a high skin crease.

Neurogenic defects

A *third nerve palsy* may be either congenital or acquired. The many causes and appropriate investigations are not detailed here. There is a ptosis and the eye is abducted by the lateral rectus and intorted by the superior oblique muscle. There may be associated neurological defects.[66] The pupil is usually but not always large with loss of accommodation if the parasympathetic supply is

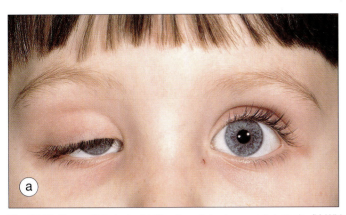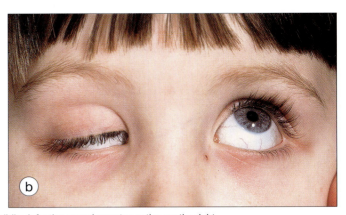

Fig. 25.23 Congenital ptosis. (a) Simple unilateral congenital ptosis. (b) With mildly defective superior rectus action on the right.

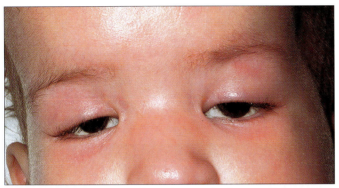

Fig. 25.24 Congenital ptosis. Bilateral severe simple congenital ptosis.

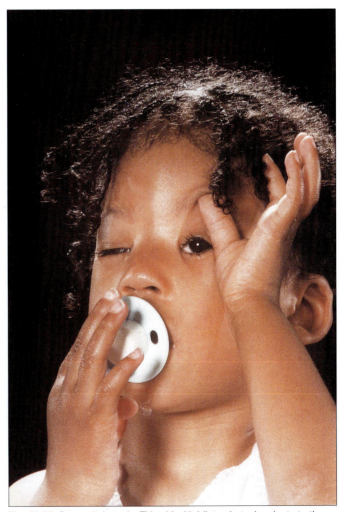

Fig. 25.25 Congenital ptosis. This girl with bilateral ptosis adapts to the condition by lifting her lid anytime she wants to see more clearly.

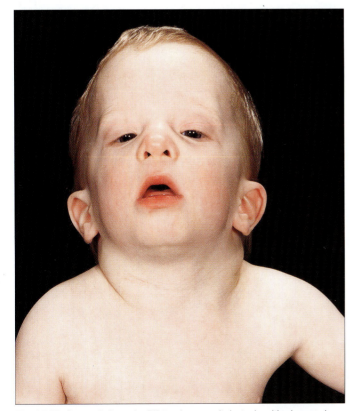

Fig. 25.26 Congenital ptosis. Bilateral congenital ptosis with abnormal head posture. The abnormal head posture is an adaptive mechanism to allow binocular vision.

involved. Recognition of the condition in its complete form is easy, but in partial form the diagnosis may be missed and investigation delayed.

Aberrant third nerve regeneration may occur after a congenital or acquired oculomotor palsy.

Marcus Gunn jaw-winking syndrome is due to an abnormal synkinesis between the levator and usually the lateral pterygoid muscle. The affected eyelid is usually ptotic but elevates when the jaw is opened and deviated to the contralateral side (Figs. 25.27, 25.28). A medial pterygoid synkinesis in which the affected eyelid elevates when the jaw is clenched or protruded is less common. The voluntary levator excursion is always decreased, and frequently there is a weakness of the superior rectus muscle. The condition is almost always congenital, sporadic, and unilateral, but acquired and familial cases may occur. There is normally a synkinesis between the lateral pterygoid and the levator muscles.

Horner syndrome comprises ptosis, miosis, and sometimes anhidrosis on the affected side of the face and neck. If the lesion is congenital, iris pigmentation may be defective (see Chapter 67).

Myogenic ptosis

Progressive external ophthalmoplegia may present in childhood with ptosis, which may initially be unilateral but becomes bilateral. There is an associated slowly progressive palsy of all the extraocular muscles, which usually limits elevation first but progresses until the eyes are practically immobile (Fig. 25.29). The pupil and accommodation are not involved. It may occur sporadically, but a familial incidence is common as a dominant trait.

Histology, electron microscopy, and electromyography suggest that it is a muscular dystrophy. Characteristic ragged red fibers may be seen on muscle biopsy stained with a modified trichrome method. It is probably due to a generalized mitochondrial abnormality and may progress to involve the orbicularis, facial, pharyngeal, and skeletal muscles, especially of the neck and shoulders. A pigmentary retinopathy and cardiomyopathy may occur, and there is an increased anesthetic risk of malignant hyperthermia.

Myasthenia gravis is a chronic disease characterized by an abnormal fatigability of striated muscles. It may be confined indefinitely to a single group of muscles or may become generalized. Ten percent of cases occur in children before puberty, and it may occur transitorily in newborns of myasthenic mothers. A familial incidence is recognized although there is no clear hereditary pattern. Many cases are associated with hyperplasia of the thymus or a thymoma. The cause is an autoimmune defect in the acetylcholine mechanism at the neuromuscular junction, to which the ocular muscles are particularly sensitive. Ptosis, which

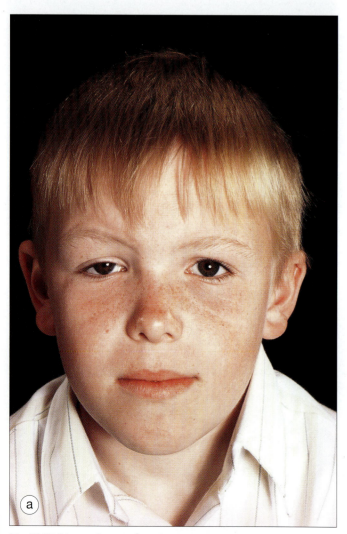
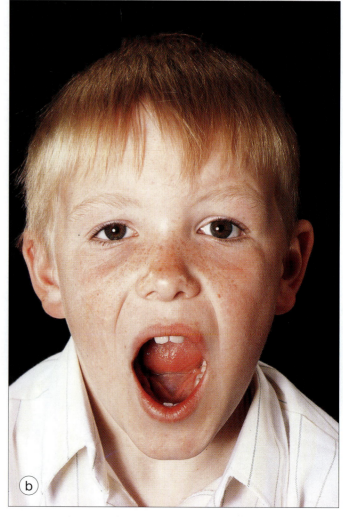

Fig. 25.27 Marcus Gunn ptosis. (a) Right ptosis. (b) With jaw open the right upper lid rises.

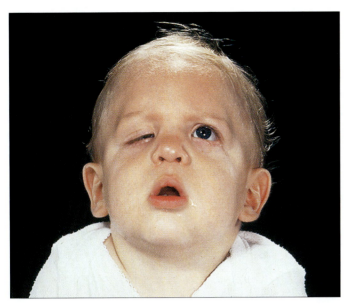 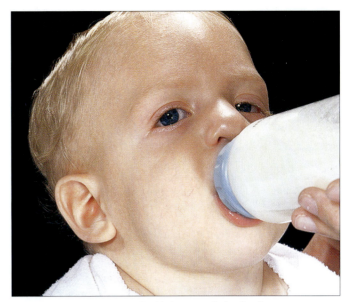

Fig. 25.28 Marcus Gunn ptosis showing marked right ptosis, which completely elevates on jaw movements; in this instance during feeding.

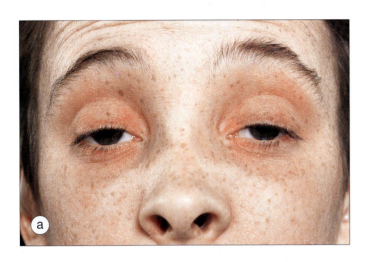

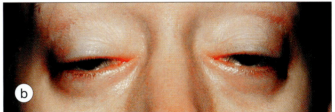

Fig. 25.29 Ptosis in chronic external ophthalmoplegia in a mitochondrial disorder.

may be unilateral and variable, but is usually worse at the end of the day, is often the presenting symptom. Diplopia commonly occurs and the child may present with an unusual squint. The orbicularis oculi is usually also weak.

Easy fatigability causes an increase in the ptosis after repeated up- and downgaze. The abnormality of neuromuscular control may be demonstrated by an overshoot of the eyelid on upgaze, and the horizontal eye movements may show hypometric saccades.

It is diagnosed:

1. Clinically;
2. By antibody studies:
   a. By finding raised levels of anticholinesterase receptor antibody (AchR); and
   b. By finding raised levels of IgG antibodies against the muscle-specific kinase (MuSK);
3. By single-fiber electromyography; probably the most sensitive test is looking for "jitter" on the EMG of an affected muscle or, if the eye muscles only are affected, another muscle; and
4. By the Tensilon test.

In an adult-sized child, 2 mg of Tensilon (edrophonium chloride) is given intravenously as a test dose followed by 8 mg given rapidly. This may produce quick relief of the ptosis.

Unless pre- and post-test parameters (such as a Hess chart or orthoptic measurements) are measured the test is often equivocal except in cases clinically obvious, and this limits the value of the test, which is used less frequently than previously. If the child is less than 10 kg in weight, the dose is reduced or prostigmin (neostigmine) can be given by intramuscular injection 20 minutes after an intramuscular injection of atropine. The test carries a significant risk and must only be carried out in circumstances where resuscitation facilities are available, appropriate to the age of the child.

Pseudoptosis

A pseudoptosis is any condition in which the eyelid margin is at the normal level but the eyelid appears ptotic. If the eye is hypotropic, there may be such an apparent ptosis, which disappears when the eye takes up fixation. In enophthalmos such as microphthalmos or with anophthalmos, the apparent ptosis can be corrected by restoring the orbital volume. Excess skin from a resolving hemangioma may overhang the lid margin and be another cause of pseudoptosis.

Syndromes with ptosis

Several genetic disorders are associated with ptosis and a few

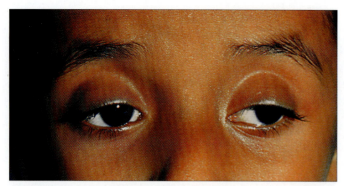

Fig. 25.30 Ptosis in Saenthre–Chotzen syndrome.

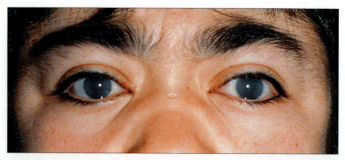

Fig. 25.31 Heavy eyebrows and coarse facies in mucopolysaccharidosis. Image courtesy of Clinique ophthalmologique des Hôpitaux Universitaires de Strasbourg.

examples are cited hereafter. Although this chapter is focused on developmental anomalies the authors emphasize that progressive ptosis in a child suggests a mitochondrial disorder.

In Noonan syndrome, defined by small stature, a webbed neck, and pulmonary stenosis, ptosis is a common feature. Ptosis is a leading feature in the Saethre–Chotzen syndrome, an autosomal dominant craniosynostosis syndrome with syndactyly[67] (Fig. 25.30).

EYEBROWS AND EYELASHES

Anomalies of the dermatological component of the eyelids is also important (see section on congenital hemangiomas) as isolated or syndromic features.

Prominent eyebrows and/or eyelashes

Prominent eyelashes with highly arched heavy eyebrows associated with down-slanting palpebral fissures and/or ptosis are found for instance in the Rubinstein–Taybi syndrome, a mental retardation syndrome associated with broad thumbs and toes.[68]

Heavy and thick eyebrows can be observed in patients with metabolic disorders (see Chapter 65), such as the mucopolysaccharidoses, mucolipidoses, and fucosidosis, usually associated with a coarse face (Fig. 25.31).

Distichiasis

Distichiasis refers to a congenital abnormality with partial or complete accessory rows of eyelashes exiting from the posterior lid margin at or near the meibomian gland orifices[69] (Fig. 25.32). It may occur as an isolated anomaly, or be inherited as an autosomal dominant trait. In the autosomal dominant distichiasis-lymphedema syndrome, it is associated with chronic lymphedema of the lower extremities[70,71] possibly associated to a webbed neck, cardiac defects, vertebral anomalies, extradural spinal cysts, and bifid uvula.[72]

In the Setleis syndrome,[73] there are bilateral temporal skin defects resembling forceps marks, absent lashes, or distichiasis, with a coarse facial appearance.[74]

Trichomegaly

Excessive growth of eyelashes defines trichomegaly. Trichomegaly can be familial or acquired noticeably with human immunodeficiency virus infection or some medical drugs such as interferon alpha treatment.[75] This feature combined with mental retardation and retinal dystrophy is characteristic of Oliver–McFarlane syndrome[76] (Fig. 25.33) (see Chapter 53).

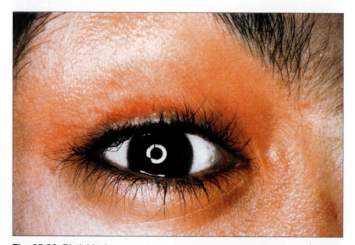

Fig. 25.32 Distichiasis.

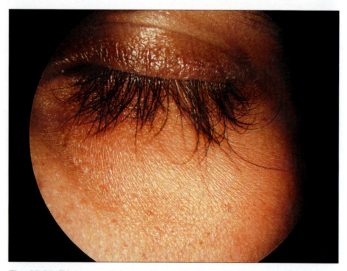

Fig. 25.33 Trichomegaly in a patient with Oliver–McFarlane syndrome (image courtesy of Dr L Santos).

Synophrys

Synophrys is when eyebrows extend to the midline, and it is commonly observed in naturally hairy persons.

Cornelia de Lange syndrome is the association of mental retardation, growth retardation, limb reduction defect, flared nostrils, and hirsutism with characteristic synophrys as well as long eyelashes[77,78] (Fig. 25.34).

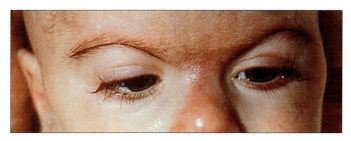

Fig. 25.34 Synophrys in Cornelia de Lange syndrome.

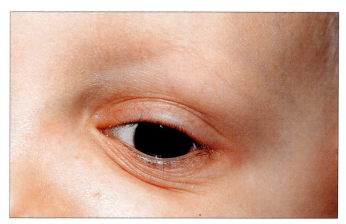

Fig. 25.35 Sparse eyebrows in anhidrotic ectodermal hypoplasia. Image courtesy of Clinique ophthalmologique des Hôpitaux Universitaires de Strasbourg.

Occasionally synophrys can be observed in Waardenburg syndrome (see the section "Telecanthus and dystopia canthorum").

An autosomal recessive condition with a cone–rod dystrophy, hairy face and eyebrows, synophrys, coarse scalp hair, and distichiasis has been described.[79]

SPARSE OR ABSENT EYEBROWS AND/OR EYELASHES

Sparse or absent eyebrows and/or eyelashes can be observed as an isolated condition or associated with other features and has been reported in many syndromes.

Alopecia universalis congenita (generalized atrichia) is an autosomal recessive condition characterized by absent scalp, pubic, and axillary hair as well as absent eyebrows and eyelashes from birth.[80]

In GAPO syndrome (growth retardation, alopecia, pseudo-anodontia, optic atrophy) the eyebrows and eyelashes are sparse or absent and can be associated with optic atrophy and/or glaucoma.[81,82]

Ectodermal dysplasia is a clinical and genetic heterogeneous group of congenital disorders characterized by abnormal development of one or several ectoderm-derived tissues. Sparse eyebrows and eyelashes are classical features.[83]

EEC syndrome is an autosomal dominant syndrome with highly variable expression characterized by sparse or absent hair, sparse eyebrows and eyelashes, brittle nails, teeth anomalies, and split hands or ectodactyly.[84,85] In this condition, the lacrimal duct system is defective in more then 90% (see Chapter 31).

Ectodermal dysplasia anhydrotic (EDA), an X-linked condition, is characterized in affected males by hypotrichosis, abnormal teeth, and absent sweat glands[86] (Fig. 25.35).

Familial conditions with hypotrichosis/alopecia and retinal degeneration,[87] as well as a syndrome associating alopecia and cataract,[88] have been reported in a few families.

Patches of hypotrichosis/alopecia at the level of the eyebrow can be observed in the progressive facial hemiatrophy syndrome or Parry–Romberg syndrome with an "en coup de sabre" appearance and ipsilateral neurologic and eye features such as enophthalmos and retinal telangiectasias[89] (Fig. 25.36).

Trichotillomania, a differential diagnosis of the previous conditions, is a chronic psychiatric condition defined by uncontrollable hair pulling, the eyelashes being the most commonly affected[90] (Fig. 25.37) (see Chapter 71).

White brows or lashes

White eyelashes and eyebrows are observed in oculocutaneous albinism (and not in ocular albinism, an X-linked condition in

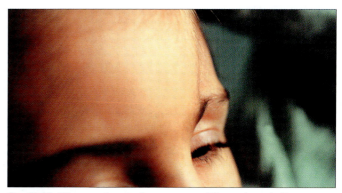

Fig. 25.36 "En coup de sabre" appearance of the eyebrow in Parry–Romberg syndrome.

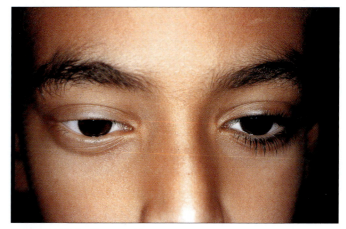

Fig. 25.37 Trichotillomania. The lashes have been plucked. A few remaining broken lashes can be seen in the upper lid.

which the skin is normally pigmented). The lashes and eyebrows are white as the hair and the skin.

Poliosis is defined as white brows or lashes in an otherwise normally pigmented individual. Poliosis has been observed in Waardenburg (Fig. 25.38) syndrome and Parry–Romberg syndrome. It is also a feature of the acquired Vogt–Koyangi–Harada syndrome.

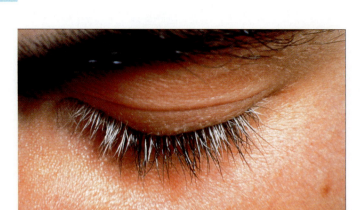

Fig. 25.38 Poliosis in a patient with Waardenburg syndrome. The poliosis can be clearly seen against the normally dark lashes.

DYSMORPHOLOGY DATABASES AND GENES INVOLVED IN SYNDROMES WITH EYELID ANOMALIES

To help the clinician in syndrome diagnosis, databases are available. Databases in dysmorphology and genetics are based on morphological analysis of the patient guiding the clinician by submitting a list of possibly corresponding syndromes.[91,92]

The clinical observation of the face remains essential. Severe or discrete anomalies may be important in diagnosis. The analysis of these features, with the help of databases, helps the clinician diagnostically and guides molecular investigations.

Table 25.2 (on p. 207) summarizes the genes identified in the syndromes with developmental anomalies of the eyelids mentioned in this chapter.

REFERENCES

1. Jones KL. Smith's Recognizable Patterns of Human Malformation. 5th ed. Philadelphia: Saunders; 1997.
2. Optiz JM. The developmental field concept in clinical genetics. J Pediatr 1982; 101: 805–9.
3. Sevel D. A reappraisal of the development of the eyelids. Eye 1988; 2: 123–9.
4. Paiva SN, Minare-Filho AM, Cruz AV. Palpebral fissure changes in early childhood. J Pediatr Ophthalmol Strabismus 2001; 38: 219–23.
5. Feingold M, Bossert WH. Normal values for selected physical parameters: an aid to syndrome delineation. Birth Defects 1974; 10: 1–16.
6. Thomas IT, Gaitantzis YA, Frias JL. Palpebral fissure length from 29 weeks gestation to 14 years. J Pediatr 1987; 111: 267–8.
7. Fries PD, Katowitz JA. Congenital craniofacial anomalies of ophthalmic importance. Surv Ophthalmol 1990; 35: 87–119.
8. Zimmermann AA, Armstrong El, Scammon RE. The change in position of the eyeballs during fetal life. Anat Re 1934; 59: 109–34.
9. Cohen MM, Richieri-Costa A, Guion-Almeida ML, et al. Hypertelorism: interorbital growth, measurements, and pathogenetic considerations. Int J Oral Maxillofac Surg 1995; 24: 387–95.
10. Costaras M, Pruzansky S, Broadbent BH Jr. Bony interorbital distance (BIOD), head size, and level of the cribriform plate relative to orbital height. II. Possible pathogenesis of orbital hypertelorism. J Craniofac Genet Dev Biol 1982; 2: 19–34.
11. Freihoffer HPM. Inner intercanthal and interorbital distances. J Max-Fac Surg 1980; 8: 324–8.
12. Laestadius ND, Aase JM, Smith DW. Normal inner canthal and outer orbital dimensions. J Pediatr 1969; 74: 465–8.
13. Pryor HB. Objective measurement of interpupillary distance. Pediatrics 1969; 44: 973–7.
14. Romanus T. Interocular-biorbital index. A gauge of hypertelorism. Acta Genet 1953; 4: 117–23.
15. Sivan Y, Merlob P, Reisner SH. Eye measurements in preterm and term newborn infants. J Craniofac Genet Dev Biol 1982; 2: 239–42.
16. Omotade OO. Facial measurements in the newborn (towards syndrome delineation). J Med Genet 1990; 27: 358–62.
17. Denis D, Genitori L, Bardot J, et al. Ocular findings in trigonocephaly. Graefe's Arch Clin Exp Ophthalmol 1994; 232: 728–33.
18. Golden JA: Holoprosencephaly: a defect in brain patterning. J Neuropathol Exp Neurol 1998; 57: 991–9
19. Johnson VP. Holoprosencephaly : a developmental field defect. Am J Med Genet 1989; 34: 258–64
20. DeMyer W, Zeman W, Palmer CG. The face predicts the brain: diagnostic significance of median facial abnormalities for holoprosencephaly. Pediatrics 1964; 34: 256–63.
21. Kjaer I, Keeling JW, Graem N. The midline craniofacial skeleton in holoprosencephalic fetuses. J Med Genet 1991; 28: 846–55.
22. Wallis D, Muenke M. Mutations in holoprosencephaly. Hum Mutat 2000; 16: 99–108.
23. Cohen MM Jr, Lemire RJ. Syndromes with cephaloceles. Teratology 1982; 25: 161–72.
24. Waardenburg PJ. A new syndrome combining developmental anomalies of the eyelids, eyebrows and nose root with pigmentary defects of the iris and head hair and with congenital deafness. Am J Hum Genet 1951; 3: 195–253
25. Read AP, Newton VE. Waardenburg syndrome. J Med Genet 1997; 34: 656–65.
26. Newton VE. Waardenburg's syndrome: a comparison of biometric indices used to diagnose lateral displacement of the inner canthi. Scand Audiol 1989; 18: 221–3.
27. Shapiro I, Borochowitz Z, Degani S, et al. Neu-Laxova syndrome. Am J Med Genet 1992; 43: 602–5.
28. McCarthy GT, West CM. Ablepharon macrostomia syndrome. Div Med Child Neurol 1977; 19: 659–63.
29. Ferraz VEF, Melo DG, Hansing SE, et al. Ablepharon-macrostomia syndrome: first report of familial occurrence. Am J Med Genet 2000; 94: 281–3.
30. Boyd PA, Keeling JW, Lindenbaum RH. Fraser syndrome (cryptophthalmos-syndactyly syndrome): a review of eleven cases with postmortem findings. Am J Med Genet 1988; 31: 159–68.
31. Slavotinek AM, Tifft CJ. Fraser syndrome and cryptophthalmos: review of the diagnostic criteria and evidence for phenotypic modules in complex malformation syndromes. J Med Genet 2002; 39: 623–33.
32. Weiss AH, Riscile G, Kousseff BG. Ankyloblepharon filiforme adnatum. Am J Med Genet 1992; 42: 69–73.
33. Hay RJ, Wells RS. The syndrome of ankyloblepharon, ectodermal defects and cleft lip and palate: an autosomal dominant condition. Br J Dermatol 1976; 94: 277–89.
34. Clark DI, Patterson A. Ankyloblepharon filiforme adnatum in trisomy 18 (Edwards's syndrome). Br J Ophthalmol 1985; 69: 471–3.
35. Seah LL, Choo CT, Fong KS. Congenital upper lid colobomas. Ophthal Plast Reconstr Surg 2002; 18: 190–5.
36. Collin JR. Congenital upper lid coloboma. Aust N Z J Ophthalmol 1986; 14: 313–7.
37. Tessier P. Anatomical classification of facial, cranio–facial and latero facial clefts. In: Symposium on Plastic Surgery in the Orbital Region. St Louis: Mosby; 1980.
38. Miller MT, Deutsch TA, Cronin C, et al: Amniotic bands as a cause of ocular anomalies. Am J Ophthalmol 1987; 104: 270–9.
39. Wang FM, Millman AL, Sidoti PA, et al. Ocular findings in Treacher Collins syndrome. Am J Ophthalmol 1990; 110: 280–6.
40. Hertle RW, Ziylan S, Katowitz JA: Ophthalmic features and visual prognosis in the Treacher–Collins syndrome. Br J Ophthalmol 1993; 77: 642–5.

41. Allanson JE, O'Hara P, Farkas LG, et al. Anthropometric craniofacial pattern profiles in Down syndrome. Am J Med Genet 1993; 47: 748–52.

42. da Cunha RP, Moreira JB. Ocular findings in Down's syndrome. Am J Ophthalmol 1996; 122: 236–44.

43. Chandler KE, Kidd A, Al-Gazali L, et al. Diagnostic criteria, clinical characteristics and natural history of Cohen syndrome. J Med Genet 2003; 40: 233–41.

44. Keipert JA. Euryblepharon. Br J Ophthalmol 1975; 59: 57–8.

45. Markowitz GD, Hsandler LF, Katowitz JA. Congenital euryblepharon and nasolacrimal anomalies in a patient with Down syndrome. J Pediatr Ophthalmol Strabismus 1994; 31: 330–1.

46. Niikawa N, Matsuura N, Fukushima Y, et al. Kabuki make-up syndrome: a syndrome of mental retardation, unusual facies, large and protruding ears, and postnatal growth deficiency. J Pediat 1981; 99: 565–9.

47. Kawame H, Hannibal MC, Hudgins L, et al. Phenotypic spectrum and management issues in Kabuki syndrome. J Pediat 1999; 134: 480–5.

48. Cunniff C, Curtis M, Hassed SJ, et al. Blepharophimosis: a causally heterogeneous malformation frequently associated with developmental disabilities. Am J Med Genet 1998; 75: 52–4.

49. Stromland K. Ocular involvement in the fetal alcohol syndrome. Surv Ophthalmol 1987; 31: 277–84.

50. Zlotogora J, Sagi M, Cohen T. The blepharophimosis, ptosis, and epicanthus inversus syndrome: delineation of two types. Am J Hum Genet 1983; 35: 1020–7.

51. Ohdo S, Madokoro H, Sonoda T, et al. Mental retardation associated with congenital heart disease, blepharophimosis, blepharoptosis and hypoplastic teeth. J Med Genet 1986; 23: 242–4.

52. Moncla A, Philip N, Mattei JF. Blepharophimosis-mental retardation syndrome and terminal deletion of chromosome 3p. J Med Genet 1995; 32: 245–6.

53. Sellar PW, Bryars JH, Archer DB. Late presentation of congenital ectropion of the eyelids in a child with Down syndrome. J Pediatr Ophthalmol Strabismus 1992; 29: 64–7.

54. Oestreicher JH, Nelson CC. Lamellar ichthyosis and congenital ectropion. Arch Ophthalmol 1990; 108: 1772–3.

55. Kronish JW, Lingua R. Pressure patch treatment for congenital upper eyelid eversion. Arch Ophthalmol 1991; 109: 767–8.

56. Khurana AK, Ahluwalia BK, Mehtani VG. Primary epitarsus: a case report. Br J Ophthalmol 1986; 70: 931–2.

57. Noda S, Hayasaka S, Setogawa T. Epiblepharon with inverted lashes in Japanese children I. Incidence and symptoms. Br J Ophthalmol 1989; 73: 126–7.

58. Tse DT, Anderson RL, Fratkin JD. Aponeurosis disinsertion in congenital entropion. Arch Ophthalmol 1983; 101: 436–40.

59. Bartley GB, Nerad JA, Kersten RC, et al. Congenital entropion with intact lower eyelid retractor insertion. Am J Ophthalmol 1991; 112: 437–41.

60. Jordan R. The lower-lid retractors in congenital entropion and epiblepharon. Ophthalmic Surg 1993; 24: 494–6.

61. Yang LL, Lambert SR, Chapman J, et al. Congenital entropion and congenital corneal ulcer. Am J Ophthalmol 1996; 121: 329–31.

62. Collin JR, Allen L, Castronuovo S. Congenital eyelid retraction. Br J Ophthalmol 1990; 9: 542–4.

63. Shields CL, Nelson LB, Carpenter GC, et al. Neonatal Grave's disease. Br J Ophthalmol 1988; 72: 424–8.

64. Stout AU, Borchert M. Etiology of eyelid retraction in children. J Pediatr Ophthalmol Strabismus 1993; 30: 96–9.

65. Zak TA. Congenital primary upper eyelid entropion. J Pediatr Ophthalmol Strabismus 1984; 21: 69–73.

66. Balkan R, Hoyt CS. Associated neurologic abnormalities in congenital third nerve palsies. Am J Ophthalmol 1984; 97: 315–9.

67. Dollfus H, Biswas P, Kumaramanickavel G, et al. Saethre–Chotzen syndrome: notable intrafamilial phenotypic variability in a large family with Q28X TWIST mutation. Am J Med Genet 2002; 109: 218–25.

68. Berry AC. Rubinstein–Taybi syndrome. J Med Genet 1987; 24: 562–6.

69. O'Donnell BA, Collin JR. Distichiasis: management with cryotherapy to the posterior lamella. Br J Ophthalmol 1993; 77: 289–92.

70. Anderson RL, Harvey JT. Lid splitting in posterior lamellar cryo-

surgery for congenital and acquired distichiasis. Arch Ophthalmol 1981; 99: 631–41.

71. Temple IK, Collin JR. Distichiasis-lymphoedema syndrome: a family report. Clin Dysmorphol 1994; 3: 139–42.

72. Kolin T, Johns K, Wadlington W, et al. Hereditary lymphedema and dystichiasis. Arch Ophthalmol 1991; 109: 980–1.

73. Frederick DR, Robb RM. Ophthalmic manifestations of Setleis forceps marks syndrome. J Pediatr Ophthalmol Strabismus 1992; 29: 127–9.

74. McGaughran J, Aftimos S. Setleis syndrome: three new cases and a review of the literature. Am J Med Genet 2002; 111; 376–80.

75. Harrison DA, Mullaney PB. Familial trichomegaly. Arch Ophthalmol 1997; 115: 1602–3.

76. Oliver GL, McFarlane DC. Congenital trichomegaly with associated pigmentary degeneration of the retina, dwarfism and mental retardation. Arch Ophthalmol 1965; 74: 169–171.

77. Levin AV, Seidman DJ, Nelson LB, et al. Ophthalmic findings in Cornelia de Lange syndrome. J Pediatr Ophthalmol Strabismus 1990; 27: 94–102.

78. Jackson L, Kline AD, Barr MA, et al. De Lange syndrome: a clinical review of 310 individuals. Am J Med Genet 1993; 47: 940–6.

79. Jalili IK. Cone–rod congenital amaurosis associated with congenital hypertrichosis: an autosomal recessive condition. J Med Genet 1989; 26: 504–10.

80. Tillman W G. Alopecia congenita: report of two families. Brit Med J 1952; 2: 428.

81. Manouvrier-Hanu S, Largilliere C, Benalioua M, et al. The GAPO syndrome. Am J Med Genet 1987; 26: 683–8.

82. Ilker SS, Ozturk F, Kurt E, et al. Ophthalmic findings in GAPO syndrome. Jpn J Ophthalmol 1999; 43: 48–52.

83. McNab AA, Potts MJ, Welham RA. The EEC syndrome and its ocular manifestations. Br J Ophthalmol 1989; 73: 261–4.

84. Moshegov CN. Ectrodactyly-ectodermal dysplasia-clefting (EEC) syndrome. Arch Ophthalmol 1996; 114: 1290–1.

85. Roelfsema NM, Cobben JM. The EEC syndrome: a literature study. Clin Dysmorph 1996; 5: 115–27.

86. Reed WB, Lopez DA, Landing B. Clinical spectrum of anhidrotic ectodermal dysplasia. Arch Derm 1970; 102: 134–43.

87. Albrectsen B, Svendsen IB. Hypotrichosis, syndactyly, and retinal degeneration in two siblings. Acta Derm Venerol 1956; 11: 96–101.

88. Wallis C, Ip FS, Beighton P. Cataracts, alopecia, and sclerodactyly: a previously apparently undescribed ectodermal dysplasia syndrome on the island of Rodrigues. Am J Med Genet 1989; 32: 500–3.

89. Lewkonia RM, Lowry RB. Progressive hemifacial atrophy (Parry–Romberg syndrome) report with review of genetics and nosology. Am J Med Genet 1983; 14: 385–90.

90. Mawn LA, Jordan DR. Trichotillomania. Ophthalmology 1997; 104: 2175–8.

91. Online mendelian inheritance in man, OMIM. McKusicks-Nathans Institute for Genetic Medicine, Johns Hopkins University (Baltimore, MD) and National Center for Biotechnology Information, National Library of Medecine (Bethesda, MD); 2000. Available at: http://www.ncbi.nlm.nih.gov/omim.

92. The London Dysmorphology Database (LDDB). Oxford Medical database. R Winter – M Baraister

93. Roessler E, Belloni E, Gaudenz K, et al. Mutations in the human Sonic Hedgehog gene cause holoproencephaly. Nat Genet 1996; 14: 357–60.

94. Wallis D E, Roessler E, Hehr U, et al. Mutations in the homeodomain of the human SIX3 gene cause holoprosencephaly. Nature Genet 1999; 22: 196–8.

95. Gripp KW, Wotton D, Edwards MC, et al. Mutations in TGIF cause holoprosencephaly and link NODAL signalling to human neural axis determination. Nat Genet 2000; 25: 205–8.

96. Brown SA, Warburton D, Brown LY, et al. Holoprosencephaly due to mutations in ZIC2, a homologue of Drosophila odd-paired. Nat Genet 1998; 20: 180–3.

97. Wilkie AM, Slaney SF, Oldridge M, et al. Apert syndrome results from localized mutations of FGFR2 and is allelic with Crouzon syndrome. Nat Genet 1995; 9: 165–72.

98. Reardon W, Winter RM, Rutland P, et al: Mutations in the fibroblast growth factor receptor 2 gene cause Crouzon syndrome. Nat Genet 1994; 8: 98–103.

99. Trivier E, De Cesare D, Jacquot S, et al. Mutations in the kinase Rsk-2 associated with Coffin–Lowry syndrome. Nature 1996; 384: 567–70.

100. Baldwin CT, Hoth CF, Macina RA, et al. Mutations in PAX3 that cause Waardenburg syndrome type I: ten new mutations and review of the literature. Am J Med Genet 1995; 58: 115–22.

101. Hughes AE, Newton VE, Liu XZ, et al. A gene for Waardenburg syndrome type 2 maps close to the human homologue of the microphthalmia gene at chromosome 3p12–p14.1. Nat Genet 1994; 7: 509–12.

102. McGregor L, Makela V, Darling SM, et al. Fraser syndrome and mouse blebbed phenotype caused by mutations in FRAS1/Fras1 encoding a putative extracellular matrix protein. Nature Genet 2003; 34: 203–8.

103. Celli J, Duijf P, Hamel BC, et al: Heterozygous germline mutations in the p53 homolog p63 are the cause of EEC syndrome. Cell 1999; 99: 143–53.

104. McGrath JA, Duijf PH, Doetsch V, et al. Hay–Wells syndrome is caused by heterozygous missense mutations in the SAM domain of p63. Hum Molec Genet 2001; 10: 221–9.

105. Wise CA, Chiang LC, Paznekas WA, et al. TCOF1 gene encodes a putative nucleolar phosphoprotein that exhibits mutations in Treacher Collins syndrome throughout its coding region. Proc Natl Acad Sci 1997; 94: 3110–5.

106. Kolehmainen J, Black GC, Saarinen A, et al. Cohen syndrome is caused by mutations in a novel gene, COH1, encoding a transmembrane protein with a presumed role in vesicle-mediated sorting and intracellular protein transport. Am J Hum Genet 2003; 72: 1359–69.

107. Crisponi L, Deiana M, Loi A, et al. The putative forkhead transcription factor FOXL2 is mutated in blepharophimosis/ptosis/epicanthus inversus syndrome. Nat Genet 2001; 27: 159–66.

108. De Baere E, Dixon MJ, Small KW, et al. Spectrum of FOXL2 gene mutations in blepharophimosis-ptosis-epicanthus inversus (BPES) families demonstrates a genotype-phenotype correlation. Hum Mol Genet 2001; 10: 1591–600.

109. el Ghouzzi V, Le Merrer M, Perrin-Schmitt F, et al. Mutations of the TWIST gene in the Saethre–Chotzen syndrome. Nat Genet 1997; 15: 42–6.

110. Howard TD, Paznekas WA, Green ED, et al. Mutations in TWIST, a basic helix-loop-helix transcription factor, in Saethre–Chotzen syndrome. Nat Genet 1997; 15: 36–41.

111. Tartaglia M, Mehler EL, Goldberg R, et al. Mutations in PTPN11, encoding the protein tyrosine phosphatase SHP-2, cause Noonan syndrome. Nature Genet 2001; 29: 465–8.

112. Petrij F, Giles RH, Dauwerse HG, et al: Rubinstein–Taybi syndrome caused by mutations in the transcriptional co-activator CBP. Nature 1995; 376: 348–51.

113. Ahmad W, Faiyaz ul Haque M, Brancolini V, et al. Alopecia universalis associated with a mutation in the human hairless gene. Science 1998; 279: 720–4.

114. Kere J, Srivastava AK, Montonen O, et al. X-linked anhidrotic (hypohidrotic) ectodermal dysplasia is caused by mutation in a novel transmembrane protein. Nature Genet 1996; 13: 409–16.

115. Bell R, Brice G, Child AH, et al. Analysis of lymphoedema-distichiasis families for FOXC2 mutations reveals small insertions and deletions throughout the gene. Hum Genet 2001; 108: 546–51.

116. Finegold DN, Kimak MA, Lawrence EC, et al. Truncating mutations in FOXC2 cause multiple lymphedema syndromes. Hum Mol Genet 2001; 10: 1185–9.

CHAPTER
26

Lids: Acquired Abnormalities and Practical Management

Hugo W A Henderson and J Richard O Collin

The main indications for eyelid surgery in children are to try to give a chance of salvaging some useful vision in severe congenital malformations, to treat sight-threatening disease, to prevent amblyopia, to control pain, to improve cosmesis, and rarely to save life. Luckily these aims are often aligned as reconstructive lid surgery usually results in both improved function and improved cosmesis.

Complex cases require a careful treatment plan, with input from all the medical and surgical teams involved in the patient's management, to plan and stage any surgery.

However, flexibility is often required in oculoplastic surgery, and the best plans may need to be modified during the procedure.

MANAGEMENT OF CONGENITAL LID CONDITIONS

Lid coloboma

The treatment of lid coloboma is directed toward treating sight-threatening corneal exposure, preventing amblyopia and ocular motility disorders by treating underlying bands, and improving cosmesis.

The coloboma is described in terms of its position using the Tessier classification, and in terms of its extent.[1] A full examination is carried out to exclude other ocular and systemic abnormalities. Treatment is directed toward firstly protection of the ocular surface with lubrication and occlusive dressing. Care is taken not to induce amblyopia with ointments or dressings. A forced duction test is performed on all children with an eyelid coloboma because of the risk of underlying bands.[2] This should be carried out as soon as possible and usually requires an examination under anesthesia. A small coloboma can be closed under the same anesthetic. If a more complicated repair is required, this can often wait until early childhood when the tissues are a little larger and the repair simpler. If corneal exposure cannot be controlled, the eyelid reconstruction must proceed urgently. If any bands limiting ocular motility are detected, they must be excised as early as possible in an attempt to avoid secondary strabismus.

A defect less than 25% of the lid length can be repaired by excision of the coloboma margins and direct closure. For defects of approximately 25–50% of lid length a lateral canthotomy and cantholysis are required to allow the wound edges to come together.

For defects of 50% or more tissue will need to be added from another location. In the lower eyelid the posterior lamellar can be reconstructed using tarsoconjunctival grafts from the upper lid, or a hard palate mucous membrane graft, together with a skin flap. Alternatively a tarsoconjunctival flap can be used from the upper lid with an overlying skin flap, or skin graft. Eyelid-sharing procedures are better for older children or eyes in which there is

no visual potential, as there is a risk of amblyopia. They may be necessary in cases of uncontrolled exposure, and in these circumstances the flap should be divided early at two weeks, and followed with aggressive occlusion therapy.

The coloboma in Treacher-Collins syndrome (see Chapter 25) is a pseudocoloboma in which there is a defect of subcutaneous tissue rather than a true eyelid discontinuity. The syndrome occurs in several degrees of severity, including an abortive form. Severe cases may require craniofacial surgery prior to lid surgery. The malar defect is closed with a composite temporal bone flap or cranial bone graft to correct the flattening of the cheeks, and the defective lateral orbital floor and wall are then reconstructed with another bone graft, lifting the eyeball and correcting the anti-mongoloid slant.

In less severe cases the lids can be built with oculoplastic surgery alone. In mild cases the lateral canthus can be repositioned with a lateral canthoplasty. In moderate cases, with absence of vertical and horizontal eyelid soft tissue, the lid can be reconstructed with the use of hard palate mucous membrane grafts or ear cartilage to support the lid, and the lateral canthus can be secured with wire fixation to bore holes in the lateral orbital rim. Moderately severe cases may require transposition flaps from the upper to lower lids with a lateral canthal strip.

Cryptophthalmos

Cryptophthalmos is a rare condition in which the globe is covered by a fold of skin that extends from the brow to the cheek. The condition can be complete, incomplete, or partial (congenital symblepharon) (see Chapter 24).

In cases of complete cryptophthalmos there is little chance of gaining useful vision even with reconstructive surgery; however, if electrodiagnostic tests suggest that there is visual potential, one may feel duty bound to consider surgery to try to give a chance of salvaging some vision.

There has been some success in treating cases of incomplete cryptophthalmos and partial cryptophthalmos, the results of surgery depending on the degree of involvement of the lid structures and the integrity of the underlying ocular structures. Thus these conditions require urgent treatment from birth with instillation of lubricants and antibiotics prior to planning surgery to reconstruct the lids. Moisture chambers with plastic wrappings or even inferior rectus section with upward rotation of the globe may help as temporary measures.

The urgency of surgery depends on whether the condition is unilateral or bilateral, the presence of any visual potential, and the degree of corneal exposure. If the condition is unilateral, no visual potential exists, and exposure is controlled, surgery should be delayed to allow for the relaxation of tissues, which occur as the infant matures.[3]

The surgery is aimed at reconstituting the components of the anterior and posterior lamellae. Pedicle rotation flaps from the cheek or brow, eyelid sharing, full-thickness skin grafts, and mucous membrane grafts are used in the reconstructions. The success of complex lid reconstruction is limited by defective tear production, a lack of healthy conjunctiva, and by underlying ocular defects associated with the condition such as corneal and anterior segment dysgenesis. The surgeon must be prepared to perform a corneal graft when reconstruction is undertaken as the lids and cornea are one continuous tissue plane and there will often be a danger of perforation.

Ablepharon

Complete failure of eyelid development is rare (see Chapter 25). As with incomplete cryptophthalmos urgent treatment is required to protect the ocular surface followed by early lid reconstruction, and again the results depend on the severity of the lid changes and the integrity of the underlying structures. Treatment of true ablepharon has poor results; however, treatment of milder cases of microblepharon, with a vertical shortening of the lid, is more successful.

Ankyloblepharon

In ankyloblepharon (see Chapter 25) the eyelid margins are partially or completely fused together with a reduction in the palpebral aperture. Ankyloblepharon filiforme adnatum is a similar condition in which one or more skin tags join the two lids and there is usually a normal horizontal palpebral aperture.

Ankyloblepharon must be differentiated from blepharophimosis in which the palpebral aperture is reduced and there is telecanthus, but the eyelid margins are normal. Recognition of ankyloblepharon necessitates careful systemic examination to detect associated abnormalities. The lids are opened along the line of fusion with either sharp scissors or a scalpel. A thin strip of skin and orbicularis is excised and an attempt made to allow the lid margin to conjunctivalize. The lid structure and tarsus are usually otherwise normal.

Euryblepharon

Euryblepharon (see Chapter 25) is a condition of congenital primary enlargement of the palpebral aperture, usually greatest in the lateral aspect. There is a localized outward and downward displacement of the lateral canthus with a downward displacement of the lower lid. Mild cases may require no treatment or simple lubrication. If there is a danger of corneal exposure the lateral canthus may be tightened and be positioned more superiorly and posteriorly. If the eyelid is short vertically, skin grafts and/or posterior lamellar grafts may be required. However, free grafts should be used with caution, as the cosmetic result in the young can be poor.

Ectropion

The initial treatment of ectropion in childhood is conservative using lubrication to prevent exposure keratitis. Indications for surgery are failure of lubrication to prevent exposure and cosmesis. Surgery is aimed at treating the underlying cause: shortage of skin or increased lid laxity (paralytic ectropion is discussed later). Ectropion associated with a shortage of skin occurs in congenital conditions such as Down syndrome,

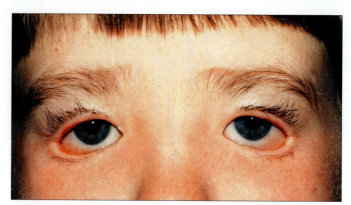

Fig. 26.1 Bilateral ectropion due to shortage of the anterior lamella in a patient with euryblepharon and blepharophimosis.

blepharophimosis (Fig. 26.1), and acquired conditions such as ichthyosis, dermatomyositis, and trauma. A localized scar can be lengthened with a Z-plasty, and a generalized shortage of skin corrected with a skin flap or graft. Increased lid laxity causing ectropion is found in congenital conditions such as mega-loblepharon and euryblepharon and can occur after trauma. It is treated with lid-shortening procedures.[4]

Eversion

Treatment of congenital eversion (see Chapter 25) is aimed at reducing chemosis, which may obstruct the visual axis, and improving ocular comfort and cosmesis. Initial treatment is by pressure patching or repositioning of the lids and taping.[5] More severe cases have been treated by intermarginal sutures, inverting sutures, tarsorrhaphy, horizontal shortening procedures, or the insertion of a skin graft.

Epiblepharon

Epiblepharon refers to the presence of a horizontal fold of skin across the upper or lower eyelid that may push the lashes against the cornea (see Chapter 25). The lid margin itself remains in a normal position. The epiblepharon usually resolves by about 2 years of age as the facial bones grow. It is usually asymptomatic and is seldom associated with keratitis (Fig. 26.2).

Surgical intervention is therefore rarely indicated except when foreign-body symptoms, photophobia, or corneal compromise persist despite conservative treatment (i.e., lubrication). Transverse sutures can be tried in milder cases, or the excision of an ellipse of skin and orbicularis muscle in more severe cases.[6,7]

Entropion

In congenital entropion (see Chapter 25) as opposed to congenital epiblepharon the eyelid margin is inverted. This often requires prompt surgical intervention to prevent corneal scarring and infection. It should be distinguished from epiblepharon, where a skin fold causes a secondary turning of the lower lid lashes. A trial of simple treatment may be worthwhile (Figs. 26.3 and 26.4); however, surgery is often required. In the Hotz-type procedure a horizontal ellipse of skin of about 2–2.5 mm vertical height is removed just below the inferior border of the lower lid tarsus. The skin edges are sutured to the lower border of the tarsus to prevent the orbicularis from again overriding the lid margin. To

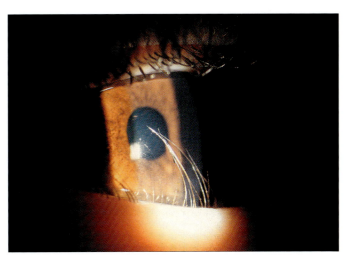

Fig. 26.2 Epiblepharon. In this child the lower lid lashes have turned in from birth, but the cornea has remained undamaged. Spontaneous improvement usually occurs.

enhance the procedure the lower lid retractors can be included in the suture.

Tarsal kink/upper lid entropion

Congenital upper lid entropion is rare but often associated with a horizontal kinking of the tarsus. As with lower lid entropion there is a risk of corneal scarring and infection. It can be corrected by repositioning of the anterior lamella of the eyelid with a simple upper lid entropion correction; alternatively a lid suture with mechanical flattening of the kink may be successful (Fig. 26.5).

Distichiasis

Distichiasis is a developmental abnormality in which a second row of cilia emerges behind the normal eyelashes from the meibomian gland orifices. Pseudo-distichiasis occurs in chronic lid disease with metaplasia and lash growth from the meibomian orifices in trachoma, Stevens-Johnson syndrome, and chronic blepharitis. The abnormal lashes may be asymptomatic or cause superficial corneal problems.

If the patients are symptomatic or show signs of significant corneal staining, treatment is indicated.

Electrolysis is the treatment of choice for a single or very few lashes, and can be combined with a posterior cutdown in which a short vertical incision is made through the tarsal plate to expose the lash root, which can be treated with electrolysis under direct vision. For larger numbers of lashes electrolysis is not very effective, takes a long time, and produces tarsal scarring. Cryotherapy is preferable with a double freeze–thaw cycle to a temperature of –20°C, under thermocouple control.[8] In the upper lid a gray line split into two lamellae is helpful to separate the normal from the distichiasis lashes. Cryotherapy can be applied directly to the tarsus, avoiding damage to the normal lash roots and, in dark-skinned patients, discoloration of the skin. The posterior lamella is then advanced, leaving the raw surface of the tarsal plate to granulate. This prevents contraction of the tarsal plate, leading to an upper lid entropion. Note that no mucous membrane graft is sutured to the anterior tarsus since it has been frozen; also note that however carefully the lid margin is split, some or all the normal lashes may be lost. A lid-split can be used in the lower lid,

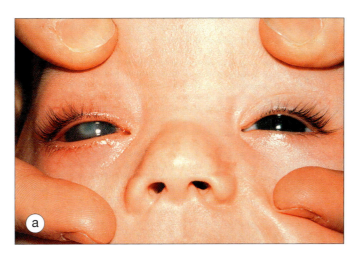

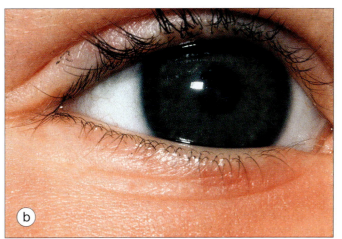

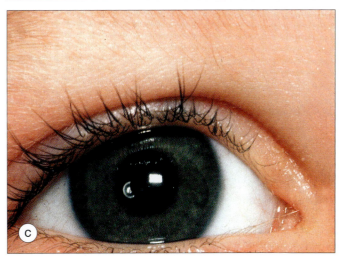

Fig. 26.3 Congenital entropion. (a) Shortly after birth this child's eye was found to be swollen. During examination under anesthetic right upper lid entropion was found with a corneal abrasion caused by the entropion. (b) After taping the lids, the entropion resolved, and (c) ultimately there was only minimal subepithelial opacity.

but the normal lashes are usually lost since it is difficult to split the lower lid and preserve the lashes. Localized areas of abnormal lashes can be excised directly. This is usually best achieved with a gray line split and excision of the tissue containing the abnormal eyelash roots.

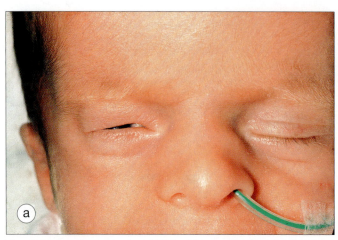
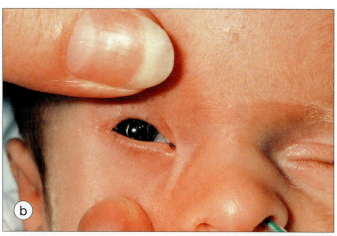

Fig. 26.4 Congenital entropion. (a) This child presented with irritability and an abnormality of the right lids, which were slightly swollen. (b) Same child with the lid everted, showing the lashes inturned and abrading the cornea without damage at this stage. It was treated with simple lid suture and resolved without complication.

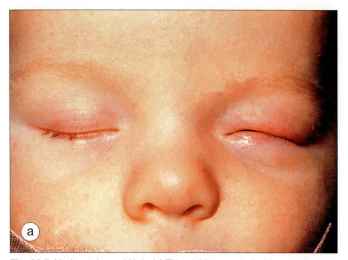
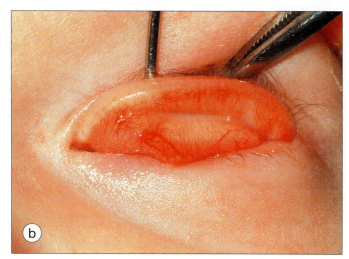

Fig. 26.5 Horizontal tarsal kink. (a) This child presented with a swollen and sore left eye with blepharospasm. (b) On eversion of the lid the horizontal kink in the tarsus can be seen. It runs the whole length of the tarsal plate, which is bent to 90°. It was treated by forced eversion using a strabismus hook to straighten the tarsus by force while the margin of the lid was held. This was followed by a week of lid suture, and the condition resolved following that treatment but there was severe corneal scarring and the eye was blind.

Epicanthic folds

Epicanthal folds are folds of skin that extend from the upper eyelid toward the medial canthus. The fundamental difference between epicanthic folds and epiblepharon is that the former are caused by a relative shortage of skin and the latter are caused by overriding tissue. Like epiblepharon, epicanthic folds only require urgent treatment if they cause trichiasis or obstruct vision. They are largely an esthetic issue, and with development of the bridge of the nose they become less prominent. As the folds represent lines of relative skin shortage, they can be broken up and lengthened with various different flaps. A simple epicanthic fold can be treated with a Z-plasty. Two separate Z-plasties can be used when a fold affects both the upper and lower lid. A mild epicanthic fold associated with telecanthus can be treated with a Y–V plasty and shortening of the underlying medial canthal tendon. If there is a marked epicanthic fold associated with telecanthus, a double Z-plasty can be combined with a Y–V plasty.[9,10]

Telecanthus

Telecanthus is an increased width between the medial canthi, with a normal interpupillary distance. If there is an overgrowth of bone with an increase in the interorbital width the condition is referred to as hypertelorism. Telecanthus can usually be improved by shortening the medial canthal tendons without involving a significant reduction in bone.[11]

Mild cases of telecanthus can be treated by medial canthal plication with a nonabsorbable or wire suture combined with a Y–V plasty. More severe cases may require transnasal wiring combined with a Y–V plasty. Posterior placement of the wire is necessary for a good cosmetic result. The thickness of the anterior lacrimal crest and medial orbital wall bone can be reduced with a burr at the same procedure. If a transnasal wire is required, it is essential to have preoperative radiological evidence of the height of the cribriform plate to avoid damage to the intracranial structures. The correction of hypertelorism requires mobilization of the orbital rims and reduction of the ethmoid bones, which involves craniofacial surgery.

Blepharophimosis

Blepharophimosis literally means small eyelids. In the blepharophimosis syndrome, the horizontal palpebral aperture is reduced and this is associated with epicanthic folds, ptosis, and telecanthus (see Chapters 5 and 25).

As with all congenital and acquired eyelid conditions, the ophthalmologist's participation is directed toward promoting visual development and improving cosmesis. Patients should be evaluated for the presence of refractive errors, amblyopia, and strabismus, which are common in this condition.[12] Resting lid position will determine the urgency of ptosis correction. If a markedly ptotic lid obstructs the visual axis and contributes to the development of amblyopia, lid elevation should proceed promptly.

The surgical treatment of blepharophimosis syndrome is staged. Hypertelorism, epicanthus, and telecanthus can be repaired at the same general anesthetic. Ptosis surgery is done as a second procedure because correcting the telecanthus may worsen the ptosis, and as levator function is usually very poor, if there is no risk of amblyopia, ptosis surgery can be delayed until the child is sufficiently developed to carry out a brow suspension with autologous fascia lata or temporalis fascia (Fig. 26.6).

MANAGEMENT OF CONGENITAL AND ACQUIRED PTOSIS

Congenital ptosis is usually associated with a dysgenesis of the levator muscle. There is a direct relationship between the levator muscle function, i.e., the excursion of the upper lid between full upgaze and downgaze, and the number of healthy striated muscle fibers. This is the main factor influencing the choice of ptosis surgery. Causes of acquired ptosis include aponeurotic defects, third nerve palsies and associated syndromes, Horner syndrome, the ocular myopathies, and myasthenia. These will influence the choice of surgery by affecting Bell's phenomenon, the variability of ptosis, etc.

History

The essential questions such as length of history, associated signs and symptoms, variability, family history, and so on are obvious from the account of the causes of ptosis in Chapter 25. With a simple congenital ptosis there is often a history that the condition seemed to improve initially after birth then become static.

Examination

A full eye examination should be performed, with particular attention to the position of the lid on downgaze, the extraocular muscle movements, any squint,[13,14] the facial appearance, evidence of jaw-winking, aberrant movements of the lid, the pupil, variability in the signs, pseudo-epicanthic folds, and so on. Associated abnormalities, such as astigmatism with hemangiomas or pigmentary retinopathy with progressive external ophthalmoplegia, may be found. Further investigations may be indicated, depending on the findings (e.g., with third nerve palsies).[15]

The degree of ptosis should be assessed both by comparing the vertical interpalpebral aperture measurements on both sides and by assessing the height of the lid above the corneal reflex from a spot source of light. This obviates inaccuracies from malposition of the lower eyelid. The levator function should be measured by

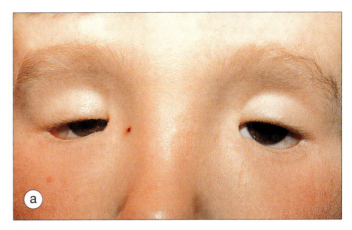

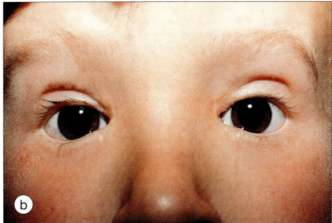

Fig. 26.6 Blepharophimosis. (a) This patient has blepharophimosis syndrome with blepharophimosis, ptosis, and telecanthus. (b) The same child after Y–V canthoplasties followed by brow suspensions with autogenous fascia lata.

pressing over the brow to prevent any frontalis action and then measuring the excursion of the lid between full up- and downgaze. The position of the skin crease on both sides and the presence or absence of Bell's phenomenon should be noted.

Treatment

This depends on the diagnosis and physical findings. Surgical correction is urgent only if there is a risk of amblyopia because the eyelid is occluding the pupil in infancy. This is rare but does occur. Even in the setting of severe unilateral ptosis, a chin-up head posture may be adopted in an attempt to maintain binocular fusion. Hence ptosis surgery usually can be delayed until the child is old enough for an accurate assessment of the levator function, which usually occurs at about the age of 4 years. However, if there is any suggestion of the lid being close to the visual axis, the child must be kept under appropriate medical supervision, and occlusion instituted whenever necessary. With a simple congenital ptosis the levator function and degree of ptosis govern the choice of operation.

In mild congenital ptosis, if there is about 2 mm of ptosis with good levator function of 10 mm or more, a Fasanella Servat procedure is very useful when surgery that is not functionally necessary is requested. The upper border of the tarsal plate with the lower border of the Muller's muscle and its overlying conjunctiva are clamped and excised and the wound edges held together by a continuous suture. The levator aponeurosis is not involved in the surgery.

In moderate congenital ptosis, a greater degree of ptosis with a levator function between 4 and 10 mm can usually be corrected with a levator resection graded according to the amount of levator function and degree of ptosis (Fig. 26.7). Either an anterior or a posterior approach to the levator can give satisfactory results. The posterior approach has the advantage that the resected levator muscle is held by pull-out sutures that are tied in the skin crease. These can be removed in the early postoperative period and the eyelid lowered if an overcorrection occurs. The anterior approach is suitable for a maximum levator resection, as it gives a slightly better exposure of the levator muscle and allows the creation of an enhanced lid fold. The disadvantage of a large levator resection is that it increases the lid lag on downgaze. If there is a weakness of the superior rectus muscle, a larger levator resection is required for any given degree of ptosis and levator function.

In severe congenital ptosis, if there is less than 4 mm of levator function, two basic techniques have been advocated. First, the eyelid can be suspended from the brow and elevated by the frontalis muscle. If it is necessary to elevate an eyelid urgently to prevent amblyopia, this can be done with a unilateral procedure using a nonautogenous material.[16] Nonautogenous materials may slip, become infected, extrude, or lead to granulation formation. If the operation does not have to be done to prevent amblyopia, it is better to wait until the child's leg is large enough to take autogenous fascia lata (usually by the age of 3 to 4 years). A unilateral sling may produce an unacceptable degree of asymmetry if the contralateral levator muscle is working normally. It is therefore reasonable to consider correcting a severe unilateral ptosis by first weakening or excising the normal levator muscle and then lifting both eyelids symmetrically with a bilateral brow suspension procedure (Fig. 26.8).

An alternative to the brow suspension procedure in a patient with a poor levator function is to excise the aponeurosis anterior to the Whitnall's ligament and suture the ligament to the tarsus, possibly combining this with a partial tarsectomy.[17] Whitnall's ligament is attached to the orbital roof in the region of the trochlea and lacrimal fossa and therefore acts as an "internal sling." This may elevate the eyelid satisfactorily in the primary position but may cause unacceptable unilateral lagophthalmos.

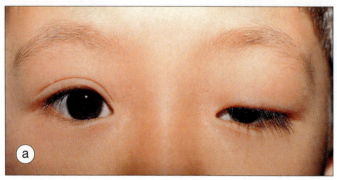
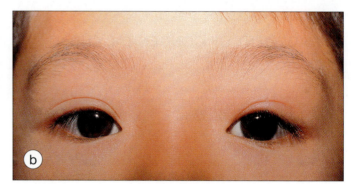

Fig. 26.7 (a) Unilateral simple congenital ptosis. (b) The same child after levator resection.

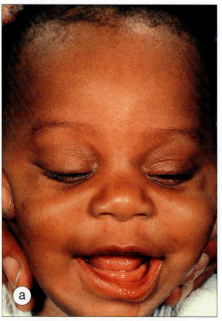
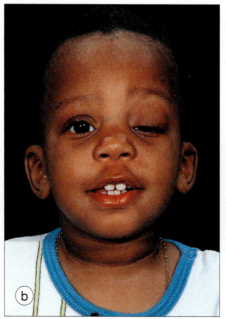
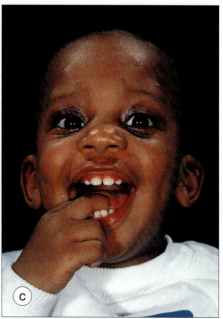

Fig. 26.8 (a) Right ptosis in a 6-month-old baby. It can be seen that there is no lid crease on the right while it is present on the left. The child is looking down during this photograph and the normally ptotic lid is slightly higher than the normal lid, suggesting a dystrophic ptosis. (b) Same child at 2 years of age preoperatively. (c) Same child postoperatively. A bilateral levator sling procedure has been carried out.

Finally, a maximal levator resection may be performed. In this technique, the levator muscle is dissected free of all attachments, including Whitnall's, and is resected such that the lid rests at the superior limbus intraoperatively.[18] If the levator muscle is very dystrophic it may stretch in time with a recurrence of the ptosis.

Specific conditions

In the blepharophimosis syndrome levator function is usually poor and bilateral autogenous fascia lata brow suspensions are required. If the levator function is good, bilateral levator resections can be performed instead. The epicanthus inversus is usually best treated with a medial canthoplasty about 6 months before the lids are lifted.

In Marcus Gunn syndrome, if the jaw-winking element is unobtrusive, the ptosis alone can be corrected based on the levator function. If the jaw-winking is severe, it can be abolished by cutting the levator muscle. The ptosis must then be corrected with a brow suspension procedure. The logical treatment is perhaps to excise both levator muscles and correct the ptosis with a bilateral autogenous fascia lata brow suspension in the interest of symmetry.[19] Some cases may become less marked with time, and it may therefore be justifiable to delay surgery until the child is old enough to help in the decision-making.

With third nerve lesions the eye should be straightened first with horizontal muscle surgery, supplemented if necessary by transplanting the superior oblique from the trochlea, and suturing it to the adjacent medial rectus muscle insertion to hold the eye just in adduction. The correction of the ptosis depends as usual on the levator function. If Bell's phenomenon is defective, there is a risk of exposure keratitis and ptosis surgery should be more conservative.

The same remarks apply to the correction of aberrant third nerve regeneration syndromes and cyclic oculomotor palsy, both of which may require excision of the levator muscle and brow suspension procedure.

Horner syndrome usually does well with a Fasanella Servat procedure.

Myasthenics should rarely be operated on. Appropriate medication and ptosis prop contact lenses usually offer a better solution, but conservative surgery may sometimes be justified.

Progressive external ophthalmoplegia is similar but autogenous fascia lata brow suspensions may be successful if the slings are left loose enough to allow the lids to be closed on the operating table. When the patient raises his eyebrows the ptosis will be improved without causing lagophthalmos and corneal exposure. There is, however, always the risk of exposure problems as the ocular movements become more limited and the orbicularis muscle becomes weaker. This may necessitate cutting the fascial bands to allow complete eyelid closure and then using ptosis props, which will be tolerated if the orbicularis muscle is sufficiently weak.

Aponeurotic defects occurring congenitally, traumatically, or in blepharochalasis should be repaired.

A hypotropia should be corrected before embarking on ptosis surgery. If it is due to mechanical restriction, this should be relieved. A superior rectus muscle resection may increase the ptosis. If the medial and lateral rectus muscles are disinserted and reattached close to the insertion of the superior rectus, the eye may be elevated. If a forced duction test shows inferior rectus restriction, the inferior rectus muscle must be recessed. Any residual ptosis can be corrected with a subsequent ptosis operation.

In the ocular fibrosis syndrome, a brow suspension with careful postoperative management to prevent exposure may give good results.

LID RETRACTION IN INFANCY

Lid retraction in infancy can be caused by a variety of conditions (see Chapter 25). Major lid retraction with corneal exposure requires urgent treatment with lubrication and early surgery to protect the cornea. Cases of mild lid retraction may benefit from cosmetic surgery that may be delayed into early childhood.

The upper lid can be lowered and the lower lid raised by recessing the lid retractors provided there is no shortage of skin or conjunctiva. Upper lid retractor recessions through a posterior approach can be used to correct a mild degree of retraction; a tenotomy will cure up to 2 mm of lid retraction and a levator recession 3 mm of lid retraction. However, posterior approach upper lid retractor recessions inevitably cause a raised skin crease. This does not matter in mild or bilateral cases but is important in severe unilateral cases. In these, the retractors should be lengthened via an anterior approach levator recession or Z-myotomy or a spacer graft and the skin crease reformed at the desired level. Lower lid retraction may be corrected by retractor recession, usually in combination with a spacer graft.[20]

SEVENTH NERVE PALSY

Congenital causes of pediatric seventh nerve palsy include the following:
1. Mononeural agenesis;
2. Facial paralysis with other defects: e.g., Möbius syndrome, hemifacial microsoma, and oculoauriculovertebral dysplasia; and
3. Drugs or infection in pregnancy: e.g., thalidomide, rubella.

Acquired causes of pediatric seventh nerve palsy include the following:
1. Birth trauma;
2. Idiopathic: e.g., Bell's palsy;
3. Systemic disease/infection: poliomyelitis, infectious mononucleosis, varicella, rubella, Lyme disease, acute otitis media, and meningitis;
4. Intracranial lesions: e.g., tumors, arteriovenous malformations, and infarcts; and
5. Invasive lesions: e.g., leukemic, and rhabdomyosarcoma.

In the newborn the incidence of facial palsy is 0.2%. Birth trauma is the cause of 78% of facial paralysis in this group, and can be caused by forceps delivery, pressure from the maternal sacrum, pressure from the fetal shoulder, or intracranial hemorrhage. As much as 89% of newborn facial palsies go on to a complete recovery without treatment; however, 11% have an incomplete recovery. Most cases will clear by 5 months of age.[21] In infancy/childhood facial palsy is most often associated with an otitis media.

Bell's palsy, a diagnosis of exclusion, is less common in children than adults. It is manifest as a paralysis of all muscle groups on one side of the face, with a sudden onset, and an absence of signs of ear or cerebellopontine angle disease. It is bilateral in 0.3% of cases, and recurrent in 9% of cases.

Bilateral facial palsy is rare, accounting for 0.3–2% of cases. The resultant disability is dramatically more severe, and can be associated with severe feeding problems. In the newborn it may be associated with Möbius syndrome (see Chapter 85). In childhood the most common cause in endemic areas is Lyme disease, followed by otitis media and idiopathic.[22]

Although facial nerve palsy in children is considered to have a good prognosis, it may be the initial manifestation of a life-threatening disorder such as an intracranial neoplasm or vascular malformation. If neurological findings in addition to facial palsy are manifested or suspected, imaging studies are indicated. Likewise, progression of facial nerve palsy is almost invariably due to a tumor, and in 20% of patients with recurrent facial weakness a tumor is eventually discovered.

The main problems caused by a seventh nerve palsy are:[23]
1. corneal exposure;
2. Paralytic ectropion;
3. Epiphora; and
4. Cosmesis.

Corneal exposure

Corneal exposure does not usually result from poor lid closure alone as the Bell's phenomenon is good in infants; there is usually an additional risk factor. This may be an inadequate Bell's phenomenon, a reduction in corneal sensation, a lower lid ectropion, treatment on a ventilator, prematurity, or a reduction in tear production if the lesion is proximal to the geniculate ganglion. A reduction in corneal sensation is more common after surgical treatment of intracranial tumors or a cerebellopontine angle tumor, or may be present in some variants of Möbius syndrome.

Initial treatment is with lubricants, taping at night, and occasionally occlusive dressings may be required. The lubricants can be stopped for 2 to 3 hours a day, or the other eye patched in order to avoid inducing amblyopia. Occasionally a temporary lateral tarsorrhaphy may be required to protect the cornea during the initial assessment. If there is continued corneal exposure after 6 months, or earlier if there is no chance of recovery, the palpebral aperture can be reduced. The vertical palpebral aperture can be reduced by raising the lower lid with a lateral tarsorrhaphy and medial canthoplasty, by lowering the upper lid with a Mullerectomy, by recession of Muller's muscle and the levator muscle, or with a blepharotomy. The horizontal palpebral aperture can be reduced by medial and lateral tarsorrhaphies. Lid closure can be improved mechanically with upper lid gold weights, springs, magnets, etc. Care is taken to avoid astigmatic amblyopia in the young using these treatments. Where severe exposure is present, lid closure can be improved dynamically with muscle grafts, temporalis muscle and fascial slings, cross-face nerve anastomosis, etc. More complex surgery requires a multidisciplinary input and careful planning to stage surgery.[24]

Paralytic ectropion

Paralytic ectropion can be treated by a medial canthoplasty, and if required this can be combined with lateral canthal shortening.

Epiphora

Epiphora is due to the loss of the lacrimal pump mechanism, and is exacerbated by lower lid ectropion. It may also occur due to the "crocodile tear syndrome" in which tearing is associated with eating due to aberrant regeneration of the parasympathetic to one or more of the salivary glands, which become misdirected

to the lacrimal glands. Persistent watering after 6 months may be improved by correction of any ectropion with a lateral canthal sling and medial canthoplasty. Crocodile tears may be improved either by repeated injections of botulinum toxin into the lacrimal gland, which requires a general anesthetic in a child, or by a posterior lacrimal gland debulking. Severe watering may require a Lester Jones tube.

Cosmesis

Cosmetic improvements may be difficult to achieve. Surgery to raise the brow, reduce the palpebral aperture, and correct ectropion may help.

LID TUMORS

Nevi

Surgery for nevi is indicated if there is concern for the development of malignant potential, for amblyopia due to lid malposition, and for cosmesis.

Large, or giant, congenital nevi are associated with a risk of malignant transformation, which is variably assessed from a few to 20%. These lesions are more common on the face or trunk, but do occur on the eyelid. The lesions are difficult to treat due to their size, and surgery may require numerous stages, with skin grafts and flaps, and the use of tissue expanders. The multiple procedures may result in marked scarring. Early dermabrasion, within the first few months and preferably weeks of life, may reduce the chance of malignant transformation, improve cosmesis, and reduce the extent of further surgery.[25]

The incidence of malignant transformation in small and medium congenital nevi is controversial but thought to be negligible. Divided nevi are a form of congenital melanocytic nevus that involves the upper and lower lids (Fig. 26.9).

The nevus of Ota is a congenital lesion characterized by a gray discoloration of the face in the distribution of the ophthalmic and maxillary divisions of the trigeminal nerve. The skin, conjunctiva, and sclera are affected and there may also be increased uveal pigmentation. In Caucasians there may be an increased risk of melanoma, and patients are given periodic eye examinations.

Acquired nevi are rarely a concern in children, but as an adult these lesions are monitored for pathologic changes.

Molluscum contagiosum and warts

Molluscum contagiosum and warts of viral origin also frequently occur on the eyelids (Fig. 26.10); they may rarely obtain large size, and "kiss" lesions may occur on the upper and lower lids (Fig. 26.11). They are often associated with a follicular conjunctivitis (Fig. 26.12), which does not resolve until the lesions near the eyelid are eradicated. Treatment modalities include curettage and diathermy of the core of the lesion, cryotherapy, and chemical ablatives.

Juvenile xanthogranuloma

Juvenile xanthogranuloma is a benign disease of children characterized by the development of small red rubbery cutaneous lesions, including eyelid lesions, of 1 to 10 mm, in the first 1 to 9 months of life. The lesions may be associated with ocular xanthogranuloma lesions, particularly in the iris, when they may

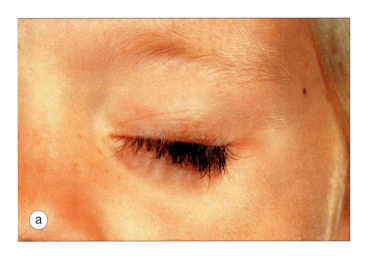
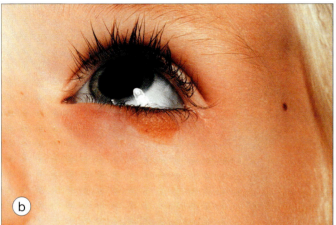

Fig. 26.9 (a, b) Divided nevus.

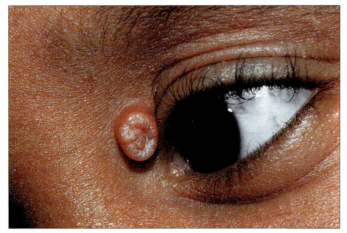

Fig. 26.10 Large molluscum contagiosum lesion. Dr Susan Day's patient.

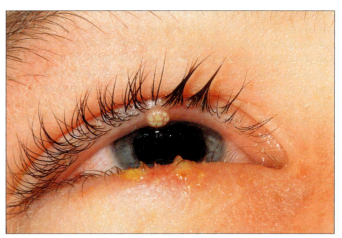

Fig. 26.11 Molluscum contagiosum showing multiple lesions and a follicular conjunctivitis.

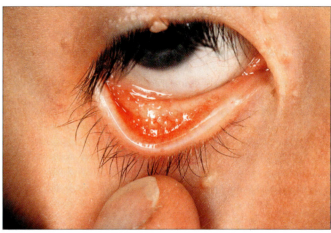

Fig. 26.12 Molluscum contagiosum showing "kiss" lesions on upper and lower lids.

present with spontaneous hyphema and glaucoma. Most lesions resolve after a year, but larger lesions may respond to steroids, cryotherapy, excision, or radiotherapy.

Complex choristoma

These are rare lid tumors that consist of variable combinations of ectopic tissues. Clinically they resemble other choristomas such as dermoids and lipodermoids. When acinar elements compose the majority of the tissue they may have a more fleshy appearance or resemble an ectopic lacrimal gland. Mild growth may occur during puberty, but malignant transformation is rare. They can invade deep into the underlying tissue; conjunctival lesions may invade deep into the globe and therefore excision is often best avoided.

Pilomatrixoma (calcifying epithelioma of Malherbe)

A small hard nodule in the eyebrow is likely to be a pilomatrixoma. The overlying skin is intact and may have a pink to purple discoloration. It may be mistaken for a chalazion or dermoid. Treatment is excision.

Carney complex

This constitutes the association of eyelid myxoma, potentially lethal cardiac myxoma, genital tumors, and other metabolic abnormalities. Myxomas are benign neoplasms of mesenchymal origin. Treatment is with a wide local excision as inadequate excision may result in recurrence.

Lid hamartoma

Lid hamartomas include hemangiomas, plexiform neurofibromas, lymphangiomas (venolymphatic malformations), and congenital nevi. The treatment of hemangiomas is covered in Chapter 42, and the treatment of congenital nevi is covered in the section "Nevi."

Indications for oculoplastic surgery for plexiform neurofibroma and lymphangioma include mechanical ptosis, occlusion amblyopia, astigmatic anisometropic amblyopia, and cosmetic deformity. Surgery for both these lesions is challenging. The lesions may be extensive, involving the lids, orbits, and surrounding facial tissues, and due to the infiltrative nature of these lesions complete excision is rarely possible. Further, the lesions continue to grow and recur after excision, and there may be a marked increase in growth around puberty. Treatment should be planned in conjunction with any allied surgical specialties. In general less surgical intervention is better than more, and multiple procedures may be necessary over the lifetime of the patient.

MEIBOMIAN GLAND DISEASES

The functions of the Meibomian glands include the following:[26]
1. Reduce tear evaporation;
2. Enhance tear stability;
3. Prevent tear spillover at the lid margin;
4. Prevent tear contamination by sebum; and
5. Sealing the apposed tear margins during sleep.

Chalazia (Meibomian cysts)

A chalazion is a lipogranuloma of the meibomian gland that results from obstruction of the gland duct and is usually located in the mid-portion of the tarsus, away from the lid border, and sometimes well away from the lid margin. It may occur on the lid margin if the opening of the duct is involved. A secondary infection of the surrounding tissue may develop with swelling of the entire lid. Chalazia may cause pressure on the globe, thereby altering refractive error. Small chalazia may resolve spontaneously. If they are large, however, or secondarily infected, treatment is usually required. This involves the use of warm compresses with topical antibiotic therapy. Incision of the conjunctival wall of the lesion and curettage is sometimes necessary; however, this is avoided whenever possible in young children since it usually necessitates a general anesthetic. Chronic meibomitis and blepharitis, which may predispose to recurrent chalazia, should be treated by lid cleaning together with antibiotic/hydrocortisone ointment for a circumscribed period before resorting to incision and curettage. Chronic chalazia should be treated with suspicion as rhabdomyosarcoma may present in this guise.

Other diseases of the meibomian glands include the following:
1. Absent or deficient glands: primary congenital ectodermal dysplasia or ichthyosis, or secondary to lid disease.
2. Replacement: primary distichiasis, or secondary distichiasis due to metaplasia.
3. Meibomian seborrhea: associated with seborrheic dermatitis and acne rosacea. The meibum is greasy and solidified.
4. Meibomitis: often occurs with blepharitis. The orifices are red and swollen and sometimes there is soreness with associated lid edema. Treatment is similar to blepharitis.

Acute blepharitis

Acute blepharitis presents with ulceration of the lid margins and is usually caused by *Staphlococcus aureus*, other organisms and viruses, including *Moraxella* species, herpes simplex, and various fungi in immunosuppressed patients (Fig. 26.13). Staphylococcal and *Moraxella* blepharitis usually respond well to antibiotic cream and lid toilet. Fungi or herpes simplex usually respond to appropriate chemotherapy.

Chronic blepharitis

Chronic blepharitis is much more common than the acute form. It presents as irritable eyelids that are red, scaly, and sometimes rather swollen (Fig. 26.14). The anterior lid margin is usually most affected, but occasionally the posterior lid margin is more red and swollen when the Meibomian glands are affected (chronic meibomitis). Infection plays a role with *S. aureus*, *Propionibacterium acnes*, or coagulase-negative staphylococcal species being important.[27] The role of yeasts like *Pityrosporum ovale* is uncertain but it seems clearer that the mite *Demodex folliculorum* plays a role, perhaps as a vector for bacteria and yeasts.

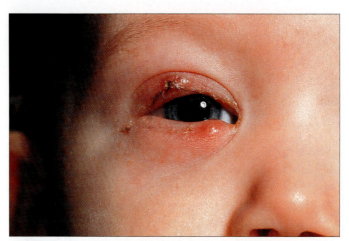

Fig. 26.13 Acute blepharitis with lid ulceration and stye formation.

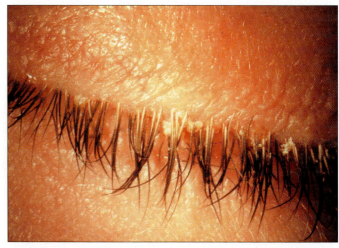

Fig. 26.14 Chronic blepharitis associated with chronic *Staphylococcus* infection.

Most of the cases of chronic blepharitis have a seborrheic element with greasy, scaly lids associated in some cases with seborrheic dermatitis of the scalp (dandruff) or elsewhere.

Treatment is by regular lid cleaning, with particular attention to the lid margins. Expression of greasy Meibomian secretion by firm pressure may also help the symptoms of burning and irritation. This simple treatment should be carried out long after the symptoms have improved. Recurrent or severe cases, which may be associated with keratoconjunctivitis, may be treated in addition by a short course of steroid–antibiotic combination ointment.

Lid lice

Lid lice are usually pubic lice rather than head lice because their body shape is more suited to the wider spacing of the lashes (Fig. 26.15). They may be found on slit-lamp examination of the lash bases or their eggs ("nits") may be found attached to the lashes. The pubic hair must be treated as well as the lashes. Lid treatment is with a topical eserine.

Trichiasis

Trichiasis is an acquired condition of the eyelash roots in which the cilia are misdirected, usually backward, causing corneal and conjunctival irritation. It differs from entropion in that the lid margin itself is in a normal position, but because of fibrosis or cicatrization, the cilia are misplaced. The most common causes of trichiasis include chronic blepharitis, Stevens-Johnson syndrome, severe burns, and pemphigus.

The treatment of trichiasis depends on the number of abnormal lashes. One or a few lashes can be treated with electrolysis or surgery either to excise the lash roots or to resect the affected portion of the eyelid margin. More numerous lashes are best treated with cryotherapy, but all the lashes in the treated area are liable to be destroyed and it may cause depigmentation. In black patients it can sometimes be combined with a lid-splitting technique as described for distichiasis.

SOCKET MANAGEMENT
Contracted socket

Early socket growth is rapid. At 3 months the face is only 40% of its adult size, and by 5½ years it is 80% of its adult size. The

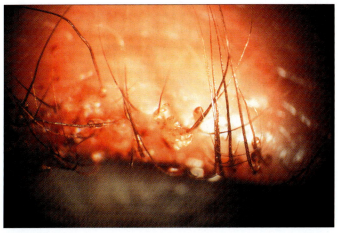

Fig. 26.15 Lid lice.

presence of an eye is necessary for normal orbital growth. The loss of an eye, microphthalmia, or anophthalmia all result in abnormal orbital growth. The aims of socket management in infants are to increase the size of the bony orbit, conjunctival space, and palpebral length, and to promote the normal development of the lid margins and lashes.

Treatment must be started early to avoid a poor esthetic result. If the patient has an orbital cyst associated with microphthalmos or anophthalmos this may be left to aid socket expansion.[28] In most cases the socket can be expanded using increasing sizes of orbital conformer. More recently a number of expandable conformers that do not require serial changes and can be increased in size by injecting saline through a port have become available. These can be placed either in the intraconal space and connected to a remote injection port under the skin (for example, over the ear) or in the conjunctival sac with an anterior port directly accessible through the palpebral fissure.

An alternative is the self-inflating hydrogel expander. This is made of a modified copolymer of methylmethacrylate and vinyl pyrrolidone (MMA-VP), similar to contact lens material but with more capacity for swelling. It swells 10–12 times in volume, taking about 2 to 6 weeks to expand to its full size in the orbit.

Orbital volume replacement

Sometimes orbital expansion results in an increase in the anteroposterior dimension of the socket without increasing the palpebral fissure length, and fornical depth. The resultant conformer is round and deep and will not promote an increase in vertical and horizontal lid length, and will be difficult to retain. In these circumstances an orbital implant can be inserted, and a thinner conformer used to improve the fornices. Alternatively, if hydrogel expanders are used, a lens-shaped expander can be used to expand the conjunctival space followed by a spherical expander for the orbit.

The lateral fornix is often difficult to promote, and it may need to be constructed surgically with a mucous membrane graft in order to retain a prosthesis.

Orbital implants available include the porous implants hydroxyapatite and polypropylethylene, nonporous implants made from silicone and acrylic, and dermis fat grafts. The porous implants have the advantage that they become integrated into the socket and so are less likely to extrude, and there may be the option of pegging the implant to improve motility at a later date. However, integration into the socket tissues makes these implants more difficult to remove, and in the pediatric population an implant may need to be replaced for a larger size at some stage in the future. They are therefore not advised in patients under 6 years old. Hydroxyapatite implants are often wrapped in donor material so that muscles can be attached to the implant, and to reduce the risk of exposure caused by abrasion of the Tenon's and conjunctiva by the hard rough material. If sclera is used there is a risk of prion transmission. Alternatively vicryl mesh can be used. Polypropylethylene implants do not require a wrapping; they are softer and muscles can be attached directly to the implant.

Silicone and acrylic implants are easier to remove, but may be more likely to extrude, and cannot be pegged. Dermis fat grafts have several advantages.[29] Whereas in the adult population they tend to atrophy, in children they can grow as the child grows, and can help with socket expansion. They have been reported to grow such that they require debulking.[30] The conjunctiva can be attached to the edge of the graft, allowing the conjunctival epithelium to grow over the surface of the graft and increase the size of the conjunctival sac. If further volume augmentation is required, an orbital implant can easily be placed posterior to the graft.[31] The main disadvantage is donor site morbidity, although this is seldom a problem.

If treatment has failed to achieve adequate orbital expansion, resulting in marked facial asymmetry, craniofacial surgery may be required to augment or repair the orbit, and vascularized flaps to increase soft tissue, for example, in cases of tissue atrophy secondary to radiotherapy.

Discharging sockets

Socket discharge is a common problem in patients with a prosthesis. The common causes are:[32]

1. Prosthesis: poor fit, mechanical irritation, hypersensitive reaction, and poor prosthetic hygiene;
2. Orbital implant: extrusion of implant, conjunctival inclusion cyst, and granuloma formation;
3. Lid: poor closure and infected focus;
4. Socket lining: mixture of skin and mucous membrane; and
5. Lacrimal system: defective tear production, defective tear drainage, and infected focus.

Management is to treat the underlying cause.

TRAUMA (see Chapter 70)

Etiology

The majority of pediatric lid and adnexal injuries are accidental in nature, most commonly occurring during domestic activity, during play time or sporting activity, and at school.[33,34] Compared to adults, injuries from dog bites and unusual projectiles occur more frequently, and injury from high-velocity projectiles and blunt trauma due to assault occurs less frequently. A Norwegian study found that the most common cause of injury was projectiles (22%), followed by toys such as balls and arrows (18%), pencils and sticks (10%), and falls (10%).[35] Injuries caused to the lids include contusions, crush injuries, abrasions, lacerations, puncture wounds, and burns. These frequently occur in combination.

Immediate management

An accurate history is taken, noting the time of the injury, nature of any projectile (was it sharp or blunt, metallic or vegetable), the speed of the projectile (was it thrown or shot), height of a fall and the type of surface the child landed on, any loss of consciousness, and any witnesses.

The assessment of the patient starts by examining and treating the patient for all injuries. Any necessary basic life support is given, and a full systemic examination may be required, including a neurological examination if there is any suspicion of intracranial injury. A full ocular examination is performed. The visual function is assessed, if possible the visual acuity is taken, or in a young child it may be simpler to look for fixation or check that the patient tolerates occlusion of the opposite eye, and check the pupil responses for a relative afferent defect.

The injury is assessed by looking for any damage not readily visible. A small lid laceration may have extensive underlying damage, possibly including intracranial injury, orbital fractures, optic neuropathy, and injury to the globe. The patient is examined for any evidence of a retained foreign body, any missing tissue, and any damage to the lacrimal system. The presence of any levator function should be noted in upper lid lacerations. If a large hematoma is present there should be a greater suspicion of damage to the orbit and globe. CT scans are used to look for retained foreign bodies and fractures, and MRI scans can be useful to look for a retained organic foreign body, or if there is likely to be repetitive scans with an unacceptable radiation dose. Photographs are taken of any injury for future reference. A tetanus toxoid booster is given as appropriate.

In principle surgery should be carried out as early as safely possible; however, the results of eyelid surgery are not prejudiced by waiting for up to 48 or 72 hours if this allows more time and better facilities to be available.[36] The wound is cleaned thoroughly to prevent subsequent tattooing and remove foreign bodies. It is examined carefully and the tissues repositioned as accurately as possible. The skin can be closed with absorbable sutures, avoiding a further anesthetic for suture removal. Tissue should not be excised or discarded as the eyelid region has an excellent blood supply, but any pedicle should be preserved if possible. It is not usually necessary to cut or "freshen" the wound. Surgery is covered with intravenous antibiotics, followed by a one-week course of oral antibiotics.

Major reconstruction should be delayed for 3 to 6 months, or even 9 months before repairing defects such as lid retraction or ptosis, unless the patient develops symptoms of corneal exposure that cannot be controlled with simple lubrication, or is at risk of developing amblyopia.[36]

Lid margin defects require careful approximation of the lash line and gray line to avoid lid notch, rotation of the lid, and lash abnormalities. The gray line and lash line sutures can be buried to avoid later removal.

Traumatic ptosis

A traumatic ptosis can be caused by the following: a direct injury or stretching of the aponeurosis or levator muscle; a loss of orbital contents or phthisical eye, causing a lowering of the fulcrum of the levator complex; injury to the third nerve or sympathetic nerve supply; or a mechanical restriction due to conjunctival, lid, or deep orbital scarring. Any obvious levator defect should be sutured at the time of the primary repair; however, minor defects can be left as they are likely to heal spontaneously and excessive surgery may lead to lid retraction. Any residual ptosis may be repaired at a later date, usually after 6 months or after any improvement has ceased. Early intervention is indicated if there is any risk of amblyopia. A temporary frontalis sling using an easily removable material such as a Prolene or Supramid suture, or a silicone rod may be required. Secondary repair is via an anterior approach. Excision of the scar tissue may leave a gap in the levator complex, requiring a spacer. A dermis fat graft can be used to prevent the reformation of dense adhesions. The treatment of ptosis due to nerve injury is described in the section on ptosis earlier in this chapter.

Lacrimal drainage injuries

In normal circumstances 30% of tear drainage is via the upper canaliculus, and 70% via the lower canaliculus. Whether damage to a single canaliculus should be repaired is a contentious issue. Some authors recommend that any damage to either canaliculus be carefully repaired, even if only one is involved, as some patients require two functioning canaliculi to avoid epiphora. Others suggest that, as it is rare to get symptoms from a blocked upper canaliculus if the lower canaliculus is functioning normally, only damage to the lower canaliculus needs to be repaired.[37]

The canaliculi can be repaired either by marsupializing the lacerated medial canaliculus into the conjunctival sac, or by suturing together the two ends of a canaliculus. It is difficult to ensure that an anastomosis remains patent after a few months. Various stents have been used, but the stents themselves may induce fibrosis.

The white color of the canalicular epithelium can usually be clearly seen with the aid of an operating microscope. Injection of fluorescein or air or viscoelastic via the opposite punctum (or directly into the sac in cases of upper and lower canalicular damage) may help to identify the canaliculus. Use of the pigtail probe is controversial as it may damage healthy tissue (especially the older hooked instruments). It is unreasonable to use this probe to repair the upper canaliculus as it may jeopardize the patency of the lower canaliculus. With the use of an operating microscope, good hemostasis, and a thorough knowledge of the anatomy, this is seldom required.

If the canaliculi are to be anastomosed, they are intubated with a self-retaining monocanalicular stent, or with Crawford tubes, and the defect closed in layers. In closing, care is taken to repair the posterior limb of the medial canthal tendon, which is immediately posterior to the medial canaliculus, as this maintains the lid in apposition to the globe. In repairing the canaliculus the sutures should be passed into the tissues immediately around the canaliculus and not through its epithelium.[38]

Common canalicular injury is repaired, or opened into the lacrimal sac, the canaliculi intubated, and a dacryocystorhinostomy performed.

Established canalicular damage near the punctum can be treated by a retrograde dacryocystorhinostomy with marsupialization of the canaliculus into the conjunctival sac. Blockage near the lacrimal sac can be treated by excision of the scar and connection of the patent canaliculus to the sac. In either case at least 8 mm of one canaliculus is necessary for success.

Medial canthal tendon injuries

The anterior limb of the medial canthal tendon seldom needs to be repaired; however, if the posterior limb is damaged and only the anterior limb is repaired the lid will be anteropositioned. The method of repair of the posterior limb depends on the posterior fixation point available. If the lacrimal drainage system is intact and there is a firm and reasonably positioned medial wall fixation point, the posterior limb and eyelid tissues can be directly attached to the medial orbital wall. If the lacrimal sac must be opened for dacryocystorhinostomy and the tissues behind the lacrimal sac are adequate, a nonabsorbable suture can be passed behind the opened lacrimal sac and used to reattach the medial canthus and eyelid tissues medially and posterior to the posterior lacrimal fascia. If there is no adequate ipsilateral fixation point a transnasal wire can be used to reposition the medial canthus.

Burns

In the acute stage burns are treated with heavy lubrication or occlusive therapy to protect the cornea. To avoid amblyopia the eye may be left for 2 to 3 hours a day without lubrication, or the other eye can be patched. In severe cases of exposure a conjunctival flap may be required. In the chronic stage, after 30 days, the lids are reconstructed. Split skin grafts may be required; lid-sharing procedures are avoided where possible to avoid the risk of amblyopia.

REFERENCES

1. Tessier P. Plastic Surgery of the Orbit and Eyelids. Chicago: Mosby; 1977.
2. Collin JRO. Congenital upper lid coloboma. Austral NZ J Ophthalmol 1986; 14: 313–17.
3. Sullivan TJ, Clarke MP, Rootman DS, et al. Eyelid and fornix reconstruction in bilateral abortive cryptophthalmos (Fraser syndrome). Austral NZ J Ophthalmol 1992; 20: 51–6.
4. Morris RJ, Collin JRO. Functional lid surgery in Down's syndrome. Br J Ophthalmol 1986; 73: 494–7.
5. Kronish J, Lingua R. Pressure patch treatment for congenital upper eyelid eversion. Arch Ophthalmol 1991; 109: 767–8.
6. Hayasaka S, Noda S, Setogawa T. Epiblepharon with inverted eyelashes in Japanese children. II. Surgical repairs. Br J Ophthalmol 1989; 73: 128–30.
7. O'Donnell BA, Collin JRO. Congenital lower eyelid deformity with trichiasis, epiblepharon and entropion. Austral NZ J Ophthalmol 1994; 22: 33–7.
8. O'Donnell BA, Collin JRO. Distichiasis; management with cryotherapy to the posterior lamella. Br J Ophthalmol 1993; 77: 289–92.
9. Mustardé JC. Epicanthic folds and the problem of telecanthus. Trans Ophthalmol Soc UK 1963; 83: 397–411.
10. Anderson RL, Nowinski TS. The five flap technique for blepharophimosis. Arch Ophthalmol 1989; 107: 448–52.
11. McCord CD. The correction of telecanthus and epicanthic folds. Ophthalmic Surg 1980; 11: 446–56.
12. Beaconsfield M, Walker JW, Collin JRO. Visual development in blepharophimosis syndrome. Br J Ophthalmol 1991; 75: 746–8.
13. Anderson L, Baumgartner A. Amblyopia in ptosis. Arch Ophthalmol 1980; 98: 1068–9.
14. Anderson L, Baumgartner A. Strabismus in ptosis. Arch Ophthalmol 1980; 98: 1062–7.
15. Collin JRO. New concepts in the management of ptosis. Eye 1988; 2: 185–9.
16. Downes RN, Collin JRO. The mersilene mesh sling – a new concept in ptosis surgery. Br J Ophthalmol 1984; 68: 524–9.
17. Holds JB, McLeish WM, Anderson RL. Whitnall's sling with superior tarsectomy for the correction of severe unilateral blepharophimosis. Arch Ophthalmol 1993; 111: 1285–91.
18. Mauriello JA, Wagner RS, Caputo AR. Treatment of congenital ptosis by maximal levator resection. Ophthalmology 1986; 93: 466–8.
19. Beard C. A new treatment for severe unilateral ptosis with jaw-winking. Am J Ophthalmol 1965; 59: 252–7.
20. Collin JRO, Castronovo S, Allen L. Congenital eyelid retraction. Br J Ophthalmol 1990; 9: 542–4.
21. Falco NA, Eriksson E. Facial nerve palsy in the newborn: incidence and outcome. Plast Reconstr Surg 1990; 85: 1–4.
22. Cook SP, Maccartney KK, Rose CD, et al. Lyme disease and seventh nerve paralysis in children. Ann J Otolaryngol 1997; 18: 320–3.
23. Collin JRO. Facial palsy, thyroid eye disease and corneal protection. In: Collin JRO, editor. A Manual of Systematic Eyelid Surgery. 2nd ed. Edinburgh: Churchill Livingstone; 1989: 139–48.
24. Seiff SR, Chang J. The staged management of ophthalmic complications of facial nerve palsy. Ophthal Plast Reconstr Surg 1990; 9: 241–9.
25. Reynolds N, Kenealy J, Mercer N. Carbon dioxide laser dermabrasion for giant congenital melanocytic nevi. Plast Reconstr Surg 2003; 111: 2209–14.
26. Bron AJ, Benjamin L, Snibson GR. Meibomian gland disease. Eye 1991; 5: 395–411.
27. Dougherty JM, McCully JP. Comparative bacteriology of chronic blepharitis. Br J Ophthalmol 1984; 68: 524–9.
28. McLean CJ, Ragge NK, Jones RB, et al. The management of orbital cysts associated with congenital microphthalmos and anophthalmos. Br J Ophthalmol 2003; 87: 860–3.
29. Piest KL, Welsh MG. Pediatric enucleation, evisceration, and exenteration techniques. In: Katowitz JA, editor. Pediatric Oculoplastic Surgery. New York. Springer-Verlag; 2002: 617–27.

30. Heher K, Katowitz J, Low J. Unilateral dermis-fat implantation in the pediatric orbit. Ophthalmic Plast Reconstr Surg 1998; 14: 81.

31. Kazim M, Katowitz JA, Fallon M, et al. Evaluation of a collagen/hydroxyapatite implant for orbital reconstructive surgery. Ophthalmic Plast Reconstr Surg 1992; 8: 94–108.

32. Jones CA, Collin JRO. A classification and review of the causes of discharging sockets. Trans Ophthal Soc UK 1983; 103: 351–3.

33. Gonnering RS. Ocular adnexal injury and complications in orbital dog bites. Ophthalmic Plast Reconstr Surg 1987; 231–5.

34. Umbeh BE, Umbeh OC. Causes and visual outcome of childhood injuries in Nigeria. Eye 1997; 11: 485–95.

35. Takvam JA, Midelfart A. Survey of eye injuries in Norwegian children. Acta Ophthalmol 1993; 71: 500–5.

36. Collin JRO. Immediate management of lid laceration. Trans Ophthal Soc UK 1982; 102: 214.

37. Reifler DM. Management of canalicular laceration. Surv Ophthalmol 1992; 36: 323–4.

38. Kersten RC, Kulwn DR. One-stitch canalicular repair. A simplified approach for repair of canalicular laceration. Ophthalmology 1997; 104: 785–9.

Conjunctiva and Subconjunctival Tissue

CHAPTER 27

Cameron F Parsa

STRUCTURE, FUNCTION, AND EMBRYOLOGY

The conjunctiva is derived from mesenchyme around the limbus that also forms the sclera, episclera, and Tenon's capsule. In childhood, Tenon's is thicker and the blood vessels are fewer, less tortuous, smaller, and less prominent. Tenon's also serves as an insertion pulley for the extraocular muscles.[1] The conjunctiva is a tougher tissue than Tenon's: it holds sutures well. In childhood, the conjunctiva is also thicker and the epithelial cells are squarer and more numerous than later. The conjunctiva contains goblet cells that produce mucus and, in the fornices, the accessory lacrimal glands of Krause and Wolfring responsible for basal aqueous tear production. At the limbus, within the palisades of Vogt, lie the stem cells of the corneal epithelium.[2] The growth of the conjunctival fornix, orbital margin, and palpebral fissure correlates with weight and gestational age of term and premature neonates.[3] Limbal episcleral circulation also subserves anterior segment structures such as the iris and cornea. Fornix, rather than limbal, incisions during strabismus surgery may spare a portion of this blood supply protecting against anterior segment ischemia.[4] Unlike brain and other ocular structures, the conjunctiva is rich in lymphatics.

VASCULAR ABNORMALITIES

Hemangioma and lymphohemangioma

Capillary and cavernous hemangiomas are common benign soft tissue tumors composed only of blood vessels: both are associated with lid, orbital (Figs. 27.1a, 27.1b), and sometimes intracranial tumors.

Capillary hemangiomas are bright red masses that blanch on pressure and may hemorrhage spontaneously or with trivial trauma. They may grow rapidly within the first few months of life, but most undergo complete spontaneous regression by five years. Large lesions producing refractive or deprivation amblyopia may require intervention such as repeated perilesional or intralesional depot steroid injections or, rarely, surgery. More extensive hemangiomas, especially those also involving less accessible sites, may require oral steroids. Interferon therapy may be used in refractive cases.[5]

Cavernous hemangiomas are rarer and larger and more frequently involve deeper structures; they exhibit growth slowly, without regression. Treatment, if necessary, is surgical. Conjunctival cavernous hemangiomas may be seen with widespread skin and organ involvement in congenital diffuse hemangiomatosis and blue-rubber-bleb-nevus-syndromes.

Lymphohemangiomas (Fig. 27.1c) are venous and lymphoid anomalies with channels that are isolated from the circulation and accumulate lymph-like protein-rich fluid. Bleeding into these channels may occur, enlarging the mass. Clinically they may be distinguished by clear fluid-filled cystic areas amongst the blood-filled hemangioma tissue. Lymphohemangiomas are usually widespread, and appear in other parts of the face: in the nose causing nose bleeds, on the palate causing bleeding when eating, or in the orbit causing increased proptosis with upper respiratory infections. Lymphohemangiomas are less prone to the cessation of

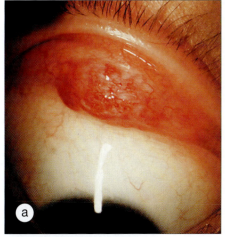
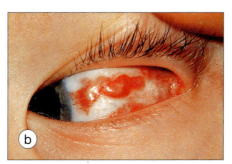
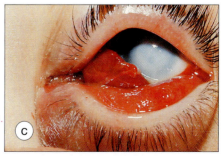

Fig. 27.1 (a) An isolated conjunctival capillary hemangioma in a 2-year-old child that disappeared by the age of 6 years. (b) Subconjunctival capillary hemangioma in an otherwise normal child. Although it had regressed spontaneously from being quite large at birth, it was prone to repeated subconjunctival hemorrhages. On this occasion the hemorrhage is contained within the subconjunctival tissue but can be seen to be spreading anteriorly. (c) This 2-year-old child had an anomalous left eye from birth; at 18 months of age the lids became swollen due to a lymphohemangioma that also involved the orbit and maxilla. The palate also contained clear and blood-filled cysts typical of lymphohemangioma.

growth capillary hemangiomas exhibit, but some may show resolution. Surgery should be restricted to those patients for whom there is a risk of amblyopia, the cosmetic appearance is extremely poor, or there appears to be no cessation of growth.

Sturge-Weber/Klippel-Trenaunay-Weber syndromes (see also Chapter 69)

Congenital facial nevus flammeus, or port-wine stains, are best termed vascular ectasias. They consist of dilated venules containing darkened, deoxygenated blood. Whenever bridging veins from cerebral cortex to dural sinuses are absent, impaired cortical drainage results in leptomeningeal thickening. Supplemental drainage via adjacent patent bridging veins may produce ectasia of scalp emissary and diploic veins. Centripetal drainage also occurs via deep cerebral veins with collaterals to cavernous sinus. Blood-flow reversing from cavernous sinus to ophthalmic veins results in orbital and periorbital facial venous ectasia. Segmental or diffuse dilatation of conjunctival and episcleral veins, choroid, and choriocapillaris may thus be noted. Dilation and expansion of the choriocapillaris obscures the deeper choroid: the "tomato ketchup" fundus. Despite alternative blood drainage pathways, cerebral venous drainage may remain impaired (as evidenced by a thickened choroidal plexus on MRI scans), reducing arterial perfusion. Cortical atrophy follows with calcification and fits: Sturge-Weber syndrome.

Conjunctiva and episcleral tissues often demonstrate vascular dilatory changes (Fig. 27.2), especially when both upper and lower eyelids are involved. Sometimes only a faint sectorial blush is visible or it may be more extensive. Glaucoma may ensue (see Chapters 48 and 69).

Obliteration of superficial port-wine stains may reduce venous outflow channels and may exacerbate both ocular hypertension and cerebral perfusion anomalies; such risks should be taken into account when considering treatment of these lesions.

Klippel-Trenaunay-Weber syndrome shares the pathophysiology with Sturge-Weber syndrome but affects other portions of the body. Venous dysplasia in non-CNS structures, where lymphatics are present, results in congestion with secondary tissue hypertrophy. Patients with both cephalic and limb involvement, along with glaucoma or seizures, may be referred to as having both Sturge-Weber and Klippel-Trenaunay-Weber syndromes, neither

of which is hereditable. Because of poor venous blood flow, thromboembolic events are common in both syndromes, exacerbating perfusion anomalies and symptoms. Aspirin thromboprophylaxis may be of benefit.

Ataxia telangiectasia (Louis-Bar syndrome)

Louis-Bar syndrome is autosomal recessively inherited and patients usually present with slowly progressive limb and truncal cerebellar ataxia after normal early development. Dysarthria and movement difficulties, including extrapyramidal disorders, become severely handicapping by 12 years of age. Mental regression is frequent, and growth retardation occurs especially in those who have recurrent infections, which are due to immunological defects. They are susceptible to neoplasms and some have abnormal carbohydrate metabolism.

The diagnosis is often not made until the appearance of conjunctival telangiectasias. These extremely tortuous and telangiectatic conjunctival venules occur first in the light-exposed bulbar conjunctiva[6] usually by age 10 years (Fig. 27.3). Initially subtle, they may become gross and they usually precede the

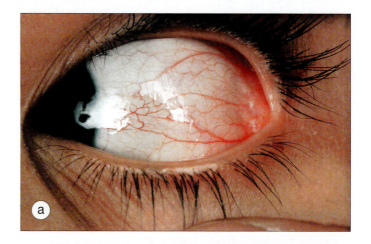

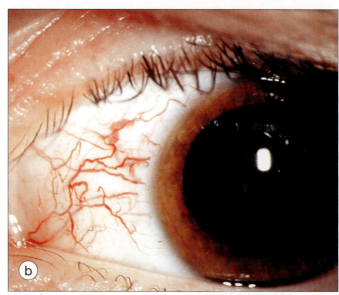

Fig. 27.3 Ataxia telangiectasia. (a) There is a group of telangiectatic and tortuous vessels only in the exposed area of the bulbar conjunctiva, especially temporally. (b) More advanced telangiectases (Courtesy of Michael X. Repka MD).

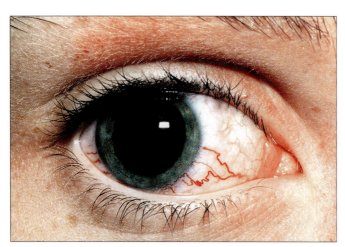

Fig. 27.2 Sturge-Weber syndrome. Dilated conjunctival and subconjunctival capillary vessels reflect increased orbital venous pressure associated with glaucoma.

ataxia. The lesions consist of a postcapillary venular link with vessels of nonuniform caliber with slow flow of red blood cells.[7] Later, telangiectases may develop on exposed areas of skin, especially on the ears and the bridge of the nose.

Other characteristic ocular findings may include movement defects consisting of pursuit abnormalities, hypometric saccades, horizontal ocular motor apraxia, deficient accommodative ability, strabismus, and nystagmus.[6]

Bloom syndrome

Bloom syndrome is a rare autosomal recessive skin disorder characterized by photosensitivity, telangiectasias, growth retardation, immune deficiencies, and malignancies.[8] In some, prominent bulbar conjunctival telangiectasias similar to those seen in ataxia telangiectasia may be seen but in Bloom syndrome there are no neurological defects.

Rendu-Osler-Weber disease (hereditary hemorrhagic telangiectasia)

Palpebral conjunctival telangiectases or retinal vascular malformations occur in about a third of patients with Rendu-Osler-Weber syndrome, a rare autosomal dominant disease characterized by capillary dilatation in multiple organs,[9] which increases after puberty. Vessel walls may be thin and friable, making them more prone to bleed. Frequent bleeds can be treated by cautery although this can result in satellite lesions.

Fabry disease (see Chapter 65)

In Fabry disease, small conjunctival vessels often show aneurysms, tortuosity, and kinking, and corneal verticillata occurs.

Carotid-cavernous sinus fistula

Children who develop a red eye days, or even weeks, after head trauma may have a direct or indirect (dural) carotid-cavernous sinus fistula. Rare in childhood, they may be severe and associated with raised intraocular pressure. Arterialization of the conjunctival and episcleral veins, with a corkscrew appearance, is pathognomonic. Interpalpebral and inferior palpebral conjunctival chemosis is often present, especially with high-flow direct fistulas. Ehlers-Danlos syndrome should be suspected in spontaneous or familial cases.

Sickle cell disease

Although no conjunctival symptoms are produced by sickle cell disease, the conjunctiva is good for observing vascular changes by slit-lamp microscopy. A decrease in vascularity gives the bulbar conjunctiva a "blanched" appearance. Vessel tortuosity, comma-shaped conjunctival capillaries formed by short columns of stationary red cells in small obstructed vessels, and slow flow (boxcarring) may be seen, with all signs exacerbated during crises.[10]

Hyperviscosity

In blood hyperviscosity states, the conjunctiva appears suffused, while the capillaries appear dilated and tortuous with slow flow seen on slit-lamp microscopy. Isolated comma or corkscrew-shaped venular segments may be observed.

Anemia

Pallor of the palpebral conjunctiva has been used as a highly specific but insensitive sign in anemia. Slit-lamp examination of the peribulbar conjunctival blood column enhances the sensitivity. Assessment of blood flow as normal, granular appearing, or discontinuous–with the latter two indicating anemia–may be used.[11]

Infantile lipemia

Pinkish discoloration of conjunctival and iris vessels may be present in infantile lipemia and is suggestive of hyperlipidemia type I or V.[12] Creamy white retinal vessels (lipemia retinalis) accompany these findings.

Conjunctival hemorrhage

Often impressive in appearance, conjunctival hemorrhage frequently occurs after minor trauma or with a rise in central venous pressure such as after a seizure, immediately after birth, or after any Valsalva-type maneuvers such as violent coughing as occurs with pertussis. The hemorrhages usually improve spontaneously within two weeks and do not require treatment.

Spontaneous conjunctival hemorrhages are common in childhood and some mythology is popularly attached to their cause: except in Rendu-Osler-Weber disease, they are not associated with any serious abnormality. Sometimes they occur repeatedly in one area, and slit-lamp examination may reveal an anomalous vessel that occasionally needs cautery to prevent recurrence.

Subconjunctival hemorrhages occur in thrombocytopenia, for instance, in leukemia. Concomitant use of aspirin or other anticoagulant agents often results in more extensive hemorrhages. Various forms of conjunctivitis may be associated with subconjunctival hemorrhage.

Conjunctival lymphangiectasia

Conjunctival lymphangiectasia, manifesting as persistent chemosis, may be associated with generalized lymphedema (Nonne-Milroy-Meige disease). It has been described with Turner syndrome,[13] and dilated subconjunctival lymph vessels may be seen adjacent to plexiform neuromas.

Linear scleroderma (morphea en coup de sabre)

A perilimbal dilated vascular network is often seen in morphea en coup de sabre.[14] Morphea appears as a linear groove in the scalp or forehead skin (hence "saber blow") and may involve the lids, orbit, and eye. Uveitis is not uncommon, and ipsilateral glaucoma may occur,[15] possibly also secondary to the development of fibrovascular episclera resulting in increased outflow resistance.

Diabetes

Readily observable conjunctival microvascular abnormalities are seen in diabetic children undergoing slit-lamp examination: comma signs, boxcarring, microaneurysms, beading, vessel wall thickening, and overall decreased vascularity.[16]

PIGMENTED LESIONS

Oculodermal melanocytosis (nevus of Ota) and ocular melanosis

Pigmentation of the conjunctiva and subconjunctival tissue is termed ocular melanosis; when the ipsilateral skin and mucous membrane are involved, the condition is known as oculodermal melanocytosis or nevus of Ota.

Ocular melanosis (Fig. 27.4) shows as a slate-blue scleral, conjunctival, and subconjunctival pigmentation associated with skin and mucous membrane hyperpigmentation usually on the same side. It is usually noticed in the first year or two of life, sometimes later. Familial occurrence is unusual. It may worsen initially and at puberty when the periorbital skin may darken. There is an increased risk of later development of uveal, though not dermal, malignant melanomas. Melanosis is far more common in black and Asian people but malignant change occurs far less frequently than in Caucasians[17] in whom the incidence of malignant change is still very low and generally occurs in adulthood.[18]

Ten percent of patients with oculodermal melanocytosis have raised intraocular pressure with or without glaucoma[19] so mainly for this reason affected children should be examined periodically.

Nevi

Nevi are the most common childhood epibulbar tumors: they usually appear after the first few years of life,[20] or later when pigmentation may develop. Slit-lamp examination can disclose

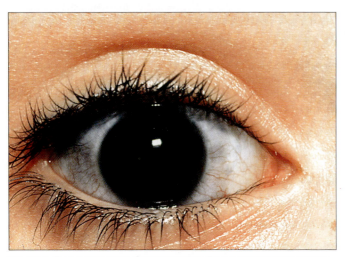

Fig. 27.4 Ocular melanosis. Congenital slate-blue episcleral pigmentation.

cystic epithelial changes not generally seen in skin lesions. Junctional nevi comprise melanocytic nevus cells located only within the epithelial layer of the conjunctiva. Compound nevi have subepithelial and epithelial nevus cells. Sometimes only subepithelial cells are found. They usually occur near the limbus and are well circumscribed, flat or slightly raised (Fig. 27.5a). Compound nevi are sometimes slightly elevated and may be cystic. Many remain lightly or nonpigmented (Fig. 27.5b).

There is scant evidence of progression of nevi into melanomas. Whereas nevi are common, melanomas of the conjunctiva are extremely rare in childhood.[21,22] Melanomas are more raised, vascular, and fleshy than nevi (Fig. 27.5c); however, even histopathologic differentiation can be difficult, with some lesions classified as indeterminate.[23]

Gaucher disease

Thickening of the exposed perilimbal conjunctiva resembling pingueculae and conjunctival pigmentation occur in the chronic forms of Gaucher disease. See Chapter 65.

Alkaptonuria

Often a presenting sign, episcleral and conjunctival pigmentation (ochronosis) occurs in the area of the horizontal rectus muscle insertions. Children with this presentation, whose urine turns black after standing, later develop bone disease with characteristic arthritis and calcific valvular and atherosclerotic heart disease secondary to homozygous mutations in the human homogentisate 1,2-dioxygenase gene. Dietary supplementation with ascorbic acid may be helpful.[24]

Kartagener syndrome

Children with the recessively inherited Kartagener syndrome may have dextrocardia, and they develop bronchiectasis, bronchitis, and respiratory tract infections. Characteristic marked perilimbal conjunctival melanosis and hypertrophy of the plica semilunaris may be present.[25]

Peutz-Jeghers syndrome

Peutz-Jeghers syndrome is a rare autosomal dominantly inherited syndrome with gastrointestinal polyposis, especially of the small bowel. The polyps bleed and may become malignant. Freckles that usually appear in infancy or early childhood and may fade with age are seen around the orifices, on the lids, and less frequently on the conjunctiva.[26]

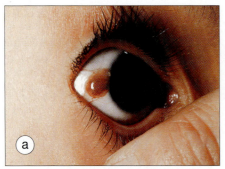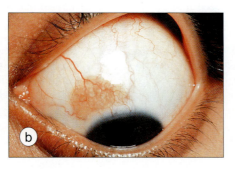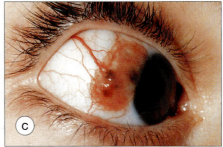

Fig. 27.5 (a) Raised pigmented limbal nevus. (b) Lightly pigmented cystic compound nevus of the conjunctiva in a 14-year-old patient. (c) A raised vascular fleshy nevus that may be a melanoma.

Tumors and infiltrates

The most common epibulbar tumors besides nevi (described above) are dermoids, inclusion cysts, and papillomas.[27]

Epibulbar dermoids

Epibulbar dermoids are choristomas that contain a combination of epithelial-derived tissues: fat, hair follicles, and sebaceous glands. They occur on the cornea or at the limbus, extending posteriorly. Corneal and limbal dermoids are yellowish-white, usually rounded, elevations sometimes with pigmentation and hair (Figs. 27.6a, 27.6b). They sometimes are associated with intraocular abnormalities. The posterior dermoids (dermolipomas) may have more fatty tissue without hairs. They extend far posteriorly, and because they may be closely related to eye muscles, surgeons need to limit their treatment aims to the safely achievable.[28]

Either type of dermoid may be associated with Goldenhar syndrome in which often bilateral epibulbar dermoids occur with a lid coloboma and with preauricular skin tags or appendages; a variety of first branchial arch abnormalities; deafness; and occasionally a neurotrophic or neuroparalytic keratitis.[29]

Occasionally, epibulbar choristomas containing other tissues such as lacrimal tissue, smooth muscle, or cartilage also occur. Such choristomas may be vascularized and have raised, translucent nodules, distinguishing them from the white, avascular appearance of dermoids, and may grow during puberty.[30]

Systemic associations for these choristomas are the linear nevus sebaceous syndrome (Schimmelpenning-Fuerstein-Mims) and encephalocraniocutaneous lipomatosis,[31] in which ipsilateral ocular, cutaneous, and intracranial choristomas and hamartomas occur.

The rarest of epibulbar choristomas, osseous choristomas are composed of mature flat bone surrounded by fibrous connective tissue in the supratemporal or temporal region with underlying attachments to sclera or muscles.[32]

Most dermoids and other choristomas can be simply excised for cosmetic reasons. When the cornea is involved, a lamellar keratectomy is carried out but the results are often only moderately good. The improvement is that the elevated mass is removed, but the remaining cornea is sometimes opalescent or may even become opaque. Freehand corneal lamellar grafting may improve the appearance in refractory cases.

Proteus syndrome

Proteus syndrome, a rare entity with broad phenotypic expression, is characterized by an asymmetric, progressive, warty overgrowth of the sole of the foot, craniofacial anomalies, visceral anomalies, intradermal nevi, variable mental retardation, and variably enlarging epibulbar and lid hamartomas.[33]

Clear cysts

Occasionally, small clear fluid-filled cysts appear in the conjunctiva in older children. They may be post-traumatic, surgical, or idiopathic. They often disappear spontaneously, but if they cause symptoms, they can be needled or simply excised.

Secondary tumors

The conjunctiva may be invaded by rhabdomyosarcoma and retinoblastoma; rarely, they may present as a conjunctival or subconjunctival swelling. Langerhans cell histiocytosis, leukemia, and juvenile xanthogranuloma occasionally involve the conjunctiva. Conjunctival neurofibromas are usually associated with a plexiform neuroma of the orbit in neurofibromatosis type 1 (NF1). They may present with a whitish or clear cystic knotted mass in the subconjunctival tissue. A Burkitt lymphoma has presented with a subconjunctival mass.[34] Isolated benign lymphoid conjunctival hyperplasia may occasionally develop in children.[35]

Xeroderma pigmentosa

Xeroderma pigmentosa is a rare, genetically complex, autosomal recessive disease in which a defect in DNA repair renders tissues sensitive to ultraviolet light. This results in pigmentation, telangiectasis, keratosis, and the development of basal cell and squamous cell carcinomas, malignant melanomas, and other tumors. Conjunctival signs include telangiectasias, xerosis, chronic congestion, pigmentation, pingueculae, and pterygia. This condition may lead to squamous cell carcinomas of the conjunctiva and, less commonly, malignant melanoma developing in childhood (Fig. 27.7).[22,36] It is also associated with progressive neurological abnormalities including deafness, ataxia, mental retardation, and cerebellar atrophy: the De Sanctis-Cacchione syndrome.

In addition to covering the skin with clothing and using sunscreen, persons with xeroderma pigmentosa should protect their eyes by wearing 100% ultraviolet barrier spectacles with side

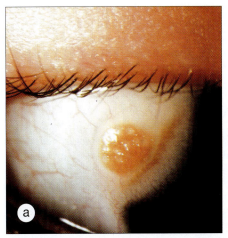
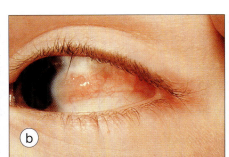
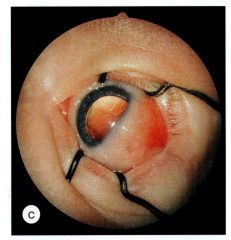

Fig. 27.6 (a) A hairy limbal dermoid. (b) A limbal dermoid encroaching on the cornea and extending back to the temporal fornix. (c) Limbal epibulbar dermoid encroaching on the lateral third of the cornea. Although later removed, leaving minimal scarring, the eye had profound amblyopia due to irregular astigmatism.

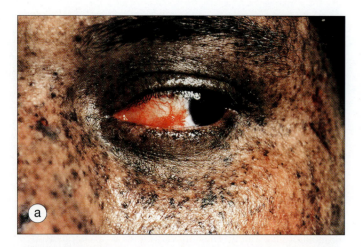

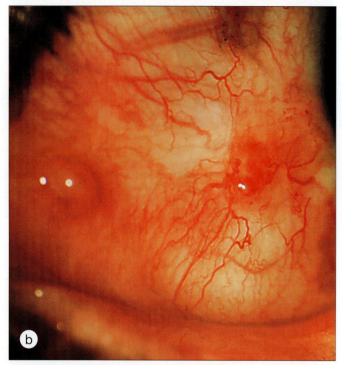

Fig. 27.7 Xeroderma pigmentosa. (a) The widespread skin pigmentation can be seen in this girl of Indian origin. (b) The conjunctiva was affected by multifocal recurrent squamous cell carcinomas.

arms. Frequent slit-lamp examinations for conjunctival and lid tumors are mandatory.

Benign hereditary epithelial dyskeratosis

Benign hereditary epithelial dyskeratosis (Witkop-von Sallman syndrome), a rare dominantly inherited condition, is marked by the presence of elevated white granular-to-gelatinous plaques of hyperkeratotic tissue with hyperemic blood vessels that produce a "bloodshot" appearance that may wax and wane in the horizontal exposed limbal areas of the conjunctiva and in the oral mucosa. Originally described in Haliwa Indians in North Carolina, it has been identified as a new mutation in European families.[37]

Papillomas

Produced by infection with human papillomavirus, conjunctival papillomas are seen in children and adults as elevated, sometimes pedunculated lesions that are usually white or yellowish, but they may be quite heavily pigmented or pink. On slit-lamp examination they consist of translucent "flesh" with small red core vessels. They may be multiple and occur in more than one member of a family. They often disappear spontaneously,[38] but if they are causing considerable trouble, then cryotherapy, surgical excision, or diathermy may be indicated.

Neurofibromas

Neurofibromas are benign, raised, solid, grey-white, or pinkish nodules often near the limbus, but they may occur at any site over the conjunctiva. They are rare and occur in patients with neurofibromatosis type 1 (NF1) or type 2 (NF2).[39] They can be treated by simple excision.

Neuromas

Multiple submucosal nodules, usually on the palpebral conjunctiva and eyelids as well as on the lips and tongue, are frequently seen in patients with multiple endocrine neoplasia type IIb (MEN IIb), and their presence may assist in earlier diagnosis of this autosomal dominant disease, notably in other family members. Although clinically similar to neurofibromas, but often multiple in number, they are histologically distinct.[39,40] Prominent perilimbal conjunctival blood vessels are frequently noted in patients with MEN. Markedly prominent corneal nerves are always present.

Sarcoidosis

The conjunctiva was thought to be frequently involved in sarcoidosis, and "blind" biopsies were carried out for diagnosis. The histology could be confused with meibomian cysts. Conjunctival biopsy is still indicated in suspected sarcoidosis if a discrete elevated lesion is seen. Scattered, white "breadcrumb-like" deposits over the bulbar conjunctiva can be the initial clinical manifestation.[41] Conjunctival sarcoidosis does not usually cause any symptoms and, if isolated, in itself requires no treatment.

Avitaminosis

Xerophthalmia, the term applied to all ocular manifestations of vitamin A deficiency, affects 1 to 5% of preschool children in undernourished populations and is one of the most common causes of blindness in the world today.[42] Night blindness, the earliest symptom, is due to insufficient vitamin A for normal rod photoreceptor function and consequent vision under low light. Often a local term exists to describe the condition, translated as "twilight blindness" or "chicken eyes" (lacking rods, chickens are genetically night blind). Conjunctival xerosis is attributed to a loss of mucus-secreting goblet cells and keratinizing metaplasia on the bulbar conjunctiva. It is most typically diagnosed as a "Bitôt's spot": a dry, lusterless, irregular lesion that may be small to large, triangular or round, bubbly, cheesy, or foamy in appearance, usually bilateral and always lying temporal to the limbus (Figs. 27.8a, 27.8b). Bubbles of carbon dioxide present within lesions are produced by saprophytic bacilli entrapped under desquamated keratinized epithelium. Advanced cases may have nasal lesions and also a wrinkled conjunctiva. Underlying pigmentation, if present, is coincidental. Night blindness and Bitôt's spots are "mild," nonblinding stages of xerophthalmia, but reflect moderate-to-severe vitamin A deficiency, carrying increased risks of infectious morbidity and child death.[42] Potentially blinding corneal xerosis, ulceration, and liquefactive necrosis ("keratomalacia") occur acutely in severely malnourished children, often following a prolonged or severe infectious illness, especially

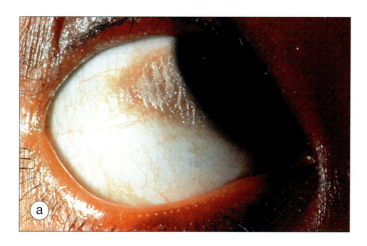
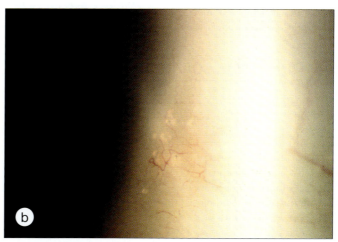

Fig. 27.8 Xerophthalmia. (a, b) Bitot's spots are flaky elevated exposed patches of desquamated pigmented, keratinized conjunctiva, entrapping bubbles of carbon dioxide formed by saprophytic bacilli. As in this case, they are often pigmented. Note lack of any inflammation. Image (a) is courtesy of Dr Keith P West, Jr. from Nutritional blindness xerophthalmia and keratomalacia by Alfred Sommer, copyright. Used by permission of Oxford University Press, Inc. Image (b) is courtesy of Michael X Repka, MD. The patient in image (b) was diagnosed with a fat-malabsorption syndrome.

measles. Case fatality can be 5 to 25% among treated, hospitalized children with corneal xerophthalmia. All children with xerophthalmia should be treated with 200,000 international units of vitamin A orally on days 1 and 2, and 1–4 weeks later. Responses to therapy usually occur within 48 hours for night blindness, a week for corneal xerophthalmia, and 2 weeks for Bitôt's spots. In older children, Bitôt's spots may sometimes persist despite adequate therapy secondary to metaplasia in situ. Prevention should consider substantial seasonality in the risk of xerophthalmia and other nutritional deficiency and disease patterns. Milder cases in otherwise well-nourished individuals should lead one to suspect a fat-malabsorption syndrome.

Xanthogranulomas

Conjunctival involvement is rare and may present as unilateral fleshy raised nodules, usually at the limbus, sometimes with a yellowish-orange color. When limbal, xanthogranulomas tend to be isolated and localized, without systemic findings. Simple excision is generally effective, but recurrences often occur if the xanthogranuloma is not fully removed. Superficial keratectomy with lamellar graft allows complete excision.[43]

Pingueculum and pterygium

Pingueculae and pterygia are rare in children, but can occur occasionally in those exposed to high levels of sunlight; they are initiated by the process of limbal burns caused by unshielded sunlight, most often from the temporal side and focused through the cornea onto the nasal limbal margin. Conversely, pseudopterygia are fairly common in children after an inflammatory corneal disease or the excision of a corneal lesion, for instance, an epibulbar dermoid. If cosmetically unsightly, they may be excised with a wide conjunctival margin and a superficial keratectomy, but occasionally a mucous membrane graft may be required.

CONJUNCTIVAL THINNING

Conjunctival thinning occurs in Degos disease, the scalded baby syndrome, epidermolysis bullosa,[44] and ectodermal dysplasia. Perilimbal conjunctival hypoplasia from absence of the palisades of Vogt occurs in aniridia.

Degos disease (malignant atrophic papulosis) is a rare, multiple-organ-system vasculitis characterized by a papular eruption, on the trunk and extremities, with atrophic white-centered lesions surrounded by a telangiectatic border. A variety of ocular manifestations may occur, such as branch or central retinal arterial occlusions together with atrophic telangiectatic conjunctival lesions due to the underlying arteritis.

In ectodermal dysplasia, conjunctival and corneal thinning may lead to spontaneous perforation. This condition may be inherited in autosomal dominant, autosomal recessive, or X-linked forms with variable expression. Eye findings include absent palisades of Vogt with corneal pannus, limbal hair follicles with hair, and Bitôt-like spots in the conjunctiva.[45]

In dystrophic epidermolysis bullosa, common eye changes include symblepharon, broadening of the limbus, corneal opacities, and recurrent erosions.[46]

CONJUNCTIVAL THICKENING

Conjunctival thickening occurs in conjunctival scarring, pemphigus, and tyrosinemia type II. In tyrosinemia type II, also known as the Richner-Hanhart syndrome, there are hyperkeratotic lesions of the palm, soles, and elbows and occasionally mental retardation occurs. The syndrome, transmitted as an autosomal recessive trait, is associated with an increase in serum and urine tyrosine. Children with this condition are photophobic and have watering eyes with thickened conjunctiva and hypertrophy of the tarsal conjunctiva. Epithelial and subepithelial opacities of the cornea and corneal ulceration appear dendritic at times and are often bilateral. The lesions on the cornea tend to heal spontaneously, but may take some time. Corneal lesions may be treated with corticosteroids and, with an appropriate diet, rapidly improve.[47]

EPITARSUS

Epitarsus refers to an apron-like fold of conjunctiva forming a bridge of tissue, usually in the upper lid, under which a probe may be passed. Although usually the end result of inadequately treated cicatrizing conjunctivitis in infants and children, it may, on rare occasions, appear as a congenital anomaly.[48,49]

CONJUNCTIVAL SCARRING

Conjunctival scarring occurs in a wide variety of conditions (see Bernauer et al.[50] for an excellent review), some of which affect children:

1. Burns:
   (a) Thermal;
   (b) Chemical; and
   (c) Ionizing radiation.
2. Traumatic, including strabismus surgery and surgery to remove dermoids, etc.
3. Infection:
   (a) Trachoma; and
   (b) Severe and prolonged bacterial and viral infections and membranous conjunctivitis.

4. Avitaminosis.
5. Inflammatory disease:
   (a) Stevens-Johnson syndrome and erythema multiforme;
   (b) Tyrosinemia type II (Richner-Hanhart syndrome);
   (c) Chronic vernal conjunctivitis;
   (d) Toxic epidermal necrolysis;
   (e) Epidermolysis bullosa acquisita; and
   (f) Linear IgA disease.
6. Dry eye.
7. Ectodermal dysplasia.
8. Congenital dyskeratosis.[51]
9. Epidermolysis bullosa.[44,46]
10. Drugs:
    (a) Systemic; and
    (b) Topical (lower fornix).

REFERENCES

1. Roth A, Mühlendyck H, De Gottrau P. La fonction de la capsule de Tenon revisitée. J Fr Opthalmol 2002; 25: 968–76.
2. Dua HS, Azuara-Blanco A. Limbal stem cells of the corneal epithelium. Surv Ophthalmol 2000; 44: 415–25.
3. Isenberg SJ, McCarty JW, Rich R. Growth of the conjunctival fornix and orbital margin in term and premature infants. Ophthalmology 1987; 94: 1276–80.
4. Fishman PH, Repka MX, Green WR, et al. A primate model of anterior segment ischemia after strabismus surgery. The role of the conjunctival circulation. Ophthalmology 1990; 97: 456–61.
5. Fledelius HC, Illum N, Jensen H, et al. Interferon-alfa treatment of facial infantile haemangiomas with emphasis on the sight-threatening varieties: a clinical series. Acta Ophthalmol Scand 2001; 79: 370–3.
6. Farr AK, Shalev B, Crawford TO, et al. Ocular manifestations of ataxia-telangiectasia. Am J Ophthalmol 2002; 134: 891–6.
7. Kulikov VV. Changes in the microvascular bed of the eye conjunctiva in ataxia-telangiectasis (Louis-Bar syndrome). Arkh Patol (Moscow) 1974; 36: 30–8.
8. Sahn EE, Hussey RH, Christmann LM. A case of Bloom syndrome with conjunctival telangiectasia. Pediatr Dermatol 1997; 14: 120–4.
9. Brant AM, Schachat AP, White RI. Ocular manifestations in hereditary hemorrhagic telangiectasia (Rendu-Osler-Weber disease). Am J Ophthalmol 1989; 107: 642–6.
10. Cheung AT, Chen PC, Larkin EC, et al. Microvascular abnormalities in sickle cell disease: a computer-assisted intravital microscopy study. Blood 2002; 99: 3999–4005.
11. Kent AR, Elsing SH, Hebert RL. Conjunctival vasculature in the assessment of anemia. Ophthalmology 2000; 107: 274–7.
12. Uwaydat S, Mansour AM. Infantile lipemia retinalis and conjunctivalis. J Pediatr Ophthalmol Strabismus 2000; 37: 47–9.
13. Perry HD, Cossari AJ. Chronic lymphangiectasis in Turner's syndrome. Br J Ophthalmol 1986; 70: 396–9.
14. Taylor P, Talbot EM. Perilimbal vascular anomaly associated with ipsilateral en coup de sabre morphoea. Br J Ophthalmol 1985; 69: 60–2.
15. Perrot H, Durand L, Thivolet J, et al. Sclérodermie en coup de sabre et glaucome chronique homo-latéral. Ann Dermatol Vénéréol 1977; 104: 381–6.
16. Cheung AT, Price AR, Duong PL, et al. Microvascular abnormalities in pediatric diabetic patients. Microvasc Res 2002; 63: 252–8.
17. Dutton JJ, Anderson RL, Schelper RL, et al. Orbital malignant melanoma and oculodermal melanocytosis: report of two cases and review of the literature. Ophthalmology 1984; 91: 497–507.
18. Roldan M, Llanes F, Negrete O, et al. Malignant melanoma of the choroid associated with melanosis oculi in a child. Am J Ophthalmol 1987; 104: 662–3.
19. Teekhasaenee C, Ritch R, Rutnin U, et al. Ocular findings in oculodermal melanocytosis. Arch Ophthalmol 1990; 108: 1114–20.

20. Jay B. Naevi and melanomata of the conjunctiva. Br J Ophthalmol 1965; 49: 169–204.
21. McDonnell JM, Carpenter JD, Jacobs P, et al. Conjunctival melanocytic lesions in children. Ophthalmology 1989; 96: 986–93.
22. Mehta C, Gupta CN, Krishnaswamy M. Malignant melanoma of conjunctiva with xeroderma pigmentosa – a case report. Indian J Ophthalmol 1996; 44: 165–6.
23. Grossniklaus HE, Margo CE, Solomon AR. Indeterminate melanocytic proliferations of the conjunctiva. Arch Ophthalmol 1999; 117: 1131–6.
24. Mayatepek E, Kallas K, Anninos A, et al. Effects of ascorbic acid and low-protein diet in alkaptonuria. Eur J Pediatr 1998; 157: 867–8.
25. Collier M. Constatations ophtalmologiques dans le syndrome de Kartagener. Bull Mem Soc Franc Ophtalmol 1961; 74: 429–47.
26. Traboulsi EI, Maumenee IH. Periocular pigmentation in the Peutz-Jeghers syndrome. Am J Ophthalmol 1986; 102: 126–7.
27. Cunha RP, Cunha MC, Shields JA. Epibulbar tumours in children: a survey of 282 biopsies. J Pediatr Ophthalmol Strabismus 1987; 24: 249–54.
28. Fry CL, Leone CR. Safe management of dermolipomas. Arch Ophthalmol 1994; 112: 1114–6.
29. Mohandessan MM, Romano PE. Neuroparalytic keratitis in Goldenhar's syndrome. Am J Ophthalmol 1978; 85: 111–3.
30. Pokorny KS, Hyman BM, Jakobiec FA, et al. Epibulbar choristomas containing lacrimal tissue: clinical distinction from dermoids and histologic evidence of an origin from the palpebral lobe. Ophthalmology 1987; 94: 1249–58.
31. Kodsi SR, Bloom KE, Egbert JE, et al. Ocular and systemic manifestations of encephalocraniocutaneous lipomatosis. Am J Ophthalmol 1994; 118: 77–82.
32. Gayre GS, Proia AD, Duton JJ. Epibulbar osseous choristoma: case report and review of the literature. Ophthalmic Surg Lasers 2002; 33: 410–5.
33. Burke JP, Bowell R, O'Doherty N. Proteus syndrome: ocular complications. J Pediatr Ophthalmol Strabismus 1988; 25: 99–102.
34. Weisenthal RW, Streeten BW, Dubansky AS, et al. Burkitt lymphoma presenting as a conjunctival mass. Ophthalmology 1995; 102: 129–34.
35. McLeod SD, Edward DP. Benign lymphoid hyperplasia of the conjunctiva in children. Arch Ophthalmol 1999; 17: 832–5.
36. Goyal J, Rao V, Srinivasan R, et al. Oculocutaneous manifestations in xeroderma pigmentosa. Br J Ophthalmol 1994; 78: 295–7.
37. Dithmar S, Stulting RD, Grossniklaus HE. Hereditäre benigne intraepitheliale Dyskeratose. Ophthalmologe 1998; 95: 684–6.
38. Wilson FM, Ostler HB. Conjunctival papillomas in siblings. Am J Ophthalmol 1974; 77: 103–7.
39. Kalina PH, Bartley GB, Campbell RJ, et al. Isolated neurofibromas of the conjunctiva. Am J Ophthalmol 1991; 111: 694–8.
40. Jacobs JM, Hawes MJ. From eyelids bumps to thyroid lumps: report of a MEN type IIb family and review of the literature. Ophthal Plas Reconstru Surg 2001; 17: 195–201.

41. Dithmar S, Waring GO, Goldblum TA, et al. Conjunctival deposits as an initial manifestation of sarcoidosis. Am J Ophthalmol 1999; 128: 361–2.

42. Sommer A, West KP Jr. Vitamin A Deficiency: Health Survival and Vision. New York: Oxford University Press; 1996.

43. Spraul CW, Lang GE, Lang GK. Juveniles Xanthogranulom am korneoskleralen Limbus: Bericht über einen Patienten sowie Literaturübersicht. Klin Monatsbl Augenheilkd 1995; 206: 467–73.

44. Iwamoto M, Haik BG, Iwamoto T, et al. The ultrastructural defect in conjunctiva from a case of recessive dystrophic epidermolysis bullosa. Arch Ophthalmol 1991; 109: 1382–6.

45. Tijmes NT, Zaal MJ, De Jong PT, et al. Two families with dyshidrotic ectodermal dysplasias associated with ingrowth of corneal vessels, limbal hair growth, and Bitôt-like conjunctival anomalies. Ophthalmic Genet 1997; 18: 185–92.

46. McDonnell PJ, Schofield OM, Spalton DJ, et al. The eye in dystrophic epidermolysis bullosa. Eye 1989; 3: 79–84.

47. Michalski A, Leonard JV, Taylor DS. The eye in inherited metabolic disease: a review. J Roy Soc Med 1988; 81: 286–90.

48. Varma BM, Garg BK. Congenital epitarsus. J All India Ophthalmol Soc 1969; 17: 163–5.

49. Khurana AK, Ahluwalia BK, Mehtani VG. Primary epitarsus: a case report. Br J Ophthalmol 1986; 70: 931–2.

50. Bernauer W, Broadway DC, Wright P. Chronic progressive conjunctival cicatrisation. Eye 1993; 7: 371–8.

51. Merchant A, Zhao TZ, Foster CS. Chronic keratoconjunctivitis associated with conjunctival dyskeratosis and erythrokeratodermia variables. Ophthalmology 1998; 105: 1286–91.

CHAPTER
28

Anterior Segment: Developmental Anomalies

Ken K Nischal and Jane Sowden

The anterior segment of the eye is an intricate arrangement of interacting tissues essential for vision. The cornea, iris, and the anterior epithelium of the lens form the boundaries of the anterior chamber. Schwalbe's line, the trabecular meshwork, and the scleral spur lie in the anterior chamber angle at the junction of the peripheral cornea and the root of the iris. Aqueous produced by the ciliary body flows into the anterior chamber through the pupil and leaves the eye through the trabecular meshwork into Schlemm's canal and the venous circulation.

A large number of clinical conditions feature abnormal development of the anterior segment. Structural changes that cause impedance of the aqueous flow at the angle may increase intraocular pressure and glaucoma, and together with developmental abnormalities may affect corneal transparency. Recent progress in the identification of gene mutations causing these conditions, combined with increased understanding of gene function through the study of protein function and of animal models, has shed new light on the normal development of the mammalian anterior segment and on disease etiology. By understanding the relationship between anterior segment developmental abnormalities (ASDAs) and the rare developmental glaucomas, one may have insight into all glaucomas.

EMBRYOLOGY OF THE ANTERIOR SEGMENT

Neural crest cells are critical for the development of the anterior segment. They originate at the edge of the neural fold. During neurulation, as the neural tube closes, the neural crest cells undergo an epithelial to mesenchymal transition and migrate away ventrally on either side of the neural tube. The different migratory pathways of the neural crest cells give rise to a wide variety of cell types including a contribution to the developing eye.

By five weeks of development in the human embryo, the lens vesicle has separated from the surface ectoderm, and mesenchyme cells of neural crest origin are migrating anteriorly around the optic cup and between the surface ectoderm and the developing lens (Fig. 28.1a). During the seventh week, the loose mesenchymal layer differentiates into two layers; the corneal stroma (keratocytes) bounded by endothelium and the anterior iris stroma. This process of cell differentiation occurs simultaneously with a separation of the two cellular layers to form the anterior chamber between the developing cornea and the iris (Fig. 28.1b). Descemet's membrane (the basement membrane of the corneal endothelium) is secreted by the corneal endothelial cells, which thin to a monolayer by the 18th week.

The trabecular meshwork and Schlemm's canal, located anterior to the trabeculae, develop from the mesenchyme at the periphery of the developing cornea adjacent to the sclera.

Schwalbe's ring, or line, is the anterior limit of the developing drainage structures and marks the posterior limit of Descemet's membrane. A sheet of mesenchyme bridging the future pupil persists until the seventh month of gestation and extends from the iris across the developing trabecular meshwork to the cornea. As the tissues at the iridocorneal angle differentiate, the angle separating the cornea and the iris extends posteriorly and become a deeper angle recess so Schlemm's canal and the trabecular meshwork gradually become exposed to the anterior chamber. The outflow of aqueous through the trabecular meshwork reaches postnatal levels by the 32nd week of gestation.[1] Maturation of the angle continues in the first year of life to give the open angle and relatively flat iris structure characteristic of the normal adult eye (Fig. 28.2).

In addition to the large contribution from neural crest-derived mesenchymal cells (Table 28.1) to tissues of the anterior segment, the neurectoderm of the optic cup and the surface ectoderm also give rise to anterior segment components. The peripheral edge of the optic cup forms the posterior iris epithelium and the ciliary body epithelium. The surface ectoderm gives rise to the corneal epithelium after the separation of the lens vesicle.

CONTROL OF DEVELOPMENT: RESPONSIBLE GENES

Gene mutations causing anterior segment dysgenesis

Molecular genetic analysis of families exhibiting Mendelian inheritance of ASDAs has led to the identification of several disease genes (Table 28.2). Animal models have illuminated the essential role of these genes in the normal molecular and cellular processes underlying the development of the anterior segment. Such work has led to better understanding of how disruption of normal developmental processes leads to the condition of anterior segment dysgenesis seen in the clinic.

The identification of genes essential for anterior segment development has made it possible to classify anterior segment dysgeneses according to their underlying gene mutation. Molecular genetic analysis has provided a simplification of the clinical classifications of conditions.

Transcription factors and anterior segment development

The genes proven to play critical roles in anterior segment dysgenesis all encode transcription factors (Table 28.2), which act by regulating the transcription of other genes, which are their downstream target genes. Hence, transcription factors coordinate programs of growth and differentiation by either enhancing or

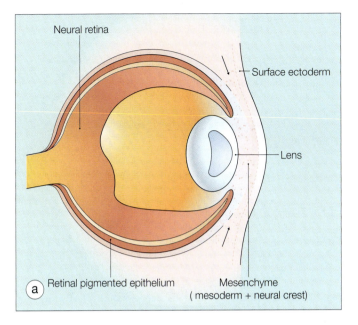

a Neural retina
Surface ectoderm
Lens
Retinal pigmented epithelium
Mesenchyme
(mesoderm + neural crest)

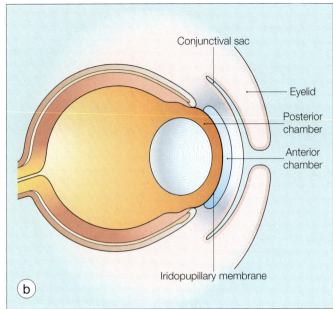

b Conjunctival sac
Eyelid
Posterior chamber
Anterior chamber
Iridopupillary membrane

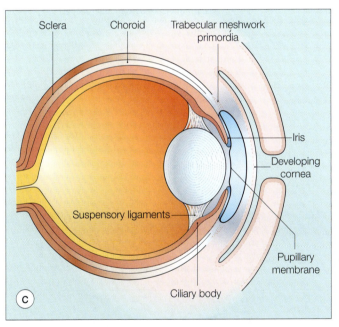

c Sclera
Choroid
Trabecular meshwork primordia
Iris
Developing cornea
Pupillary membrane
Suspensory ligaments
Ciliary body

Fig. 28.1 Early development of the anterior segment.
(a) By five weeks of development in the human embryo, the lens vesicle has separated from the surface ectoderm and neural crest cells are migrating around the optic cup and between the surface ectoderm and the developing lens. (b) During the seventh week, the mesenchymal layer gives rise to the corneal stroma, bounded by an endothelium, and the anterior iris stroma. This process of differentiation occurs simultaneously with a separation of the two layers to form the anterior chamber between the developing cornea and the iris. (c) A sheet of mesenchyme bridging the future pupil remains until the seventh month of gestation. The edges of the optic cup form the posterior iris epithelium and the ciliary body epithelium.[1a,1b]

Table 28.1 Origin of tissue of the anterior segment and sites of expression of important genes[5,7,9]

Embryonic tissue contributing to the anterior segment	Gene expression in early embryonic tissue	Anterior segment tissues (other ocular tissues)	Gene expression in developing angle tissues
Neural crest-derived periocular mesenchymal tissue	Pitx2 Foxc1 Lmx1b	Corneal endothelium Corneal stroma Anterior iris stroma Angle structures: Trabecular meshwork Ciliary muscle (Extraocular muscles) (Sclera) (choroid)	Foxc1, Pitx2 Foxc1, Pitx2 Foxc1, Pax6 (Pitx2) (Foxc1)
Neurectoderm of the optic cup	Pax6	Pigmented iris epithelium Ciliary epithelium (retina)	Pax6 Pax6 (Pax6)
Surface ectoderm	Pax6	Lens Corneal epithelium	Pax6, Foxe3, Maf Pax6, Pitx2

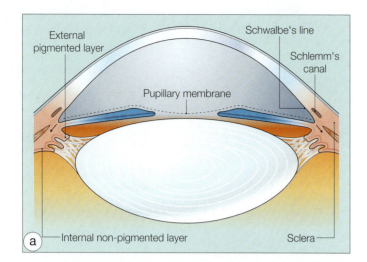

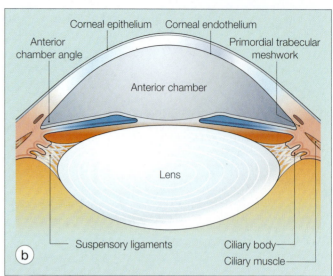

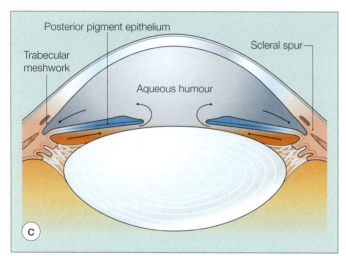

Fig. 28.2 Maturation of the angle of the anterior segment. (a) By five months the iris insertion is anterior to the trabecular meshwork primordia. (b) Realignment of the iris insertion gradually uncovers the developing trabecular meshwork. (c) At birth the iris insertion has reached the level of the scleral spur uncovering the angle.[30,36,41]

Table 28.2 Genes essential for the normal development of the anterior segment and whose mutation causes ASDAs

Human gene	Type	Chromosome location	Human disease	OMIM number
CYP1B1	Enzyme	2p22	Congenital glaucoma	601771
EYA1	Transcription factor	8q13	Branchiootorenal dysplasia ASDA	601653
FOXC1	Transcription factor	6p25	ASDA (iridogoniodysgenesis anomaly, iris hypoplasia, Axenfeld Rieger anomaly, Axenfeld-Rieger syndrome) Congenital glaucoma	601090
FOXE3	Transcription factor	1p23	ASDA and cataracts Peters anomaly	601094
LMX1B	Transcription factor	9q34	Nail-patella syndrome	602575
MAF	Transcription factor	16q23	ASDA and cataracts	177075
PAX6	Transcription factor	11p13	Aniridia Peters anomaly Cataracts ASDA Keratitis Optic nerve hypoplasia and glaucoma Foveal hypoplasia	106210
PITX2	Transcription factor	4q25	ASDA (Axenfeld-Rieger syndrome, iris hypoplasia, iridogoniodysgenesis) Glaucoma	601542
PITX3	Transcription factor	10q25	ASDA and cataracts	602669

repressing the expression of their target genes. Each transcription factor has a different type of DNA-binding domain for the purpose of interacting with the regulatory DNA sequence of its target genes. These DNA-binding domains are highly conserved throughout the animal kingdom, and this is partly why animal models have proved to be so useful for understanding the function of human genes. *PAX6* and *PITX2* encode proteins containing a paired-type and bicoid-type homeodomain, respectively, whereas *FOXC1* encodes a forkhead domain containing protein. These genes are closely related to genes called paired, bicoid, and forkhead, first shown to be essential for development and patterning the body of *Drosophila melanogaster*, an invaluable model system for the discovery of many genes important for human development and disease.

Gene expression in the developing anterior segment: sites of gene action

The sites of gene expression during development of the anterior segment pinpoint their site of action (Fig. 28.1 and Table 28.1). Knowledge of sites of gene expression derives mainly from study of the mouse as a model for mammalian development combined with limited expression data from human studies and other animal model or experimental systems. This information helps understand the origin of the abnormalities observed in patients with gene mutations.

The patterns of expression of genes whose mutation causes ASDAs can be considered as three types:
1. Those expressed within migrating periocular neural crest cells (*Foxc1*, *Pitx2*, *Lmx1b*);
2. Those expressed only within the developing lens (*Foxe3*, *Maf*); and
3. Those with a more panocular expression including the lens, of which *Pax6* is the only example.

Pax6 is expressed from the earliest stages of eye development. During early embryogenesis its expression pattern within the developing telencephalon defines the regions that evaginate to form the optic vesicle. It is expressed within the inner (future neural retina) and outer layer (future retinal pigmented epithelium) of the optic cup and within the lens vesicle during formation of the anterior segment. Expression within the early eye field and the lack of eye (and forebrain) development in the absence of *Pax6*, combined with the ability of *Pax6* to direct development of ectopic (inappropriately positioned) eyes in fruit flies, has earned *Pax6* the title of an eye master control gene. *Pax6* expression continues throughout eye development in cells deriving from the neurectoderm of the optic cup and from the anterior surface ectoderm. *Pax6* is expressed in the developing lens, inner and pigmented layers of the iris and ciliary body, the corneal epithelium, and the developing retina. Significantly it is also expressed later in the mesenchymally derived developing trabecular meshwork.

In contrast to the widespread expression of *Pax6*, *Foxc1* and *Pitx2* have a more restricted expression within the developing eye. Both genes are expressed within the mesenchyme around the developing optic cup (the periocular mesenchyme) including the prospective cornea. Their expression is downregulated as the mesenchyme differentiates with expression persisting, in structures of the developing angle. *Foxc1* and *Pitx2* are both expressed in the forming iris, but not within the neurectoderm of the optic cup or in the lens vesicle.

Understanding gene function through study of animal models

Each human gene whose mutation causes ASDA has a highly related and equivalent gene (a homologous gene) in the mouse genome. Mice lacking functional copies of these genes show anterior segment abnormalities similar to clinical conditions. Their analysis provides better understanding of the underlying normal and abnormal developmental processes highly conserved between humans and mice. The phenotype of mice heterozygous for a mutation and carrying only one functional gene copy provide models of dominantly inherited clinical conditions. Information from homozygous mouse mutations, although rare in patients, is useful for defining the essential role of key genes. Differences in the genetic regulation of human and mouse eye development exist but the mouse is the best available model and is proving particularly valuable for understanding ASDAs and glaucoma.

Foxc1 and *Pitx2* are essential for corneal development

Developmental arrest and abnormal retention and contraction of the embryonic endothelial layer on portions of the iris and anterior chamber angle has been proposed as the cause of the iris changes, tissue strands, and the abnormalities of Schwalbe's line found in ASDAs.[30] Study of the phenotypes of mouse models carrying specific gene mutations has refined our understanding of the disruption to normal tissue differentiation that underlies these conditions.

Heterozygous mutation of the *Foxc1* gene in mice causes ocular abnormalities with marked variable expressivity, which are very similar to patient conditions and the widely variable ocular defects sometimes seen within families sharing the same mutation.[2,3] The most common anterior segment defect observed is corectopia, mostly bilateral but sometimes unilateral. Iridocorneal adhesion is observed ranging in size from broad sheets to thread-like strands, and some animals show prominent Schwalbe's line (posterior embryotoxon).

Several important insights have been gained from study of this disease model. Careful observation has shown that the ocular defects in the heterozygotes are progressive with a gradual worsening of the corectopia and with the peripheral iridocorneal adhesions becoming more evident over time. The iris stroma thins with age, and later, multiple iris holes (polycoria) develop in opposite quadrants of the displaced pupil. In addition, some juvenile mice showed mild corneal opacity progressing to a high incidence of corneal opacification, with neovascularization and cataracts, in older animals.

Studies with mice have also demonstrated that the genetic background influences the penetrance of ocular defects in heterozygotes and is likely to cause some of the variation seen between families carrying the same mutations. However, as a high level of variability is often seen in genetically identical mice, the variation must to a large extent stem from developmental events and may reflect stochastic events relating to levels of key molecules at critical moments of development. The asymmetric phenotypes often observed between eyes in the same patient also likely reflect such stochastic events. Identifying the role of the causative gene in normal development is key to understanding how its disruption can cause a wide spectrum of observable phenotypes.

Mice that are homozygous for mutation of *Foxc1* (called the congenital hydrocephalus, ch, or Mf1 gene-targeted mouse) show a more severe dysgenesis of the anterior segment.[4,5] The primary defect is failure of development of the neural crest-derived corneal tissue. Histological analysis shows that the cornea fails to separate from the lens, resulting in the complete absence of an anterior chamber. The outer corneal epithelium is thicker than normal and the stroma is disorganized. There is no differentiation of the inner corneal endothelial layer, and there is a failure to form tight occluding junctions between these posterior endothelial cells necessary for normal physiological barrier function. Descemet's membrane, the basal lamina secreted by the corneal endothelium, is thus absent. Hypoplasia of the iris stromal mesenchyme and the pigmented layer accompanies the corneal abnormalities, and the eye is typically microphthalmic.

The phenotype of these mice gives insight into the role of *Foxc1* in development of the anterior segment. It suggests that *Foxc1* is essential for conversion of mesenchymal neural crest cells to an endothelium phenotype.

The phenotype of the mice homozygous for *Foxc1* mutation is strikingly similar to that of those mice carrying homozygous mutation of another gene implicated in human ASDAs, the *Pitx2* gene. Mice homozygous for mutation of *Pitx2* have displaced, irregular pupils, and this condition is also present in some heterozygotes. In homozygotes, the anterior chamber and the corneal endothelium are absent, and the corneal epithelium is thickened (hypercellular) with undifferentiated mesenchymal cells lying between this epithelium and the optic cup.[6] *Pitx2* appears essential for differentiation of both the mesenchymal and epithelial components of the cornea, tissues derived from the cranial neural crest-derived periocular mesenchyme and the surface ectoderm, respectively. *Pitx2* expression but not *Foxc1* expression has been reported in the corneal ectoderm (derived from the surface ectoderm).[7] It is thought that in human congenital hereditary endothelial dystrophy (CHED) the corneal endothelium degenerates and the stroma become edematous with the collagen fibers losing their highly regular organization. This has interesting similarities to the phenotype resulting from a lack of endothelial formation in the absence of *Foxc1* and *Pitx2*.

Lack of *Pitx2* in mice also causes failure of extraocular muscle development, reduced eye size (microphthalmia), and delay in optic fissure closure (optic nerve coloboma). These conditions have not been observed in patients with *PITX2* mutation, although the optic fissure defects could be related to the prevalence of early onset glaucoma in these patients.

Another important role for the murine models of ASDA is their use for understanding the interactions between key genes. By analyzing how the lack of a single gene affects the activity of other genes, the common genetic pathways underlying these related conditions will be discovered. It is of interest that the expression pattern of *Pitx2* is not affected by the absence of *Foxc1* in mice, suggesting that Pitx2 is regulated independently of *Foxc1* and indeed may lie upstream of *Foxc1*. Certainly both genes appear to play an essential and nonredundant role in the differentiation and delamination of the corneal endothelial layer from the presumptive corneal mesenchyme. The idea that they act in the same genetic pathway responsible for differentiation of the neural crest-derived mesenchyme is consistent with the similarity of the patient conditions caused by their mutation.

Mice that lack *Pitx2* also have abnormalities in multiple organs that are essential sites of *Pitx2* gene activity. These include roles for *Pitx2* in left–right asymmetry involved in cardiac positioning and lung asymmetry and pituitary, craniofacial, and tooth development. Only eye and tooth abnormalities are apparent in heterozygote animals,[8] and these are consistent with the dental abnormalities found in patients with *PITX2* mutation. Knowledge of other organs critically affected by lack of *Pitx2* is useful for understanding other systemic features often identified in patients with anterior segment dysgenesis.

Pax6 and other genes expressed in the developing lens cause ASDAs

It is now well established that mutation or deletion of the *PAX6* gene and/or chromosomal rearrangements involving the *PAX6* gene on 11p13 underlies many cases of aniridia (absence of the iris).[9,96] *PAX6* is also more widely implicated in anterior segment malformations. Mice with heterozygous mutations of the *Pax6* gene help in understanding the role of *Pax6* in anterior segment dysgenesis as their phenotype resembles the patient conditions associated with *PAX6* mutation. Heterozygous *Pax6* (small-eye (Sey)) mice have a reduced eye size (microphthalmia) and a wide spectrum of anterior eye defects including iris hypoplasia, iridocorneal adhesions and corneal opacification, incomplete separation of the lens from the cornea (keratolenticular adhesion), vascularized cornea, and cataracts.[10,11]

Peters anomaly is a genetically heterogeneous condition characterized by keratolenticular adhesion. A proportion of cases of Peters anomaly have *PAX6* mutations, and the phenotype of the Sey heterozygous mice resembles that of Peters anomaly.[12] *FOXC3* mutation has been identified in a patient with Peters anomaly, and mice heterozygous for *Foxe3* mutation also have central corneal opacity and keratolenticular adhesion similar to Peters anomaly.[13]

PAX6 mutation may also cause autosomal dominant keratitis (ADK), which is characterized by corneal opacification and vascularization and by foveal hypoplasia. ADK and aniridia show overlapping clinical findings, and improved understanding of aniridia-related keratopathy and ADK has been gained by study of the corneal abnormalities in *Pax6* (SeyNeu) mice. The corneal epithelium was abnormally thin, and the stroma was irregular and hypercellular during development. In the adult, the thin corneal epithelium was repopulated by goblet cells from the conjunctival epithelium, which may reflect impaired function of limbal stem cells.[14]

The lens plays an essential role in the induction of anterior segment differentiation.[15,16] Analysis of heterozygous *Pax6* eyes indicates that haploinsufficiency of *Pax6* causes primary defects in the lens and that these underlie secondary complex defects of the anterior segment iris and cornea. *Pax6* is highly expressed in anterior lens epithelium and may act indirectly on neural crest-derived mesenchymal cells of the developing anterior segment by regulating the production of lens-derived signaling molecules. Two other genes are implicated in causing ASD by affecting the inductive properties of the lens. *MAF* and *FOXE3* mutation both cause ASD with cataracts. In the mouse the *Maf* and the *Foxe3* genes are both primarily expressed in the developing lens and not within the neural crest-derived mesenchymal cells of the developing anterior segment.

Considering the different roles of the genes implicated in ASDAs suggests a model in which *Pax6* and possibly *Maf* and *Foxe3* are involved in the production of secreted signaling factors from the lens important for organizing the anterior segment development. *Pitx2*, *Foxc1*, and *Lmx1b* are essential for the differentiation of the neural crest-derived mesenchymal tissue, which happens in response to factors secreted by the lens. Without these mesenchymally expressed genes the separation between the cornea and the lens to form the anterior chamber, as well as differentiation of the angle drainage structures, does not take place or is incomplete, depending on the gene dosage.

Insights into the etiology of developmental glaucoma from mouse models of ASDA

The relationships between gene mutations, structural abnormalities of the angle, and the high incidence of glaucoma in ASDAs are not well understood. Histology of the anterior chamber angle from patients has shown failure of the intertrabecular spaces and Schlemm's canal to develop. Analysis of mouse models of the human conditions is now conclusively demonstrating that single-gene mutations cause abnormalities in the trabecular meshwork tissue, which obstruct aqueous flow.

In *Foxc1* homozygous mice, histological analysis of the iridocorneal angle identified abnormalities, including small or absent Schlemm's canal, hypoplastic or absent trabecular meshwork, and hypoplastic ciliary body with short and thin ciliary processes.[2] The development of the chamber angle has also been studied in *Pax6* heterozygotes. Mesenchymal cells at the angle that normally express *Pax6* and differentiate into trabecular meshwork cells next to Schlemm's canal remain undifferentiated, demonstrating that *Pax6* is directly required for differentiation of the angle.[11]

In addition to the ASDAs, which have overt abnormalities in the anterior segment associated with glaucoma, new understanding is being gained of the similarities between primary congenital glaucoma and the common genetic pathways that may underlie these related disease etiologies. Primary congenital glaucoma occurs in about 1 in 10,000 births and has a higher incidence in populations where intermarriage is common. Mutation in the *CYP1B1* gene, which encodes a cytochrome P450 enzyme, is a common cause of primary congenital glaucoma. Mice lacking *Cyp1b1* have developmental abnormalities of the angle similar to those reported in patients. Although much of the angle has normal morphology, focal defects were also present. These defects were small or absent Schlemm's canal, basal lamina (resembling Descemet's membrane) extending from the cornea over the trabecular meshwork, and attachments of the iris to the trabecular meshwork and peripheral cornea (synechiae).

The finding that albino mice showed more severe angle abnormalities than pigmented mice led to the identification of tyrosinase, *Tyr* (the rate-limiting enzyme in the pigment production pathway), as a gene that modifies the severity of abnormalities in mice with *Cyp1b1* mutations or those with *Foxc1* mutation.[17] Indeed, administering the tyrosinase product L-dopa (dihydroxyphenylalanine) to embryos lacking *Cyp1b1* and *Tyr* alleviated the severe dysgenesis. These findings implicate an L-dopa pathway in angle development and may provide an avenue for future therapeutic intervention to reduce developmental glaucoma.

CLINICAL CONDITIONS DUE TO ANTERIOR SEGMENT DEVELOPMENTAL ANOMALIES

ASDAs may be considered in terms of their embryological origin. Therefore they may be:
- of neural crest cell origin;
- of ectodermal origin; or
- of global origin.

Anterior segment developmental anomalies of neural crest cell origin

Posterior embryotoxon

This is a prominent, anteriorly displaced Schwalbe's line, which may be seen in 8–15% of the normal population and may be inherited in an autosomal dominant fashion.[18,19] In isolation, it is not associated with an increased risk of glaucoma. It is often incomplete and appears on slit-lamp examination as a whitish, irregular ridge up to several millimeters from the limbus.

Ocular associations may include iris adhesions with or without iris changes such as hypoplasia, pseudopolycoria, and/or corectopia, in which case it forms part of the spectrum of the Axenfeld-Rieger anomaly (Fig. 28.3).

The main systemic association is in a jaundiced neonate, in which case its presence may be suggestive of Alagille syndrome (arteriohepatic dysplasia).[20–22] This is an autosomal dominant condition characterized by intrahepatic cholestasis, peripheral pulmonary artery stenosis, peculiar facies, and butterfly vertebral arch defects. Posterior embryotoxon is seen in 90% of all cases and 77% of cases also have iris strands.[20,21]

There is no need for treatment of isolated posterior embryotoxon or for regular review.

Iris hypoplasia

Iris stromal hypoplasia may be isolated or associated with angle maldevelopment (goniodysgenesis or goniodysplasia) or with iris

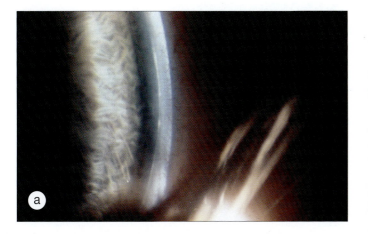
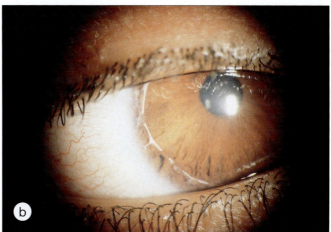

Fig. 28.3 Posterior embryotoxon. (a) Posterior embryotoxon with no associated ocular anomalies is a common but subtle anomaly seen on slit-lamp examination. (b) Marked posterior embryotoxon with iris strands attached (Axenfeld anomaly).

strands attached to a prominent Schwalbe's line (Axenfeld-Rieger anomaly, ARA, Fig. 28.3b). These ocular anomalies may be associated with nonocular features (iridogoniodysgenesis syndrome or Axenfeld-Rieger syndrome, ARS). The overlap between the above conditions is both phenotypic and genotypic. There are two main genetic loci involved: 6p25 and 4q25.[23–28]

Locus 6p25

FOXC1 are the gene, mutations of which have been shown to cause the allelic conditions of ARA,[24] familial glaucoma iridogoniodysplasia (FGI), and iridogoniodysgenesis anomaly (IGDA). Both IGDA and FGI have also been classified as iridogoniodysgenesis I. FGI has been described in one pedigree and entails marked iris hypoplasia, iridocorneal angle anomalies, and frequently, glaucoma.[26]

IGDA is an uncommon condition that consists of iridocorneal angle anomalies, iris stromal hypoplasia, and glaucoma in 50% of cases.

ARA is an uncommon condition with a posterior embryotoxon to which there are attached iris processes with iris hypoplasia, or pseudopolycoria or large defects in the iris (Fig. 28.4). Glaucoma may occur in 50% of cases.[24] Occasionally the pupil corectopia is severe enough to warrant surgical pupilloplasty. The pupil may still progress over years to become even more eccentric in placement despite surgery.

Locus 4q25

PITX2 mutations cause the allelic conditions of iris hypoplasia with glaucoma, iridogoniodysgenesis syndrome (IGDS), and Axenfeld-Rieger syndrome. *In vitro* studies have shown that the arg 53-to-pro mutation results in nonfunctional *PITX2* proteins, which results in the Axenfeld-Rieger syndrome.[27] Other mutations, however, arg 46-to-trp and arg 31-to-his result in reduced *PITX2* proteins activity, resulting in iris hypoplasia and iridogoniodysgenesis, respectively. Both iris hypoplasia with glaucoma and IGDS have been classified as iridogoniodysgenesis II.

Iris hypoplasia with glaucoma is a rare condition whereby there is marked iris stromal hypoplasia giving the eyes a slate gray color, and glaucoma develops by the second decade of life in 60% of all affected individuals.[23]

IGDS is a rare condition in which iris hypoplasia and iridocorneal angle anomalies are associated with nonocular features such as jaw and dental abnormalities.[27]

Axenfeld-Rieger syndrome (ARS) is an uncommon autosomal dominant condition that has ocular and nonocular features. The ocular features consist of posterior embryotoxon with iris strands attached, some of which may be very broad and thick and others thread-like. Historically if these were the only findings the term Axenfeld anomaly was used. If in addition iris defects are present then historically this was termed Rieger anomaly. Axenfeld-Rieger anomaly encompasses both now. Iris findings range from

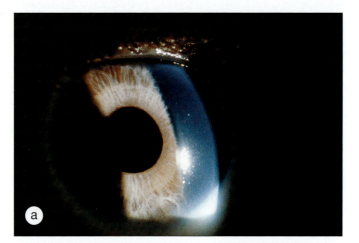
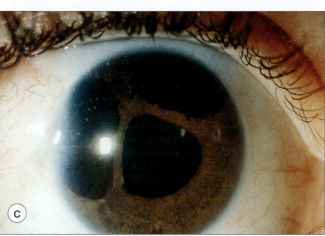
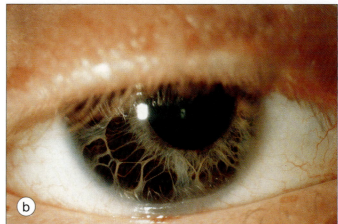
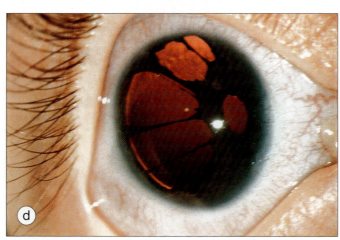

Fig. 28.4 Iris hypoplasia. (a) Iris hypoplasia showing the loss of stroma giving rise to prominence of the sphincter muscle. (b) Marked stromal hypoplasia revealing the posterior pigmented epithelium. (c) Marked stromal hypoplasia giving rise to pseudopolycoria in Axenfeld-Rieger anomaly (ARA). (d) Pseudopolycoria in ARA seen in retroillumination.

stromal hypoplasia, pseudopolycoria, corectopia (pupil displaced toward a thick peripheral iris strand) (Fig. 28.5), and ectropion uveae. The anterior chamber angle is usually open though there may be a high insertion of the iris into the posterior portion of the trabecular meshwork.[24,29,30]

Developmentally, these clinical features can be explained by an arrest in normal development. First, abnormal retention of the primordial endothelium on the iridogonioscopic surface, with subsequent contraction, is thought to explain the iris changes and the tissue strands in the anterior chamber angle, while basement membrane deposition by these cells is felt to result in a posterior embryotoxon. Secondly, a failure/delay in the posterior recession of the iris root during the third trimester results in a high insertion into the posterior aspect of the trabeculum.

Angle and iris changes are usually stable but there may be continued distortion of the pupil in some cases. Glaucoma develops in 50 to 60% of patients with ARS, usually manifesting itself in childhood or young adulthood. Incomplete development of the trabecular meshwork and Schlemm's canal is thought to occur again due to development arrest occurring during the third trimester, causing obstruction to aqueous outflow and hence glaucoma.[24,30]

Other less frequently occurring ocular features include strabismus, cataracts, limbal dermoids, retinal detachment, macular degeneration, chorioretinal colobomas, and choroidal and optic nerve head hypoplasia.

The characteristic nonocular features of ARS are maxillary hypoplasia, mild prognathism, hypodontia (decreased but evenly spaced teeth), anodontia/oligodontia (focal absence of teeth), microdontia (reduction in crown size), cone-shaped teeth (Fig. 28.6), and excess periumbilical skin (Fig. 28.7) with or without hernia. Hypertelorism, telecanthus, and a broad flat nose have also been described. Other systemic features that have been reported include growth hormone deficiency and short stature, heart defects, middle ear deafness, mental deficiency, oculocutaneous albinism, hypospadias, abnormal ears, and in one pedigree, myotonic dystrophy and Peters anomaly.[30,31]

Management depends on the presenting complication of the structural anomalies. Occasionally there is severe pupillary stenosis for which pupilloplasty is required. Care needs to be exercised because lens damage may occur during pupilloplasty. A large pupilloplasty needs to be performed because it tends to contract with time. Severe corectopia without severe stenosis can be adequately treated with occlusion therapy of the less affected eye.

Glaucoma can be difficult to treat in these cases. Medical therapy is used before surgical intervention with the exception of infantile cases where goniotomy/trabeculotomy is first choice of treatment. Miotics should be used with caution, since they may cause trabecular meshwork collapse, with a reduction in aqueous outflow. Beta-blockers and carbonic anhydrase inhibitors may be more effective.

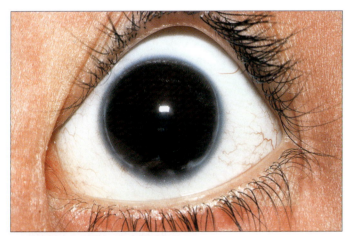

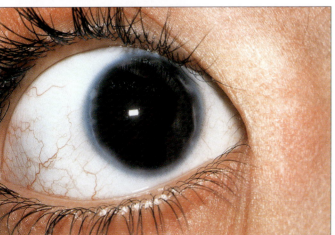

Fig. 28.5 Axenfeld-Rieger anomaly. There is iris hypoplasia, posterior embryotoxon, pseudopolycoria (top picture), and corectopia with the pupil drawn peripherally.

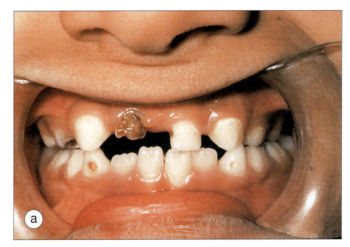

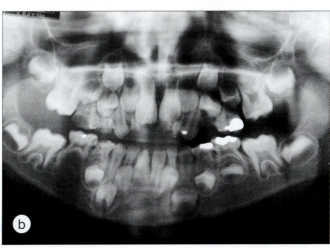

Fig. 28.6 Axenfeld-Rieger syndrome (a) Widely spaced, some conical, teeth; partial anodontia and caries. (b) Dental X-ray of a patient with ARS.

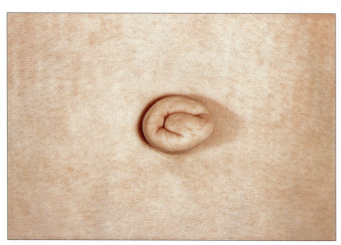

Fig. 28.7 Axenfeld-Rieger syndrome. Excess periumbilical skin in ARS.

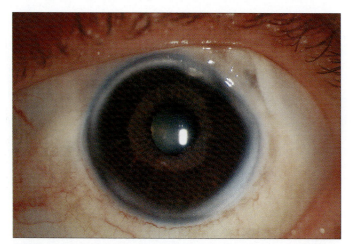

Fig. 28.8 Axenfeld-Rieger syndrome. Trabeculectomy bleb in a child with ARS. There is iris hypoplasia.

Trabeculectomy with antimetabolite augmentation appears to be the procedure of choice for most patients with glaucoma secondary to ARS, especially in older children (Fig. 28.8). The use of cycloablation should be considered in cases where, because of cooperation of the child, a drainage procedure would be unsuitable. Draining procedures other than trabeculectomy include the use of drainage tubes with or without antimetabolite augmentation.[32–35]

Congenital iris ectropion

This is a rare usually unilateral condition in which there is a congenital, nonprogressive ectropion of the posterior pigment iris epithelium onto the anterior surface of the iris. This is due to a nontractional hyperplasia of the posterior pigment epithelium of the iris. The child is often thought to have anisocoria because of the dark nature of the posterior pigment epithelium with the affected eye thought to have mydriasis. The ectropion may be circumferential (Fig. 28.9) or appear as an apron in one segment. Other ocular features include iris stromal hypoplasia, a high iris insertion into trabeculum with trabecular meshwork, and Schlemm canal dysgenesis and secondary glaucoma.

The clinical features are thought to result from an arrest in development with abnormal retention of primordial endothelium, which explains the central iris and angle changes. Although the affected pupil reacts to light and accommodation it may not do so at the same speed as the unaffected eye.[36–38] Glaucoma occurs in the majority of these patients usually between early childhood and puberty.

Systemic associations that should be excluded include neurofibromatosis I and Prader-Willi syndrome.

Management of the glaucoma can be difficult with medical therapy often being unsuccessful. Goniotomy/trabeculotomy is often unsuccessful and augmented trabeculectomy is often the surgical operation of choice.[36–38]

Congenital hereditary endothelial dystrophy

This condition appears to result from abnormal endothelial cell development late in gestation. There are two types of CHED: CHED I is autosomal dominant and CHED II is autosomal recessive[39,40] (see Chapter 30).

Posterior polymorphous dystrophy (PPD)

It is thought that neural crest cells destined to form the corneal endothelium fail to undergo final differentiation late in gestation, causing these cells to retain a degree of pluripotentiality and retain some characteristics of epithelial cells. The iridocorneal peripheral attachments seen in PPD are not the same as those seen in ARS (see Chapter 30).

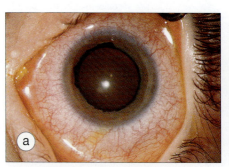
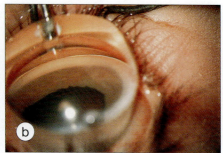
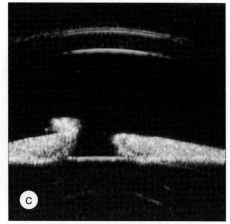

Fig. 28.9 Congenital ectropion uveae. (a) Ectropion uveae, shown as a wide, irregular, dark brown margin to the pupil in a child with glaucoma. (b) Gonioscopic view showing high iris insertion. (c) High-frequency ultrasound image of a child with congenital iris ectropion. Note the frill of posterior pigment epithelium displaced anteriorly.

Primary congenital glaucoma (PCG)

PCG represents an anterior segment developmental anomaly of neural crest cell origin. Histologically, Barkan's membrane (thought to cover the angle and restrict aqueous outflow) has never been found;[6] instead, compactness of the trabecular plates under tension has been demonstrated, which are thought to be released by goniotomy.[41,42] Developmental arrest of the posterior recession of the iris is felt to cause iridotrabecular tissue "hang-up." CYP1B1 is a gene involved with the P450 enzyme system. Mutations in CYP1B1 may result in reduced enzyme activity with a resultant decreased energy production, which results in late developmental arrest. Primordial endothelium is not retained, and the trabecular meshwork and Schlemm's canal are usually fully developed, which would explain the success of goniotomy/trabeculotomy as a treatment modality for this condition. (See Chapter 48.)

ICE syndromes

The iridocorneal endothelial (ICE) syndromes represent a spectrum of disease involving a primary abnormality of the cornea. They include progressive essential iris atrophy, Chandler syndrome, and the iris–nevus syndrome (also known as Cogan-Reese syndrome).[43–45]

These rare syndromes are typically clinically unilateral with females affected more than males and are almost exclusively found in whites. However, specular microscopy almost always reveals mild corneal and iris abnormalities in the "unaffected" eye.[46] The time of onset of these conditions is unknown but they are often diagnosed in early to middle adulthood, although a few cases have been seen in young children.

The ICE syndromes may be the result of a primary neural crest cell abnormality, resulting in a late arrest of final differentiation of the corneal endothelium with retention of these cells of a degree of pluripotentiality. This is thought to have resulted in a capacity of these cells to multiply and/or migrate. Specular microscopy studies[47] have shown two types of population of endothelial cells in early cases of ICE syndromes (one normal, the other dystrophic), which suggests that a subpopulation of corneal endothelial cells are congenitally abnormal and subsequently migrate/proliferate at a slow rate, resulting in a delayed onset of symptoms or diagnosis. These cells may migrate over the angle and onto the iris to cause different signs.

The main features of the ICE syndromes are corneal endothelial abnormalities, peripheral anterior synechiae, unilateral glaucoma, varying degrees of iris atrophy and hole formation, and iris nodules. Peripheral anterior synechiae and glaucoma occur if the abnormal cells migrate over the angle, pulling the peripheral iris up and reducing aqueous outflow, whereas iris holes and thinning occur due to contraction of the membrane formed by the migrating cells. The relative prominence of these features varies widely among the three different subclassifications of ICE syndrome, and is the reason for the original distinction between them.[43–45,48]

Progressive iris atrophy shows a progressive iris atrophy, corectopia, iris ectropion, and pseudopolycoria. Peripheral anterior synechiae often form and gradually become very broad based. The cornea can appear normal in this condition or have an appearance at the endothelial level similar to that of Fuchs dystrophy. Glaucoma is not uncommon in this condition and may develop before extensive iris changes.

Chandler syndrome is usually associated with corneal edema due to corneal endothelial changes, but iris changes if present are much milder than those seen in progressive essential iris atrophy, with glaucoma if present also being more easily controlled medically.[43–45,48]

Iris–nevus syndrome consists of iris changes either of a nodular type or a flattish pigmented type. These lesions may be associated with varying degrees of iris atrophy and/or corneal endothelial changes.

Older patients present with visual disturbance whereas younger ones usually present due to the finding of pupil disturbance, pseudopolycoria, or pigmentary change of the iris.

Management is purely of any glaucoma that may occur in the first instance. Children are unlikely to require corneal grafting but may do so in their adult lives.[49] Glaucoma management should be attempted initially with aqueous production-suppressing topical treatment but filtering surgery may be needed. Usually antimetabolite augmented trabeculectomy is favored, whereas some authors also advocate the use of drainage tubes.

Anterior segment developmental anomalies of ectodermal origin

The two main conditions in this category are limbal and corneal dermoids, which may be associated with Goldenhar syndrome with up to 30% of patients being affected[50–52] (see Chapter 29 and Figs. 29.2–29.6).

If assessed bilaterally with electrophysiology, ultrasound (high frequency and normal ocular) should be performed before considering penetrating keratoplasty.

ANTERIOR SEGMENT DEVELOPMENTAL ANOMALIES OF A GLOBAL ORIGIN

The anomalies in this category include megalocornea, microcornea, aniridia, autosomal dominant keratitis, Peters anomaly, cornea plana, sclerocornea, microphthalmos, and anophthalmos. Of these, microphthalmos and anophthalmos will be discussed in Chapter 24.

Congenital megalocornea

This rare, usually bilateral, condition is thought to be due to defective growth of the optic cup, which results in the cornea growing larger in an attempt to close the gap. It is usually inherited as an X-linked recessive trait in most instances, so that 90% of patients are males. The condition maps to Xq21.3–q22. Female carriers may have slightly enlarged corneal diameters. The remaining cases are autosomal dominant or occasionally autosomal recessive. It is defined as a nonprogressive, enlarged cornea with a horizontal diameter of more than 13 mm, in the absence of congenital glaucoma (Fig. 28.10). Myopia is the most common refractive disorder associated with this condition, often accompanied by with-the-rule astigmatism. Associated ocular features include Krukenberg's spindle, increased pigmentation in the trabecular meshwork, iris stromal hypoplasia with iris trans-illumination, cataracts, ectopia lentis, mosaic corneal dystrophy, and later onset glaucoma. This can be difficult to assess because the cornea is usually thinner than it should be centrally, which can result in artificially lower intraocular pressure measurements using applanation tonometry. Reported systemic associations include Alport syndrome, craniosynostosis, dwarfism, Down syndrome, facial hemiatrophy, Marfan syndrome, Mucolipidosis type II, and megalocornea-mental retardation syndrome.[53–57]

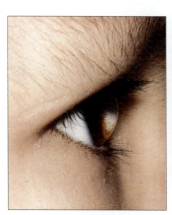
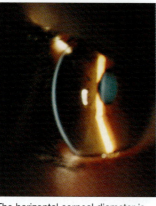

Fig. 28.10 Congenital megalocornea. The horizontal corneal diameter is 13.5 mm, and the anterior chamber is deep as seen in the right-hand picture. On the left it is possible to see into the iridocorneal angle without a gonioscope.

Management consists of careful observation for complications such as cataract formation, dislocated lens and glaucoma. The iris transillumination can result in difficulty in bright light (usually outdoors), and some patients benefit from tints in their spectacles. Lagophthalmos can be a problem due to improper closure of the eyelids at night, and a lubricating eye ointment may be used nightly to prevent exposure problems. Contact lenses can be considered for children with high astigmatism.

Microcornea

This is an uncommon condition defined as any cornea less than 10 mm in horizontal diameter. It may be the result of overgrowth of the tips of the optic cup and may be inherited in an autosomal dominant or recessive manner. If it is an isolated finding with the rest of the eye normal, it is called microcornea, whereas if the anterior segment and the rest of the eye is small, the term is microphthalmos.

Microcornea may be unilateral or bilateral and is usually associated with hypermetropia. Associated ocular findings may include iris colobomas, corectopia, cataracts, microphakia, persistent hyperplastic primary vitreous, retinopathy of prematurity, angle closure glaucoma, infantile glaucoma, and chronic open-angle glaucoma (occurring in up to 20% of patients later in life) (Fig. 28.11).

Systemic associations include Ehlers-Danlos syndrome, Marfan syndrome, Rieger syndrome, Norrie syndrome, Trisomy 21, rubella, Turner syndrome, Waardenburg syndrome, Weil-Marchesani syndrome, Warburg microsyndrome, cataract-microcornea syndrome, and acrorenoocular syndrome and microsyndrome.[58–61]

Visual acuity may be normal if it is an isolated finding and if any refractive error is corrected early to avoid amblyopia.

Cornea plana

Cornea plana may be due to an arrest in development at the 4-month embryo stage, which results in a bilateral or unilateral flattening of the corneal curvature with a curvature of less than 43 D (Fig. 28.12). The cornea may be clear or associated with sclerocornea (see later). If there is a large amount of sclerocornea, visual acuity may be reduced. There is usually hypermetropia and microcornea may also be seen. The recessive and dominant forms share clinical signs such as reduced corneal curvature, indistinct limbus, and arcus lipoides at an early age. The two forms are distinguished by a central, round, and opaque thickening, approximately 5 mm in width, only seen in recessive cases.[62]

Autosomal recessive cornea plana (CNA2) may be caused by mutations in the *KERA* gene (12q22), which encodes for keratocan. Keratocan, lumican, and mimecan are keratan sulfate proteoglycans (KSPGs), which are important to the transparency of the cornea.[63]

Associated ocular findings include sclerocornea, infantile glaucoma, angle closure glaucoma and chronic open-angle glaucoma, retinal aplasia, anterior synechiae, aniridia, congenital cataracts, ectopia lentis, choroidal and iris coloboma (Fig. 28.13), blue sclera, pseudoptosis, and microphthalmos. Systemic associations include osteogenesis imperfecta and epidermolysis bullosa.[64]

Management consists of cycloplegic refraction and correction of any refractive error and surveillance for glaucoma. In those cases where there is associated bilateral sclerocornea there may be an indication to consider at least unilateral penetrating keratoplasty.

Sclerocornea

In this uncommon, noninflammatory, nonprogressive condition there is extension of opaque scleral tissue and fine vascular conjunctival and episcleral tissue into the peripheral cornea,

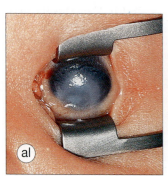
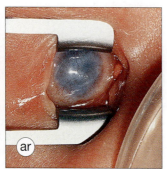
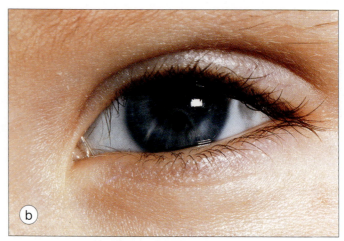

Fig. 28.11 Microcornea. (a) Microcornea in a child with ASDA. (b) Microcornea with iris and pupil anomalies.

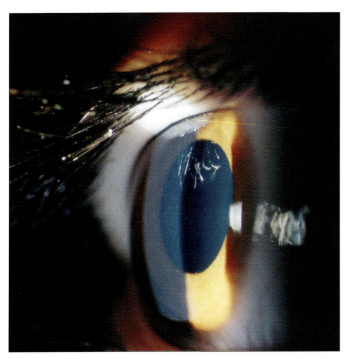

Fig. 28.12 Cornea plana. In profile, the flat nature of the cornea is clearly seen.

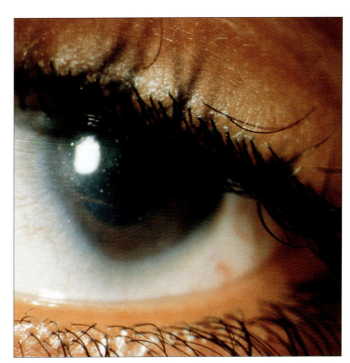

Fig. 28.14 Sclerocornea. Peripheral type III sclerocornea with peripheral scleralization.

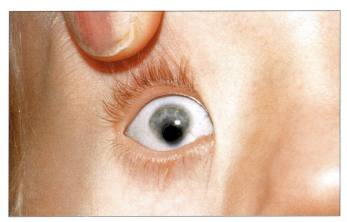

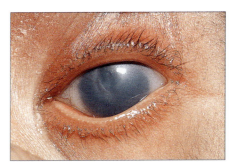

Fig. 28.15 Type II sclerocornea with diffuse, noninflammatory opacity of the normal-sized cornea.

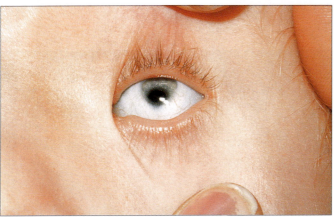

Fig. 28.13 Cornea plana associated with coloboma.

obscuring the limbus. It is bilateral in 90% of cases. Visual acuity is reduced only if the central cornea is involved. Sclerocornea may be autosomal dominant or recessive (more severe) with 50% of cases being sporadic.

Sclerocornea has been divided into three types:

Type I is peripheral and associated with cornea plana;

Type II is peripheral or central with disorganization and microphthalmos; and

Type III is mild and peripheral only (Fig. 28.14).

Histologically Bowman's layer is absent in the affected areas, and the corneal epithelium shows secondary changes with interstitial vascularization without inflammation (Fig. 28.15). The stromal collagen fibrils are comparable to scleral collagen in size and organization. There may be irregular absence of both endothelium and Descemet's membrane or an abnormally thinned Descemet's membrane composed of multilaminar basement membrane.[65-69]

Ocular associations include glaucoma, cataract, iris and choroidal colobomas, blue sclera, cornea plana (in 80% of cases), aniridia, angle abnormalities, and microphthalmos.

Systemic associations include spina bifida occulta, cerebellar abnormalities, cranial abnormalities, decreased hearing, limb deformities, cryptorchidism, Hallermann-Streiff syndrome, Mietens syndrome, Smith-Lemli-Opitz syndrome, osteogenesis imperfecta, and hereditary osteonychodysplasias.[66,67,70]

Management consists of careful refraction if possible and surveillance for glaucoma or cataract. In bilateral cases with central involvement, penetrating keratoplasty may be performed but postoperative glaucoma is a major problem. Preoperative assessment with high-frequency ultrasound is advisable to assess the presence of iridocorneal and keratolenticular adhesions.[71,72]

Peters anomaly

The prevalence of congenital corneal opacity, including Peters anomaly, sclerocornea, CHED, and posterior polymorphous dystrophy is approximately 3/100,000.[73]

The pathogenesis of Peters' anomaly is controversial. There may be at least four different developmental defects that may result in Peters anomaly:

(a) Intrauterine keratitis, commonly referred to as the "internal corneal ulcer of von Hippel";

(b) Defective separation of the lens vesicle from the surface ectoderm resulting in a posterior corneal defect caused by a persistent keratolenticular adhesion blocking the ingrowth of secondary mesenchyme;

(c) Incomplete central migration and differentiation of mesenchymal tissue destined to form the corneal endothelium and Descemet's membrane; and

(d) Secondary anterior displacement of lens–iris diaphragm, causing forward displacement of the lens, which in turn causes passive pressure against the cornea at a time in development when Descemet's membrane is absent or still a delicate, thin structure. This results in a posterior corneal defect.[68,69,74–79]

None of these theories adequately explains all the clinical and histopathologic findings in all forms of Peters anomaly. Peters anomaly should be regarded as a heterogenous group of congenital anomalies with a similar clinical appearance.

At least three developmental genes, *PAX6*, *PITX2*, and *PITX3*, are involved in the development of the anterior segment of the eye,[80,81] and mutations in each one have been shown to be associated with different cases of Peters anomaly. Mutations in the mouse *Pax6* gene are responsible for human aniridia, and it has been suggested that no other locus other than chromosome 11p13 has been implicated in aniridia.[80] *PITX2* is a transcription factor gene, mutations in which have been shown to cause Axenfeld-Rieger syndrome type 1, iris hypoplasia with glaucoma, and iridogoniodysgenesis syndrome.[24] *PITX3* is a transcription factor gene located on 10q25 that has been shown to be responsible for some cases of anterior segment mesenchymal dysgenesis (ASMD). ASMD is an autosomal dominant inherited condition with clinical findings ranging from an anterior Schwalbe line with mild cataract to severe corneal opacification with moderate cataract, while visual acuity can vary from 20/20 to hand motion only.[82,83]

Peters anomaly represents a spectrum of morphologic abnormalities and probably results from several pathogenic mechanisms, including genetic and/or environmental factors.

It is likely that in those cases where a genetic basis is responsible, accompanying ocular conditions may point to the likely mutation; e.g., aniridia and Peters anomaly is likely to be due to a *PAX6* mutation whereas Axenfeld-Rieger anomaly/syndrome with Peters anomaly is likely to be due to *PITX2* mutations.[31,84] Most cases are sporadic, but autosomal recessive and dominant inheritance have been reported.

Peters anomaly is defined as a congenital central corneal opacity with corresponding defects in the posterior corneal stroma, Descemet's membrane, and endothelium. Eighty percent of cases are bilateral. Glaucoma is present in 50% to 70% of cases.

Peters anomaly is often classified into three groups:

1. Posterior corneal defect with leukoma alone (Fig. 28.16);
2. Posterior corneal defect with leukoma and adherent iris strands (Fig. 28.17); and
3. Posterior corneal defect with leukoma, adherent iris strands, and keratolenticular contact or cataract (Fig. 28.18).

Posterior corneal defect with leukoma alone is the simplest form of Peters anomaly and the least documented in the literature. The iris and lens are normal, but a defect in the posterior cornea has produced an overlying opacity, which varies from a mild haze to an elevated vascularized lesion, and may decrease in the first few years of life. Occasionally the defect is so severe as to cause relative clearing centrally with opacification in the mid-periphery of the cornea (Fig. 28.19). The peripheral cornea is usually clear, allowing visualization of the lens–cornea adhesion with a gonioscope (Fig. 28.20), although scleralization of the limbus is common.[68,69,75–79]

If there are iridocorneal adhesions these usually arise from the collarette and vary from fine strands to broad bands. Kerato-

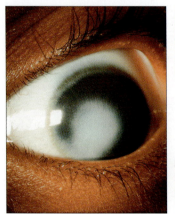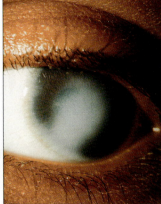

Fig. 28.16 Bilateral Peters anomaly with central opacification. The limbus also is scleralized inferonasally. This may be evidence that sclerocornea and Peters anomaly are part of the same spectrum of ASDA.

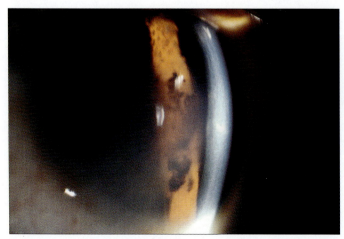

Fig. 28.17 Peters anomaly. Congenital leucoma, which has cleared to reveal iris strands to the posterior surface of the cornea.

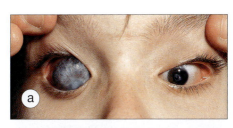

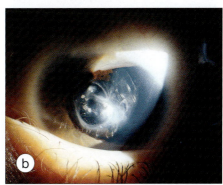

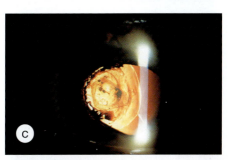

Fig. 28.18 Peters anomaly. (a) Severe bilateral Peters' anomaly with glaucoma of the right eye. (b). The left eye has lens-cornea and iris-cornea attachments and iris hypoplasia. The eye is slightly small. (c) The left eye in retroillumination.

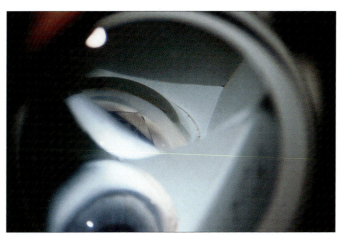

Fig. 28.20 Peters anomaly. A gonioscopic view of lens–cornea adhesion (arrow).

lenticular adhesions may occur and can be described as one of the following types:

(a) The lens may be adherent to the corneal stroma with absence of Descemet's membrane and lens capsule;

(b) The lens may be located in a forward position, but only opposed and not adherent to the posterior surface of the cornea;

(c) The lens may be in place but with a portion of the anterior capsule and lens cortex in contact or imbedded in the posterior corneal surface;

(d) The lens is in place but has a cone-shaped pyramidal cataract axially aligned with a posterior corneal defect; and

(e) The lens may be in place but has an axial anterior polar or nuclear cataract.

Associated ocular features include Axenfeld-Rieger syndrome or aniridia, microphthalmia, persistent hyperplastic primary vitreous (PHPV), and retinal dysplasia.[31,84]

Systemic associations include craniofacial anomalies, congenital heart disease, pulmonary hypoplasia, syndactyly, ear anomalies, genitourinary disorders, central nervous system abnormalities, dwarfism, fetal alcohol syndrome, and chromosomal abnormalities. Peters plus syndrome[85] is a rare autosomal recessive disorder comprising short-limb dwarfism, smooth philtrum with thin upper lip, hearing loss, cleft lip/palate, brachymorphism, with short hands and tapering brachydactyly, mental retardation, and bilateral Peters anomaly.

Histologically findings may vary but include diffuse thickening of Bowman's layer, mild atrophic changes in the overlying epithelium, normal anterior stroma, compressed posterior stromal lamellae partially replaced by fibrous tissue, and a broad central defect of Descemet's membrane and endothelium. The periphery of the cornea usually has an intact Descemet's membrane and endothelium. The anterior chamber is usually deep, except in areas of iridocorneal or keratolenticular adhesions. In other cases absence of Bowman's layer with anterior stromal edema and posterior corneal defect has been described.[72,86]

Management of congenital corneal opacification is quite difficult, and despite early diagnosis and prompt medical treatment or surgery, many of these cases have a poor outcome. Early penetrating keratoplasty, within the first 3 months, offers the infant the best hope for good vision. Suture removal after 4 to 6 weeks, followed by contact lens fitting and treatment of any amblyopia, is only successful if all involved are committed and

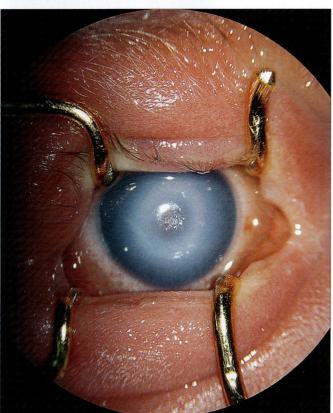

Fig. 28.19 A variant of Peters anomaly where the posterior corneal defect is so great so as to give relatively clear appearance centrally.

motivated. Alternatives to allograft penetrating keratoplasty include broad iridectomies and autorotational keratoplasty.[87,88]

Autosomal dominant keratitis

This rare recurrent stromal keratitis and corneal vascularization has been shown to be due to mutations in *PAX6*, which are also known to cause aniridia.

The child usually presents with an irritated red eye and is photophobic. It may be associated with foveal hypoplasia. Being autosomal dominant, there is variable expressivity and penetrance within the same pedigree with the mildest phenotype resulting in a 1- or 2-mm circumferential band of corneal opacification and vascularization contiguous with the limbus.[89–91]

Management is difficult and examination under anesthesia may be needed to clinch the diagnosis. Lubrication with artificial tears and ointments is essential. The role of limbal stem cell transplantation is unclear in this condition but early recurrence after penetrating keratoplasty has been noted. It is thought that this condition may be a variant of aniridia. If this is so, limbal stem cell transplantation might be a viable option.[90]

Aniridia

Aniridia has a prevalence of 1 in 50,000.[81] Mutations in *PAX6* are responsible for human aniridia, and it has been suggested that no other locus other than chromosome 11p13 has been implicated in aniridia and that *PAX6* may be the only gene responsible.[80] Inadequate gene dosage may thus lead to global impairment of morphogenesis. It is suggested that the aniridia trait may be lethal in the homozygous state.

Aniridia is a misnomer since at least a rudimentary iris is always present (Figs. 28.21 and 28.22). It is a panocular, bilateral disorder with absence of much (Fig. 28.23) or most of the iris tissue, although iris hypoplasia may also be seen. Foveal and optic nerve hypoplasia are variably present (Fig. 28.24), resulting in a congenital sensory nystagmus and leading to reduced visual acuity to 6/30 or worse. Associated ocular features include anterior polar cataracts, often with attached persistent papillary membrane strands, cortical cataract (Fig. 28.25), glaucoma, and corneal opacification, all of which often develop later in childhood (Fig. 28.26). Glaucoma occurs in up to half of all cases. Corneal opacification occurs secondary to limbal stem cell

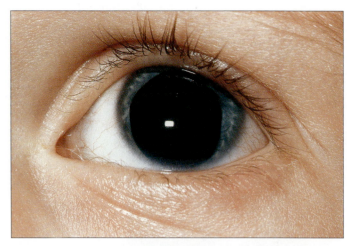

Fig. 28.22 Partial aniridia in a member of an autosomal dominant pedigree.

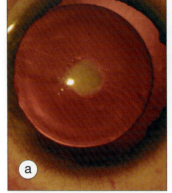
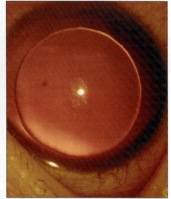

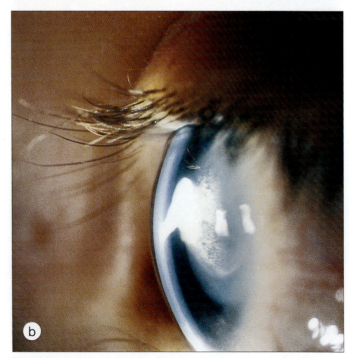

Fig. 28.23 Aniridia. (a) Aniridia with anterior polar cataract. (b) Aniridia with anterior extension of an anterior polar cataract with attachment to the cornea.

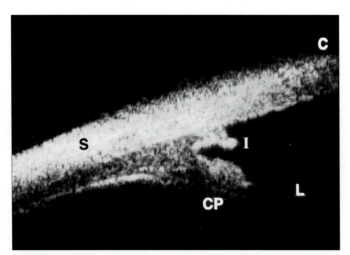

Fig. 28.21 Aniridia. A high-frequency ultrasound of an adolescent with aniridia. Note the iris stump (I), ciliary processes (CP), cornea (C), sclera (S), and lens (L).

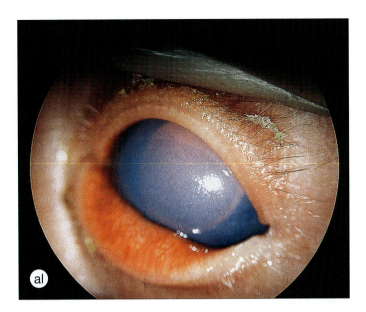

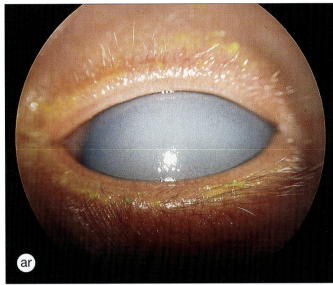

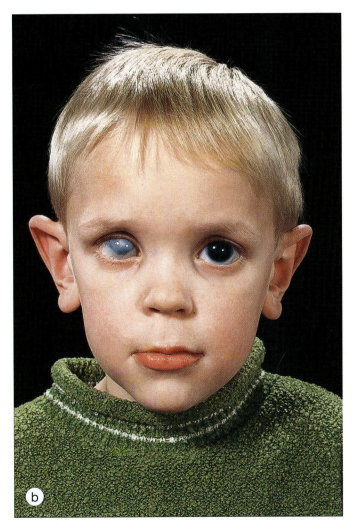

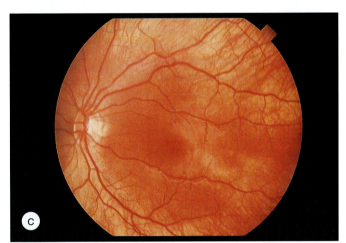

Fig. 28.24 Aniridia. (a) Bilateral severe congenital glaucoma in aniridia. (b) Same patient after multiple surgery showing uncontrolled glaucoma in the right eye and controlled glaucoma in the left. (c) Left fundus of the same patient showing mild foveal hypoplasia. The acuity was 6/18.

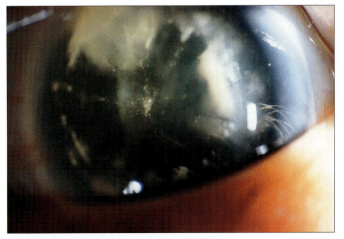

Fig. 28.25 Axenfeld-Rieger anomaly. There is iris hypoplasia, posterior embryotoxon, pseudopolycoria (top of picture), and corectopia with the pupil drawn peripherally.

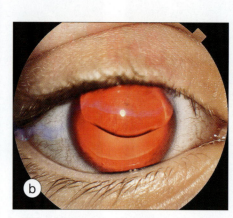
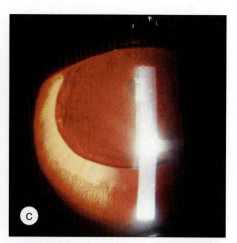

Fig. 28.26 Aniridia. (a) Aniridia with lens subluxation in 1979. (b) Same patient in 1985, showing progressive subluxation. (c) In 1995 there is further subluxation and corneal vascularization.

deficiency in aniridia (Fig. 28.16). Lens subluxation (Fig. 28.26) can also be associated with aniridia, often with glaucoma.[81,92,93]

The typical presentation is a baby with nystagmus who has the appearance of absent irides or dilated unresponsive pupils. Photophobia may be present.

Variable expressivity complicates the diagnosis of aniridia. So-called "aniridia with preserved ocular function" has been described as type II aniridia.[92] Visual acuity is more normal and nystagmus is usually not present. The incidence of cataracts, glaucoma, and corneal opacification is less. Type II aniridia has also been linked to 11p13.

Aniridia can be sporadic or familial. The familial form is autosomal dominant with complete penetrance, but variable expressivity. Two-thirds of all aniridia children have affected parents. It is said that sporadic aniridia is associated with Wilms tumor in up to one-third of cases.[94]

The Wilms tumor gene *WT1* locus lies close to the *PAX6* gene locus on 11p13. A chromosomal deletion involving both loci results in the association of Wilms tumor with aniridia. In Denmark,[94] patients with sporadic aniridia have a relative risk of 67 (confidence interval: 8.1-241) of developing Wilms tumor. Among patients investigated for mutations, Wilms tumor developed in only 2 patients out of 5 with the Wilms tumor gene (*WT1*) deleted. *None of the patients* with smaller chromosomal deletions or intragenic mutations were found to develop Wilms tumor. Familial aniridia patients are said not to be at risk for Wilms tumor. However, one case of Wilms tumor has been reported in a child with familial aniridia, but this probably represents a familial 11p13 deletion.[95]

When associated with aniridia, Wilms tumor is diagnosed before the age of 5 in 80% of cases. The median age at diagnosis is 3 years.

Sporadic aniridia has also been associated with genitourinary abnormalities and mental retardation (AGR triad), a constellation that has been linked with a deletion of the short arm of chromosome 11 (11p-). Some but not all of these patients get Wilms tumor (WAGR association). Aniridia can also rarely be associated with ataxia and mental retardation (Gillespie syndrome). Multisystem syndromes and chromosomal abnormalities such as ring chromosome 6 can also include aniridia.[96,97] Ocular associations of aniridia include Peters anomaly, microcornea, and ectopia lentis.

Management includes genetic analysis to exclude chromosomal deletion. Until this is done and the result known, all children with sporadic aniridia should have repeated abdominal ultra-sonographic and clinical examinations. One protocol advised that the child be seen every 3 months until the age of 5, every 6 months until the age of 10, and once a year until the age of 16. However, the examinations are best continued until chromosomal and then intragenic mutational analyses have confirmed a *PAX6* mutation only. If chromosomal deletion is found then 3-monthly scans should be performed and the child transferred to the care of a nephrologist.

Management of the ocular condition consists of conservative measures such as correction of any refractive errors with filter lenses to reduce glare, and surveillance for onset of glaucoma. These patients often suffer from chronic angle closure glaucoma, which usually develops later and is difficult to treat. For this reason[98] prophylactic goniotomy in cases of aniridia is sometimes advocated. Cyclodiode laser, drainage tubes, and trabeculectomy with antimetabolite (usually mitomycin) have all been advocated for treatment of established glaucoma uncontrolled by topical medication alone. Usually corneal opacification occurs in adulthood but may occur in children. This may necessitate limbal stem cell transplant and corneal graft.[99]

Penetrating keratoplasty for anterior segment developmental anomalies

Infant penetrating keratoplasty has historically been thought to be a thankless endeavor with poor results.[100,101] However, 35% graft survival at 7 years post graft has been reported in cases of Peters anomaly,[102] and good visual results have been reported following early penetrating keratoplasty (PKP).[103–105]

Crucial to penetrating keratoplasty in children is the acknowledgment that pediatric ocular tissue behaves differently from that of the adult. The age at which the child's eye becomes more like that of an adult is controversial, but experience suggests that a child over the age of 10 years will have ocular tissue that behaves almost like that of an adults.

High-frequency ultrasound is a well-established tool for the examination of the anterior segment, especially in eyes with corneal opacity.[106–108] It is one of the most challenging conditions to treat surgically,[105] but the use of high-frequency ultrasound evaluation helps determine a more appropriate entry into the anterior chamber.

All cases require a Flieringa ring because the sclera is much less rigid than that of an adult (Fig. 28.27). This is sutured using 8/0 nylon in four quadrants, and the suture is left long so as to stabilize the eye with the long suture ends using Steri-Strips. A

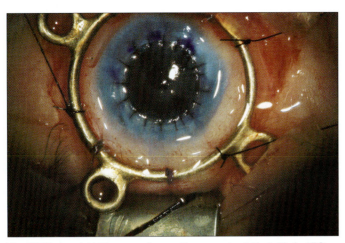

Fig. 28.27 Axenfeld-Rieger syndrome. Excess periumbilical skin in ARS.

pediatric radial corneal marker is used to mark the cornea and allow centration, which aids placement of the trephine. A small paracentesis is made and the anterior chamber hyperinflated with viscoelastic usually Healon GV.

Prior to trephination of the host, mannitol is infused according to the weight and age of the child to reduce the intraocular pressure and reduce the risk of expulsive hemorrhage.

A manual trephine is used and if keratolenticular adhesions or extensive iridocorneal adhesions are present, the anterior chamber is not entered with the trephine. Vacuum trephines such as the Barron-Hessburg are usually not manufactured to a small enough diameter.

The host button is fashioned after initial trephination with a 15° disposable blade so as to avoid excessive damage to the iris and/or lens. In cases of keratolenticular adhesion the lens may be carefully peeled off the cornea but this usually results in cataract formation within a few weeks of the graft. Therefore there is an argument for lens aspiration with sparing of the posterior capsule; this needs surgical capsulectomy through a pars plicata approach usually within a few weeks also, but at least the donor cornea is a little more protected from trauma since the capsulectomy occurs a little deeper in the eye away from the corneal endothelium. All cases of Peters anomaly or sclerocornea have an iridectomy in four quadrants to try and reduce the incidence of glaucoma. The donor corneal button is oversized by 1 mm in all these cases also to increase the anterior chamber depth There is evidence that this improves outcome.[109] Grafts are sutured using at least 16 10/0 nylon interrupted sutures.

All cases receive subconjunctival antibiotic and steroid injection at the end of the procedure. Intracameral dexamethasone is not routinely used by these authors.

The commonest causes of congenital corneal opacification include sclerocornea and Peters anomaly, both of which are probably part and parcel of the same spectrum of an ASDA. UBM imaging is more reliable in making a definitive diagnosis than just clinical examination alone in such cases.[20] Assessment of presence or absence of the lens, the iris, keratolenticular adhesions, and iridocorneal adhesions all help with surgical planning and also with assessment of surgical prognosis.

Histologically, absence of Bowman's layer has been named as a poor prognosticator of penetrating keratoplasty in Peters anomaly as has absence of Descemet's membrane; both of these can be detected using UBM.

The presence or absence of glaucoma must be assessed. If glaucoma is present preoperatively, this again is a poor prognosticator. In these circumstances and if the corneal opacification is bilateral, laser cycloablation (usually cyclodiode laser) is used under UBM guidance to treat the inferior half of the eye. This allows control of the glaucoma with appropriate topical medication, and penetrating keratoplasty can then be performed with the clear understanding that drainage will probably be needed to be placed at a later stage to control the glaucoma. Simultaneous PKP and drainage tube placement in infant eyes is not a route favored by this author.

The tissue reactivity in infants is such that intensive topical steroid/antibiotic preparations are a necessity to prevent fibrin formation, synechiae, and rejection. These are applied half-hourly for the first 24 hours with cycloplegic drops three times daily and antibiotic/steroid ointment at night to allow the infant to sleep. The intensity of drops is tailed off over 2 months, and cycloplegia may continue for the same period. Infants are reviewed twice weekly for the first 6 weeks because the slightest hint of a loose suture or suture vascularization necessitates removal of the offending suture under anesthesia within 24 hours (Fig. 28.28). Failure to do so results in rapid epithelial rejection. In any case, all sutures are removed in infants at the latest by 6 weeks postoperatively.

After two weeks, topical cyclosporin A (CsA) eye drops (2% in corn oil) are used twice daily indefinitely to prevent rejection of the corneal graft. There is evidence that topical cyclosporin A reaches adequate levels for immunosuppression within the cornea but not necessarily within the eye, and that the combined use of CsA and steroid drops reduces the rate of rejection in high-risk corneal grafts compared to topical steroids only.

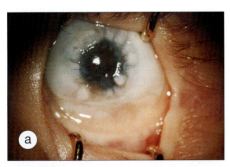 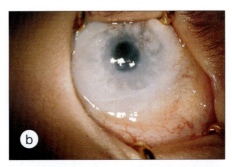 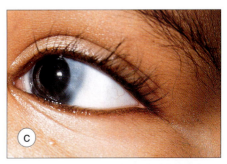

Fig. 28.28 Infant keratoplasty. (a) There is mucus plug formation around loose sutures only 4 weeks post PKP for this case of complete sclerocornea. (b) The same case as in (a) 4 months later. There is peripheral opacification and scarring encroaching on the visual axis. (c) Two years post PKP for Peters' anomaly. The child remains on cyclosporin nightly.

In 1977 Waring and Laibson[101] stated "We do not recommend PK in patients with unilateral, congenital corneal opacities. However, those with bilateral cloudy corneas should have an attempt at keratoplasty as early in life as possible." These authors agree with this statement almost in its entirety; the only point of contention is that in some cases the so-called "normal" eye is not normal, only less affected. In these cases the parents should be given the option of keratoplasty with the clear understanding that

the prognosis for vision is poor due to the physiological phenomenon of amblyopia on top of the risks of rejection, infection, and glaucoma.

There is no doubt that if it is understood that the aim of surgery is to give functional vision and not perfect vision and that a partially clear graft that allows delivery of functional vision is still a successful outcome, then infant PKP can be very rewarding for the patient and the surgeon[100–116] (Figs. 28.20 and 28.21).

REFERENCES

1. Kupfer, C, Ross K. The development of outflow facility in human eyes. Invest Ophthalmol 1971; 10: 513–7.
1a. Larsen WJ. Human Embryology. New York, Edinburgh, Churchill Livingstone. 2001.
1b. O'Rahilly R. The prenatal development of the human eye. Exp Eye Res 1975; 21: 93–112.
2. Smith RS, Zabaleta A, Kume T, et al. Haploinsufficiency of the transcription factors FOXC1 and FOXC2 results in aberrant ocular development. Hum Mol Genet 2000; 9: 1021–32.
3. Hong, HK, Lass JH, Chakravarti A. Pleiotropic skeletal and ocular phenotypes of the mouse mutation congenital hydrocephalus (ch/Mf1) arise from a winged helix/forkhead transcription factor gene. Hum Mol Genet 1999; 8: 625–37.
4. Kume T, Deng KY, Winfrey V, et al. The forkhead/winged helix gene Mf1 is disrupted in the pleiotropic mouse mutation congenital hydrocephalus. Cell 1998; 93: 985–96.
5. Kidson SH, Kume T, Deng K, et al. The forkhead/winged-helix gene, Mf1, is necessary for the normal development of the cornea and formation of the anterior chamber in the mouse eye. Dev Biol 1999; 211: 306–22.
6. Kitamura K, Miura H, Miyagawa-Tomita S, et al. Mouse Pitx2 deficiency leads to anomalies of the ventral body wall, heart, extra- and periocular mesoderm and right pulmonary isomerism. Development 1999; 126: 5749–58.
7. Hjalt TA, Semina EV, Amendt BA, et al. The Pitx2 protein in mouse development. Dev Dyn 2000; 218: 195–200.
8. Gage PJ, Suh H, Camper SA. Dosage requirement of Pitx2 for development of multiple organs. Development 1999; 126: 4643–51.
9. van Heyningen V, Williamson KA. PAX6 in sensory development. Hum Mol Genet 2002; 11: 1161–67.
10. Hogan BL, Hirst EM, Horsburgh G, et al. Small eye (Sey): a mouse model for the genetic analysis of craniofacial abnormalities. Development 1988;103(Suppl): 115–9.
11. Baulmann, DC, Ohlmann A, Flugel-Koch C, et al. Pax6 heterozygous eyes show defects in chamber angle differentiation that are associated with a wide spectrum of other anterior eye segment abnormalities. Mech Dev 2002; 118: 3–17.
12. Hanson IM, Fletcher JM, Jordan T, et al. Mutations at the PAX6 locus are found in heterogeneous anterior segment malformations including Peters anomaly. Nat Genet 1994; 6: 168–73.
13. Ormestad M, Blixt A, Churchill A, et al. Foxe3 haploinsufficiency in mice: a model for Peters anomaly. Invest Ophthalmol Vis Sci 2002; 43: 1350–7.
14. Ramaesh T, Collinson JM, Ramaesh K, et al. Corneal abnormalities in Pax6 small eye mice mimic human aniridia-related keratopathy. Invest Ophthalmol Vis Sci 2003; 44: 1871–8.
15. Beebe DC, Coats JM. The lens organizes the anterior segment: specification of neural crest cell differentiation in the avian eye. Dev Biol 2000; 220: 424–31.
16. Thut CJ, Rountree RB, Hwa M, et al. A large-scale in situ screen provides molecular evidence for the induction of eye anterior segment structures by the developing lens. Dev Biol 2001; 231: 63–76.
17. Libby RT, Smith RS, Savinova OV, et al. Modification of ocular defects in mouse developmental glaucoma models by tyrosinase. Science 2003; 299: 1578–81.
18. Burian HM, Braley AE, Allen L. External and gonioscopic visibility of the ring of Schwalbe and the trabecular zone: an interpretation of the posterior corneal embryotoxon and the so-called congenital hyaline membranes on the posterior corneal surface. Trans Am Ophthalmol Soc 1955; 52: 389–428.
19. Axenfeld T. Embryotoxon cornea posterius. Ber Deutsch Ophthalmol Ges 1920; 42: 301–2.
20. Raymond WR, Kearney JJ, Parmsley VC. Ocular findings in arteriohepatic dysplasia (Alagille's syndrome). Arch Ophthalmol 1989; 107: 1077.
21. Johnson BL. Ocular pathologic features of arteriohepatic dysplasia (Alagille's syndrome). Am J Ophthalmol 1990; 110: 504–12.
22. Hingorani M, Nischal KK, Davies A, et al. Ocular abnormalities in Alagille syndrome. Ophthalmology 1999; 106: 330–7.
23. Heon E, Sheth BP, Kalenak JW, et al. Linkage of autosomal dominant iris hypoplasia to the region of the Rieger syndrome locus (4q25). Hum Molec Genet 1995; 4: 1435–9.
24. Alward WL. Axenfeld-Rieger syndrome in the age of molecular genetics. Am J Ophthalmol 2000; 130: 107–15.
25. Alward WL, Semina EV, Kalenak JW, et al. Autosomal dominant iris hypoplasia is caused by a mutation in the Rieger syndrome (RIEG/PITX2) gene. Am J Ophthalmol 1998; 125: 98–100.
26. Jordan T, Ebenezer N, Manners R, et al. Familial glaucoma iridogoniodysplasia maps to a 6p25 region implicated in primary congenital glaucoma and iridogoniodysgenesis anomaly. Am J Hum Genet 1997; 61: 882–8.
27. Kozlowski K, Walter MA. Variation in residual PITX2 activity underlies the phenotypic spectrum of anterior segment developmental disorders. Hum Molec Genet 2000; 9: 2131–9.
28. Fryns JP, van den Berghe H. Rieger syndrome and interstitial 4q26 deletion. Genetic Counseling 1992; 3: 153–4.
29. Shields MB. Axenfeld-Rieger syndrome: A theory mechanism and distinctions from the iridocorneal endothelial syndrome. Trans Am Ophthalmol Soc 1983; 81: 736–84.
30. Shields MB, Buckley E, Klintworth GK, et al. Axenfeld-Rieger syndrome: a spectrum of developmental disorders. Surv Ophthal 1985; 29: 387–409.
31. Doward W, Perveen R, Lloyd IC, et al. A mutation in the RIEG1 gene associated with Peters anomaly. Genet 1999; 36: 152–5.
32. Mandal AK, Prasad K, Naduvilath TJ. Surgical results and complications of mitomycin C-augmented trabeculectomy in refractory developmental glaucoma. Ophthalmic Surg Lasers 1999; 30: 473–80.
33. Plager DA, Neely DE. Intermediate-term results of endoscopic diode laser cyclophotocoagulation for pediatric glaucoma. J AAPOS 1999; 3: 131–7.
34. Spencer F, Vernon S. "Cyclodiode": results of a standard protocol. Br J Ophthalmol 1999; 83: 311–6.
35. Guerrero AH, Latina MA. Complications of glaucoma drainage implant surgery. Int Ophthalmol Clin 2000; 40: 149–63.
36. Wilson ME. Congenital iris ectropion and a new classification for anterior segment dysgenesis. J Pediatr Ophthalmol Strabismus 1990; 27: 48–55.
37. Ritch R, Forbes M, Hetherington J, et al. Congenital ectropion uveae with glaucoma. Ophthalmology 1984; 91: 326–31.
38. Dowling JL, Albert DM, Nelson LB, et al. Primary glaucoma associated with iridotrabecular dysgenesis and ectropion uveae. Ophthalmology 1985; 92: 912–21.
39. Judisch GF, Maumenee IH. Clinical differentiation of recessive congenital hereditary endothelial dystrophy and dominant hereditary endothelial dystrophy. Am J Ophthalmol 1978; 85: 606–12.
40. Toma NM, Ebenezer ND, Inglehearn CF, et al. Linkage of congenital hereditary endothelial dystrophy to chromosome 20. Hum Molec Genet 1995; 4: 2395–8.
41. Kupfer C, Kaiser-Kupfer MI. Observations on the development of the anterior chamber angle with reference to the pathogenesis of congenital glaucomas. Am J Ophthalmol 1979; 88: 424–6.

42. Maumenee AE. The pathogenesis of congenital glaucoma: A new theory. Am J Ophthalmol 1959; 47: 827–59.

43. Chandler P. Atrophy of the stroma of the iris: endothelial dystrophy, corneal edema and glaucoma. Am J Ophthalmol 1956; 41: 607–15.

44. Cogan DG, Reese AB. A syndrome of iris nodules, ectopic Descemet's membrane and unilateral glaucoma. Doc Ophthalmol 1969; 26: 424–33.

45. Campbell DG, Shields MB, Smith TR. The corneal endothelium and the spectrum of essential iris atrophy. Am J Ophthalmol 1978; 86: 317–24.

46. Kupfer C, Kaiser-Kupfer MI, Datiles M, et al. The contralateral eye in the iridocorneal endothelial (ICE) syndrome. Ophthalmology 1983; 90: 1343–50.

47. Hirst LW, Quigley HA, Stark WJ, et al. Specular microscopy of iridocorneal endothelial syndrome. Am J Ophthalmol 1980; 89: 11–21.

48. Shields MB, Campbell DG, Simmons RJ. The essential iris atrophies. Am J Ophthalmol 1978; 85: 749–59.

49. Alvim PT, Cohen Et, Rapuano CT, et al. Penetrating keratoplasty in iridocorneal endothelial syndrome. Cornea 2001; 20: 134–40.

50. Baum JL, Feingold M. Ocular aspects of Goldenhar's syndrome. Am J Ophthalmol 1953; 75: 250.

51. Shields JA, Laibson PR, Augsburger JJ, et al. Central corneal dermoid: a clinicopathologic correlation and review of the literature. Can J Ophthalmol 1986; 21: 23–6.

52. Igbal MA, Chitayat D, Hahm SY, et al. Linkage of gene for corneal dermoids with the DXS43 (Xp22.2–p22.1) locus. (Abstract) Am J Hum Genet 1987; 41: A171.

53. Rogers GL, Polomeno RC. Autosomal-dominant inheritance of megalocornea associated with Down's syndrome. Am J Ophthalmol 1974; 78: 526–9.

54. Raas RA, Berkenstadt M, Goodman RM. Megalocornea and mental retardation syndrome [letter]. Am J Med Genet 1988; 29: 221–3.

55. Prapaitrakul W, Sprockel OL, Shivanand P. Megalocornea in nonketotic hyperglycinemia. J Pediatr Ophthalmol Strabismus 1978; 15: 85–8.

56. Roche O, Dureau P, Uteza Y, et al. [Congenital megalocornea.] J Fr Ophtalmol 2002; 25: 312–8.

57. Meire FM. Megalocornea. Clinical and genetic aspects. Doc Ophthalmol 1994; 87: 1–121.

58. Salmon JF, Wallis CE, Murray AD. Variable expressivity of autosomal dominant microcornea with cataract. Arch Ophthalmol 1988; 106: 505–10.

59. Polomeno RC, Cummings C. Autosomal dominant cataracts and microcornea. Can J Ophthalmol 1979; 14: 227–9.

60. Ainsworth JR, Morton JE, Good P, et al. Micro syndrome in Muslim Pakistan children. Ophthalmology 2001; 108: 491–7.

61. Fukuchi T, Ueda J, Hara H, et al. [Glaucoma with microcornea; morphometry and differential diagnosis.] Nippon Ganka Gakkai Zasshi 1998; 102: 746–51.

62. Forsius H, Damsten M, Eriksson AW, et al. Autosomal recessive cornea plana. A clinical and genetic study of 78 cases in Finland. Acta Ophthalmol Scand 1998; 76: 196–203.

63. Kao WW, Liu CY. Roles of lumican and keratocan on corneal transparency. Glycoconj J 2002; 19: 275–85.

64. Gavin MP, Kirkness CM. Cornea plana–clinical features, videokeratometry, and management. Br J Ophthalmol 1998; 82: 329–30.

65. Rodrigues MM, Calhoun J, Weinreb S. Sclerocornea with an unbalanced translocation (17p, 10q). Am J Ophthalmol 1974; 78: 49–53.

66. Stanley JA. Congenital anomalies of the peripheral cornea. Int Ophthalmol Clin 1986; 26: 15–28.

67. Babel J. [Sclerocornea.] Klin Monatsbl Augenheilkd 1985; 186: 180–3.

68. Townsend WM. Congenital corneal leukomas 1. Peters central defect in Descemet's membrane. Am J Ophthalmol 1974; 77: 80–6.

69. Townsend WM, Font RL, Zimmerman LE. Congenital corneal leukomas 2. Histopathologic findings in 19 eyes with central defect in Descemet's membrane. Am J Ophthalmol 1974; 77: 192–206.

70. Schanzlin DJ, Goldberg DB, Brown SI. Hallermann-Streiff syndrome associated with sclerocornea, aniridia, and a chromosomal abnormality. Am J Ophthalmol 1980; 90: 411–5.

71. Wood T, Kaufman HE. Penetrating keratoplasty in an infant with sclerocomea. Am J Ophthalmology 1970; 70: 609–13.

72. Nischal KK, Naor J, Jay V, et al. Clinicopathological correlation of congenital corneal opacification using ultrasound biomicroscopy. Br J Ophthalmol 2002; 86: 62–9.

73. Bermejo E, Martinez-Frias ML. Congenital eye malformations: clinical epidemiological analysis of 1,124,654 consecutive births in Spain. Am J Med Genet 1998; 75: 497–504.

74. Kivlin JD, Fineman RM, Crandall AS, et al. Peters anomaly as a consequence of genetic and nongenetic syndromes. Arch Ophthalmol 1986; 104: 61–4.

75. Stone DL, Kenyon KR, Green WR, et al. Congenital corneal leukoma anomaly. Am J Ophthalmol 1976; 81: 173–93.

76. Waring GO, Rodrigues MM, Laibson PR. Anterior chamber cleavage syndrome: a stepladder classification. Surv Ophthalmol 1975; 20: 3–27.

77. Peters A. Ueber angeborene Defektbildung der Descemetschen membrane Klein Monatsbl Augenheilkd 1906; 44: 2740.

78. Polack FM, Grau EL. Scanning electron microscopy of congenital corneal leukomas (Peters anomaly). Am J Ophthalmol 1979; 88: 169–78.

79. Polack FM, Graue EL. Scanning electron microscopy of congenital corneal leukomas (Peters anomaly). Am J Ophthalmol 1979; 88: 169–78.

80. Prosser J, van Heyningen V. PAX6 mutations reviewed. Human Mutat 1998; 11: 93–108.

81. Churchill A, Booth A. Genetics of aniridia and anterior segment dysgenesis. Br J Ophthalmol 1996; 80: 669–73.

82. Hittner HM, Kretzer FL, Antoszyk JH, et al. Variable expressivity of autosomal dominant anterior segment mesenchymal dysgenesis in six generations. Am J Ophthalmol 1982; 93: 57–70.

83. Semina EV, Ferrell RE, Mintz-Hittner HA, et al. A novel homeobox gene PITX3 is mutated in families with autosomal-dominant cataracts and ASMD. Nat Genet 1998; 19: 167–70.

84. Koster R, van Balen AT. Congenital corneal opacity (Peters anomaly) combined with buphthalmos and aniridia. Ophthalmic Paediatr Genet 1985; 6: 241–6.

85. de Almeida JC, Reis DF, Llerena J Jr, et al. Short stature, brachydactyly, and Peters anomaly (Peters-plus syndrome): confirmation of autosomal recessive inheritance. J Med Genet 1991; 28: 277–9.

86. Kupfer C, Kuwabara T, Stark WJ. The histopathology of Peters anomaly. Am J Ophthalmol 1975; 80: 653–60.

87. Zaidman GW, Rabinowitz Y, Forstot SL. Optical iridectomy for corneal opacities in Peter's anomaly. Cataract Refrac Surg 1998; 24: 719–22.

88. Haumann GO, Volcker HE, Gackle D. Ipsilateral rotational autokeratoplasty. Klinische Monatsblatter fur Augenheilkunde 1977; 170: 488–93.

89. Mirzayans F, Pearce WG, MacDonald IM, Walter MA. Mutation of the PAX6 gene in patients with autosomal dominant keratitis. Am J Hum Genet 1995; 57: 539–48.

90. Pearce WG, Mielke BW, Hassard DT, et al. Autosomal dominant keratitis: a possible aniridia variant. Can J Ophthalmol 1995; 30: 131–7.

91. Kivlin JD, Apple DJ, Olson RJ, et al. Dominantly inherited keratitis. Arch Ophthal 1986; 104: 1621–3.

92. Elsas FJ, Maumenee IH, Kenyon KR, et al. Familial aniridia with preserved ocular function. Am J Ophthal 1977; 83: 718–24.

93. Traboulsi EI. Ocular malformations and developmental genes. J AAPOS 1998; 2: 317–23.

94. Gronskov K, Olsen JH, Sand A, et al. Population-based risk estimates of Wilms tumor in sporadic aniridia. A comprehensive mutation screening procedure of PAX6 identifies 80% of mutations in aniridia. Hum Genet 2001; 109: 11–8.

95. Breslow NE, Beckwith JB. Epidemiological features of Wilms' tumor: results of the National Wilms' Tumor Study. J Natl Cancer Inst 1982; 68: 429–36.

96. Crolla JA, van Heyningen V. Frequent chromosome aberrations revealed by molecular cytogenetic studies in patients with aniridia. Am J Hum Genet 2002; 71: 1138–49.

97. Nelson LB, Spaeth GL, Nowinski TS, et al. Aniridia. A review. Surv Ophthalmol 1984; 28: 621–42.

98. Chen TC, Walton DS. Goniosurgery for prevention of aniridic glaucoma. Arch Ophthalmol 1999; 117: 1144–8.

99. Dua HS, Saini JS, Azuara-Blanco A, et al. Limbal stem cell deficiency: concept, aetiology, clinical presentation, diagnosis and management. Indian J Ophthalmol 2000; 48: 83–92.

100. Alberth B. Keratoplasty in infants and children. Klin Monatsbl Augenheild 1980; 177: 802–4.

101. Pavlin CJ, Sherar MD, Foster FS. Subsurface ultrasound microscopic imaging of the intact eye. Ophthalmology 1990; 97: 244–50.

102. Frucht-Pery J, Chayet AS, Feldman ST, et al. The effect of corneal grafting on vision in bilateral amblyopia. Acta Ophthalmol (Suppl) 1989; 192: 20–3.

103. Yang LL, Lambert SR, Lynn MJ, et al. Long-term results of corneal graft survival in infants and children with Peters anomaly. Ophthalmology 1999; 106: 833–48.

104. Pavlin CJ. Practical application of ultrasound biomicroscopy. Can J Ophthalmol 1995; 30: 225–9.

105. Joseph A, Fernandez ST, Ittyerah TP, et al. Keratoplasty in congenital corneal opacity. Indian J Ophthalmol 1980; 28: 79–80.

106. Brown SI, Salomon SM. Wound healing of grafts in congenitally opaque infant corneas. Am J Ophthalmol 1983; 95: 641–4.

107. Waring GO III, Parks MM. Successful lens removal in congenital corneolenticular adhesion (Peters anomaly). Am J Ophthalmol 1977; 83: 526–9.

108. Hertle RW, Orlin SE. Successful visual rehabilitation after neonatal penetrating keratoplasty. Br J Ophthalmol 1997; 81: 644–8.

109. Frueh BE, Brown SL. Transplantation of congenitally opaque corneas. Br J Ophthalmol 1997; 81: 1064–9.

110. Waring GO 3d, Laibson PR. Keratoplasty in infants and children. Trans Am Acad Ophthalmol Otolaryngol 1977; 83: 283–96.

111. Dana MR, Moyes AL, Games JA, et al. The indications for and outcome in pediatric keratoplasty. A multicenter study. Ophthalmology 1995; 102: 1129–38.

112. Cameron JA. Good visual result following early penetrating keratoplasty for Peters anomaly. J Pediatr Ophthalmol Strabismus 1993; 30: 109–12.

113. Erlich CM, Rootman DS, Morin JD. Corneal transplantation in infants, children and young adults: experience of the Toronto Hospital for Sick Children, 1979–88. Can J Ophthalmol 1991; 26: 206–10.

114. Pavlin CJ, Harasiewicz K, Sherar MD, et al. Clinical use of ultrasound biomicroscopy. Ophthalmology 1991; 98: 287–95.

115. Vajpayee RB, Ramu M, Panda A, et al. Oversized grafts in children. Ophthalmology 1999; 106: 829–32.

116. Cowden JW. Penetrating keratoplasty in infants and children. Ophthalmology 1990; 97: 324–9.

CHAPTER
29

Corneal Abnormalities in Childhood

Creig S Hoyt

Corneal disease is still the most common cause of blindness in the world. It is not surgery but the combination of better nutrition, public and private health measures, and antibiotics that have made corneal disease an unusual cause of blindness in the Western world. Nonetheless corneal diseases are a small but significant cause of disability from visual defect, glare, or pain, and corneal abnormalities may form important clues to the nature of systemic diseases.

TRISOMY 18 AND TRISOMY 8 MOSAIC

In trisomy 18, the eyelid may be abnormal, and the eye frequently is colobomatous. The cornea may be diffusely opaque at birth. Discrete corneal opacities caused by breakdown of the corneal epithelium occasionally occur.

In trisomy 8 mosaic syndrome geographical corneal opacities are characteristic.[1] These opacities consist of richly vascularized fibrous tissue in the superficial layers of the cornea (Fig. 29.1).

DERMOIDS (CHORISTOMAS)

Choristomas are benign congenital overgrowths of abnormally located tissue; in the eye they consist of masses of skin, hair follicles, hair, and sebaceous glands (Figs. 29.2–29.4). They may be multiple. These tissues were originally destined to become skin but were displaced onto the eye.

Single-tissue choristomas contain ectopic tissues of mesenchymal or ectodermal origin,[2] i.e., dermis, lacrimal gland, fat, respiratory epithelium, brain, nerve, bone, teeth, and so on. Complex choristomas contain two or more tissues of mesenchymal or ectodermal origin.

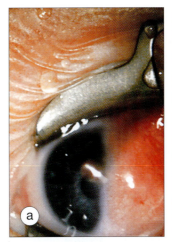
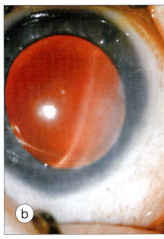

Fig. 29.2 (a) Limbal dermoid that covered half of the cornea and extended posteriorly in the fornix. (b) Same patient, 1 year following lamellar keratectomy carried out at 2 months of age. Although the cosmetic appearance was satisfactory and remained so for 5 years after this photograph the eye was deeply amblyopic due to high astigmatism and the corneal opacity.

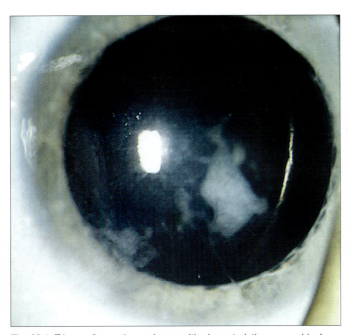

Fig. 29.1 Trisomy 8 mosaic syndrome with characteristic geographical corneal opacity.

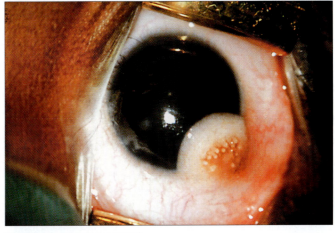

Fig. 29.3 Hairy limbal dermoid.

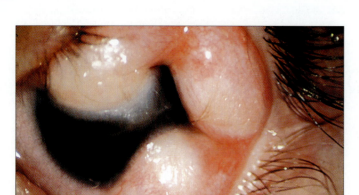

Fig. 29.4 Multiple corneal dermoids in a patient with Goldenhar syndrome.

A dermoid (or lipodermoid) is a congenital, solid mass of dermis-like and pilosebaceous material covered with keratinized, often hairy squamous epithelium. They are usually found at the corneoscleral junction, in the inferotemporal quadrant, but they may be much more widespread and overlie a microphthalmic or staphylomatous eye.[3] Dermoids can involve the entire thickness of the cornea and sclera.[4] They reduce vision by occlusion (if they occur across the cornea) or by distorting the contour of the cornea, giving astigmatism and amblyopia. They may sometimes cover the cornea. A recent study suggests that corneal dermoids can be mapped to Xq24-qter.[5]

Dermolipomas are similar to dermoids but have a large amount of fat and few or no pilosebaceous glands. Some are inherited in an autosomal dominant fashion, though X-linked recessive inheritance has also been described.[6] Dermoids and dermolipomas also occur in Goldenhar syndrome,[7] encephalocraniocutaneous lipomatosis,[8] congenital generalized fibromatosis,[9] and the linear nevus sebaceous syndrome.[10]

Treatment is usually necessary on cosmetic grounds alone but must be preceded by a full ocular examination including gonioscopy (Fig. 29.5) and/or high-resolution biomicroscopy to assess the extent of the mass.[11] Lamellar keratectomy is sufficient in most cases (Fig. 29.6) and improves the appearance by not only removing the white-yellow appearance and any hairs but also the elevation. Many cases reopacify but the appearance is often adequate postoperatively. Some authors now prefer lamellar keratoplasty as the initial treatment.[12] Full-thickness dermoids may be treated by excision and corneal (not scleral) grafting but the prognosis is guarded. Enucleation is occasionally the best option for widespread dermoids. This should be delayed for as long as possible to allow for orbital growth.

CORNEAL STAPHYLOMA

In congenital corneal staphyloma the cornea is enlarged, ectatic, opaque, and the Descemet's membrane is missing (Fig. 29.7).[13] The posterior segment of the eye is usually normal, but glaucoma occurs and may cause buphthalmos. Corneal metaplasia is a similar condition, and like sclerocornea and staphyloma may be caused by a neural crest cell migration defect. Intraocular defects sometimes coexist, and the cornea may become opaque and keratinized with time.[14] Corneoscleral staphyloma may coexist with Peters anomaly.[15]

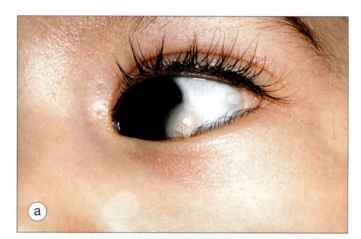

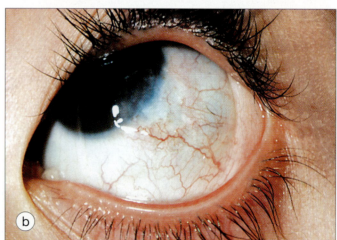

Fig. 29.6 Limbal dermoid. (a) The indication for surgery was the cosmetic appearance. It can be seen that the dermoid is raised and pale colored. (b) Same case as in (a) after lamellar keratectomy. Although there is still some residual corneal opacity the lesion is now flat and cosmetically acceptable.

Fig. 29.5 Limbal dermoid: gonioscopic view. Through the gonioscope it can just be seen that the dermoid involves the inner part of the cornea, indicating that caution should be taken during surgery. A full-thickness corneal graft may be the only way to treat this sort of problem and may not be indicated unless the cosmetic appearance is extreme.

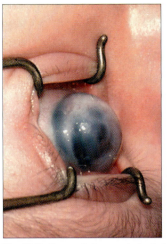
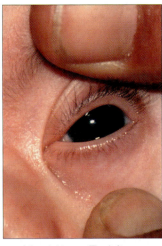

Fig. 29.7 Congenital corneal staphyloma of the right eye. The left eye was normal.

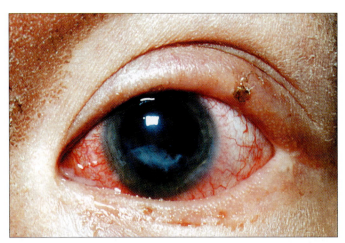

Fig. 29.8 Keratitis resulting from a combination of exposure, drying, and the direct effects of irradiation for orbital rhabdomyosarcoma.

AMNIOTIC BANDS

Amniotic bands may be associated with congenital corneal leukomas or with exposure keratitis from lid defects.[16]

TREATMENT OF THE CONGENITALLY OPAQUE CORNEA (see Chapter 28)

Unilateral cases are usually treated as a cosmetic problem with a tattoo, cosmetic shell or contact lens. The eye is enucleated if painful or excessively large or ugly. In bilateral cases, if the infant is blind in both eyes corneal grafting may be indicated, with occasional good results.[17,18] The possibility of spontaneous improvement, and secondary complications in failures leads most experienced surgeons to prefer conservatism. Grafts in infants are often followed by myopia, especially if infant donor material is used.[19] This may be used to advantage in aphakic cases.

KERATITIS

Allergic

See Chapter 19.

Infection

See Chapter 19.

EXPOSURE KERATITIS

Exposure keratitis is a disorder of the ocular surface due to failure to maintain adequate lubrication and protection of the corneal epithelium, which results in its breakdown (Fig. 29.8). The cornea loses its luster, and this may be followed by punctate loss of corneal epithelium. Larger areas of epithelial loss are followed by thinning of the corneal stroma. In severe cases, corneal perforation can occur. Usually these cases are associated with a bacterial infection, which occurs because of the loss of protection afforded by the normal spread of tears.

Eyelid abnormalities may cause exposure keratitis.[16] An ectropion, for example, can result in poor eyelid apposition; the cornea, then, is relatively unprotected. Disorders of the lacrimal gland (e.g., tumors, congenital malfunctions, central nervous system disease, and radiation necrosis) result in poor lubrication of the corneal surface. Exophthalmos from orbit disease results in poor lid closure. Seventh nerve palsies affect closure of the eyelids (Fig. 29.9). Fifth nerve palsies also result in keratitis and combined fifth and seventh cranial nerve palsies cause the most serious problems especially if the eye is also dry. Sensory innervation of the cornea may play an important role in maintaining its integrity.[20] Blinking is also influenced by sensory input.

ACCIDENTAL AND NONACCIDENTAL INJURY

A spectrum of corneal injuries can occur in child abuse.[21] The corneal epithelium may be abraded, producing a characteristic stain when fluorescein is placed on the eye. Deeper injuries are produced when the object striking the eye is sharp. This has been reported to be self-inflicted in the ocular Munchausen syndrome.[22] Corneal perforation with flattening of the anterior chamber occurs rarely. The presence of lid ecchymoses

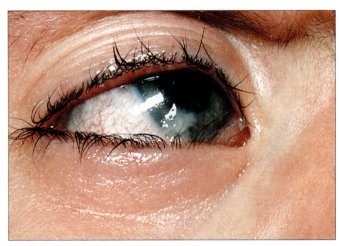

Fig. 29.9 Dry and exposed eye giving rise to keratitis in a patient with seventh nerve palsy associated with the CHARGE association.

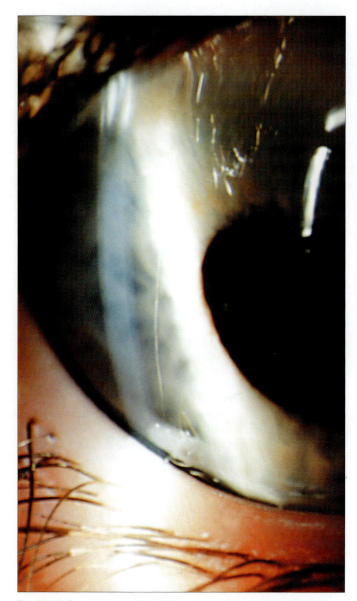

Fig. 29.10 Forceps injury. This child was born with an opalescent right cornea in a normal-sized eye. After a few months the cornea cleared, revealing vertical breaks in Descemet's membrane. The other eye was normal.

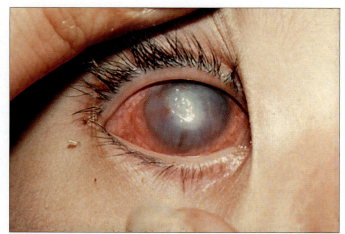

Fig. 29.11 Presumed nonaccidental chemical injury to the cornea. This child suddenly developed a profoundly severe keratitis in one eye on the day that his mother's boyfriend left home.

accompanying the corneal injury should arouse suspicion of abuse. A careful history and physical examination should be conducted, searching for other unexplained injuries.

Forceps injuries (Fig. 29.10) cause ruptures of Descemet's membrane usually in a vertical direction and are associated with high astigmatism in the axis of the ruptures, myopia, and deep amblyopia.[23] Chemical injuries, sometimes repeated, may be due to nonaccidental injury by the parents[24] (Fig. 29.11).

COGAN SYNDROME

Cogan syndrome consists of interstitial keratitis and audio-vestibular disease.[25] The cornea shows bilateral patchy stromal infiltrates, with vascularization and uveitis. Eventually, vascularization of the cornea occurs. The eighth nerve impairment may precede or follow corneal involvement. An association of this syndrome with polyarteritis nodosa has been described, and there are many case reports of this and other systemic associations.[26] The cause is unknown although immunological factors,[27] viral agents,[28] and vasculitis[29] have been implicated. The associated uveitis is treated with topical steroids or cyclosporin A.[30]

VITAMIN A DEFICIENCY AND MEASLES
(see Chapters 28 and 72)

Deficiency of vitamin A damages the cornea. The surface loses its normal luster, even though the eye is not always excessively dry. The tears show abnormal electrophoretic responses to measles infection, especially in malnourished children.[31] Corneal vascularization, keratinization, and edema can occur. When vitamin deficiency is accompanied by malnourishment and protein deficiency, an acute liquefactive necrosis of the cornea can occur (Fig. 29.12).

This is particularly marked when associated with measles infection, herpes simplex, or the use of traditional eye medicines.[32] If diagnosed early, some of these problems are reversible with vitamin A replacement and may be prevented by dietary measures, vitamin A replacement, and measles vaccination.[33] Higher doses of vitamin A are necessary when the child has worms or diarrhea.[34] The Bitot's spot is a triangular foamy-appearing lesion that occurs over the conjunctiva in vitamin A deficiency; its presence on the temporal side of the eye suggests active deficiency.[35] Vitamin A deficiency also causes night-blindness.

ECTODERMAL DYSPLASIA

Ectodermal dysplasia is a very rare (1:100,000 live births), usually X-linked or autosomal recessive, condition, with abnormal eccrine glands, wispy or absent hair, and abnormal teeth or nails. Innumerable syndromes make up the ectodermal dysplasia group, the two main groups being the hidrotic and the anhidrotic (or hypohidrotic) forms. Ocular involvement is usually limited to the anhidrotic forms.[36] General management poses numerous problems.[36,37]

Occasionally, corneal changes occur. Epithelial corneal cysts and opacities best seen with a slit lamp develop (Fig. 29.13). Pannus, the abnormal growth of superficial blood vessels onto the cornea, occurs. A dry-eye state may result from deficient tear

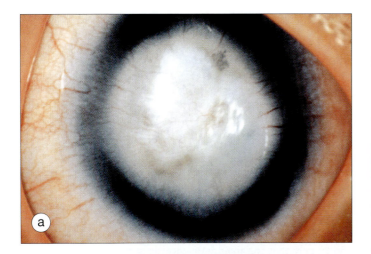

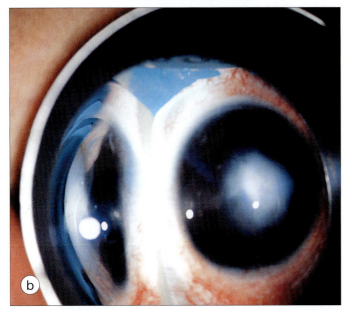

Fig. 29.12 (a) Keratomalacia showing the large axial scar. (b) Gonioscopic view showing the iris attached to the posterior surface of the cornea—leucoma adherens.

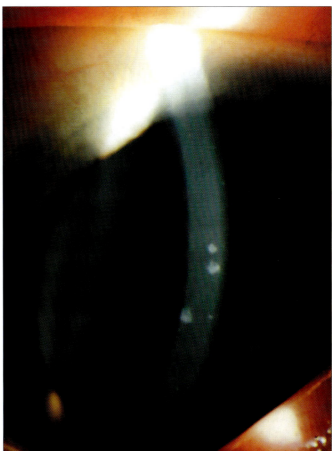

Fig. 29.13 Ectodermal dysplasia with small superficial corneal opacities.

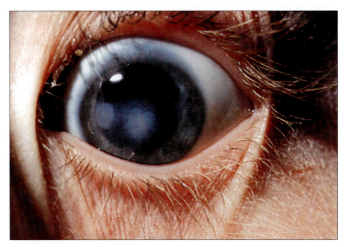

Fig. 29.14 Ectodermal dysplasia with an axial keratopathy: the acuity was 6/24.

production. A more severe keratopathy with severe visual consequences occurs in some cases (Fig. 29.14). This may be due to the combination of the underlying dysplasia, tear film abnormalities, and infection.[38] If the tear film is adequate, grafting may help but recent reports suggest that conjunctival limbal allograft may be most effective in addressing the deficiencies.[39]

EPIDERMOLYSIS BULLOSA

Severe corneal abnormalities are surprisingly infrequent in epidermolysis bullosa, but changes include limbal broadening, corneal reticular opacities at the level of Bowman's capsule, and symblepharon.[40] Symblepharon is more frequent in dystrophic epidermolysis bullosa.[41,42] Although the lesions are usually small and anterior, they may develop widespread corneal epithelial erosions and abrasions (Fig. 29.15).[42] In dystrophic epidermolysis bullosa, there are absent anchoring fibrils at the conjunctival dermoepidermal junction[43] and abnormal attachment complexes between the corneal epithelium and its basement membrane.[44] Laminin-5 is the major adhesion ligand for epithelial cells, and a

missense mutation in the adhesion G domain of Laminin-5 may be important in the pathogenesis of epidermolysis bullosa.[45]

ICHTHYOSIS

The ichthyosiform dermatoses are a group of disorders characterized by scaling. "Harlequin baby" and "collodion baby" are extreme congenital forms that may have congenital ectropion.[46] They frequently succumb to skin infections in the

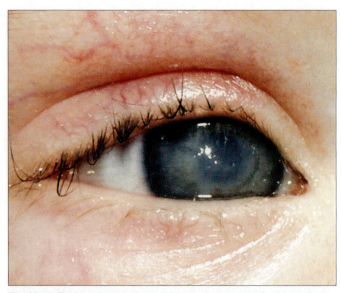

Fig. 29.15 Epidermolysis bullosa. Although many cases of epidermolysis bullosa do not have corneal changes, some, like this patient, develop acute epithelial erosions as a result of minor trauma, which if repeated result in permanent corneal opacity and vascularization.

neonatal period. Ichthyosis vulgaris is the most common form, inherited as an autosomal dominant trait, with scaling of the extensor surfaces and back. No eye problems occur.

X-linked ichthyosis is congenital and occurs in one in 6000 men.[47] Afflicted individuals note scaling of the scalp, face and neck, abdomen, and limbs; palms and soles are spared. Corneal nerves may be thickened and band keratopathy occurs as an isolated abnormality.[48] Superficial corneal lesions, which stain with fluorescein (Fig. 29.16a), occur; they are usually transient but recur and eventually cause superficial scarring. The scarring and superficial lesions may be caused by eyelid abnormalities, or may occur independently of eyelid problems.

Posterior corneal opacities are also known to occur. These opacities are small and located in deep corneal stroma or Descemet's membrane. Seldom do corneal lesions diminish visual acuity.[48]

Lamellar ichthyosis and ichthyosis linearis circumflexa are severe autosomal recessive disorders that give rise to ectropion

and keratoconjunctivitis mainly due to exposure.[49] Epidermolytic hyperkeratosis and erythrokeratoderma variabilis are two autosomal-dominant varieties. Ichthyosis also occurs in the Sjögren-Larsson syndrome, Netherton syndrome (ichthyosis, sparse hair, eyebrows, and eyelashes, and atopic diathesis), Refsum disease, chondrodysplasia punctata (see Chapter 65), IBIDS syndrome (ichthyosis, brittle hair, impaired intelligence, decreased fertility, and short stature), and the KID syndrome of ichthyosis, deafness, and keratitis (Fig. 29.16b).[50]

CORNEAL ANESTHESIA AND HYPOESTHESIA

Defective corneal sensation may give rise to a keratitis that is chronic, recurrent, and often severe. Although termed neurotropic, implying that the lack of some nerve factor is important, it is most likely that the main etiological factors are drying, reduced blinking, and repeated trivial trauma. Defective corneal sensation may arise from any cause of fifth nerve damage. As in adults, it occurs with trauma, herpes zoster ophthalmicus, developmental or acquired brain stem lesions, and tumors, in particular cerebellopontine angle or pontine tumors. It may occur with herpes simplex keratitis.[51]

In addition, corneal hypoesthesia has been described in leprosy, Goldenhar syndrome,[52] and other oculofacial syndromes.[53] It occurred in a family of Navajo Indians with an acromutilating neuropathy.[54] It can be found in a subclinical form in Adie pupil,[55] and in some corneal dystrophies.[56] It is common in the Riley-Day syndrome (Fig 29.17). It has been described in the MURCS association—Mullerian duct aplasia/hypoplasia, renal agenesis or ectopy, and cervicothoracic somite dysplasia.[57]

It may be unilateral,[58] familial,[59] and occasionally associated with fifth nerve motor involvement.[60] A proportion of these children have other neurological disorders. An interesting feature in some is an element of self-mutilation, which can be difficult to treat—elbow splinting being the most satisfactory method.[61]

Congenital corneal hypoesthesia may occur as an isolated abnormality, or with an associated trigeminal (usually first division) hypoesthesia. Because it is unusual it is often diagnosed late. When it is severe it may give rise to blinding keratitis.

Although in many cases the corneal anesthesia is part of a more widespread anesthesia,[54,62] it is most often confined to the cornea.[63] It may be unilateral. Familial cases have been recorded.[64]

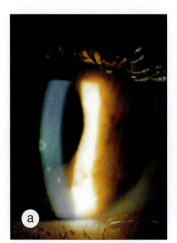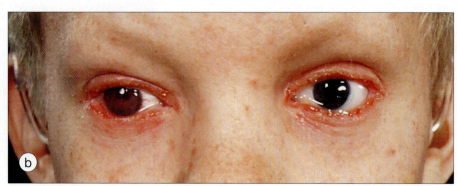

Fig. 29.16 (a) Ichthyosis with fluorescein-staining superficial corneal lesions. (b) KID syndrome with deafness (the patient is using hearing aids) and severe bilateral keratopathy. The left eye has been enucleated.

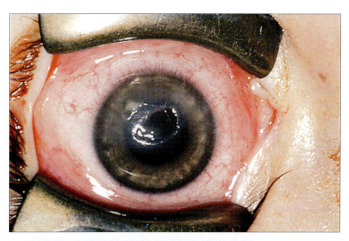

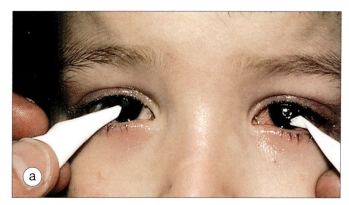

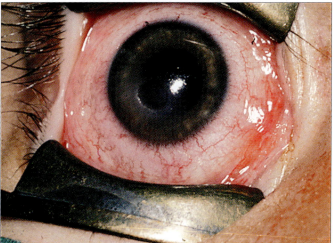

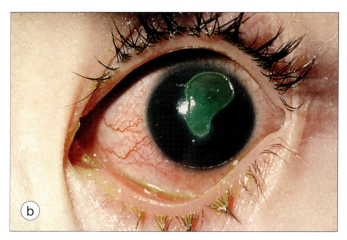

Fig. 29.17 Riley-Day syndrome. This child had a combination of anesthetic corneas and dry eyes that had been treated for several months by topical wetting agents without success. He responded well to a bilateral tarsorrhaphy and lubricant ointment. Later, punctal occlusion allowed enough wetting of his eyes to allow the tarsorrhaphies to be undone.

Children with neurotrophic keratitis (Fig. 29.18) are rarely diagnosed when they first present. It is the recurrent nature of the disease, and to a certain extent their relative lack of symptoms, that draws attention to the real cause. They have several attacks of redness, watering, and sometimes discharging eye. Pain may be present from an associated uveitis. Sometimes the presence of scars on the forehead gives the clue to trigeminal anesthesia. Care should be taken over the diagnosis, remembering that in almost any severe keratitis the corneal sensation may be reduced. As a general rule, unless combined with lagophthalmos or a dry eye, the corneal anesthesia must be profound to assure the diagnosis. The child is usually insensitive to any corneal stimulus; therefore care needs to be taken to avoid causing an abrasion. Repeated trauma may cause hypertrophic corneal scars.

Cases with lagophthalmos or defective tears (most anesthetic corneas are associated with reduced reflex tearing because an afferent of the tearing reflex is missing) are much more severe. This combination is seen in the Riley-Day syndrome, leprosy, and some brain stem lesions.

Treatment in small children is very difficult but it improves with age; it may require dedicated parents to avoid blindness. There are a variety of regimes, but the following regimes have been successful in most cases.

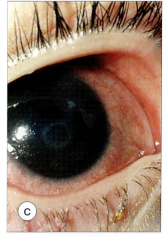

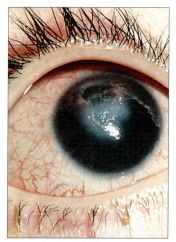

Fig. 29.18 (a) Profound corneal anesthesia that allows the eye to be touched and for keratitis to occur without pain. There are faint scars on the nose and forehead from painless recurrent trauma. (b) In this child acute episodes of erosion due to direct trauma resulted in corneal scarring. (c) Repeated corneal ulceration and keratitis gave rise to bilateral scarring.

Treatment in infancy

Acute cases are treated with frequent antibiotic drops (without preservative) and ointment with temporary taping of the eye. Frequent use of lubricant drops in mild cases is sufficient, but once keratitis has occurred more than once, the child must have the exposed area of the cornea reduced. Taping or gluing the lids or using protective bubble shields or spectacles is good as a temporary measure, but an early tarsorrhaphy is the most effective measure in the long term. An outer half or third tarsorrhaphy is used, remembering that it is easier to undo than to increase the procedure. Simple eye ointment (containing no antibiotic) is used at night, or day and night in severe cases. This can blur vision and may cause amblyopia in young children, so it should be used sparingly. Rubbing the eye may be a problem in infants and young children, especially if they are developmentally delayed: elbow splinting may be the only solution here.

Treatment in childhood

Children can usually be treated with simple ointment and antibiotics in the acute phase but more severe cases require a tarsorrhaphy, which is better done early than late.

CORNEAL TRAUMA

A condition mistaken for trauma is spontaneous corneal perforation in premature infants.[65]

KERATOCONUS

Keratoconus is a condition causing usually bilateral, central thinning of the cornea. It occurs with a frequency of 1:2000 in the general population.[66] It usually starts in adolescence and may progress rapidly or stabilize. The younger the presentation and the occurrence in black people are poor prognostic factors.[66] Keratoconus is occasionally familial; it may occur with atopy, floppy lids, Down syndrome, Marfan syndrome, retinal dystrophies, congenital cone/rod dystrophy, aniridia, Ehlers-Danlos syndrome, congenital rubella, and mitral valve prolapse.[66] Posterior polymorphous dystrophy (PPMD) is a condition characterized by vesicular lesions of the posterior cornea and by epithelialization of corneal endothelium. Keratoconus may occasionally occur in PPMD.[67] Recent studies suggest that a common gene may account for some cases of both PPMD and keratoconus.[68]

First symptoms are usually related to visual impairment. Corneal thinning leads to increasing amounts of astigmatism (Fig. 29.19). Ultimately, contact lens use becomes necessary to compensate for irregular corneal curvature because spectacle correction is inadequate.

When Descemet's membrane is stretched beyond its breaking point, it may rupture. This condition is called acute hydrops (Fig. 29.20). The symptoms of hydrops are blurred vision, caused by corneal edema, and pain. Hydrops resolves in several months, leaving variable corneal scarring; treatment is usually conservative, as padding and bandaging the eye are successful even in severe cases, although where neovascularization occurs, early grafting may be indicated.[69] Videokeratography has proven to be a very useful tool in establishing the diagnosis early in the course of this disorder.[66,70]

Most cases of keratoconus can be managed conservatively, with contact lenses.[66] Occasionally corneal transplant is indicated. Both lamellar and penetrating keratoplasty have been used to treat keratoconus.[71] Other less orthodox therapies include intrastromal corneal rings[72] and astigmatic keratotomy and intraocular lenses.[73]

Although the pathophysiology of keratoconus is incompletely understood, it appears that degradative enzymes (lysosomal acid phosphatase and cathepsin B) are upregulated and inhibitory enzymes (alpha-1 proteinase inhibitor and alpha-2 macroglobulin) are downregulated.[66,74] The interleukin-1 system may also be involved.[66]

KERATOGLOBUS

In keratoconus, the stromal thinning occurs in the center of the cornea; in keratoglobus, which may occur in families with keratoconus, the thinning is in the mid-periphery. The result is that the cornea takes on a globular rather than conical appearance. This can often be appreciated by standing over the patient's head and looking down on the protruding cornea. Keratoglobus may be associated with blue sclerae,[75] joint hyperextensibility, deafness, and mottled teeth.[76] The collagen defect in these patients may give rise to perforation of the eye after minimal trauma.

Acute keratoglobus is a form of hydrops, as in keratoconus; it occurs in Down syndrome and the Rubinstein-Taybi syndrome.

METABOLIC DISEASES AND THE CORNEA
(see Chapter 65)

Metabolic diseases, by abnormal accumulation of enzymatic byproducts, can stain the cornea. Systemic medications, like

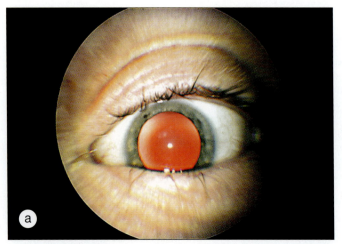
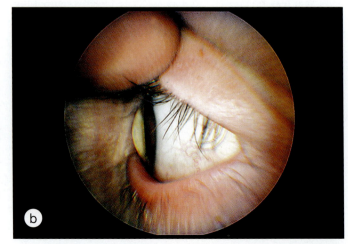

Fig. 29.19 Keratoconus. (a) The retinoscopy reflex in keratoconus is abnormal with no clear end point. (b) Side view showing the conical corneal and the outward bowing of the lower lid (Munson's sign).

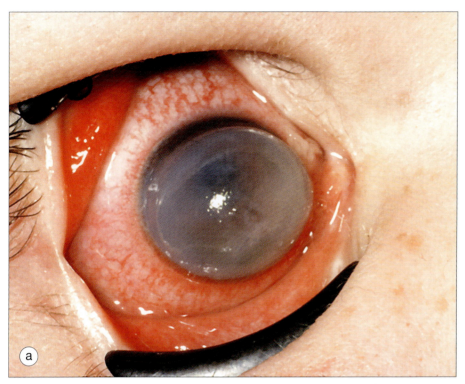

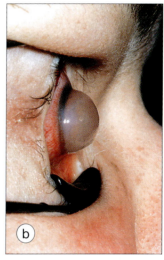

Fig. 29.20 (a) Acute hydrops in a child with Down syndrome and keratoconus. (b) Same patient. Side view showing extreme keratoglobus. After using elbow restraints to stop her rubbing her eyes, bilateral tarsorrhaphies, and padding of the eye, the keratoglobus resolved and became asymptomatic but vision was reduced by axial scarring.

chloroquine and amiodarone, form deposits in the cornea. Sometimes the cornea is secondarily altered by ocular disease (band keratopathy). Occasionally, the degree of accumulation is enough to degrade vision. Some toxic diseases can be diagnosed by the pattern of corneal involvement.

The corneal epithelium may be stained by toxins. Chloroquine diphosphate and hydroxychloroquine sulfate are used to treat malaria and systemic lupus erythematosus. These compounds stain the corneal epithelium and form whorl-like opacities. Amiodarone, Fabry disease, and mucolipidosis type IV (Fig. 29.21) also induce a vortex pattern of corneal epithelium staining although in the case amiodarone changes are also seen in the stroma and endothelium.[77] Indometacin can cause fine opacities

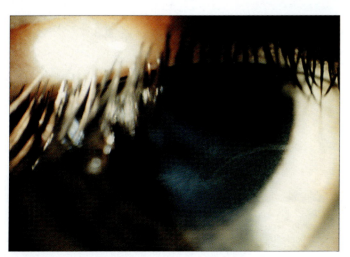

Fig. 29.21 Corneal verticillata in mucolipidosis type IV.

in the corneal epithelium. A vortex-like pattern is sometimes seen in corneal edema.

Wilson disease is an inherited disorder of copper metabolism. Low levels of the copper-transporting protein, ceruloplasmin, accompany low serum and high tissue levels of copper. More than two-hundred mutations of the gene, ATP7B (which is on chromosome 13q143 and encodes a P-type ATPase), have been identified.[78]

Wilson disease usually presents in the second decade of life. Four organ systems are involved. Central nervous system involvement leads to basal ganglia degeneration with tremor, choreoathetosis, and neuropsychiatric changes. Renal tubular damage causes aminoaciduria. The liver is affected by nodular cirrhosis. The cornea often develops staining of the peripheral Descemet's membrane, most marked in the 12 and 6 o'clock positions (Kayser-Fleischer ring, see Chap. 65, Fig. 65.24). The stain, which is due to copper deposition, is brown-green and is best seen at the slit lamp. Gonioscopy may be necessary for visualization in some cases. The ring is not absolutely pathognomonic of Wilson disease; other causes of liver failure, carotenemia, and multiple myeloma may lead to a similar ring.[79]

In Wilson disease, a rare but characteristic abnormality is the "sunflower" subcapsular cataract. Penicillamine is the drug of choice, but trientine and zinc may be safe and effective; liver transplant may be necessary.[80] Abnormalities of both the electroretinogram and visual-evoked potentials suggest that the retina and/or optic nerve may also be affected.[81]

Acrodermatitis enteropathica is associated with radial, subepithelial lines in the superior portion of the cornea. The lines are whorl-like and pass from the corneoscleral junction toward the center of the cornea. Keratomalacia may be associated.[82] This rare dermatitis is characterized by an asymmetrical rash that begins in infancy. The nails are dystrophic. A gastrointestinal disturbance causes diarrhea and poor growth; it is treated successfully with zinc dietary supplements.

In cystinosis (see Chapter 65), a defect in lysosomal transport leads to accumulation of cystine in lysosomes. Mutations in the gene that codes for cystinosin, the integral membrane protein responsible for membrane transport of cystine, are responsible.[83] Growth retardation, renal failure, decreased skin and hair pigmentation, and corneal crystalline deposits occur. Infantile cystinosis causes renal failure and early death. Corneal crystals are detected as early as 2 months of age. They start anteriorly, progressing posteriorly.[84] A pigmentary retinopathy also develops. Congenitally narrowed angles and a ciliary body configuration similar to plateau iris syndrome coupled with crystalline deposits in the trabecular meshwork apparently account for the increased risk of glaucoma.[85] An adult form of cystinosis (nonnephropathic) causes corneal deposits but no systemic manifestations. The adolescent form resembles the infantile form, with the absence of growth retardation and skin hypopigmentation.

Although corneal crystals in cystinosis are mainly in the anterior stroma (Fig. 29.22), they occur in all tissues and the cornea is thick.[84] They seldom reduce visual acuity, but photophobia is frequent. The glare disability may be profound. Patients may also have an abnormal contrast sensitivity and reduced corneal sensitivity.[86] A superficial punctate keratopathy and recurrent erosions occur. The crystals have different morphologies depending on the site.[87] Cysteamine treatment has been shown to have beneficial effects.[88,89] Corneal grafts may remain clear at least in the medium term.[90]

Photic sneezes have been described in cystinosis.[91] They may also be autosomal dominantly inherited.[92]

CORNEAL CRYSTALS

Crystalline corneal deposits or crystal-like deposits occur under the following conditions:

1. Cystinosis.
2. Crystalline corneal dystrophy (Schnyder dystrophy):
   (a) This may present in infancy;
   (b) There are anterior central corneal ring-like aggregations of stromal crystals that may be yellowish and hard; they are composed of cholesterol;[93]
   (c) They are usually asymptomatic, it does not affect the epithelium;
   (d) It may be autosomal dominant;[93]
   (e) It may be accompanied by an arcus lipoides and white limbus girdle; and
   (f) There are not usually systemic associations.[94]
3. Lecithin cholesterol acyltransferase (LCAT) deficiency disease.
4. Uric acid crystals (brownish-colored).
5. Granular dystrophy and Bietti marginal dystrophy.[95]
6. Multiple myeloma. In the monoclonal gammopathies, crystals are rare.[96]
7. Calcium deposition.
8. Dieffenbachian plant keratoconjunctivitis.[97]
9. A syndrome of corneal crystals, myopathy, and nephropathy.[98]
10. Keratopathy in mesoendemic onchocercal communities.[99]
11. Tyrosinemia type II—the Richner-Hanhart syndrome (see Chapter 65):
    (a) Plaque-like pseudodendritic lesions with crystalline edges that are intra- and subepithelial, raised, bilateral, and conjunctival occur; thickening also occurs;
    (b) Children usually present with photophobia and watering eyes;
    (c) Ulceration occurs;
    (d) Steroid treatment may help corneal lesions;
    (e) A low-tyrosine, low-phenylalanine diet may rapidly abolish the symptoms[100] and prevent recurrence;
    (f) Mental and physical retardation may be present;
    (g) The skin lesions occur particularly on the pressure areas of the palms and soles (Fig. 29.23);[101] and
    (h) Significant intrafamilial phenotypic variation occurs.

BAND KERATOPATHY

Band keratopathy is the result of ocular inflammation or systemic disease. The band (Fig. 29.24) occurs in the region between the

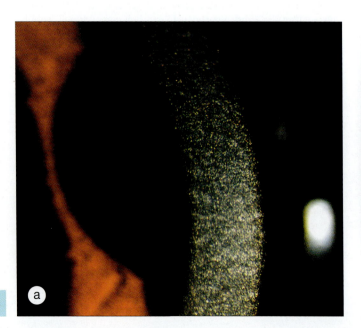

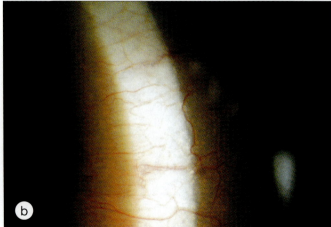

Fig. 29.22 Cystinosis. (a) Corneal crystals can be seen by slit-lamp microscopy. The children are often blonde, fair-skinned, and very photophobic. (b) Crystal deposition occurs in many tissues throughout the body, including the conjunctiva, which can be seen here on slit-lamp biomicroscopy.

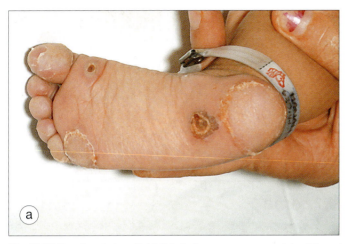
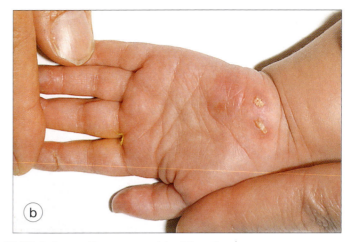

Fig. 29.23 Tyrosinemia type II. (a) Skin lesions on pressure points of the sole. (b) Skin lesions on the pressure points of the palms.

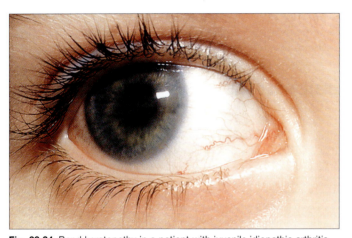

Fig. 29.24 Band keratopathy in a patient with juvenile idiopathic arthritis (see Chapter 44)

mutations in the LCAT gene are associated with fish-eye disease.[104] Premature arcus senilis develops in heterozygotes. LCAT esterifies free cholesterol for use in the synthesis of cell membranes. Its absence causes proteinuria, renal failure, anemia, and hyperlipidemia.

CORNEAL ARCUS

Arcus lipoides is due to a deposition of a variety of phospholipids, low-density lipoproteins, and triglycerides in the stroma of the peripheral cornea (Fig. 29.25). Unlike xanthomas, corneal arcus is not invariably associated with hyperlipidemia, but when corneal arcus appears in youth it is highly suggestive of raised plasma low-density lipoproteins. Arcus is not correlated with plasma high-density lipoprotein or very-low-density lipoprotein. Arcus appears in youth in familial hypercholesterolemia (Fredrickson type II) and in familial hyperlipoproteinemia (type III).

Arcus lipoides may also occur in children adjacent to areas of corneal disease including vernal keratopathy (Fig. 29.26), herpes simplex, and limbal dermoid.

Disorders of high-density lipoprotein metabolism tend to cause diffuse corneal clouding; these include LCAT disease, Tangier disease, fish-eye disease, and apoprotein A1 absence; occasionally, however, an arcus-like peripheral condensation occurs.

Primary lipoidal degeneration of the cornea is an arcus that occurs in a healthy cornea in a person with normal plasma lipids.

eyelids (interpalpebral region), usually with a clear region between the band and the corneoscleral limbus. Bowman's membrane is infiltrated with calcium and eventually will be destroyed. The deposits of calcium take on a "Swiss-cheese" appearance, which helps distinguish this condition from simple corneal calcific degeneration. This latter condition is the end product of phthisis bulbi or a necrotic ocular tumour and may involve all corneal layers.

Any condition causing systemic hypercalcemia can cause band keratopathy. Thus, sarcoidosis, parathyroid disease, and multiple myeloma are occasionally associated with a band. Chronic ocular inflammation also causes band keratopathy. This is most characteristic in juvenile idiopathic arthritis in its pauciarticular form (Chapter 44). Prolonged corneal edema and glaucoma rarely lead to band formation. Toxic mercury vapors or eye drops and gout are uncommonly associated with band keratopathy. Gouty band keratopathy differs from other causes by being brown. Band keratopathy may occur with some forms of ichthyosis.[48] A rare band-shaped spheroidal keratopathy has been reported in China.[102]

LECITHIN CHOLESTEROL ACYLTRANSFERASE DEFICIENCY

LCAT deficiency is a rare autosomal recessive condition that causes a central corneal haze in homozygotes.[103] At least two

WHITE OR CLOUDY CORNEA AT BIRTH

The white cornea at birth poses an important differential diagnosis. The first consideration is that the newborn suffers congenital glaucoma. The corneal diameter will be large (due to expansion of the globe from increased pressure). Ruptures in Descemet's membrane that are limbus parallel may be present. Intraocular pressure is elevated. The optic nerves will show increased cupping. Urgent intervention in the form of surgery is usually indicated if vision is to be preserved.

In most countries the most common cause of a congenitally opaque cornea is a developmental abnormality of the anterior segment. The next possibility is a forceps injury. Forceps marks may be visible on the lids or cheek. A linear, usually vertical, rupture of Descemet's membrane will be present. This causes

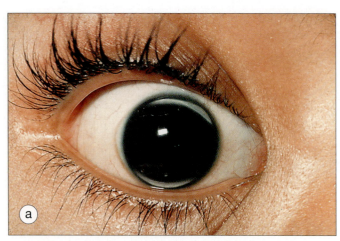
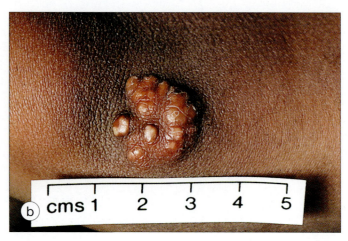

Fig. 29.25 (a) Corneal arcus in a patient with hyperlipidemia. (b) Skin xanthoma in hypercholesterolemia.

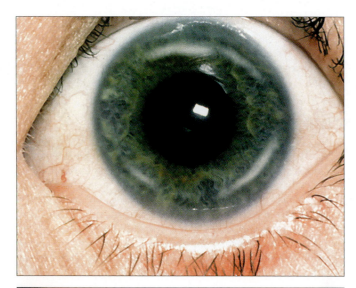

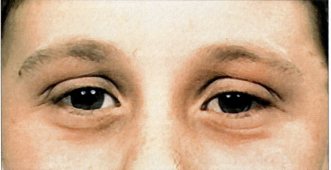

Fig. 29.26 Corneal arcus remaining in a child who had had severe vernal catarrh.

corneal edema. Edema always resolves, leaving varying degrees of astigmatism. Late corneal decompensation is possible.

Certain metabolic conditions are in the differential diagnosis. Cystinosis rarely causes a cloudy cornea at birth. Mucopolysaccharidoses, occasionally present as congenital cloudy cornea, and rare conditions such as acromesomelic dysplasia may have congenital scarring.[105]

Congenital hereditary corneal dystrophy usually presents in the first months of life. A rare Bowman's layer dysgenesis may cause congenital corneal clouding.

Infection of the cornea will also cause it to turn white. Rubella keratitis should be considered. Neonatal infection with *Gonococcus* is also in the differential diagnosis.

BLUE SCLERAE

Hereditary conditions that cause a defect in the mesodermal structures will produce a blue-appearing sclera. The characteristic blue discoloration is probably related to thinning of the sclera. In a study by Chan et al., a defect in the fine structure of collagen fibrils was the morphological abnormality that explained blue sclera.[106] Blue sclera is a consistent finding in osteogenesis imperfecta. This condition is associated with brittle bones and a conductive hearing loss. Six types of osteogenesis imperfecta have been described; four of these are autosomal dominantly inherited and two are recessive. Autosomal recessive osteogenesis imperfecta is characterized by early infant death or severe growth retardation.

Blue sclera also occurs in the Ehlers-Danlos syndrome. The Ehlers-Danlos syndrome is a heterogeneous group of disorders with characteristics such as fragile skin and hypermobile joints. At least 10 types have been described, all of which may show blue sclera. Ocular findings in Ehlers-Danlos include spontaneous corneal rupture, keratoglobus, cornea plana, peripheral sclerocornea, and microcornea.[76,107]

Rarely, blue sclera occurs in the Hallermann-Streiff syndrome and Marfan syndrome and in association with brittle corneas[108] or ectodermal dysplasia.[37] In infancy many normal children have blueish corneas and some myopic children also have the same appearance.

HYPHEMA AND CORNEAL BLOOD STAINING

Blood staining of the cornea is an important and devastating complication of hyphema. Generally, duration of hyphema, degree of elevation of intraocular pressure, the integrity of the corneal endothelium, and the occurrence of secondary hemorrhages are the factors associated with staining. The doctor should observe the patient with hyphema at least daily, administering non-aspirin-containing analgesics and acetazolamide if the intraocular pressure is raised, and, when staining of the cornea is suspected, an anterior chamber lavage may be recommended; the efficacy of antifibrinolytic drugs is not established.[109] Corneal blood staining may occur within 3 days if the intraocular pressure is high.

The incidence in one series was 17 per 100,000 pediatric population per year.[110] Rebleeds occurred in 7.6% but did not correlate with age or the use of cycloplegics or steroids. Ninety-one percent of this series achieved acuity of 20/30 or better. Amblyopia occurred in the two children who required cataract extraction of the 316 in the series.

CORNEAL NERVES

Corneal nerves are visible in the periphery of the cornea in normal people but they may be more visible under certain conditions, including the following:[111]

1. Dystrophies: Fuchs corneal dystrophy, keratoconus;
2. Buphthalmos;
3. Inflammatory disease: leprosy; after corneal grafts; corneal trauma;
4. Refsum disease;
5. Ichthyosis;
6. Multiple endocrine neoplasia (MEN) type IIb (Fig. 29.27); and
7. Neurofibromatosis—rare, may have MENIIb.[112]

MULTIPLE ENDOCRINE NEOPLASIA

There are three main syndromes in which tumours occur in a variety of endocrine organs at a young age. For the ophthalmologist the most prominent of these is MEN type IIb. Patients show a marfanoid habitus, full and fleshy lips, and nodular neuromas on the tip and edges of the tongue and on the margins of the eyelids.[113] Pes cavus, constipation, and peroneal muscular atrophy are due to neuroma formation.[114] It is autosomal

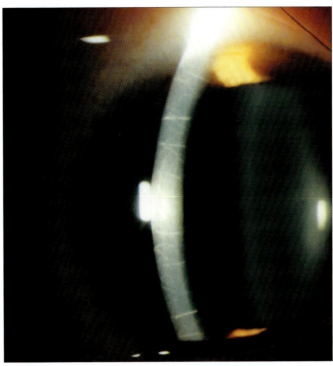

Fig. 29.27 Multiple endocrine neoplasia type IIb. Thickened corneal nerves can be seen crossing even the axial area of the cornea.

dominantly inherited. Prominent corneal nerves within an otherwise normal cornea and nodular subconjunctival tumors are an important diagnostic feature.[113] Because of a very high incidence of thyroid medullary carcinoma in MEN type IIb, prophylactic thyroidectomy may be recommended in childhood. Pheochromocytoma also occurs. Somewhat enlarged corneal nerves may occur in MEN type Ia.[115]

REFERENCES

1. Frangoulis M, Taylor D. Corneal opacities—a diagnostic feature of the trisomy 8 mosaic syndrome. Br J Ophthalmol 1983; 67: 619–22.
2. Mansour AM, Barber JC, Reinecke RD, Wang FM. Ocular choristomas. Surv Ophthalmol 1989; 33: 339–58.
3. Murata T, Ishibashi T, Ohnishi Y, Inomata H. Corneal choristoma with microphthalmos. Arch Ophthalmol 1991; 109: 1130–3.
4. Oakman J, Lambert S, Grossniklaus H. Corneal dermoid: case report and review of classification. J Pediatr Ophthalmol Strabismus 1993; 30: 388–91.
5. Dar P, Javed AA, Ben-Yashay A, et al. Potential mapping of corneal dermoids Xq24-qter. J Med Genet 2001; 38: 719–23.
6. Topilow HW, Cykiert RC, Goldman K, et al. Bilateral corneal dermis-like choristoma: an X-chromosome-linked disorder. Arch Ophthalmol 1981; 99: 1387–91.
7. Mansour AM, Wang F, Henkind P, et al. Ocular findings in facio-auriculovertebral sequence (Goldenhar-Gerlin syndrome). Am J Ophthalmol 1985; 100: 555–9.
8. Kodsi SR, Bloom KE, Egbert JE, et al. Ocular and systemic manifestations of encephalocraniocutaneous lipomatosis. Am J Ophthalmol 1994; 118: 77–82.
9. Vangsted P, Limpaphayom P. Dermoid of the cornea in association with congenital generalized fibromatosis. A case report. Acta Ophthalmol 1983; 61: 927–33.
10. Mansour AM, Laibson P, Reinecke R, et al. Bilateral total corneal and conjunctival choristomas associated with epidermal nevus. Arch Ophthalmol 1986; 104: 245–8.

11. Hoops JP, Ludwig K, Boergen KP, Kampik A. Preoperative evaluation of limbal dermoids using high-resolution biomicroscopy. Graefes Arch Clin Exp Ophthalmol 2001; 23: 459–61.
12. Watts P, Michaeli-Cohen A, Abdoleil M. Outcome of lamellar keratoplasty for limbal dermoids in children. J AAPOS 2002; 6: 209–15.
13. Schanzlin DJ, Robin JB, Erickson G, et al. Histopathologic and ultrastructural analysis of congenital corneal staphyloma. Am J Ophthalmol 1983; 95: 506–14.
14. Klauss V, Reidel K. Bilateral and unilateral mesodermal corneal metaplasia. Br J Ophthalmol 1983; 67: 320–3.
15. Miller MM, Butrus S, Hidayat A, et al. Corneoscleral transplantation in congenital corneal staphyloma and Peter's anomaly. Ophthalmic Genet 2003; 24: 59–63.
16. Miller MT, Deutsch TA, Cronin C, Keys CL. Amniotic bands as a cause of ocular anomalies. Am J Ophthalmol 1987; 104: 270–9.
17. Hertle RW, Orlin SE. Successful rehabilitation after neonatal penetrating keratoplasty. Br J Ophthalmol 1997; 81: 644–8.
18. Cowden JW. Penetrating keratoplasty in infants and children. Ophthalmology 1990; 97: 324–8.
19. Gloor P, Keech RV, Krachmer JH. Factors associated with high postoperative myopia after penetrating keratoplasties in infants. Ophthalmology 1992; 99: 775–9.
20. Schimmelpfennig B, Beurman RW. Evidence for neurotropism in the cornea (abstract). Invest Ophthalmol Vis Sci 1979; 18: 125.
21. Levine LM. Pediatric ocular trauma and shaken infant syndrome. Pediatr Clin North AM 2003; 50: 137–48.
22. Voutilanen R, Tuppurainen K. Ocular Munchausen syndrome induced by incest. Acta Ophthalmol (COPENH) 1989; 67: 319–21.

23. Angell LK, Robb RM, Benson FG. Visual prognosis in patients with ruptures in Descemet's membrane due to forceps injuries. Arch Ophthalmol 1981; 99: 2137–9.

24. Taylor D, Bentovim A. Recurrent nonaccidentally inflicted chemical eye injuries to siblings. J Pediatr Ophthalmol Strabismus 1976; 13: 238–42.

25. Cogan DG. Syndrome of non-syphilitic interstitial keratitis and vestibular auditory symptoms. Arch Ophthalmol 1945; 33: 144–9.

26. Orsoni JG, Zavota L, Pellistri I, et al. Cogan syndrome. Cornea 2002; 21: 356–9.

27. Cogan DG, Sullivan WR. Immunologic study of non-syphilitic interstitial keratitis with vestibuloauditory symptoms. Am J Ophthalmol 1975; 80: 491–5.

28. Darougar S, John AC, Viswalingam M, et al. Isolation of Chlamydia psittaci from a patient with interstitial keratitis and uveitis associated with otological and cardiovascular lesions. Br J Ophthalmol 1978; 62: 709–13.

29. Podder S, Shepherd R. Cogan syndrome: a rare systemic vasculitis. Arch Dis Child 1994; 71: 163–4.

30. Shimura M, Yashuda K, Fuse N, et al. Effective treatment with topical cyclosporin A of a patient with Cogan syndrome. Opthalmologica 2000; 214: 429–32.

31. Kogbe O, Listet S. Tear electrophoretic changes in Nigerian children after measles. Br J Ophthalmol 1987; 71: 326–30.

32. Foster A, Sommer A. Corneal ulceration, measles and childhood blindness in Tanzania. Br J Ophthalmol 1987; 71: 331–43.

33. Kello AB, Gilbert C. Causes of severe visual impairment and blindness in children in schools for the blind in Ethiopia. Br J Ophthalmol 2003; 87: 526–30.

34. Gujral S, Abbi R, Golpaldas T. Xerophthalmia, vitamin A supplementation and morbidity in children. J Trop Pediatr 1993; 39: 89–92.

35. Sommer A. Renewed interest in the ancient scourge xerophthalmia (editorial). Am J Ophthalmol 1978; 86: 284–5.

36. Donahue SP, Shea CJ, Taravella MJ. Hidrotic ectodermal dysplasia with corneal involvement. J AAPOS 1999; 3: 372–5.

37. Wilson FM, Grayson M, Pieroni D. Corneal changes in ectodermal dysplasia: case report, histopathology and differential diagnosis. Am J Ophthalmol 1973; 75: 17–27.

38. Mawhorter LG, Ruttum MS, Koenig SR. Keratopathy in a family with the ectrodactyly ectodermal dysplasia clefting syndrome. Ophthalmology 1985; 92: 1427–31.

39. Daya SM, Ilari FA. Living related conjunctival limbal allograft for the treatment of stem cell deficiency. Ophthalmology 2001; 108: 126–33.

40. McDonnell PJ, Spalton DJ. The ocular signs and complications of epidermolysis bullosa. J Roy Soc Med 1988; 81: 576–8.

41. Deplus S, Bremond-Gignac D, Blanchet-Bardon C. Review of ophthalmological complications in hereditary bullous epidermalysis. J Fr Ophthalmol 1999; 22: 760–5.

42. Lin A, Murphy F, Brodie S, Carter DM. Review of ophthalmic findings in 204 patients with epidermolysis bullosa. Am J Ophthalmol 1994; 118: 384–90.

43. Iwamoto M, Haik BG, Iwamoto T, et al. The ultrastructural defect in conjunctiva from a case of recessive dystrophic epidermolysis bullosa. Arch Ophthalmol 1991; 109: 1382–6.

44. Adamis AP, Schein OD, Kenyon KR. Anterior corneal disease of epidermolysis bullosa simplex. Arch Ophthalmol 1993; 111: 499–502.

45. Scaturro M, Posteraro P, Mastrogiacomo A, et al. A missense mutation (G1506E) in the adhesion G domain of laminin-5 causes mild junctional epidermolysis bullosa. Biochem Biophys Res Comun 2003; 309: 96–103.

46. Orth DH, Fretzin DF, Abramson V. Collodian baby with transient bilateral upper lid ectropion. Review of ocular manifestations in ichthyosis. Arch Ophthalmol 1974; 91: 206–7.

47. Wells RS, Kerr CB. Clinical features of autosomal dominance in sex-linked ichthyosis in an English population. Br Med J 1966; 1: 947.

48. Jay B, Blach RK, Wells RS. Ocular manifestations of ichthyosis. Br J Ophthalmol 1968; 52: 217–26.

49. Katowitz JA, Yolles EA, Yanoff M. Ichthyosis congenita. Arch Ophthalmol 1974; 91: 208–10.

50. Derse M, Wannke E, Payer H. Successful topical cyclosporin A in the therapy of progressive vascularising keratitis in keratitis-ichythosis-deafness (KID) syndrome. Kiln Monatsbl Augenhilkd 2002; 219: 383–6.

51. Shields JA, Waring GO, Monte LG. Ocular findings in leprosy. Am J Ophthalmol 1974; 77: 880–90.

52. Mohandessan MM, Romano PE. Neuroparalytic keratitis in Goldenhar-Gorlin syndrome. Am J Ophthalmol 1978; 85: 111–3.

53. Bowen DI, Collum LM, Rees DO. Clinical aspects of oculo-auriculo-vertebral dysplasia. Br J Ophthalmol 1971; 55: 145–54.

54. Appenzeller O, Kornfeld M, Snyder R. Acromutilating paralyzing neuropathy with corneal ulceration in Navajo children. Arch Neurol 1976; 33: 733–8.

55. Purcell JJ, Krachmer JH, Thompson HS. Corneal sensation in Adie's pupil. Am J Ophthalmol 1977; 84: 496–500.

56. Birndorff LA, Ginsberg SP. Hereditary fleck dystrophy associated with decreased corneal sensitivity. Am J Ophthalmol 1972; 73: 670–2.

57. Esakowitz L, Yates JR. Congenital corneal anaesthesia and the MURCs association: a case report. Br J Ophthalmol 1988; 72: 236–9.

58. Hennis HL, Saunders RA. Unilateral corneal anesthesia. Am J Ophthalmol 1989; 108: 331–2.

59. Keys C, Sugar J, Mafee M. Familial trigeminal anesthesia. Arch Ophthalmol 1990; 108: 1720–3.

60. Heath JD, Long G. Neurotropic keratitis presenting in infancy with involvement of the motor component of the trigeminal nerve. Br J Ophthalmol 1993; 77: 679–80.

61. Trope GE, Jay JL, Dudgeon J, Woodruff G. Self-inflicted corneal injuries in children with congenital anaesthesia. Br J Ophthalmol 1985; 69: 551–4.

62. Manfredi M, Bini G, Cruccu G, et al. Congenital absence of pain. Arch Neurol 1981; 38: 507–11.

63. Carpel EF. Congenital corneal anesthesia. Am J Ophthalmol 1978; 85: 357–9.

64. Wong VA, Cline RA, Dubord PJ, Rees M. Congenital trigemimal anesthesia in two siblings and their long-term followup. Am J Ophthalmol 2000; 129: 96–8.

65. Bachynski BN, Andreu R, Flynn JR. Spontaneous corneal perforation and extrusion of intraocular contents in premature infants. J Pediatr Ophthalmol Strabismus 1986; 23: 25–8.

66. Rabinowitz YG. Keratoconus. Surv Ophthalmol 1998; 42: 297–319.

67. Driver PJ, Reed JW, Davis RH. Familial cases of keratoconus associated with posterior polymorphous dystrophy. Am J Ophthalmol 1994; 118: 256–7.

68. Heon E, Greenberg A, Kopp KK, et al. VSX1: a gene for posterior polymorphous dystrophy and keratoconus. Hum Mol Genet 2002; 11: 1029–36.

69. Rowson N, Dart J, Buckley R. Corneal neovascularisation in acute hydrops. Eye 1992; 6: 404–6.

70. Totan Y, Hepsen IF, Cekic O, et al. Incidence of keratoconus in subjects with vernal keratoconjunctivitis: a video keratographic study. Ophthalmology 2001; 108: 824–7.

71. Coombs AG, Kirnan JF, Rostron CK. Deep lamellar keratoplasty with lophilised tissue in the management of keratoconus. Br J Ophthalmol 2001; 85: 788–91.

72. Colin J, Simonpoli-Velou S. The management of keratoconus with intrastromal corneal rings. Int Ophthalmol Clin 2003; 43: 65–80.

73. Rowsey JJ, Gills JP, Gills P. Treating keratoconus with astigmatic keratotomy and intraocular lenses. Int Ophthalmol Clin 2003; 43: 81–92.

74. Maruyama Y, Wang X, Li Y, et al. Involvement of Sp1 elements in the promoter activity of genes affected in keratoconus. Invest Ophthalmol Vis Sci 2001; 42: 1980–5.

75. Hyams SW, Kar H, Neumann E. Blue sclerae and keratoglobus. Ocular signs of a systemic connective tissue disorder. Br J Ophthalmol 1969; 53: 53–8.

76. Biglan AW, Brown SI, Johnson BL. Keratoglobus and blue sclerae. Am J Ophthalmol 1977; 83: 225–33.

77. Ciancaglini M, Carpineto P, Zuppardi E, et al. In vivo confocal microscopy of patients with amiodarone-induced keratopathy. Cornea 2001; 20: 368–73.

78. Ferenci P, Caca K, Loudianos G, et al. Diagnosis and phenotypic classification of Wilson disease. Liver Int 2003; 23: 139–42.

79. Liu M, Cohen EJ, Brewer GJ, Laibson PR. Kayser-Fleischer ring as

presenting sign of Wilson disease. Am J Ophthalmol 2002; 133: 832–4.

80. Yarze JC, Martin P, Munoz SJ, Friedman LS. Wilson's disease: current status. Am J Med 1992; 92: 643–54.

81. Satishchandra P, Ravishankar Naik K. Visual pathway abnormalities in Wilson's disease: an electrophysiological study using electroretinography and visual evoked potentials. J Neuro Sci 2000; 176: 13–20.

82. Feldberg R, Yassur Y, Ben-Sira I, et al. Keratomalacia in acrodermatitis enteropathica. Metab Pediatr Ophthalmol 1981; 5: 207–11.

83. Mason S, Pepe G, Dall'Amico R, et al. Mutational spectrum of CTNS gene in Italy. Eur J Hum Genet 2003; 11: 503–8.

84. Grupcheva CN, Omonde SE, McGhee C. In vivo confocal microscopy of the cornea in nephropathic cystinosis. Arch Ophthalmol 2002; 120: 1742–5.

85. Mungan N, Nischal KK, Heon E, et al. Ultrasound biomicroscopy of the eye in cystinosis. Arch Opthalmol 2000; 118: 1329–33.

86. Katz B, Melles RB, Schneider JA. Corneal sensitivity in nephropathic cystinosis. Am J Ophthalmol 1987; 104: 413–16.

87. Frazier PD, Wong VG. Cystinosis. Histologic and crystallographic examination of crystals in eye tissues. Arch Ophthalmol 1968; 80: 87–91.

88. Gahl WA, Kuehl EM, Iwath F, et al. Corneal crystals in nephropathic cystinosis. Natural history and treatment with cysteamine eye drops. Mol Genet Metab 2000; 71: 100–20.

89. Kaiser-Kupfer MI, Gazzo MA, Datiles MB, et al. A randomized placebo-controlled trial of cysteamine eye drops in nephropathic cystinosis. Arch Ophthalmol 1990; 108: 689–93.

90. Kaiser-Kupfer MI, Caruso RC, Minkler DS, Gahl WA. Long-term ocular manifestations in nephropathic cystinosis. Arch Ophthalmol 1986; 104: 706–11.

91. Katz B, Melles RB, Swenson MR, Schneider JA. Photic sneeze reflex in nephropathic cystinosis. Br J Ophthalmol 1990; 74: 706–8.

92. Peroutka SJ, Peroutka LA. Autosomal dominant transmission of the 'photic sneeze reflex'. N Engl J Med 1984; 310: 599–600.

93. Vesaluoma MH, Linna TU, Sankila EM, et al. In vivo confocal microscopy of a family with Schnyder crystalline dystrophy. Ophthalmology 1999; 106: 94–51.

94. Lisch W, Weidle EG, Lisch C, et al. Schnyder's dystrophy. Progression and metabolism. Ophthalmol Pediatr Genet 1986; 7: 45–56.

95. Wilson DJ, Weleber RG, Klein M, et al. Bietti's crystalline dystrophy: a clinicopathologic correlative study. Arch Ophthalmol 1989; 107: 213–21.

96. Bourne WM, Kyle RA, Brubaker RF, Greipp PR. Incidence of corneal crystals in the monoclonal gammopathies. Am J Ophthalmol 1989; 107: 192–3.

97. Ellis W, Barfort P, Mastman GJ. Keratoconjunctivitis with corneal crystals caused by the dieffenbachian plant. Am J Ophthalmol 1973; 76: 143–7.

98. Arnold RW, Stickler G, Bourne W, Mellinger JF. Corneal crystals, myopathy and nephropathy: a new syndrome? J Pediatr Ophthalmol Strabismus 1987; 24: 151–5.

99. Babalola OE, Murdoch IE. Corneal changes of uncertain etiology in mesoendemic onchocercal communities of Northern Nigeria. Cornea 2001; 20: 183–6.

100. Michalski A, Leonard JV, Taylor DS. The eye and inherited metabolic disease. J Roy Soc Med 1988; 82: 286–90.

101. Paige D, Clayton P, Bowron A, Harper JI. Richner-Hanhart syndrome (oculocutaneous tyrosinaemia, tyrosinaemia type II). J Roy Soc Med 1992; 85: 759–60.

102. Cohen KL, Bouldin TW. Familial, band-shaped, spheroidal keratopathy. Histopathology in ethnic Chinese siblings. Cornea 2002; 21: 774–7.

103. Viestenz A, Seitz B. Ocular manifestations in LCAT deficiency—a clinicopathological correlation. Kiln Monatsbl Augenheilkd 2003; 220: 499–502.

104. Klein HG, Lohse P, Pritchard PH, et al. Two different allelic mutations in lecithin-cholesterol acyltransferase gene associated with fish-eye syndrome. J Clin Invest 1992; 89: 499–506.

105. Clarke WN, Munro S, Brownstein S, et al. Ocular findings in acromesomelic dysplasia. Am J Ophthalmol 1994; 118: 797–804.

106. Chan CC, Green WR, de la Cruz ZC, Hillis A. Ocular findings in osteogenesis imperfecta. Arch Ophthalmol 1982; 100: 1458–63.

107. Cameron JA. Corneal abnormalities in Ehlers-Danlos syndrome type VI. Cornea 1993; 12: 54–9.

108. Zlotogora J, BenEzra D, Cohen T, Cohen E. Syndrome of brittle cornea, blue sclera and joint hyperextensibility. Am J Med Genet 1990; 36: 269–72.

109. Dinakaran S. Outpatient management of traumatic hyphemia. Sur Ophthalmol 2003; 48: 2472.

110. Agapitos PJ, Noel L-P, Clarke WN. Traumatic hyphemia in children. Ophthalmology 1987; 94: 1238–42.

111. Mensher JH. Corneal nerves. Surv Ophthalmol 1974; 19: 1–18.

112. Arigon V, Binaghi M, Sabouret C, et al. Usefulness of systemic of opthalmologic investigation in neurofibromatosis 1: a cross-sectional study of two hundred eleven patients. Eur J Ophthalmol 2002; 12: 413–8.

113. Eter N, Klingmuller D, Hoppner W, Spitznas M. Typical ocular findings in a patient with multiple endocrine neoplasia type 2b syndrome. Graeffes Arch Clin Exp Ophthalmol 2001; 239: 391–4.

114. Dyck PJ, Carney JA, Sizemore GW, et al. Multiple endocrine neoplasia type 2b: phenotype recognition, neurological features and their pathological basis. Ann Neurol 1979; 6: 302–14.

115. Kinoshita S, Tanaka F, Ohashi Y, et al. Incidence of prominent corneal nerves in multiple endocrine neoplasia type 2a. Am J Ophthalmol 1991; 111: 307–11.

CHAPTER
30 Corneal Dystrophies

Hans Ulrik Møller

Corneal dystrophies are Mendelian-inherited conditions that exhibit bilateral and usually symmetrical corneal changes.

No two reviews on corneal dystrophies are the same. Nomenclature has been difficult because of controversies about the phenotype. The literature from the first half of the past century was in German and was misinterpreted in the English and American literature. Grayscale clinical pictures were often of poor quality. Valid information on many got lost among insubstantial papers, and many authors published different sorts of patients under the same headings. An excellent survey[1] summarized the recent advances on the subject.

In this chapter the focus will be on a few classic dystrophies, highlighting the clinical presentation in the young patient and emphasizing differences from the adult. Slit-lamp pictures of the often very subtle changes of the young cornea dystrophy patient are difficult to take.

A comprehensive list of well-known and rare corneal dystrophies is available in the database GENEEYE.[2]

DEFINITION AND CLASSIFICATION

The term dystrophy is derived from the Greek words *dys* (meaning "wrong" or "difficult") and *trophe* ("nourishment"). A dystrophy is the process and consequence of hereditary progressive affections of specific cells in one or more tissues that initially show normal function.[3] This definition comprises most diseases traditionally named corneal dystrophies, with or without systemic manifestations.

The classical subdivision of corneal dystrophies according to the layer of their main involvement, e.g., stromal dystrophies, has historical interest but little practical importance; often the classification antedates the slit lamp.

Dystrophies should be distinguished from corneal degenerations, which are secondary, nongenetic processes resulting from aging or previous corneal inflammation.

MUTATION RATE

The prevalence and importance of the different conditions vary. The founder effect has, in some countries, given rise to large pedigrees and publications of cases that may be almost nonexistent elsewhere. As the mutation rates for many of the corneal dystrophies are probably very low, it is important to be cautious when diagnosing apparently sporadic cases, and a family history and examination of parents are mandatory. Phenocopies do exist although they may be rare in children; paraproteinemic crystalline keratopathy is an example of a disease mimicking granular dystrophy, and mucolipidosis IV can cause cornea verticillata similar to granular dystrophy I.

Dystrophies related to mutations in the TGFBI gene

An example of the emerging genetic information bringing order out of chaos is the different allelic mutations within the TGFBI (transforming growth factor-beta induced) gene (called, by some, the "BIGH3" gene) on chromosome 5q22–q32. It comprises two of the classic corneal dystrophies. Thus new genetic knowledge is bringing order to this field of ophthalmology, although naming the diseases according to mutation number has not gained universal recognition. For practical purposes most ophthalmologists rely on genetic analysis to distinguish between the rarer varieties.

Granular dystrophies
Granular dystrophy type I (Groenouw type I)
Granular dystrophy type I is an autosomal dominant dystrophy of the TGFBI gene. It is distinguished by discrete granular-appearing corneal opacities in an otherwise clear cornea. One type has several hundred granules in one cornea (mutation R555W).

The opacities are white in direct illumination, and transparent, like a crack in glass, by retroillumination. At 5 years of age or so, these may be brownish and superficial to Bowman's membrane and present in a verticillata configuration (Fig. 30.1a). The granules increase in number and size and progress into the stroma during early adulthood. There is always a 2-mm clear, limbal zone. One striking feature is that unlike most dominant disorders the expressivity is constant in all generations.[4]

Grafting is rarely required until the fifth or sixth decade when visual acuity may drop below 6/12 in patients with many granules; recurrence in the graft is the rule. It has no extra ocular signs or symptoms.

A so-called superficial, unusual variety (Fig. 30.1b) with a very severe clinical outcome in young children has been described. They have an almost white central cornea before the age of 10 years. These patients are homozygous for the dominant gene; different mutations have been described.

Granular dystrophy type II
Granular type II (Avellino) corneal dystrophy named from an Italian village is universally known (mutation R124H). It is probably the most frequent one worldwide; the author has seen these patients in 6 countries. Clinically as well as on electron microscopy this mutation looks like a mixture of granular and lattice dystrophies with fewer, often larger elements in the cornea. It rarely is possible to diagnose until the late teens and thus parents carrying this mutation need genetic analysis to know whether their children inherited the trait.

Lattice dystrophies
Lattice dystrophy (type I, mutation R124C) is also an autosomal

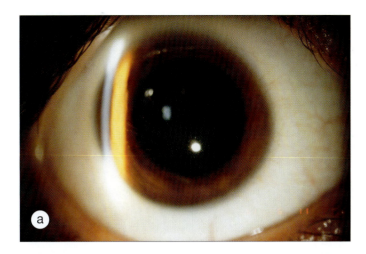

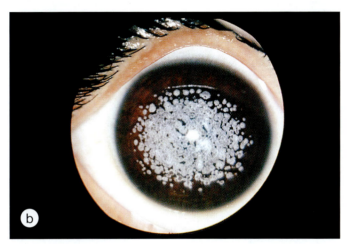

Fig. 30.1 Granular dystrophy. (a) A verticillata-like configuration of the corneal opacities. (b) A 7-year-old homozygous patient.

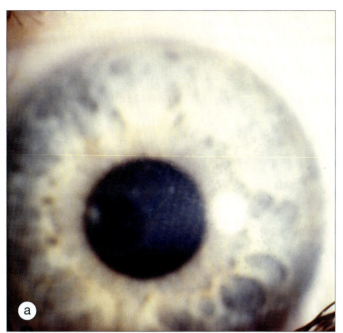

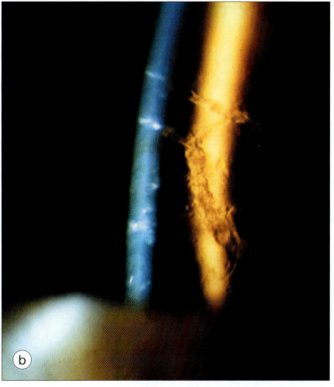

Fig. 30.2 Lattice dystrophy. (a) Early changes showing nonrefractile round spots just visible in the pupil (Mr A E A Ridgway's patient). (b) Later changes showing filamentary lines.

dominant condition of the TGFBI gene. The deposition of amyloid is the hallmark of this condition, and the opacities of the child's cornea are recognized by three distinct slit-lamp observations:[5]

1. Tiny nonrefractile, whitish spots, round or ovoid (Fig. 30.2a);
2. A diffuse axial, anterior stromal haze; and
3. White, anterior, stromal dots as well as (in the somewhat older patient) filamentary lines that are refractile on indirect illumination (Fig. 30.2b).

The deposition may be symmetrical or asymmetrical. The intervening stroma becomes increasingly hazy in the adult. The lattice lines giving rise to the name of the condition only become evident in adulthood. Many patients experience recurrent erosions, and corneal grafting may be necessary in early adult life due to visual impairment. Recurrence in the graft is the rule.

Subtypes due to several different mutations exist; only one mutation, the Meretoja variation, has systemic manifestations but is a disease of the adult.

Reis–Bücklers and Thiel–Behnke dystrophies

Mutations in that same gene also give rise to Reis–Bücklers dystrophy (mutation R124L) and Thiel–Behnke honeycomb dystrophy (probably mutation R555Q and maybe others). Both have early onset recurrent erosions. Reis–Bücklers has confluent irregular subepithelial opacities showing rod-shaped bodies on electron microscopy, as does granular dystrophy. The Thiel–

Behnke dystrophy has a honeycomb look in the slit lamp and curly fibers on electron microscopy.

Dystrophy due to mutations in the CHST6 gene

Macular dystrophy (Groenouw type II)

Not many ophthalmologists will diagnose macular dystrophy in a very young child; the first subtle findings are very discrete. They comprise nebulous, whitish opacities in the center of the cornea (Fig. 30.3), which itself is very thin. However, over the years it increases in thickness and the corneal stroma becomes increasingly hazy between the opacities with an irregular surface. Deposits of glycosaminoglycan cause the opacification. Two subtypes are described. As it is inherited as a recessive trait, consanguinity is frequent. The high prevalence of macular dystrophy in Iceland is an example of the founder effect in a particular geographical area.[6] Macular dystrophy has been linked to chromosome 16; several mutations exist.

Visual deterioration is symmetrical and inevitable, but patients do not usually require corneal grafting until late in the second or third decade. Patients experience no systemic symptoms.

Dystrophies due to mutations in the COL8A gene

Posterior polymorphous dystrophy (Schlichting)

This is also an autosomal dominant dystrophy that may be seen in the very young. It is asymmetrical and slowly progressive. Slit-lamp appearances show small, round, discrete, transparent, vesicular lesions (Fig. 30.4) surrounded by a ring of opacity deep

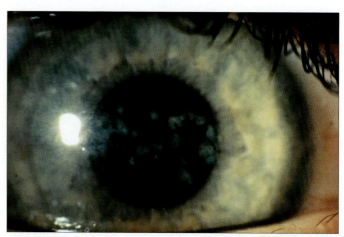

Fig. 30.3 Macular dystrophy in a 13-year-old girl. Typical macular corneal opacities. What cannot be seen in a picture is the opaque ground substance between opacities and the thin cornea.

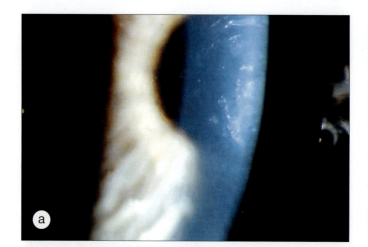

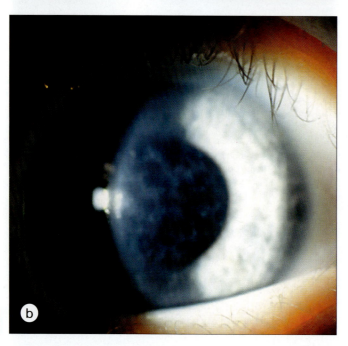

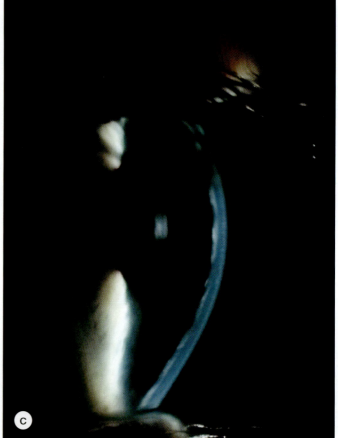

Fig. 30.4 Posterior polymorphous dystrophy. (a) Deep transparent vesicular lesions. (b) Direct illumination showing geographical opacities. (c) Slit-lamp picture showing deep posterior stromal-endothelial ring-like opacities.

in the cornea at the level of Descemet's membrane; the deep involvement is in contrast to most other corneal dystrophies. The opacities are best seen on retroillumination. Geographical and band varieties exist as well. It is difficult to distinguish between posterior polymorphous dystrophy and iridocorneal endothelial syndrome (ICE).[7]

Posterior polymorphous dystrophy has been linked to chromosomes 20q11 and 1p34–p32.2.

The symptoms are often mild and vision unaffected, and most patients do not require corneal grafting.

Dystrophy due to mutations in the KRT3/KRT12 gene

Juvenile epithelial dystrophy (Meesmann)

This condition has a varied expression.[8] Although often asymptomatic it may present in early childhood with symptoms of ocular irritation and photophobia due to recurrent erosions and a mild blur of vision. The typical patient has a huge number of tiny epithelial vesicles (Fig. 30.5). In the young child, small areas may be spared.

The mutation rate is probably very low indeed for this disease, and a family history is important. The best-documented pedigree is traced back to 1620 in northern Germany, counting probably hundreds of patients.

Treatment may be with soft contact lenses, corneal abrasion, or excimer laser treatment, the indication being a decrease in visual acuity caused by basement membrane changes. Recurrence will follow soon, however.

Vision is rarely severely affected in childhood, and the patients are otherwise healthy. Mutations in two loci, 12q13 and 17q12, have been published.

Dystrophies mapped but with unidentified genes

Central crystalline dystrophy (Schnyder)

This autosomal dominant corneal dystrophy[9] can be diagnosed in children and may have a variable expression. The central anterior cornea has a slowly progressing, disc-like central opacification with or without polychromatic crystals (Fig. 30.6). It may be visible from a few years of age. In their twenties patients develop an arcus lipoides and a diffuse stromal haze. Vision is variably affected and keratoplasty may be necessary in the adult. The crystals comprise cholesterol and other lipids. Gene locus is 1p34.1–p36.

Congenital hereditary endothelial dystrophy

This important but rare corneal disease was clearly described by Maumenee,[10] a name still used as an eponym, although sometimes it is called by the acronym CHED. Strictly speaking it may not be a true dystrophy according to the above-mentioned definition as it is congenital. However, it is usually included among the dystrophies. Autosomal dominant as well as recessive inheritance patterns exist. It has been described in association with nail hypoplasia.

The recessive form (chromosome 20p13) is the more severe, and usually the presentation is at birth with a variable diffuse avascular haziness, ground-glass, bluish-white opacity of the cornea (Fig. 30.7). Nystagmus is seen. The dominant form (chromosome 20p11.2–q11.2) develops during the first or second year of life and progression is slow. The cornea is thicker than normal. Outcome varies; it is suggested that congenital hereditary endothelial dystrophy patients should be observed rather than operated on in early life. A pressure-lowering treatment to yield subnormal levels of intraocular pressure may be considered. If grafting is necessary, it carries a relatively good prognosis. Differentiation from congenital glaucoma is important but often difficult.

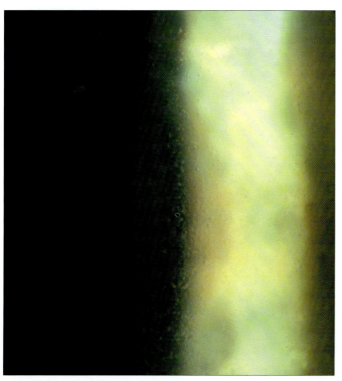

Fig. 30.5 Juvenile epithelial dystrophy showing multiple epithelial vesicles (Dr Wittebol-Post's patient).

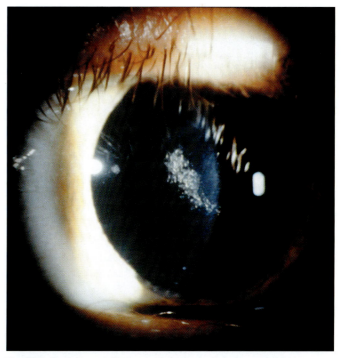

Fig. 30.6 Central crystalline corneal dystrophy in a young patient. Crystals in a clear cornea without any arcus (Dr. Weiss' patient).

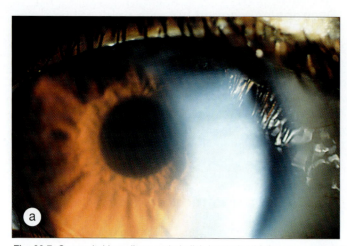

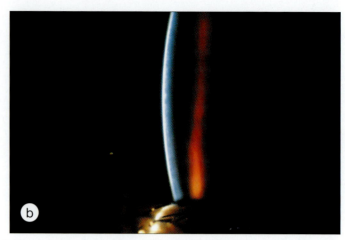

Fig. 30.7 Congenital hereditary endothelial dystrophy. (a) Opaque cornea. (b) Opaque and thickened cornea on slit-lamp illumination.

REFERENCES

1. Klintworth GK. The molecular genetics of the corneal dystrophies – current status. Front Biosci 2003; 8: d687–713.
2. Baraitser M, Winter RM, Russell-Eggitt I et al. GENEEYE. Institute of Child Health, London 2003.
3. Warburg M, Møller HU. Dystrophy. A revised definition. J Med Genet 1989; 26: 769–71.
4. Møller HU. Granular corneal dystrophy Groenouw type I. Acta Ophthalmol (Suppl) 1991; 69(198): 1–40.
5. Dubord PJ, Krachmer JH. Diagnosis of early lattice corneal dystrophy. Arch Ophthalmol 1982; 100: 788–90.
6. Jonasson F, Johannsson H, Garner A, Rice NSC. Macular corneal dystrophy in Iceland. Eye 1989; 3: 446–54.
7. Anderson NJ, Badawi DY, Grossniklaus HE, Stulting RD. Posterior polymorphous membranous dystrophy with overlapping features of iridocorneal endothelial syndrome. Arch Ophthalmol 2001; 119: 624–25.
8. Thiel HJ, Behnke H. Über die Variationsbreite der hereditären Hornhautepitheldystrophie Typ Meesmann-Wilke. Ophthalmologica 1968; 155: 81–6.
9. Weiss JS. Schnyder's dystrophy of the cornea. A Swede-Finn connection. Cornea 1992; 11: 93–101.
10. Maumenee AE. Congenital hereditary corneal dystrophy. Am J Ophthalmol 1960; 50: 1114–24.

CHAPTER
31 The Lacrimal System

Caroline J MacEwen

INTRODUCTION

The lacrimal system consists of a secretory portion and a drainage system. The secretory portion is made up of the lacrimal and accessory lacrimal glands, which, together with the meibomian glands and the goblet cells, secrete the components of the tear film. The tear film is trilaminar: the inner mucin layer secreted by the conjunctival goblet cells, the intermediate aqueous layer by the lacrimal and accessory lacrimal glands, and the outer, oily layer by the meibomian glands. The accessory lacrimal glands produce basal tear secretion, and the lacrimal gland is largely responsible for reflex tearing in response to noxious or emotional stimuli.

The drainage system consists of the lacrimal puncta, canaliculi, lacrimal sac, and the nasolacrimal duct. This active system pumps tears from the conjunctival sac into the inferior meatus of the nose.

Tears flow along the lid margins and conjunctival fornices and are spread across the surface of the eye by blinking. Tears protect the eye in a number of ways: surface lubrication; provision of oxygen and antibacterial substances such as IgA, IgG, and lysozyme; and mechanical removal of irritating substances and cellular debris.

Clinical problems with the lacrimal system in children usually relate to either the underproduction of tears, causing dry eyes, which is rare but potentially sight-threatening, or the reduced drainage of tears, which is much more common but less serious.

LACRIMAL GLAND

Embryology

The lacrimal gland develops from the same ectoderm as the conjunctiva. It is supported by mesodermal connective tissue. The accessory lacrimal glands have common origins but remain within the lids rather than migrating with the main lacrimal gland. The lacrimal gland continues to grow 3–4 years after birth. Basal tearing is present in infants from birth, and reflex tearing begins at any time from birth to several months of age.[1]

Anatomy

The main lacrimal gland is an exocrine gland in the anterior aspect of the supratemporal orbit within the bony lacrimal fossa. The majority of the gland lies within this fossa but the lateral horn of the levator palpebrae superioris separates this orbital part from the palpebral lobe, which extends anteriorly into the supratemporal conjunctival cul-de-sac. The ducts of the gland pass through the palpebral lobe and open on to the conjunctiva in the superior fornix. The lacrimal gland is innervated via the facial (afferent) and trigeminal (efferent) nerves. The accessory glands of Kraus and Wolfring sit in the superior conjunctival fornix.

Congenital abnormalities

Congenital absence of the lacrimal gland is rare and usually occurs in conditions with reduced conjunctiva: anophthalmus, cryptophthalmus, and the lacrimo-auriculo-dento-digital (LADD) syndrome.[2] Anomalous lacrimal ductules that secrete tears on to the skin rather than the conjunctival sac may be found near the lacrimal gland, around the lateral canthus or in the preauricular region. These are rare but may require dissection and excision.[3]

As the embryology of the lacrimal gland is closely linked to that of the conjunctival epithelium, this explains the common supra-temporal position of dermoid cysts, near the lacrimal gland.

Other congenital anomalies include orbital ectopic lacrimal gland tissue. A drainage system may not be present in such cases and an enlarging orbital mass may develop. Neoplasms occur with such ectopic tissue: recognition is important.

Crocodile tears occur from congenital aberrant innervation between the fifth and seventh cranial nerves and cause tearing with chewing or sucking.[4] Crocodile tears may be associated with other types of aberrant innervation such as Marcus Gunn jaw winking or Duane retraction syndrome.[5]

Dry eyes in children

Congenital causes

Congenital alacrima, or hyposecretion of tears, is relatively rare. This may be due to absence of the lacrimal gland or to the lacrimal gland being ectopic, deep in the orbit. Alacrima may be associated with systemic conditions such as the Riley–Day syndrome (familial dysautonomia),[6] anhydrotic ectodermal dysplasia, and Allgrove syndrome (familial alacrima, achalasia of the cardia and glucocorticoid deficiency).[7]

Acquired causes

Acquired tear deficiency may be due to pathology of the lacrimal gland, causing failure of tear production, or to conjunctival damage, leading to ductule obliteration. It may be damaged by Epstein–Barr infection,[8] as the result of HIV infection, or in patients with bone marrow transplantation (often associated with graft versus host disease).[9] The conjunctiva may be affected by injury (commonly burns), infection, the sequelae of trachoma, Stevens–Johnson syndrome, or toxic epidermal necrolysis.[10]

Sjögren syndrome is rare in children; it can be a primary auto-immune event or secondary, associated with rheumatoid arthritis or SLE. Children with Sjögren syndrome often have lacrimal gland enlargement, and they may have recurrent parotid gland swelling and salivary gland involvement. Sjögren should be considered in any child with recurrent parotiditis, kerato-conjunctivitis sicca, and early tooth decay due to xerostomia.[11]

Chronic blepharitis is uncommon; it usually presents with recurrent chalazia, although the lids may appear relatively normal. The associated poor quality tear film causes patches of dryness and may lead to peripheral corneal vascularization and scarring which can be serious.

Isotretinoin treatment for acne is a cause of dry eyes in adolescence. This is usually reversible at cessation of the drug, and affected teenagers should be treated symptomatically.

Children with dry eyes present with irritable, uncomfortable, gritty eyes, which may be diffusely injected. On examination a reduced tear meniscus is evident with punctate keratopathy, particularly affecting the interpalpebral zone. Staining occurs with fluorescein and Rose Bengal dyes; the latter is very uncomfortable when instilled into dry eyes. Severe keratopathy due to concomitant corneal hypoesthesia can be a problem in the Riley–Day syndrome.[6]

Treatment of dry eyes involves copious use of artificial tears and temporary or permanent punctal occlusion in severe cases. Immunomodulation may have a role to play in secondary lacrimal gland failure including that due to infections. Blepharitis should be treated with lid hygiene, lubricants, and systemic antibiotics such as erythromycin or azithromycin. Oral tetracyclines should be avoided in children prior to their second dentition.

Dacryoadenitis

Dacryoadenitis is commonly bilateral and associated with generalized systemic upset. Causes include mumps,[12] infectious mononucleosis, herpes zoster, tuberculosis, brucella, histoplasmosis, or gonococcal infection.[13] Lacrimal gland swelling may rarely be a sign of childhood Sjögren disease, which must be differentiated from true dacryoadenitis.

The clinical features of dacryoadenitis are the "S sign" in which there is drooping of the lateral aspect of the upper lid. In acute inflammatory cases, the overlying skin is inflamed. Neuroimaging confirms enlargement and helps rule out other orbital masses if the dacryoadenitis does not resolve. In the long-term, dacryoadenitis may damage the lacrimal gland and cause reduced tear secretion.

Dacryoadenitis must be differentiated from a lacrimal gland infarct, which occurs in children with a sickle cell crisis. The onset is rapid and may resemble acute dacryoadenitis.

Treatment of acute dacryocystitis is aimed at the underlying cause.

Lacrimal tumors

Lacrimal tumors are extremely rare in children. Pseudotumor causing painful swelling is rare, but may affect the lacrimal gland.[14] Malignant epithelial tumors, including mixed cell adenocystic and other carcinomas, have been recorded in childhood.[15]

Lacrimal gland prolapse

Prolapse of the lacrimal gland, commonly bilateral, may present as a subconjunctival mass in the upper outer fornix. Uncommon before puberty, it is more frequent in black people than other races. It may occur with craniofacial anomalies due to reduced orbital volume and increased orbital pressure. Children with lacrimal gland prolapse should be imaged to exclude enlargement from conditions such as sarcoidosis, tumors, or leukemia. Depending on the extent, the gland may need to be reduced surgically.

THE LACRIMAL DRAINAGE SYSTEM

Embryology

The lacrimal outflow system develops between the maxilla and the lateral nasal process from a cord of surface ectoderm. By the end of the first trimester this tissue begins, piecemeal, to canalize. The puncta usually open with the eyelids during the sixth month of gestation. The nasolacrimal duct opens into the inferior meatus of the nose just before or after term birth. There may be a failure of this canalization process at any part of the system, but this is most frequent at the lower end.[16]

Anatomy

A clear understanding of the lacrimal outflow system is important for the pediatric ophthalmologist, especially for performing probing.

The puncta should be touching the globe at the medial aspect of the upper and lower lids in order to collect tears. The proximal part of the canaliculus is the ampulla, which is a slightly dilated vertical portion 1 mm in length in the young child. The canaliculus then turns 90° to run medially in a horizontal direction. The upper and lower canaliculi join to form the common canaliculus that enters the lateral wall of the lacrimal sac. Rosenmüller's valve prevents reflux of tears from the sac into the canaliculus. The lacrimal sac sits in the bony lacrimal fossa, separated from the middle meatus of the nose by the maxilla and lacrimal bone. The lacrimal sac extends superiorly under the medial canthal ligament to form its fundus. The nasolacrimal duct exits from the lower end of the sac and passes in a downward, lateral, and slightly posterior direction. This duct is surrounded by bone in its upper part but becomes membranous inferiorly. The nasolacrimal duct opens into the medial wall of the inferior meatus of the nose via the valve of Hasner. This ostium is found under the inferior turbinate of the nose, sitting approximately 1 cm directly behind the entrance of the nose in the baby.

Lacrimal pumping mechanism

Tears are actively pumped through the outflow system. During blinking, when the lids close, the canaliculi are shortened and narrowed by contraction of the pretarsal orbicularis muscles. Simultaneously the same muscles pull the lateral sac wall, creating negative pressure inside the sac. These changes suck fluid into the expanded sac. Further lid closure causes contraction of the orbicularis oculi muscle, which squeezes the tears from the sac into the nasolacrimal duct. At the end of each blink, the sac is empty and as the lids open, the canaliculi and the sac elastically expand, causing a vacuum within the system into which tears enter via the puncta, and the cycle begins again.

Congenital abnormalities

Abnormalities, which are common, include narrowing (stenosis), blockage (atresia), complete absence (agenesis), or duplication (accessory channels) of any part of the system. A membranous obstruction at the distal end of the nasolacrimal duct is the commonest abnormality, causing congenital nasolacrimal duct obstruction.[16] Obstruction at other sites is very rare but may become more relevant in older children as cases of congenital nasolacrimal duct obstruction spontaneously resolve.

Children with craniofacial abnormalities, particularly clefting syndromes, have complex anomalies of the lacrimal outflow system that may involve large areas being either blocked or absent.

Congenital dacryocystocele

A dacryocystocele is a congenital swelling located at the medial canthus due to trapped fluid inside the lacrimal sac and nasolacrimal duct.[17] The fluid is unable to escape from either the upper or lower end of the drainage system as both are blocked. This usually presents as a tense, blue, nonpulsatile swelling below the medial canthus that is evident at, or shortly after, birth (Fig. 31.1a). The inferior end of the dacryocystocele projects into the nose (Fig. 31.1b) and in some cases may be responsible for breathing difficulties due to nasal block of the newborn.[18] If respiratory compromise occurs, urgent treatment is required.

The clinical appearance is classic, but care must be taken to differentiate congenital dacryocystocele from a meningo-encephalocele, a meningocele, a mid-line nasal dermoid cyst, or a capillary hemangioma. If there is any doubt about the diagnosis an MRI scan is helpful in identifying the dilated sac and nasolacrimal duct and in excluding other pathology. Routine imaging, however, is not necessary and the diagnosis is usually made clinically.

Treatment of a dacryocystocele involves observation during the first two weeks of life, during which time most spontaneously improve. If it has not settled by this stage or if acute dacryocystitis (Fig. 31.2) or respiratory difficulties develop, then surgical treatment is required. Treatment involves drainage of the dacryocystocele into the nose using an endoscopic approach. The nasal mucosa over the dacryocystocele should be excised. If acute dacryocystitis has intervened, intravenous antibiotics should be given prior to surgery.

Congenital nasolacrimal duct obstruction

Congenital nasolacrimal duct obstruction represents a delay in maturation of the lacrimal system where it enters the nose,

resulting in a persistent membranous obstruction at the valve of Hasner. The diagnosis is made on a clear history, from the parents, of a watery eye that has been present from the first few weeks of birth (Table 31.1). This is usually unilateral but may be bilateral and, if so, commonly asymmetrical. Some children develop a mucopurulent discharge that may be constant or intermittent. The eye remains "white" without evidence of active infection, although attacks of conjunctivitis may complicate the condition. The child is well with no evidence of irritation or photophobia. The skin around the eye becomes red and may become excoriated. Although usually an isolated abnormality, congenital nasolacrimal duct obstruction may be more frequent in certain conditions (Table 31.2).

On examination there is an increased tear meniscus and there may be stickiness or crusting on the lashes. A mucocele, with swelling at the medial canthus, may develop: the contents can be expressed into the conjunctival sac.

Table 31.1 Watery eyes in children

Excess tear production (lacrimation)
Allergic rhinitis
Upper respiratory tract infection
Epiblepharon
Subtarsal foreign body
Iritis
Corneal abrasion/ulceration
Conjunctivitis
Glaucoma
Drainage failure (epiphora)
Congenital nasolacrimal duct obstruction
Skeletal and sinus abnormalities
Lid malposition
Punctal malposition
Punctal occlusion
Anomalous drainage system

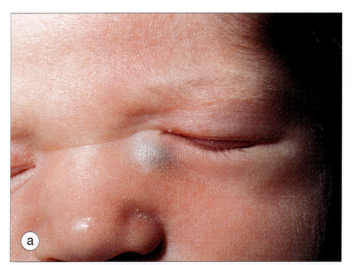

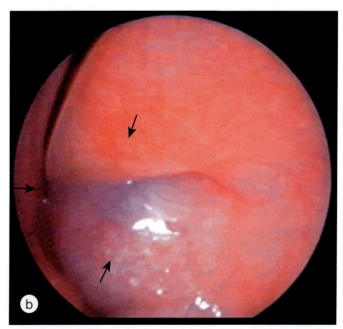

Fig. 31.1 Congenital dacryocystocele. (a) A bluish swelling is seen below the medial canthal tendon. It can present as nasal obstruction. (b) Dacryocystocele viewed from inside the nose, demonstrating the dilated nasolacrimal duct protruding into the nasal cavity, which may cause respiratory distress (left nostril).

Table 31.2 Systemic associations of nasolacrimal duct obstruction in young children
EEC syndrome (ectrodactyly, ectodermal dysplasia, clefting) (Fig. 31.3) Branchio-oculo facial syndrome[19] Craniometaphyseal or craniodiaphysial dysplasia[20] Down syndrome[21] Lacrimo-auriculo-dento-digital (LADD) syndrome[22] The CHARGE association[23]

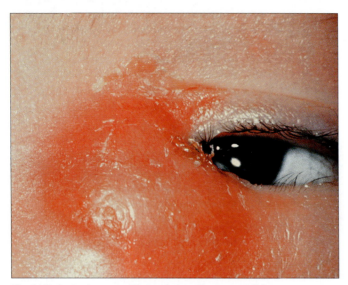

Fig. 31.2 Acute dacryocystitis in a baby with a congenital dacryocystocele. A dacryocystocele is not normally inflamed.

A fluorescein disappearance test (FDT) should be performed on all children with epiphora as it provides evidence to support a diagnosis of lacrimal outflow obstruction.[24] Fluorescein 1% is instilled into each lower conjunctival fornix. The child sits on the parent's lap while the cobalt blue light from the slit lamp illuminates the eyes. The slit lamp can be some distance from the child so as not to frighten. The tear meniscus is evaluated at 2 and 5 minutes—it is also reviewed at 10 minutes in equivocal cases. Each eye is graded at 0, 1, 2, or 3 (0 = fluorescein completely disappeared, 3 = no fluorescein disappeared at all) (Fig. 31.4). Normally, the fluorescein disappears by 5 minutes (graded 0 or 1), but remains present in children with obstruction. Pressure on the lacrimal sac produces regurgitation of fluorescein-stained tears, particularly striking in those with mucoceles. This test illustrates clearly the nature of the problem to the parents and provides useful time to discuss the etiology and management.

Natural history

Congenital nasolacrimal duct obstruction is clinically evident in up to 20% of infants, of which the vast majority become symptomatic during the first month (Fig. 31.5a). The natural history is to spontaneously resolve with maturation.[25–28] Spontaneous resolution is rapid with more than 50% better by 3 months, more than 80% by 6 months, and about 95% by the age of one year[26–28] (Figs. 31.5b, 31.5c). Resolution continues and by 24 months of age a further 60–79% of children will have no symptoms[29,30] (Fig. 31.5d). Older children have not been studied, but spontaneous improvement can occur at any age.[25,29]

Conservative treatment

Because of the high rate of spontaneous resolution, observation is recommended until the child is at least one year old and even older if this is the parent's preference. The most important aspect of conservative treatment is parental education, providing reassurance and information about the etiology and natural history. Printed leaflets that provide information for the parent are very useful.

Parents should be encouraged to cleanse the lids and lashes with cooled boiled water and to gently express the contents of the lacrimal sac proximally into the conjunctival sac.[31] This maintains flow in the system and prevents stagnation, reducing any sticky discharge. Massage of the sac may also increase hydrostatic pressure within the lacrimal system, and this has been reported to increase patency by rupturing the membranous obstruction.[32,33] Parents find this difficult and need clear instructions. They should press on the sac below the medial canthus with their little finger 2–3 times per day if possible. Vaseline (or liquid paraffin) should be applied to the periocular skin to protect and treat any areas of redness or broken skin.

Antibiotics are not required and should be avoided unless there is evidence of conjunctivitis (red, irritable, sticky eyes). Swabs for bacterial growth should also only be performed under these conditions as "pathogenic" bacteria are frequently commensals in the conjunctival sacs of normal infants and children and do not require antibiotic treatment in quiet watering eyes.[34]

Syringing and probing

If epiphora persists, syringing and probing of the lacrimal drainage system is the treatment of choice. The optimum time to intervene has long been a topic of controversy. Originally probing was advocated at presentation or after a short period of conservative treatment.[35,36] However, with better understanding of the natural history of the condition, especially during the first year of life, this has become less favored. It has been shown that the

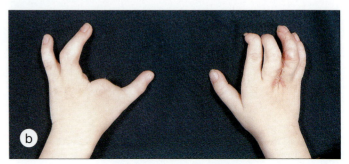

Fig. 31.3 (a) The ectrodactyly, ectodermal dysplasia, clefting (EEC) syndrome is associated with nasolacrimal duct obstruction and (b) "lobster claw" deformity of the hands.

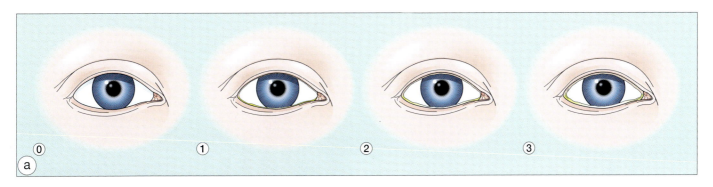

⓪ ① ② ③

a

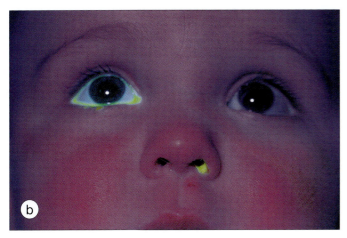

b

Fig. 31.4 (a) The fluorescein disappearance test—grading the test is usually performed at 5 minutes, or 10 minutes in doubtful cases.[24] (b) This child has evidence of a delayed fluorescein disappearance test from the right eye, and a patent left system is confirmed by the presence of fluorescein in the nostril.

earlier probing is performed, the greater is the success rate.[37,38] However, other work has shown that the higher failure rate in older children is probably unrelated to the age of the child but is due to a process of natural selection:[39-42] as children grow older, more complex and severe obstructions become commoner as cases of simple membranous obstruction spontaneously resolve; this reduces the success rate of probing in older children and increases the requirement for more extensive surgery. This thesis is supported by a controlled prospective trial in which probing and syringing between 12 and 14 months of age was found to be more successful than the spontaneous resolution rate in a control group at 15 months.[29] However, by 2 years of age, continued spontaneous resolution in the control group meant that there was no statistical difference in the outcome between those probed and those not probed at this stage (Fig. 31.5d). This indicates that observation is as effective as probing in children up to the age of 2, but that probing provides a more rapid result if performed at, or just after, 12 months of age.

The decision to probe is based on the natural history, severity, and informed parental request. Timing should be based on these considerations with no particular age being considered sacred. It is usually recommended that probing under 12 months of age is not indicated, and there is no evidence that it is detrimental to wait until 2 years of age[29,39-43] and probably later if desired.

"Office probing," carried out on awake, restrained babies, which is favored in the USA, is less popular elsewhere because it must be performed on babies no older than 4–6 months of age, and at this stage there is still a very high chance of spontaneous resolution. In addition, the danger of iatrogenic damage to the friable nasolacrimal duct, with possible false passage formation, has made this unpopular. The use of this type of probing is influenced by medical economics, as it avoids the expense of a general anesthetic.[44] However, at least 50% of those undergoing probing would not require intervention if left until 1 year of age.

After informed consent, probing should be carried out in a pediatric environment with the child anesthetized so that attention can be paid to the site and nature of the obstruction. Probing should be viewed as diagnostic, as well as therapeutic, so that in the small number of cases that remain symptomatic the cause of failure can be identified and a clear management plan formed. These conditions can only be achieved under general anesthesia using a laryngeal mask following full nasal preparation. Probing should be carried out in a step-wise fashion, identifying the patency or obstruction of each area between the puncta and end of the nasolacrimal duct. Probing is a blind procedure and depends on awareness of resistance to the probe as it passes through the system. The use of a nasal endoscope permits direct visualization of the lower end of the nasolacrimal duct, which is the commonest area of abnormality. This assists in the diagnosis, and management and knowledge of endonasal techniques is useful for anyone undertaking probing.[45]

Probing and syringing should be carried out paying attention to the anatomy of the lacrimal drainage system. Each punctum is dilated using a Nettleship dilator. This is introduced firstly in a vertical direction for approximately 1 mm and then rotated through 90° in a medial direction to run horizontally parallel to the lid margin to dilate the proximal canaliculus. This is easier if the lid is held taut by pulling the eyelid laterally during this process as this straightens out the canaliculus. The lacrimal system should be syringed with fluorescein-stained saline using a disposable cannula. Syringing takes place via each punctum and note is made of any areas of resistance to the cannula and to any regurgitation of fluid or mucus. The inside of the nose should be inspected with an endoscope or fluorescein retrieved via a nasal

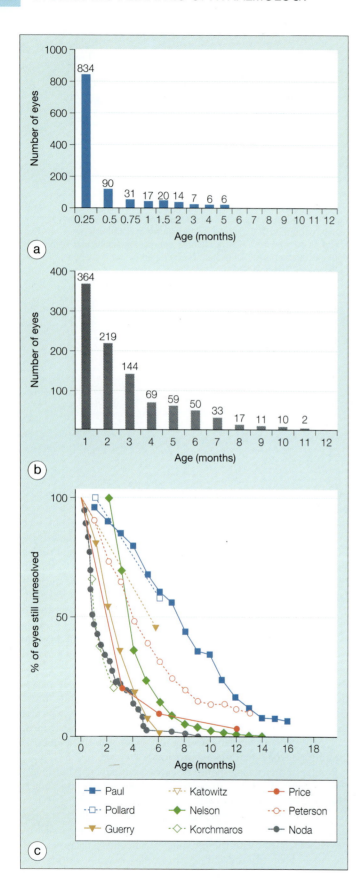

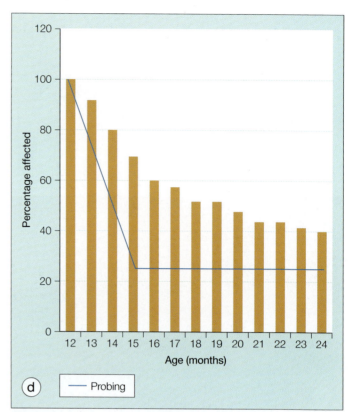

Fig. 31.5 (a) Age of onset of epiphora. In 95%, the epiphora presented during the first month of life.[28] (b) Spontaneous resolution. Each column demonstrates the number of eyes that spontaneously resolved during that month of life.[28] (c) The rate of spontaneous resolution of nasolacrimal duct obstruction expressed as a percentage of those still unresolved at a given age in months.[44] (d) Success of probing compared with spontaneous resolution during the second year of life. Probing is more successful than spontaneous resolution at 15 months, but by 24 months there is no statistically significant difference between the two treatments.[29,30]

or pharyngeal aspirate. Fluid should pass freely in a normal system and any resistance should be noted. The passage of fluorescein and the amount of resistance are important factors in deciding the site (canaliculus, sac, upper or lower nasolacrimal duct) and nature (agenesis, atresia, stenosis) of any abnormality of the lacrimal outflow system.

In children with atresia at the lower end of the nasolacrimal duct regurgitation of mucus via the other punctum is usually noted on syringing and no fluorescein is retrieved from the nose. Fluorescein is identified in the nose of children who have stenosis at the valve of Hasner, or in those with a narrow inferior meatus caused by a tight inferior turbinate. Difficulty in injecting the fluid may be evident in such instances. Infracture of the inferior turbinate opens up the inferior meatus and may stretch a stenosed valve. Free and easy flow of fluorescein into the nose may occur in symptomatic children, indicating a normal anatomical pathway. This suggests physiological or functional blockage.

If a nasal endoscope is being used, it should be introduced into the inferior meatus at this stage after gentle "infracture" of the cartilaginous inferior turbinate–bending it inwards. This maneuver itself is often therapeutic as it opens up a narrow inferior meatus and may stretch a stenotic ostium.[46] The fluorescein–stained fluid should be syringed through the system and observed through the endoscope. Atresia is identified as ballooning of the submucosa with no passage of fluorescein and stenosis appears as a poor flow through the narrow valve (Fig. 31.6a). A clear free flow indicates either that the infracture has been effective or that the patient has "functional epiphora."

The system should then be probed via the upper canaliculus using the smallest probe available (usually a Bowman's size 0000). The probe is passed in the same manner as the dilator until it reaches a hard stop that indicates the medial wall of the sac. The probe is then withdrawn slightly and rotated through 90° so that its tip is pointing downward. The probe is then advanced very gently downward but also slightly posteriorly and laterally to follow the path of the nasolacrimal duct. During passage of the probe the operator should feel for and note the level of any resistance. If the probe perforates a persistent membrane at the valve of Hasner this may be felt as it enters the inferior meatus. If being performed with endonasal control, the probe should be observed entering the inferior meatus (Fig. 31.6b). Problems may be encountered if the probe fails to perforate the mucosa (Fig. 31.6c), misses the valve of Hasner, and carries on in a submucosal plane to the floor of the nose or enters the meatus through a false and usually ineffective passage. In the first instance, a cut down onto the probe may be required, and in the other instances it may be possible to steer the probe under direct visualization toward and through the valve of Hasner. If the perforation is inadequate and felt to be tight, the probe size should be increased to a maximum size 1. Larger probes should be avoided as they may induce canalicular damage. After probing, the syringing should be repeated with fluorescein-stained saline and patency confirmed by directly viewing the valve of Hasner or aspirating the fluid from the nose or throat with a soft suction tube in those without endoscopic assistance.

Postoperatively a steroid/antibiotic combination should be instilled topically for 2 weeks. The patient is reviewed one month after surgery when the parents should be asked to report any change and the fluorescein disappearance test is repeated to confirm the outcome. Improvement is usually noted within a few

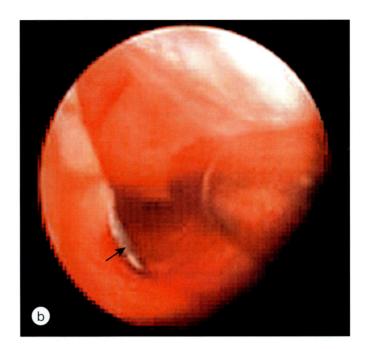

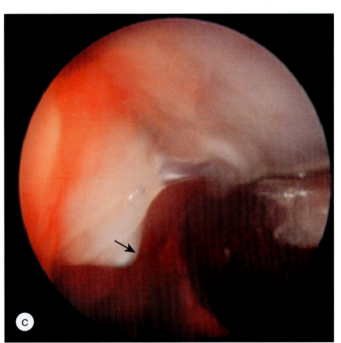

Fig. 31.6 (a) Stenotic flow through the valve of Hasner–right nostril. (b) Probe entering the inferior meatus via the valve of Hasner–right nostril. (c) Probe distending, but not perforating, the mucosa in a case of atresia of the lower end of the nasolacriminal duct–right nostril. (With thanks to Paul White.)

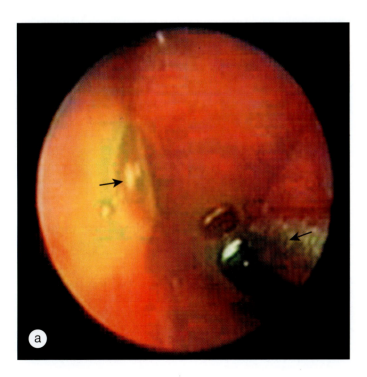

days of the probing. If there has been no improvement by the review appointment it is unlikely that the treatment has been successful.

What to do if probing fails

If probing fails, it is important to identify the reason for failure. Failure is generally due to one of three causes:

1. Failure to create an anatomically patent passage:
   –a tight inferior meatus due to a large inferior turbinate;

–failure to perforate the mucosa;
–submucosal passage of the probe;
–false passage formation; or
–inadequate size of the perforation.

2. Physiological (functional) epiphora.

Functional epiphora is persistent watering despite a clear, patent, free-flowing syringing, observed endoscopically in the inferior meatus, with no resistance felt on probing. All other causes of lacrimation or epiphora must be eliminated. The fluorescein disappearance test demonstrates delay. The cause of functional epiphora is probably physiological pump failure but such children may have an upper respiratory cause, such as large adenoids, for their symptoms, and a careful history regarding nasal symptoms should be taken.

3. Complex abnormalities of the outflow system.

Abnormalities of the canaliculi or the proximal nasolacrimal duct become commoner in older children. These abnormalities may be very complex, especially in children with abnormal facial skeletons.[47]

A major advantage of endoscopic probing over "blind" probing is that these common causes of failure can be identified and treated accordingly at the first probing, improving the success rate of the procedure.[48]

If endoscopic probing was not performed on the first occasion then this approach is useful in reprobings as it will identify the most frequent causes of failure and permit appropriate treatment.[48] If the initial procedure was an endoscopic procedure then subsequent treatment is dependent on the original findings. Another option then is intubation of the system with silicone tubes;[49] however, intubation carries more risk of damage to the canaliculi, may not be required (e.g., in functional cases), and is probably no more effective than endoscopic probing in repeat cases.[50]

Intubation

Indications to pass silicone tubes are for upper nasolacrimal duct obstruction and canalicular stenosis.[49] Some recommend intubation for "failed probings"[51] but the etiology of the failure should be clarified prior to performing intubation.

Intubation should take place under general anesthetic after the nose has been prepared with decongestant. It requires nasal endoscopic guidance to view the inferior meatus. The lacrimal system should be probed first to ensure that the tubes have an anatomical passage. Tubes come with a metal introducer and one end should be placed through the system via the upper canaliculus, into the sac, and down the nasolacrimal duct into the inferior meatus from where it should be retrieved under direct vision. The other end of the tube is inserted in exactly the same way through the lower canaliculus. The ends are tied securely with multiple square knots inside the nose and trimmed. Postoperative treatment consists of a topical antibiotic and steroid preparation into the conjunctival sac.

Possible complications of intubation include cheese-wiring through the canaliculi, dislocation superiorly or inferiorly, infection, and scarring of any part of the drainage system.[52]

The optimum time to leave tubes in place is not known, but 3–6 months is usually recommended.[52] Tubes should be removed under general anesthetic via the nose. The tube is cut at the medial canthus and removed under direct vision to prevent aspiration of the tube. This system is then irrigated to remove debris and to confirm patency.

Balloon catheter dilatation of the lacrimal system is a possible alternative to intubation in patients with failed probing.[53] This

has a high success rate similar to intubation, but is significantly more expensive,[54] and the role of balloon dacryoplasty in the management of congenital nasolacrimal duct obstruction has not been fully evaluated.

Dacryocystorhinostomy (DCR)

Children rarely require a dacryocystorhinostomy (DCR), but may do so for persistent epiphora despite probing and intubation, for complex congenital abnormalities of the lacrimal outflow apparatus, particularly involving the canaliculi or upper nasolacrimal duct, or for acquired disease, usually caused by infection or trauma.[55] External and endoscopic routes are possible, and excellent success rates, comparable to those of adult DCRs, have been reported for both.[56,57]

Children with complex craniofacial abnormalities or clefting syndromes may have complicated facial skeletons and must be considered separately. A high success rate can be achieved by specialists with skills to adapt surgical techniques to meet the specific needs of individuals.[20]

Congenital fistulae of the lacrimal outflow system

Fistulae of the lacrimal system are rare anomalies in which tracts open onto the skin directly from the puncta, canaliculi, lacrimal sac, or nasolacrimal duct. They may appear as double puncta, or appear in the region of the medial canthus or below it (Fig. 31.7). They usually pass unnoticed as they are nonfunctioning and should be left untreated unless they allow flow of tears onto the face or result in epiphora (this is rare). Treatment involves excision of the fistula after ensuring that the remaining outflow system is patent.

Punctal and canalicular abnormalities

Failure of the proximal end of the lacrimal drainage system to canalize may result in punctal stenosis or atresia. This is often asymptomatic especially if only one punctum is abnormal. Narrow puncta should be dilated with a Nettleship dilator. Membranous obstruction should be pierced with a needle and dilated. These cases do very well but are often associated with distal abnormalities and a probing should always be performed.

Overall, abnormalities proximal to the sac result in surprisingly few symptoms. Agenesis should be suspected if the papilla is not readily obvious.[58] If only one punctum is missing, syringing via the other one detects the extent of the damage. Surgery to construct these areas is specialized. Retrograde probing from an external DCR incision may be attempted through the sac; otherwise, a Jones tube is required. This type of surgery may be left until the child is in their teens when referral to a specialist should be made.

Acquired conditions of the lacrimal drainage apparatus

Canaliculitis

Canaliculitis in children is uncommon but may be due to bacterial or primary herpes simplex infection. Management involves obtaining viral and bacterial cultures and treating with antibiotics or antiviral agents depending on the clinical and laboratory findings. Probing in the active phase should be avoided.

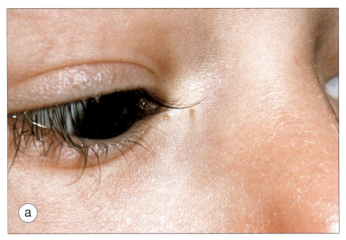 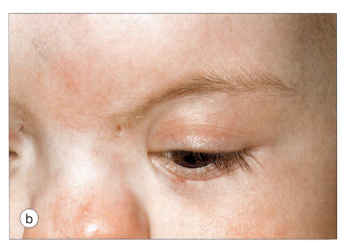

Fig. 31.7 Congenital fistula of the nasolacrimal system. (a) A fistula can be seen as a tiny mark below the medial canthus. (b) A fistula can be seen as a tiny mark above the medial canthus on the side of the nose.

Acute dacryocystitis

Acute dacryocystitis may accompany nonpatent nasolacrimal systems or may occur as a primary event. This is particularly common in infants with dacryocystocele.[59] This requires intravenous antibiotic treatment promptly as retrobulbar abscesses may occur. Cultures should be taken of any pus that can be expressed through the punctum. Probing should not be performed as damage to the congested epithelium may cause false passage formation and lead to orbital cellulitis and fistula formation.[60] Similarly skin incisions should not be made during the acute phase as an external fistula may occur. If a mass remains after resolution, evacuation can be performed through the skin with a needle through the lower pole of the sac, although the pus may be inspissated or loculated, preventing a successful outcome. Once the infection has resolved, probing should be performed although, if completely asymptomatic, this may be avoided.

Acquired nasolacrimal duct obstruction

Acquired nasolacrimal duct obstruction may be caused by diseases of the nose or paranasal sinuses, especially chronic allergic rhinitis or persistent upper respiratory tract infections with enlarged adenoidal lymphoid tissue. These are commoner in older children and adolescents.[43] Rarely acquired obstruction may herald a more sinister cause such as fibrous dysplasia, cranial metaphysial or cranial diaphysial dysplasia, or tumor formation. Treatment should be aimed at the underlying cause.

REFERENCES

1. Sevel D. Development and congenital abnormalities of the nasolacrimal apparatus. J Pediatr Ophthalmol Strabismus 1981; 18: 13–9.
2. Thompson E, Pembury M, Graham JM. Phenotypic variation in the LADD syndrome. J Med Genet 1985; 22: 382–5.
3. Blanksma IJ, Pol BAE. Congenital fistulae of the lacrimal gland. Br J Ophthalmol 1980; 64: 515–7.
4. Chorobski J. Syndrome of crocodile tears. Arch Neurol Psychiatr 1951; 65: 299–318.
5. Ramsay J, Taylor D. Congenital crocodile tears: a key to the aetiology of Duane's syndrome. Br J Ophthalmol 1980; 64: 518–22.
6. Riley CM. Familial autonomic dysfunction. J Am Med Assoc 1952; 149: 1532–5.
7. Houlden H, Smith S, De Carvalho M, et al. Clinical and genetic characterization of families with triple A (Allgrove) syndrome. Brain 2002; 125: 2681–90.
8. Merayo-Lloves J, Baltatzis Z, Foster CS. Epstein Barr virus dacryoadenitis resulting in keratoconjunctivitis sicca in a child. Am J Ophthalmol 2001; 132: 922–3.
9. Suh DW, Ruttum MS, Stuckenschneider BJ, et al. Ocular findings after bone marrow transplantation in a pediatric population. Ophthalmology 1999; 106: 1564–70
10. Prendiville JS, Hebert AA, Greenwald MJ, Esterly NB. Management of Stevens Johnson syndrome and toxic epidermal necrolysis in children. J Pediatr 1989; 115: 881–7.
11. Stiller M, Golder W, Doring E, Biedermann T. Primary and secondary Sjogren's syndrome in children–a comparative study. Clin Oral Investig 2000; 4: 176–82.
12. Riffenburgh RS. Ocular manifestations of mumps. Arch Ophthalmol 1961; 66: 739–43.
13. Duke Elder S, MacFaul PA. The ocular adnexae. In: Duke-Elder S, editor. System of Ophthalmology. St Louis: Mosby; 1974: 605–10. (vol 8, Part 1.)
14. Chavis RM, Garner A, Wright JE. Inflammatory orbital pseudotumour. A clinicopathologic study. Arch Ophthalmol 1978; 96: 1817–22.
15. Wright JE, Stewart WB, Krohel GB. Clinical presentation and management of lacrimal gland tumours. Br J Ophthalmol 1979; 63: 600–6.
16. Cassady JV. Developmental anatomy of the nasolacrimal duct. Arch Ophthalmol 1952; 47: 141–58.
17. Harris GJ, DiClementi D. Congenital dacryocystocoele. Arch Ophthalmol 1982; 100: 1763–5.
18. Edmond JC, Keech RV. Congenital nasolacrimal sac mucocoele associated with respiratory distress. J Pediatr Ophthalmol Strabismus 1991; 28: 287–9.
19. Lin AE, Losken HW, Jaffe R, Biglan AW. The branchio-oculo-facial syndrome. Cleft Palate Craniofac J 1991; 28: 96–102.
20. McHugh DA, Rose GE, Garner A. Nasolacrimal obstruction and facial bone histopathology in craniodiaphyseal dysplasia. Br J Ophthalmol 1994; 78: 501–3.
21. Markowitz GD, Handler LF, Katowitz JA. Congenital euryoblepharon and nasolacrimal duct abnormalies in a patient with Down syndrome. J Pediatr Ophthalmol Strabismus 1994; 31: 330–1.
22. Heinz GW, Bateman JB, Barrett DJ, et al. Ocular manifestations of the lacrimo-auriculo-dento-digital syndrome. Am J Ophthalmol 1993; 115: 243–8.
23. Bowling BS, Chandna A. Superior lacrimal canalicular atresia and nasolacrimal duct obstruction in the CHARGE association. J Pediatr Ophthalmol Strabismus 1994; 31: 336–7.

24. MacEwen CJ, Young JD. The fluorescein disappearance test (FDT): an evaluation of its use in infants. J Pediatr Ophthalmol Strabismus 1991; 28: 302–5.

25. Price HW. Dacryostenosis. J Pediatr 1947; 30: 302–5.

26. Petersen RA, Robb RM. The natural course of congenital obstruction of the nasolacrimal duct. J Pediatr Ophthalmol Strabismus 1978; 15: 246–50.

27. Paul TO. Medical management of congenital nasolacrimal duct obstruction. J Pediatr Ophthalmol Strabismus 1985; 22: 68–70.

28. MacEwen CJ, Young JD. Epiphora during the first year of life. Eye 1991; 5: 596–600.

29. Young JD, MacEwen CJ, Ogston SA. Congenital nasolacrimal duct obstruction in the second year of life: a multicentre trial of management. Eye 1996; 10: 485–91.

30. Nucci P, Capoferri C, Alfarano R, Brancato R. Conservative management of congenital nasolacrimal duct obstruction. J Pediatr Ophthalmol Strabismus 1989; 26: 39–43.

31. Jones LT, Wobig JL. Surgery of the Eyelids and the Lacrimal System. Birmingham, AL: Aesculapius; 1976: 96–104.

32. Kushner BJ. Congenital nasolacrimal system obstruction. Arch Ophthalmol 1982; 100: 597–600.

33. Noda S, Hayasaka S, Setogawa T. Congenital nasolacrimal duct obstruction in Japanese infants; its incidence and treatment with massage. J Pediatr Ophthalmol Strabismus 1991; 28: 20–2.

34. MacEwen CJ, Phillips MG, Young JD. Value of bacterial culturing in the course of congenital nasolacrimal duct (NLD) obstruction. J Pediatr Ophthalmol Strabismus 1994; 31: 246–50.

35. Ffookes OO. Dacryocystitis in infancy. Br J Ophthalmol 1962; 46: 422–34.

36. Baker JD. Treatment of congenital nasolacrimal duct obstruction. J Pediatr Ophthalmol Strabismus 1985; 22: 34–6.

37. Katowitz JA, Welsh MG. Timing of initial probing and irrigation in congenital nasolacrimal duct obstruction. Ophthalmology 1987; 94: 698–705.

38. Mannor GE, Rose GE, Frimpong-Ansah K, Ezra E. Factors affecting the success of nasolacrimal duct probing for congenital nasolacrimal duct obstruction. Am J Ophthalmol 1999; 127: 616–7.

39. Robb RM. Probing and irrigation for congenital nasolacrimal duct obstruction. Arch Ophthalmol 1986; 104: 378–9.

40. el-Mansoury J, Calhoun JH, Nelson LB, Harley RD. Results of late probing for congenital nasolacrimal obstruction. Ophthalmology 1986; 93: 1052–4.

41. Nelson LB, Calhoun JH, Menduke H. Medical management of congenital nasolacrimal duct obstruction. Pediatriacs 1985; 76: 172–5.

42. Kashkouli MB, Kassaee A, Tabatabaee Z. Initial nasolacrimal duct probing in children under age 5: cure rate and factors affecting success. J AAPOS 2002; 6: 360–3.

43. Sturrock SM, MacEwen CJ, Young JD. Long term results after probing for congenital naso-lacrimal duct obstruction. Br J Ophthalmol 1994; 78: 892–4.

44. Paul TO, Shepherd R. Congenital nasolacrimal duct obstruction: natural history and the timing of optimal intervention. J Pediatr Ophthalmol Strabismus 1994; 31: 362–7.

45. Ram B, Barras CW, White PS, et al. The technique of nasendoscopy in the evaluation of nasolacrimal duct obstruction in children. Rhinology 2000; 38: 83–6.

46. Wesley RE. Inferior turbinate fracture in the treatment of congenital nasolacrimal duct obstruction and congenital nasolacrimal duct anomaly. Ophthalmic Surg 1985; 16: 368–71.

47. Hicks C, Pitts J, Rose GE. Lacrimal surgery in patients with congenital cranial or facial anomalies. Eye 1994; 8: 583–91.

48. MacEwen CJ, Young JD, Barras CW, et al. Value of nasal endoscopy and probing in the diagnosis and management of children with congenital epiphora. Br J Ophthalmol 2001; 85: 314–8.

49. Crawford JA, Pashby RC. Lacrimal system disorders. Int Ophthalmol Clin 1984; 24: 39–53.

50. Gardiner JA, Forte V, Pashby RC, Levin AV. The role of nasal endoscopy in repeat paediatric naso-lacrimal duct probings. JAAPOS 2001; 5: 148–52.

51. Aggarwal RK, Misson GP, Donaldson I, Willshaw HE. The role of nasolacrimal intubation in the management of childhood epiphora. Eye 1993; 7: 760–2.

52. Welsh MG, Katowitz JA. Timing of Silastic tubing removal after intubation for congenital nasolacrimal duct obstruction. Ophthal Plast Resconstr Surg 1989; 5: 43–8.

53. Becker BB, Berry FD. Balloon catheter dilatation in pediatric patients. Ophthalmic Surg 1991; 22: 750–2.

54. Kushner BJ. Balloon catheter dilatation for congenital nasolacrimal duct obstruction. Am J Ophthalmol 1996; 122: 598–9.

55. Billson FA, Taylor HR, Hoyt CS. Trauma to the lacrimal system in children. Am J Ophthalmol 1978; 86: 828–33.

56. Welham RA, Hughes S. Lacrimal surgery in children. Am J Ophthalmol 1985; 99: 27–34.

57. Hakin KN, Sullivan TJ, Sharma A, Welham RA. Paediatric dacryocystorhinostomy. Aust NZ J Ophthalmol 1994; 22: 231–5.

58. Lyons CJ, Rosser PM, Welham RA. The management of punctal agenesis. Ophthalmology 1993; 100: 1851–5.

59. Pollard ZF. Treatment of acute dacryocystitis in neonates. J Pediatr Ophthalmol Strabismus 1991; 28: 341–3.

60. Weiss GH, Leib ML. Congenital dacryocystitis and retrobulbar abscess. J Pediatr Ophthalmol Strabismus 1993; 30: 271–2.

CHAPTER 32 Orbital Disease in Children

Christopher J Lyons, Wilma Chang, and Jack Rootman

Abnormalities of the orbit in childhood may be developmental or acquired. Developmental abnormalities can be confined to the orbit or be part of a more widespread craniofacial malformation. A shallow or small orbit can result in proptosis. The relationship between the orbits may be disturbed; hypertelorism results in wide separation while conversely in hypotelorism, they are set close together. Part of the orbital walls may be deficient, allowing prolapse of intracranial tissue, a cause of pulsating exophthalmos, or sometimes pulsating enophthalmos. Normally, the orbits continue to develop throughout childhood but congenital absence of the globe, enucleation, or radiotherapy can result in failure of the orbit to grow normally.

Children with acquired orbital disease most commonly present with signs and symptoms of a mass effect, leading to proptosis or nonaxial displacement, soft tissue signs, and/or a palpable orbital mass. Other presenting symptoms and signs include reduced vision, restriction of ocular movements, pain, and inflammation. Occasionally, enophthalmos may be a presenting sign, for instance, following orbital trauma resulting in a blowout fracture.

The relative frequencies of the conditions causing proptosis in childhood have varied considerably in previous series,[1–8] depending, in part, on the source of the material. Series from eye hospitals[3] are different from those from neurosurgical[2] or pediatric units.[6] Geographical factors are also important. For example, the major causes of proptosis in African children[4] are different from those seen in Europe and North America. Series that have relied solely on histopathological examination of biopsy specimens[1,5,7,8] reflect the incidence of lesions encountered surgically. However, biopsy-based studies do not represent the many conditions that can be diagnosed and treated without biopsy or surgery, such as capillary hemangioma, or those in which biopsy may be more conveniently obtained at another site of involvement, such as neuroblastoma or histiocytosis. In that sense, they are not helpful in formulating the differential diagnosis of a child with proptosis.

ORBITAL DISEASE AND AGE

The reviews mentioned above have stressed the major differences between childhood and adult orbital disease. However, even within the childhood years, defined here as ages up to and including 16 years, there are trends in the incidence of the causative disorders that, when understood, can usefully contribute to the diagnostic process.

We have reviewed the clinical data of 326 children seen by the orbital service in Vancouver, Canada since 1976 (Table 32.1). This period postdates the introduction of the computed tomography (CT) scan, a watershed in the noninvasive investigation of orbital disease. It is clear from Fig. 32.1 that neoplasia and

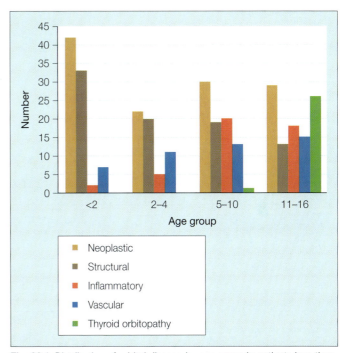

Fig. 32.1 Distribution of orbital disease by age group in patients less than 17 years of age.

structural abnormalities (including cysts) account for the great majority of children presenting with orbital disease. This is quite different from the adult pattern of orbital disease, in which over 60% of presentations are due to inflammatory causes and structural abnormalities account for less than 15% of cases.[9] The distribution of orbital disease in children aged over 11 years largely conforms to the adult pattern (Fig. 32.2).

Surprisingly, only a small proportion of the neoplasia can be considered malignant, which concurs with previously published series.[6,7,10] Under 2 years of age, the major causes of proptosis are capillary hemangioma and lymphangioma, inclusion and dermoid cysts, and other structural abnormalities. Figure 32.3, which shows the distribution of the major diagnostic groups by age at presentation, indicates that while some lesions are distributed evenly throughout childhood (lymphangioma, varices, and arteriovenous malformations), others tend to occur within a specific age range. Seven patients with rhabdomyosarcoma were seen, whose ages ranged from 2 to 11 years. The seven patients with Langerhans cell histiocytosis ranged in age from 3 to 9 years. Capillary hemangiomas did not present after the age of 15 years. The incidence of inflammatory conditions increased over the age of 5 years, especially orbital cellulitis, nonspecific orbital inflammatory syndromes (6 years and over), and thyroid orbitopathy

Table 32.1 Orbital disease in children—multiseries data comparison

	Rootman[9]		Bullock et al.[10]		Crawford[6]		All series	
	No.	% of series	No.	% of series	No.	% of series	No.	% of all series
Neoplasia								
Optic nerve glioma	17	5.2	5	3.6	17	3.0	39	3.8
Meningioma	2	0.6	2	1.4			4	0.4
Other neurogenic tumor	6	1.8					1	0.1
PNS tumors	19	5.8	9	6.4	14	2.5	42	4.1
Lymphocytic	1	0.3	1	0.7	3	0.5	5	0.5
Other lymphocytic	3	0.9	4	2.9	20	3.6	27	2.6
Histiocytic	7	2.1	1	0.7	20	3.6	28	2.7
Vascular	36	11.0	14	13.6	14	2.5	64	6.2
Secondary/metastatic	5	1.5	4	2.9	21	3.8	30	2.9
Mesenchymal								
Rhabdomyosarcoma	7	2.1	3	2.1	11	2.0	21	2.0
Fibrous	1	0.3	3	2.1	1	0.2	5	0.5
Histiocytic	2	0.6	2	1.4			4	0.4
Bone	3	0.9					3	0.3
Neoplasia	6	1.8	2	1.4	5	0.9	13	1.3
Other	2	0.6	1	0.7			3	0.3
Unknown neoplasia			1	0.7	3	0.5	4	0.4
Lacrimal	2	0.6					2	0.2
Teratoma					1	0.2	1	0.1
Structural								
Cystic	60	18.4	59	42.1	6	1.1	122	11.9
Bone anomalies	9	2.8			50	8.9	59	5.8
Ectopia	13	4.0	11	7.9			24	2.3
Other	3	0.9			2	0.4	4	0.4
Inflammatory								
Infectious diseases	21	6.4			232	41.5	253	24.7
NSOIS	14	4.3	6	4.3	5	0.9	25	2.4
Other–inflammatory	10	3.1	3	2.1			13	1.3
Thyroid orbitopathy	27	8.3			107	19.1	134	13.1
Vascular	46	14.1	9	2.9	14	2.5	69	6.7
Atrophy/degeneration	2	0.6					2	0.2
Unknown	2	0.6			13	2.3	15	1.5
Total	326		140		559		1025	

NSOIS, nonspecific orbital inflammatory syndrome
PNS, peripheral nerve sheath

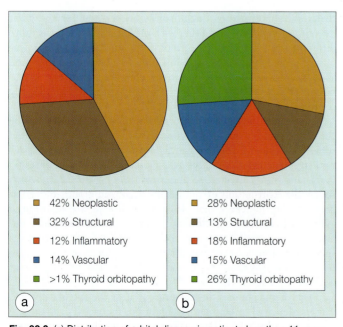

(a)   (b)

Legend (a):
- 42% Neoplastic
- 32% Structural
- 12% Inflammatory
- 14% Vascular
- >1% Thyroid orbitopathy

Legend (b):
- 28% Neoplastic
- 13% Structural
- 18% Inflammatory
- 15% Vascular
- 26% Thyroid orbitopathy

Fig. 32.2 (a) Distribution of orbital disease in patients less than 11 years of age. (b) Distribution of orbital disease in patients 11–17 years.

(11 years and over). The small numbers involved do not allow hard and fast rules to be stated since, for example, histiocytosis is well known to occur in infancy and early childhood, but this series may provide clinicians with a framework for the working diagnosis of a child with mass effect. It is also noteworthy that there were two cases of lacrimal gland carcinoma and four of Wegener granulomatosis in this series, a reminder that, although rare, these potentially lethal conditions do occur in children.

CLINICAL ASSESSMENT

When assessing a child with orbital disease, a careful history, examination, and differential diagnosis in the context of the child's age are essential before investigations can be planned.

History

The age of onset, laterality (unilateral or bilateral), and the tempo of onset are important clues to the underlying diagnosis. As with adult orbital disease, the duration may be difficult to determine accurately. A review of old photographs may be helpful to identify the time of onset of an orbital problem.

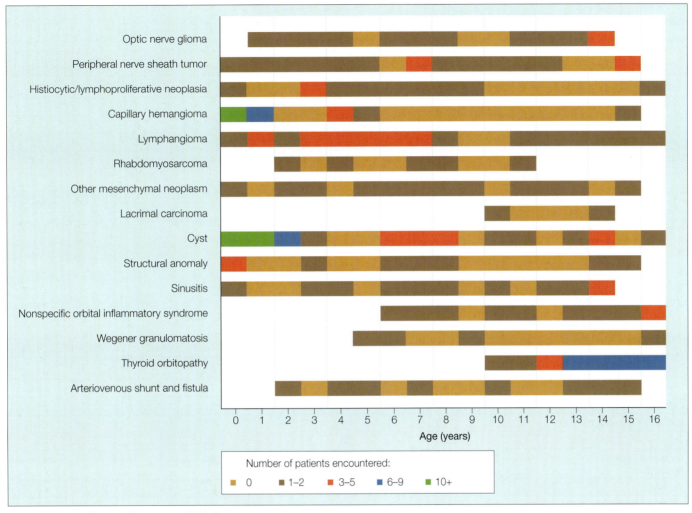

Fig. 32.3 Age distribution of common orbital diseases.

Bilateral proptosis in early infancy is often due to orbital shallowing in craniofacial malformations. This can occasionally be unilateral, as in plagiocephaly. Usually, however, unilateral proptosis is due to the globe being displaced forward by a mass within the orbit.

Some masses such as optic nerve glioma or dermoid cyst grow slowly. Rapidly increasing proptosis suggests a metastatic deposit or rapidly growing tumor such as rhabdomyosarcoma. Rapid tumor growth may be associated with necrosis, resulting in periorbital ecchymosis. The presence of bilateral ecchymosis is suggestive of metastatic neuroblastoma. The causes of proptosis in our series are listed in Table 32.2.

A catastrophic onset (within hours) implies a bleed within an (often unsuspected) preexisting lesion such as a lymphangioma. Occasionally, the onset of orbital cellulitis may also be very sudden. Here, it is usually accompanied by pain, local inflammation, and limitation of ocular motility in a child who is generally ill and febrile. The presence of clinically detectable orbital and periorbital inflammatory symptoms and signs in childhood is overwhelmingly associated with either infection or nonspecific orbital inflammatory disease. Although inflammation is part of the classical description of rhabdomyosarcoma, this sign was absent in all six patients with this diagnosis in our series, all of which did, however, have rapid onset.

Most round-cell tumors in childhood, including rhabdomyosarcoma, granulocytic sarcoma (chloroma), and Ewing sarcoma, present as a mass developing over weeks in a subacute manner, except neuroblastoma, which can present with onset of proptosis over days.

An increase in proptosis with crying or straining is suggestive of capillary hemangioma, varices, or absence of the sphenoid wing (as in neurofibromatosis type 1, NF1). This sign is useful in the neonate, where crying is almost invariably elicited by a thorough examination. When very obvious, its presence helps to exclude malignancy as a cause of the proptosis.

Pulsating exophthalmos may be associated with congenital defects of the orbital wall (as seen in NF1) or encephalocele. Occasionally, large capillary hemangiomas may pulsate due to their rich arterial blood supply, as may high-flow arteriovenous malformations, although the latter are rare in childhood and more commonly present in adolescence or young adulthood.

Skin discoloration may offer a clue to the underlying etiology. Red is suggestive of the arterial supply of capillary hemangioma, which, when superficial to the septum, almost invariably involves the overlying skin. When deep, these may have a blueish or purple hue. Lesions derived from venous anlage, such as varices or lymphangiomas, appear blue or purple, as do some cystic lesions, such as lacrimal or conjunctival cysts. The brownish cutaneous discoloration of hemosiderin is usually caused by previous bleeds into a lymphangioma or, rarely, by neuroblastoma. Both of these may present with spontaneous ecchymosis.

Table 32.2 Causes of proptosis in children (excluding thyroid orbitopathy)

	All years		0–2 years		3–10 years		11+ years	
	Number	%	*Number*	%	*Number*	%	*Number*	%
Optic nerve gliomas	8	2.5	1	0.3	3	0.9	4	1.2
Peripheral nerve sheath tumors	4	1.2	1	0.3	1	0.3	2	0.6
Lymphoproliferative	5	1.5	1	0.3	4	1.2	1	0.3
Capillary hemangiomas	7	2.2	6	1.8	1	0.3	1	0.3
Bone/mesenchymal tumors	7	2.2	3	0.9	3	0.9	1	0.3
Sinusitis	9	2.8	0	0.0	8	2.5	1	0.3
Lymphangiomas	20	6.2	5	1.5	10	3.1	5	1.5
All causes	81	24.9	21	6.5	41	12.6	19	5.8

Number of patients in series with nonthyroid orbital disease, *n*=325.

Table 32.3 Causes of mass effect in children (excluding thyroid orbitopathy)

	All years			0–2 years			3–10 years			11–16 years		
	No.	% series	% cohort	No.	% series	% cohort	No.	% series	% cohort	No.	% series	% cohort
Optic nerve gliomas	8	2.5	3.9	1	0.3	1.2	3	0.9	3.7	4	1.2	10.5
Peripheral nerve sheath tumors	8	2.5	3.9	2	0.6	2.4	4	1.2	4.9	2	0.6	5.3
Lymphoproliferative	8	2.5	3.9	1	0.3	1.2	6	1.8	7.3	1	0.3	2.6
Capillary hemangiomas	30	9.2	14.8	22	6.8	26.5	5	1.5	6.1	1	0.3	2.6
Bone/mesenchymal tumors	15	4.6	7.4	3	0.9	3.6	8	2.5	9.8	4	1.2	10.5
Congenital cysts and dermolipomas	62	19.1	30.5	37	11.4	44.6	17	5.2	20.7	8	2.5	21.1
Sinusitis	9	2.8	4.4	0	0.0	0.0	8	2.5	9.8	1	0.3	2.6
Lymphangiomas	26	8.0	12.8	6	1.8	7.2	14	4.3	17.1	7	2.2	18.4
All causes of mass effect	203	62.5		83	25.5		82	25.2		38	11.7	

Number of patients in series with nonthyroid orbital disease, *n* = 325.

Examination

Children with proptosis must have a visual acuity assessment. In infants, this may be limited to observing the fixation of the two eyes; resentment to covering the contralateral eye suggests poor vision. The 10-prism-diopter base-down test may be useful if poor vision is suspected in a child with straight eyes. A cover test should be performed and ocular ductions and versions assessed. Limitation of ductions may be due to mechanical restriction by tumor, muscle infiltration, inflammation, edema, or entrapment. Third, fourth, and sixth cranial nerve function should be tested, as well as sensory testing in the V_1 and V_2 distribution in patients old enough to cooperate. Occasionally, as in an older child with a blowout fracture, a forced duction test may be useful in detecting muscle restriction.

The site of an orbital mass may be indicated by the direction in which the eye is displaced. A posterior or intraconal tumor will result in axial proptosis, whereas a tumor placed more anteriorly may displace the eye vertically or laterally. For example, in fibrous dysplasia of the orbit, which most commonly affects the frontal bone, the globe is usually displaced downward and forward. Orbital cellulitis secondary to ethmoidal sinus infection usually displaces the globe laterally. Although the globe is dis-

placed away from most mass lesions, it can occasionally be displaced toward them, as in the case of cicatrizing metastasis to the orbit (Table 32.3).

Enophthalmos

Enophthalmos, or a relative recession of the eyeball in the orbit, may occur in the following cases:
1. Following radiotherapy (Fig. 32.4);
2. Sphenoid wing dysplasia and other bone dysplasias;
3. Parry-Romberg syndrome or morphea (Fig. 32.5);
4. Developmental tumors (Fig. 32.6); and
5. Orbital blowout fracture.

Globe position should be recorded using an exophthalmometer, and a transparent ruler is used to measure the amount of vertical and horizontal displacement. Eyelid position should also be recorded; retraction or lag may suggest thyroid orbitopathy, but may also be indicative of tethering by tumors such as Langerhans cell histiocytosis.

Slit-lamp examination may show dilated dysmorphic venous channels in the conjunctiva of patients with varices. Lymphangioma may be associated with visible conjunctival lymphangiectasis or

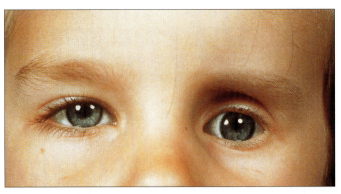

Fig. 32.4 Left enophthalmos following radiotherapy for retinoblastoma. Patient of the University of British Columbia.

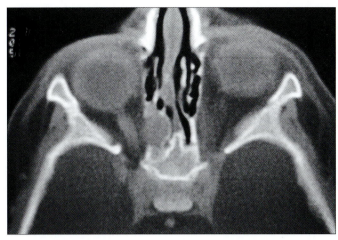

Fig. 32.6 Acquired enophthalmos caused by an astroglial tumor involving the paranasal sinuses.

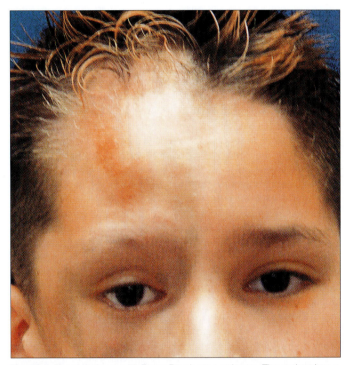

Fig. 32.5 Enophthalmos with Parry-Romberg syndrome. The patient has a chronic right-sided uveitis, atrophy of the subcutaneous tissues, pigmentary changes, and hair loss on the affected side. Patient of the University of British Columbia.

cysts, which occasionally contain a meniscus of blood (see Fig. 42.13b). The presence of Lisch nodules on the iris is one of the earliest diagnostic signs of NF1, suggesting plexiform neurofibroma or sphenoid wing dysplasia with encephalocele as causes of proptosis. Optic nerve glioma is thought to run a relatively benign course in the presence of NF1, and identification of Lisch nodules in an affected patient may suggest a relatively good visual prognosis, but a poorer prognosis for survival due to the risk of developing other central nervous system tumors. Juvenile cataract is increasingly recognized as an early marker for NF2, and its presence may suggest meningioma or schwannoma as a cause of orbital mass effect, possibly prompting audiological assessment for vestibular schwannoma.

The existence of an afferent pupillary defect indicates optic neuropathy, which may be due to intrinsic disease, as in glioma, or to extrinsic compression, as in fibrous dysplasia involving the optic canal (rare). In the cooperative child, the use of neutral density filters allows accurate comparison of the affected nerve with its fellow. In this situation, field testing might reveal the central scotoma of optic neuropathy; chiasmal involvement, for example by glioma, may show bitemporal field loss. In the older age group, color vision can be assessed using subjective red desaturation or an Ishihara chart to confirm the presence of a subtle optic neuropathy.

Cycloplegic refraction is important for detecting astigmatism due to distortion of the globe by an orbital mass. Retrobulbar lesions tend to result in a hyperopic shift, whereas lesions at or anterior to the equator produce astigmatism. Left untreated, these changes are important causes of amblyopia.[11] Occasionally, myopia may mimic proptosis, particularly when unilateral. Long-term occlusion of an eye, as in uncorrected unilateral ptosis due to capillary hemangioma, results in ipsilateral axial myopia.

Optic disc swelling or atrophy can appear in patients with optic nerve compression or glioma. If the mass is close behind the globe, choroidal folds may be present. Opticociliary shunt vessels, classically associated with meningioma, may much less frequently be noted in optic nerve glioma.

Palpation of the orbit reveals the consistency of a localized mass. Capillary hemangiomas feel firm and spongy, and their contents cannot be expelled by palpation, whereas orbital varices are easily drained of blood, even with gentle pressure. Dermoids should be carefully examined for mobility and the presence of a tail extending into the posterior orbit or temporalis fossa. A posterior extension or extension through the lateral wall of the orbit is more likely to be present in dermoids situated inside the orbital rim than in those directly overlying the rim.

Although the orbit does not have true lymphatics, the preauricular and submandibular lymph nodes should be palpated to exclude enlargement from metastasis, as in rhabdomyosarcoma involving the eyelids, or infection, as in orbital cellulitis.

The evaluation of children with orbital disease should include systemic examination, since this may give useful clues to the diagnosis. Café-au-lait spots may suggest a diagnosis of neuro-fibromatosis, and skin pigmentation may also be seen in fibrous dysplasia. Characteristic skin lesions may also be present in Langerhans cell histiocytosis and juvenile xanthogranuloma. Capillary hemangioma of the orbit is often associated with cutaneous capillary hemangiomas elsewhere. In suspected metastatic disease there may be other involved sites such as an abdominal mass in neuroblastoma or skin, scalp, or bony lesions in Langerhans cell histiocytosis. Thyroid orbitopathy may be accompanied by systemic signs or history of hyperthyroidism suggestive of this diagnosis.

Opinions from other specialists, particularly general pediatricians and ENT surgeons, may help to determine the cause of unexplained proptosis in a child.

INVESTIGATIONS

Investigating children with proptosis should be guided by the history and clinical findings and tailored to each individual case. In some instances, such as craniofacial abnormalities, the abnormalities fit a clear pattern and further investigations are not warranted. In others, further tests will be necessary to confirm the suspected diagnosis or to assess the degree of orbital involvement. When other systems are involved, such as extension of tumor into the brain or sinuses or systemic involvement in malignancy, investigation of the child should be planned from the outset with the other specialists who may become involved in the child's care.

Radiology

Plain X-rays
Although CT scan is the initial radiological investigation in most patients with orbital disease, plain X-rays are still useful in certain circumstances. These include the assessment of orbital bony trauma, localization of a radio-opaque orbital foreign body, and assessment of systemic disease (such as absence of the sphenoid wing in neurofibromatosis).

Sinus X-rays in suspected sinus disease with orbital cellulitis should be interpreted with care, since sinus anatomy is variable under the age of 10 years. Although the finding of bony distortion on the affected side suggests a long-standing or slow-growing process in adults, this sign is unreliable in children, where it may be seen with rapidly enlarging lesions (see Fig. 37.4).

The principal merits of plain X-rays are the ubiquity of the equipment, low cost, and the fact that sedation is rarely required. Although the dose of radiation delivered in a CT scan of the orbit is higher than that used in a plain X-ray, the diagnostic yield per unit of radiation exposure is much greater with CT.[12]

Computed tomography and magnetic resonance imaging
Diagnostic imaging of orbital structures was revolutionized by the development of CT in the early 1970s. Optimal imaging requires 1.5- to 3.0-mm slice thickness and both direct coronal and axial images, but may be tailored to the clinical need.[13] Thin slices are indicated for optic nerve and foreign body imaging. Recent scanners allow high-resolution coronal reformatting of axial images, avoiding repositioning of the patient to obtain coronal views. CT will provide information about intracranial as well as orbital structures.[13] It yields more information on the presence of

calcification and on bony detail; soft tissue and "bone window" settings can be specifically requested.[14] CT can also be used when a ferromagnetic foreign body is suspected. The differential diagnostic yield is increased by the use of contrast in selected cases,[15] since vascular lesions, inflammations, and some malignancies are enhanced after contrast injection. Sedation is usually necessary under the age of 5 years. Other disadvantages include the relatively high dose of radiation delivered to the eye.

Magnetic resonance imaging (MRI) provides higher resolution of soft tissue without exposure to ionizing radiation.[13] This is particularly important if repeat imaging is necessary, for example, a child with NF1 and optic nerve glioma who is being followed regularly. Any desired plane can be chosen at the time of the examination, for example, directly along the optic nerve. Orbital views may be obtained with a 0.5- to 3.0-T field, and surface coils should be used to increase the surface-to-noise ratio. Contrast enhancement can be obtained for indications similar to those outlined above for CT, using Gadolinium, which results in T_1 shortening. Because fat has a bright signal on T_1-weighted images, fat saturation techniques must be used to maximize the conspicuity of contrast enhancement in the orbit. Multiple image sequences can provide characteristic signal patterns, such as the fluid/fluid levels typical of low- or no-flow vascular malformations and aneurysmal bone cysts. Identification and dating of blood within hemorrhagic lesions such as lymphangiomas, presence or absence of flow within mass lesions, and contrast enhancement of the optic nerve in optic neuritis are further strengths of this technique in the orbit.

Disadvantages include the time taken to image an orbit (30–45 minutes) compared with CT, which takes less than 5 minutes; the actual image acquisition time for the latter is even shorter, so CT can be used without sedation for much younger patients who can lie still for 2 or 3 minutes. Conversely, most patients under the age of 8 require sedation for MRI because of the noise and duration of the procedure. Other drawbacks include a contraindication for patients with ferromagnetic foreign bodies, including aneurysm clips. A more specific problem of MRI for orbital work is its relative inability to image bone and calcification clearly,[14] which may be important when differentiating glioma from meningioma in the orbit. Also, specific fat-suppression techniques are needed to mask the bright signal from fat to image orbital structures such as the optic nerve.

The texts by Newton and Bilaniuk,[16] Bilaniuk and Farber,[17] and Som and Curtin[18] are useful for readers seeking further information on imaging of the orbit in childhood.

SURGERY

The surgical approach for access to the child's orbit differs markedly from that taken in adult orbital disease. This is due to the relative shallowness of the orbit in childhood. Lateral orbitotomy, with lateral orbital wall removal, is unnecessary in most cases since the lesions can usually be reached via the relatively atraumatic anterior approach.

REFERENCES

1. Porterfield JF. Orbital tumors in children: a report on 214 cases. Int Ophthalmol Clin 1962; 2: 319–26.
2. MacCarty CS, Brown DN. Orbital tumors in children. Clin Neurosurg 1982; 11: 76–84.
3. Youseffi B. Orbital tumors in children: a clinical study of 62 cases. J Pediatr Ophthalmol Strabismus 1969; 6: 177–81.
4. Templeton AC. Orbital tumours in African children. Br J Ophthalmol 1971; 55: 254–61.
5. Eldrup-Jorgensen P, Fledelius H. Orbital tumours in infancy: an analysis of Danish cases from 1943–1962. Acta Ophthalmol 1975; 53: 887–93.
6. Crawford JS. Diseases of the orbit. In: Crawford JS, Morin JD, editors. The Eye in Childhood. New York: Grune and Stratton; 1983: 361–94.
7. Shields JA, Bakewell B, Augsburger JJ, et al. Space occupying orbital masses in children. A review of 250 consecutive biopsies. Ophthalmology 1986; 93: 379–84.
8. Kodsi SR, Shetlar DJ, Campbell RJ, et al. A review of 340 orbital tumors in children during a 60-year period. Am J Ophthalmol 1994; 117: 177–82.
9. Rootman J. Diseases of the Orbit: a Multidisciplinary Approach. 2nd ed. Philadelphia: Lippincott Williams and Wilkins; 2003.
10. Bullock JD, Goldberg SH, Rakes SM. Orbital tumors in children. Ophthal Plast Reconstr Surg 1989; 5: 13–6.
11. Bogan S, Simon JW, Krohel GB, et al. Astigmatism associated with adnexal masses in infancy. Arch Ophthalmol 1987; 105: 1368–70.
12. Weiss RA, Haik BG, Smith ME. Introduction to diagnostic imaging techniques in ophthalmology. Int Ophthalmol Clin 1986; 26: 1–24.
13. Mafee MF, Mafee RF, Malik M, et al. Medical imaging in pediatric ophthalmology. Pediatr Clin N Am 2003; 50: 259–86.
14. Mafee MF. The orbit proper. In: Som PM, Bergeron RT, editors. Head and Neck Imaging. 2nd ed. St. Louis: Mosby; 1991: 747–813.
15. Moseley IF, Sanders MD. Computerized Tomography in Neuro-ophthalmology. London: Chapman and Hall; 1982.
16. Newton TH, Bilaniuk LT, editors. Radiology of the Eye and Orbit. New York: Raven Press; 1990.
17. Bilaniuk LT, Farber M. Imaging of developmental anomalies of the eye and orbit. Am J Neuroradiol 1992; 13: 793–803.
18. Som PM, Curtin HD, editors. Head and Neck Imaging. 4th ed. St. Louis: Mosby; 2003.

CHAPTER 33   Neurofibromatosis

Christopher J Lyons

The term "neurofibromatosis" originally described a condition that is now known to be a group of genetically distinct neurocristopathies. Although they have a number of similar features, their clinically significant manifestations are largely different. It is the overlap in their cutaneous manifestations, including neurofibromas, café-au-lait patches and plexiform neurofibromas which gave rise to the common name. Affected patients also have a propensity to develop hamartomas and central nervous system tumors, and there also appears to be some overlap in their type. Nevertheless, these diseases are separate entities. The most common are neurofibromatosis types 1 and 2 (NF1 and NF2), as well as type 5 (segmental, NF5). Up to seven distinct entities have been identified.[1] Since each name denotes a specific disease entity with a predictable range of manifestations, each may require a different screening and follow-up protocol. The numeric suffix is therefore important.

NEUROFIBROMATOSIS TYPE 1

This disease, described by von Recklinghausen in 1882[2] and eponymous thereafter, has also been called peripheral neurofibromatosis in contrast to the central form, which is now known as NF2. The National Institutes of Health (NIH) diagnostic criteria are listed in Table 33.1. These are by no means the only findings in NF1 and many others are described below.

Genetic aspects

NF1 is a progressive disease whose final manifestations are extremely variable. With time, however, existing lesions tend to enlarge gradually and new lesions develop. The parents of a newly diagnosed child will wish to know the likely severity of their NF1 manifestations and their potential effects on life, sight and cosmesis. They will also enquire about the likelihood of further children being affected. Careful counseling is important to allay the fears of gross physical deformity, which folklore has often incorrectly attributed to this diagnosis.

NF1 is probably the most common single gene disorder affecting the nervous system, occurring in approximately 1 in 3000 people. It is autosomal dominantly inherited. Although it has 100% penetrance, its expressivity is highly variable from generation to generation. There is a high spontaneous mutation rate, possibly related to the very large size of the gene, which is situated in the pericentromeric region of the long arm of chromosome 17. The absence of a family history therefore does not preclude the diagnosis of NF1.

The NF1 gene encodes a large cytoplasmic protein called neurofibromin expressed in a variety of tissues including, in the brain, neurons, astrocytes, oligodendrocytes and in the periphery, Schwann cells and peripheral nerves. Part of the protein is thought to down-regulate Ras molecules, which promote astrocyte proliferation and malignant transformation. Loss of neurofibromin expression increases Ras activity. NF1 is therefore thought to function as a tumor suppressor gene.

The genetic mechanism through which NF1 mutations give rise to malignant tumors may be similar to that of retinoblastoma formation,[3] which results from the deletion of both copies of a tumor-suppressor gene. The first "hit" is the germ-line mutation of one copy of the gene and the second hit corresponds to a spontaneous mutation within a specific cell, allowing tumor development.[4] Loss of both alleles of the NF1 gene has been identified in neurofibrosarcoma[5] and bone marrow cells of children with myeloid leukemia.[6]

Clinical presentation

The NIH diagnostic criteria for NF1 (Table 33.1) include the ocular finding of Lisch nodules and orbital findings of plexiform neurofibroma, sphenoid wing dysplasia and optic nerve glioma.

Lisch nodules

These dome-shaped, discrete lesions may occur anywhere on the anterior surface of the iris, including the angle where they may only be seen with a gonioscope. They are usually orange-brown, the color of burnt sienna (Fig. 33.1), appearing darker than blue irides but paler than brown irides (Fig. 33.2). Most are round and evenly distributed on the iris. Their size varies from a pinpoint to involvement of a segment of iris. They are usually bilateral. Histologically, they are melanocytic hamartomas. They may be confluent.

In NF1, they are present in one-third of 2.5 year olds, half of 5 year olds, three-quarters of 15-year-olds and almost all adults over 30.[7] Lubs et al.[8] found them in 100% of the 65 patients with

---

Table 33.1 Diagnostic criteria for NF1

The diagnostic criteria are met if two or more of the following are found:
1. Six or more café-au-lait macules over 5 mm in greatest diameter in prepubertal individuals and over 15 mm in greatest diameter in postpubertal individuals
2. Two or more neurofibromas of any type or one plexiform neurofibroma
3. Freckling in the axillary or inguinal regions
4. Optic glioma
5. Two or more Lisch nodules (iris hamartomas)
6. A distinctive osseous lesion such as sphenoid dysplasia or thinning of long bone cortex, with or without pseudoarthrosis
7. A first-degree relative (parent, sibling or offspring) with NF1 by the above criteria

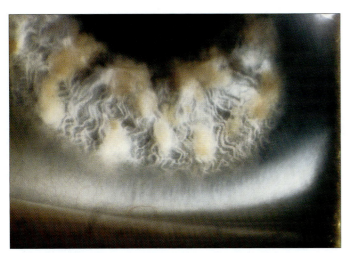

Fig. 33.1 Multiple Lisch nodules in neurofibromatosis.

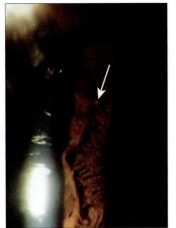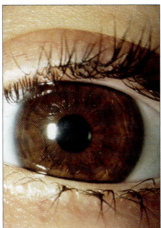

Fig. 33.2 Very small Lisch nodule, but of diagnostic importance in neurofibromatosis. In brown irides, Lisch nodules appear light brown (arrow).

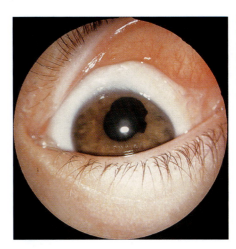

Fig. 33.3 Ectropion uveae, another iris abnormality occurring in NF1.
Patient of Dr Andrew McCormick, University of British Columbia.

NF1 aged 21 or above who were examined with a slit lamp. Although patients with NF2 have been reported to have iris nodules,[9,10] true Lisch nodules are overwhelmingly more common in NF1. They occur earlier than neurofibromas in children[8] and are therefore a useful marker for NF1. Since their recognition can trigger the early detection of central nervous system tumors and contribute to genetic counseling of other family members, it is important for ophthalmologists to recognize them, and be able to distinguish them from iris nevi.

Anterior segment and uvea

Prominent nerves have been reported in the cornea, although it is likely that they are not a sign of NF1 but of multiple endocrine neoplasia (MEN) syndrome,[11] another neurocristopathy which is genetically distinct from NF1. Neurofibromas may occur in the perilimbal conjunctiva.[12] Buphthalmos from congenital glaucoma is well recognized in NF1,[13–15] particularly in association with a plexiform neurofibroma involving the ipsilateral upper lid. It is virtually always unilateral. Grant and Walton[13] suggested the major cause was involvement of the angle by neurofibroma, although other causes such as angle obstruction by neurofibromatous thickening of the ciliary body and failure of differentiation of the angle structures have been invoked.

Brownstein and Little[16] also reported synechial angle closure and endothelialization of the iris in one case of congenital glaucoma with NF1. Congenital ectropion uveae (Fig. 33.3), iris heterochromia, angle abnormalities and posterior embryotoxon may predispose to later onset glaucoma. Cataract is not a feature of NF1.

Pigmentary hamartomas may also involve the posterior uveal tract. Huson et al.[17] found choroidal nevi in 35% of their patients with NF1. Rarely, the whole uveal tract may be involved by diffuse thickening that can give rise to glaucoma.[16,18] Malignant melanoma may arise within these pigmentary hamartomas, as in one of our patients with NF1 in whom a contralateral optic nerve glioma was also present.

Retina and optic disc

Retinal manifestations are rare in NF1. They may include astrocytic hamartomas, like those found in tuberous sclerosis but occasionally much more extensive.[19] Combined hamartoma of the retina and pigment epithelium has also been described in NF1. Retinal detachment may complicate these lesions. Retinal hemangiomas with exudation may require treatment with laser photocoagulation.[19] Central retinal vein obstruction by optic nerve glioma can give rise to clinical findings of central retinal vein occlusion or venous stasis retinopathy, and rubeosis has been described in this context.[20] Retinal arterial vascular occlusive disease with low flow retinopathy and retinal ischemia has been described in a 4-year-old boy with NF1 and no evidence of glioma on computed tomography (CT) scan.[21] Gliomas limited to the optic disc may occur[22] although some of the cases reported as having optic disc glioma with von Recklinghausen disease may actually have had NF2.[23] Pallor of the optic disc may suggest optic nerve or chiasmal glioma. Optic disc swelling may be due to optic nerve glioma (Fig. 33.4), or may be secondary to increased cerebrospinal fluid pressure from tumor or congenital anomalies such as aqueductal stenosis.

Skin, lids and orbits

Café-au-lait spots are hyperpigmented macular lesions which are usually present at birth, and will all have appeared by the age of 1 year.[1] They tend to enlarge at puberty. They are particularly common on the trunk but are absent from the scalp and eyebrows as well as the palms and soles. Histologically, there is melanocytic hyperplasia with increased pigmentation in the basal layer of epidermis. The presence of six café-au-lait spots after the age of 1 year is one of the diagnostic criteria for NF1.[24]

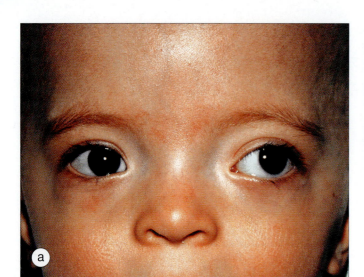

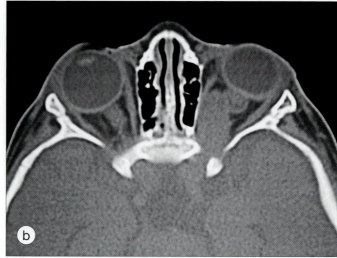

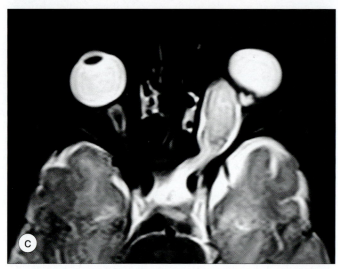

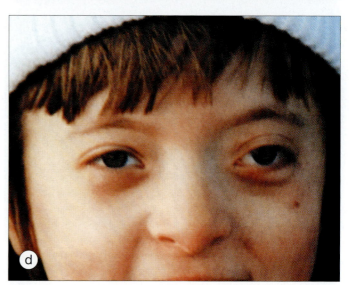

Fig. 33.4 Optic nerve glioma. (a) This 13-month-old girl presented with a history of intermittent exotropia since age 6 months, increasing numbers of café-au-lait spots and increasing proptosis on the left side. She had a left afferent pupillary defect with a raised gliotic disc, and the pupil was larger on that side. She appeared to be blind on the left. (b) CT scan on bone setting demonstrates an enlarged left optic canal with an optic nerve tumor, showing kinking of the distal end. (c) A T2-weighted MRI done 6 months later showed a fusiform tumor of the optic nerve extending up to and involving the chiasm, and the distal end of the right optic nerve appeared enlarged. It was decided to observe the patient and over the next 4 years, she developed significant left proptosis. This required a lateral orbitotomy for removal of the left intraorbital optic nerve, which revealed optic nerve glioma with perineural gliomatosis and meningeal hyperplasia. (d) Photograph 4 years postsurgery shows relative symmetry following alignment surgery. Patient of the University of British Columbia.

Neurofibromas

The old-fashioned name "neuroma" has now been replaced by the correct histopathological terms (Fig. 33.5). These masses arising from peripheral nerves are usually neurofibromas in NF1 and usually schwannomas in NF2[25] although some overlap is possible. The "acoustic neuromas" of NF2 are actually vestibular schwannomas.

Four types of neurofibroma are recognized.[1] First, the discrete cutaneous neurofibroma occurs in the epidermis and dermis, moves with the skin and may be blueish-tinged. Second, subcutaneous neurofibromas in contrast are deep to the dermis. Skin moves over them, they feel firm and rounded and tend to occur along the course of peripheral nerves. Third, nodular plexiform neurofibromas interdigitate with normal tissues in a localized manner. Classically, they feel like a "bag of worms" when palpated (Figs 33.6, 33.7). Fourth, diffuse plexiform

neurofibromas infiltrate widely and deeply into surrounding tissues, resulting in a smooth, slightly irregular thickening of the skin. They are always congenital but may only manifest clinically later in life. They usually are ipsilateral to congenital dysplasia of the greater wing of the sphenoid, although this can also occur without this tumor.[1] Although the overlying skin is often deeply pigmented, this is not a true café-au-lait spot.

The presence and growth pattern of neurofibromas is age-related; in infancy and early childhood, diffuse plexiform neurofibromas are most active and give rise to cosmetic and visual problems within the orbit. Manifestations of cutaneous or subcutaneous neurofibromas are rare in this age group; these develop and grow fastest at puberty, the late teens (Fig. 33.6c), and during pregnancy.

The medial portion of the upper lid is often the first site for a neurofibroma to develop, giving rise to the classically-described

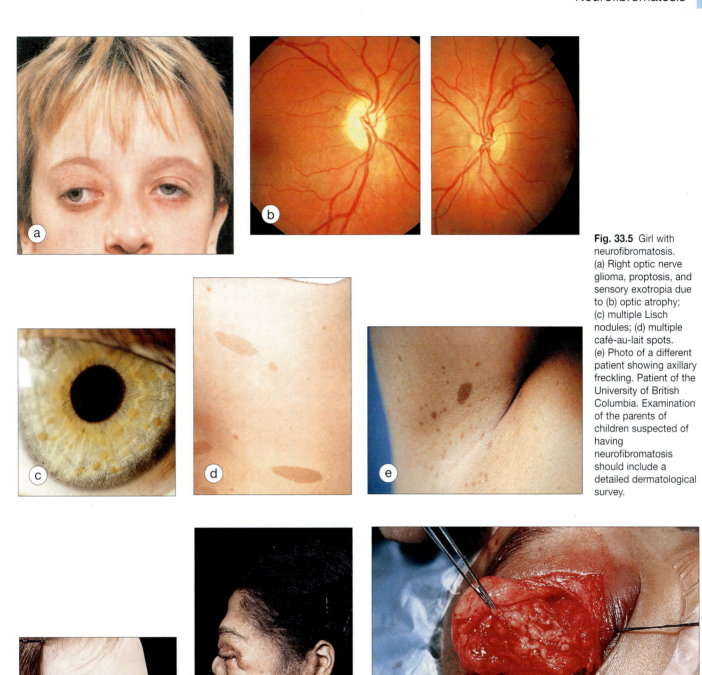

Fig. 33.5 Girl with neurofibromatosis. (a) Right optic nerve glioma, proptosis, and sensory exotropia due to (b) optic atrophy; (c) multiple Lisch nodules; (d) multiple café-au-lait spots. (e) Photo of a different patient showing axillary freckling. Patient of the University of British Columbia. Examination of the parents of children suspected of having neurofibromatosis should include a detailed dermatological survey.

Fig. 33.6 Plexiform neurofibroma. (a) Plexiform neurofibroma of the lid. There is a high incidence of congenital glaucoma in association with lid plexiform neurofibromas. (b) Large plexiform neurofibromas of the face in neurofibromatosis. (c) At surgery the worm-like consistency of an orbital plexiform neurofibroma can be seen. Patient of the University of British Columbia.

sinusoid lid margin or a diffusely swollen appearance. Its growth may cause a mechanical ptosis and distort the globe. Amblyopia may result from this or from induced astigmatism. Orbital involvement by plexiform neurofibromas may give rise to early complications as the tumor tends to grow rapidly in the first 3 years of life. Growth may be directed backwards, expanding the orbital walls and fissures into the middle cranial fossa, producing enophthalmos or exophthalmos which may be pulsatile (Fig. 33.8). It is not clear whether the sphenoid defect is dysplastic or secondary to the plexiform neurofibroma. They may also grow forwards onto the face[26] giving rise to disfigurement that may require surgical repair. Plexiform neurofibroma appears on CT scan as a nonencapsulated, poorly defined, infiltrating mass with moderate contrast enhancement.[27,28]

Neurofibromas are not radiosensitive[29] and are difficult to treat surgically. Plexiform lesions tend to be diffuse, enveloping the orbital structures such as the optic nerve, extraocular muscles, vessels and lacrimal gland. When extensive, they cannot usually

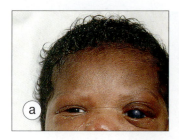
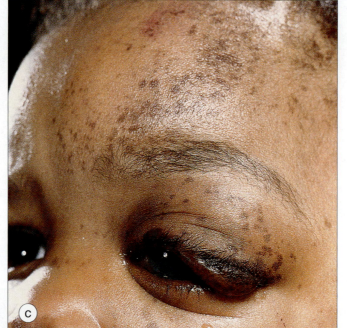

Fig. 33.7 Neurofibroma. (a) Neonate with enlarged glaucomatous left eye and thickened pigmented lid. (b) Same patient showing axillary freckling suggesting NF1. (c) Same patient 2 years later showing S-shaped lid with plexiform neurofibroma. The glaucoma failed to respond to treatment.

be completely excised, so multiple subtotal resections may be required and recurrence after partial removal is typical. Moreover, these tumors tend to bleed profusely at surgery. Where an eye sees poorly (due to amblyopia resulting from lid involvement or to optic atrophy) and the cosmetic defect is considerable, exenteration with orbital bone grafting is a possibility.[30,31] Lid neurofibroma can be reduced by plastic surgical procedures.[32]

In some cases orbital enlargement is not associated with an intraorbital mass and is due instead to bony malformation. Other sphenoid bone defects occur, such as hypoplasia of the greater and lesser wings, elevation of the lesser wing, widening of the superior orbital fissure, and lateral displacement of the oblique line of the orbit.[33] There may be absence of the lateral wall of the orbit, resulting in masticatory oscillopsia, as was noted in one of our patients.

In addition to their mechanical effects, neurofibromas may interfere with cranial nerve function. Thus, third, fourth, fifth and sixth nerve palsies may occur, as may Horner syndrome. Neurofibroma affecting the trigeminal nerve may give rise to symptoms of aching pain in the orbital region.

Central nervous system

The commonest consequence of NF1 in childhood and often the major concern of parents of a child with NF1 is cognitive impairment. The children are not usually mentally retarded but often display a wide range of learning disabilities manifesting as academic underachievement, and behavioral problems.[4] Vascular anomalies are common and may contribute to the seizures. Hydrocephalus may occur as a complication of congenital or tumoral aqueductal stenosis.[34,35] It may present with headache or dorsal midbrain syndrome, and should be remembered as a cause of sixth nerve palsy in NF1. Arachnoid cysts arising from the

meninges are a common incidental finding in NF1. These rarely produce clinical features of space-occupying lesions.

The incidence of strabismus is said to be higher than in the general population.[1] Strabismus may be the presenting sign of optic nerve glioma.

Optic nerve and chiasmal glioma with and without NF1 is considered in the section on neurogenic tumors.

Other systems

Tumors of the spinal cord, sympathetic nerves and adrenals may occur in patients with neurofibromatosis. The patient may first present with malignant hypertension from pheochromocytoma. There may be multiple neurofibromas of the gastrointestinal tract and various osseous abnormalities including abnormal vertebrae, scoliosis, pseudoarthrosis of long bones and subperiosteal changes.

However, it is the other central nervous system tumors associated with NF1 which are of greatest importance in reducing the life-expectancy of these patients.

NEUROFIBROMATOSIS TYPE 2

NF2, formerly known as central neurofibromatosis, is characterized by the development of vestibular schwannomas (acoustic neuromas). Other features include meningiomas, spinal nerve root schwannomas and presenile lens opacities. The severe disease features of NF2 are limited to the central nervous system, in contrast to NF1 where any system may be affected. Two patterns of presentation exist: the severe subtype presents early and progresses rapidly, and the milder type has a later onset and less aggressive course.[36]

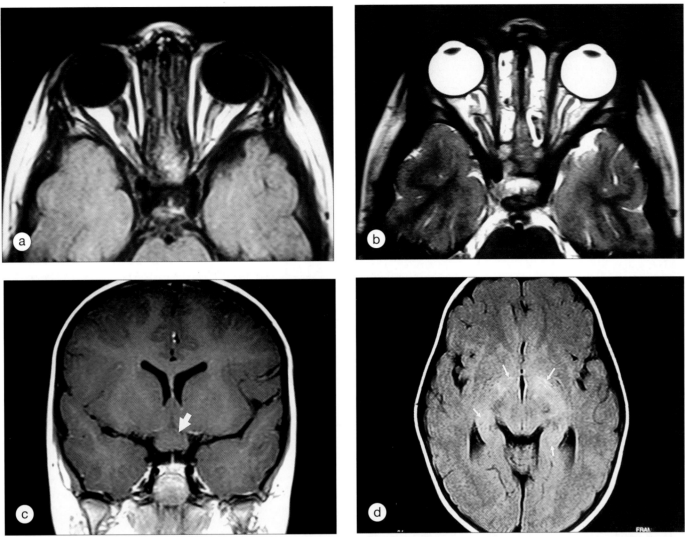

Fig. 33.8 This 4-year-old girl presented with the clinical stigmata of, and a mother with, neurofibromatosis type 1. She appeared to have relatively normal vision, full range of ocular movement, bilateral Lisch nodules and bilateral temporal pallor of her optic nerves. (a) The T1-weighted MRI demonstrates bilateral enlargement of the optic nerves, confirmed in (b), the T2-weighted MRI, which shows characteristic enlargement of the subarachnoid space due to perineural gliomatosis. (c) The coronal view demonstrates enlargement of the chiasmatic optic nerve (arrow) and the axial view of the brain (d) shows involvement of the optic radiations (arrows). Patient of the University of British Columbia.

Genetics

This autosomal dominantly transmitted defect is about 10 times rarer than NF1, since it is found only in 1 in 37 000 of the population. Like NF1 the gene has almost complete penetrance and there is considerable interindividual variation in the phenotypic manifestations of NF2, but unlike NF1 the phenotype of NF2 seems to "breed true" within affected families. A negative family history does not preclude the diagnosis of NF2 since at least half of patients with NF2 have a new mutation.[1] A maternal effect has been suggested, with earlier onset of clinical manifestations among patients born to a mother with NF2 than those whose father was affected.[37] It seems that virtually all gene carriers develop tumors of the central nervous system with significant morbidity and mortality.[25]

Genetic studies have shown that the gene for NF2 is situated on chromosome 22, coding for a membrane organizing protein known as Merlin.[38–40] This protein is related to the membrane cytoskeleton associated proteins.[41] The gene implicated in NF2 is

another tumor suppressor, therefore subject to the "two hit" mechanism operating in tumor-genesis in this context. The NF2 gene has been implicated in meningiomas, schwannomas,[42,43] several human malignancies[44] as well as retinal and optic nerve lesions in NF2 patients.[45] The two patterns of disease discussed above could be explained by the tendency for nonsense or frameshift mutations to produce earlier more aggressive disease than splice-site mutations.[46]

Systemic findings

Patients with NF2 often have a few café-au-lait spots, and cutaneous lesions that are usually schwannomas. There are usually less than six café-au-lait spots, often on the trunk, and axillary and groin freckling is absent. Deep plexiform neurofibromas rarely occur and were not found in 120 patients reviewed by Evans et al.[25]

The hallmark of NF2 is the presence of bilateral vestibular schwannomas ("acoustic neuromas") which may only be evident

Table 33.2 Diagnostic criteria for NF2

NF2 may be diagnosed when one of the following is present:

1. Bilateral eighth nerve masses seen by appropriate imaging techniques (e.g. CT scan or MRI). Preferably MRI with gadolinium*

2. A parent, sibling or child with NF2 and either unilateral eighth nerve mass or any two of the following:
   (a) neurofibroma
   (b) meningioma
   (c) glioma
   (d) schwannoma
   (e) juvenile posterior subcapsular lens opacity

Borrowed with permission from the National Institutes of Health. National Institutes of Health Consensus Development Conference Statement: neurofibromatosis. Bethesda, MD, USA, July 13–15, 1987. Neurofibromatosis 1988; 1(3): 172–178.
*Mulvihill JJ, Parry DM, Sherman JL, et al. NIH Conference. Neurofibromatosis 1 (Recklinghausen disease) and neurofibromatosis 2 (bilateral acoustic neurofibromatosis). An update. Ann Intern Med 1990; 113(1): 39–52.

on CT scan. Gadolinium-enhanced MRI is the modality of choice for imaging schwannomas in NF2. It is thought that the gene for NF2 can produce either bilateral vestibular schwannomas if there is a germ-line mutation or unilateral schwannomas if the mutation is somatic. The origin of the trigeminal nerve is another frequent intracranial site for schwannomas,[1] and they have been noted on multiple cranial nerves in affected patients.[47] The NIH criteria necessary to reach a diagnosis of NF2 are shown in Table 33.2.

In Kanter et al.'s[37] study, the most common presenting symptom was bilateral hearing loss (50%), followed by unilateral hearing loss (21%), usually presenting in the mid-teens to twenties. Vestibular problems (10%), tinnitus (9%), and other presentations including headache, visual symptoms and facial nerve paresis (10%) accounted for most of the remainder.

Whereas patients with NF1 tend to develop neural or astrocytic tumors (astrocytomas and optic nerve "gliomas"), the nervous system tumors of NF2 typically involve neural coverings or linings (meningiomas, optic nerve sheath meningiomas, schwannomas, and ependymomas).[48] Astrocytomas are rare in the brain in NF2, especially involving the optic pathways, but are relatively common in the spinal cord. Although usually of low histological grade, they may have serious sequelae if they occur in the brainstem or spinal cord. Spinal cord meningiomas are also commonly seen, with a predilection for the exit point of foramina, perhaps due to the stretching of the nerves that occurs at these sites.[1]

Ocular findings

Bouzas et al.[49] reviewed 54 patients with NF2 and found decreased vision (20/40 or worse) in 18, five bilaterally. Nineteen per cent of the affected eyes had vision of 20/100 or worse. Visual loss is particularly significant in NF2 since progressive bilateral hearing loss is so common in this condition: in this series of 54 patients, whose mean age was 36 years, 26 patients had bilateral profound hearing loss, and nine others had profound hearing loss in one ear and moderate hearing loss in the other. Only eight patients had normal hearing.

Anterior segment

As in NF1, the ocular changes of NF2 are early markers of the disease which may be of diagnostic importance. In particular, 55–87% of affected patients have presenile central posterior subcapsular lens opacities.[50–52] Cataracts (Fig. 33.9) were present in 44 of the 54 patients reviewed by Bouzas et al.,[49] but they only interfered significantly with vision in seven of these, and produced symptomatic glare in a further six. Evans et al.[25] reported that 16 (18%) of their 90 patients had cataracts in the pediatric period, congenital in five. Cataracts presented before any other feature in 11 of 97 patients. Meyers and colleagues[53] reported lens opacities in 12 of the 15 patients with NF2 in their study. Lens opacities may therefore suggest a predisposition to develop bilateral vestibular schwannomas since they often precede the development of these tumors. The types of cataract that are most suggestive of NF2 are plaque-like posterior subcapsular or capsular cataract and cortical cataract with onset under the age of 30 years.[54] Juvenile onset peripheral cortical lens opacities have also been described in NF2.[50,51,55] Corneal hypoesthesia from trigeminal nerve schwannoma, and decreased tear production, reduced blinking and lagophthalmos from facial nerve palsy may adversely affect the outcome of cataract extraction in patients requiring surgery. These causes resulted in corneal opacification and visual impairment (20/40 or less) in six of the 54 patients reviewed by Bouzas et al.[49]

Lisch nodules are rare but have been reported in NF2.[9,10,51]

Several patients with NF2 with childhood third nerve palsies (Fig. 33.10) have been reported.[48,51,56] Tonsgard and Oesterle[47] reported a patient with epiretinal membrane noted at the age of 4 years, who developed an ipsilateral third nerve palsy when aged 10 years and whose vestibular schwannomas were identified after symptomatic hearing loss at the age of 17 years. We have seen

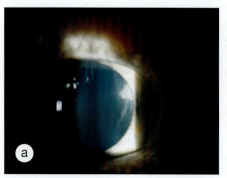
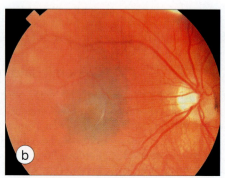
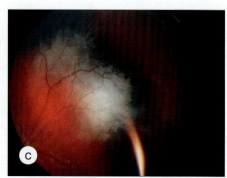

Fig. 33.9 Neurofibromatosis type 2. (a) Cataract in a patient with NF2. (b) Epiretinal membrane in the same patient. The membrane is distorting the vessel running below the macula. (c) Combined hamartoma in another patient with NF2.

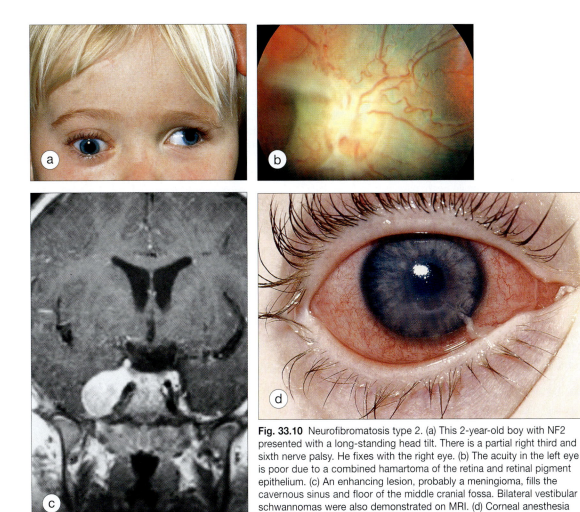

Fig. 33.10 Neurofibromatosis type 2. (a) This 2-year-old boy with NF2 presented with a long-standing head tilt. There is a partial right third and sixth nerve palsy. He fixes with the right eye. (b) The acuity in the left eye is poor due to a combined hamartoma of the retina and retinal pigment epithelium. (c) An enhancing lesion, probably a meningioma, fills the cavernous sinus and floor of the middle cranial fossa. Bilateral vestibular schwannomas were also demonstrated on MRI. (d) Corneal anesthesia developed on the right side due to trigeminal involvement. There was corneal ulceration due to repeated trauma to the right eye.

one patient with congenital third nerve palsy and NF2 whose other eye was blind due to combined hamartoma of the retina and pigment epithelium (Fig. 33.10). Fourth and sixth nerve involvement have also been described in NF2.[47,55]

Posterior segment

Combined retinal and pigment epithelial hamartomas (CRPEH) have been reported in NF2.[55,57] They were present in two of the 54 patients with NF2 reported by Bouzas et al.[58] They may be bilateral[59] and familial.[58] They typically occur at the posterior pole and their characteristic appearance is shown in Fig. 33.10. The severity of the abnormality ranges from mild, with a visual acuity of 20/80,[57] to severe, as in Landau et al.'s[55] patient whose acuity was "finger-counting" and the case we present here who did not take up fixation with the affected eye. There may be co-existing epiretinal membranes.[60]

Epiretinal membranes may occur alone in NF2, usually affecting the posterior pole. They may represent an abortive form of CRPEH and may occasionally be seen in the contralateral eye of a patient with CRPEH.[53] They were reported in seven of the nine patients with NF2 studied by Kaye et al.,[51] four of the six patients by Landau and Yasargil[55] and 12 of the 15 patients reported by Meyers et al.[53] The severity of these membranes ranged from cellophane maculopathy (two eyes) to macular pucker (three eyes) with visual acuities ranging from 20/20 to 20/200, respectively. Histologically, intraretinal glial proliferation is seen, with an overlying membrane consisting of astrocytic glial fibrillary acidic protein (GFAP)-staining cells.[51] It is interesting that uncontrolled glial proliferation, a process which is widely implicated in the other central nervous system manifestations of NF2, should be seen in the retina.

Other rare fundus abnormalities have been described in NF2, including astrocytic hamartomas[51,55] and optic disc gliomas.[23,55,61]

Optic nerve sheath meningiomas, which may be bilateral, can also cause visual loss in NF2. These are described in the chapter on neurogenic tumors. They may easily be missed on MRI unless fat suppression techniques are used.

Progress

The progression of vestibular schwannoma (acoustic neuroma) is unpredictable but is more rapid with NF2 than without, and appears to be hastened by pregnancy. The use of estrogens is contraindicated in NF2.[1] Others have questioned the effect of pregnancy on the progression of NF2-related tumors.[25] The mere presence of a vestibular schwannoma on MRI scan is not an indication for its removal, since many of these tumors remain unchanged for years.[62]

Patients with NF2 were perhaps most often seen by ophthalmologists for the ocular management of their facial nerve paresis following vestibular schwannoma excision. The incidence of this complication is higher for larger tumors, but is reduced by the use of the operating microscope and intraoperative physiological monitoring of facial nerve function. Recent series, possibly reflecting a trend towards earlier surgery, suggest that anatomical preservation of the facial nerve is possible in up to 97% of cases, with good function in three-quarters of these.[63] Unfortunately, hearing preservation after vestibular schwannoma excision is only possible in a minority of patients. Small preoperative tumor size is a favorable prognostic factor, but hearing preservation is less likely for bilateral tumors.[64] The "gamma knife" or highly collimated radiotherapy is currently under evaluation for the noninvasive treatment of vestibular schwannoma.

Since morbidity from the excision of vestibular schwannoma increases with tumor size, early diagnosis and surgery may be advantageous. Early evaluation of the offspring of parents with NF2 for vestibular schwannoma is essential. Nine children who had either one parent with NF2 or skin or spinal tumors suggestive of NF2 were studied by Mautner et al.[56] Vestibular schwannomas were identified in seven of these by MRI scanning with gadolinium. Six of these, whose age ranged from 9 to 16 years, had no clinical signs or symptoms. Slit-lamp examination revealed posterior subcapsular cataracts in four of these, two of whom were 10 years old. In retrospect, the first signs of NF2 were present in infancy in four of the nine children, and by age 5 years in six of the nine. Although NF2 is generally considered a disease of teenage and adulthood, it is becoming evident that this gene defect gives rise to manifestations occurring much earlier in life. Evans et al.[25] have suggested ophthalmological screening with a slit-lamp examination is indicated in early childhood, and screening for vestibular schwannoma with annual brainstem evoked responses should start in the early teens. A genetic screening test for at-risk relatives will help to determine whether the germ-line mutation is present or not.[65]

Pediatric ophthalmologists should remain alert to the possibility of NF2 and initiate investigations such as hearing tests and gadolinium-enhanced MRI scans of the cerebellopontine angle and vestibular nerves in patients with characteristic ocular findings. These include combined hamartomas of the retina and pigment epithelium, apparently idiopathic juvenile posterior subcapsular cataracts and, possibly, unexplained third nerve palsy in a child. Moreover, a child who has too few café-au-lait spots and neurofibroma-like cutaneous lesions to meet the criteria for a diagnosis of NF1 may actually have NF2.

Affected patients and their at-risk relatives should be warned of the risks associated with this diagnosis. In particular, drowning or near-drowning due to loss of direction under water, occurred in eight of 73 patients studied by Kanter et al.[37] and two others died in accidents related to insidious hearing loss such as being hit by cars or trains.

OTHER FORMS OF NEUROFIBROMATOSIS

NF3 is a mixed form of neurofibromatosis in which features of both NF1 and NF2 are present. Palmar neurofibromas are characteristic lesions. Café-au-lait spots occur but are few in number. Intracranial, spinal or paraspinal tumors occur commonly. Lisch nodules are absent, as are optic pathway gliomas. The tumors tend to behave aggressively and life prognosis is poor.[1]

NF4 or variant neurofibromatosis designates a group of patients whose phenotypic features do not fit into any other group of neurofibromatosis. This is really a "sorting" category, devised to prevent these patients from masking the relative uniformity found in other groups for investigational purposes.

NF5 is segmental. Café-au-lait spots, freckling, and other signs of NF1 are restricted to one side or quadrant of the body, strictly respecting the midline. The possibility of this form of neurofibromatosis being due to a somatic mutation is called into question by Weleber and Zonana's[66] report of Lisch nodules and the report of NF1 in the offspring of an affected patient.[67]

NF6 and NF7 describe "café-au-lait spots only" and "late onset" neurofibromatosis, respectively. NF1, NF2 and NF5 are the most common types in childhood.

CONCLUSION

The ophthalmologist may have a pivotal role in making the diagnosis of NF1, by correctly identifying Lisch nodules, orbital plexiform neurofibromas, characteristic sphenoid wing defects, and optic nerve gliomas. In NF2 also, ocular findings such as juvenile posterior subcapsular cataract, idiopathic epiretinal membrane and combined hamartoma of the retina and pigment epithelium are important in making a presymptomatic diagnosis.

In both cases, ocular findings may precede other, sometimes sight- or even life-threatening manifestations of NF1 or NF2. It is therefore essential for pediatric ophthalmologists to be aware of their ocular features, and refer early and appropriately for audiological, neuroradiological or other relevant investigations.

As our understanding improves, and gene probes become freely available for diagnostic testing and genetic counseling, we will be better able to define the phenotype of each gene defect.

REFERENCES

1. Riccardi VM. Neurofibromatosis: Phenotype, Natural History, and Pathogenesis. 2nd edn. Baltimore: Johns Hopkins University; 1992.
2. von Recklinghausen FD. Ueber die multiplen Fibrome der Haut und ihre Beziehung zu den multiplen Neuromen. Festschrift zur Feier des 25 Jährigen Bestchens des Pathologischen Instituts zu Berlin. Berlin: Herrn Rudolf Virchow Dargebracht; 1882.
3. Knudson AG, Jr. Mutation and cancer: statistical study of retinoblastoma. Proc Natl Acad Sci USA 1971;68:820-3.
4. Gutmann DH. Neurofibromin in the brain. J Child Neurol 2002;17:592–601.
5. Legius E, Marchuk DA, Hall BK, et al. NF1-related locus on chromosome 15. Genomics 1992;13:1316–8.
6. Shannon KM, O'Connell P, Martin GA, et al. Loss of the normal NF1 allele from the bone marrow of children with type 1 neurofibromatosis and malignant myeloid disorders. N Engl J Med 1994; 330: 637–9.
7. Ragge NK, Falk R, Cohen WE, et al. Images of Lisch nodules across the spectrum. Eye 1993; 7: 95–101.

8. Lubs ML, Bauer MS, Formas ME, et al. Lisch nodules in neurofibromatosis type 1. N Engl J Med 1991; 324: 1264–6.

9. Charles SJ, Moore AT, Yates JR, et al. Lisch nodules in neurofibromatosis type 2. Case report. Arch Ophthalmol 1989; 107: 1571–2.

10. Garretto NS, Ameriso S, Molina HA, et al. Type 2 neurofibromatosis with Lisch nodules. Neurofibromatosis 1989; 2: 315–21.

11. Knox DL, Payne JW, Hartmann WH. Thickened corneal nerves and eyelids as signs of neurofibromatosis and medullary thyroid carcinoma. In: Progress in Neuro-ophthalmology, No 176. Amsterdam: Exerpta Medica; 1969: 262–6.

12. Insler MS, Helm C, Napoli S. Conjunctival hamartoma in neurofibromatosis. Am J Ophthalmol 1985; 99: 731–3.

13. Grant WM, Walton DS. Distinctive gonioscopic findings in glaucoma due to neurofibromatosis. Arch Ophthalmol 1968; 79: 127–34.

14. Castillo M, Quencer RM, Glaser J, et al. Congenital glaucoma and buphthalmos in a child with neurofibromatosis. J Clin Neuro-ophthalmol 1988; 9: 69–71.

15. Tripathi BJ, Tripathi RC. Neural crest origin of human trabecular meshwork and its implications for the pathogenesis of glaucoma. Am J Ophthalmol 1989; 107: 583–90.

16. Brownstein S, Little JM. Ocular neurofibromatosis. Ophthalmology 1983; 90: 1595–9.

17. Huson S, Jones D, Beck L. Ophthalmic manifestations of neurofibromatosis. Br J Ophthalmol 1987; 71: 235–9.

18. Kurosawa A, Kurosawa H. Ovoid bodies in choroidal neurofibromatosis. Arch Ophthalmol 1982; 100: 1939–41.

19. Destro M, D'Amico DJ, Gragoudas ES, et al. Retinal manifestations of neurofibromatosis. Diagnosis and management. Arch Ophthalmol 1991; 109: 662–6.

20. Buchanan TA, Hoyt WF. Optic nerve glioma and neovascular glaucoma: report of a case. Br J Ophthalmol 1982; 66: 96–8.

21. Moadel K, Yannuzzi LA, Ho AC, et al. Retinal vascular occlusive disease in a child with neurofibromatosis (letter). Arch Ophthalmol 1994; 112: 1021–3.

22. Malbrel C, Hecart JF, Malbrel G, et al. Gliome de la papille. Bull Soc Ophtalmol Fr 1986; 86: 289–91.

23. Dossetor FR, Landau K, Hoyt WF. Optic disk glioma in neurofibromatosis type 2. Am J Ophthalmol 1989; 108: 602–3.

24. National Institutes of Health. National Institutes of Health Consensus Development Conference Statement: neurofibromatosis. Bethesda, MD, USA, July 13–15, 1987. Neurofibromatosis 1988; 1: 172–8.

25. Evans DG, Huson SM, Donnai D, et al. A genetic study of type 2 neurofibromatosis in the United Kingdom. II. Guidelines for genetic counselling. J Med Genet 1992; 29: 847–52.

26. Savino PJ, Glaser JS, Luxenberg MN. Pulsating enophthalmos and choroidal hamartomas: two rare stigmata of neurofibromatosis. Br J Ophthalmol 1977; 61: 483–8.

27. Linder B, Campos M, Schafer M. CT and MRI of orbital anomalies in neurofibromatosis and selected craniofacial anomalies. Radiol Clin N Am 1987; 25: 787–802.

28. Reed D, Robertson WD, Rootman J, et al. Plexiform neurofibromatosis of the orbit. CT evaluation. Am J Neuroradiol 1986; 7: 259–63.

29. Font RL, Ferry AP. The phakomatoses. Int Ophthalmol Clin 1972; 12: 1–50.

30. Hoyt CS, Billson FA. Buphthalmos in neurofibromatosis: is it an expression of regional giantism? J Pediatr Ophthalmol Strabismus 1977; 14: 228–34.

31. Jackson IT, Laws ER, Martin RD. The surgical management of orbital neurofibromatosis. Plast Reconstr Surg 1983; 71: 751–8.

32. Tenzel RR, Boynton JR, Miller GR, et al. Surgical treatment of eyelid neurofibromatosis. Arch Ophthalmol 1977; 95: 479–83.

33. Binet E, Keiffer SA, Martin SH, et al. Orbital dysplasia in neurofibromatosis. Radiology 1969; 93: 829–33.

34. Riviello JJ, Jr, Marks HG, Lee MS, et al. Aqueductal stenosis in neurofibromatosis. Neurofibromatosis 1988; 1: 312–7.

35. Senveli E, Altinors N, Kars Z, et al. Association of von Recklinghausen's neurofibromatosis and aqueduct stenosis. Neurosurgery 1989; 25: 318–9.

36. Parry DM, Eldridge R, Kaiser-Kupfer MI, et al. Neurofibromatosis 2 (NF2): clinical characteristics of 63 affected individuals and clinical evidence for heterogeneity. Am J Med Genet 1994; 52: 450–61.

37. Kanter WR, Eldridge R, Fabricant R, et al. Central neurofibromatosis with bilateral acoustic neuroma: genetic, clinical and biochemical distinctions from peripheral neurofibromatosis. Neurology 1980; 30: 851–9.

38. Rouleau GA, Merel P, Lutchman M, et al. Alteration in a new gene encoding a putative membrane-organizing protein causes neurofibromatosis type 2. Nature 1993; 363: 515–21.

39. Trofatter JA, MacCollin MM, Rutter JL, et al. A novel moesin-, ezrin-, radixin-like gene is a candidate for the neurofibromatosis 2 tumor suppressor. Cell 1993; 75: 826.

40. Xiao GH, Chernoff J, Testa JR. NF2: the wizardry of merlin. Genes Chromosomes Cancer 2003; 38: 389–99.

41. McClatchey AI. Merlin and ERM proteins: unappreciated roles in cancer development? Nat Rev Cancer 2003; 3: 877–83.

42. Bolger GB, Stamberg J, Kirsch IR, et al. Chromosome translocation t(14;22) and oncogene (c-sis) variant in a pedigree with familial meningioma. N Engl J Med 1985; 312: 564–7.

43. Sainz J, Huynh DP, Figueroa K, et al. Mutations of the neurofibromatosis type 2 gene and lack of the gene product in vestibular schwannomas. Hum Mol Genet 1994; 3: 885–91.

44. Bianchi AB, Hara T, Ramesh V, et al. Mutations in transcript isoforms of the neurofibromatosis 2 gene in multiple human tumour types. Nature Genet 1994; 6: 185–92.

45. Chan CC, Koch CA, Kaiser-Kupfer MI, et al. Loss of heterozygosity for the NF2 gene in retinal and optic nerve lesions of patients with neurofibromatosis 2. J Pathol 2002; 198: 14–20.

46. Parry DM, MacCollin MM, Kaiser-Kupfer MI, et al. Germ-line mutations in the neurofibromatosis 2 gene: correlations with disease severity and retinal abnormalities. Am J Hum Genet 1996; 59: 529–39.

47. Tonsgard JH, Oesterle CS. The ophthalmologic presentation of NF2 in childhood. J Pediatr Ophthalmol Strabismus 1993;30:327–30.

48. Ragge NK. Clinical and genetic patterns of neurofibromatosis 1 and 2. Br J Ophthalmol 1993; 77: 662–72.

49. Bouzas EA, Parry DM, Eldridge R, et al. Visual impairment in patients with neurofibromatosis 2. Neurology 1993; 43: 622–3.

50. Bouzas EA, Freidlin V, Parry DM, et al. Lens opacities in neurofibromatosis 2: further significant correlations. Br J Ophthalmol 1993; 77: 354–7.

51. Kaye L, Rothner A, Beauchamp G, et al. Ocular findings associated with neurofibromatosis type 2. Ophthalmology 1992; 99: 1424–9.

52. Kaiser-Kupfer MI, Freidlin V, Datiles MB, et al. The association of posterior capsular lens opacities with bilateral acoustic neuromas in patients with neurofibromatosis type 2. Arch Ophthalmol 1989; 107: 541–4.

53. Meyers SM, Gutman FA, Kaye LD, et al. Retinal changes associated with neurofibromatosis 2. Trans Am Ophthalmol Soc 1995; 93: 245–52.

54. Ragge NK, Baser ME, Klein J, et al. Ocular abnormalities in neurofibromatosis 2. Am J Ophthalmol 1995; 120: 634–41.

55. Landau K, Yasargil GM. Ocular fundus in neurofibromatosis type 2. Br J Ophthalmol 1993; 77: 646–9.

56. Mautner VF, Tatagiba M, Guthoff R, et al. Neurofibromatosis 2 in the pediatric age group. Neurosurgery 1993; 33: 92–6.

57. Sivalingam A, Augsburger J, Perilongo G, et al. Combined hamartoma of the retina and retinal pigment epithelium in a patient with neurofibromatosis type 2. J Pediatr Ophthalmol Strabismus 1991; 28: 320–2.

58. Bouzas EA, Parry DM, Eldridge R, et al. Familial occurrence of combined pigment epithelial and retinal hamartomas associated with neurofibromatosis 2. Retina 1992; 12: 103–7.

59. Good WV, Erodsky MC, Edwards MS, et al. Bilateral retinal hamartomas in neurofibromatosis type 2. Br J Ophthalmol 1991; 75: 190.

60. Schachat AP, Shields JA, Fine SL, et al. Combined hamartomas of the retina and retinal pigment epithelium. Ophthalmology 1984; 91: 1609–5.

61. Stallard HB. A case of intra-ocular neuroma (von Recklinghausen's disease) of the left optic nerve head. Br J Ophthalmol 1938; 21: 11.

62. Mulvihill JJ, Parry DM, Sherman JL, et al. NIH Conference. Neurofibromatosis 1 (Recklinghausen disease) and neurofibromatosis 2 (bilateral acoustic neurofibromatosis). An update. Ann Intern Med 1990; 113: 39–52.

63. Kartush JM, Lundy LB. Facial nerve outcome in acoustic neuroma surgery. Otolaryngol Clin North Am 1992; 25: 623–47.

64. Shelton C. Hearing preservation in acoustic tumor surgery. Otolaryngol Clin North Am 1992; 25: 609–21.

65. Merel P, Hoang-Xuan K, Sanson M, et al. Screening for germ-line mutations in the NF2 gene. Genes Chromosomes Cancer 1995; 12: 117–27.

66. Weleber RG, Zonana J. Iris hamartomas (Lisch nodules) in a case of segmental neurofibromatosis. Am J Ophthalmol 1983; 96: 740–3.

67. Boltshauser E, Stocker H, Machler M. Neurofibromatosis type 1 in a child of a parent with segmental neurofibromatosis (NF5). Neurofibromatosis 1989; 2: 244–5.

CHAPTER
34 Neurogenic Tumors

Christopher J Lyons and Jack Rootman

OPTIC NERVE TUMORS

Glioma

Gliomas (astrocytomas) are the most common intracranial tumors in neurofibromatosis type 1 (NF1), occurring most frequently in the anterior visual pathways, brainstem, and posterior fossa.[1] They rarely affect the brain in neurofibromatosis type 2 (NF2) but are found in the spinal cord. Conversely, Friedman and Riccardi[2] have questioned whether meningiomas and schwannomas are part of the NF1 phenotype, and suggested that these tumors are more typical of NF2.

Anterior pathway gliomas

The overall prevalence has been estimated at 19% of patients with NF1.[3] Depending on the series, between 10 and 70% of patients with anterior pathway glioma have been said to have NF1.[4] Glioma shows no particular predilection for any part of the anterior visual pathway and may arise in one or both optic nerves, the chiasm, or the chiasm and either or both nerves. Bilateral optic nerve glioma is one of the diagnostic criteria of NF1. Patients with anterior pathway gliomas should be examined for signs of neurofibromatosis in the eye (Lisch nodules, ectropion uveae, glaucoma, fundus lesions), orbit (neurofibromas, sphenoid defects), and skin (café-au-lait spots, neurofibromas). Family members should also be examined.

Many clinicians[3,5–7] have commented that glioma occurring in the presence of NF1 has a relatively good visual prognosis compared to sporadic optic nerve gliomas, but the survival is worse in these patients as they develop other central nervous system tumors. This clinical impression is supported by recent comparative studies.[8,9] The differences between these will be highlighted to outline a practical management of glioma with and without NF1.

It is important to distinguish optic nerve glioma, where the chiasm is not involved, from chiasmal glioma, where the optic nerves may be involved since they are managed differently.

Optic nerve glioma
Presentation

The reported age of presentation ranges from birth to 79 years, mostly between 4 and 12 years; the vast majority have presented by 20 years of age and the overall mean from several large combined series was 8.8 years.[10] Females are affected more often than males. Optic nerve glioma is occasionally bilateral, especially in patients with neurofibromatosis,[11] but florid outward signs of NF1 such as orbital plexiform neurofibromas are no more common in patients with a glioma than in other patients with NF1.[3] Indeed, they may be altogether absent even in the presence of the NF1 mutation so the comparison of glioma behavior with and without NF1 is sometimes confused.

The site of the tumor determines its presentation. Gliomas involving the intraorbital portion of the nerve commonly present with axial proptosis[12] (Fig. 34.1). This may be quite sudden in onset or recognition and is occasionally rapidly progressive. The eye is painless and uninflamed unless there is corneal exposure or neovascular glaucoma.[13] Limitation of elevation was present in almost half of Wright et al.'s[12] 31 patients. Strabismus associated with unilateral visual loss can be the presenting feature.[14] Occasionally, older patients may complain of visual loss, and color vision deficits with central field defects[12] may be identified. Other visual field abnormalities such as altitudinal defects may occur, depending on the relationship of the tumor to the nerve and its blood supply. In patients with unilateral or asymmetrical optic nerve involvement, there is usually an afferent pupillary defect on the worse-affected side.

Poor vision, disc swelling, or more commonly pallor may be noted at a routine examination of an asymptomatic patient. Opticociliary shunt vessels may be found and involvement of the disc by tumor is occasionally seen. However, many series have shown these tumors to be silent in as many as 10% of patients with NF1.[1] In the absence of visual symptoms, optic nerve glioma is rarely identified by fundus examination alone. Listernick et al.[15] have suggested that routine neuroimaging is of value at the time of presentation with NF1 in order to detect asymptomatic glioma. It is arguable that this may help to secure the diagnosis of NF1 but rarely alters the patient's management.

Patients with the stigmata of NF1 often present with relatively good visual acuity, which may fluctuate at follow-up. Conversely, visual loss patients with NF1 can occasionally progress rapidly and are worse if the visual pathway involvement is extensive.[16] The major features of glioma with and without NF1 are described in Table 34.1.

Radiographic features

In patients with a suggestive history, the radiographic appearances of optic nerve glioma are so characteristic that biopsy is not needed to make a diagnosis. Indeed, biopsy carries a risk of ocular or visual morbidity and is frequently misleading in optic nerve glioma since reactive changes in the arachnoid can mimic meningioma.[12] Although optic canal enlargement on plain X-ray suggests a diagnosis of glioma, this modality has largely been abandoned since it yields insufficient information for diagnostic and management purposes. Computed tomography (CT) scanning reveals a smooth fusiform optic nerve enlargement with variable contrast enhancement. The optic nerve is commonly kinked in the immediate retrobulbar zone, due to its elongation[17] and the soft nature of the tumor, a finding which helps to differentiate glioma from the rarer but more aggressive childhood optic nerve sheath meningioma.[18] Nevertheless, these two entities are easily confused radiologically.[5,19] Calcification rarely

313

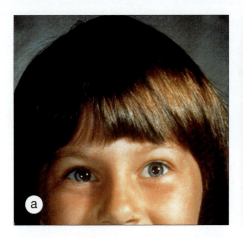
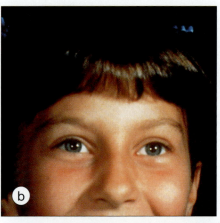
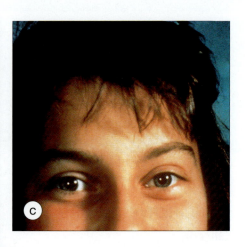
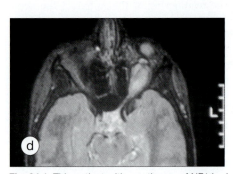
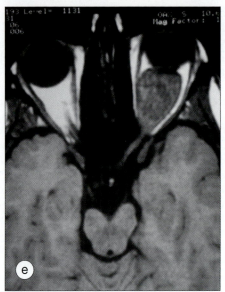

Fig. 34.1 This patient with no stigmas of NF1 had progressive left proptosis due to an optic nerve glioma since childhood and was followed to the age of 17 (a–c) when her vision deteriorated from 20/80 to 20/200 and she developed unsightly proptosis. As the chiasm appeared to be free of tumor on MRI (d, e), she underwent excision of the optic nerve and the tumor had histologically clear margins. There has been no recurrence with 7 years of follow-up.

Table 34.1	Characteristics of optic nerve glioma with and without neurofibromatosis type 1 (NF1)	
	NF1	**No NF1**
Associated features	Café-au-lait spots; Lisch nodules; other tumors (see text)	None
Presentation	Asymptomatic; routine examination finding; visual loss	Visual loss; strabismus; proptosis
Tumor distribution	Multifocal, diffuse bilateral	Discrete, unilateral
Progression	Stable–slow progression; fluctuating vision	Stable–slow progression; occasionally rapid
Histology	Arachnoid gliomatosis; perineural gliomatous and mucinous accumulation	Obliteration of perineural space by expanding optic nerve
Radiographic high signal	Fusiform optic nerve enlargement; intensity of perineural arachnoid gliomatosis on T_2-weighted MRI; kinking of intraorbital nerve	Fusiform optic nerve enlargement; loss of perineural space
Visual prognosis	Good	Poor
Life expectancy	Reduced	Normal

occurs in glioma, whereas it is a typical feature of meningioma. There is smooth enlargement of the optic canal when this area is involved.

Magnetic resonance imaging (MRI) (Fig. 34.2) is the modality of choice for evaluation and follow-up of anterior pathway gliomas since this has superior definition in distinguishing involved from uninvolved tissue (especially T_2 weighting), axial views along the nerve can easily be acquired, and there is no exposure to radiation. In Wright et al.'s series,[19] 2 of 31 patients with optic nerve glioma were found to have chiasmal involvement on MRI, which had been unsuspected clinically and had not been detected by visual-evoked potentials (VEP) and CT scan.

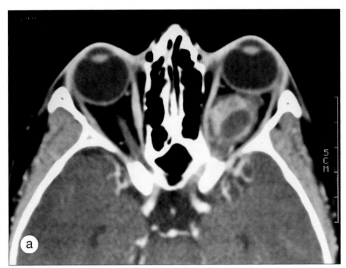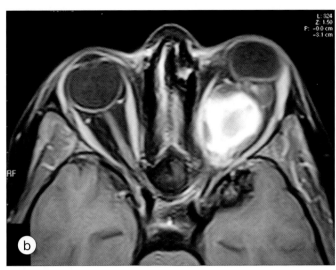

Fig. 34.2 Optic nerve glioma. (a) CT scan demonstrates a large, partially cystic appearing intraconal lesion in the plane of the optic nerve. Note retrobulbar kinking of the optic nerve. (b) T_1-weighted postcontrast MRI demonstrates marked enhancement with a central radiolucency that proved on excision to be cystic degenerative changes in an optic nerve glioma. Note the lesion extends up to but not beyond the optic canal. The patient has been tumor free for 4 years. (Patient of the University of British Columbia.)

The optic nerve gliomas found in NF1 are thought to differ histopathologically from others: arachnoid gliomatosis with mucinous accumulation in the perineural subarachnoid space is a characteristic feature, whereas obliteration of the subarachnoid space with replacement of the nerve is typical of gliomas in the absence of NF1.[20] T_2-weighted images of NF1 gliomas show an area of high signal intensity (corresponding to the mucinous element) surrounding a central core of lower signal intensity (the intraneural tumor).[17,21,22] The presence of gadolinium enhancement may further define the extent of the tumor.

Screening for anterior visual pathway gliomas

A child with a unilateral optic nerve glioma, good vision, and no evidence of chiasmal involvement on MRI scan or contralateral VEP studies should be followed up regularly with visual acuity and color vision tests, as well as visual field testing as soon as this is feasible. The NF1 Optic Pathway Glioma Task Force[23] has recommended annual screening for children with asymptomatic NF1 until age 6 and examinations every 2 to 4 years thereafter, though others[16] argue the follow-up intervals should be shorter, particularly initially, in view of the occasionally rapid progression of glioma even in the context of NF1.

VEPs may provide a low-cost and safe alternative to the general anesthetic necessary for MRI of children under the age of 6 years. Delay and reduction in amplitude on pattern VEP and, in patients with worse visual acuity, an increased latency on flash VEP are characteristic. Reviewing their experience and the literature on the subject, Ng and North[24] reported a 100% sensitivity for VEP testing in optic glioma, with specificities ranging from 60 to 83%. One paper[25] reporting normal pattern reversal VEPs in six children with documented optic nerve gliomas was out of keeping with six other studies that confirmed VEP testing to be much more sensitive than ophthalmological examination. On this basis, they suggested that MRI could be limited to those children with NF1 whose VEPs are found to be abnormal using pattern reversal and hemifield techniques.

The National Institutes of Health (NIH) conference on neurofibromatosis stated that tests such as CT, MRI, and VEPs are unlikely to be of value in asymptomatic patients with NF1. Annual ophthalmological follow-up was recommended for patients with NF1 and those with gliomas of the optic pathways documented to have stable findings. Many would now argue that baseline imaging of the optic pathways is indicated for all patients with NF1.[3,26]

Groswasser et al.[27] recorded VEPs in 25 patients with optic nerve glioma. The mean age in their study group was 11.3 years (range 2–29 years). They reported delay and reduction in amplitude from eyes with optic nerve gliomas in which there was moderate visual impairment. In severe visual impairment, the pattern reversal VEP was unrecordable but flash VEP showed an increase in latency. They also described de novo involvement and subsequent deterioration of the contralateral temporal hemifield VEP in a patient with clinically unsuspected progressive chiasmal involvement from optic nerve glioma with, later, spontaneous improvement.

Biological behavior and management

Optic nerve gliomas are low-grade pilocytic astrocytomas. Their behavior parallels the behavior of these tumors elsewhere in the central nervous system. The vast majority have little potential for growth, and their management is therefore conservative wherever possible. Static findings or slow growth is usually documented at annual follow-up. Fluctuation of visual acuity is known to occur, and improvement of vision is well documented.[4,14,19,28] Tumor regression was recently documented radiologically in a group of 13 patients, 9 of whom did not have NF1.[29] Ten of the 13 demonstrated improved visual function. Bilaterality (see Fig. 33.8a) and multifocal optic nerve/chiasmatic involvement is relatively common. Patients without NF1 tend to present with an isolated localized lesion, more abnormalities of the ocular fundus, and worse visual acuity on the affected side.[9] However, rare cases run a more aggressive course.[4,19] Enlargement, which can be rapid and substantial, takes place by a combination of glial proliferation, mucoid degeneration, and meningeal hyperplasia.[12,30] The difficulty is in identifying which patient is going to progress. Disc edema (as opposed to atrophy), restriction of movement, and the absence of neurofibromatosis were identified as risk factors for rapid progression by Wright et al.[19]

Overall, however, patients with NF1 are more likely to have stable findings and an indolent course, diffuse or multifocal involvement of their visual pathways, and chiasmal involvement. They also tend to have good preservation of visual function, and fluctuation of vision is well known to occur (see above). The emphasis of management in this group is therefore conservative. Visual deterioration without fluctuation may be an indication for treatment with low-dose chemotherapy, as advocated by Packer et al.,[31] or, more recently, as a cisplatin/etoposide regimen[32] or conformal radiotherapy.[33] If the tumor is associated with visual obscurations due to mucoid accumulation within the nerve sheath, nerve sheath decompression can be considered.

Patients without evidence of NF1 tend to present with worse visual acuity and localized involvement of the optic nerve. These gliomas also behave in a very benign way with slow or no progression at annual assessment. However, tumors situated anterior to the chiasm showing progression and threatening to involve this structure, or evidence of steady enlargement on sequential MRIs with disfiguring proptosis or globe luxation as well as poor vision are indications for surgical excision. This is performed through a lateral orbitotomy if the tumor is restricted to the intraorbital portion of the nerve, or a temporofrontal panoramic orbitotomy if extension beyond the orbit is noted. The affected nerve is divided posterior to the tumor, with frozen section control to ensure complete removal. In cases where there is intracranial extension, the nerve is divided just anterior to the chiasm. The globe is usually spared after tumor excision, even if the central retinal and posterior ciliary arteries appear to be involved. Dissection of the posterior ciliary vessels prior to resection of the nerve prevents postoperative ocular ischemia,[34] which was previously reported to be a common complication after glioma excision.[19] Obviously, vision is sacrificed in the ipsilateral eye. Orbitotomy has minimal effect on the subsequent growth of the facial and orbital bones.

It is important to stress that excision is only indicated in the absence of chiasmal involvement by tumor, although accurate assessment of this remains problematic even with the most modern techniques. Nevertheless, Wright et al.[19] reported no evidence of recurrent chiasmal disease in all six patients in whom the proximal end of the excised optic nerve was histologically free of tumor, with a mean follow-up of 6.5 years. It is not clear whether these patients had NF1 or not. Enlargement of glioma proximal to the cut end of the optic nerve is well recorded.

Chiasmal glioma
Presentation
Glioma affecting predominantly the chiasm is more common than optic nerve glioma.[35,36] Unlike optic nerve glioma, which is more common in girls, there is no gender predilection. They are seen in a slightly older age group than children with optic nerve glioma.[36] The usual presentation to the ophthalmologist is with bilateral visual loss (Figs. 34.3 and 34.4), although chiasmal glioma may be discovered during investigation of hydrocephalus or endocrine dysfunction[14] or in a hitherto asymptomatic patient by neuroimaging studies.[3] The history is usually of slowly deteriorating vision, but sudden visual loss mimicking optic neuritis may occur as a result of hemorrhage within the tumor, a complication called "chiasmal apoplexy."[37]

Strabismus may occur. Unilateral or asymmetrical (dissociated) nystagmus caused by chiasmal glioma may mimic spasmus nutans.[38] Neuroradiological studies are therefore indicated in any child with asymmetrical nystagmus, particularly in the presence of optic atrophy, poor feeding, or hydrocephalus since this is suggestive of chiasmal glioma with or without posterior extension.[39]

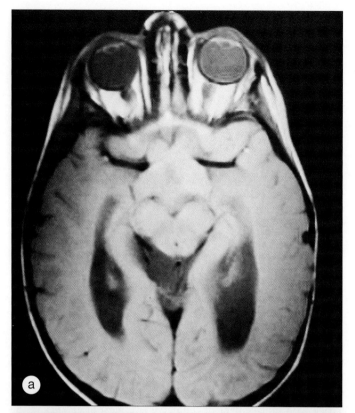

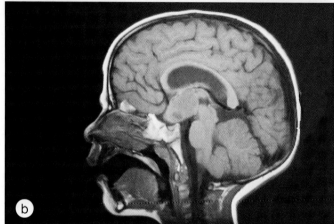

Fig. 34.3 (a, b) Chiasmal and hypothalamic glioma with thickened intracranial optic nerves.

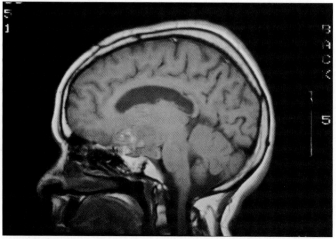

Fig. 34.4 Large, vascular, chiasmal, and hypothalamic glioma.

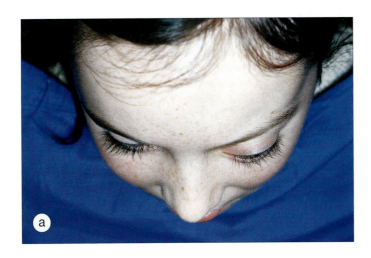

Proptosis is an unusual presenting sign (Fig. 34.5), although the tumor often extends forward into one or both optic nerves and occasionally into the orbit. The tumor can also extend into the optic tracts and the visual field findings are therefore variable,[40] but bitemporal loss is common.[36] The discs may be normal but are more likely to be atrophic or, more rarely, swollen.[36]

Extension of the lesion into the hypothalamus produces various endocrine abnormalities. Precocious puberty was reported in 7 of 18 children with chiasmal glioma, with ages ranging from 4.8 to 5.9 years.[3] Reduced growth and sexual maturation, diabetes insipidus, and obesity may also occur. In some cases, there may be extreme wasting, reduced development, and often vertical or rotary nystagmus, an association known as Russell diencephalic syndrome.[35,41]

Radiologically, chiasmal glioma is seen as a suprasellar mass that may be accompanied by a diagnostic contiguous enlargement of

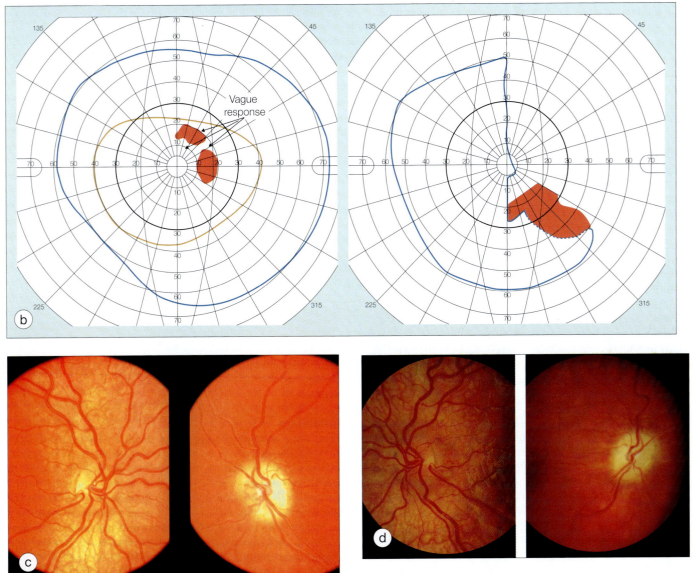

Fig. 34.5 (a) Chiasmal and left optic nerve glioma with left proptosis. (b) Right visual fields done 17 months apart show increasing chiasmal involvement. A clear-cut temporal field loss is unusual in chiasmal glioma because there are frequently associated tract and optic nerve lesions. (c) In November 1974, the patient had poor vision on the left with optic atrophy, disc swelling, and visible shunt vessels. The right eye shows mild band atrophy. (d) Seventeen months later the left optic nerve had become completely atrophic, and the patient was blind on that side. The shunt vessels were no longer visible. There was right-sided papilledema due to raised intracranial pressure. This was bilobed in nature ("twin peaks" papilledema) due to the previous band atrophy. There was an associated temporal field defect.

the optic nerve or tract.[42] Minor degrees of chiasmal enlargement are relatively difficult to detect with CT. MRI is better for studying the chiasm, intracranial optic nerves, and optic tract.[43–45]

The diagnosis can be made on the basis of neuroimaging studies, and tissue diagnosis is rarely necessary for lesions that appear intrinsic to the chiasm.

Biological behavior and management

Several long-term studies have documented stability in the majority of chiasmal gliomas.[14,40,46] Surgery may be of benefit in gliomas in which a significant exophytic component is compressing the chiasm or either optic nerve.[47] Surgery on the chiasm carries an appreciable risk of hypothalamic syndrome and sudden death. Moreover, surgical removal of intrinsic chiasmal glioma is not possible without sacrificing vision bilaterally. Management options are observation, radiotherapy, and possibly, chemotherapy. The management plans suggested by Packer et al.[31] and reinforced by Kennerdell and Garrity[48] seem logical.

In view of remaining uncertainty about the natural history of chiasmal glioma, no treatment is given if the tumor is confined to the chiasm at the time of diagnosis. These patients are reviewed regularly with clinical evaluation of acuity, fields, and regular MRI.

There is no single accepted indication for treatment of chiasmal glioma. If there is involvement of the hypothalamus or third ventricle or gross enlargement of the optic tract, treatment by radiotherapy is advised. Although the effectiveness of radiotherapy for chiasmal glioma is still in doubt,[36,46] some authors consider that disease control in up to 50% of patients is possible.[31,49] Radiotherapy therefore appears the best treatment option available, especially when visual loss has been rapid and recent. However, radiotherapy can have numerous adverse effects on the developing brain, including mental and growth retardation, psychiatric problems, and the induction of second tumors. Chemotherapy may delay radiation and its unwanted side effects, but 60% of children eventually relapse.[7] Endocrine abnormalities associated with chiasmal glioma require assessment and treatment. Hydrocephalus may require ventricular shunting.

Malignant gliomas of the anterior visual pathway that behave aggressively, also known as glioblastoma multiforme, are recognized in adults[50,51] and may occasionally occur in children.[35,36]

MENINGIOMAS

Meningiomas are very rare in childhood, but become slightly more common in the teenage years. They result from proliferation of meningothelial cap cells of the arachnoid villi and may arise in association with NF1 or NF2. They may occur within the sheath of the optic nerve or from the dura of the sphenoid bone, affecting the sphenoid wing and/or parasellar region. The site of origin determines the pattern of presentation: tumors arising from the lateral third of the greater wing of the sphenoid present with mass effect with relative preservation of vision, whereas those situated at the medial third tend to present with visual loss with or without cranial nerve palsies. Optic nerve sheath tumors, particularly when intracanalicular, present with early visual loss and relatively little mass effect.

Optic nerve sheath meningiomas

Like other meningiomas, these tend to affect females, most commonly in middle-age.[52] However, they are seen in childhood,

usually presenting in the teens with slowly progressive visual loss; proptosis is generally mild[53] but their tendency to grow through the dura makes extraocular muscle involvement relatively frequent[5] and diplopia may also occur as a result of splinting of the optic nerve by the tumor. Compression of the optic nerve results in an optic neuropathy. Duction-induced obscurations may occur at first, followed by visual loss as the tumor enlarges. There is progressive constriction of the visual field. An afferent pupillary defect, as well as disc swelling or pallor and opticociliary shunt vessels, may be present. Although the latter may also occur with optic nerve gliomas, their presence is more suggestive of meningioma. A recent combined-center study of optic nerve meningioma has emphasized that these tumors grow faster in younger patients and are associated with more frequent intracranial involvement.[52]

Investigation

Routine MRI of the intraorbital portion of the optic nerve may not reveal the classical findings of "tramline" calcification and tubular sheath enlargement that would be evident on a CT scan (Figs 34.6a and 36.6b).[18] A diagnosis of optic nerve sheath meningioma can be missed for this reason in a patient with progressive visual loss and disc swelling or atrophy, something we have witnessed in teenagers on two occasions. Nevertheless, MRI with fat suppression and gadolinium enhancement is the modality of choice for defining the extent of the tumor[54] since it demonstrates intracanalicular and intracranial extension more clearly.

CT scanning may show the classical findings described above or the tumor may form an excrescence through the dura;[55] the nerve is seen as a radiolucent region within the tumor on axial and coronal scans.[18,55] Since meningiomas may be quite vascular, enhancement with intravenous contrast and tumor blush on angiography are common features, unlike glioma where they are rare.[35] Furthermore, kinking of the nerve, a common feature in glioma, is not seen. Dutton and Anderson[56] have drawn attention to the radiological similarity of the perineural variant of nonspecific orbital inflammation and optic nerve sheath meningioma. MRI may clearly define nerve and tumor margins.

Biopsy is not very helpful in differentiating meningioma from glioma, due to the presence of meningeal hyperplasia in the latter, which appears similar to meningioma. It should be possible to distinguish these two entities on clinical and radiological grounds.[18,55]

Treatment

The tumor may only progress very slowly or even remain stable in size for an extended period of time; since there is no metastatic potential, observation to establish the pattern of growth in individual cases appears a reasonable option. Left alone in the long term, it almost always results in complete visual loss in the affected eye, and its clinical course is more aggressive in children.[18]

The main choice lies between observation and surgical excision, although radiotherapy may also be considered.[48,52] Recently, encouraging results have been reported from treatment with stereotactic fractionated irradiation,[57] with a total dose of 54 Gy. Improvement in visual acuity and visual field was noted with a mean follow-up of 37 months. The value of this technique has not been reported for children.

If surgery is required, a lateral orbitotomy is used to approach a tumor involving the anterior two-thirds of the intraorbital nerve. Tumors extending to the posterior orbit or intracranially require a combined orbital–neurosurgical approach via a

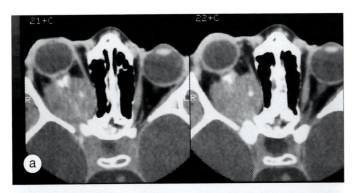

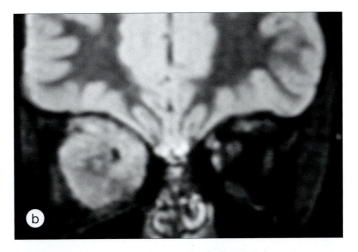

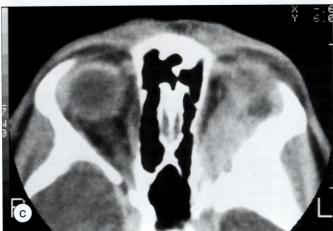

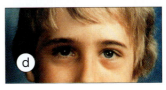

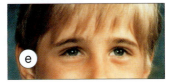

Fig. 34.6 (a) Optic nerve meningioma in a 5-year-old boy. CT scan showing calcification around the optic nerve and orbital expansion on the right. (b) MRI of same patient showing the clear differentiation between the peripheral tumor and the axial optic nerve. The calcium is not demonstrated. (c) Sphenoid wing meningioma in a 9-year-old boy: CT scan showing marked hyperostosis on the left. (d) Sphenoid wing meningioma (same patient) aged 9 years, showing lid swelling and proptosis. (e) Sphenoid wing meningioma: same patient aged 13 years after resection and radiotherapy. At age 25 years, his meningioma recurred as a petrus-clival mass anterior to the brainstem with extension into the suprachiasmic cistern and left cavernous sinus. The patient died of his disease 1 year later. (Patient of the University of British Columbia.)

panoramic orbitotomy. The eye will be blind but cosmetically satisfactory.[5,58] Intracranial involvement in young patients should prompt either very close observation or total excision of the lesion.

Extraoptic meningioma

This type of meningioma is slightly more common in childhood than optic nerve tumors, with a tendency to occur during the teenage years. The sites of ophthalmic relevance are the sphenoid wing (Figs 34.6c–34.6e), suprasellar area, and olfactory groove. The ophthalmic features reflect the position of the tumor, since those situated medially present with visual loss, cranial nerve palsies, and symptoms and signs of venous obstruction at the orbital apex, while those arising laterally cause mass effect, and swelling in the temporalis fossa. Very rarely, meningiomas can arise at extradural sites in children.[59]

The best diagnostic modality for bony change is CT scan, which demonstrates the hyperostosis underlying the tumor. The lesion is of homogeneously increased density, and enhances evenly after contrast injection. Fine calcification may be present in psammomatous tumors. The full extent of the soft tissue component is best defined with contrast-enhanced MRI.

Since tumor growth is slow, observation is warranted in most cases. The course tends to be more aggressive in childhood. Excision is indicated for cosmesis or visual loss, but encasement

of orbital structures or bone invasion may preclude complete clearance. Debulking may be sufficient to improve cosmesis and decompress the orbital apex, with improvement of optic neuropathy. Encouraging results have been reported with radical excision followed by radiotherapy to any residual tumor.[60]

RARE OPTIC NERVE TUMORS IN CHILDHOOD

Leukemic infiltration of the optic nerve traditionally has a grave systemic prognosis, although with combined radiotherapy and chemotherapy the prognosis is greatly improved when the infiltration is prelaminar and the optic disc has a fluffy appearance with edema and hemorrhage without marked visual loss. Retrolaminar involvement results in moderate disc swelling but profound visual loss.[61,62]

Tumors of the optic disc such as melanocytoma, angiomatous malformations, or glial hamartoma (as seen in tuberous sclerosis) may involve the very anterior parts of the optic nerve. Ganglioma, ganglioglioma,[63] inflammatory lesions, aneurysms, histiocytosis, sarcomas, and other rare entities have also been described.[11,64] Medulloepithelioma is a tumor that arises from the medullary epithelium of the optic vesicle and is much more commonly found in the ciliary body. It can affect the optic nerve head and may extend into the substance of the optic nerve. Both benign and malignant forms have been described. Margo and

Kincaid[65] found a vascular malformation in the retrolaminar portion of two eyes removed for suspicion of retinoblastoma; one eye had a neuroblastic tumor and the other a form of retinal dysplasia.

The importance of many of these rare optic nerve tumors is in the differential diagnosis of the much more common optic nerve glioma, for which biopsy is rarely performed.

SCHWANNOMA

Schwannomas (formerly known as neurilemomas or neurinomas) are tumors that arise from the Schwann cells of peripheral nerve sheath (Fig. 34.7). They are rare in childhood, generally occurring in middle-aged patients. They are more common in NF1 and NF2. The sensory nerves are much more frequently affected but schwannomas of the ocular motor nerves, particularly the third nerve, are well recognized.

Orbital schwannoma generally presents with proptosis. Since the trigeminal nerve is often involved, facial paraesthesia may be a feature. Diplopia may result from third nerve involvement or compression by a tumor in the trigeminal ganglion (Fig. 34.8). Progression tends to be slow and sometimes intermittent over a period of years. Schwannoma may also occur in the eyelid.[66] Orbital schwannomas tend to be localized and can be excised or their contents can be evacuated without undue difficulty.[5,66,67]

The tumor is composed of proliferating Schwann cells, without significant admixture of axons and endoneural cells, in a collagenous matrix[68] and is circumscribed by a fibrous capsule. The tumors are S-100 protein positive. Two cellular patterns, which may occur in the same tumor, are recognized. The Antoni A pattern consists of compactly arranged spindle cells with long oval nuclei, frequently orientated with their long axes parallel. The Antoni B-type pattern consists of Schwann cells with twisted and elongated shapes widely separated by a featureless collagen matrix.

Transformation into a malignant Schwann cell tumor is exceedingly rare in childhood but Miller[4] described a 6-week-old infant with increasing proptosis from birth and NF1 stigmata who was

affected bilaterally. Eviatar et al.[69] reported a 15-month old who was followed up for 9 years with no recurrence after excision of a malignant schwannoma.

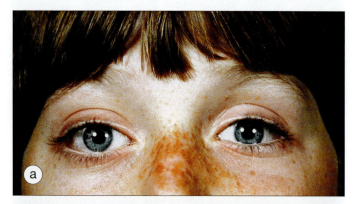

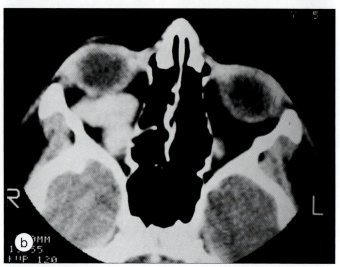

Fig. 34.7 (a) This 12-year-old boy presented with progressive right proptosis and hyperopia with indentation of the posterior pole. (b) The well-defined orbital tumor was completely excised and proved to be a schwannoma. (Patient of the University of British Columbia.)

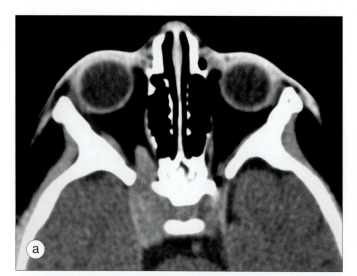

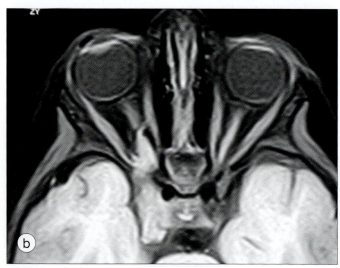

Fig. 34.8 (a–d) These CT and MRI scans demonstrate a lesion of the Gasserian ganglion in a child that presented at 19 months of age with right exotropia, partially dilated right pupil, and a slight afferent pupillary defect. In addition, he had stigmata of neurofibromatosis type 1. He had reduced vision due to amblyopia. The images support a diagnosis of schwannoma versus neurofibroma. He developed a ptosis as part of his third nerve palsy, and he has been observed and followed clinically and with imaging without progression for 4 years. (Patient of the University of British Columbia.)

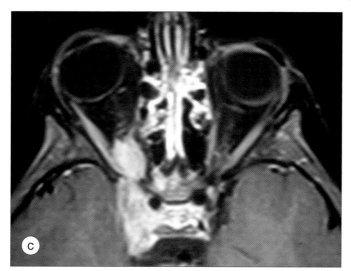
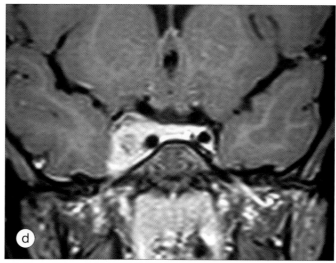

Fig. 34.8 (a–d) (Cont'd)These CT and MRI scans demonstrate a lesion of the Gasserian ganglion in a child that presented at 19 months of age with right exotropia, partially dilated right pupil, and a slight afferent pupillary defect. In addition, he had stigmata of neurofibromatosis type 1. He had reduced vision due to amblyopia. The images support a diagnosis of schwannoma versus neurofibroma. He developed a ptosis as part of his third nerve palsy, and he has been observed and followed clinically and with imaging without progression for 4 years. (Patient of the University of British Columbia.)

REFERENCES

1. Lewis RA, Gerson LP, Axelson KA, et al. Von Recklinghausen neurofibromatosis II: incidence of optic glioma. Ophthalmology 1984; 91: 929–35.

2. Friedman JM, Riccardi VM. Neurofibromatosis: Phenotype, Natural History, and Pathogenesis. 3rd ed. Baltimore: Johns Hopkins University Press; 1999.

3. Listernick R, Charrow J, Greenwald M, et al. Natural history of optic pathway tumors in children with neurofibromatosis type 1: a longitudinal study. J Pediatr 1994; 125: 63–6.

4. Hedges TR III. Tumors of neuroectodermal origin. In: Miller NR, Newman NJ, editors. Walsh and Hoyt's Clinical Neuro-ophthalmology. 5th ed. Baltimore: Williams and Wilkins; 1998: 1919–2016.

5. Rootman J. Diseases of the Orbit: a Multidisciplinary Approach. 2nd ed. Philadelphia: Lippincott Williams & Wilkins; 2002.

6. Wilson ME, Parker PL, Chavis RM. Conservative managment of childhood adult lymphangioma. Ophthalmology 1989; 96: 484–9.

7. Janss AJ, Grundy R, Cnaan A, et al. Optic pathway and hypothalamic/chiasmatic gliomas in children younger than age 5 years with a 6-year follow-up. Cancer 1995; 75: 1051–9.

8. Singhal S, Birch JM, Kerr B, et al. Neurofibromatosis type 1 and sporadic optic gliomas. Arch Dis Child 2002; 87: 65–70.

9. Czyzyk E, Jozwiak S, Roszkowski M, et al. Optic pathway gliomas in children with and without neurofibromatosis 1. J Child Neurol 2003; 18: 471–8.

10. Dutton JJ. Gliomas of the anterior visual pathway. Surv Ophthalmol 1994; 38: 427–52.

11. Eggers H, Jakobiec FA, Jones IS. Tumors of the optic nerve. Doc Ophthalmol 1976; 41: 43–128.

12. Wright JE, McDonald WI, Call NB. Management of optic nerve gliomas. Br J Ophthalmol 1980; 64: 545–52.

13. Buchanan TA, Hoyt WF. Optic nerve glioma and neovascular glaucoma: report of a case. Br J Ophthalmol 1982; 66: 96–8.

14. Hoyt WF, Baghdassarian SA. Optic glioma of childhood. Natural history and rationale for conservative management. Br J Ophthalmol 1969; 53: 793–8.

15. Listernick R, Charrow J, Greenwald MJ, et al. Optic gliomas in children with neurofibromatosis type 1. J Pediatr 1989; 114: 788–92.

16. Balcer LJ, Liu GT, Heller G, et al. Visual loss in children with neurofibromatosis type 1 and optic pathway gliomas: relation to tumor location by magnetic resonance imaging. Am J Ophthalmol 2001; 131: 442–5.

17. Imes RK, Hoyt WF. Magnetic resonance imaging signs of optic nerve glioma in neurofibromatosis 1. Am J Ophthalmol 1991; 111: 729–34.

18. Jakobiec FA, Depot MJ, Kennerdell J, et al. Combined clinical and computed tomographic diagnosis of orbital glioma and meningioma. Ophthalmology 1984; 91: 137–55.

19. Wright JE, McNab AA, McDonald WI. Optic nerve glioma and the management of optic nerve tumours in the young. Br J Ophthalmol 1989; 73: 967–74.

20. Stern J, Jakobiec FA, Housepian EM. The architecture of optic nerve gliomas with and without neurofibromatosis. Arch Ophthalmol 1980; 98: 505–11.

21. Seiff SR, Brodsky MC, MacDonald G, et al. Orbital optic glioma in neurofibromatosis. Magnetic resonance diagnosis of perineural arachnoidal gliomatosis. Arch Ophthalmol 1987; 105: 1689–92.

22. Brodsky MC. The "pseudo-CSF" signal of orbital optic glioma on magnetic resonance imaging: a signature of neurofibromatosis. Surv Ophthalmol 1993; 38: 213–8.

23. Listernick R, Louis DN, Packer RJ, et al. Optic pathway gliomas in children with neurofibromatosis 1: consensus statement from the NF1 Optic Pathway Glioma Task Force. Ann Neurol 1997; 41: 143–9.

24. Ng YT, North KN. Visual-evoked potentials in the assessment of optic gliomas. Pediatr Neurol 2001; 24: 44–8.

25. Rossi LN, Pastorino G, Scotti G, et al. Early diagnosis of optic glioma in children with neurofibromatosis type 1. Childs Nerv Syst 1994; 10: 426–9.

26. Riccardi VM. Neurofibromatosis: Phenotype, Natural History, and Pathogenesis. 2nd ed. Baltimore: Johns Hopkins University; 1992.

27. Groswasser Z, Kriss A, Halliday AM, et al. Pattern- and flash-evoked potentials in the assessment and management of optic nerve gliomas. J Neurol Neurosurg Psychiatry 1985; 48: 1125–34.

28. Frohman LP, Epstein F, Kupersmith MJ. Atypical visual prognosis with an optic nerve glioma. J Clin Neuroophthalmol 1985; 5: 90–4.

29. Parsa CF, Hoyt CS, Lesser RL, et al. Spontaneous regression of optic gliomas: thirteen cases documented by serial neuroimaging. Arch Ophthalmol 2001; 119: 516–29.

30. Spencer WH. Primary neoplasms of the optic nerve and its sheaths. Trans Am Ophthalmol Soc 1972; 70: 490–505.

31. Packer RJ, Savino PJ, Bilaniuk LT, et al. Chiasmatic gliomas of childhood. A reappraisal of natural history and effectiveness of cranial irradiation. Childs Brain 1983; 10: 393–403.

32. Massimino M, Spreafico F, Cefalo G, et al. High response rate to cisplatin/etoposide regimen in childhood low-grade glioma. J Clin Oncol 2002; 20: 4209–16.

33. Debus J, Kocagöncü KO, Hoss A, et al. Fractionated stereotactic radiotherapy (FSRT) for optic glioma. Int J Radiat Oncol Biol Phys 1999; 44: 243–8.

34. Rootman J, Stewart B, Goldberg RA. Orbital Surgery: a Conceptual Approach. Philadelphia: Lippincott-Raven; 1995.

35. Moseley IF, Sanders MD. Computerized Tomography in Neuro-ophthalmology. London: Chapman and Hall; 1982.

36. Rush JA, Younge BR, Campbell RJ, et al. Optic glioma: long-term follow-up of 85 histopathologically verified cases. Ophthalmology 1982; 89: 1213–9.

37. Maitland CG, Abiko S, Hoyt WF, et al. Chiasmal apoplexy: report of four cases. J Neurosurg 1982; 56: 118–22.

38. Farmer J, Hoyt CS. Monocular nystagmus in infancy and early childhood. Am J Ophthalmol 1984; 98: 504–9.

39. Lavery MA, O'Neill JF, Chu FE, et al. Acquired nystagmus in early childhood: a presenting sign of intracranial tumor. Ophthalmology 1984; 91: 425–34.

40. Glaser JS, Hoyt WF, Corbett J. Visual morbidity with chiasmal glioma. Long-term studies of visual fields in untreated and irradiated cases. Arch Ophthalmol 1971; 85: 3–12.

41. Russell A. A diencephalic syndrome of emaciation in infancy and childhood. Arch Dis Child 1951; 26: 274.

42. Fletcher WA, Imes RK, Hoyt WF. Chiasmal gliomas: appearance and long-term changes demonstrated by computerized tomography. J Neurosurg 1986; 65: 154–9.

43. Holman RE, Grimson BS, Drayer BP, et al. Magnetic resonance imaging of optic gliomas. Am J Ophthalmol 1985; 100: 596–601.

44. Haik BG, Saint Louis L, Bierly J, et al. Magnetic resonance imaging in the evaluation of optic nerve gliomas. Ophthalmology 1987; 94: 709–18.

45. Savino PJ. The present role of magnetic resonance imaging in neuro-ophthalmology. Can J Ophthalmol 1987;22:4–12.

46. Imes RK, Hoyt WF. Childhood chiasmal gliomas: update on the fate of patients in the 1969 San Francisco study. Br J Ophthalmol 1986; 70: 179–82.

47. Venes JL, Latack J, Kandt RS. Postoperative regression opticochiasmic astrocytoma: a case for expectant therapy. Neurosurgery 1984; 15: 421–3.

48. Kennerdell JS, Garrity JA. Tumors of the optic nerve. In: Lessell S, Van Dalen JTW, editors. Current Neuro-ophthalmology. Chicago: Year Book Medical Publishers; 1988: 25–32.

49. Horwich A, Bloom HJG. Optic gliomas: radiation therapy and prognosis. Int J Radiat Oncol Biol Phys 1985; 11: 1067–79.

50. Hoyt WF, Meshel LG, Lessell S, et al. Malignant optic glioma of adulthood. Brain 1973; 96: 121–32.

51. Spoor TC, Kennerdell JS, Martinez AJ, et al. Malignant gliomas of the optic pathways. Am J Ophthalmol 1980; 89: 284–92.

52. Saeed P, Rootman J, Nugent RA, et al. Optic nerve sheath meningiomas. Ophthalmology 2003; 110: 2019–30.

53. Dutton JJ. Optic nerve sheath meningiomas. Surv Ophthalmol 1992; 37: 167–83.

54. Lindblom B, Truwit C, Hoyt WF. Optic nerve sheath meningioma. Definition of intraorbital, intracanalicular and intracranial components with magnetic resonance imaging. Ophthalmology 1992; 99: 560–6.

55. Rothfus WE, Curtin HD, Slamovits TL, et al. Optic nerve/sheath enlargement. Radiology 1984; 150: 409–15.

56. Dutton JJ, Anderson RL. Idiopathic inflammatory perioptic neuritis simulating optic nerve sheath meningioma. Am J Ophthalmol 1985; 100: 424–30.

57. Pitz S, Becker G, Schiefer U, et al. Stereotactic fractionated irradiation of optic nerve sheath meningioma: a new treatment alternative. Br J Ophthalmol 2002; 86: 1265–8.

58. Wolter JR. Ten years without orbital optic nerve: late clinical results after removal of retrobulbar gliomas with preservation of blind eyes. J Pediatr Ophthalmol Strabismus 1988; 25: 55–60.

59. Johnson TE, Weatherhead RG, Nasr AM, et al. Ectopic (extradural) meningioma of the orbit: a report of two cases in children. J Pediatr Ophthalmol Strabismus 1993; 30: 43–7.

60. Maroon JC, Kennerdell JS, Vidovich DV, et al. Recurrent spheno-orbital meningioma. J Neurosurg 1994; 80: 202–8.

61. Kincaid MC, Green WR. Ocular and orbital involvement in leukemia. Surv Ophthalmol 1983; 15: 123–6.

62. Rosenthal AR. Ocular manifestations of leukemia. A review. Ophthalmology 1983; 90: 899–905.

63. Bergin DJ, Johnson TE, Spencer WH, et al. Ganglioglioma of the optic nerve. Am J Ophthalmol 1988; 105: 146–50.

64. Brown GC, Shields JA. Tumors of the optic nerve head. Surv Ophthalmol 1985; 29: 239–64.

65. Margo CE, Kincaid MC. Angiomatous malformation of the retrolaminar optic nerve. J Pediatr Ophthalmol Strabismus 1988; 25: 37–40.

66. Reese AB. Tumors of the Eye. 3rd ed. Hagerstown: Harper and Row; 1976.

67. Nicholson DH, Green WR. Pediatric Ocular Tumors. New York: Masson; 1981.

68. Harkin J, Reed R. Tumors of the peripheral nervous system. In: Atlas of Tumor Pathology, 2nd series, fascicle 3. Washington: Armed Forces Institute of Pathology; 1969.

69. Eviatar JA, Hornblass A, Herschorn B, et al. Malignant peripheral nerve sheath tumor of the orbit in a 15-month-old child. Nine-year survival after local excision. Ophthalmology 1992; 99: 1595–9.

CHAPTER
35 Rhabdomyosarcoma

Christopher J Lyons and Jack Rootman

Primary malignant orbital lesions are a very rare cause of proptosis in children but rhabdomyosarcoma is the most common of these. In the combined clinical series presented (see Table 32.1), it accounted for 2% of all children with orbital problems. In Shields' biopsy-based series,[1] it accounted for 4% of pediatric orbital space-occupying lesions.

Rhabdomyosarcoma is a tumor of primitive connective tissue (mesenchyme), which has the capacity to differentiate toward striated muscle. Interestingly, childhood rhabdomyosarcomas usually arise from orbital connective tissue rather than extraocular muscle. The prognosis has vastly improved over the past 40 years as treatment has evolved from radical surgery to biopsy, radiotherapy, and chemotherapy.[2]

EPIDEMIOLOGY AND GENETICS

There are about 250 new cases of rhabdomyosarcoma in the United States and 60 in the United Kingdom per year. Almost half arise from the head and neck, and about a third of these are primary orbital tumors.[2] The peak incidence is at 7–8 years of age[3] and approximately three-quarters present in the first decade of life. However, they can occur at any age and have been reported in newborns,[4–6] in infancy (with a worse prognosis in this age group)[7] (Fig. 35.1), and in old age, since Kassel et al.[8] reported one case in a 78-year-old. Overall, males are more likely to be affected than females by a ratio of 5:3.[9]

Familial cases have been reported. Li and Fraumeni[10] and Li et al.[11] described families with a positive history of malignancy, in which pairs of offspring of young mothers with carcinoma developed rhabdomyosarcoma. The Li–Fraumeni syndrome is associated with germline mutations of the p53 tumor-suppressor gene. Rhabdomyosarcoma is also more common in patients with neurofibromatosis type 1.[12]

Like other malignancies, rhabdomyosarcoma is associated with an increased prevalence of congenital malformations. One-third of the 115 children and adolescents with rhabdomyosarcoma reviewed at autopsy by Ruymann et al.[13] had malformations, most commonly involving the genitourinary, gastrointestinal, and central nervous systems.

Although the exact etiology of rhabdomyosarcoma is unknown, molecular analysis has implicated chromosome 11 in the pathogenesis of the embryonal cell type, through loss of tumor

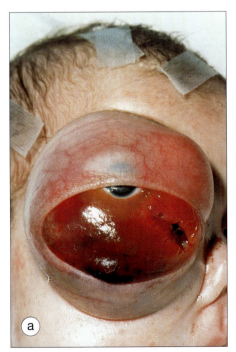
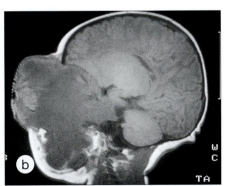
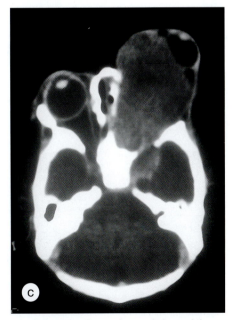

Fig. 35.1 Congenital rhabdomyosarcoma. (a) This child was born with a massive orbital tumor and proptosis. The eye itself was of normal size and the lids can be seen to be stretched by the huge tumor. (b) MRI scan showing extensive extraorbital maxillary and intracranial involvement. (c) CT scan showing bony destruction, intracranial involvement, and the gross distortion of the globe. The main differential diagnosis is with orbital teratoma.

suppressor genes.[14-16] Alveolar rhabdomyosarcoma is characterized by chromosome translocations, t(2;13)(q35;q14) in 55% of cases and t(1;13(p36;q14) in 22% of cases, which involve *PAX3* and *PAX7* on chromosomes 2 and 1, respectively, resulting in abnormal muscle development.[17-19] These translocations result in fusion genes between the undisrupted *PAX3* and 7 DNA binding domains and the *FKHR* gene on chromosome 13, which provide a useful diagnostic marker for alveolar rhabdomyosarcoma.

Cytogenetic studies of pleomorphic rhabdomyosarcoma, which is generally an adult disease, show chromosomal imbalances similar to those reported for malignant fibrous histiocytoma, suggesting that pleomorphic rhabdomyosarcoma, which has a much better prognosis than other rhabdomyosarcoma types, could (from a genetic point of view) be part of that disease spectrum.[20]

CLINICAL FEATURES

The most common presentation is with proptosis (Figs. 35.2–35.4), which may appear suddenly and progress over a few days or weeks[21,22] often with eyelid erythema and edema, as well as increasing ophthalmoplegia. The lid signs may occasionally precede the proptosis.[23] The absence of local heat, pyrexia, and general malaise help to distinguish this entity from orbital cellulitis.

Ptosis and palpable lid mass (Fig. 35.5) are other common modes of presentation.[3,24] Almost half of the 58 patients in one series[25] presented in this way. Since the lid lump can be mistaken for a chalazion, it is important to consider rhabdomyosarcoma in the differential diagnosis of any childhood lid lump or unexplained

acquired ptosis. Rarely, rhabdomyosarcoma can present as grape-like (botryoid variant), papillomatous conjunctival nodules, or circumscribed episcleral lesions,[2] or with periorbital swelling (Fig. 35.6). Intraocular origin, from the iris (possibly mimicking xanthogranuloma)[26] or from the ciliary body, has also been recorded but is very rare.[2]

The location of the tumor affects the direction of displacement of the globe. In Jones et al.'s review of 62 patients,[22] half of the tumors were retrobulbar and one-quarter were situated superiorly. Twelve percent were inferior, 6% nasal, and 6% temporal. Although the tumors are commonly retrobulbar, visual symptoms are unusual.[21] Sohaib et al.[27] found two-thirds of orbital rhabdomyosarcomas to be situated superonasally. Shields et al.[24] reported a similar propensity for superior or supranasal presentation.

Rhabdomyosarcoma spreads early by rapid local invasion. It is usually confined to the orbit at the time of diagnosis, but may later extend into the anterior or middle cranial fossa (parameningeal spread), pterygopalatine fossa, or the nasal cavity. The latter may give rise to nasal stuffiness or nosebleeds. Metastasis is typically blood-borne, to the lungs or bones.[3] Although there are no lymphatics within the orbit, involvement of the eyelids may be complicated by spread to the cervical or preauricular lymph nodes, especially in alveolar rhabdomyosarcoma.

Not uncommonly, the orbit is secondarily involved by local spread from a contiguous lesion in the paranasal sinuses, nasal cavity, pterygopalatine fossa, or parapharyngeal space. It can also arise within the cranial cavity, resulting in proptosis when orbital involvement occurs.[28] Orbital deposition of metastatic tumor from distant sites may also occur in end-stage dissemination.[29]

DIAGNOSIS

Rhabdomyosarcoma is one of the causes of rapidly progressive proptosis in childhood. As discussed above, it is rare under the

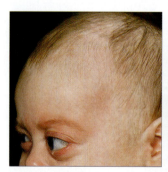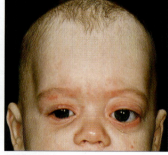

Fig. 35.2 Rhabdomyosarcoma. This 3-month-old boy had a 2-week history of proptosis.

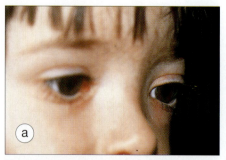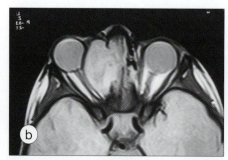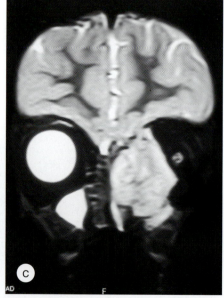

Fig. 35.3 (a) This 20-month-old girl had a 3-week history of left proptosis, nasal discharge, and nosebleeds. There is 7 mm of proptosis of the left eye with 5-mm lateral globe displacement. (b) On MRI, an ethmoidal mass had eroded through the medial orbital wall and displaced the orbital contents anteriorly and laterally. The mass has also obstructed the nasal cavity. Intranasal biopsy demonstrated rhabdomyosarcoma of alveolar type. (c) Coronal view of the same patient showing the medial orbital mass and considerable globe displacement. Patient from the University of British Columbia.

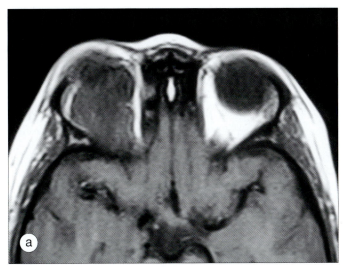 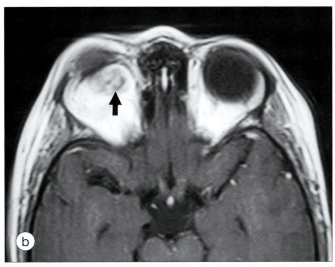

Fig. 35.4 This 9-year-old boy presented with diplopia and swelling of his right upper lid. (a) On T₁-weighted MRI, a large superior nonhomogeneous orbital lesion was noted. (b) A T₁-weighted MRI post-Gadolinium showed an area of irregular uptake of dye (arrow), suggesting focal necrosis. The mass was biopsy-proven to be rhabdomyosarcoma. Patient from the University of British Columbia.

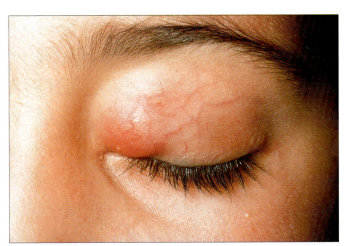

Fig. 35.5 A localized swelling in this 8-year-old girl's left upper lid was clinically diagnosed as a chalazion. Pathological examination was not requested at the time of incision and curettage. The mass recurred and a biopsy confirmed the diagnosis of rhabdomyosarcoma, which was treated with radio- and chemotherapy.

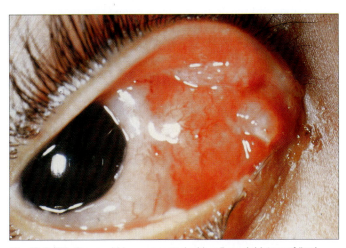

Fig. 35.6 This 8-year-old boy presented with a 5-week history of "red eye." Examination revealed the grape-like configuration of botryoid rhabdomyosarcoma. Patient from the University of British Columbia.

age of 4 years. In this age group, capillary hemangioma (Fig 35.7), lymphangioma, orbital cellulitis, metastatic neuroblastoma, leukemia, and granulocytic sarcoma are more likely to cause this clinical picture. Rarely, retinoblastoma that has spread into the orbit may present in this way. It is also relatively rare over the age of 10 years, where orbital cellulitis, inflamed dermoid cyst, secondary tumor, nonspecific orbital inflammation, and sudden hemorrhage into a preexisting lymphangioma are predominant

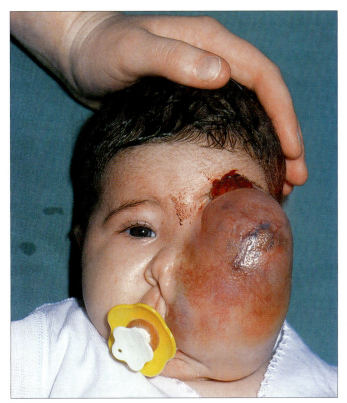

Fig. 35.7 Rhabdomyosarcoma. This 15-month-old child had a tumor that had previously been treated as a hemangioma—it involved only the soft tissues of the face.

325

causes of rapidly increasing proptosis. Nevertheless rhabdomyosarcoma can present outside the typical age group, and early identification and treatment of this tumor can be life-saving. Since its diagnosis is based on histopathological examination of tissue, the clinician dealing with rapidly progressive proptosis in childhood should keep a high index of suspicion and biopsy where indicated.

Computed tomography (CT) scanning or magnetic resonance imaging (MRI) is the best investigation in this context.[27,30] CT typically shows a nonenhancing poorly defined mass of homogeneous tissue density. There may be low-density areas within the tumor. Bone windows on CT are important to determine whether there is invasion of the orbital walls, a finding associated with a poorer prognosis.

CT or MRI will delineate the tumor in order to plan the best approach for biopsy. If these modalities are not available, plain orbital X-ray may show increased soft tissue density in the orbit or evidence of bone erosion by the tumor, and orbital ultrasound may contribute to the imaging of anteriorly situated tumors.

Since tumor seeding along the biopsy tract is well recognized,[22] the most direct approach for obtaining a biopsy should be taken and the transcranial route should be avoided. Knowles et al.[3] have stressed the importance of taking a large biopsy for accurate histopathological diagnosis. Fine needle aspiration biopsy is not appropriate.[2] The largest amount of tumor that can be safely removed is taken at surgery; it is completely excised if the surgeon feels that this will not result in permanent functional or cosmetic sequelae. The tumor may be debulked with the aid of CUSA (cavitational ultrasonic surgical aspirator), an ultrasonic suction device similar in principle to a phacoemulsifier, and often used by neurosurgeons. Since irradiation and chemotherapy are started almost immediately following surgery, the incision should be closed with particular care.

PATHOLOGY

Rhabdomyosarcoma originates in undifferentiated mesenchyme, which is either prospective muscle or capable of differentiation into muscle.[3,31] Orbital rhabdomyosarcomas are classified on the basis of their histopathological features into embryonal, alveolar, or pleomorphic types.[32] Embryonal tumors are the most common in the orbit,[33] accounting for roughly two-thirds of childhood rhabdomyosarcomas. The alveolar type, which has the worst prognosis,[3] often arises in the inferior orbit or nasopharynx and is the next most common in childhood. Pleomorphic rhabdomyosarcomas are the rarest, accounting for only 1% of rhabdomyosarcomas. They occur in teenagers and adults, arising from differentiated muscle. These have the best prognosis.[32,34]

The histopathological features of the various types overlap and diagnosis by light microscopy alone may be difficult. The pathological differential diagnosis is highlighted in Table 35.1. In particular, cross-striations, which are a helpful light microscopic feature, are only seen in about 50% of embryonal rhabdomyosarcomas and about 30% of alveolar tumors. Nevertheless, other light microscopic features such as abundant eosinophilic cytoplasm and vacuolated web-like cytoplasm may be used to characterize rhabdomyoblasts. Electron microscopy is extremely useful in confirming the diagnosis, since identification of myofilamentary differentiation can be diagnostic.[35] The presence of 150-Å diameter-thick myosin filaments is particularly significant. Immunohistochemical stains (e.g., for desmin, actin, and myoglobin) may also be contributory.[36–38] Increasingly,

Table 35.1 Pathological differential diagnosis of poorly differentiated small cell tumors

Tissue of origin	Differential diagnosis
Epithelial or presumed epithelial rhabdoid tumor	Undifferentiated carcinoma; oat cell carcinoma; rhabdoid tumor
Mesenchymal rhabdomyosarcoma	Embryonal Ewing sarcoma; small cell osteosarcoma; mesenchymal chondrosarcoma; thoracopulmonary small cell tumor; undifferentiated sarcoma; synovial sarcoma; epithelial sarcoma; mesothelioma
Neural or presumed neural crest	Neuroblastoma; retinoblastoma; glioblastoma; medulloblastoma; melanoma; alveolar soft part sarcoma
Lymphoreticular sarcoma	Lymphoma; leukemia: granulocytic; plasmacytoma

genetic mutation analysis will be used to help characterize and predict outcomes in these tumors (see above).

MANAGEMENT

Historical aspects

Orbital rhabdomyosarcoma was treated by surgery alone until the mid-1960s.[22] Frayer and Enterline[21] reported recurrence requiring orbital exenteration in all five patients treated by local tumor resection in a series of 12 patients. Exenteration remained the treatment of choice, the best published results being those of Jones et al.[22] with 32% 3-year and 29% 5-year survival. Even extensive and mutilating surgery was therefore associated with a poor prognosis.

In 1968, Cassady et al.[39] reported five patients treated by surgery and primary radiotherapy rather than radical surgery. All five patients were alive at follow-up varying from 15 months to 5 years. Reports of improved survival with radiotherapy and the benefits of adjuvant chemotherapy followed.[25,40,41]

It is now widely recognized that excellent survival rates can be achieved with biopsy followed by different combinations of radiotherapy and chemotherapy, depending on the extent of the disease.[3,42] Currently, the 5-year survival is 71% if tumors arising in all sites of the body are considered together.[43] Orbital tumors have a better prognosis,[44,45] because of their earlier symptomatic presentation and the orbit's poorly developed lymphatic system. In addition, the majority of orbital tumors are of embryonal cell type, which carries a 94% 5-year-survival as opposed to alveolar tumors whose 5-year survival is 74%.[7]

Treatment

Once the diagnosis has been confirmed histopathologically, the patient's tumor is staged. In conjunction with the surgeon's opinion regarding the amount of residual tumor and the clinical findings on examination, the CT or MRI scans are reviewed for evidence of local spread. The patient should also be worked up for metastases, with a chest X-ray, full blood count, renal and liver function tests, bone marrow aspiration for cytology, and bone scan. The cerebrospinal fluid should be examined for cytology if there is any suggestion of meningeal spread. Orbital rhabdomyosarcoma tends to metastasize to lung and bone.

There are several different methods of staging rhabdomyosarcoma. The Intergroup Rhabdomyosarcoma Study system[46]

Table 35.2 Staging of rhabdomyosarcoma (Intergroup Rhabdomyosarcoma Study)		Survival %
Group 1	Localized disease, completely excised, no microscopic residual tumor	91
–A	Confined to site of origin, completely resected	
–B	Infiltrating beyond site of origin, completely resected	
Group 2	Gross resection with evidence of microscopic local residual tumor	86
–A	Gross resection with evidence of microscopic residual tumor	
–B	Regional disease with involved lymph nodes, completely resected with no microscopic residual tumor	
–C	Microscopic local and/or nodal residual tumor	
Group 3	Incomplete resection or biopsy with gross residual tumor	35
Group 4	Distant metastases	32

Table 35.3 Late effects of therapy for rhabdomyosarcoma in 94 patients	
Ocular complications	Percentage (%)
Exenteration/enucleation for tumor control	11
Exenteration/enucleation for treatment complications	3
Cataract	82
Decreased visual acuity	70
Orbital hypoplasia	59
Dry eye	30
Chronic keratoconjunctivitis	27
Ptosis, enophthalmos	27
Retinopathy	6
Decreased growth	24
From Raney et al.[48]	

is presented in Table 35.2. The Intergroup Rhabdomyosarcoma Studies (IRS) I, II, and III were large prospective studies in which patients were randomized to treatment groups that differed according to the stage of their disease. Since 1972, the first three consecutive studies recruited and randomized over 2700 patients. The results of IRS III were published in 1995,[43] and IRS IV is presently ongoing but the 5-year outcome results are not yet available.

Patients in whom complete resection has been achieved are treated with chemotherapy alone; if there is micro- or macroscopic residual disease, lymph node involvement, or distant metastases, radiotherapy of 4500 to 5000 cGy is given over 4–5 weeks. Intrathecal chemotherapy and cranial radiotherapy is given for cases with intracranial spread.

In Europe, the International Society of Pediatric Oncology (SIOP) has been coordinating multicenter trials since 1984 with similar trend outcomes, maintaining excellent survival rates while demonstrating a reduction in morbidity from therapy. There has been a gradual divergence of philosophies between the two groups: the IRS has tended to use aggressive therapy and routine radiotherapy except for tumors that had been completely excised at the time of diagnosis, followed by prolonged chemotherapy for up to 2 years. To minimize the serious sequelae of radiotherapy, the SIOP has used chemotherapy to obtain complete remission before using surgery and radiotherapy for local control. The overall chemotherapy regime is much shorter.[17] Discussion between the groups shows that the answer lies somewhere between the different approaches.[47]

Complications of treatment

Although much effort has been devoted to avoiding mutilating surgery in rhabdomyosarcoma, Abramson et al.[25] reported that in one-third of 58 treated orbits, the eye eventually had to be enucleated due to treatment-related morbidity. Raney et al.[48] reviewed the complications of treatment by radiotherapy and chemotherapy in patients from IRS III, which are presented in Table 35.3.

Cataract, keratoconjunctivitis (Figs. 35.8 and 35.9), dry eye, and radiation retinopathy are common sequelae. Facial asymmetry from bony hypoplasia is present in many cases, its severity generally inversely related to the age of the patient at the time of

treatment. Enophthalmos, lacrimal duct stenosis, dental defects, and growth reduction from incidental irradiation of the pituitary gland are other relatively frequent sequelae. It is likely that the avoidance of radiotherapy and of prolonged treatment with

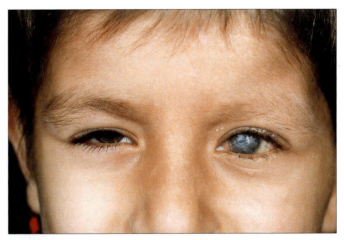

Fig. 35.8 Rhabdomyosarcoma. Radiation keratitis and dry eye.

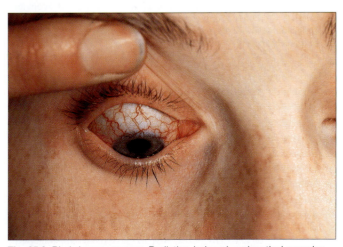

Fig. 35.9 Rhabdomyosarcoma. Radiation-induced conjunctival vascular changes.

cyclophosphamide recommended by the IRS will result in a reduction in the ocular morbidity associated with treatment.

Heyn et al.[49] reviewed the incidence of secondary malignant neoplasms in 1770 patients treated on IRS I and II. They found 22 cases; the most common secondary neoplasm was osteogenic sarcoma, followed in frequency by acute nonlymphoblastic leukemia. The affected patients were more likely to have been treated with alkylating agents and radiotherapy. Most patients had neurofibromatosis or a family history suggestive of the Li–Fraumeni syndrome (see Epidemiology and Genetics).

CONCLUSION

Rhabdomyosarcoma is the most common orbital tumor of childhood. Its onset is typically rapid with features that may mimic inflammatory orbital disease. Its diagnosis and assessment has been helped by the availability of CT and MRI scans and increasingly by cytogenetic studies, but still ultimately depends on histopathological examination of biopsy tissue. The prognosis of patients with orbital rhabdomyosarcoma has dramatically improved with newer treatment modalities. The next challenge, as in other areas of ocular oncology, is to reduce the ocular morbidity associated with treatment so that useful vision may be retained.

REFERENCES

1. Shields JA, Bakewell B, Augsburger JJ, et al. Space occupying orbital masses in children. A review of 250 consecutive biopsies. Ophthalmology 1986; 93: 379–84.
2. Shields JA, Shields CL. Rhabdomyosarcoma: review for the ophthalmologist. Surv Ophthalmol 2003; 48: 39–57.
3. Knowles DM, Jakobiec FA, Jones IS. Rhabdomyosarcoma. In: Duane TD, editor. Clinical Ophthalmology. Philadelphia: Harper and Row; 1983.
4. Jakobiec FA, Bilyk JR, Font RL. Orbit. In: Spencer WH, editor. Ophthalmic Pathology. 4th ed. Philadelphia: Saunders; 1996: 2438–933.
5. Himmel S, Siegel H. Congenital embryonal orbital rhabdomyosarcoma in a newborn. Arch Ophthalmol 1967; 77: 662–5.
6. Gormley PD, Thompson J, Aylward GW, et al. Congenital undifferentiated sarcoma of the orbit. J Pediatr Ophthalmol Strabismus 1994; 31: 59–61.
7. Kodet R, Newton WA, Jr, Hamoudi AB, et al. Orbital rhabdomyosarcomas and related tumors in childhood: relationship of morphology to prognosis–an Intergroup Rhabdomyosarcoma Study. Med Pediatr Oncol 1997; 29: 51–60.
8. Kassel SH, Copenhaver R, Arean VM. Orbital rhabdomyosarcoma. Am J Ophthalmol 1965; 60: 811–8.
9. Knowles DM 2nd, Jackobiec FA, Potter GD, et al. Ophthalmic striated muscle neoplasms. Surv Ophthalmol 1976; 21: 219–61.
10. Li FP, Fraumeni JF Jr. Rhabdomyosarcoma in children: epidemiologic study and identification of a familial cancer syndrome. J Natl Cancer Inst 1969; 43: 1365–73.
11. Li FP, Fraumeni JF Jr, Mulvihill JJ, et al. A cancer family syndrome in 24 kindreds. Cancer Res 1988; 48: 5358–62.
12. Riccardi VM. Neurofibromatosis: Phenotype, Natural History, and Pathogenesis. 2nd ed. Baltimore: Johns Hopkins University; 1992.
13. Ruymann FB, Maddux HR, Ragab A, et al. Congenital anomalies associated with rhabdomyosarcoma: an autopsy study of 115 cases. A report from the Intergroup Rhabdomyosarcoma Study Committee (representing the Children's Cancer Study Group, the Pediatric Oncology Group, the United Kingdom Children's Cancer Study Group, and the Pediatric Intergroup Statistical Center). Med Pediatr Oncol 1988; 16: 33–9.
14. Scrable HJ, Witte DP, Lampkin BC, et al. Chromosomal localization of the human rhabdomyosarcoma locus by mitotic recombination mapping. Nature 1987; 329: 645–7.
15. Loh WE Jr, Scrable HJ, Livanos E, et al. Human chromosome 11 contains two different growth suppressor genes for embryonal rhabdomyosarcoma. Proc Natl Acad Sci USA 1992; 89: 1755–9.
16. Mastrangelo D, Sappia F, Bruni S, et al. Loss of heterozygosity on the long arm of chromosome 11 in orbital embryonal rhabdomyosarcoma (OERMS): a microsatellite study of seven cases. Orbit 1998; 17: 89–95.
17. McDowell HP. Update on childhood rhabdomyosarcoma. Arch Dis Child 2003; 88: 354–7.
18. Pappo AS, Shapiro DN, Crist WM, et al. Biology and therapy of pediatric rhabdomyosarcoma. J Clin Oncol 1995; 13: 123–39.
19. Sorensen PH, Lynch JC, Qualman SJ, et al. PAX3-FKHR and PAX7-FKHR gene fusions are prognostic indicators in alveolar rhabdomyosarcoma: a report from the children's oncology group. J Clin Oncol 2002; 20: 2672–9.
20. Gordon A, McManus A, Anderson J, et al. Chromosomal imbalances in pleomorphic rhabdomyosarcomas and identification of the alveolar rhabdomyosarcoma-associated PAX3-FOXO1A fusion gene in one case. Cancer Genet Cytogenet 2003; 140: 73–7.
21. Frayer WC, Enterline HT. Embryonal rhabdomyosarcoma of the orbit in children and young adults. Arch Ophthalmol 1959; 62: 203–10.
22. Jones IS, Reese AB, Krout J. Orbital rhabdomyosarcoma: an analysis of 62 cases. Trans Am Ophthalmol Soc 1965; 63: 223–51.
23. Lederman M, Wybar K. Embryonal sarcoma. Proc Roy Soc Med 1976; 69: 895–903.
24. Shields CL, Shields JA, Honavar SG, et al. Clinical spectrum of primary ophthalmic rhabdomyosarcoma. Ophthalmology 2001; 108: 2284–92.
25. Abramson DH, Ellsworth RM, Tretter P, et al. The treatment of orbital rhabdomyosarcoma with irradiation and chemotherapy. Ophthalmology 1979; 86: 1330–5.
26. Elsas FJ, Mroczek EC, Kelly DR, et al. Primary rhabdomyosarcoma of the iris. Arch Ophthalmol 1991; 109: 982–4.
27. Sohaib SA, Moseley I, Wright JE. Orbital rhabdomyosarcoma–the radiological characteristics. Clin Radiol 1998; 53: 357–62.
28. Shuangshoti S, Phonprasert C. Primary intracranial rhabdomyosarcoma producing proptosis. J Neurol Neurosurg Psychiatry 1976; 39: 531–5.
29. Walton RC, Ellis GS Jr, Haik BG. Rhabdomyosarcoma presumed metastatic to the orbit. Ophthalmology 1996; 103: 1512–6.
30. Mafee MF, Pai E, Philip B. Rhabdomyosarcoma of the orbit. Evaluation with MR imaging and CT. Radiol Clin N Am 1998; 36: 1215–27.
31. Harry J. Pathology of rhabdomyosarcoma. Mod Probl Ophthalmol 1975; 14: 325–9.
32. Porterfield JT, Zimmerman LE. Rhabdomyosarcoma of the orbit: a clinicopathologic study of 55 cases. Virchows Arch A Pathol Anat Histopathol 1962; 335: 329.
33. Ashton N, Morgan G. Embryonal sarcoma and embryonal rhabdomyosarcoma of the orbit. J Clin Pathol 1965; 18: 644–714.
34. Charles NC. Pathology and incidence of orbital disorders: an overview. In: Hornblass A, editor. Tumors of the Ocular Adnexa and Orbit. St. Louis: Mosby; 1979: 190–3.
35. Ghafoor SY, Dudgeon J. Orbital rhabdomyosarcoma: improved survival with combined pulsed chemotherapy and irradiation. Br J Ophthalmol 1985; 69: 557–61.
36. Kahn HJ, Yeger H, Kassim O, et al. Immunohistochemical and electron microscopic assessment of childhood rhabdomyosarcoma. Increased frequency of diagnosis over routine histologic methods. Cancer 1983; 51: 1897–903.
37. Garrido CM, Arra A. Immunohistochemical study of embryonal rhabdomyosarcomas. Ophthalmologica 1986; 193: 154–9.
38. Weiss SW, Goldblum JR. Rhabdomyosarcoma. In: Weiss SW, Goldblum JR, Enzinger FM, editors. Enzinger and Weiss's Soft Tissue Tumors. 4th ed. St. Louis: Mosby; 2001: 785–835.
39. Cassady JR, Sagerman RH, Tretter P, et al. Radiation therapy for rhabdomyosarcoma. Radiology 1968; 91: 116–20.

40. Heyn RM, Holland R, Newton WA Jr, et al. The role of combined chemotherapy in the treatment of rhabdomyosarcoma in children. Cancer 1974;34:2128–42.

41. Weichselbaum RR, Cassady JR, Albert DM, et al. Multimodality management of orbital rhabdomyosarcoma. Int Ophthalmol Clin 1980; 20: 247–59.

42. Ellsworth RM. Discussion. Localized orbital rhabdomyosarcoma. An interim report of the Intergroup Rhabdomyosarcoma Study Committee. Ophthalmology 1987; 94: 254.

43. Crist W, Gehan EA, Ragab AH, et al. The third Intergroup Rhabdomyosarcoma Study. J Clin Oncol 1995; 13: 610–30.

44. Rodary C, Rey A, Olive D, et al. Prognostic factors in 281 children with nonmetastatic rhabdomyosarcoma (RMS) at diagnosis. Med Pediatr Oncol 1988; 16: 71–7.

45. Maurer HM, Gehan EA, Beltangady M, et al. The Intergroup rhabdomyosarcoma study–II. Cancer 1993; 71: 1904–22.

46. Crist WM, Anderson JR, Meza JL, et al. Intergroup rhabdomyosarcoma study–IV: results for patients with nonmetastatic disease. J Clin Oncol 2001; 19: 3091–102.

47. Oberlin O, Rey A, Anderson J, et al. Treatment of orbital rhabdomyosarcoma: survival and late effects of treatment—results of an international workshop. J Clin Oncol 2001; 19: 197–204.

48. Raney RB, Anderson JR, Kollath J, et al. Late effects of therapy in 94 patients with localized rhabdomyosarcoma of the orbit: Report from the Intergroup Rhabdomyosarcoma Study (IRS)–III, 1984–1991. Med Pediatr Oncol 2000; 34: 413–20.

49. Heyn R, Haeberlen V, Newton WA, et al. Second malignant neoplasms in children treated for rhabdomyosarcoma. Intergroup Rhabdomyosarcoma Study Committee. J Clin Oncol 1993; 11: 262–70.

CHAPTER
36

Other Mesenchymal Abnormalities

Christopher J Lyons and Jack Rootman

Rhabdomyosarcoma was discussed in a separate chapter (see Chapter 35) since this is a relatively common and important orbital disease of childhood. Every mesenchymal component of the orbit can give rise to sarcomatous tumors, but these are exceedingly rare and will not be discussed. Nevertheless they are part of the differential diagnosis of rhabdomyosarcoma.

DYSPLASIAS

Fibrous dysplasia of the orbit

Fibrous dysplasia is a rare disorder of unknown etiology characterized by the replacement of normal bone by a cellular fibrous stroma containing islands of immature bone and osteoid. It has been reported in a 9-month-old infant[1] but usually presents in childhood although its onset is extremely insidious, and it may remain asymptomatic until adult life. Progression usually slows in the second or third decade, when "bone maturity" is reached, though there is evidence that growth may continue into the fourth decade in some cases. It is important to distinguish it from meningioma[2] and osteosarcoma.

Fibrous dysplasia may be confined to a single site (monostotic form) or, more rarely, involve multiple bony sites (polyostotic form). Polyostotic fibrous dysplasia, which coexists with cutaneous pigmentation and endocrine abnormalities, is known as the McCune-Albright syndrome.[3]

Clinical features

Approximately three-quarters of patients with orbital fibrous dysplasia have the monostotic form of the disease; several contiguous bones are usually affected but the disease usually remains unilateral. The craniofacial area is affected in 20% of patients, with a predilection for the frontal, sphenoid, and ethmoid bones. Typically, there is a painless firm bony swelling with contour distortion; in the orbit, there is accompanying mass effect. The clinical presentation depends on the predominant wall involved, the most common being the roof. This results in proptosis and downward displacement of the globe and orbit.[4–7] The lacrimal fossa may be affected, mimicking a lacrimal gland tumor.[8] Maxillary disease (Fig. 36.1) displaces the eye upward, with persistent epiphora if the bony nasolacrimal duct is affected.[5,9] Sphenoid involvement may cause narrowing of the optic canal (Fig. 36.2), resulting in optic nerve compression[4,10,11] occurring in up to 50% of patients.[7] The optic nerve may also be compressed by an associated sphenoid sinus mucocele.[12,13] Rarely, involvement of the sella turcica may result in chiasmal compression, bitemporal hemianopia, or bilateral visual failure.[14] Other uncommon neuro-ophthalmic complications include cranial nerve palsies,[15,16] trigeminal neuralgia,[15] and raised intracranial pressure and papilledema.[5,17] Extensive craniofacial involvement can result in severe cosmetic deformity. Pain may occur, either localized to the orbit or as a diffuse ipsilateral headache. Visual loss was a feature in 3 of 10 cases reported by Rootman[18] and 2 of Moore et al.'s 16 cases.[4] Malignant transformation to osteosarcoma, fibrosarcoma, chondrosarcoma, and giant cell sarcoma occurs in approximately 0.5% of cases, increasing to 15% with prior radiotherapy.[18] The accompanying signs are rapid progression, worsening pain, and infiltration of surrounding structures.

The main radiographic feature of fibrous dysplasia is expansion of bone. The lesions may be sclerotic, with a dense ground-glass

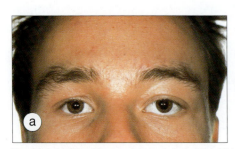
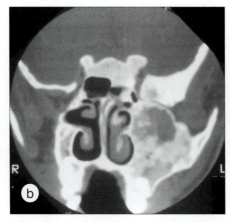
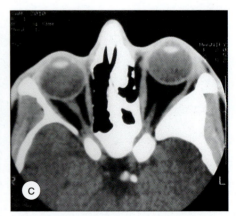

Fig. 36.1 (a) This 16-year-old presented with a history of progressive facial distortion and decreasing left visual acuity to 20/40. Compressive optic neuropathy was diagnosed secondary to fibrous dysplasia. (b) CT scan of the same case showing cystic fibrous dysplasia involving the orbital apex. (c) Axial CT scan shows optic canal involvement. This was surgically decompressed. Patient of the University of British Columbia.

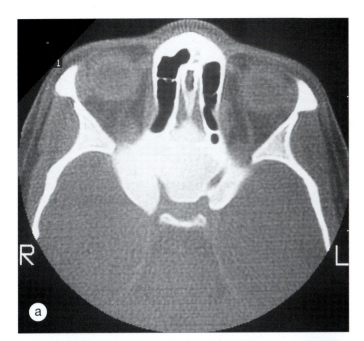

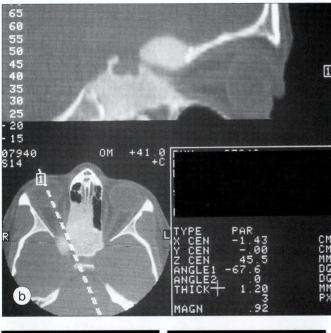

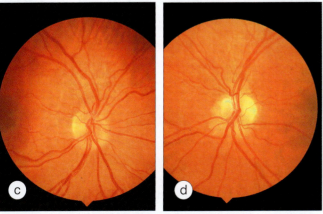

Fig. 36.2 Fibrous dysplasia. (a, b) CT scan showing sphenoid involvement. The optic canals are narrowed. (c, d) Same patient: there was chronic compressive optic neuropathy with atrophy on the left. This patient presented with decreased vision at 12 years of age, and she showed no deterioration 2 years later with minimal residual signs or symptoms; she was not treated.

homogeneity, lytic, with increased lucency, or show a mixed picture with alternating areas of lucency and increased density.[11,19,20] Fortunately most orbital cases are easily diagnosed since they are of the sclerotic type.[5] The main radiological differential diagnosis includes Langerhans cell histiocytosis, hyperostotic meningioma, Paget's disease (both rare in children), and some bone tumors. On magnetic resonance imaging (MRI), there is a correlation between T_1 and T_2 signal intensity and clinical and pathological activity of the lesion.[21] Occasionally, large cystic lesions form in the orbital wall.[4] These may contain blood (Fig. 36.3) and necrotic debris and can be mistaken for aneurysmal bone cysts.[18] Computed tomography (CT) scanning is the best modality to evaluate the extent of cranial and orbital involvement. The optic canal and chiasmal region should be assessed carefully for signs of compression.

Management

Fibrous dysplasia is a benign, self-limiting condition. However, the final extent and time of arrest of the lesion are unpredictable. The aim of treatment is to prevent complications such as optic

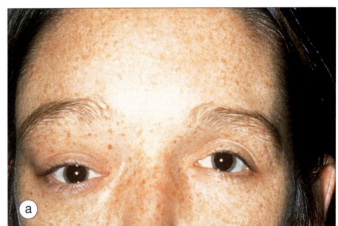

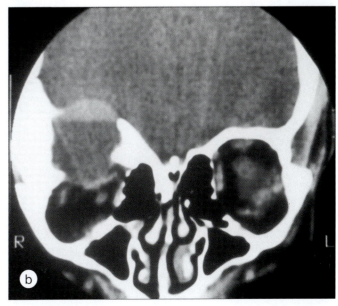

Fig. 36.3 (a) This 22-year-old developed sudden proptosis after a history of slowly progressive facial asymmetry from early childhood. (b) CT scan showed the fluid level of a hemorrhage within the cystic dysplastic bone. The diagnosis was fibrous dysplasia. Patient of the University of British Columbia.

nerve compression, and minimize any cosmetic defect while waiting for spontaneous arrest to occur.

When there is little doubt about the diagnosis, as in the case of a child with a typical sclerotic lesion on X-ray, an initial period of observation and repeat radiological assessment is mandatory. If the lesion in the orbital wall is lytic or cystic, biopsy is usually necessary to confirm the diagnosis. Outside the orbit, the risk of malignant change after radiotherapy has been reported to be high.[22,23] This modality is therefore not used.

The recommended treatment is surgical. Surgery is indicated for cosmetic disfigurement, intractable pain, or evidence of optic nerve compression. Since dysplastic bone can be very vascular and hemorrhagic at surgery, preoperative cross-matching is advisable. Resection of dysplastic bone around the optic canal can reverse the visual loss of early compressive optic neuropathy.[12,18] Steroids may also be useful in this context.[24] When decompressing the optic nerve, rongeurs rather than high-speed drills (heat producing) should be used so trauma to the nerve can be minimized.[25] Surgery has traditionally consisted of debulking of the lesion. However, the margins of the affected bone are difficult to define clinically and recurrence after this "limited" form of surgery is common.[7] In the past 20 years there has been a shift toward more aggressive surgery with radical excision of all diseased bone and immediate facial and orbital reconstruction using bone grafts[4,26,27] by combined ophthalmology/craniofacial teams. Although some groups report no visual function deterioration following optic canal decompression prior to the development of severe ocular morbidity, there have been two reports of blindness complicating prophylactic nerve decompression.[28,29] Visual loss is not usually the result of progressive optic canal stenosis but from the rapid expansion of cystic components, fibrous dysplasia, mucoceles, or hemorrhage.[30] Similarly, we feel that prophylactic optic canal decompression is not indicated and that a conservative approach is warranted, reserving optic canal decompression for patients with documented progressive or sudden deterioration of visual function.

BONE TUMORS

Reparative granuloma

Reparative granuloma and aneurysmal bone cyst are both part of a spectrum of reactive giant cell lesions, and it may be difficult to distinguish between them histologically.

Reparative granulomas (also known as giant cell granuloma) are rare. They tend to affect patients in the first and second decades of life (range 5–54 years, mean=18.6) and occur in the mandible, maxilla, and phalanges.[18,31] The lesion may spread to the maxilla, ethmoid,[32] and sphenoid bones, involving the orbit (Fig. 36.4) and causing proptosis.[33,34] The presentation may be catastrophic if intralesional hemorrhage occurs.[18] Histopathologically, there is a spindle cell stroma with profuse hemorrhagic and hemosiderin content. Osteoblastic giant cells are present within the stroma and new bone may be laid down at the edge of the lesion.

The course is usually benign. The treatment is by surgical curettage, after which healing occurs by new bone formation. The curettage may need to be repeated or the bony margins resected if the lesion recurs. Radiotherapy is rarely necessary but was required to cure a 5-year-old boy's locally aggressive lesion after it had failed to respond to surgery on two occasions.[33]

Aneurysmal bone cyst

This uncommon lesion usually affects the metaphysis of long bones or the spine. A history of trivial trauma frequently precedes presentation. The skull is affected in less than 1% of cases and about one-quarter of these affect the orbit.[35] It is a benign lesion that can usually be differentiated from reparative granuloma by the presence of large blood-filled channels lined by multinucleate giant cells and fibroblasts. Occasionally, however, they can be solid, making this differentiation difficult. The two may also coexist.[36]

Aneurysmal bone cysts of the orbit (Fig. 36.5) have been reviewed periodically.[37–39] The majority of cases present in the second decade; there is a 5:3 female:male ratio. The history is

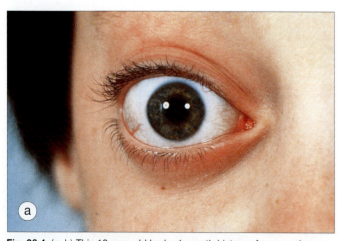

Fig. 36.4 (a, b) This 10-year-old had a 1-month history of progressive proptosis and lateral displacement of the globe. There was gradual loss of vision. Reparative granuloma was diagnosed by intranasal biopsy, and the patient underwent lateral rhinotomy and excision of lesion via the ethmoid and maxillary sinuses. Patient of the University of British Columbia.

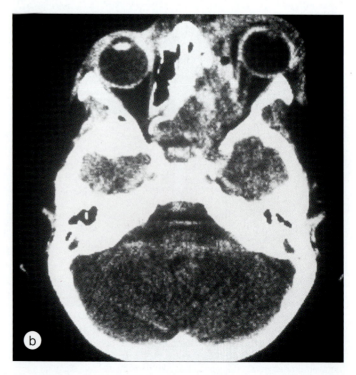

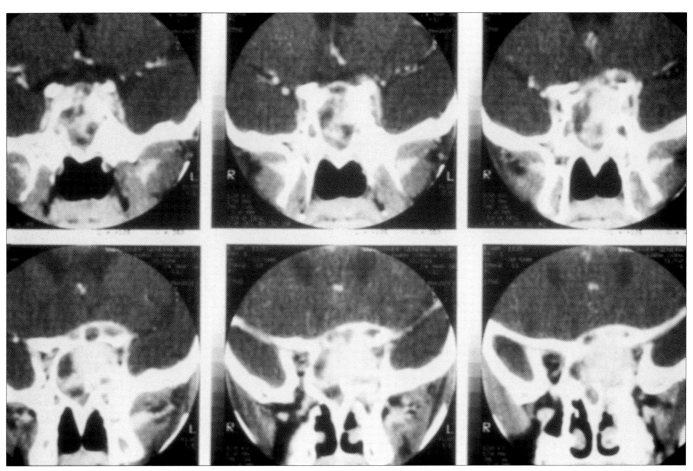

Fig. 36.5 This 12-year-old girl presented with gradual loss of vision. A sphenoid and ethmoid mass was apparent on CT. This was shown to be an aneurysmal bone cyst by intranasal biopsy, and she underwent cranio-orbitotomy. Patient of the University of British Columbia.

usually shorter than 3 months and presenting features may include proptosis, diplopia, ptosis, headache, visual deterioration due to optic nerve compression, nasal congestion,[35] and epistaxis.[40] Most cases involve the orbital roof and result in gradually increasing unilateral proptosis and downward displacement of the globe.[41] The medial and lateral orbital walls can also be involved. Like reparative granulomas, intralesional hemorrhage may occur, leading to a sudden presentation with signs related to mass effect, occasionally mimicking orbital malignancy in early childhood.[42] Large cysts with intracranial extension may give rise to raised intracranial pressure and papilledema.[43] Optic nerve compression may also occur.[18,44]

Radiologically, irregular expansion with destruction of bone is seen on CT scan, with a thin shell of bone outlining the limits of the lesion. There may be patchy enhancement of the mass or its rim. Hemorrhage and multiple fluid–fluid levels[39] may be evident on MRI or ultrasound when the patient is kept immobile for several minutes.

The treatment of choice is surgical excision or curettage with frozen section[18] and grafting with autogenous bone chips or repair of the orbital wall defect with a plate.[39] Craniofacial reconstruction may be indicated at the time of surgery.[37,38] The prognosis is good despite a recurrence rate that can be as high as 66%,[45] usually within 2 years of treatment. Cryotherapy and irradiation have also been used, although the latter carries a risk of osteosarcoma as a late sequel.

NEOPLASIAS

Juvenile ossifying fibroma of the orbit

This is an uncommon disorder that arises in the bony wall of the orbit and gives rise to slowly progressive proptosis. Although there are clinical and pathological similarities to fibrous dysplasia, it is probably a distinct entity.[18,46]

It usually presents in adolescence or early adulthood, although younger cases have been reported, usually with slowly progressive painless globe displacement. The orbital roof (Fig. 36.6) and ethmoid bone are the most common sites[46,47] although rarely maxillary involvement may cause upward displacement of the globe.[48] There may be massive enlargement with considerable morbidity and cosmetic disfigurement.[46] Diplopia may occur, and posterior tumors may cause apical crowding.

CT scan, which is preferable to MRI in this context,[49] shows a homogeneous central zone with a sclerotic margin expanding a single bone. The lesion is usually clearly demarcated but may occasionally grow to involve surrounding bones, sometimes crossing the midline to the other orbit.

Histopathologically the predominant feature is a central whorled, cellular, vascular stroma surrounded by varying amounts of bone. The psammomatoid variant contains islands of lamellar bone or "ossicles" surrounded by a rim of osteoid and osteoblasts resembling the psammoma bodies of meningioma. This variant is clinically more aggressive.

333

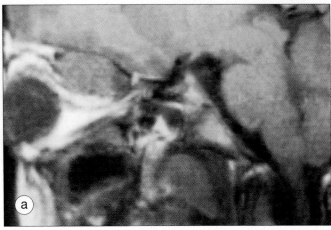

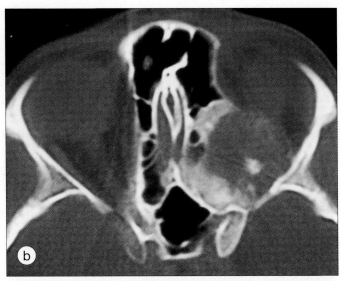

Fig. 36.6 Ossifying fibroma. (a) This 7-year-old child presented with progressive proptosis and downward displacement of the globe. The MRI scan shows a mass in the orbital roof displacing the levator-superior rectus complex, the globe, and the optic nerve downward. (b) CT scan of same patient showing the sclerotic margin of the fibroma.

The tumors tend to enlarge insidiously, and surgery becomes necessary for most cases. The treatment of choice is careful complete excision since recurrence is common. This is made more likely by the presence of residual tumor, as well as psammomatoid histopathology,[46] and regular follow-up is therefore indicated. A multidisciplinary approach is best.[50]

Extragnathic cementomas are tumors that behave in a similar fashion;[51] genetic mutations in the X chromosome and chromosome 2 have been identified in the cemento-ossifying fibromas of 3 patients.[52]

OTHER MESENCHYMAL TUMORS

Osteoblastoma

This benign tumor rarely involves the orbit[53,54] but can originate from the orbital roof and ethmoid sinuses. Clinically, it presents with mass effect and globe displacement.[53] Radiologically, they are well circumscribed and may have a lucent center with foci of calcification. The treatment of choice is surgical, with either curettage or more radical excision and reconstruction, although both of these may be associated with profuse bleeding due to the vascularity of the tumor. Histologically, they resemble osteoid osteomas but are larger and more vascular. The postoperative prognosis is reasonably good. These tumors are more common in the spine and the long bones where they have a 10–15% recurrence rate after curettage.[55] Since sarcomatous transformation has been reported in the skull,[56] complete excision, by a multidisciplinary team if necessary, is indicated.

Postirradiation osteosarcoma of the orbit
(see Chapter 50)

Survivors of the familial form of retinoblastoma are at greater risk of developing a second tumor[57,58] even in the absence of radiotherapy due to their genetic predisposition. Most of these tumors are osteosarcomas,[57] which may occur within the field of radiation given to treat the retinoblastoma, or at a distant site. Of 693 patients with bilateral retinoblastoma 89 developed second tumors;[57] 58 occurred within the radiation field and 31 outside. The latent period from completion of radiotherapy to develop-

ment of the second tumor ranged from 10 months to 23 years (mean 10.4 years). The prognosis of osteosarcoma of the orbit is extremely poor; most patients die within a year of diagnosis.

Infantile cortical hyperostosis (Caffey disease)

This uncommon disorder of unknown etiology affects infants in the first few months of life. It is characterized by sudden onset of fever, irritability, and soft tissue swelling. The soft tissue over the involved bone is swollen and tender, and plain X-rays show subperiosteal new bone formation and cortical thickening. There is usually a leucocytosis and raised erythrocyte sedimentation rate. The mandible is the most common bone to be involved, in which case the infants have a characteristic facial appearance with swollen cheeks. The condition is generally self-limiting, and the radiological appearance reverts to normal within a few months. Involvement of the facial and skull bones may lead to periorbital edema and even proptosis.[59,60] The management is generally conservative with an initial period of observation and follow-up radiological examination of the involved bones. Systemic steroids may be used for persistent disease, or to hasten remission if there is gross swelling.

Osteopetrosis

This is a rare disorder, thought to be due to defective bone resorption by osteoclasts. As a result, there is narrowing of the marrow cavity and bony foramina of the skull (Fig. 36.7) as well as impaired bony remodeling. It is characterized by increased bony thickness and density. There is an increased susceptibility to fracture. Three types are recognized:[61]
(i) Infantile autosomal recessive malignant osteopetrosis, which is fatal within the first few years of life if left untreated;
(ii) Intermediate autosomal recessive, which appears during the first decade and whose course is more benign; and
(iii) Autosomal dominant osteopetrosis in which life expectancy is normal albeit with numerous orthopedic problems.
The latter is often discovered incidentally on routine radiography and is not associated with ophthalmic complications.

The malignant form presents in infancy with failure to thrive, anemia, and thrombocytopenia; extramedullary hematopoiesis results in hepatosplenomegaly and lymphadenopathy. It is a cause of neonatal hypocalcemia, causing seizures, which may be overlooked, leading to delay in diagnosis. This is due to unopposed osteoblastic function.[62] Bony involvement in the autosomal recessive forms may result in small orbits with proptosis,[63] narrowing of the cranial foramina, temporal bossing, and nasolacrimal duct obstruction.[64] Optic atrophy follows narrowing of the optic canal and optic nerve compression.[65–69] Compression of other cranial nerves may result in facial palsy and deafness.

The bone density on X-ray is seen to be uniform without corticomedullary demarcation (Fig. 36.7). There is broadening of the metaphyses, and pathological fractures are common.

Visual function may be preserved or improved by early decompression of the optic canal.[65,70,71] This can be performed transethmoidally.[72] However, there appears to be a subgroup of patients with infantile malignant osteopetrosis in whom visual loss results from a retinal degeneration rather than optic nerve compression.[73–75] Keith[74] reported rod and cone degeneration in one such patient. This may be clinically evident as a macular chorioretinal abnormality[75] or may only be detected by electrophysiological testing.[73] The possibility of retinal disease should be borne in mind when evaluating a child with osteopetrosis with visual loss, particularly if optic nerve decompression is being considered!

Ocular involvement by a median age of 2 months was present in half of the 33 patients with autosomal recessive osteopetrosis studied by Gerritsen et al.[76] Retinal degeneration was identified in 3 of their patients. Other ophthalmic complications include exophthalmos,[65,77] nystagmus secondary to bilateral visual loss, and cranial nerve palsies.[67] Medical treatment involves high-dose calcitriol to stimulate osteoclast differentiation and bone marrow transplantation to provide monocytic osteoclast precursors.[61,78,79]

Other bone dysplasias

Other bone dysplasias include craniometaphyseal dysplasia, cranioepiphyseal dysplasia, X-linked hypophosphatemic rickets (Fig. 36.8), and many others that may be characterized by bone thickening, foraminal occlusion, and orbital narrowing.

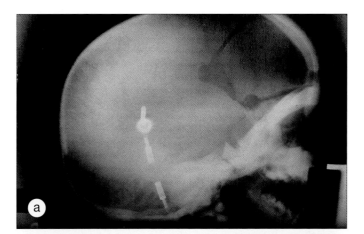

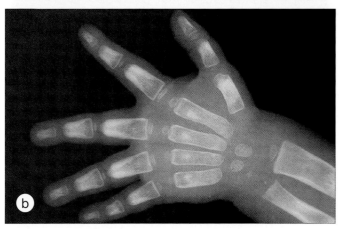

Fig. 36.7 Osteopetrosis. (a) This infant had a bilateral compressive optic neuropathy that failed to respond to optic nerve decompression. He also has a shunt *in situ*. Bone marrow transplantation has been successful in some cases. (b) X-ray of the same patient's hands showing increased density of distal ends of the phalanges.

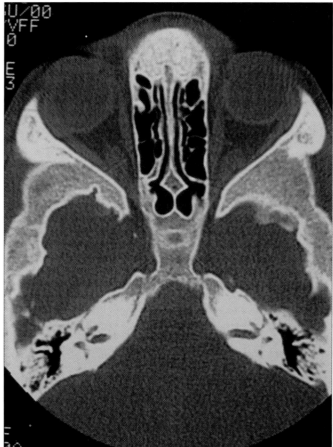

Fig. 36.8 X-linked hypophosphatemic rickets. CT scan showing increased bone density, especially of the cortical bone. There was chronic optic nerve compression, which did not deteriorate over a 10-year period while it was monitored by measuring acuity, color vision, pupil reactions, visual fields, and VEPs.

REFERENCES

1. Joseph E, Kachhara R, Bhattacharya RN, et al. Fibrous dysplasia of the orbit in an infant. Pediatr Neurosurg 2000; 32: 205–8.
2. Hansen-Knarhoi M, Poole MD. Preoperative difficulties in differentiating intraosseous meningiomas and fibrous dysplasia around the orbital apex. J Craniomaxillofac Surg 1994; 22: 226–30.
3. Albright F, Butler AM, Hampton AO, et al. Syndrome characterised by osteitis fibrosa disseminata, areas of pigmentation and endocrine dysfunction, with precocious puberty in females; report of five cases. N Engl J Med 1937; 216: 727–46.
4. Moore AT, Buncic JR, Munro I. Fibrous dysplasia of the orbit in childhood. Ophthalmology 1985; 92: 12–20.
5. Moore RT. Fibrous dysplasia of the orbit. Surv Ophthalmol 1969; 13: 321–34.
6. Gass JD. Orbital and ocular involvement in fibrous dysplasia. South Med J 1965; 58: 324–9.
7. Bibby K, McFadzean R. Fibrous dysplasia of the orbit. Br J Ophthalmol 1994; 4: 266–70.
8. McCluskey P, Wingate R, Benger R, et al. Monostotic fibrous dysplasia of the orbit: an unusual lacrimal fossa mass. Br J Ophthalmol 1993; 77: 54–6.
9. Moore AT, Pritchard J, Taylor DS. Histiocytosis X: an ophthalmological review. Br J Ophthalmol 1985; 69: 7–14.
10. Sassin JF, Rosenberg RN. Neurological complications of fibrous dysplasia of the skull. Arch Neurol 1968; 18: 363–9.
11. Jan M, Dweik A, Destrieux C, et al. Fronto-orbital sphenoidal fibrous dysplasia. Neurosurgery 1994; 34: 544–7.
12. Weisman JS, Hepler RS, Vinters HV. Reversible visual loss caused by fibrous dysplasia. Am J Ophthalmol 1990; 110: 244–9.
13. Liakos GM, Walker CB, Carruth JA. Ocular complications in craniofacial fibrous dysplasia. Br J Ophthalmol 1979; 63: 611–6.
14. Weyand RD, Craig WM, Rucker CW. Unusual lesions involving the optic chiasm. Proc Staff Mtg Mayo Clin 1952; 27: 505–11.
15. Finney HL, Roberts TS. Fibrous dysplasia of the skull with progressive cranial nerve involvement. Surg Neurol 1976; 6: 341–3.
16. Fernandez E, Colavita N, Moschini M, et al. "Fibrous dysplasia" of the skull with complete unilateral cranial nerve involvement. Case report. J Neurosurg 1980; 52: 404–6.
17. Ameli NO, Rahmat H, Abbassioun K. Monostotic fibrous dysplasia of the cranial bones: report of fourteen cases. Neurosurg Rev 1981; 4: 71–7.
18. Rootman J. Diseases of the Orbit: A Multidisciplinary Approach. 2nd ed. Philadelphia: Lippincott Williams & Wilkins; 2003.
19. Fries JW. The roentgen features of fibrous dysplasia of the skull and facial bones; a critical analysis of 39 pathologically proved cases. Am J Roentgenol Radium Ther Nucl Med 1957; 77: 71–88.
20. Leeds N, Seaman WB. Fibrous dysplasia of the skull and its differential diagnosis. A clinical and roentgenographic study of 46 cases. Radiology 1962; 78: 570–82.
21. Casselman JW, De Jonge I, Neyt L, et al. MRI in craniofacial fibrous dysplasia. Neuroradiology 1993; 35: 234–7.
22. Huvos AG, Higinbotham NL, Miller TR. Bone sarcomas arising in fibrous dysplasia. J Bone Joint Surg Am 1972; 54: 1047–56.
23. Schwartz DT, Alpert M. The malignant transformation of fibrous dysplasia. Am J Med Sci 1964; 247: 1–20.
24. Arroyo JG, Lessel S, Montgomery WW. Steroid-induced visual recovery in fibrous dysplasia. J Clin Neuroophthalmol 1991; 11: 259–61.
25. Munro IR. Discussion. Treatment of craniomaxillofacial fibrous dysplasia: how early and how extensive? Plast Reconstr Surg 1990; 86: 843–4.
26. Posnick JC, Wells MD, Drake JM, et al. Childhood fibrous dysplasia presenting as blindness: a skull base approach for resection and immediate reconstruction. Pediatr Neurosurg 1993; 19: 260–6.
27. Papay FA, Morales L, Jr, Flaharty P, et al. Optic nerve decompression in cranial base fibrous dysplasia. J Craniofac Surg 1995; 6: 5–10.
28. Edelstein C, Goldberg RA, Rubino G. Unilateral blindness after ipsilateral prophylactic transcranial optic canal decompression for fibrous dysplasia. Am J Ophthalmol 1998; 126: 469–71.
29. Frodel JL, Funk G, Boyle J, et al. Management of aggressive midface and orbital fibrous dysplasia. Arch Facial Plast Surg 2000; 2: 187–95.
30. Michael CB, Lee AG, Patrinely JR, et al. Visual loss associated with fibrous dysplasia of the anterior skull base. Case report and review of the literature. J Neurosurg 2000; 92: 350–4.
31. Cook HP. Giant-cell granuloma. Br J Oral Surg 1965; 3: 97–100.
32. deMello DE, Archer CR, Blair JD. Ethmoidal fibro-osseous lesion in a child. Diagnostic and therapeutic problems. Am J Surg Pathol 1980; 4: 595–601.
33. Sood GC, Malik SR, Gupta DK, et al. Reparative granuloma of the orbit causing unilateral proptosis. Am J Ophthalmol 1967; 63: 524–7.
34. Hoopes PC, Anderson RL, Blodi FC. Giant cell (reparative) granuloma of the orbit. Ophthalmology 1981; 88: 1361–6.
35. Hunter JV, Yokoyama C, Moseley IF, et al. Aneurysmal bone cyst of the sphenoid with orbital involvement. Br J Ophthalmol 1990; 74: 505–8.
36. Levy WM, Miller AS, Bonakdarpor A, et al. Aneurysmal bone cyst secondary to other osseous lesions: report of 57 cases. Am J Clin Pathol 1975; 64: 1–8.
37. Powell J, Glaser J. Aneurysmal bone cysts of the orbit. Arch Ophthalmol 1975; 93: 340–2.
38. Ronner HJ, Jones IS. Aneurysmal bone cyst of the orbit: a review. Ann Ophthalmol 1983; 15: 626–9.
39. Menon J, Brosnahan DM, Jellinek DA. Aneurysmal bone cyst of the orbit: a case report and review of literature. Eye 1999; 13: 764–8.
40. Patel BC, Sabir DI, Flaharty PM, et al. Aneurysmal bone cyst of the orbit and ethmoid sinus. Arch Ophthalmol 1993; 111: 586–7.
41. Johnson TE, Bergin DJ, McCord CD. Aneurysmal bone cyst of the orbit. Ophthalmology 1988; 95: 86–9.
42. Bealer LA, Cibis GW, Barker BF, et al. Aneurysmal bone cyst: report of a case mimicking orbital tumor. J Pediatr Ophthalmol Strabismus 1993; 30: 199–200.
43. Costantini FE, Iraci G, Benedetti A, et al. Aneurysmal bone cyst as an intracranial space-occupying lesion. Case report. J Neurosurg 1966; 25: 205–7.
44. Yee RD, Cogan DG, Thorp TR, et al. Optic nerve compression due to aneurysmal bone cyst. Arch Ophthalmol 1977; 95: 2176–9.
45. Biesecker JL, Marcove RC, Huvos AG, et al. Aneurysmal bone cysts. A clinicopathologic study of 66 cases. Cancer 1970; 26: 615–25.
46. Margo CE, Ragsdale BD, Perman KI, et al. Psammomatoid (juvenile) ossifying fibroma of the orbit. Ophthalmology 1985; 92: 150–9.
47. Blodi FC. Pathology of orbital bones. The XXXII Edward Jackson Memorial Lecture. Am J Ophthalmol 1976; 81: 1–26.
48. Shields JA, Peyster RG, Handler SD, et al. Massive juvenile ossifying fibroma of maxillary sinus with orbital involvement. Br J Ophthalmol 1985; 69: 392–5.
49. Fakadej A, Boynton JR. Juvenile ossifying fibroma of the orbit. Ophthal Plast Reconstr Surg 1996; 12: 174–7.
50. Hartstein ME, Grove AS Jr, Woog JJ, et al. The multidisciplinary management of psammomatoid ossifying fibroma of the orbit. Ophthalmology 1998; 105: 591–5.
51. Vivian AJ, Harkness W, Kriss AJ, et al. Extragnathic cementoma. J Pediatr Ophthalmol Strabismus 1994; 31: 399–400.
52. Sawyer JR, Swanson CM, Koller MA, et al. Centromeric instability of chromosome 1 resulting in multibranched chromosomes, telomeric fusions, and "jumping translocations" of 1q in a human immunodeficiency virus-related non-Hodgkin's lymphoma. Cancer 1995; 78: 1142–4.
53. Lowder CY, Berlin AJ, Cox W, et al. Benign osteoblastoma of the orbit. Ophthalmology 1986; 93: 1351–4.
54. Abdalla MI, Hosni F. Osteoclastoma of the orbit. Case report. Br J Ophthalmol 1966; 50: 95–8.
55. Jackson RP. Recurrent osteoblastoma: a review. Clin Orthop 1978; 131: 229–33.
56. Figarella-Branger D, Perez-Castillo M, Garbe L, et al. Malignant transformation of an osteoblastoma of the skull: an exceptional occurrence. Case report. J Neurosurg 1991; 75: 138–42.
57. Abrahamson DH, Ellsworth RM, Kitchin D, et al. Second non-ocular tumours in retinoblastoma survivors. Ophthalmology 1984; 91: 1351–5.
58. Strong LC, Knudson AG, Jr. Second cancers in retinoblastoma (letter). Lancet 1973; 2: 1086.
59. Iliff C, Ossofsky H. Infantile cortical hyperostosis: an unusual case of proptosis. Am J Ophthalmol 1962; 53: 976–80.
60. Minton LR, Elliott JH. Ocular manifestations of infantile cortical hyperostosis. Am J Ophthalmol 1967; 64: 902–7.
61. Shapiro F. Osteopetrosis. Current clinical considerations. Clin Orthop 1993; 294: 34–44.

62. Chen CJ, Lee MY, Hsu ML, et al. Malignant infantile osteopetrosis initially presenting with neonatal hypocalcemia: case report. Ann Hematol 2003; 821: 64–7.

63. Bartynski WS, Barnes PD, Wallman JK. Cranial CT of autosomal recessive osteopetrosis. Am J Neuroradiol 1989; 10: 543–50.

64. Ainsworth JR, Bryce IG, Dudgeon J. Visual loss in infantile osteopetrosis. J Pediatr Ophthalmol Strabismus 1993; 30: 201–3.

65. Ellis PP, Jackson WE. Osteopetrosis: a clinical study of optic nerve involvement. Am J Ophthalmol 1962; 53: 943–53.

66. Riser RO. Marble bones and optic atrophy. Am J Ophthalmol 1941; 24: 874–8.

67. Klintworth GK. The neurologic manifestations of osteopetrosis (Albers-Schonberg's disease). Neurology 1963; 13: 512–9.

68. Hill BG, Charlton WS. Albers-Schonberg disease. Med J Aust 1965; 2: 365–7.

69. Aasved H. Osteopetrosis from the ophthalmological point of view. A report of two cases. Acta Ophthalmol 1970; 48: 771–8.

70. Al-Mefty O, Fox JL, Al-Rodhan N, et al. Optic nerve decompression in osteopetrosis. J Neurosurg 1988; 68: 80–4.

71. Haines SJ, Erickson DL, Wirts JD. Optic nerve decompression for osteopetrosis in early childhood. Neurosurgery 1988; 23: 407–50.

72. Schmoger E, Gerhardt HJ, Burgold R. Zur operativen Optikusdekompression bei Marmorknochenkrankheit (Albers-Schonbergsche Krankheit). Klin Monatsbl Augenheilkd 1983; 183: 273–7.

73. Hoyt CS, Billson FA. Visual loss in ostopetrosis. Am J Dis Child 1979; 133: 955–8.

74. Keith CG. Retinal atrophy in osteopetrosis. Arch Ophthalmol 1968; 79: 234–41.

75. Ruben JB, Morris RJ, Judisch GF. Chorioretinal degeneration in infantile malignant osteopetrosis. Am J Ophthalmol 1990; 110: 1–5.

76. Gerritsen EJ, Vossen JM, van Loo IH, et al. Autosomal recessive osteopetrosis: variability of findings at diagnosis and during the natural course. Pediatrics 1994; 93: 247–53.

77. Patel PJ, Kolawole TM, al-Mofada S, et al. Osteopetrosis: brain ultrasound and computed tomography findings. Eur J Pediatr 1992; 151: 827–8.

78. Ballet JJ, Griscelli C, Coutris C, et al. Bone-marrow transplantation in osteopetrosis. Lancet 1977; 2: 1137.

79. Gerritsen EJ, Vossen JM, Fasth A, et al. Bone marrow transplantation for autosomal recessive osteopetrosis. A report from the Working Party on Inborn Errors of the European Bone Marrow Transplantation Group. J Pediatr 1994; 125: 896–902.

Metastatic, Secondary and Lacrimal Gland Tumors

Christopher J Lyons and Jack Rootman

Neuroblastoma and Ewing sarcoma account for most childhood orbital metastatic disease.[1] Other tumors occasionally metastasize to the orbit, including Wilms tumor,[2] testicular embryonal sarcoma, ovarian sarcoma and renal embryonal sarcoma.[3]

Jakobiec and Jones[4] are careful to differentiate between blood-borne deposits of a malignant tumor (metastatic disease) and extension of a tumor into the orbital tissues from an adjacent structure (secondary disease). Retinoblastoma extending into the optic nerve or orbital structures is the most important source of secondary orbital disease in children, but spread of rhabdomyosarcoma from the sinuses is also relatively common and is discussed in Chapter 35.

METASTATIC DISEASE

Neuroblastoma

Neuroblastoma is a malignant tumor of undifferentiated neuro-ectodermal cells derived from the neural crest anywhere within the postganglionic sympathetic nervous system. It is the most common solid tumor of childhood, accounting for 9% of all childhood cancers and 28–39% of neonatal malignancies. There are 7.5 cases for every 100 000 infants.[5] It is also the most common source of orbital metastasis in children, accounting for 41 of 46 cases of orbital metastatic disease reported by Albert et al.[1] Nevertheless, neuroblastoma remains a rare cause of orbital disease since it represents only 1.5% of 214 orbital tumors reported by Porterfield[6] and 3% of 307 orbital tumors in children quoted by Nicholson and Green.[3]

Genetics

Approximately 1–2% of cases have a family history. The genetic characteristics of each tumor have important prognostic significance; in particular, MYCN (N-*myc*) proto-oncogene amplification, is associated with worse outcome for each tumor stage.[5] Hyperdiploidy of tumor cell DNA content confers an improved prognosis for infants under 1 year of age at diagnosis. Many genetic abnormalities have been identified, including allelic deletions at multiple gene loci in 1p, 2q, 3p, 4p 11q, 14q, 16p and 19q. Also, there may be a translocation of 1p and 17q. This 17q gain is a negative prognostic factor; it is thought that this could confer a growth advantage to the tumor cells.[5,7] Knudson and Strong[8] suggested that, as in the case of retinoblastoma, two genetic hits, with the loss of function of both alleles are necessary for neuroblastoma to occur. However careful studies of the regions involved and gene mutation analyses have not uncovered any consistent mutation pattern identifying the putative "neuroblastoma suppressor gene".

Overall, it seems that cellular genetic aberrations are a better prognostic predictor of the tumor's biological behavior than are clinical factors such as age and stage at diagnosis. This is important for treatment planning since these same tumors have a propensity for spontaneous regression and, if identified, these infants can be spared harmful therapy.

Clinical presentation

The vast majority of cases occur by the age of 3 years[9] and 90% are diagnosed by age 5, but the onset may range from birth to the late teens. The adrenals are the site of primary involvement in 51% of cases, but the tumor can also arise in the cervical sympathetic chain, mediastinum or pelvis.[10,11] Localized primary orbital neuroblastoma has also been reported, but tends to occur in adults.[12,13] Neuroblastoma is more common in patients with neurofibromatosis type 1 (NF1).

The clinical features vary according to the different sites of origin, tendency for multiple metastases, features related to its hormone secretion and the accompanying paraneoplastic syndrome. Pain, fever and weight loss are common symptoms; cerebellar encephalopathy (ataxia, myoclonic jerks, opsoclonus of unknown cause), diarrhea (from tumor vasoactive peptide production), Horner syndrome (sympathetic chain involvement) and hypertension with flushing episodes (catecholamine production) are classic signs that are highly indicative of neuroblastoma.

The diagnosis is often not made until late when the patient has widespread metastases;[14,15] overall, 40% of patients with neuroblastoma have metastases at presentation, a proportion which rises to 55% if patients over the age of 1 year are considered separately. Surprisingly, about 10% of tumors and their metastases (stages 1 to 4s) undergo spontaneous regression, something which occurs 100 times more commonly than for any other cancer.[16] This fact underlies the cautious treatment approach outlined below.

There is a spectrum of tumor histology, ranging from undifferentiated (neuroblastoma) to tumors with mature ganglion cells (ganglioneuroblastoma or ganglioneuroma). The histopathological characteristics such as the amount of stroma, degree of differentiation and number of mitotic figures, reflected in the Shimada classification, do have some prognostic value.

Ninety per cent of patients have abnormally high levels of vanillylmandelic acid (VMA) in their urine due to catecholamine secretion by the tumor. The urinary VMA concentration can be useful both for diagnosis and to monitor treatment.

Ophthalmic features

The presence of neuroblastoma in the mediastinum or cervical sympathetic chain may first manifest with Horner syndrome. This was the underlying diagnosis in two of 10 children with Horner syndrome reviewed by Woodruff et al.[17] Gibbs et al.[18] described congenital Horner syndrome in an infant with non-cervical neuroblastoma, suggesting that the two conditions might indicate a widespread dysgenesis of the sympathetic nervous system. Tonic pupils have also been reported as a paraneoplastic effect of adrenal neuroblastoma.[19,20] Iris[21] and choroidal[22] metastases from abdominal neuroblastoma have also been described. The presence of opsoclonus (see Chapter 73), a striking large amplitude erratic ocular flutter also known as "dancing eyes syndrome", with or without ataxia and myoclonus suggests occult localized neuroblastoma.[15] The primary tumor in these cases is in the chest or abdomen and not the brain. It is usually associated with a good prognosis (see below), possibly because in many of these patients, only single copies of the N-*myc* oncogene are present within the tumor cells.[23] Nevertheless opsoclonus can also be present with multiple N-*myc* copies, signaling a poor outcome.[24]

Presentation

In 93% of the 46 cases reported by Albert et al.,[1] the primary tumor had been diagnosed prior to presentation with orbital signs. Ninety per cent of the 60 patients with orbital metastases reviewed by Musarella et al.[15] had a primary tumor in the abdomen. Orbital metastases commonly present with sudden onset and rapid progression of proptosis (Fig. 37.1) that may be unilateral or bilateral. Ecchymosis (Fig. 37.2) is present in 25% of cases.[15,25,26] The lesion is most commonly found in the superolateral orbit and zygoma but may occur anywhere within the orbit. Bony lesions give rise to swelling of overlying tissues so periorbital swelling and ptosis may be present. This presentation may be confused with orbital cellulitis or other rapidly progressive orbital tumors such as rhabdomyosarcoma, Ewing sarcoma, medulloblastoma, Wilms tumor and acute lymphoblastic leukemia.[27] A bleed into a pre-existing but clinically unsuspected lymphangioma may also present with sudden onset of proptosis with ecchymosis. The presence of ecchymosis can lead to erroneous investigation of child abuse resulting in diagnostic delay.[28]

Treatment

The main prognostic (risk) factors are the age at diagnosis, stage of disease (Table 37.1), MYCN status, Shimada histology and ploidy for infants. Best published survival rates for low risk groups are 90–100%, whilst those for high risk group survival range from 20–60%.

Low-risk neuroblastoma at stages 1 and 2 is treated surgically. The cure rate is greater than 90% for stage 2 neuroblastomas with no further treatment even if small residual amounts of tumor

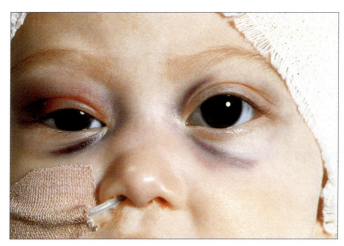

Fig. 37.2 Periorbital ecchymoses in a patient with orbital neuroblastoma.

Table 37.1 International neuroblastoma staging system (INSS)

Stage	Description
1	Tumor confined to organ or origin
2	Tumor extends beyond organ of origin but not beyond midline
2a	No lymph node involvement
3	Tumor extends beyond midline with or without bilateral lymph note involvement
4	Tumor disseminated to distant sites
4s	Children younger than 1-year-old with dissemination to liver, skin, or bone marrow without bone involvement and a primary tumor that would otherwise be stage 1 or 2

remain after surgical excision.[29] Chemotherapy or radiation can be curative in the event of local recurrence. As noted above, stage 4s has a favorable prognosis, and the survival rate is 92% with observation and supportive care only since there is spontaneous regression of the tumor.[30] Treatment for intermediate risk neuroblastoma includes surgery and chemotherapy with agents including carboplatin, cyclophosphamide, cisplatin, etoposide and doxorubicin over several months. Radiotherapy is used for incomplete response to chemotherapy. Children with stage 3 and infants with stage 4 under 1 year of age and otherwise favorable

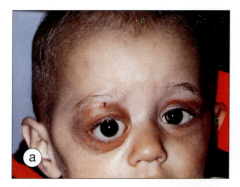
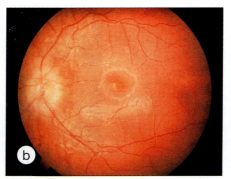
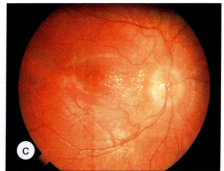

Fig. 37.1 Neuroblastoma. (a) This child presented with bilateral orbital bruising and right proptosis. Patient of Dr S. Day. (b, c) The patient had widespread orbital and cranial bone involvement with raised intracranial pressure and papilledema.

features have an excellent prognosis of more that 90% survival with moderate treatment of this type. It is important to obtain sufficient material for histopathological and genetic study to determine these patients' moderate risk and spare them the high doses necessary for higher risk groups. High-risk patients receive induction chemotherapy followed by high-dose chemotherapy and bone marrow transplantation with additional *cis*-retinoic acid treatment.[31]

Ewing sarcoma

Ewing sarcoma is a highly malignant tumor present in the bone marrow. This group of neuroectoderm-derived neoplasms includes Ewing sarcoma, Askin tumor (in the chest wall) and peripheral primitive neuroectodermal tumors.[32] It usually arises in the axial skeleton, but may occasionally occur in soft tissues. Primary orbital involvement or spread from contiguous structures such as the sinuses may also occur. Four percent of primary tumors are in the head and neck, usually the maxilla or mandible, but the orbital roof may also be primarily involved.[33] There is a marked tendency to spread to adjacent soft tissues, other bones and the lungs.[4] The usual age of onset is 10–25 years, especially the first half of the second decade, and the tumor is very rare in African and Chinese people.

Immunohistochemical characteristics help to differentiate Ewing from other small round cell tumors such as rhabdomyosarcoma, neuroblastoma and lymphoma. Ewing sarcomas are often S-100, neuron-specific enolase and surface glycoprotein MIC-2 positive and negative for muscle markers such as desmin or actin. A reciprocal translocation, t(11:22)(q24;q12) is present in 83% of tumors.[34] There is a cytogenetic rearrangement on the long arm of chromosome 22 fusing the EWS gene (whose function is unknown) and members of the ETS family of transcription factors (FLI-1, ERG). This causes deregulation of other genes within the cell and development of the malignant phenotype.[35,36] In undifferentiated tumors, the diagnosis may be secured by cytogenetic analysis for the translocation or PCR for chimeric fusion gene products EWS/FLII or EWS/ERG.

Albert et al.[1] reported five patients with Ewing sarcoma metastatic to the orbit. Orbital presentation occurred on average 14 months after diagnosis of the primary tumor. The usual presenting signs were rapidly progressive proptosis and orbital hemorrhage. There are 16 reports of primary Ewing sarcoma involving the orbit, arising from the ethmoid and sphenoid sinuses, roof of the orbit, lesser wing of sphenoid and temporal bone. A short history is typical, featuring swelling, globe displacement from mass effect, strabismus with diplopia and duction limitation, headache, visual loss, pain and localized bony tenderness.[37,38]

On computed tomography (CT) scan, there is a "moth-eaten" unevenly enhancing appearance of the involved bone, associated with a soft tissue mass. The clinical differential diagnosis includes neuroblastoma, rhabdomyosarcoma (if extraskeletal), Langerhans cell histiocytosis and osteomyelitis.

In apparently primary orbital tumors, the patient should be evaluated for metastatic disease with a chest CT, radionuclide scan, bone marrow aspirate and tissue biopsies. Adequate amounts of fresh tissue should be obtained for histopathological and cytogenetic studies.[39] Treatment of the primary tumor is with multiagent chemotherapy to shrink the tumor before attempting local control. Vincristine, doxorubicin and cyclophosphamide are the main treatments with, in addition, ifosfamide and etoposide. Although these tumors are radiosensitive and local

control may be achieved by radiotherapy, surgery is preferable due to the risk of late osteosarcoma from radiotherapy. Histologically clear margins are essential. The prognosis for metastatic disease remains poor, approximately one-third surviving in the long term. Since there is an appreciable risk of late recurrence or development of a second malignancy such as osteogenic sarcoma, prolonged scrupulous follow-up is indicated.

SECONDARY DISEASE

Retinoblastoma

See also Chapter 50.

Retinoblastoma confined within the eye poses little threat to life and is a curable disease.[4,40] The prognosis is greatly worsened by extension into the orbit or central nervous system or the presence of widespread metastatic disease. The consequences of trans-scleral involvement of the orbital tissues (orbital spread) and extension of the tumor into the optic nerve (optic nerve spread) are considered in this section.

Orbital spread

Orbital involvement with retinoblastoma was observed in 8% of patients reported by Jakobiec and Jones[4] but in only nine out of 268 (3.5%) cases reported by Lennox et al.[41] This is made more likely by delay in diagnosis.

Clinical signs (Fig. 37.3) include proptosis, a palpable orbital mass, swelling and ecchymosis. Spread may also be encouraged by neovascular glaucoma resulting in scleral thinning.[42] Orbital spread may be apparent on ultrasound, CT or MRI prior to surgery or may be evident at the time of enucleation. Pathological examination of an enucleated eye may reveal microscopic transscleral spread. Orbital disease may also be signaled by a mass arising in the orbit after enucleation. Biopsy is helpful to confirm that this is indeed retinoblastoma rather than a second tumor, such as an osteosarcoma, arising in the field of previous radiotherapy.[43]

The mainstay of management is a combination of radiotherapy and early adjuvant chemotherapy.[44]

Optic nerve spread

This is the most common route by which retinoblastoma extends beyond the globe.[45] Following invasion of the optic nerve, the neoplasm may gain access to the cerebrospinal fluid and cause widespread central nervous system deposits. Optic nerve spread

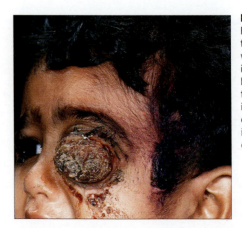

Fig. 37.3
Retinoblastoma. This tragic picture of a child with extensive orbital involvement with lymphatic spread (note the preauricular gland involvement) is a common presentation in developing countries.

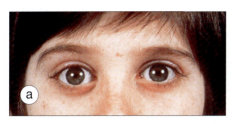 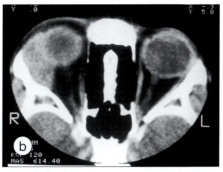 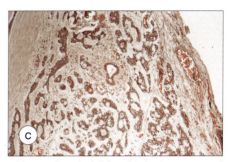

Fig. 37.4 Adenoid cystic carcinoma of the lacrimal gland. (a) This 10-year-old boy presented with a 1-year history of gradual right orbital enlargement and upper lid swelling. There was no pain or sensory loss. (b) CT scan showed a lacrimal gland mass excavating the frontal bone, without erosion. Even rapidly growing lesions may cause excavation in childhood. (c) It was an adenoid cystic carcinoma of the lacrimal gland. The patient is alive and well 17 years later. Patient of the University of British Columbia.

was identified in 12.7% of the series quoted by Jakobiec and Jones[4] and 15% of the patients reported by Lennox et al.[41] Extension into the nerve is most commonly a histological finding.

Eyes enucleated for phthisis bulbi may harbor an unsuspected viable retinoblastoma. Two of 10 such cases reported from Saudi Arabia[46] had optic nerve extension and both subsequently died of widespread retinoblastoma. Children with phthisis bulbi whose history is unclear in whom enucleation is considered should undergo a careful preoperative workup including ocular ultrasound and possibly CT scan, careful enucleation obtaining a maximal length of optic nerve, and thorough histopathological examination both of the globe and the cut end of the nerve.

Treatment

Biopsy-proven orbital retinoblastoma carries 100% mortality following surgical treatment alone.[47] Irradiation of the orbital lesions is effective but most patients develop widespread disease within 18 months if radiation is used alone.[40] Present treatment of biopsy-proven orbital retinoblastoma therefore involves irradiation and systemic chemotherapy with agents such as vincristine, cyclophosphamide, actinomycin D or doxorubicin.[40,48] A 3-year survival of 46.7% has been reported with newer chemotherapeutic regimens for orbital retinoblastoma without clinically evident metastasis.[49] If optic nerve involvement suggests central nervous system spread, treatment of the central nervous system with radiation or chemotherapy or both is also indicated.[48,50,51]

Malignant melanoma

Intraocular melanoma very rarely occurs in infancy and childhood. Occasionally, it is seen in the neonatal period, and extensive involvement of the orbital and other facial tissues is noted at presentation.

LACRIMAL GLAND TUMORS

The most common cause of a lacrimal gland fossa mass in

childhood is dermoid cyst, since these lesions tend to occur in the upper outer quadrant of the orbit.[3] In our center, we have seen 16 lacrimal masses in childhood, seven of which were inflammatory, including nonspecific lacrimal inflammation, Wegener granulomatosis, sclerosing inflammation, and angiolymphoid hyperplasia. Cystic lesions encountered in this age group include four dermoid cysts and one lacrimal cyst. In terms of neoplasia, we have seen two patients with adenoid cystic carcinoma and one chloroma of the lacrimal gland.

Primary epithelial tumors of the lacrimal gland are rare in young children (Fig. 37.4), but increase in frequency over the age of 10 years. Benign mixed tumor of the lacrimal gland is unusual and accounted for only one of the 214 childhood orbital tumors reported by Porterfield.[6] Cure is effected by complete removal of the tumor, with a tendency to recurrence if excision is incomplete. They can usually be recognized by their slow progression and the certainty of diagnosis is increased by CT scanning prior to removal.[52]

Adenoid cystic carcinoma is also uncommon in childhood, although Galliani et al.[53] reported this in a 6-year-old girl and cases have been reported by Porterfield,[6] Font and Gamel,[54] Dagher et al.,[55] Shields et al.[56] and ourselves.[57]

These tumors have a tendency to develop rapidly and to be associated with pain and paresthesia due to perineural invasion. The latter often extends microscopically beyond the tumor mass, which is in part responsible for the poor prognosis and recurrence after excision.

Radiologically, bone erosion is highly suggestive of malignancy. However, it is important to note that absence of erosion does not exclude malignancy; since bony remodeling occurs rapidly in childhood, localized bony expansion may be seen even with rapidly growing masses such as adenoid cystic carcinoma[57] whereas in adults, this sign would indicate a slow-growing mass such as pleomorphic adenoma.

These tumors may be difficult to distinguish clinically from other lacrimal lesions such as low-grade infections, nonspecific inflammation[58] or leukemic deposits[59] and biopsy may be required for confirmation.

Adenoid cystic carcinoma is invasive and carries a poor prognosis despite surgery, radiotherapy and chemotherapy.[60]

REFERENCES

1. Albert DM, Rubenstein RA, Scheie HG. Tumor metastasis to the eye. II. Clinical study in infants and children. Am J Ophthalmol 1967; 63: 727–32.
2. Apple DJ. Wilms' tumor metastatic to the orbit. Arch Ophthalmol 1968; 80: 480–3.
3. Nicholson DH, Green WR. Pediatric Ocular Tumors. New York: Masson; 1981.
4. Jakobiec FA, Jones IS. Metastatic and secondary tumors. In: Duane TD, ed. Clinical Ophthalmology. Hagerstown: Harper and Row; 1983.
5. Schwab M, Westermann F, Hero B, et al. Neuroblastoma: biology and molecular and chromosomal pathology. Lancet Oncol 2003; 4: 472–80.
6. Porterfield JF. Orbital tumors in children: a report on 214 cases. Int Ophthalmol Clin 1962; 2: 319–26.
7. Riley RD, Burchill SA, Abrams KR, et al. A systematic review and evaluation of the use of tumor markers in paediatric oncology: Ewing's sarcoma and neuroblastoma. Health Technol Assess 2003; 7: 1–162.
8. Knudson AG, Jr, Strong LC. Mutation and cancer: neuroblastoma and pheochromocytoma. Am J Hum Genet 1972; 24: 514–32.
9. Davis S, Rogers MAM, Pendergrass TW. The evidence and epidemiologic characteristics of neuroblastoma in the United States. Am J Epidemiol 1987; 126: 1063–74.
10. DeLorimier AA, Bragg KU, Linden G. Neuroblastoma in childhood. Am J Dis Child 1969; 118: 441–50.
11. Gross RE, Farber S, Martin LW. Neuroblastoma sympatheticum; a study and report of 217 cases. Pediatrics 1959; 23: 1179–91.
12. Bullock JD, Goldberg SH, Rakes SM, et al. Primary orbital neuroblastoma. Arch Ophthalmol 1989; 107: 1031–3.
13. Jakobiec FA, Klepach GL, Crissman JD, et al. Primary differentiated neuroblastoma of the orbit. Ophthalmology 1987; 94: 255–66.
14. Anonymous. Neuroblastoma (letter). Lancet 1975; 1: 379–80.
15. Musarella MA, Chan HS, DeBoer G, et al. Ocular involvement in neuroblastoma: prognostic implications. Ophthalmology 1984; 91: 936–40.
16. Pritchard J, Hickman JA. Why does stage 4s neuroblastoma regress spontaneously? Lancet 1994; 345: 992–3.
17. Woodruff G, Buncic JR, Morin JD. Horner's syndrome in children. J Pediatr Ophthalmol Strabismus 1988; 25: 40–4.
18. Gibbs J, Appleton RE, Martin J, et al. Congenital Horner syndrome associated with non-cervical neuroblastoma. Dev Med Child Neurol 1992; 34: 642–4.
19. Fisher PG, Wechsler DS, Singer HS. Anti-Hu antibody in a neuroblastoma-associated paraneoplastic syndrome. Pediatr Neurol 1994; 10: 309–12.
20. West CE, Repka MX. Tonic pupils associated with neuroblastoma. J Pediatr Ophthalmol Strabismus 1992; 29: 382–3.
21. Sekimoto M, Hayasaka S, Setogawa T, et al. Presumed iris metastasis from abdominal neuroblastoma. Ophthalmologica 1991; 203: 8–11.
22. Cibis GW, Freeman AI, Pang V, et al. Bilateral choroidal neonatal neuroblastoma. Am J Ophthalmol 1990; 109: 445–9.
23. Cohn SL, Salwen H, Herst CV, et al. Single copies of the N-myc oncogene in neuroblastomas from children presenting with the syndrome of opsoclonus-myoclonus. Cancer 1988; 62: 723–6.
24. Hiyama E, Yokoyama T, Ichikawa T, et al. Poor outcome in patients with advanced stage neuroblastoma and coincident opsomyoclonus syndrome. Cancer 1994; 74: 1821–6.
25. Alfano JE. Ophthalmological aspects of neuroblastomatosis: a study of 53 verified cases. Trans Am Acad Ophthalmol Otolaryngol 1968; 72: 830–48.
26. Mortada A. Clinical characteristics of early orbital metastatic neuroblastoma. Am J Ophthalmol 1967; 63: 1787–93.
27. Slamovits TL, Rosen CE, Suhrland MJ. Neuroblastoma presenting as acute lymphoblastic leukemia but correctly diagnosed after orbital fine-needle aspiration biopsy. J Clin Neuro-ophthalmol 1991; 11: 158–61.
28. Timmerman R. Images in clinical medicine. Raccoon eyes and neuroblastoma. N Engl J Med 2003; 349: E4.
29. Perez CA, Matthay KK, Atkinson JB, et al. Biologic variables in the outcome of stages I and II neuroblastoma treated with surgery as primary therapy: a children's cancer group study. J Clin Oncol 2000; 18: 18–26.
30. Nickerson HJ, Matthay KK, Seeger RC, et al. Favorable biology and outcome of stage IV-S neuroblastoma with supportive care or minimal therapy: a Children's Cancer Group study. J Clin Oncol 2000; 18: 477–86.
31. Matthay KK, Villablanca JG, Seeger RC, et al. Treatment of high-risk neuroblastoma with intensive chemotherapy, radiotherapy, autologous bone marrow transplantation, and 13-cis-retinoic acid. Children's Cancer Group. N Engl J Med 1999; 341: 1165–73.
32. Sandberg AA, Bridge JA. Updates on cytogenetics and molecular genetics of bone and soft tissue tumors: Ewing sarcoma and peripheral primitive neuroectodermal tumors. Cancer Genet Cytogenet 2000; 123: 1–26.
33. Alvarez-Berdecia A, Schut L, Bruce DA. Localized primary intracranial Ewing's sarcoma of the orbital roof. Case report. J Neurosurg 1979; 50: 811–3.
34. Turc-Carel C, Aurias A, Mugneret F, et al. Chromosomes in Ewing's sarcoma. I. An evaluation of 85 cases of remarkable consistency of t(11;22)(q24;q12). Cancer Genet Cytogenet 1988; 32: 229–38.
35. Delattre O, Zucman J, Plougastel B, et al. Gene fusion with an ETS DNA-binding domain caused by chromosome translocation in human tumors. Nature 1992; 359: 162–5.
36. Shing DC, McMullan DJ, Roberts P, et al. FUS/ERG gene fusions in Ewing's tumors. Cancer Res 2003; 63: 4568–76.
37. Dutton JJ, Rose JG, Jr, DeBacker CM, et al. Orbital Ewing's sarcoma of the orbit. Ophthal Plast Reconstr Surg 2000;16:292–300.
38. Bajaj MS, Pushker N, Sen S, et al. Primary Ewing's sarcoma of the orbit: a rare presentation. J Pediatr Ophthalmol Strabismus 2003; 40: 101–4.
39. Wilson DJ, Dailey RA, Griffeth MT, et al. Primary Ewing sarcoma of the orbit. Ophthal Plast Reconstr Surg 2001; 17: 300–3.
40. Abramson DH. Treatment of retinoblastoma. In: Blodi FC, ed. Retinoblastoma. Edinburgh: Churchill Livingstone; 1985: 86–8.
41. Lennox EL, Draper GJ, Sanders BM. Retinoblastoma: a study of natural history and prognosis of 268 cases. Br Med J 1975; 3: 731–4.
42. Finger PT, Harbour JW, Karcioglu ZA. Risk factors for metastasis in retinoblastoma. Surv Ophthalmol 2002; 47: 1–16.
43. Abramson DH, Ellsworth RM, Kitchin FD, et al. Second nonocular tumors in retinoblastoma survivors. Are they radiation-induced? Ophthalmology 1984; 91: 1351–5.
44. Rootman J, Ellsworth RM, Hofbauer J, et al. Orbital extension of retinoblastoma: a clinicopathological study. Can J Ophthalmol 1978; 13: 72–80.
45. Henderson JW. Miscellaneous tumors of presumed neuroepithelial origin. In: Henderson JW, ed. Orbital Tumors. 3rd edn. New York: Raven Press; 1994: 239–68.
46. Mullaney PB, Karcioglu ZA, al-Mesfer S, et al. Presentation of retinoblastoma as phthisis bulbi. Eye 1997; 11: 403–8.
47. Ellsworth RM. Orbital retinoblastoma. Trans Am Ophthalmol Soc 1974; 72: 79–88.
48. White L. The role of chemotherapy in the treatment of retinoblastoma. Retina 1983; 3: 194–9.
49. Svegberg-Winholt H, Al-Moster SA, Riley FC. Survival trends of retinoblastoma patients with extraocular extension. Abstract 502. In: XIIth Congress of the European Society of Ophthalmology, June 27–July 1; 1999; Stockholm, Sweden; 1999.
50. Keith CG, Ekert H. The management of retinoblastoma. Aust NZ J Ophthalmol 1987; 15: 359–63.
51. Zelter M, Gonzalez G, Schwartz L, et al. Treatment of retinoblastoma. Results obtained from a prospective study of 51 patients. Cancer 1988; 61: 153–60.
52. Wright JE. Symposium on orbital tumors. Methods of examination. Trans Ophthalmol Soc UK 1979; 99: 216–9.
53. Galliani CA, Faught PR, Ellis FD. Adenoid cystic carcinoma of the lacrimal gland in a six-year-old girl. Pediatr Pathol 1993; 13: 559–65.
54. Font RL, Gamel JW. Epithelial tumors of the lacrimal gland: an analysis of 256 cases. In: Jakobiec FA, ed. Ocular and Adnexae Tumors. Birmingham: Aesculapius; 1978.
55. Dagher G, Anderson RL, Ossoinig KC, et al. Adenoid cystic carcinoma of the lacrimal gland in a child. Arch Ophthalmol 1980; 98: 1098–1100.
56. Shields JA, Bakewell B, Augsburger JJ, et al. Space occupying orbital masses in children. A review of 250 consecutive biopsies. Ophthalmology 1986; 93: 379–84.
57. Rootman J. Diseases of the Orbit: A Multidisciplinary Approach. 2nd edn. Philadelphia: Lippincott Williams & Wilkins; 2003.

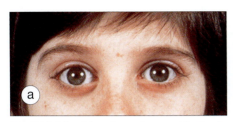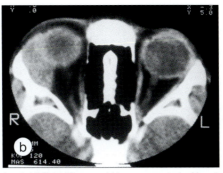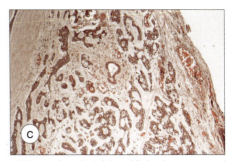

Fig. 37.4 Adenoid cystic carcinoma of the lacrimal gland. (a) This 10-year-old boy presented with a 1-year history of gradual right orbital enlargement and upper lid swelling. There was no pain or sensory loss. (b) CT scan showed a lacrimal gland mass excavating the frontal bone, without erosion. Even rapidly growing lesions may cause excavation in childhood. (c) It was an adenoid cystic carcinoma of the lacrimal gland. The patient is alive and well 17 years later. Patient of the University of British Columbia.

was identified in 12.7% of the series quoted by Jakobiec and Jones[4] and 15% of the patients reported by Lennox et al.[41] Extension into the nerve is most commonly a histological finding.

Eyes enucleated for phthisis bulbi may harbor an unsuspected viable retinoblastoma. Two of 10 such cases reported from Saudi Arabia[46] had optic nerve extension and both subsequently died of widespread retinoblastoma. Children with phthisis bulbi whose history is unclear in whom enucleation is considered should undergo a careful preoperative workup including ocular ultrasound and possibly CT scan, careful enucleation obtaining a maximal length of optic nerve, and thorough histopathological examination both of the globe and the cut end of the nerve.

Treatment

Biopsy-proven orbital retinoblastoma carries 100% mortality following surgical treatment alone.[47] Irradiation of the orbital lesions is effective but most patients develop widespread disease within 18 months if radiation is used alone.[40] Present treatment of biopsy-proven orbital retinoblastoma therefore involves irradiation and systemic chemotherapy with agents such as vincristine, cyclophosphamide, actinomycin D or doxorubicin.[40,48] A 3-year survival of 46.7% has been reported with newer chemotherapeutic regimens for orbital retinoblastoma without clinically evident metastasis.[49] If optic nerve involvement suggests central nervous system spread, treatment of the central nervous system with radiation or chemotherapy or both is also indicated.[48,50,51]

Malignant melanoma

Intraocular melanoma very rarely occurs in infancy and childhood. Occasionally, it is seen in the neonatal period, and extensive involvement of the orbital and other facial tissues is noted at presentation.

LACRIMAL GLAND TUMORS

The most common cause of a lacrimal gland fossa mass in childhood is dermoid cyst, since these lesions tend to occur in the upper outer quadrant of the orbit.[3] In our center, we have seen 16 lacrimal masses in childhood, seven of which were inflammatory, including nonspecific lacrimal inflammation, Wegener granulomatosis, sclerosing inflammation, and angiolymphoid hyperplasia. Cystic lesions encountered in this age group include four dermoid cysts and one lacrimal cyst. In terms of neoplasia, we have seen two patients with adenoid cystic carcinoma and one chloroma of the lacrimal gland.

Primary epithelial tumors of the lacrimal gland are rare in young children (Fig. 37.4), but increase in frequency over the age of 10 years. Benign mixed tumor of the lacrimal gland is unusual and accounted for only one of the 214 childhood orbital tumors reported by Porterfield.[6] Cure is effected by complete removal of the tumor, with a tendency to recurrence if excision is incomplete. They can usually be recognized by their slow progression and the certainty of diagnosis is increased by CT scanning prior to removal.[52]

Adenoid cystic carcinoma is also uncommon in childhood, although Galliani et al.[53] reported this in a 6-year-old girl and cases have been reported by Porterfield,[6] Font and Gamel,[54] Dagher et al.,[55] Shields et al.[56] and ourselves.[57]

These tumors have a tendency to develop rapidly and to be associated with pain and paresthesia due to perineural invasion. The latter often extends microscopically beyond the tumor mass, which is in part responsible for the poor prognosis and recurrence after excision.

Radiologically, bone erosion is highly suggestive of malignancy. However, it is important to note that absence of erosion does not exclude malignancy; since bony remodeling occurs rapidly in childhood, localized bony expansion may be seen even with rapidly growing masses such as adenoid cystic carcinoma[57] whereas in adults, this sign would indicate a slow-growing mass such as pleomorphic adenoma.

These tumors may be difficult to distinguish clinically from other lacrimal lesions such as low-grade infections, nonspecific inflammation[58] or leukemic deposits[59] and biopsy may be required for confirmation.

Adenoid cystic carcinoma is invasive and carries a poor prognosis despite surgery, radiotherapy and chemotherapy.[60]

REFERENCES

1. Albert DM, Rubenstein RA, Scheie HG. Tumor metastasis to the eye. II. Clinical study in infants and children. Am J Ophthalmol 1967; 63: 727–32.

2. Apple DJ. Wilms' tumor metastatic to the orbit. Arch Ophthalmol 1968; 80: 480–3.

3. Nicholson DH, Green WR. Pediatric Ocular Tumors. New York: Masson; 1981.

4. Jakobiec FA, Jones IS. Metastatic and secondary tumors. In: Duane TD, ed. Clinical Ophthalmology. Hagerstown: Harper and Row; 1983.

5. Schwab M, Westermann F, Hero B, et al. Neuroblastoma: biology and molecular and chromosomal pathology. Lancet Oncol 2003; 4: 472–80.

6. Porterfield JF. Orbital tumors in children: a report on 214 cases. Int Ophthalmol Clin 1962; 2: 319–26.

7. Riley RD, Burchill SA, Abrams KR, et al. A systematic review and evaluation of the use of tumor markers in paediatric oncology: Ewing's sarcoma and neuroblastoma. Health Technol Assess 2003; 7: 1–162.

8. Knudson AG, Jr, Strong LC. Mutation and cancer: neuroblastoma and pheochromocytoma. Am J Hum Genet 1972; 24: 514–32.

9. Davis S, Rogers MAM, Pendergrass TW. The evidence and epidemiologic characteristics of neuroblastoma in the United States. Am J Epidemiol 1987; 126: 1063–74.

10. DeLorimier AA, Bragg KU, Linden G. Neuroblastoma in childhood. Am J Dis Child 1969; 118: 441–50.

11. Gross RE, Farber S, Martin LW. Neuroblastoma sympatheticum; a study and report of 217 cases. Pediatrics 1959; 23: 1179–91.

12. Bullock JD, Goldberg SH, Rakes SM, et al. Primary orbital neuroblastoma. Arch Ophthalmol 1989; 107: 1031–3.

13. Jakobiec FA, Klepach GL, Crissman JD, et al. Primary differentiated neuroblastoma of the orbit. Ophthalmology 1987; 94: 255–66.

14. Anonymous. Neuroblastoma (letter). Lancet 1975; 1: 379–80.

15. Musarella MA, Chan HS, DeBoer G, et al. Ocular involvement in neuroblastoma: prognostic implications. Ophthalmology 1984; 91: 936–40.

16. Pritchard J, Hickman JA. Why does stage 4s neuroblastoma regress spontaneously? Lancet 1994; 345: 992–3.

17. Woodruff G, Buncic JR, Morin JD. Horner's syndrome in children. J Pediatr Ophthalmol Strabismus 1988; 25: 40–4.

18. Gibbs J, Appleton RE, Martin J, et al. Congenital Horner syndrome associated with non-cervical neuroblastoma. Dev Med Child Neurol 1992; 34: 642–4.

19. Fisher PG, Wechsler DS, Singer HS. Anti-Hu antibody in a neuroblastoma-associated paraneoplastic syndrome. Pediatr Neurol 1994; 10: 309–12.

20. West CE, Repka MX. Tonic pupils associated with neuroblastoma. J Pediatr Ophthalmol Strabismus 1992; 29: 382–3.

21. Sekimoto M, Hayasaka S, Setogawa T, et al. Presumed iris metastasis from abdominal neuroblastoma. Ophthalmologica 1991; 203: 8–11.

22. Cibis GW, Freeman AI, Pang V, et al. Bilateral choroidal neonatal neuroblastoma. Am J Ophthalmol 1990; 109: 445–9.

23. Cohn SL, Salwen H, Herst CV, et al. Single copies of the N-myc oncogene in neuroblastomas from children presenting with the syndrome of opsoclonus-myoclonus. Cancer 1988; 62: 723–6.

24. Hiyama E, Yokoyama T, Ichikawa T, et al. Poor outcome in patients with advanced stage neuroblastoma and coincident opsomyoclonus syndrome. Cancer 1994; 74: 1821–6.

25. Alfano JE. Ophthalmological aspects of neuroblastomatosis: a study of 53 verified cases. Trans Am Acad Ophthalmol Otolaryngol 1968; 72: 830–48.

26. Mortada A. Clinical characteristics of early orbital metastatic neuroblastoma. Am J Ophthalmol 1967; 63: 1787–93.

27. Slamovits TL, Rosen CE, Suhrland MJ. Neuroblastoma presenting as acute lymphoblastic leukemia but correctly diagnosed after orbital fine-needle aspiration biopsy. J Clin Neuro-ophthalmol 1991; 11: 158–61.

28. Timmerman R. Images in clinical medicine. Raccoon eyes and neuroblastoma. N Engl J Med 2003; 349: E4.

29. Perez CA, Matthay KK, Atkinson JB, et al. Biologic variables in the outcome of stages I and II neuroblastoma treated with surgery as primary therapy: a children's cancer group study. J Clin Oncol 2000; 18: 18–26.

30. Nickerson HJ, Matthay KK, Seeger RC, et al. Favorable biology and outcome of stage IV-S neuroblastoma with supportive care or minimal therapy: a Children's Cancer Group study. J Clin Oncol 2000; 18: 477–86.

31. Matthay KK, Villablanca JG, Seeger RC, et al. Treatment of high-risk neuroblastoma with intensive chemotherapy, radiotherapy, autologous bone marrow transplantation, and 13-cis-retinoic acid. Children's Cancer Group. N Engl J Med 1999; 341: 1165–73.

32. Sandberg AA, Bridge JA. Updates on cytogenetics and molecular genetics of bone and soft tissue tumors: Ewing sarcoma and peripheral primitive neuroectodermal tumors. Cancer Genet Cytogenet 2000; 123: 1–26.

33. Alvarez-Berdecia A, Schut L, Bruce DA. Localized primary intracranial Ewing's sarcoma of the orbital roof. Case report. J Neurosurg 1979; 50: 811–3.

34. Turc-Carel C, Aurias A, Mugneret F, et al. Chromosomes in Ewing's sarcoma. I. An evaluation of 85 cases of remarkable consistency of t(11;22)(q24;q12). Cancer Genet Cytogenet 1988; 32: 229–38.

35. Delattre O, Zucman J, Plougastel B, et al. Gene fusion with an ETS DNA-binding domain caused by chromosome translocation in human tumors. Nature 1992; 359: 162–5.

36. Shing DC, McMullan DJ, Roberts P, et al. FUS/ERG gene fusions in Ewing's tumors. Cancer Res 2003; 63: 4568–76.

37. Dutton JJ, Rose JG, Jr, DeBacker CM, et al. Orbital Ewing's sarcoma of the orbit. Ophthal Plast Reconstr Surg 2000;16:292–300.

38. Bajaj MS, Pushker N, Sen S, et al. Primary Ewing's sarcoma of the orbit: a rare presentation. J Pediatr Ophthalmol Strabismus 2003; 40: 101–4.

39. Wilson DJ, Dailey RA, Griffeth MT, et al. Primary Ewing sarcoma of the orbit. Ophthal Plast Reconstr Surg 2001; 17: 300–3.

40. Abramson DH. Treatment of retinoblastoma. In: Blodi FC, ed. Retinoblastoma. Edinburgh: Churchill Livingstone; 1985: 86–8.

41. Lennox EL, Draper GJ, Sanders BM. Retinoblastoma: a study of natural history and prognosis of 268 cases. Br Med J 1975; 3: 731–4.

42. Finger PT, Harbour JW, Karcioglu ZA. Risk factors for metastasis in retinoblastoma. Surv Ophthalmol 2002; 47: 1–16.

43. Abramson DH, Ellsworth RM, Kitchin FD, et al. Second nonocular tumors in retinoblastoma survivors. Are they radiation-induced? Ophthalmology 1984; 91: 1351–5.

44. Rootman J, Ellsworth RM, Hofbauer J, et al. Orbital extension of retinoblastoma: a clinicopathological study. Can J Ophthalmol 1978; 13: 72–80.

45. Henderson JW. Miscellaneous tumors of presumed neuroepithelial origin. In: Henderson JW, ed. Orbital Tumors. 3rd edn. New York: Raven Press; 1994: 239–68.

46. Mullaney PB, Karcioglu ZA, al-Mesfer S, et al. Presentation of retinoblastoma as phthisis bulbi. Eye 1997; 11: 403–8.

47. Ellsworth RM. Orbital retinoblastoma. Trans Am Ophthalmol Soc 1974; 72: 79–88.

48. White L. The role of chemotherapy in the treatment of retinoblastoma. Retina 1983; 3: 194–9.

49. Svegberg-Winholt H, Al-Moster SA, Riley FC. Survival trends of retinoblastoma patients with extraocular extension. Abstract 502. In: XIIth Congress of the European Society of Ophthalmology, June 27–July 1; 1999; Stockholm, Sweden; 1999.

50. Keith CG, Ekert H. The management of retinoblastoma. Aust NZ J Ophthalmol 1987; 15: 359–63.

51. Zelter M, Gonzalez G, Schwartz L, et al. Treatment of retinoblastoma. Results obtained from a prospective study of 51 patients. Cancer 1988; 61: 153–60.

52. Wright JE. Symposium on orbital tumors. Methods of examination. Trans Ophthalmol Soc UK 1979; 99: 216–9.

53. Galliani CA, Faught PR, Ellis FD. Adenoid cystic carcinoma of the lacrimal gland in a six-year-old girl. Pediatr Pathol 1993; 13: 559–65.

54. Font RL, Gamel JW. Epithelial tumors of the lacrimal gland: an analysis of 256 cases. In: Jakobiec FA, ed. Ocular and Adnexae Tumors. Birmingham: Aesculapius; 1978.

55. Dagher G, Anderson RL, Ossoinig KC, et al. Adenoid cystic carcinoma of the lacrimal gland in a child. Arch Ophthalmol 1980; 98: 1098–1100.

56. Shields JA, Bakewell B, Augsburger JJ, et al. Space occupying orbital masses in children. A review of 250 consecutive biopsies. Ophthalmology 1986; 93: 379–84.

57. Rootman J. Diseases of the Orbit: A Multidisciplinary Approach. 2nd edn. Philadelphia: Lippincott Williams & Wilkins; 2003.

58. Kennerdell JS, Dresner SC. The nonspecific orbital inflammatory syndromes. Surv Ophthalmol 1984; 29: 93–103.
59. Kincaid MC, Green WR. Ocular and orbital involvement in leukemia. Surv Ophthalmol 1983; 15: 123–6.
60. Krohel GB, Stewart WB, Chavis RM. Orbital Disease–a Practical Approach. New York: Grune and Stratton; 1981.

CHAPTER 38 Histiocytic, Hematopoietic and Lymphoproliferative Disorders

Christopher J Lyons and Jack Rootman

The term "histiocytosis" describes an abnormal proliferation of cells derived from the monocyte-phagocyte system in different tissues of the body. It is divided into two main groups; in Langerhans cell histiocytosis (histiocytosis X) the abnormal histiocytes are derived from Langerhans cells, which are involved in antigen presentation.[1,2] These cells have characteristic inclusions which are visible on electron microscopy. Non-Langerhans histiocytosis results from proliferation of histiocytes of different origin which lack these inclusion granules.

Our understanding of the histiocytic disorders is evolving. It is a monoclonal proliferation of dendritic cells that are the basis of a Langerhans cell histiocytosis, the (granular) Langerhans cell being affected through a monoclonal proliferation. Another class of dendritic cell, the dermal dendrocyte, which lacks the characteristic inclusion granules, is responsible for juvenile xanthogranuloma. The macrophage system, a third type of histiocytic cell, gives rise, through a polyclonal proliferation, to sinus histiocytosis which is also known as Rosai–Dorfman disease.[3] These three histiocytic disorders will be discussed in this chapter.

LANGERHANS CELL HISTIOCYTOSIS (HISTIOCYTOSIS X)

Langerhans cell histiocytosis (LCH) is an uncommon disorder, characterized by focal proliferation of abnormal histiocytes. Langerhans cells are dendritic histiocytes with minimal phagocytic capacity, involved in immune surveillance. Normally situated in the epidermis, they migrate to regional lymph nodes after antigen encounter, where they participate in antigen presentation.[4,5] LCH lesions are destructive and space-occupying producing a clinical picture that varies with site and the tissue involved. In children, the disease most commonly affects bones, especially those involved in hematopoiesis, and skin. Lesions tend also to occur in the other organs which normally contain histiocytes and macrophages such as the spleen, liver, lymph nodes and lung. Molecular techniques have demonstrated that this is a monoclonal neoplastic disorder[6] arising from a somatic mutation in a Langerhans cell or its precursor. The resultant clinical picture might vary according to the number of mutations within the cell, the role of immune surveillance and the site of origin of the affected cell.

Alfred Hand[7] first reported polyuria, exophthalmia and skull destruction in a 3-year-old in 1893. Over time, conditions describing the spectrum of histiocytic disease were given eponymous names with a complex nomenclature. Eventually, three different clinical disorders were described. The first was eosinophilic granuloma, in which the lesions were confined to bone, typically in children 4–7 years of age. The second, usually affecting younger patients, was a more widespread and aggressive disorder named Hand–Schuller–Christian disease. Multifocal lesions at the skull base resulted in the triad of diabetes insipidus (from infiltration of the hypothalamus and/or posterior pituitary), exophthalmos and bony defects of the skull. The third, often affecting children under 2 years of age, was characterized by multisystem involvement including cutaneous, lymph node, visceral, ocular and orbital disease. This, the most aggressive end of the LCH spectrum, was known as Letterer–Siwe disease and was frequently fatal. Since the histopathological changes found in the three groups were indistinguishable,[8] and there was also considerable clinical overlap between them, Lichtenstein[9] recognized these were different clinical expressions of a single disease process. To emphasize the common cell of origin as well as the unknown etiology, he called the whole group "histiocytosis X". The term "Langerhans cell histiocytosis" replaced histiocytosis X in 1987, differentiating conditions in which the abnormal histiocytes are derived from the Langerhans cell from the other histiocytic disorders. LCH has been subdivided clinically into (1) single system disease, which may be limited to a single site, or involve multiple sites and (2) multisystem disease.[10,11]

Ophthalmic involvement

The most common ophthalmic presentation of LCH is with orbital involvement (Fig. 38.1),[12,13] but disease of the ocular structures and brain may also lead to ophthalmic consultation. Intraocular lesions, with infiltration of the uveal tract, are seen most frequently in infants with disseminated LCH.[14,15] Intracranial involvement may give rise to visual field defects due to infiltration of the optic nerves, chiasm or tracts. Cranial neuropathy or raised intracranial pressure[16–18] are occasional presentations.

Orbital involvement

The orbit is involved in about 20% of cases of LCH,[12,13] usually with the localized form of the disease (eosinophilic granuloma), and is rare in patients whose disease is limited to soft tissue, suggesting that the lesion usually arises in the bone.[13] They are usually situated supertemporally, with a predilection for the frontal and parietal bones as well as the greater wing of the sphenoid.[19,20] Radiologically, the lesions have a lytic appearance, with a soft tissue component causing expansion of the surrounding tissues (Figs 38.1, 38.2, 38.3). Occasionally, lytic bony lesions may be seen radiologically in the absence of any clinical signs.

Clinical features

The usual presentation is with unilateral or bilateral proptosis in a child with known LCH. Rarely, the proptosis may be extreme

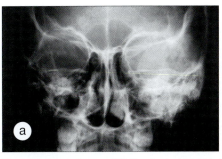 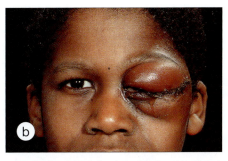 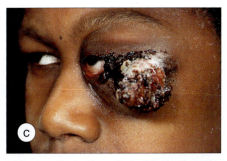

Fig. 38.1 Langerhans cell histiocytosis. (a) LCH with extensive bone hypertrophy around a chronic lesion. (b) Same patient with marked orbital involvement. The vision was unaffected. (c) Same patient with ulcerated skin lesion which ultimately responded to steroid injection, limited surgery and curettage.

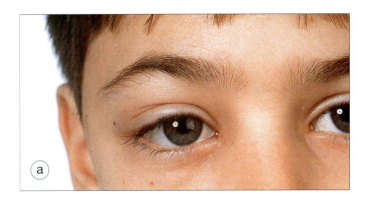 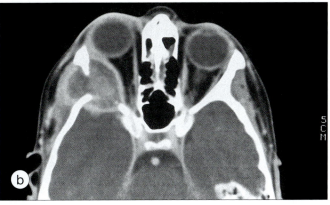

Fig. 38.2 Langerhans cell histiocytosis (LCH). (a) This 9-year-old boy presented with swelling and erythema of the right upper lid of 2 weeks duration. There was 4 mm proptosis. The CT scan (b) showed a mass which had eroded the posterolateral wall of the orbit, into the temporal fossa. Fine needle biopsy was consistent with LCH. The lesion was excised surgically and irrigated locally with corticosteroid. There was a good response to a tapering course of systemic prednisolone given in addition. Patient of the University of British Columbia.

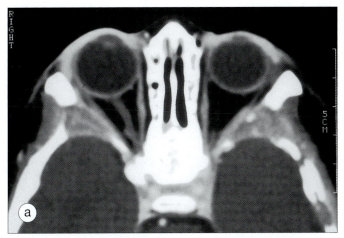 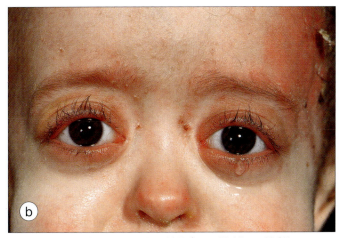

Fig. 38.3 Langerhans cell histiocytosis. (a) CT scan demonstrates extensive orbital involvement with bony erosion. (b) Patient with bilateral LCH, proptosis and obstructed nasolacrimal duct.

enough to precipitate luxation of the globe.[21] Less commonly the presentation is with isolated orbital involvement in a previously healthy child, in which case the disease is usually unilateral. Initially, the course may be evanescent and relapsing. An isolated lesion of the superior orbital wall may present with unilateral ptosis or inferonasal globe displacement. The lesions, if superficial, are generally soft to palpation. Optic nerve compression and cranial nerve palsies are rare but may be seen with extensive orbital involvement.[13,22] Skin tethering (Fig. 38.4), erythema and erosion may occur. Visual loss may be caused by optic nerve compression,[13,22] optic atrophy due to chronically raised intracranial pressure,[13] chiasmal disease[16–18] or intraocular infiltration.[15,23,24] Chronic disseminated LCH (Hand–Schuller–Christian disease) may initially present with polyuria and polydipsia, and can be associated with growth, thyroid and gonadotrophic hormone deficiencies.

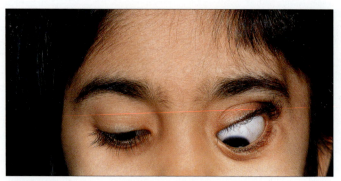

Fig. 38.4 Skin and lid tethering with orbital LCH.

Investigation

In most children with orbital disease, plain X-rays (Fig. 38.5) will demonstrate a lytic lesion of the bone. Computed tomography (CT) scan demonstrates an enhancing mass often with a low density center (Fig. 38.2b), and this, together with magnetic resonance imaging (MRI) will delineate the extent of intraorbital and intracranial involvement (Fig. 38.6). On MRI, most bony LCH lesions are hypointense on T_1-weighted images with intermediate to high signal intensity on T_2-weighted images. After contrast, most lesions show moderate to intense contrast enhancement. MRI is preferable for evaluation of intracranial extension.[25] Orbital lesions usually remain extraconal but may spread into the muscle cone.

The diagnosis is confirmed by histological examination of involved tissue. In children with multisystem disease, an accessible site such as skin or a peripheral bony site should be biopsied, but in cases with solitary orbital involvement, orbital biopsy cannot be avoided. Fine needle aspiration may be useful in these circumstances.[26] Children who present initially to the ophthalmologist should be referred to a pediatric oncologist to define the extent of any systemic involvement. Further investigations may include chest X-ray, skeletal survey, lung and liver function tests and specific gravity of early morning urine.

Examination of tissue by light microscopy reveals granulomatous infiltration consisting of histiocytes and multinucleated lipid-laden giant cells, together with eosinophils (particularly numerous in single-site bone-based lesions or "eosinophilic granulomas"), lymphocytes, plasma cells and neutrophils. Electron microscopy of the histiocytes demonstrates the presence of typical Langerhans granules also known as Birbeck or racket bodies, in about 50% of cases[27] indicating that the proliferating histiocytes are derivatives of the Langerhans cells, part of the mononuclear-phagocyte system.[28] Immunohistochemical techniques may also be helpful to secure the diagnosis.[2]

Management and prognosis

Children with LCH and orbital involvement are best managed by a pediatric oncologist in collaboration with the ophthalmologist. Advice from other specialties such as ENT and orthopedic surgery may be needed for specific problems.

The management of orbital lesions depends on whether there is single system involvement or multisystem disease.[29] Conservative management with careful observation only may be justified in patients with single site orbital onvolvement, where complete spontaneous resolution after incisional biopsy[30] or even fine needle aspiration[31] has been reported. Usually, patients with a

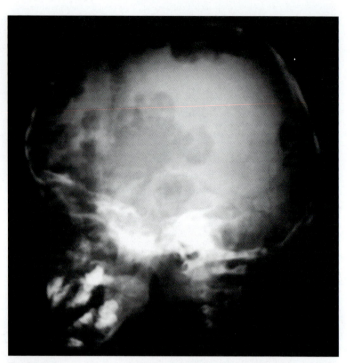

Fig. 38.5 Disseminated Langerhans cell histiocytosis with punched-out skull lesion.

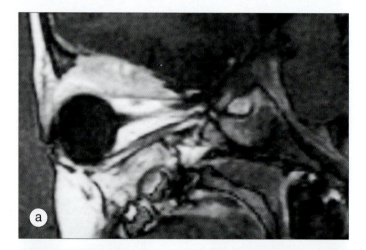

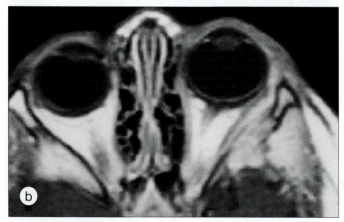

Fig. 38.6 Langerhans cell histiocytosis. (a, b) LCH showing extensive involvement of the left orbital bones.

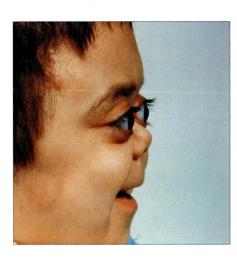

Fig. 38.7 Langerhans cell histocytosis. This patient has shallow orbits and exophthalmos due to the arrest of bony development following treatment for orbital Langerhans cell histiocytosis. Patient of the University of British Columbia. (With permission from Rootman J. Diseases of the Orbit: A Multidisciplinary Approach. 2nd edn. Philadelphia: Lippincott Williams and Wilkins; 2003: 411.)

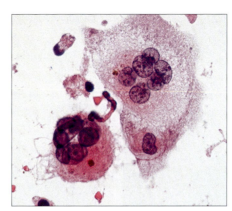

Fig. 38.8 Juvenile xanthogranuloma. Touton giant cell.

single orbital lesion are treated by biopsy and curettage resulting in resolution.[13] Intralesional steroids may also be used to hasten remission[13,32,33] or reduce pain.[34] If there is marked proptosis or evidence of optic nerve compression, a short course of systemic steroids or radiotherapy may be used to induce remission. A radiation dose of 500–600 cGy is usually sufficient. The total dose should not exceed 1000 cGy because of the risk of radiation-induced malignancies occurring in later life. Cosmetically disfiguring lesions of the orbital wall may be removed surgically with curettage of the affected bone. Orbital bone involvement frequently results in arrested growth of the walls with shallowing. This feature is not related to the use of radiotherapy (Fig. 38.7).

In patients with generalized LCH, orbital involvement will generally respond to systemic chemotherapy. Local radiotherapy may be used in addition if there is progressive proptosis or optic nerve compression. The most frequently used systemic agents are prednisolone, etoposide, VP16 and vinblastine.[29,35]

Children with single system disease, for example of the bone, have a good prognosis.[36,37] Conversely, the prognosis is poor in multisystem or visceral disease, especially if there is infiltration and failure of key organs such as the bone marrow, liver, and lungs, which may be fatal. Children under the age of 2 years have a mortality rate of 55–60%, but death is rare after the age of 3 years.[38,39] Although some authors have stressed age as the most important prognostic factor,[40] it is really the tendency of infants to develop multisystem disease rather than their age which dictates the poorer prognosis of children aged 2 years and under.[41] Response to the initial treatment of multisystem LCH appears to be a good predictor of eventual outcome.[35]

NON-LANGERHANS CELL HISTIOCYTOSIS

Juvenile xanthogranuloma

Juvenile xanthogranuloma (JXG) is a disorder of unknown etiology in which there is abnormal proliferation of non-Langerhans histiocytes. These, like Langerhans histiocytes, are probably a group of dendritic cells.[42,43] It is characteristically seen as a benign skin disorder in infants and young children and has a tendency to undergo spontaneous regression. It is more common in children with neurofibromatosis type 1 (NF1)[44] and can be the first sign of this disorder.[45] This group could be more liable to develop leukemias.[46] The skin lesions are occasionally accompanied by ocular involvement but ocular involvement can occur without cutaneous lesions. Visceral and bony involvement occurs less commonly than in LCH.[47]

Histopathology

The JXG lesion consists of a mixture of lymphocytes, plasma cells, histiocytes, giant cells and occasional eosinophils. The distinctive histological feature, however, is the presence of Touton giant cells, in which a central ring of nuclei encloses an area of eosinophilic cytoplasm surrounded by a foamy cytoplasm (Fig. 38.8). An important electron microscopic feature is the absence of Langerhans (Birbeck) granules in the histiocytes, distinguishing these lesions from LCH. Immunohistochemistry of JXG is positive for vimentin, CD 68 and factor XIIIa immunostains and negative for S100 protein, helping to differentiate this condition from other histiocytic proliferations.[42]

Ocular involvement

As its name suggests, JXG predominantly occurs in infancy and early childhood; in Zimmerman's series[47] 85% of patients with ocular involvement were less than 1 year old and 64% less than 8 months. It has been reported in neonates.[48,49] Patients with ocular disease may also occasionally present in adult life.[50,51] Most have unilateral disease although a few cases with bilateral involvement have been reported.[52,53] Cutaneous lesions are relatively benign and often self-limited whilst ocular involvement can result in glaucoma and visual loss from optic nerve damage or amblyopia; however, since only three or four patients of every 1000 with cutaneous JXG develop ocular complications, routine eye screening would not be productive.[54] Chang et al.[54] argued that this could be limited to children with cutaneous involvement under 2 years of age, whose risk of ocular involvement is highest.

Uveal involvement

The iris is infiltrated in the majority of cases[47,51,53,55–57]; the ciliary body,[47,52,55] or rarely the choroid and retina,[58,59] may also be affected. Rarely, juvenile xanthogranuloma can masquerade as uveitis in childhood in the absence of skin lesions.[58,60]

Zimmermann[47] has reviewed the main presenting signs. Typically, a localized or diffuse yellow or fluffy-white iris lesion is evident in one eye of an infant, (Fig. 38.9) accompanied by hyphema (Fig. 38.10). Glaucoma, with corneal edema, photophobia, ocular enlargement and circumcorneal flush are frequently present. There may be some uveitis and a xanthochromic flare. In some cases, iris heterochromia is the only presenting sign.

Although typically yellow or creamy-white, the iris lesion may occasionally be very vascular and can therefore be mistaken for a

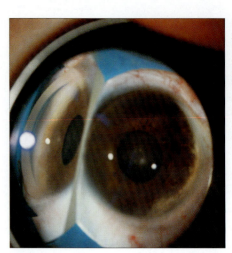

Fig. 38.9 Juvenile xanthogranuloma. Gonioscopy view showing the angle filled with yellowish xanthogranuloma material. It can also be seen in the bottom right of the picture directly.

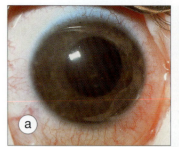
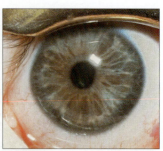
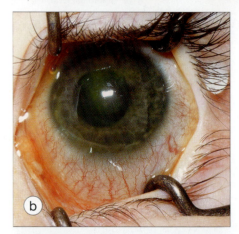
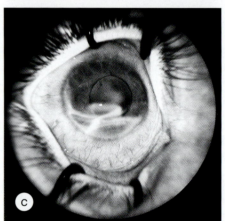
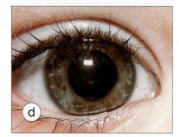
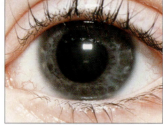

hemangioma. The main differential diagnosis of spontaneous hyphema in childhood includes the following:

1. Trauma (unrecognized or with abuse).
2. Tumor (retinoblastoma, dictyoma, LCH, leukemia, neuroblastoma).
3. Rubeosis (secondary to retinopathy of prematurity, retinal dysplasia, persistent hyperplastic primary vitreous (PHPV)).
4. Iris arteriovenous malformation.

Management

If cutaneous lesions are present in a patient with an iris lesion, a diagnosis of JXG is best confirmed by skin biopsy. In cases without cutaneous involvement of eye lesions, examination of aqueous from a paracentesis may show typical histiocytes. Diagnostic iris biopsy should be avoided if possible because of the risk of hemorrhage.

Several different methods of treatment have been advocated for uveal lesions, including topical and systemic steroids,[48] radiotherapy and surgical excision. Medical treatment is preferable because of the risk of extensive hemorrhage following excision. A reasonable approach is to try a short course of topical,[61] subconjunctival[62] and/or systemic steroids[63] to induce remission, adding a topical beta-blocker or carbonic anhydrase inhibitor if the intraocular pressure is raised. If there is no response to steroids, radiotherapy (at a dose not exceeding 500 cGy) should be used.[63]

Optic nerve and retinal involvement

Wertz et al.[59] reported a 20-month-old infant who presented with iris heterochromia in the absence of skin lesions. Hemorrhagic infarction of the retina was accompanied by rubeosis. Histological examination of the enucleated eye revealed massive infiltration of the optic nerve, disc, retina and choroid with histiocytes. Touton giant cells, diagnostic of JXG, were also present.

Epibulbar lesions

Conjunctival (Fig. 38.11), episcleral and corneal involvement in JXG is uncommon. This presents as a limbal nodule whose color has been described as yellow, orange or pink.[64] This may grow to some extent over as well as around the cornea, and may accompany intraocular involvement.[65] It may also appear as a yellowish or yellowish-pink subconjunctival mass, which could be mistaken for subconjunctival lymphoma.[47] Progressive lesions may be

Fig. 38.10 Juvenile xanthogranuloma. (a–c) Presumed juvenile xanthogranuloma. The patient had presented because of recurrent left hyphema resulting in glaucoma. There was iris vascularization with profuse fluorescein leakage but no frank mass formation. (d) One year later. After 350 cGy radiotherapy there was a very marked improvement and after a period of occlusion of the right eye the acuity was 6/6. No recurrence occurred over the next 9 years.

treated in the same way as uveal lesions, with topical or systemic steroids or radiotherapy. Bleeding is occasionally troublesome if the lesion is excised[66] and recurrence is a possibility; Collum et al.[66] recommended keratectomy with lamellar grafting for these.

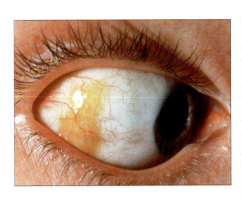

Fig. 38.11 Juvenile xanthogranuloma. A slowly enlarging yellowish lesion was noticed in the conjunctiva of this 15-year-old boy. Histology showed Touton giant cells, characteristic of juvenile xanthogranuloma. Patient of the University of British Columbia.

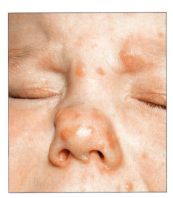

Fig. 38.12 Juvenile xanthogranuloma with skin lesions. Both eyes were glaucomatous (see Chapter 40).

Involvement of the ocular adnexae

The typical skin lesions (Fig. 38.12) early in the course of the disease are tense yellow to reddish-brown papules. Later, these become softer and orange or yellow-brown in color. Since they have a predilection for the face, neck and trunk, it is not surprising that they are common on the eyelids. Occasionally, a single lid lesion is the only manifestation of JXG and biopsy may be necessary to make a diagnosis. The nodules usually regress spontaneously within a year but may occasionally persist for several years.

Orbital involvement in JXG is uncommon,[47,58,67–70] and is one of the causes of unilateral proptosis in infancy. Most of the cases have presented within the first 6 months of life, often in the absence of cutaneous findings. JXG has been described arising in the lacrimal sac fossa as a mass causing nasolacrimal duct obstruction in a 2-year-old.[71] The extraocular muscles may be infiltrated, resulting in strabismus and limitation of ocular movement.[47,68] In contrast to LCH, bony destruction is unusual but may occur.[70] Intracranial involvement is also well-documented, with a clinical course which ranges from spontaneous regression to fatal progression.[43,72,73] If there are no other systemic features it may be difficult to differentiate between JXG and LCH clinically, but light and electron microscopy are diagnostic. The lungs, liver, spleen, gastrointestinal tract and pericardium may also be affected.[74] Freyer et al.[43] have reviewed systemic involvement in JXG and stress that, unlike its cutaneous form, significant complications may arise from this disease.

As JXG has a tendency to undergo spontaneous remission, patients with orbital involvement should initially be observed. Patients with progressive proptosis or marked restriction of ocular motility should be given a short course of systemic steroids to induce remission.[70] If there is no response to this, low-dose radiotherapy (500 cGy) should be given. The visual and systemic prognosis are usually excellent.

SINUS HISTIOCYTOSIS WITH MASSIVE LYMPHADENOPATHY (ROSAI–DORFMAN DISEASE)

Rosai and Dorfman first used the name "sinus histiocytosis with massive lymphadenopathy" in 1969 to describe a group of patients. Known since then as sinus histiocytosis or Rosai–Dorfman disease, this idiopathic disorder mainly affects children and young adults. In the series of 113 patients reported by Foucar et al.,[75] the average age was 8.6 years. The cause is unknown. Massive painless cervical lymphadenopathy is present in the vast majority of patients, often with enlargement of other lymph node groups. About 43% of patients have involvement of extranodal sites;[76] in a newer Foucar et al. series,[76] 8.5% of patients with sinus histiocytosis had orbital or eyelid involvement. The upper respiratory tract, salivary gland, skin, testes and bone can also be affected. The lymphadenopathy is accompanied by fever, neutrophil leukocytosis, polyclonal hypergammaglobulinemia and a raised erythrocyte sedimentation rate.[77] The signs and symptoms may persist for months or years before recovery.[78]

Patients with ophthalmic involvement usually present with unilateral or bilateral proptosis. The condition infiltrates the soft tissues of the orbit, without bony involvement[75,79,80] occasionally affecting both lacrimal glands[81] or all four eyelids.[82] The tumor mass usually remains extraconal so optic nerve compression is rare but there may be a duction deficit.[77] Less commonly there is an epibulbar mass without proptosis.[80,83] Progressive proptosis may lead to corneal exposure, ulceration and even endophthalmitis.[75,79] Involvement of the lids is common and rarely there may be intraocular lesions with infiltration of the uveal tract by histiocytes.[75] Relapsing uveitis is an occasional feature which may precede the lymphadenopathy by years.[84] The lack of bony and visceral involvement helps to differentiate this condition from LCH.

Histopathological examination of orbital biopsy specimens show a dense cellular infiltrate of histiocytes, lymphocytes and plasma cells surrounded by connective tissue. The histiocytes often show intracellular phagocytosed lymphocytes and plasma cells, possibly suggesting a macrophage-related cell line of origin.[3] Electron microscopy fails to demonstrate the typical Birbeck inclusion granules of Langerhans cells, differentiating this condition from LCH, though, like Langerhans cells, the cells are S100-positive and may express CD1a antigen.[3] Malignant lymphoma is an important differential diagnosis.

There is no general agreement regarding the treatment of this disorder; high-dose systemic steroids, systemic chemotherapeutic agents such as vinblastine and methotrexate, and radiotherapy[85] have all been used without consistent success. The management of orbital involvement should include frequent assessment of vision and the maintenance of adequate corneal care. Progressive proptosis causing exposure keratitis may require orbital decompression.[75,79] The orbital disease tends to be chronic with occasional recurrences, but overall the systemic prognosis is good; there was one death in Foucar et al.'s series[75] which may have been related to complications from systemic chemotherapy. Involvement of kidneys, lungs, liver or associated immunological disease may be poor prognostic features.[76]

LEUKEMIA

The eye, like the brain, is a relative "pharmacological sanctuary" in the treatment of leukemia. It is not surprising therefore that recurrent disease frequently manifests within the eye or central nervous system. Orbital involvement may be the first manifestation or part of disseminated leukemia.

Leukemia accounted for 11% of the 27 cases of unilateral proptosis in children reported by Oakhill et al.[86] It was second only to rhabdomyosarcoma in frequency of childhood malignant orbital disease in Porterfield's[87] series. The orbit is more commonly involved in acute than chronic leukemia and, in children, by myeloblastic than lymphoblastic tumors. Ridgway et al.[88] examined 657 children with acute leukemia and found clinical evidence of orbital involvement in 1%. Kincaid and Green[89] found post mortem evidence of orbital involvement in 10% of 384 patients.

The clinical features of orbital leukemic involvement include proptosis, lid edema, chemosis and pain.[90] Both orbits are involved in 2% of patients with orbital leukemia. The proptosis may be due either to a mass of leukemic cells or to orbital hemorrhage,[91] which may also appear subconjunctivally and cause eyelid discoloration (Fig. 38.13).[92] Other diseases which may present with rapidly increasing proptosis, chemosis and hemorrhage must be considered in the differential diagnosis. These include rhabdomyosarcoma, neuroblastoma, Ewing sarcoma and orbital cellulitis.[89,91] Leukemia may present with intraocular involvement in childhood, with conjunctival injection, hypopyon and glaucoma.[93]

Orbital leukemic deposits are often associated with meningeal involvement[88] and are part of terminal disease,[87,88] although in some cases orbital signs may be the presenting feature of leukemia (chloroma) and biopsy provides the diagnosis. The lacrimal gland[94] or, more rarely, the extraocular muscles[89] may be infiltrated and contiguous sinus disease is a common post mortem finding. The orbit is occasionally the site of opportunistic infection by bacteria or fungi in immunosuppressed leukemic children.[95] Iatrogenic complications include ptosis and extraocular muscle palsy from the use of cytotoxic agents such as vincristine.[96]

Leukemic deposits consist of cells derived either from lymphoblasts or myeloblasts. A localized form of acute myeloblastic leukemia has a predilection for the orbit where it presents as a rapidly expanding tumor. This was initially called "chloroma", a reference to its greenish color from the pigmented enzyme myeloperoxidase. The terms "myeloblastoma" and "granulocytic sarcoma" are now preferred. Granulocytic sarcoma may appear at any time in the course of myeloblastic leukemia and occasionally may precede the generalized leukemic process by weeks or months.[97–99] Histologically, it is a poorly differentiated high-grade malignancy which should be distinguished from the other round cell tumors of childhood. Its main diagnostic differential, large B-cell lymphoma (also referred to as histiocytic lymphoma or reticulum cell sarcoma) is very much rarer in children. If necessary, esterase stains may be useful to identify myelocytic differentiation in granulocytic sarcoma.[100]

Granulocytic sarcoma carries a poor prognosis: 19 of 32 affected patients reported by Zimmerman and Font[94] had died within 30 months of the onset of ophthalmic signs.

Treatment of orbital leukemia is by systemic chemotherapy and local irradiation, although the dose and effect of the latter (reviewed by Kincaid and Green[89]) are not clearly defined. Orbital disease in children with acute leukemia still carries a poor prognosis despite chemotherapy and radiotherapy.[89]

LYMPHOMA

Knowles et al.[101] stated in 1983 that they had never seen orbital lymphoma as part of systemic nodal disease in children, attesting to the rarity of this disorder in childhood. It seems however that the incidence of lymphoma is increasing in the general population for reasons which are currently not understood.[102] There are individual case reports of childhood orbital involvement by B, T and null cell lymphomas[103–105] and the orbit is recognized as a site for post-transplantation lymphoproliferative disorders[106], but the only lymphoma with a predilection for the child, and in particular the head and neck region is Burkitt lymphoma.

This high-grade undifferentiated lymphocytic tumor most commonly affects children in tropical Africa but occurs sporadically worldwide. The Epstein–Barr virus acts as an oncogene in patients who have been immunologically stimulated by chronic exposure to malaria organisms.[107] The tumor affects males more commonly than females (2:1 ratio), with a median age of 7 years at presentation. In 60% of African cases, there is a maxillary tumor causing massive proptosis, but this may only appear late in the disease, since only 13% of patients present with exophthalmos. Non-African cases tend to present later (median age 11 years)

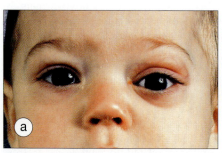
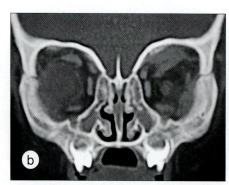
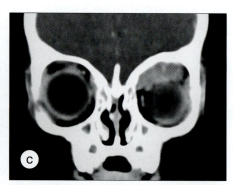

Fig. 38.13 Leukemia. (a) This 10-month-old boy presented with 3-week history of cough, irritability and puffy eyes. X-rays showed pneumonia, and CBC revealed pancytopenia. He had bilateral palpebral lid masses with downward displacement of the left globe and blue-yellow discoloration of the lid. (b, c) CT scan demonstrates a left irregular orbital mass superiorly and inferolaterally, extending to the apex where the bone was irregular. Biopsy demonstrated chloroma and cytogenetics confirmed a diagnosis of AML M5 with marrow involvement. Patient of the University of British Columbia.

with a greater propensity for abdominal involvement, although the head and neck region can be involved in this group.[108,109] Burkitt lymphoma may also present with cranial nerve palsies or papilledema from central nervous system involvement. Younger patients, and those with localized disease have a better prognosis. The tumor responds to chemotherapy with prolonged remission and some patients are reported to show immunological self-cure.[100]

REFERENCES

1. Rowden G. The Langerhans cell. Crit Rev Immunol 1981; 3: 95–180.
2. Pinkus GS, Lones MA, Matsumura F, et al. Langerhans cell histiocytosis immunohistochemical expression of fascin, a dendritic cell marker. Am J Clin Pathol 2002; 118: 335–43.
3. Favara BE, Feller AC, Pauli M, et al. Contemporary classification of histiocytic disorders. The WHO Committee on Histiocytic/Reticulum Cell Proliferations. Reclassification Working Group of the Histiocyte Society. Med Pediatr Oncol 1997; 29: 157–66.
4. Schmitz L, Favara BE. Nosology and pathology of Langerhans cell histiocytosis. Hematol/Oncol Clin North Am 1998; 12: 221–46.
5. Herzog KM, Tubbs RR. Langerhans cell histiocytosis. Adv Anat Pathol 1998; 5: 347–58.
6. Willman CL, Busque L, Griffith BB, et al. Langerhans'-cell histiocytosis (histiocytosis X)–a clonal proliferative disease. N Eng J Med 1994; 331: 154–60.
7. Hand AR. Polyuria and tuberculosis. Arch Pediatr 1893; 10: 673–5.
8. Risdall RJ, Dehner LP, Duray P, et al. Histiocytosis X (Langerhans' cell histiocytosis). Prognostic role of histopathology. Arch Pathol Lab Med 1983; 107: 59–63.
9. Lichtenstein L. Histiocytosis X; integration of eosinophilic granuloma of bone, Letterer–Siwe disease, and Schuller–Christian disease as related manifestations of a single nosologic entity. AMA Arch Pathol 1953; 56: 84–102.
10. Broadbent V, Gadner H, Komp DM, et al. Histiocytosis syndromes in children: II. Approach to the clinical and laboratory evaluation of children with Langerhans cell histiocytosis. Clinical Writing Group of the Histiocyte Society. Med Pediatr Oncol 1989; 17: 492–5.
11. Chu T, D'Angio GJ, Favara BE, et al. Histiocytosis syndromes in children. Lancet 1987; 2: 41–2.
12. Oberman HA. A clinicopathologic study of 40 cases and review of the literature on eosinophilic granuloma of bone. Hand–Schuller–Christian disease and Letterer–Siwe disease. Pediatrics 1961; 28: 307–27.
13. Moore AT, Pritchard J, Taylor DS. Histiocytosis X: an ophthalmological review. Br J Ophthalmol 1985; 69: 7–14.
14. Lahav M, Albert DM. Unusual ocular involvement in acute disseminated histiocytosis X. Arch Ophthalmol 1974; 91: 455–8.
15. Epstein DL, Grant WM. Secondary open-angle glaucoma in histiocytosis X. Am J Ophthalmol 1977; 84: 332–6.
16. Goodman RH, Post KD, Molitch ME, et al. Eosinophilic granuloma mimicking a pituitary tumor. Neurosurgery 1979; 5: 723–5.
17. Kepes JJ, Kepes M. Predominantly cerebral forms of histiocytosis-X. A reappraisal of "Gagel's hypothalamic granuloma", "granuloma infiltrans of the hypothalamus" and "Ayala's disease" with a report of four cases. Acta Neuropathol 1969; 14: 77–98.
18. Bernard JD, Aguilar MJ. Localized hypothalamic histiocytosis X. Report of a case. Arch Neurol 1969; 20: 368–72.
19. Kramer TR, Noecker RJ, Miller JM, et al. Langerhans cell histiocytosis with orbital involvement. Am J Ophthalmol 1997; 124: 814–24.
20. Rootman J. Diseases of the Orbit: A Multidisciplinary Approach. 2nd edn. Philadelphia: Lippincott Williams & Wilkins; 2003.
21. Wood CM, Pearson AD, Craft AW, et al. Globe luxation in histiocytosis X. Br J Ophthalmol 1988; 72: 631–3.
22. Beller AJ, Kornbleuth W. Eosinophilic granuloma of the orbit. Br J Ophthalmol 1951; 35: 220–5.
23. Mozziconacci P, Offret G, Forest A, et al. Histiocytose X avec lesions oculaires etude anatomique. Ann Pediatr 1966; 13: 348–55.
24. Rupp RH, Holloman KR. Histiocytosis X affecting the uveal tract. Arch Ophthalmol 1970; 84: 468–70.
25. Koch BL. Langerhans histiocytosis of temporal bone: role of magnetic resonance imaging. Top Magn Reson Imaging 2000; 11: 66–74.
26. Harbour JW, Char DH, Ljung BM, et al. Langerhans cell histiocytosis diagnosed by fine needle biopsy. Arch Ophthalmol 1997; 115: 1212–3.
27. Nezelof C, Frileux-Herbet F, Cronier-Sachot J. Disseminated histiocytosis X: analysis of prognostic factors based on a retrospective study of 50 cases. Cancer 1979; 44: 1824–38.
28. Katz SI, Tamaki K, Sachs DH. Epidermal Langerhans cells are derived from cells originating in bone marrow. Nature 1979; 282: 324–6.
29. Broadbent V, Gadner H. Current therapy for Langerhans cell histiocytosis. Hematol/Oncol Clin North Am 1998; 12: 327–38.
30. Glover AT, Grove AS, Jr. Eosinophilic granuloma of the orbit with spontaneous healing. Ophthalmology 1987; 94: 1008–12.
31. Smith JH, Fulton L, O'Brien JM. Spontaneous regression of orbital Langerhans cell granulomatosis in a three-year-old girl. Am J Ophthalmol 1999; 128: 119–21.
32. Wirtschafter JD, Nesbit M, Anderson P, et al. Intralesional methylprednisolone for Langerhans' cell histiocytosis of the orbit and cranium. J Pediatr Ophthalmol Strabismus 1987; 24: 194–7.
33. Kindy-Degnan NA, Laflamme P, Duprat G, et al. Intralesional steroid in the treatment of an orbital eosinophilic granuloma. Arch Ophthalmol 1991; 109: 617–8.
34. Egeler RM, Thompson RC, Jr, Voute PA, et al. Intralesional infiltration of corticosteroids in localized Langerhans' cell histiocytosis. J Pediatr Orthop 1992; 12: 811–4.
35. Minkov M, Grois N, Heitger A, et al. Response to initial treatment of multisystem Langerhans cell histiocytosis: an important prognostic indicator. Med Pediatr Oncol 2002; 39: 581–5.
36. Pritchard J. Histiocytosis X: natural history and management in childhood. Clin Exp Dermatol 1979; 4: 421–33.
37. Broadbent V. Favourable prognostic features in histiocytosis X: bone involvement and absence of skin disease. Arch Dis Child 1986; 61: 1219–21.
38. Lucaya J. Histiocytosis X. Am J Dis Child 1971; 121: 289–95.
39. Lahey ME. Histiocytosis X–comparison of three treatment regimens. J Pediatr 1975; 87: 179–83.
40. Greenberger JS, Crocker AC, Vawter G, et al. Results of treatment of 127 patients with systemic histiocytosis. Medicine 1981; 60: 311–38.
41. Nezelof C, Barbey S. Histiocytosis: nosology and pathobiology. Pediatr Pathol 1985; 3: 1–41.
42. Dehner LP. Juvenile xanthogranulomas in the first two decades of life: a clinicopathologic study of 174 cases with cutaneous and extracutaneous manifestations. Am J Surg Pathol 2003; 27: 579–93.
43. Freyer DR, Kennedy R, Bostrom BC, et al. Juvenile xanthogranuloma: forms of systemic disease and their clinical implications. J Pediatr 1996; 129: 227–37.
44. Morier P, Merot Y, Paccaud D, et al. Juvenile chronic granulocytic leukemia, juvenile xanthogranulomas, and neurofibromatosis. Case report and review of the literature. J Am Acad Dermatol 1990; 22: 962–5.
45. Algros MP, Laithier V, Montard M, et al. Juvenile xanthogranuloma of the iris as the first manifestation of a neurofibromatosis. J Pediatr Ophthalmol Strabismus 2003; 40: 166–7.
46. Riccardi VM. Neurofibromatosis: Phenotype, Natural History, and Pathogenesis. 2nd edn. Baltimore: Johns Hopkins University; 1992.
47. Zimmerman LE. Ocular lesions of juvenile xanthogranuloma. Nevoxanthoedothelioma. Am J Ophthalmol 1965; 60: 1011–35.
48. Casteels I, Olver J, Malone M, et al. Early treatment of juvenile xanthogranuloma of the iris with subconjunctival steroids. Br J Ophthalmol 1993; 77: 57–60.
49. Raz J, Sinnreich Z, Freund M, et al. Congenital uveal xanthogranuloma. J Pediatr Ophthalmol Strabismus 1999; 36: 344–6.

50. Rouhiainen H, Nerdrum K, Puustjarvi T, et al. Xanthogranuloma juvenile–a rare cause of orbital swelling in adulthood. Ophthalmologica 1992; 204: 162–5.

51. Brenkman RF, Oosterhuis JA, Manschot WA. Recurrent hemorrhage in the anterior chamber caused by a (juvenile) xanthogranuloma of the iris in an adult. Doc Ophthalmol 1977; 42: 329–33.

52. Smith ME, Sanders TE, Bresnick GH. Juvenile xanthogranuloma of the ciliary body in an adult. Arch Ophthalmol 1969; 81: 813–4.

53. Hadden OB. Bilateral juvenile xanthogranuloma of the iris. Br J Ophthalmol 1975; 59: 699–702.

54. Chang MW, Frieden IJ, Good W. The risk intraocular juvenile xanthogranuloma: survey of current practices and assessment of risk. J Am Acad Dermatol 1996; 34: 445–9.

55. Sanders TE. Intraocular juvenile xanthogranuloma (nevoxanthogranuloma): a survey of 20 cases. Trans Am Ophthalmol Soc 1960; 58: 59–74.

56. Gass JD. Management of juvenile xanthogranuloma of the iris. Arch Ophthalmol 1964; 71: 344–7.

57. Smith JLS, Ingram RM. Juvenile oculodermal xanthogranuloma. Br J Ophthalmol 1968; 52: 696–703.

58. DeBarge LR, Chan CC, Greenberg SC, et al. Chorioretinal, iris, and ciliary body infiltration by juvenile xanthogranuloma masquerading as uveitis. Surv Ophthalmol 1994; 39: 65–71.

59. Wertz FD, Zimmerman LE, McKeown CA, et al. Juvenile xanthogranuloma of the optic nerve, disc, retina, and choroid. Ophthalmology 1982; 89: 1331–5.

60. Zamir E, Wang RC, Krishnakumar S, et al. Juvenile xanthogranuloma masquerading as pediatric chronic uveitis: a clinicopathologic study. Surv Ophthalmol 2001; 46: 164–71.

61. Clements DB. Juvenile xanthogranuloma treated with local steroids. Br J Ophthalmol 1966; 50: 663–5.

62. Treacy KW, Letson RD, Summers CG. Subconjunctival steroid in the management of uveal juvenile xanthogranuloma: a case report. J Pediatr Ophthalmol Strabismus 1990; 27: 126–8.

63. Harley RD, Romayananda N, Chan GH. Juvenile xanthogranuloma. J Pediatr Ophthalmol Strabismus 1982; 19: 33–9.

64. Yanoff M, Perry HD. Juvenile xanthogranuloma of the corneoscleral limbus. Arch Ophthalmol 1995; 113: 915–7.

65. Rad AS, Kheradvar A. Juvenile xanthogranuloma: concurrent involvement of skin and eye. Cornea 2001; 20: 760–2.

66. Collum LM, Power WJ, Mullaney J, et al. Limbal xanthogranuloma. J Pediatr Ophthalmol Strabismus 1991; 28: 157–9.

67. Sanders TE, Miller JE. Infantile xanthogranuloma of the orbit. Trans Am Acad Ophthalmol Otolaryngol 1965; 69: 458–64.

68. Sanders TE. Infantile xanthogranuloma of the orbit. A report of three cases. Am J Ophthalmol 1966; 61: 1299–306.

69. Shields CL, Shields JA, Buchanon HW. Solitary orbital involvement with juvenile xanthogranuloma. Arch Ophthalmol 1990; 108: 1587–9.

70. Gaynes PM, Cohen GS. Juvenile xanthogranuloma of the orbit. Am J Ophthalmol 1967; 63: 755–7.

71. Mruthyunjaya P, Meyer DR. Juvenile xanthogranuloma of the lacrimal sac fossa. Am J Ophthalmol 1997; 123: 400–2.

72. Bostrom J, Janssen G, Messing-Junger M, et al. Multiple intracranial juvenile xanthogranulomas. Case report. J Neurosurg 2000; 93: 335–41.

73. Okubo T, Okabe H, Kato G. Juvenile xanthogranuloma with cutaneous and cerebral manifestations in a young infant. Acta Neuropathol 1995; 90: 87–92.

74. Webster SB, Reister HC, Harman LE, Jr. Juvenile xanthogranuloma with extracutaneous lesions. A case report and review of the literature. Arch Dermatol 1966;93:71–6.

75. Foucar E, Rosai J, Dorfman RF. The ophthalmologic manifestations of sinus histiocytosis with massive lymphadenopathy. Am J Ophthalmol 1979; 87: 354–67.

76. Foucar E, Rosai J, Dorfman R. Sinus histiocytosis with massive lymphadenopathy (Rosai–Dorfman disease): review of the entity. Semin Diag Pathol 1990; 7: 19–73.

77. Brau RH, Sosa IJ, Marcial-Seoane MA. Sinus histiocytosis with massive lymphadenopathy (Rosai–Dorfman disease) and extranodal involvement of the orbit. P R Health Sci J 1995; 14: 145–9.

78. Rosai J, Dorfman RF. Sinus histiocytosis with massive lymphadenopathy: a pseudolymphomatous benign disorder. Analysis of 34 cases. Cancer 1972; 30: 1174–88.

79. Friendly DS, Font RL, Rao NA. Orbital involvement in "sinus" histiocytosis. A report of four cases. Arch Ophthalmol 1977; 95: 2006–11.

80. Karcioglu ZA, Allam B, Insler MS. Ocular involvement in sinus histiocytosis with massive lymphadenopathy. Br J Ophthalmol 1988; 72: 793–5.

81. Lee-Wing M, Oryschak A, Attariwala G, et al. Rosai–Dorfman disease presenting as bilateral lacrimal gland enlargement. Am J Ophthalmol 2001; 131: 677–8.

82. Levinger S, Pe'er J, Aker M, et al. Rosai–Dorfman disease involving four eyelids. Am J Ophthalmol 1993; 116: 382–4.

83. Stopak SS, Dreizen NG, Zimmerman LE, et al. Sinus histiocytosis presenting as an epibulbar mass. A clinicopathologic case report. Arch Ophthalmol 1988; 106: 1426–8.

84. Pivetti-Pezzi P, Torce C, Colabelli-Gisoldi RA, et al. Relapsing bilateral uveitis and papilledema in sinus histiocytosis with massive lymphadenopathy (Rosai–Dorfman disease). Eur J Ophthalmol 1995; 5: 59–62.

85. Childs HA, 3rd, Kim RY. Radiation response of Rosai–Dorfman disease presenting with involvement of the orbits. Am J Clin Oncol 1999; 22: 526–8.

86. Oakhill A, Willshaw H, Mann JR. Unilateral proptosis. Arch Dis Child 1981; 56: 549–51.

87. Porterfield JF. Orbital tumors in children: a report on 214 cases. Intern Ophthalmol Clin 1962; 2: 319–26.

88. Ridgway EW, Jaffe N, Walton DS. Leukemic ophthalmopathy in children. Cancer 1976; 38: 1744–9.

89. Kincaid MC, Green WR. Ocular and orbital involvement in leukemia. Surv Ophthalmol 1983; 15: 123–6.

90. Cavdar AO, Gozdasoglu S, Arcasoy A, et al. Chlorama-like ocular manifestations in Turkish children with acute myelomonocytic leukaemia. Lancet 1971; 1: 680–2.

91. Jha BK, Lamba PA. Proptosis as a manifestation of acute myeloid leukaemia. Br J Ophthalmol 1971; 55: 844–7.

92. Rosenthal AR. Ocular manifestations of leukemia. A review. Ophthalmology 1983; 90: 899–905.

93. Ells A, Clarke WN, Noel LP. Pseudohypopyon in acute myelogenous leukemia. J Pediatr Ophthalmol Strabismus 1995; 32: 123–4.

94. Zimmerman LE, Font RL. Ophthalmologic manifestations of granulocytic sarcoma (myeloid sarcoma or chloroma). The third Pan American Association of Ophthalmology and American Journal of Ophthalmology Lecture. Am J Ophthalmol 1975; 80: 975–90.

95. Rubinfeld RS, Gootenberg JE, Chavis RM, et al. Early onset acute orbital involvement in childhood acute lymphoblastic leukemia. Ophthalmology 1988; 95: 116–20.

96. Nicholson DH, Green WR. Pediatric Ocular Tumors. New York: Masson; 1981.

97. Rajantie J, Tarkkanen A, Rapola J, et al. Orbital granulocytic sarcoma as a presenting sign in acute myelogenous leukemia. Ophthalmologica 1984; 189: 158–61.

98. Puri P, Grover AK. Granulocytic sarcoma of orbit preceding acute myeloid leukaemia: a case report. Eur J Cancer Care 1999; 8: 113–5.

99. Davis JL, Parke DW 2nd, Font RL. Granulocytic sarcoma of the orbit. A clinicopathologic study. Ophthalmology 1985; 92: 1758–62.

100. Jakobiec FA, Jones IS. Lymphomatous, plasmacytic, histiocytic and haemopoietic tumors. In: Duane TD, ed. Clinical Ophthalmology. Hagerstown: Harper and Row; 1983, v. 2.

101. Knowles DM, Jakobiec FA, Jones IS. Rhabdomyosarcoma. In: Duane TD, ed. Clinical Ophthalmology. Philadelphia: Harper and Row; 1983.

102. Margo CE, Mulla ZD. Malignant tumors of the orbit. Analysis of the Florida Cancer Registry. Ophthalmology 1998; 105: 185–90.

103. King AJ, Fahy GT, Brown L. Null cell lymphoblastic lymphoma of the orbit. Eye 2000; 14: 665–7.

104. Johnson DA, Rosen D. B-cell lymphoma presenting as a periorbital mass in a child. J Pediatr Ophthalmol Strabismus 2000; 37: 244–6.

105. Leidenix MJ, Mamalis N, Olson RJ, et al. Primary T-cell immunoblastic lymphoma of the orbit in a pediatric patient. Ophthalmology 1993; 100: 998–1003.

106. Douglas RS, Goldstein SM, Katowitz JA, et al. Orbital presentation of posttransplantation lymphoproliferative disorder: a small case series. Ophthalmology 2002; 109: 2351–5.

107. Henle W, Henle G. Epstein–Barr virus and human malignancies. Cancer 1974; 34(4 Suppl): 1368–74.
108. Edelstein C, Shields JA, Shields CL, et al. Non-African Burkitt lymphoma presenting with oral thrush and an orbital mass in a child. Am J Ophthalmol 1997; 124: 859–61.
109. Banthia V, Jen A, Kacker A. Sporadic Burkitt's lymphoma of the head and neck in the pediatric population. Int J Pediatr Otorhinolaryngol 2003; 67: 59–65.

CHAPTER
39 Craniofacial Abnormalities

Christopher J Lyons

These disorders fall into three groups:
(i) Craniosynostoses, in which an abnormally shaped skull results from premature closure of sutures (for example, Crouzon and Apert syndromes);
(ii) The clefting syndromes, in which there is failure of apposition or fusion of tissues *in utero*, and
(iii) The mandibulofacial dysostoses, a group which includes Treacher Collins and Goldenhar syndromes.

CRANIOSYNOSTOSIS SYNDROMES

Normal development of the face and cranial vault requires coordinated growth of all the bones of the skull. Approximately one in 2100–3000 infants has craniosynostosis, in which premature fusion of one or more sutures results in abnormalities of the face and cranial vault.

Genetics

Over 100 syndromes with craniosynostosis are recognized. Classification is based on the suture involved and the resultant craniofacial features, the other associated defects such as limb and other organ systems involved, and the inheritance pattern. This may be autosomal dominant, recessive, or X-linked.[1] Mutation analysis is also helpful to define each disorder and to identify mildly affected carrier parents.

Causative heterozygous mutations of single genes can be identified in approximately 20% of cases; the majority involve the transcription factor *TWIST* and three fibroblast growth factor receptors (*FGFR1*, *FGFR2*, and *FGFR3*). The latter are transmembrane signal-transduction molecules crucial in conveying intercellular signals regarding the proliferation, migration, differentiation, and survival of cells. Mutations of *FGFR2*, on the long arm of chromosome 10 (10q26), have been described in Crouzon, Apert, Pfeiffer, and other syndromes. The mutations most commonly affect the extracellular component of the transmembrane protein, although mutations affecting the intracellular region also rarely occur.[2] The mutations most commonly involve an extracellular immunoglobulin-like molecule, consisting of mis-sense substitutions; the mutation causing Apert syndrome has the highest rate currently known for trans-versions in the human genome. The mutations are activating.[1]

There is a strong association between de novo mutations and advanced paternal age in Apert[3] as well as Crouzon and Pfeiffer syndromes.[4] Advanced paternal age has also been implicated in *FGFR3* mutations causing achondroplasia. The magnitude of the observed increase in *FGFR* mutation frequency in sperm with paternal age is insufficient to account for the increased likelihood of having an affected child. Another factor, such as selection for mutation-carrying sperm, might be the cause of this observation.[5]

Pathogenesis

The basic structure of the head and face is established in the first 7 weeks of embryonic life. Since most congenital craniofacial anomalies represent an arrest in the development of specific structures at one point of development, here is a brief reminder of the relevant embryology.

Development of the face
The mandible and maxilla are formed from the first branchial arch. As the maxilla develops around week 6, the eyes are gradually brought from the lateral surfaces of the head to face progressively more anteriorly, a process helped by the growth of the nose and mostly completed by week 16. Arrest of this process results in a lateral orientation of the orbits, a defect known as exorbitism. Late in week 6, the maxillary processes cover the nasal groove and fuse with the medial nasal fold, enclosing the future nasolacrimal duct. The eyelids develop from mesodermal collections covered by surface ectoderm. Fusion of the lids occurs at week 9 and separation at week 25.

Development of the cranial vault
The vault of the skull arises from neural crest cells that condense at the site of the future crista galli, lesser wings of the sphenoid, and the petrous ridges.[6] These condensations grow to surround the enlarging brain, and the sites at which these sheets of cells meet determine the future sites of the cranial sutures. The bone of the cranium is produced from osteoblastic centers at the suture sites. The undifferentiated state of a suture, allowing bony expansion, is determined by a complex process coordinated by the underlying dura mater and complex genetic interactions. Failure of this process results in fusion or synostosis (Fig. 39.1).

Premature closure of a suture inhibits growth perpendicular to it. The skull grows in a direction parallel to the suture to accommodate the enlarging brain. Thus, premature closure of the sagittal suture results in an elongated, boat-shaped skull (scaphocephaly). If anteroposterior growth is restricted by premature fusion of the coronal suture, the head becomes short and wide (brachycephaly). If both anteroposterior and lateral growth are restricted, growth is directed vertically and the head becomes peaked (acrocephaly) or pointed (oxycephaly). When the skull is excessively high as well as short the term turricephaly (tower head) is used. Lastly, closure of any single suture may result in considerable distortion of the skull and face, with flattening of the forehead on the affected side (plagiocephaly).

The bones of the skull base are formed from differentiation of cartilage surrounding the notochord. Premature closure of skull base sutures, especially sphenozygomatic and sphenoethmoidal, results in reduced midfacial growth and shallow orbits. The cartilage destined to form the bones of the base of the skull also

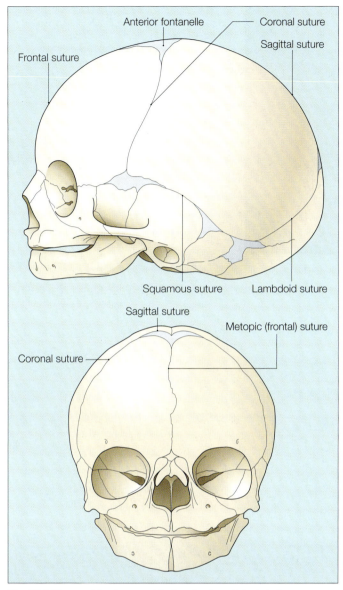

Fig. 39.1 The cranial sutures and fontanelles in an infant skull.

contributes to the nasal septum, which, as discussed above, plays an important role in reducing the wide interorbital distance and "exorbitism" of the embryonic face.

Prenatal ultrasound diagnosis is possible for many types of craniosynostosis from the second trimester onward;[7] it cannot be detected by routine ultrasound screening in the first trimester.

The classification of craniosynostosis was reviewed by Howell,[8] Blodi,[9] Duke-Elder,[10] Cohen,[11] Marchac and Renier,[12] and Fries and Katowitz.[13] Understanding the genetic mutations underlying craniosynostosis has given rise to a reappraisal of the various syndromes involved, and was reviewed by Muenke and Wilkie in 2001.[1]

Common ophthalmic features in craniosynostosis syndromes

The ocular manifestations of the craniosynostoses share a number of similarities. These will be discussed first, and the specific features of each of the common craniosynostoses will then be highlighted.

Amblyopia

Khan et al.[14] reviewed visual outcome in 141 children with craniosynostosis. Anisometropia greater than 1 D was present in 18% of patients, horizontal strabismus in 70%, and a visual acuity inferior to 6/12 in their better eye in 40%. High degrees of astigmatism and ptosis also occur.[15] The detection and early correction of these abnormalities is an important aspect of the care of these patients. This is often complicated by difficulties patching markedly exophthalmic eyes, or fitting glasses in patients whose nasal bridge is hypoplastic.[16] Hypertelorism also complicates the centering of spectacle lenses, particularly important when correcting high astigmatic errors.

Structural abnormalities

Visual failure due to optic atrophy is a relatively common finding. In a series of 244 patients with craniosynostosis, Dufier et al.[17] observed optic disc pallor or atrophy in 50% of patients with Crouzon syndrome, in 34% of those with oxycephaly, and in 24% of those with Apert syndrome. Disc swelling was observed at some stage in assessment in 31% of patients with Crouzon syndrome, in 23% of those with oxycephaly, and in 9.5% of those with Apert syndrome.

The mechanism of optic nerve damage implicated for each particular patient is often ambiguous. Optic atrophy secondary to chronic papilledema is one possible cause. Hydrocephalus occurs more frequently in the complex forms of craniosynostosis–Apert and Crouzon syndromes and cloverleaf skull–than in single-suture synostosis.[18] A disproportion between the rates of brain and skull growth with resultant increase in intracranial pressure has often been suggested as the cause of papilledema.[8,12,18,19] Papilledema (Fig. 39.2) may also result from central nervous abnormalities such as Chiari malformation or stenosis of the jugular foramina. Since these could be remedied by shunting or calvarial remodeling, regular fundoscopic examination of patients with craniosynostosis is important. Other possible mechanisms such as narrowing of the optic canals[19] and kinking or stretching of the optic nerves[10] have also been suggested to explain the high incidence of optic atrophy.

Many patients with craniofacial disorders, in particular Apert, Pfeiffer, and Goldenhar spectrum patients, are prone to respiratory obstruction and present an anesthetic challenge; fiberoptic intubation equipment may be required for some of these patients.

Exophthalmos

Orbital shallowing, maxillary hypoplasia, and retrusion of the lower forehead contribute to the exophthalmic appearance of many patients with craniofacial synostosis. Patients with Crouzon, Pfeiffer, or cloverleaf skull syndrome are particularly severely affected (see Fig. 39.8). Maxillary hypoplasia results in lower lid retraction, and inferior scleral shows with a risk of spontaneous prolapse of the globe.[9,10] Lagophthalmos with exposure of the conjunctiva and cornea may be complicated by vascularization or infection, descemetocele formation, and perforation, unless preventative measures are instituted early. These may include the frequent use of topical lubricants and application of ointment at night, the temporary use of moisture chambers, and in severe cases, lateral (and possibly medial) tarsorrhaphies (see Fig. 39.6).

Strabismus

Dufier et al.[17] identified strabismus in 73 of 200 patients (36.5%) with craniofacial anomalies, whereas Cheng et al.[20] found this in

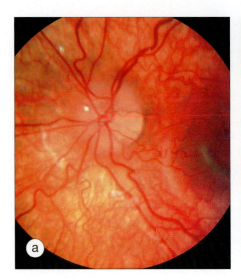
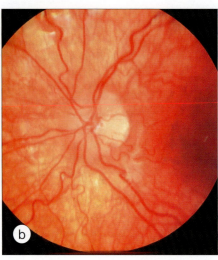

Fig. 39.2 Crouzon syndrome. (a) Left eye showing mild papilledema. (b) Same patient 4 years later. Mild papilledema in Crouzon syndrome may remain stable for many years but careful follow-up is necessary for monitoring of optic nerve function. Serial VEPs may be helpful to detect early optic atrophy.

68% of 63 patients. Morax[21] found exotropia or a vertical deviation in 89% of his series. V-pattern exotropia (Fig. 39.3) is the most commonly reported abnormality, with marked updrift of the adducting eye. When unilateral, as in plagiocephaly, the patient may present with a head tilt to the opposite side.[22] A number of explanations to account for this pattern, including divergent orbital axes or exorbitism,[17] shortening of the antero-posterior orbital dimensions resulting in mechanical disadvantage of the superior oblique muscle,[22] and hypertelorism have been suggested. All of these could contribute to the development of exodeviations. In addition, absence or abnormal insertion of one or more extraocular muscles has been described.[17,23,24] Cheng et al.[20] observed excyclorotation of the orbits (and extraocular muscles) on the magnetic resonance imaging (MRI) and computed tomography (CT) scans of five patients with cranio-synostosis. This is in fact a frequent feature accompanying V-pattern exotropia in craniofacial disorders, and the ocular motility abnormalities result from uncoupling of yoke pairs due to displacement of the extraocular muscles relative to the vertical and horizontal meridians. Herring's law acting on the horizontal recti in right gaze would normally couple the right lateral rectus with the left medial rectus. Orbital excyclotorsion with inferior shift of the lateral rectus and superior shift of the medial rectus results in depression of the abducting eye with simultaneous elevation of the adducting eye, mimicking a left superior oblique palsy pattern. This is further suggested by the pronounced V-pattern due to the laterally shifted superior recti acting in upgaze and medially shifted inferior recti in downgaze (Fig. 39.3).

"Missing muscles" have been reported complicating strabismus surgery in craniofacial disorders; as a result strabismus surgeons should be prepared to modify their surgical plan in patients with associated craniofacial disorders. It is likely, however, that in many cases the muscles are actually present but situated in abnormally rotated positions; Cheng et al.[20] described one such patient in whom the inferior rectus and superior oblique muscles were thought to be absent at the time of surgery but were later shown by MRI to be present, but in abnormally excyclorotated positions. Preoperative review of coronal CT scans or MRIs is helpful when planning strabismus surgery in patients with craniofacial disorders, and may show both rotational displacement of muscles and their abnormal differentiation into distinct muscle groups.

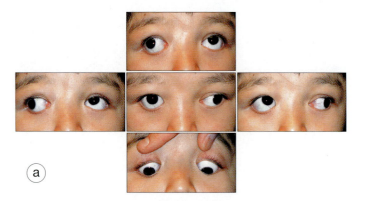

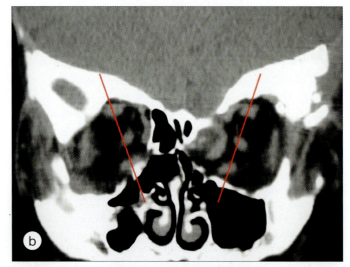

Fig. 39.3 Strabismus in Crouzon syndrome. (a) This 8-year-old girl had undergone three craniofacial operations. She has the V-pattern esotropia characteristic of Crouzon, Apert, and many other craniofacial syndromes. There is also marked updrift of each eye in adduction, mimicking bilateral superior oblique palsies. (b) The coronal CT scan shows extorsion of both orbits and their contents, which has been emphasized by lines drawn between the centers of the superior and inferior rectus muscles on each side. Patient of the University of British Columbia.

Various techniques for strabismus correction, many addressing the characteristic pattern outlined above primarily through oblique muscle surgery[25] with or without rectus transposition,[26] have been advocated. Most surgeons and authors agree that this is a particularly demanding area of strabismus surgery with suboptimal results, probably because of the complexity of the decoupling of yoke pairs, which affects all the extraocular muscles and their interrelations. A surgical incyclorotation of all the orbital contents, which would be a desirable theoretical goal, is not technically feasible at this stage, although leaving the anterior periorbita attached to the orbital bone at the time of surgical incyclorotation of the orbit has been tested on a cadaveric model. This helped to correct the excyclorotation of the globe. In the long run, this avenue could contribute to a correction of the underlying motility problem.[27]

Hypertelorism

Wide separation of the orbits, or hypertelorism, occurred in 45% of the patients with craniosynostosis reviewed by Dufier et al.[17] The diagnosis is best made on the basis of radiographic findings, although telecanthus is a fairly good indicator of underlying hypertelorism in most craniofacial syndromes.[13] The normal intercanthal distance is 20 ± 2 mm in infants, less than 26 ± 1.5 mm in 2 year olds, and less than 30 mm in adults. The normal interpupillary distance is 39 ± 3 mm at birth, increasing to 48 ± 2 by the age of 2 years.[28] Hypotelorism (abnormal proximity of the orbits) was a common feature of trigonocephaly, and it may occur in midline facial clefting (see Midline Facial Clefts).

Description of conditions

Ophthalmic complications are likely in oxycephaly and Crouzon and Apert syndromes; these conditions are outlined in this section. Pfeiffer and Carpenter syndromes, conditions similar to Apert, are also mentioned. Hypertelorism is discussed.

Oxycephaly

This condition is characterized by a high, narrow, pointed, or dome-shaped skull.[29] The forehead is high (Fig. 39.4), and the supraorbital ridges are poorly developed. There is hypertelorism. Proptosis is due to orbital shallowing from medial and forward displacement of the greater wing of the sphenoid and to a lesser extent the vertical orientation of the orbital plate of the frontal bone. The orbital roof is thus almost vertical, continuing the line of the forehead.[10]

There is superior prognathism,[30] and the palatal arch is high and narrow. The deformity results from premature synostosis of all the skull sutures, particularly the coronal suture. Intracranial hypertension is common in oxycephaly[12] and may give rise to visual failure, headache, and vomiting. Skull X-ray may show marked digital impression reflecting chronically elevated intracranial pressure. Mental ability in these patients may fluctuate, being inversely related to intracranial pressure.[18] Occasionally, there is a history of convulsions in infancy[29] and the electroencephalogram (EEG) may be abnormal.[9]

Ocular problems, including visual failure, proptosis, strabismus, restricted eye movements, and nystagmus, tend to become evident in the 2- to 5-year-old age group.

Crouzon syndrome

This was first described by Crouzon in 1912 and is one of the more common craniosynostosis syndromes with an incidence of 1 in 65,000.[31] Half the cases are familial, with complete

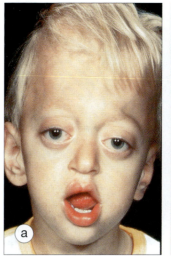
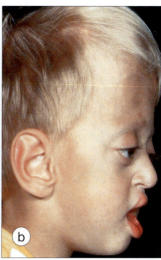
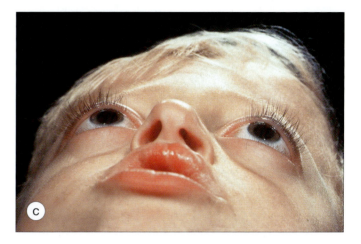
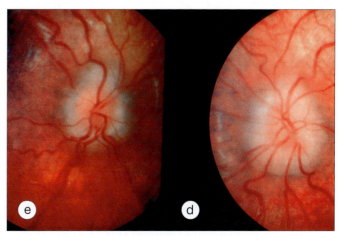

Fig. 39.4 Oxycephaly. (a–c) Oxycephaly showing the high narrow skull with increased height of the skull, shallow orbits, superior prognathism, and poorly developed superciliary ridges. (d, e) Same patient. Oxycephaly showing papilledema secondary to craniosynostosis. Marked papilledema may be an indication for early craniectomy.

penetrance but variable expressivity,[32,33] and the other half are new mutations with evidence of advanced paternal age.[1] It consists of premature craniosynostosis, midfacial hypoplasia (Fig. 39.5), and exophthalmos. Although occasionally noted at birth, the synostosis of the coronal or multiple sutures usually develops

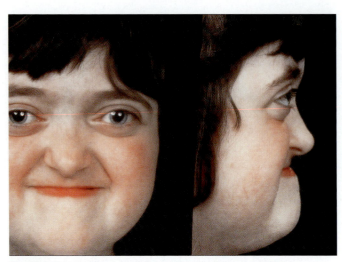

Fig. 39.5 Crouzon syndrome. This girl has the features of inferior prognathism, maxillary hypoplasia, and a prominent forehead, while her nose is quite straight—it often is more "hooked" in this condition.

during the first year of life and is complete by the age of 2 or 3 years. As a result, the shape of the calvarium is highly variable.[11] Some affected children have no vault deformity, but the majority have anteroposterior shortening of the skull with a steep forehead and occiput due to the predominantly coronal synostosis.

The facial appearance is more characteristic, with orbital shallowing resulting in proptosis. The orbits are also widely separated and their axes are laterally rotated (exorbitism). The bridge of the nose is flattened and, as in Apert syndrome, its tip is often shaped like a parrot's beak.[10] The flattened appearance of the midface is emphasized by the prominence of the lower jaw. In addition, the palatal arch is often high and the mouth characteristically held half open.[30]

Orbital shallowing may be extreme, leading to severe problems with corneal exposure. Spontaneous prolapse of the globe, often provoked by a fit of coughing, is a distressing event, which can be complicated by ischemic changes as well as exposure problems. The globe should be repositioned using traction on the lids, which may have to be accompanied by gentle pressure on the anesthetized eye using a wet gauze square. It can precipitate the need to proceed with lateral tarsorrhaphy or maxillary advancement surgery.

Optic nerve complications were present in 80% of Bertelsen's series.[34] Intracranial hypertension may be related to herniation of the cerebellar tonsils following craniofacial surgery.[35]

V-pattern exotropia is commonly present, as described already. Other reported associations include iris coloboma, aniridia, corectopia, microcornea, megalocornea, cataract, ectopia lentis, blue sclera, glaucoma, and nystagmus. Associated physical abnormalities include mild to moderate hearing impairment in 50% of cases, cervical spine fusions usually involving C2–C3, and epilepsy. The hands and feet are clinically normal although there are subtle radiological differences in the metacarpophalangeal pattern. Mental retardation was present in 13% of Bertelsen's patients. Airway obstruction and visceral abnormalities are rare compared with those in Apert and Pfeiffer syndromes. It is occasionally associated with skin hyperpigmentation, hyperkeratosis with verrucous hyperplasia, and melanocytic nevi, which constitute a diagnosis of acanthosis nigricans. This association is due to an *FGFR3* mutation[1] and may be accompanied by narrow-

ing of the foramen magnum and spinal canal, causing distal paraesthesia.

Acrocephalosyndactyly

Wheaton[36] preceded Apert by 8 years with his description of two children with congenital cranial deformity associated with fusion of the fingers and toes. The association of craniofacial synostosis with syndactyly was termed "acrocephalosyndactyly" by Apert.[37] Five types are now recognized.[38] Apert syndrome (type I), Saethre-Chotzen (type III), and Pfeiffer syndrome (type V) are the most common. In Carpenter syndrome (type II), craniofacial synostosis is associated with syndactyly as well as supernumerary digits. Goodman syndrome (type IV) is similar to Carpenter.

Apert syndrome

This condition, closely allied to Crouzon syndrome, is characterized by craniosynostosis, broad thumbs and great toes, and symmetrical syndactyly involving the second to fourth or fifth fingers and toes (Fig. 39.6). As well as syndactyly, there is fusion of the corresponding nails.

The estimated frequency of occurrence is one in 65,000 live births[39] and 4% of all cases of craniosynostosis. The vast majority of Apert syndrome cases are sporadic, due to an *FGFR2* mutation; this occurrence is closely correlated with increased paternal age as discussed already.

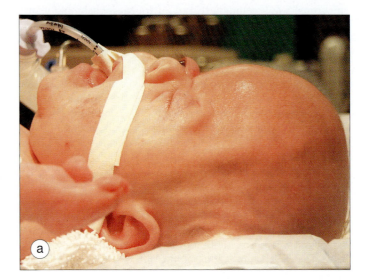

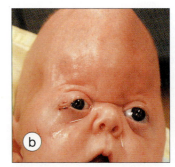

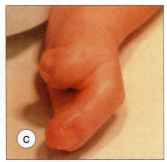

Fig. 39.6 This infant is one of twins with Apert syndrome. There is marked asymmetrical proptosis (a) with recurrent spontaneous globe luxation. The characteristic hypoplasia of the brow and maxilla is apparent in profile. A lateral tarsorrhaphy was performed to prevent the globe luxation (b). (c) There is characteristic symmetrical syndactyly affecting the second to fifth digits of hands and feet. The nails are fused. Patient of the University of British Columbia.

Clinical findings in Apert syndrome tend to be more severe than those of in most of the other craniosynostosis syndromes. As with Crouzon and Pfeiffer syndromes, patients with Apert syndrome may first be seen in the special care nursery, with neonatal respiratory difficulties related to shortening of the nasopharyngeal space. The palate, which is usually highly arched, is also cleft in approximately one-third of cases. Other associations such as tracheoesophageal fistula and congenital heart disease may contribute to the neonatal problems.

The typical facial appearance includes turribrachycephaly due to predominant involvement of the coronal suture, a markedly deficient supraorbital ridge, which is replaced by a horizontal groove, and midfacial hypoplasia with upward tilting. The lower jaw is protuberant. Dental abnormalities are common, as are ear anomalies, which may include conductive deafness.

There are few differences between the ophthalmic findings of Apert and Crouzon syndromes. Proptosis is often less marked in Apert syndrome. Severe proptosis was only present in 3 of 33 patients with Apert syndrome reviewed by Hanieh and David.[40] Hypertelorism is also relatively mild.[40] The palpebral fissures have an antimongoloid slant. Rare associations that have been reported include keratoconus, ectopia lentis, and congenital glaucoma. The optic discs may be normal, edematous, or atrophic.

Brain abnormalities include corpus callosum, septum pellucidum, or limbic abnormalities, cerebral white matter hypoplasia, or heterotopic gray matter as well as ventriculomegaly.[41] The assessment of intracranial pressure in complex craniosynostosis, and particularly Apert syndrome, presents a challenge for the neurosurgeon.[42,43] Ventriculomegaly on CT scan or MRI may be primary or secondary to hydrocephalus from aqueductal stenosis, to synostosis at the skull base impeding cerebrospinal fluid flow from the fourth ventricle, or to defective cerebrospinal fluid reabsorption due to stenosis of the basal foramina impeding drainage from the venous sinuses. Hanieh and David[40] found true hydrocephalus to be uncommon in Apert syndrome. When the intracranial pressure is raised, neurosurgeons may opt for either vault reshaping or shunting. Murovic et al.[44] noted ventriculomegaly in 60% of 25 patients with Apert syndrome but only opted to shunt 3 of these patients. They suggested that shunting is indicated only in the presence of documented progressive ventriculomegaly or ventriculomegaly in association with clinical signs of raised intracranial pressure (bulging fontanelles, papilledema, optic atrophy, apnea) unrelieved by cranial vault suture release, decompression, and reshaping. Nevertheless, since head circumference is a poor indicator of the need for shunting in a patient with craniosynostosis and since hydrocephalus can be present without any symptoms of raised intracranial pressure, careful examination of the optic nerves is an essential part of the follow-up of patients, especially after closure of the fontanelles.

Mental retardation, often thought to be invariably associated with Apert syndrome, is common but not always present. Normal intelligence has often been reported,[11,45] but 52% of 29 patients with Apert syndrome reviewed by Patton et al.[46] had an IQ below 70. Various theories to account for its frequent occurrence have been postulated. Premature closure of the sutures may limit brain growth and therefore intelligence. However, early craniectomy did not lead to a significant reduction in its incidence.[46] Hydrocephalus is another possible cause, and Renier et al.[18] found a statistically significant relationship between intracranial pressure and IQ, although there was a great deal of variation. Lastly, low cortical neurone numbers have been reported in postmortem analysis of a macroscopically normal brain from a patient with Apert syndrome;[47] mental retardation may be a further manifestation of the central nervous system anomalies that often accompany this syndrome.[41]

Pfeiffer syndrome

This disorder is very much rarer than Apert syndrome; the coronal suture is most severely affected, resulting in acrocephaly with midfacial hypoplasia and exorbitism with downslanting palpebral fissures. The syndactyly is mild and the thumbs and great toes are characteristically broad (Fig. 39.7) with various deformities. The fingers are often short with soft tissue syndactyly, and X-rays may show missing phalanges or reduplicated metatarsals. There may also be vertebral abnormalities.

Although the facial and ophthalmic features are similar to those of Apert syndrome, mental retardation is less common in Pfeiffer syndrome. Transmission is autosomal dominant with complete penetrance but variable expressivity,[48] the most extreme of which is cloverleaf skull (see Cloverleaf Skull).

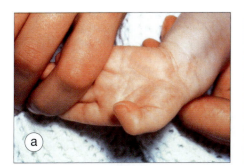
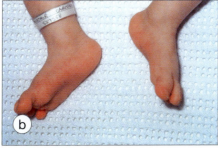
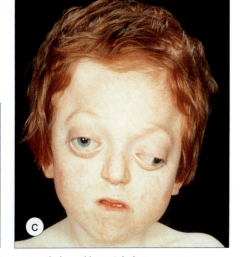

Fig. 39.7 Pfeiffer syndrome. (a, b) Broad thumb and great toes. (c) Same patient at a later date showing acrocephaly and hypertelorism.

Pfeiffer syndrome was considered to be a single clinical entity, and increasing degrees of involvement were called types 1, 2, and 3. Discovery of the causal gene mutations involved revealed a genetically heterogeneous condition, caused by mutations coding for *FGFR1* (chromosome 8) and *FGFR2* (chromosome 10). The latter result in severely affected phenotypes, including cloverleaf skull (Kleeblattschädel)[11] in sporadic cases.[1]

Cloverleaf skull

There is a spectrum of variation in the expression of Crouzon, Carpenter, and Pfeiffer syndromes. At their most marked these disorders may present as cloverleaf skull (Fig. 39.8) syndrome (Kleeblattschädel).[11] This is much more common in Pfeiffer than in Crouzon syndrome, and it tends to occur more commonly in sporadic than familial cases, perhaps because of the reduced fitness of the affected individual.[49]

The skull has a flat, trilobed appearance from synostosis of the coronal and lambdoid sutures–hence the term cloverleaf. Hydrocephalus and airway problems are common and difficult to treat.[50] The orbits are extremely shallow, and proptosis with globe subluxation and repeated corneal damage may occur.[51] The definitive treatment of the subluxation is by frontal bone advancement. In the first instance, however, reposition of the globes followed by moist chambers with medial and lateral tarsorrhaphies may be necessary to protect the ocular surface. Life expectancy is limited.

Saethre-Chotzen syndrome

Variable skull and facial asymmetry, short fingers with cutaneous syndactyly, and a low-set frontal hairline characterize this rare syndrome. The diagnosis may be missed as the facial changes are often subtle; there is very little midfacial hypoplasia and the eyes are not proptosed. Instead, ptosis is common as are tear duct abnormalities, including bony obstruction of the nasolacrimal duct, which are present in up to 50% of cases.[13] There is partial cutaneous syndactyly, frequently between the second and third fingers and toes. The genetic defect does not involve the *FRFR* genes but the *TWIST* gene at 7p21, and patients with large deletions may be mentally retarded. The disorder is autosomal dominantly transmitted with incomplete penetrance and variable expression. Because the phenotypic changes are highly variable and overlap with Muenke syndrome, the two have often been mistaken.

Muenke syndrome

This has also been called *FGFR3*-associated coronal synostosis syndrome, and was first described in 1996; it has a wide spectrum of clinical manifestations and was often confused with other craniosynostosis syndromes. It is relatively common, and the mutation is found in sporadic or familial patients with uni- or bicoronal synostosis whose findings are not typical of the classic syndromes. Other features of the syndrome include midface hypoplasia (59%), downslanting palpebral fissures, and ptosis in almost one-third of cases. Some carriers do not show any of these features and simply have macrocephaly or even normal head size. About one-third have hearing impairment, and developmental delay affects a similar proportion of patients. Hand abnormalities, including short fingers with characteristic radiographic changes of thimble-like middle phalanges, coned epiphyses, and carpal fusions, are common but not invariable. Unlike *FGFR3*-associated achondroplasia, height is normal.[1]

Carpenter syndrome

This rare syndrome consists of craniosynostosis, polysyndactyly of the feet, and syndactyly of the hands, with shortening of the fingers. The craniosynostosis is severe, affecting multiple sutures and resulting in a markedly shrunken and distorted skull vault. Mental retardation is usually present. The ocular findings include hypertelorism, epicanthic folds, and telecanthus.[11]

Hypertelorism

This term describes a condition in which the two orbits are widely separated. It may be difficult to distinguish the point at which wide orbital separation ceases to be a normal variant (morphogenetic hypertelorism) and becomes a condition determined by anomalous development of the face and head, as described by Greig (embryonic hypertelorism). The latter condition involves characteristic broadening of the nasal bridge with a prominent forehead. The orbits are widely displaced and there is commonly a divergent strabismus. Visual function is usually good. François[30] considered transmission to be either dominant (mild form) or recessive (pronounced form). Hypertelorism may also be due to other disorders, including basal encephalocele, or previous trauma. Hypertelorism may also be associated with facial clefting.[52]

Management of craniosynostoses

Children with craniofacial abnormalities are best managed by a team consisting of a pediatrician and ophthalmologist, together with a plastic surgeon, ENT specialist, and neurosurgeon. Other specialists may need to be consulted, including oral surgeons and orthodontists, speech therapists, audiologists, and psychologists. Families with an affected child should also be offered genetic counseling. The patient's progress should be monitored by periodic visits followed by multidisciplinary planning conferences.

The role of the ophthalmologist may be to coordinate referral to these various specialists. Generally, the main function of the ophthalmologist is to ensure that ocular structures are adequately protected, that visual development proceeds normally, and that orbital anatomy is respected during reconstruction surgery. Specifically, the most important duty is to ensure that the optic discs are examined regularly and frequently.

Surgical approaches to the skull (Fig. 39.9) include decompressive osteotomy when intracranial pressure is raised early in life and, later, combined craniofacial techniques as described by Tessier.[19] The timing of this surgery remains controversial but early surgery

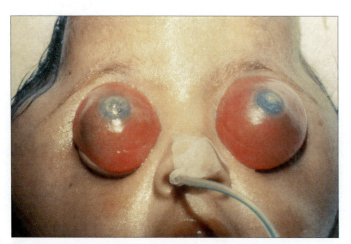

Fig. 39.8 Cloverleaf skull with trilobed flattened skull appearance, subluxated globes, exposure keratitis, and chemotic conjunctiva.

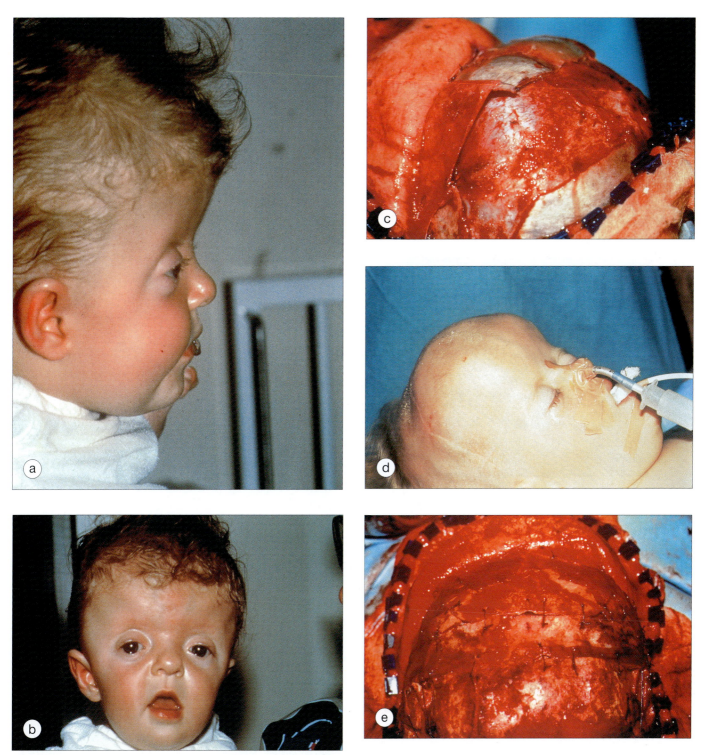

Fig. 39.9 (a, b) This 5-month-old girl with Apert syndrome has pronounced brow and lower forehead retrusion. (c) The forehead and supraorbital margin are advanced for cosmetic purposes and to increase the intracranial volume; the vault is divided by a coronal incision and a horizontal incision divides the orbital roof and the root of the nose. (d) Fifteen months later turricephaly has developed due to vault expansion at the previous operative site. (e) At 20 months of age frontal and parietal bone is removed. The forehead is created from parietal bone on a Marchac template.

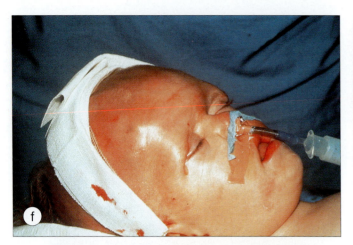

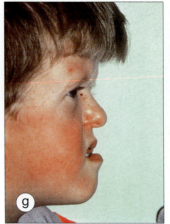

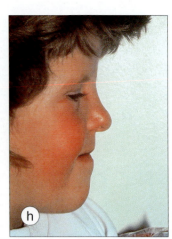

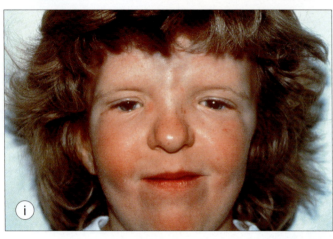

Fig. 39.9 (*Cont'd*) (f) Postoperatively the forehead retrusion has been corrected and a brow has been created. (g) At the age of 5.5 years, maxillary retrusion gives the patient a remarkably prognathic appearance. (h, i) A Le Fort III procedure has corrected the maxillary retrusion. Photos courtesy of Dr Don Fitzpatrick and Dr Paul Steinbok. Patient of the University of British Columbia.

may be indicated if vision is threatened by optic atrophy or corneal exposure.

Generally, the first step in reconstructive surgery is a forehead advancement, if this is necessary (as in Apert syndrome). The effect of this procedure may be short-lived if it is performed in infancy, especially in Apert syndrome. Midfacial hypoplasia can be addressed by midface advancement surgery at preschool age. This surgery results in considerable cosmetic improvement but is associated with significant morbidity if carried out earlier in life. A Le Fort III "monobloc" maxillary osteotomy with advancement of the forehead, orbital margins, nose, and maxillae results in expansion of the restricted intracranial space and improves the child's cosmesis in a single procedure. However, this procedure creates direct continuity between the nasal and intracranial spaces and therefore a risk of meningitis. Many surgeons would opt for a staged procedure in which the forehead advancement precedes the Le Fort III maxillary advancement. Finally, surgery during the teenage years is aimed at correcting any residual midfacial abnormality, including the bridge of the nose.

Facial reconstructive surgery often involves elevation of the periorbita and fracture/mobilization of the anterior two-thirds of the orbital walls. Ocular complications that may arise include intraorbital hemorrhage, direct trauma to the optic nerve or globe during surgery, or pressure on these structures by a malpositioned bone graft. Although ocular alignment was found to be relatively unaffected by orbital procedures in craniofacial reconstruction,[23]

we have found strabismus to be relatively common following facial reconstruction involving the orbits.

CLEFTING SYNDROMES

The second major group of craniofacial abnormalities is known as the clefting syndromes. These result from defective apposition or failure of fusion of neighboring structures during embryonic development. Tessier[52] classified facial clefts in a purely descriptive manner, numbering them from 0 to 14 in clockwise rotation about the right eye. Thus, clefts involving the midline structures of the nose and forehead are numbered 0 and 1 below the level of the medial canthus and 13 and 14 above. Nasolacrimal and medial canthal clefts are numbered 2, 3, and 4 below and 10, 11, and 12 above, and so on (Fig. 39.10).

This descriptive system gives no clue to the underlying mechanism; clefts with etiologies as diverse as failure of embryonic closure of the nasolacrimal furrow, amniotic bands, and Goldenhar syndrome are simply numbered according to their location relative to the eye. Nevertheless, it is a logical method of expressing a facial defect and it is widely used.

Although Tessier's system encompasses the syndromes grouped together as mandibulofacial dysostoses by François,[30] their eponymous names are so well known that they are useful. They include a number of congenital disorders of the face due primarily to retarded differentiation of the first branchial arch

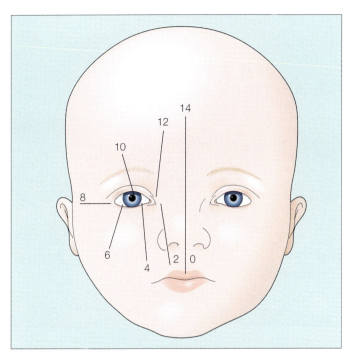

Fig. 39.10 Sites of facial clefts. Modified from Tessie P. Anatomical classification facial, cranio-facial and laterofacial clefts. J Maxillofac Surg 1976; 4: 69–92. With permission from Georg Thieme Verlag KG, Stuttgart, Germany.

mesoderm. Treacher Collins and Goldenhar syndromes are the most common syndromes in this category.

Treacher Collins syndrome

This syndrome was described by Treacher Collins in 1900 but is also associated with the names of Franceschetti and Zwahlen,

who provided a detailed description in 1944. The incidence is 1 in 50,000 live births.[53] The mode of inheritance is autosomal dominant with complete penetrance but variable expressivity.

The gene responsible was mapped to the long arm of chromosome 5 (5q32–33.3);[54,55] this has since been refined with identification of the *TCOF1* gene coding for a 1411 amino acid molecule named treacle, expressed at peak levels in the first and second branchial arches whose role is likely to involve intracellular transport.[56–58]

The complete form of Treacher Collins syndrome involves clefts 6, 7, and 8 on Tessier's classification; the facial characteristics (Fig. 39.11) include malar hypoplasia and hypoplastic zygomas with deficient inferolateral orbital angles. Absence of the nasofrontal angle results in a birdlike or fishlike profile. The lower jaw is hypoplastic with abnormal dentition. Choanal atresia and mandibular retrusion may cause respiratory problems. Malformations of the external ear are common and may be associated with middle or inner ear abnormalities, causing deafness. Accessory auricular appendages as well as blind fistulae occur anywhere between the angle of the mouth and the ear.

The palpebral fissures have an antimongoloid slant and colobomas of the lateral third of the lower lid are common. These may be pseudocolobomas, where cilia, subcutaneous tissues, and muscle are hypoplastic. Canthal dystopia, nasolacrimal obstruction, and limbal or orbital dermoids also occur frequently.[59,60] High degrees of astigmatism are present in severely affected cases. This, together with the conductive hearing loss in 50% of cases due to ossicular chain malformation often combined with meatal atresia,[61] will not only make it difficult to fit glasses in the presence of hearing aids and external ear abnormalities but, if not identified early, could place an affected infant at risk of cognitive deprivation.

Treatment involves oculoplastic repair of the lid colobomas and, where appropriate, surgery to correct the underdevelopment of the zygoma, maxillae, and mandible by bone or cartilage grafts.[62] Early audiological assessment is important.

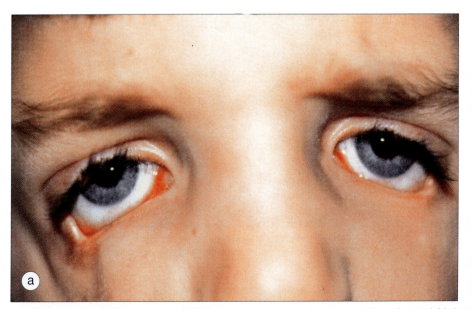
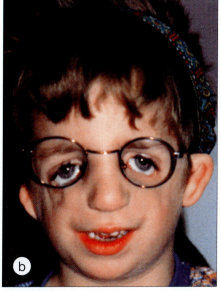

Fig. 39.11 Treacher Collins syndrome. (a) This 4-year-old boy has malar hypoplasia, antimongoloid slanted lid fissures, and lower lid colobomas. The ocular surfaces are healthy despite the marked lagophthalmos. (b) There is a degree of mandibular hypoplasia and macrostomia. He has severe conductive hearing loss and 6 D of astigmatism on the right, 3 D on the left. To prevent amblyopia, glasses were custom-designed for his increased interpupillary distance and ear changes. Patient of the University of British Columbia.

Goldenhar syndrome

In 1952, Goldenhar described a syndrome consisting of epibulbar dermoids, preauricular appendages, and mandibular hypoplasia,[63] which was also termed hemifacial microsomia. Gorlin et al.[53] expanded this to the "oculoauriculovertebral spectrum" to encompass the wide range of abnormalities seen with this condition. Expression is extremely variable[53] and may range from a few preauricular appendages only to pronounced facial asymmetry, and even bilateral clefting extending from the angles of the mouth to the tragus as well as of the palate and either side of the frontonasal process to the medial canthi. Microphthalmos is common. The "expanded Goldenhar complex" in which vertebral, cardiac, renal, and central nervous system abnormalities are present may include severe hydrocephalus, and mental retardation.[64] Most cases are sporadic but familial cases have been reported; the genetic basis of the disorder is not clear.

The facial abnormalities may be bilateral, but are usually more severe on one side. The preauricular appendages are usually anterior to the tragus, with or without fistulae to the ear. Vertebral, cardiac, or pulmonary anomalies are common. Ocular findings include ptosis (12%), nasolacrimal duct obstruction and fistula, and coloboma of the middle third of the upper lid (20%), which is often associated with an epibulbar lesion on the ipsilateral eye. This may be a dermoid (white, solid) or dermolipoma (yellow, often conjunctival). Dermoids may occur unilaterally (50%) or bilaterally (25%), at any location on the globe or within the orbit. The most common site is the inferotemporal limbus (Fig. 39.12). The vision may be impaired if they encroach on the visual axis or cause astigmatism and amblyopia. They can be excised using Vannas scissors and a rounded Beaver blade to decrease the astigmatism; gonioscopy at the start of surgery can help determine the depth of corneal involvement since perforation is a recognized complication. A diamond bur can be used to polish the base of the dermoid tissue after excision, and some surgeons replace the dermoid with a lamellar graft. Reepithelialization can be problematic if the dermoid was extensive. Others prefer to tattoo the base of the dermoid if an obvious leukoma persists.[65]

Dermolipomas are famous for the problems that result from overenthusiastic attempts at complete excision, which may include ptosis, diplopia, and dry eye.[66-68] Ocular motility disorders are common in Goldenhar syndrome. Duane syndrome, esotropia, and exotropia are found in approximately one-quarter of patients.[53] The syndrome shares a number of features with Treacher Collins syndrome, and combinations of the two have been reported.[30,63]

Midline facial clefts

These may combine midline bifid nose, cleft lip and palate, and midline encephalocele together with intracranial abnormalities (Fig. 39.13) (see Chapter 63). The signs of an underlying cleft may be rather subtle. A small notch in the upper lip or in the middle of the nose may alert the clinician to an underlying defect.

Amniotic bands

Amniotic bands are thought to occur when bands of amnion encircle parts of the developing fetus, locally restricting growth. The clefts that result do not conform to developmental patterns. They may cause minor deformities, such as ring constriction of fingers, but major craniofacial malformations may occur (Fig. 39.14). The condition is sporadic and both sexes are affected equally.[13]

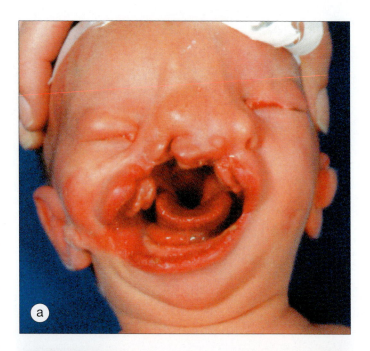

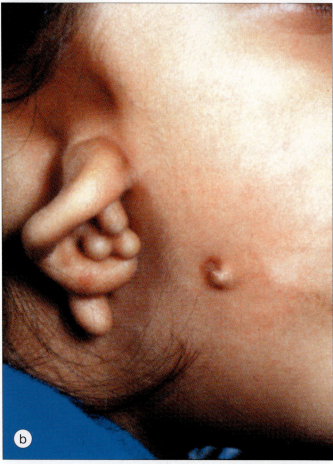

Fig. 39.12 Goldenhar syndrome. (a) Extreme manifestation of Goldenhar syndrome (auriculo-oculovertebral spectrum) in an infant. There is severe clefting with absent fusion between the structures of the embryonic frontonasal process and maxilla and between the mandible and maxilla. The patient died at 18 months of age. Photo courtesy of Dr Andrew McCormick. Patient of the University of British Columbia. (b) Preauricular tags and microtia associated with hemifacial microsomia in Goldenhar syndrome. There is ipsilateral conductive hearing loss. Pits and preauricular tags occur in a line connecting the ear to the angle of the mouth.

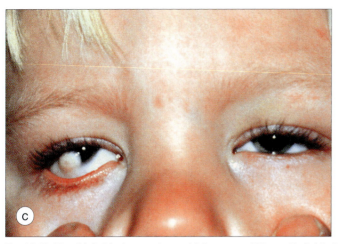
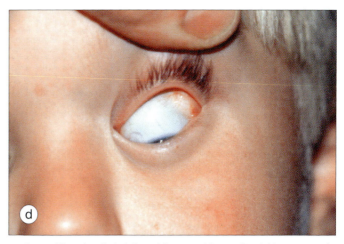

Fig. 39.12 (*Cont'd*) Goldenhar syndrome. (c) Four-year-old boy with Goldenhar syndrome. There is a limbal dermoid encroaching on the right cornea and a left-sided dermolipoma (d).

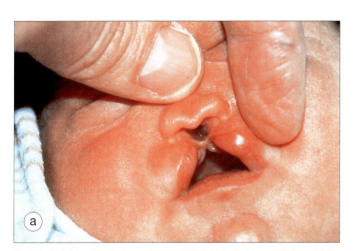
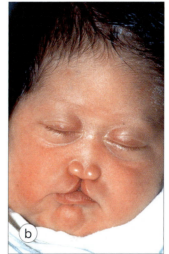
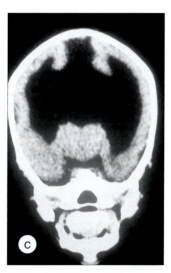

Fig. 39.13 (a) Midline facial and nose cleft. (b) Marked hypotelorism. (c) Associated severe holoprosencephaly. This would be classified as a 0/14 cleft on Tessier's classification.[52] Patient of the University of British Columbia.

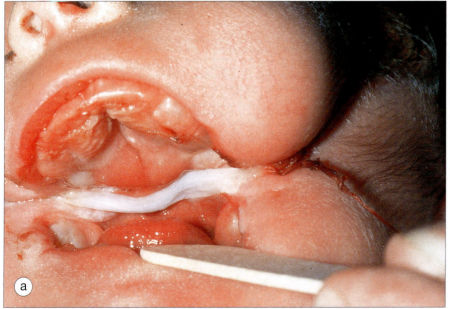
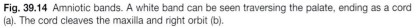
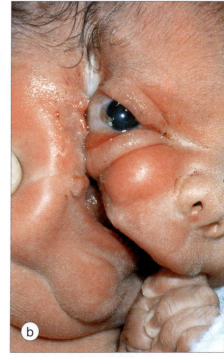

Fig. 39.14 Amniotic bands. A white band can be seen traversing the palate, ending as a cord (a). The cord cleaves the maxilla and right orbit (b).

REFERENCES

1. Muenke M, Wilkie AOM. Craniosynostosis syndromes. In: Scirver CR, Beaudet AL, Sly W, et al, editors. The Metabolic and Molecular Bases of Inherited Disease. 8th ed. New York: McGraw-Hill; 2001: 6117–46.
2. Kan SH, Elanko N, Johnson D, et al. Genomic screening of fibroblast growth-factor receptor 2 reveals a wide spectrum of mutations in patients with syndromic craniosynostosis. Am J Hum Genet 2002; 70: 472–86.
3. Moloney DM, Slaney SF, Oldridge M, et al. Exclusive paternal origin of new mutations in Apert syndrome. Nat Genet 1996; 13: 48–53.
4. Glaser RL, Jiang W, Boyadjiev SA, et al. Paternal origin of FGFR2 mutations in sporadic cases of Crouzon syndrome and Pfeiffer syndrome. Am J Hum Genet 2000; 66: 768–77.
5. Tiemann-Boege I, Navidi W, Grewal R, et al. The observed human sperm mutation frequency cannot explain the achondroplasia paternal age effect. Proc Natl Acad Sci USA 2002; 99: 14, 952–7.
6. Smith DW, Tondury G. Origin of the calvaria and its sutures. Am J Dis Child 1978; 132: 662–6.
7. Miller C, Losken HW, Towbin R, et al. Ultrasound diagnosis of craniosynostosis. Cleft Palate Craniofac J 2002; 39: 73–80.
8. Howell SC. The craniostenoses. Am J Ophthalmol 1954; 37: 359–79.
9. Blodi FC. Developmental anomalies of the skull affecting the eye. Arch Ophthalmol 1957; 57: 593–610.
10. Duke-Elder S. Normal and abnormal development: congenital deformities. In: Duke-Elder S, editor. System of Ophthalmology, Part 2. London: Henry Kimpton; 1964: 1037–57.
11. Cohen MM Jr. An etiologic and nosologic overview of craniosynostosis syndromes. Birth Defects Orig Artic Ser 1975; 11: 137–89.
12. Marchac D, Renier D. Craniofacial Surgery for Craniosynostosis. Boston: Little, Brown; 1982.
13. Fries PD, Katowitz JA. Congenital craniofacial anomalies of ophthalmic importance. Surv Ophthalmol 1990; 35: 87–119.
14. Khan SH, Nischal KK, Dean F, et al. Visual outcomes and amblyogenic risk factors in craniosynostotic syndromes: a review of 141 cases. Br J Ophthalmol 2003; 87: 999–1003.
15. Hertle RW, Quinn GE, Minguini N, et al. Visual loss in patients with craniofacial synostosis. J Pediatr Ophthalmol Strabismus 1991; 28: 344–9.
16. Buncic JR. Ocular aspects of Apert syndrome. Clin Plast Surg 1991; 18: 315–9.
17. Dufier JL, Vinurel MC, Renier D, et al. Ophthalmologic complications of craniofacial stenoses. Apropos of 244 cases. J Fr Ophtalmol 1986; 9: 273–80.
18. Renier D, Sainte-Rose C, Marchac D, et al. Intracranial pressure in craniostenosis. J Neurosurg 1982; 57: 370–7.
19. Tessier P. The definitive plastic surgical treatment of the severe facial deformities of craniofacial dysostosis. Crouzon's and Apert's diseases. Plast Reconstr Surg 1971; 48: 419–42.
20. Cheng H, Burdon MA, Shun-Shin GA, et al. Dissociated eye movements in craniosynostosis: a hypothesis revived. Br J Ophthalmol 1993; 77: 563–8.
21. Morax S. Oculo-motor disorders in craniofacial malformations. J Maxillofac Surg 1984; 12: 1–10.
22. Bagolini B, Campos EC, Chiesi C. Plagiocephaly causing superior oblique deficiency and ocular torticollis. A new clinical entity. Arch Ophthalmol 1982; 100: 1093–6.
23. Diamond GR, Katowitz JA, Whitaker LA, et al. Variations in extraocular muscle number and structure in craniofacial dysostosis. Am J Ophthalmol 1980; 90: 416–8.
24. Coats DK, Ou R. Anomalous medial rectus muscle insertion in a child with craniosynostosis. Binocul Vis Strabismus Q 2001; 16: 119–20.
25. Coats DK, Paysse EA, Stager DR. Surgical management of V-pattern strabismus and oblique dysfunction in craniofacial dysostosis. J AAPOS 2000; 4: 338–42.
26. Clement R, Nischal K. Simulation of oculomotility in craniosynostosis patients. Strabismus 2003; 11: 239–42.
27. Liew S, Poole M, Kenton-Smith J, et al. Orbital and globe rotation: the role of the periorbita. J Craniomaxillofac Surg 1999; 27: 7–10.
28. Feingold M, Bossert WH. Normal values for selected physical parameters: an aid to syndrome delineation. Birth Defects Orig Artic Ser 1974; 10: 1–16.
29. Mann I. Developmental Abnormalities of the Eye. London: British Medical Association; 1957.
30. Francois J. Heredity of the craniofacial dysostoses. Mod Probl Ophthalmol 1975; 14: 5–48.
31. Cohen MM Jr, Kreiborg S. Birth prevalence studies of the Crouzon syndrome: comparison of direct and indirect methods. Clin Genet 1992; 41: 12–5.
32. Cohen MM Jr. Syndromes with craniosynostosis. In: Cohen MM Jr, editor. Craniosynostosis: Diagnosis, Evaluation and Management. New York: Raven Press; 1986: 413–990.
33. Kreiborg S, Cohen MM, Jr. Germinal mosaicism in Crouzon syndrome. Hum Genet 1990; 84: 487–8.
34. Bertelsen TI. The premature synostosis of the cranial sutures. Acta Ophthalmol 1958; 36: 1–176.
35. Francis PM, Beals S, Rekate HL, et al. Chronic tonsillar herniation and Crouzon's syndrome. Pediatr Neurosurg 1992; 18: 202–6.
36. Wheaton SW. Two specimens of congenital cranial deformity in infants associated with fusion of the fingers and toes. Trans Pathol Soc London 1894; 45: 238–50.
37. Apert E. De l'acrocephalsyndactylie. Bull Soc Med Paris 1906; 23: 1310–37.
38. Temtamy SA, McKusick VA. The genetics of hand malformations. Birth Defects Orig Artic Ser 1978; 14: i–xviii, 1–619.
39. Cohen MM Jr, Kreiborg S, Lammer EJ, et al. Birth prevalence study of the Apert syndrome. Am J Med Genet 1992; 42: 655–9.
40. Hanieh A, David DJ. Apert's syndrome. Childs Nerv Syst 1993; 9: 289–91.
41. Cohen MM Jr, Kreiborg S. The central nervous system in the Apert syndrome. Am J Med Genet 1990; 35: 36–45.
42. Taylor WJ, Hayward RD, Lasjaunias P, et al. Enigma of raised intracranial pressure in patients with complex craniosynostosis: the role of abnormal intracranial venous drainage. J Neurosurg 2001; 94: 377–85.
43. Humphreys RP. Apert syndrome. Diagnosis and treatment of cranio-stenosis and intracranial anomalies. Clin Plast Surg 1991; 18: 231–5.
44. Murovic JA, Posnick JC, Drake JM, et al. Hydrocephalus in Apert syndrome: a retrospective review. Pediatr Neurosurg 1993; 19: 151–5.
45. Cohen MM Jr, Pantke H, Siris E. Nosologic and genetic considerations in the aglossy-adactyly syndrome. Birth Defects Orig Artic Ser 1971; 7: 237–40.
46. Patton MA, Goodship J, Hayward R, et al. Intellectual development in Apert's syndrome: a long term follow up of 29 patients. J Med Genet 1988; 25: 164–7.
47. Crome L. A critique of current views on acrocephaly and related conditions. J Ment Sci 1961; 107: 459–74.
48. Goodman RM. Atlas of the Eye in Genetic Disorders. St. Louis: Mosby; 1977.
49. Rutland P, Pulleyn LJ, Reardon W, et al. Identical mutations in the FGFR2 gene cause both Pfeiffer and Crouzon syndrome phenotypes. Nat Genet 1995; 9: 173–6.
50. Lodge ML, Moore MH, Hanieh A, et al. The cloverleaf skull anomaly: managing extreme cranio-orbitofaciostenosis. Plast Reconstr Surg 1993; 91: 1–9.
51. Watters EC, Hiles DA, Johnson BL. Cloverleaf skull syndrome. Am J Ophthalmol 1973; 76: 716–20.
52. Tessier P. Anatomical classification facial, cranio-facial and latero-facial clefts. J Maxillofac Surg 1976; 4: 69–92.
53. Gorlin RJ, Cohen MM Jr, Hennekam RCM. Syndromes of the Head and Neck. New York: Oxford University Press; 2001.
54. Dixon MJ, Dixon J, Houseal T, et al. Narrowing the position of the Treacher Collins syndrome locus to a small interval between three new microsatellite markers at 5q32–33.1. Am J Hum Genet 1993; 52: 907–14.
55. Dixon MJ, Read AP, Donnai D, et al. The gene for Treacher Collins syndrome maps to the long arm of chromosome 5. Am J Hum Genet 1991; 49: 17–22.
56. Marszalek B, Wojcicki P, Kobus K, et al. Clinical features, treatment and genetic background of Treacher Collins syndrome. J Appl Genet 2002; 43: 223–33.
57. Dixon J, Edwards SJ, Anderson I, et al. Identification of the complete coding sequence and genomic organization of the Treacher Collins syndrome gene. Genome Res 1997; 7: 223–34.

58. Dixon J, Hovanes K, Shiang R, et al. Sequence analysis, identification of evolutionary conserved motifs and expression analysis of murine tcof1 provide further evidence for a potential function for the gene and its human homologue, TCOF1. Hum Mol Genet 1997; 6: 727–37.

59. Wang FM, Millman AL, Sidoti PA, et al. Ocular findings in Treacher Collins syndrome. Am J Ophthalmol 1990; 110: 280–6.

60. Hertle RW, Ziylan S, Katowitz JA. Ophthalmic features and visual prognosis in the Treacher-Collins syndrome. Br J Ophthalmol 1993; 77: 642–5.

61. Marres HA. Hearing loss in the Treacher-Collins syndrome. Adv Otorhinolaryngol 2002; 61: 209–15.

62. Tulasne JF, Tessier PL. Results of the Tessier integral procedure for correction of Treacher Collins syndrome. Cleft Palate J 1986; 23: 40–9.

63. Goldenhar M. Associations malformatives de l'oeil et del'oreille; en particulier le syndrome dermöide epibulbaire – appendices auriculaires – fistula auris congenita et ses relations avec la dysostose mandibulo-faciale. J Genet Hum 1952; 1: 243.

64. Cohen MS, Samango-Sprouse CA, Stern HJ, et al. Neuro-developmental profile of infants and toddlers with oculo-auriculo-vertebral spectrum and the correlation of prognosis with physical findings. Am J Med Genet 1995; 60: 535–40.

65. Kaufman A, Medow N, Phillips R, et al. Treatment of epibulbar limbal dermoids. J Pediatr Ophthalmol Strabismus 1999; 36: 136–40.

66. Crawford JS. Benign tumors of the eyelid and adjacent structures: should they be removed? J Pediatr Ophthalmol Strabismus 1979; 16: 246–50.

67. Fry CL, Leone CR. Safe management of dermolipomas. Arch Ophthalmol 1994; 112: 1114–6.

68. McNab AA, Wright JE, Caswell AG. Clinical features and surgical management of dermolipomas. Aust N Z J Ophthalmol 1990; 18: 159–62.

CHAPTER
40 Cystic Lesions and Ectopias

Christopher J Lyons and Jack Rootman

CYSTIC LESIONS

Cystic lesions of the orbit in childhood include dermoid cyst, microphthalmos with cyst, lacrimal ductal cyst, congenital cystic eyeball, encephalocele, sinus mucocele, and teratoma. In some parts of the world parasitic cysts involving organisms such as *Echinococcus* and *Schistosoma* are common, but these are rare in Europe and North America.[1] Hemorrhage within orbital lymphangiomas may give rise to the so-called "chocolate" cysts. Cystic lesions of the orbital bones may be seen in fibrous dysplasia, ossifying fibroma, and aneurysmal bone cyst. Cystic lesions of the orbit and bone were reviewed by Lessner et al.[2]

Lacrimal ductal cyst

Lacrimal ductal cysts are rare but important since they are part of the differential diagnosis of ocular adnexal masses in childhood, particularly in the lacrimal gland region. Bullock et al.[3] suggested that lacrimal cysts should be classified according to their site of origin, that is, palpebral lobe (simple dacryops), orbital lobe, accessory glands, or ectopic lacrimal gland. The first three are considered here, and ectopic lacrimal gland is discussed later. Clinically, they may be confused with superficial dermoid cysts and inclusion and parasitic cysts.

Overall, lacrimal ductal cysts most commonly arise in the palpebral lobe. These tend to occur in adulthood but may be seen in the teenage years. There is sometimes a history of trauma or inflammation. A smooth, transilluminating mass slowly enlarges in the lateral aspect of the upper lid (Fig. 40.1) and may be evident on lid eversion as a blueish cyst. They may enlarge with crying and pain or tenderness may occur, spontaneously resolving as the cyst decompresses itself with a gush of tears. Careful surgical excision of the intact cyst is curative if the patient is symptomatic. Marsupialization of larger cysts may be necessary.

Cysts in the orbital lobe are rare but usually present in infancy or early childhood as a tense mass of the lacrimal fossa. They tend to be larger than their palpebral counterparts and many enlarge, sometimes quite suddenly due to inflammation or hemorrhage, causing proptosis and inferonasal displacement of the globe. Globe subluxation may occur.[4] Deep extension into the posterior orbit may be seen on CT scan. Once again, excision of the intact cyst is desirable. A lateral orbitotomy may be necessary if there is posterior extension. Histologically, ductal cysts of the palpebral lobe are lined by an outer layer of myoepithelium and inner layer of cuboidal cells, unlike congenital orbital lobe cysts whose lining epithelium is cuboidal.

Cysts of the accessory glands of Krause and Wolfring may also occur, resulting in swelling in the conjunctival fornix. These can be excised via a conjunctival approach.

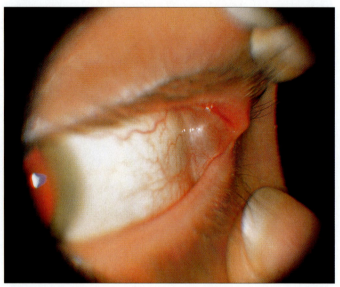

Fig. 40.1 Lacrimal ductal cyst showing as a transilluminating mass in the lateral fornix revealed by pulling the lid away from the globe. Patient of the University of British Columbia.

Lacrimal tissue may occasionally occur ectopically within the eye and orbit, often with an associated cystic component (see Ectopic Lacrimal Gland).

Dermoid cyst

Dermoid cysts of the orbit and periorbital region are common in childhood, accounting for 3–9% of orbital masses in most series.[5,6] They are developmental choristomas, which are thought to arise from ectodermal rests trapped at suture lines or within mesenchyme during orbital development.

Histologically, the cysts are lined by keratinized stratified squamous epithelium. Dermal appendages, including hair follicles and sebaceous glands, are found in their wall. Cyst leakage or rupture may give rise to a chronic granulomatous reaction.

Dermoids may be superficial or deep.[7] Conjunctival dermoids are variants, occurring posterior to the septum in the orbit. Most dermoids seen in childhood are superficial.

Superficial dermoids

These often present in infancy as a rounded mass, typically at the superotemporal (Fig. 40.2) margin of the orbit.[8,9] About one-quarter of superficial dermoids arise in the medial orbit[8,10,11] (Fig. 40.3), and these tend to be lined by stratified squamous epithelium.[10] They are painless, nontender, firm, nonfluctuant, and often immobile when fixed by deep attachment to the bone.

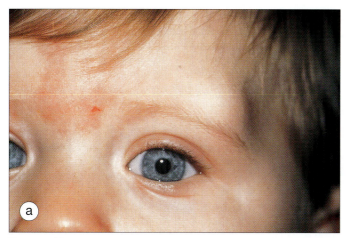
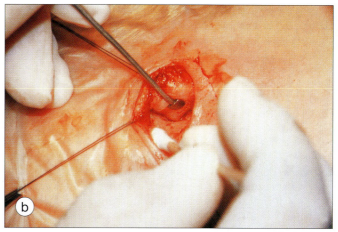

Fig. 40.2 (a) Typical superficial dermoid cyst on the brow of an 18-month-old boy. No intraorbital extension was noted preoperatively, although a small tail was seen to insert into bone at the time of surgery (b). This was divided and cauterized. The cyst was removed intact. Patient of the University of British Columbia.

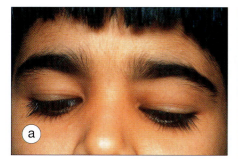
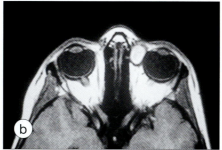
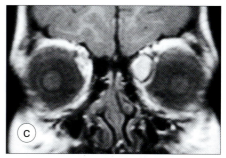

Fig. 40.3 (a) This 10-year-old boy had a gradually enlarging mass in his left upper lid for several years. (b) T_1-weighted MRI shows that this is situated anteriorly and its contents are isodense with orbital fat. (c) On coronal view, the mass is seen indenting the globe. It was excised completely and found to be a dermoid cyst. Patient of the University of British Columbia.

Since, strictly speaking, they are situated outside the orbit, they cause no displacement of the globe and the orbital rim is palpable behind their posterior edge. Unsuspected deep extension into the temporalis fossa, posterior orbit, or even intracranial space is not an uncommon finding in the apparently superficial dermoid cysts of childhood. These "dumbbell" dermoids may present with the typical signs of superficial dermoid but extend into the temporalis fossa in an hourglass configuration (Fig. 40.4). This finding was present in 24 of 70 patients with outer canthus dermoids reviewed at Moorfields[12] and 2 of the 17 cases reported by Gotzamanis et al.[13] Only one of the 65 patients reported by Ruszkowski et al.[14] had a deep extension. Very rarely, proptosis with or without visual impairment triggered by mastication (masticatory oscillopsia) can result from pressure on a communicating cyst by temporalis contraction with chewing.[15,16] Simultaneous orbital and temporalis fossa dermoid cysts without communication have also been described.[17]

The radiological appearance of a dermoid cyst is characteristic: on CT scan, a rounded discrete mass is seen, associated with thinning and smooth erosion of the underlying bone. The contents are often of heterogeneous density. Although fat lucency is not universally present, it was noted in 71% of the 70 patients reviewed by Sathananthan et al.[12] Its presence within the cyst is often considered diagnostic.[18]

Clearly, preoperative assessment of any dermoid cyst is essential to rule out deep extension of a superficial dermoid. If the cyst is small, mobile, and easily palpable for its entire extent,

imaging may not be necessary; large cysts with ill-defined, deep margins are best assessed preoperatively with a CT scan using 2-mm slices through the lesion, preferably with coronal cuts.

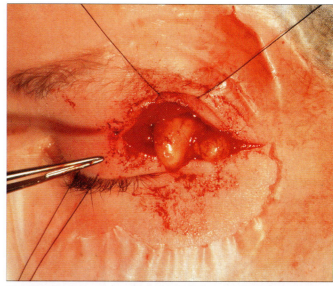

Fig. 40.4 Surgical excision of a "dumbbell" dermoid. The intervening bone has been removed. Patient of the University of British Columbia.

Excision of superficial dermoid cysts is relatively simple and should, in our opinion, be performed by the age of 5 years or so to avoid accidental rupture or inflammatory episodes related to spontaneous leakage.[19] The incision may be situated directly over the lesion above, below, or through the eyebrow. A skin-crease approach may be used to avoid a conspicuous postoperative scar,[14,20,21] and for the same reason, endoscopic removal has also been advocated in children.[22–24]

Although excision of the intact cyst is desirable, intraoperative rupture is not disastrous if the contents and all of the cyst wall are carefully removed. Decompression of the cyst may be helpful to expose the bony floor. Failure to excise the cyst wall completely or residual cyst contents in the operative site can elicit a chronic inflammatory reaction with sinus formation and persistent discharge. Surprisingly, cyst rupture is often not associated with dramatic inflammatory signs; these were present in only 4 of 17 patients with ruptured cysts reported by Satorre et al.[25] A chronic lipogranulomatous response was more common.

Deep dermoids

Although deep dermoid typically present in adolescence and adulthood with gradual enlargement and consequent displacement of orbital contents, they can occasionally present in infancy in a similar way.[26] Typically only their smooth and rounded anterior margin can be palpated although they may extend to the orbital apex.[27] The lesion may not be palpable at all (Fig. 40.5), as in the intraconal dermoid cyst reported by Wilkins and Byrd.[28] Proptosis and/or globe displacement predominate in the clinical picture but ocular motility[8,29] or visual disturbances and pain may occur. Dermoid cysts have been reported within[29,30] or attached to the lateral rectus muscle.[13]

The CT findings of deep dermoids are similar to those of superficial dermoids except for the frequent presence of irregular orbital wall defects as well as sclerosis, irregular scalloping, or notching of the underlying bone. The walls of large dermoid cysts may calcify.

The management of deep dermoids is complicated[9,27,31] since total surgical excision is necessary to prevent complications. A careful preoperative clinical and radiological assessment is essential to plan the appropriate surgical approach, which may involve combined anterior and lateral orbitotomies.[27] Although it was felt that this surgery was best delayed until bone growth had ceased,[31] the craniofacial literature suggests that delay is not necessary to safeguard facial bony growth.

Conjunctival dermoids

Almost one-half of these arise in the medial orbit in relation to the caruncle, usually in teenagers and adults.[27] They are not attached to the orbital bones, and are lined by typical conjunctival epithelium with goblet cells and adnexal structures with mucinous content in the cyst. They are managed by complete excision.

Orbital encephalocele

These rare abnormalities may be congenital or acquired. The congenital lesions arise from a presumed defective separation of neuroectoderm from surface ectoderm, resulting in a bony dehiscence with a "cystic" herniation of dura into the orbit, either alone (meningocele) or with brain tissue (meningoencephalocele). They may present in association with an optic disc anomaly,[32] and basal encephalocele should always be excluded in a child with an optic nerve anomaly such as coloboma or morning glory disc, especially if there is also a midline facial anomaly such as hypertelorism, cleft lip, or palate.[33] Orbital encephaloceles may be acquired as a result of head injury and orbital fracture, with herniation of the dura with or without brain tissue through the resulting bony defect.[34–36]

Orbital encephaloceles may be anterior or posterior.[37] Anterior orbital encephaloceles herniate through the region of the sutures dividing the frontal, ethmoid, lacrimal, and maxillary bones. The bony openings may be multiple.[38] They usually present as a congenital cystic swelling of the medial orbit extending onto the face, accompanied by telecanthus and, frequently, epiphora. They may also present in infancy and early childhood with gradually increasing proptosis and lateral globe displacement. The medial canthal tendon is usually displaced in an inferolateral direction. Atypical presentations are also encountered, such as a 10-mm blueish cystic mass in the superonasal fornix of a 1-month-old patient, which was found to be a meningoencephalocele.[39]

Classically, the size of the cyst increases on straining or crying.[4,40–42] It may be fluctuant, pulsatile, reducible with gentle pressure, and may transilluminate. Anterior encephaloceles are important in the differential diagnosis of any medial canthal swelling, and have been mistaken for sinus mucoceles, dermoid cysts, or even nasolacrimal duct mucoceles.[43] A bony defect is usually evident on X-ray and intracranial communication can be confirmed by CT scan. Three-dimensional CT reconstruction may be helpful in planning surgery,[44] which is usually performed by neurosurgical and/or maxillofacial teams.[45]

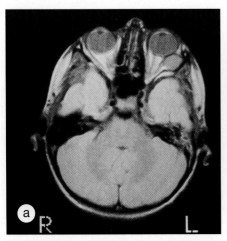
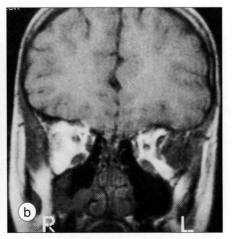

Fig. 40.5 Deep orbital dermoid. (a, b) MRI scans show a laterally-situated lesion behind the left globe.

Posterior encephaloceles herniate into the orbit via the optic foramen, orbital fissures, or a bony defect. They present with slowly progressive proptosis, which may be pulsatile. Occasionally, posterior encephaloceles may present during the teenage years or in adulthood.

Typically, the eye is displaced forward and downward[4] and the proptosis increases on straining or crying. Plain X-rays demonstrate enlarged foramina or a bony defect of the posterior orbit. CT scan demonstrates the size and content of the cyst. Posterior encephaloceles are particularly associated with the sphenoid wing dysplasia of neurofibromatosis type 1 (NF1). This type of defect can also be associated with enophthalmos.

Sinus mucocele

The paranasal sinuses are of clinical relevance to childhood orbital disease, and it is important to be familiar with their development. All the sinuses are present at birth in a rudimentary form, except the frontal sinus, which first appears at the age of 2 years. There are two spurts of enlargement: at the age of 6 or 7 years, coinciding with the eruption of the second dentition, and again at puberty.[46] Since the frontal sinus is the source of most mucoceles, it is not surprising that this disorder is rare in childhood. Ethmoidal sinus mucoceles, however, may present in early life,[47,48] particularly in association with cystic fibrosis. Their incidence is increasing in adulthood and, probably, childhood too.

A mucocele is a cystic expansion of a paranasal sinus, which results from obstruction of its ostium. The normal mucous secretions of the respiratory epithelial lining accumulate within the sinus, leading to a gradual expansion with loss of its internal bony structure. With further expansion, the cystic mass transgresses the orbital wall and displaces the orbital contents. It may also erode into the intracranial space.[49] Eventually, the cyst contents consist of viscous material, which may be white, yellow, or brown and contained by a fibrous capsule.

Most mucoceles arise anteriorly, affecting frontal or anterior ethmoid sinuses. The usual presentation is therefore with gradually increasing proptosis (Fig. 40.6) with inferolateral or lateral displacement of the globe, which may appear clinically as hypertelorism. A firm cystic noncompressible swelling may be palpable in the medial orbit. Its extension above the medial

canthal tendon should differentiate it from a mucocele of the lacrimal sac. Inflammatory signs are absent. The absence of pulsation, expansion with straining, and bony skull defect all differentiate it from an encephalocele. Sphenoid sinus mucoceles are rare in childhood, though Casteels et al.[50] reported a 10-year-old girl presenting with sudden blindness from optic nerve compression by a previously unsuspected sphenoid sinus mucocele.

Plain X-rays will show a markedly enlarged sinus on the affected side. On CT scan, a smooth-walled cystic lesion, often with eggshell calcification of the margins, is noted arising from the affected sinus. In childhood, this is most commonly the ethmoid, and expansion into the medial orbit is noted along with thinning of the wall and destruction of the internal septa.

Management is surgical, aiming to completely remove the cyst walls and reestablish sinus drainage. Collaboration with an ENT surgeon is essential; excision or drainage of the mucocele is increasingly performed endoscopically.[51] The transcaruncular approach has also been recommended for the management of frontoethmoidal mucoceles.[52] In cases where a Lynch incision is used, Lund and Rolfe[53] have stressed the importance of carefully repositioning the trochlea to avoid postoperative superior oblique underaction. Incomplete excision of the cyst wall is frequently followed by recurrence. Other cystic lesions arising in the sinuses may also cause proptosis, including dentigerous cysts.

Congenital cystic eyeball (anophthalmos with cyst)

True anophthalmia is very rare. More commonly, complete or partial failure of invagination of the optic vesicle before the 7-mm stage results in a congenital cystic eye or "anophthalmos with cyst."[54,55] No recognizable globe is present within the orbit. The congenital cystic "eye" is lined by neuroglial tissue without any of the normal ocular structures such as lens, ciliary body, or retina. The wall of the cyst is fibrous connective tissue with attached extraocular muscles. The absence of surface ectoderm-derived ocular structures is a common feature that may help with correct diagnosis of this condition. Congenital cystic eyeball is rare compared to microphthalmos with cyst, which represents a later defect in embryogenesis.[56]

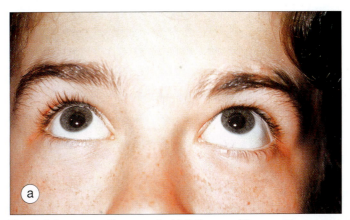

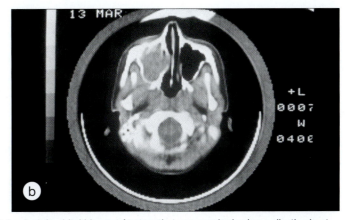

Fig. 40.6 Post-traumatic mucocele. (a) At the age of 9 years, this patient sustained a left orbital blowout fracture that was repaired using a silastic sheet. He is seen here at the age of 14 years; there is proptosis and upward displacement of the globe. (b) CT scanning showed the silastic implant had caused maxillary sinus obstruction and secondary mucocele. The implant was removed and the sinus opened surgically to allow drainage into the nose. Patient of the University of British Columbia.

It presents at birth as a large cystic swelling within the affected orbit. In contrast to microphthalmos with cyst, the cystic eyeball is usually centrally placed or distends the upper lid[54,55] though the cyst may occasionally be inferior.[56] The fellow eye is usually normal, though contralateral microphthalmos with cyst,[57] persistent hyperplastic primary vitreous (PHPV), or even bilateral congenital cystic eyes have been reported.[56]

The histology is similar to the cystic portion of microphthalmos with cyst: multiple cavities filled with proliferating glial tissue.[54,56] These cystic orbital lesions, occurring in neonates, should be distinguished from teratomas.

Microphthalmos with cyst

Incomplete closure of the fetal fissure between the 7- and 14-mm stage of embryonic development may result in a variety of colobomatous defects of the eye.[58] Eyes with severe colobomas are often microphthalmic and proliferation of neuroectoderm at the lips of the persistent fetal fissure may result in the formation of an orbital cyst that communicates with the eye. The size of the cyst varies from microscopic to massive. SOX2 mutations have recently been implicated in some cases of microphthalmia.[59]

Clinical presentation

The manifestations are variable, ranging from an apparently normal eye with a clinically unapparent cyst, an obvious cyst in association with a deformed eye, to an invisible eye displaced by an obvious cyst occupying the whole orbit. Typically, a blueish cystic transilluminating lesion (Fig. 40.7) bulges inferiorly into the lower fornix and lid, displacing a microphthalmic or rudimentary eye under the upper lid.[60,61] Rarely the cyst may be present in the upper lid and the eye is displaced downward.[62] Occasionally, the eye cannot be identified clinically,[60] even at examination under anesthesia. Bilateral microphthalmos with cyst has been reported.[63] The cyst communicates with the eye via a narrow stalk. The microphthalmic eye usually has extremely poor vision and an associated optic nerve and retinal coloboma. The eye, though often very small, has achieved differentiation with cornea, iris, ciliary body, and lens as well as retina. The other eye may be normal or may also have an optic nerve or retinal coloboma.[60,61] Ocular coloboma may be associated with a variety of systemic malformations.[58,60] The extent of the cystic component is best delineated by CT scan, although B-scan ultrasound can also be useful (Fig. 40.8). Small asymptomatic cysts may occasionally be found incidentally on CT scan. The glial nature of the cyst lining can be clearly demonstrated by immunohistochemistry.[64]

Management

In most cases no active intervention is needed.[61] The presence of the cyst contributes to socket expansion and a good cosmetic outcome is likely.[57] If cyst enlargement results in an unsightly appearance it may be managed by aspiration. Recurrence is

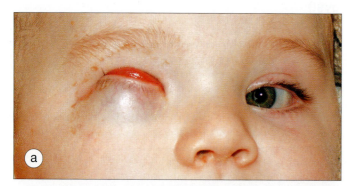

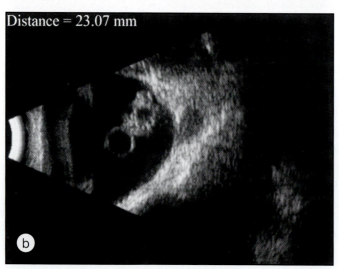

Distance = 23.07 mm

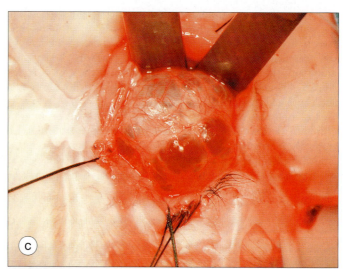

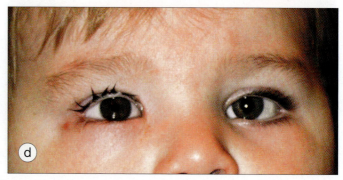

Fig. 40.7 Microphthalmos with cyst. (a) This boy was born with a blueish swelling of the right lower lid, which gradually enlarged. At 6 months, a massive cyst fills the right orbit and distorts the lower lid, leading to conjunctival prolapse and exposure. (b) Imaging showed an expanded orbit with a multilocular cyst and a possible residual eye superior and posterior to the cyst. (c) The mass was excised along with the microphthalmic eye. (d) Postoperative result with prosthesis. Patient of the University of British Columbia.

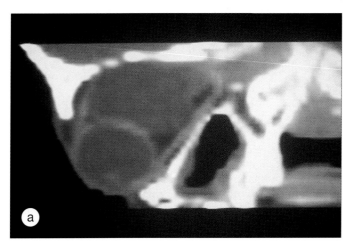

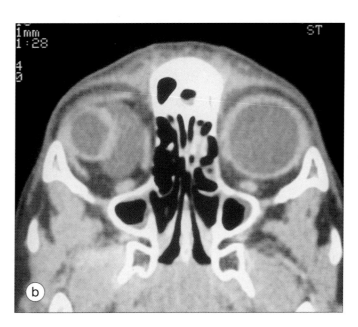

Fig. 40.8 (a, b) CT scans showing the superior and medial orbital cyst.

common and repeated aspiration may be necessary. When there is recurrence of the cyst after multiple aspirations, surgery may be indicated. Although it may be difficult to excise the cyst without sacrificing the globe, this can be achieved in patients with mild microphthalmos, with a satisfactory cosmetic outcome.[65]

The presence of an eye is thought to be important in inducing normal bony orbital growth. A congenitally anophthalmic socket is known to run into problems with delayed orbital growth as well as conjunctival contraction, which may prevent satisfactory prosthetic fitting later. Early orbital volume replacement with an appropriate implant and/or prosthesis is therefore advocated if the globe is small or absent. Various types of conformers and socket expanders can be used to maintain the conjunctival fornices and palpebral fissures and, perhaps, promote normal orbital growth.[66-71]

Early enucleation also produces a bony volume reduction; good cosmetic results are generally recognized from the currently accepted practice of using a large orbital implant at the time of enucleation.[70] Surprising evidence comes from recent CT three-dimensional reconstruction and volumetric analysis on a group of patients enucleated in childhood (8 patients) or adult life (21 patients), with or without orbital implants. These demonstrated a bony orbital volume reduction of up to 15%, less than generally thought, and clinically imperceptible. Although the numbers were too small for statistical analysis, no facial asymmetry was apparent whether an orbital implant was used or not at the time of enucleation in early childhood (0.4–8.0 years), with a follow-up ranging from 25 to 52 years.[72]

Orbital teratoma

Teratomas are tumors that arise from pluripotential embryonic stem cells and consist of elements derived from more than one germ cell layer. Although classically all three layers should be represented within the tumor, only mesoderm is invariably seen, and ectodermal or endodermal elements can be absent. Strictly speaking, such tumors should be called "teratoid." The extent of the tumor can be limited to the orbit (primary orbital teratoma), or it may involve the intracranial compartment and/or nasal and sinus cavities (combined orbital and extraorbital teratoma). Cavernous sinus teratoma has also been reported.[73] Occasionally,

a much larger primary intracranial tumor invades the orbit (secondary orbital teratoma). This usually manifests prenatally as polyhydramnios and is rarely compatible with life.[74]

The usual presentation of a primary orbital teratoma is unilateral, often massive proptosis in a newborn child.[75-78] Teratomas are more common in females by a ratio of 2:1. Surprisingly, the globe itself is usually of normal size or slightly smaller (Fig. 40.9), but it is surrounded by intensely chemotic conjunctiva. It is displaced by a large cystic mass that is often fluctuant and transilluminates but may also appear solid. The mass is often intraconal, giving rise to axial displacement with indentation by the four recti. Superior or inferior teratomas can also occur. Typically there is rapid growth after birth as secretions from the epithelial elements of the tumor accumulate within its cystic spaces. Exposure keratopathy, ulceration, and even perforation can complicate the resultant lagophthalmos. The tumor may stretch and adhere to the optic nerve, giving rise to secondary optic atrophy. Occasionally, teratomas grow slowly over a number of years.[77]

On ultrasound, the tumor is of heterogeneous density and may contain foci of calcification. Plain X-rays will show an enlarged orbit on the affected side, and the extent of the lesion is easily delineated on CT scan. This modality is particularly useful for excluding intracranial extension.

The treatment of choice is surgical excision within the first month, with preservation of the globe.[75-77] Many cases where some vision was preserved in the affected eye have been reported.[78] Intraoperative aspiration of fluid from the cystic mass may facilitate tumor removal. Unlike teratomas arising from other sites, malignant change is very rare in the orbit.[79] However, it is recorded in combined orbital and intracranial teratoma, where a bony defect allows the tumor to extend into the intracranial space. In these cases, a combined orbitotomy and craniotomy is necessary to remove the tumor. Total excision can be difficult, and the residual tumor can give rise to problems of late recurrence and malignancy.[80]

Parasitic cysts

Echinococcosis (hydatid cyst)

The tapeworm *Echinococcus* is an intestinal parasite of dogs and foxes. Sheep, cattle, or rodents may ingest contaminated feces

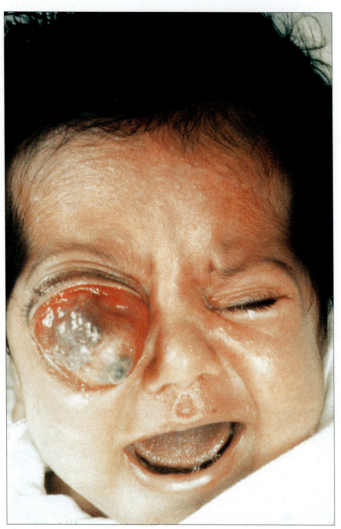

Fig. 40.9 Orbital teratoma.

throughout the body, settling in various end-organs to form slowly enlarging, fluid-filled cysts full of larvae. Due to the distribution of blood from the portal tract, there is a predilection for the right lobe of the liver. Orbital involvement is well recognized.[81–83] Approximately 1% of infestations involve the orbit,[84] especially the superior and posterior orbit.

Most sheep- and cattle-rearing areas of the world have a high prevalence. Clinically, orbital echinococcosis presents with insidious signs of mass effect, which may be accompanied by chemosis, diplopia, and restricted ocular motility. Pressure on the optic nerve can result in visual loss and optic atrophy. Rupture of the cyst can result in an acute inflammatory episode.

The diagnosis of orbital echinococcosis is made by ultrasonography, CT (Fig. 40.10), or magnetic resonance imaging (MRI) scanning, which show a cystic mass whose wall is occasionally calcified and which contains fluid that is isodense with vitreous. Other confirmatory findings include eosinophilia on a blood film, and positive enzyme-linked immunosorbent assay (ELISA) testing for echinococcal antibodies–this has a sensitivity and specificity of over 90% for *Echinococcus*.

Systemic treatment with albendazole is effective and a suitable alternative to surgery in uncomplicated cases.[85] Orbital cysts may be excised intact via a direct or lateral orbitotomy. Intraoperative rupture should be avoided since it may be complicated by inflammation and implantation of daughter cysts within the surgical site, although this is sometimes technically difficult.[86] Surgery should be accompanied by treatment with albendazole. Other parasitic infestations of the orbit include cysticercosis and trichinosis, both acquired from pork.

ECTOPIAS

Dermolipoma

These congenital lesions arise as a result of sequestration of skin within the conjunctiva at the time of embryonic development of the eyelids. They are frequently mistaken for true orbital dermoids. They may occur alone or as part of the Goldenhar spectrum, with lid coloboma, preauricular skin tags, hemifacial microsomia, and palatal and hearing abnormalities. They are situated laterally on the bulbar surface, are pink and skin-like due to their keratinization (Fig. 40.11), and may have surface hairs, which can cause irritation. Rarely, they may contain bony tissue.[87] Their frequent superior and

and become hosts, and dogs become infected by eating their carcasses. Humans are drawn accidentally into the cycle by ingesting ova in contaminated meat, berries, or feces from poor hand hygiene. The ova hatch in the intestine, and larvae migrate

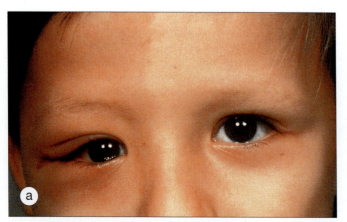

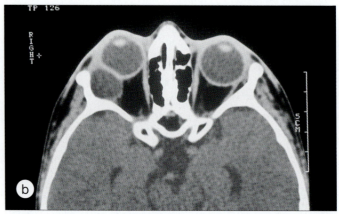

Fig. 40.10 (a) This 9-year-old refugee, who had no access to sanitation for 2 years, presented with a 6-month history of increasing right upper lid swelling. He has 4 mm of right proptosis, downward displacement of the globe, and lateral ptosis. (b) On CT scan a cystic lesion is found situated posterolaterally to the globe; this was an echinococcal cyst, which was excised intact. Patient of the University of British Columbia.

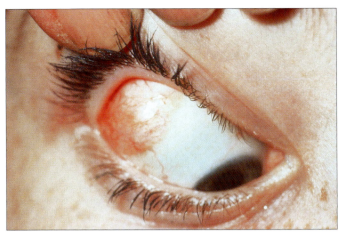

Fig. 40.11 This 16-year-old girl has a long-standing lesion in the upper fornix of the right eye, which is consistent with a dermolipoma.

posterior extension are closely associated with the lacrimal ducts and levator muscle.[88] Surgery should be conservative, in response to symptoms of irritation, and should be performed with the microscope and limited to excision of the hair-bearing surface tissues or the interpalpebral lesion.[84,89] Care should be taken to identify and preserve the lacrimal ducts, and to avoid the lateral rectus and levator muscles. There are numerous reports of complications from attempts at complete excision of dermolipoma with aggressive orbital dissection. These include dry eye, restrictive symblepharon, strabismus, and ptosis.[87,90]

Ectopic lacrimal gland

Lacrimal gland tissue may occasionally occur at ectopic sites within the orbit. Most commonly, it is found in the eyelid or conjunctiva, but it may occur on the cornea or even the iris and choroid.[91] Green and Zimmerman[92] reported eight such cases and more have since been added to the literature, often in children or teenagers. The ectopic tissue may be situated intra- or extraconally. Typically, the patients present with proptosis; double vision is a common symptom due to muscle restriction from the inflammatory response, which the ectopic tissue often incites. The differential diagnosis includes true orbital neoplasms. Investigation, including CT scan, often shows a cystic component.[93] The treatment of choice is surgical excision; if this is incomplete, proptosis may recur.[92] The aberrant tissue may also give rise to tumors such as pleomorphic adenoma[94] or adenocarcinoma.[92]

Conjunctival and inclusion cyst

Conjunctival tissue may be sequestered as a primary embryological malformation or as a result of trauma or surgery. This may occur anywhere on the conjunctiva and may be seen as a blister-like conjunctival swelling, filled with clear fluid. Occasionally, a posterior extension is present, with mass effect. Recurrence is common if the cyst is punctured, and complete excision of the wall is indicated for a cure (Fig. 40.12). Histologically, this is conjunctival epithelium. Inclusion cysts may also occur on the skin of the eyelids after trauma or surgery.

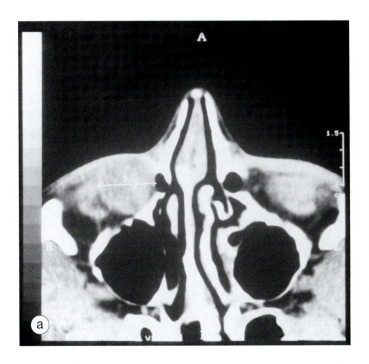

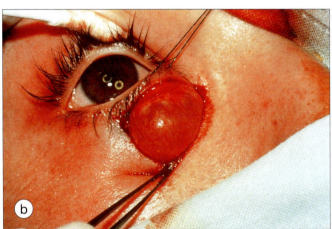

Fig. 40.12 (a) This child had a lower lid swelling, found to be cystic on CT scanning. (b) A conjunctival cyst was excised via a skin incision. The differential diagnosis includes conjunctival dermoid, ductal cyst, lymphangioma, and respiratory cyst. Dr Alan McNab's patient.

Other cystic lesions

A variety of other very rare, developmental cysts of neural origin may occur (Fig. 40.13).

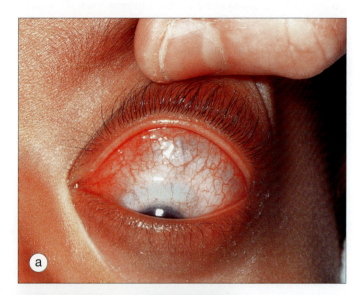

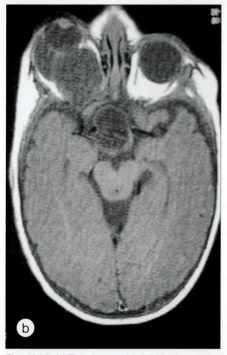

Fig. 40.13 (a) This 1-year-old child had a congenital proptosis with a cystic lesion seen almost surrounding the eye. (b) MRI scanning showed the cystic lesion to be contiguous with a cyst in the suprasellar cistern. Total excision revealed that this was an ectopic neural cystic hamartoma. The lesion was removed *en bloc*.

REFERENCES

1. Jakobiec FA, Jones IS. Orbital inflammation. In: Duane TD, editor. Clinical Ophthalmology. Hagerstown: Harper and Row; 1983: 60–5.
2. Lessner AM, Antle CM, Rootman J, et al. Cystic lesions of the orbit and radiolucent defects of bone. In: Margo CE, Hamed LM, Mames RN, editors. Diagnostic Problems in Clinical Ophthalmology. Philadelphia: Saunders; 1994: 87–98.
3. Bullock JD, Fleishman JA, Rosset JS. Lacrimal ductal cysts. Ophthalmology 1986; 93: 1355–60.
4. Duke-Elder S. Congenital deformities of the orbit. In: Duke-Elder S, editor. System of Ophthalmology. London: Kimpton; 1964: 949–56.
5. Youseffi B. Orbital tumors in children: a clinical study of 62 cases. J Pediatr Ophthalmol Strabismus 1969; 6: 177–81.
6. Crawford JS. Diseases of the orbit. In: Crawford JS, Morin JD, editors. The Eye in Childhood. New York: Grune and Stratton; 1983: 361–94.
7. Grove AS, Jr. Orbital Disorders: Diagnosis and Management. New York: Raven Press; 1981.
8. Bonavolonta G, Tranfa F, de Conciliis C, et al. Dermoid cysts: 16-year survey. Ophthal Plast Reconstr Surg 1995; 11: 187–92.
9. Pfeiffer RL, Nichol RJ. Dermoid and epidermoid tumors of the orbit. Arch Ophthalmol 1948; 40: 639–64.
10. Shields JA, Kaden IH, Eagle RC, Jr, et al. Orbital dermoid cysts: clinicopathologic correlations, classification, and management. The 1997 Josephine E. Schueler Lecture. Ophthal Plast Reconstr Surg 1997; 13: 265–76.
11. Chawda SJ, Moseley IF. Computed tomography of orbital dermoids: a 20-year review. Clin Radiol 1999; 54: 821–5.
12. Sathananthan N, Moseley IF, Rose GE, et al. The frequency and clinical significance of bone involvement in outer canthus dermoid cysts. Br J Ophthalmol 1993; 77: 789–94.
13. Gotzamanis A, Desphieux JL, Pluot M, et al. Les kystes dermoides. Epidemiologie, aspects cliniques et anatomo–pathologiques, prise en charge therapeutique. J Fr Ophtalmol 1999; 22: 549–53.
14. Ruszkowski A, Caouette-Laberge L, Bortoluzzi P, et al. Superior eyelid incision: an alternative approach for frontozygomatic dermoid cyst excision. Ann Plast Surg 2000; 44: 591–4.
15. Emerick GT, Shields CL, Shields JA, et al. Chewing-induced visual impairment from a dumbbell dermoid cyst. Ophthal Plast Reconstr Surg 1997; 13: 57–61.
16. Whitney CE, Leone CR, Kincaid MC. Proptosis with mastication: an unusual presentation of an orbital dermoid cyst. Ophthal Surg 1986; 17: 295–8.
17. Perry JD, Tuthill R. Simultaneous ipsilateral temporal fossa and orbital dermoid cysts. Am J Ophthalmol 2003; 135: 413–5.
18. Nugent RA, Lapointe JS, Rootman J, et al. Orbital dermoids: features on CT. Radiology 1987; 165: 475–8.
19. Abou-Rayyah Y, Rose GE, Konrad H, et al. Clinical, radiological and pathological examination of periocular dermoid cysts: evidence of inflammation from an early age. Eye 2002; 16: 507–12.
20. Kersten RC. The eyelid crease approach to superficial lateral dermoid cysts. J Pediatr Ophthalmol Strabismus 1988; 25: 48–51.
21. Kronish JW, Dortzbach RK. Upper eyelid crease surgical approach to dermoid and epidermoid cysts in children. Arch Ophthalmol 1988; 106: 1625–7.
22. Steele MH, Suskind DL, Moses M, et al. Orbitofacial masses in children: an endoscopic approach. Arch Otolaryngol Head Neck Surg 2002; 128: 409–13.
23. Paige KT, Eaves FF 3rd, Wood RJ. Endoscopically assisted plastic surgical procedures in the pediatric patient. J Craniofac Surg 1997; 8: 164–8.
24. Mulhern M, Kirkpatrick N, Joshi N, et al. Endoscopic removal of periorbital lesions. Orbit 2002; 21: 263–9.
25. Satorre J, Antle M, O'Sullivan R, et al. Orbital lesions with granulomatous inflammation. Can J Ophthalmol 1991; 26: 174–5.
26. Leonardo D, Shields CL, Shields JA, et al. Recurrent giant orbital dermoid of infancy. J Pediatr Ophthalmol Strabismus 1994; 31: 50–2.
27. Sherman RP, Rootman J, Lapointe JS. Orbital dermoids: clinical presentation and management. Br J Ophthalmol 1984; 68: 642–52.
28. Wilkins RB, Byrd WA. Intraconal dermoid cyst. Ophthal Reconstr Surg 1986; 2: 83–7.
29. Gatzonis S, Charakidas A, Papathanassiou M, et al. Multiple orbital dermoid cysts located within the latera rectus muscle, clinically

mimicking Duane syndrome type II. J Pediatr Ophthalmol Strabismus 2002; 39: 324.

30. Howard GR, Nerad JA, Bonavolonta G, et al. Orbital dermoid cysts located within the lateral rectus muscle. Ophthalmology 1994; 101: 767–71.

31. Lane CM, Erlich WW, Wright JE. Orbital dermoid cyst. Eye 1987; 1: 504–11.

32. Pollock JA, Newton TH, Hoyt WF. Trans-sphenoidal and transethmoidal encephaloceles. Radiology 1968; 90: 442–53.

33. Caprioli J, Lesser RL. Basal encephalocoele and morning glory syndrome. Br J Ophthalmol 1983; 67: 349–51.

34. Antonelli V, Cremonini AM, Campobassi A, et al. Traumatic encephalocele related to orbital roof fractures: report of six cases and literature review. Surg Neurol 2002; 57: 117–25.

35. Martello JY, Vasconez HC. Supraorbital roof fractures: a formidable entity with which to contend. Ann Plast Surg 1997; 38: 223–7.

36. Kumar R, Verma A, Sharma K, et al. Post-traumatic pseudo-meningocele of the orbit in a young child. J Pediatr Ophthalmol Strabismus 2003; 40: 110–2.

37. Duke-Elder S. System of Ophthalmology, part 2, Normal and Abnormal Development: Congenital Deformities. London: Kimpton; 1964.

38. Boonvisut S, Ladpli S, Sujatanond M, et al. Morphologic study of 120 skull base defects in frontoethmoidal encephalomeningoceles. Plast Reconstr Surg 1998; 101: 1784–95.

39. Terry A, Patrinely JR, Anderson RL, et al. Orbital meningoencephalocele manifesting as a conjunctival mass. Am J Ophthalmol 1993; 115: 46–9.

40. Mortada A, E-Toraei I. Orbital meningo-encephalocoele and exophthalmos. Br J Ophthalmol 1960; 44: 309–14.

41. Consul BN, Kulshrestha OP. Orbital meningocoele. Br J Ophthalmol 1965; 49: 374–6.

42. Leone CR, Marlowe JF. Orbital presentation of an ethmoidal encephalocele. Arch Ophthalmol 1970; 83: 445–7.

43. Rashid ER, Bergstrom TJ, Evans RM, et al. Anterior encephaloceles presenting as nasolacrimal obstruction. Ann Ophthalmol 1986; 18: 132–6.

44. David DJ, Sheffield L, Simpson D, et al. Frontoethmoidal meningo-encephalocoeles: morphology and treatment. Br J Plast Surg 1984; 37: 271–84.

45. Lello GE, Sparrow OC, Gopal R. The surgical correction of fronto-ethmoidal meningo-encephaloceles. J Craniomaxillofac Surg 1989; 17: 293–8.

46. Last RJ. Anatomy. Regional and Applied. Edinburgh: Churchill Livingstone; 1978.

47. Alberti PW, Marshall HF, Munro-Black JI. Frontal ethmoidal mucocoele as a cause of unilateral proptosis. Br J Ophthalmol 1968; 52: 833–8.

48. Robertson DM, Henderson JW. Unilateral proptosis secondary to orbital mucocele in infancy. Am J Ophthalmol 1969; 68: 845–7.

49. Delfini R, Missori P, Iannetti G, et al. Mucoceles of the paranasal sinuses with intracranial and intraorbital extension: report of 28 cases. Neurosurgery 1993; 32: 901–6.

50. Casteels I, De Loof E, Brock P, et al. Sudden blindness in a child: presenting symptom of a sphenoid sinus mucocoele. Br J Ophthalmol 1992; 76: 502–4.

51. Conboy PJ, Jones NS. The place of endoscopic sinus surgery in the treatment of paranasal sinus mucocoeles. Clin Otolaryngol 2003; 28: 207–10.

52. Lai PC, Liao SL, Jou JR, et al. Transcaruncular approach for the management of frontoethmoid mucoceles. Br J Ophthalmol 2003; 87: 699–703.

53. Lund VJ, Rolfe ME. Ophthalmic considerations in front ethmoidal mucocoeles. J Laryn Otol 1989; 103: 667–9.

54. Dollfus MA, Langlois J, Clement JC, et al. Congenital cystic eyeball. Am J Ophthalmol 1968; 66: 504–9.

55. Helveston EM, Malone E, Lashmet MH. Congenital cystic eye. Arch Ophthalmol 1970; 84: 622–4.

56. Hayashi N, Repka MX, Ueno H, et al. Congenital cystic eye: report of two cases and review of the literature. Surv Ophthalmol 1999; 44: 173–9.

57. McLean CJ, Ragge NK, Jones RB, et al. The management of orbital cysts associated with congenital microphthalmos and anophthalmos. Br J Ophthalmol 2003; 87: 860–3.

58. Pagon RA. Ocular coloboma. Surv Ophthalmol 1981; 25: 223–36.

59. Fantes J, Ragge NK, Lynch SA, et al. Mutations in SOX2 cause anophthalmia. Nat Genet 2003; 33: 461–3.

60. Waring GO, Roth AM, Rodrigues M. Clinicopathologic correlation of microphthalmos with cyst. Am J Ophthalmol 1976; 82: 714–21.

61. Weiss A, Martinez C, Greenwald M. Microphthalmos with cyst. Clinical presentation and computed tomographic findings. J Pediatr Ophthalmol Srabismus 1985; 22: 6–12.

62. Nicholson DH, Green RW. Microphthalmos with cyst. In: Nicholson DH, Green RW, editors. Pediatric Ocular Tumors. New York: Masson; 1981: 219–21.

63. Arstikaitis M. A case report of bilateral microphthalmos with cysts. Arch Ophthalmol 1969; 82: 480–2.

64. Lieb W, Rochels R, Gronemeyer U. Microphthalmos with colobomatous orbital cyst: clinical, histological, immunological, and electronmicroscopic findings. Br J Ophthalmol 1990; 74: 59–62.

65. Polito E, Leccisotti A. Colobomatous ocular cyst excision with globe preservation. Ophthal Plast Reconstr Surg 1995; 11: 288–92.

66. Price E, Simon JW, Calhoun JH. Prosthetic treatment of severe microphthalmos in infancy. J Pediatr Ophthalmol Strabismus 1986; 23: 22–4.

67. O'Keefe M, Webb M, Pashby RC, et al. Clinical anophthalmos. Br J Ophthalmol 1987; 71: 635–8.

68. Dootz GL. The ocularist's management of congenital microphthalmos and anophthalmos. Adv Ophthalmic Plast Reconstr Surg 1992; 9: 41–56.

69. Downes R, Lavin M, Collin R. Hydrophilic expanders for the congenital anophthalmic socket. Adv Ophthalmic Plast Reconstr Surg 1992; 9: 57–61.

70. Fountain TR, Goldberger S, Murphree AL. Orbital development after enucleation in early childhood. Ophthal Plast Reconstr Surg 1999; 15: 32–6.

71. Tucker SM, Sapp N, Collin R. Orbital expansion of the congenitally anophthalmic socket. Br J Ophthalmol 1995; 79: 667–71.

72. Hintschich C, Zonneveld F, Baldeschi L, et al. Bony orbital development after early enucleation in humans. Br J Ophthalmol 2001; 85: 205–8.

73. Tobias S, Valarezo J, Meir K, et al. Giant cavernous sinus teratoma: a clinical example of a rare entity: case report. Neurosurgery 2001; 48: 1367–70.

74. Kivela T, Tarkkanen A. Orbital germ cell tumors revisited: a clinico-pathological approach to classification. Surv Ophthalmol 1994; 38: 541–54.

75. Hoyt WF, Joe S. Congenital teratoid cyst. Arch Ophthalmol 1962; 68: 197–201.

76. Barber JC, Barber LF, Guerry D, et al. Congenital orbital teratoma. Arch Ophthalmol 1974; 91: 45–8.

77. Levin M, Leone CR, Kincaid MC. Congenital orbital teratoma. Am J Ophthalmol 1986; 102: 476–81.

78. Chang DF, Dallow RL, Walton DS. Congenital orbital teratoma: report of a case with visual preservation. J Pediatr Ophthalmol Strabismus 1980; 17: 88–95.

79. Soares E, Lopes K, Adrade J, et al. Orbital malignant teratoma. A case report. Orbit 1983; 2: 235–40.

80. Garden JW, McManus J. Congenital orbital-intracranial teratoma with subsequent malignancy. Br J Ophthalmol 1986; 70: 111–4.

81. Morales GA, Croxatto JO, Crovetto L, et al. Hydatid cysts of the orbit. A review of 35 cases. Ophthalmology 1988; 95: 1027–32.

82. Alparslan L, Kanberoglu K, Peksayar G, et al. Orbital hydatid cyst: assessment of two cases. Neuroradiology 1990; 32: 163–5.

83. Chaabouni M, Ben Zina Z, Ben Ayez H, et al. Kyste hydatique de l'orbite: localisation intra-orbitaire unique. A propos d'une observation. J Fr Ophtalmol 1999; 22: 329–33.

84. Rootman J. Diseases of the Orbit: a Multidisciplinary Approach. 2nd ed. Philadelphia: Lippincott Williams & Wilkins; 2002.

85. Gil-Grande LA, Rodriguez-Caabeiro F, Prieto JG, et al. Randomised controlled trial of efficacy of albendazole in intra-abdominal hydatid disease. Lancet 1993; 342: 1269–72.

86. Ergun R, Okten AI, Yuksel M, et al. Orbital hydatid cysts: report of four cases. Neurosurg Rev 1997; 20: 33–7.

87. Fry CL, Leone CR. Safe management of dermolipomas. Arch Ophthalmol 1994; 112: 1114–6.

88. Eijpe AA, Koornneef L, Bras J, et al. Dermolipoma: characteristic CT appearance. Doc Ophthalmol 1990; 74: 321–8.

89. McNab AA, Wright JE, Caswell AG. Clinical features and surgical management of dermolipomas. Aust N Z J Ophthalmol 1990; 18: 159–62.

90. Crawford JS. Benign tumors of the eyelid and adjacent structures: should they be removed? J Pediatr Ophthalmol Strabismus 1979; 16: 246–50.

91. Hunter WS. Aberrant intraocular lacrimal gland tissue. Br J Ophthalmol 1960; 44: 619–25.

92. Green WR, Zimmerman LE. Ectopic lacrimal gland tissue. Report of eight cases with orbital involvement. Arch Ophthalmol 1967; 78: 318–27.

93. Rush A, Leone CR. Ectopic lacrimal gland cyst of the orbit. Am J Ophthalmol 1981; 92: 198–201.

94. Boudet G, Bertezene M. Exophthalmie par adenome lacrymal en position ectopique (angiographie de l'orbite). Bull Soc Ophtalmol Fr 1964; 64: 624.

CHAPTER
41 Inflammatory Disorders

Christopher J Lyons and Jack Rootman

The orbit in childhood can be affected by a variety of inflammatory disorders. As discussed in Chapter 32, these become more common in the second decade of life, when causes of orbital disease increasingly resemble those found in adulthood.

The principal causes of inflammation in our series can be divided into nonspecific orbital inflammatory syndromes (NSOIS) (previously known under the umbrella term of "inflammatory pseudotumor") and specific causes such as sarcoidosis and Wegener granulomatosis, both of which are rare but potentially life-threatening. The incidence of thyroid orbitopathy increases with age in the teenage years, and this subject is discussed briefly.

Infective orbital cellulitis in early childhood is most commonly related to dacryocystitis or trauma. Over the age of 6 years, and particularly in the second decade, the fully-formed sinuses become the most common source of orbital cellulitis (see Chapter 20).

NONSPECIFIC ORBITAL INFLAMMATORY SYNDROMES (INFLAMMATORY PSEUDOTUMORS)

The child's orbit is occasionally the site of acute or subacute inflammation of unknown cause.[1–4] This entity was previously known as "orbital inflammatory pseudotumor",[5] a term which, with the advent of computed tomography (CT) and magnetic resonance imaging (MRI), has been abandoned in favor of terminology describing the site of inflammation.[6–8] Thus, anterior, diffuse, apical, myositic and lacrimal types are recognized. Children tend to develop the anterior and diffuse types, but myositis and lacrimal inflammation are also well recognized. Apical involvement is rare. Sclerosing inflammation of the orbit is a specific inflammation and is very rare in childhood.

Definition

These syndromes present acutely or subacutely with inflammatory signs. Although apparently idiopathic, they have many features of an orbital immune reaction.[9] Histologically, there is an influx of neutrophils, lymphocytes, plasma cells and macrophages. Inflammatory mediators cause edema, vascular dilatation and pain without systemic malaise. In contrast, chronic inflammations and granulomatous diseases cause mass effect as their predominant feature without signs of acute inflammation. The common imaging feature of acute or subacute NSOIS is the presence of a poorly defined margin to the inflammatory focus, as well as contrast enhancement.[10,11]

Anterior idiopathic orbital inflammation: acute and subacute

This is the most common type of NSOIS found in childhood. The inflammatory process is centered on the anterior orbit and adjacent globe (Fig. 41.1). Pain, proptosis, lid swelling, conjunctival injection and decreased vision are the main presenting features, with an onset over days or occasionally weeks. Of particular note in the pediatric age group is the presence of associated anterior and posterior uveitis, which can lead to erroneous treatment with topical steroid due to misdiagnosis.[4,12,13] The optic nerve head may be elevated.[14] Systemically, the erythrocyte sedimentation rate may be raised, and there is often cerebrospinal fluid pleocytosis.[14] Disturbances in thyroid function tests and frank hypothyroidism have also been reported in association with NSOIS.[15,16] CT scans shows diffuse anterior orbital inflammation centered on the globe, producing scleral and choroidal thickening with or without serous retinal detachment. The junction of the globe and optic nerve is characteristically obscured on CT scan with inflammatory changes extending along

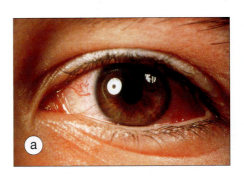
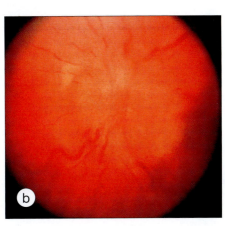

Fig. 41.1 Nonspecific orbital inflammatory syndrome. Anterior NSOIS in a 6-year-old boy who presented with a red eye (a), pain on eye movement and decreased vision of 3 days duration. Fundoscopy (b) shows choroidal swelling and papillitis. Patient from the University of British Columbia.

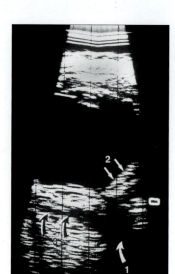

Fig. 41.2 Ultrasound scan of anterior NSOIS showing the T-sign. There is doubling of the optic nerve shadow,[1] shallow retinal detachment[2] and accentuation of Tenon's space.[3] Patient from the University of British Columbia.

the nerve sheath. On ultrasound, there is a uniform-density infiltrate corresponding to sclerotenonitis, with accentuation of the sub-Tenon space and doubling of the optic nerve shadow, which produces a T-shaped shadow (or T-sign) (Fig. 41.2).

Diffuse idiopathic orbital inflammation: acute and subacute

This is clinically similar to the anterior form described above, although the symptoms and clinical signs tend to be more severe (Fig. 41.3). Restriction of eye movements is more pronounced and the visual acuity is worse due to retinal detachment and/or optic neuropathy. Inflammatory soft tissue changes permeate all the orbital components on CT scan, with a white-out appearance whose density is proportional to the severity of the clinical signs, and which resolves as the condition settles. Again, the T-sign is evident on ultrasonography.

Anterior and diffuse nonspecific orbital inflammatory syndromes: differential diagnoses and management

The differential diagnosis includes infection such as orbital cellulitis, scleritis, sudden enlargement of a pre-existing lesion as in a ruptured dermoid or hemorrhage into a lymphangioma, or malignancy which, in childhood, may be rhabdomyosarcoma, neuroblastoma, Ewing sarcoma or leukemic infiltration. Anterior and diffuse NSOIS are also part of the differential diagnosis of uveitis and serous retinal detachment in childhood. Biopsy of involved orbital tissues should be considered in all but the most typical cases.

Treatment with nonsteroidal anti-inflammatory drugs such as flurbiprofen is tried first. Systemic steroids may be used in addition, or as an alternative in doses of 1–1.5 mg/kg per day. There is usually a rapid improvement in symptoms, especially pain, as well as clinical signs. Progress can be monitored by resolution of the clinical, CT and ultrasound features. This disease may have a recalcitrant course, with frequent recurrences and steroid dependence. High-dose steroid is restarted for recurrence and tapered as quickly as clinical progress will allow, usually over a few weeks. Failure to respond suggests the need for biopsy of involved tissues and the renewed search for a specific etiology. Low-dose radiotherapy has been advocated for biopsy-proven cases that do not respond to steroids. In addition, combined steroids and immunosuppressives may be necessary.

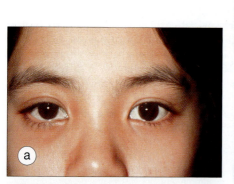

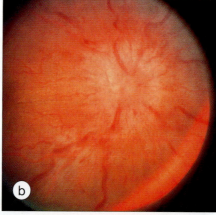

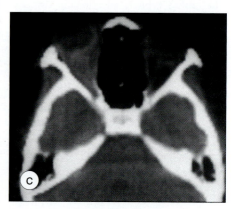

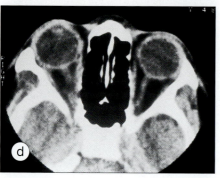

Fig. 41.3 Diffuse NSOIS. A 12-year-old girl presented with a right-sided retrobulbar ache, associated with ptosis (a), and pain on eye movement. There was right-sided uveitis with marked disc swelling (b). On CT scanning (c), there was a "white-out" appearance of the right orbit (similar patient) that resolved after treatment with systemic steroids (d). Patient from the University of British Columbia.

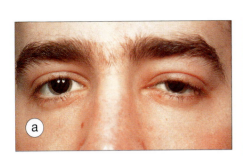
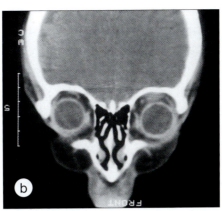

Fig. 41.4 Left superior rectus myositis in a 16-year-old boy. Ptosis (a), pain and limitation of upgaze with diplopia were the presenting signs; this was due to left superior rectus myositis shown as (b) a thickened muscle complex on CT scan. Patient from the University of British Columbia.

Idiopathic orbital myositis: acute and subacute

This is characterized by pain and limitation of eye movement, diplopia, ptosis, lid edema and conjunctival chemosis. Proptosis was present in five of six cases reported by Hankey et al.[17] Strabismus is often present in the primary position, with duction limitation in the direction of action of the involved muscle(s).[18] Spasm of the affected muscle also causes restriction of the ipsilateral antagonist with a positive forced duction test. Globe retraction and narrowing of the lid fissure similar to Duane syndrome is a frequent finding.[19,20]

CT scan shows diffuse muscle enlargement with irregular margins (Fig. 41.4). The muscle enlargement frequently extends forward to involve the tendon,[21] in contradistinction to thyroid orbitopathy where the tendon is typically spared. The superior rectus-levator complex or medial rectus are the most common muscles to be involved, but any muscle can be affected, including the obliques.[22] More than one muscle may simultaneously be involved and bilateral disease is well recognized.[2]

The cause of orbital myositis is unknown but a number of associations have been reported in the literature, including upper respiratory tract infection,[23] Lyme disease,[24] Whipple disease[25] and other autoimmune diseases.[26]

The differential diagnosis includes thyroid orbitopathy, which differs from idiopathic orbital myositis in that a preceding or concurrent history of thyroid disorder is commonly present, pain is absent, the inferior recti tend to be the first muscles involved (although any muscle may be involved) and sparing of the tendon is apparent on CT scan (see above). In some cases, differentiating between these two conditions can be very difficult[27] and mis-diagnosis is not uncommon.[4] Early orbital cellulitis, orbital metastasis, and trichinosis are other differential diagnoses.

Nonsteroidal anti-inflammatory treatment has been advocated by some,[28] but the rapid and dramatic response to steroids is almost diagnostic. We recommend an initial dose of 0.5–1 mg/kg per day, tapering to nothing over 2–4 weeks. Delay in diagnosis and initiation of therapy is associated with recurrence and incomplete resolution of signs.

Idiopathic lacrimal inflammation: acute and subacute

Pain, tenderness and swelling over the lateral aspect of the upper lid are typical presenting features of this disorder. The lid may have an S-shaped configuration with ptosis, which is more marked laterally than medially, and the globe is often slightly displaced downward and medially. Slit-lamp examination shows supero-temporal conjunctival chemosis and pouting of the lacrimal duct orifices. There is no uveitis. On CT scans, the inflammation is seen to be centered on the lacrimal gland, often extending diffusely into the lateral orbit and involving the adjacent globe. The differential diagnosis includes bacterial and viral dacryoadenitis, the latter often occurring in association with childhood infections such as mumps or mononucleosis. In this situation, the child is likely to be ill, and generalized lymphadenopathy or salivary gland enlargement may be noted, along with lymphocytosis. Inflammation related to leakage from a dermoid cyst and neoplasia is another rare possibility. Lacrimal gland involvement in orbital sarcoid tends to be a chronic process, presenting with signs and symptoms of dry eyes, and is rare in childhood.

Acute or subacute lacrimal gland swellings in childhood do not need biopsy if they are related to an obvious viral illness such as mumps or if there are other findings suggestive of mononucleosis. A high index of suspicion should be held for atypical lesions with early biopsy in patients whose signs and symptoms fail to respond to treatment.

Treatment of idiopathic lacrimal inflammation is with moderate-dose steroids, tapering with resolution of symptoms and signs.

SPECIFIC CAUSES OF ORBITAL INFLAMMATION

The most common cause of orbital inflammation in childhood is infective orbital cellulitis (see Chapter 20). Other orbital inflammatory diseases encountered in childhood are comparatively rare. We refer to them as "specific" since they have a defined clinical, radiological, biochemical and histopathological spectrum, though their underlying cause has not been clearly determined. Wegener's granulomatosis, sarcoidosis and thyroid orbitopathy will be discussed.

Wegener granulomatosis

This is a necrotizing granulomatous vasculitis that has a predilection for the airways and the kidneys. There is a limited form of the disease in which the kidneys are spared and has a better prognosis. Both forms have the same incidence of ocular and orbital involvement, ranging in different studies from 28 to 45%.[29] Before the introduction of cyclophosphamide, over 90% of affected patients died within 2 years.[30] Although this is not a common disease of childhood, it does occur under the age of 18.[4,31]

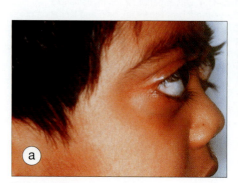
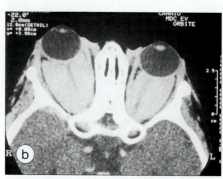
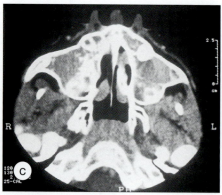

Fig. 41.5 Wegener granulomatosis. A 7-year-old boy presented with a 3-month history of progressive bilateral proptosis (a). He has positive ANCA titers. CT (b) shows widespread involvement of the orbital soft tissues and (c) maxillary sinuses. Patient from the University of British Columbia.

Clinical features

The onset of orbital Wegener granulomatosis is often preceded by a history of subacute or chronic low-grade disease, with sudden aggravation leading to presentation. The main features are proptosis, which is frequently bilateral, with ocular and facial pain that may be severe. An orbital mass usually develops (Fig. 41.5), displacing the globe, even in patients who initially present with scleritis. The latter is typically nodular and necrotizing, accompanied by characteristic marginal corneal infiltration, which can progress to ulceration. Decreased vision is a common finding, that can be related to optic neuropathy.

We have seen five children or adolescents with Wegener's granulomatosis affecting the orbit; lacrimal gland involvement with lid swelling and brawny discoloration occurred in two of these. The orbital disease was bilateral in two patients; midline disease and lacrimal gland involvement was present in the remaining three. All our patients had ENT symptoms in the 3 months prior to presentation, including nasal blockage, discharge or bleeds, pain over the paranasal or mastoid sinuses and hearing loss or tinnitus.

CT scans show an orbital mass with infiltrative margins obscuring fat and adjacent muscles. Midline bony erosion and sinus involvement may also be evident. Histological changes include areas of fat disruption and focal necrosis with lipid-laden macrophages, giant cells and evidence of acute inflammatory cells. Vasculitis is often difficult to find in these specimens.[32,33] Fibrosis is a common feature. Stains for fungi and mycobacteria should be performed to exclude these causes of granulomatous inflammation.

Septra (Septrin), an antibiotic combination of trimethoprim and sulfamethoxazole, is a first-line treatment for this condition. Azathioprine is a second-line drug. Cyclophosphamide is known to be effective in Wegener granulomatosis[34] but is reserved for children who have not responded to the above, due to its oncogenic potential. Antineutrophil cytoplasmic antibodies (cANCA) are specific markers for Wegener if there is a "cytoplasmic" staining pattern. Their plasma level correlates with disease activity and severity. Failure of these to return to normal after clinical improvement with treatment indicates a high risk of relapse.[35]

Wegener granulomatosis is rare but well recognized in childhood and clinicians should remain alert for this potentially lethal disorder. Their suspicion should increase in patients with bilateral orbital involvement, particularly with scleritis accompanied by characteristic marginal corneal infiltration (Fig. 41.6). Respiratory tract or sinus (including the mastoid sinuses) involvement is further evidence supporting this diagnosis.

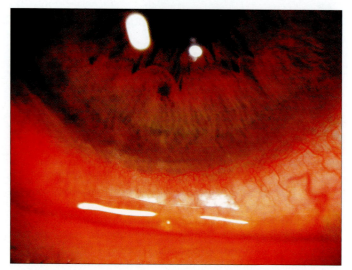

Fig. 41.6 Wegener granulomatosis. Photograph or cornea demonstrates marginal infiltration with a clear zone between the infiltrate and limbus, a feature characteristic of the disease. Patient from the University of British Columbia.

Sarcoidosis

This chronic granulomatous inflammatory disease of unknown cause is more commonly seen in the orbit as a cause of dacryoadenitis in females aged 30 years and over. Nevertheless children are occasionally affected; several hundred cases have been documented in children under the age of 15 years; the incidence of the disease rapidly increases in the late teens, peaking in the third decade. The risk is increased 3–10 times in African-Americans versus Caucasians, with a slight female preponderance. Age defines to some extent the pattern of systemic involvement: children aged 5 years or less develop uveitis, arthropathy and skin rash, while those aged 8–15 have lung involvement with ocular, skin and spleen involvement in approximately one third.[36]

Anterior uveitis, which may be chronic and granulomatous or acute, is the commonest finding at presentation, affecting one quarter to one half of patients. The eyelid, conjunctiva, sclera, episclera and lacrimal glands may be involved. Orbital infiltration causing unilateral proptosis has been reported in a 5-year-old child in the setting of arthritis.[37] Cornblath et al.[38] reported a 15-year-old white boy with pain, diplopia and ophthalmoplegia from generalized involvement of the extraocular muscles. There was diffuse enlargement of all the muscles on CT, suggesting

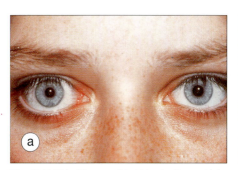 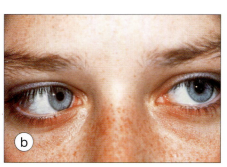 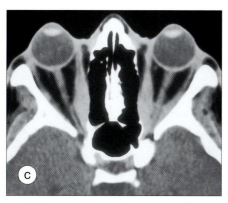

Fig. 41.7 This 12-year-old girl had a 6-year history of double vision at the extremes of gaze. Her past medical history included autoimmune hepatitis and hyperthyroidism, treated with radioiodine. There is lid retraction (a), lid lag, and restriction of abduction with esotropia in lateral gaze (b). Bilateral medial rectus enlargement involving the muscle belly but sparing the tendons is evident on CT scanning (c). Patient from the University of British Columbia.

orbital myositis or thyroid orbitopathy. Unlike the latter,[39] the muscle insertions were enlarged on CT scan.

Thyroid orbitopathy

Approximately 2.5% of all cases of Graves disease occur in children,[40] and about half of these develop ophthalmic signs.[41,42] In the series from the Toronto Hospital for Sick Children,[43] it was the second most common cause of proptosis in children (orbital cellulitis was first). Neonatal thyroid orbitopathy is well recognized, affecting the infant of a hyperthyroid mother. It is otherwise rare before puberty and the age of onset is generally from 12 years onwards. As in adulthood, this disorder is more prevalent in girls, with a 6:1 sex ratio.[44] There is commonly a family or past history of

hyperthyroidism. Associations with other autoimmune disorders, diabetes[44] and Down syndrome have been reported.

Orbital involvement is mild, often limited to lid edema or retraction. There may be proptosis, sometimes asymmetrical, which is occasionally significant enough to warrant orbital decompression.[45]

A few patients develop severe thyroid orbitopathy with marked restriction of ductions[45] (Figs 41.7a and b) and proptosis with inflammatory signs. The severity of the orbitopathy tends to increase with the age of involvement.[42] Optic neuropathy and sight-threatening corneal problems have not been described in children. Orbital imaging may show enlarged muscles (Fig. 41.7c) with characteristic sparing of the tendons.

REFERENCES

1. Mottow LS, Jakobiec FA. Idiopathic inflammatory orbital pseudotumor in childhood I. Clinical characteristics. Arch Ophthalmol 1978; 96: 1410–17.
2. Slavin ML, Glaser JS. Idiopathic orbital myositis. A report of six cases. Arch Ophthalmol 1982; 100: 1261–5.
3. Grossniklaus HE, Lass JH, Abramowsky CR, et al. Childhood orbital pseudotumor. Ann Ophthalmol 1985; 17: 372–7.
4. Rootman J. Diseases of the Orbit: A Multidisciplinary Approach. 2nd edn. Philadelphia: Lippincott Williams & Wilkins; 2003.
5. Blodi FC, Gass DJM. Inflammatory pseudotumor of the orbit. Br J Ophthalmol 1968; 2: 79–93.
6. Jakobiec FA, Jones IS. Orbital inflammation. In: Duane TD, ed. Clinical Ophthalmology. Hagerstown: Harper and Row; 1983.
7. Rootman J, Nugent RA. The classification and management of acute orbital pseudotumors. Ophthalmology 1982; 89: 1040–8.
8. Rootman J. Why pseudotumor is no longer a useful concept [editorial]. Br J Ophthalmol 1998; 82: 339–40.
9. Kennerdell JS, Dresner SC. The nonspecific orbital inflammatory syndromes. Surv Ophthalmol 1984; 29: 93–103.
10. Moseley IF, Sanders MD. Computerized Tomography in Neuro-ophthalmology. London: Chapman and Hall; 1982.
11. Atlas SW, Grossman RI, Savino PJ, et al. Surface coil MRI of orbital pseudotumor. Am J Roentgenol 1987; 148: 803–8.
12. Bloom JN, Graviss ER, Byrne BJ. Orbital pseudotumor in the differential diagnosis of pediatric uveitis. J Pediatr Ophthalmol Strabismus 1992; 29: 59–63.
13. Hertle RW, Granet DB, Goyal AK, et al. Orbital pseudotumor in the differential diagnosis of pediatric uveitis [letter]. J Pediatr Ophthalmol Strabismus 1993; 30: 61.
14. Mottow-Lippa L, Jakobiec FA, Smith M. Idiopathic inflammatory orbital pseudotumor in childhood II. Results of diagnostic tests and biopsies. Ophthalmology 1981; 88: 565–74.
15. Atabay C, Tyutyunikov A, Scalise D, et al. Serum antibodies reactive with eye muscle membrane antigens are detected in patients with nonspecific orbital inflammation. Ophthalmology 1995; 102: 145–53.
16. Uddin JM, Rennie CA, Moore AT. Bilateral non-specific orbital inflammation (orbital "pseudotumor"), posterior scleritis, and anterior uveitis associated with hypothyroidism in a child. Br J Ophthalmol 2002; 86: 936.
17. Hankey GJ, Silbert PL, Edis RH, et al. Orbital myositis: a study of six cases. Aust NZ J Med 1987; 17: 585–91.
18. Pollard ZF. Acute rectus muscle palsy in children as a result of orbital myositis. J Pediatr 1996; 128: 230–3.
19. Timms C, Russell-Eggitt IM, Taylor DS. Simulated (pseudo-) Duane's syndrome secondary to orbital myositis. Binoc Vis Q 1989; 4: 109–12.
20. Moorman CM, Elston JS. Acute orbital myositis. Eye 1995; 9: 96–101.
21. Trokel SL, Hilal SK. Recognition and differential diagnosis of enlarged extraocular muscles in computed tomography. Am J Ophthalmol 1979; 87: 503–12.
22. Wan WL, Cano MR, Green RL. Orbital myositis involving the oblique muscles: an echographic study. Ophthalmology 1988; 95: 1522–8.
23. Purcell JJ, Jr, Taulbee WA. Orbital myositis after upper respiratory tract infection. Arch Ophthalmol 1981; 99: 437–8.
24. Seidenberg KB, Leib ML. Orbital myositis with Lyme disease. Am J Ophthalmol 1990; 109: 4713–6.
25. Orssaud C, Poisson M, Gardeur D. Myosite orbitaire, recidive d'une maladie de Whipple. J Fr Ophtalmol 1992; 15: 205–8.
26. Weinstein GS, Dresner SC, Slamovits TL, et al. Acute and subacute orbital myositis. Am J Ophthalmol 1983; 96: 209–17.
27. Jellinek EH. The orbital pseudotumor syndrome and its differentiation from endocrine exophthalmos. Brain 1969; 92: 35–58.

28. Noble AG, Tripathi RC, Levine RA. Indomethacin for the treatment of idiopathic orbital myositis. Am J Ophthalmol 1989; 108: 336–8.

29. Robin JB, Schanzlin DJ, Meisler DM, et al. Ocular involvement in the respiratory vasculitides. Surv Ophthalmol 1985; 30: 127–40.

30. Hollander D, Manning RT. The use of alkylating agents in the treatment of Wegener's granulomatosis. Ann Intern Med 1967; 67: 393–8.

31. Fechner FP, Faquin WC, Pilch BZ. Wegener's granulomatosis of the orbit: a clinicopathological study of 15 patients. Laryngoscope 2002; 112: 1945–50.

32. Satorre J, Antle CM, O'Sullivan R, et al. Orbital lesions with granulomatous inflammation. Can J Ophthalmol 1991; 26: 174–95.

33. Perry SR, Rootman J, White VA. The clinical and pathologic constellation of Wegener's granulomatosis of the orbit. Ophthalmology 1997; 104: 683–94.

34. Fauci AS, Haynes BF, Katz P, et al. Wegener's granulomatosis: prospective clinical and therapeutic experience with 85 patients for 21 years. Ann Intern Med 1983; 98: 76–85.

35. Power WJ, Rodriguez A, Neves RA, et al. Disease relapse in patients with ocular manifestations of Wegener's granulomatosis. Ophthalmology 1995; 102: 154–60.

36. Hoover DL, Khan JA, Giangiacomo J. Pediatric ocular sarcoidosis. Surv Ophthalmol 1986; 30: 215–28.

37. Khan JA, Hoover DL, Giangiacomo J, et al. Orbital and childhood sarcoidosis. J Pediatr Ophthalmol Strabismus 1986; 23: 190–4.

38. Cornblath WT, Elner V, Rolfe M. Extraocular muscle involvement in sarcoidosis. Ophthalmology 1993; 100: 501–5.

39. Trokel SL, Jakobiec FA. Correlation of CT scanning and pathologic features of ophthalmic Graves' disease. Ophthalmology 1981; 88: 553–64.

40. Bram I. Exophthalmic goiter in children: comments based upon 128 cases in patients of 12 and under. Arch Pediatr 1937; 54: 419–24.

41. Young LA. Dysthyroid ophthalmopathy in children. J Pediatr Ophthalmol Strabismus 1979; 16: 105–7.

42. Uretsky SH, Kennerdell JS, Gutai JP. Graves' ophthalmopathy in childhood and adolescence. Arch Ophthalmol 1980; 98: 1963–4.

43. Crawford JS. Diseases of the orbit. In: Crawford JS, Morin JD, eds. The Eye in Childhood. New York: Grune and Stratton; 1983: 361–94.

44. Hayles AB, Kennedy RL, Beahrs OH, et al. Exophthalmic goiter in children. J Clin Endocrinol Metab 1959; 19: 138–51.

45. Liu GT, Heher KL, Katowitz JA, et al. Prominent proptosis in childhood thyroid eye disease. Ophthalmology 1996; 103: 779–84.

CHAPTER
42 Vascular Disease

Christopher J Lyons and Jack Rootman

Vascular lesions of the orbit include tumors such as capillary and cavernous hemangiomas and hemangiopericytomas as well as malformations such as lymphangiomas, orbital varices, and arteriovenous malformations. Capillary hemangiomas are common, usually present in early childhood and characteristically undergo spontaneous regression.[1,2] Cavernous hemangiomas and hemangiopericytomas are predominantly seen in adults but may rarely cause proptosis in childhood. Lymphangiomas are vascular malformations that may present in early childhood and are complicated by bouts of hemorrhage and progressive enlargement. Both varices and arteriovenous malformations tend to present in the second and third decades.

We feel that there is a spectrum of vascular abnormalities, ranging from the isolated lymphatic lymphangioma to the "high flow varix". Reports of patients with concurrent lymphangioma and orbital varices as well as patients with concurrent lymphangioma with arteriovenous malformation suggest that a fundamental problem with vasculogenesis may be at the root of all these lesions.

TUMORS

Capillary hemangioma

Capillary hemangioma is the most common orbital tumor of childhood. It occurs more frequently in females than males by a ratio of 3:2[3] with no apparent familial inheritance pattern. Its incidence is increased by prematurity and it is distinguished from other orbital vascular lesions by its tendency to regress spontaneously. An accurate diagnosis is therefore important to plan treatment which is appropriate for a self-limiting condition and, sometimes, to reassure the parents of a child with a cosmetically obvious lesion that no treatment is indicated.

The histopathological appearance of this vascular hamartoma varies with its clinical phase; in its early proliferative phase, the tumor consists mostly of numerous dividing endothelial cells and vascular spaces are rare. Also, it is surprisingly rich in mast cells,[4] whose function is not clear. There may be numerous mitotic figures at this stage, which could lead to an incorrect diagnosis of malignancy in rapidly enlarging lesions. The characterization of poorly differentiated lesions may be helped by reticulin stains or by the identification of factor VIII, which is produced by the endothelial cells, using peroxidase or fluorescein antibody techniques.[3] In more mature tumors, vascular spaces are larger, with fewer flattened endothelial cells. The tumor is not encapsulated and usually tends to infiltrate surrounding structures. In the involutional phase, there is often deposition of fibrous and adipose tissue around and within the lesion.

The natural history of capillary hemangioma, with rapid enlargement followed by spontaneous involution, is unique for vascular tumors. North et al.[5] in 2001 found that their vascular

endothelium expressed placenta-associated antigens that were not expressed by control tissues such as vascular malformations, granulation tissue, pyogenic granuloma or the vasculature of malignant tumors of nonvascular origin. They suggested that capillary hemangiomas in the infant could be sequestered tissue of placental origin that grows rapidly due to the post-natal escape from the intra-uterine factors, controlling placental growth. This novel finding could offer therapeutic avenues to control growth and hasten their resolution.

Clinical features

Approximately one-third of capillary hemangiomas (Fig. 42.1) are present at birth, and they will all have appeared by the age of

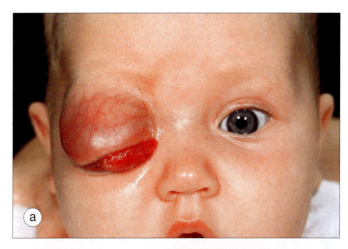

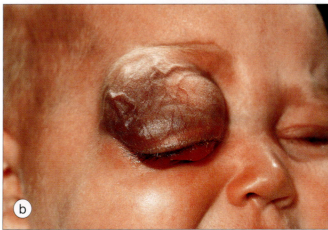

Fig. 42.1 Capillary hemangioma. (a) Capillary hemangioma of the anterior orbit and lid. (b) Same patient when crying showing engorgement and mild increase in size.

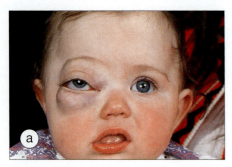 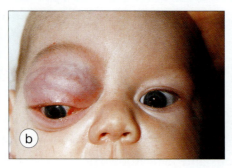 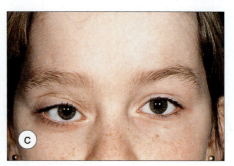

Fig. 42.2 Orbital capillary hemangioma. (a) As sometimes happens, the mother of this child was accused, on several occasions, of having injured her child. (b) Orbital capillary hemangioma in a child aged 2 months. (c) Same patient as (b) aged 9 years after some spontaneous resolution and surgery. Surgery is often not necessary and best avoided in most instances (see text).

6 months. The appearance of the tumor may be preceded by a faint cutaneous flush. Rapid growth lasting 3–6 months is followed by a period of stabilization and then usually regression (Fig. 42.2). Margileth and Museles[1] found that 30% of 336 hemangiomas had regressed by the age of 3 years, 60% by 4 years, and 76% by 7 years.

Capillary hemangiomas are most commonly situated in the upper lid or orbit (Figs 42.2a, b). Their appearance varies according to the depth of involvement (Fig. 42.2a); superficial cutaneous lesions have the red lobulated appearance, which gave rise to the name "strawberry" nevus (see Fig. 42.8a), and they may enlarge and become blueish in color with crying. Subcutaneous hemangiomas are often blueish in color. Lesions situated deep to the orbital septum may present with proptosis only with no cutaneous discoloration. Occasionally, the proptosis is severe enough to cause corneal exposure. About one-third of hemangiomas involve several levels of depth.[6] A deeply situated lesion causing proptosis only with no overlying cutaneous signs may present a diagnostic dilemma. Helpful diagnostic signs include the increase in proptosis with crying (Fig. 42.1). In approximately 30% of patients, "strawberry" nevi are found at other cutaneous sites.[2] Occasionally, enormous growth occurs obliterating facial structures (Fig. 42.3).

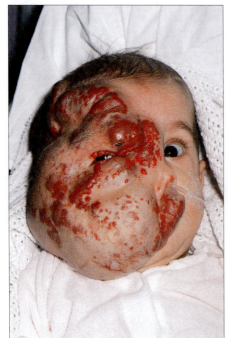

Fig. 42.3 Massive facial and orbital capillary hemangioma.

Amblyopia is common in patients with orbital capillary hemangiomas, with a prevalence ranging between 43 and 60% in published series of affected verbal children.[2,7,8] This may result from occlusion of the visual axis by a bulky tumor. More often, however, it results from distortion of the globe by tumor causing corneal astigmatism. The axis of the corrective plus cylinder is directed toward the tumor. This may persist after the hemangioma has regressed,[7] but usually resolves at least partially,[9] particularly if the hemangioma resolves or is removed early.[10] Lastly, prolonged occlusion can result in ipsilateral myopia[11] and the resultant anisometropia may be another contributory factor in the development of amblyopia. Secondary strabismus is common as a result of the interruption of binocularity.

Systemic complications of capillary hemangiomas are rare.[3] The Kasabach–Merritt syndrome is a coagulopathy resulting from consumption of fibrinogen and platelet entrapment within a large vascular hemangioma, often in the viscera. It usually responds to treatment with platelet replacement and corticosteroids.

Investigation

In the majority of children presenting with proptosis, lid involvement or other cutaneous hemangiomas allow a clinical diagnosis to be made.

Plain X-ray of the orbit may show enlargement of the affected side but is otherwise unhelpful. Doppler ultrasound can help to secure the diagnosis.[12] The extent of the lesion can be assessed by computed tomography (CT) scanning. A soft tissue density mass is seen to infiltrate the orbit, frequently with smooth or nodular margins, often crossing boundaries between compartments such as the muscle cone or orbital septum. Enhancement is variable, according to the vascularity of the lesion and its stage of growth or involution. T_2-weighted magnetic resonance imaging (MRI) is useful to delineate the tumor since the lesion is hyperintense due to its intrinsic blood flow (Fig. 42.4). T_1-weighted gadolinium-enhanced views with fat suppression to improve contrast give the best assessment of the anatomical relationships of the tumor. Lesions confined to the posterior orbit, especially during a period of growth, may occasionally be mistaken for a malignant tumor such as rhabdomyosarcoma, and biopsy may then be indicated.

A thorough fundus examination is necessary to exclude the presence of optic disc abnormalities such as "morning glory disc" with its negative visual implications.[13]

An association exists between large facial capillary hemangioma, cerebral and ocular malformations, reported with individual cases since 1984.[14–16] Recently, Frieden et al.[17] coined the acronym PHACE syndrome (Posterior fossa malformations, Hemangiomas,

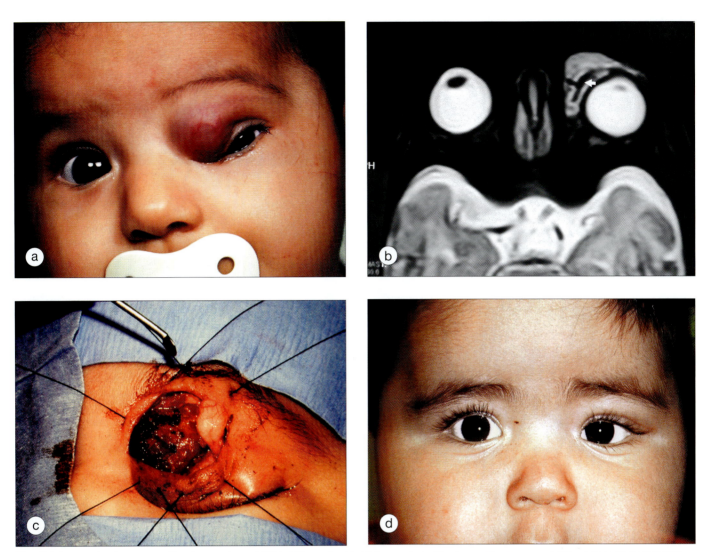

Fig. 42.4 Large subcutaneous capillary hemangioma. (a) This 2.5-month-old child presented with a large subcutaneous capillary hemangioma that was unresponsive to steroids and inducing significant astigmatism. (b) T2-weighted MRI demonstrated a relatively well-defined anterior orbital mass with a large central flow void (arrow). (c) Operative photo of the same lesion during excision. (d) After surgery, she had minimal ptosis, and her astigmatism regressed. Patient of the University of British Columbia. (Figs 42.4a & b with permission from Rootman J. Diseases of the Orbit: A Multidisciplinary Approach. 2nd edn. Philadelphia: Lippincott Williams and Wilkins; 2002:542.)

Arterial anomalies, Coarctation of the aorta and other cardiac defects and Eye abnormalities) to describe this. They suggested that a careful ocular, cardiac and neurological examination is necessary for patients with extensive facial capillary hemangiomas.[18] Neuroimaging can be indicated in patients in whom capillary hemangioma, cardiac and eye abnormalities co-exist.

Management

As discussed above, most capillary hemangiomas undergo spontaneous regression and three-quarters disappear by the age of 7 years.[1] Management should therefore be conservative if possible, with treatment of significant refractive error and amblyopia while awaiting spontaneous regression (Fig. 42.5). The appearance of superficial pale stellate areas of scarring on a typical "strawberry lesion (herald spots)" is a useful early indicator of spontaneous regression, which can be reassuring to anxious parents. Occlusion of the contralateral eye for amblyopia therapy should be accompanied by correction of the astigmatic error of the affected eye with appropriate glasses (Fig. 42.6).

Active treatment to reduce the size of the tumor is only indicated if there is occlusion of the visual axis or if a posterior lesion results in progressive proptosis with evidence of optic nerve compression, corneal exposure, and significant or progressive amblyopia brought about by obscuration of vision or astigmatism. Methods of treatment have included local or systemic steroids,[19] surgical excision, radiotherapy and injection of sclerosing agents. Kushner[20] has reported good results with injection of local steroid into the hemangioma. We have similarly obtained good results with this technique and recommend the injection of methylprednisolone 25–40 mg and triamcinolone 40 mg into the hemangioma. Tumor regression should be noted within 2–4 weeks, and further injections may be necessary (Fig. 42.7). The steroid should be given by slow injection throughout the tumor while the needle is withdrawn to reduce the risk of central retinal artery embolization,[21,22] a rare but devastating complication which was reported to have occurred bilaterally in one case.[23] Other reported complications include local fat atrophy, eyelid necrosis and adrenal suppression with Cushingoid features.[3] Ultrasound guidance may be helpful for posteriorly

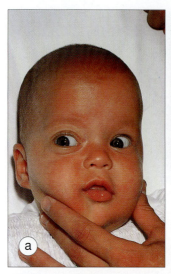
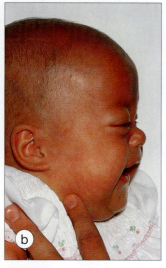

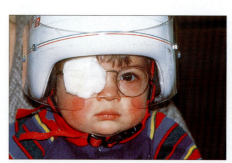

Fig. 42.6 Deep capillary hemangioma in a 6-month-old boy. A faint blueish tinge is evident in the left lower lid. There is a +4.0 diopter-induced cylinder. Occlusion is vital in virtually every case and, in this child, his inventive parents have devised a novel method of preventing him from removing the patch. Eighteen months later the lesion had resolved, as had the cylinder. Patient of the University of British Columbia.

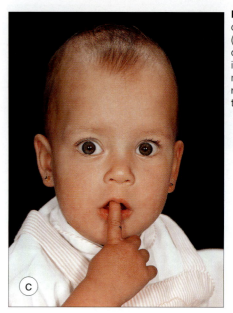

Fig. 42.5 Right orbital capillary hemangioma. (a, b) Right orbital capillary hemangioma in a child aged 5 months. (c) Complete resolution without treatment.

situated lesions.[24] The whitish skin discoloration that is sometimes noted from superficial accumulation of depot steroid after injection is usually transient.

Systemic steroids in doses of 1.5–5.0 mg/kg/day may be preferable for very extensive or posteriorly situated lesions (Fig. 42.8). The exact dose necessary is still debated, but the response of over 90% for doses greater than 3 mg/kg/day falls to less than 70% for doses of 2 mg/kg/day and less.[25] The side-effects of growth retardation, adrenal suppression and Cushingoid changes, which should be discussed with the parents, may make this form of therapy relatively undesirable, though these can also occur after intralesional injection. A rebound phenomenon has been noted after discontinuation of oral steroid, with an increase in size of the capillary hemangioma

Sight-threatening lesions which have failed to respond to steroids may be amenable to treatment with interferon alpha 2a, although the response to this treatment may be slow.[26] Fledelius et al.[27] recently reported arrest of tumor growth and accelerated shrinkage with this technique on a series of nine infants. Daily injections were necessary for an average of 22 weeks in this series, something which most families would find quite demanding. Loughnan et al.[28] reported a rapid regression of a massive steroid-unresponsive orbital capillary hemangioma after systemic injections of interferon alpha 2b.

The carbon dioxide, argon, yttrium–aluminum–garnet (YAG) and dye lasers have all been used to treat hemangiomas. Their use

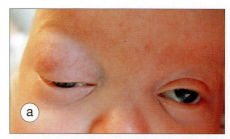
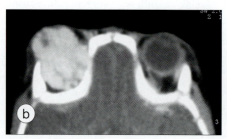
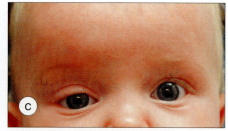

Fig. 42.7 Capillary hemangioma. This infant was born at 27 weeks' gestation. (a) Right upper lid swelling was noted at age 6 weeks, and she was seen in our clinic at 16 weeks of age. (b) CT scan confirmed capillary hemangioma, showing a poorly defined, enhancing lesion in the superior orbit. An intralesional injection of 40 mg triamcinolone and 20 mg methylprednisolone was given at this time. Repeat injection was planned for 8 weeks later but was deferred due to her clinical improvement. Part-time occlusion of the left eye was used. (c) Three months later, she was equally visually attentive with each eye. No further treatment is planned. Patient of the University of British Columbia.

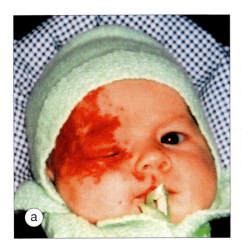
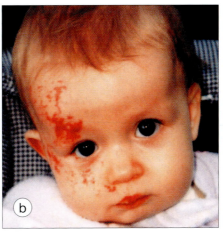
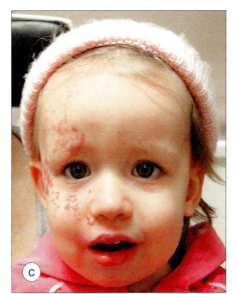

Fig. 42.8 Capillary hemangioma. (a) This 6-week old infant was noted to have right upper lid swelling and discoloration from the second week of life, increasing on crying. There is complete closure of the right eye. Oral steroids were started at 6 weeks of age at 5 mg/kg/day, tapering to nothing over 6 months. (b) By 9 months of age, her Cushingoid features have resolved; the capillary hemangioma no longer obstructs the right visual axis. (c) At 11 months, the cutaneous changes have largely disappeared. There is no amblyopia. Patient of the University of British Columbia.

is limited by the scarring they induce, although the dye laser tuned to 577 or 585 nm with a 10 ms pulse duration may allow selective thermal damage of capillary tissue with minimal scarring and accelerated regression.[29] The use of lasers to treat these lesions is still not widely accepted. Radiotherapy and sclerosing agents should no longer be used.

In the past, surgical excision was usually deferred until the lesion stopped regressing, often after 6 or 7 years of age when any residual cosmetic defect may be corrected.[30] However, it is important to note that well-defined lesions that cause significant obstruction or more particularly, significant astigmatism, can be removed safely and thereby facilitating reversal of amblyopia cause. The technique requires meticulous hemostasis, but the

tumor is readily removed using microsurgical techniques. These are indicated after failure to respond to treatment with steroids or as a primary therapeutic approach.[31,32] We have had very good results in reversing astigmatism in this manner (Fig. 42.9).

In summary, numerous techniques are available to manage this common, usually benign but potentially disfiguring and even blinding disorder. There is no "one size fits all" approach, since the behavior of the tumor is so unpredictable; it could be argued that single patients whose lesion resolves rapidly with intralesional or systemic corticosteroids would have done so anyway. Conversely, the family and treating physicians are always fearful of uncontrolled growth, as seen in Fig. 42.3. In anticipation of a

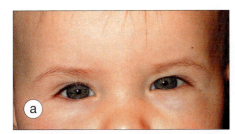
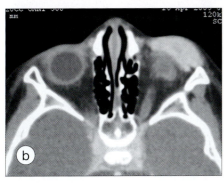
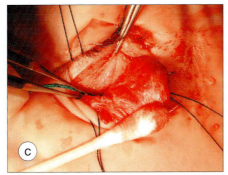
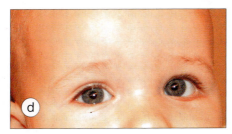

Fig. 42.9 Capillary hemangioma. (a) Clinical photograph of an 8-month-old child who presented with a progressive mass of the left lower left lid, causing astigmatism (+2.50 cylinder at 90°) and upward displacement of the left globe. (b) Contrast-enhanced CT scan demonstrates a relatively well defined anterior orbital mass involving the left lid and inferior orbit. (c) Intraoperative photo of the same patient at the time of excision of the capillary hemangioma. (d) One month after surgery, his astigmatism resolved. Patient of the University of British Columbia.

good randomized trial, our policy has been to treat visually threatening lesions whose extent is limited to the orbit immediately with an intralesional steroid injection. We rarely inject more than a total of 1.5 ml into any lesion. The patient is reviewed 6 weeks later and parents sometimes report early shrinkage with renewed enlargement in the previous 2 weeks. If so, a further injection is given, and repeated at 6-weekly intervals until stabilization is achieved and the visual axis is clear, with an acceptable amount of astigmatism. Lesions not limited to the orbital region are treated in conjunction with the dermatologists at our institution, who, after thorough counseling regarding the likelihood of Cushingoid side-effects and the other issues discussed above, institute a regimen of oral prednisone ranging up to 5 mg/kg. Once again, early treatment appears to be more effective. We have not used interferon, but have done surgical excision early for localized nonresponsive lesions in 12 cases, with excellent visual and cosmetic results. Interferon may have a role in the treatment of extensive lesions that have not responded to systemic steroids.

Hemangiopericytoma

This rare tumor, whose character ranges from benign to malignant, is derived from the pericyte. It is usually seen in adults but has been reported to affect children as young as 20 months.[33,34] Its pattern of behavior is unpredictable, but the usual presentation is with gradually increasing proptosis and mass effect related to a tumor that is usually superiorly placed. On CT scan, it is a well-circumscribed lesion showing marked, homogeneous contrast enhancement. There is a pronounced, early blush on angiography. It is usually a locally invasive tumor that recurs locally unless carefully and completely excised within its pseudocapsule. Unfortunately this is often technically challenging as the tumor is very friable. Ten to 15% may develop distant metastasis. Occasionally, these tumors behave very aggressively. In these cases, exenteration may be necessary to control local tumor progression.[6]

VASCULAR MALFORMATIONS

Vascular malformations of the orbit are derived from venous (varices and lymphangiomas) and arterial (arteriovenous malformations) vascular anlage and constitute an important cause of orbital tumor in childhood. They are best understood in the context of their hemodynamics and can be divided into three types on this basis.[6,35,36] Type 1 (no flow) lesions have little connection to the vascular system and include the entity of lymphangiomas, or combined venous lymphatic malformations. Type 2 (venous flow) lesions appear clinically as either distensible, with a direct and significant communication to the venous system, or nondistensible, which have minimal communication with the venous system. Both types 1 and 2 can be combined, with features both of distensibility and non-distensible hemodynamics. Type 3 lesions are arterial flow and include arteriovenous malformations that are characterized by an antegrade high-flow through the lesion to the venous system.

Lymphangioma

These vascular anomalies usually arise in childhood and are often difficult to manage. They may enlarge gradually but usually their expansion is sudden, from hemorrhage into the lesion. Unlike capillary hemangiomas, they do not undergo spontaneous regression. Deeply situated lesions are difficult to excise

surgically as their margins are poorly defined and they arborize widely throughout the orbital tissues.

Lymphangiomas accounted for 3% of the 600 orbital tumors on file at Wills Hospital in Iliff and Green's series[37] and 8.1% of 326 pediatric orbital tumors in our series. In approximately one-third of cases, the lymphangioma is apparent at birth or within the first weeks of life,[38,39] and over three-quarters of patients present in the first decade of life.[37] The average age of onset in Jones' series[38] of 29 patients was 6.2 years. A female preponderance (ratio 2–3:1) has been reported.[37,39]

Their frequency of occurrence within the orbit is puzzling in view of the absence of lymphatic drainage from the retroseptal tissues. It is likely that lymphangiomas arise from primitive vascular elements within the orbit.[40] Unlike capillary hemangiomas, they do not appear to grow by cellular proliferation. Instead, the full extent of the malformation is present at birth, insinuating itself within the normal orbital tissues.[39] Since the vascular channels have characteristics of both lymphatic and venous vessels, the histological differentiation of lymphangiomas from orbital varices has been a source of debate.[41–43] Hemodynamically, lymphangiomas and varices are part of a continuum of venous-derived lesions, which are differentiated according to the presence or lack of connection to the venous system. Whereas varices are typically connected and therefore expand with Valsalva maneuver or supine posture, lymphangiomas are isolated and therefore do not. Lesions may be mixed with both venous and lymphatic components represented within a single mass. The extremes of the spectrum can also be differentiated histo-pathologically, since the lymphangiomatous element has distinctive electron microscopic features.[44] Overall, the pathogenesis of these lesions relate to the lack of blood flow and the tendency for sludging, neovascularization, and hemorrhage with recurrent inflammatory episodes and the formation of isolated chocolate cysts.[36]

Histopathologically, they consist of diaphanous, serous fluid-filled channels lined by endothelium. These have characteristics of true lymphatic channels as well as areas of dysplastic channels.[6] Lymphoid follicles are often present in the stromal components. Hemorrhage into the tumor is common giving rise to so-called chocolate cysts.

The clinical features of lymphangiomas vary with the extent and depth of orbital involvement.

Superficial

Isolated superficial involvement is comparatively rare and may consist of multiple conjunctival cysts filled with clear or xanthochromic fluid, or a subcutaneous blueish cystic swelling of the eyelid. The latter may transilluminate and may occasionally present with an abrupt localized change in color due to hemorrhage into a pre-existing lesion.[45] Superficial lymphangiomas are easily accessible and, if unsightly, may be excised surgically with good results.

Deep

The hallmark of deeply situated orbital lymphangiomas is proptosis (Figs 42.10 and 42.11). Deep lymphangiomas may present with gradually increasing proptosis with or without ptosis. In contrast to capillary hemangiomas the proptosis is said to be variable. An increase with upper respiratory tract infections and other generalized inflammatory states[38] has been ascribed to lymphoid activity within the lesion.[35]

The most typical presentation, however, is with sudden proptosis resulting from hemorrhage into a hitherto unsuspected

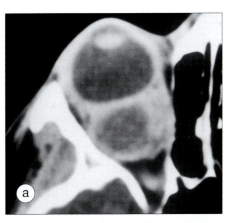

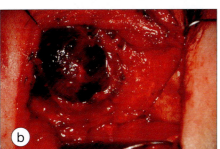

Fig. 42.10 Lymphangioma. Previously asymptomatic 8-year-old presenting with sudden onset axial proptosis overnight, decreased vision, afferent pupillary defect and optic disc swelling. (a) CT shows a cystic mass indenting the globe posteriorly. (b) At surgery, the "chocolate" cyst was identified and decompressed. Patient of the University of British Columbia.

lesion. In these cases, the differential diagnoses include other causes of rapidly increasing proptosis such as rhabdomyosarcoma, neuroblastoma, and so on. In this situation, examination of the nasal and palatal mucosa may be helpful if it reveals the characteristic mixed clear fluid and blood-filled blebs of widespread lymphangioma (Fig. 42.12). Optic nerve compression may occur with a rapidly expanding blood-filled chocolate cyst[46] (Fig. 42.10) and can result in decreased visual acuity with disc swelling. It is an indication for urgent orbital intervention to decompress or excise the lesion.

Combined lesions

These usually present in infancy, gradually enlarging over many years. Long-standing lesions may be associated with orbital enlargement. The presence of tell-tale conjunctival and lid changes is helpful in making the diagnosis of lymphangioma (Fig. 42.12). Hemorrhage into superficial lesions may result in the striking appearance of blood menisci within the conjunctival cysts (Fig. 42.13). These may be accompanied by generalized recurrent subconjunctival hemorrhage and lid ecchymosis. Deep hemorrhage results in proptosis which is commonly associated with compressive optic neuropathy. Combined lesions may be large enough to simultaneously involve every orbital space and can give rise to gross proptosis and facial deformity. Katz et al.[47] reported a series of seven patients, four of whom were children. All had extension of the lymphangiomatous lesion through the

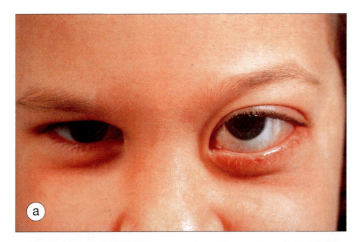

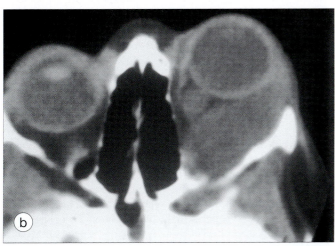

Fig. 42.11 Orbital lymphangioma. (a) Sudden onset of proptosis in the left eye of a previously asymptomatic 5-year-old child. (b) CT scan shows diffuse soft tissue density lesion arborizing through the retrobulbar tissues. Patient of the University of British Columbia.

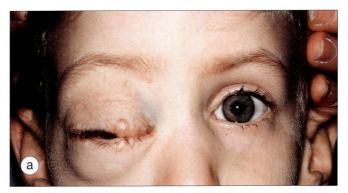

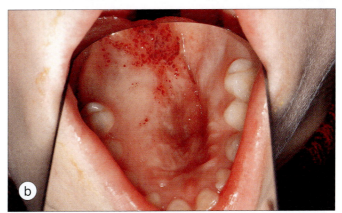

Fig. 42.12 Lymphangioma. (a) This 4-year-old boy was born after a 32-week gestation. Right proptosis developed by 4 weeks and was progressive despite orbital surgery, until the age of 3 years. It has been static since then. The diagnosis was a lymphangioma. (b) Same patient showing clear and blood-filled cystic lesions on the palate.

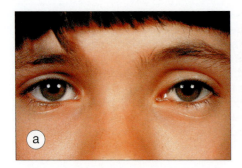

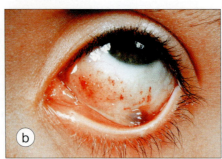

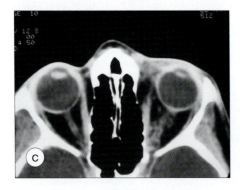

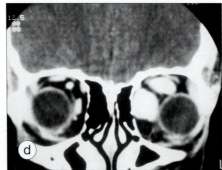

Fig. 42.13 Lymphangioma. (a) This 12-year-old child presented with an epibulbar lesion on the left side associated with fullness of the upper and lower lids and slight ptosis. (b) The epibulbar surface demonstrates a gelatinous-appearing lesion medially containing many clear fluid-filled cysts along with focal blood cysts, many of which appear to have menisci. In addition, in the inferolateral fornix, there appears to be a dark varix. The conjunctival lesion was proven on biopsy to be consistent with a lymphangioma histologically and by electron microscopy. It was noted also that the superior sulcus appeared somewhat deepened on the left. (c) Postcontrast CT scan in the axial view shows an irregular lesion occupying the anteromedial orbit around and behind the caruncle. On direct coronal view (d), there is evidence of a posterior orbital varix that appeared with increased venous pressure. This lesion represents a combined lymphangioma and varix. Patient of the University of British Columbia. (Reproduced with permission from Rootman J. Vascular malformations of the orbit: hemodynamic concepts. Orbit 2003; 22: 103–20.)

superior orbital fissure and noncontiguous intracranial vascular abnormalities. Since the latter are also at risk of bleeding, imaging of the brain is indicated in patients with orbital lymphangioma.

Investigation

CT scanning shows a soft tissue density mass with poorly defined margins and inhomogeneous enhancement after injection of contrast medium. Bony destruction is absent but large lesions can result in smooth enlargement of the orbit (Fig. 42.11b). The presence of a cystic component may be helpful in differentiating lymphangiomas from capillary hemangiomas. Since hemoglobin has paramagnetic qualities which change as blood denatures after hemorrhage, blood-containing chocolate cysts are particularly well visualized by MRI scanning[46,48] (Fig. 42.14). The age of intralesional hemorrhages can also be assessed with this modality since oxyhemoglobin in fresh hemorrhage is hypointense on T_1- and T_2-weighted images, gradually becoming hyperintense as this is converted to methemoglobin. Later still, degradation to ferritin and hemosiderin once again produces a hypointense image. Intravenous contrast in the case of CT scan or gadolinium in MRI may be helpful in imaging the component of the lesion that is most active and takes up the dye. That is the component that should be removed if surgical intervention is contemplated. A careful review of brain images is indicated in view of the possibility of associated noncontiguous intracranial vascular anomalies.[47]

Management

A conservative approach should be adopted if possible, since complete excision is difficult in all but the most superficial lesions and since hemorrhagic cysts tend to shrink with time. In addition, surgery itself can precipitate further hemorrhage.[49] Wilson et al.[50] have stressed that bed rest alone or with the use of cold compresses can be associated with a good outcome even in cases with acute proptosis of up to 10 mm. None of their six patients had an afferent pupillary defect, but biopsy was

performed in the acute stage in three of these patients, which might have contributed to the resolution of the problem.

Surgery is indicated if there is evidence of optic nerve dysfunction, corneal exposure, pain and nausea from raised orbital pressure or the risk of amblyopia from induced astigmatism or strabismus. It is possible to temporize by aspirating the cyst contents through a needle under ultrasound guidance. Poor results and frequent morbidity have been reported from attempts at subtotal excision. We feel that surgery when indicated should be aimed at excising as much of the lymphangioma as is safe, particularly removing the offending focus of active tissue as well as draining blood cysts with release of their contents. Unlike dermoid or sebaceous cysts, excision of the whole cyst wall is not necessary to avoid recurrence. The carbon dioxide laser may be useful in reducing the hemorrhagic complications associated with conventional subtotal excision surgery.[51]

Congenital orbital varices

Varices may be divided into high and low flow types. Low flow varices are clinically similar to lymphangiomas, with a tendency for sudden, often recurrent hemorrhage,[52] while high flow varices expand with increased jugular venous pressure and rarely bleed.[6,36]

Distensible orbital varices expand only slowly during childhood and rarely give rise to visual problems. There is often a subconjunctival component (Fig. 42.13). They often present in adolescence with an awareness of discomfort on bending over and the slow development of enophthalmos and deepening superior sulcus due to fat atrophy and enlargement of the orbit, which may be seen on plain X-rays, along with phleboliths. The main indications for surgical excision might be removal of the superficial component for cosmetic reasons or removal of deeper lesions in instances of grave, persistent pain. A recently described combined neuroradiologic method with gluing followed by

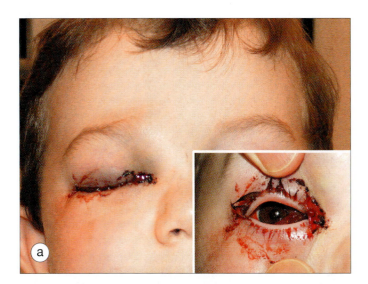

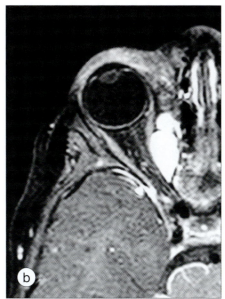

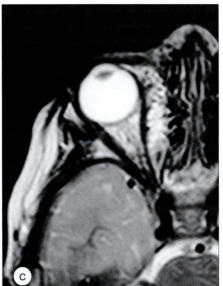

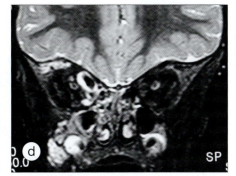

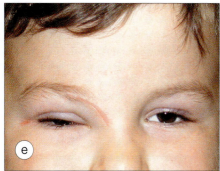

Fig. 42.14 Lymphangioma. (a) This 2.5-year-old boy was born with a swollen right eye. At age 1, he developed spontaneous bruising and a gelatinous lesion on the surface of the right globe, treated at the time with steroids with improvement. He continued, however, to have constant bleeding from the epibulbar surface, progressive lid closure and swelling. (b–d) MRI scans demonstrate an extraconal medial lesion that involves the lid and forehead and extends to the apex of the right orbit. Posteriorly, note the cystic components consistent with lymphangioma. The patient underwent excision of his lymphangioma. (e) He did well postoperatively (seen here at 1 month following surgery) with a residual ptosis and persistent lid involvement, which will require future surgery. Patient of the University of British Columbia.

excision may be worthwhile on a limited number of cases that demonstrate an isolated relationship to the venous system and that does not share out-flow with critical orbital structures.[53] Some orbital varices may be associated with extensive intracranial varicosities (Fig. 42.15).

Arteriovenous malformations

Arteriovenous malformations are characterized clinically by the development of pulsating exophthalmos with occasional episodes of hemorrhage, thrombosis, or a caput medusae effect secondary to arterialization of out-flow venous channels. They may have an audible bruit and can cause pain when engorged, secondary to Valsalva maneuver. Typically, these present in late adolescence or early adult life.

Imaging, arteriovenous malformations are characterized by the presence of irregular, rapidly enhancing masses. On Doppler studies and CT or MR angiography, they demonstrate high-flow characteristics. With selective angiography, the lesions consist of engorged proximal arterial supply, a tangled malformation, and a distal venous out-flow (Fig. 42.16).

In terms of management, arteriovenous malformations can largely be observed. The indications for intervention might be recurrent hemorrhage or persistent pain. The malformations can be removed using a combination of selective gluing of in-flow vessels followed by excision.

Sturge–Weber syndrome

See Chapters 27, 69, and 48.

Sturge-Weber syndrome consists of facial port-wine stain, with leptomeningeal angiomatosis. The facial lesion is classically unilateral, involving the dermatome of the ophthalmic branch of the trigeminal nerve (Fig. 42.17). The maxillary and mandibular divisions may also be involved. Hypertrophy of the underlying tissues is common and frequently causes greater disfigurement

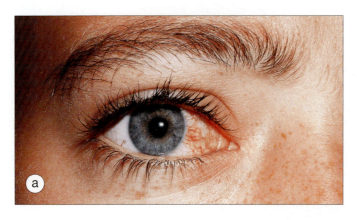
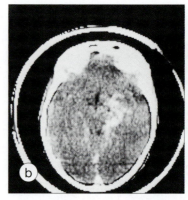
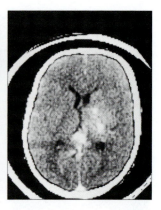

Fig. 42.15 Congenital orbital varices. (a) Subconjunctival varicosities in a patient with an orbital and intracranial hemangioma. (b) Contrast-enhanced CT scans showing the intracranial lesion (same patient).

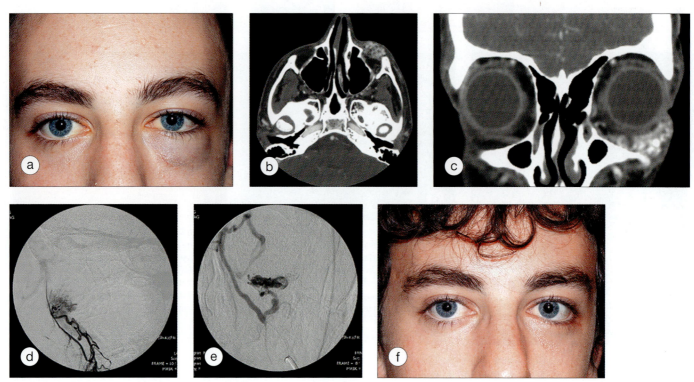

Fig. 42.16 Arteriovenous malformations. (a) This 15-year-old boy presented first at age 12 with a fullness of the left lower lid and transient visual obscuration episodes on exertion, due to an arteriovenous malformation. He was observed for 2.5 years, during which time the lesion progressed, and it was decided to intervene. He underwent combined embolization and excision of his mass. (b, c) CT angiograms demonstrate the tangle of the arteriovenous malformation in the left inferior orbit and lid. (d) Selective external carotid angiogram shows the external maxillary supply, while the anterior-posterior venous phase angiogram (e) reveals the venous outflow to the facial and superior ophthalmic veins with facial compression. (f) Photograph of the patient 4 months after his surgery shows his postoperative result. Patient of the University of British Columbia.

than the cutaneous discoloration. Angiomatous malformations may involve other tissues including the eye, respiratory and gastrointestinal tracts, ovary and pancreas. Cerebral involvement may give to seizures, hemiplegia and mental retardation. Not all patients, however, have the complete syndrome and there is wide variability in expression.

The ophthalmic manifestations include unilateral glaucoma, which may be congenital but is often juvenile.[54] Episcleral and conjunctival vascular anomalies are ommon; their presence seems to indicate an increased risk of developing glaucoma. Diffuse choroidal hemangiomas are also common, recognized by a diffusely red fundus with loss of choroidal markings. These may be complicated by serous retinal detachment. Orbital involvement is rare; Hofeldt et al.[55] described two patients with ipsilateral nevus flammeus and a unilateral orbital vascular malformation causing proptosis. In each case there was no evidence of any intracranial lesion.

The use of pulsed dye lasers for nevus flammeus have been encouraging. In the long term, this treatment may reduce the disfiguring hypertrophy that accompanies the port-wine stain. Regular follow-up is indicated for intraocular pressure monitoring.

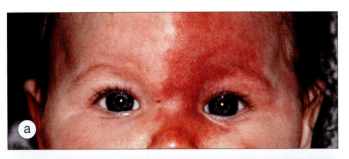

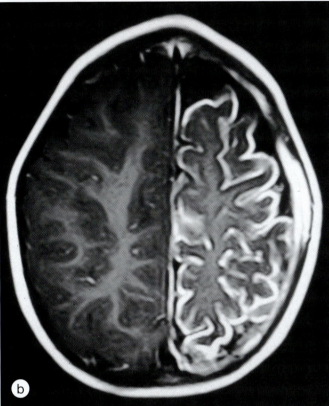

Fig. 42.17 Sturge-Weber syndrome. (a) This 3-month-old infant with left-sided facial port-wine stain, seizures and contralateral weakness has left-sided leptomeningeal involvement with underlying cerebral atrophy, which is seen clearly on T_2-weighted MRI (b). She later developed left-sided glaucoma. Patient of the University of British Columbia.

Rare vascular lesions of the orbit

Klippel–Trenaunay–Weber syndrome

See Chapter 69.

This syndrome comprises multiple cutaneous nevi associated with various angiomas of one or more limbs, which may show hypertrophy of the soft tissues. Rathbun et al.[56] described a 15-year-old girl with the classical features of the syndrome who developed intermittent proptosis from an orbital varix. This was ligated and excised with good results.

Blue rubber bleb nevus syndrome

This rare syndrome usually presents in childhood. It consists of multiple blueish cutaneous cavernous hemangiomas, associated with angiomas of the gastrointestinal tract, lung, heart and central nervous system. The cutaneous lesions are soft, rubbery and compressible. Most cases are sporadic but autosomal dominant inheritance has been reported in several families. Conjunctival, iris and retinal angiomas may occur.[57] McCannel et al.[58] reported a 7-year-old girl with the syndrome who developed unilateral proptosis on Valsalva maneuver from a vascular malformation at the orbital apex.

The main systemic complication is gastrointestinal bleeding, which may lead to iron-deficiency anemia or even a consumption coagulopathy[59] whose mechanism is probably similar to that of the Kasabach-Merritt syndrome of capillary hemangiomas.[60]

REFERENCES

1. Margileth AM, Museles M. Cutaneous hemangiomas in children. Diagnosis and conservative management. JAMA 1965; 194: 135–8.
2. Haik BG, Jakobiec FA, Ellsworth RM, et al. Capillary hemangioma of the lids and orbit: an analysis of the clinical features and therapeutic results in 101 cases. Ophthalmology 1979; 86: 760–89.
3. Haik BG, Karcioglu ZA, Gordon RA, et al. Capillary hemangioma (infantile periocular hemangioma). Surv Ophthalmol 1994; 38: 399–426.
4. Glowacki J, Mulliken JB. Mast cells in hemangiomas and vascular malformations. Pediatrics 1982; 70: 48–51.
5. North PE, Waner M, Mizeracki A, et al. A unique microvascular phenotype shared by juvenile hemangiomas and human placenta. Arch Dermatol 2001; 137: 559–70.
6. Rootman J. Diseases of the Orbit: A Multidisciplinary Approach. 2nd edn. Philadelphia: Lippincott Williams & Wilkins; 2003.
7. Robb R. Refractive errors associated with hemangiomas of the eyelids and orbit in infancy. Am J Ophthalmol 1977; 83: 52–7.
8. Stigmar G, Crawford JS, Ward CM, et al. Ophthalmic sequelae of infantile hemangiomas of the eyelids and orbit. Am J Ophthalmol 1978; 85: 806–13.
9. Morrell AJ, Willshaw HE. Normalisation of refractive error after steroid injection for adnexal haemangiomas. Br J Ophthalmol 1991; 75: 301–5.
10. Plager DA, Snyder SK. Resolution of astigmatism after surgical resection of capillary hemangiomas in infants. Ophthalmology 1997; 104: 1102–6.
11. Hoyt CS, Stone RD, Fromer C, et al. Monocular axial myopia associated with neonatal eyelid closure in human infants. Am J Ophthalmol 1981; 91: 197–206.
12. Sleep TJ, Fairhurst JJ, Manners RM, et al. Doppler ultrasonography to aid diagnosis of orbital capillary haemangioma in neonates. Eye 2002; 16: 316–9.

13. Holmstrom G, Taylor D. Capillary haemangiomas in association with morning glory disc anomaly. Acta Ophthalmol Scand 1998; 76: 613–6.

14. Atkin JF, Patil S. Apparently new oculo–cerebro-acral syndrome. Am J Med Genet 1984; 19: 585–7.

15. Deady JP, Willshaw HE. Vascular hamartomas in childhood. Trans Ophthalmol Soc UK 1986; 105: 712–6.

16. Fernandez GR, Munoz FJ, Padron C, et al. Microphthalmos, facial capillary hemangioma and Dandy-Walker malformation. Acta Ophthalmol Scand 1995; 73: 173–5.

17. Frieden IJ, Reese V, Cohen D. PHACE syndrome. The association of posterior fossa brain malformations, hemangiomas, arterial anomalies, coarctation of the aorta and cardiac defects, and eye abnormalities. Arch Dermatol 1996; 132: 307–11.

18. Coats DK, Paysse EA, Levy ML. PHACE: a neurocutaneous syndrome with important ophthalmologic implications: case report and literature review. Ophthalmology 1999; 106: 1739–41.

19. Hiles D, Pilchard WA. Corticosteroid control of neonatal hemangiomas of orbit and ocular adnexae. Am J Ophthalmol 1971; 71: 1003–8.

20. Kushner BJ. Intralesional corticosteroid injection for infantile adnexal hemangioma. Am J Ophthalmol 1982; 92: 496–506.

21. Egbert JE, Schwartz GS, Walsh AW. Diagnosis and treatment of an ophthalmic artery occlusion during an intralesional injection of corticosteroid into an eyelid capillary hemangioma. Am J Ophthalmol 1996; 121: 638–42.

22. Egbert JE, Paul S, Engel WK, et al. High injection pressure during intralesional injection of corticosteroids into capillary hemangiomas. Arch Ophthalmol 2001; 119: 677–83.

23. Ruttum MS, Abrams GW, Harris GJ, et al. Bilateral retinal embolization associated with intralesional corticosteroid injection for capillary hemangioma of infancy. J Pediatr Ophthalmol Strabismus 1993; 30: 4–7.

24. Neumann D, Isenberg SJ, Rosenbaum AL, et al. Ultrasonographically guided injection of corticosteroids for the treatment of retroseptal capillary hemangiomas in infants. J AAPOS 1997; 1: 34–40.

25. Bennett ML, Fleischer AB, Jr, Chamlin SL, et al. Oral corticosteroid use is effective for cutaneous hemangiomas: an evidence-based evaluation. Arch Dermatol 2001; 137: 1208–13.

26. Ezekowitz RA, Mulliken JB, Folkman J. Interferon alpha-2a therapy for life-threatening hemangiomas of infancy. N Engl J Med 1992; 326: 1456–63.

27. Fledelius HC, Illum N, Jensen H, et al. Interferon-alfa treatment of facial infantile haemangiomas: with emphasis on the sight-threatening varieties. A clinical series. Acta Ophthalmol Scand 2001; 79: 370–3.

28. Loughnan MS, Elder J, Kemp A. Treatment of a massive orbital capillary hemangioma with interferon alpha-2b: short-term results [letter]. Arch Ophthalmol 1992; 110: 1366–7.

29. Garden JM, Bakus AD, Paller AS. Treatment of cutaneous hemangiomas by the flashlamp-pumped pulsed dye laser: prospective analysis. J Pediatr 1992; 120: 555–60.

30. Boyd MJ, Collin JRO. Capillary haemangiomas: an approach to their management. Br J Ophthalmol 1991; 75: 298–300.

31. Deans RM, Harris GJ, Kivlin JD. Surgical dissection of capillary hemangiomas. An alternative to intralesional corticosteroids. Arch Ophthalmol 1992; 110: 1743–7.

32. Walker RS, Custer PL, Nerad JA. Surgical excision of periorbital capillary hemangiomas. Ophthalmology 1994; 101: 1333–40.

33. Kapoor S, Kapoor MS, Aurora AL, et al. Orbital hemangio-pericytoma: a report of a 3-year-old child. J Pediatr Ophthalmol Strabismus 1978; 15: 40–2.

34. Croxatto JO, Font RL. Hemangiopericytoma of the orbit: a clinicopathological study of 30 cases. Hum Pathol 1982; 13: 210–8.

35. Harris GJ. Orbital vascular malformations: a consensus statement on terminology and its clinical implications. Orbital Society. Am J Ophthalmol 1999; 127: 453–5.

36. Rootman J. Vascular malformations of the orbit: hemodynamic concepts. Orbit 2003; 22: 103–20.

37. Iliff WJ, Green WR. Orbital lymphangiomas. Ophthalmology 1979; 86: 914–929.

38. Jones IS. Lymphangiomas of the ocular adnexia: an analysis of 62 cases. Trans Am Ophthalmol Soc 1959; 57: 602–65.

39. Harris GJ, Sakol PJ, Bonavolonta G, et al. An analysis of thirty cases of orbital lymphangioma. Pathophysiologic considerations and management recommendations. Ophthalmology 1990; 97: 1583–92.

40. Jakobiec FA, Bilyk Jr, Font RL. Orbit. In: Spencer WH, ed. Ophthalmic Pathology. 4th edn. Philadelphia: WB Saunders; 1996: 2438–933.

41. Garrity JA. Orbital venous anomalies: a long-standing dilemma [editorial]. Ophthalmology 1997; 104: 903–4.

42. Wright JE, Sullivan TJ, Garner A. Orbital venous anomalies. Ophthalmology 1997; 104: 905–13.

43. Rootman J. Orbital venous anomalies [letter]. Ophthalmology 1998; 105: 387–88.

44. Rootman J, Hay E, Graeb D, et al. Orbital-adnexal lymphangiomas: a spectrum of hemodynamically isolated vascular hamartomas. Ophthalmology 1986; 93: 1558–70.

45. Pang P, Jakobiec FA, Iwamoto T, et al. Small lymphangiomas of the eyelids. Ophthalmology 1984; 91: 1278–84.

46. Kazim M, Kennerdell JS, Rothfus W, et al. Orbital lymphangioma. Correlation of magnetic resonance images and intraoperative findings. Ophthalmology 1992; 99: 1588–94.

47. Katz SE, Rootman J, Vangveeravong S, et al. Combined venous lymphatic malformations of the orbit (so-called lymphangiomas): association with noncontiguous intracranial vascular anomalies. Ophthalmology 1998; 105: 176–84.

48. Bond JB, Haik BG, Taveras JL, et al. Magnetic resonance imaging of orbital lymphangioma with and without gadolinium contrast enhancement. Ophthalmology 1992; 99: 1318–24.

49. Henderson JW. Orbital Tumors. 3rd edn. Philadelphia: Lippincott-Raven Press; 1994.

50. Wilson ME, Parker PL, Chavis RM. Conservative management of childhood adult lymphangioma. Ophthalmology 1989; 96: 484–9.

51. Kennerdell JS, Maroon JC, Garrity JA, et al. Surgical management of orbital lymphangioma with the carbon dioxide laser. Am J Ophthalmol 1986; 102: 308–14.

52. Kremer I, Nissenkorn I, Feuerman P, et al. Congenital orbital vascular malformation complicated by massive retrobulbar hemorrhage. J Pediatr Ophthalmol Strabismus 1987; 24: 190–3.

53. Lacey B, Rootman J, Marotta TR. Distensible venous malformations of the orbit. Clinical and hemodynamic features and a new technique of management. Ophthalmology 1999; 106: 1197–1209.

54. Sujansky E, Conradi S. Sturge-Weber syndrome: age of onset of seizures and glaucoma and the prognosis for affected children. J Child Neurol 1995; 10: 49–58.

55. Hofeldt AJ, Zaret CR, Jakobiec FA, et al. Orbitofacial angiomatosis. Arch Ophthalmol 1979; 97: 484–8.

56. Rathbun JE, Hoyt WF, Beard C. Surgical management of orbitofrontal varix in Klippel-Trenaunay-Weber syndrome. Am J Ophthalmol 1970; 70: 109–12.

57. Crompton JL, Taylor D. Ocular lesions in the blue rubber naevus syndrome. Br J Ophthalmol 1981; 65: 133–7.

58. McCannel CA, Hoenig J, Umlas J, et al. Orbital lesions in the blue rubber bleb nevus syndrome. Ophthalmology 1996; 103: 933–6.

59. Oranje AP. Blue rubber bleb nevus syndrome. Pediatr Dermatol 1986; 3: 304–10.

60. Moodley M, Ramdial P. Blue rubber bleb nevus syndrome: case report and review of the literature. Pediatrics 1993; 92: 160–2.

CHAPTER
43 The Uveal Tract

Creig S Hoyt

The uveal tract consists of iris, ciliary body and choroid, each of which has a rich vascular supply and pigment. Its colorful grape-like appearance gives rise to its name "uvea". The structure contains two apertures–the pupil and the region of the optic nerve.

The uveal tract's functions are diverse–its pigment acts as a filter; iris musculature forms an "F-stop" for the eye; the ciliary body secretes aqueous, provides the skeleton for the zonular suspension of the lens as well as the power for focusing, and provides nutrition for the lens. The choroid with its rich vascular supply provides nutrition for 65% of the outer retinal layers.[1] Bruch's membrane forms a boundary between retina and choroid; abnormalities in this layer play an important role in various choroidal and retinal disorders.[2]

EMBRYOLOGY

The uveal tract includes contributions from the neural ectoderm, neural crest and mesoderm. The neural ectoderm gives rise to the iris sphincter and dilator muscles, posterior iris epithelium, pigmented and nonpigmented ciliary epithelium. Neural crest cells contribute to iris and choroidal stroma as well as ciliary smooth muscle. Mesodermal tissue forms the endothelium for the many blood vessels.

The neural ectoderm differentiation occurs within 6–10 weeks of conception whilst definition of the vasculature and pigment migration span the final two trimesters.

Iris formation commences with closure of the fetal cleft at approximately 35 days of gestation. The sphincter is first evidenced by neuroectodermal pigment at the optic cup's margin by 10 weeks of gestation[3] and differentiation into myofibril occurs at 11–12 weeks of gestation. The dilator forms at approximately 24 weeks gestation.

The neuroectoderm also gives rise to both pigmented and nonpigmented ciliary epithelium. Once the optic cup has invaginated, creating the inner and outer layers of neuro-ectoderm, pigmentation of only the outer layer occurs. At 10–12 weeks, longitudinal ridges form from the outer layer and adhere to the inner layers, and the ciliary processes form. More posteriorly, the two layers adhere to each other without folding, giving rise to the pars plana.

After the neuroectoderm invaginates, neural crest cells are derived from within the space between the neuroectoderm and surface ectoderm. Neural crest cells may be to the head and neck as mesoderm is to somites of the body, since no true somites exist in the head and neck region. Tissue derived from these cells is referred to as mesectoderm and its connection to the neuro-epithelium remains loose into adulthood, accounting for the porosity of the iris to particles of 50–200 mm by diffusion. The ciliary smooth muscle is first evident at nearly 4 months gestation just posterior to the precursors of the iris stroma. The fibers connect anteriorly to the developing scleral spur during the fifth month, and further increase in size and structure continues after birth.

Finally, neural crest cells also give rise to pigment cell precursors of the uveal tract (in contradistinction to neuroectoderm-derived retinal pigment epithelium). Pigmented cells surrounding the optic cup are visible at 10 weeks gestation. Pigment appears in the peripapillary region after 24 weeks. Migration occurs anteriorly and is nearly complete at birth as mostly mature melanosomes.[4]

The mesoderm gives rise solely to the endothelium of blood vessels whereas the muscular and support structures of the vessels arise from neural crest cells. These two components combine to form the "mesenchyme" or connective tissue elements of the head and neck region.

The iris vasculature primordia are present by 6 weeks gestation as loops extending over the anterior surface of the anterior chamber (tunica vasculosa lentis), in association with the development of the ciliary body vasculature. By the end of the third month, indentations are created by the radially oriented vessels. The long posterior ciliary arteries are present in the ciliary body, and their terminal branches unite with the peripheral parts of the tunica vasculosa lentis to form the major arterial circle. As the tunica vasculosa lentis regresses, a residual pupillary membrane is created. During the fifth month of gestation the major arterial circle gives rise to radial vessels and branches to the ciliary body.

The choroidal vasculature first differentiates from mesenchymal elements during the second month of gestation, with precursors of the short posterior ciliary arteries which connect posteriorly with the developing choriocapillaris at 3 months, at which time the long posterior ciliary arteries anastomose with the anterior circulation. Further differentiation with intermediate-size vessels occurs during the fourth month. The arterial and venous systems undergo further differentiation into the forerunners of the middle or Sattler's layer during the fifth month. The foveal circulation differentiates at approximately the third to fourth month.[5]

POSTNATAL DEVELOPMENT

At birth, the uveal tract is well differentiated. Two features which are very well-scrutinized by the parents are iris color and pupil size. Of particular concern is the color of the eyes. The ophthalmologist might best observe that (i) the neonate's eyes will never be lighter than they are at birth; (ii) pigmentation is usually defined by 6 months of age and always by 1 year; and (iii) it is possible for brown-eyed but heterozygous parents to have a blue-eyed child.

At birth, Caucasians often have blue eyes because there are few melanocytes present with sparse pigment. More darkly pigmented races have irides with already pigmented melanocytes. The pigmentation in all races increases over the first 6 months to 1 year of life.

Pupil size is relatively small at birth, especially in darkly pigmented eyes. As the iris dilator muscle develops postnatally, the pupil correspondingly enlarges. The pupil margin may be accentuated by a prominent ectropion uveae, creating unnecessary concern by the parents or pediatrician.

In the full-term infant, the residual pupillary membrane may rarely alter the red reflex, resulting in referral from the primary care physician for further evaluation. In the preterm infant, assessment of the degree of atrophy of the pupillary membrane and its precursor, the tunica vasculosa lentis, has been used to estimate gestational age.

The ciliary muscle is incompletely developed at birth, the increase in accommodation over 3–6 months supports further development postnatally.[6] An autopsy study of 76 infant eyes has documented this development with 75% of the final adult ciliary body length being achieved by 2 years of age.[6]

The clinically significant effects of prematurity on the development of retinal circulation are not matched by any effect on choroidal circulation. Choroidal development and pigmentation is relatively complete at birth[4]; the changing fundus pigmentation is more due to changes in the retinal pigment epithelium.

DEVELOPMENTAL ABNORMALITIES

Coloboma

See Chapter 50.

Congenital iris and ciliary body cysts

These occur when fluid fills an epithelium-lined cyst of the iris. The two types of cyst are iris stromal cysts (Figs 43.1, 43.2) and pigment epithelial cysts (Fig. 43.3). They consist of a squamous epithelial or neuroepithelial lining, respectively[7,8] and are probably congenital in origin.

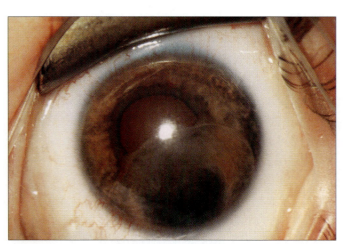

Fig. 43.1 Iris cyst. This stromal cyst recurred after local removal and eventually required a sector iridectomy.

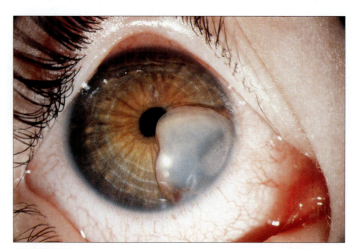

Fig. 43.2 Iris stromal cyst.

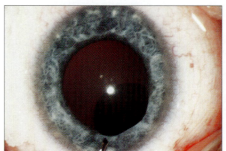

Fig. 43.3 Posterior iris cyst consisting of pigment epithelium. Cysts of this type tend not to recur after simple removal with a vitrectomy machine or puncture with a YAG laser.

Iris stromal cysts occur on the anterior surface of the iris, and have a transparent wall with a visible vascular lining. Pigment epithelial cysts occur at or behind the pupillary margin (Fig. 43.3) and have a nontransparent lining. If the size and location impairs the visual axis, surgical intervention may be necessary. Complications include glaucoma and spontaneous detachment intraocularly.[9] Iris pigment epithelial cysts are usually stationary.[10]

Stromal cysts appear to enlarge progressively as they may recur if incompletely excised – a wide excision is recommended. Suggested treatments have included photocoagulation, injection of sclerosants and radiation. However, surgical excision with sector iridectomy apparently gives best results.[7] Pigment epithelial cysts often require no treatment, but may be treated by simple excision or puncture with a yttrium–aluminum–garnet (YAG) laser.

The differential diagnoses of iris cysts include secondary cyst formation from epithelial implantation due to surgery or penetrating trauma, and solid iris or ciliary body tumors.

Ciliary body cysts may cause astigmatism and amblyopia (see Fig. 43.4).

Brushfield spots

These are typically found with Down syndrome at least in a European population.[11] However, studies of Asian children suggest that Brushfield spots occur only rarely in Down syndrome or unaffected children.[12,13] Histologically, the spots correlate with a normal to hypercellular area of iris tissue with surrounding relative stromal hypoplasia.

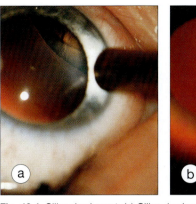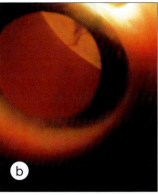

Fig. 43.4 Ciliary body cyst. (a) Ciliary body cyst in direct illumination. It appears brown and solid. (b) Ciliary body cyst in transillumination: it is semi-transparent and fluid filled.

Persistent pupillary membranes

Persistent pupillary membranes represent an incomplete involution of the anterior tunica vasculosa lentis. The membranes are attached to the collarette (Fig. 43.5) and may be free floating, span the pupil to attach on its opposite side, or attach to the anterior surface of the lens (Figs 43.6–43.8) with or without an associated cataract. Autosomal dominant inheritance has been reported.[14] The membranes have been noted to occur in conjunction with other ocular anomalies including microcornea, megalocornea, microphthalmos and coloboma.[15]

They may be substantial but even then may not impair vision. The vast majority of cases do not have visual consequences. However, there is a group which take on the appearances of a hyperplastic membrane.[16] With these more extensive membranes (Fig. 43.9a), the red reflex may be altered, despite pharmacological dilation, and they may impair vision.

It is important to realize that the tunica vasculosa lentis does not normally involute until the beginning of the third trimester, and it may be seen in normal, but very premature babies (Fig. 43.9b,c).

The membranes may have fibrous remnants with extensive attachments to the lens (Fig. 43.10); surgical management has included attempts to improve vision with iridectomy, some of which have been unsuccessful,[14] removal of the membrane[17] and laser therapy to the persistent strands to the collarette.[18] On the whole, those pupillary membranes that require treatment respond to medical therapy alone, i.e. pupillary dilation and occlusion therapy.

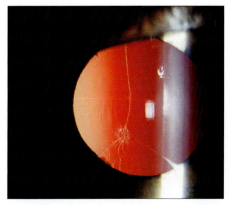

Fig. 43.5 Persistent pupillary membrane with vascularized attachments to the collarette and anterior to the lens.

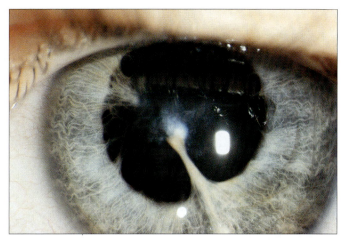

Fig. 43.6 Hyperplastic persistent pupillary membrane. The visual acuity was 6/12. Patient of Dr John Crompton.

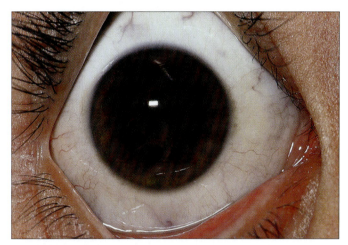

Fig. 43.7 Persistent pupillary membrane attached to the lens.

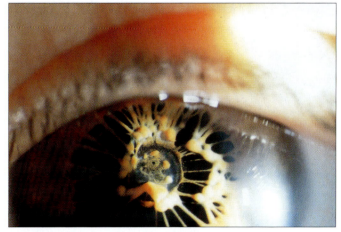

Fig. 43.8 Persistent pupillary membrane.

Congenital idiopathic microcoria

Microcoria is a small pupil with a diameter of less than 2 mm when the patient looks at a distant object. It may be transmitted as an autosomal dominant trait.[19] In this predominantly unilateral anomaly the pupil is microscopically small so that the pupil is nearly or actually obliterated (Fig. 43.11); it is often eccentric. It

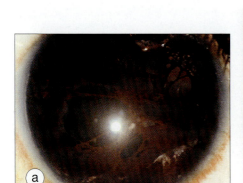
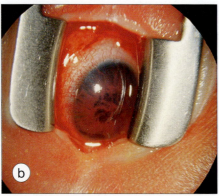
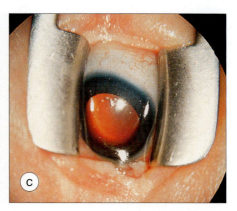

Fig. 43.9 Persistent pupillary membrane. (a) Marked persistent hyperplastic pupillary membrane. (b) Prominent tunica vasculosa lentis in a very premature baby. There is no hemorrhage. (c) Same patient as (b) 11 days later. A persistent tunica vasculosa lentis is barely visible, and disappeared to leave a perfectly normal eye. Patient of Mr Robert Morris.

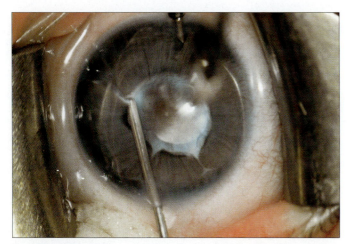

Fig. 43.10 Hyperplastic pupillary membrane stretching across the pupil attached to the collarette. It also involves the anterior capsule of the lens.

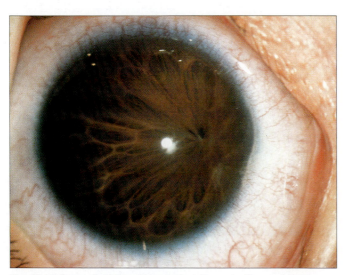

Fig. 43.11 Congenital idiopathic extreme microcoria. The pupil in this case was so small that the eye was potentially amblyopic and a pupil was created surgically.

is probably related to an abnormality of the development of the fetal pupillary membrane and its main effect is to cause amblyopia and put the eye at risk from glaucoma. An accurate refraction is essential as the condition is associated with myopia and astigmatism.[19] Early surgical treatment and occlusion therapy can result in useful vision.

Bilateral microcoria has been reported in association with microphthalmos and more posterior anomalies.[20]

Aniridia

Aniridia represents a spectrum of disorders with iris hypoplasia. Its incidence has been estimated between 1:64 000 and 1:96 000.[21] Both hereditary and sporadic forms exist. The usual mode of inheritance is as an autosomal dominant trait but autosomal recessive transmission is suggested in the rarer, Gillespie syndrome, i.e. aniridia associated with mental retardation and cerebellar ataxia.[22] One-third of cases arise spontaneously and they may have the 11p13 deletion.

Aniridia is caused by a haploinsufficiency of PAX6 gene of which abnormalities include base alterations and deletions.[23] When a deletion involves its adjacent genes, those in the PAX6-WT1 critical region (WTCR) patients are predisposed to Wilms tumor.[23] PAX6 function was first identified through aniridia-associated null mutations. Since then this transcription factor has also been found to be essential in the development of the olfactory system and forebrain and cerebellum.[24]

Histologically, the iris is reduced to a small stub, and smooth muscle is usually absent. The angle may be poorly developed, and the retina may be present over portions of the pars plana and pars plicata of the ciliary body. Later changes include development of peripheral anterior synechiae with corneal endothelial growth into the angle.[25] Other corneal irregularities include epithelial and Bowman's layer abnormalities and a thick fibrovascular pannus in patients with glaucoma. Incursion of goblet cells suggest impaired function of limbal stem cells, abnormal expression of cytokeratin 12 may result in greater epithelial fragility and corneal opacification may reflect poor wound-healing responses to accumulated environmental insults.[26]

Aniridia is a bilateral condition but can show marked asymmetry between the two eyes in patients with a family history of aniridia. In the screening of other family members for evidence of aniridia, it is important to recognize the variable expressivity of this condition. Aniridia is not only associated with poor vision, glaucoma and cataract but also with systemic abnormalities. Decreased vision is usual, with multiple contributory factors including light scatter, corneal and lenticular opacities, severe glaucoma, optic nerve hypoplasia, foveal hypoplasia and nystagmus. Pedigree studies have found approximately 60% with vision better than 6/9 (20/30) and 5% with vision worse than 6/60 (20/200).[27] Others have reported as high an incidence as 86% with vision 6/30 (20/100) or worse.[28] A lot of the variation in the various studies is accounted for by different inclusion criteria.

Although glaucoma is not typically present at birth, the incidence of childhood glaucoma has been reported between 6 and 75%.[1,27,29] The delay in the onset of glaucoma is probably due to progressive changes in the angle. The glaucoma is due either to angle anomalies leading to an open angle glaucoma or angle closure glaucoma from obstruction of the angle by the rudimentary iris stump.[30]

Cataract formation is present in 50–85% of patients by the age of 20 years.[27,31] The changes are usually progressive. Ectopia lentis may also occur in conjunction with aniridia,[21] due to an abnormality of the zonular structure.[30]

The corneal abnormalities are also progressive;[26] peripheral corneal epithelial irregularities spread to involve the entire cornea. Microcornea has also been reported in association with aniridia.

Optic nerve hypoplasia was found in nine of 12 patients by Layman et al.,[31] contributing to reduced vision.

Aniridia with systemic disease

The WAGR syndrome (Wilms tumor, aniridia, genitourinary abnormalities and mental retardation). Between one-quarter and one-third of children with sporadic aniridia will develop Wilms tumor prior to 3 years of age.[23] Frequently, mental retardation, genitourinary abnormalities, craniofacial abnormalities, microcephaly and growth retardation are also present. In the triad of aniridia, genitourinary abnormalities and mental retardation, in which an extensive deletion of the short arm of chromosome 11 has been demonstrated,[32] there is also a high incidence of bilateral Wilms tumors.[33]

There may be other systemic manifestations.[23] Until the molecular genetic identification of the deletion is routinely available, patients with sporadic aniridia need to be screened for Wilms tumor by abdominal palpation (this can also be done by the parents), or ultrasound studies every 3 months for 5 years.
Gillespie syndrome. Aniridia with cerebellar ataxia and mental retardation.[22,34]
Aniridia in association with absent patellae.[35]
Dominant aniridia with ptosis, obesity and mental retardation.[36]
Aniridia, anophthalmos and microcephaly.[37] There may be some similarities between this condition and that of the case described by Glaser et al.[38] suggesting PAX6 gene dosage effect in a child, both of whose parents had aniridia.

Gene mapping has supported the 11p13 deletion locus in patients with aniridia and Wilms tumor. The majority of patients with the 11p13 deletion are sporadic. It now appears that chromosomes 1 and 2 do not play an important role in dominant congenital aniridia with linkage studies supporting the existence of a single map position for aniridia at the 11p13 position involving the PAX6 gene.[24,38] PAX6 gene mutations have been shown to give rise to many associated ocular anomalies in conjunction with aniridia.[38]

Elevated intraocular pressure may be better tolerated in aniridic eyes.[30] When surgery is required, a higher percentage of patients require tube implantation.[39]

Infants with aniridia and glaucoma may not have a normal Schlemm's canal, making goniotomy an unlikely choice for surgery. Walton[40] advocated at least yearly gonioscopy to assess for the presence of increasing iris processes and angle closure with a view to prophylactic goniotomy. Laser trabeculoplasty is not helpful and trabeculectomy may be a better procedure in older patients.[30]

Cataract extraction in aniridia patients must also require extra preparation since the lens zonules do not support the lens in a normal fashion; the issue of intraocular lens implantation has met with some success[41] but, because of potential lens dislocation with time, intraocular lenses are probably not indicated in the young. Penetrating keratoplasty may help severe cases of associated corneal involvement but visual expectations must be limited. Corneal surgery in such patients has warranted caution due to the high rate of graft rejection.[42]

Optical correction of significant refractive errors, and a shift to an aphakic refractive error after lens subluxation may be of great help to some affected children. Even though the "pupil" is large, cycloplegic agents must be used for refraction in young patients since active accommodation is present. The use of occluder contact lenses with a pupillary aperture has been advocated for infants but is not warranted in most cases. Recently black iris-diaphragm intraocular lenses have been implanted in some aniridics.[43]

Heterochromia iridis

A difference in iris color can be congenital or acquired, the abnormal eye being either darker or lighter than the other eye, and it may be difficult to decide which is the abnormal eye. Skin pigmentation, parental eye color, assessment of earlier photographs and the history usually resolve this question.

Congenital

Congenital heterochromia with the involved iris being darker, may point to ocular melanocytosis or oculodermal melanocytosis, or to a sector iris hamartoma syndrome. An iris pigment epithelial hamartoma creates a jet-black superficial lesion which consists of iris pigment epithelium with clumped smooth muscle cells and melanocytes.[44]

Horner syndrome. Congenital Horner syndrome results in ipsilateral hypopigmentation, miosis and ptosis (see Chapter 59).

Waardenburg syndrome. Waardenburg syndrome is transmitted as an autosomal dominant trait. There are four clinical types. Type 1 (Fig. 43.12) includes lateral displacement of the inner canthi, prominent root of the nose and unusual brows. Type 2 (Fig. 43.13) does not include the facial dysmorphism. Both types 1 and 2 include sensorineural deafness, a white forelock and heterochromia iridis. Fundus pigmentary heterochromia may also be present. Type 1 is caused by a mutation in the PAX3 gene located on chromosome 2q35.[45] More recently type 2 Waardenburg syndrome has been isolated to 3p12-p14.1, close to

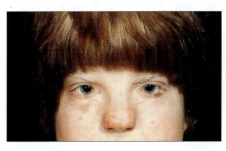

Fig. 43.12
Waardenburg syndrome type 1. Shows poliosis, lateral displacement of the inner canthi and a prominent root of the nose.

401

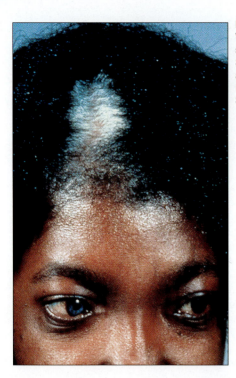

Fig. 43.13 Waardenburg syndrome type 2. Shows heterochromia and white forelock. Patient of Dr Dai Stephens.

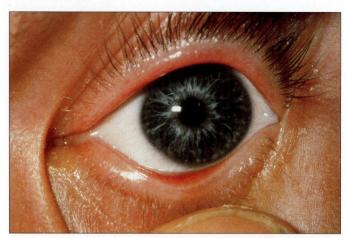

Fig. 43.15 Williams syndrome showing the characteristic stellate iris pattern.

the homologue of the microphthalmia gene.[45] Type 3 (Klein–Waardenburg syndrome) is very rare and it represents an extreme form of type 1 associated with musculoskeletal abnormalities.[45] Type 4 (Waardenburg–Hirschsprung disease) is comprised of sensorineural deafness, hypopigmentation of skin, hair and irides and Hirschsprung disease. It may be associated with central or peripheral nervous system disorders. Mutations in the endothelian B receptor (EDNRB) gene have been identified in this type.[46]

Acquired

Acquired heterochromia with the involved iris darker results from infiltrative processes–such as nevi (Fig. 43.14) and melanomatous tumors–and deposition of material within the iris.

Siderosis results from iron deposition within the dilator muscles of the iris.[47] Heterochromia may be the presenting feature of an intraocular foreign body, which may only be found on a computed tomography (CT) scan. Hemosiderosis results

from deposition of iron derived from blood products, as in heterochromia from long-standing hyphema.

With an acquired lighter colored iris, Fuchs heterochromic iridocyclitis must be strongly considered (see below); more rarely infiltrations such as juvenile xanthogranuloma, metastatic malignancies and leukemia can be responsible. Acquired Horner syndrome early in the first year of life can also lead to heterochromia.

William syndrome

William syndrome is a rare autosomal dominantly inherited disorder that is a segmental aneusomy syndrome that results from heterozygous mild deletions of 20 continuous genes at 7g11.23.[48] Its general features are aortic valvular disease, hypercalcemia, physical and developmental delay, elfin or pixie-like facial features with prominent lips, hyperacusis and a predisposition to developing otitis media.[48] Ophthalmic involvement comprises a typical iris pattern (Fig. 43.15) which takes on a stellate appearance.[49] Other ocular features include strabismus, mainly esotropia, hypermetropia and retinal vessel tortuosity.[50]

Iris ectropion and flocculi

When the posterior pigment epithelium of the iris extends onto the front of the iris it is known as ectropion uveae or, more correctly, as iris ectropion (Fig. 43.16a,b). It may be congenital. It is sometimes associated with glaucoma (see Chapter 40), neurofibromatosis type 1 (NF1) or anterior segment dysgenesis. Iris flocculi are small excrescences of pigment epithelium at the pupil margin; whilst normally isolated and of no significance, they may act as a marker for familial aortic dissection.[51]

UVEAL TUMORS

With the exception of iris nevi, tumors involving the uveal tract are rare in children. Presentation of tumors may be as heterochromia, glaucoma, hyphema or decreased vision, with or without squint in the case of more posterior masses.

Iris nevi and freckles

Iris nevi consist of localized nests of melanocytes which vary in size and shape: spindle (the most common), epithelioid and

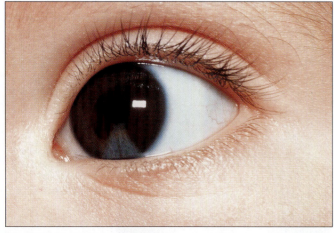

Fig. 43.14 Iris sector hypopigmentation.

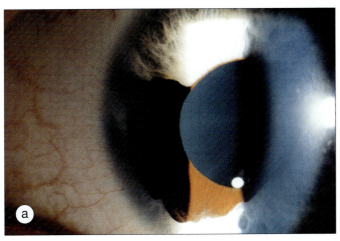

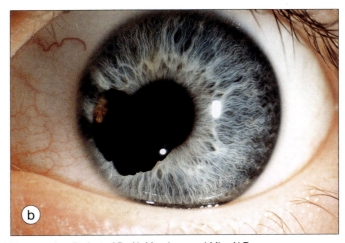

Fig. 43.16 Iris ectropion. (a) Iris ectropion. The pupil functions were normal. (b) Iris ectropion. Patient of Dr AL·Murphree and Miss N·Ragge.

polyhedral. They are common and their association with posterior choroidal melanomas is debatable. Rarely, involvement of angle structures can lead to glaucoma.[52] Glaucoma has also been described in association with an aggressive form of iris nevi in children.[53] Iris nevi may also create an irregular pupil, be associated with a sectoral cataract, or seed into the anterior chamber. None of these has any prognostic significance, as iris nevi are benign.

Iris nevi should be distinguished from iris freckles, which are on the anterior surface of the iris without altering the iris structures. Histologically, iris freckles are a cluster of normal iris melanocytes.

Iris melanosis and iris mamillations

Iris melanosis is a condition in which the iris is hyperpigmented. It is commonly associated with scleral pigmentation and choroidal hyperpigmentation; the surface of the iris is smooth. It may be familial, occurring in sibships[54] or as an autosomal dominant trait.

Iris mamillations (Fig.·43.17) are villiform protuberances that can cover much of the anterior surface of the iris and are sometimes associated with an iris nevus.

The incidence of glaucoma in both conditions is uncertain, but affected people should be followed for life.

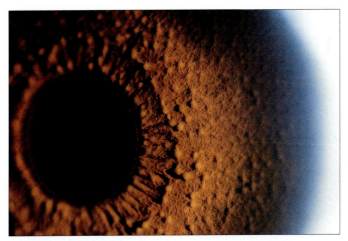

Fig. 43.17 Iris mamillations.

Cogan–Reese syndrome

Within the spectrum of iridocorneal endothelial syndrome is the Cogan–Reese syndrome that consists of iris nevus with peripheral iris–corneal attachments. Glaucoma is strongly associated with this syndrome.[55]

Iris and choroidal melanoma

These are uncommon in children.[56] Iris melanomas are relatively nonaggressive,[57] and all melanomas are rare in black people. Iris melanomas present 10–20 years earlier than choroidal melanomas due to their visibility. Whereas less than 10% of all malignant melanomas in the general population arise in the iris, 40–50% of such tumors arise in the iris in patients 29 years of age or younger.[58] In Shields' series, 12% of malignant uveal tumors arose from the iris in patients under 20 years of age.[59]

Iris melanomas have a strong bias for presentation inferiorly. Due to their vascularity, their presentation may be as a hyphema.

Iris melanoma differs histologically from that of ciliary body and choroidal melanomas; approximately 60% are spindle cell, 33% are mixed cell and the remainder epithelioid. Only the spindle cell type behaves in a malignant fashion. A more detailed histological classification has been made by Jakobiec and Silbert[57] which includes their view of appropriate treatment.

The differential diagnoses of iris melanomas include juvenile xanthogranuloma, iris rhabdomyosarcoma, iris foreign body, segmental melanosis oculi, iris abscess, and Fuchs' adenoma in adults.[60] Differentiation must also be made from a ciliary body mass since the prognosis differs for this location.

Uveal melanomas are exceedingly rare during childhood. Childhood uveal melanomas represent between 0.6 and 1.1% of all patients with uveal melanoma.[59] Two cases reports exist of a uveal melanoma in neonates[61,62] both with infants having multiple skin nevi. The slow growth of these tumors may account for their relatively late presentation due to refractive changes and lens distortion, narrowed anterior chamber, prominent episcleral vessels and slightly reduced intraocular pressure. Later, extension into the anterior chamber, cataracts and glaucoma may be the presenting features.

Choroidal melanomas are rare in childhood but failure to consider this diagnosis may lead to a delay in treatment.[58] There have been two reports of this tumor in two 5-year-old children.[63] A review by Shields et al. of 40 patients less than 20 years of age demonstrates the need to consider this rare but potentially fatal tumor.[59] The differential diagnoses include choroidal nevi, which are characterized as having a diameter of 7 mm or less, an elevation of 2 mm or less, overlying drusen in older patients, and sparse lipofuscin; they are asymptomatic and have no or slow growth. Choroidal nevi may give rise to malignant melanoma. Photographic documentation with careful follow-up is appropriate.

Childhood uveal malignant melanomas do not seem to have a poorer prognosis than adult tumors. A recent review has shown 5-year survival rates to be 96%.[59] Poorer prognostic indicators include extraocular extension at the time of diagnosis, base diameter greater than 10 mm, and mixed or epithelioid cell type.[64]

Certain congenital disorders are felt to predispose to uveal melanomas. In addition to previously mentioned choroidal melanomas,[65] neurofibromatosis may be associated with a greater number of melanocytic nevi and of uveal melanomas.[65]

Although familial occurrences of malignant melanoma are known,[66] the inverse relationship with skin and eye pigmentation has been much more apparent to clinicians.[67]

Medulloepithelioma

Medulloepithelioma is usually a unilateral, solid or cystic tumor of the ciliary body nonpigmented epithelium; it is a congenital lesion derived from embryonic retina which occasionally includes cartilage, brain, striated muscle and other elements and are called teratomedulloepitheliomas. Ordinarily they are comprised of membranes, tubules and rosettes. The arrangement of such networks accounts for their initial designation as dictyomas. They may undergo malignant transformation.[68] Other structures such as the optic nerve may rarely be involved.

They usually present within the first decade as a visible iris tumor, leukocoria, abnormally shaped pupil, glaucoma, hyphema or decreased vision with or without strabismus.[69] Extraocular extension at the time of enucleation was the most important prognostic indicator with an excellent prognosis for tumor confined to the eye. Other series have implied a more benign nature.[68]

Occurrence with other tumors has been reported including retinoblastoma and pinealoblastoma.

Enucleation is the recommended treatment unless well localized anteriorly, when local excision or cryotherapy may play a role.[68] The differential diagnoses include juvenile xanthogranuloma and retinoblastoma, but the cystic nature, the origin from the ciliary body, the rather felt-like appearance and the unilaterality speak heavily for medulloepithelioma (see Chapter 42).

Choroidal and iris hemangioma

Choroidal hemangiomas may be divided into diffuse and localized lesions. The localized form is a minimally growing lesion which is usually asymptomatic. They are characteristically orange-red in color, located usually within two disc diameters of the optic disc. They may include both capillary and cavernous components. Superficial changes, including pigmentation, have resulted in a misdiagnosis with subsequent enucleation for malignant melanoma.[71]

The diffuse choroidal hemangiomas (tomato ketchup fundus) are associated with Sturge–Weber syndrome and carry a risk of associated glaucoma.[72] Episcleral vascular hamartomas may be the cause of the increased intraocular pressure.

Retinal detachment may also occur and laser treatment has been advocated for this. Localized hemangiomas are associated with a poor visual prognosis with subfoveal involvement. Extrafoveal tumors may be associated with a better prognosis with usage of scatter photocoagulation. For small solitary tumors, radiotherapy, using a lens-sparing technique, may be indicated. Low-dose stereotactic radiotherapy may provide the best treatment for symptomatic circumscribed lesions.[73] No treatment is effective for diffuse or large solitary tumors.

Iris hemangiomas are rare lesions. They have been described as occurring in conjunction with a more generalized diffuse neonatal hemangiomatosis.[74] They have also been reported in association with infants who have more typical lid hemangiomas.[75]

Uveal adenoma and adenocarcinoma

Rare cases of adenomas involving the iris[76] and ciliary body[77] have been reported. Adenomas and adenocarcinomas of the iris and ciliary body may arise from the pigmented or nonpigmented ciliary epithelium.

Adenocarcinoma of the ciliary nonpigmented epithelium in children has been documented following ocular trauma.[78]

Choroidal osteoma

Choroidal osteomas, though typically unilateral, rarely present bilaterally. The clinical presentation and course may vary. They are a benign ossifying tumor of the choroid which is typically found in the peripapillary region (Fig. 43.18a–b). There is a suggestion that the tumor tendency may be inherited as an autosomal dominant trait.[79] The exact pathogenesis is unclear.

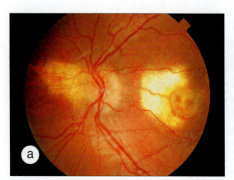
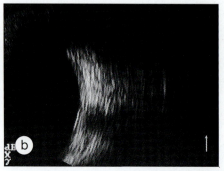

Fig. 43.18 Choroidal osteoma with submacular hemorrhage. (a) The acuity had deteriorated to 6/60. (b) Same patient. Ultrasound showing increased echoes from the osteoma.

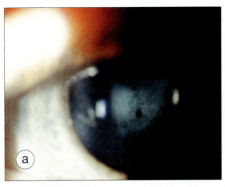 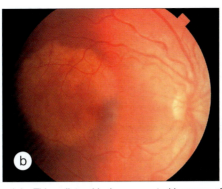 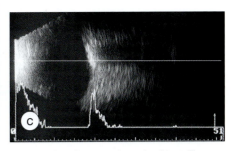

Fig. 43.19 Choroidal osteoma probably of traumatic origin. This unilateral lesion presented because of poor vision found at a routine school test. There was also a posterior subcapsular cataract (a) and the pale fundus lesion (b) had high echogenicity on ultrasound (c).

They may represent a choristoma, i.e. a primary congenital tumor of an embryonic tissue nest, or may represent a secondary calcification of an area affected by inflammatory disease or trauma (Fig. 43.19a–c).[80] Clinically, choroidal osteomas are yellow-white in color. B-scan ultrasonography confirms the presence of calcification. These tumors may not exhibit any growth. Complications include visual loss secondary to extension of the osteoma onto the foveal region, subretinal neovascular membrane formation and exudative retinal detachment.[81]

Iris rhabdomyosarcoma

This rare mass has been described as a light fleshy tumor of the iris.

Juvenile xanthogranuloma

See Chapter 33.

Lisch nodules and neurofibromatosis

See Chapter 28.

Leiomyoma

Leiomyomas of the iris and ciliary body are benign slow-growing tumors of smooth muscle that may arise from pericytes, ciliary or intrascleral heterotropic muscle.[82] They are rare tumors that are more prevalent in females.

Iris leiomyomas take on a pale or pink appearance and are well-circumscribed lesions. The presenting features may include pupillary distortion, hyphema, with complications of secondary glaucoma and cataract formation.[82]

Ciliary body lesions may present as a result of enlargement onto adjacent structures. The increasing mass can result in iris distortion, secondary local cataract formation or glaucoma from angle occlusion.[82]

The appearances of both iris and ciliary body leiomyomas are indistinguishable from melanoma. It has been suggested that many previously diagnosed leiomyomas may in fact be melanocytic lesions.[83] The tumors may not enlarge in size. If there is definite evidence of enlargement then surgical excision is indicated.

Other tumors

There have been sporadic reports of rare forms of uveal tumors both primary and secondary. These include hemangiopericytomas of the ciliary body,[84] neuroblastoma of the choroid[85] and choristoma of the iris and ciliary body.[86]

Spontaneous hyphema

Trauma is the leading cause of hyphema and even when there is no history of trauma other signs of trauma, such as recessed angle or contralateral retinal hemorrhages, must be carefully sought. Nonaccidental injury may also cause hyphema.

Truly spontaneous hyphemas can occur and indicate either underlying pathology of the uveal tract or a bleeding diathesis. Vascular tumors such as juvenile xanthogranuloma, medulloepithelioma, and retinoblastoma are important. Retinoschisis, retinopathy of prematurity, persistent hyperplastic primary vitreous, blood dyscrasias such as leukemia, and postcontusion injury or postsurgical intervention have all been implicated.[87] In older children and adults, scurvy, purpura, severe iritis, rubeosis and migraine may also cause apparently spontaneous hyphema.

Spontaneous hyphemas deserve immediate concern about elevated intraocular pressure and corneal blood staining, but equal importance must be paid to determination of the underlying cause, including studies such as ultrasound and CT scanning. A careful general physical examination may reveal other clues, as might hematological screening for blood dyscrasias.

Uveal manifestations (noninflammatory) of systemic disease

Direct leukemic infiltration of the iris may lead to heterochromia, spontaneous hyphema, glaucoma or hypopyon.[88] However, a study of 657 children with leukemia revealed only nine children with anterior segment abnormalities.[89]

Burkitt lymphoma, with its close association with Epstein–Barr virus, commonly affects children from tropical countries.[90] Although orbital involvement is most common, choroidal findings have been seen on postmortem cases. This tumor may gain further clinical significance since it has been reported in association with acquired immunodeficiency syndrome.[91]

Uveitic processes that fail to respond to routine therapy should raise the suspicion of other underlying pathological processes. Focal lesions giving rise to inflammatory diseases may include intraocular tumors, primary or secondary. Adjacent orbital inflammatory processes giving rise to a secondary uveitis, such as pseudotumors, may also need to be considered.[92]

REFERENCES

1. Alm A, Bill A. The oxygen supply to the retina II. Effects of high intraocular pressure and of increased arterial carbon dioxide tension on uveal and retinal blood flow in cats. Acta Physiol Scand 1972; 84: 306–19.
2. Hogan M. Ultrastructure of the choroid. Its role in the pathogenesis of chorioretinal disease. Trans Pacific Coast Ophthalmol Soc 1961; 42: 61.
3. Mund ML, Rodrigues MM, Fine BS. Light and electron microscopic observations on the pigmented layers of the developing human eye. Am J Ophthalmol 1972; 73: 167–82.
4. Rodrigues MM, Hackett J, Donohon P. Iris. In: Jakobiec FA, ed. Ocular Anatomy, Embryology and Teratology. Philadelphia: Harper & Row; 1982: 285–302.
5. Heimann K. The development of the choroid in man: choroidal vascular system. Ophthalmic Res 1972; 3: 257–73.
6. Aiello AL, Tran VT, Narsing AR. Postnatal development of the ciliary body and pars plana: a morphometric study in childhood. Arch Ophthalmol 1992: 110: 802–5.
7. Naumann GO, Rummelt V. Congenital nonpigmented epithelial iris cyst removed by block excision. Graef Arch Clin Exp Ophthamol 1990; 228: 392–7.
8. Paridaens AD, Deuble K, McCartney AC. Spontaneous congenital non-pigmented epithelial cysts of the iris stroma. Br J Ophthalmol 1992; 76: 39–42.
9. Watts MT, Rennie IG. Detached iris cyst presenting as an intraocular foreign body. J Roy Soc Med 1991; 84: 172–3.
10. Shields JA, Kline MU, Augsburger JJ. Primary iris cysts: a review of the literature and report of 62 cases. Br J Ophthalmol 1984; 68: 152–66.
11. Berk AT, Saatci AO, Ercal MD, et al. Ocular findings in 55 patients with Down's syndrome. Ophthalmic Genet 1996; 17: 15–9.
12. Kim JH, Hwang JM, Kim HS, et al. Characteristic ocular findings in Asian children with Down syndrome. Eye 2002; 16: 710–4.
13. Wong V, Ho D. Ocular abnormalities in Down syndrome: an analysis of 140 children. Pediatr Neurol 1997; 16: 311–14.
14. Merin S, Crawford JS, Cardarelli J. Hyperplastic persistent pupillary membrane. Am J Ophthalmol 1971; 72: 717–19.
15. Cassady JR, Light A. Familial persistent pupillary membranes. Arch Ophthalmol 1957; 58: 438.
16. Jacobs M, Jaouni Z, Crompton J, et al. Persistent pupillary membranes. J Pediatr Ophthalmol Strabismus 1991; 28: 215–18.
17. Reynolds JD, Hiles DA, Johnson BL, et al. Hyperplastic persistent pupillary membrane: surgical management. J Pediatr Ophthalmol Strabismus 1983; 20: 149–52.
18. Gupta R, Kumar S, Sonika S. Laser and surgical management of hyperplastic pupillary membrane. Ophthalmic Surg Lasers Imaging 2003; 34: 136–139.
19. Toulemont PJ, Urvoy M, Coscus G, et al. Association of congenital microcoria with myopia and glaucoma. Ophthalmology 1995; 102: 193–8.
20. Maden A, Buyukgebiz B, Gunenc U, et al. Bilateral congenital absence of pupillary aperture. Am J Ophthalmol 1991; 112: 608–9.
21. Shaw MW, Falls HF, Neel JV. Congenital aniridia. Am J Hum Genet 1960; 12: 389–415.
22. Crawfurd M d'A, Harcourt RB, Shaw PA. Non-progressive cerebellar ataxia, aplasia of pupillary zone of iris, and mental subnormality (Gillespie's syndrome) affecting three members of a non-consanguineous family in two generations. J Med Genet 1979; 16: 373–8.
23. Muto R, Yamomori S, Ohashi H, et al. Prediction by FISH analysis of the occurrence of Wilms tumor in aniridia patients. Am J Med Genet 2002; 108: 285–9.
24. van Heyningen V, Williamson KA. PAX6 in sensory development. Hum Mol Genet 2002; 11: 1161–7.
25. Margo CE. Congenital aniridia: a histopathologic study of the anterior segment in children. J Pediatr Ophthalmol Strabismus 1983; 20: 192–8.
26. Ramesh T, Collinson JM, Remesh K, et al. Corneal abnormalities in Pax6+/− small eye mice mimic human aniridia related keratopathy. Invest Ophthalmol Vis Sci 2003; 44: 1871–8.
27. Elsas TJ, Maumenee IH, Kenyon KR, et al. Familial aniridia with preserved ocular function. Am J Ophthalmol 1977; 83: 718–24.
28. Jesberg DO. Aniridia with retinal lipid deposits. Arch Ophthalmol 1962; 68: 331–6.
29. Grant WM, Walton DS. Progressive changes in the angle in congenital aniridia, with development of glaucoma. Am J Ophthalmol 1974; 18: 842–7.
30. Nelson LB, Spaeth GL, Nowinski TS et al. Aniridia, a review. Surv Ophthalmol 1984; 28: 621–42.
31. Layman PR, Anderson DR, Flynn JT. Frequent occurrence of hypoplastic optic discs in patients with aniridia. Am J Ophthalmol 1974; 77: 573–6.
32. Riccardi VM, Borges W. Aniridia, cataracts, and Wilms' tumor. Am J Ophthalmol 1978; 86: 577–99.
33. Warburg M, Mikkelsen M, Andersen SR, et al. Aniridia and interstitial deletion of the short arm of chromosome 11. Metab Pediatr Ophthalmol 1980; 4: 97–102.
34. Gillespie FD. Aniridia, cerebellar ataxia, and oligophrenia. Arch Ophthalmol 1965; 73: 338–41.
35. Mirkinson AE, Mirkinson NK. A familial syndrome of aniridia and absence of the patella. Birth Defects 1975; 11: 129–31.
36. Hamming NA, Miller MT, Rabb M. Unusual variant of familial aniridia. J Pediatr Ophthalmol Strabismus 1986; 23: 195–200.
37. Edwards J, Lampert R, Hammer M, et al. Ocular defects and dysmorphic features in three generations. J Clin Dysmorphol 1984; 2: 8–12.
38. Glaser T, Jepeal L, Edwards JG, et al. Pax 6 gene dosage effect in a family with congenital cataracts, aniridia, anophthalmia and central nervous system defects. Nat Genet 1994; 7: 463–71.
39. Wiggins RE, Tomey KF. The results of glaucoma surgery in aniridia. Arch Ophthalmol 1992; 110: 503–5.
40. Chew TC, Walton DS. Goniosurgery for prevention of aniridic glaucoma. Arch Ophthalmol 1999; 117: 1144–8.
41. Johns KJ, O'Day DM. Posterior chamber intraocular lenses after extracapsular cataract extraction in patients with aniridia. Ophthalmology 1991; 98: 1698–702.
42. Kremer I, Rajpal R, Rapuano C, et al. Results of penetrating keratoplasty in aniridia. Am J Ophthalmol 1993; 115: 317–20.
43. Tanzer DJ, Smith RF. Black iris-diaphragm intraocular lens for aniridia and aphakia. J Cataract Refract Surg 1999; 25: 1548–51.
44. Quigley HA, Stanish FS. Unilateral congenital iris pigment epithelial hyperplasia associated with late onset glaucoma. Am J Ophthalmol 1978; 86: 182–4.
45. Wollnik B, Tukel T, Uyguner O, et al. Homozygous and heterozygous inheritance of PAX3 mutations cause different types Waardenburg syndrome. Am J Med Genet 2003; 122A: 42–5.
46. Inoue K, Shilo K, Boerkoel CF, et al. Congenital hypomyelinating neuropathy, central dismyelination and Waardenburg-Hirschsprung disease. Ann Neurol 2002; 52: 836–42.
47. Burger PC, Klintworth GK. Experimental retinal degeneration in the rabbit produced by intraocular iron. Lab Invest 1974; 30: 9–19.
48. Bayes M, Magano LF, Rivera N, et al. Mutational mechanisms of Williams-Beuren syndrome deletions. Am J Human Genet 2003; 73: 131–51.
49. Holmstrom G, Almond G, Temple K, et al. The iris in Williams' syndrome. Arch Dis Child 1990; 65: 987–9.
50. Greenberg F, Lewis RA. The Williams' syndrome: spectrum and significance of ocular features. Ophthalmology 1988; 95: 1608–12.
51. Lewis RA, Merin LM. Iris flocculi and familial aortic dissection. Arch Ophthalmol 1995; 113: 1330–1.
52. Nik NA, Hidayat A, Zimmerman LE, et al. Diffuse iris nevis manifested by unilateral open angle glaucoma. Arch Ophthalmol 1981; 99: 125–7.
53. Carlson DW, Wallace LM, Folberg R. Aggressive nevus of the iris with secondary glaucoma in a child. Am J Ophthalmol 1995; 119: 367–8.
54. Joondeph BC, Goldberg MF. Familial iris melanosis – a misnomer? Br J Ophthalmol 1989; 73: 289–94.
55. Teekhasaenee C, Rich R. Irido corneal endothelium syndrome in Thai patients: clinical variations. Arch Ophthalmol 2000; 118: 187–192.
56. Castillo BV, Kaufman L. Pediatric tumors of the eye and orbit. Pediatr Clin North Am 2003; 50149–72.
57. Jakobiec FA, Silbert G. Are most iris "melanomas" really nevi? Arch Ophthalmol 1981; 99: 2117–32.
58. Apt L. Uveal melanoma in children and adolescents. Int Ophthalmol Clin 1963; 2: 403–10.
59. Shields JA, Eagle R, Shields C, et al. Natural course and

histopathologic findings of lacrimal gland choristoma of the iris and ciliary body. Am J Ophthalmol 1995; 119: 219–24.

60. Ferry AP. Lesions mistaken for malignant melanoma of the iris. Arch Ophthalmol 1965; 74: 9–18.

61. Greer CH. Congenital melanoma of the anterior uvea. Arch Ophthalmol 1966; 76: 77–8.

62. Broadway D, Lang S, Harper J, et al. Congenital malignant melanoma of the eye. Cancer 1991; 67: 2642–52.

63. Rosenbaum PS, Boniuk M, Font R. Diffuse uveal melanoma in a 5-year-old child. Am J Ophthalmol 1988; 106: 601–6.

64. Barr CC, McLean IW, Zimmerman LE. Uveal melanoma in children and adolescents. Arch Ophthalmol 1981; 99: 2133–6.

65. Yanoff M, Zimmerman LE. The relationship of congenital ocular melanocytosis and neurofibromatosis to uveal melanomas. Arch Ophthalmol 1967; 77: 331–6.

66. Walker JP, Weiter JJ, Albert DM, et al. Uveal malignant melanoma in three generations of the same family. Am J Ophthalmol 1979; 88: 723–6.

67. Vajdic CM, Kricker A, Giblin M. Eye color and cutaneous nevi predict risk of ocular melanoma in Australia. Int J Cancer 2001; 92: 906–12.

68. Zimmerman LE, Broughton WL. A clinicopathologic and follow-up study of 56 intraocular medulloepitheliomas. In: Jakobiec FA, ed. Ocular and Adnexal Tumors. Alabama: Aesculapius, 1978: 181–5.

69. Apt LA, Heller MD, Moskovitz M, et al. Dictyoma (embryonal medulloepitheliomas). Recent review and case report. J Pediatr Ophthalmol Strabismus 1973; 10: 30–7.

70. Canning CR, McCartney AC, Hungerford J. Medulloepithelioma (dictyoma). Br J Ophthalmol 1988; 72: 764–8.

71. Witschel H, Font RL. Hemangioma of the choroid. A clinicopathologic study of 71 cases and a review of the literature. Surv Ophthalmol 1975; 20: 415–31.

72. Susac JO, Smith JL, Scelfo R. The "tomato catsup" fundus in Sturge-Weber syndrome. Arch Ophthalmol 1974; 92: 69–70.

73. Kivela T, Tenhunen M, Joensuu T. Stereotactic radiotherapy of symptomatic circumscribed choroidal hemangiomas. Ophthalmology 2003; 110: 1977–82.

74. Naidoff MA, Kenyon KR, Green WR. Iris haemangioma and abnormal retinal vasculature in a case of diffuse congenital haemangiomatosis. Am J Ophthalmol 1971; 72: 633–44.

75. Ruttum MS, Mittelman D, Singh P. Iris hemangiomas in infants with periorbital capillary hemangiomas. J Pediatr Ophthalmol Strabismus 1993; 30: 331–3.

76. Rennie IG, Parsons MA, Palmer CA. Congenital adenoma of the iris and ciliary body: light and electron microscopic observations. Br J Ophthalmol 1992; 76: 563–6.

77. Campochiaro PA, Gonzalez-Fernandez F, Newman SA, Conway BP, Feldman PS. Ciliary body adenoma in a 10-year-old girl who had a rhabdomyosarcoma. Arch Ophthalmol 1992; 110: 681–3.

78. Margo CE, Brooks HL Jr. Adenocarcinoma of the ciliary epithelium in a 12-year-old black child. J Pediatr Ophthalmol Strabismus 1991; 28: 232–5.

79. Cunha SL. Osseous choristoma of the choroid. Arch Ophthalmol 1984; 102: 1052–4.

80. Katz RS, Gass JD. Multiple choroidal osteoma developing in association with recurrent orbital inflammatory pseudotumor. Arch Ophthalmol 1983; 101: 1724.

81. Grand MG, Burgess DR, Singerman LJ, et al. Choroidal osteoma. Treatment of associated subretinal neovascular membranes. Retina 1984; 4: 84.

82. Heegaard S, Jensen PK, Scherfig E, et al. Leiomyoma of the ciliary body. ACTA Ophthalmol Scand 1999; 77: 709–12.

83. Foss AJ, Pecorella I, Alexander RA, et al. Are most intraocular "leiomyomas" really melanocytic lesions? Ophthalmology 1994; 101: 919–24.

84. Brown HH, Brodsky MC, Hembree K, et al. Supraciliary hemangiopericytoma. Ophthalmology 1991; 98: 378–82.

85. Cibis GW, Freeman AI, Pang V, et al. Bilateral choroidal neonatal neuroblastoma. Am J Ophthalmol 1990; 109: 445–9.

86. Shields CL, Shields JA, Milite J, et al. Uveal melanoma in teenagers and children. A report of 40 cases. Ophthalmology 1991; 98: 1662–6.

87. Misra A, Watts P. Neonatal hyphema in precipitous delivery with dynoprostone. J AAPOS 2003; 7: 213–4.

88. Kincaid MC, Green WR. Ocular and orbital involvement in leukemia. Surv Ophthalmol 1983; 27: 211–13.

89. Ridgeway EW, Jaffe N, Walton DS. Leukemic ophthalmopathy in children. Cancer 1976; 38: 1744–9.

90. Makata AM, Toriyama K, Kamidigo NO, et al. The pattern of pediatric solid malignant tumors in western Kenya in East Africa, 1979–1994. Am J Trop Med Hyg 1996; 54: 343–7.

91. Fujikawa LS, Schwartz LK, Rosenbaum EH. Acquired immunodeficiency syndrome associated with Burkitt's lymphoma presenting with ocular findings. Ophthalmology 1983; 90: 50–1.

92. Bloom JN, Graviss RE, Byrne BJ. Orbital pseudotumor in the differential diagnosis of pediatric uveitis. J Pediatr Ophthalmol Strabismus 1992; 29: 59–63.

CHAPTER 44 Uveitis

Clive Edelsten

NOMENCLATURE

Uveitis describes inflammation arising from the iris, ciliary body, or choroid including conditions where the retina and retinal pigment epithelium are primarily involved. The terms *intraocular inflammation* and *uveoretinitis* include both retinal and uveal inflammation, and *ocular inflammation* includes scleritis and keratitis, which may cause adjacent uveoretinitis.

It is sometimes difficult to determine whether vascular signs are due to vasculitis or extravascular inflammation. *Retinal vasculitis* is used to describe all types of inflammation involving the retinal vessels as well as inflammation specifically arising from the vessel wall.

This chapter will describe the conditions causing endogenous childhood ocular inflammation, including uveitis, and the vasculitides.

The differential diagnosis of childhood uveitis includes hereditary anatomical abnormalities and degenerations that may be accompanied by inflammation and tumors specific to childhood (Table 44.1).

ORGANIZATION

Childhood uveitis requires a specific diagnostic approach. Therapeutic decisions with lifelong consequences for visual function and general health may need to be made within the first months of disease. Their management depends on efficient referral patterns from primary care. Improvements in outcome depend on public health measures as well as effective immunosuppressants and surgical techniques. General ophthalmologists need information about the threshold for starting systemic immunosuppression, contemporary indications and methods of surgical treatment, and the patterns of ocular inflammation indicating severe systemic disease.

EVALUATION

Ocular inflammation may herald systemic disease (Table 44.2). Children may not report symptoms and the ophthalmologist may be the only one in the position to uncover them. The follow-up of abnormal investigations needs to be directed by the ophthalmologist's differential diagnosis. Symptoms of systemic disease need to be repeatedly sought in idiopathic ocular inflammation.

Neurological inflammation may accompany ocular inflammation in many diseases. Central nervous system (CNS) inflammation is difficult to diagnose if it presents with behavioral changes, deafness, retrobulbar optic neuritis, headaches, or movement disorders in preverbal toddlers.

Optic disc edema is frequent childhood ocular inflammation, and congenital disc abnormalities may first be noticed when children present with inflammatory disease. The diagnosis of optic disc changes may therefore be challenging (Table 44.3) and may require lumbar puncture and neuroimaging under sedation. Judgment to balance the risks of investigations with the failure to treat CNS inflammation is required.

The immune system develops during childhood when most infections are encountered. The response to infection and the expression of many autoinflammatory diseases can be different to that of adults. Congenital infection and immunodeficiency may first present in childhood and broadens the differential diagnosis of ocular inflammation. Uveitis occurs in immunodeficiency states, and immunodeficiency predisposes to autoinflammatory disease (Table 44.4). It is important to enquire about a family history of both autoimmune disease and recurrent or unusual infection.

EPIDEMIOLOGY

Childhood uveitis is uncommon. In 0–4 year olds it is 3/100 000, in 10–14 year olds 6/100 000, and in adults 17–25/100 000. Childhood uveitis comprises 5% of most uveitis series.

It is frequently idiopathic with no diagnostic features. Specific signs define many uveitis syndromes, but these are exceptionally rare in children. Uveitis is a feature of several localized autoinflammatory diseases but does not occur more frequently in organ-specific autoimmune diseases. Ocular inflammation is also seen accompanying vasculitides, following infection ("reactive uveitis"), with immunodeficiency and systemic autoinflammatory diseases.

Table 44.1 Differential diagnosis of childhood uveitis—including cells, posterior segment edema, and retinochoroidal scars

Trauma or intraocular foreign body
Neoplasia
    Diffuse retinoblastoma
    Juvenile xanthogranuloma
    Relapse of leukemia
    Rosai-Dorfman disease
Photoreceptor dystrophy, especially where RPE changes have not yet developed or where RPE changes resemble choroiditis
Retinochoroidal dysgenesis
Vitreoretinal degeneration
Retinal vascular abnormalities that leak or bleed
Congenital disc abnormalities especially with secondary vascular complications
Infection, especially in the congenitally or iatrogenically immunodeficient

Table 44.2 Inflammatory disease associated with childhood uveitis

Systemic autoinflammatory diseases

Disease	Systemic disease	Ocular disease	Gene	Inheritance
Familial Mediterranean fever	Peritonitis, rash, arthritis	Uveitis	*MEFV*	Recessive
Hyperimmunoglobulin D syndrome	Peritonitis, rash, arthralgia		*MVK*	Recessive
Tumor necrosis factor receptor-associated periodic syndrome	Rash, myalgia	Conjunctivitis	*TNFRSFIA*	Dominant
Chronic infantile neurological cutaneous articular syndrome	Rash, arthritis, hepatosplenomegaly, deafness, chronic meningitis	Disc edema, uveitis	*CIAS1*	Dominant
Muckle-Wells syndrome	Rash, arthralgia, deafness	Conjunctivitis, disc edema	*CIAS1*	Dominant
Blau syndrome	Rash, arthritis	Panuveitis	*CARD15*	Dominant

Localized autoinflammatory diseases

Disease	Systemic disease	Common type of uveitis	Gene associations	Ethnicity
Juvenile idiopathic arthritis	Joint	Chronic anterior	*DRB*0801, 1101, 1301, DPB1*02*	
Behçet disease	Mucosa, skin, vasculitis	Pan	*B51*	Eastern Mediterranean to Orientals
Enthesis-related arthritides	Joint	Acute anterior	*B27*	N. Europeans
Sarcoidosis	Skin, joints, lung	Pan	*DR3*	N. Europeans, Afro-Caribbeans
Ulcerative colitis	Colon, joints	Acute anterior	*DRB1*150 2, 0103*	
Crohn disease	Bowel, joints	Acute anterior	*CARD15*	
Vogt Koyanagi Harada syndrome	Skin, CNS	Pan	*DRB1*04*	Native Americans, Orientals, Asians
Tubulointerstitial nephritis and uveitis syndrome	Kidney	Chronic anterior	*DRB1*0102*	
Multiple sclerosis	CNS	Intermediate	*DR1501*	N. Europeans
Psoriasis	Skin, joints	All	*Cw6, CARD15*	

Idiopathic uveitis and juvenile idiopathic arthritis (JIA)-associated uveitis are the most frequent.[1-3] Idiopathic uveitis is most frequent in general practice. JIA-uveitis is most common in referral series followed by idiopathic uveitis, enthesis (ligament–bone junction)-related arthritis (ERA), sarcoidosis, and Behçet disease. Other diagnoses are rare even in countries with a high prevalence in adulthood (Table 44.5).

Differences between childhood and adult uveitis derive from the unexplained mean age of onset of systemic diseases associated with uveitis, which generally start between 25 and 45 years. In contrast, diseases such as JIA, Kawasaki disease, and hereditary conditions usually present in childhood. This results in major differences not only between adult and childhood disease but also between early and late childhood (Table 44.6).

Table 44.3 Causes of disc swelling

Severe anterior uveitis
  Hypotony
Posterior uveitis
Papillitis
Neuroretinitis
Optic neuritis
CNS disease
  Raised ICP
    Mass lesion
    Communicating or obstructive hydrocephalus
    Secondary to drugs including steroid withdrawal
  Inflamed CSF from meningoencephalitis
  Venous sinus thrombosis

Table 44.4 Immunodeficiency disease associated with uveitis

Chronic granulomatous disease of childhood
X-linked lymphoproliferative disease with EBV and hypogammaglobulinemia
Common variable immunodeficiency
IgG2 deficiency
Hyper IgM disease with hypogammaglobulinemia

Table 44.5 Classification and frequency of endogenous childhood uveitis recorded in recent published series

Type of Systemic disease	Localised autoinflammatory disease	Systemic autoimflammatory disease	Vasculitides	Clinical uveitis syndromes	Para infectious
The frequency of idiopathic uveitis without systemic disease or defined uveitis syndrome is 29%. Only four localised autoinflammatory diseases are found in >1% of cases of childhood uveitis overall. No cases of uveitis associated with immunodeficiency states have been recorded in series of childhood uveitis. [see refs 1 and 2].					
Frequency >/=1%					
JIA 62% Behcet 3% ERA 2% Sarcoid 1%					
Frequency <1%					
VKH MS UC Psoriasis diabetes	CINCA		Kawasaki Cogan SLE	Fuchs APMMPE Lens-induced	Post streptococcal

Table 44.6 Age related changes in the relative frequency of patterns of uveitis

	0–6 years	7–12 years	13–16 years	Adult
Common	Chronic anterior (JIA)	Posterior		Acute anterior (ERA, IBD, psoriasis)
			Posterior (sarcoid)	Posterior (sarcoid, MS, Behçet)
		Chronic anterior (idiopathic)		
		Acute anterior (reactive)	Acute anterior (ERA)	
	Posterior		Chronic anterior	
Very rare	Acute anterior			Chronic anterior

GEOGRAPHICAL AND ETHNIC VARIATIONS

The differential diagnosis of ocular inflammation depends on the patient's genetic and environmental background. Behçet's disease, VKH syndrome, and Kawasaki disease are 10–100 times more common in some Oriental, Asian, and Mediterranean groups than in Caucasians. HLA-B27-related diseases, multiple sclerosis, and sarcoidosis are more common in North Europeans. One must also consider not only the environment of the mother during pregnancy, but the environment and close contacts of the patient in early childhood and their ethnicity.

Uveitis is rarely familial. It usually has multifactorial causes and a polygenic background. Human leukocyte antigen (HLA) genes are associated with many localized autoinflammatory diseases and some uveitis syndromes. The association of HLA-B27 with ankylosing spondylitis and acute anterior uveitis was one of the earliest reported and the association of HLA-A29 with birdshot retinochoroidopathy one of the strongest. However, most HLA associations are weak and not disease-specific: the

many reports of autoinflammatory disease associations reflect this. Similar polymorphisms of genes controlling the inflammatory response are associated with both autoinflammatory disease and response to infection.

IDIOPATHIC UVEITIS

Ocular inflammation produces a variety of signs that evolve over time (Table 44.7), and as there is a paucity of histology, classification depends heavily on descriptive reports.

Classification is best made on the basis of the site of visible inflammation, whether it is unilateral or bilateral, whether its course is acute or chronic, and whether attacks are accompanied by pain and redness. Chronic unilateral uveitis is less frequently associated with systemic disease but should not preclude a search for it.

Table 44.7 Complications of uveitis characteristic of children

Chronic anterior
Band keratopathy
Early irreversible ciliary body damage with hypotony and phthisis
Iris hyperemia and persistent flare
Early cataract formation
Pupillary membranes
Cyclitic membranes
Marked disc edema in the absence of significant vitreitis
Diffuse posterior pole edema
Disc neovascularization
Unexplained hyphema and vitreous hemorrhage
Sudden profound loss of vision with absent ERG
Early severe postsurgical uveitis
Rapid posterior synechiae and IOL membrane formation
Universal posterior capsular opacification
Membrane formation following capsulotomy

Intermediate uveitis
Extensive pars planitis
Minimal macular edema despite persistent vitreitis
Marked disc edema despite mild vitreitis and absent macula edema
Vitreous hemorrhage

ACUTE ANTERIOR UVEITIS (AAU)

Unilateral painful AAU is most frequently associated with HLA-B27-related diseases, which first present in later childhood, and painful AAU is very rare in children under 6. A search for an infective or posterior segment cause is a priority in this age group. Bilateral painful AAU is the most frequent uveitis type following infection or systemic inflammation. Painless AAU is rare and mainly seen in the elderly.

Glaucomatocyclitic crises

This is a hypertensive, relatively painless unilateral AAU.[4] There are usually a handful of small KPs with mydriasis. It is rare in childhood.

Chronic anterior uveitis (CAU)

Unilateral and bilateral CAU are most frequently associated with JIA. It is almost always painless unless the onset is severe. Occasionally JIA develops after CAU: the arthritis is usually mild. Older children with CAU are more likely to have idiopathic disease identical to that seen in JIA.

There is a second pattern of idiopathic CAU that differs from JIA-uveitis with attacks accompanied by pain, insignificant posterior synechiae or band keratopathy, and a more benign outcome. Recurrent, painful CAU is rare in adults and is usually a sclero-uveitis. Idiopathic CAU in children probably has an increased association with antinuclear antibodies (ANA), HLA-B27, and raised antistreptolysin (ASO) titers, but none of these laboratory findings consistently define a discrete pattern of disease. [Figs 44.1 and 44.2]

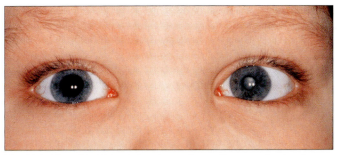

Fig. 44.2 Idiopathic bilateral chronic anterior uveitis presenting in a four-year-old girl with left cataract.

Fuchs heterochromic cyclitis

There is a chronic anterior uveitis with diffuse KPs and lack of posterior synechiae and iris atrophy. Pain, iris heterochromia, bilaterality, vitreitis, and chorioretinal scars are variably reported. It is rare in childhood.

Intermediate uveitis

This refers to vitreitis with a variable amount of retinal inflammation and a minimal amount of anterior segment inflammation. Children present late, and there may be floaters and complications including vitreous hemorrhage and retinal detachment. Children may be less likely to develop macular edema with chronic vitreitis than adults but, once developed, it is more difficult to control. Peripheral vascular abnormalities are difficult to detect and may only be suspected when they cause hemorrhage. Neovascularization of the optic disc and retina may be caused solely by inflammation and subside with immunosuppression.

The average age of onset in childhood is 9–13 and it is rare in very young children.

Changing signs in the inferior fundus are useful to monitor disease progression as the level of vitreitis is difficult to monitor in children and visual acuity may be maintained despite progressive extramacular damage. Sarcoidosis usually produces aggregates of white cells in the inferior vitreous (snowballs) rather than pars planitis (snow bank), and intermediate uveitis associated with multiple sclerosis (MS) rarely produces significant vitreous opacities. Pars planitis may constitute a subgroup of patients in whom systemic disease is less likely and idiopathic intermediate uveitis is thought to be a more frequent diagnosis in childhood. Focal retinal pigment epithelial scars can develop inferiorly at sites of previous retinal inflammation and do not necessarily indicate the development of choroiditis.

Panuveitis

As children present late, severe anterior uveitis may be complicated by retinal edema and vitreous opacification, in the absence of significant vitreous cells. If the fundus cannot be visualized children with anterior uveitis must initially be assumed to have panuveitis: ultrasound may demonstrate optic disc edema, retinal detachment, or tumor. Very young children with panuveitis are rare and have a wide differential diagnosis: they usually present with a red eye, which may be the sign of severe posterior disease, which should be evaluated while anterior segment signs are managed.

Reactive uveitis may have equally severe anterior and posterior inflammation. Most reports of post-streptococcal uveitis are of a

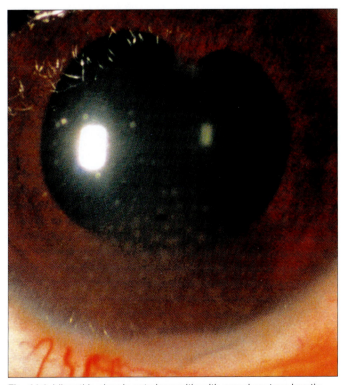

Fig. 44.1 Idiopathic chronic anterior uveitis with granulomatous keratic precipitates and limbal inflammation.

painful acute or chronic panuveitis. Clusters of severe acute panuveitis in children have been reported from Tanzania and Nepal; in the former the incidence was 540/100 000 in the under 9's.[5-8]

Retinal vascular leakage and periphlebitis may be marked in cases of childhood idiopathic uveitis but are not diagnostic of any specific cause.

Panuveitis is a feature of many inflammatory diseases, and unless there is an obvious acute infectious trigger, there should be a rigorous search for autoinflammatory disease and masquerade syndromes.

Occlusive retinal vasculopathy with uveitis

Retinal vascular changes may accompany all types of inflammation. Neovascularization of the optic disc and peripheral retina is frequently seen in intermediate uveitis or CAU and is not usually due to retinal ischemia. Vaso-occlusive retinal inflammation is a feature of severe sarcoidosis and Behçet disease and may result in secondary neovascularization. Occasionally retinal vaso-occlusion occurs with little inflammation: the process may occur in venules, as in Eale disease, or arterioles with aneurysm formation.

Neuroretinitis

Neuroretinitis describes swelling of the neuroretina, maximal at the optic disc, out of proportion to other signs of posterior segment inflammation (Chapter 61). Exudates may collect around the fovea, forming a macular star. Children are more likely to develop edema in response to infections that trigger optic neuritis and neuroretinitis. Cat-scratch fever typically involves the posterior segment in this manner.

Retinitis

Focal infiltrates of the inner retina with little overlying vitreitis are typical of acute viral infections. They are more discrete and persistent and yellower than cotton-wool spots. Retinal infiltrates in Behçet disease are invariably accompanied by signs of retinal vasculitis.

Choroiditis

Choroiditis distinguishes posterior uveitis from intermediate uveitis and may be part of a panuveitis. Unifocal, unilateral choroiditis suggests infection such as toxoplasmosis. Multifocal, bilateral disease suggests systemic disease or a white spot syndrome, which are exceptionally rare in childhood. As with adults, many children with multifocal choroiditis and vitreitis resemble sarcoidosis, with no evidence of extraocular disease. Some infections such as brucellosis, borreliosis, and varicella may also mimic sarcoid choroiditis. [Figs 44.3 and 44.4]

POST-TRAUMATIC UVEITIS

Trauma may provoke an autoimmune response to ocular antigens. Children are as prone as adults to these rare conditions.

Sympathetic ophthalmia

There is a bilateral chronic panuveitis with peripheral multifocal choroiditis with many clinical and histological similarities to

VKH and sarcoidosis. Vitreitis may be severe. By definition it follows unilateral penetrating trauma, cycloablation, or intraocular surgery. It may co-exist with lens-induced uveitis.

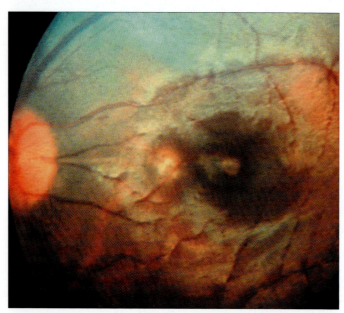

Fig. 44.3 Idiopathic bilateral choroiditis and panuveitis complicated by a choroidal neovascular membrane in the papillomacular bundle.

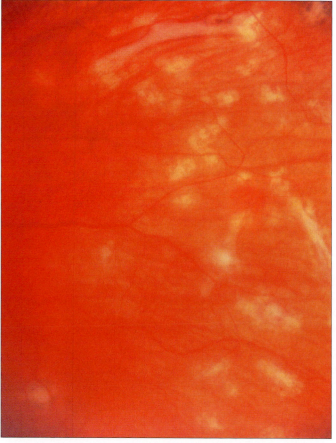

Fig. 44.4 Idiopathic unilateral choroiditis and panuveitis with patchy subretinal fibrosis.

Lens-induced uveitis

This is a granulomatous panuveitis that may occur hours to months after the release of lens material and can complicate severe uveitis from other causes.

INFECTIOUS OR PARAINFECTIOUS UVEITIS

Childhood is a time when common airborne pathogens are frequently first encountered and transient ocular inflammation may result. Varicella and streptococci are most frequently reported as antecedents. The maximum incidence of many infections coincides with the maximum incidence of idiopathic childhood uveitis, and many of the reported associations may be coincidental.

AAU is the most common ocular inflammation following varicella but mild retinal vasculitis, a self-limiting retinitis, and multifocal choroiditis can occur, usually within 4 weeks. [Fig. 44.5] Chronic inflammation and progressive retinitis is an absolute indication for antiviral treatment but it may not be necessary for AAU.

Enteric infections known to trigger reactive arthritis may cause a reactive uveitis: HLA-B27 positivity is a potent risk factor. Classical Reiter syndrome with urethritis is rare in children.

LOCALIZED AUTOINFLAMMATORY DISEASES
Juvenile arthritis

Nomenclature
The term juvenile idiopathic arthritis now replaces juvenile chronic arthritis, used in Europe, and juvenile rheumatoid arthritis, used in America. JIA is a diagnosis of exclusion to describe chronic joint inflammation starting before 16 years.

Ankylosing spondylitis refers to a severe spinal arthritis that causes joint fusion. The initial inflammation is in the ligament attachments and milder cases may only involve peripheral joints: the generic term for these conditions is now enthesis-related arthritides.

The differential diagnosis of childhood arthritis is large and differs significantly between early and late childhood. Early-onset rheumatoid arthritis, vasculitides, and ERA are extremely rare causes of arthritis under the age of 7.

Epidemiology
The incidence of juvenile arthritis is 10/100 000. Only half are patients with oligoarticular or polyarticular JIA, and the incidence of JIA-uveitis is 1/100 000.

Diagnosis of JIA
Oligoarticular ("pauciarticular") JIA is defined by the involvement of less than five joints at the onset of disease. If more joints are later involved the classification becomes extended oligoarticular JIA. Minimal arthritis can occur–one hypertrophied toe joint may be the sole evidence. All children with CAU need a rheumatological examination to screen for such minor abnormalities and exclude other systemic diseases.

Routine laboratory testing in CAU can be limited to white count, serum angiotensin converting enzyme (sACE), antinuclear antibody, immunoglobulins, antistreptolysin titers, electrolytes, and C-reactive protein. There is no antinuclear antibody of diagnostic specificity. Other autoantibodies, such as anticardiolipin and perinuclear antineutrophil cytoplasmic, may occur. High titers of ANA or specific ANA such as double-stranded DNA or extractable nuclear antigens warrant further investigation. Raised sACE, immunoglobulins, and a lymphopenia suggest granulomatous disease. There is no need for repeated physical examination after the initial review but new symptoms need to be repeatedly sought.

Expert advice is required for rashes and fever, which are often transient, and skin biopsy is often the least invasive way to provide a diagnosis of other systemic diseases.

ERA presents with peripheral arthritis and enthesitis in children, rather than sacroiliitis. In younger children it may be indistinguishable from JIA. A family history of ERA is more suggestive of the diagnosis than HLA-B27 positivity.

Psoriasis present in a family member of a child with arthritis changes the rheumatological classification, but the accompanying arthritis may initially be indistinguishable from JIA. Skin changes may develop ten years after the onset of arthritis and uveitis.[9] Psoriasis does not reduce the risk of uveitis and patients should undergo JIA screening protocols.

The risk of uveitis
In those developing uveitis, arthritis typically starts at 28 months and uveitis 13 months later: 86% have oligoarticular onset JIA, 75% are female, and 80% are ANA positive.[10]

The risk factors for uveitis are young age at onset of arthritis, ANA positivity, and oligoarticular rather than polyarticular onset JIA. Uveitis occurs in 20% of oligoarticular JIA and 5% of polyarticular JIA. Those at highest risk are those with ANA positive, oligoarticular JIA that commences before the age of 3 where 65% may eventually develop uveitis. In contrast, uveitis is extremely rare in oligoarticular JIA commencing after the age of 12 and polyarticular JIA commencing after the age of 8.

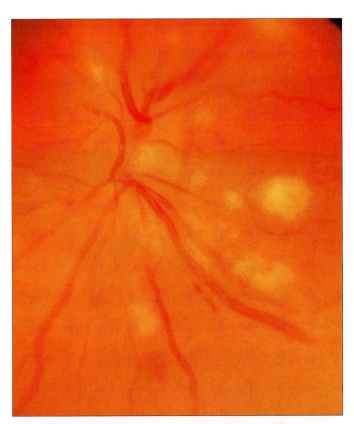

Fig. 44.5 Acute post-viral retinitis with retinal infiltrates and flame hemorrhages. The acuity was 6/6.

The period of risk of developing uveitis depends on the age at onset of the arthritis. Those developing arthritis below the age of 3 remain at risk for 7 years. Those developing arthritis after the age of 6 are at risk for 3 years.

The population at risk should primarily be defined by the age at onset of arthritis and the type of JIA. The presence or absence of ANA does not change the risk sufficiently to determine screening policy.

Clinical signs

The course of uveitis has a wide range of severity and chronicity. Late presentation has a profound effect on the severity of long-term complications. There are wide variations in the aggressiveness of disease. Mild disease is a painless CAU; severe disease may cause a chronic panuveitis and a red eye at presentation from severe CAU or acute glaucoma. A red eye occurring at each relapse warrants reconsideration of the diagnosis.

Minimal disease may produce dusting of the corneal endothelium and a few anterior chamber (AC) cells. A severe cellular reaction with 4+, cells, hypopyon, or fibrin is unusual. Band keratopathy accompanying mild uveitis is characteristic but not universal. Progression of keratopathy on treatment indicates aggressive disease. Keratic precipitates may appear granulomatous. [Figs 44.6, 44.7, 44.8 and 44.9]

Flare, iris hyperemia, and an intraocular pressure (IOP) less than 10 are signs of severe disease and may be reversible if treated aggressively.[11] These signs are not always accompanied by a dramatic increase in AC cells on treatment. Severe iris hyperemia may be mistaken for rubeosis.

Fibrovascular sheets may progress from the iris to cover the pupil and impede a clear view of the posterior segment despite a clear lens. Iris bombé is not uncommon due to the frequency of posterior synechiae. Sometimes posterior synechiae are not obvious without mydriasis.

AC cells rarely "spill over" into the vitreous as with adult AAU but fibrin clumps and dense vitreous haze that takes several weeks of systemic steroids to clear may occur. It can be difficult to determine the cause of media opacities with severe disease at presentation. Some lens opacities at presentation can reverse with treatment.

Posterior segment edema occurs with severe CAU: co-existent hypotony may contribute. Macular edema can be more extensive than that in adults. Disc edema can be profound and persistent and mimic papilledema or sarcoid papillitis.

Outcome

Rates of blindness have reduced from 30–40% in series more than 30 years ago to 7% in recent series. Outcome is profoundly influenced by severity at presentation.[10]

The proportion of those with severe disease at presentation will depend on referral patterns. It is found in 5% of JIA patients screened at Great Ormond Street Hospital.[12] Severe disease at presentation is largely caused by delays in diagnosis but males are at greater risk. Severe onset uveitis is less likely the longer the interval from the onset of arthritis.

Five percent of patients with mild disease at presentation will develop cataracts within 5 years, but 75% will enter long-term

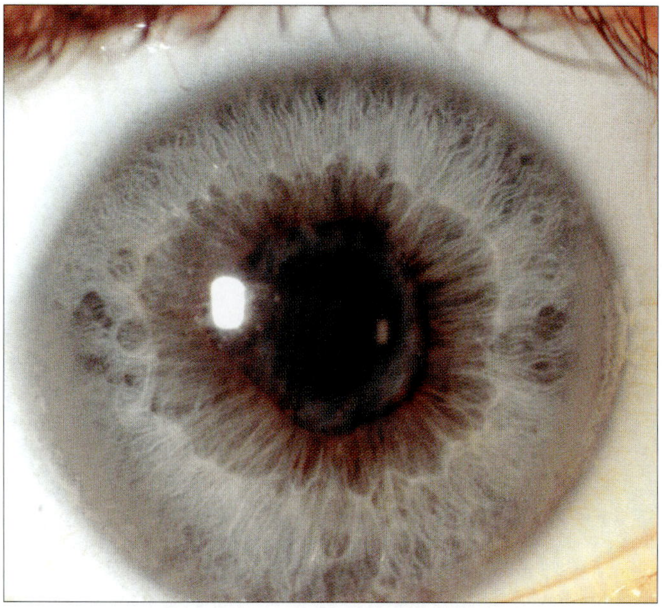

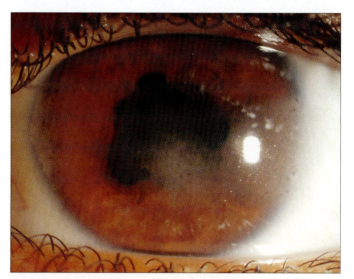

Fig. 44.7 JIA-uveitis. Mild band keratopathy not affecting acuity and posterior synechiae.

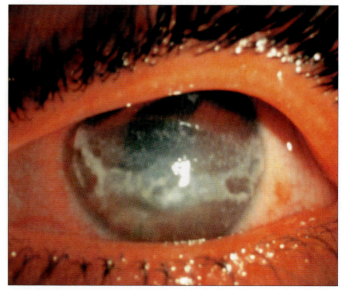

Fig. 44.8 JIA-uveitis. Severe band keratopathy.

Fig. 44.6 JIA-uveitis. Pupillary membrane extending from the iris margin.

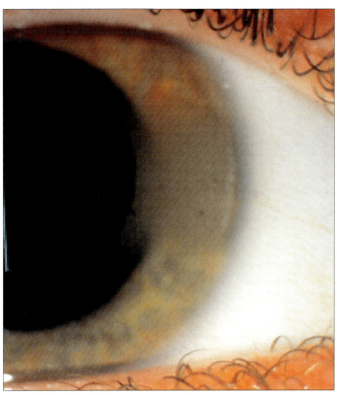

Fig. 44.9 JIA-uveitis. Peripheral band keratopathy after clearance of visual axis with excimer laser.

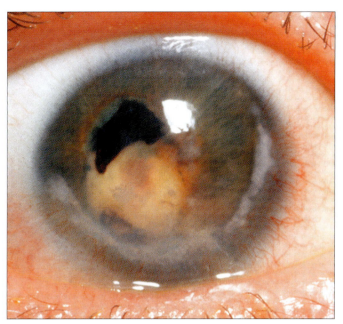

Fig. 44.10 JIA-uveitis. Severe untreated disease with cataract formation and phthisis.

remission within 15 years. In contrast, those with severe disease have an 80% risk of cataract surgery within 5 years and 21% of eyes will go blind: only 10% will enter long-term remission. The rate of cataracts has stayed at 20% in the past 20 years. Cataracts are virtually all caused by inflammation now that chronic oral steroids are rarely given to treat arthritis. Patients may take topical steroids for several years with no cataract formation although their long-term use clearly adds some risk.

Glaucoma occurs in 13% of recent studies and this may have reduced since earlier reports. Steroid-induced ocular hypertension (OHT) and aphakia are the main causes; inflammatory glaucoma may contribute to both or be the sole cause and usually develops after 2 or 3 years of CAU. It is not found at presentation. Steroid-induced OHT is expected in 5% and is usually evident within a few months. Angle-closure glaucoma can occur if the early presentation was complicated by iris bombé but rarely develops in treated eyes. The cause of intraocular pressure changes is usually complex in severely damaged eyes as outflow obstruction may be combined with severe ciliary body damage with aqueous hyposecretion.

The course of disease may be very prolonged despite trivial anterior chamber activity. Patients continue to be at risk of hypotony for at least 15 years, and dramatic loss of vision can occur after years of visually insignificant CAU from phthisis and sudden loss of retinal function accompanied by an absent ERG. Pathological specimens show the iris and ciliary body replaced with plasma cells and lymphocytes and granulation tissue. Treatment of all patients with severe disease should be vigorous to prevent irreversible uveal damage. [Fig. 44.10]

Genetic background

JIA is found in all races; JIA-uveitis may be more common in Caucasians.

Several genes, including *HLA*, are associated with different clinical types of JIA.[13,14] Oligoarticular onset JIA is associated with *HLA* genes common to polyarticular JIA (*DRB1*08*), psoriatic arthropathy (*DRB1*1301*), and systemic onset JIA (*DRB1*11*), as well as unique associations such as *DPB1*02*. Uveitis appears to be associated primarily with the *DRB1*13* haplotype, which is most frequent in oligoarticular JIA, and *DPB1*02*. ERA and early-onset rheumatoid arthritis are clinically and genetically distinct from the types of JIA associated with CAU.

Screening

All children with arthritis should be provided with an urgent initial ophthalmic examination to aid the diagnosis and rule out severe ocular disease.[15] Rheumatologists should be encouraged to dilate new cases and check for posterior synechiae and media opacities in order that severe uveitis is detected as early as possible.

Screening reduces the complication rate, and all doctors need to facilitate early ophthalmic referral and not wait until a definitive rheumatological diagnosis has been made. Ophthalmologists must provide urgent slit-lamp examination when JIA is suspected.

The youngest children most at risk of severe uveitis are most difficult to examine, and experienced personnel should perform the initial examinations until the child is cooperative; it is best not to frighten the child at the early visits as this may delay an adequate examination, even if this means not performing slit-lamp examination at the first visits. Initial screening might need to be repeated weekly, with dilated pupils if it is not possible to determine that minimal uveitis is definitely absent, as disease may progress rapidly in the first year between 3-month checks.

It should be provided for all those at risk of visually disabling uveitis, at a rate preventing the development of severe disease, and continue for the period of risk of developing severe disease. None of these parameters have been determined with precision.

Screening of patients on systemic immunosuppression for arthritis is problematic, as it is impossible to know whether uveitis is absent or masked by the treatment. Patients with uveitis that has entered remission while on systemic treatment should be monitored for the length of the treatment and for 3 years thereafter. Uveitis may recur vigorously when systemic immunosuppression is reduced, and patients should be checked within a few weeks of every dose reduction. Monitoring is especially needed in those with previously controlled uveitis when systemic immunosuppression is abruptly withdrawn because of side-effects.

Where uveitis has entered remission, off all treatment, monitoring needs to be maintained to ensure that recurrence is detected. This should continue for at least 3 years.

When patients are old enough to cooperate with an adequate slit-lamp examination and can reliably report blurring and floaters, monitoring can be devolved to less specialist practitioners. The age at which this is possible depends on each individual child and local facilities.

Patients also require screening for glaucoma. In order to reduce the need for examination under anesthetic, children need to be trained to accept contact tonometry as soon as possible after the diagnosis of uveitis. Most can tolerate this within a few visits. Air-puff tonometry is less well tolerated. Disc appearances must be documented at the initial visit and changes photographed. There should be a low threshold for examination under anesthesia as inflammatory glaucoma can progress rapidly.

OTHER LOCALIZED AUTOINFLAMMATORY DISEASES

Behçet disease

Systemic features

Recurrent, painful, oropharyngeal, and genital ulceration with uveitis are major criteria for the diagnosis. Ulceration may precede the full expression of disease by 2 years. Mild symptoms such as arthralgia, erythema nodosum, gastrointestinal inflammation, and ulceration are nonspecific. Acne and folliculitis, epididymitis, and intestinal ulcers are more specific. Spondylitis may occur in one-third of cases.

Vascular thrombosis and CNS disease are the major causes of morbidity. Venous thrombosis is more common than arterial. CNS inflammation can be primary, with demyelination, or secondary to thrombosis. The pyramidal brain stem is commonly involved but there may be diffuse, acute meningoencephalitis with behavioral changes.

Children may have milder disease and more delay to the complete syndrome: arthritis may be more common and ulceration less common. Neonatal onset has been reported.

Ocular features

There is a panuveitis with explosive relapses, hypopyon formation, and sudden small and large retinal vein occlusion with characteristic white patches of retinitis. Retinal arteries may be involved; macular edema occurs in a minority. Retinal ischemia frequently leads to neovascular complications.

A nongranulomatous CAU may occur but chronic intermediate uveitis is unusual. Conjunctivitis and episcleritis or scleritis may occur. Choroidal involvement is rare. The optic nerve may be involved by inflammatory optic neuropathy, and papilledema from CNS involvement, particularly sinus venous thrombosis, can occur. Secondary optic atrophy is common. The natural course of retinal vasculitis and ischemia leads to a high risk of bilateral blindness and a quarter of eyes may eventually lose vision.

Enthesis-related arthritis (ERA)

Systemic features

The usual onset of arthritis is in the early twenties. The majority have mild arthritis that never results in hospital referral. Disabling ankylosis of the spine is unusual. There is a strong association with HLA-B27. It is associated with psoriasis, inflammatory bowel disease, and Behçet disease. Early-onset disease is rare before the age of 8 although children with oligoarticular JIA that starts before this age sometimes later develop ERA. Spinal involvement is unusual before the mid-teens.

Enthesitis and spondyloarthropathy are also seen following infection, typically *Enterobacter*, and can be accompanied by urethritis or conjunctivitis. Classical Reiter syndrome is very rare in children.

Ocular features

The most frequent type of uveitis is AAU, which typically starts 20 years after the onset of arthritis and eventually develops in 25% of adults with ERA. About 10% of HLA-B27-positive patients will have a uni- or bilateral CAU or chronic panuveitis that is painless. It is possible that patients who first develop JIA that later shows features of ERA can have a chronic anterior uveitis. AAU associated with ERA is very rare in children under 8: its incidence steadily increases through the next 30 years.

Sarcoidosis

Systemic features

There is a chronic granulomatous inflammation that can affect any part of the body. Histology shows a noncaseating epithelioid cell granuloma with an accumulation of CD4+ T-lymphocytes. In adults, sarcoid involves the lung in 90% of cases. In two-thirds of patients the disease remits, usually within 2 years, the majority requiring no treatment.

Sarcoidosis presents very differently in those under 8 as it rarely involves the lung.[16] Skin, joint, and eye involvement are the common sites of presentation and therefore it can be difficult to differentiate from JIA, and an aggressive biopsy policy is warranted. Diagnostic biopsies are most frequently obtained from skin, synovium, and liver. Joints develop synovial hypertrophy with little pain or restriction in early stages. Skin involvement consists of a persistent follicular or nodular rash. Renal involvement is not uncommon. In one series of childhood sarcoid arthritis, 44/53 developed uveitis. Serum ACE may be elevated in only a third of cases and Gallium-67 scanning can aid the diagnosis. CNS involvement is common in those with posterior segment inflammation and may require CSF analysis and neuroimaging to detect meningeal involvement.

Childhood sarcoidosis is more common in Caucasians. Familial disease occurs in 4%, and this must be distinguished from Blau syndrome, which is also familial and lung involvement also does not occur.

Ocular features

Anterior uveitis may start with pain and redness and become chronic and painless. Iris and angle granulomas may distinguish the CAU from JIA-uveitis; band keratopathy is less common and inflammatory ocular hypertension more common than other types of CAU.

Sarcoid rarely causes chronic intermediate uveitis without other features. Panuveitis can develop with multifocal choroiditis that may be very widespread. Visual loss may result from choroidal neovascular membranes arising from macular scars. Optic disc swelling is frequent and may have multiple causes including a granulomatous optic neuropathy or raised intracranial pressure or may be secondary to uveitis. There may be a necrotizing vasculitis. Unilateral posterior segment or optic nerve disease may occur.

As young children may present with uveitis, disease may be very advanced at presentation and blindness frequently results. Uveitis frequently requires more prolonged and intensive immunosuppression than extraocular sarcoid.

Inflammatory bowel disease

Crohn disease and ulcerative colitis are associated with ocular inflammation in a minority of patients. Both may present with a mild arthritis in childhood. [Fig. 44.11]

AAU and episcleritis are the most frequent presentations: 6% of children with Crohn disease were found to have asymptomatic anterior uveitis, but none in those with ulcerative colitis. Rarely, there may be a severe retinal vasculitis, and anterior uveitis may produce an acute hypopyon.

Vogt Koyanagi Harada syndrome (VKH)

Systemic features

There is an acute onset meningoencephalitis with headache, vitiligo, poliosis, tinnitus, and dysacusis. The skin may be painful to touch in the acute phase. In one series, 3% began in childhood and all presented with painful panuveitis with vitiligo developing later.[17]

Ocular features

There is a painful bilateral panuveitis with granulomatous anterior uveitis. Ciliary body edema may shallow the anterior chamber and increase or lower the intraocular pressure. Scleral perforation may occur. Serous retinal detachments are characteristic, especially inferiorly. Disc edema and peripheral choroiditis are frequent and angiography may demonstrate widespread pinpoint sites of leakage at the RPE. After repeated inflammation, depigmentation of the RPE and choroid leads to a "sunset glow fundus."

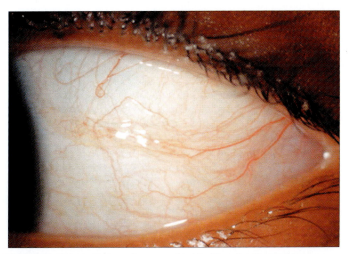

Fig. 44.11 Episcleritis in a nine-year-old girl with polyarticular JIA who subsequently developed ulcerative colitis.

Children are more likely to have severe ocular disease because of late presentation with 61% of eyes losing sight compared to 26% in adults.

Tubulointerstitial nephritis and uveitis syndrome (TINU)

Systemic features

Acute tubulointerstitial nephritis and uveitis occur together. The commonest symptoms are fever, malaise, and weight loss: a third have signs of ocular inflammation.

Twenty percent present with uveitis occurring up to 2 months before renal involvement.[18] The median age of onset is 15 years: the youngest reported is 9 years. Renal disease consists of an eosinophilic and mononuclear infiltrate but granulomas can also been found in the lymph nodes and marrow. Interstitial nephritis occurs in other conditions associated with uveitis such as sarcoidosis, Behçet disease, Sjögren syndrome, and postviral syndromes. Uveitis has also been reported with IgA nephropathy.

Ocular features

There is a CAU with pain at onset; there may be granulomatous features. Posterior involvement occurs in one-fifth with retinal periphlebitis, hemorrhages, and multifocal choroiditis. The mean length is 2 years and visual outcome is usually good.

Multiple sclerosis

Multiple sclerosis is rare in childhood. It can occasionally present with uveitis, usually a mild intermediate uveitis.

Rasmussen syndrome

This is chronic unilateral epilepsy associated with an ipsilateral chronic uveitis that may present in childhood. It has been associated with cytomegalovirus infection.[19]

Psoriasis

Psoriasis is associated with ERA, inflammatory bowel disease, and Behçet disease. It may also be an independent risk factor for uveitis.[9] A family history of psoriasis is often the only risk factor found in idiopathic uveitis. It is associated with JIA and also causes a distinctive arthropathy; 8% of children with psoriatic arthritis develop uveitis.

The pattern of uveitis varies with the other systemic diseases that may be present. Psoriasis itself can be associated with AAU, CAU, and chronic panuveitis.

SYSTEMIC AUTOINFLAMMATORY DISORDERS

These are rare, familial, inflammatory disorders that present with transient fevers, rashes, and joint or muscle pain. Ocular inflammation may be restricted to the episodes of systemic inflammation but occasionally can be chronic. Several genetic associations have now been determined and involve genes dealing with the control of inflammation (see Table 44.2).

Blau syndrome (familial juvenile systemic granulomatosis)

Systemic features

Blau syndrome is a familial, early onset granulomatous disorder with many features resembling childhood sarcoidosis. There is a transient punctate erythematous rash and a nonerosive arthropathy with giant synovial cysts starting in first 3 years. Granulomas are found on synovial or tendon biopsy. The hands may show curving of the little fingers: camptodactyly. Hepatic and renal involvement may occur but not the lung. A vasculopathy may develop involving small and large vessels.

There is earlier onset in successive generations and incomplete forms may occur.

Ocular features

Uveitis develops on average at 8 years, 4 years after arthritis; the youngest recorded is 18 months.[20] A JIA-like CAU with band keratopathy is the most frequent presentation. Multifocal choroiditis is common later. The vasculopathy may affect the optic nerve, retina, and cranial nerves. The outcome is severe: in one series 11/16 had cataracts, 6/16 developed glaucoma, and half required immunosuppression.

CINCA (Chronic infantile neurological cutaneous articular) syndrome

Systemic features

CINCA starts with a neonatal, evanescent, urticarial rash that is histologically a neutrophilic eccrine hidradenitis. Arthritis of large joints develops with diagnostic epiphyseal radiological changes. There may also be developmental delay, chronic meningitis, lymphadenopathy, hepatosplenomegaly, eosinophilia, and hyperglobulinemia.

Ocular features

The chronic meningitis is associated with a cellular CSF and raised intracranial pressure, both of which may cause chronic disc swelling and subsequent optic atrophy.[21] A mild CAU develops around 7 years of age without synechiae formation.

VASCULITIDES

Vasculitis is uncommon in childhood and ocular involvement in most types of vasculitis is rare. However, they are of major clinical importance as life-threatening disease may present with benign ophthalmic signs and sight-threatening disease may require rapid and intensive treatment (Table 44.6). Their treatment may require prolonged immunosuppression, which may result in drug-associated ocular complications and the risk of infection from iatrogenic immunodeficiency.

Epidemiology

The UK incidence of childhood systemic vasculitis is 23/100 000.[22] The incidence of SLE is 0.8/100 000 and juvenile dermatomyositis 0.4/100 000. Childhood polyarteritis nodosa, Wegener granulomatosis, Behçet disease, and microscopic polyangiitis are very rare–each less than 0.1/100 000.

Takayasu disease and Kawasaki disease are more common in Asians and Orientals. In Japan the incidence of Kawasaki disease in under 5's is 110/100 000.

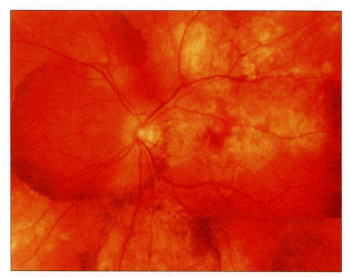

Fig. 44.12 Choroidopathy associated with polyarthritis and Sjögren syndrome.

Ocular involvement in vasculitis

Vasculitis can affect the visual system in several ways. The diseases are defined by the common pathology of inflammation of the vessel wall; signs will vary, depending on the size of the vessel involved, the frequency of vascular occlusion, and the propensity for extravascular inflammation. Severe local ocular involvement may occur in the absence of systemic disturbance, and trivial ocular involvement may accompany severe systemic disease.

There are few diagnostic signs when vasculitis involves the eye as there are pathological processes common to several diseases. Vasculitis is found in 2% of adult uveitis series and is usually a monoepisodic or recurrent AAU. Prolonged uveitis is most uncommon apart from mild vitreitis when retinal vasculitis is active. Choroidal vasculitis may be asymptomatic and unaccompanied by retinal inflammation. [Fig. 44.12]

An acute red eye is unusual in very young children and the risk of it being associated with systemic disease is higher than that in adults. It needs full evaluation although it may appear to be of low priority when life-threatening disease is present. Episcleritis appears more likely to be accompanied by systemic disease in childhood than in adults; in contrast reported cases of childhood posterior scleritis are idiopathic.[23]

Types of ocular involvement

1. Bilateral signs of severe systemic disturbance: conjunctivitis, episcleritis, scleritis, anterior uveitis, retinopathy, and optic disc edema;
2. Localized vasculitis-causing inflammation, which may indicate systemic activity: peripheral ulcerative keratitis, focal scleritis and episcleritis, retinal vasculitis, choroidopathy optic neuropathy, focal orbital inflammation;
3. CNS inflammation, which may be diffuse or focal;
4. Hypertensive retinopathy from renal vasculitis; and
5. Acute and chronic ischemic complications within the eye and CNS.

Classification of vasculitis

The vasculitides are classified by the size of vessels involved and the nomenclature has been developed from adult disease (Table

Table 44.8 The vasculitides

Type	Diagnosis	Childhood arthritis	Systemic features	Main ocular features	Relevant investigations
Primary vasculitides **Large, medium, and small vessels**					
	Takayasu disease		Chronic ischemia of aortic branches	Ocular ischemia	Angiography
Medium and small vessels					
	Kawasaki disease		Fever, rash, coronary aneurysms	Conjunctivitis, AAU	Echocardiogram
	Cogan syndrome		Deafness, aortitis	Keratitis, uveitis, scleritis	
	Polyarteritis nodosa	Yes	Rash, neuropathy, abdominal pain, renal failure	Episcleritis, scleritis, optic neuropathy	Nerve biopsy, angiography, streptococcal and hepatitis titers
Small blood vessels					
	Henoch Schönlein purpura		Purpura, glomerulonephritis		
	Wegener granulomatosis	Yes	Respiratory tract granulomas, glomerulonephritis	Scleritis, orbitopathy	cANCA, biops
	Churg-Strauss syndrome		Asthma, neuropathy	Orbitopathy	pANCA, eosinophilia
	Microscopic polyangiitis		Glomerulonephritis	Retinopathy	pANCA
Vasculitis secondary to connective tissue disease					
	Scleroderma	Yes	Raynaud's, skin tightness, pulmonary fibrosis, esophageal dysfunction, renal failure	Uveitis, choroidopathy	ANA speckled, nucleolar anticentromere
	Dermatomyositis	Yes	Muscle pain and weakness, rash	Retinopathy	Muscle biopsy, creatine kinase
	Polychondritis		Inflamed cartilage of upper respiratory tract and ear	Scleritis, keratitis	
	Systemic lupus erythematosus	Yes	Fever, rash, renal failure, encephalitis	Dry eye, episcleritis, acute retinopathy	dsDNA
	Mixed connective tissue disease	Yes		Optic neuropathy	ENA-U1 small nuclear RNP
	Sjögren syndrome		Dry eyes and mouth, neuropathy	Dry eyes, optic neuropathy	ENA-Ro and La

44.8). Vasculitis may be significant in other autoinflammatory conditions such as sarcoidosis, inflammatory bowel disease, and Behçet disease and can be secondary to infection or drugs.

Types of vasculitides with childhood onset

Kawasaki disease
Systemic features
There is an acute onset of conjunctivitis, a red tongue, and erythema of the trunk, palms, and soles. There may be marked edema of hands and feet. The skin of the soles and hands desquamate on recovery. Later one-third develop cardiac involvement with coronary artery aneurysms. CNS involvement is uncommon.

AAU and conjunctivitis occur in the majority in the acute phase and appear to be benign: disc edema and congested retinal vessels may occur.[24]

Urticarial vasculitis
There is a leukocytoclastic vasculitis that mostly occurs in middle-aged women; half have reduced complement. It has been associated with uveitis, scleritis, and idiopathic intracranial hypertension.

Cogan syndrome
Systemic features
The typical syndrome consists of acute interstitial keratitis, deafness, and systemic vasculitis with onset in the third decade.[25,26] Acute hearing loss and keratitis can occur in many systemic diseases that need to be excluded. Aortitis is more common in typical disease, whereas other vessels are more frequently involved in atypical disease. There may be an autoantigen shared between the cornea, large vessels, and the inner ear. Several cases have been recorded with childhood onset with delays in diagnosis due to the difficulties of distinguishing progressive inflammatory sensorineural hearing loss from congenital causes. In one series three children presented initially with ocular involvement diagnosed as conjunctivitis. CNS involvement from vasculitis occurs in a small minority.

Ocular features
Interstitial keratitis is found in two-thirds of cases. Episcleritis and scleritis are found in 36% and retinal vasculitis in 24%. Uveitis and conjunctivitis may be the sole manifestation in a minority. Keratitis can be severe, leading to corneal perforation and extensive neovascularization.

Polyarteritis nodosa (PAN)
Systemic features
PAN is a necrotizing segmental vasculitis of small and medium arteries with frequent aneurysm formation. Tissue or angiographic diagnosis is usually needed. Thrombosis of involved arteries is frequent. It can be secondary to infections such as hepatitis and streptococci as well as neoplasia. Half of children with PAN present with the systemic form with fever, rashes, and musculoskeletal pain. Seizures from CNS involvement are more frequent than peripheral neuropathy.

Conjunctivitis, episcleritis and necrotizing scleritis, and peripheral ulcerative keratitis are found in up to 20%. AAU and bilateral panuveitis are rare. Choroidal vasculitis is a common histological change but is usually asymptomatic; retinal involvement is usually an arteriolitis but veins may also be involved.

Wegener granulomatosis
Tissue damage from respiratory tract granulomas can be extensive. Subglottic stenosis and nasal deformity are more common in children.

Ocular involvement may occur eventually in the majority of patients and is the presenting site in 10% of cases. Focal, necrotizing scleritis with adjacent keratitis is the most common presentation. Orbital inflammation may be diffuse or from adjacent sinus involvement. A panuveitis or AAU can occur rarely.

Vasculitis accompanying connective tissue disease

Scleroderma
Limited forms start with skin involvement of the extremities but may progress to the diffuse form with proximal limb and organ involvement (systemic sclerosis). The mean age of onset in childhood is 9 years and the majority are female. Localized scleroderma is more common in young females and may involve isolated patches of skin (morphea) or a linear patch on the face (en coup de sabre). Thirteen percent of those with localized scleroderma have eye involvement, and it is not always related to the site of skin disease.

Choroidopathy is relatively common, arising from choroidal capillary closure and perivascular mucopolysaccharide deposition. Uveitis may occur, especially where scleroderma en coup de sabre involves the orbit. The retinal circulation is usually spared but hypertensive changes may occur.[27]

Dermatomyositis and polymyositis
Dermatomyositis is the commonest inflammatory myopathy of childhood presenting with gradual muscle weakness. A characteristic heliotrope rash on the eyelids commonly precedes the myopathy. Extramuscular features are more common in children, including subcutaneous calcification and vasculitis. A retinal microangiopathy may occur.[28,29]

Relapsing polychondritis
Systemic features
There is recurrent inflammation of cartilage in the ear, nose, trachea and larynx, and joints with an adjacent dermal vasculitis. One-quarter of patients have other connective tissue disease particularly rheumatoid arthritis. It is rare in childhood.

Ocular features
Up to 60% have ocular involvement and 25% present with ocular symptoms. Episcleritis and scleritis are the most frequent patterns with keratitis, uveitis, and retinal vasculitis occurring rarely. A CNS vasculitis may occur.

Systemic lupus erythematosus (SLE)
The vasculopathy involves small arteries, arterioles, and capillaries, resulting in fibrinoid necrosis. A hypersensitivity vasculitis occurs in 28% of cases. Thrombosis is more likely in the presence of anticardiolipin antibodies, and these may also occur as an independent phenomenon in the antiphospholipid syndrome, or precede the development of SLE for several years. CNS disease may be caused by diffuse vasculopathy and localized thrombosis exacerbated by the presence of anticardiolipin antibodies.

Five percent of children with SLE have ocular involvement. The most frequent ocular involvement is dry eye: chronic inflammation is unusual. Lupus retinopathy is a sign of severe systemic vasculopathy and may be complicated by simultaneous hypertensive changes. AAU, scleritis, episcleritis, and keratitis are uncommon and may indicate uncontrolled systemic disease.

TREATMENT

Visual loss may cause lifelong restriction in employment and mobility. It may be far more disabling than arthritis. Visually significant uveitis needs as aggressive management as severe arthritis but families need to participate with full knowledge of the efficacy of treatment on reducing visual loss as well as the side-effects of treatment.[30]

The management of most patients with systemic disease will be determined by the risk of life-threatening complications. Where ocular inflammation is the major problem, management of children has certain differences to adults. One can rarely rely on symptoms or acuity as a guide to disease control, and because of the long periods of asymptomatic disease in childhood chronic uveitis, treatment is more often required to prevent future complications rather than react to symptomatic relapse.

The initial treatment of most patients with endogenous uveitis is with topical and systemic steroids and cycloplegic agents. Steroids are especially effective at rapidly controlling inflammation causing tissue edema from vascular leakage and some cases of neovascularization. Their short-term disadvantages must be balanced against their ease of administration and dosage; these include steroid-induced ocular hypertension, behavioral changes, infection (especially varicella), and weight gain. Diabetes and hypertension are rare in children.

Steroid-sparing immunosuppressants are essential for patients who require long-term, high-dose steroids to control disease as they inevitably cause growth retardation and osteoporosis. They have an equally long list of potential side-effects whose frequency may vary enormously between patients, they rarely have proven superiority to high-dose steroids in achieving initial disease control, and they have rarely been compared with each other in formal trials, especially in rare conditions such as those causing childhood ocular inflammation. Methotrexate has been most frequently used because of its use in JIA. It may be inadequate in 25% of patients and half may relapse despite inducing short-term disease remission. Azathioprine has a low rate of side-effects in children compared to ciclosporine and mycophenolate mofetil. Cyclophosphamide is frequently needed in severe vasculitis and may be useful in uveitis unresponsive to less toxic immunosuppressants.

In the absence of formal treatment trials in childhood ocular inflammation, one must use information from comparable adult disease as well as the experience of drug dosage, interactions, and safety profile. As many children with childhood uveitis are under the care of several specialties, each with experience of a different range of drugs, frequent communication is needed to determine a consensus on the optimum treatment.

Analogies from adult disease are not always helpful. There is no adult equivalent of JIA-uveitis and the safety profile, dosage, and tolerability of some drugs such as methotrexate are very different in adults. The analogy of extraocular disease response is also limited. Diseases such as multiple sclerosis and ankylosing spondylitis often have uveitis that responds well to short courses of steroids, whereas the chronic course of extraocular disease is unaffected. Ciclosporin may be far more effective in neuro-ophthalmic sarcoidosis than in pulmonary disease. Some of the new biologic agents appear to have a profound effect on the course of chronic arthritis, yet minimal effect on the uveitis associated with these conditions.

Cataracts

The indications for cataract surgery are:
1. The prevention of amblyopia;
2. To allow the management of posterior segment disease; and
3. To improve visual function with an acceptable risk.

It should not be embarked upon lightly.[31] Children with mild bilateral cataracts and persistent inflammation may easily complete their education with 6/18 vision and surgery deferred until disease activity subsides. A single aphakic amblyopic eye rarely adds to the visual function, but failing to quickly remove a rapidly forming unilateral cataract during the first years of life will not only produce amblyopia, but also prevent adequate monitoring of posterior segment disease. In these circumstances the family must be informed that in some circumstances all one can aim for is an eye of normal appearance.

Disease activity must be rigorously controlled as postoperative inflammation can be unpredictable and severe. When cataract surgery appears likely, patients should be started on systemic immunosuppression in order to see whether disease can be completely controlled without topical medication. Treatment should be increased at the time of surgery and for at least 2 months thereafter. Some patients with preoperative macular edema require 4 or 5 months of systemic steroids as well as second-line immunosuppression before maximum postoperative acuity is achieved.

In order to reduce the load of systemic steroid in the perioperative period then periocular steroids should be routinely given intraoperatively and repeated on two or three further occasions.

Visibility may be compromised by band keratopathy and pre-operative excimer laser, or EDTA scrub may be performed prior to intraocular surgery. Posterior synechiae can be more extensive than is apparent on slit-lamp examination. Pupillary membranes may be vascularized and bleed intraoperatively but may be simply peeled off the anterior capsule without jeopardizing the capsulorrhexis.

Techniques of lens removal depend on the possibility of capsulorrhexis, visibility, and hardness of the lens. Often the lens is aspiratible, even if white. Occasionally there are calcified lumps at sites of synechiae.

Posterior capsule opacification is universal and a posterior capsulorrhexis is advisable especially if the child will need laser treatment under GA. An anterior vitrectomy may reduce the risk of posterior IOL membrane formation but a more extensive vitrectomy may add the risk of other complications.

Intraocular lenses are easy to put in but are very difficult to take out. JIA-uveitis is an inflammation unlike most other uveitis syndromes with a high rate of IOL cocooning and synechiae and membrane formation. Some patients develop unexpected post-operative complications despite adequate preoperative systemic immunosuppression and uncomplicated surgery. It may be prudent to delay IOL implantation until months after lens extraction. The drawbacks of aphakia are trivial compared to the profound visual loss that may result from complications of IOL implantation so families should be fully informed of the added risk to the visual outcome that IOL implantation provides.

Glaucoma

See Chapter 48.

REFERENCES

1. Edelsten C, Reddy MA, Stanford MR, et al. Visual loss associated with pediatric uveitis in English primary and referral centres. Am J Ophthalmol 2003; 135: 676-80.
2. De Boer J, Wulffratt N, Rothova A. Visual loss in uveitis of childhood. Br J Ophthalmol 2003;87:879-84.
3. Paivonsalo-Hietanen T, Tuominen J, Saari KM. Uveitis in children: population-based study in Finland. Acta Ophthalmol Scand 2000; 78: 84-8.
4. Burnestein Y, Shelton K, Higginbotham EJ. Glaucomatocyclitic crisis in a child. Am J Ophthalmol 1998; 126: 136-7.
5. Upadhyaya MP, Rai NC, Ogg JE, et al. Seasonal hyperacute panuveitis of unknown aetiology. Ann Ophthalmol 1984; 16: 38-44.
6. Foster A, Yorston D. Unusual childhood uveitis in Tanzania. Lancet 1989; 1: 226.
7. Ito Y, Nakano M, Kyu N, et al. Frosted branch angiitis in a child. Jpn J Clin Ophthalmol 1976; 30: 797-803.
8. Matsuo T, Matsuo N. Bilateral iridocyclitis with retinal capillaritis in juveniles. Ophthalmology 1997; 104: 939-44.
9. Twilt M, Swart Van Den Berg M, Van Meurs JC, et al. Persisting uveitis antedating psoriasis in two boys. Eur J Pediatr 2003; 162: 607-9.
10. Edelsten C, Lee V, Bentley CR, et al. An evaluation of baseline risk factors predicting severity in juvenile idiopathic arthritis associated uveitis and other chronic anterior uveitis in early childhood. Br J Ophthalmol 2002; 86: 51-6.
11. Davis JL, Dacany LM, Holland GN, et al. Laser flare photometry and complications of chronic uveitis in children. Am J Ophthalmol 2003; 135: 763-71.
12. Chia A, Lee V, Graham EM, et al. Factors related to severe uveitis at diagnosis in children with juvenile idiopathic arthritis in a screening program. Am J Ophthalmol 2003; 135: 757-62.
13. Thompson W, Barrett LH, Donn R, et al. Juvenile idiopathic arthritis classified by the ILAR criteria HLA associations in UK patients. Rheumatology 2002; 41: 1183-9.
14. Thomas E, Barrett JH, Donn RP, et al. British Paediatric Rheumatology Group. Subtyping of juvenile idiopathic arthritis using latent class analysis. Arth Rheum 2000; 43: 1010-5.
15. Kanski JJ. Screening for uveitis in juvenile chronic arthritis. Br J Ophthalmol 1989; 73: 225-8.
16. Fink CW, Cimaz R. Early onset sarcoidosis: not a benign disease. J Rheumatol 1997; 24: 174-7.
17. Rathinam SR, Vijayalakshmi P, Namperumalsamy P, et al. Vogt-Koyanagi-Harada syndrome in children. Ocul Immunol Inflamm 1998; 6: 155-61.
18. Mandeville JTH, Levinson RD, Holland GN. The tubulointerstitial nephritis and uveitis syndrome. Surv Ophthalmol 2001; 46: 195-208.
19. Fukuda T, Oguni H, Yanagaki S, et al. Chronic localized encephalitis (Rasmussen's syndrome) preceded by ipsilateral uveitis: a case report. Epilepsia 1994; 35: 1328-31.

20. Latakny PA, Jabs DA, Smith JR, et al. Multifocal choroiditis in patients with familial juvenile systemic granulomatosis. Am J Ophthalmol 2002; 134: 897–904.

21. Kuo IC, Fan J, Cunningham ET. Ophthalmic manifestations of neonatal onset multisystem inflammatory disease. Am J Ophthalmol. 2000; 130: 856–8.

22. Gardner-Medwin JMM, Dolezalova P, Cummins C, et al. Incidence of Henoch-Schönlein purpura, Kawasaki disease, and rare vasculitides in children of different ethnic origins. Lancet 2002; 360: 1197–202.

23. Read RW, Weiss AH, Sherry DD. Episcleritis in childhood. Ophthalmology 1999; 106: 2377–9.

24. Burns JC, Joffe L, Sargent RA, et al. Anterior uveitis associated with Kawasaki syndrome. Pediatr Infect Dis 1985;4:258-61.

25. Olfat M, Al-Mayouf SM. Cogan's syndrome in childhood. Rheumatol Int 2001; 20: 246–9.

26. Ndiaye IC, Rassi SJ, Wiener-Vacher SR. Cochleovestibular impairment in pediatric Cogan's syndrome. Pediatrics 2002; 109: E38.

27. David J, Wilson J, Woo P. Scleroderma "en coup de sabre." Ann Rheum Dis 1991; 50: 260–2.

28. Lenoble P, Desprez P, Fischbach M, et al. Ocular involvement in dermatomyositis. Apropos of the case of a 15-year old girl. J Fr Ophtalmol 1995; 18: 312–6.

29. Erdol H, Elmas R, Alioglu Z, et al. Retinopathy due to juvenile polymyositis. J Pediatr Ophthalmol Strabismus 2001; 38: 41–3.

30. Holland GN, Stiehm ER. Special considerations in the evaluation and management of uveitis in children. Am J Ophthalmol 2003; 135: 867–78.

31. Lam LA, Lowder CY, Baerveldt G, et al. Surgical management of cataracts in children with juvenile rheumatoid arthritis-associated uveitis. Am J Ophthalmol 2003; 135: 772–8.

CHAPTER
45 Albinism

Isabelle M Russell-Eggitt

More than 100 genes influence the pigmentation of the hair, skin and eyes of mice and it is likely at least as many genes are involved in man.[1] Mutation of these genes may be associated with either generalized or localized hypopigmentation of hair, skin and eyes. The hypopigmentation disorder is then only classified as albinism if there is an underdevelopment of the retina and visual pathways and this is usually associated with nystagmus.

THE MAIN PIGMENTATION GENES

1. The largest set of pigment genes control development and differentiation of the pigment cells. Mutation of these genes, such as MITF, may be associated with deafness, but usually not with ocular defects.
2. The second set encode protein components of the melanosome, the pigment producing organelle within the melanocyte, and mutations in these genes often affect both skin and eyes to produce oculocutaneous albinism.
3. The third set control the biogenesis of lysosome-related organelles including the melanosome and are associated with the Hermansky–Pudlak and Chediak Higashi syndromes and have ocular features of albinism.
4. The fourth set is involved in organelle transport and are associated with disorders such as Griscelli syndrome with normal eyes.
5. Genes such as melanocortin 1 receptor protein, are involved in the switching between eumelanin (brown and black pigment) and pheomelanin (red and yellow pigment).

Hair, skin and iris color are not inherited as simple Mendelian traits. Genes from the different sets interact with each other to give a wide variety of pigmentation both in normal individuals as well as those with albinism. The phenotype varies with ethnic group.

Albinism is a common heterogeneous disorder of melanin metabolism resulting in all genotypes in misrouting of the optic nerve fibers during embryogenesis, underdevelopment of the neuroretina and in varying degrees of hypopigmentation of eyes, skin and hair. Albinism is associated either with an abnormality in the enzymes of the melanosomes, the melanin producing organelles within the melanin producing cells (melanocytes), or in an abnormality of melanosome maturation, numbers or distribution with the melanocytes and keratinocytes. The albinism phenotype results from the mutations in at least 13 different genes inherited either in an autosomal or an X-linked manner.

VISUAL SYSTEM PHENOTYPE

The ocular features are important for distinguishing albinos from other hypopigmented individuals. In humans the classification of "albinism" is only applied to hypomelanotic conditions that have accompanying ocular features of reduced vision, nystagmus, iris translucency, macular hypoplasia and anomalous optic chiasm. Rarely one or two of these features may be absent in an individual yet a diagnosis is made, particularly if there is a supporting pedigree.

Reduced visual acuity

Various factors contribute to poor visual acuity in albinos.[2] The retinal image is degraded by refractive error, light scatter and by nystagmus. Resolving power is limited by foveal hypoplasia. Refractive error and strabismus are causes of amblyopia. Acuity may be close to normal or reduced to 4/60, but this is not a degenerative group of disorders and acuity may even improve over the first two decades. An exception is the retinal dystrophy that may be associated with CHS.

Refractive error

Emmetropia is rare in albinism.[3,4] Albino children with myopia and astigmatism often dislike wearing spectacles, whilst those with hypermetropia benefit from a correction which improves their near vision.

Delayed visual maturation (DVM type 3)

DVM is common with a marked improvement in behavioral acuity occurring at about 4–6 months of age.[5] In some cases immature nystagmus is misinterpreted as roving eye movements. The infant can see but has difficulty in directing their eyes towards an object of interest.

Foveal hypoplasia

Even if the nystagmus of an albino subject could be damped they would have subnormal acuity due to the foveal anatomy.[6] The features characterizing the albino macular region are absence of the foveal pit,[7] reduction in the usual foveal hyperpigmentation (Fig. 45.1), lack of macular xanthophylls (lutein and zeaxanthin) and occasionally retinal vessels cross the central area of the macula.[8] A minority of albinos increase their foveal pigment (Fig. 45.2) with slowly improving acuity into the second decade.[2]

Iris translucency

Normal blue-eyed individuals may have mild transillumination of their irides. In a blue-eyed albino, irides are usually grossly transilluminant (Fig. 45.3), the lens edge often being visible when the iris is retroilluminated[9]: the transilluminance can often be

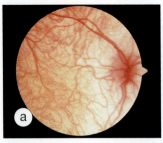
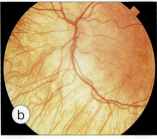

Fig. 45.1 Albinism. (a) Albinism showing marked choroidal and retinal pigmentation and foveal aplasia. (b) Albino fundus showing hypopigmentation.

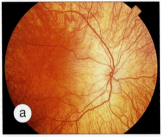
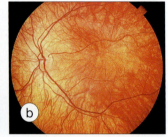

Fig. 45.2 Albinism showing moderate hypopigmentation and macular hypoplasia. (a, b) Some cases with moderate hypopigmentation may show a limited increase in acuity measurements as they grow older.

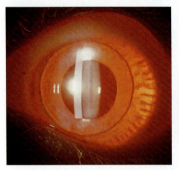
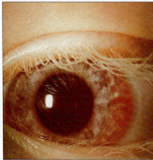

Fig. 45.3 Albinism showing iris transillumination in direct light (on the right) and in retroillumination (on the left). The retroillumination picture shows details of the lens and ciliary processes seen through the transilluminant iris with the pupil dark in the center of the picture. The marked red reflex through the sclera is due to the lack of pigmentation. The lashes are white and the iris pink-blue on direct illumination.

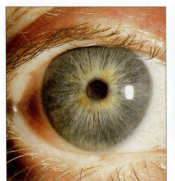
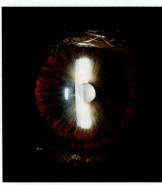

Fig. 45.4 Moderate transillumination on retroillumination in a blue-eyed albino carrier.

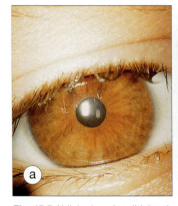
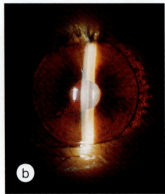

Fig. 45.5 X-linked ocular albinism in a boy of Indian origin who presented with nystagmus and poor vision. (a) Showing a brown iris, but (b) marked transillumination.

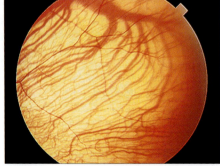

Fig. 45.6 Marked fundus hypopigmentation in an albino revealing the choroidal vessels.

seen with the naked eye. With increasing pigmentation, the transillumination increasingly requires slit-lamp examination (Fig. 45.4) in a darkened room. The irides of brown-eyed albinos (Fig. 45.5) are not always translucent.

Strabismus and stereoacuity

Both esotropia and exotropia occur in albinism, orthophoria being uncommon.

Albinos have anomalous visual pathway anatomy, which in the majority of cases precludes high-grade stereoacuity. However, within each phenotype there is a spectrum.[10] Rarely there is only mild impairment of acuity and high-grade stereoacuity.[11]

Fundus hypopigmentation

The fundus is hypopigmented to a variable degree (Figs 45.1, 45.2 and 45.6). In lightly pigmented Caucasians lack of macular

pigment is a useful clinical sign of albinism. The globe may be translucent in OCA1 and OCA2.

Reduced photoreceptor numbers

Photoreceptor numbers are reduced especially the rods. However albinos are not night-blind.

Electroretinogram

The ERG may be of larger amplitude with shorter implicit time than in normal individuals. The ERG changes seem to correlate with the degree of ocular hypopigmentation with light scatter, iris and eye wall translucency being factors.

Optic disc abnormalities

See Chapter 59.

Anomalous optic chiasm

The higher visual projections are anomalous. There is a paucity of ipsilaterally projecting temporal retinal fibers resulting in almost all optic fibers decussating, whilst in normal individuals only about 50% fibers cross. The optic chiasm is smaller in albinos.[12]

Visual evoked potentials

Visual pathway misrouting can be detected by recording of the visual evoked potential with uniocular stimulation and comparing the response from electrodes either side of the midline and by functional MRI imaging and comparison of projections with hemifield stimulation.[13] This VEP crossed asymmetry (Fig. 45.7) is a feature of all forms of albinism. Similar findings have been reported in cases with incomplete congenital stationary night-blindness, CSNB2.[14] However it may be difficult to distinguish clinically and electrophysiologically between OA1 and CSNB2.

Lateral geniculate body (LGB)

There is reduction in the size and disruption of laminar structures of the LGB nucleus in cats with OCA1 and HPS.[15]

Primary visual cortex

There is a severe disruption of binocular driven neurons in cortical areas 17, 18 and 19. Functional MRI scanning of normal individuals during binocular stimulation results in activation of the two hemispheres from the occipital pole to deep in the calcarine fissure. In albinos the most superficial parts of either occipital pole are not activated.

Nystagmus

Nystagmus usually develops over several weeks after birth and initially with a large amplitude pendular nystagmus. There is no characteristic waveform. The eyes often appear steadier and nystagmus may even disappear later in childhood.[16] Tiredness, stress and bright lighting may all increase the intensity or change the direction of the nystagmus with a decrease in acuity as a result of this. Although foveal hypoplasia is a major limiting factor, nystagmus characteristics add to the reduction in acuity.[6] The larger the proportion of the waveform spent with the eye relatively steady and with central fixation the better the acuity. A few albinos do not have nystagmus. Lack of nystagmus is often associated with better acuity than other albinos in the same pedigree. These individuals may have a slow involuntary micro-drift off fixation.

Head nodding

Head nodding may occur in association with nystagmus in albinism and often resolves after infancy.[17]

Contrast sensitivity

The overall shape of the contrast sensitivity function graph is similar in albinos to controls but the peak in maximum sensitivity shifted towards 1 cycle per degree.

Perceptual difficulties

The dysgraphia and dyspraxia that Dr Spooner (famous for "Spoonerisms") suffered from may have been related to his albinism.[18]

Behavioral problems

Generally individuals with albinism have normal or even above normal levels of intelligence. Early education may be difficult with some young children with albinism having a short attention span. Relationships with other children may be more difficult due to a combination of factors including their different appearance, approaching others very closely, not allowing personal space, and not recognizing friends at a distance. Unlike attention deficit disorder this problem becomes less late in childhood and individuals with albinism are often high achievers at school.

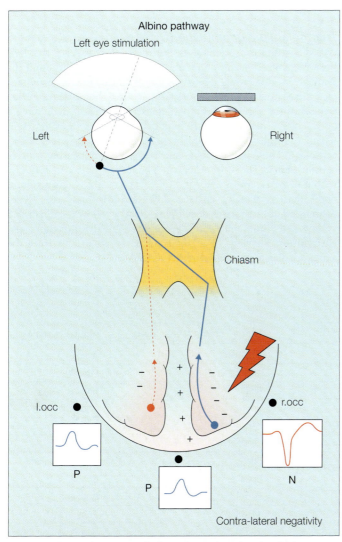

Fig. 45.7 "Crossed asymmetry" of the electrophysiology in albinism results from a larger than normal crossing of fibers in the chiasm. When the left eye is stimulated with a bright flash, the majority of the resulting electrical activity takes place in the right visual cortex with the largest positivity detected over the left occiput. When the right eye is stimulated, the opposite occurs, i.e. it crosses over.

Susceptibility to hearing damage

Unless another gene is involved hearing is normal. However some albino animals may be more sensitive to noise induced hearing loss and to ototoxic drugs such as gentamicin.

MOLECULAR DEFECTS CAUSING ALBINISM
(Table 45.1)

OCA1 tyrosinase related albinism

OCA1 is associated with mutation of both alleles of the TYR gene encoding tyrosinase and accounts for approximately 40% of OCA worldwide. The enzyme tyrosinase within the melanosomes is important in the early steps of the pathway forming melanins from the amino acid tyrosine. At least 100 mutations spanning all parts of the gene have been reported.[19] The majority of affected individuals, not born within a consanguinous family, are compound heterozygotes, with different maternal and paternal alleles. OCA1 includes albinos previously classified as tyrosinase negative and some that are weakly positive on the hairbulb incubation test of tyrosinase activity or on the electron microscopic dihydroxyphenylalanine reaction test.[20] Most albinos born with snow white hair at birth have mutations in the tyrosinase gene although a minority will have OCA2.[21] OCA1 is divided into OCA1A and OCA1B by the activity of the tyrosinase produced.

OCA1A tyrosinase negative albinism

Most mutations of the tyrosinase gene produce a protein with no enzyme activity. If both alleles have null mutations the individual will manifest the clinical type OCA1A oculocutaneous albinism in which there is snow-white hair, no skin pigmentation, gross iris translucency and reduced best-corrected distance acuity of the order 3/60–6/60. Rarely OCA1 individuals may have single pigmented hairs explained by spontaneous mutation resulting in locally active enzyme.

OCA1B tyrosinase related albinism

At least one allele produces partially active enzyme. Various phenotypes have been described within OCA1B.

Yellow mutant type
A single base substitution within the gene is prevalent in the Amish community and results in tyrosinase with 90% reduction in activity.[22] Individuals have white hair at birth, which becomes yellow red during infancy. The iris may develop some brown pigment and their skin may tan in later life.

Minimal pigment type (OCA1MP)
This albinism phenotype has been described in Caucasians with some residual tyrosinase activity. Children are born with white scalp hair and skin, but over the 1st decade they develop some pigmentation and may develop pigmented nevi. They have nystagmus and acuity ranges from 20/50 to 20/200.[23] Vision rarely improves over the first two decades.[23] Irides are blue and translucent in infancy, but often pigment increases. There is foveal hypoplasia, nystagmus and marked hypopigmentation of the fundus.

Thermolabile pigment type (OCA1ts)
OCA1ts mutant tyrosinase is thermolabile. OCA1ts has long been recognized in furry animals such as the Siamese cat and the Himalayan guinea-pig. The first fur of both Himalayan guinea pigs and Siamese kittens is pure white (due to higher intrauterine temperature). The pure-bred Siamese adult has a light cream body color and dark brown "points" (face, ears, feet and tail) which is similar to the Himalayan guinea pig (ears, feet, nose, testicles). The irides are blue and translucent appearing ruby in certain lights. The differences in phenotype between OCA1A with null tyrosinase activity and OCA1ts are subtle in humans, as body hair is usually sparse.[24] These individuals are hypopigmented at birth, later developing slightly yellow head hair and yellow/red limb hair and pigmented nevi on truck and extremities. Shavings of leg hair are darker than hair from the axilla. Ocular features resemble OCA1A.

Table 45.1 Types of albinism and their genes

Type of albinism	Gene	Human chromosome locus	Mouse homolog
OCA1	TYR tyrosinase	11q14–q21	Albino
OCA2	P	15q11.2–q12	Pink eye
OCA3	TRP1 dopachrome tautomerase	9p23	Brown
OCA4	MATP membrane associated transporter protein	5p	Underwhite
WS2-OA	TYR tyrosinase + MITF microphthalmia associated transcription factor	11q14–q21 + 3p14.1–p12.3	
HPS1	HPS1	10q23	Pale ear
HPS2	ADTB3A adaptor complex 3 β3A subunit	5q13	Pearl
HPS3	HPS3	3q24	Cocoa
HPS4	HPS4	22q11.2–q12.2	Light ear
HPS5	HPS5	11p15–p13	Ruby eye 2
HPS6	HPS6	10q24.32	Ruby eye
HPS7	DTNBP1 dysbindin	6p22.3	Sandy
CHS1	LYST lysosomal trafficking regulator	1q42–q44	Beige
OA1	OA1	Xp22.3	
ADFN	del OA1, TBL1	Xp22.3	

Interaction of the tyrosinase gene with other genes

Red-haired albinism OCA1-MC1R

Caucasian albinos with red hair are uncommon. Those with strawberry blonde or red hair have a classic oculocutaneous albinism, but their phenotype has been modified by a mutation in the melanocortin 1 receptor gene which controls the switch between eumelanin and pheomelanin.[25]

MITF-OA1

Waardenburg syndrome is a clinically and genetically heterogeneous disease accounting for >2% of the congenitally deaf population. Waardenburg syndrome is divided clinically into two subtypes: WS1 and WS2. Mutation in the MITF gene is associated with WS2 and accounts for 20% of WS. Hearing loss is variable and depigmentation often patchy. Tietz syndrome is now known to be a severe variant with profound congenital sensorineural deafness, generalized cutaneous hypomelanosis with complete lack of melanin on biopsy and not a distinct disorder.[26] MITF is a transcription factor that is required to induce the expression of melanogenic enzymes including tyrosinase, TRP1, MATP and melanocortin 1 receptor in the melanosome.[27] In some pedigrees there is a digenic interaction between MITF and tyrosinase that results in individuals with only one mutant and one partially active polymorphism tyrosinase allele manifesting as albinos with congenital deafness.[28]

BADS (ermine phenotype), ABCD and Shah–Waardenburg syndromes

Black locks with congenital profound sensorineural deafness and hypopigmentation is inherited as an autosomal recessive. The skin is pale with brown spots and the hair white with small patches of black.[29] The term ermine phenotype is also used to describe the phenotype of white hair with black tufts and sensorineural hearing loss.[30] Cell migration disorder of the gut (Hirschsprung disease)[31] also occurs with these features and then the phenotype is called ABCD. ABCD is thought to be part of the Shah–Waardenburg syndrome and may also be due to mutation of the endothelin B receptor gene.[32] This group of disorders may rarely be associated with a true albinism with translucent irides, nystagmus and reduced vision.[29] The mechanism may be due to digenic interaction as in MITF-OCA1.

Cross syndrome (oculocerebral syndrome with hypopigmentation: OCSH)

It is not certain whether Cross syndrome should be classified as a true albinism or a hypopigmentation syndrome with ocular abnormalities. Cross syndrome is a very rare autosomal recessive syndrome and reported cases may not all have the same condition. Ocular features include: optic atrophy, microphthalmia, spastic ectropion, corneal opacification, iris translucency, cataracts, peripapillary pigmented "scars" and absence of the electroretinogram. Systemic features include[33]: severe global retardation, hypopigmentation of skin and grey silvery blond hair or mixed pattern of hair pigmentation, spasticity, athetoid movements, dental defects, gingival fibromatosis, Dandy–Walker malformation, urinary tract abnormality, inguinal hernia, focal interventricular septal hypertrophy of the heart and vacuolization of myeloid series cells. Microphthalmia mouse has been suggested to have a similar disorder. Mutations in the human homologue of the mouse microphthalmia gene have Waardenburg syndrome type 2.

OCA2 "tyrosinase positive" albinism

OCA2 is the commonest form of oculocutaneous albinism and account for about 50% of OCA worldwide. The prevalence of OCA2 in the United States is approximately 1/36 000.[34] However prevalence is higher in Navajo Americans (>1/2000)[35] and in certain African communities due to founder effects (1/1100 in the Ibo of Nigeria).[36] In southern and central African populations there is a frequent 2.7 Kb deletion that removes one exon of the gene. OCA2 is autosomal recessive and non-allelic with OCA1.[37] There is a mutation of the "P" gene on chromosome 15 that was identified by homology to the mouse pink-eyed dilution or "p" gene.[38] There is no assay to assess the activity of the OCA2 P gene product to subdivide OCA2 into those with homozygous null mutations and those with partially active protein and the function of the gene product is uncertain.

OCA2A

Individuals with OCA2, particularly in Caucasians, may have a similar phenotype to OCA1, but often develop some pigmentation with age. An individual who is of African origin with the classic phenotype of OCA2 has hair that ranges in color from white through yellow to ginger, hypopigmented skin that tans poorly, is prone to the development of freckles, lentigines, pachyderma, keratosis and skin cancers in ultraviolet exposed areas.[39] There is nystagmus and reduced acuity. Iris pigment often increases with age, but iris translucency is almost invariable. Retinal pigment also accumulates but does not reach racially normal levels.[39]

OCA2B

Some Caucasian individuals with OCA2 are pigmented from birth and may be mistyped as having ocular albinism. A "brown albinism" phenotype (BOCA) has been described in individuals of African origin and is caused by mutation of the P gene.[40] The phenotype is not as hypopigmented as classic OCA2 associated with homozygosity for the common deletion of part of the "P" gene in an African. The skin and hair is light brown, but pigment diluted as compared with their parents. The skin tans and freckles in exposed areas, but lentigines are not prevalent.[39] Almost all cases have nystagmus. Iris color varies from blue to brown and translucency is common.

Interaction of P gene with other genes

The Prader–Willi syndrome (PWS) is a congenital disorder characterized by infantile hypotonia, hyperphagia with obesity, hypogonadism, mental retardation, short stature with small hands and feet and is due to a gene defect on the long arm of chromosome 15 in the region of the P gene.[41] There is a deletion of a portion of the paternally derived chromosome, mutation of the imprinting control center, chromosomal translocation or uniparental disomy of the maternal chromosome 15. Many individuals have translucent irides and hypopigmented skin. Angelman syndrome (AS) is characterized by severe developmental delay, severe speech impairment, ataxia, microcephaly, seizures and a happy disposition that includes frequent inappropriate laughing. AS may be associated with VEP evidence of chiasm misrouting without other ocular features of albinism.[42] AS is caused by deletion of a portion of the maternally derived chromosome in the same region as is affected in PWS, uniparental disomy, an imprinting defect, or mutation of the UBE3A gene.

In both AS and PWS hypopigmentation of the hair skin and eyes occurs where the P gene is deleted. Albinism occurs if the other P gene is mutant.[43] Parental hemizygotes with a mutation of the P gene have normal tyrosinase activity and pigmentation, yet hemizygotes with Angelman and Prader–Willi have reduced tyrosinase function and are hypopigmented. There may more than one gene, which plays a role in pigmentation in this region of chromosome 15.[44] Trisomy of a portion of chromosome 15 that includes the P gene has been associated with hyperpigmentation.[45]

OCA3 rufous "albinism"

OCA3 is a rare form of albinism. The phenotype of OCA3 in Caucasians is unknown and may be difficult to recognize if reduction in pigmentation is mild and if the eyes may be normal. A gene on the short arm of chromosome 9 encodes tyrosinase related protein 1 (TRP-1) a melanocyte specific member of the tyrosinase family.[46] The gene is homologous to the mouse "*brown*" gene. When the "*brown*" gene is mutant murine coat color is brown rather than black. The first human in whom a mutation in this gene was identified was a lightly pigmented African-American boy with light brown hair, skin and blue-gray irides and nystagmus.[46] The same deletion as well as other mutations of TRP-1 have been found in South African rufous phenotype (ROCA)[47] and OCA3 is referred to as rufous albinism but includes individuals with a brown phenotype (BOCA). The prevalence of the ROCA phenotype in Southern Africa is about 1/8500.[47] Affected individuals form some skin pigment unlike most red-headed individuals with OCA1 and OCA2. Many individuals said to have rufous albinism clinically do not have nystagmus, iris translucency, strabismus, or foveal hypoplasia. They are just abnormally pigmented for their race. Many rufous albinos probably do not have misrouting of their optic fibers and many of these cases may not have true albinism. The gene products tyrosinase and tyrosinase related protein 1 are shown to interact and mutation in one influences the maturation and stability of the other.[48]

OCA4

OCA4 is caused by mutation in both alleles of the MATP gene.[49]

Vesiculo-organellar disorders associated with albinism

This group of disorders includes the eponymous syndromes of Hermansky–Pudlak and Chediak–Higashi. These conditions are heterogeneous. HPS2 straddles the classic phenotype of each condition. In this group of disorders there is abnormal vesicle trafficking (protein sorting and vesicle docking and fusion) in various organelles; melanosomes, platelets, lysosomes and pneumocytes. Individuals with albinism should be questioned for a history of easy bruising and bleeding after minor procedures such as dental extractions. Standard screening tests for a bleeding disorder may fail to diagnose HPS. Investigation includes a full blood count to screen for neutropenia and electron microscopy of a thin blood film to look for deficiency of platelet dense bodies. The diagnosis is then confirmed on analysis of platelet storage and release.

Hermansky–Pudlak syndrome

Hermansky–Pudlak syndrome (HPS) is not a single disorder, but a group of related disorders that have in common oculocutaneous albinism with a platelet storage disorder, ceroid-lipofuscin lysosomal storage disease and autosomal recessive inheritance with variable expression even within a pedigree. There are defects in the biogenesis or function of multiple cytoplasmic organelles: melanosomes, platelet dense granules, and lysosomes. The HPS gene products are part of distinct protein complexes: the adaptor complex AP-3 and six different BLOCs (biogenesis of lysosome-related organelles complex).[50]

AP-3

Within the melanosome enzymes are transported from the Golgi apparatus. The transport package is a vesicular body with a protein shell. The shell is the mailing address. If the protein coat is mutated then they misdirect through the melanosome or stay in the perinuclear region and fail to reach the melanosomal dendrites. Adaptor complex-3 (AP-3) is involved in endosomal– lysosomal protein trafficking.[51] The gene product of HPS2, ADTB3A, codes for the beta 3A subunit of AP-3. Mocha mouse has a deletion in the delta subunit[52] and has a platelet storage pool deficiency, pigment dilution, and deafness and in some strains seizures.

BLOC-1

Regulates trafficking to lysosome-related organelles and includes the proteins dysbindin, pallidin, muted and cappuccino.[53] Mice with mutations in these proteins have an HPS phenotype. Human HPS7 is caused by mutation of the dysbindin gene.

BLOC-2

HPS5 and HPS6 gene products interact and form BLOC-2.[54]

BLOC-3

The gene products of HPS1 and HPS4 are part of a protein complex that regulates the intracellular localization of lysosomes and late endosomes.[55]

HPS1

In north-western Puerto Rico the incidence of HPS1 is 1/1800 due to a founder mutation. HPS1 mutations are found in about 50% non-Puerto Rican HPS patients.[56] There is a wide variation in pigmentation, ocular abnormalities and the severity of bleeding disorder in HPS1 between Puerto Ricans who have same gene defect and even within sibships of HPS. Nystagmus is rarely absent and acuity varies between 20/80 and 20/250.[16] The HPS1 and HPS4 phenotypes include progressive lung fibrosis and a granulomatous colitis resembling Crohn disease that are the cause of death at 30 to 50 years of age in 60% of cases.[57] Rarely there is cardiomyopathy and renal failure.[58]

HPS2

HPS2 is a rare form of HPS. The first cases reported were two brothers of Dutch origin[59] with white hair at birth that became blonde, easy bruising, recurrent epistaxis, absent platelet dense bodies, mild pulmonary fibrosis, neutropenia, persistent recurrent upper respiratory tract infection and otitis media. Their visual acuity was reduced with nystagmus, marked iris transillumination, iris hypopigmentation, and radial opacities of both lenses. Both had congenital dysplastic acetabulae of the hip and a mild balance defect but this is not thought to be part of HPS2 as subsequent reports lack these features.

HPS3

Amazingly the Island of Puerto Rico not only has a high incidence of HPS1 due to a founder effect, but also of HPS3 due to a second founder effect[60] and mutations have also been identified in non-Puerto Ricans.[61] The pigmentation and bleeding defect is mild. Nystagmus and iris translucency are reported and acuity is impaired but often is 20/100 or better. Granulomatous colitis occurs in HPS3 but there are no reports of associated lung or immune dysfunction.

HPS4

HPS4 phenotype is severe and similar to HPS1 with iris transillumination, variable hair and skin pigmentation, absent platelet dense bodies, and occasional pulmonary fibrosis and granulomatous colitis.[62]

HPS5

HPS5 was first reported in a Turkish boy with mild oculocutaneous albinism and easy bruising.[54]

HPS6

The first reported cases of HPS6 were Belgian siblings with bleeding tendency and rare platelet-dense granules.[54]

HPS7

HPS7 is a disorder of melanosome and lysosome biogenesis.[63]

Chediak–Higashi syndrome

Chediak–Higashi syndrome (CHS) is a rare autosomal recessive vesiculo-organellar disorder associated with albinism and has features in common with HPS especially HPS2. Vesicular transport to and from the lysosome and late endosome is defective. There are abnormal giant melanosomal complexes with defective melanin pigmentation, large inclusion bodies in the myeloblasts and promyelocytes of the bone marrow, giant lysosomes in monocytes and neutrophils with neutropenia. CHS usually presents in early childhood with recurrent skin and mucosal infections. Additional features are hypopigmentation of the skin, eyes and hair, prolonged bleeding times, easy bruising. Photophobia, nystagmus, reduced stereoacuity, strabismus and asymmetry of the VEP are reported, but not invariably present.[64] Rarely there is retinal degeneration associated with progressive loss of vision, constriction in visual field and deterioration of the ERG[65] and loss of rods receptors has also been reported in a cat model of CHS.[66] In some individuals pallor of the fundi may be the only unusual ocular finding.

In aggressive forms patients succumb in the first decade to frequent bacterial infections or to an "accelerated phase" of lymphohistiocytic proliferation into major organs.[67] Bone marrow transplantation improves the immunological status but does not affect the albinism features. Milder phenotypes survive into adulthood. The full spectrum of phenotypes have been shown to be associated with mutation of the lysosomal trafficking regular gene.[68] Null mutations are associated with severe phenotype whilst missense mutations have a better prognosis.[69] If the first decade is survived neurological degeneration occurs; Parkinsonism, dementia, spinocerebellar degeneration and peripheral neuropathy have all been reported. Beige mouse has the homologous defect.

"ADOC": autosomal dominant oculocutaneous albinism

ADOC is not thought to be a distinct form of albinism and most examples are due to pseudodominance.

OA1 X-linked ocular albinism

X-linked ocular albinism (OA1) is caused by mutations in *OA1* gene, which encodes an integral transmembrane glycoprotein localized to melanosomes.[70] There is pigment dilution of skin and hair compared with unaffected relatives and affected individuals may have brown iris and hair coloration. The visual acuity is usually reduced to between 20/30 and 20/400 with most seeing 20/100 or better. There is often a wide variation in acuity even within a pedigree. Carriers of OA1 may have diaphanous irides (Fig. 45.8) and normal acuity. However affected males do not always have iris translucency and may be misdiagnosed as having X-linked idiopathic congenital nystagmus.[71,72] Examination of the fundus of the mother and other close female relatives and ocular electrophysiology may aid diagnosis.[73] A typical mosaical fundus pigmentation, a "mud-splattered" appearance, (Fig. 45.9) is present in more than 90% of obligate heterozygotes and may be diagnostic.[71] Giant spherical macromelanosomes are found within the skin and the eyes of ocular albinos suggesting a disorder of the melanin secretion from the melanosome into keratocytes rather than a defect in melanin synthesis.[74] Macromelanosomes are found on skin biopsy in 85% of obligate carriers,[71] in some individuals with Hermansky–Pudlak and Chediak–Higashi syndromes but not in OCA1 or OCA2. However, macromelanosomes are found in a wide variety of non-albino disorders such as neurofibromatosis, nevus spilus and lentigoses.

Interaction of the OA1 gene with contiguous genes

Most individuals with OA1 have a mutation within the OA1 gene. Some individuals have a contiguous gene syndrome with a deletion that spans OA1 and other genes. OA1 features may be associated with steroid sulfatase deficiency causing ichthyosis of the skin[75] with Kallmann syndrome (hypogonadotropic hypogonadism and anosmia)[76] and with X-linked recessive chondrodysplasia punctata.[77] Albinism-deafness syndrome (ADFN) is another contiguous gene syndrome with involvement of the transducin (beta)-like 1 gene. Late onset sensorineural deafness occurs in these OA1 families.[78]

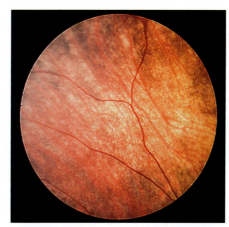

Fig. 45.8 Female carrier of X-linked ocular albinism showing the peripheral retina with mottled areas of hypopigmentation.

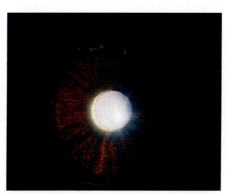

Fig. 45.9 Female carrier of ocular albinism showing the iris in direct illumination. The iris is barely, but definitely transilluminant on retroillumination.

"OA2" CSNB2

The disorder reported by Forsius and Eriksson as prevalent in the Aland Islands is now classified as a form of congenital stationary night-blindness.[79]

"OA3" autosomal recessive ocular albinism

Autosomal recessive ocular albinism (OA3/AROA) is now not thought to be a distinct entity. Many have "P" gene mutations and should be classified as having OCA2.[34]

Website

Mutation and polymorphism data on the genes available on the International Center Albinism Database website (*http://www.cbc.umn.edu/tad*).

Support groups

NOAH (http://www.albinism.org)
UK Albinism fellowship (http://www.albinism.org.uk)

REFERENCES

1. Bennett DC. IL-12 The colors of mice and men: 100 genes and beyond? Pigment Cell Res 2003; 16: 576–7.
2. Summers CG. Vision in albinism. Trans Am Ophthalmol Soc 1996; 94: 1095–155.
3. Sampath V, Bedell HE. Distribution of refractive errors in albinos and persons with idiopathic congenital nystagmus. Optom Vis Sci 2002; 79: 292–9.
4. Wildsoet CF, Oswald PJ, Clark S. Albinism: its implications for refractive development. Invest Ophthalmol Vis Sci 2000; 41: 1–7.
5. Fielder AR, Russell-Eggitt IM, Dodd KL, et al. Delayed visual maturation. Trans Ophthalmol Soc UK 1985; 104: 653–61.
6. Abadi RV, Pascal E. Visual resolution limits in human albinism. Vision Res 1991; 31: 1445–7.
7. Meyer CH, Lapolice DJ, Freedman SF. Foveal hypoplasia in oculocutaneous albinism demonstrated by optical coherence tomography. Am J Ophthalmol 2002; 133: 409–10.
8. Spedick MJ, Beauchamp GR. Retinal vascular and optic nerve abnormalities in albinism. J Pediatr Ophthalmol Strabismus 1986; 23: 58–63.
9. Wirtschafter JD, Denslow GT, Shine IB. Quantification of iris translucency in albinism. Arch Ophthalmol 1973; 90: 274–7.
10. Summers CG, Oetting WS, King RA. Diagnosis of oculocutaneous albinism with molecular analysis. Am J Ophthalmol 1996; 121: 724–6.
11. Lee KA, King RA, Summers CG. Stereopsis in patients with albinism: clinical correlates. J AAPOS 2001; 5: 98–104.
12. Schmitz B, Schaefer T, Krick CM, et al. Configuration of the optic chiasm in humans with albinism as revealed by magnetic resonance imaging. Invest Ophthalmol Vis Sci 2003; 44: 16–21.
13. Morland AB, Hoffmann MB, Neveu M, et al. Abnormal visual projection in a human albino studied with functional magnetic resonance imaging and visual evoked potentials. J Neurol Neurosurg Psychiatr 2002; 72: 523–6.
14. Tremblay F, De Becker I, Cheung C, et al. Visual evoked potentials with crossed asymmetry in incomplete congenital stationary night blindness. Invest Ophthalmol Vis Sci 1996; 37: 1783–92.
15. Creel D, Collier LL, Leventhal AG, et al. Abnormal retinal projections in cats with the Chediak-Higashi syndrome. Invest Ophthalmol Vis Sci 1982; 23: 798–801.
16. Gahl WA, Brantly M, Kaiser-Kupfer MI, et al. Genetic defects and clinical characteristics of patients with a form of oculocutaneous albinism (Hermansky-Pudlak syndrome). N Engl J Med 1998; 338: 1258–64.
17. Abadi RV, Bjerre A. Motor and sensory characteristics of infantile nystagmus. Br J Ophthalmol 2002; 86: 1152–60.
18. Jay B. What was the matter with Dr Spooner? Br Med J (Clin Res Ed) 1987; 295: 942–3.
19. Camand O, Marchant D, Boutboul S, et al. Mutation analysis of the tyrosinase gene in oculocutaneous albinism. Hum Mutat 2001; 17: 352.
20. Takizawa Y, Kato S, Matsunaga J, et al. Electron microscopic DOPA reaction test for oculocutaneous albinism. Arch Dermatol Res 2000; 292: 301–5.
21. King RA, Pietsch J, Fryer JP, et al. Tyrosinase gene mutations in oculocutaneous albinism 1 (OCA1): definition of the phenotype. Hum Genet 2003; 113: 502–13.
22. Giebel LB, Tripathi RK, Strunk KM, et al. Tyrosinase gene mutations associated with type IB ("yellow") oculocutaneous albinism. Am J Hum Genet 1991; 48: 1159–67.
23. Summers CG, King RA. Ophthalmic features of minimal pigment oculocutaneous albinism. Ophthalmology 1994; 101: 906–14.
24. King RA, Townsend D, Oetting W, et al. Temperature-sensitive tyrosinase associated with peripheral pigmentation in oculocutaneous albinism. J Clin Invest 1991; 87: 1046–53.
25. King RA, Willaert RK, Schmidt RM, et al. MC1R mutations modify the classic phenotype of oculocutaneous albinism type 2 (OCA2). Am J Hum Genet 2003; 73: 638–45.
26. Smith SD, Kelley PM, Kenyon JB, et al. Tietz syndrome (hypopigmentation/deafness) caused by mutation of MITF. J Med Genet 2000; 37: 446–8.
27. Gaggioli C, Busca R, Abbe P, et al. Microphthalmia-associated transcription factor (MITF) is required but is not sufficient to induce the expression of melanogenic genes. Pigment Cell Res 2003; 16: 374–82.
28. Morell R, Spritz RA, Ho L, et al. Apparent digenic inheritance of Waardenburg syndrome type 2 (WS2) and autosomal recessive ocular albinism (AROA). Hum Mol Genet 1997; 6: 659–64.
29. Witkop CJ. Depigmentations of the general and oral tissues and their genetic foundations. Ala J Med Sci 1979; 16: 330–43.
30. O'Doherty NJ, Gorlin RJ. The ermine phenotype: pigmentary-hearing loss heterogeneity. Am J Med Genet 1988; 30: 945–52.
31. Gross A, Kunze J, Maier RF, et al. Autosomal-recessive neural crest syndrome with albinism, black lock, cell migration disorder of the neurocytes of the gut, and deafness: ABCD syndrome. Am J Med Genet 1995; 56: 322–6.
32. Verheij JB, Kunze J, Osinga J, et al. ABCD syndrome is caused by a homozygous mutation in the EDNRB gene. Am J Med Genet 2002; 108: 223–5.
33. Cross HE, McKusick VA, Breen W. A new oculocerebral syndrome with hypopigmentation. J Pediatr 1967; 70: 398–406.
34. Lee ST, Nicholls RD, Bundey S, et al. Mutations of the P gene in oculocutaneous albinism, ocular albinism, and Prader-Willi syndrome plus albinism. N Engl J Med 1994; 330: 529–34.
35. Yi Z, Garrison N, Cohen-Barak O, et al. A 122.5-kilobase deletion of the P gene underlies the high prevalence of oculocutaneous albinism type 2 in the Navajo population. Am J Hum Genet 2003; 72: 62–72.
36. Okoro AN. Albinism in Nigeria. A clinical and social study. Br J Dermatol 1975; 92: 485–92.
37. Trevor-Roper PD. Symposium on metabolic diseases of the eye. Albinism. Proc R Soc Med 1963; 56: 21–3.
38. Rinchik EM, Bultman SJ, Horsthemke B, et al. A gene for the mouse pink-eyed dilution locus and for human type II oculocutaneous albinism. Nature 1993; 361: 72–6.
39. King RA, Creel D, Cervenka J, et al. Albinism in Nigeria with delineation of new recessive oculocutaneous type. Clin Genet 1980; 17: 259–70.
40. Manga P, Kromberg J, Turner A, et al. In Southern Africa, brown oculocutaneous albinism (BOCA) maps to the OCA2 locus on chromosome 15q: P-gene mutations identified. Am J Hum Genet 2001; 68: 782–7.
41. Gardner JM, Nakatsu Y, Gondo Y, et al. The mouse pink-eyed dilution gene: association with human Prader-Willi and Angelman syndromes. Science 1992; 257: 1121–4.
42. Thompson DA, Kriss A, Cottrell S, et al. Visual evoked potential evidence of albino-like chiasmal misrouting in a patient with Angelman syndrome with no ocular features of albinism. Dev Med Child Neurol 1999; 41: 633–8.

43. Fridman C, Hosomi N, Varela MC, et al. Angelman syndrome associated with oculocutaneous albinism due to an intragenic deletion of the P gene. Am J Med Genet 2003; 119A: 180–3.

44. Spritz RA, Bailin T, Nicholls RD, et al. Hypopigmentation in the Prader-Willi syndrome correlates with P gene deletion but not with haplotype of the hemizygous P allele. Am J Med Genet 1997; 71: 57–62.

45. Akahoshi K, Fukai K, Kato A, et al. Duplication of 15q11.2-q14, including the P gene, in a woman with generalized skin hyperpigmentation. Am J Med Genet 2001; 104: 299–302.

46. Boissy RE, Zhao H, Oetting WS, et al. Mutation in and lack of expression of tyrosinase-related protein-1 (TRP-1) in melanocytes from an individual with brown oculocutaneous albinism: a new subtype of albinism classified as "OCA3." Am J Hum Genet 1996; 58: 1145–56.

47. Manga P, Kromberg JG, Box NF, et al. Rufous oculocutaneous albinism in southern African Blacks is caused by mutations in the TYRP1 gene. Am J Hum Genet 1997; 61: 1095–101.

48. Toyofuku K, Wada I, Valencia JC, et al. Oculocutaneous albinism types 1 and 3 are ER retention diseases: mutation of tyrosinase or Tyrp1 can affect the processing of both mutant and wild-type proteins. FASEB J 2001; 15: 2149–61.

49. Newton JM, Cohen-Barak O, Hagiwara N, et al. Mutations in the human orthologue of the mouse underwhite gene (uw) underlie a new form of oculocutaneous albinism, OCA4. Am J Hum Genet 2001; 69: 981–8.

50. Huizing M, Helip-Wooley A, Dorward H, et al. IL-25 Hermansky-Pudlak syndrome: a model for abnormal vesicle formation and trafficking. Pigment Cell Res 2003; 16: 584.

51. Zhen L, Jiang S, Feng L, et al. Abnormal expression and subcellular distribution of subunit proteins of the AP-3 adaptor complex lead to platelet storage pool deficiency in the pearl mouse. Blood 1999; 94: 146–55.

52. Kantheti P, Diaz ME, Peden AE, et al. Genetic and phenotypic analysis of the mouse mutant mh2J, an Ap3d allele caused by IAP element insertion. Mamm Genome 2003; 14: 157–67.

53. Ciciotte SL, Gwynn B, Moriyama K, et al. Cappuccino, a mouse model of Hermansky-Pudlak syndrome, encodes a novel protein that is part of the pallidin-muted complex (BLOC-1). Blood 2003; 101: 4402–7.

54. Zhang Q, Zhao B, Li W, et al. Ru2 and Ru encode mouse orthologs of the genes mutated in human Hermansky-Pudlak syndrome types 5 and 6. Nat Genet 2003; 33: 145–53.

55. Martina JA, Moriyama K, Bonifacino JS. BLOC-3, a protein complex containing the Hermansky-Pudlak syndrome gene products HPS1 and HPS4. J Biol Chem 2003; 278: 29376–84.

56. Hermos CR, Huizing M, Kaiser-Kupfer MI, et al. Hermansky-Pudlak syndrome type 1: gene organization, novel mutations, and clinical-molecular review of non-Puerto Rican cases. Hum Mutat 2002; 20: 482.

57. Witkop CJ, Townsend D, Bitterman PB, et al. The role of ceroid in lung and gastrointestinal disease in Hermansky-Pudlak syndrome. Adv Exp Med Biol 1989; 266: 283–96.

58. Witkop CJ, Jr, Wolfe LS, Cal SX, et al. Elevated urinary dolichol excretion in the Hermansky-Pudlak syndrome. Indicator of lysosomal dysfunction. Am J Med 1987; 82: 463–70.

59. Shotelersuk V, Dell'Angelica EC, Hartnell L, et al. A new variant of Hermansky-Pudlak syndrome due to mutations in a gene responsible for vesicle formation. Am J Med 2000; 108: 423–7.

60. Anikster Y, Huizing M, White J, et al. Mutation of a new gene causes a unique form of Hermansky-Pudlak syndrome in a genetic isolate of central Puerto Rico. Nat Genet 2001; 28: 376–80.

61. Huizing M, Anikster Y, Fitzpatrick DL, et al. Hermansky-Pudlak syndrome type 3 in Ashkenazi Jews and other non-Puerto Rican patients with hypopigmentation and platelet storage-pool deficiency. Am J Hum Genet 2001; 69: 1022–32.

62. Anderson PD, Huizing M, Claassen DA, et al. Hermansky-Pudlak syndrome type 4 (HPS-4): clinical and molecular characteristics. Hum Genet 2003; 113: 10–7.

63. Li W, Zhang Q, Oiso N, et al. Hermansky-Pudlak syndrome type 7 (HPS-7) results from mutant dysbindin, a member of the biogenesis of lysosome-related organelles complex 1 (BLOC-1). Nat Genet 2003; 35: 84–9.

64. Creel D, Boxer LA, Fauci AS. Visual and auditory anomalies in Chediak-Higashi syndrome. Electroencephalogr Clin Neurophysiol 1983; 55: 252–7.

65. Sayanagi K, Fujikado T, Onodera T, et al. Chediak-Higashi syndrome with progressive visual loss. Jpn J Ophthalmol 2003; 47: 304–6.

66. Collier LL, King EJ, Prieur DJ. Tapetal degeneration in cats with Chediak-Higashi syndrome. Curr Eye Res 1985; 4: 767–73.

67. Ahluwalia J, Pattari S, Trehan A, et al. Accelerated phase at initial presentation: an uncommon occurrence in Chediak-Higashi syndrome. Pediatr Hematol Oncol 2003; 20: 563–7.

68. Barbosa MD, Nguyen QA, Tchernev VT, et al. Identification of the homologous beige and Chediak-Higashi syndrome genes. Nature 1996; 382: 262–5.

69. Karim MA, Suzuki K, Fukai K, et al. Apparent genotype-phenotype correlation in childhood, adolescent, and adult Chediak-Higashi syndrome. Am J Med Genet 2002; 108: 16–22.

70. Schiaffino MV, d'Addio M, Alloni A, et al. Ocular albinism: evidence for a defect in an intracellular signal transduction system. Nat Genet 1999; 23: 108–12.

71. Charles SJ, Moore AT, Yates JR. Genetic mapping of X linked ocular albinism: linkage analysis in British families. J Med Genet 1992; 29: 552–4.

72. Faugere V, Tuffery-Giraud S, Hamel C, et al. Identification of three novel OA1 gene mutations identified in three families misdiagnosed with congenital nystagmus and carrier status determination by real-time quantitative PCR assay. BMC Genet 2003; 4: 1.

73. Rudolph G, Meindl A, Bechmann M, et al. X-linked ocular albinism (Nettleship-Falls): a novel 29-bp deletion in exon 1. Carrier detection by ophthalmic examination and DNA analysis. Graefes Arch Clin Exp Ophthalmol 2001; 239: 167–72.

74. O'Donnell FE, Jr, Green WR, Fleischman JA, et al. X-linked ocular albinism in Blacks. Ocular albinism cum pigmento. Arch Ophthalmol 1978; 96: 1189–92.

75. Schnur RE, Trask BJ, van den EG, et al. An Xp22 microdeletion associated with ocular albinism and ichthyosis: approximation of breakpoints and estimation of deletion size by using cloned DNA probes and flow cytometry. Am J Hum Genet 1989; 45: 706–20.

76. Punnett HH, Zakai EH. Old syndromes and new cytogenetics. Dev Med Child Neurol 1990; 32: 824–31.

77. Meindl A, Hosenfeld D, Bruckl W, et al. Analysis of a terminal Xp22.3 deletion in a patient with six monogenic disorders: implications for the mapping of X linked ocular albinism. J Med Genet 1993; 30: 838–42.

78. Bassi MT, Ramesar RS, Caciotti B, et al. X-linked late-onset sensorineural deafness caused by a deletion involving OA1 and a novel gene containing WD-40 repeats. Am J Hum Genet 1999; 64: 1604–16.

79. Wutz K, Sauer C, Zrenner E, et al. Thirty distinct CACNA1F mutations in 33 families with incomplete type of XLCSNB and Cacna1f expression profiling in mouse retina. Eur J Hum Genet 2002; 10: 449–56.

CHAPTER
46 The Lens

Ian C Lloyd

ANATOMY

The crystalline lens, in conjunction with the cornea, plays a critical role in the refraction of the eye. Its structure reflects this purpose. It is a transparent, biconvex, avascular mass of uniquely differentiated epithelial cells. It lies immediately posterior to the iris and is held in position behind the pupil by zonular fibers from the ciliary body.

The lens has an equatorial diameter of 6.5 mm at birth and a maximum anteroposterior thickness of 3.5 mm at the poles. It has a single layer of cuboidal epithelium lying beneath its anterior surface and is completely enveloped by a collagenous capsule, the basement membrane of the epithelium. The epithelial nuclei associated with the posterior part of the capsule lie deeper within an area of the lens known as the nuclear bow. This configuration results from cellular migration during embryogenesis. The cuboidal cells at the equatorial region of the lens develop throughout life to form spindle-shaped secondary lens fibers. Lens fiber elongation is accompanied by an increase in cell volume and decrease in intercellular space within the lens.[1] This addition of secondary lens fibers at the equatorial region slowly changes the morphology of the lens from an almost spherical fetal shape to an elliptical biconvex shape in childhood and early adulthood. Newly formed lens fibers have a complicated architectural form. They are arranged into zones where fibers growing from different directions meet and form sutures. The oldest cells are most central whereas the younger are more peripheral. The embryonic and fetal nuclei are present at birth. The fetal nucleus is demarcated from the embryonic nucleus by Y-shaped upright sutures anteriorly and inverted Y-shaped sutures posteriorly. Successive nuclear zones are laid down as development proceeds. Lens fibers developing after birth contribute to the adult nucleus. Thus the lens nucleus is made up of densely compacted lens fibers with the more peripheral lens cortex less densely packed. Individual lens fibers have been shown to be identifiable by specular microscopy of the superficial layers of the lens.[2] Further lens growth mostly affects anteroposterior depth so that by early adulthood the lens has a stable equatorial diameter of approximately 9 mm and an anteroposterior depth of 5 mm.

EMBRYOLOGY

Lens development has been shown to be induced by factors present before the appearance of the optic vesicle,[3] although the lens develops as a thickening of the surface ectoderm overlying the optic vesicle. This thickening or "lens placoid" begins early on day 26–27 of gestational age in the human. In the chick, a tight extracellular matrix-mediated adhesion occurs between the optic vesicle and the surface ectoderm.[4] The mitotically active surface ectoderm is thus fixed in place, resulting in cell crowding, elongation, and thickening of the placoid. Adhesion of the optic vesicle to the lens placoid ensures eventual alignment of the lens and retina in the visual axis. However, there is no direct cellular contact between the basement membranes of the optic vesicle and surface ectoderm.[5] The lens placoid then invaginates to form the lens pit. This in turn becomes the lens vesicle. Lens vesicle detachment is the initial event leading to eventual formation of the anterior segment of the eye (day 33). It is accompanied by migration of epithelial cells via a keratolenticular stalk, cellular necrosis, and basement membrane breakdown.[6] Disruption to this process by teratogens or faulty transcription factors can result in anterior segment dysgenesis. The detached lens vesicle is lined by a single layer of columnar epithelial cells surrounded by a basal lamina, the future lens capsule. Primary lens fiber formation occurs in the epithelial cells lining the posterior surface of the lens vesicle. This is promoted by the adjacent retinal primordium.[7] The lens is thus dependent upon the retinal primordium for cytodifferentiation. The primary fibers fill the lumen of the lens vesicle. Elongation of lens cells adjacent to the retina forms the embryonal lens nucleus. The anterior lens cells nearest the corneal primordium remain as a cuboidal mono-layer and become the lens epithelium. This remains mitotically active for life-providing future lens fiber cells. Epithelial cells differentiate into secondary lens fibers at the lens equator (lens bow). These fibers elongate both anteriorly and posteriorly and insert over the primary lens fibers. They exhibit surface inter-digitations and have little extracellular space between them. They are thickest at the equator. This produces preferential growth of the equatorial diameter of the fetal lens. Secondary lens fibers meet anteriorly and posteriorly at the Y sutures (as described above).

Zonular fibers are derived from the nonpigmented ciliary epithelium during the fifth month of gestation. The glycoprotein fibrillin is the main component of the ciliary zonule. There are two isoforms, fibrillin-1 and fibrillin-2. Fibrillin-1 polymers form, without any significant additional elastin, a structural scaffold of extensible microfibrils. These are arranged in parallel bundles to form the zonular fibers. Disorders affecting the structure or function of these fibrillin-rich microfibrils result in zonular problems, in particular ectopia lentis.[8]

The tunica vasculosa lentis is a vascular network derived from the hyaloid artery posteriorly and a parallel radial palisade of anastomoses with the annular blood vessel laterally. It envelops the developing lens and nourishes it at a time when aqueous production and formation of the anterior chamber have not yet begun. This intraocular network of vessels begins development in the first month of gestation, is maximal in the second to third month, and begins to regress by the fourth month. It has largely disappeared by birth.[9]

Developmental anomalies

Anomalous lens development can produce a wide range of abnormalities. These include complete absence of the lens (primary aphakia) and anomalies of lens size, shape, position, and transparency.

Congenital aphakia results from failure of induction of embryonic surface ectoderm to form a lens placoid and lens vesicle. This can result from a variety of teratogenic events in the first four weeks of embryogenesis and usually results in coexistent microphthalmos, severe anterior segment dysgenesis, and posterior segment colobomata.[10] Rubella in the first trimester of pregnancy is also a known cause of congenital aphakia. Secondary congenital aphakia occurs as a result of spontaneous absorption or expulsion of the developing lens. It is associated with less severe ocular anomalies. Both primary and secondary congenital aphakia arise in association with severe ocular dysgenesis. Visual function in such eyes is usually extremely poor.

The size of the lens vesicle is determined by the area of contact between the optic vesicle and the overlying surface ectoderm. Anomalies causing microphakia (small lens) may occur early in gestation during neural plate formation.

Microspherophakia (Fig. 46.1) is a developmental anomaly referring to a spherically shaped lens of reduced size and diameter. It may also result from abnormal or arrested development of secondary lens fibers. It arises as a sporadic (probably recessive) abnormality or more commonly in association with other ocular anomalies including ectopia lentis, myopia, and retinal detachment. It is seen as part of a systemic disorder, particularly Weill-Marchesani syndrome[11] (see "Weill Marchesani syndrome (WMS)").

Duplication of the lens is a very rare anomaly associated with corneal metaplasia,[12] uveal coloboma, and cornea plana.[13] It is presumed that metaplastic changes in the surface ectoderm prevent normal lens placoid formation and thus lead to multiple lens vesicles.

Lens colobomas (Fig. 46.2) occur in areas where there is a failure of zonular development. Lens indentations or scalloped defects in the lens edge demarcate areas of absent zonules. They may occur unilaterally as an isolated anomaly or bilaterally as part of a uveoretinal coloboma phenotype. Lens colobomas may be seen secondary to zonular damage by the congenital ciliary body tumor medulloepithelioma.[14] A localized opacity is often found in the region of the lens coloboma, and this is particularly true

where it is associated with a ciliary body medulloepithelioma. Most lens colobomas occur inferiorly or inferotemporally.

Lenticonus (Fig. 46.3) and lentiglobus are developmental malformations of the anterior or posterior lens surfaces. Posterior surface abnormalities are more common than anterior surface

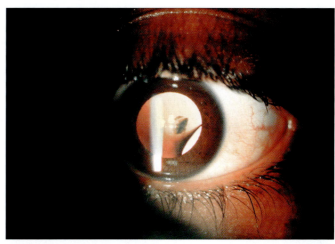

Fig. 46.2 Lens coloboma. Note small cataract adjacent to the coloboma. (Patient of Dr S Day.)

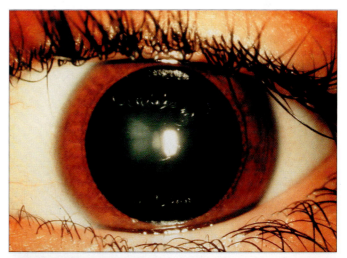

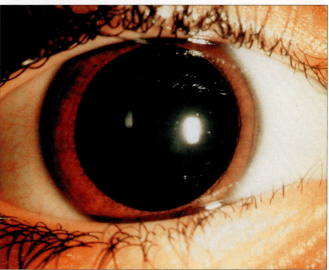

Fig. 46.3 Lenticonus with cataract. The characteristic reflex is only visible on retroillumination as in Fig. 46.4.

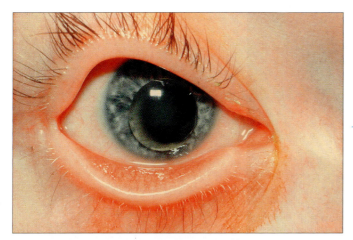

Fig. 46.1 Microspherophakia with anterior dislocation.

anomalies. Both are usually axial. The resulting refractive error through the central lens is often much more myopic and astigmatic than through the peripheral lens. Lentiglobus was thought to be more common than lenticonus and usually unilateral.[15] Lenticonus is more common than previously thought.[16] It may be familial with dominant or X-linked recessive inheritance (Figs. 46.4 and 46.5). It may also be seen with Down syndrome or in the presence of a persistent hyaloid artery remnant (Fig. 46.6). Management of posterior lenticonus is covered in Chapter 47.

Anterior lenticonus occurs secondary to an abnormally thin anterior capsule centrally and is frequently associated with nephropathy and deafness in Alport syndrome.[17] Retinoscopy can be a useful tool for its detection. Alport syndrome is probably not a single condition. Deafness is a strong feature in some affected families but not in others, suggesting heterogeneity. The renal abnormality in affected males is progressive degeneration of the glomerular capillary basement membrane, usually resulting in eventual renal failure. It is typically inherited as an X-linked dominant trait although a separate autosomal dominant "Alport-like" syndrome associated with cataracts is recognized. Carrier females of X-linked Alport syndrome usually demonstrate microscopic hematuria. They may also have anterior lenticonus and macular flecks. Mutations have been shown in the alpha5(IV) collagen gene (COL4A5) at Xq21–q22.[18] Alpha5(IV) collagen is a component of glomerular basement membrane. Autosomal recessive pedigrees have also been described and have had mutations demonstrated in the COL4A3 gene at chromosome 2qter. At least 13% of sporadic or non-X-linked Alport syndrome cases also map to this locus.[19]

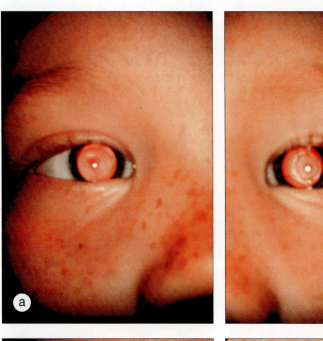
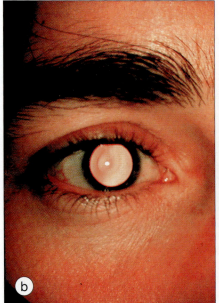
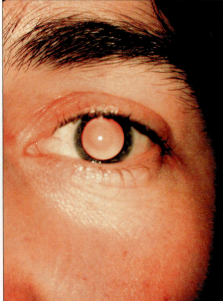

Fig. 46.4 Lenticonus. (a) Although the reflex is a dynamic phenomenon seen on retinoscopy, it can be seen here as a static change in the homogeneity of the red reflex. (b) Mother of patient in (a). Posterior lenticonus is more frequent in boys and may be X-linked.

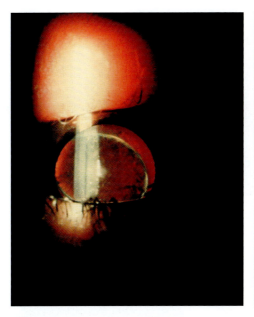

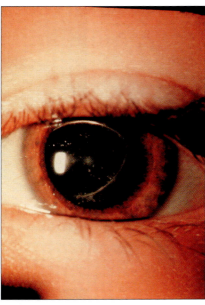

Fig. 46.5 (Left) Lenticonus with posterior extension and cataract formation occurring in a healthy girl. (Right) Operative photograph with retroillumination on the left showing the defect in the posterior capsule (same patient).

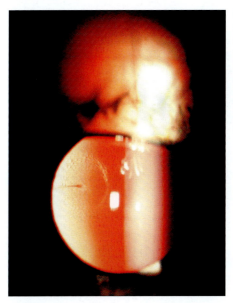

Fig. 46.6 Lenticonic area on the posterior surface of the lens associated with a hyaloid remnant. The presence of the persistent hyaloid remnant suggested that it was important in the pathogenesis.

Persistence of components of the fetal lens vasculature system (tunica vasculosa lentis and hyaloid artery) can lead to a variety of congenital lens abnormalities. These incorporate the spectrum of disorders known as PHPV/PFV (persistent hyperplastic primary vitreous/persistent fetal vasculature). This spectrum includes persistent pupillary membranes, epicapsular stars, iridohyaloid blood vessels, persistence of the posterior fetal fibrovascular sheath (most commonly called anterior PHPV), and Mittendorff dots[9] (see Chapter 47).

Ectopia lentis

Ectopia lentis or lens dislocation is most commonly due to disorders that disrupt the fibrillin-rich microfibrils of the ciliary zonule and thus affect its structure and function. The lens may in consequence become displaced. It may remain within the pupil but if eventual total dislocation occurs, this is as a result of break-age of most or all of the zonular attachments. Ectopia lentis usually results in reduced visual acuity due to induced refractive error.

Marfan syndrome (MFS)

Mutations in the gene for fibrillin-1 (*FBN1*) result in the connective tissue disorder Marfan syndrome (MFS) as well as "simple" ectopia lentis. *FBN1* has been mapped to chromosome 15q 21.1. Microfibril abnormalities have been shown to lie behind the spectrum of diseases produced by *FBN1* mutations, collectively termed fibrillinopathies. They range from the severe condition neonatal Marfan syndrome (usually fatal by age 2) to "simple" ectopia lentis, which is not associated with systemic disease. However, there is little genotype–phenotype correlation of *FBN1* mutations. Over 2230 mainly unique mutations have been published to date and with the exception of a clustering of *FBN1* mutations associated with neonatal Marfan syndrome, no clear pattern emerges. There is also significant intrafamilial variability of individuals with a specific mutation in *FBN1*. MFS has an incidence of approximately 1 in 10,000 births[20] and is an autosomal dominant disorder. The criteria for diagnosis include positive family history and skeletal, cardiac, and ocular abnormalities. Two of the four criteria must be present for diagnosis. Associated skeletal abnormalities include tall stature (Fig. 46.7), arachnodactyly (Fig. 46.8), chest wall deformities, and scoliosis. The typical cardiac abnormalities are dilation of the aortic root, mitral valve prolapse, and aortic aneurysm formation. The most common ocular abnormality is ectopia lentis. This affects approximately 60% of patients with MFS.[21] Lenses in MFS can luxate in any direction but most commonly displace upward (Fig. 46.9). Zonular fibers in ectopia lentis are fewer in number, thin, stretched, and irregular in diameter.[8] They are also inelastic and more easily broken than normal fibers. The insertion and ultrastructure of zonular fibers attached to the lens capsule in MFS is also abnormal. The microfibrils of the fibers are loosely arranged and disorganized. They exhibit fragmentation and interbead periodicity. It is thought that reduced synthesis of fibrillin-1 combined with proteolytic degradation of microfibrils lies behind the variable and occasionally progressive nature of some of the clinical manifestations of MFS.[8]

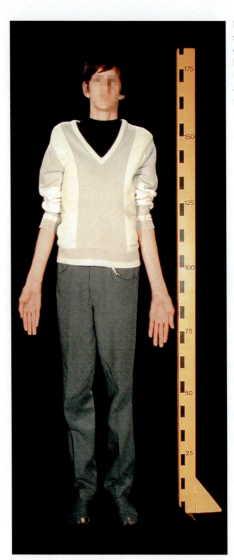

Fig. 46.7 Marfan syndrome. At 15 years of age he is 1.75 m in height. He has very long limbs, arachnodactyly, and pectus excavatum.

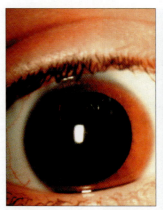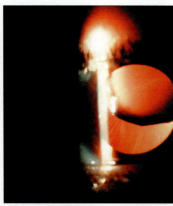

Fig. 46.9 Marfan syndrome. Upward and nasal dislocation of the lens with intact zonules.

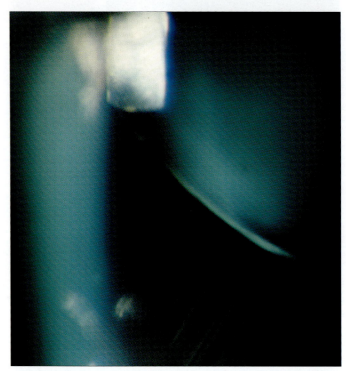

Fig. 46.10 Marfan syndrome. Dislocated lens with intact stretched zonules. The shadow on the left is the slit beam (out of focus) passing through the cornea.

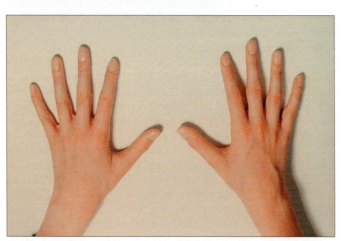

Fig. 46.8 Marfan syndrome. Arachnodactyly.

Early lens luxation can be seen as a flattening or scalloped notching of one lens sector. Zonular fibers typically elongate (Fig. 46.10) and accommodation may be unaffected. Progression of subluxation is relatively unusual.[21]

Familial (simple) ectopia lentis occurs in patients in whom the clinical criteria for MFS are not fulfilled although some affected individuals may also exhibit arachnodactyly and tall stature. Both MFS and familial ectopia lentis are associated with other ocular abnormalities. These include axial myopia, corneal flattening, cataract, hypoplasia of the ciliary muscle and iris, open angle glaucoma, elongation of the ciliary processes, and strabismus.

Homocystinuria

Homocystinuria is a disorder of methionine catabolism. Most homocystine, an intermediate compound of methionine degradation, is normally remethylated to methionine. This reaction is catalyzed by the enzyme methionine synthase. Homocysteine (and its dimer homocystine) is thus not ordinarily detectable in plasma or urine. There are three major forms of homocystinemia and homocystinuria recognized. Classic homocystinuria (type 1) is due to a deficiency of cystathionine-beta-synthetase. It is the most prevalent inborn error of methionine metabolism and is an autosomal recessive condition. It is estimated to occur in 1 in 300,000 to 1 in 500,000 live births. It is more common in Ireland where there is an incidence of 1 in 52,000. The gene for cystathionine-beta-synthetase (*CBS*) lies on chromosome 21 q 22.3. The majority of mutations in *CBS* are missense mutations. Affected individuals are normal at birth but during early childhood may show neurodevelopmental delay and failure to thrive. Ectopia lentis is a later sign along with osteoporosis, fits, psychiatric problems, and thromboembolic phenomena. However, diagnostic delay is common[22] with one study indicating a delay of on average 11 years after the first onset of major signs of the disease. Untreated 90% of individuals develop progressive ectopia lentis.[23] Slit-lamp examination of affected individuals with ectopia lentis reveals broken and matted zonular fibers (Fig. 46.11). The lens typically subluxates inferiorly or anteriorly and may cause pupil block glaucoma (Fig. 46.12). Patients with homocystinuria are usually tall with elongated limbs and arachnodactyly. They have fair complexions, blue irides, and a malar flush (Fig. 46.13). Kyphoscoliosis, pectus excavatum, high arched palate, and generalized osteoporosis are also common. Other ophthalmic features include progressive myopia (often seen prior to the onset of ectopia lentis), iridodonesis, cataract, iris atrophy, retinal detachment, central retinal arteriole occlusion, optic atrophy, anterior staphylomas, and corneal opacities.[24] Screening for this disorder is carried out by the urinary cyanide-nitroprusside test, but testing of urinary levels of homocystine after a methionine "load" provides more definitive diagnosis.

Early diagnosis and medical treatment significantly improves outcome. Forty to 50% of individuals respond to high doses of Vitamin B6, whereas dietary treatment (methionine restriction and cysteine supplementation) aimed at good biochemical control of plasma homocystine prevents lens luxation and mental retardation.[25] Anesthesia can be complicated by thromboembolic events, and precautions should include optimal biochemical control together with preoperative aspirin, intravenous hydration, and compressive stockings. Lens dislocation into the anterior chamber is the most common indication for surgery followed by pupil block glaucoma.[24]

Weill Marchesani syndrome (WMS)

Weill Marchesani syndrome (WMS) is a rare systemic connective tissue disorder. Affected individuals exhibit microspherophakia, ectopia lentis, lenticular myopia, and glaucoma in association with short stature, brachydactyly, and joint stiffness. The lens commonly dislocates into the anterior chamber, causing pupil

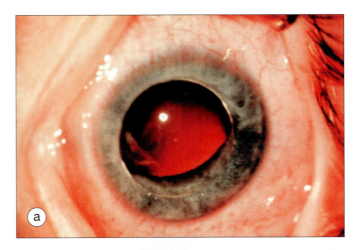

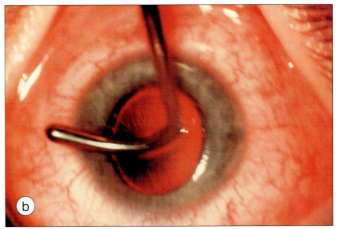

Fig. 46.12 Homocystinuria. (a) Anterior/inferior dislocation of the lens, which is jammed in the pupil. (b) Homocystinuria with anterior dislocation and glaucoma. The lens is being repositioned under local anesthetic with a strabismus hook.

block glaucoma. Presenile vitreous liquefaction is also reported.[26] It is usually an autosomal recessive disorder that has been mapped to chromosome 19p13.2–p13.3. Linkage analysis of an autosomal dominant pedigree of Weill-Marchesani individuals suggests a gene for this form of the condition maps to 15q 21.1, an area that also maps for fibrillin-1 and microfibril-associated protein 1,[11] suggesting that AD WMS and Marfan syndrome are allelic conditions at the fibrillin-1 locus.

Aniridia and congenital glaucoma

Aniridia is rarely complicated by ectopia lentis. This may be secondary to associated advanced infantile glaucoma and buphthalmos. Surgical removal of the cataracts often found in such individuals may compromise the subsequent success of glaucoma procedures. Sturge-Weber syndrome may also cause secondary ectopia lentis by the same mechanism.

Megalocornea

Ectopia lentis in association with megalocornea (in the absence of raised intraocular pressure) has been described. Cataract may coexist.[27]

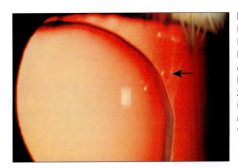

Fig. 46.11 Homocystinuria. Inferiorly dislocated lens with broken, short, and curly zonules. In homocystinuria, the zonules tend to break in their central portion and curl up adjacent to the lens (arrow).

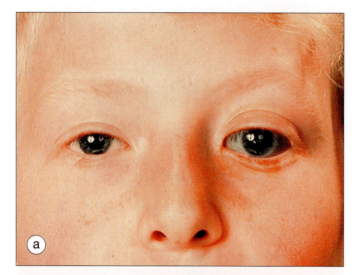

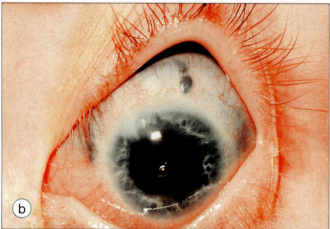

Fig. 46.13 Homocystinuria. (a) Fair-haired boy with chronic glaucoma following unreported anterior dislocation of the lens. (b) Despite his age the left eye had become buphthalmic.

Ehlers Danlos syndrome

Ectopia lentis may rarely occur in association with high myopia in Ehlers Danlos syndrome.

Ectopia lentis et pupillae (ELeP)

Ectopia lentis et pupillae (ELeP) is a rare condition that usually exhibits an autosomal recessive inheritance pattern, although a dominant pedigree has been described.[28] Lenticular and pupillary ectopia occur in opposite directions, resulting in an oval- or slit-shaped pupil. Poor pupillary dilatation, axial myopia, glaucoma, megalocornea, and iris transillumination defects are also described. A case of ELeP has recently been described in association with patchy skin and hair depigmentation. Ultrasound biomicroscopy studies indicate that the pathogenesis of this condition is mechanical tethering of the pupil by a membranous structure with coexistent zonular disruption.[29]

Trauma

Trauma to the eye may result in zonular damage and ectopia lentis.[30] Rarely this may occur as a result of nonaccidental injury.

Sulfite oxidase deficiency

This is a rare autosomal recessive condition that is difficult to diagnose on clinical presentation alone. The diagnosis is suggested in neonates by the association of seizures and severe neuro-developmental delay with ectopia lentis. Affected children usually die in early childhood.[31]

Molybdenum cofactor deficiency

This is a very rare metabolic disorder characterized by early ectopia lentis, epilepsy, and urinary excretion of sulfite, xanthine, hypoxanthine, and S-Sulfocysteine.[32]

Xanthine oxidase deficiency

This is a very rare cause of ectopia lentis. It is associated with low serum uric acid levels.

MANAGEMENT OF ECTOPIA LENTIS

The ophthalmologist's primary aims for eyes affected by ectopia lentis are restoration of visual function, avoidance/treatment of amblyopia (in those children within the sensitive period of visual development), and the appropriate management of any complications such as glaucoma. In many children, all that is necessary to correct acquired myopia/astigmatism are optical measures alone. Spectacles can provide very satisfactory optical correction particularly where there is a relatively symmetrical refractive error. However, where there is asymmetrical (or unilateral) ectopia lentis, the use of a contact lens may be necessary to avoid aniseikonia. If the crystalline lens is extensively subluxed, correction of the refractive error of the aphakic zone of the pupil should be tried. Coexistent pharmacological pupillary dilatation can aid acceptance of this.

Bilateral ametropic amblyopia has been reported as occurring in up to 50% of individuals with ectopia lentis despite good conservative management.[33] This was found to be particularly evident where the lens edge was adjacent to the center of the pupil but where the visual axis was still primarily phakic. Axial high myopia is common in such cases and is thought to be secondary to amblyopia.[33] This study associated retinal detachment with high myopia rather than lens surgery. It is postulated that early lens surgery may avoid induced myopia and a subsequent higher risk of retinal detachment. Thus, surgical removal of the lens is indicated in individuals with poor visual acuity due to the pupil being bisected by the lens edge. It is also indicated in those individuals with anterior dislocation of the lens or persistent uveitis due to friction of the displaced lens on the iris. Posteriorly dislocated lenses may be managed conservatively but should be monitored. Signs of glaucoma, uveitis, or retinal degenerative changes are indications for vitreo-lensectomy. The lens is most likely to dislocate anteriorly in homocystinuria. Lens repositioning can often be carried out after pupillary dilatation by using direct mechanical pressure on the cornea with a squint hook. The pupil is then miosed (Fig. 46.12b).

Modern microsurgical techniques yield very good results following either limbal or pars plana approach lensectomy for ectopia lentis.[34,35] If the limbal technique is adopted, the vitreous cutter should be introduced into the area of greatest subluxation (Fig. 46.14). Aspiration of the lens material from within the capsular bag prior to completing the capsulectomy ensures lens material is not displaced into the vitreous cavity. Retinal detachment, a frequent problem prior to lensectomy procedures using vitreous cutting instruments, is now a rare complication.[36] Contact lens or spectacle correction of subsequent aphakia is effective and relatively straightforward. In one large study the best-corrected visual acuity of approximately 90% of eyes with ectopia lentis was improved by 2 Snellen lines or more following lensectomy.[36]

YAG laser zonulysis has been described as an alternative technique for moving a lens edge out of the pupillary axis[37] and allowing subsequent aphakic correction. Damage to the lens may occur during this procedure, necessitating subsequent lensectomy.

Intraocular lens implantation (sclerally fixated and "in the bag"

fixation) has been described in a small series of children aged 8 to 11 with Marfan syndrome. Short-term follow-up suggests initially good functional results with improved postoperative acuities. However, anterior dislocation of one intraocular lens into the anterior chamber was reported.[38] Most pediatric ophthalmologists currently feel that, given the abnormal zonule in children with ectopia lentis and the limited capsular support for an intraocular lens, the postoperative refractive correction of those undergoing lens surgery should remain contact lenses or spectacles.

Visual improvement occurs in nearly all cases but it should be noted that it may be delayed (often reflecting long-established ametropic amblyopia).[39]

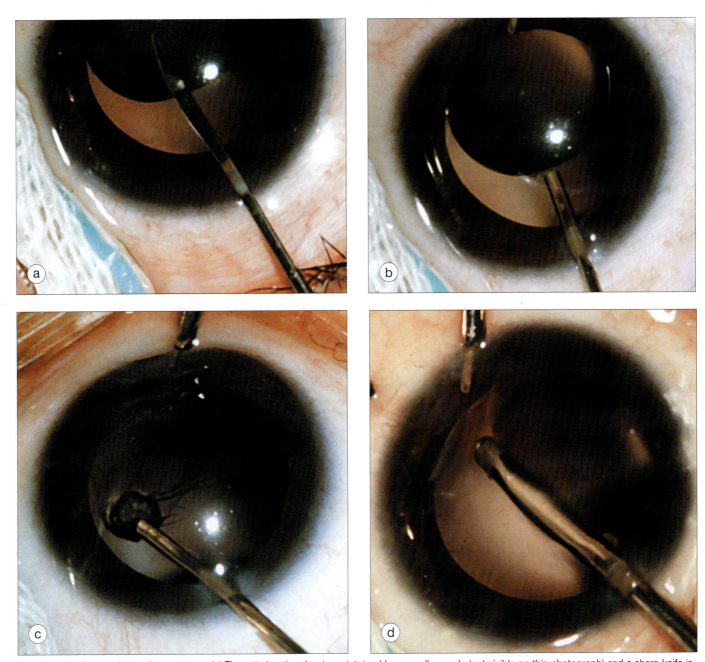

Fig. 46.14 Marfan syndrome. Lens surgery. (a) The anterior chamber is maintained by a small cannula (not visible on this photograph) and a sharp knife is being used to penetrate the lens capsule. (b) A simple aspiration cannula is inserted into the lens through the capsular incision. (c) All of the lens material is aspirated. (d) A vitrectomy machine is used to clear the remains of the capsule.

REFERENCES

1. Beebe DC, Compart PJ, Johnson MC, et al. The mechanism of cell elongation during lens fiber cell differentiation. Devel Biol 1982; 92: 54–9.
2. Bron AJ, Lambert S. Specular microscopy of the lens. Ophthalmic Res 1984; 16(suppl): 209.
3. Grainger RM, Henry JJ, Saha MS, et al. Recent progress on the mechanisms of embryonic lens formation. Eye 1992; 6: 117–22.
4. Hendrix RW, Zwaan J. Changes in the glycoprotein concentration of the extracellular matrix between lens and optic vesicle associated with early lens differentiation. Differentiation 1974; 2: 357–62.
5. Hunt HH. A study of the fine structure of the optic vesicle and lens placode of the chick embryo during incubation. Devel Biol 1961; 3: 175–209.
6. Garcia-Porrero JA, Colvee E, Ojeda JL. The mechanisms of cell death and phagocytosis in the early chick lens morphogenesis: A scanning electron microscopy and cytochemical approach. Anat Rec 1984; 208: 123–36.
7. Coulombre JL, Coulombre AJ. Lens development: IV. Size, shape and orientation. Invest Ophthalmol 1969; 8: 251–7.
8. Ashworth JL, Kielty CM, McLeod D. Fibrillin and the eye. Br J Ophthalmol 2000; 84: 1312–17.
9. Goldberg MF. Persistent fetal vasculature (PFV): an integrated interpretation of signs and symptoms associated with persistent hyperplastic primary vitreous (PHPV). LIV Edward Jackson Memorial Lecture. Am J Ophthalmol 1997; 124: 587–626.
10. Johnson BL, Cheng KP. Congenital aphakia: a clinicopathologic report of three cases. J Pediatr Ophthalmol Strabismus 1997; 34: 208–9.
11. Faivre L, Gorlin RJ, Wirtz MK, et al. In frame fibrillin-1 gene deletion in autosomal dominant Weill-Marchesani syndrome. J Med Genet 2003; 40: 34–6.
12. Evans AK, Hickey-Dwyer MU. Cleft anterior segment with maternal hypervitaminosis. Br J Ophthalmol 1991; 75: 691–2.
13. Hemady RK, Blum S, Sylvia BM. Duplication of the lens, hour-glass cornea and cornea plana. Arch Ophthalmol 1993; 111: 303.
14. Singh A, Singh AD, Shields CL, et al. Iris neovascularisation in children as a manifestation of underlying medulloepithelioma. J Pediatr Ophthalmol Strabismus 2001; 38: 224–8.
15. Crouch ER Jr, Parks MM. Management of posterior lenticonus complicated by unilateral cataract. Am J Ophthalmol 1978; 85: 503–8.
16. Russell-Eggitt IM. Non-syndromic posterior lenticonus a cause of childhood cataract: evidence for X-linked inheritance. Eye 2000; 14: 861–3.
17. Streeten BW, Robinson MR, Wallace R, et al. Lens capsule abnormalities in Alport's syndrome. Arch Ophthalmol 1987; 105: 1693–7.
18. Knebelmann B, Breillat C, Forestier L, et.al. Spectrum of mutations in the COL4A5 collagen gene in X-linked Alport syndrome. Am J Hum Genet 1996; 59: 1221–32.
19. Flinter F. Alport's syndrome. J Med Genet 1997; 34: 326–30.
20. Fuchs J. Marfan syndrome and other systemic disorders with congenital ectopia lentis. A Danish national survey. Acta Paediatr 1997; 86: 947–52.
21. Maumenee IH. The eye in Marfan syndrome. Trans Am Ophthalmol Soc 1981; 79: 684–733.
22. Cruysberg JR, Boers GH, Trijbels JM, et al. Delay in diagnosis of homocystinuria: retrospective study of consecutive patients. BMJ 1996; 313: 1037–40.
23. Cross HE, Jensen AD. Ocular manifestations in the Marfan syndrome and homocystinuria. Am J Ophthalmol 1973; 75: 405–20.
24. Harrison DA, Mullaney PB, Mesfer SA, et al. Management of ophthalmic complications of homocystinuria. Ophthalmology 1998; 105: 1886–90.
25. Yap S, Rushe H, Howard PM, et al. The intellectual abilities of early-treated individuals with pyridoxine-nonresponsive homocystinuria due to cystathionine beta-synthase deficiency. J Inherit Metab Dis 2001; 24: 437–47.
26. Evereklioglu C, Hepsen IF, Er H. Weill-Marchesani syndrome in three generations. Eye 1999; 13: 773–7.
27. Saatci AO, Soylev M, Kavukcu S, et al. Bilateral megalocornea with unilateral lens subluxation. Ophthalmic Genet 1997; 18: 35–8.
28. Cruysberg JR, Pinckers A. Ectopia lentis et pupillae syndrome in three generations. Br J Ophthalmol 1995; 79: 135–8.
29. Byles DB, Nischal KK, Cheng H. Ectopia lentis et pupillae. A hypothesis revisited. Ophthalmology 1998; 105: 1331–6.
30. Jarrett WH. Dislocation of the lens. A study of 166 hospitalised cases. Arch Ophthalmol 1967; 78: 289–96.
31. Edwards MC, Johnson JL, Marriage B, et al. Isolated sulfite oxidase deficiency: review of two cases in one family. Ophthalmology 1999; 106: 1957–61.
32. Lueder GT, Steiner RD. Ophthalmic abnormalities in molybdenum cofactor deficiency and isolated sulfite oxidase defiency. J Pediatr Ophthalmol Strabismus 1995; 32: 334–7.
33. Romano PE, Kerr NC, Hope GM. Bilateral ametropic functional amblyopia in genetic ectopia lentis: its relation to the amount of subluxation, an indicator for early surgical management. Binocul Vis Strabismus 2002; 17: 235–41.
34. Salehpour O, Lavy T, Leonard J, et al. The surgical management of non-traumatic lenses. J Pediatr Ophthalmol Strabismus 1996; 33: 8–13.
35. Reese PD, Weingeist TA. Pars plana management of ectopia lentis in children. Arch Ophthalmol 1987; 105: 1202–4.
36. Halpert M, BenEzra D. Surgery of the hereditary subluxated lenses in children. Ophthalmology 1996; 103: 681–6.
37. Tchah H, Larson RS, Nichols BD, et al. Neodymium:Yag laser zonulysis for treatment of lens subluxation. Ophthalmology 1989; 96: 230–5.
38. Vadala P, Capozzi P, Fortunato M, et al. Intraocular lens implantation in Marfan's syndrome. J Pediatr Ophthalmol Strabismus 2000; 37: 206–8.
39. Speedwell L, Russell-Eggitt I. Improvement in visual acuity in children with ectopia lentis. J Pediatr Ophthalmol Strabismus 1995; 32: 94–7.

CHAPTER
47

Cataract and Persistent Hyperplastic Primary Vitreous (PHPV)

Scott R Lambert

Cataracts are opacities of the crystalline lens. Because they frequently interfere with normal visual development, they represent an important problem in pediatric ophthalmology (Fig. 47.1). Up to one-third of children with unilateral congenital cataracts remain legally blind even after surgical and optical treatment, and eyes with monocular congenital cataracts often do not develop useful vision in the affected eye. Incidence varies from country to country but in the UK the adjusted cumulative incidence at 5 years was 3.18 per 10,000, increasing to 3.46 per 10,000 by 15 years:[1] other, retrospective, studies have concurred.[2] Bilateral cataract is more common than unilateral. Since early treatment is probably the most important factor in determining the visual outcome of these eyes, prompt detection and treatment of cataracts in all neonates is the aim;[3] however, that aim is difficult to achieve by screening.[4]

ETIOLOGY

The etiology of congenital cataracts can be established in many children by careful assessment. The most common etiologies include autosomal dominant hereditary cataracts, metabolic disorders, genetically transmitted syndromes, and intra-uterine infections (Table 47.1). In an otherwise healthy child, an

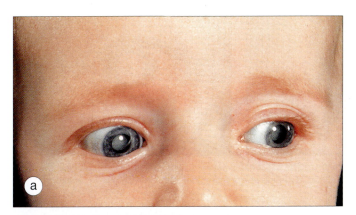
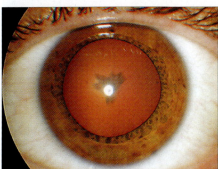
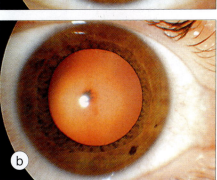

Fig. 47.1 Familial cataracts. (a) Three-month-old infant with bilateral cataracts. (b) His mother also has bilateral cataracts.

Table 47.1 Etiology of cataracts in childhood	
Idiopathic	**Inherited with systemic abnormalities**
Intrauterine infection	**Chromosomal**
Rubella	Trisomy 21
Varicella	Turner syndrome
Toxoplasmosis	Trisomy 13
Herpes simplex	Trisomy 18
Uveitis or acquired infection	Cri du chat syndrome
Pars planitis	**Craniofacial syndromes**
Juvenile idiopathic arthritis	COFS syndrome
Toxocara canis	**Renal disease**
Drug-induced	Lowe syndrome
Corticosteroids	Alport syndrome
Chlorpromazine	Hallermann–Streiff–François
Metabolic disorders	**Skeletal disease**
Galactosemia	Smith–Lemli–Opitz
Galactokinase deficiency	Conradi syndrome
Hypocalcemia	Weill–Marchesani syndrome
Hypoglycemia	Stickler syndrome
Diabetes mellitus	Syndactyly, polydactyly or digital anomalies
Mannosidosis	Bardet–Biedl syndrome
Hyperferritinemia	Rubinstein–Taybi syndrome
Trauma	**Neurometabolic disease**
Accidental	Zellweger syndrome
Laser photocoagulation	Meckel–Gruber syndrome
Non-accidental	Marinesco–Sjögren syndrome
Radiation-induced	Infantile neuronal ceroid-lipofuscinosis
Other diseases	**Muscular disease**
Microphthalmia	Myotonic dystrophy
Aniridia	**Dermatological**
Retinitis pigmentosa	Crystalline cataract and uncombable hair
PHPV	Cockayne syndrome
Retinopathy of prematurity	Rothmund–Thomson
Endophthalmitis	Atopic dermatitis
Inherited	Incontinentia pigmenti
Autosomal dominant	Progeria
Autosomal recessive	Congenital ichthyosis
X-linked	Ectodermal dysplasia
Mental retardation	Werner syndrome
See text	

extensive evaluation is not usually necessary. A pediatrician and an ophthalmologist working together can detect most of the associated ocular and systemic diseases with only a few simple urine and blood tests, and dysmorphic cases may be diagnosed with the help of a database such as "Possum" or "GENEEYE."[5]

Inherited cataracts

Congenital cataracts are frequently inherited as an autosomal dominant trait (Fig. 47.1) often accompanied by microphthalmos. Parents and siblings should be examined using biomicroscopy for clinically insignificant cataracts since phenotypic heterogeneity is a characteristic of autosomal dominantly inherited cataracts.[6,7] In addition to intrafamilial morphological variability (Fig. 47.2), there can also be marked interocular variability in the morphology of these cataracts.[8] Anterior polar cataracts may also be inherited as an autosomal dominant trait (Fig. 47.3).

Autosomal recessive inheritance is less common, but should be suspected if there is consanguinity or multiply affected offspring and unaffected parents. Galactosemia is a notable autosomal recessive condition causing cataracts.

Lowe syndrome (Fig. 47.4) is the most common X-linked condition causing cataracts. Children with Lowe's syndrome have hypotonia, mental retardation, aminoaciduria, and an abnormal facial appearance with frontal bossing and chubby cheeks.[9] The lens typically has a reduced anterior–posterior diameter, and there is mesenchymal dysgenesis and glaucoma; despite perfect management the prognosis must be guarded.[9] Carriers have multiple fine peripheral cortical punctate lens opacities or posterior subcapsular cataracts, which can progress to visually significant cataracts.[10]

X-linked inheritance also occurs in the Nance–Horan syndrome (Fig. 47.5) in which cataract, supernumerary teeth, and prominent ears with anteverted pinnae are associated

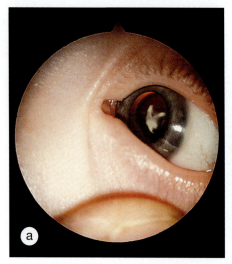
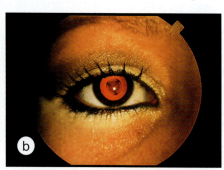
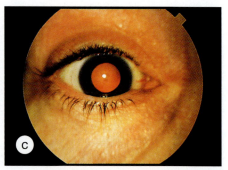

Fig. 47.2 Heterogeneity in autosomal dominant cataract. (a) Dominant lamellar cataract. The infant had presented because his parents had seen the white pupils. (b) His asymptomatic mother, who has vision good enough to drive a car. (c) His asymptomatic grandmother who had tiny lamellar cataracts.

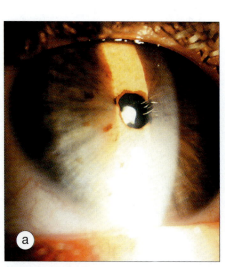
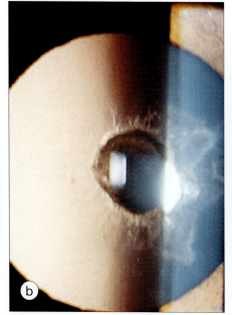
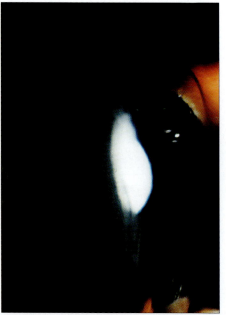

Fig. 47.3 Anterior polar and pyramidal cataracts. (a) The acuity is 0.0 logMAR: the cataracts are unlikely to increase or affect vision. (b) Anterior pyramidal cataracts project forward from the anterior lens capsule and may progressively affect the anterior cortex.

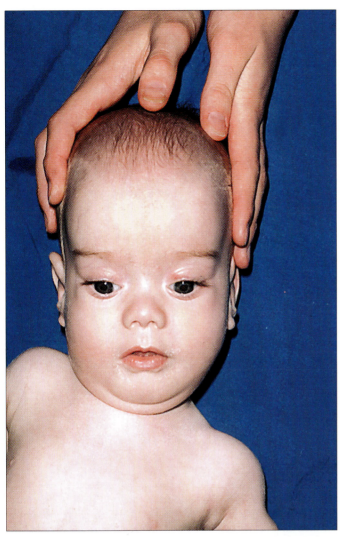

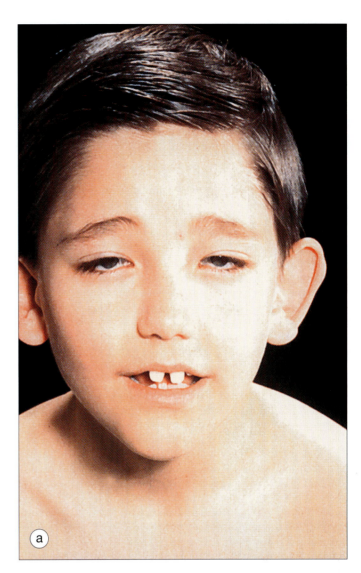

Fig. 47.4 Lowe syndrome. "Chubby" cheeks and rounded forehead. He has bilateral cataracts.

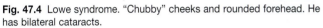

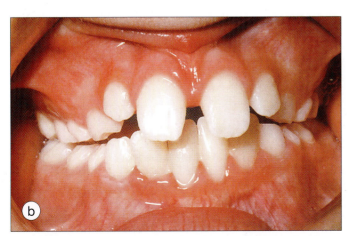

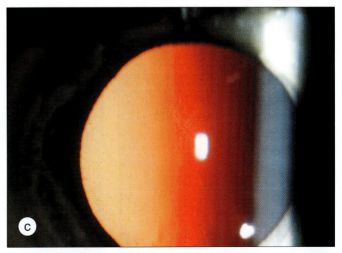

Fig. 47.5 Nance–Horan syndrome. (a) Nance–Horan syndrome showing prominent ears and teeth. (b) Nance–Horan syndrome showing supernumerary and abnormal teeth. (c) Asymptomatic cataract in the mother.

with developmental delay. Obligate carriers have sutural cataracts and abnormal teeth. The gene has been mapped to Xp22.2–p22.3.[11]

The X-linked recessive Lenz syndrome may also be associated with cataracts; other features of this syndrome include microphthalmos (colobomatous in 75%), prominent simple ears, and dental anomalies.[12] Developmental delay is very frequent as are ptosis, skeletal abnormalities, and urogenital anomalies and clefts.

Metabolic disorders (see Chapter 65)

Classic galactosemia is caused by a mutation of the gene on the short arm of chromosome 9 coding for the enzyme galactose-1-phosphate uridyl-transferase (GALT). More than 60% of patients with classical galactosemia have a mutation on exon 6 (Q188R) of the GALT gene. Homozygotes for this mutation have no GALT activity and present during infancy with diarrhea, vomiting, jaundice, hepatomegaly, and Gram-positive septicemia. Heterozygotes for classical galactosemia are also at increased risk of developing cataracts during early adulthood. Reducing substances are present in the urine of patients with both classical galactosemia and galactokinase deficiency after a galactose-containing meal (milk). Enzymatic assays using erythrocytes and DNA studies can then be used to distinguish between the different types of galactosemia.

Infants with classical galactosemia develop "oil droplet" cataracts (Fig. 47.6), which are not true cataracts but refractive changes in the lens nucleus that appear as a drop in the center of the lens in retroillumination like an oil droplet floating in water. If left untreated, these oil droplet cataracts progress to lamellar and then total cataracts due to the accumulation of galactitol in the lens. However, if galactose is eliminated from the diet of these children early in life, the lenses may become transparent again (Fig. 47.6b).[13] Galactose-1-phosphate levels in the serum can be used to monitor dietary compliance.

Inherited mitochondrial diseases, with skeletal muscle involvement, cardiomyopathy, and other manifestations may be associated with cataract:[14] see Chapter 65.

In Wilson disease there may be subcapsular "sunflower" cataracts.

Cerebrotendinous xanthomatosis is an autosomal recessive sterol storage disorder due to lack of mitochondrial hydroxylase; the gene is on chromosome 2. Affected children have dementia, ataxia, and tendon xanthomas. Bilateral, irregular, corticonuclear, anterior polar, or posterior capsular cataracts occur sometimes in the first decade.[15]

Children with hypocalcemia usually have seizures, failure-to-thrive, and irritability. Many also develop cataracts as a result of the altered permeability of the lens capsule. These cataracts generally begin as fine white punctate opacities scattered throughout the lens cortex that may then progress to lamellar cataracts. Serum calcium and phosphorus levels should be measured in infants with bilateral cataracts.

Cataracts occur infrequently in children with diabetes mellitus. When they do develop, they usually occur in the teenage years. They frequently begin as cortical opacities but may rapidly progress to total cataracts.

Hypoglycemia during the perinatal period or in early infancy may result in lens opacities. These opacities are reversible in most cases but occasionally may develop into total cataracts.

In hyperferritinemia, crumb-like, sometimes colored, nuclear, and cortical lens opacities may occur as an autosomal dominant trait.[16,17]

Intrauterine infection

An intrauterine infection should be suspected in infants with dense unilateral or bilateral (Fig. 47.7) central cataracts (see Chapter 18). A history of a maternal illness accompanied by a rash during the pregnancy is particularly suggestive of an intrauterine rubella or varicella infection. Rubella immunoglobulin G (IgG) and IgM antibody titers should be obtained from the mother and the child. At the time of surgery, the lens aspirate can also be cultured for rubella virus. Even with sophisticated management the prognosis remains poor.[18]

Toxoplasmosis, varicella, and other intrauterine infections may also result in congenital cataracts but if cataracts are present in such cases it suggests widespread damage to the eye (Fig. 47.8).

Chromosomal and other syndromes

Cataracts are manifest in a large number of syndromes (see Table 47.1), the most common being trisomy 21 (Fig. 47.9). Children

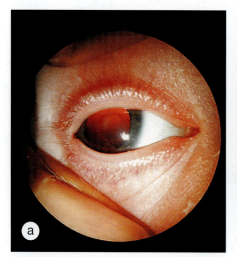
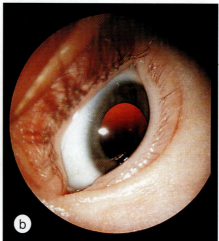
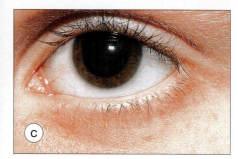

Fig. 47.6 Galactosemia. (a) "Oil droplet" cataract. It is a change in the refractive index in the nucleus of the lens. (b) After early dietary treatment the "cataract" had disappeared (same patient). (c) If treatment is late and compliance poor, a lamellar cataract may develop, seen here as a faint central opalescence.

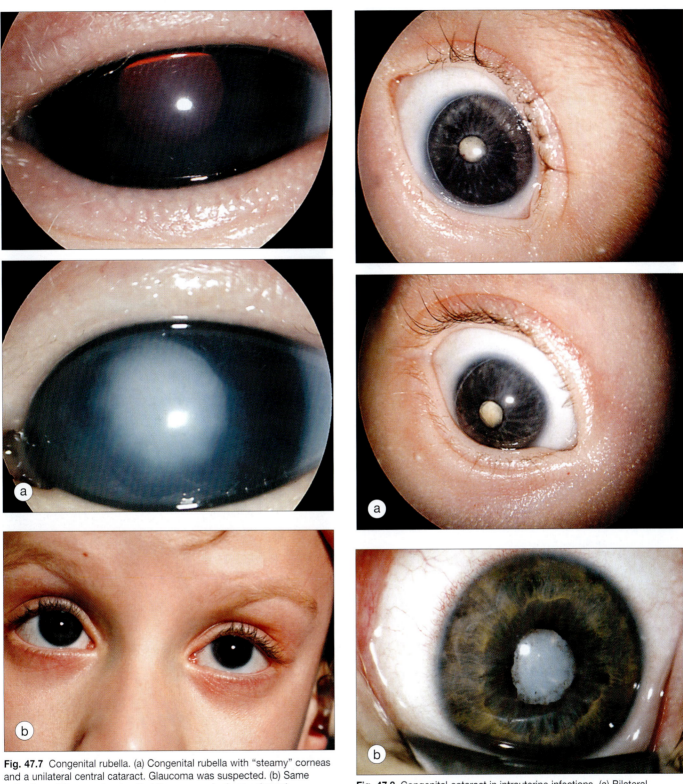

Fig. 47.7 Congenital rubella. (a) Congenital rubella with "steamy" corneas and a unilateral central cataract. Glaucoma was suspected. (b) Same patient aged 6 years showing that the corneas had not enlarged. Buphthalmos does occur in congenital rubella but it is important to be sure that the intraocular pressure is raised because corneal edema also occurs from a transient keratopathy.

Fig. 47.8 Congenital cataract in intrauterine infections. (a) Bilateral cataracts and microphthalmos in a child with severe intrauterine toxoplasmosis. A posterior embryotoxon is present. (b) Congenital cataract in a child with intrauterine varicella. If there is a cataract in a child with an intrauterine infection, it is very likely that there is severe intraocular damage.

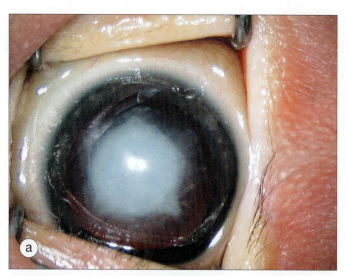
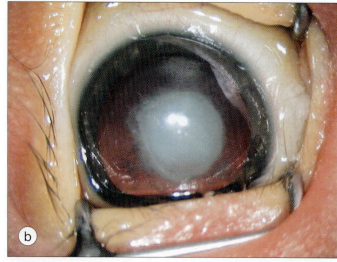

Fig. 47.9 Down syndrome. Dense bilateral cataracts in an infant with trisomy 21.

with trisomy 21 usually develop cataracts later in childhood, but less commonly they may develop during infancy.[19]

Cataracts have also been reported in children with reciprocal translocations of chromosomes 3 and 4 with a familial 2;14 translocation and the Cri du chat syndrome caused by a partial deletion of the short arm of chromosome 5.

Cataracts may also be the presenting sign of the Hallermann–Streiff–François syndrome;[20] it comprises the following (Fig. 47.10):
1. Dyscephaly with a beak-shaped nose and micrognathia;
2. Short stature;
3. Hypotrichosis;
4. Dental abnormalities;
5. Blue sclerae; and
6. Congenital cataract.

Cataracts with mental retardation

Cataracts occur with mental retardation in the following conditions:
1. Martsolf syndrome: micrognathia, brachycephaly, flat maxilla, broad sternum, talipes, clefts.[21]
2. The Marinesco–Sjögren syndrome: cerebellar ataxia and myopathy.[22]
3. The peroxisomal disorders and mitochondrial cytopathies (see Chapter 65).
4. Chondrodysplasia punctata. This occurs in three main forms:
   (a) An autosomal recessive "rhizomelic," lethal form with rhizomelia (short limbs), mongoloid eye-slant, ichthyosis, flat nasal bridge.
   (b) An X-linked dominant form: shortened leg bones; scaly, "orange peel" skin; alopecia. The cataracts may be sectorial, a possible lyonization effect.
   (c) A possible autosomal dominant form similar to (b).
5. X-linked cataract, spasticity, and mental retardation.
6. Autosomal cerebro-oculofacial skeletal syndrome (COFS, Pena-Shokeir II). These infants have microcephaly, joint contractures, rocker-bottom feet, micrognathia, sloping forehead, and prominent nasal root.[23]

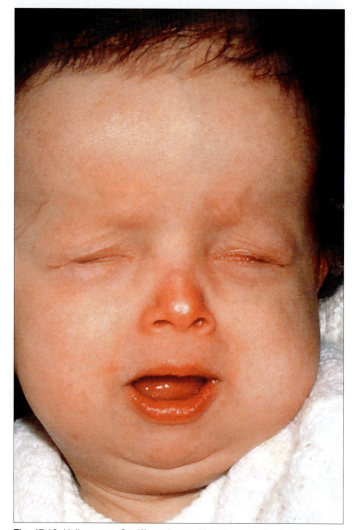

Fig. 47.10 Hallenmann–Streiff syndrome. Note the receding hairline and the vascular, small, upturned nose.

7. Czeizel–Lowry syndrome. Affected children have cataract, microcephaly, mental retardation, and Perthes disease of the hip.[24] It is probably autosomal recessive.

8. The Killian–Pallister mosaic syndrome. The syndrome is associated with tetrasomy of the short arm of chromosome 12, coarse facial features with a broad forehead hypertelorism, saggy cheeks and mouth, and sparse hair. The condition is diagnosed by skin chromosome studies and can be made prenatally.[25]

9. Progressive spinocerebellar ataxia, deafness, and a peripheral neuropathy.[26]

10. A syndrome with proximal myopathy with facial, ocular, and bulbar weaknesses, hypogonadism, and ataxia.[27]

11. IBIDS, TAY, BIDS, or Pollitt syndrome. In this autosomal recessive syndrome, cataract and mild to moderate mental retardation are associated with short stature and scaly skin with trichorrhexis nodosa.[28]

12. The Schwartz–Jampel syndrome associated with a congenital myotonic myopathy, ptosis, and skeletal defects with microphthalmos and cataract.

13. Cataract, mental retardation, microdontia, pectus excavation, and hypertrichosis.[29]

14. The velocardiofacial (Shprintzen) syndrome is an autosomal dominant syndrome with cardiac anomalies, a prominent nose with square tip, notched alae nasae, micrognathia, and a cleft palate. These individuals have 22q11 deletions, and there is an overlap with di George syndrome. These and some other syndromes with conotruncal cardiac defects have been given the catchy acronym CATCH 22.[30]

15. Cataracts and mental retardation also occur in the following conditions described elsewhere in this book: aniridia, Lowe syndrome, Bardet–Biedl syndrome, Cockayne syndrome, vitamin A toxicity, Hallgren syndrome, and many other retinal and vitreous degenerations.

Persistent fetal vasculature (PFV)
(see also Chapter 49)

The term PFV is used to describe a wide spectrum of congenital anomalies.[31] These abnormalities most commonly consist of a retrolental plaque (Fig. 47.11) in a microphthalmic eye with prominent blood vessels on the iris, a shallow anterior chamber, elongated ciliary processes, and occasionally intralenticular hemorrhages.[32] They are unilateral in 90% of patients. Nystagmus may be present even in unilateral cases and strabismus is common. Although the lens may be clear initially, with time they usually become cataractous. In some instances, the lens cortex and nucleus may undergo spontaneous absorption through a break in the posterior lens capsule while in others the lens becomes swollen, resulting in the loss of the anterior

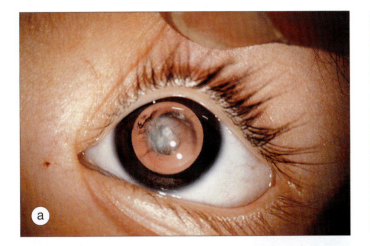
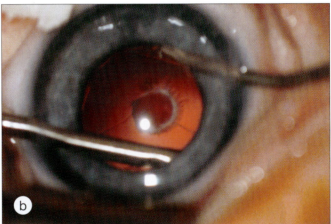
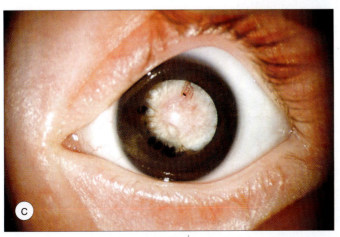
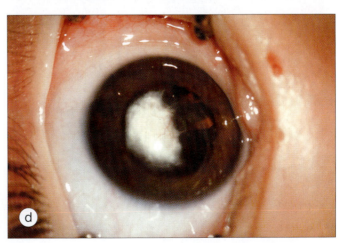

Fig. 47.11 PFV (PHPV). (a) A small PFV with a hyaloid vessel (block arrow) and vessels anterior to the iris (open arrow). (b) Small vascular PFV with a "blood lake" representing a low-flow shunt centrally. (c) Marked vascular PFV with multiple vessels between the fibrous plaque, lens, and the iris. (d) Marked PFV with ciliary processes stretched to the membrane.

chamber and an elevation in the intraocular pressure. The retrolental fibrovascular plaque may be vascular and may bleed if cut surgically. In early infancy, the ciliary processes are often stretched. Retinal involvement usually occurs secondary to contraction of the retrolental plaque, resulting in traction on the vitreous base and peripheral retina.

Whereas in many instances the posterior pole is normal, fibrous tissue arising from the remnant of the hyaloid vessels may occur and occasionally result in peripapillary tractional retinal detachments. Other conditions that can mimic PFV include retinoblastoma, retinopathy of prematurity, retinal dysplasia, posterior uveitis, and congenital cataracts. The presence of microphthalmos, a shallow anterior chamber, long ciliary processes, a cataract, and a retrolental opacity with a persistent hyaloid artery are all helpful in distinguishing PFV from these other conditions. Good visual results may be obtained in some eyes with mild PFV after early surgery; however, eyes with severe PFV usually have a poor visual outcome secondary to amblyopia, glaucoma, or retinal detachment.[33]

Steroid cataracts

Chronic corticosteroid therapy, even when given in low doses systemically, may result in the formation of posterior subcapsular cataracts. The progression of these cataracts may be arrested if the corticosteroids are promptly discontinued. However, since the systemic conditions that prompted the initial steroid therapy are often life-threatening, cessation of steroid therapy may not be possible. Steroid-induced posterior subcapsular cataracts are frequently associated with little if any visual disability and may progress quite slowly. Posterior subcapsular cataracts also commonly develop in children treated with external beam radiation to the orbital region.

Uveitis

Posterior subcapsular cataracts also develop in children with uveitis secondary to juvenile idiopathic arthritis (JIA) and pars planitis.[34] Children with JRA-associated cataracts also characteristically develop band keratopathy and posterior synechiae. Cystoid macular edema is a common accompaniment of both conditions.

Prematurity

Transient cataracts have been noted in some premature infants. They are usually bilateral and symmetrical opacities beginning as vacuoles along the posterior lens suture. Only rarely do they persist and result in permanent lens opacities. They may occur as a result of treatment of retinopathy of prematurity.

MORPHOLOGY

The morphology of cataract is important: it can give a clue to the age of onset and to the visual prognosis, it may suggest heritability, and it may give a lead to the etiology.[35] Although it may be technically difficult in infants and young children, slit-lamp examination is necessary to define the morphology and location of cataracts. The morphology of the cataract is largely determined by the anatomy of the lens, its embryology, and the timing and nature of the insult that caused the abnormality. Some morphological types have a better prognosis than others in surgical series,[36] with smaller, less dense, anterior polar, lamellar (Fig. 47.12), sutural (Fig. 47.13), and posterior lenticonus-associated cataracts doing relatively well and larger (Fig. 47.14), more dense, central, and posterior cataracts having a relatively poor prognosis.[36] The cataracts associated with posterior lenticonus (Fig. 47.15) are believed to be acquired in most instances and as such are associated with better visual prognosis.[37]

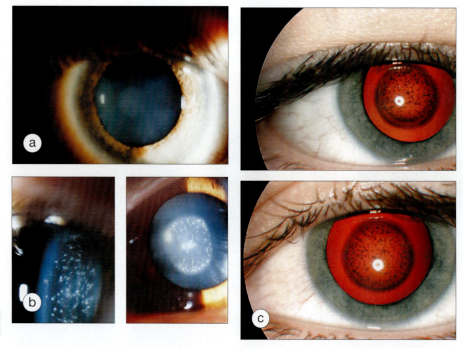

Fig. 47.12 a) Asymptomatic, familial, central pulverulent ("Coppock") cataracts.
(b) Asymptomatic central "ant-egg" cataract.
(c) Bilateral symmetrical lamellar cataracts in retroillumination. The acuity is 6/9 in both eyes.

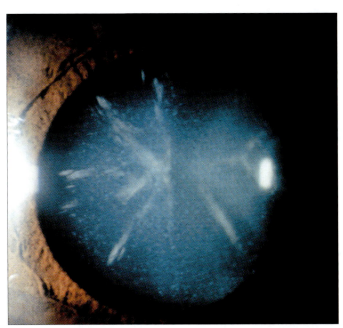

Fig. 47.13 Sutural cataracts. The visual acuity was 0.0 logMAR and the patient complained of glare.

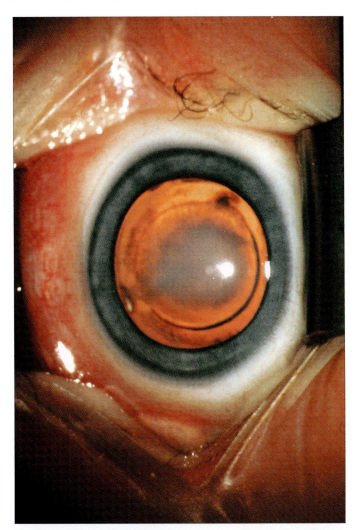

Fig. 47.14 Diffuse cataract. Although there is a moderately sized lamellar cataract, there are also widespread diffuse cataractous changes and a dense central opacity that caused visual deprivation and nystagmus in this three-month-old child.

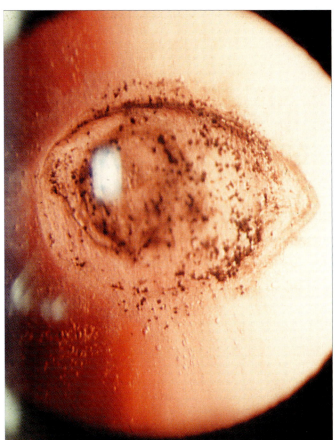

Fig. 47.15 Posterior lenticonus. Operative photograph of posterior lenticonus in a child noted to suddenly develop leukocoria in the left eye when 12 months of age. There is an oblique defect in the posterior capsule around which there are numerous white opacities.

Certain types of cataracts are also frequently associated with other ocular abnormalities. For instance, nuclear cataracts are often associated with microphthalmos (Fig. 47.7) while autosomal dominantly inherited anterior polar cataracts are associated with corneal guttata or astigmatism. Anterior subcapsular and anterior capsular cataracts are usually acquired in children with severe skin diseases (syndermatotic cataract).

Cerulean cataracts are progressive blue-white nuclear or cortical cataracts. Wedge-shaped or sectional cataracts may occur with Stickler syndrome and Conradi syndrome. That this may be a manifestation of lyonization.

Nearly thirty genes had been mapped by the end of 2003.[38]

VISUAL EFFECTS

Because of the significant visual deprivation that occurs with both monocular and binocular cataracts in early infancy, success requires early detection and immediate referral for definitive treatment. The red light reflex should be assessed by direct ophthalmoscopy in the newborn nursery at 6 weeks and 6 months of age by a general practitioner or pediatrician. If an abnormality is detected, a prompt referral should be made to an ophthalmologist. Pupillary dilation may be necessary to detect incomplete cataracts in some children.

Children with visually significant monocular cataracts often present with strabismus, which may not develop until irreparable visual loss has occurred. Rarely monocular nystagmus may be the presenting sign of a monocular congenital cataract. In most instances, visual behavior will be unaffected by a monocular cataract, and parents are not aware of the problem. In contrast, dense binocular cataracts are usually associated with delayed development and obviously impaired visual behavior. If manifest nystagmus does develop, the visual prognosis is worse although on occasion it may be reversed by prompt treatment. Children with manifest nystagmus in primary gaze during the first year of life should be carefully evaluated for cataracts.

MANAGEMENT

Assessment

Although dense bilateral congenital cataracts should be removed as early as possible, partial cataracts should only be removed after a careful assessment of the morphology of the lens opacity and the visual behavior of the child. Conservative management is indicated at least until the child's visual status can be accurately assessed. The visual prognosis of bilateral incomplete cataracts correlates better with the density than with the size of the opacity. Hence nuclear cataracts, although smaller in size than lamellar cataracts, may have a poorer visual prognosis. If the major blood vessels of the fundus cannot be distinguished through the central portion of the cataract, significant visual deprivation can be expected from even a moderately sized partial cataract.

The systemic investigation should usually be carried out in collaboration with a pediatrician who has an interest in dysmorphology and metabolic disease and who will carry out further tests as appropriate, such as plasma electrolytes and amino acid studies. Further investigations, such as galactose enzyme studies, can be carried out when appropriate. Clearly some cataracts, such as posterior lentiglobus and unilateral PFV, are purely ocular problems and do not require a pediatric investigation.

An attempt should be made to evaluate the integrity of the retina and optic nerve in all children with significant cataracts. If the density of the cataracts precludes an adequate view of the fundus, an ultrasound examination may be carried out prior to any surgical intervention. It is also important to assess the pupillary reflexes. An afferent pupillary defect suggests a structural defect of the optic disc or retina and is associated with a poor visual prognosis. A visual assessment should also be performed using patterns of fixation and supplemented when possible by forced choice preferential looking and/or pattern visual-evoked potentials. Surgery for visually significant bilateral cataracts should be carried out as soon as possible without jeopardizing the general health of the child. Only a short interval should elapse between the removal of the right and left lenses to prevent relative amblyopia of the fellow eye.

Surgery

The surgical treatment of children's cataracts has evolved considerably. At present, most authorities prefer to perform a lensectomy and anterior vitrectomy utilizing a closed eye system in infant eyes.[39] By creating a primary posterior capsulotomy or primary posterior capsulorrhexis and vitrectomy,[40] the number of secondary operations can be greatly reduced. Moreover, the clear

visual axis thus created facilitates retinoscopy. However, since the latent period for retinal detachment is long, the incidence of retinal detachment following a lensectomy may prove to be higher with longer term follow-up.

In some infants without other eye disease (microphthalmos, microphakia, or anterior segment abnormalities) and in older children, who are less susceptible to amblyopia and in whom posterior capsular opacification is less likely to occur, a simple lens aspiration with the implantation of an intraocular lens is the preferred procedure. Phacoemulsification is not necessary to remove a pediatric cataract.

If the posterior capsule opacifies, a YAG laser can be used to create a posterior capsulotomy. It is important that the procedure not be delayed because of the danger of amblyopia and the increased difficulty of opening a thickened posterior capsule. Posterior capsule opacification is due largely to proliferation and migration of residual lens epithelial cells, which may need to be removed by a pars plicata approach capsulectomy with a vitrectomy machine.

Correction of aphakia

One of the major obstacles confronting ophthalmologists and the families of infants requiring cataract extraction is the optical correction of the induced aphakia.

Contact lenses

Contact lenses remain the standard method of optically correcting aphakia during infancy (Fig. 47.16). Rigid gas-permeable contact lenses are well suited for correcting aphakia during infancy because of their wide range of available powers, low cost, ability to correct large astigmatic errors, and greater ease of insertion and removal.[41] Their biggest disadvantage is the greater expertise required to fit them. Silicone lenses have the advantage of being worn on an extended wear basis, but are more expensive and associated with a higher rate of complications. Aphakic soft lenses are relatively inexpensive and easy to fit, but have the disadvantage of being more difficult to insert and can only correct small astigmatic errors.[42]

The frequent loss of lenses and the need to change regularly the lens power as the eye elongates necessitates frequent lens replacements, particularly during the first 2 years of life.[43] Parents are strongly advised to remove the lenses if the child's eye becomes inflamed or irritated or if excessive discharge develops. Inadequate care can result in ulcerative keratitis and corneal scarring. Poor compliance with contact lens wear is most commonly due to poor vision in the aphakic eye or poor patient cooperation rather than complications arising from use. With persistence, contact lenses can be successfully worn by most infants.

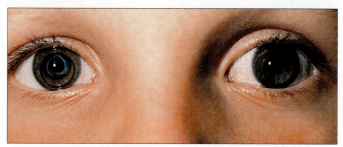

Fig. 47.16 Aphakic contact lenses. This child had successfully worn contact lenses since lens aspiration at three weeks of age.

Spectacles

Aphakic spectacles (Fig. 47.17) are better tolerated than contact lenses by some children with bilateral aphakia. This is particularly true of children between 18 months and 4 years of age. Aphakic spectacles sometimes have the cosmetic advantage of improving the appearance of mildly microphthalmic eyes because of the magnification they induce. In addition, a secondary strabismus may be manipulated by the prismatic effect of spectacles.

Intraocular lenses

Intraocular lenses are being used increasingly to optically correct aphakia in children with good visual results;[44] however, their use during early infancy remains controversial[45] because of the difficulty of accurately predicting the most appropriate lens power to insert and the increased incidence of complications in these eyes.[46,47] Most authorities recommend implanting an intraocular lens with a power that will undercorrect a child 6 years of age or less, but fully correct a child 6 years of age or older (Table 47.2). While it is generally better to implant an intraocular lens "in the bag" at the same time a cataract is removed (Fig. 47.18), intraocular lenses can also be implanted as a secondary procedure if there is enough residual lens capsule for support. Multifocal lenses remain experimental in children.

In older children, intraocular lenses have become the standard of care.[48] They offer the advantage of a constant optical correction superior to that achieved with contact lenses or spectacles. However, leaving a younger child undercorrected necessitates that this child wear an overcorrection with either spectacles or contact lenses for a period of time until a myopic shift has developed. In some cases this myopic shift does not fully correct the residual hyperopia.[49-51]

Table 47.2 Guidelines for intraocular lens power selection in children (undercorrection in diopters or % from emmetropia)

Age	Dahan and Drusedau[70]	Enyedi et al.[49] (diopters)	Flitcroft et al.[51] (diopters)
<1	20% undercorrection	–	+6
1–2 years	20% undercorrection	+6 to +5	+3
3–4 years	10% undercorrection	+4 to +3	+3
5–6 years	10% undercorrection	+2 to +1	+1
7–8 years	10% undercorrection	Plano	+1

Management of amblyopia

No matter what form of aphakic correction is chosen, frequent reevaluations are necessary. Each examination should include a careful analysis of fixation behavior to screen for amblyopia. If amblyopia is suspected, occlusion therapy of the preferred eye should be initiated. Frequent retinoscopic measurements of the refractive error and adjustments in the power of the aphakic correction are imperative. The intraocular pressure should also be periodically assessed, particularly if other signs or symptoms of glaucoma develop. This may require general anesthesia in an infant. The importance of encouragement and support for the parents of aphakic children cannot be overemphasized if a successful rehabilitation program is to be established.

Unilateral cataract

The management of a unilateral congenital cataract is particularly challenging. Although eyes with unilateral congenital cataracts may be successfully rehabilitated on occasion, most do not achieve a visual acuity compatible with reading.[52]

Before a decision is made to perform surgery on a unilateral congenital cataract, the importance of occlusion therapy should be described in detail to the parents.

If a decision is made to perform surgery on a unilateral congenital cataract, prompt surgical intervention is critical. Most studies suggest that surgery after the first 6 weeks of life is less likely to result in good visual acuity.[53] Immediate and continued optical correction of the unilateral aphakia and occlusion therapy of the phakic eye is crucial in the visual rehabilitation of these eyes.

Occluding the fellow eye 50–70% of all waking hours throughout early childhood is associated with the best visual outcomes in aphakic eyes. Excessive patching may result in the development of subtle visual deficits in the fellow eye and impaired binocularity.[54,55] Although "binocular vision" is unusual in children treated for unilateral cataracts, it may rarely be achieved.[56]

Bilateral and traumatic cataracts

Occlusion therapy is often not necessary in children with bilateral congenital cataracts or children with unilateral traumatic cataracts who are treated promptly.

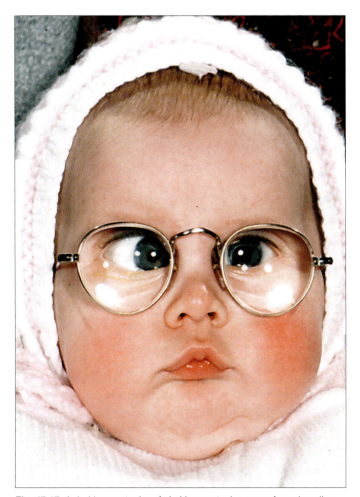

Fig. 47.17 Aphakic spectacles. Aphakic spectacles are safe and easily changed but have optical and cosmetic disadvantages.

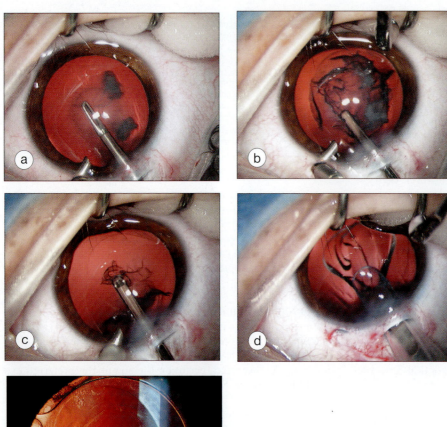

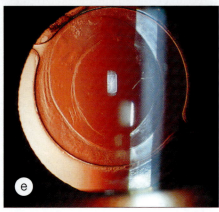

Fig. 47.18 Intraocular lens surgery. Extracapsular cataract extraction is performed in a 3-year-old child with a lamellar cataract. After performing a manual anterior capsulorrhexis (a), the lens cortex is aspirated (b, c) and a SA-60 Acrysof IOL is injected into the eye and then positioned in the capsular bag (d). An "in the bag" PMMA intraocular lens (e) in an infant shows the anterior and posterior capsulorrhexis. Intraocular lenses for infants are controversial and should be implanted only in units performing a large number of infant cataract operations.

COMPLICATIONS OF CATARACT SURGERY

A much higher incidence of complications occurs in children after cataract surgery than in adults. Whereas some complications are preventable by meticulous attention to surgical technique and postoperative care, others arise due to the intrinsic abnormalities of these eyes or the more exuberant inflammatory response associated with surgery on an immature eye.

Amblyopia

Amblyopia is a nearly universal finding in children with congenital cataracts, and a common finding in children with developmental cataracts during the first 7 years of life. It is particularly a problem in children with unilateral congenital cataracts. It arises as a consequence of the retina receiving a defocused image during the critical period of visual development. Uncorrected aphakia or induced anisometropia can exacerbate this amblyopia even after the removal of a cataract. In most cases forced visual deprivation of the fellow eye using occlusion therapy, optical defocus, or atropinization is required.

Glaucoma

Glaucoma (see Chapter 48), which may arise during the early postoperative period or as a late complication years later, is a serious and difficult-to-manage complication.[57] Pupil block glaucoma has a higher incidence in neonates following lensectomy due to vitreous prolapse or pupillary membrane formation. Affected patients usually have ocular pain, corneal edema, and iris bombé. Performing a deep anterior vitrectomy, creating a peripheral iridectomy, and dilating the pupil of an infant for several weeks after a lensectomy can prevent this complication.

Glaucoma is also one of the most common late complications of cataract surgery, occurring in up to one-third of all children after cataract extraction.[58] Its prevalence is particularly high in children with microphthalmos and nuclear cataracts and may be more frequent in eyes operated on during infancy. IOL implantation may reduce the incidence of glaucoma following cataract surgery by either stabilizing the trabecular meshwork or preventing the anterior migration of a substance toxic to the trabecular meshwork from the vitreous chamber.[59] Unlike infantile onset glaucoma, which is usually associated with readily detectable signs and symptoms such as buphthalmos, photophobia, and corneal edema, juvenile onset glaucoma is usually more protean in its manifestations. Although an elevation of the intraocular pressure and optic disc cupping may be present, it is frequently difficult to obtain a reliable measurement of intraocular pressure until later in childhood. For this reason, particular attention should be paid to any cupping of the optic disc, increase in eye size, or rapid loss of hypermetropia.

Strabismus

Strabismus is often the presenting sign of a child with a unilateral cataract and is also frequently present preoperatively in children with bilateral cataracts. Esotropias are more commonly observed in children with congenital cataracts while exotropias are observed more frequently in children with acquired cataracts. An even higher percentage of children develop strabismus after surgical and optical treatment of their cataracts. Strabismus is a particularly troubling problem in older children with acquired cataracts if there is a delay in the removal of the cataract or the optical correction of the induced aphakia. In some cases, these patients can develop diplopia, which will persist even after the eyes are surgically aligned secondary to a disturbance of central fusion.[60]

Capsular opacification

Capsular opacification occurs to a varying degree in all infants after cataract surgery. The incidence is reduced by anterior and posterior capsulorrhexis especially with a vitrectomy.[40] Regrown lens fibers are ubiquitous in children's eyes after cataract surgery unless the lens capsule is completely removed at the time of surgery. If marked, they are known as Soemmerring's rings. Although in most cases they remain confined to the retroiridial space, on occasion reproliferating lens material can extend into the pupillary aperture. In these instances, a reoperation is usually necessary to create a clear visual axis. Anterior capsulorrhexes that are too small may undergo phimosis (Fig. 47.19), which can be treated by surgery or YAG laser.

Irregular pupil

An irregular pupil is a fairly common complication of cataract surgery during infancy. In some instances, the iris sphincter muscle is damaged intraoperatively by the vitreous-cutting instrument. In other instances, the iris may prolapse out of the scleral incision during surgery and become atrophic thereafter. This is particularly a problem in children with lightly colored irides.

Strands of vitreous extending to the surgical incision may also cause peaking of the pupil. This complication may be averted by turning off the infusion line before removing the vitreous-cutting instrument from the eye, maintaining a low flow of irrigating solution, and minimizing the number of times the vitreous-cutting instrument is inserted and removed from the eye.

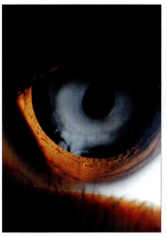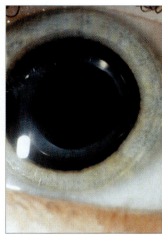

Fig. 47.19 Anterior capsular opacification and phimosis. On the right is an anterior capsule with a good, central capsulorrhexis, which is smaller than the IOL optic holding it in place. On the left, the capsulorrhexis is too small and has undergone progressive phimosis, which complicates retinoscopy—important in the management of amblyopia.

Even when the pupil remains round after cataract surgery, it frequently is less reactive to light and pharmacological dilation. Rigid pupils are particularly common in children who undergo a lensectomy during infancy.

Heterochromia iridis

Cataract surgery during infancy is frequently associated with increased iris pigmentation in the operative eye (Fig. 47.20). This likely occurs due to the release of prostaglandins following cataract surgery.[61]

Secondary membranes

Secondary membranes may arise from fibrin forming a pupillary membrane or opacification of the residual posterior lens capsule. If they obstruct the visual axis, they may be opened with a YAG laser or surgical discission. Because of the high incidence of these complications in infants a primary posterior capsulotomy is usually recommended coupled with atropinization of the pupil for at least 2 weeks after surgery.

Postoperative inflammation and endophthalmitis

Fibrinous uveitis is common after intraocular lens implantation; its severity and frequency can be reduced by the use of heparin-coated IOLs, intracameral heparin, and subconjunctival and intensive postoperative steroid drops. Although rare but particularly possible when iris-fixed IOLs are used, any cataract surgery can give rise to bilateral uveitis.

Persistent uveitis after cataract surgery is a potentially very serious complication (Figs. 47.21, 47.22).

Bacterial endophthalmitis is an uncommon, but devastating complication after cataract extraction.[61] A concurrent naso-lacrimal duct obstruction, upper respiratory infection, or periorbital skin disease increases the risk of this complication developing. The most common organisms causing postoperative

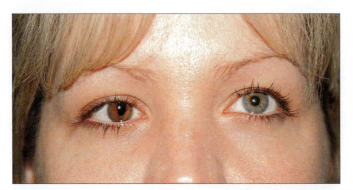

Fig. 47.20 Heterochromia iridis in a 32-year-old woman who underwent cataract surgery at one year of age in the right eye.

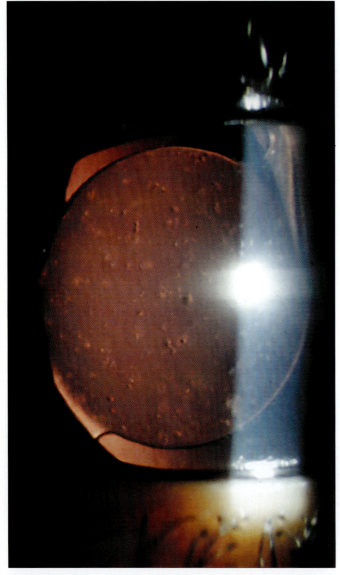

Fig. 47.21 Chronic uveitis after infant lens surgery. An anterior chamber lens (the haptic can be seen top right) was implanted at the time of lensectomy, and postoperatively the eye showed persistent inflammation (KPs can be seen all over the lens surface) with glaucoma. The acuity was 2/60.

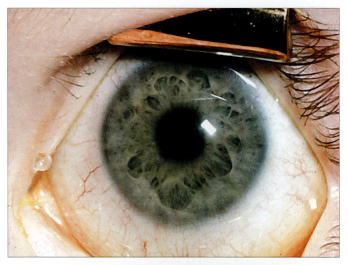

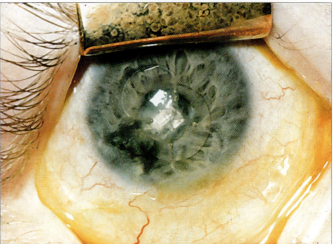

Fig. 47.22 Blinding uveitis after iris-clip IOL. A secondary iris-clip IOL (bottom picture) was implanted at the age of 18 months: by 2.5 years there was bilateral blinding uveitis.

endophthalmitis in children are *Staphylococcus aureus* and *Streptococcus pneumoniae*.

Even though most cases are diagnosed during the first 3 postoperative days, the visual prognosis is still quite poor. In one series, 65% of affected eyes ended up with no light perception vision despite aggressive treatment with intravitreal and systemic antibiotics.[62] Although bilateral simultaneous cataract extractions may be justified in infants with increased anesthetic risks,[63] the risk of bilateral endophthalmitis developing in these patients is the strongest argument against this practice.

Nystagmus

Nystagmus is present in 50% of children with bilateral congenital cataracts. Nystagmus may also develop in children with monocular cataracts, although this occurs less frequently. In some cases, it may become the limiting factor in the visual rehabilitation of children after cataract extraction. Early treatment may reduce the incidence, but very early and excessive patching may make it worse.

Retinal hemorrhages and detachments

A hemorrhagic retinopathy develops in a significant percentage of infants after a lensectomy and anterior vitrectomy. In most cases this consists of flame-shaped hemorrhages in the posterior pole that resolve without sequelae in several weeks. Occasionally, a hemorrhage may occur in the fovea and result in a severe reduction of vision. In these cases, even after the hemorrhage has resolved, the visual acuity may remain reduced secondary to amblyopia.

Retinal detachments usually occur decades after the removal of a congenital cataract[64] but may be a result of associated myopia and trauma in developmentally delayed children with cataracts (Fig. 47.23). Retinal detachments frequently occur bilaterally, and the visualization of the retinal breaks may be hampered by miotic pupils and Soemmerring's rings.

Cystoid macular edema

Cystoid macular edema is a common complication after cataract extraction in adults, but a rare complication in children. In one series no cases of cystoid macular edema occurred in 25 children who underwent fluorescein angiography after cataract extraction.[65]

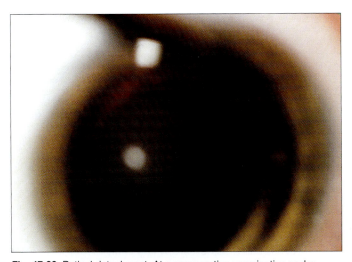

Fig. 47.23 Retinal detachment. At a preoperative examination under anesthetic of a severely developmentally delayed child with bilateral congenital cataract, high myopia and bilateral retinal detachments (seen as a gray line below the lamellar lens opacity) were found.

Corneal edema

Corneal edema can occur after cataract surgery, but usually resolves within a few days. Although in most cases it is probably caused by prolongation of the surgical procedure, it may occur secondary to detergent left on surgical instruments or cannulas.[66] It also commonly occurs after the removal of rubella cataracts.

VISUAL RESULTS

The visual results after the surgical removal of pediatric cataracts have improved dramatically. Improvements in visual results may be attributed to better surgical techniques, the increased implantation of intraocular lenses in children, and the improved screening of children for cataracts by pediatricians and general practitioners at an earlier age.

The visual results obtained after cataract extraction in infants and children depend on a number of factors including:

1. The age of onset of the cataracts;
2. The age when surgery is performed;[67]
3. Associated ocular and systemic conditions; and
4. Compliance with optical and patching therapy.

There may be a late improvement in their tested vision[68] so caution needs to be exercised when giving a prognosis in a young child. Children who develop cataracts after the completion of normal visual development usually have an excellent visual prognosis.

Many children with early onset bilateral cataracts also have an excellent visual outcome if treatment is initiated immediately; however, if treatment is delayed, many of these children will remain legally blind secondary to amblyopia.

Early onset unilateral cataracts continue to be associated with the worse visual prognosis, although even they can be associated with a good visual outcome on occasion.

Concomitant ocular abnormalities such as corneal opacities, glaucoma, retinal abnormalities, and nystagmus worsen the visual prognosis of children with cataracts. Mental retardation is also associated with a poor visual prognosis. Although mental retardation per se is not a contraindication to cataract surgery, the postoperative care and visual rehabilitation of these children is much more difficult. Whereas gross stereopsis may develop on rare occasions in a child after cataract surgery, in most instances the disruption of normal binocular input to the central nervous system during the critical period of visual development precludes this outcome.

REFERENCES

1. Rahi JS, Dezateaux C. Measuring and interpreting the incidence of congenital ocular anomalies: lessons from a national study of congenital cataract in the UK. Invest Ophthalmol Vis Sci 2001; 42: 1444–8.

2. Holmes JM, Leske DA, Burke JP, Hodge DO. Birth prevalence of visually significant infantile cataract in a defined U.S. population. Ophthalmic Epidemiol 2003; 10: 67–74.

3. Committee on Practice and Ambulatory Medicine, Section on Ophthalmology, et al. Eye examination in infants, children, and young adults by pediatricians. Pediatrics 2003; 111: 902–7.

4. Rahi JS, Dezateaux C. National cross sectional study of detection of congenital and infantile cataract in the United Kingdom: role of childhood screening and surveillance. The British Congenital Cataract Interest Group BMJ 1999; 318: 362–5.

5. Baraitser M, Winter RM. GENEEYE–a database of genetic disorders with ophthalmological features. Bushey: London Medical Databases Ltd; 2003. Available at: http://www.lmdatabases.com.

6. Ionides A, Francis P, Berry V et al. Clinical and genetic heterogeneity in autosomal dominant cataract. Br J Ophthalmol 1999; 83: 802–8.

7. Gibbs ML, Jacobs M, Wilkie AO, Taylor D. Posterior lenticonus: clinical patterns and genetics. J Pediatr Ophthalmol Strabismus 1993; 30: 171–5.

8. Scott MH, Hejtmancik JF, Wozencraft LA et al. Autosomal dominant congenital cataract. Interocular phenotypic variability. Ophthalmology 1994; 101: 866–71.

9. Kruger SJ, Wilson ME Jr, Hutchinson AK et al. Cataracts and glaucoma in patients with oculocerebrorenal syndrome. Arch Ophthalmol 2003; 121: 1234–7.

10. Cibis GW, Waeltermann JM, Whitcraft CT et al. Lenticular opacities in carriers of Lowe's syndrome. Ophthalmology 1986; 93: 1041–5.

11. Lewis RA, Nussbaum RL, Stambolian D. Mapping X-linked ophthalmic diseases: provisional assignment of the locus for X-linked congenital cataracts and microcornea (the Nance-Horan syndrome) to Xp22.2-p22.3. Ophthalmology 1992; 97: 110–20.

12. Traboulsi EI, Lenz W, Gonzales-Ramos M et al. The Lenz microphthalmia syndrome. Am J Ophthalmol 1988; 105: 40–5.

13. Beigi B, O'Keefe M, Bowell R et al. Ophthalmic findings in classical galactosaemia – prospective study. Br J Ophthalmol 1993; 7: 162–4.

14. Cruysberg JR, Sengers RC, Pinckers A et al. Features of a syndrome with congenital cataract and hypertrophic cardiomyopathy. Am J Ophthalmol 1986; 102: 740–9.

15. Cruysberg JR, Wevers RA, van Engelen BG et al. Ocular and systemic manifestations of cerebrotendinous xanthomatosis. Am J Ophthalmol 1995; 120: 597–604.

16. Chang-Godinich A, Ades S, Schenkein D et al. Lens changes in hereditary hyperferritinemia-cataract syndrome. Am J Ophthalmol 2001; 132: 786–8.

17. Mumford AD, Cree IA, Arnold JD et al. The lens in hereditary hyperferritinaemia cataract syndrome contains crystalline deposits of L-ferritin. Br J Ophthalmol 2000; 84: 697–700.

18. Vijayalakshmi P, Srivastava KK, Poornima B, Nirmalan P. Visual outcome of cataract surgery in children with congenital rubella syndrome. J AAPOS 2003; 7: 91–5.

19. Cunha R, Moreira JB. Ocular findings in Down's syndrome. Am J Ophthalmol 1996; 122: 236–44.

20. Cohen MM. Hallermann-Streiff syndrome: a review. Am J Med Genet 1991; 41: 488–99.

21. Hennekam RC, van de Meeberg AG, van Doorne JM et al. Martsoff syndrome in a brother and sister: clinical features and pattern of inheritance. Eur J Pediatr 1988; 147: 539–43.

22. Zimmer C, Gosztonyi G, Cervos-Navarro J et al. Neuropathy with lysosomal charges in Marinesco-Sjogren syndrome: fine structural findings in skeletal muscle and conjunctiva. Neuropediatrics 1992; 23: 329–35.

23. Jonas JB, Mayer U, Budde WM. Ocular findings in cerebro-oculo-facial-skeletal syndrome (Pena-Shokeir-II syndrome). Eur J Ophthalmol 2003; 13: 209–11.

24. Czeizel A, Lowry RB. Syndrome of cataract, mild microcephaly, mental retardation and Perthes-like changes in sibs. Acta Paed Hung 1990; 30: 343–9.

25. Bernert J, Bartels I, Gatz G et al. Prenatal diagnosis of the Pallister-Killian mosaic aneuploidy syndrome. Am J Med Genet 1992; 42: 747–50.

26. Begeer J, Scholte F, van Essen A. Two sisters with mental retardation, cataract, ataxia, progressive hearing loss, and polyneuropathy. J Med Genet 1991; 28: 884–5.

27. Lundberg PO. Hereditary myopathy, oligophrenia, cataract, skeletal abnormalities and hypergonadotrophic hypogonadism: a new syndrome. Acta Genet Med Gemel 1974; 23: 245–7.

28. Pollitt RJ, Vamos E. Trichothiodystrophy, mental retardation, short stature, ataxia and gonadal dysfunction in three Moroccan siblings. Am J Med Genet 1990; 35: 566–73.

29. Temtamy SA, Sinbawy AH. Cataract, hypertrichosis, and mental retardation (CAHMR): a new autosomal recessive syndrome. Am J Med Genet 1991; 41: 432–3.

30. Hall J. Catch 22 (editorial). J Med Genet 1993; 30: 801–2.

31. Goldberg MF. Clinical manifestations of ectopia lentis et pupillae in 16 patients. Ophthalmology 1988; 95: 1080–7.

32. Reese AB. Persistent hyperplastic primary vitreous. Am J Ophthalmol 1955; 40: 317–31.

33. Karr DJ, Scott WE. Visual acuity results following treatment for persistent hyperplastic primary vitreous. Arch Ophthalmol 1986; 104: 662–7.

34. Foster CS, Barrett F. Cataract development and cataract surgery in patients with juvenile rheumatoid arthritis-associated iridocyclitis. Ophthalmology 1993; 100: 809–17.

35. Amaya L, Taylor D, Russell-Eggitt I et al. The morphology and natural history of childhood cataracts. Surv Ophthalmol 2003; 48: 125–44.

36. Parks MM, Johnson DA, Reed GW. Long-term visual results and complications in children with aphakia. A function of cataract type. Ophthalmology 1993; 100: 826–41.

37. Cheng KP, Hiles DA, Biglan AW, Pettapiece MC. Management of posterior lenticonus. J Pediatr Ophthalmol Strabismus 1991; 28: 143–9.

38. Hejtmancik JF, Smaoui N. Molecular genetics of cataract. Dev Ophthalmol 2003; 37: 67–82.

39. Lambert SR, Amaya L, Taylor DS. Detection and treatment of infantile cataracts. Int Ophthalmol Clin 1989; 29: 51–6.

40. O'Keefe M, Fenton S, Lanigan B. Visual outcomes and complications of posterior chamber intraocular lens implantation in the first year of life. J Cataract Refract Surg 2001; 27: 2006–11.

41. Amos CF, Lambert SR, Ward MA. Rigid gas permeable contact lens correction of aphakia following congenital cataract removal during infancy. J Pediatr Ophthalmol Strabismus 1992; 29: 243–5.

42. Amaya L, Speedwell L, Taylor DS. Contact lenses for infant aphakia. Br J Ophthalmol 1990; 74: 150–4.

43. Moore BD. Pediatric aphakic contact lens wear: rates of successful wear. J Pediatr Ophthalmol Strabismus 1993; 30: 253–8.

44. Lambert SR, Drack AV. Infantile cataracts. Surv Ophthalmol 1996; 40: 427–58.

45. Taylor D, Wright KW, Amaya L et al. Should we aggressively treat unilateral congenital cataracts? Br J Ophthalmol 2001; 85: 1120–6.

46. Lambert SR, Buckley EG, Plager DA et al. Unilateral intraocular lens implantation during the first six months of life. J AAPOS 1999; 3: 344–9.

47. Lambert SR, Lynn M, Drews-Botsch C et al. A comparison of grating visual acuity, strabismus, and reoperation outcomes among children with aphakia and pseudophakia after unilateral cataract surgery during the first six months of life. J AAPOS 2001; 5: 70–5.

48. Cassidy L, Rahi J, Nischal K et al. Outcome of lens aspiration and intraocular lens implantation in children aged 5 years and under. Br J Ophthalmol 2001; 85: 540–2.

49. Enyedi LB, Peterseim MW, Freedman SF, Buckley EG. Refractive changes after pediatric intraocular lens implantation. Am J Ophthalmol 1998; 126: 772–81.

50. Plager DA, Kipfer H, Sprunger DT et al. Refractive change in pediatric pseudophakia: 6-year follow-up. J Cataract Refract Surg 2002; 28: 810–5.

51. Flitcroft DI, Knight-Nanan D, Bowell R et al. Intraocular lenses in children: Changes in axial length, corneal curvature, and refraction. Br J Ophthalmol 1999; 83: 265–9.

52. Neumann D, Weissman BA, Isenberg SJ et al. The effectiveness of daily wear contact lenses for the correction of infantile aphakia. Arch Ophthalmol 1993; 111: 927–30.

53. Birch EE, Stager DR. The critical period for surgical treatment of dense congenital unilateral cataract. Invest Ophthalmol Vis Sci 1996; 37: 1532–8.

54. Lewis TL, Maurer D, Tytla ME et al. Vision in the "good" eye of children treated for unilateral congenital cataract. Ophthalmology 1992; 99: 1013–7.

55. Shawkat FS, Harris CM, Taylor DS et al. The optokinetic response differences between congenital profound and non-profound unilateral visual deprivation. Ophthalmology 1995; 102: 1615–22.

56. Gregg F, Parks M. Stereopsis after congenital monocular cataract extraction. Am J Ophthalmol 1992; 114: 314–7.

57. Papadopoulos M, Khaw PT. Meeting the challenge of glaucoma after paediatric cataract surgery. Eye 2003; 17: 1–2.

58. Simon JW, Mehta N, Simmons ST et al. Glaucoma after pediatric lensectomy/vitrectomy. Ophthalmology 1991; 98: 670–4.

59. Asrani S, Freedman S, Hasselblad V et al. Does primary intraocular lens implantation prevent "aphakic" glaucoma in children? J AAPOS 2000; 4: 33–9.

60. Pratt-Johnson JA, Tillson G. Intractable diplopia after vision restoration in unilateral cataract. Am J Ophthalmol 1989; 107: 23–7.

61. Lenart TD, Drack AV, Tarnuzzer RW et al. Heterochromia after pediatric cataract surgery. JAAPOS 2000; 4: 40–5.

62. Wheeler DT, Stager DR, Weakley DR. Endophthalmitis following pediatric intraocular surgery for congenital cataracts and congenital glaucoma. J Pediatr Ophthalmol Strabismus 1992; 29: 139–41.

63. Guo S, Nelson LB, Calhoun J, Levin A. Simultaneous surgery for congenital cataracts. J Pediatr Ophthalmol Strabismus 1990; 27: 23–5.

64. Jagger JD, Cooling RJ, Fison LG et al. Management of retinal detachment following congenital cataract surgery. Trans Ophthalmol Soc UK 1983; 103: 103–7.

65. Poer DV, Helveston EM, Ellis FD. Aphakic cystoid macular edema in children. Arch Ophthalmol 1981; 99: 249–52.

66. Nuyts RM, Edelhauser HF, Pels E, Breebaart AC. Toxic effects of detergent on the corneal endothelium. Arch Ophthalmol 1990; 108: 1158–62.

67. Lambert SR. Treatment of congenital cataract. BJO 2004; In press.

68. Magnusson G, Abrahamsson M, Sjostrand J. Changes in visual acuity from 4 to 12 years of age in children operated for bilateral congenital cataracts. Br J Ophthalmol 2002; 86: 1385–9.

69. Lambert SR, Lynn M, Drews-Botschc et al. Optotype acuity and reoperation rate after unilateral cataract surgery during the first six months of life with or without IOL implantation. BJO 2004; In press.

70. Dahan E, Drusedau MU. Choice of lens and dioptric power in pediatric pseudophakia. J Cataract Refract Surg 1997; 23: 618–23.

CHAPTER 48 Childhood Glaucoma

Maria Papadopoulos and Peng Tee Khaw

INTRODUCTION

Glaucoma in children is a rare, potentially blinding condition. There are many causes but elevated intraocular pressure (IOP) is what they all have in common. The clinical manifestations of raised IOP are variable. Successful control of IOP is crucial and challenging and most often achieved surgically, with medical therapy playing a supportive role. The correction of ametropia and amblyopia therapy are also integral in management. Developing a trusting relationship with the child and their parents plays a key role in achieving the goal of preserving a lifetime of vision.

CLASSIFICATION

Childhood glaucoma can be classified as *primary*, where an isolated developmental abnormality of the anterior chamber angle exists, and *secondary,* where aqueous outflow is reduced due to congenital or acquired ocular diseases or systemic disorders (Table 48.1). The classifications will change as we learn more about each condition.

CLINICAL FINDINGS

A child suspected of having glaucoma usually presents in one of three ways:
1. Clinical manifestations of elevated IOP;
2. With a condition that predisposes them to glaucoma, e.g., aphakia; and
3. As part of screening when there is a family history of pediatric glaucoma.

The clinical manifestations are largely determined by the magnitude of the elevated IOP and the age of onset. Very high IOP can present dramatically in a newborn with cloudy, enlarged corneas. However, a slower rise in IOP results in a less acute presentation of an infant with buphthalmos but no corneal clouding or photophobia. Furthermore, the timing of the pressure rise influences the clinical features owing to the limited potential of the young eye to deform.

Glaucoma from any cause in a neonate and infant is synonymous with the *classic triad of lacrimation, blepharospasm, and photophobia* due to corneal edema from elevated IOP. These signs are not specific but are suggestive of glaucoma and may appear before the hazy cornea (the most frequent physical sign) and buphthalmos become obvious. Glaucoma should be excluded in any newborn or infant who presents with these signs. After the age of 3 years, children are more likely to present with progressive myopia or strabismus or after having failed routine school vision testing. In late-onset presentations, the child may

Table 48.1 Classification of childhood glaucoma

PRIMARY
(a) **Primary congenital glaucoma (*isolated trabeculodysgenesis*)**
(b) **Juvenile open angle glaucoma**

SECONDARY
(a) **Anterior segment dysgenesis**
  Iridodysgenesis: Iris hypoplasia, aniridia, congenital ectropion uveae
  Corneodysgenesis
    Peripheral: Axenfeld anomaly
    Midperipheral: Reiger anomaly
    Central: Peter anomaly
    Corneal size: Microcornea, megalocornea
(b) **Other ocular disease/treatment**
  Aphakia following congenital cataract surgery
  Persistent hyperplastic primary vitreous
  Retinopathy of prematurity
  Lens related: Ectopia lentis, microspherophakia
  Microphthalmos
  Trauma related: hyphema, angle recession
(c) **Phacomatoses**
  Sturge-Weber syndrome (Enchephalotrigeminal angiomatosis)
    Facial nevus flammeus (Port wine stain)
    Klippel Trenaunay Weber syndrome (combined form)
  Neurofibromatosis (von Recklinghausen disease)
  Oculodermal melanocytosis (Nevus of Ota)
  von-Hippel Lindau syndrome
(d) **Inflammatory/infective disease**
  Juvenile chronic arthritis
  Congenital rubella
  Congenital syphilis
  Cytomegalovirus disease
  Herpes simplex disease
(e) **Ocular tumors**
  Benign: iris cysts, juvenile xanthogranuloma
  Malignant: retinoblastoma, leukemia
(f) **Metabolic disease**
  Oculocerebrorenal syndrome (Lowe syndrome)
  Homocystinuria
  Mucopolysaccharidoses, e.g., Hurlers
  Cystinosis
(g) **Chromosomal disorders**
  Down syndrome (trisomy 21)
  Patau syndrome (trisomy 13-15)
  Turner syndrome (XO)
  Prader–Willi syndrome
(h) **Connective tissue abnormalities**
  Marfan syndrome
  Weil–Marchesani syndrome
  Homocystinuria
  Ehler Danlos syndrome
  Sulfite oxidase deficiency
  Osteogenesis imperfecta
(i) **Other systemic congenital disorders**
  Rubinstein–Taybi syndrome
  Pierre Robin syndrome
  Cutis marmorata telangiectasia congenita

be asymptomatic until they become aware of visual field defects or start bumping into objects.

Unique features of glaucoma in infancy

Generalized ocular enlargement

Buphthalmos is a descriptive term that refers to a prominent, enlarged eye due to elevated IOP from any cause in infancy (Fig. 48.1). It is due to corneal and scleral collagen immaturity. The potential for corneal enlargement usually ceases by the age of 3 although the sclera remains deformable up until the age of 10. As the IOP rises, Descemet's membrane eventually ruptures with the edges usually retracting as a scroll to form a ridge known as *Haab's striae* (Fig. 48.2). They are typically horizontal and linear centrally but concentric with the limbus in peripheral cornea. They rarely occur after 18 months of age or with corneal diameters less than 12.5 mm. As the underlying endothelium is damaged, localized or diffuse corneal edema results from the influx of aqueous into the stroma between the ruptured edges, causing a sudden increase in cloudiness. With lowering of the IOP, corneal clouding typically begins clearing in the periphery first. The photophobia may persist with normalization of IOP due to the Haab's striae. However, it is usually reduced and so may be an indicator of success.

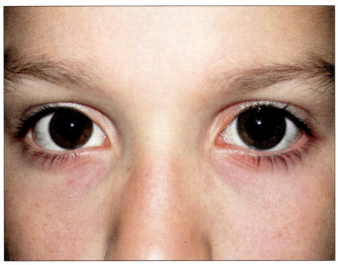

Fig. 48.1 Child with unilateral buphthalmos.

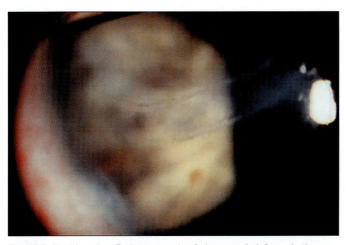

Fig. 48.2 Haab's striae. Pathognomonic of glaucoma in infancy in the presence of enlarged corneas.

Reversible optic nerve cupping

Changes of the optic nerve in children due to glaucoma are similar to those that occur in adults and are just as important in making a diagnosis and evaluating progression.

Glaucomatous optic disc cupping in infants differs from adults in two major ways:

1. It occurs *earlier and more rapidly*, with severe excavation possible even at birth.
2. It is often *reversible* if IOP reduction occurs before irreversible nerve atrophy.

DIFFERENTIAL DIAGNOSIS

The differential diagnosis of glaucoma in children is broad and should always be borne in mind to distinguish a potentially blinding condition from a relatively benign one. An extensive list of differential diagnoses is outlined in Table 48.2.

Corneal enlargement

Megalocornea

Megalocornea (anterior megalophthalmos) is a bilateral developmental anomaly where the anterior segment of the eye is larger than normal in the absence of raised IOP. It is a rare, congenital, usually X-linked recessive condition (90% males), which is bilateral, symmetrical, and nonprogressive. It is characterized by marked corneal enlargement (12–18 mm) *but the IOP, optic disc, and axial length are normal and there are no Haab's striae.* The diagnosis is made by careful exclusion based on repeated examination and should not be made unless all signs for glaucoma are negative. They must be followed up to detect glaucoma and refractive amblyopia.

Table 48.2 Differential diagnosis of childhood glaucoma
Cornea enlargement **(No Descemet's membrane splits, corneal edema, nor progression in these conditions)** Megalocornea Megalophthalmos Axial myopia Osteogenesis imperfecta Connective tissue disorders (i.e., fibrillinopathies)
Corneal splits **(No corneal enlargement in these conditions)** Birth trauma (history) Hydrops (history)
Corneal edema or opacity **(Usually no corneal enlargement unless associated with glaucoma, which is uncommon in these conditions)** Birth trauma Congenital corneal dystrophies Sclerocornea Metabolic, e.g., mucopolysaccharidoses, cystinosis Infective, e.g., congenital rubella, herpes simplex keratitis
Watering and "red eye" **(No Descemet's membrane splits, edema, nor corneal enlargement in these conditions)** Conjunctivitis Nasolacrimal duct obstruction Corneal epithelial defect, very occasionally dystrophy Ocular inflammation
Optic nerve abnormalities Congenital optic nerve pits Optic disc colobomata Physiological cupping in large optic discs

Congenital high myopia

Corneal enlargement may be present but the posterior pole findings such as tilted optic nerve insertion, peripapillary scleral crescent, and choroidal mottling characteristic of axial myopia serve to distinguish this condition from glaucoma.

Corneal clouding

Sclerocornea

Sclerocornea is a congenital, bilateral, often asymmetric disease that may be sporadic or autosomal dominant. It is characterized by predominantly *peripheral corneal opacification with vascularization*. Glaucoma may be associated due to goniodysgenesis.

Congenital corneal dystrophies

Corneal dystrophies are characterized by being congenital, hereditary, and symmetrical. Normal corneal diameters and IOP along with a positive family history are useful in differentiating these from glaucoma. Congenital hereditary endothelial dystrophy (CHED) typically presents at birth or in the first few years of life characterized by bilateral diffuse, corneal edema with significant stromal thickening; the latter is not a feature of congenital hereditary stromal dystrophy (CHSD). Posterior polymorphous dystrophy can also present at birth (occasionally in infancy) with corneal edema but is characterized by diffuse irregular thickening and opacification at the level of Descemet's membrane best seen on retroillumination. Photophobia and epiphora are unusual. Meesman corneal dystrophy usually becomes evident in the first few months with ocular irritation from the ruptured epithelial cysts, which typify this condition.

Obstetric trauma

Compression of the globe with forceps at the time of delivery can result in Descemet's membrane breaks and corneal edema that may mimic Haab's striae, but it is rare. They are usually located centrally with a smooth, fusiform appearance and often vertically orientated and parallel if multiple. Although there is no definite way of differentiating between the two, obstetrical corneal trauma is usually unilateral and left-sided and there is *no corneal enlargement*, which is significant considering that ruptures of Descemet's membrane almost never occur without corneal enlargement in glaucoma.

Inflammatory/infectious diseases

Inflammatory disease, such as *keratitis* and *iridocyclitis*, can cause corneal edema and enlargement (if IOP is raised) but there are often prominent inflammatory signs. *Intrauterine infection with rubella* virus may result in transient or permanent corneal clouding with or without elevated pressure. Infection in the first trimester can result in glaucoma, which closely resembles primary congenital glaucoma (PCG) both in gonioscopic appearance and in its response to goniotomy.

Metabolic disorders

Lowe syndrome, the *mucopolysaccharidoses*, *cystinosis*, and *corneal lipidosis* can produce corneal clouding mimicking the corneal edema of glaucoma.

Epiphora, photophobia, and "red eye"

Nasolacrimal duct obstruction

By far the most common cause of epiphora is nasolacrimal duct obstruction. Although it can also be associated with blepharospasm, photophobia is not associated with this condition and should make the examiner consider the diagnosis of glaucoma.

Conjunctivitis

Glaucoma may present as a "red eye" mimicking conjunctivitis. Any cause of conjunctivitis can cause redness and watering. Corneal abrasions are common causes of acute ocular irritation and are often diagnosed from the history and examination.

Optic nerve abnormalities

Congenital malformations of the disc such as *congenital pits* and *colobomata* may be difficult to differentiate from glaucomatous optic neuropathy. Distinguishing *large physiological cupping* is more of a problem in children over 3 years who may be too young for visual fields and in whom globe enlargement is not obvious. In these cases it may be helpful to examine family members as they may have similar optic discs.

CLASSIFICATION

Primary

Primary congenital glaucoma (PCG)

PCG is typically bilateral (70–80%) and usually manifests in the first year of life. Presentation at or within a few days of birth is thought to be associated with a more severe angle anomaly, a worst prognosis, and greater likelihood of an inherited disease. Diagnosis is based on the finding of *isolated trabeculodysgenesis*.

Demographics

PCG is the commonest glaucoma in infancy but has a reported incidence of only about 1 in 10,000–20,000 live births in Western countries.[1] The incidence in the Middle East is 1:8200 live births in Palestinian Arabs and 1:2500 live births in Saudi Arabians. The highest reported incidence is 1:1250 in Slovakian gypsies. Parental consanguinity is thought to be responsible for the higher prevalence in certain ethnic and religious groups.

In Europe, the United States, and Japan, PCG occurs more frequently in males than females at a ratio of between 2–25:1. Familial cases in both the Middle East and the Slovak Romany population tend to have an equal sex distribution.

Genetics

Most cases of PCG are sporadic. A family history of glaucoma is reported in 10–40% of cases associated with autosomal recessive inheritance and variable penetrance ranging from 40 to 100%. Insufficient data exist to confirm or reject multifactorial or dominant forms of the disease.

GCL3A is the major locus for PCG, accounting perhaps for 85–90% of all familial cases. It has been mapped to the short arm of chromosome 2p21 and the GLC3B locus to chromosome 1p36. At least one more locus is believed to exist. Molecular genetic studies suggest the primary molecular defect underlying the majority of cases of PCG (87% of familial and 27% of sporadic cases) is related to mutations of the *CYP1B1 gene* associated with the GLC3A locus.[2] It encodes for enzyme cytochrome P4501B1, which is postulated to participate in the development and function of the eye.

With regards sibling risk, Jay and Rice, in their series of predominantly Caucasian patients with PCG (low parental consanguinity), found a family history in only 4% and the risk of another affected child to be as low as 3% if a male child and almost zero if a girl.[3] Even though the occurrence of PCG in siblings and offspring is low, it is prudent to examine the siblings and offspring of patients, especially in the first 6 months of life.

Pathogenesis

The pathogenesis of PCG remains disputed. Pathology studies suggest that the appearance of an immature angle results from the developmental arrest of tissues derived from cranial neural crest cells in the third trimester of gestation. With regards to the mechanism of glaucoma, obstruction to outflow was classically thought to be due to the presence of an impermeable membrane (*Barkan's membrane*) related to mesoblastic remnants but this has never been verified histopathologically nor clinically. It is now thought to be due to thick, compacted trabecular sheets. It seems likely that the way forward in understanding the pathogenesis of this condition will be to identify the responsible gene(s) and protein(s).

Gonioscopic findings

The characteristic gonioscopic appearance includes a flat iris insertion into the trabecular meshwork and the absence of an angle recess. There is usually no obvious membrane visible in the angle but instead a pale amorphous tissue known as "Lister's morning mist." Changes due to the physical stretching of structures from elevated IOP include a thin and hypopigmented iris stroma, peripheral scalloping of the posterior pigmented iris layer, and easily visible, hyperemic, iris vessels with circumferential vessels running tortuously in the peripheral iris or on the ciliary body. In unilateral disease, fellow eyes usually have abnormal angles or corneal diameters and may represent drainage angles that have opened late, leading to *spontaneous arrest* of the disease.

Treatment

The principal treatment is surgery that aims to eliminate or bypass the obstruction to aqueous outflow. Preoperatively, pilocarpine 0.5–1% every 6–8 hours may allow corneal edema to clear by reducing IOP and so improve visualization of the angle at the time of surgery. Its IOP lowering effect, however, is limited by the abnormal angle. Postoperatively, it may enhance aqueous outflow and prevent anterior synechiae following goniotomy. Conventional angle surgery, goniotomy and trabeculotomy, are the procedures of choice in PCG but require an experienced surgeon and often more than one operation to achieve IOP control. They enjoy a high rate of success in favorable cases such as unoperated eyes before the age of 1. The surgical prognosis may relate more to the severity of the disease than the surgical technique. The options in children that fail angle surgery are either enhanced filtering or tube drainage surgery.

In the past this diagnosis was synonymous with a poor visual result. However, earlier detection, improved surgical techniques with better IOP control along with aggressive amblyopia treatment has resulted in an improved visual prognosis. Over 50% of eyes will see 6/15 or better.[4]

Juvenile open angle glaucoma (JOAG)

Juvenile glaucoma is a nonspecific term that traditionally describes a group of patients presenting after the first few years of life but before the age of 35. However, there is a distinct group of patients who have no anterior segment abnormalities and present late in childhood with glaucoma. Often there is a strong family history of glaucoma. Several of these families have mutations of the *myocilin/TIGR (trabecular meshwork inducible glucocorticoid response) gene* at the GLC1A locus on chromosome 1q21–q31.[5] These patients typically have high pressures (40–50 mmHg) and do not respond well long term to medical or laser treatment, often requiring enhanced filtration surgery.

Secondary

Anterior segment dysgenesis (ASD)

ASD represents a spectrum of developmental disease involving neural crest mesenchyme. *Axenfeld anomaly* refers to the presence of posterior embryotoxon (anteriorly displaced, prominent Schwalbe's line) with attached iris strands. When these peripheral abnormalities are associated with iris changes such as corectopia or atrophy it is called *Rieger anomaly* (Fig. 48.3). In association with systemic anomalies such as abnormal teeth and facial abnormalities, particularly hypertelorism, it is referred to as *Rieger syndrome*. Families with Axenfeld/Rieger anomaly show an autosomal dominant pattern of inheritance. With regards to Reiger syndrome two loci have been identified, RIEG1 at chromosome 4q25 associated with the *RIEG/PITX2* gene[6] and RIEG2 at 13q14 with an unidentified gene. It is also associated with abnormalities in *FOXC1* gene and *PAX6* gene. Patients with segmental duplication of the *FOXC1* gene may have increased central corneal thickness, potentially leading to overestimation of IOP.[7]

Peter anomaly is characterized by a congenital central corneal opacity with underlying defects in stroma, Descemet's membrane, and endothelium with iris strands and sometimes lens attachment to the periphery of this opacity. It is usually bilateral (80%) and sporadic. Peter anomaly may result from abnormalities of the *PAX6* gene on chromosome 11p13 and *RIEG/PITX2* and *FOXC1* genes.

There is a subgroup of patients with a distinctive hypoplastic iris stroma who are probably part of the anterior segment dysgenesis spectrum. *Iris hypoplasia* is associated with a characteristic maldevelopment of the anterior stromal layer of the iris and early onset glaucoma and can have the same systemic features as Axenfeld/Rieger syndrome. Autosomal dominant iris hypoplasia is associated with *RIEG/PITX2* gene mutations.

The risk of glaucoma with these anomalies is approximately 50–70% so lifelong surveillance is indicated. Glaucoma usually occurs in childhood or young adulthood, very rarely in infancy. The IOP is typically labile. The cause of outflow obstruction is believed to be due to the arrested maturation of angle structures. Angle surgery has a success rate lower than that in PCG. Medical therapy is recommended first, followed by enhanced filtering surgery. It is the authors' impression that the more disorganized the anterior segment, the greater the risk of failure and the more

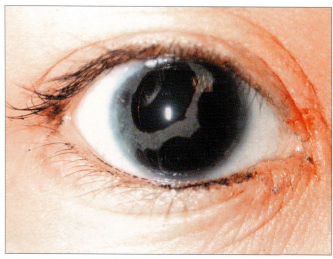

Fig. 48.3 Rieger anomaly with corectopia and posterior embryotoxon.

potent the antiscarring agent required. A potent antimetabolite is also more likely to achieve IOP in the low teens and so significantly reduce corneal opacification (Figs. 48.4, 48.5).

Chronic pupil dilation or an optical iridectomy (via a scleral approach to prevent further corneal scarring) should be considered rather than penetrating keratoplasty, which is associated with disappointing results.[8] Primary tube drainage surgery may be indicated in the most severe cases.

Aniridia

Aniridia is characterized by bilateral variable absence of the iris with findings such as photophobia, nystagmus, foveola hypoplasia, amblyopia, and strabismus. Visual loss is further compounded by a high incidence of glaucoma, cataract, ectopia lentis, and corneal surface abnormalities due to corneal epithelial stem cell failure. Minimally affected patients demonstrate vascular abnormalities on iris and retinal fluorescein angiography. Aniridia results from abnormal neuroectodermal development secondary to *PAX6* gene mutations at chromosome 11p13. Inheritance is usually autosomal dominant although recessive transmission is possible. Sporadic aniridia is associated with Wilms tumor, genitourinary abnormalities, and mental retardation (WAGR) related to large deletions of 11p13, which encompasses *PAX6* and the adjacent Wilms tumor locus.

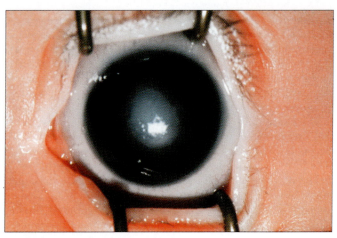

Fig. 48.4 Uncontrolled IOP and dense central corneal opacification before antimetabolite trabeculectomy.

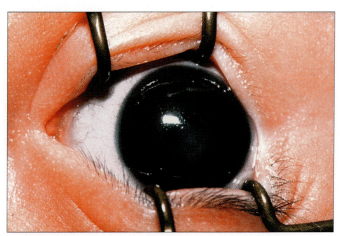

Fig. 48.5 Same eye with controlled IOP in low teens and improved corneal clarity after surgery.

Glaucoma associated with aniridia is usually due to progressive angle closure from the iris stump, presenting often in preadolescence or early adulthood with an incidence ranging from 6 to 75%. Medical therapy should always be the first line of treatment in aniridia as this is the safest but surgery is often inevitable. Goniotomy both as therapy and prophylaxis[9] has been described but not widely practiced due to the potential risks. Trabeculotomy may be safer but is associated with a success rate poorer than that in PCG. Enhanced filtration surgery with MMC is indicated but hypotony should be avoided due to the danger of lens–corneal touch, which will cause both cataract and corneal decompensation. Tube drainage surgery is associated with favorable results and is indicated if trabeculectomy fails or as a primary procedure if future surgery such as lensectomy is contemplated.[10] Symptomatic relief of photophobia can be achieved with tinted spectacles or contact lenses which can be painted with an artificial iris.

Phakomatoses

The commonest phakomatosis associated with glaucoma is *Sturge–Weber* syndrome (encephalotrigeminal angiomatosis; see Chapter 69), a sporadic condition characterized by a facial cutaneous angioma (port wine stain) present at birth, which affects the regions innervated by the first and second divisions of the trigeminal nerve. Choroidal hemangiomas occur in 40% of patients of whom 90% develop glaucoma. They are usually diffuse and can be easily missed on examination. Upper lid involvement is usually present when patients present with elevated IOP. It can occur at any time from birth to adulthood. Glaucoma can arise from elevated episcleral venous pressure and goniodysgenesis.

Other phakomatoses can be associated with glaucoma although with an incidence lower than that of Sturge–Weber syndrome. *Klippel–Trenaunay–Weber syndrome* is characterized by a triad of cutaneous hemangioma and varicosities involving one limb and hypertrophy of bone and soft tissue. Most cases with glaucoma also have a facial nevus (*combined form*). *Neurofibromatosis* is an autosomal dominant condition, which may first present with iris abnormalities, e.g., ectropion uveae and glaucoma, before the systemic disease is apparent. Glaucoma occurs in 50% of patients with plexiform neuroma so these patients must be followed for life. It is typically unilateral and usually presents at or shortly after birth. *Congenital ectropion uveae* is a rare nonprogressive condition strongly associated with glaucoma and may occur with neurofibromatosis.

Surgery is indicated when medical treatment fails. This is more likely with congenital presentation, which responds to angle surgery if there is evidence of goniodysgenesis, but less well than PCG.[11] Otherwise, filtration surgery with antimetabolites is the treatment of choice. However, the potential for serious complications is high. Choroidal hemangiomas may give rise to expulsive choroidal hemorrhage if rapid decompression of the globe occurs or to choroidal effusions if there is prolonged hypotony. Choroidal effusions occur at an IOP relatively higher than expected in these patients. It follows that surgery in these patients must be coupled with measures to minimize hypotony.

Aphakic glaucoma

Aphakic glaucoma is one of the most serious causes of late visual loss following congenital cataract surgery. Early, acute angle closure from pupil block is now rare but open angle aphakic glaucoma may complicate initial uneventful surgery at any stage. Its pathogenesis is uncertain; both chemical (inflammatory cells, lens remnants, and vitreous-derived factors) and mechanical (lack of ciliary body tension and trabecular meshwork collapse) theories have been proposed. The incidence of glaucoma following childhood cataract surgery varies with duration of follow-up and ranges from 5% with simple aspiration[12] to as high as 41% with lensectomy and vitrectomy with at least a 5-year follow-up.[13] Risk factors for aphakic glaucoma such as microcornea, poor pupil dilation, early surgery, the need for secondary surgery, and nuclear cataract are well documented. The role of posterior capsule integrity and intraocular lens implantation is less clear. Certainly following meticulous cataract surgery, irrespective of the method chosen, lifelong surveillance for glaucoma is crucial. If IOP measurement is difficult, it is essential to frequently monitor the optic disc for progressive cupping. Excessive loss of hyperopia may also be a useful sign.

Aphakic glaucoma presents a therapeutic challenge, as it is notoriously refractory to treatment. Angle surgery does not provide good long-term control. Cyclodiode laser treatment provides temporizing treatment with occasional long-term control.[14] Filtration surgery with MMC not only has a poor success rate[15] but also often excludes postoperative contact lens use due to the risk of endophthalmitis. Drainage tube implants probably have the highest chance of long-term success particularly when combined with antifibrotic therapy.[16] However, aphakic eyes have higher rates of complications when hypotony occurs, particularly if buphthalmic. Thus, techniques to avoid catastrophic hypotony are essential.

Inflammatory glaucoma

Glaucoma may arise following inflammation from any cause but is most commonly seen in juvenile chronic arthropathies (30%) and congenital infective conditions. It is multifactorial due to chronic cellular trabecular obstruction, trabeculitis, peripheral anterior synechiae, pupil block, being secondary to cataract removal, and following chronic topical steroid usage. If chronic steroid usage is an essential part of the disease management, then the intraocular pressure should be managed within this context rather than constantly changing the steroid regimen to reduce intraocular pressure. The glaucoma that develops is characteristically refractory to treatment and warrants a MMC trabeculectomy. Angle surgery often requires medical treatment to control IOP.[17] Primary tube drainage surgery is indicated if lensectomy is contemplated in the future or if aphakia is present.[18] The risk of postoperative hypotony is high due to potentially brittle aqueous production. It is essential that these patients are adequately immunosuppressed systemically, particularly with steroids, before surgery to maximize success and reduce complications.

Miscellaneous conditions

A wide variety of other conditions are associated with childhood glaucoma, including syndromes and congenital malformations (Table 48.1 on p. 458). For many of these rare conditions there is very little precedent in the literature as to the appropriate treatment of glaucoma. Determining the mechanism of the glaucoma by a thorough history and examination along with an assessment of risk factors for surgical failure results in the best treatment plan. For instance, a variety of diseases such as *Marfan syndrome*, *Weil Marchesani syndrome*, *homocystinuria*, and *high myopia* may give rise to childhood glaucoma, which is usually associated with lens displacement and secondary pupil block. A prophylactic iridectomy and chronic miosis may be required to prevent pupil block glaucoma or dislocation of the lens into the anterior chamber.

It is important to mention childhood tumors such as *leukemia* or *retinoblastoma*, which may give rise to glaucoma from outflow obstruction by tumor cells or secondary hemorrhage. The diagnosis of these rare conditions is important as inadvertent surgery and release of malignant cells external to the globe may worsen the prognosis for life. The treatment is generally conservative and involves treating the primary disorder along with topical medical treatment and cyclodestruction.

MANAGEMENT

Assessment

The suspicion of glaucoma in a child should always be treated seriously and with urgency to minimize visual impairment. This requires examination either in the clinic or office or under anesthesia, depending on the child's age and ability to cooperate. The initial consultation and assessment is a vital part of management as it is the beginning of what may potentially be a lifetime relationship between the ophthalmologist, patient, and their parents. The aim of the initial assessment in a neonate or infant is either to rule out glaucoma or to establish that enough evidence for glaucoma exists to justify examination under anesthesia (EUA) for a more complete examination and possible surgery. If there is any doubt as to the diagnosis it is advisable to proceed with an EUA. If glaucoma is the presumptive diagnosis it may be preferable to have the initial anesthetic examination performed by the surgeon who will proceed with surgery to avoid unnecessary anesthesia and delay in surgery.

Examination in clinic/office

With regards to history it is important to determine the age of clinical onset for prognosis, associated congenital defects for anesthetic risk, problems during pregnancy (rubella), a family history of pediatric glaucoma and parental consanguinity.

Reducing the level of ambient illumination often allows the child to open their eyes, permitting a more complete examination. By just observing an infant it may be possible to assess the presence of corneal edema, lacrimation, photophobia, blepharospasm, and the relative and actual size of both eyes. If a neonate has recently been fed, a thorough examination including applanation tonometry with a Perkins tonometer or a Tono-Pen is possible. When indicated, it is important to examine the patient's parents as the presence of subtle signs of anterior segment dysgenesis in the parents may change the genetic advice given and alter the management of subsequent siblings.

Examination under anesthesia
Anesthesia

As a general rule, all anesthetics lower the IOP with the possible exception of ketamine, chloral hydrate, and nitrous oxide. Inhalation anesthetics, such as sevoflurane, may substantially lower the IOP. This makes an appropriate anesthetic vital in the assessment of these patients, especially in subtle cases where it can have a profound impact on the timing of the diagnosis and the visual prognosis. Furthermore, it follows that the finding of a normal IOP with the use of agents known to reduce IOP does not exclude glaucoma.

Ketamine hydrochloride is given intravenously following the use of local anesthetic patches. Children are premedicated with atropine, which reduces bronchial secretions and oral midazolam. Ketamine can cause a transient rise in IOP, which may last 3 to 4 minutes so the timing of IOP measurement is critical. Its duration is short, usually lasting 10 to 15 minutes. Its use in children is not universally accepted by pediatric anesthetists.

Ocular examination

Intraocular pressure measurement

The gold standard for tonometry in children is the Perkins handheld tonometer with a blue filter after installation of fluorescein. Preferably, the eyes should be in the primary position and motionless as pressure readings may be altered by eye movements. The IOP should always be measured several times in both eyes. The Tono-Pen has the advantage of requiring only a small area of contact and therefore useful with large central corneal opacities. Accurate IOP measurement can be difficult as the type of anesthetic, instrumentation, corneal thickness, and opacities affects it. Hence, tonometry under anesthesia generally provides only an approximation of the true tension. *It should never be the sole method by which the presence or control of glaucoma is assessed.*

Corneal diameter measurement

The horizontal corneal diameter is measured with calipers from limbus to limbus and checked with a graduated ruler with estimation to the nearest 0.25 mm. The normal horizontal neonatal diameter is up to 10.5 mm increasing by about 1 mm in the first year of life. *A diameter greater than 11 mm in a newborn and 12 mm in an infant less than 1 year is very suggestive of raised IOP, but with Haab's striae it is diagnostic.* A measurement of greater than 13 mm in a child of any age and asymmetrical corneal diameters is abnormal. An increasing corneal diameter in a vulnerable eye may indicate inadequate control of IOP, requiring further treatment.

Corneal thickness

Increased corneal thickness may lead to an overestimation of the IOP e.g., a 750-μm-thick cornea may overestimate the IOP by about 10 mmHg. However, the exact relationship between corneal thickness and IOP in children is uncertain. Pachymetry is indicated to avoid unnecessary treatment.

Anterior segment examination

The cornea can be examined with a portable slit lamp for edema, opacities, and Haab's striae. Oblique illumination and magnification are necessary as the signs can sometimes be subtle. The presence of *corneal enlargement with splits, with or without edema, indicates raised IOP at some stage in infancy.* Persistent corneal edema may be a sign of poorly controlled glaucoma.

When a deep anterior chamber in infants is associated with an enlarged cornea, glaucoma should be strongly suspected. Detecting coexisting lens opacities is important as they may require treatment and influence the choice of glaucoma surgery. Furthermore, lens subluxation should be identified as it increases the likelihood of vitreous prolapse during surgery and worsens the prognosis.

Gonioscopy

Direct gonioscopy with a *Koeppe* lens is crucial in making the correct diagnosis, which determines the most appropriate operation and prognosis.

Posterior segment examination

Optic disc The appearance of the optic disc is by far the most important and sensitive parameter for both diagnosis and progression of disease, as it is influenced by neither anesthesia nor the effect of growth. The pupil is not dilated preoperatively as this may alter the angle appearance, spuriously increase IOP,

and increase the risk of lens damage if surgery is required. An indirect ophthalmoscope with a small pupil facility can be very useful in obtaining a view of the disc. The optic disc is carefully recorded with a drawing or photograph if possible. Richardson noted a cup:disc ratio (CDR) of greater than 0.3 in only 3% of 468 normal newborn eyes,[19] in contrast to Shaffer who found a CDR of greater than 0.3 in 61% of 85 eyes in infants less than one year with congenital glaucoma.[20] *A CDR > 0.3 in an infant less than 1 year or > 0.5 in a child and disc asymmetry should greatly increase suspicion of glaucoma.* An increase in disc cupping is definite evidence of poorly controlled glaucoma and the need for further treatment, regardless of the IOP measurement obtained.

Retina and vitreous

The remainder of the fundus should be examined for any associated abnormalities such as foveal hypoplasia associated with aniridia, choroidal hemangiomas in Sturge–Weber syndrome, and pigmentary retinopathy associated with rubella.

Retinoscopy

If satisfactory cycloplegic refraction is not possible in the outpatient setting, retinoscopy will need to be performed during the EUA if corneal clarity allows. Progressive myopia may suggest inadequate IOP control.

Systemic examination

While the patient is under anesthesia, a general examination that is not possible while the patient is awake and venesection for laboratory investigation (e.g., screening for infective agents and chromosome studies) can be performed. If necessary, other investigations such as keratometry, pachymetry, and ultrasonography can also be performed.

Interpretation of findings

The diagnosis and decision to treat is based on the overall clinical findings, especially on the three most important signs: IOP, corneal enlargement, and optic disc changes. When the IOP reading is discordant with other findings one should remember that it may be unreliable. For example, when the IOP is normal but buphthalmos, corneal enlargement with Haab's striae, and pathological optic cupping are present, it may be a case of either falsely low IOP related to anesthesia, measurement error, or "arrested" glaucoma. If the diagnosis is unclear but there is a high risk of glaucoma, then clearly further examinations under anesthesia are necessary to confirm pathology before committing the patient to surgery. If glaucoma is confirmed, it is important to explain early to the parents the chronic nature of the condition, the possible need for repeat surgery, and the definite lifelong follow-up as glaucoma can relapse at any stage and may develop in the fellow eye of unilateral glaucoma. The majority of children require an EUA up until about the age of 5.

Ultrasound investigations

Axial length measurement and anterior chamber depth

(see Chapter 12)

Serial axial lengths can be useful adjuncts in infants when the distensible eye is still vulnerable to IOP. In glaucoma, axial length measurements are usually asymmetrical in contrast to megalocornea and normal eyes. There usually is a slight decrease in axial length following successful lowering of IOP. Anterior chamber depth is usually increased in infants with glaucoma.

B-scan and ultrasound biomicroscopy (UBM)
(see Chapter 12)
High-resolution contact B-scan may be a useful adjunct in the preoperative evaluation of an eye with opaque media to detect the presence of severe cupping or exclude posterior segment pathology. UBM can identify details of the structure of the angle, ciliary body, cornea, and lens.

Treatment

The treatment of primary and secondary childhood glaucoma differs. Primary glaucoma is basically surgical conditions. In secondary glaucoma, medical treatment is usually first line followed by surgery if ineffective and angle surgery is usually associated with limited success.

Medical therapy
Long-term medical therapy is sometimes necessary if surgery is significantly high risk or not possible due to risk of anesthesia. As a general principle, we do not persist with prolonged, suboptimal medical treatment as it results in progressive optic nerve damage and has a deleterious effect on conjunctival wound healing after glaucoma filtration surgery.

Although drugs used in childhood glaucoma are similar to those in adults, great care must be exercised when prescribing in children as they are at a higher risk of systemic, potentially fatal side effects from topical administration. Blood levels from drops can approach or even exceed oral therapeutic levels. To reduce systemic toxicity parents should be instructed to use punctal occlusion for 3–5 minutes after instilling drops.

Parasympathomimetics
Parasympathomimetic agents, such as pilocarpine 1–4%, act at parasympathetic receptors to increase outflow via the trabecular meshwork. Systemic toxicity is rarely a problem but symptoms of gastrointestinal upset, sweating, bradycardia, hypotension, bronchospasm, and central nervous system stimulation can occur. *Pilocarpine gel* may cause less side effects with daily nocturnal use and so be better tolerated by children. Parasympathomimetic agents are first-line treatment in PCG.

β blockers
Beta blockers reduce aqueous humor production through β_2 and possibly β_1 ciliary body receptors. Use in premature or newborn infants and in children with asthma or any cardiac problems including arrhythmias should be avoided. It is important to inquire about asthma symptoms, which may manifest with nocturnal cough in children rather than wheezing. *Betaxolol, timolol 0.1%,* and *long-acting timolol 0.25%* are the β blockers of choice due to their superior risk profile.

Carbonic anhydrase inhibitors
Carbonic anhydrase inhibitors reduce ciliary body production of aqueous humor. Local side effects are more common than systemic with corneal decompensation potentially the most serious. Although *oral acetazolamide* is more potent in reducing IOP than dorzolamide, its use in children is limited by serious systemic side effects such as metabolic acidosis, failure to thrive, disturbed hyperactive behavior and bed-wetting. Therefore, it should be considered only on a short-term basis prior to surgery. *Dorzolamide*, which is as efficacious as betaxolol but safer or less irritant, and *brinzolamide* are useful as second-line drugs or when β blockers are contraindicated.

Prostaglandin agonists
Prostaglandin analogues reduce IOP primarily by enhancing uveoscleral outflow. PGF2α receptors are also found in the trabecular meshwork, suggesting a secondary effect on outflow. *Latanoprost* may be less efficacious in children compared to adults both as monotherapy and in combination with other medications.[21] Parents should be advised about the possibility of longer, thicker hyperpigmented eyelashes and the potential for permanent iris color change, which has been reported in a one-year-old child with blue-gray irides following 5.5 months of treatment.[22] Its role in childhood glaucoma is unclear largely due to the unknown long-term effects on melanocytes.

Sympathomimetics
Topical alpha agonists are thought to reduce IOP by initially decreasing aqueous production via the cAMP pathway and consequently increasing outflow. *Brimonidine* can cause drowsiness to the point of coma and apnea in infants due to its lipophilic properties, which allow it to readily penetrate the cornea and the blood–brain barrier once it is absorbed systemically. Brimonidine has also been associated with bradycardia, hypotension, and apnea in neonates. The use of *apraclonidine* in children is theoretically safer as it is less lipophilic. It should be considered when β blockers are contraindicated.

Surgical therapy
The principal treatment modality of childhood glaucoma is surgical. The available surgical procedures have varying indications with both advantages and disadvantages and potentially good success rates, especially when performed at referral centers where there is sufficient volume to ensure both skilful surgery and safe anesthesia. Lack of familiarity with buphthalmic eyes can lead to severe complications related to difficult access in small orbits, distorted limbal anatomy, thin sclera with low rigidity, lens subluxation from stretched zonules and syneretic vitreous. The procedure of choice is largely determined by the type of glaucoma, associated ocular disease and the surgeon's experience, but may further be influenced by the corneal clarity, degree of optic nerve damage, race, history of previous surgery, and the state of the fellow eye.

As reoperation is frequent, owing to the patient's long life expectancy, devising a long-term surgical strategy that will prolong the child's visual life for as long as possible is crucial. Making the right choice initially is paramount as the first operation has the greatest chance of success. In eyes that have undergone multiple procedures it is important to make the next operation the definitive one; otherwise, these eyes are at risk of a downward spiral from repetitive unsuccessful procedures. Once the procedure has been chosen, surgery must be meticulous to minimize complications.

Angle surgery
Goniotomy
Goniotomy is considered to be the treatment of choice in PCG where the cornea allows satisfactory visualization of the angle. By incising angle tissue the operation restores the natural pathway of aqueous outflow. The exact mechanism of action remains unknown. The advantages and disadvantages of goniotomy are summarized in Table 48.3.

Although goniotomy is simple in concept and brief in execution, it is a difficult procedure to perform requiring considerable experience and rare surgical skills. *Adequate*

Table 48.3 Advantages and disadvantages of goniotomy

Advantages
- Direct visualization of angle allows precise location of incision
- Less traumatic and safer
- Does not violate conjunctiva and prejudice success of future surgery
- Rapid
- Can be repeated
- No long-term risk of bleb-related complications

Disadvantages
- Works mainly for primary congenital glaucoma
- Not possible if details of angle structures not visible
- Considerable surgical experience required
- Technically demanding
- Requires special instruments
- Complications include corneal endothelial, angle, and lens trauma
- Discomfort for first few days if epithelium has been stripped

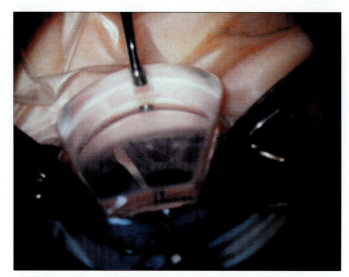

Fig. 48.6 Goniotomy performed in primary congenital glaucoma.

visualization of the angle is the key to successfully performing this procedure. The cornea may be cleared by the use of glycerol 20% drops immediately before surgery; if unsuccessful, epithelial debridement with absolute alcohol provides an adequate view of the angle to allow goniotomy in more than 90% of Caucasian patients.[23] To be performed safely, general anesthesia, an operating microscope, a contact lens (e.g., Barkan lens), and a tapered goniotomy blade are required (Fig. 48.6). Preoperative pilocarpine is useful to open the angle and protect the lens by constricting the pupil. The angle is gently engaged by the blade tip halfway between the root of the iris and Schwalbe's line and is gently swept across the angle, resulting in a superficial incision of the nasal trabecular meshwork over 90°–120°. A mild hyphema on withdrawal of the knife from the anterior chamber is typical and perhaps a favorable sign, indicating a correctly placed incision. A corneal suture is recommended to maintain a deep anterior chamber post-operatively. Viscoelastic agents can be used to maintain the anterior chamber during the procedure but they must be thoroughly removed to prevent a severe rise in IOP. If there has been a reasonable but suboptimal lowering of IOP after the first goniotomy, it can be repeated in the nonoperated part of the angle. Direct visualization of the angle allows precise location of the incision, making it less traumatic and safer than trabeculotomy. However, potential complications

include lens and corneal damage, inadvertent iridodialysis or cyclodialysis, and scleral perforation.

Goniotomy is a very effective operation, with success following multiple goniotomies usually ranging from 70 to 90% with medium-term follow-up.[4,23] However, these eyes are at risk of relapsing at any stage. The moorfield's experience showed a 20% relapse rate over a 30-year period with no peak age of relapse,[23] emphasizing the importance of lifelong follow-up.

The surgical prognosis of goniotomy is influenced by the age of manifestation with infants presenting between the ages of 3 to 6 months having the best prognosis. Although the prognosis may be poorer over the age of 1 (especially > 4 years) and with a corneal diameter greater than 14 mm, goniotomy may still be worthwhile considering because of its safety. Other risk factors for failure include family history and being female. Response in black children has been reported to be as good as Caucasians.

Trabeculotomy

Trabeculotomy is the procedure of choice for surgeons more familiar with the required surgical approach to the limbus than the technique of goniotomy. Since corneal opacification does not prevent its performance it has greater application and more relevance in populations where this is a common finding. The advantages and disadvantages of trabeculotomy are summarized in Table 48.4.

An operating microscope and special trabeculotome are essential for conventional trabeculotomy. A limbal or fornix-based conjunctival flap is dissected, preferably in the inferotemporal quadrant to preserve the superior conjunctiva for future filtration surgery if necessary. A trabeculectomy scleral flap is fashioned and Schlemm's canal located by slowly deepening a small radial incision. The trabeculotome is gently threaded into the canal and swept into the anterior chamber, rupturing trabecular meshwork and the internal wall of Schlemm's canal and directly exposing it to aqueous humor. This is then repeated on the other side of the canal. The scleral flap is closed sufficiently tightly to ensure a formed anterior chamber. *Accurate localization of Schlemm's canal is the key to the successful performance of this operation.* However, abnormally stretched limbal anatomy in buphthalmic eyes makes it difficult to identify, and it may not be found at all in many patients, especially if the anterior chamber is inadvertently entered before the canal is found. A mild to

Table 48.4 Advantages and disadvantages of trabeculotomy

Advantages
- Can be performed even when cornea is opaque
- Many components of technique similar to trabeculectomy
- ? Higher success rate when combined with trabeculectomy

Disadvantages
- Angle not directly visualized, leading potentially to significant complications
- Damages conjunctiva and prejudices success of future filtering surgery
- Requires special trabeculotomy probes
- Schlemm's canal is not found in 4–20% of cases
- Entry site closer to iris base to enable cannulation of Schlemm's canal increases risk of iris and ciliary body incarceration
- When combined with trabeculectomy may be technically more difficult
- Converting a trabeculotomy entry site to trabeculectomy places the sclerostomy very close to the iris root predisposing to iris incarceration
- Hypotony is possible as it may be more difficult to secure scleral flap because of posterior position–particularly a problem if antimetabolites are used
- Undesirable external filtration is possible

moderate hyphema is a regular occurrence. Mendicino et al. have described a 360° suture trabeculotomy using 6/0 polypropylene, with results suggesting greater success than goniotomy.[24] However, success is not always possible with a single incision, and severe hypotony has been reported.

Complications are seldom serious but may be more frequent than goniotomy because of the inability to directly visualize the angle structures and often the presence of distorted limbal anatomy increases the risk of trauma. Potential complications include stripping of Descemet's membrane, iris prolapse, iridodialysis, cyclodialysis with persistent hypotony, lens subluxation, false passages, significant hyphema, bleb formation and a prolonged flat anterior chamber.

Success rates in PCG following multiple operations have been reported to be greater than 90% with medium- to long-term follow up similar to that of goniotomy.[25,26] Success may be reduced in different racial groups.[27] Factors similar to those for goniotomy influence prognosis following trabeculotomy.

Trabeculotomy combined with trabeculectomy

Trabeculotomy has the added advantage of being combined with trabeculectomy to provide, in theory, two major outflow pathways. In practice the clinical benefit is unclear with some authors reporting greater success than either procedure performed alone, especially in populations at high risk of failure such as in East Asia and the Middle East.[28,29] Others have found no difference in success between the three procedures. Technically it is a more complex procedure with potentially significant complications especially with antimetabolite use.

Filtering surgery
Trabeculectomy

One of the main indications for trabeculectomy is failed angle surgery. It may be the primary procedure of choice when the surgeon has limited experience with angle surgery, the patient is unlikely to respond sufficiently to angle surgery (very early or late presentations), very low target pressures are required (improved cornea clarity, advanced disc cupping), or for secondary glaucoma. The advantages and disadvantages of trabeculectomy are summarized in Table 48.5.

Table 48.5 Advantages and disadvantages of trabeculectomy (with antimetabolites)

Advantages
- Familiarity with technique—more surgeons perform trabeculectomy on a regular basis and can deal with complications
- Postoperative pressures "titratable" compared with angle surgery by using techniques such as adjustable, releasable sutures, and postoperative antimetabolites
- Lower pressures achievable with antimetabolites
- Trabeculectomy with antimetabolites may significantly clear cloudy corneas

Disadvantages
- Damages conjunctiva compared to goniotomy and increases risk of failure with secondary surgery
- Greater risk of hypotony with choroidal effusion and hemorrhage than angle surgery particularly with MMC
- Greater risk of endophthalmitis than angle surgery particularly with MMC and limbus-based flaps
- Risk of intraocular damage if antimetabolites enter eye
- Poor results due to scarring in high-risk eyes particularly early onset cases and those with previous surgery
- Poor results in aphakic glaucoma even with MMC

Technically it is a more demanding procedure and more likely to fail in children than in adults. A superior fornix-based conjunctival flap allows adequate exposure, reduces surgical trauma to the conjunctiva and episclera, and improves bleb morphology reducing the risk of blebitis.[30] It is vital in buphthalmic eyes that the scleral flap be large and as thick as possible to be able to control flow and avoid sutures from cheese-wiring. Scleral flap closure should be very tight as these eyes are prone to develop complications of hypotony. Intraoperative hypotony can be minimized with the use of preplaced scleral flap sutures before the sclerostomy is performed and with an anterior chamber maintainer. For a summary of the technique refer to Table 48.6. Complications that may be more serious with antimetabolites include moderate hyphema, shallow or flat anterior chamber, iris incarceration, lens dislocation, choroidal effusions, vitreous loss, vitreous and suprachoroidal hemorrhage, staphyloma, retinal detachment, phthisis, chronic bleb leak, and endophthalmitis. Postoperatively, if the IOP is increased then sutures can be adjusted, removed, or cut. If significant conjunctival inflammation is present at the drainage site, subconjunctival 5FU (0.1–0.2 ml of 5FU 50 mg/ml) can be injected adjacent to the bleb with care taken to avoid intraocular entry as 5FU has a pH of 9.0. Subconjunctival steroids such as betamethasone can be given in combination with 5FU.

Trabeculectomy has a variable success rate influenced by factors such as racial group and previous surgery. Unenhanced trabeculectomies performed as a primary procedure in Caucasian children with medium to long-term follow-up have reported success rate (IOP < 18 mmHg ± medications) of between 87 and 100% with multiple operations.[31–33] This falls to approximately 60% with shorter follow-up (< 2 years) in children from the Middle East.[27,34,35]

Moderate success rates (IOP < 22 mmHg without medication) ranging from 40 to 95% are reported for secondary MMC trabeculectomies (0.2–0.4 mg/ml) with a mean follow-up ranging from 18 months to just under 2 years in non-Caucasians.[36–39] Sidoti et al. reported the use of MMC 0.5 mg/ml in a mixed racial group with a success of 73% with medical therapy over 21 months of follow-up but with the highest reported rate of endophthalmitis (17%).[40]

Deep sclerectomy for congenital glaucoma has been performed in an attempt to avoid potential trabeculectomy-related complications but is associated with poor results and high complication rates.[41]

Antifibrosis treatment

The long-term success rate of glaucoma filtering surgery in children is reduced compared to adults because of both a thicker Tenon's capsule, which impedes filtration and contains a large reservoir of fibroblasts responsible for scarring, and a more vigorous wound-healing response. This is further compounded by difficult postoperative management in the very young, which may delay the implementation of adjunctive measures that prolong bleb survival. Single intraoperative application regimens according to risk factors are the most appropriate in children. However, the potential for intraoperative and postoperative complications after trabeculectomy with antifibrosis therapy, especially MMC, cannot be overstated in children. *MMC should not be used unless clearly indicated especially in primary surgery.* To prevent postoperative fibrosis and failure a number of antifibrosis treatments are available.

β Irradiation

Intraoperative β irradiation has been shown to have a beneficial effect on the prognosis of glaucoma filtering surgery in children

Table 48.6 Important surgical points in pediatric trabeculectomy

Point	Action	Rationale
Exposure	Corneal traction suture (7/0 mersilk) Fornix-based conjunctival flap	Allows maximum inferoduction of globe and adequate exposure Allows better visualization of limbal anatomy Easier placement of sutures in scleral flap Less likely to limit posterior flow Limbal flap may not be possible in neonate
Hemostasis	Corneal traction suture Wet field cautery	Avoids hemorrhage from superior rectus suture Avoids scleral shrinkage (very important in thin sclera)
Prevention of scarring	Antimetabolites	See text
Scleral flap	Anterior placement Large and thick (5 × 4 mm) Anterior pocket valve (radial cuts not all the wa to limbus)	Avoids iris, ciliary body, and vitreous incarceration Easier to suture without cheese-wiring thin sclera Greater resistance to aqueous outflow (vital in buphthalmic eyes, especially with antimetabolites) Valve effect to prevent hypotony Directs aqueous posteriorly to prevent cystic blebs
Paracentesis	Oblique, long tunnel	Reduces risk of inadvertent lens damage during maneuver and less likely to leak Allows assessment of scleral flap opening pressure Allows reformation of the AC postoperatively For AC maintainer
Maintenance of intraoperative IOP	Anterior chamber maintainer	Prevents eye from becoming hypotonous and choroidal effusions forming during surgery Can be used to gauge flow through the scleral flap and ensure adequate closure
Sclerostomy	Small (500-μm bite) with special punch Anterior as possible	Increased control of aqueous outflow intra- and postoperatively Quick, therefore less intraoperative hypotony Prevents iris, ciliary body, vitreous incarceration
Scleral flap closure	Preplaced sutures before sclerostomy Tight releasable/adjustable sutures Releasable loop buried in cornea Adjustable knots	Easier to place with formed globe Faster to tie therefore reduced period of intraoperative hypotony Allows control of opening pressures (vital with antimetabolite use) Sutures can be left indefinitely Can be removed under anesthetic without need for laser Allows tight closure but can be easily loosened without need for complete removal using special forceps
Conjunctival closure (Fornix-based)	10/0 nylon purse string at edges	Retains tension longer than dissolvable sutures Minimal associated inflammation Ends of nylon buried under conjunctiva
Postoperative prevention of hypotony	Viscoelastic in anterior chamber	May be necessary if flow rate too high despite maximal suturing Can be repeated

without serious complications.[42] A semicircular Strontium-90 probe is gently applied to the conjunctiva in the filtration area at the end of the operation until it delivers a dose of 1000 cGy. The resultant blebs tend to be diffuse, less cystic, slightly elevated, and uninflamed. Beta irradiation is equivalent in cell culture to the effect of intraoperative 5FU.

Antimetabolites

Despite potential complications, the use of antimetabolites to enhance success in refractory or difficult cases appears unavoidable in children. The successful use of multiple perioperative subconjunctival 5FU injections in congenital glaucoma has been reported. However, given the marked tendency of children to scar and the generally poor cooperation with postoperative examination, a single application of the more potent MMC is preferable to 5FU, especially for those with a combination of high-risk characteristics. Its greater potency can result in significant IOP reduction with a dramatic effect on corneal clarity (Figs 48.4 and 48.5). Regimens ranging from 0.2 to 0.5 mg/ml intraoperative MMC for 1.5–5 minutes are reported. The safest and most effective dose (concentration and

exposure time) of antimetabolite is unknown as are the long-term effects of antimetabolites.

Early postoperative complications usually relate to hypotony, whereas late complications largely relate to progressive bleb thinning, putting the child at a lifetime risk of endophthalmitis and bleb rupture, leading to chronic leak and hypotony.[40,43] However, recent modifications to the intraoperative application of MMC based on clinical observation and subsequent laboratory research seems to result in more favorable bleb morphology[30] (Fig. 48.7).

Tube drainage surgery

Tube drainage surgery remains an important part of the therapeutic repertoire in childhood glaucoma as it offers the best chance of long-term IOP control in a small proportion of patients whose disease relentlessly progresses despite conventional surgical treatment. Furthermore, it is indicated when future intraocular surgery such as cataract extraction is contemplated, as it is more likely to control IOP postoperatively than filtering surgery. The prevailing current opinion is that tubes are best implanted sooner rather than later in the hope of achieving early, definitive IOP

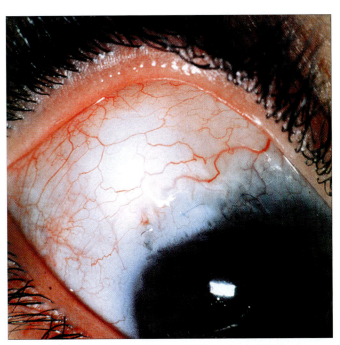

Fig. 48.7 Mitomycin C trabeculectomy following a fornix based conjunctival flap and large antimetabolite treatment area.

Table 48.7 Advantages and disadvantages of tube surgery (with antimetabolites)
Advantages
▪ Very effective in reducing IOP long term even if previously failed antimetabolite trabeculectomy
▪ Most likely to survive future intraocular surgery e.g. penetrating keratoplasty, lensectomy, vitrectomy therefore best drainage option in these circumstances
▪ Contact lens wear possible in aphakic glaucoma
Disadvantages
▪ Longest surgical time
▪ Highest short term complication rate, particularly hypotony related complications including sight-threatening complications
▪ Longest rehabilitation period
▪ Long-term complications include tube extrusion, tube blockage, endothelial damage, and plate encapsulation
▪ Risk of infection with use of foreign patch graft (sclera, pericardium, dura mater)
▪ ? Higher rate of corneal graft rejection

control and in doing so optimizing long-term visual prognosis. The advantages and disadvantages of tube drainage surgery are summarized in Table 48.7.

Common to all studies, regardless of the implant, is the ongoing decline in success with duration of follow-up and the requirement for adjunctive topical medication to control IOP. Plate encapsulation is a major cause of late failure. Success rates of approximately 80% are reported with a mean follow-up of 2 years or less,[44–46] falling to between 31 and 45% after around 4 years.[47,48] This improves to 78–95% with the use of systemic antifibrotic therapy in the form of systemic prednisolone, flufenamic acid, and colchicine.[16,49,50]

Although it may be argued that drainage devices offer the most effective long-term treatment for IOP control, they all have a relatively high complication rate. The problems usually relate to hypotony or to the tube itself (e.g., occlusion, retraction, exposure, corneal or iris touch), resulting in visual loss as high as 61% in some

studies.[45,48,51] Buphthalmic eyes are especially prone to hypotony-related complications because reduced scleral rigidity allows leakage around the tube at its entry site, making subsequent problems such as choroidal effusions and suprachoroidal hemorrhage more likely, even with the use of valved implants. Modifications to protect from intra- and postoperative hypotony (mandatory when using MMC in a buphthalmic eye) include an anterior chamber maintainer (Lewicky cannula); a relatively long and "snug" limbal tunnel incision (25-G needle for Molteno and Baerveldt implants); the use of an intraluminal suture (3/0 Supramid); an external ligating suture (6/0 vicryl) with a venting "Sherwood" slit;[52] and viscoelastic or intraocular gases such as 20% C_3F_8 in the anterior chamber if required. Tube surgery in an aphakic eye should be combined with a complete anterior and partial core vitrectomy to prevent tube blockage even if no vitreous is present in the anterior chamber at the time of surgery. A high surgical revision rate of up to 83% has been reported with the majority of complications being tube related (15–44%), especially tube–cornea touch, which may be avoided with accurate angle of entry of the tube into the anterior chamber and secure implant fixation.

Cyclodestruction

The indications for cyclodestruction are blind painful eyes, those with poor visual potential or in whom surgery either has a poor prognosis or is technically impossible (e.g., severely scarred conjunctiva). It is also worth contemplating when the risk of surgery is high, or as a temporizing measure when the fellow eye has undergone recent drainage surgery. The advantages and disadvantages of diode laser cyclodestruction are summarized in Table 48.8.

A contact transscleral semiconductor diode laser (810 nm) has become increasingly more popular than a Nd:YAG laser and cyclocryotherapy as a method of ciliary body ablation because it is better tolerated and associated with less complications. As buphthalmic eyes often have distorted anatomical landmarks, transillumination of the eye is essential to ensure accurate placement of the laser burns (Fig. 48.8). Care must be taken to avoid areas of pigmentation, hemorrhage, and scleral thinning, as scleral perforation in a buphthalmic eye has been reported.[53]

Diode laser seems to be moderately effective in the short term with a success rate of over 50% on medical therapy. These results have been achieved with total energy doses of between 74 and

Table 48.8 Advantages and disadvantages of diode laser cyclodestruction
Advantages
▪ Short surgical time
▪ Low complication rate
▪ Rapid rehabilitation
▪ Good short-term response rate
▪ Very useful where surgery has high risks particularly in only eyes
▪ Technically less demanding than other procedures in difficult eyes
Disadvantages
▪ Often needs to be repeated in more than 50% of cases due to recovery of ciliary body
▪ Most patients remain on medical therapy
▪ Pressure control is worse than drainage surgery (pressures in the low teens usually not achieved)
▪ Danger of long-term phthisis with recurrent treatment due to recurrent damage to ciliary body
▪ ? May affect future drainage surgery: hypotony due to hyposecretion, and fibrotic failure due to destruction of blood aqueous barrier releasing stimulatory cytokines into aqueous and drainage site

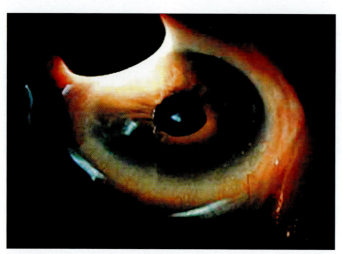

Fig. 48.8 Cyclodiode laser. Transillumination is crucial for correct placement of burns on the ciliary body.

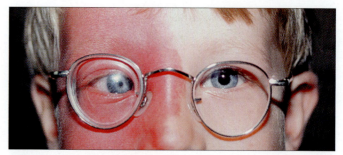

Fig. 48.9 Sturge–Weber syndrome patient with myopic-affected eye requiring optical correction.

113 J and a variable retreatment rate of 33–70%.[14,54,55] Overall visual loss rates of up to 18% have been reported, usually in eyes with preexisting poor vision.[54]

Refractive correction and amblyopia therapy

The ultimate aim of preserving lifelong vision in children with glaucoma is dependent not only on IOP control but also on several interrelated factors such as the treatment of ametropia, strabismus, and amblyopia. Children with glaucoma are at a particular risk of amblyopia due to a combination of corneal pathology, strabismus, astigmatism, and anisometropia from unilateral or asymmetric bilateral disease. Cataracts and aniseikonia as a result of abnormal anatomy of the buphthalmic globe can also contribute to amblyopia. Anisometropia greater than 6 diopters has been found to be associated with significant amblyopia, unresponsive to occlusion (Fig. 48.9).

All children with glaucoma should be examined regularly for the presence of strabismus and amblyopia. Refraction should be part of the periodic examination with glasses prescribed as appropriate when the cornea clears and is practical. Occlusion therapy for amblyopia should be attempted in all patients in whom there is potential for visual improvement however young the child.

THE ROLE OF PENETRATING KERATOPLASTY

The results of penetrating keratoplasty in children with glaucoma are poor.[8,56–58] Ariyasu et al. recommended penetrating keratoplasty in only bilateral, visually disabling congenital glaucoma along with a dedicated, reliable caregiver to deal with the postoperative management.[59] It is important to remember that the use of antimetabolites can achieve lower IOP to levels that can clear corneal opacities (Figs. 48.4, 48.5).

PROGNOSIS

Visual loss in children with glaucoma occurs from a combination of intractable glaucoma and optic nerve damage, corneal pathology, uncorrected refractive errors, and amblyopia. They remain susceptible to visual loss from lens subluxation, cataract, corneal decompensation, retinal detachment, strabismus, and phthisis. Parents and, later, patients should be warned that minor blunt trauma in buphthalmic eyes may be complicated by lens dislocation, intraocular hemorrhage, globe rupture, and retinal detachment. Protective eyewear should be recommended, especially in monocular patients.

Visual prognosis depends on many factors but the most important are:

1. The time between the first clinical manifestation, diagnosis, and surgery;
2. Successful control of IOP to a level where progression is unlikely; and
3. Correction of ametropia and amblyopia therapy.

There are some patients in whom, despite all efforts, the prognosis for long-term vision is poor but it is worth persisting because the longer the child is kept seeing, the better they will function as an adult.

Periodic examination must continue throughout life. Not only because an increase in IOP can occur at any stage, but also because complications can occur many years after a seemingly successful operation.

REFERENCES

1. François J. Congenital glaucoma and its inheritance. Ophthalmologica 1980; 181: 61–73.
2. Stoilov I, Akarsu AN, Sarfarazi M. Identification of three different truncating mutations in cytochrome P4501B1 (CYP1B1) as the principle cause of primary congenital glaucoma (buphthalmos) in families linked to the GLC3A locus on chromosome 2p21. Hum Mol Genet 1997; 6: 641–7.
3. Jay MR, Rice NS. Genetic implications of congenital glaucoma. Metab Ophthalmol 1978; 2: 257–8.
4. Shaffer RN. Prognosis of goniotomy in primary infantile glaucoma (trabeculodysgenesis). Trans Am Ophthalmol Soc 1982; 80: 321–5.
5. Stone EM, Fingert JH, Alward WL, et al. Identification of a gene that causes primary open angle glaucoma. Science 1997; 275: 668–70.
6. Semina EV, Reiter R, Leysens NJ, et al. Cloning and characterization of a novel bicoid-related homeobox transcription factor gene, RIEG, involved in Rieger syndrome. Nat Genet 1996; 14: 392–9.
7. Lehmann OJ, Tuft S, Brice G, et al. Novel anterior segment phenotypes resulting from forkhead gene alterations: evidence for cross-species conservation of function. Invest Ophthalmol Vis Sci 2003; 44: 2627–33.

8. Yang LL, Lambert SR. Peters anomaly. A synopsis of surgical management and visual outcome. Ophthalmol Clin North Am 2001; 14: 467–77.
9. Chen TC, Walton DS. Goniosurgery for the prevention of aniridic glaucoma. Arch Ophthalmol 1999; 117: 1144–8.
10. Arroyave CP, Scott IU, Gedde SJ, et al. Use of glaucoma drainage devices in the management of glaucoma associated with aniridia. Am J Ophthalmol 2003; 135: 155–9.
11. Olsen KE, Huang AS, Wright MM. The efficacy of goniotomy/trabeculotomy in early-onset glaucoma associated with the Sturge-Weber syndrome. J AAPOS 1998; 2: 365–8.
12. François J. Late results of congenital cataract surgery. Ophthalmol 1979; 86: 1586–98.
13. Simon JW, Mehta N, Simmons ST, et al. Glaucoma after pediatric lensectomy/vitrectomy. Ophthalmology 1991; 98: 670–4.
14. Kirwan JF, Shah P, Khaw PT. Diode laser cyclophotocoagulation: role in the management of refractory pediatric glaucomas. Ophthalmol 2002; 109: 316–23.
15. Mandal AK, Bagga H, Nutheti R, et al. Trabeculectomy with or without mitomycin-C for paediatric glaucoma in aphakia and pseudophakia following congenital cataract surgery. Eye 2003; 17: 53–62.
16. Cunliffe IA, Molteno AC. Long-term follow-up of Molteno drains used in the treatment of glaucoma presenting in childhood. Eye 1998; 12: 379–85.
17. Freedman SF, Rodriguez-Rosa RE, Rojas MC, Enyedi LB. Goniotomy for glaucoma secondary to chronic childhood uveitis. Am J Ophthalmol 2002; 133: 617–21.
18. Molteno AC, Sayawat N, Herbison P. Otago glaucoma surgery outcome study: long-term results of uveitis with secondary glaucoma drained by Molteno implants. Ophthalmology 2001; 108: 605–13.
19. Richardson KT. Optic cup symmetry in normal newborn infants. Invest Ophthalmol 1968; 7: 137–40.
20. Shaffer RN. New concepts in infantile glaucoma. Can J Ophthalmol 1967; 2: 243–8.
21. Enyedi LB, Freedman SF, Buckley EG. The effectiveness of latanoprost for the treatment of pediatric glaucoma. J AAPOS 1999; 3: 33–9.
22. Brown SM. Increased iris pigment in a child due to latanoprost. Arch Ophthalmol 1998; 116: 1683–4.
23. Russell-Eggitt IM, Rice NS, Jay B, Wyse RK. Relapse following goniotomy for congenital glaucoma due to trabecular dysgenesis. Eye 1992; 6: 197–200.
24. Mendicino ME, Lynch MG, Drack A, et al. Long-term surgical and visual outcomes in primary congenital glaucoma: 360 degrees trabeculotomy versus goniotomy. J AAPOS 2000; 4: 205–10.
25. Martin BB. External trabeculotomy in the surgical treatment of congenital glaucoma. Aust N Z J Ophthalmol 1989; 17: 299–301.
26. Akimoto M, Tanihara H, Negi A, Nagata M. Surgical results of trabeculotomy ab externo for developmental glaucoma. Arch Ophthalmol 1994; 112: 1540–4.
27. Elder MJ. Congenital glaucoma in the West Bank and Gaza Strip. Br J Ophthalmol 1993; 77: 413–6.
28. Elder MJ. Combined trabeculotomy-trabeculectomy compared with primary trabeculectomy for congenital glaucoma. Br J Ophthalmol 1994; 78: 745–8.
29. Mandal AK, Bhatia PG, Gothwal VK, et al. Safety and efficacy of simultaneous bilateral primary combined trabeculotomy-trabeculectomy for developmental glaucoma. Indian J Ophthalmol 2002; 50: 13–9.
30. Wells AP, Cordeiro MF, Bunce C, Khaw PT. Cystic bleb formation and related complications in limbus- versus fornix-based conjunctival flaps in pediatric and young adult trabeculectomy with mitomycin C. Ophthalmology 2003; 110: 2192–7.
31. Burke JP, Bowell R. Primary trabeculectomy in congenital glaucoma. Br J Ophthalmol 1989; 73: 186–90.
32. Fulcher T, Chan J, Lanigan B, et al. Long term follow up of primary trabeculectomy for infantile glaucoma. Br J Ophthalmol 1996; 80: 499–502.
33. Dureau P, Dollfus H, Cassegrain C, Dufier JL. Long term results of trabeculectomy for congenital glaucoma. J Pediatr Ophthalmol Strabismus 1998; 35: 198–202.
34. Debnath SC, Teichmann KD, Salamah K. Trabeculectomy versus trabeculotomy in congenital glaucoma. Br J Ophthalmol 1989; 73: 608–11.
35. Marrakchi S, Nacef L, Kamoun N, et al. Results of trabeculectomy in congenital glaucoma. J Fr Ophthalmol 1992; 15: 400–4.
36. Susanna R Jr, Oltrogge EW, Carani JCE, Nicolela MT. Mitomycin as adjunct chemotherapy with trabeculectomy in congenital and developmental glaucomas. J Glaucoma 1995; 4: 151–7.
37. al-Hazmi A, Zwaan J, Awad A, et al. Effectiveness and complications of mitomycin C use during pediatric glaucoma surgery. Ophthalmology 1998; 105: 1915–20.
38. Mandal AK, Walton DS, John T, Jayagandan A. Mitomycin C-augmented trabeculectomy in refractory congenital glaucoma. Ophthalmol 1997; 104: 996–1001.
39. Mandal AK, Prasad K, Naduvilath TJ. Surgical results and complications of mitomycin C-augmented trabeculectomy in refractory developmental glaucoma. Ophthalmic Surg Lasers 1999; 30: 473–80.
40. Sidoti PA, Belmonte SJ, Liebmann JM, Ritch R. Trabeculectomy with mitomycin-C in the treatment of pediatric glaucomas. Ophthalmology 2000; 107: 422–9.
41. Luke C, Dietlein TS, Jacobi PC, et al. Risk profile of deep sclerectomy for the treatment of refractory congenital glaucomas. Ophthalmology 2002; 109: 1066–71.
42. Miller MH, Rice NS. Trabeculectomy combined with β irradiation for congenital glaucoma. Br J Ophthalmol 1991; 75: 584–90.
43. Waheed S, Ritterband DC, Greenfield DS, et al. Bleb-related ocular infection in children after trabeculectomy with mitomycin C. Ophthalmology 1997; 104: 2117–20.
44. Fellenbaum PS, Sidoti PA, Heuer DK, et al. Experience with the Baerveldt implant in young patients with complicated glaucomas. J Glaucoma 1995; 4: 91–7.
45. Morad Y, Donaldson CE, Kim YM, et al. The Ahmed drainage implant in the treatment of pediatric glaucoma. Am J Ophthalmol 2003; 135: 821–9.
46. Netland PA, Walton DS. Glaucoma drainage implants in pediatric patients. Ophthalmic Surg 1993; 24: 723–9.
47. Lloyd MA, Sedlak T, Heuer DK, et al. Clinical experience with the single plate Molteno implant in complicated glaucoma. Ophthalmol 1992; 99: 679–87.
48. Eid TE, Katz LJ, Spaeth GL, Augsburger JJ. Long-term effects of tube-shunt procedures on management of refractory childhood glaucoma. Ophthalmology 1997; 104: 1011–6.
49. Billson F, Thomas R, Aylward W. The use of two-stage Molteno implants in developmental glaucoma. J Pediatr Ophthalmol Strabismus 1989; 26: 3–8.
50. Molteno AC, Ancker E, Van Biljon G. Surgical technique for advanced juvenile glaucoma. Arch Ophthalmol 1984; 102: 51–7.
51. Djodeyre MR, Calvo JP, Gomez JA. Clinical evaluation and risk factors of time to failure of Ahmed Glaucoma Valve implant in pediatric patients. Ophthalmology 2001; 108: 614–20.
52. Sherwood MB, Smith MF. Prevention of early hypotony associated with Molteno implants by a new occluding stent technique. Ophthalmology 1993; 100: 85–90.
53. Sabri K, Vernon SA. Scleral perforation following trans-scleral cyclodiode. Br J Ophthalmol 1999; 83: 502–3.
54. Bock CJ, Freedman SF, Buckley EG, Shields MB. Transscleral diode laser cyclophotocoagulation for refractory pediatric glaucomas. J Ped Ophthalmol Strabismus 1997; 34: 235-9.
55. Hamard P, May F, Quesnot S, Hamard H. Trans-scleral diode laser cyclophotocoagulation for the treatment of refractory pediatric glaucoma. J Fr Ophthalmol 2000; 23: 773–80.
56. Waring GO, Laibson PR. Keratoplasty in infants and children. Trans Am Acad Ophthalmol Otolaryngol 1977; 83: 283–96.
57. Frueh BE, Brown SI. Transplantation of congenitally opaque corneas. Br J Ophthalmol 1997; 81: 1064–9.
58. Erlich CM, Rootman DS, Morin JD. Corneal transplantation in infants, children and young adults: experience of the Toronto Hospital for Sick Children, 1979–88. Can J Ophthalmol 1991; 26: 206–10.
59. Ariyasu RG, Silverman J, Irvine JA. Penetrating keratoplasty in infants with congenital glaucoma. Cornea 1989; 13: 521–6.

CHAPTER 49 Vitreous

Anthony Moore and Michel Michaelides

INTRODUCTION

The vitreous, a transparent gelatinous structure that fills the posterior four-fifths of the globe, is firmly attached to the pars plana and loosely to the retina and optic nerve posteriorly. In childhood there is a firm attachment to the lens.

The development of the vitreous body and zonule can be divided into three stages[1]:

1. The **primary** vitreous is formed during the first month and is a vascularized mesodermal tissue separating the developing lens vesicle and the neuroectoderm of the optic cup. It contains branches of the hyaloid artery that later regress.
2. The **secondary** vitreous starts at 9 weeks (410mm stage)[2] and develops throughout embryonic life, most rapidly in early infancy. It ultimately forms the established vitreous body, is avascular and transparent, and displaces the primary vitreous, which becomes Cloquet's canal from the optic disc to the lens. By the third month (70mm stage) the secondary vitreous fills most of the developing vitreous cavity.
3. The **tertiary** vitreous starts when the vitreous lying between the ciliary body and lens becomes separated from the secondary vitreous as well-formed fibrils that later develop into the zonule.

DEVELOPMENTAL ANOMALIES OF THE VITREOUS

Persistence of the primary vitreous or part of its structure may give rise to a number of congenital abnormalities.

Persistent hyaloid artery

Persistence of all or part of the hyaloid artery is a common congenital abnormality. Hyaloid artery remnants occur in about 3% of full-term infants but are commonly seen in premature infants.[3] Most regress and persistence of the whole artery is uncommon. Rarely, the whole artery may run from the disc to the lens. Posterior remnants may give rise to a single vessel running from the center of the disc or to an elevated bud of glial tissue – the Bergmeister's papilla. Anterior remnants of the hyaloid system may be seen as a small white dot on the posterior lens capsule – the Mittendorf's dot. They do not interfere with vision and do not progress.

Vitreous cysts

Acquired cysts occur with inflammatory disease, and rarely with juvenile retinoschisis.[4]

Congenital cysts are usually found in otherwise normal eyes.[5–7] Their origin is unknown but, as blood vessels are sometimes seen

within them, they may develop from hyaloid artery remnants.[5] No histopathology is available.

Cysts may lie in the anterior vitreous immediately behind the lens[8,9] (Fig. 49.1) or in the posterior vitreous.[5–7] They may be mobile[6,7,9,10] or attached to the lens[9] or optic disc.[5] Mostly, intervention is not required; occasionally laser treatment helps when they are symptomatic.[11–13] Nd:YAG and argon laser both give good results.[11,12] However, repeat Nd:YAG therapy of an anterior pigmented cyst has resulted in a cataract.[13]

Persistent fetal vasculature (PFV)

Persistent hyperplastic primary vitreous (PHPV) (see also Chapter 47)

PFV (PHPV) is caused by failure of the primary vitreous to regress. Most are sporadic and unilateral although there may be minor abnormalities in the fellow eye. Bilateral and familial cases have been reported,[14–16] but these are probably cases of vitreoretinal dysplasia.

For anterior PFV see Chapter 47.

Posterior PHPV, in which the ocular abnormality is confined to the posterior segment, may present with leukocoria, strabismus, microphthalmia, or nystagmus. The lens is usually clear. There is often a fold of condensed vitreous and retina running from the optic disc to the ora serrata (Fig. 49.2), with a retinal detachment.[17,18] Ultrasound and CT scan help in differentiating PHPV from retinoblastoma.[19]

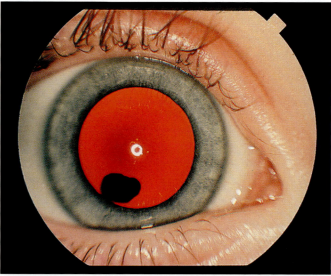

Fig. 49.1 Anterior vitreous cyst seen with retroillumination.

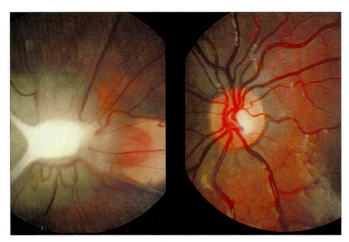

Fig. 49.2 Posterior PHPV. A fold of condensed vitreous running from the optic disc can be seen. The left optic disc is normal.

Histopathologically, there is variable vascularization and fat, smooth muscle and cartilage may also be present.[20,21]

Posterior PHPV is usually associated with poor vision in the affected eye and is not amenable to treatment. In anterior PHPV a limbal or pars plicata approach may be used to remove the lens and retrolental tissue,[18,22] clear the visual axis, improve cosmesis, deepen the anterior chamber, and prevent angle closure glaucoma caused by anterior chamber shallowing. Enucleation should be avoided because a prosthesis is less acceptable cosmetically and may result in decreased growth of the orbit and facial asymmetry.[23] The management of anterior PHPV is covered in Chapter 47.

VITREORETINAL DYSPLASIA

Maldevelopment of the vitreous and retina is either an isolated abnormality[24,25] or associated with systemic abnormalities. Syndromes such as Norrie disease,[26–28] incontinentia pigmenti,[29–33] and Warburg syndrome[34,35] may have bilateral vitreoretinal dysplasia. It also occurs in trisomy 13, trisomy 18, and triploidy and in association with cerebral malformations.[36,37] In animals, virus infections can induce it.[38]

There appears to be no relationship between the histological findings[24] and the various syndromes in which retinal dysplasia is reported. The dysplastic retina contains rosettes that resemble retinoblastoma rosettes but actually contain Müller cells with an abnormal relationship between the retina and retinal pigment epithelium (RPE).[36]

Norrie disease

Clinical and histological findings

Norrie disease is an X-linked recessive disorder in which affected males are blind at birth or early infancy.[26–28] About 25% of affected males are developmentally delayed and about one-third develop cochlear deafness at any time from infancy to adult life.[39] There are bilateral retinal folds, retinal detachment, vitreous hemorrhage, and bilateral vitreoretinal dysplasia (Fig. 49.3). The retinal detachments are usually of early onset and have been observed *in utero* by abdominal ultrasonography.[40] Most cases progress to an extensive vitreoretinal mass and bilateral blindness.

Angle closure glaucoma may develop in some infants, and this is best managed by limbal or pars plicata lensectomy. Late signs

include corneal opacification, band keratopathy, and phthisis bulbi.

A more severe phenotype is seen in patients who have large chromosomal deletions, including profound mental retardation, disruptive behavior, abnormal sexual maturation, atonic seizures, and hypotonia.[41]

Vitreoretinal biopsy histopathology suggested an arrest of normal retinal development during the third or fourth months of gestation,[42] but the eyes of an aborted 11-week fetus with Norrie disease showed no evidence of primary neuroectodermal maldevelopment of the retina, suggesting a later disorder.[43]

Carrier females do not usually show any ocular abnormality and electroretinography (ERG) is normal.[44] Woodruff et al. reported an affected female, born to a carrier mother, who had a retrolental mass in the right eye and a retinal fold with a tractional retinal detachment in the left.[45] Molecular genetic testing confirmed that she was a manifesting heterozygote, and she showed skewed X-inactivation in her peripheral blood lymphocytes, suggesting nonrandom inactivation, with inactivation occurring more frequently in the normal rather than in the mutant X chromosome.[46–48] A female with Norrie disease, with an X autosome translocation, has also been described.[49]

Molecular genetics and pathogenesis

The Norrie disease gene, *NDP*, was cloned in 1992;[50,51] there are more than 100 mutations.[52–55] The gene has three exons (the first of which is not translated) and is expressed in the neural layers of the retina, throughout the brain, and in the spiral ganglion and stria vascularis of the cochlea.[47] The predicted protein, norrin, consists of 133 amino acid residues and is similar in structure to the mucins and to growth factors, especially transforming growth factor (TGF),[56,57] suggesting that norrin is involved in ocular development and differentiation.[58] The identification of the Norrie disease gene has allowed molecular genetic diagnosis of the carrier state and prenatal diagnosis.

Norrie disease may be associated with chromosomal deletions involving the *NDP* locus, located at Xp11.3, the adjacent monoamine oxidase genes *MAOA* and *MAOB*, and additional genetic material. Children with such deletions have a more severe ("atypical") phenotype.[41] In addition to the characteristic retinal dysplasia, the atypical phenotypes include all or some of the following: mental retardation, involuntary movements, atonic seizures, hypertensive crises, and hypogonadism.[41]

Mutations of the Norrie disease gene may also be responsible for another rare vitreoretinal disorder, X-linked familial exudative vitreoretinopathy (see below). Sequence changes in the Norrie gene have also been reported in infants with retinopathy of prematurity (ROP)[59–61] and assomatic mutations in eyes with Coats disease[62] (see Chapter 55), suggesting that norrin may be involved in normal retinal angiogenesis, a suggestion supported by the association of Norrie disease with peripheral vascular disease in one large Costa Rican family.[63]

Coats disease may be caused by somatic mutations (present in retinal tissue of the affected eye and not in nonretinal tissue) in *NDP*;[62] the somatic mutations result in deficiency of norrin with consequent abnormal retinal vascular development, the hallmark of Coats disease.

The possible role of the *NDP* gene in ROP is controversial. Sequence changes in the *NDP* gene may predispose to stage 5 ROP. There are as many reports supporting this suggestion[59–61] as have failed to demonstrate any association of ROP with *NDP* mutations.[64–66] *NDP* mutations may only account for 3% of cases of advanced ROP.[60]

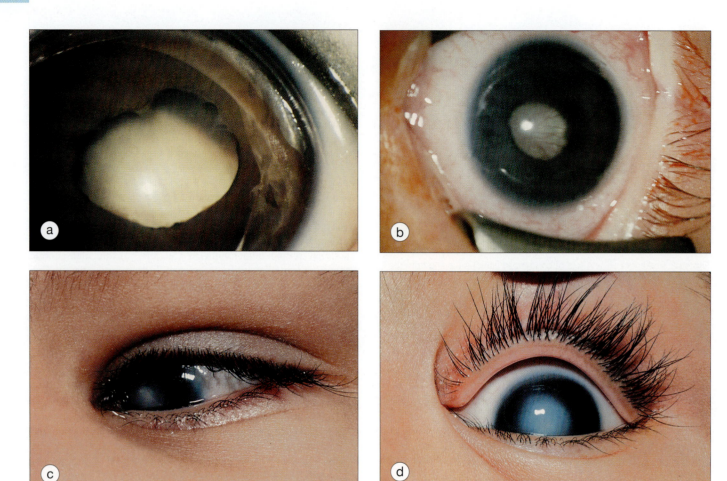

Fig. 49.3 Norrie disease. (a) Posterior synechiae, shallow anterior chamber, and retrolental white mass. (b) Brother of patient in (a) showing vascularized white retrolental mass. (c, d) Flat anterior chambers and lens–cornea adhesions.

Knockout mouse models have a similar ocular phenotype to humans with fibrous masses in the vitreous cavities, disorganization of retinal ganglion cells, and sporadic degeneration of other retinal cell types.[67] Their retinal vasculature is abnormal by postnatal day 9, with abnormal vessels in the inner retina and few vessels in the outer retina.[68] As in humans, the knockout mice had progressive hearing loss leading to profound deafness.[69] The primary lesion was in the stria vascularis, where the main vasculature of the cochlea is found; there was abnormal vasculature and eventual loss of most of the vessels, suggesting that a principal function of norrin in the ear is to regulate the interaction of the cochlea with its vasculature, further evidence of its angiogenic role.

Trisomy 13

Clinical and histological findings

Trisomy 13 (Patau syndrome)[70] is the chromosomal abnormality most consistently associated with severe ocular defects. Systemic abnormalities include microcephaly, cleft palate, congenital cardiac defects, polydactyly, skin hemangiomas, umbilical hernia, and malformation of the central nervous system.[70,71] Most infants with Trisomy 13 die within the first few months of life.

Bilateral ocular abnormalities are seen in almost all cases of trisomy 13;[71] the common ocular findings are detailed in Table 49.1. Affected infants often show total disorganization of the vitreous and retina, and histology shows extensive retinal dysplasia.[72,73] Intraocular cartilage is frequent and may be characteristic.[73]

Table 49.1 Ocular abnormalities in trisomy 13
Microphthalmos
Coloboma of the uveal tract
Cataract
Corneal opacities
Retinal dysplasia
PHPV
Dysplastic optic nerves
Cyclopia

Incontinentia pigmenti (Bloch–Sulzberger syndrome)

Clinical and histological findings

Incontinentia pigmenti is an uncommon familial disorder affecting the skin, bones, teeth, central nervous system, and eyes.[32,74] It is thought to be an X-linked dominant disorder that is usually lethal in the male, leading to a marked female preponderance. The characteristic skin lesions appear soon after birth with a linear eruption of bullae predominantly affecting the extremities (Fig. 49.4a). The bullae gradually resolve to leave a linear pattern of pigmentation[29,32] (Fig. 49.4b).

Ocular abnormalities including amblyopia, strabismus, nystagmus, cataract, optic atrophy, and retinal changes are common.[30,33,75,76] Corneal abnormalities include whorl-like

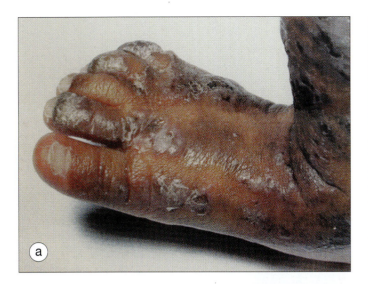

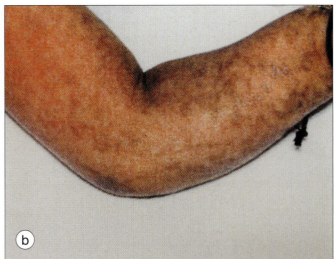

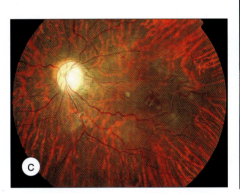

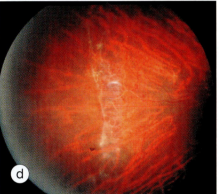

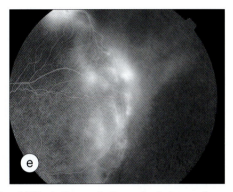

Fig. 49.4 Incontinentia pigmenti. (a) The characteristic skin bullae predominantly affecting the extremities. (b) The bullae gradually resolve to leave a linear pattern of pigmentation. (c) Retinal vascular tortuosity. (d) Capillary closure in the temporal peripheral retina. (e) Fundus fluorescein angiogram at 2 minutes showing peripheral retinal nonperfusion. Figures used with the permission of *Ophthalmic Genetics*. (Cates et al. Opthalmic Genetics 2003; 24: 247–52).

epithelial keratitis, with fluorescein-staining epithelial microcysts and mild mid-stromal "haziness,"[77] and corneal subepithelial anterior stromal opacities, resembling small white "bubbles" of differing sizes.[78]

The most serious, rare, complication is retinal detachment, which may lead to severe visual impairment. Retinovascular abnormalities are common and include retinal vascular tortuosity, capillary closure, and peripheral arteriovenous shunts[31,33,75,79] (Figs. 49.4c–49.4e). These are most marked in the temporal periphery and may be associated with preretinal fibrosis. Tractional retinal detachments occur in a minority.[33,75] Fluorescein angiography demonstrates areas of nonperfusion in the temporal periphery (Fig. 49.4e): they may be an early stage in the development of retinal detachment and "pseudoglioma".[33,75]

Affected females should be assessed by an ophthalmologist as soon after diagnosis as possible and at regular intervals during early childhood, in order to detect strabismus, refractive errors, amblyopia, and retinovascular abnormalities. Cryotherapy or photocoagulation of the retinovascular abnormalities may prevent progression,[79,80] but the natural history is not well established and treatment should be reserved for cases showing progression. Established retinal detachment presents a difficult management problem.[75]

Molecular genetics and pathogenesis

The gene for the familial form of incontinentia pigmenti was mapped by linkage studies to the Xq28 region, and the causative gene, *NEMO* (NF-κB essential modulator) was identified.[81] *NEMO* is a ubiquitously expressed 23kb gene composed of 10 exons. The NEMO protein is the regulatory component of the IκB kinase (IKK) complex, a central activator of the NF-κB transcriptional signaling pathway.[82,83] In incontinentia pigmenti, loss-of-function mutations in *NEMO* lead to a susceptibility to cellular apoptosis in response to TNF-α.[81,83]

In 357 affected individuals, an identical genomic deletion within *NEMO* accounted for 90% of the mutations (248 of 277 patients with mutations).[84] This deletion eliminated exons 4 to 10 (*NEMOΔ4–10*) and abolished protein function. The remaining mutations were small duplications, substitutions, and deletions. Most *NEMO* mutations caused premature protein truncation, which may cause cell death. In families transmitting the recurrent deletion, the rearrangement usually occurred in the paternal germline, suggesting intrachromosomal misalignment during meiosis.[84] Expression analysis of human and mouse *NEMO/nemo* showed that the gene becomes active early during embryogenesis and is expressed ubiquitously,[84] suggesting a vital role in embryonic and postnatal development.

Whatever mutation causes incontinentia pigmenti, X-inactivation is likely to modulate the severity in females and account for phenotypic variation. Some females carry the common deletion but are clinically normal,[84] suggesting that selection against mutant cells may have commenced very early in prenatal development as in mouse models, in which surviving *nemo*$^{+/-}$ female mice show marked skewing of X-inactivation.[85,86] Although X-inactivation may account for the female phenotypic variation, a role for modifier genes cannot be excluded. In males, X-inactivation is not an issue, and most *NEMO* mutations are lethal because they abolish NF-κB activity, making cells susceptible to TNF-α-induced apoptosis,[81] a finding also demonstrated in *nemo*-null male mice.[85,86]

Less deleterious mutations can give rise to surviving males and an ectodermal dysplasia-like phenotype with immunodeficiency.[87] Males with skin, dental, and ocular abnormalities typical of those seen in female patients with incontinentia pigmenti are rare; four have been investigated.[88] All carried the common deletion *NEMOΔ4–10*, normally associated with male death *in utero*. Survival in one patient was explained by a 47,XXY karyotype and skewed X-inactivation. The three other patients had a normal 46,XY karyotype, and they had both wild-type and deleted copies of the *NEMO* gene and are therefore somatic mosaics for the common mutation: they acquired the deletion at a postzygotic stage.[88] There are therefore three mechanisms for survival of males carrying a *NEMO* mutation: mild mutations, a 47,XXY karyotype, and somatic mosaicism.

Walker–Warburg syndrome (WWS) (HARD ± E) and related syndromes

Clinical and histological findings

The acronym HARD ± E stands for hydrocephalus, agyria, retinal dysplasia with or without encephalocele (Fig. 49.5). This autosomal recessive syndrome is characterized by type II lissencephaly (absence of cortical gyri), retinal dysplasia, cerebellar malformation, and congenital muscular dystrophy.[34,35] Hydrocephalus is common, which is helpful in prenatal diagnosis by ultrasonography. Other variable features of the Walker–Warburg syndrome (WWS) include Dandy–Walker malformation and encephalocele. Neonatal death is common and survivors are severely developmentally delayed.[34,35] The ocular features in this disorder are variable and include microphthalmia, Peters anomaly, cataract, retinal coloboma, and retinal dysplasia.

There are two other rare autosomal recessive disorders characterized by the combination of congenital muscular dystrophy and brain malformations, including a neuronal migration defect: muscle–eye–brain disease (MEB) and Fukuyama congenital muscular dystrophy (FCMD). Ocular abnormalities are a constant feature in MEB and WWS, but not in FCMD.[89] The distinction between MEB and WWS is difficult due to the overlap in their clinical characteristics.[89] Survival past 3 years of age is far more likely in MEB, whereas death in infancy is more usual in WWS. MRI findings can also be helpful in differentiating between MEB and WWS: an absent corpus callosum suggests WWS.[89]

Genetic linkage studies have shown that WWS is not allelic to MEB.[89] The molecular genetics of these three disorders is likely to be helpful in distinguishing between them when the clinical diagnosis is unclear.[90–92]

Molecular genetics and pathogenesis

MEB and FCMD have many similarities to WWS. The causative genes have already been cloned in MEB[90] and FCMD;[91] their protein products are implicated in protein glycosylation. Candidate genes in 15 consanguineous families with WWS were selected on the basis of the role of the FCMD and MEB genes.[92] Analysis of the locus for O-mannosyltransferase 1 (*POMT1*) revealed homozygosity in 5 of 15 families. Sequencing of *POMT1* (located on chromosome 9q) revealed mutations in 6 of the 30

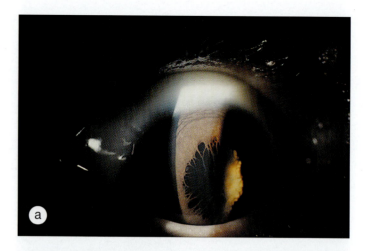

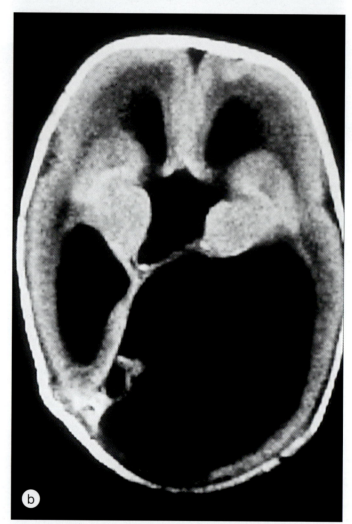

Fig. 49.5 Walker–Warburg syndrome. (a) Shallow anterior chamber and a retrolental mass. (b) CT scan showing hydrocephalus, lissencephaly, and colpocephaly.

unrelated patients with WWS. Of the five mutations identified, four were nonsense mutations and one was a missense mutation. Immunohistochemical analysis of muscle from patients with *POMT1* mutations corroborated the O-mannosylation defect, as judged by the absence of glycosylation of α-dystroglycan, with the lack of such glycosylation believed to be sufficient to explain

the muscular dystrophy in WWS.[92] The brain and eye phenotypes in WWS may involve defective glycosylation of other
proteins. Further genetic heterogeneity in WWS is likely since of
the 30 patients tested only 6 (20%) were found to have *POMT1*
mutations. Loci on 5q and 6q are suggested by a baby with WWS
who had a de novo reciprocal translocation between chromosomes
5 and 6, t(5;6)(q35;q21).[93]

Autosomal recessive vitreoretinal dysplasia

Vitreoretinal dysplasia may occur as an isolated abnormality in an
otherwise healthy child.[24,25] The inheritance is presumed to be
autosomal recessive. The Norrie disease gene (*NDP*) must be
excluded. Presentation is with bilateral poor vision in early
infancy, a shallow anterior chamber, and white retrolental mass.
Progressive shallowing of the anterior chamber may lead to pupil-
block glaucoma, which, following failure to respond to medical
therapy, may require lensectomy.

Osteoporosis–pseudoglioma–mental retardation syndrome

Clinical findings

This autosomal recessive syndrome associates osteoporosis,
mental retardation, and vitreoretinal dysplasia[94,95] (Fig. 49.6).
Multiple fractures, often after minor trauma, are commonplace,
but are not usually diagnosable at the time of presentation. Eye
features include vitreoretinal dysplasia with retrolental masses,
microphthalmia, anterior chamber anomalies, cataract, and
phthisis bulbi, although these are variable. Usually congenitally
blind, a few patients have useful vision into their teenage years.

Molecular genetics and pathogenesis

The gene locus has been mapped to chromosome 11q12-13.[96]
Mutation in the gene encoding the low-density lipoprotein
receptor-related protein 5 (*LRP5*)[1] has been identified.[97] Studies
of *LRP5* indicate that it affects bone accrual during growth by
regulating osteoblastic proliferation. Transient expression of
LRP5 by normal vitreous cells may initiate regression of the
primary vitreous[2]; loss of this function in patients with *LRP5*
mutations may result in vitreoretinal dysplasia.[97]

Oculopalatal-cerebral dwarfism

Three siblings of consanguineous parents were described with
vitreoretinal dysplasia and systemic abnormalities including
microcephaly, mental retardation, cleft palate, and short
stature.[98] The ocular abnormalities, which were like those seen in
PHPV, were bilateral in one child and unilateral in the others. It
is probably autosomal recessive.

Unilateral retinal dysplasia

Lloyd et al. reported a unique and unusual family in which three
affected members had unilateral retinal dysplasia without any
systemic abnormalities.[99]

Genetic counseling in the vitreoretinal dysplasias

The vitreoretinal dysplasias are genetically heterogeneous
disorders, which result in a similar ocular abnormality; it is
impossible to subdivide them on the clinical or pathological
ocular findings,[24] so the diagnosis depends on the systemic find-

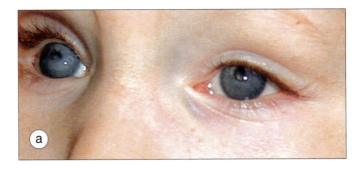
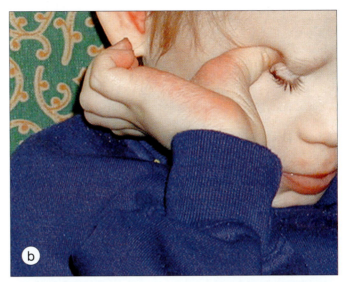
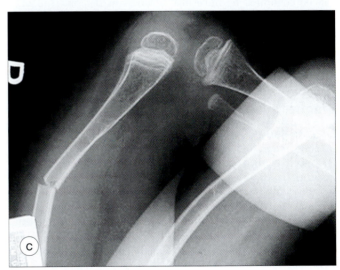

Fig. 49.6 Osteoporosis–pseudoglioma–mental retardation syndrome.
(a) Bilateral leukocoria secondary to retrolental masses. (b) Eye poking in
children with blindness due to retinal disease is common. (c) X-ray of
femur showing fracture and bone demineralization. Osteoporosis takes
some years to develop. Figures reproduced with the permission of the
British Journal of Ophthalmology.[95]

ings or molecular genetics, although the family history may
suggest the mode of inheritance.

For the purposes of genetic counseling, families fall into two
groups. In the first group the diagnosis (and hence the mode of
inheritance) of the affected child is clear. In the second are those
families in which a child is born without a family history and with
isolated retinal dysplasia and no associated systemic findings.

In the first group counseling is straightforward. When one child has been born with a trisomy the risk of a similar affected child in a future pregnancy is about 1%, but may be higher if one of the parents has a structural chromosome abnormality or mosaicism.[100] Such parents may be offered prenatal diagnosis.

In children with the systemic features of Walker–Warburg syndrome or the osteoporosis–pseudoglioma–mental retardation syndrome the inheritance is autosomal recessive.

In Norrie disease there are no detectable clinical abnormalities in the carrier female to aid counseling. When there is another affected male relative the mother can be assumed to be a carrier. In isolated boys, the status of the mother is uncertain, but can usually be resolved by molecular genetics. If the mutation has been identified in the affected child, the mother and other at-risk female members can be screened for the mutation. Most mothers will be identified as carriers. However, some mothers will not carry the identified Norrie gene mutation: their affected child may have a new mutation. However, germ line mosaicism is possible but rare. In this situation, the mother will need to be counseled that there is an increased, but low, risk of having a further child with Norrie disease.

Counseling a family with an otherwise normal child with bilateral retinal dysplasia is more difficult. Isolated retinal dysplasia is sufficiently rare that there are insufficient empirical data to aid counseling. If the affected child is female, retinal dysplasia may be autosomal recessive or nongenetic; since autosomal recessive dysplasia is rare, so long as there is no parental consanguinity the recurrence risk is likely to be low. In an affected male child the retinal dysplasia may be autosomal recessive, X-linked, or nongenetic. Most affected males will have Norrie disease, which can be confirmed by molecular genetics. In the small minority without identifiable mutations in the *NDP* gene, so long as there is no parental consanguinity and other multisystem disorders have been excluded, the recurrence risk is probably low.

INHERITED VITREORETINAL DYSTROPHIES

Wagner syndrome (see also Chapter 56)

Clinical and histological findings

Wagner syndrome[101] is an autosomal dominant vitreoretinal dystrophy with low myopia and vitreous and retinal abnormalities.[102] The vitreous appears optically empty apart from scattered translucent membranes: there is usually a posterior vitreous detachment with a thickened posterior hyaloid. Peripheral vascular sheathing is common and is normally associated with perivascular RPE atrophy and pigment deposition. The ERG is subnormal and parallels the chorioretinal pathology and poor night vision. Cataract develops after the second decade and causes visual loss. Rhegmatogenous retinal detachment is infrequent, whereas peripheral tractional retinal detachment occurs in most of the elderly affected.[102]

Wagner syndrome should be reserved for families without systemic abnormalities.[101,102]

Molecular genetics and pathogenesis

Wagner syndrome and erosive vitreoretinopathy are linked to 5q13-14; they may be allelic disorders, distinct from Stickler syndrome.[103] A phenotypically distinct vitreoretinopathy has been described with early-onset retinal detachments and anterior segment developmental abnormalities, without systemic features, that maps to 5q13-q14, to a 5-cM region already implicated in both Wagner syndrome and erosive vitreoretinopathy.[104]

Erosive vitreoretinopathy

Clinical findings

Erosive vitreoretinopathy is characterized by autosomal dominant inheritance, night blindness, progressive field loss, vitreous abnormalities, progressive RPE atrophy, and combined tractional and rhegmatogenous retinal detachment.[105] ERG shows widespread rod and cone dysfunction. Peripheral RPE atrophy, field loss, and ERG abnormalities are evident in childhood. The vitreous is syneretic with areas of condensation but without inflammatory signs. There are no systemic abnormalities.

Dragged retinal vessels and macular ectopia occur and tractional or rhegmatogenous retinal detachment happens in most affected adults. Twenty percent of affected eyes become blind from retinal detachment.[105]

Molecular genetics and pathogenesis

Erosive vitreoretinopathy, Wagner syndrome, and the syndrome referred to above have been mapped to 5q13-q14, suggesting they may be allelic.[103,104]

Stickler syndrome (see also Chapter 56)

Clinical and histological findings

In Stickler[106] syndrome, abnormalities of vitreous gel architecture are a pathognomonic feature, usually associated with congenital and nonprogressive high myopia.[107] Other eye features include paravascular pigmented lattice degeneration, cataracts, and retinal detachment. Nonocular features are very variable: deafness, a flat mid-face with depressed nasal bridge, short nose, anteverted nares, and micrognathia that can become less pronounced with age. Midline clefting, if present, ranges from a submucous cleft to Pierre-Robin sequence, while joint hypermobility declines with age. Osteoarthritis may develop after the third decade. Stature and intellect are normal.[107]

Molecular genetics and pathogenesis

The *COL2A1* gene encodes type II procollagen, a precursor of components of secondary vitreous and articular cartilage;[108] several mutations occur in families with Stickler[109,110] and Kniest syndrome.[111] There is phenotypic variability with presence or absence of systemic features and locus heterogeneity with about two-thirds of families showing linkage to *COL2A1*.

Stickler syndrome can be divided into two types by slit-lamp biomicroscopy of the vitreous:[112] families with Stickler type 1 vitreous anomaly are associated with mutations of the *COL2A1* gene, whereas those without this anomaly are designated type 2. Mutations in *COL11A1* (encoding α1 chain of type XI collagen)[113] and *COL11A2* (encoding α2 chain of type XI collagen)[114] have been reported in type 2 families. Mutations in exon 2 of the *COL2A1* gene may produce a Stickler phenotype with predominantly ocular manifestations.[115]

Myelinated nerve fibers, vitreoretinopathy, and skeletal malformations

Severe vitreoretinal degeneration, high myopia, myelinated nerve fibers, and skeletal abnormalities were described in a mother and daughter[116] that were distinct from those seen in Stickler syndrome. Both had severe visual impairment and roving eye movements, and electrophysiological testing in the mother showed an abnormal scotopic and photopic ERG.

Juvenile X-linked retinoschisis

(see also Chapter 54)

Clinical and histological findings

This X-linked disorder is almost exclusive to males. Macular abnormalities, usually foveal schisis, are virtually invariable, and are often the only abnormality (Fig. 49.7a–49.7c). Most children present between 5 and 10 years either with reading difficulties or when they fail the school eye test. The visual acuity is 6/12–6/36 at presentation, and strabismus, hypermetropia, and astigmatism are common. If the macular changes are subtle, the disorder is often misdiagnosed as strabismic or ametropic amblyopia or functional visual loss.[117]

About 50% of affected males show peripheral retinal changes including peripheral retinoschisis, a peripheral pigmentary retinopathy (Fig. 49.7d), perivascular sheathing, capillary closure, gray-white dendriform appearance on the inner surface of the retina, and even frank neovascularization[117] (Table 49.2). Retinal detachment and vitreous hemorrhage may complicate X-linked retinoschisis (Fig. 49.8).

The EOG is normal but the ERG shows a reduced or absent b-wave with a normal a-wave, the "negative ERG." Carriers have a normal fundus appearance and normal EOG and ERG. Histo-pathologically there is a split in the nerve fiber layer.

The visual prognosis is relatively good.[117] Central vision deteriorates slowly with most patients retaining stable vision until the fifth or sixth decade when macular atrophy may develop. Peripheral fields are usually normal unless there is peripheral retinoschisis or detachment. Most children require conservative management with correction of refractive errors, treatment of amblyopia, and sometimes, low-vision aids. Vitreoretinal surgery may occasionally be indicated for persistent vitreous hemorrhage or retinal detachment.

Molecular genetics and pathogenesis

Juvenile X-linked retinoschisis (XLRS) has been linked to Xp22.2, and mutations in the *XLRS1* (*RS1*) gene have been

Table 49.2 Fundus abnormalities in X-linked juvenile retinoschisis[117]
Macular changes Foveal schisis "Blunted" foveal reflex Macular atrophy Macular coloboma Pigment line
Peripheral retinal abnormalities Peripheral schisis Vitreous veils Inner leaf breaks
Vascular abnormalities Vascular sheathing Capillary closure Optic disc neovascularization Peripheral retinal neovascularization "Dendriform figures" "Dragged" retinal vessels
Pigmentary retinopathy **Flecked retina** **Inner retinal reflex**

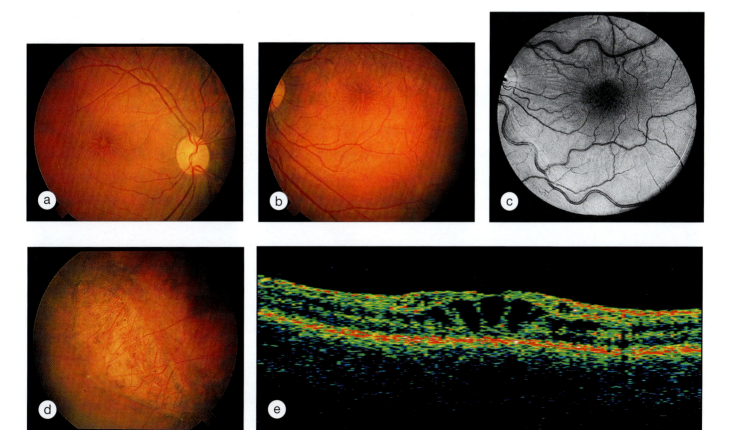

Fig. 49.7 Juvenile X-linked retinoschisis. (a, b) Bilateral foveal schisis. (c) The foveal schisis is best seen with ophthalmoscopy using a red free light. (d) Peripheral pigmentary changes in an area of schisis. (e) OCT study of retinoschisis demonstrating the optically empty spaces in the macula (image courtesy of Dr Dorothy Thompson).

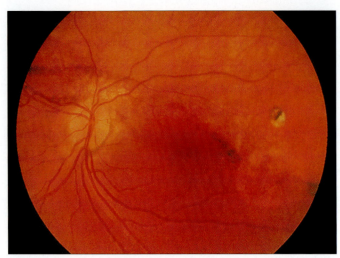

Fig. 49.8 Juvenile X-linked retinoschisis. Fundus appearance after a bullous retinoschisis cyst involving the macula has resolved, leaving a flat retina with a pigment demarcation line.

identified.[118] *XLRS1* encodes a protein, retinoschisin (*RS1*), with a discoidin domain implicated in cell–cell adhesion and cell–matrix interactions, correlating well with retinal splitting in XLRS.

Familial exudative vitreoretinopathy (FEVR)

FEVR describes inherited disorders in which there is evidence of abnormal retinal vascularization, sometimes associated with exudation, neovascularization, and tractional retinal detachment, with some clinical similarities to cicatricial ROP.

Three main forms are recognized:

1. Autosomal dominant familial exudative vitreoretinopathy (AD-FEVR);
2. X-linked familial exudative vitreoretinopathy (XL-FEVR); and
3. Autosomal recessive familial exudative vitreoretinopathy (AR-FEVR).

Autosomal dominant familial exudative vitreoretinopathy (AD-FEVR)

Clinical and histological findings

Early reports were of a progressive vitreoretinopathy like cicatricial ROP,[119] autosomal dominant inheritance, and a variable clinical expression[120] (Table 49.3).

Histopathology in FEVR has been performed on cases too advanced to help our understanding.[121] Clinically there is a widespread abnormality of the retinal vasculature, due to arrest of normal vasculogenesis.[122] In the asymptomatic form, fundoscopy and fluorescein angiography reveal peripheral retinal retinovascular abnormalities, particularly temporally (Fig. 49.9). These include vascular dilatation and tortuosity, A-V shunting, capillary closure, and peripheral retinal neovascularization (Fig. 49.10). Optic disc neovascularization is less common. Vitreoretinal adhesions are frequently seen at the border between vascularized and nonvascularized retina, and other peripheral retinal changes include retinal pigmentation and intraretinal white deposits.

More advanced cases show vascular leakage, cicatrization with macular ectopia, tractional retinal detachment, and macular edema (Fig. 49.11). Vitreous hemorrhage and secondary rhegmatogenous retinal detachment are also recognized complications. The retinal

changes may progress throughout childhood, rarely after the age of 20. In children who show progression from stage I disease cryotherapy of peripheral ischemic retina may be indicated.[120] In advanced cases, vitreoretinal surgery may be beneficial.[123]

The majority of FEVR gene carriers are asymptomatic and have only minor retinovascular abnormalities. The gene is highly penetrant, and in counseling, it is important to perform a careful

Table 49.3 Classification of autosomal dominant familial exudative vitreoretinopathy[120]
Stage I Mild peripheral retinal changes with abnormal vitreous traction but no evidence of retinal vascular or exudative change.
Stage II Dilated tortuous vessels between the equator and ora serrata with subretinal exudates and localized retinal detachment. Dragging of disc vessels and macular ectopia is often present.
Stage III Advanced disease with total retinal detachment and extensive vitreoretinal traction. There may be secondary cataract and rubeosis iridis.

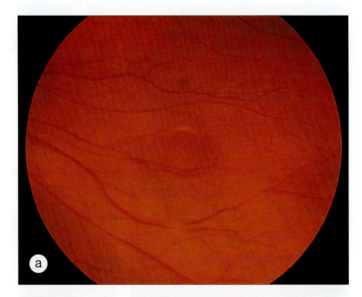

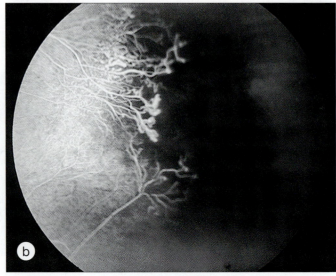

Fig. 49.9 Autosomal dominant familial exudative vitreoretinopathy. (a, b) Vascular dilatation, shunting, and capillary closure.

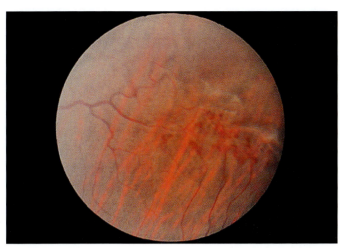

Fig. 49.10 Autosomal dominant familial exudative vitreoretinopathy. Peripheral vascular dilatation, tortuosity, and shunting with some preretinal changes.

fundoscopic examination, preferably with fluorescein angiography, before excluding carrier status.

Molecular genetics and pathogenesis

AD-FEVR has been mapped to 11q[124] as has ADNIV (see below).[125] Linkage to the 11q13-23 locus has been confirmed, with mutations detected in FZD4 (encoding the Wnt receptor frizzled-4) in affected individuals.[126] Further genetic heterogeneity in FEVR has been demonstrated by a second locus for AD-FEVR, on 11p12-13.[127]

X-linked familial exudative vitreoretinopathy (XL-FEVR)

Clinical findings

The phenotype may be similar to the severe form of dominant exudative vitreoretinopathy[128] and may also resemble congenital falciform retinal folds. Affected males have severe early-onset visual impairment, and prominent retinal folds from the disc to the ora serrata are characteristic.

Molecular genetics and pathogenesis

The X-linked form of FEVR, which has an earlier age of onset, has been shown to map to Xp,[128] to a region which includes the gene for Norrie disease (NDP). Point mutations in (NDP), in an XL-FEVR family with the mutation segregating with disease[52] and in XL-FEVR simplex cases[129] have been identified, suggesting that XL-FEVR and Norrie disease are allelic (different mutations of the same gene give rise to a different but well-defined phenotype).

Autosomal recessive familial exudative vitreoretinopathy (AR-FEVR)

Two unrelated families with FEVR showed apparent autosomal recessive inheritance.[130] Compared with the other modes of inheritance, the clinical features included a congenital onset and more severe progression.

Autosomal dominant vitreoretinochoroidopathy (ADVIRC)

Clinical and histological findings

This rare dystrophy has abnormal chorioretinal pigmentation in a 360° circumference between the vortex veins and the ora serrata, which are present in childhood and usually progress. There are areas of hypo- and hyperpigmentation, and scattered yellow dots may be seen in the peripheral retina and at the posterior pole. There are usually retinovascular changes with arteriolar narrowing, venous occlusion, and widespread leakage.[131] A demarcation line is seen between the normal and abnormal retina. The vitreous is liquefied with peripheral condensation. Presenile cataract occurs frequently. Fluorescein angiography shows areas of capillary dilatation and diffuse vascular leakage; peripheral neovascularization may develop in a small proportion of cases.[131]

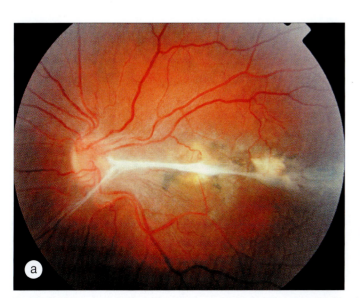

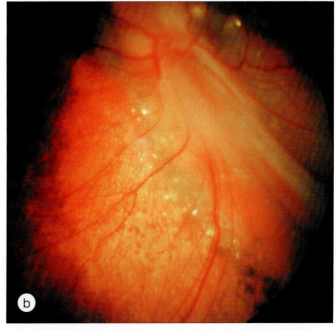

Fig. 49.11 Autosomal dominant familial exudative vitreoretinopathy. (a) Cicatrization with macular ectopia. (b) Severe retinal fold secondary to FEVR.

Visual symptoms are rare in childhood but may occur in adults from cataract, macular edema, vitreous hemorrhage, and retinal detachment. Nyctalopia is not prominent and the ERG is normal, sometimes becoming abnormal with age.[132] The EOG is usually suggesting abnormal widespread RPE defect[133] but can be normal.[134] There are no consistent systemic abnormalities.

Light and electron microscopy showed similar findings in a young[135] and an old patient,[136] suggesting that ADVIRC is an early-onset peripheral retinal dystrophy with minimal subsequent progression, characterized by a RPE response that includes marked intraretinal migration and extracellular matrix deposition.

Autosomal dominant neovascular inflammatory vitreoretinopathy (ADNIV)

Clinical findings

This rare autosomal dominant disorder is characterized by panocular inflammation, peripheral retinal pigment deposition, retinal vascular occlusion and neovascularization, vitreous hemorrhage, and tractional retinal detachment.[137] Presenile cataract is common. The ERG shows early selective loss of the b-wave ("negative ERG"), which differentiates it from the other vitreoretinopathies with vascular closure. Night-blindness is a late feature, and the ERG may become totally extinguished in advanced disease. There are no reported systemic abnormalities.

The earliest signs are vitreous cells, mild peripheral retinal ischemia, and reduced b-wave amplitudes on ERG.

Molecular genetics and pathogenesis

It has been mapped to 11q close to the 11q locus for autosomal dominant familial exudative vitreoretinopathy,[125] suggesting they may be allelic.

Autosomal dominant snowflake degeneration

This disorder is characterized by extensive "white-with-pressure" change in the peripheral retina, multiple minute "snowflake" retinal deposits, and sheathing of the peripheral retinal vessels.[138] Later, there may be peripheral vascular occlusion and retinal pigmentation. The vitreous is degenerate and liquefied. Psychophysical studies show abnormal rod and cone function, and although ERG may be normal initially, the b-wave amplitude is later reduced.[139] There is an increased risk of retinal tears and detachment. The retinal changes may be seen in childhood, more often in the teens or later.[139] There are no systemic abnormalities.

ACQUIRED DISORDERS OF THE VITREOUS

Acquired disorders of the vitreous are uncommon in childhood and generally occur when there is vitreous opacification caused by hemorrhage or inflammation. Less commonly tumor or infection may involve the vitreous cavity.

Vitreous hemorrhage (see Table 49.4)

The management of vitreous hemorrhage is relatively straightforward in older children who have reached the age of visual maturity. A conservative approach is preferred with surgery only indicated if the hemorrhage is persistent or if there is an associated retinal detachment. In infants and young children, vitreous hemorrhage may lead to amblyopia and may also affect emmetropization.[141,142] If, after a short period of observation, there is no resolution and if there is no underlying retinal abnormality that may herald a poor prognosis, early lens-sparing vitrectomy may be considered. Occlusion needs to be started as soon as possible.

Inflammatory disease of the vitreous

(see Chapter 44)

Vitreous opacity due to tumor

Vitreous seeding is a well-recognized complication of retinoblastoma;[143] clumps of tumor cells float in the vitreous but rarely give rise to diagnostic problems as there is also usually a typical retinoblastoma. Occasionally, when there are clumps of cells in the anterior vitreous in an inflamed eye with an opaque vitreous there may be doubt as to whether the underlying etiology is inflammatory or neoplastic. Ultrasound or CT scan usually demonstrates a retinoblastoma, but not in the rare diffuse infiltrating forms.

Tumor cells may also be found in the vitreous in leukemia but there is almost always associated retinal infiltration (see Chapter 68). Other intraocular tumors are rare.

Table 49.4 Some causes of vitreous hemorrhage in children

Trauma
    Blunt
    Penetrating

X-linked juvenile retinoschisis
Vitreoretinal dystrophies
    FEVR
    ADVIRC
    ADNIV

Stickler syndrome ROP PHPV Retinal dysplasias Retinal hemangioblastoma Cavernous hemangioma[140] Eales disease Coats disease NAI/child abuse Birth-related hemorrhages Optic disc drusen

Hematological disorders
    Leukemia
    Thrombocytopenia
    Hemophilia
    von Willebrand disease
    Protein C deficiency

REFERENCES

1. Duke-Elder S, editor. System of Ophthalmology. London: Henry Kimpton; 1963: 141–52. (vol. 3.)
2. Spencer WH. Vitreous. In: Ophthalmic Pathology. An Atlas and Textbook. London: Saunders; 1985: 554–6.
3. Jones HE. Hyaloid remnants in the eyes of premature babies. Br J Ophthalmol 1963; 47: 39–44.
4. Lusky M, Weinberger D, Kremer L. Vitreous cyst combined with bilateral juvenile retinoschisis. J Paediatr Ophthalmol Strabismus 1988; 25: 75–7.
5. François J. Prepapillary cysts developed from remnants of the hyaloid artery. Br J Ophthalmol 1950; 34: 365–8.
6. Bullock JD. Developmental vitreous cysts. Arch Ophthalmol 1974; 91: 83–4.
7. Feman SS, Straatsma BR. Cyst of the posterior vitreous. Arch Ophthalmol 1974; 91: 328–9.
8. Hilsdorf C. Uber einen fall einer einseitigen glaskorpercyste. Ophthalmologica (Basel) 1965; 149: 12–20.
9. Lisch W, Rochels R. Pathogenesis of congenital vitreous cysts. Klin Monatsbl Augenheilk 1989; 195: 375–8.
10. Elkington AR, Watson DM. Mobile vitreous cysts. Br J Ophthalmol 1974; 58: 103–4.
11. Ruby AJ, Jampol LM. Nd:YAG treatment of a posterior vitreous cyst. Am J Ophthalmol 1990; 110: 428–9.
12. Awan KJ. Biomicroscopy and argon laser photocystotomy of free-floating vitreous cysts. Ophthalmology 1985; 92: 1710–1.
13. Gupta R, Pannu BK, Bhargav S, et al. Nd:YAG laser photocystotomy of a free-floating pigmented anterior vitreous cyst. Ophthalmic Surg Lasers Imaging 2003; 34: 203–5.
14. Menchini U, Pece A, Alberti M, et al. Hyperplastic primary vitreous with persistent hyaloid artery in two non twin brothers. J Ophthalmol 1987; 10: 241–5.
15. Storimans CW, van Schooneveld MJ. Rieger's eye anomaly and persistent hyperplastic primary vitreous. Ophthalmol Paediatr Genet 1989; 10: 257–62.
16. Lin AE, Biglan AW, Garver KL. Persistent hyperplastic primary vitreous with vertical transmission. Ophthalmol Pediatr Genet 1990; 11: 121–2.
17. Pruett RC, Schepens CL. Posterior hyperplastic primary vitreous. Am J Ophthalmol Strabismus 1970; 69: 535–43.
18. Pollard Z. Treatment of persistent hyperplastic primary vitreous. J Pediatr Ophthalmol 1985; 22: 180–3.
19. Goldberg MF, Mafee M. Computed tomography for the diagnosis of persistent hyperplastic primary vitreous. Ophthalmology 1983; 90: 442–51.
20. Reese AB. Persistent hyperplastic primary vitreous. Am J Ophthalmol 1955; 40: 317–31.
21. Font RL, Yanoff M, Zimmerman LE. Intraocular adipose tissue and persistent hyperplastic primary vitreous. Arch Ophthalmol 1969; 82: 43–50.
22. Stark WJ, Lindsey P, Fagadau WR, Michels RG. Persistent hyperplastic primary vitreous; surgical treatment. Ophthalmology 1983; 90: 452–7.
23. Kennedy RE. The effect of early enucleation on the orbit in animals and humans. Am J Ophthalmol 1965; 60: 277–306.
24. Lahav M, Albert DM, Wyand S. Clinical and histopathologic classification of retinal dysplasia. Am J Ophthalmol 1973; 75: 648–67.
25. Ohba N, Watanabe S, Fujital S. Primary vitreoretinal dysplasia transmitted as an autosomal recessive disorder. Br J Ophthalmol 1981; 65: 631–40.
26. Norrie G. Causes of blindness in children; 25 years experience of Danish Institutes for the Blind. Acta Ophthalmol l927; 5: 357–86.
27. Warburg M. Norrie disease, a new hereditary bilateral pseudotumour of the retina. Acta Ophthalmol 1961; 39: 757–72.
28. Warburg M. Norrie disease (atrofia bulborum hereditaria). Acta Ophthalmol 1963; 41: 134–46.
29. Carney RG, Carney RG Jr. Incontinentia pigmenti. Arch Dermatol 1970; 102: 157–62.
30. Carney RG. Incontinentia pigmenti: a world statistical analysis. Arch Dermatol 1976; 112: 535–42.
31. François J. Incontinentia pigmenti (Bloch-Sulzberger syndrome) and retinal changes. Br J Ophthalmol 1984; 68: 19–25.
32. Landy SJ, Donnai D. Incontinentia pigmenti (Bloch-Sulzberger syndrome). J Med Genet 1993; 30: 53–9.
33. Goldberg MF, Custis PH. Retinal and other manifestations of incontinentia pigmenti (Bloch-Sulzberger syndrome). Ophthalmology 1993; 100: 1645–54.
34. Warburg M. The heterogeneity of microphthalmia in the mentally retarded. Birth Defects Orig Artic Ser 1971; 7: 136–54.
35. Pagon RA, Clarren SK, Milam DF Jr, Hendrickson AE. Autosomal recessive eye and brain anomalies: Warburg syndrome. J Pediatr 1983; 102: 542–6.
36. Fulton AB, Craft JL, Howard RO, Albert DM. Human retinal dysplasia. Am J Ophthalmol 1978; 85: 690–8.
37. Bernado AI, Kirsch LS, Brownstein S. Ocular anomalies in anencephaly: a clinicopathological study of 11 globes. Can J Ophthalmol 1991; 26: 257–63.
38. Silverstein AM, Parshall CJ, Osburn BI, Pendergast RA. An experimental virus induced retinal dysplasia in the fetal lamb. Am J Ophthalmol 1971; 72: 22–34.
39. Parving A, Warburg M. Audiological findings in Norrie's disease. Audiology 1977; 16: 124–31.
40. Redmond R, Vaughan J, Jay M, Jay B. In utero diagnosis of Norrie's disease by ultrasonography. Ophthalmic Paediatr Genet 1993; 141: 1–3.
41. Suarez-Merino B, Bye J, McDowall J, et al. Sequence analysis and transcript identification within 1.5 MB of DNA deleted together with the NDP and MAO genes in atypical Norrie disease patients presenting with a profound phenotype. Hum Mutat 2001; 17: 523.
42. Enyedi L, de Juan E, Gaiton A. Ultrastructural study of Norrie's disease. Am J Ophthalmol 1991; 111: 439–46.
43. Parsons MA, Curtis D, Blank CE, et al. The ocular pathology of Norrie disease in a fetus of 11 weeks' gestational age. Graefes Arch Clin Exp Ophthalmol 1992; 230: 248–51.
44. Joos KM, Kimura AE, Vandenburgh K, et al. Ocular findings associated with a Cys39Arg mutation in the Norrie disease gene. Arch Ophthalmol 1994; 112: 1574–9.
45. Woodruff G, Newbury-Ecob R, Plaha D, Young ID. Manifesting heterozygosity in Norrie's disease. Br J Ophthalmol 1993; 77: 813–4.
46. Chen ZY, Battinelli EM, Woodruff G, et al. Characterisation of a mutation within the NDP gene in a family with a manifesting female carrier. Hum Mol Genet 1993; 2: 1727–9.
47. Black G, Redmond RM. The molecular biology of Norrie's disease. Eye 1994; 8: 491–6.
48. Yamada K, Limprasert P, Ratanasukon M, et al. Two Thai families with Norrie disease (ND): association of two novel missense mutations with severe ND phenotype, seizures, and a manifesting carrier. Am J Med Genet 2001; 100: 52–5.
49. Ohba N, Yamashita T. Primary vitreoretinal dysplasia resembling Norrie's disease in a female: associated with X autosome chromosomal translocation. Br J Ophthalmol 1986; 70: 64–71.
50. Berger W, van de Pol D, Warburg M, et al. Mutations in the candidate gene for Norrie disease. Hum Mol Genet 1992; 1: 461–5.
51. Chen Z, Hendriks RW, Jobling MA, et al. Isolation and characterisation of a candidate gene for Norrie disease. Nature Genet 1992; 1: 203–9.
52. Chen ZY, Battinelli EM, Fielder A, et al. A mutation in the Norrie disease gene (NDP) associated with X-linked familial vitreoretinopathy. Nature Genet 1993; 5: 180–3.
53. Chen ZY, Battinelli EM, Hendriks RW, et al. Norrie disease gene: characterisation of deletions and possible functions. Genomics 1993; 16: 533–5.
54. Wong F, Goldberg MF, Hao Y. Identification of a nonsense mutation at codon 128 of the Norrie's disease gene in a male infant. Arch Ophthalmol 1993; 111: 1553–7.
55. Zhu D, Maumenee IH. Mutation analysis of the Norrie disease gene in 11 families. Invest Ophthalmol Vis Sci 1994; 35: 1265.
56. Meindl A, Berger W, Meitinger T, et al. Norrie disease is caused by mutations in an extracellular protein resembling C-terminal globular domain of mucins. Nature Genet 1992; 2: 139–43.
57. Meitinger T, Meindl A, Bork P, et al. Molecular modelling of the Norrie disease protein predicts cysteine knot growth factor tertiary structure. Nature Genet 1993; 5: 376–80.
58. Matsuo T. The genes involved in the morphogenesis of the eye. Jpn J Ophthalmol 1993; 37: 215–51.

59. Shastry BS, Pendergast SD, Hartzer MK, et al. Identification of missense mutations in the Norrie disease gene associated with advanced retinopathy of prematurity. Arch Ophthalmol 1997; 115: 651–5.

60. Hiraoka M, Berinstein DM, Trese MT, Shastry BS. Insertion and deletion mutations in the dinucleotide repeat region of the Norrie disease gene in patients with advanced retinopathy of prematurity. J Hum Genet 2001; 46: 178–81.

61. Talks SJ, Ebenezer N, Hykin P, et al. De novo mutations in the 5' regulatory region of the Norrie disease gene in retinopathy of prematurity. J Med Genet 2001; 38: E46.

62. Black GC, Perveen R, Bonshek R, et al. Coats disease of the retina (unilateral retinal telangiectasis) caused by somatic mutation in the NDP gene: a role for norrin in retinal angiogenesis. Hum Mol Genet 1999;8:2031–5.

63. Rehm HL, Gutierrez-Espeleta GA, Garcia R, et al. Norrie disease gene mutation in a large Costa Rican kindred with a novel phenotype including venous insufficiency. Hum Mutat 1997; 9: 402–8.

64. Haider MZ, Devarajan LV, Al-Essa M, et al. Missense mutations in norrie disease gene are not associated with advanced stages of retinopathy of prematurity in Kuwaiti arabs. Biol Neonate 2000; 77: 88–91.

65. Kim JH, Yu YS, Kim J, Park SS. Mutations of the Norrie gene in Korean ROP infants. Korean J Ophthalmol 2002; 16: 93–6.

66. Haider MZ, Devarajan LV, Al-Essa M, et al. Retinopathy of prematurity: mutations in the Norrie disease gene and the risk of progression to advanced stages. Pediatr Int 2001; 43: 120–3.

67. Berger W, van de Pol D, Bachner D, et al. An animal model for Norrie disease (ND): gene targeting of the mouse ND gene. Hum Mol Genet 1996; 5: 51–9.

68. Richter M, Gottanka J, May CA, et al. Retinal vasculature changes in Norrie disease mice. Invest Ophthalmol Vis Sci 1998; 39: 2450–7.

69. Rehm HL, Zhang DS, Brown MC, et al. Vascular defects and sensorineural deafness in a mouse model of Norrie disease. J Neurosci 2002; 22: 4286–92.

70. Patau K, Smith DW, Therman E, et al. Multiple congenital anomalies caused by an extra autosome. Lancet 1960; i: 790–3.

71. Smith DW, Patau K, Therman E, et al. The D1 trisomy syndrome. J Pediatr 1963; 62: 326–41.

72. Hoepner J, Yanoff M. Ocular anomalies in trisomy 13–15: an analysis of 13 eyes with two new findings. Am J Ophthalmol 1972; 74: 729–37.

73. Cogan DG, Kuwubara T. Ocular pathology of the 13–15 trisomy syndrome. Arch Ophthalmol 1964; 72: 346–53.

74. Berlin AL, Paller AS, Chan LS. Incontinentia pigmenti: a review and update on the molecular basis of pathophysiology. J Am Acad Dermatol 2002; 47: 169–87.

75. Wald KJ, Mehta MC, Katsumi O, et al. Retinal detachments in incontinentia pigmenti. Arch Ophthalmol 1993; 111:614–7.

76. Holmstrom G, Thoren K. Ocular manifestations of incontinentia pigmenti. Acta Ophthalmol Scand 2000; 78: 348–53.

77. Ferreira RC, Ferreira LC, Forstot L, King R. Corneal abnormalities associated with incontinentia pigmenti. Am J Ophthalmol 1997; 123: 549–51.

78. Mayer EJ, Shuttleworth GN, Greenhalgh KL, et al. Novel corneal features in two males with incontinentia pigmenti. Br J Ophthalmol 2003; 87: 554–6.

79. Watzke RC, Stevens TS, Carney RG. Retinal vascular changes of incontinentia pigmenti. Arch Ophthalmol 1976; 94: 743–6.

80. Rahi J, Hungerford J. Early diagnosis of the retinopathy of incontinentia pigmenti: successful treatment by cryotherapy. Br J Ophthalmol 1990; 74: 377–9.

81. Smahi A, Courtois G, Vabres P, et al. Genomic rearrangement in NEMO impairs NF-?B activation and is a cause of incontinentia pigmenti. The International Incontinentia Pigmenti (IP) Consortium. Nature 2000; 405: 466–72.

82. Karin M, Ben-Neriah Y. Phosphorylation meets ubiquitination: the control of NF- κB activity. Annu Rev Immunol 2000; 18: 621–63.

83. Aradhya S, Nelson DL. NF-κB signaling and human disease. Curr Opin Genet Dev 2001; 11: 300–6.

84. Aradhya S, Woffendin H, Jakins T, et al. A recurrent deletion in the ubiquitously expressed NEMO (IKK-κ) gene accounts for the vast majority of incontinentia pigmenti mutations. Hum Mol Genet 2001; 10: 2171–9.

85. Schmidt-Supprian M, Bloch W, Courtois G, et al. NEMO/IKKG-deficient mice model incontinentia pigmenti. Mol Cell 2000; 5: 981–92.

86. Makris C, Godfrey VL, Krahn-Senftleben G, et al. Female mice heterozygous for IKKκ/NEMO deficiencies develop a dermatopathy similar to the human X-linked disorder incontinentia pigmenti. Mol Cell 2000; 5: 969–79.

87. Aradhya S, Courtois G, Rajkovic A, et al. Atypical forms of incontinentia pigmenti in male individuals result from mutations of a cytosine tract in exon 10 of NEMO (IKK-κ). Am J Hum Genet 2001; 68: 765–71.

88. Kenwrick S, Woffendin H, Jakins T, et al. Survival of male patients with incontinentia pigmenti carrying a lethal mutation can be explained by somatic mosaicism or Klinefelter syndrome. Am J Hum Genet 2001; 69: 1210–7.

89. Cormand B, Pihko H, Bayes M, et al. Clinical and genetic distinction between Walker–Warburg syndrome and muscle-eye-brain disease. Neurology 2001; 56: 1059–69.

90. Yoshida A, Kobayashi K, Manya H, et al. Muscular dystrophy and neuronal migration disorder caused by mutations in a glycosyltransferase, POMGnT1. Dev Cell 2001; 1: 717–24.

91. Kobayashi K, Nakahori Y, Miyake M, et al. An ancient retrotransposal insertion causes Fukuyama-type congenital muscular dystrophy. Nature 1998; 394: 388–92.

92. Beltran-Valero de Bernabe D, Currier S, Steinbrecher A, et al. Mutations in the O-mannosyltransferase gene POMT1 give rise to the severe neuronal migration disorder Walker-Warburg syndrome. Am J Hum Genet 2002; 71: 1033-43.

93. Karadeniz N, Zenciroglu A, Gurer YK, et al. De novo translocation t(5;6)(q35;q21) in an infant with Walker-Warburg syndrome. Am J Med Genet 2002; 109: 67–9.

94. Neuhauser G, Kaveggia EG, Opitz JM. Autosomal recessive syndrome of pseudogliomatous blindness, osteoporosis and mild mental retardation. Clin Genet 1976; 9: 324–32.

95. Wilson G, Moore A, Allgrove J. Bilateral retinal detachments at birth: the osteoporosis pseudoglioma syndrome. Br J Ophthalmol 2001; 85: 1139.

96. Gong Y, Vikkula M, Boon L, et al. Osteoporosis-pseudoglioma syndrome, a disorder affecting skeletal strength and vision, is assigned to chromosome region 11q12-13. Am J Hum Genet 1996; 59: 146–51.

97. Gong Y, Slee RB, Fukai N, et al. LDL receptor-related protein 5 (LRP5) affects bone accrual and eye development. Cell 2001;107:513–23.

98. Frydman M, Kauschansky A, Leshem I, Savir H. Oculo-palato-cerebral dwarfism. Clin Genet 1985; 27: 414–9.

99. Lloyd I, Colley A, Tullo A, Bonshek R. Dominantly inherited unilateral retinal dysplasia. Br J Ophthalmol 1993; 77: 378–80.

100. Steve J, Steve E, Mikkelson M. Risk for chromosome abnormality at aminiocentesis following a child with a non-inherited chromosome aberration. Prenat Diagn 1984;4:81–5.

101. Wagner H. Ein Bisher Unbekanntes Erbleiden des Auges (Degeneration Hyaloideo Retinalis Hereditaria), Beobachtet im Karifon Zurich. Klin Monatsebl Augenheilkd 1938; 100: 840–56.

102. Graemiger RA, Niemeyer G, Schneeberger SA, Messmer EP. Wagner vitreoretinal degeneration. Follow–up of the original pedigree. Ophthalmology 1995; 102: 1830–9.

103. Brown DM, Graemiger RA, Hergersberg M, et al. Genetic linkage of Wagner disease and erosive retinopathy to chromosome 5q13-14. Arch Ophthalmol 1995; 113: 671–5.

104. Black GC, Perveen R, Wiszniewski W, et al. A novel hereditary developmental vitreoretinopathy with multiple ocular abnor-malities localizing to a 5-cM region of chromosome 5q13-q14. Ophthalmology 1999; 106: 2074–81.

105. Brown DM, Kimura AE, Weingeist TA, Stone EM. Erosive vitreoretinopathy. A new clinical entity. Ophthalmology 1994; 101: 694–704.

106. Stickler GB, Belau PG, Farrel FJ, et al. Hereditary progressive ophthalmo-arthropathy. Mayo Clin Proc 1965; 40: 433–95.

107. Snead MP, Yates JR. Clinical and molecular genetics of Stickler syndrome. J Med Genet 1999; 36: 353–9.

108. Francomano C, Liberfarb RM, Hirose T, et al. The Stickler syndrome: evidence for close linkage to the structural gene for type II collagen. Genomics 1987; 1: 293–6.

109. Ahmad NN, Ala-Korkho L, Knowlton RG, et al. Stop codon in the procollagen II gene (COL2A1) 3 prime variable region in the family with Stickler's syndrome (arthro-ophthalmopathy). Proc Natl Acad Sci USA 1991; 88: 6624–7.

110. Brown DM, Vandenburgh K, Nichols BE, et al. Incidence of frameshift mutations in the procollagen II gene in Stickler syndrome and identification of four new mutations. Invest Ophthalmol Vis Sci 1994; 35: 1717.

111. Wilkin DJ, Weiss MA, Gruber HE, et al. An exon skipping mutation in the type II collagen gene (COL2A1) produces Kneist dysplasia. Am J Hum Genet 1993; 53: A210.

112. Snead MP, Payne SJ, Barton DE, et al. Stickler syndrome: correlation between vitreoretinal phenotypes and linkage to COL2A1. Eye 1994; 8: 414–8.

113. Richards AJ, Yates JR, Williams R, Payne SJ, et al. A family with Stickler syndrome type 2 has a mutation in the COL11A1 gene resulting in the substitution of glycine 97 by valine in a1 (XI) collagen. Hum Mol Genet 1996; 5: 1339–43.

114. Sirko-Osadsa DA, Murray MA, Scott JA, et al. Stickler syndrome without eye involvement is caused by mutations in COL11A2, the gene encoding the a2(XI) chain of type XI collagen. J Pediatr 1998; 132: 368–71.

115. Donoso LA, Edwards AO, Frost AT, et al. Clinical variability of Stickler syndrome: role of exon 2 of the collagen COL2A1 gene. Surv Ophthalmol 2003; 48: 191–203.

116. Traboulsi EI, Lim JI, Pyeritz R, et al. A new syndrome of myelinated nerve fibres, vitreoretinopathy and skeletal malformations. Arch Ophthalmol 1993; 111: 1543–5.

117. George NG, Yates JRW, Moore AT. Clinical features of affected males in juvenile X-linked retinoschisis. Arch Ophthalmol 1996; 114: 274–80.

118. Sauer CG, Gehrig A, Warneke-Wittstock R, et al. Positional cloning of the gene associated with X-linked juvenile retinoschisis. Nat Genet 1997; 17: 164–170.

119. Criswick VG, Schepens CL. Familial exudative vitreoretinopathy. Am J Ophthalmol 1969; 68: 578–94.

120. Gow J, Oliver GL. Familial exudative vitreoretinopathy, an expanded view. Arch Ophthalmol 1971; 86: 150–5.

121. Boldrey EE, Egbert P, Gass JD, Friberg T. The histopathology of familial exudative vitreoretinopathy. A report of two cases. Arch Ophthalmol 1985; 103: 238–41.

122. van Nouhuys CE. Signs, complications, and platelet aggregation in familial exudative vitreoretinopathy. Am J Ophthalmol 1991; 111: 34–41.

123. Pendergast SD, Trese MT. Familial exudative vitreoretinopathy. Results of surgical management. Ophthalmology 1998; 105: 1015–23.

124. Li Y, Muller B, Fuhrmann C, et al. The autosomal dominant familial exudative retinopathy maps on 11q and is closely linked to D11S533. Am J Hum Genet 1992; 51: 749–54.

125. Stone EM, Kimura AE, Folk JC, et al. Genetic linkage of autosomal dominant neovascular inflammatory vitreoretinopathy to chromosome 11q13. Hum Mol Genet 1992; 1: 685–9.

126. Robitaille J, MacDonald ML, Kaykas A, et al. Mutant frizzled-4 disrupts retinal angiogenesis in familial exudative vitreoretinopathy. Nat Genet 2002; 32: 326–30.

127. Downey LM, Keen TJ, Roberts E, et al. A new locus for autosomal dominant familial exudative vitreoretinopathy maps to chromosome 11p12-13. Am J Hum Genet 2001; 68: 778–81.

128. Fullwood P, Jones J, Bundey S, et al. X-linked exudative vitreoretinopathy: clinical features and genetic linkage analysis. Br J Ophthalmol 1993; 77: 168–70.

129. Shastry BS. Identification of a recurrent missense mutation in the Norrie disease gene associated with a simplex case of exudative vitreoretinopathy. Biochem Biophys Res Commun 1998; 246: 35–8.

130. de Crecchio G, Simonelli F, Nunziata G, et al. Autosomal recessive familial exudative vitreoretinopathy: evidence for genetic heterogeneity. Clin Genet 1998; 54: 315–20.

131. Kaufman SJ, Goldberg MF, Orth DH, et al. Autosomal dominant vitreoretino-choroidopathy. Arch Ophthalmol 1982; 100: 272–8.

132. Lafaut BA, Loeys B, Leroy BP, et al. Clinical and electro-physiological findings in autosomal dominant vitreoretino-choroidopathy: report of a new pedigree. Graefes Arch Clin Exp Ophthalmol 2001; 239: 575–82.

133. Han D, Lewandowski M. Electro-oculography in autosomal dominant vitreoretinochoroidopathy. Arch Ophthalmol 1992; 110: 1563–7.

134. Kellner U, Jandeck C, Kraus H, Foerster MH. Autosomal dominant vitreoretinochoroidopathy with normal electrooculogram in a German family. Graefes Arch Clin Exp Ophthalmol 1998; 236: 109–14.

135. Han DP, Burke JM, Blair JR, Simons KB. Histopathologic study of autosomal dominant vitreoretinochoroidopathy in a 26-year-old woman. Arch Ophthalmol 1995; 113: 1561–6.

136. Goldberg MF, Lee FL, Tso MO, Fishman GA. Histopathologic study of autosomal dominant vitreoretinochoroidopathy. Peripheral annular pigmentary dystrophy of the retina. Ophthalmology 1989; 96: 1736–46.

137. Bennett SR, Folk JC, Kimura AE, et al. Raphtis EM. Autosomal dominant neovascular inflammatory vitreoretinopathy. Ophthalmology 1990; 97: 1125–35.

138. Hirose T, Lee KY, Schepens CL. Snowflake degeneration in hereditary vitreoretinal degeneration. Am J Ophthalmol 1974; 77: 143–53.

139. Pollack A, Uchenik D, Chemke J, Oliver M. Prophylactic laser photocoagulation in hereditary snowflake vitreoretinal degeneration: a family report. Arch Ophthalmol 1983; 101: 1536–9.

140. Yamaguchi K, Yamaguchi K, Tamai M. Cavernous haemangioma of the retina in a pediatric patient. Ophthalmologica 1988; 197: 127–9.

141. Miller-Meeks MJ, Bennett SR, Keech RV, Blodi CF. Myopia induced by vitreous haemorrhage. Am J Ophthalmol 1990; 109: 199–203.

142. Mohney BG. Axial myopia associated with dense vitreous haemorrhage of the neonate. J AAPOS 2002 6: 348–53.

143. Rosenthal AR. Ocular manifestations of leukemia: a review. Ophthalmology 1983; 16: 899–905.

CHAPTER

50 Retinoblastoma

Brenda L Gallie, Vasudha Erraguntla, Elise Héon and Helen S L Chan

Retinoblastoma is the commonest malignant ocular tumor of childhood, but is quite rare at one in 20 000 live births.[1] Untreated, the tumor is almost uniformly fatal, but with modern methods of treatment the survival rate is over 90%. An integrated team approach of clinical specialists with imaging specialists, play therapists, parents and others is the most effective way to manage this disease. The tumor arises from primitive retinal cells so the majority of cases occur in children under the age of 4 years. Until recently, treatment included only enucleation or/and radiation. Children with mutations in the *RB1* tumor suppressor gene may develop secondary tumors when exposed to radiation so, since the 1990s, the combination of systemic chemotherapy and focal therapy have been widely used, in order to avoid these very serious side-effects.

The study of retinoblastoma has led to a revolution in the understanding of cancer in general: studies revealed that both hereditary and nonhereditary tumors are initiated by the loss of both alleles of the tumor suppressor gene, *RB1*.[2] The existence of specific genes that normally act to suppress cancer was predicted from clinical studies of retinoblastoma,[3,4] which opened up the knowledge of events that led to the predisposition of cancer in humans. The *RB1* gene was the first tumor suppressor gene to be cloned,[5] and the knowledge about the function of this gene revealed its critical role in cell cycle regulation in cancer.

PATHOGENESIS OF RETINOBLASTOMA

Heritable and nonheritable retinoblastoma

Nearly 50% of retinoblastoma cases are heritable, due to a mutation in the *RB1* gene, which predisposes a child to develop retinal tumors. The hallmark of the majority of hereditary cases is the occurrence of bilateral or multifocal tumors, but 15% of children with unilateral tumors also have a mutation of one allele of the *RB1* gene in their germ cells, that will be inherited by one half of their children. Less than 25% of all cases have a family history of retinoblastoma,[6] since usually the affected child, even those with bilateral disease, has suffered a *new* germline mutation. In familial cases, the predisposition to retinoblastoma is transmitted as an autosomal dominant trait.

Nonheritable retinoblastoma is caused by mutations in the same *RB1* gene. In nonheritable retinoblastoma, somatic mutations in both alleles of the *RB1* gene occur in a single primitive retinal cell, which gives rise to a solitary, unilateral tumor. Since no germ cell mutation is involved, the disease is not transmitted to the offspring.

Loss of both *RB1* alleles induces retinoblastoma

The simple clinical observation that the children with bilateral retinoblastoma tended to be diagnosed at a younger age than those with nonhereditary retinoblastoma was analyzed mathematically by Knudson. He predicted that two mutational events (M1 and M2) were required to initiate retinoblastoma.[3] The ages at diagnosis of children with bilateral and unilateral retinoblastoma plotted in a semi-log curve against the proportion not yet diagnosed fitted a simple exponential equation which suggested that it was a single second mutation (M2) in one developing retinal cell that initiated tumor development (heritable retinoblastoma), in the presence of a predisposing first mutation (M1) in the germline. However, two or more mutations (M1 and M2) had to occur in one single developing retinal cell in order to initiate retinoblastoma in the absence of a predisposing germline mutation (nonheritable retinoblastoma).

This "two-hit" hypothesis was expanded by Comings who proposed that the two events could be mutations that occurred on the two different alleles of the predisposing *RB1* gene, which as long as one normal allele was present, would normally have "suppressed" tumor formation in the retina.[4] The chance of two or more primitive retinal cells bearing germline M1 undergoing additional M2 events is sufficiently high that multiple tumors are a common occurrence in hereditary retinoblastoma (Fig. 50.1). However, the chance that both M1 and M2 events would occur in the same retinal cell is so extremely small that it is virtually impossible for nonhereditary cases to have multiple tumors. Perhaps because time is required for two mutational events to occur, or because two affected eyes come to attention sooner than one affected eye, children with nonhereditary retinoblastoma tend to be diagnosed at an older age than children with hereditary retinoblastoma.

In about half of the cases, the M2 event in the tumor is loss and reduplication of large chromosomal regions surrounding *RB1*, which could be detected by loss of heterozygosity, or homozygosity for the M1 mutation (Fig. 50.2). In such tumors, the two mutant alleles are identical and the normal allele is missing.[2,7] In the remaining tumors, the second *RB1* allele acquires a completely different mutation.[8]

Function of the retinoblastoma protein

pRB is a 110 kDa phosphoprotein that inhibits cell proliferation by altering the expression of genes which promote cell division, through interaction with the transcription factor E2F family and many other modifying proteins.[9] DNA tumor viruses that induce cancer, such as human papilloma virus, do so in part by binding to pRB through the "pocket" region of pRB. The active form of pRB is underphosphorylated, and for the cell cycle to proceed, pRB has to be inactivated by phosphorylation mediated by protein complexes of cyclins and cyclin-dependent kinases.

Why does mutation of a cell cycle regulatory gene lead specifically to the development of retinoblastoma? Germline

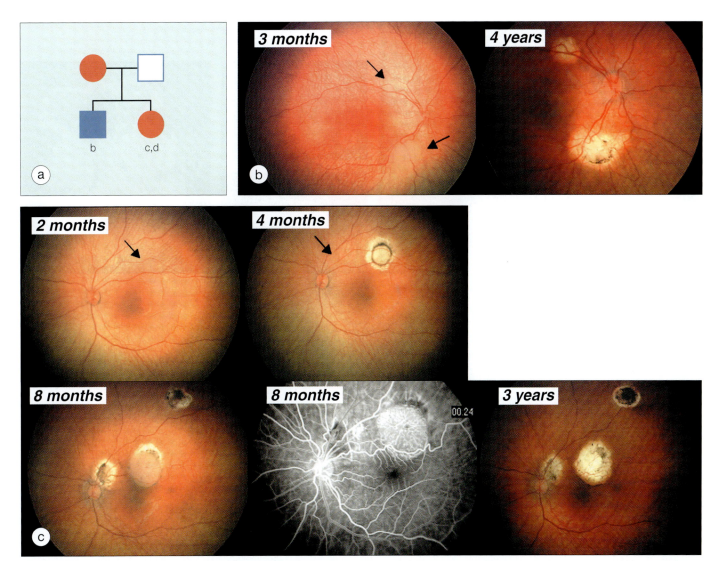

Fig. 50.1 Hereditary retinoblastoma. (a) Family tree: mother was cured of bilateral retinoblastoma by enucleation of one eye and external beam radiation of the other eye. Both children were delivered at 36 weeks gestation to facilitate early treatment of tumors and developed bilateral tumors. Mother and both children carry a germline *RB1* mutation (M1, deletion of ATTTC starting at bp 778, reading to a STOP, 9 codons away) that results in no pRB when the normal *RB1* allele is lost (M2) from a developing retinal cell, initiating a tumor. RetCam® images: (b) prior to treatment, right eye IIRC Group A, more than 1.5 mm from optic disc) of the boy at 3 months, showing two tumors; stable right eye of boy age 4 years after laser, two cycles of CEV with cyclosporine A chemotherapy, and more laser treatments. (c) prior to treatment, left eye (IIRC Group B, tumor less than 3 mm from fovea) of the girl at 2 months; laser scar and new tumor above nerve at 4 months of age; recurrence in original scar extending toward fovea, with tumor vascularization showing on fluorescein angiography; flat scars at age 3 years after laser, two cycles of CEV with cyclosporine A chemotherapy to control recurrence threatening vision chemotherapy and more laser. (Images by Leslie MacKeen, Cynthia Vandenhoeven and Carmelina Trimboli.)

mutation of *RB1* leads to a 40 000-fold relative risk (RR) for retinoblastoma, a 500-fold RR for sarcoma that is increased up to 2000-fold by therapeutic radiation, but no increase in the RR for leukemia.[10] Although pRB is present in all cycling cells, its function in development is highly tissue-specific. Thus, mice constructed to have no pRB die *in utero* of trophoblast failure,[11] even though many other tissues have apparently formed normally. If the mice are rescued by the provision of a wild-type placenta, they still die at birth from inadequate muscle development.[12] The retina may be uniquely dependent on pRB in order to be able to differentiate terminally into adult, functioning retina. In the absence of pRB, proliferation of the susceptible cell continues when terminal differentiation or cell death should normally have occurred. Further mutations in oncogenes and other tumor suppressor genes (M3-Mn) result in a retinal tumor.[13,14]

Spectrum of *RB1* mutations

The majority of *RB1* mutations are unique to each affected individual in a family, and are distributed throughout the *RB1* gene with no real hot spots.[8] Sensitive mutation identification requires determination of the copy number of each exon and the gene promoter in order to reveal large deletions and duplications, scanning and sequencing for point mutations, examining the mRNA to detect or confirm splice variants, and assay for the methylation status of the promoter in tumor samples. Exon scanning and sequencing reveals approximately 70% of the *RB1* mutations. Application of all these techniques, combined with a gene disease-specific focused expertise, identifies over 90% of the *RB1* mutations. When tumor or blood samples are submitted to a clinical test laboratory, it is critical to know that such a

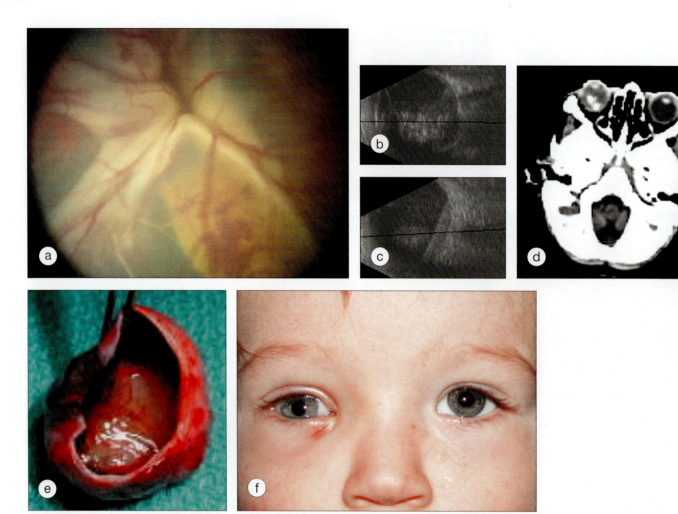

Fig. 50.2 Exophytic retinoblastoma (IIRC Group D). (a) With retinal detachment in a unilaterally affected 3-year-old boy. (b) B-scan ultrasound showing calcification in a single tumor beside the optic nerve. (c) B-scan ultrasound showing subretinal hemorrhage and no tumor involvement of optic nerve. (d) CT scan showing intraocular calcification, normal-sized optic nerve. (e) The eye was opened immediately after enucleation, in order to obtain live tumor cells in order to determine the two *RB1* mutations (M1, M2) (homozygous exon 16 deletion C-1450, insertion AT). This mutant *RB1* allele was not detected in the child's blood, eliminating risk for his siblings. His future offspring will be checked for this mutant allele since he could still be mosaic. (f) The child two days after enucleation, wearing the temporary prosthetic conformer inserted at the time of surgery. The exon 16 *RB1* mutation of the tumor is not detected in blood, indicating high likelihood that the retinoblastoma is not heritable, eliminating risk for siblings. Due to the remaining possibility that the affected child is mosaic for the *RB1* mutation, his future offspring will be tested for this mutation. (Images by Cynthia Vandenhoeven and Carmelina Trimboli.)

laboratory does have the state-of-the-art test sensitivity, and that the turn-around-time in that particular laboratory is optimal, since these prerequisites greatly impact on care of the entire retinoblastoma family.

Genetic counseling for retinoblastoma

Without the knowledge of which *RB1* allele is mutant, the risk for the relatives of retinoblastoma patients can be estimated.[15] Offspring of patients with a family history of retinoblastoma or bilateral tumors have a 50% risk of inheriting the mutant allele and a 45% risk of developing retinoblastoma. When two affected children are born to apparently normal parents, one parent must be carrying but not expressing the mutant allele, and hence there is also a 45% risk that any subsequent child born will develop retinoblastoma. The risk that other relatives have inherited the mutant allele depends on the number of intervening "apparently normal" individuals, each of which have a 10% chance of carrying but not expressing the mutant allele. The risk therefore falls by a factor of 0.1 for each intervening unaffected generation.

Since 15% of patients with unilateral retinoblastoma have a germinal mutation, it is evident that the offspring of individuals with unilateral retinoblastoma have a 7.5% risk of carrying the abnormal gene. The probability of other relatives developing retinoblastoma can be calculated in a similar way.[15]

Infants born with the above-calculated risks for developing retinoblastoma are examined electively at regular intervals to detect early tumors that can be treated to obtain the best visual result (Fig. 50.1). This includes an awake-examination of the entire retina of infants less than 3 months of age, and examinations under anesthesia subsequently every 3–6 months until they reach the age of 3 years and several years of further clinic examinations.

Impact of genetic testing

Timely and sensitive molecular diagnosis of *RB1* mutations enables earlier treatment, lower risk and better health outcomes for retinoblastoma patients, empowers families to make informed family-planning decisions, and costs less than conventional surveillance.[8,16] New tumors occurred in 24% of children with retinoblastoma, much more frequently in the peripheral retina,[17] emphasizing the importance of a careful fundoscopic examination with indentation to obtain a clear view of the periphery. Accurate molecular analysis allows definitive identification of those family members who carry the same mutation found in the proband (Fig. 50.1). The unaffected children (otherwise previously considered to be at-risk) avoid further surveillance examinations under anesthetic and or in the clinic. The savings in direct costs from incurred by at-risk children in these families avoiding such repeated examinations substantially exceeds the one-time cost of molecular testing. Moreover, health care savings continue to accrue as succeeding generations avoid the unnecessary examinations and usually do not need molecular analysis.

The result of the *RB1* mutations is usually truncation of the expected protein, which is so unstable that no mutant protein is detectable. Such mutations show high penetrance (>95% of offspring affected) and expressivity (average of seven tumors per child). More uncommon *RB1* mutations cause much lower penetrance and expressivity[18]: "in frame" deletions or insertions that result in a stable but defective pRB[19]; promoter mutations that result in a reduced amount of otherwise normal protein[20] and splice mutations that may be additionally altered by unlinked "modifier genes".[21]

Other manifestations of *RB1* mutations

Mutations of *RB1* also predispose to benign retinal tumors, retinoma,[22] ectopic intracranial retinoblastoma (trilateral retinoblastoma), and second nonocular malignancies.[23,24]

Retinoma

A retinoma is a nonmalignant manifestation of the *RB1* mutation.[22] Three features characterize these nonprogressive lesions: an elevated grey retinal mass, calcification, and surrounding retinal pigment epithelium (RPE) proliferation and pigmentation (Fig. 50.3a, b). Such features are also seen after radiation treatment for retinoblastoma. If documented at all in childhood, which is very rare, retinoma is observed as a quiescent tumor that has not progressed to full malignancy. Retinoma may develop when the M2 mutation occurs in a nearly developed retinal cell, that therefore, has a reduced potential for acquiring the M3-Mn mutations that are necessary for full malignancy, resulting in a benign disordered growth in the retina.[13] The importance of finding a retinoma lies in its significance for genetic counseling (Fig. 50.3). The presence of one retinoma puts an individual at risk to carry an *RB1* mutation. With a family history of retinoblastoma, or multiple retinomas, the individual definitely carries a *RB1* mutation; other family members that carry the same mutation may develop a fully malignant retinoblastoma.

Second nonocular malignancies

Children with the hereditary form of retinoblastoma are at increased risk of developing second nonocular malignancies,[24] which may occur within or outside the radiation field (Fig. 50.4). Radiation, particularly of infants under one year of age, increases the risk of sarcomas and other cancers within the radiation field.[23] Osteosarcoma is the commonest second primary tumor in persons with *RB1* mutations, but a wide variety of other neoplasms have been reported. Since these radiation-induced tumors are very difficult to treat, more children with *RB1* mutations have died of their second tumor following the cure of intraocular retinoblastoma by radiotherapy, than those that have died of the consequences of retinoblastoma.

Ectopic intracranial retinoblastoma (trilateral retinoblastoma)

Trilateral retinoblastoma refers to a midline intracranial tumor or a primary pineal tumor associated with hereditary retinoblastoma, that is not a metastasis.[25] The tumors are neuroblastic in origin and resemble a poorly differentiated retinoblastoma. They arise in the vestigial "third eye". Pineal tumors are estimated to occur in 2% of cases of retinoblastoma,[26] but the frequency may have decreased since chemotherapy has replaced radiation as primary treatment. Since, in most cases, the retinoblastoma is familial or bilateral, it is assumed that the pineal gland, like the developing retina, also has a risk for malignant transformation in the presence of an *RB1* mutation. Affected children usually present with symptoms and signs of raised intracranial pressure and are found to have a pineal or parasellar mass on CT scan. Routine screening by MRI for tumors may be useful to detect pineal tumors at a stage when they can be cured.[25]

Histopathology

Retinoblastomas are poorly differentiated malignant neuroblastic tumors, composed of cells with large hyperchromatic nuclei and scanty cytoplasm. Mitotic figures are common. In some tumors, more differentiated cells form the typical Flexner–Wintersteiner rosettes in which columnar cells are uniformly arranged in spheres around a lumen containing the primitive inner segments of photoreceptors.[27]

Tumor cells often outgrow their blood supply leading to necrosis. A true spontaneous regression of retinoblastoma, which is very rare, is probably due to extensive tumor necrosis resulting in phthisis bulbi.[22,28] Programmed cell death or apoptosis is also evident in the tumors that generally lacked pRB or functional pRB, supporting the idea that the normal function of pRB is to promote differentiation over apoptosis in response to differentiation signals. Calcification is almost pathognomonic of retinoblastoma, but the origin of this calcification is not understood.

Two main patterns of retinoblastoma growth are seen within the eye. Endophytic tumors (Figs 50.5 and 50.6) tend to push into the vitreous with only a delicate inner limiting membrane separating tumor from vitreous. When the inner limiting membrane of the retina breaks, "seeds" float in the vitreous cavity, where they are hypoxic and relatively resistant to therapy. When the seeds fall onto the retinal surface, they can attach and grow (Fig. 50.6). Spread of tumor into the anterior chamber may lead to hypopyon, rubeosis iridis and glaucoma, with increased risk of metastasis. Exophytic tumors (Figs 50.2, 50.7) grow into the subretinal space leading to retinal detachment over the tumor. Bruch's membrane may be breached and spread into the

Fig. 50.3 (*Facing page*) Multifocal unilateral retinoma. (a) Discovered at age 16 years, followed for 30 years without change. Note the apparent "seed" in the vitreous when the two images are viewed in stereo. Patient carries a "null" *RB1* germline mutation (deletion of one copy from the promoter to exon 7), inherited by one of his two daughters who developed bilateral retinoblastoma. (b & c) Multifocal bilateral retinoma discovered in the grandfather when his granddaughter developed unilateral retinoblastoma. His daughter had bilateral retinoblastoma and meningioma at age 40. (d) All affected members carry a "null" germline *RB1* mutation (heterozygous point mutation in exon 17 resulting in a STOP codon).

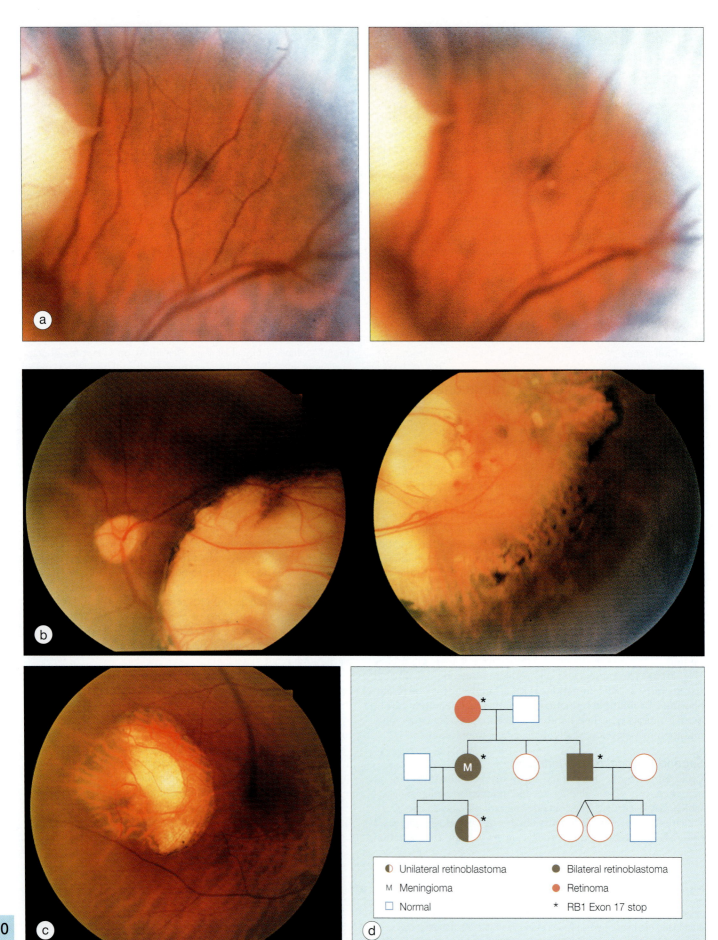

◖ Unilateral retinoblastoma	● Bilateral retinoblastoma
M Meningioma	● Retinoma
☐ Normal	* RB1 Exon 17 stop

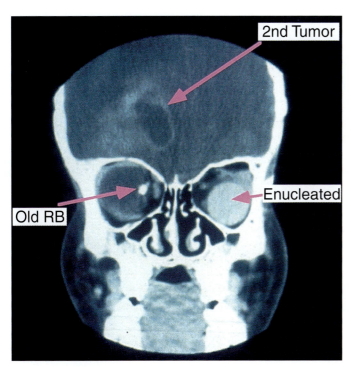

Fig. 50.4 Glioblastoma multiforme. Arising within the radiation field, 10 years after enucleation of the left eye and irradiation of the right eye for bilateral retinoblastoma.

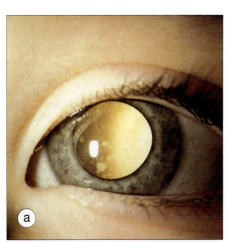

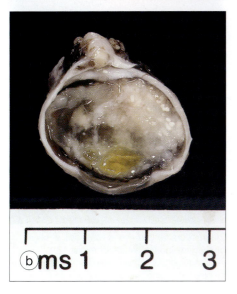

Fig. 50.5 Endophytic retinoblastoma. (a) The tumor has invaded the vitreous and seeds can be seen on the back of the lens (IIRC Group E). (b) Calotte of enucleated eye with tumor filling the eye (same patient).

choroid can occur, which, when extensive, increases the risk of spreading outside the eye and systemic metastasis. Diffusely infiltrating retinoblastoma is uncommon, and since there is no solid, calcified tumor mass or retinal detachment, diagnosis may be difficult.[29]

If retinoblastoma metastasizes, it is generally becomes evident within 18 months of the last active tumor in the eye, and is rare beyond 3 years without evidence of active tumor in the eye.[1] The most common and dangerous route of metastasis of retinoblastoma is direct extension into the optic nerve. The tumor can grow toward the optic chiasm and beyond, or into the subarachnoid space with extensive leptomeningeal involvement (Figs 50.8 and 50.9).[30] Direct extension into optic nerve or via the choroidal vessels, or spread along the ciliary vessels and nerves into the orbit, may occur in advanced cases (Fig. 50.10). True systemic metastasis may occur via the choroidal circulation or aqueous drainage, particularly if glaucoma is present.[30,31] The bone marrow is the preferred site for retinoblastoma metastasis, and only terminally are bone, lymph node, and liver involved. Lung metastases are rare.

CLINICAL MANAGEMENT OF RETINOBLASTOMA

Presentation

The majority of children with retinoblastoma without a family history are first noticed because of leukocoria (Table 50.1).[32] Worldwide, parents have glimpsed an odd appearance in their child's eye, which depends on the source of illumination being in line with the viewer's gaze. So, unless the pediatrician or family physician is aware of the importance of this symptom and refers the child appropriately to a specialist, the diagnosis may be delayed. The parent's description is usually very accurate, and should stimulate full investigation of the eyes but it is still common for diagnosis to be delayed because the primary care physician is not aware of the implication of what the parents are telling them. Frequently snapshots of the baby show the white pupil, "photoleukocoria," before even the parents have noticed it (Fig. 50.11).[33] In nonfamilial retinoblastoma, earlier diagnosis is dependent on this appearance of the eyes on photographs. A similar appearance can result from various benign conditions including: myelinated nerve fibers, optic nerve coloboma, high myopia, congenital cataract, or even normal optic nerves if the camera angle is directed at the normal optic nerve.

The next most common presenting sign is strabismus (esotropia or exotropia).[32] The strabismus is constant and unilateral rather than alternating, and vision in the strabismic eye is poor. All young children with a constant unilateral strabismus should have a careful fundus examination to rule out this diagnosis. Other presenting symptoms and signs (Table 50.1) include a painful red eye from glaucoma, and orbital cellulitis secondary to extensive necrosis of the intraocular tumor (Figs 50.8 and 50.12),[28] unilateral mydriasis, heterochromia, hyphema, hypopyon uveitis, and "searching" nystagmus (due to blindness from bilateral macular involvement).[32] In countries with limited medical services, many children present late often with extraocular and systemic extension, so that extensive unilateral or bilateral proptosis with orbital extension of the tumors is a common presentation (Figs 50.8 and 50.10).

Retinoblastoma in babies and children that are relatives of patients with heritable retinoblastoma should be looked for specifically by screening examinations, long before any symptoms occur (Fig. 50.1). For most families, it is possible to detect

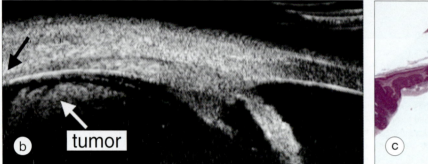
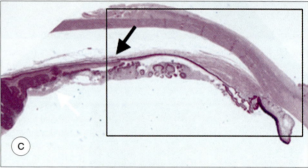

Fig. 50.6 Unilateral endophytic IIRC Group E retinoblastoma. (a) With massive vitreous seeding (left); and (right) extension of tumor for 180° inferiorly, anterior to the ora serrata (arrows) to lie on the pars plana. (b) Ultrasound biomicroscopy of tumor on pars plana and pars plicata of ciliary body. HaE staining of ciliary region showing tumor anterior to ora serrata (arrow); box corresponds to area imaged in (b). (RetCam®) images by Carmelina Trimboli.)

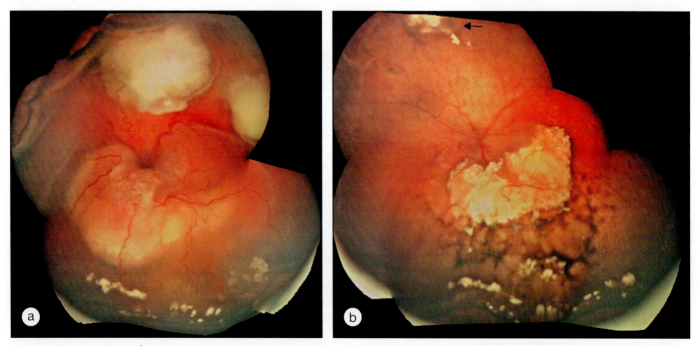

Fig. 50.7 Collage of RetCam® images of the whole retina. The ora serrata is visualized for 360° by scleral depression. (a) Left eye at diagnosis of child with bilateral multifocal exophytic IIRC Group D retinoblastoma, no family history, and a "null" *RB1* mutation (heterozygous deletion of exons 18 to 23) in blood. (b) Excellent regression after 3 of 7 cycles of CEV with cyclosporine A chemotherapy, with arrow indicating residual tumor treated by laser and cryotherapy. Similar appearance of residual tumor and tented retina near the macula was not treated to optimize vision and has not changed over 1 year off treatment. (Images and collage by Cynthia Vandenhoeven.) This child had excellent response in both IIRC Group D eyes.

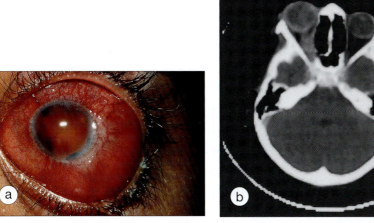 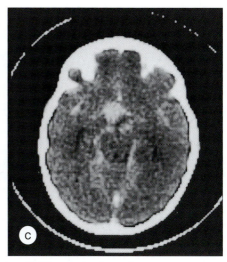

Fig. 50.8 Extraocular retinoblastoma. (a) With iris invasion, glaucoma, subconjunctival and orbital extension. (b) CT scan showing optic nerve involvement. (c) CT scan showing suprasellar and cerebral extension from optic nerve invasion.

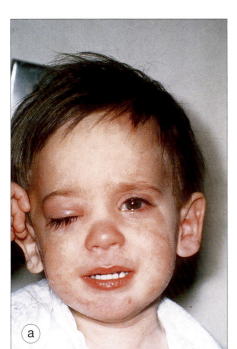 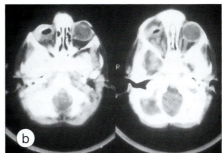

Fig. 50.9 Unilateral retinoblastoma. (a) Unilateral retinoblastoma that presented as orbital cellulitis (IIRC Group E, suggestive of extraocular tumor). (b) Extensive intraocular necrosis and replacement of the optic nerve with tumor. (c) Despite therapy, the brain was covered with meningeal retinoblastoma four months later and the child died.

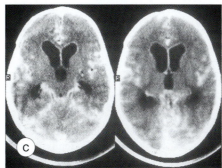

molecularly the precise *RB1* mutation of the proband, check the relatives for that mutation, identify those carrying the mutant allele, and diagnose and initiate treatment early when the tumors are still small. Such small tumors can often be cured by laser therapy alone, or with short cycles of chemotherapy.

Diagnosis

When a child is referred with a possible diagnosis of retinoblastoma, a careful history and thorough ocular and systemic examination may exclude some important differential diagnoses (Table 50.2).[32] Referral of a child with possible retinoblastoma is considered urgent, namely, within one week.

Initial visit

Leukocoria (Fig. 50.11) requires that a careful history be obtained of the pregnancy, labor and delivery of the mother, and birth weight and neonatal period of the child. Maternal illnesses in early pregnancy, premature labor and oxygen usage in the neonatal period may be relevant. For older infants, the parents should be asked about exposure to kittens, puppies, and other animals. A careful family history of any eye disorder should be obtained. The retinas of the parents, the siblings, and any other family members with a history of similar eye disorder should also be examined. The discovery of a retinoma in a relative will significantly alter the understanding of disease and management of the child and the family.

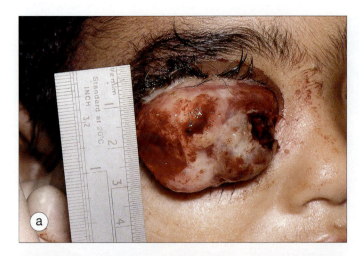

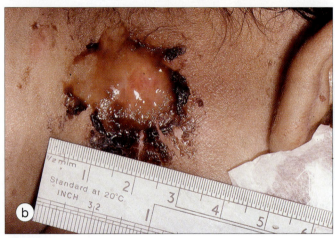

Fig. 50.10 Late diagnosed retinoblastoma. (a) With destruction of the globe and orbital extension. (b) Ulcerating malignant occipital lymph nodes in the same patient.

Table 50.1 Presenting symptoms and signs of retinoblastoma (Ellsworth 1969)

White reflex	56%
Strabismus	20%
Glaucoma	7%
Poor vision	5%
Routine examination	3%
Orbital cellulitis	3%
Unilateral mydriasis	2%
Heterochromia iris	1%
Hyphema	1%
Other	2%

The initial clinical examination of the child will provide a short-list of differential diagnoses, and an estimation of the extent of disease involvement (the staging) if the diagnosis is retinoblastoma. Imaging studies such as CT scan or MRI may be ordered prior to the examination under anesthesia (EUA). If chemotherapy might be indicated, a surgery consultation for the concurrent placement of a central venous line should be arranged prior to the first EUA. The whole multidisciplinary team (ophthalmology, oncology, nursing, social work, cytogenetics) should be aware of the patient and each will play a role from the beginning and throughout the management of each patient.

Table 50.2 Differential diagnosis of retinoblastoma. Modified from Shields and Augsburger (1981)

Hereditary conditions	Inflammatory conditions
Norrie disease	Toxocariasis
Warburg syndrome	Toxoplasmosis
Autosomal recessive retinal dysplasia	Metastatic endophthalmitis
Dominant exudative vitreoretinopathy	Viral retinitis
Juvenile X-linked retinoschisis	Vitritis
Orbital cellulitis	

Developmental anomalies	Tumors
Persistent hyperplastic primary vitreous	Astrocytic hamartoma
Cataract	Medulloepithelioma
Coloboma	Choroidal hemangioma
Congenital retinal fold	Combined hamartoma
Myelinated nerve fibers	
High myopia	
Morning glory syndrome	

Others	
Coats disease	
Retinopathy of prematurity	
Rhegmatogenous retinal detachment	
Vitreous hemorrhage	
Leukemic infiltration of the iris	

Examination under anesthesia (EUA)

For anterior segment examination, fundus examination, and imaging to be performed completely, general anesthesia is required for infants and young children. The pupils must be widely dilated and scleral depression used in order to visualize the whole retina up to the ora serrata. A wide-angle camera, the RetCam® (Massie Laboratories, Inc.), has become standard equipment in many retinoblastoma centers, since it provides excellent 130° wide-field imaging of the retina and anterior segment, including the anterior chamber angle (Figs 50.1, 50.6–50.7, 50.13–50.16). Some small retinoblastoma tumors, visualized as an alteration of the pattern of the retinal pigment epithelium, are actually more easily seen on RetCam® images than with indirect ophthalmoscopy (Fig. 50.1, 50.16).

Children presenting with suspected retinoblastoma may be divided into three broad groups:

Group 1

There is a clear view of the tumor.

Endophytic tumor growth gives rise to a creamy white mass (Figs 50.5, 50.6) projecting into the vitreous with large irregular blood vessels running on the surface and penetrating the tumor. Hemorrhage may be present on the surface of the tumor. Clumps of tumor cells in the vitreous ("seeding") is pathognomonic of retinoblastoma (Fig. 50.6). Some tumors are surrounded by a halo of proliferating retinal pigment epithelium, suggesting that they may be slow-growing and have a retinoma component. Calcification within the tumor mass is common and resembles white, "cottage cheese" (Figs 50.3b, 50.7 and 50.17). Such tumors leave no doubt as to the diagnosis of retinoblastoma. Less commonly, retinoblastoma may present as an avascular white mass in the periphery of the retina.

Group 2

The tumor is poorly seen due to vitreous opacity or extensive retinal detachment (Fig. 50.2a). The presence of calcification confirmed by ultrasonography or CT scan (Figs 50.2b,c,d, 50.6, 50.8, 50.12), may be critical in establishing the diagnosis of retinoblastoma. Other aspects of the examination may support or

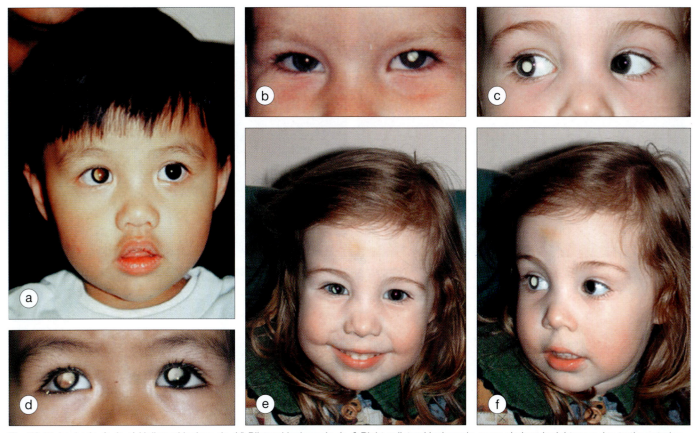

Fig. 50.11 Leukoria. (a, b, c) Unilateral leukocoria. (d) Bilateral leukocoria. (e, f) Right unilateral leukocoria, more obvious in right gaze due to the anterior temporal location of tumor. (Images by Leslie MacKeen.)

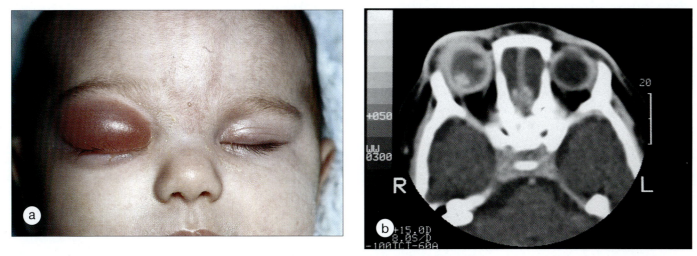

Fig. 50.12 Retinoblastoma presenting as orbital cellulitis (IIRC Group E). (a) At referral the patient was ill but not apyrexial. The globe could not be seen due to lid swelling, which reduced after 2 days of systemic steroid treatment. A small noncalcified tumor was present in the left eye and a calcified retinoblastoma was present in the right eye, (b) shown on CT scan.

help exclude the diagnosis of retinoblastoma. For example, retinoblastoma generally occurs in normal-sized eyes, whereas microphthalmos is more likely to be associated with a developmental abnormality. Examination of the other eye is very important. The presence of small tumors in the other eye confirms the diagnosis of retinoblastoma. Dragged retinal vessels suggests retinopathy of prematurity. Peripheral vitreoretinal changes suggest a dominant exudative vitreoretinopathy.

Group 3
Unusual presentations: heterochromia, hypopyon (Fig. 50.8), uveitis or orbital cellulitis (Fig. 50.12). Here, the diagnosis may be difficult and specialized investigations are helpful, particularly CT scan or MRI.

Once the diagnosis of retinoblastoma is clear, bone marrow aspiration and lumbar puncture to screen for metastatic disease, are performed at the initial EUA, especially if one or both of the

Fig. 50.13 Unilateral retinoblastoma. (a) At diagnosis. (b) The subretinal seed (arrow) inferiorly at the 6 o'clock position places this eye in IIRC Group D (subretinal seeding more than 3 mm from the tumor). (c) Response to chemotherapy (four cycles of carboplatin, etoposide, vincristine with high dose cyclosporine) and laser and cryotherapy. (d) Fluorescein angiography shows active tumor vessels in the scar, which were successfully ablated by 532 nm and 810 nm laser treatments. (Images by Leslie MacKeen and Cynthia Vandenhoeven.)

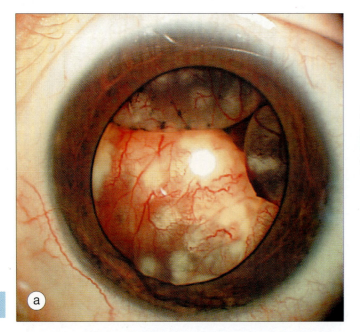

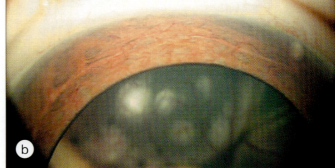

Fig. 50.14 Right eye prior to enucleation for IIRC Group E retinoblastoma. (a) Large retinoblastoma, total retinal detachment, large subretinal seeds, neovascular glaucoma and (b) anterior chamber seeding, arrow, visualized by RetCam® anterior segment and anterior chamber angle photography through gel. (Images by Leslie MacKeen.)

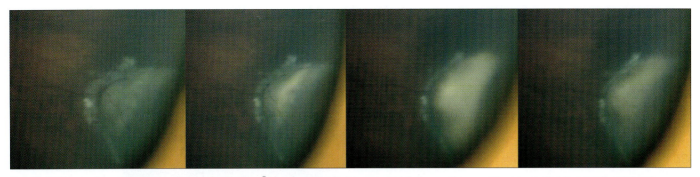

Fig. 50.15 Freeze–thaw cryotherapy. Sequential RetCam® images of the first freeze of triple freeze–thaw cryotherapy applied to a small peripheral retinoblastoma after placement of a 532 nm laser barrier line to limit serous effusion.

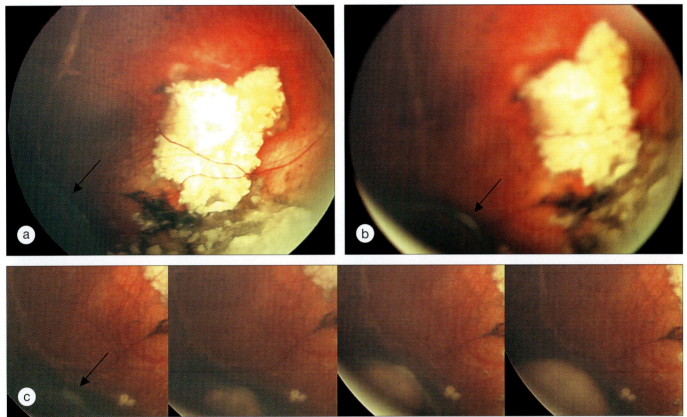

Fig. 50.16 New tumor in a previously treated eye. (a) Arrow indicates no tumor 8 months after initiation of CEV chemotherapy with cyclosporine for IIRC Group D retinoblastoma in the right of the child whose left eye is shown in Fig. 50.7. (b) New peripheral small tumor 2 months later, 10 months after diagnosis. (c) Triple freeze–thaw cryotherapy for the small new tumor, encasing the tumor in ice, thawing for one minute, and refreezing. (RetCam® images by Cynthia Vandenhoeven).

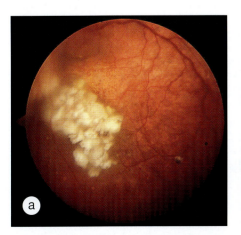 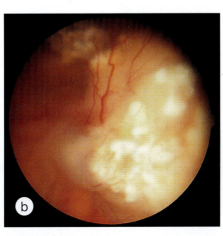

Fig. 50.17 Retinoblastoma regression following external beam radiation. (a) Calcified "cottage cheese" appearance. (b) Mixed, suspicious regression, but after 4 years follow-up, no recurrence occurred.

optic nerves are not visible or there are other adverse risk features (Figs 50.5, 50.8–10 and 50.14). These tests are not necessary if the tumors are small and require only focal therapy.

Differential diagnosis

Conditions which may simulate retinoblastoma are detailed in Table 50.2. In North America, Coats disease, ocular toxocariasis, and persistent hyperplastic primary vitreous (PHPV) are the three commonest conditions confused with retinoblastoma.[34]

Coats disease

See Chapter 55.

Coats disease is almost always unilateral and usually affects boys. It may present with loss of vision and the leukocoria is yellowish due to exudate at the macula whereas in retinoblastoma it is white. Intraocular calcification is rare in Coats disease, and ultrasonography shows a diffuse uniform increase in opacity of the vitreous with no mass. Later there is an exudative detachment with telangiectatic vessels, subretinal lipid and cholesterol crystals (Fig. 50.18). Treatment of early Coats disease with cryotherapy or laser coagulation may arrest the disease or result in improvement of the retinal exudate[35,36]

Ocular toxocariasis

Ocular inflammation due to toxocariasis presents either as chronic endophthalmitis with an opaque vitreous, or a solitary retinal granuloma in an otherwise healthy child.[37] Several features help to differentiate this condition from retinoblastoma. Toxocariasis may show marked vitreous inflammation, with yellow-grey strands extending into the vitreous from the chorioretinal lesions. Such findings are rarely seen in retinoblastoma. CT scan shows calcification in retinoblastoma but not in toxocariasis. Solitary granulomas may resemble retinoblastoma but often show a small translucent center (Fig. 50.19). If there is doubt about the diagnosis, a period of observation with regular fundus examination may be indicated. A positive serological test for toxocariasis is supportive, but not diagnostic, since exposure to the organism is common.

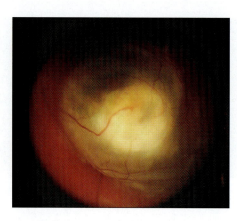

Fig. 50.19 Solitary granuloma in the macula, with a cilioretinal arteriole, masquerading as a retinoblastoma.

Persistent hyperplastic primary vitreous (PHPV)

See Chapter 47.

PHPV is congenital and is almost always unilateral. The affected eye is microphthalmic and there is a dense retrolental mass which may be vascularized. The ciliary processes are often prominent and drawn towards the center of the pupil. PHPV eyes may develop pupillary block glaucoma, vitreous hemorrhage, retinal detachment or phthisis bulbi. In one report, an infant presenting with unilateral leukocoria has been found to have both PHPV and a diffuse infiltrating retinoblastoma.[38]

Retinal dysplasia

See Chapter 49.

Retinal dysplasia presents as bilateral retrolental masses at birth or soon afterwards, unrelated to prematurity or oxygen use. There may be serious systemic abnormalities (see Chapter 49). There may be a shallow anterior chamber, a clear lens, and a relatively avascular retrolental mass without any inflammatory signs. There is no calcification on ultrasonography or CT scan.

Retinopathy of prematurity (ROP)

See Chapter 51.

Advanced cicatricial ROP may give rise to dense unilateral or bilateral retrolental masses. It is seen predominantly in very low birth weight infants who have been exposed to oxygen. It is seldom mistaken for retinoblastoma.

Metastatic endophthalmitis

Metastatic endophthalmitis results from hematogenous spread of infection from a distant infective locus such as meningitis, endocarditis or intra-abdominal sepsis. *Streptococcus, Staphylococcus,* and *Meningococcus* are the most commonly involved organisms. The condition may cause marked vitreous opacification but the presence of other inflammatory signs and systemic infection usually distinguishes this condition from retinoblastoma.[39]

Medulloepithelioma (diktyoma)

This tumor arises from the ciliary epithelium and is always unilateral. It generally occurs at a later age than retinoblastoma. It is located anterior to the ciliary body and has a cystic structure.[40] The tumor is white and friable, sometimes with a felt-like texture (Fig. 50.20). These tumors are best treated by enucleation since local excision is not usually successful.[41] A course of medulloblastoma-type chemotherapy is recommended. Life expectancy is good.

Other disorders

Occasionally, chronic granulomatous uveitis with a hypopyon

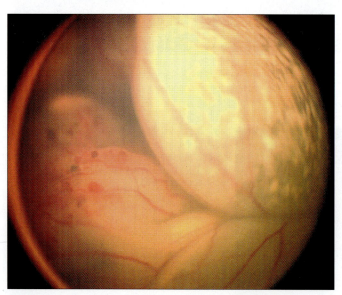

Fig. 50.18 Coats disease presenting with leukocoria. Note yellow appearance, not white as in retinoblastoma, total retinal detachment and the characteristic aneurysmal vascular malformations in the peripheral retina.

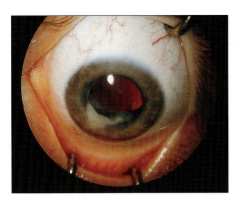

Fig. 50.20
Medulloepithelioma (diktyoma) presenting as a felt-like structure arising in the ciliary body and involving the iris.

may simulate retinoblastoma, especially if the posterior segment cannot be visualized.

Investigations

CT scan is helpful in confirming the diagnosis, but also for excluding intracranial involvement and pineal tumor. Not only is the intraocular mass and its pathognomonic calcification well visualized on CT scan (Figs 50.2d and 50.8b), but the optic nerves can be assessed, and the pineal region imaged. Since avoidance of radiation, even the small doses incurred on CT scanning, is desirable for children with *RB1* mutations, magnetic resonance imaging (MRI) may be preferred since it provides similar information, and is particularly good for delineating the anatomy of the optic nerve and pineal gland. However, MRI is not effective for delineating calcification, if the diagnosis is in question.[42]

Fluorescein angiography (FA) may be helpful in distinguishing some retinoblastoma tumors from Coats disease or dominant exudative vitreoretinopathy. Tiny early retinoblastoma tumors are not vascularized and are best seen on color images. However, fluorescein angiography can play an important role in the management of retinoblastoma. The FA attachment of the RetCam® facilitates the follow-up of retinoblastoma after focal therapy, by helping to detect vascularity and residual activity within tumors, and recurrences within laser scars (Figs 50.1c, 50.13d and 50.21b).

Two-dimensional ultrasound (B-scan) may be useful in diagnosis of some retinoblastoma tumors (Fig. 50.2b,c) and in monitoring the height of the tumor, but its major role may be in following regression after therapy, particularly when the tumor cannot be directly visualized due to radiation keratopathy or cataract. The 3D ultrasound can also play a role by monitoring tumor volume.[43]

Ultrasound biomicroscopy (UBM) is the only way to detect anterior disease beyond the ora and in the region of the ciliary body, which cannot be viewed by indirect ophthalmoscopy, nor by RetCam® and conventional ultrasonography (Fig. 50.6b). It is critical to detect the presence of anterior disease. Anterior disease is an indication for immediate enucleation because the chance of salvaging the eye is small, but risk for systemic metastasis is increased.

Since the survival of patients is normal if retinoblastoma remains intraocular (96% of cases), but the disease is very difficult to cure once it becomes metastatic, the **biopsy of retinoblastoma is strictly contraindicated** due to its incurring an increased risk for tumor spread outside the eye. In cases of suspected retinoblastoma with anterior segment involvement, when the diagnosis remains unclear despite all investigations, an

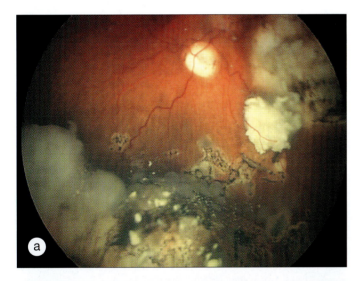

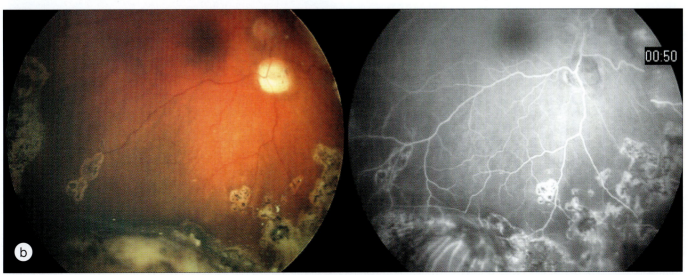

Fig. 50.21 Bilateral retinoblastoma treatment. Bilateral retinoblastoma was treated with enucleation of the left eye and CEV chemotherapy without cyclosporine for the right eye with IIRC Group D disease. (a) Extensive recurrence with vitreous seeding. (b) No detectable active tumor 3 months after four cycles of CEV chemotherapy with cyclosporine A with prechemo cryotherapy and sub-Tenon's carboplatin; fluorescein angiogram showing no tumor vessels in the location of recurrent tumor. (RetCam® images by Cynthia Vandenhoeven).

aqueous tap through clear cornea may be cautiously performed for a cytological diagnosis. However, a vitreous biopsy should be avoided unless the likelihood of retinoblastoma is extremely small because biopsy of retinoblastoma risks extraocular spread of tumor.[44]

Treatment

The treatment of retinoblastoma is best delivered in specialized centers where multidisciplinary teams have been developed, special expertise and equipment are available, and specific treatment protocols are used. This cancer is much too rare for individual ophthalmologists and oncologists to remain up-to-date and manage each patient in an *ad hoc* manner, or to have required the expertise necessary for optimizing outcomes for the children and their families. In addition, overall outcomes will only improve if each affected child is treated systematically on defined protocols, such that the knowledge gained from analyzing treatment results can be built on for designing more effective future treatment protocols.

Classification

Optimized care and outcome for intraocular retinoblastoma depend on use of the therapy with the least morbidity that is most likely to cure the tumor. The informed selection of therapy depends on classification of the disease severity in a way that is meaningful for predicting outcomes from current therapies. The Reese–Ellsworth (R-E) Classification of the 1960s was devised for predicting prognosis when intraocular retinoblastoma was treated with external beam radiotherapy. The International Intraocular Retinoblastoma Classification (IIRC) has been developed for predicting outcomes from current therapy (predominantly chemotherapy and focal therapy, with radiation as a salvage modality for recurrence) (Figs 50.1, 50.2, 50.5–50.7, 50.9, 50.12–50.14, 50.16 and 50.21).[45] The IIRC has been validated by correlating disease severity at presentation with outcomes from primary therapy, and eventual outcomes after salvage therapy, through a two-step Internet Survey that collected information on more than 1000 affected eyes treated world-wide in retinoblastoma centers.[46,47] At diagnosis, it is valuable to record both the R-E and IIRC classification stages for comparison with previous data. Current treatment protocols may also be recommended based on IIRC staging (Table 50.3).

IIRC general principles:

Group A: eyes with small tumors away from the macula and the optic nerve are primarily treated with focal therapy only (Fig. 50.1).

Group B: eyes with medium-sized tumors or tumors at the macula and the optic nerve may be first shrunk with a small number of chemotherapy cycles before applying focal therapy to optimize the visual potential (Fig. 50.1).

Group C: eyes with large tumors with limited vitreous and/or subretinal seeding are primarily treated with chemotherapy followed by focal therapy.

Group D: eyes with large tumors with extensive vitreous and/or subretinal seeding are also primarily treated with chemotherapy and focal therapy (Figs 50.2, 50.7, 50.13, 50.16 and 50.21). Most centers, but not all, now use external beam irradiation only as a salvage modality for Groups B, C and D eyes that have failed chemotherapy and focal therapy, rather than as initial elective therapy.

Group E: eyes (Figs 50.5, 50.6, 50.9, 50.12, 50.14) with high-risk features such as tumor touching the lens, neovascular

Table 50.3 International Intraocular Retinoblastoma Classification
Group A Small intraretinal tumors away from foveola and disc All tumors 3 mm or smaller in greatest dimension, confined to the retina *and* All tumors located further than 3 mm from the foveola and 1.5 mm from the optic disc
Group B All remaining discrete tumors confined to the retina All tumors confined to the retina not in Group A Any tumor-associated subretinal fluid less than 3 mm from the tumor with no subretinal seeding
Group C Discrete local disease with minimal subretinal or vitreous seeding Tumor(s) discrete Subretinal fluid, present or past, without seeding, involving up to 1/4 retina Local subretinal seeding, present or past, less than 3 mm (2 DD) from the tumor Local fine vitreous seeding close to discrete tumor
Group D Diffuse disease with significant vitreous or subretinal seeding Tumor(s) may be massive or diffuse Subretinal fluid, present or past, without seeding, involving up to total retinal detachment Diffuse subretinal seeding, present or past, may include subretinal plaques or tumor nodules Diffuse or massive vitreous disease may include "greasy" seeds or avascular tumor masses
Group E Presence of any one or more of these poor prognosis features Tumor touching the lens Neovascular glaucoma Tumor anterior to anterior vitreous face involving ciliary body or anterior segment Diffuse infiltrating retinoblastoma Opaque media from hemorrhage Tumor necrosis with aseptic orbital cellulitis Phthisis bulbi

glaucoma, orbital cellulitis (Figs. 50.9 and 50.12), anterior segment, anterior chamber (Fig. 50.14), iris or ciliary involvement (Fig. 50.6), total hyphema, suspected choroid, optic nerve or orbital involvement (Fig. 50.8) on ultrasonography, MRI and CT scans, are enucleated.

Enucleation

Initial enucleation is indicated for all Group E eyes since a trial of chemotherapy prior to enucleation may create a sense of false security by obscuring those adverse factors that puts the child's life at risk. Such adverse risk factors may be indications for further intensive therapy such as bone marrow or peripheral stem cell transplantation. Enucleation is an excellent way to cure retinoblastoma that is confined to the eye, such as in the case of unilateral retinoblastoma at diagnosis, or when the other eye is Group A for which chemotherapy is not necessary. Then the Group C or D fellow eye may be enucleated to avoid ever giving the child chemotherapy. Enucleation is also indicated for recurrent tumor that has failed all other treatment modalities.

It is rare now for both eyes to be primarily enucleated, except if both eyes are Group E, since attempts to save such severely involved Group E eyes may put the child's life in jeopardy from possible development of difficult-to-treat, poor-prognosis systemic metastasis. However, some Group E eyes can be cured, but very little vision is usually retained in such a severely damaged eye. Additionally, chemotherapy has short-term morbidity, and radiation, significant long-term complications, and such therapy may not in the best interest of a child with bilateral Group E eyes.

Bilateral retinoblastoma most commonly presents with one eye full of tumor, with smaller tumors in the fellow eye. If both eyes require chemotherapy for Groups B, C or D disease, then neither eye needs to be enucleated primarily (Figs 50.7 and 50.16).

Enucleation should be performed with a minimum of manipulation of the globe, with great care not to spill tumor inadvertently. A long optic nerve (8–12 mm) should be obtained in order to ensure that the surgical margin is tumor-free. For enucleation in unilaterally affected children, the tumor is very important for *RB1* mutation studies, in order to determine whether the child has heritable or nonheritable retinoblastoma (Figs 50.2e and 50.22). An orbital implant is placed within the muscle cone, with the muscles sutured onto the implant to prevent its subsequent migration out of the muscle cone. Implants of porous material such as hydroxyapatite or ceramic that allow vascularization will give a better long-term cosmetic effect. The attachment of the muscles onto the implant will allow consensual movement of the artificial eye with the retained fellow eye. A conformer is placed under the eyelids. We use a simple prosthetic eye, so that when the patch is removed 48 hours later, the child will look good and does not need to continue to wear an eye-patch[48] (Fig. 50.2f). This preliminary artificial eye may not fit perfectly, but will allow healing to be completed over several months before a final artificial eye is made.

Chemotherapy

Systemic chemotherapy has become the standard primary treatment for IIRC Groups B, C and D. Following an initial response to the first few cycles of chemotherapy, focal therapy with cryotherapy or laser therapy is initiated to destroy residual or recurrent tumor[49] (Figs 50.1, 50.15 and 50.16). Chemotherapy is best given on a rigorous protocol, ideally part of a research study. The most commonly used chemotherapy drugs include carboplatin, etoposide and vincristine (CEV) given every 3 weeks through a central venous access line.[50] However, different retinoblastoma centers have administered the chemotherapy using a variation of the CEV protocol.

The Toronto protocol suggests that the addition of short 3-hour infusions of high-dose cyclosporine A enhances the effectiveness of the chemotherapy by blocking the P-glycoprotein that mediates multidrug resistance by acting as a plasma membrane drug-efflux pump, which is commonly over-expressed in retinoblastoma tumors.[51] Cyclosporine may also act through the circumvention of other non-P-glycoprotein drug resistance mechanisms, such as by the reduction of carboplatin induction of expression of *c-fos* or *c-myc* oncogene,[52,53] or genes required for repair of drug-induced DNA damage.[54] Furthermore, *in vitro* data suggest that cyclosporine might augment the efficacy of etoposide even in nonresistant tumor cells, by modulating another undefined non- multidrug resistance mechanism.[55] Laboratory studies suggest that cyclosporine levels up to 5000 ng/ml do not block the function of another protein that mediates multidrug resistance, MRP, which we have identified in relapsed retinoblastoma tumors.[56,57] However, it is not known if the really high cyclosporine peak levels of >20 000 ng/ml that we have achieved in our protocol might be capable of inhibiting MRP.

On the Toronto protocol, Groups C and D eyes are treated with seven cycles of CEV chemotherapy modulated with high-dose cyclosporine, and Group B eyes with four cycles. Since

1991, even with standard-dose CEV/high-dose cyclosporine, followed by focal cryotherapy and laser therapy, our 6-year cure rates (avoidance of both enucleation and external beam radiation) are excellent for Groups B and C eyes, and we have not seen a significant increase in the toxicity of chemotherapy given with high-dose cyclosporine. With the addition of high-dose cyclosporine, long-term results are better than previous published results with chemotherapy, radiotherapy, and even chemotherapy plus radiotherapy. Furthermore, the Toronto protocol has successfully salvaged eyes that have already failed previous chemotherapy and/or radiotherapy. The current Toronto protocol uses higher carboplatin and etoposide dosages with standard dose vincristine, with high-dose cyclosporine, and cytokine granulocyte- stimulating factor (Neupogen) support of the myeloid bone marrow. Preliminary results show good avoidance of both enucleation and external beam radiation for many Group D eyes (Figs 50.2, 50.7, 50.13, 50.16, 50.21).[58,59] Local recurrence is expected approximately 2–6 months after finishing the chemotherapy, which can often be controlled by focal therapy given when recurrence first appears (Fig. 50.16). This requires vigilant EUAs with appropriate focal therapy every 4–6 weeks for at least one year after any sign of active tumor.

Short-term side effects of chemotherapy that are easily managed with present day oncological supportive therapy include myelosuppression (ameliorated by administration of the cytokine granulocyte-stimulating factor, Neupogen) with requirement for hospital admissions for fever-and-neutropenia or infections, low platelet counts requiring platelet transfusions, anemia requiring blood transfusions, nausea and vomiting prevented by potent antiemetic drugs, and hair loss which grows back after completion of chemotherapy. We have found that the addition of high-dose cyclosporine does not significantly increase the toxicity due to chemotherapy. Unlike radiation, no long-term cosmetic deformity of the orbit and upper face results from chemotherapy, and no radiation-induced cataracts and ocular complications. Although chemotherapy was undertaken in order to avoid the known and large risk of induction of second primary tumor by radiation, (estimated to be as high a 51% risk at 50-year follow-up[60]), we recommend the cautious use of chemotherapy, particularly etoposide, which carries a small risk of induction of a specific type of acute myelogenous leukemia with 11q23 or 21q22 translocations or myelodysplastic syndrome. The cumulative dosage of etoposide used for treating retinoblastoma is less than the higher dosages that have been estimated to carry a 2–3% risk of inducing leukemia, generally in the 1–2 years after completion of etoposide chemotherapy.[61] Adequate follow-up on retinoblastoma children is not yet available to provide evidence of the precise risk. Furthermore, the leukemia-induction risk may be increased by the concurrent usage of carboplatin chemotherapy, and in the case of relapsed patients, the subsequent use of salvage radiation or anthracycline (doxorubicin) and alkylating agents (ifosfamide, cyclophosphamide) salvage chemotherapy.

We have also shown that increased intraocular concentrations of the chemotherapy drugs (e.g. carboplatin) may be induced in eyes with vitreous seeding by the application of a single-freeze cryotherapy ("prechemo cryotherapy") at the peripheral retina in the vicinity of the seeds.[62] The concurrent usage of high-dose cyclosporine apparently can further increase the intraocular concentrations of chemotherapy,[62] possibly by inhibiting the P-glycoprotein expressed in the blood–eye barrier. Local chemotherapy with instillation of carboplatin into Tenon's space may be used to achieve increased vitreous concentration of carboplatin,[63] to accentuate the levels attained by systemic carboplatin therapy.

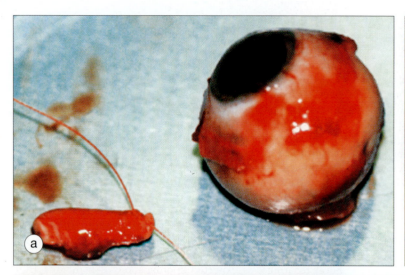
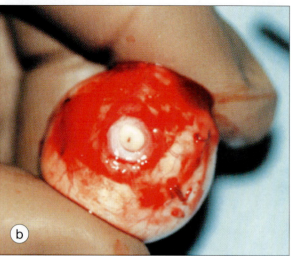
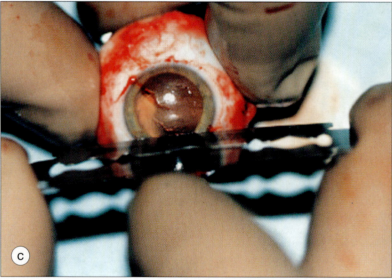
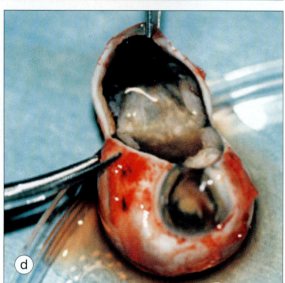

Fig. 50.22 Harvest of fresh tumor for determination of the *RB1* mutant alleles in unilateral tumor. (a) Optic nerve (8–12 mm) is excised from the globe and the distal end marked with a suture. The nerve is submitted as a separate specimen in a separate formalin container so that it is not contaminated by tumor from the opened eye. (b) Optic nerve just beyond the cribriform plate appears normal on gross inspection, to be confirmed microscopically. (c) Globe is opened with a razor incision in a pupillary-optic nerve plane, superior or inferior, at the limbus, in order to access intraocular live tumor. (d) Superior or inferior callotte allows harvest of large amount of intraocular tumor for adequate molecular studies. Optic nerve and choroid are not interfered with, since these are important for pathological assessment for risk of extraocular spread. Tumor for molecular studies is sent to the lab in sterile tissue culture medium. The *RB1* mutations (M1 and M2) in this unilateral tumor were a heterozygous exon 14 CGA to TGA (R445X) and a heterozygous intron 16 G to A (cDNA 1498+5) causing a splice mutation. Neither M1 or M2 were detected in blood of the child. (Images by Cynthia Vandenhoeven.)

However, sub-Tenon's carboplatin instillation should be used only for certain well-defined indications because of the local toxicity, including orbital fat necrosis that may limit ocular motility and cause enophthalmos, and fibrosis that may complicate any subsequent eye enucleation.[64]

Cryotherapy

Cryotherapy is used for small anteriorly placed tumors (IIRC Groups A and B eyes), or more posterior tumors when visual damage will not result.[65] Since the tumor cells are killed when they thaw, a triple freeze-thaw technique is used, with care to allow a full minute for thawing between the successive freezes (Figs 50.15 and 50.16). Cryotherapy almost always has to be repeated at several EUAs 4–6 weeks apart, until no residual active tumor remains. Cryotherapy may be used either as a primary procedure or to treat residual or

recurrent tumors. When superiorly placed, moderately sized tumors must be treated with cryotherapy, a laser barrier placed posterior to the tumor may protect the retina from detachment by the serous exudate of the acute freeze (Fig. 50.18).

Laser

Laser coagulation is used for small tumors (Groups A and B eyes) (Fig. 50.1), for tumors that have been initially shrunk by chemotherapy, or for recurrences following chemotherapy. Traditionally small tumors (Group A eyes) behind the equator are treated by encircling the tumor with a double row of contiguous laser burns. The small avascular tumor can then be directly coagulated, starting with power/duration settings that barely blanch or opacify the tumor, and gradually increasing the power to make the tumor turn opaque white. Larger or visually threatening tumors (Groups B and C eyes) are treated first with chemo-therapy while residual disease and recurrent tumors after stopping chemotherapy are treated with laser coagulation. For Group D eyes, laser is used only after a good response has occurred with chemotherapy, to eliminate any residual or recurrent tumor before it has a chance to regrow (Fig. 50.7). The diode 810 nm laser is most widely available and is the cheapest. 'Thermotherapy' with the 810 nm laser has been promoted, using the laser to gently heat tumor over a long period of time. However, this technique offers no special benefit for tumor cell-kill, and results in a high frequency of edge recurrence and produces scars that extend gradually over time.[66,67] For small Group A tumors, green lasers (argon or frequency-doubled YAG at 532 nm) are used effectively without drifting of the scars. Infrared lasers (diode 810 nm or 1064 nm YAG) can be applied after chemotherapy to larger, thicker tumors. With all lasers, it is important to NOT use too much power at any one treatment, and to expect to re-treat at frequent intervals until only flat scars remain. Fluorescein angiography is useful for catching potential spots of recurrences in a laser scar early (Figs 50.1c, 50.13d and 50.21b).

Focal irradiation

Solitary tumors less than 15 mm in diameter which are not adjacent to the disc or macula may be treated with an episcleral radioactive plaque,[125] iodine or ruthenium.[68] Plaques are also useful for treating single recurrences after chemotherapy or external beam irradiation where a second course of radiation to the whole eye would be prohibited because it will lead to severe radiation retinopathy or optic neuropathy. Under general anesthesia, the tumor is localized and the plaque is sutured to the sclera and left *in situ* until the prescribed dose of radiation has been delivered to the apex of the tumor.

External beam irradiation

Historically radiation was the first approach to curing intraocular retinoblastoma, resulting in saving many eyes with useful vision, but with severe side-effects. Most commonly, there is significant calcification ("cottage cheese-like") or a combination of calcification and translucent residual tumor after radiation (Fig. 50.17). Most importantly, the risk of second primary tumors within the radiation field in children with a germline *RB1* mutation is very significant, and most children died of these second tumors[24,69] (Fig. 50.4). The risk may be greatest with infants that are irradiated under one year of age.[23] Additional complications of external irradiation, which are not a problem with chemotherapy, include cosmetic deformity due to growth retardation of the orbit (worse the younger the child is at the time of irradiation), cataract (reduced by lens-sparing radiation portals), reduced tearing effectiveness, and dry-eye syndromes. In addition, recurrences following irradiation was commonly seen with large tumors and vitreous seeding (R-E Group IV, Va and b, IIRC Groups C and D).

External beam radiotherapy is now mostly used for treatment of postchemotherapy recurrences that are too large or extensive for focal therapy, or unresponsive to focal therapy. Focused radiation such as stereotactic radiation may avoid radiation of adjacent tissues for treatment of localized disease. However, whole eye radiation may be the only choice in chemoresistant retinoblastoma with extensive vitreous or subretinal seeding.

A total dose of 3500–4000 cGy has been traditionally given for primary or secondary irradiation of eyes with retinoblastoma, in divided fractions over a 3–4 week period.[70] A temporal portal excluding the lens is used whenever possible to avoid a radiation-induced cataract,[71] but when it is important to irradiate the ora serrata, or when vitreous seeds are present, an anterior approach must be used despite the certainty of cataract induction. Corneal damage can be reduced by irradiating with the eyelid opened with a speculum, to move the increased entry dose 5 mm below surface, deeper into the eye.

Extraocular retinoblastoma

Extraocular retinoblastoma results in a precipitous drop in the prognosis for life. Until recently, metastatic retinoblastoma was considered fatal. Local orbital recurrence is generally treated with 4000–5000 cGy orbital radiation and systemic chemotherapy. Metastatic retinoblastoma to bone marrow or other sites may be treated with intensive chemotherapy with cyclosporine to counter multidrug resistance, and if remission is attained, autologous or allogeneic bone marrow or peripheral stem cell transplantation is performed. Meningeal spread of retinoblastoma is treated with the addition of intrathecal and intraventricular chemotherapy via an Ommaya reservoir. Long-term follow-up in these patients suggests that such approaches may be curative.[72]

Prophylactic radiation is considered when histopathological examination of the enucleated globe with optic nerve shows involvement of the cut end of the optic nerve. When marked choroidal invasion and involvement of the optic nerve past the cribriform plate are noted on histopathology, extra therapy may be advised to treat spread of tumor beyond the eye. However, lesser involvement of the optic nerve may be managed adequately by close follow-up with regular MRI, bone marrow and cerebrospinal fluid examinations, applying treatment only when disease is documented. Otherwise, many children may be treated unnecessarily. Evidence to support these treatment recommendations is pending a multicenter trial of prophylactic treatment for adverse histology.

LONG-TERM FOLLOW-UP

Following the initial management and resolution of active tumor, assessment of the response to treatment will require frequent general anesthesia, especially in the first year following diagnosis with completion of chemotherapy, when recurrence or new tumors are most likely to occur. Regular EUAs will be necessary until the child is old enough to co-operate for a full-dilated eye examination in the clinic, variably at about 3 years of age. Follow-up can then be continued on an outpatient basis. However, children with Groups C and D eyes may need a much longer follow-up with EUA in order to assess adequately peripheral tumors for recurrence. Likewise, patients who have been treated with chemotherapy and/or radiation will require oncological follow-up for early detection and appropriate management of possible long-term complications of their previous therapy. It is particularly important for retinoblastoma patients to retain contact with their oncologist because of the risk of secondary malignancies, whether sporadic or induced by radiation or chemotherapy. In long-term follow-up, it is also important to ensure that accurate genetic counseling is available to the parents, and to the child when he or she reaches maturity.

PROGNOSIS

With modern methods of diagnosis and treatment the prognosis for retinoblastoma is excellent. The 3-year survival for both unilateral and bilateral retinoblastoma approaches 96%.[1] In fact, more patients with germline *RB1* mutations die of their second tumor than from uncontrolled retinoblastoma.[24]

The prognosis for vision is excellent in unilateral retinoblastoma, but depends on the size and location of the tumors in bilateral cases. Overall treatment with chemotherapy and focal therapy has improved results such that bilateral enucleation is now rare. Extra-foveal tumors have a good visual prognosis but when the macular region is directly involved, the visual result may be poor, despite tumor control. The most important impact on further improving visual outcome for retinoblastoma children lies in the earlier recognition of the presenting signs by the primary care givers. This requires enhanced awareness and understanding that retinoblastoma does exist, and enhanced receptiveness to parental complaints, with a solid ophthalmological and oncological network for urgent referral to facilitate diagnosis and appropriate treatment as early as possible.

REFERENCES

1. Sanders BM, Draper GJ, Kingston JE. Retinoblastoma in Great Britain 1969–80: incidence, treatment, and survival. Br J Ophthalmol 1988; 72: 576–83.

2. Cavenee WK, Dryja TP, Phillips RA, et al. Expression of recessive alleles by chromosomal mechanisms in retinoblastoma. Nature 1983; 305: 779–84.

3. Knudson AG. Mutation and cancer: statistical study of retinoblastoma. Proc Natl Acad Sci USA 1971; 68: 820–23.

4. Comings DE. A general theory of carcinogenesis. Proc Natl Acad Sci USA 1973; 70: 3324–8.

5. Friend SH, Bernards R, Rogelj S, et al. A human DNA segment with properties of the gene that predisposes to retinoblastoma and osteosarcoma. Nature 1986; 323: 643–6.

6. Jay M, Cowell J, Hungerford J. Register of retinoblastoma: preliminary results. Eye 1988; 2: 102–5.

7. Godbout R, Dryja TP, Squire J, et al. Somatic inactivation of genes on chromosome 13 is a common event in retinoblastoma. Nature 1983; 304: 451–3.

8. Richter S, Vandezande K, Chen N, et al. Sensitive and efficient detection of RB1 Gene mutations enhances care for families with retinoblastoma. Am J Hum Genet 2003; 72: 253–69.

9. DiCiommo D, Gallie BL, Bremner R. Retinoblastoma: the disease, gene and protein provide critical leads to understand cancer. Semin Cancer Biol 2000; 10: 255–69.

10. Phillips RA, Gill RM, Zacksenhaus E, et al. Why don't germline mutations in RB1 predispose to leukemia? [Review]. Curr Top Microbiol Immunol 1992; 182: 485–91.

11. Wu L, de Bruin A, Saavedra HI, et al. Extra-embryonic function of Rb is essential for embryonic development and viability. Nature 2003; 421: 942–7.

12. Zacksenhaus E, Jiang Z, Chung D, et al. pRb controls proliferation, differentiation, and death of skeletal muscle cells and other lineages during embryogenesis. Genes Dev 1996; 10: 3051–64.

13. Gallie BL, Campbell C, Devlin H, et al. Developmental basis of retinal-specific induction of cancer by RB mutation. Cancer Res 1999; 59: 1731s–35s.

14. Chen D, Pajovic S, Duckett A, et al. Genomic amplification in retinoblastoma narrowed to 0.6 megabase on chromosome 6p containing a kinesin-like gene, RBKIN. Cancer Res 2002; 62: 967–71.

15. Musarella MA, Gallie BL. A simplified scheme for genetic counseling in retinoblastoma. J Pediatr Ophthalmol Strabismus 1987; 24: 124–5.

16. Noorani HZ, Khan HN, Gallie BL, et al. Cost comparison of molecular versus conventional screening of relatives at risk for retinoblastoma [see comments]. Am J Hum Genet 1996; 59: 301–7.

17. Abramson DH, Greenfield DS, Ellsworth RM. Bilateral retinoblastoma. Correlations between age at diagnosis and time course for new intraocular tumors. Ophthalmic Paediatr Genet 1992; 13: 1–7.

18. Lohmann D, Gallie BL. Retinoblastoma: revisiting the model prototype of inherited cancer. Am J Med Genet (in press).

19. Bremner R, Du DC, Connolly-Wilson MJ, et al. Deletion of RB exons 24 and 25 causes low-penetrance retinoblastoma. Am J Hum Genet 1997; 61: 556–70.

20. Sakai T, Ohtani N, McGee TL, et al. Oncogenic germ-line mutations in Sp1 and ATF sites in the human retinoblastoma gene. Nature 1991; 353: 83–86.

21. Klutz M, Brockmann D, Lohmann DR. A parent-of-origin effect in two families with retinoblastoma is associated with a distinct splice mutation in the RB1 gene. Am J Hum Genet 2002; 71: 174–9.

22. Gallie BL, Ellsworth RM, Abramson DH, et al. Retinoma: spontaneous regression of retinoblastoma or benign manifestation of the mutation? Br J Cancer 1982; 45: 513–21.

23. Abramson DH, Frank CM. Second nonocular tumors in survivors of bilateral retinoblastoma: a possible age effect on radiation-related risk [see comments]. Ophthalmology 1998; 105: 573–9; discussion 579–80.

24. Eng C, Li FP, Abramson DH, et al. Mortality from second tumors among long-term survivors of retinoblastoma. J Natl Cancer Inst 1993; 85: 1121–8.

25. Kivela T. Trilateral retinoblastoma: a meta-analysis of hereditary retinoblastoma associated with primary ectopic intracranial retinoblastoma. J Clin Oncol 1999; 17: 1829–37.

26. Kingston JE, Plowman PN, Hungerford JL. Ectopic intracranial retinoblastoma in childhood. Br J Ophthalmol 1985; 69: 742–8.

27. Tso MO. Clues to the cells of origin in retinoblastoma. Int Ophthalmol Clin 1980; 20: 191–211.

28. Valverde K, Pandya J, Heon E, et al. Retinoblastoma with central retinal artery thrombosis that mimics extraocular disease. Med Pediatr Oncol 2002; 38: 277–9.

29. Bhatnagar R, Vine AK. Diffuse infiltrating retinoblastoma. Ophthalmology 1991; 98: 1657–61.

30. Messmer EP, Heinrich T, Hopping W, et al. Risk factors for metastases in patients with retinoblastoma. Ophthalmology 1991; 98: 136–41.

31. Shields CL, Shields JA, Baez KA, et al. Choroidal invasion of retinoblastoma: metastatic potential and clinical risk factors [see comments]. Br J Ophthalmol 1993; 77: 544–8.

32. Ellsworth RM. The practical management of retinoblastoma. Trans Am Ophthalmol Soc 1969; 67: 462–534.

33. MacKeen LD, Panton RL, Héon E, et al. In: The 14th International Symposium for Genetic Eye Diseases (ISGED) and 11th The International Symposium on Retinoblastoma (ISR), Paris, France, 2003.

34. Shields JA, Parsons HM, Shields CL, et al. Lesions simulating retinoblastoma. J Pediatr Ophthalmol Strabismus 1991; 28: 338–40.

35. Budning AS, Heon E, Gallie BL. Visual prognosis of Coats' disease. J AAPOS 1998; 2: 356–9.

36. Ridley ME, Shields JA, Brown GC, et al. Coats' disease: evaluation of management. Ophthalmology 1982; 89: 1381–7.

37. Zygulska-Mach H, Krukar-Baster K, Ziobrowski S. Ocular toxocariasis in children and youth. Doc Ophthalmol 1993; 84: 145–54.

38. Liang JC, Augsburger JJ, Shields JA. Diffuse infiltrating retinoblastoma associated with persistent primary vitreous. J Pediatr Ophthalmol Strabismus 1985; 22: 31–3.

39. Shields JA, Shields CL, Parsons HM. Differential diagnosis of retinoblastoma. Retina 1991; 11: 232–43.

40. Broughton WL, Zimmerman LE. A clinicopathologic study of 56 cases of intraocular medulloepitheliomas. Am J Ophthalmol 1978; 85: 407–18.

41. Canning CR, McCartney AC, Hungerford J. Medulloepithelioma (diktyoma). Br J Ophthalmol 1988; 72: 764–7.

42. Schueler AO, Hosten N, Bechrakis NE, et al. High resolution magnetic resonance imaging of retinoblastoma. Br J Ophthalmol 2003; 87: 330–5.

43. Finger PT, Khoobehi A, Ponce-Contreras MR, et al. Three dimensional ultrasound of retinoblastoma: initial experience. Br J Ophthalmol 2002; 86: 1136–8.

44. Stevenson KE, Hungerford J, Garner A. Local extraocular extension of retinoblastoma following intraocular surgery. Br J Ophthalmol 1989; 73: 739–42.

45. Murphree AL. In: Singh A, editor. International Congress of Ocular Oncology Hyderabad, India, 2004.

46. Gallie BL, Truong TH, Shields C, et al. In: Singh A, ed. International Congress of Ocular Oncology Hyderabad, India, 2004.

47. Gallie BL, Truong TH, Shields C, et al. In: Singh A, ed. International Congress of Ocular Oncology Hyderabad, India, 2004.

48. Vincent AL, Webb MC, Gallie BL, et al. Prosthetic conformers: a step towards improved rehabilitation of enucleated children. Clin Exp Ophthalmol 2002; 30: 58–9.

49. Gallie BL, Budning A, DeBoer G, et al. Chemotherapy with focal therapy can cure intraocular retinoblastoma without radiation. Arch Ophthalmol 1996; 114: 1321–9.

50. Chan HSL, DeBoer G, Thiessen JJ, et al. Combining cyclosporin with chemotherapy controls intraocular retinoblastoma without radiation. Clin Cancer Res 1996; 2: 1499–1508.

51. Chan HS, Lu Y, Grogan TM, et al. Multidrug Resistance Protein (MRP) expression in retinoblastoma correlates with rare failure of chemotherapy despite cyclosporine for reversal of P-glycoprotein. Cancer Res 1997; 57: 2325–30.

52. Kashani-Sabet M, Lu Y, Leong L, et al. Differential oncogene amplification in tumor cells from a patient treated with cisplatin and 5-fluorouracil. Eur J Cancer 1990; 26: 383–90.

53. Scanlon KJ, Wang WZ, Han H. Cyclosporin A suppresses cisplatin-induced oncogene expression in human cancer cells. Cancer Treat Rev 1990; 17 Suppl A: 27–35.

54. Muller MR, Seiler F, Thomale J, et al. Capacity of individual chronic lymphatic leukemia lymphocytes and leukemic blast cells for repair of O6-ethylguanine in DNA: relation to chemosensitivity in vitro and treatment outcome. Cancer Res 1994; 54: 4524–31.

55. Slater LM, Cho J, Wetzel M. Cyclosporin A potentiation of VP-16: production of long-term survival in murine acute lymphatic leukemia. Cancer Chemother Pharmacol 1992; 31: 53–6.

56. Cole SP, Sparks KE, Fraser K, et al. Pharmacological characterization of multidrug resistant MRP-transfected human tumor cells. Cancer Res 1994; 54: 5902–10.

57. Twentyman PR. Modifiers of multidrug resistance. Br J Haematol 1995; 90: 735–7.

58. Chan HL, Heon E, Budning A, et al. In: The 14th International Symposium for Genetic Eye Diseases (ISGED) and 11th The International Symposium on Retinoblastoma (ISR), Paris, 2003.

59. Chan HL, Heon E, Budning A, et al. Excellent long-term outcome in extraocular and metastatic retinoblastoma treated with cyclosporine-modulated chemotherapy. The 14th International Symposium for Genetic Eye Diseases (ISGED) and 11th International Symposium on Retinoblastoma (ISR), Paris, 2003.

60. Wong FL, Boice JD, Jr., Abramson DH, et al. Cancer incidence after retinoblastoma. Radiation dose and sarcoma risk [see comments]. JAMA 1997; 278: 1262–7.

61. Smith MA, Rubinstein L, Anderson JR, et al. Secondary leukemia or myelodysplastic syndrome after treatment with epipodophyllotoxins. J Clin Oncol 1999; 17: 569–77.

62. Wilson TW, Chan HSL, Moselhy GM, et al. Penetration of chemotherapy into vitreous is increased by cryotherapy and cyclosporin in rabbits. Arch Ophthalmol 1996; 114: 1390–5.

63. Abramson DH, Frank CM, Dunkel IJ. A phase I/II study of sub-conjunctival carboplatin for intraocular retinoblastoma. Ophthalmology 1999; 106: 1947–50.

64. Mulvihill A, Budning A, Jay V, et al. Ocular motility changes after subtenon carboplatin chemotherapy for retinoblastoma. Arch Ophthalmol 2003; 121: 1120–4.

65. Shields JA, Shields CL, De Potter P. Cryotherapy for retinoblastoma. Int Ophthalmol Clin 1993; 33: 101–5.

66. Deegan WF. Emerging strategies for the treatment of retinoblastoma. Curr Opin Ophthalmol 2003; 14: 291–5.

67. Schueler AO, Jurklies C, Heimann H, et al. Thermochemotherapy in hereditary retinoblastoma. Br J Ophthalmol 2003; 87: 90–5.

68. Shields CL, Shields JA, Cater J, et al. Plaque radiotherapy for retinoblastoma: long-term tumor control and treatment complications in 208 tumors. Ophthalmology 2001; 108: 2116–21.

69. Draper GJ, Sanders BM, Kingston JE. Second primary neoplasms in patients with retinoblastoma. Br J Cancer 1986; 53: 661–71.

70. Harnett AN, Hungerford J, Lambert G, et al. Modern lateral external beam (lens sparing) radiotherapy for retinoblastoma. Ophthalmic Paediatr Genet 1987; 8: 53–61.

71. Schipper J, Imhoff SM, Tan KE. Precision megavoltage external beam radiation therapy for retinoblastoma. Front Radiat Ther Oncol 1997; 30: 65–80.

72. Chan H, Pandya J, Valverde K, et al. Metastatic retinoblastoma in the CSF that responded to intensive systemic and intraventricular multi-drug resistance-reversal chemotherapy. Proc Am Assoc Cancer Res 2002; 43: 3720.

51 Retinopathy of Prematurity

Alistair R Fielder and Graham E Quinn

PREMATURITY: THE BACKGROUND

Continuing dramatic improvements in the resuscitation and care of very small premature infants has resulted in increased survival rates even in those infants with a birth weight of 1000g or less. Regrettably, this increased survival has also led to increased levels of disability and associated defects. Retinopathy of prematurity (ROP), its presence or absence, occupies much of the attention of ophthalmologists caring for premature children, but other ocular, neurological, or developmental difficulties may ultimately be more important in defining the disability of the child.

About 30% of very preterm infants suffer from chronic lung disease. The incidence of neurological sequelae in infants with chronic lung disease has been reported to be much higher than in low-birth-weight infants without chronic lung complications (40% versus 6%). It should be noted, however, that the impaired development of premature babies with chronic lung disease is linked to the associated intraventricular hemorrhage (with or without hydrocephalus and periventricular leukomalacia) rather than the lung disease per se. Long-term longitudinal developmental studies suggest that these account for the increased incidence of poor hand–eye difficulties in visuomotor and other perceptual problems and reduced intelligence.

Specific eye disorders are also found with increased frequency in premature infants who have developed intraventricular hemorrhage or who have periventricular leukomalacia. In infants with low-grade intraventricular hemorrhage, strabismus developed just as frequently as in cases of high-grade intraventricular hemorrhage–around 40%. In contrast, optic atrophy occurs much more commonly in infants with high-grade intraventricular hemorrhage than in those with low-grade intraventricular hemorrhage (32% versus 16%). In infants with periventricular leukomalacia, tonic downgaze, esotropia, nystagmus, optic nerve hypoplasia, and atrophy occur more frequently than in normal-birth-weight infants. For those interested in the neuropathophysiology of strabismus it is important to note that the presence of thinning of the corpus callosum correlates best to which infant with periventricular leukomalacia is likely to develop strabismus.

The increased risk of strabismus in premature infants of low birth weight cannot be entirely attributed to the presence of periventricular leukomalacia. At least 20% of premature infants with a birth weight less than 1700g will develop strabismus. There is a relative increase in the occurrence of constant exotropia in low-birth-weight infants. It appears that retinopathy of prematurity, birth weight, cerebral palsy, anisometropia, and refractive error are all independently associated with strabismus.

Considerable interest surrounds the development of refractive errors in low-birth-weight prematures. Several studies have documented an increased risk of myopia in premature infants even if they do not develop retinopathy of prematurity (Chapter 6). Premature infants without retinopathy of prematurity are myopic early in life but become emmetropic as they approach full-term. As they age, they become more hypermetropic. Premature babies were found to have shorter axial lengths, shallower anterior chambers, and more high curved corneas.

In contrast, premature babies with ROP have higher rates of myopia than those without retinopathy of prematurity. Surprisingly, the treatment of retinopathy of prematurity with cryotherapy has only a minor effect on the developing refractive error. There is no difference in the incidence of refractive error from +8 diopter hypermetropia to 8 diopter myopia. There was, however, a higher rate of 8 diopters of myopia or more in the treated group. There is currently no consensus concerning the assertion that laser therapy has less effect on the developing refractive error than does cryotherapy.

RETINOPATHY OF PREMATURITY

Retinopathy of prematurity was first reported in 1942 by Terry,[1] who published a description of the histological findings of what would now be considered end-stage cicatricial disease. As more cases were reported, it became evident that this condition, by then known as retrolental fibroplasia, was confined to premature infants and is a disorder of the immature retinal vasculature. Retrospective studies showed it to be extremely rare before the 1940s.[2] Owens and Owens showed that the retinopathy developed postnatally in infants who had a normal fundus examination at birth.[3] ROP subsequently became the leading cause of blindness in children in the USA, and a similar epidemic of ROP was seen in certain countries in Europe during the 1940s and 1950s.

Following Campbell's suggestion that the appearance of this condition at this time might be related temporally to the introduction of oxygen therapy into the premature nursery,[4] evidence accumulated to support the concept of a toxic effect of oxygen on the immature retinal vasculature. This clinical observation was supported by experimental studies,[5-7] and the cumulative evidence led to the restriction of oxygen use in preterm neonates. Although this resulted in a dramatic fall in incidence, ROP was not eradicated completely, and it is now clear that even though oxygen remains center stage, many other factors play a role in the pathogenesis of ROP.[8-11] The history of the scientific investigation of the pathogenesis of ROP makes fascinating reading and has been comprehensively reviewed.[8,12-15]

Retinal vascular development

Our understanding of vascular development has advanced recently, both in general[16] and with respect of the retinal circulation.[17] As a rule, the retinal vasculature develops to meet retinal metabolic demand, with the exception of the foveal region, which has a very different vascular pattern,[17] so that very early in development when the retina is thin it receives all its nutrients from the underlying choroid. The choroid is vascularized from about 6 weeks gestational age (GA),[18] but with increasing neural density and retinal thickness, the choroidal circulation alone cannot meet *all* the needs of the retina and a separate retinal circulation is required. Consequently at 14–15 weeks of gestation, retinal vascularization commences. This comprises two main processes: vasculogenesis and angiogenesis.[17] The former is the formation of primary vessels from undifferentiated precursor cells on the retinal surface, while angiogenesis is the sprouting from these vessels to create a secondary vasculature in the deep retina. Vascular endothelial cells, microglia, pericytes, and astrocytes all migrate centrifugally from the optic disc, proliferate, and become aligned into vascular cords that develop lumina and further differentiate into a capillary network. Newly formed capillaries later remodel and form a mature retina vascular network with capillary-free areas,[19] which in modern parlance indicates that retinal tissue responds to excess or lack of oxygen by trimming or inducing growth in its microvasculature so that oxygen supply matches the metabolic requirements of the retina.[20]

Normal maturational increase of retinal thickness generates local "physiological" hypoxia just in advance of the developing retinal vessels. Astrocytes in this hypoxic region respond by secreting vascular endothelial growth factor (VEGF) that subsequently stimulates endothelial migration, differentiation, and proliferation. Oxygen-dependent VEGF plays a part in all stages of vascular development; however, factors other than VEGF are also involved.[16] One of these is oxygen-independent insulin-like growth factor (IGF-1) that controls VEGF activation of the Akt endothelial cell survival pathway, so that low levels result in reduced survival and growth of vascular endothelial cells.[21]

The nasal retina is vascularized by about 32 weeks GA and the temporal retina by just after term.[22] The ophthalmoscopic appearance of the unvascularized retina is gray-white, its extent being related to the degree of immaturity. The retinal vessels in the preterm infant are slender, relatively straight, and taper as they terminate toward the gray, avascular periphery (Fig. 51.1). The foveal region is only differentiated ophthalmoscopically at around term and the foveolar reflex develops later.[23]

Pathogenesis

The realization that the introduction of oxygen therapy for preterm infants played a major role in the epidemic of ROP in the 1940s and 1950s led to a period of oxygen restriction and to the anticipation of the demise of this blinding condition. Unfortunately, this proved not to be so–"that a single maneuver would abolish ROP seems naive in the light of our current understanding of the condition."[24] There has been an unwritten swing of opinion away from the view that oxygen is the single causative factor in ROP toward almost the opposite view that oxygen plays little or no part in its development: both are incorrect. It is now evident that many factors can be involved in its pathogenesis, but oxygen remains center stage. Currently ROP is not entirely preventable, but the evidence presented below shows that meticulous medical control is vital not only for the general well being of the baby, but also to keep ROP, especially severe ROP, to a minimum.

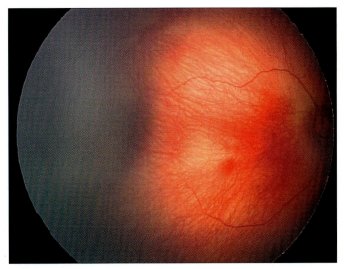

Fig. 51.1 Normal retinal vasculature and optic disc of a preterm baby without retinopathy. Note the straightness and fine calibre of retinal vessels - the arterioles are hardly visible. The vessels taper into the grey nonvascularized periphery. Macular area poorly defined. This and many other figures were obtained using wide field digital imaging (RetCam 130).

An exhaustive review of the vast literature on this subject is outside the scope of this chapter but some of the more important factors related to the development of ROP are discussed. Several excellent articles have been published.[8–11,14,24–30]

First we must mention two theories of ROP pathogenesis that are now largely historical. According to the first–"classic" theory–developed by Ashton[7] and Patz,[6] ROP (then called RLF) consists of two phases of equal importance. First, there is a hyperoxic phase, the phase in oxygen that causes retinal arteriolar constriction and irreversible vaso-obliteration and dissolution of the retinal capillary endothelial cells. This is followed by the second phase, on removal from the hyperoxic environment, the phase in air which is characterized by a vasoproliferative response induced by the ischemia due to the capillary closure of the first phase.

The second–"gap junction"–theory, proposed by Kretzer and Hittner,[31] is based on the activity of the mesenchymal spindle cell precursors of the retinal capillaries. These authors were unable to identify either endothelial cell necrosis, as would be expected from vaso-obliteration, or evidence of retinal ischemia. Mesenchymal spindle cells migrate centrifugally from the optic disc, and those cells canalize to form capillaries just behind the advancing vanguard. Under normal *in utero* conditions this process proceeds unimpeded, but under relative hyperoxic extrauterine conditions, gap junctions appear between adjacent spindle cells. Gap junction formation interferes with normal migration and vascular formation, and the angiogenic factors secreted by damaged spindle cells trigger the neovascular response.

Current concepts of ROP pathogenesis are a logical extension to both classic and gap junction theories, but with greater understanding of events at a cellular level. As mentioned, VEGF is secreted in response to physiological hypoxia of the maturing avascular retina just anterior to the advancing vanguard of retinal vessels. Hyperoxia causes cessation of vessel growth and shut-down of parts of the retinal vasculature by apoptosis and excessive capillary regression with consequent retinal ischemia. This retinal ischemia has the effect of stimulating overproduction of VEGF, resulting in neovascularization known as ROP.[32–34] Recently two VEGF-A phases have been differentiated. First, there is its vessel sustaining role, which is reduced by hyperoxia, causing down-regulation of VEGF-A with cessation of vessel growth and capillary regression. Second is upregulation of VEGF-A by hypoxia, consequent on phase one, and the resultant vasoproliferation known as ROP. There are two VEGF-A receptors in the mouse retina (VEGFR-1 and VEGFR-2). VEGFR-1 receptor is concerned with supporting retinal vessel survival (phase 1), but not with endothelial permeability and proliferation (vasoproliferation), which is mediated by VEGFR-2.[35]

Other factors, such as IGF-1, a somatic growth factor, have also been implicated in controlling VEGF activation for when IGF-1 is low, vessels do not grow. Fetal IGF-1, whose levels rise in the second and third trimesters, is provided mainly by the placenta, so that levels fall after preterm birth. Oxygen-independent IGF-1 and oxygen-dependent VEGF are complementary and synergistic, and IGF-1 permits VEGF to function maximally at low levels. A low serum IGF-1 is said to predict ROP,[21] but IGF-1 is expressed by many tissues and a low serum level therefore could be a general marker of a sick baby at risk of ROP rather than a specific marker for retinal disease.[36] The experimental studies alluded to earlier offer a number of exciting therapeutic options, such as stimulating selectively VEGFR-1 but not VEGFR-2 receptors,[37] or replacing IGF-1 in preterm infants. Application to human infants is awaited.

Rather than completely eschew the classic and gap junction theories it is pertinent to consider their similarities with the current VEGF theory. In all three, normal vasculogenesis is impeded, and also pivotal to all is an oxidative insult. Recent research explains why hyperoxia is important in the initial phase and how vascular shutdown is the consequence of VEGF downregulation rather than a direct cytotoxic action on the retinal vessels. Perhaps Kretzer and Hittner were unable to find endothelial cell necrosis, as this is not a feature of apoptosis, which is the process, consequent upon VEGF downregulation, by which capillary retraction occurs. Not all features of the early theories of ROP pathogenesis can be incorporated into our current concepts. The temporal separation of the "oxygen" and "air" phases pivotal to the classic theory based on the hypothesis that ROP vasoproliferation only developed after removal from oxygen does not reflect the situation for the human infant, an observation important for screening protocol design.

Risk or associated factors

Many factors have been implicated in the development of this condition, but whether each is independently significant in ROP causation or simply an associated factor indicative of an ill neonate has in many instances yet to be determined. The enormous problem of recording, collecting, and analyzing data intermittently obtained from sick neonates whose state can fluctuate widely and unpredictably, from minute to minute, must not be underestimated.

So many factors have been associated with ROP that they cannot be individually considered here, but they include:
(i) maternal factors such as complications of pregnancy or the use of beta-blockers; and
(ii) fetal factors including hypercarbia, sepsis, vitamin E deficiency, intraventricular hemorrhage, recurrent apnea, respiratory distress syndrome, surfactant, indomethacin treatment for patent ductus arteriosus, light, and the type of neonatal unit. Some, but not all of these factors are considered below. The mechanism by which some of these factors generate ROP may not be directly causal. For instance, acidosis, which has been reported as an independent risk factor for ROP,[26,38] may act by

causing retinovascular dilatation, thereby increasing oxygen delivery to the retinal tissues.

Birth weight and gestational age

The major ROP risk factor is the degree of immaturity as measured by either birth weight or GA. Although these two parameters are highly correlated, this relationship is not linear as in intrauterine growth retardation. Furthermore, the assessment of GA, especially for the most immature neonate is prone to inaccuracy. As stated earlier both the incidence and severity of ROP are inversely related to birth weight and GA,[14,39–43] with the first being the more powerful predictor.[27,30,44,45]

Oxygen

Campbell was the first to suggest that supplemental oxygen was the cause for the sudden increase in the numbers of infants developing RLF in the early 1940s.[4] Subsequently, Ashton et al.[5] and Patz[6] using animal models were able to demonstrate the toxic effect of oxygen on immature vessels. Although several controlled trials comparing high and low supplemental oxygen in premature infants later confirmed the relationship between oxygen therapy and ROP,[46–48] it has not been possible over the ensuing 40 years to define safe levels of oxygen usage for clinical practice. The lower oxygen levels used in the mid- to late 1950s reduced the incidence but ROP was not eliminated, and there was an increase in both neonatal mortality[49] and neurological morbidity.[50] Indeed it was estimated that for each case of blindness prevented by the restriction of oxygen, about 16 infants died because of inadequate oxygenation.[51] Although this figure has since been debated,[24] the point is that both hypoxia and hyperoxia can have serious consequences for the preterm neonate.

When arterial blood gas monitoring became available, a multi-center study using intermittent umbilical artery oxygen analysis was mounted, but it failed to demonstrate any relationship between ROP and arterial blood oxygen tension.[39] More recently, a randomized controlled trial comparing continuous transcutaneous oxygen monitoring with standard neonatal care failed to show any reduction in ROP in the continuously monitored group, except in the older larger infants in whom ROP is less severe.[52] However, a re-analysis of these data specifically studied the relationship between arterial oxygen tensions and retinopathy and found a significant association between the duration of transcutaneous PO_2 over 80 mmHg and the incidence and severity of ROP.[53] It is worth emphasizing that this study alone used continuous rather than the intermittent monitoring employed in previous studies. Saito et al.'s conclusion that extremely premature infants with fluctuating arterial oxygen probably have a higher risk of developing progressive ROP[54] was confirmed by Cunningham et al.[55] and York et al.,[56] and the clinical implication from these four studies is that, with respect to ROP development, arterial oxygen levels are particularly critical within the first weeks after birth (probably 4–6 weeks).

ROP may develop in preterm infants who have never received oxygen and in premature infants with cyanotic heart disease.[8] Furthermore, some studies have suggested a relationship between neonatal hypoxia and ROP,[8,57] and in an animal model retinal ischemia may lead to the same retinal changes as hyperoxia.[58]

That hyperoxia and hypoxia may be associated with ROP is not entirely contradictory.[59] It is postulated that whereas relative hyperoxia may lead to initial retinal capillary damage it is the subsequent ischemia that acts as a stimulus for vasoproliferation. This mechanism would explain the association of recurrent apnea and cerebral ischemic events with ROP and provide the rationale for the administration of oxygen to treat ROP in the experimental animal.[60] Extending this idea to the human infant, a clinical trial in the USA designed to determine the efficacy and risks of using supplemental oxygen therapy for children whose eyes had moderate stages of ROP (pre-threshold disease) was reported in 2000.[61] At the diagnosis of pre-threshold disease in one or both eyes, the infants were randomly assigned to receive conventional oxygen treatment with pulse oximetry targets of 89 to 94% saturation or to receive supplemental oxygen treatment with pulse oximetry targets of 96 to 99%. With 649 infants enrolled during the 5-year study, the rate of progression to threshold disease (defined as in the CRYO-ROP study below) was 48% in the eyes of children assigned to conventional oxygen treatment, compared to 41% in the eyes of children in the supplemented group. Supplemental oxygen treatment also increased the risk of adverse pulmonary events including pneumonia and chronic lung disease.

After four decades of clinical research, although no direct relationship has been demonstrated between arterial oxygen levels and ROP, reviewing past and recent literature[60] shows that oxygen remains firmly center stage in ROP pathogenesis. Current neonatal research is exploring the safe upper and lower limits of oxygen arterial saturation. Looking first at higher levels, a randomized controlled trial, comparing oxygen saturation ranges of 91–94% against 95–98%, reported no difference in infant growth, neurodevelopment, or rates of ROP.[62] Exploring "what constitutes the lower safe limit" was stimulated, in part, by a recent study showing that babies with target saturation levels of 94–98% (but not measured) had a much higher incidence of ROP requiring treatment compared to those reared in target oxygen levels of 70–90%, with no increase in neurological morbidity in the latter.[63,64] A fall in the incidence of ROP stage 3 following the introduction of a strict oxygen management regimen that included minimizing fluctuations of inspired oxygen and avoiding high saturation levels was reported.[65]

Carbon dioxide

In the experimental animal, respiratory or metabolic acidosis induced either by hypercarbia[66] or acetazolamide[67] respectively induce retinal neovascularization. In the human, acidosis has been associated with the development of ROP,[26,38] whereas hypercarbia has not.[68,69]

Steroids

Prenatal steroids have been reported to be protective for the development of ROP,[70,71] but no such benefit has been reported with the use of steroids administered after birth.[72]

Ethnic origin

How ROP affects different ethnic groups has attracted relatively little interest. One study in the UK showed that although Asians (Indo-Pakistani) infants were not smaller than their Caucasian counterparts, and had similar incidence of acute ROP, they were significantly more likely to develop severe ROP.[42] Afro-Caribbean infants are less likely to develop any ROP.[44,73–75]

Genetic factors

In addition to the ethnic factors mentioned above other genetic factors have been implicated in severe ROP, notably the Norrie disease gene. Mutations of the Norrie gene have been found in some patients in the USA with advanced ROP.[76,77] However, in Kuwait no such mutations were detected although C597A

polymorphisms of the Norrie gene were higher in the advanced stages of ROP.[78] Although this did not alter the Norrie gene amino acid sequence, it may influence protein expression and possibly play a role in ROP severity. Although this line of investigation is potentially of great interest, it has yet to yield results that contribute to greatly to our understanding of ROP pathogenesis.[11]

Multiple birth

Although multiple birth per se does not increase the risk of developing ROP[79] and concordant twins behave similarly,[80] it has been reported that for discordant twins the smaller baby has a greater risk of developing this condition.[81,82]

Antioxidants and vitamin E

It has been suggested that the relative hyperoxic extrauterine environment causes free oxygen radical production, which inhibits spindle cell migration and stimulates these cells to produce angiogenic factors responsible for ROP.[31] It has been argued that vitamin E can suppress this free-radical damage and this is the basis for vitamin E therapy in ROP. Certainly a suppressive effect has been shown in an animal model.[83]

Vitamin E is a naturally occurring antioxidant important in maintaining cell integrity,[84] and the preterm neonate has low levels compared to either the adult or full-term infant.[31] For this substance to be delivered to the inner retinal tissues the carrier protein interstitial retinal binding protein (IRBP) is necessary. Yet IRBP is not present in the peripheral retina until around 29 weeks gestation.[85] Theoretically selenium-dependent glutathione peroxidase, which is active before 29 weeks gestation, might be the appropriate agent to offer free-radical protection for the very immature neonate acting through the vitamin C antioxidant system.[31] Another free-radical scavenger that may act as an antioxidant is bilirubin[86] although its protective effect has not been agreed upon.[87–89]

The use of vitamin E in ROP was first suggested by Owens and Owens[3] in the late 1940s and taken up again by Johnson et al.[85,90] A flurry of clinical trials in the 1980s demonstrated that although vitamin E does not appear to reduce the frequency of ROP, it may reduce its severity.[90–93] Despite these findings, concern was expressed about the side-effects of vitamin E and methods of administration, including sepsis and necrotizing enterocolitis,[90] retinal hemorrhage,[94] and intraventricular hemorrhage.[93] The use of Vitamin E as a prophylactic agent is not now recommended,[84] although Raju et al.[95] conducted a meta-analysis of RCTs of vitamin E prophylaxis, reported a 52% reduction in the incidence of stage 3+ ROP, and made a plea for the role of this substance to be re-evaluated.

Blood transfusions

Preterm infants given blood transfusions receive adult hemoglobin. As the latter binds oxygen less avidly than fetal hemoglobin the oxygen dissociation curve is shifted so that more oxygen is delivered up, rendering tissues relatively hyperoxic. This could increase the risk of ROP and although several studies have demonstrated an association between ROP and blood transfusion,[96–99] this association was not confirmed by Brooks et al.[100] It is still unclear whether repeated blood transfusion is an independent ROP risk factor or simply yet another indicator of a very ill neonate.

Surfactant

The use of this agent has reduced mortality, the severity of respiratory distress syndrome, and chronic lung disease in very immature neonates.[101] Studies have not shown any difference between treated and nontreated infants.[102–105]

Standard of care

Infants born in large, tertiary referral neonatal units have been reported to have a lower incidence[27] and severity[45] of ROP. Mindful that these are the units caring for the most sick and most immature neonates, for them to have disproportionately less ROP is surprising and is attributed by Darlow et al.[27] to the better quality of care they provide. Tentative support for this theory comes from the finding that in middle-income communities babies with a wider range of birth weights and gestational age are at risk of developing severe ROP,[106] perhaps reflecting the availability of neonatal intensive care facilities but paucity of appropriate level of resources.

Light

Early exposure to light was suggested as a causative factor in the first descriptions of this condition by Terry.[1,107] Studies by Hepner et al.[108] and Locke and Reese[109] did not provide supportive evidence, but at this time supplemental oxygen could well have swamped any effect of light. It was proposed that light could, by damaging retinal tissues, generate free radicals and thereby cause ROP. Interest in light reawakened with the report by Glass et al.[110] that reduction in the neonatal unit illumination reduced the incidence and severity of ROP. This finding was later supported[111] but not universally.[112,113] A prospective randomized clinical trial, the LIGHT-ROP study, was designed to examine the effect on incidence of ROP by limitation of light exposure early in life and thereby decreasing oxidant radical formation in the eyes of premature infants.[114] Goggles were placed over the eyes of randomly selected infants, all of whom had gestational ages of <31 weeks and birth weights of <1251g. Goggles were maintained until 4 weeks after birth or 31 weeks post-conceptional age, whichever was later. Among the 188 surviving infants who wore goggles during the neonatal period, 54% developed ROP, compared to 58% of the 100 babies in the group that did not have goggles. In this study, it did not appear that light reduction early in life decreased the likelihood of developing ROP, but the study did not have enough babies who developed severe ROP to determine the effect of light limitation on severe disease.

CLASSIFICATION

The international classification of the acute stages of ROP was published in 1984,[115] and in 1987 was expanded to include a classification of retinal detachment and ROP sequelae,[116] thus replacing that of Reese et al.[117] All stages of ROP are now covered by this single classification (Table 51.1). For the first time, direct comparison between centers and countries became possible, and this stimulated a flurry of clinical research that has had major impact on clinical practice worldwide. A revision of the international classification is nearing completion.

The classification involves describing ROP by four parameters:
(i)   Severity by stage;
(ii) Location by zone;
(iii) Extent by clock hour of circumferential retinal involvement at the junction between the vascularized and avascular retina; and
(iv) Plus disease.

A number of charts on which to record clinical findings have been devised (Fig. 51.2). The normal fundus of the extremely pre-

Table 51.1 Stages of ROP

Stage 1	Demarcation line
Stage 2	Ridge
Stage 3	Ridge with extraretinal fibrovascular proliferation
Stage 4	Subtotal retinal detachment
	Extrafoveal
	Retinal detachment including fovea
Stage 5	Total retinal detachment

Funnel	
Anterior	**Posterior**
Open	Open
Narrow	Narrow
Open	Narrow
Narrow	Open

From Committee for Classification of Retinopathy of Prematurity.[116]

mature baby can be difficult to visualize in detail (Figs. 51.1, 51.3, and 51.4). The retinal blood vessels are thin and straight. With time they increase normally in caliber and tortuosity, but abnormally with active ROP.

Severity of disease

ROP has been divided into five stages.

Stage 1

In stage 1 ROP there is a flat gray-white demarcation line separating the vascularized from nonvascularized retina. Often feint it can be difficult to identify. Retinal vessels may run up to the line but do not cross it (Figs. 51.5, 51.6).

Stage 2

In stage 2 the demarcation line has increased in volume and extends out of the plane of the retina (Figs. 51.6–51.9). The color of the ridge may be white or pink and small neovascular tufts may be seen posterior to the ridge. Differentiating stage 1 and early stage 2 is not always simple.

Stage 3

Stage 3 exhibits the features of stage 2, but is characterized by extraretinal neovascularization (Figs. 51.8 and 51.10). The new vessels may be continuous with, or disconnected from, the posterior border of the ridge, or extend into the vitreous.

Stage 4

This stage is characterized by subtotal retinal detachment, exudative or tractional, which may (stage 4b) or may not (stage 4a) involve the fovea.

Stage 5

In stage 5 there is a funnel-shaped total retinal detachment (Figs. 51.11, 51.12). This stage is further divided according to the characteristics of the funnel, whether it is open or narrowed anteriorly and posteriorly.

Plus disease

This is a constellation of signs indicating ROP activity (Figs. 51.13–51.16). The first signs of plus are tortuosity of the retinal arterioles and congestion of the retinal veins close to the optic

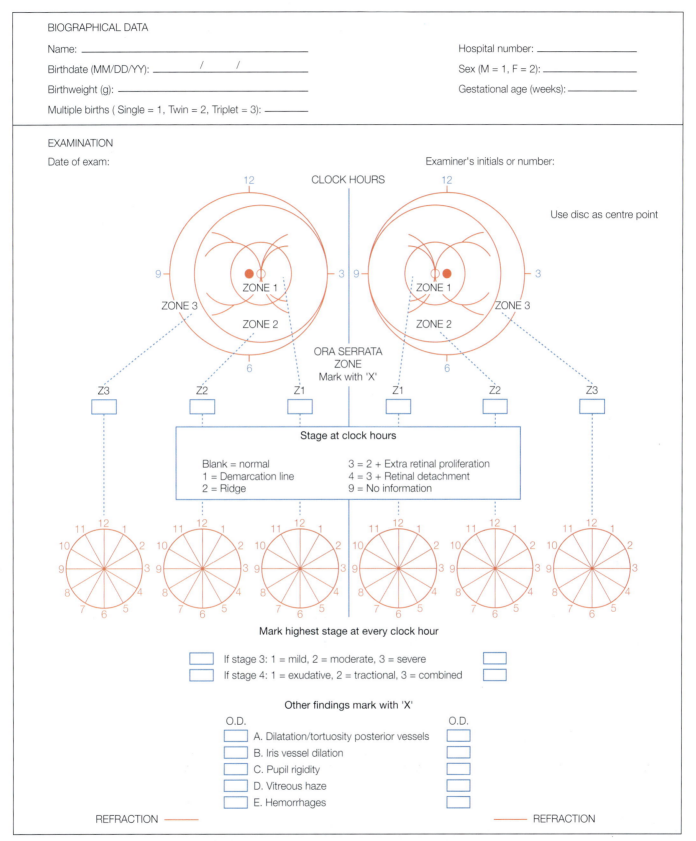

Fig. 51.2 A chart for recording fundus details and staging ROP. Five stages are recorded (see text).

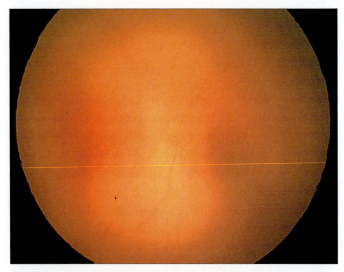

Fig. 51.3 Immature retinal vessels in an extremely immature baby - the view is hazy. Note how thin and straight are the retinal vessels

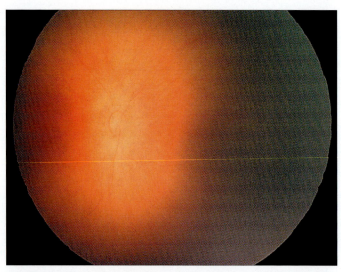

Fig. 51.4 Immature retinal vessels one week after figure in Figure 51.3. No ROP.

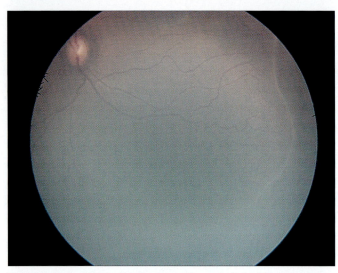

Fig. 51.5 Stage 1 ROP – thin line separating vascularized from avascular retinal regions. The bluish tint is due to dark fundus

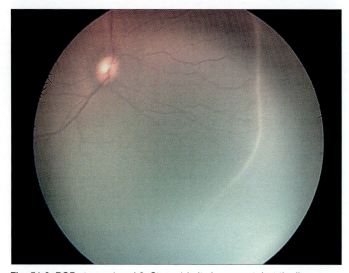

Fig. 51.6 ROP stages 1 and 2. Stage 1 in its lower part, but the line becomes thicker (ridge) towards the top of the image. Differentiating stages 1 and 2 is not always easy - or necessarily important.

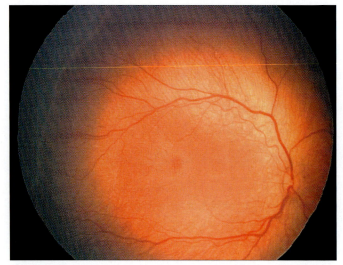

Fig. 51.7 Stage 2 ROP

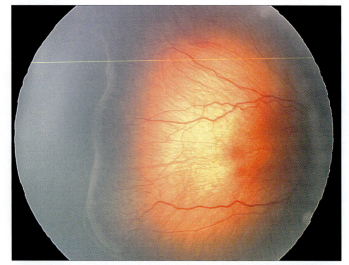

Fig. 51.8 Stage 2 and 3 ROP. Stage 2 at top and bottom of the image with about one clock hour of mild stage 3 disease that curls away from the ridge at its lower edge.

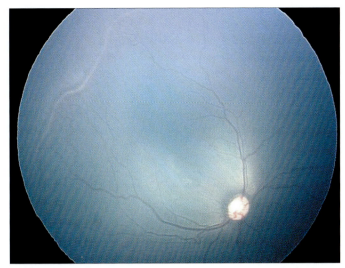

Fig. 51.9 Stage 2 ROP in a black baby.

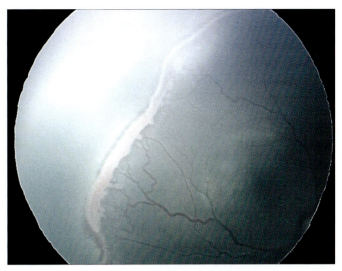

Fig. 51.0 Stage 3 ROP that has developed in the eye with stage 2 disease shown in Figure 51.7. Note the peripheral tortuosity and dilation as the vessels become close to the ROP lesion (compare with Fig 51.7). The shadow, just behind the lesion, indicates that the lesion is off the retinal surface.

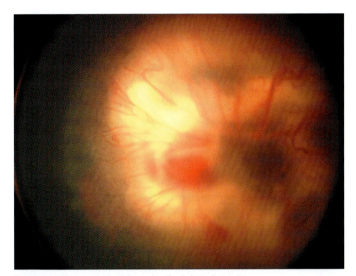

Fig. 51.11 Acute stage 5 funnel retinal detachment.

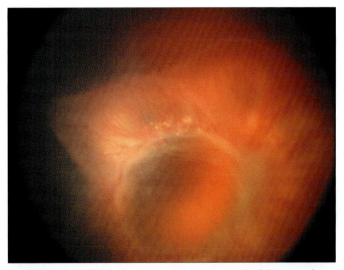

Fig. 51.12 Acute stage 5 funnel retinal detachment - the fellow eye of Figure 51.11.

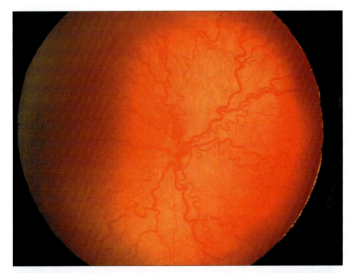

Fig. 51.13 Plus disease in zone 1 ROP. This is extreme plus disease, and the ROP lesion in the periphery of the picture is not well differentiated (compare with figure 51.10). This lack of differentiation is characteristic of severe zone 1 ROP and is one of the driving forces for early treatment. (Reproduced by kind permission of Dr Anna Ells, Calgary, Canada.)

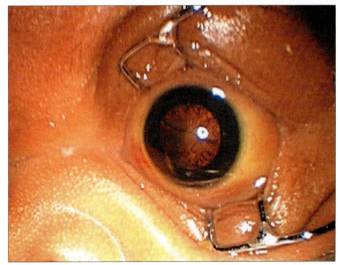

Fig. 51.14 Plus disease involving the anterior segment, with iris engorgement and persistence of the tunica vasculosa lentis seen in silhouette. Plus disease of the anterior segment indicates very active and severe ROP.

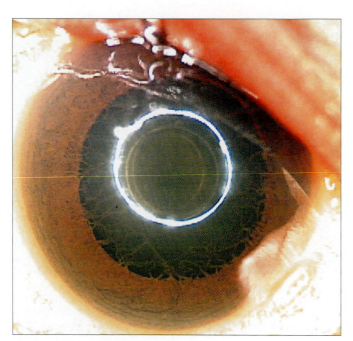

Fig. 51.15 Plus disease close up of Figure 51.14.

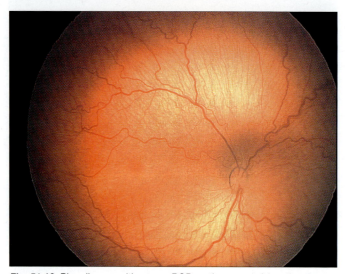

Fig. 51.16 Plus disease with severe ROP on the zone 1–2 junction, in same baby as Figures 51.13 and 51.14, 2 weeks after the last. This baby progressed from no ROP to requiring treatment over a 5 week period. The ROP lesion is to the extreme left of the picture and appears relatively innocuous, but is not.

disc. Later, the vessels of the iris become engorged and the pupil fails to dilate to mydriatics (pupil rigidity; Figs 51.14, 51.15). Eventually the vitreous becomes hazy. Signs of plus disease may appear at any ROP stage and even occasionally as a precursor. The diagnosis of plus disease is against a standard photograph, and for the diagnosis at least two quadrants must be involved. When less than two quadrants are involved the term pre-plus can be used. It is also pertinent to note the plus disease does not refer to vascular changes in the retinal periphery. It is acknowledged that the diagnosis of plus disease is critical and is an important indicator of eyes that have severe ROP,[118] may require treatment,[119] and are of unfavorable outcome.[45]

Location

The retina is divided into three zones centered on the optic disc, in contrast to retinal neural organization, which centers on the fovea. Zone 1 is a circle whose radius is twice the disc–foveal distance about 30°. Zone 2 extends from the edge of zone 1 to the ora serrata on the nasal side and encircles the anatomical equator. Zone 3 includes all retina temporally, superiorly, and inferiorly anterior to zone 2. With no anatomical landmarks identifying zone 3, only when the directly nasal retina is fully vascularized can it be stated that zone 3 has been entered. As described below, ROP in zone 1 has an atypical appearance and does not usually progress through stages 1 to 3.

Extent

The extent of disease is described in clock hours or by 30° sectors. As the examiner looks at the eyes the 3 o'clock position is on the right, i.e., on the nasal side of the right eye and temporal side of the left eye.

Regression and resolution

The time course of resolution of acute phase retinopathy has been less well studied, largely because once the need for surgical intervention has passed there is less need for frequent surveillance and meticulous recording of clinical detail.[116] The rate of regression reflects postmenstrual age (PMA)[120] with the first signs of regression being failure to progress (stabilization) and the lessening of any signs of plus disease. The ridge thins and breaks up. Later vessels grow through the ridge into the peripheral avascular retina.[121] Involution is characterized by vascular remodeling with gradual movement of vessels toward the retinal periphery, although in some eyes that have had acute phase retinopathy, vascularization to the ora serrata does not occur. The acute ROP lesion becomes white and vessels may be seen extending beyond the lesion into the periphery. Vasoproliferative lesions become fibrotic.[116] All stage 1 and 2 ROP, provided that is the maximum stage reached, undergo complete resolution. Stage 3 may or may not resolve, depending on its severity, and one sign of failure of complete resolution is retinal dragging (Figs. 51.17, 51.18). Repka et al.[120] reported that the mean time of

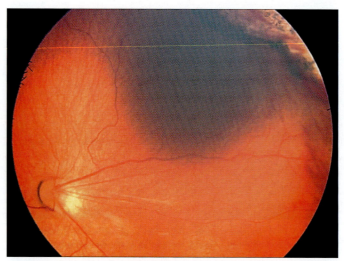

Fig. 51.17 Mild dragging of the retinal vessels - note response to cryotherapy on upper border of picture.

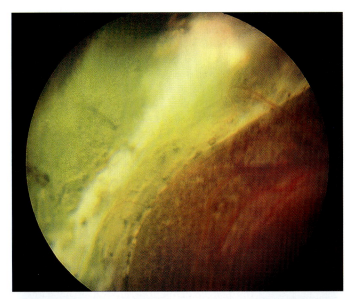

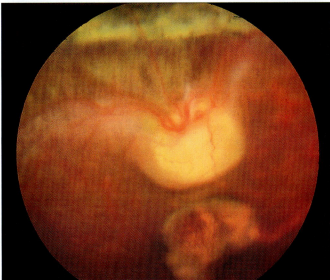

Fig. 51.18 Marked retinal dragging towards an area of chorioretinal atrophy and vitreoretinal fibrosis in the area of what was probably stage 3 zone 1 disease.

Table 51.2 Cicatricial changes in retinopathy of prematurity

Peripheral changes	Posterior changes
Vascular Failure to vascularize peripheral retina Abnormal, nondichotomous branching of retinal vessels Vascular arcades with circumferential interconnection Telangiectatic vessels	**Vascular** Vascular tortuosity Straightening of blood vessels in temporal arcade Decrease in angle of insertion of major temporal arcade
Retinal Pigmentary changes Vitreoretinal interface changes Thin retina Peripheral folds Vitreous membranes with or without attachment to retina	**Retinal** Pigmentary changes Distortion or ectopia of macula Stretching and folding of retina in macular region leading to periphery Vitreoretinal interface changes Vitreous membrane
Lattice-like degeneration Retinal breaks Traction/rhegmatogenous retinal detachment	Dragging of retina over disc Traction/rhegmatogenous retinal detachment

From Committee of Classification of Retinopathy of Prematurity.[116]

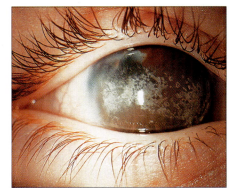

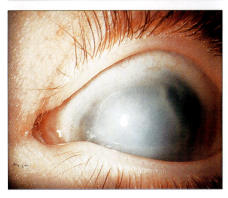

Fig. 51.19 Cicatricial ROP with bilateral obliteration of the anterior chamber and angle closure glaucoma with secondary corneal degenerative changes.

onset of signs of involution of disease in children with birth weights of less than 1251g was 38.6 weeks, and 74% of all ROP had begun to involute by 40 weeks of postmenstrual age and in 90% by 44 weeks.

Advanced cicatricial changes involving the anterior vitreous and retina (Table 51.2) may push the lens/iris diaphragm forward and cause shallowing of the anterior chamber, glaucoma, and corneal decompensation (Fig. 51.19). In such cases lensectomy is indicated to relieve narrow angle glaucoma.

INCIDENCE AND PREVALENCE

Acute phase ROP

There was a plethora of publications on this topic mostly in the 1980s and early 1990s.[15,43,122] Most reports came from single centers, but there were three prospective geographically based studies from New Zealand,[123] England,[42] and Sweden,[124] the last named being undertaken after treatment was introduced.

The largest report thus far detailing the natural history of acute phase ROP is based on data obtained during the multicenter study of cryotherapy for retinopathy of prematurity (CRYO-ROP study) conducted in 23 nurseries in the USA and enrolled babies from January 1986 through November 1987.[73] Over 4000 children with birth weights of less than 1251g underwent detailed serial eye examinations. ROP was observed in one or both eyes of 65.8% of these infants, with ROP observed in 90% of children with birth weights of less than 750g, in 78% of those with birth weights of 751–1000g, and in 47% of those with birth weights of 1001–1250g. In addition, as part of the natural history of ROP, the CRYO-ROP study also reported on the residua of ROP (the cicatricial phase in the eyes of 2759 children at age 1 year). None of these eyes had undergone cryotherapy. There was advanced, serious scarring involving the posterior pole in approximately 4%, with 2% likely to have severe visual loss due to severe posterior pole scarring or retinal detachment.[125]

Some publications have reported on the declining incidence of ROP,[64,126–128] but this is not a universal experience.[129,130] There are several inherent biases in single-center studies,[131] including survival rates,[132] ethnic issues, and standard of care. Studies into the incidence of mild ROP need to be rigorously controlled for examination technique and frequency. Thus, studying secular changes in ROP is fraught with difficulty. Despite these caveats it is not in doubt that both the incidence and severity of ROP rise with the degree of prematurity, and more than 50% babies under 1000g birth weight will develop some ROP while babies under 1251g birth weight have an incidence of stage 3 ROP of around 18%, of whom 6% reached "threshold" stage (see below) and required treatment.[133]

Hussain et al., in a review of their intensive care nursery experience from 1989 to 1997, found that both the incidence and severity of acute retinopathy was decreased, compared to the results of the CRYO-ROP study.[127] The overall incidence of ROP in infants with birth weights of less than 1251g was 34% compared to 65.8% for CRYO-ROP study patients. For infants with birth weights of less than 1000g, they found an incidence rate for ROP of 46%, compared to 81.6% for CRYO-ROP patients in the same birth weight group. Much larger scale studies are needed to confirm what may be a promising trend toward lower prevalence of ROP.

In industrialized countries, ROP is largely confined to infants with birth weights of less than 1000g and gestational age of 31 weeks or less, and blinding disease is rarely seen in larger babies.[134] However, the prevalence of retinopathy in developing countries appears to be increasing in Latin America and urban regions of industrializing countries such as India, Malaysia, and Thailand, and blinding disease is not confined to the very-low-birth-weight infant. As infant mortality rates fall between 10 and 50 per 1000 births in industrializing countries, the risk for blindness due to ROP increases dramatically, whereas the risk is very low in those countries with infant mortality rates more than 50 per 1000 births.[135] Table 51.3 summarizes risk factors that may be responsible for the varying rates of blinding disease among countries and may help explain why larger babies are

developing ROP as survival rates and neonatal outcomes improve in industrializing countries. The table shows that, in settings where only the larger-birth-weight premature babies survive (as in the epidemic of the 1940–1950s), extent of prematurity and low birth weight have minimal contributions. In this setting, oxygen supplementation as a surrogate for the level of neonatal care is a prominent risk factor. As the smallest-birth-weight babies survive due to improvements in neonatal and perinatal care (as in the nursery of the 1990s and 2000s), then the extent of the infant's prematurity becomes more important.

ROP disability: the two epidemics

An overview of the past 50 years shows two ROP epidemics.[136–138] The first, which commenced in the early 1940s, was due to high unrestricted unmonitored oxygen and was brought to an end about a decade later by oxygen restriction, which followed the discovery that oxygen supplementation was a factor in ROP causation. The second epidemic began in the late 1960s and is ongoing. During the first epidemic, the survival of neonates of <1000g birth weight was around 5–8%, and most of the babies blinded during this period were of heavier birth weight. Advances in neonatal care have largely eliminated the risk of severe ROP in these larger babies (>1000g birth weight).[139] Thus, these same advances that terminated the first epidemic and increased the survival of the very immature neonate (now around 50–60% <1000g birth weight) resulted in the second epidemic, which involves mainly the very immature neonate who previously was unlikely to survive. In retrospect, the first epidemic could now be considered largely preventable, whereas currently the second is not.

We have presented the two epidemics as discrete, historically separated, entities–this greatly oversimplifies the situation. The work of Gilbert and colleagues has provided important worldwide insight into contemporary ROP-induced visual disability. Countries can be subdivided according to health–socioeconomic criteria into high-, middle-, or low-income communities, and these determine the health provision to each community. Thus, there may be diverse health-socioeconomic communities within a single country. In high-income countries such as the USA, and much of Europe, wealth and technology permit high-quality health care and neonatal intensive care. In these countries ROP-induced disability accounts for 3–8% of childhood vision impairment.[140–143] In

Table 51.3 Risk factors for retinopathy of prematurity; historical perspective		"First epidemic" (1940–1950s)	"Second epidemic" (1970–1980s), and "third epidemic" in middle-income countries	ROP in NICU of 21st century
Risk factors				
Prematurity		+	++	++++
Low birth weight		+	++	++++
High oxygen supplementation		++++	+++	+
Illness		+	+	+/–
Babies at risk				
<1,000 g	Survival rate	+	++	++++
	Risk of ROP	+	++	+++
1,000–1,500 g	Survival rate	+++	++++	++++
	Risk of ROP	+++	+	+/–
Ocular outcomes		Poor	Moderate	Good

Adapted from Gilbert et al.,[135] p. 275, Table 16.11, used with permission.

middle-income communities (Latin America, Eastern Europe, and other countries) technology permits the increased survival of the preterm baby, but limited health resources limit the standard of care.[144] Consequently babies with a wider range of birth weights and gestational ages are at risk of developing severe ROP, and ROP-induced blindness contributes up to 39% childhood vision impairment. In effect, the current epidemic occurring in middle-income countries (sometimes called the third epidemic) contains elements from the first and second epidemics: increased survival, but associated with limited resources that do not permit high-quality neonatal care. By way of complete contrast, in low-income countries, such as many countries in Africa, Albania, etc., there are not the facilities to permit the survival of preterm babies. Very few babies in low-income communities survive to develop ROP.[144]

The evidence that ROP-induced disability has been reduced by treatment since it was introduced in 1988 comes from two sources. First, from the CRYO-ROP Study, which demonstrated that the beneficial effects of treatment is maintained 10 years after treatment. Second, epidemiological studies from the UK show that as a proportion of childhood vision impairment, between 1976 and 1985 ROP contributed 5%. This rose to 8% between 1986 and 1990[141] but fell to 3% by 2000.[143] Although these studies are not directly comparable, given the increase in survival of the most immature babies,[145] in the absence of a treatment effect, a considerable increase could have been anticipated.

NATURAL HISTORY

Understanding the natural history of ROP has both theoretical and practical implications as it provides clues to underlying mechanisms and is vital for the screening and management of ROP. There are five important elements to the natural history of retinopathy of prematurity:

(i)   Age at onset;
(ii) Site of onset;
(iii) Rate of progression;
(iv) Plus disease; and
(v)   Resolution.

Age at onset

ROP affects only the immature retinal vessels and does not develop after retinal vascularization is complete. Instinctively one would expect the most premature, often ill neonate, with a very immature retinal vascular system, to develop ROP sooner postnatally than his or her larger and more mature counterpart. However, this is not so (Fig. 51.20) and ROP develops over a relatively narrow PMA range.[44,73,146,147] Thus ROP onset is linked more to the stage of development of the infant, by PMA, than neonatal events. However, ROP is not present at birth, and this event is clearly necessary for its development, which is of course influenced by neonatal events.

Zone of involvement

The propensity for severity is governed to a large extent by the state of retinal vascularization, so that zone is perhaps the most important predictor of outcome.[45,125,148] Thus incomplete vascularization in zone 1 carries a 54% risk of reaching threshold but this falls to only 8% when vessels have reached zone 2. For ROP developing in zone 3 the risk of an adverse outcome is almost nil.[149]

Site of onset by clock hour

ROP commences in the temporal retina in the more mature neonates when the nasal retina is already vascularized. However, in the more immature neonate, frequently seen nowadays, ROP commences preferentially in the nasal retina (Fig. 51.21) and later extends to other regions.[44,150] Although the zones of vascular development are depicted by the international classification as being circular, in practice they are elliptical so that retinopathy in

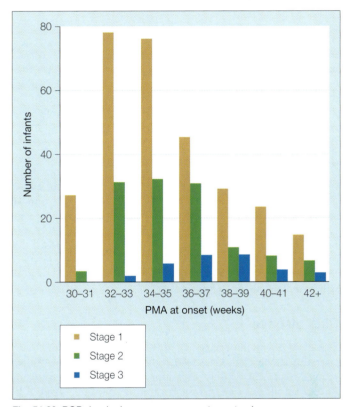

Fig. 51.20 ROP developing over narrow postmenstrual age.

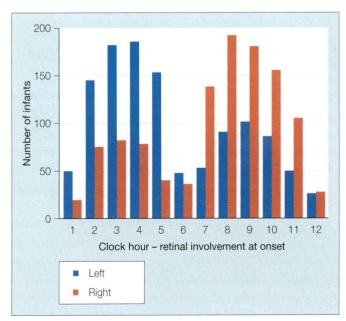

Fig. 51.21 Retinal location at ROP onset.

the nasal retina is frequently closer to the optic disc than ROP in the temporal retina.[151] The vertical retinal regions are less likely to be involved at onset and are only involved when ROP involves most of the circumference. The finding of ROP in these regions early in the course of the disease is a useful indicator of the possibility of future severity. The more premature the neonate, the more posterior by zone the location of the retinopathy and the greater the potential for progression. Thus zone 1 disease is very likely to progress to stage 3, but for ROP always confined entirely to zone 3 this rarely if ever happens.

Rate of progression

As with onset, the rate of progression is also governed predominantly by the stage of development (PMA) rather than by postnatal age, or neonatal events such as oxygen therapy or illnesses.[44,73] Of course the latter contribute to ROP severity. The median PMA at which the various stages develop is as follows:
(i)   Stage 1, 34 weeks;
(ii) Stage 2, 35 weeks;
(iii) Stage 3, 36 weeks; and
(iv) Threshold ROP, 37 weeks.
In the CRYO-ROP study babies were randomized for treatment (i.e., within 72 hours of diagnosis of threshold ROP) at a mean age of 37.7 weeks PMA (range 32–50 weeks)).[152] This was confirmed by comparing the rate of progress in CRYO-ROP and LIGHT-ROP trials.[153] It is important to note the extremes of this range, as Subhani et al. reported threshold ROP at 31 weeks PMA, but almost all babies (99%) that will develop severe ROP will have done so by 46.3 weeks PMA.[154]

Plus disease

Plus disease is an important sign of ROP activity and as discussed later this is one of the key features that indicates an eye might require treatment.[119] Plus disease may be superimposed on any ROP stage and is a sign that ROP is, or may become, severe.[45,118] Advanced plus disease is obvious, but unfortunately if mild, is the least robust aspect of ROP to diagnose. To overcome this, attempts are being made to quantify some components of plus disease by digitized[155] or digital images.[156,157]

Summary of retinopathy of prematurity natural history

ROP affects only immature retinal vessels, and the greater the degree of prematurity, the higher the incidence and the greater the propensity for severe disease to develop. Intriguingly, ROP onset and progression are determined mainly by postmenstrual and not postnatal age. Whereas ROP develops in the temporal retina of larger babies, in the most immature babies retinopathy frequently commences in the nasal retina. Acute phase ROP exhibits a high degree of symmetry between the two eyes.[44,158]

CLINICAL ASPECTS

Concepts of screening

Since the demonstration in 1988 that severe ROP can be successfully treated,[133] the ophthalmologist has had a duty to screen. Advances in our understanding of its natural history have provided the basis for a logical and relatively simple screening protocol that

is cost-effective.[159,160] There are a number of published reviews and recommendations that do not differ greatly.[121,161–164]

With four randomized controlled trials and several epidemiological studies, ROP screening is one of the most evidence-based activities we undertake in ophthalmology. Naturally it takes time for advances to be incorporated into national screening guidelines, but in recognition of this evolution here we deal with the concepts of screening that can be flexibly applied to the communities of the world that have significant differences in their neonatal populations.

The purpose of screening

The purpose of screening is to identify severe ROP (stage 3), which may require treatment, mindful that the indications for treatment changed very recently.[119] Apart from the need to diagnose ROP requiring treatment, babies with stage 3 ROP have a high risk of developing strabismus, myopia, and vision deficits, and in themselves merit ophthalmic surveillance.

Which infants should be screened

In high-income communities, severe ROP (stage 3 or more) is virtually confined to infants of birth weight <1501g and <32 weeks GA and only these babies need to be examined. Accordingly, in the UK, there is no indication to include a sickness criterion or to screen larger babies who have required prolonged oxygen therapy. This is in contrast to the USA where screening is recommended for all babies <1501g or with a gestational age of <29 weeks. Infants between 1500 and 2000g birth weight who had an unstable clinical course and are considered at risk of ROP should also be examined. In essence, the difference between UK and USA criteria is small.

For high-income countries, the UK criteria include most, if not all, babies who develop severe ROP (stage 3 or more).[165–170] However, there is debate as to whether it is possible to safely reduce the number of babies screened for ROP because many of the larger and more mature babies currently screened are not at risk of developing severe ROP. A study from Canada of more than 16,000 babies reported only one baby over 1200g with severe ROP.[171] Two studies from the UK have shown that the criteria of <1251g BW and or <30 weeks GA included all babies with stage 3;[165,166] however, a few US studies have reported stage 3 in larger babies.[167,168,172] It should be noted that by using both birth weight and gestational age the number of babies to be screened can be reduced.

For low- and middle-income countries, larger babies also develop severe ROP, and the UK and US criteria may not include all babies at risk.[144] It is essential therefore in these communities for the screening net to be cast wider, based on local data.

Time of examinations

Examinations can be timed on the principle that the onset and progression of ROP are both predominantly determined by PMA rather than by neonatal events. So while most guidelines recommend commencing screening examinations between 4 and 7 weeks, Reynolds et al.[154] recently developed an algorithm for examining the most immature baby later postnatally than the more mature baby. Timing examinations is critical, as there is only a narrow, albeit imperfectly determined, window of opportunity for treatment–up to about one week. Onset is rare before 30 weeks PMA, and ROP commencing once vascularization has entered zone 3 and/or after 36 weeks PMA is most unlikely to reach stage 3. Because of the predetermined timescale it is sometimes necessary to examine the very sick neonate who may be ventilated.

Two-weekly examinations are generally recommended as a routine but if ROP is severe, then more frequent examinations will be required. On a practical basis a weekly visit to the neonatal intensive care unit (NICU) saves the need to recall most infants discharged to home between visits, and consequently promotes concordance between clinicians and families.[173] The vast majority of examinations can and should be undertaken in hospital. Visits to outpatients greatly inconvenience the family, and failure to attend at the appropriate time may have disastrous consequences. For the infant discharged to another hospital while still at risk, arrangements for the completion of the screening program need to be made–this is a significant cause of failure to diagnose severe ROP at the appropriate time.

In the absence of ROP, screening can cease when the retinal vessels have grown well into zone 3. This can only be ascertained with certainty when the nasal retina is vascularized so that there is no doubt of the extent of vascularization.

Screening protocol

The next paragraph is written with countries like the UK in mind and carries the important caveat mentioned in the previous sections that this may not be fully applicable to all preterm populations.

All infants <1501g birth weight and <32 weeks GA should be examined 6–7 weeks postnatally and then every 2 weeks until 36 weeks PMA or until vascularization has progressed well into zone 3 and the risk of stage 3 has passed. It is not necessary to review infants until the retina is fully vascularized. Some larger babies may be discharged to home before screening is due to commence at 6 weeks. In such situations an examination before discharge is recommended as this can indicate the potential for ROP and frequently obviate the need for review, thus simplifying life for parents and clinician alike.

Methods of examination

Eye examinations are stressful for the preterm baby,[174–176] and this can be reduced by nesting. Infants should be handled gently and it is helpful if a trained nurse is in attendance to help and to monitor the infant's well-being. The ophthalmic examination should be performed using the indirect ophthalmoscope, with a 28-diopter lens, through dilated pupils, achieved by instilling 1 drop each of cyclopentolate 0.5% and phenylephrine 2.5% 30 minutes prior to examination and repeated once if necessary. A pediatric lid speculum and scleral indenter (for ocular rotation rather than indentation), after the instillation of 0.5% proxymetacaine hydrochloride or sodium benoxinate 0.4% eye drops, is used by many to permit complete evaluation of the peripheral retina. Although it can be argued that very peripheral disease so observed is of no clinical importance, identifying peripheral nasal retinopathy can be a clue to later progression and only by observing the state of vascularization of the nasal retina can the ophthalmologist determine whether zone 3 has been entered.

Clinical findings

The ophthalmoscopic appearance of the neonate is different in a number of respects from that of the older infant.[177] Before examining the retina it is important to use the indirect lens as a simple magnifier to examine the anterior segment, which may contain useful information. For instance the amount of regression of the tunica vasculosa lentis is an indicator of maturity (regressing between 28 and 34 weeks GA),[178] and also of ROP activity as it may persist in the presence of severe disease. Transient lens vacuoles are not infrequently observed.

The retinal periphery is white-gray in its nonvascularized regions, the extent of this depending on the degree of immaturity (Fig. 51.1). The optic disc frequently has a grayish and a doubling-ring appearance, almost akin to mild optic nerve hypoplasia. The macular area is relatively ill defined, there being no macular or foveolar reflexes until around 36 and 42 weeks PMA, respectively.[23] The retinal arterioles in the early neonatal period are not tortuous, but tend to become so later, and this is in part related to ROP severity.[44]

Acute phase retinopathy of prematurity

The purpose of screening is to identify severe ROP, which might require treatment. The four parameters by which ROP is classified, according to the international classification, should be noted at every examination: location by zone, severity by stage, extent by clock hour or sector, and the presence of plus disease.

The extent of retinal vascularization and ROP location indicate the likelihood of future progression. For instance, the more posterior the retinopathy, the greater the propensity to become severe. Thus zone 1 retinopathy very frequently progresses to stage 3, whereas zone 3 disease does not. Also ROP frequently starts in the nasal retina in the most immature neonate and has a propensity greater than that of ROP with temporal onset to become severe. Similarly greater circumferential involvement is a poor prognostic sign.

Only if the advancing edge of the peripheral retinal vessels can be visualized can one determine whether ROP is present. Another diagnostic aid is vessels that dilate slightly rather than taper as they traverse the retina toward the periphery. Pay particular attention to the nasal and temporal peripheries. Use a scleral indenter to rotate rather than indent, but be careful that the indent does not obscure the early signs; looking to either side of the indent is helpful. In the mildest form of ROP (stage 1) a white line is seen at the junction between vascularized and nonvascularized retina, and with stage 2 the line becomes thicker and extends just out of the plane of the retina. In practice it can be difficult to distinguish between stage 1 and 2. Abnormal arborization and circumferential arcading are often seen in the vessels running up to the ridge.

Look for signs of plus disease in the posterior pole as this alerts the clinician at the start of the examination that ROP is present and active and may require treatment–even if the ROP lesion itself is not in the field of view.

Acute phase ROP has a strong tendency for symmetry between the two eyes, in marked contrast to its residua, which are characteristically asymmetrical.[44,158] The stage 3 lesion is an arteriovenous shunt that contains blood with rapid flow and marked vascular leakage on fluorescein angiography,[31,121] which can be seen histopathologically.[179] With more advanced disease new vessels grow forward into the vitreous (stage 3) and retinal detachment may be seen, which can be partial (stage 4) or total (stage 5).

Recent advances in screening

An exciting recent innovation has been contact wide-field digital imaging of the neonatal retina. This opens up a range of opportunities for the study of ROP and the developing retina. Because the image is presented on a monitor at the cotside, the retinal image can be viewed by trainee and nontrainee ophthalmologists, so reducing the need for multiple examinations. The retinal picture can also be seen by the neonatal team and the parents. Digital ocular imaging, which provides high-quality retinal images (bitmap stills or video), has several advantages:

(i) Examinations can be performed by nonophthalmologists;

(ii) Images can be transmitted via the Internet to local or distant centers for expert opinion (telemedicine);

(iii) Images can be stored for immediate or subsequent analysis, permitting quantification of changes; and

(iv) Images have the potential to be analyzed semi-automatically.

Preliminary studies, which used using nurses or pediatricians to obtain the images, show considerable promise.[180–183] Although there remains some debate about its sensitivity to detect mild peripheral ROP, in the study by Roth et al. while there were 12 false-negative results, none of these affected the decision to treat.[181] The value of digital imaging in detecting severe ROP is acknowledged. There is some uncertainty in its ability to detect mild peripheral ROP. Until this is clarified, in cases of uncertainty the ophthalmologist might consider backing digital imaging by an indirect ophthalmoscopic assessment so that the baby can be discharged from screening with certainty. Ells et al. demonstrated that this technique can be used for telemedicine.[184]

Digital imaging therefore opens opportunities for ROP screening to be undertaken by professionals other than ophthalmologists to perform ROP screening. This is pertinent in the UK, for instance, where less than 2% babies examined require treatment[185] and one could debate whether this is optimal use of ophthalmic expertise, and even more in middle-income countries where expertise is in even shorter supply and yet there are more babies to be screened.

As mentioned elsewhere, plus disease is recognized as being critically important in diagnosing the eye that might require treatment. Yet diagnosing plus disease is not easy and remains the least robust aspect of ROP diagnosis.[186] Early studies have demonstrated that some components of plus disease can be quantified from digitized photographs[155] or semi-automatically directly from digitally acquired images.[156,157] There is still some way to go, but it may well be that in the foreseeable future, an automatic objective measure of plus disease can be obtained from one digital image of the vessels close to the optic disc. Screening could then be undertaken by nonmedical personnel[187] and the expert ophthalmologist consulted only, via telemedicine, when plus disease is present. This may be an example of how technological advance can promote access to health in middle-income countries with limited health resources.

TREATMENT

There have been several overviews of ROP treatment to which the reader is directed for detailed information.[162,163,188,189]

Prophylaxis

Although there is no obvious prophylactic treatment on the horizon there are a number of factors that might either minimize the incidence and severity of ROP or reduce the rate of progression, thus possibly improving outcome. As already discussed these include the standard of neonatal care, oxygen administration, and vitamin E.

Acute phase retinopathy of prematurity

Cryotherapy and xenon arc photocoagulation were first used for acute ROP in the late 1960s[190,191] with argon laser soon entering the picture. However, it was not until 1988 that retinal ablative therapy was proven to have a beneficial effect on severe retinopathy following the publication of the preliminary report of the US-based Multicenter Trial of Cryotherapy for Retinopathy of Prematurity.[133] This study has had such impact that it merits a detailed review here.

The Multicenter Trial of Cryotherapy for Retinopathy of Prematurity set out primarily to determine prospectively whether cryotherapy is effective in the treatment of severe acute ROP, and second to study the natural history of this condition. Study design will not be considered here.[133,152] Infants of less than 1251g birth weight ($n = 9751$) were enrolled at 23 centers in the USA over a 23-month period commencing 1 January 1986. Ophthalmic examinations commenced at 6 weeks postnatally and were continued at fortnightly intervals until vascularization was complete. A total of 291 infants participated in a randomized trial. Eyes of infants that reached threshold stage (defined as 5 continuous or 8 cumulative clock hours of stage 3 in zone 1 or 2 with plus disease) were randomly allocated to either treatment (cryotherapy) or control groups. In infants who reached threshold disease at the same time, one eye was randomized to treatment and the fellow eye to observation (control). Cryotherapy was then performed within 72 hours.

Results showed that cryotherapy produced a significant reduction in the unfavorable structural outcome of threshold ROP of 49.3% at 3 months[133,152] and 45.8% at 12 months,[192] as judged by fundus photographs and clinical examination. The beneficial effect of cryotherapy has persisted with a 43.2% reduction with unfavorable structural outcomes at the 10-year follow-up study examinations.[193]

Visual acuity was added as an important outcome in this trial beginning at the 1-year study examinations. At 1 year, treated infants had significantly better visual acuity (using the acuity card procedure) than controls.[194] At the $5^1/_2$-year study examination, the rates of unfavorable visual acuity outcomes (a Snellen score of 20/200 or worse using the Early Treatment Diabetic Retinopathy chart (Lighthouse, Inc., New York, NY)) were 47.1% in the treated group and 61.7% in controls.[195] Unfavorable structural outcomes had remained stable at 26.9% (treated) and 45.4% (control). In the control group of eyes, 20% achieved a visual acuity of 20/40 or better whereas only 13% of the treated group reached this level ($p = 0.06$). This possible detrimental effect of cryotherapy was not substantiated at the 10-year follow-up examination. With a high rate of follow-up of eligible children (97%; 36 of the original cohort of 291 children had died), 25.2% of treated eyes achieved visual acuity of 20/40 or better, compared to 23.7% of control eyes.[193]

Not all eyes treated behaved identically: zone 2 disease had a significantly better outcome than zone 1 ROP. Indeed zone predicted the beneficial effect of cryotherapy better than any other parameter such as birth weight.[45]

Thus after two decades of small-scale inconclusive clinical studies, the Multicenter Trial of Cryotherapy for Retinopathy of Prematurity study has shown conclusively that cryotherapy for threshold ROP produces a significant benefit for structural status of the eye[196] and for visual function.[193,197] However, retinal ablation in eyes with severe ROP does not necessarily result in normal retinal structure or the development of visual acuity in the normal range. Interestingly, in eyes that have previously had severe ROP the correlation between posterior retinal structure and visual function is good, although not invariably so,[198] whereas in eyes with mild to moderate residua of ROP the prediction of function according to structure is poor, and ophthalmoscopy is no substitute for acuity measurement.[199]

After the Multicenter Trial of Cryotherapy for Retinopathy of Prematurity Study

This important study has dramatically changed clinical practice worldwide and ROP screening is now required. However, cryotherapy performed using the study protocol is no panacea as at 10 years after treatment 45.4% eyes had a visual acuity of 6/60 or worse. This raised the issue of treatment criteria. Threshold as employed in this study was defined as the stage where the risk of blindness if untreated is 50%. Perhaps this threshold is set too high and should be lowered, especially for zone 1 disease[200–202] as was performed in the STOP-ROP Study.[61] This had to be balanced against the possibility that some eyes that would otherwise undergo spontaneous resolution might be treated.

Two recently reported treatment studies have addressed the timing of intervention for sight-threatening ROP. The first involved the use of supplemental oxygen to determine whether the incidence of progression from moderate (pre-threshold) stages to severe (threshold) stages of ROP could be altered.[61] At the diagnosis of pre-threshold disease in one or both eyes, the infants were randomly assigned to receive conventional oxygen treatment with pulse oximetry targets of 89 to 94% saturation or to receive supplemental oxygen treatment with pulse oximetry targets of 96 to 99%. With 649 infants enrolled during the 5-year study, the rate of progression to threshold disease (defined as in the CRYO-ROP study below) was 48% in the eyes of children assigned to *conventional* oxygen treatment, compared to 41% in the eyes of children in the *supplemented* oxygen group (p = NS). Supplemental oxygen treatment also increased the risk of adverse pulmonary events including pneumonia and chronic lung disease.

A second recent study examined the possibility that some eyes with ROP of less than threshold severity might benefit from treatment. The multicenter Early Treatment for Retinopathy of Prematurity Randomized Trial[119] was conducted at 26 clinical sites in the USA. This study used a risk model (RM-ROP2) including patient demographic characteristics, pace of disease, and severity of retinopathy to predict the likelihood of eyes with pre-threshold ROP going on to retinal detachment.[203] Pre-threshold ROP was defined as:

(i) Zone 1, any ROP less than threshold;
(ii) Zone 2, stage 2 with plus disease and stage 3 without plus disease; and
(iii) Stage 3 with plus disease but less than threshold.

In this trial, eyes found to have a risk of 0.15 or greater of progressing to unfavorable structural outcome were randomized to receive peripheral retinal ablation at the diagnosis of "high-risk pre-threshold" or to conventional management. Conventional management consisted of observation with treatment if threshold ROP developed, or simply observation if regression occurred. Among the 828 infants identified as having pre-threshold ROP in one or both eyes, 401 of the 499 with high-risk ROP participated in the randomized trial. The recent report of the structural and visual function outcomes, which showed that early treatment of high-risk pre-threshold eyes significantly reduced unfavorable outcomes.[119] At 9 months, grating acuity was assessed by masked testers using the Teller Acuity Card procedure and showed a reduction in unfavorable visual acuity outcomes from 19.5 to 14.5% (p = 0.01). Structural outcomes also benefited from early treatment with a reduction in unfavorable structural outcomes from 15.6% of conventionally treated eyes to 9.1% for earlier-treated eyes ($p<0.001$).

The ET-ROP investigators also developed a clinical algorithm based on the International Classification of ROP that provides the clinician with useful information concerning whether an eye should be considered for earlier treatment. Two types of pre-threshold disease are defined: type 1, which should be considered for earlier treatment, and type 2, which can be followed conservatively and treated if progression to type 1 or threshold is observed. Details of these two types are given in the next section. Using this ICROP-based algorithm approximately 38% fewer high-risk pre-threshold eye would be treated with no increase in unfavorable outcomes.

Treatment practicalities

The issues to be considered in the rapidly changing field of ROP treatment are dealt with very briefly here. Treatment details can be obtained from articles referenced here.[133,162,163,204,205,212,222]

Rationale and criteria for treatment

The aim of treatment is to remove the stimulus for vessel growth by ablating the peripheral avascular retina. Either cryotherapy or laser can be used, and although both are effective,[205–212] laser is now the modality of choice by the vast majority of ophthalmologists (93% in STOP-ROP Study).[61] Although in most instances treatment is applied to the entire 360° of the retinal circumference partial ablation is sometimes considered for highly localized disease.[213,214]

Indications for treatment

The indications for ROP treatment changed at the end of 2003 with the publication of the results of ET-ROP Study (see Table 51.4). Until that time the sole indication for treatment was threshold ROP, but because the outcome of some eyes treated at that stage has been so poor, treatment is now recommended *also* for certain categories of pre-threshold ROP.

Threshold ROP

If there are at least 5 continuous or 8 cumulative clock hours of stage 3 ROP in zones 1 or 2, in the presence of plus disease, such eyes should be treated.

Pre-threshold–type 1

Pre-threshold type 1 ROP is defined as:
(i) Zone 1, any stage of ROP with plus disease;
(ii) Zone 1, stage 3 with or without plus disease; or
(iii) Zone 2, stage 2 or 3 with plus disease.

These eyes have highly active ROP and should be considered for early treatment.

Pre-threshold–type 2

Pre-threshold type 2 ROP is defined as:
(i) Zone 1, stage 1 or 2 with no plus disease; or
(ii) Zone 2, stage 3 with *no* plus disease.

These eyes may be followed conservatively unless they become pre-threshold type 1 or reach threshold ROP.

It is critical to remember that the window for treatment probably is a maximum of 1 week and treatment should be undertaken as soon as possible–within 2–3 days of threshold identification. Clearly determining the urgency of treatment requires clinical judgment as some eyes with posterior ROP with severe plus disease require very urgent treatment whereas some eyes progress more slowly and the degree of urgency is less. Treatment should ideally be performed in the neonatal intensive care unit where there are full neonatal support facilities.

Table 51.4 Treatment algorithm based on results of ET-ROP Study[a]

			Treatment considerations
Zone 1	Plus disease	Any stage ROP	Consider treatment
	No plus disease	Stage 1 or 2	Observe very closely for progression or presence of plus
		Stage 3	Consider treatment
Zone 2	Plus disease	Stage 1	Observe for progression
		Stage 2 or 3	Consider treatment
	No plus disease	Stage 1	Observe for progression or presence of plus
		Stage 2	Observe for progression or presence of plus
		Stage 3	Observe very closely for progression or presence of plus
Zone 3[b]	Plus disease	Any stage ROP	Observe closely for progression
	No plus disease	Any stage ROP	Observe for progression or presence of plus

[a] The ET-ROP study defined type 1 ROP as ROP of sufficient severity to warrant treatment and type 2 as ROP that should be very closely monitored for progression or development of plus disease. For the purpose of this study, plus disease was defined as sufficient dilation and tortuosity of the posterior poles vessels in two or more quadrants. No recommendations based on the results of the ET-ROP study were made for ROP less severe or ROP in zone 3 and the recommendations in this instance are the authors' own.
[b] ROP in zone 3 cannot by definition reach threshold severity and treatment must be tailored to the individual patient.

Cryotherapy is painful and systemic complications can occur,[215] and laser treatment can be lengthy and take an hour to perform. Both modalities can be performed under either sedation or full anesthesia, but the important components are good analgesia and facilities for artificial ventilation. A neonatologist, or an experienced neonatal anesthetist, will help in this decision. Resuscitation equipment must be available, and an intravenous line must be in place before starting the administration of sedation or resuscitation agents.

Cryotherapy

Cryotherapy is applied transsclerally to the avascular zone anterior to, and avoiding, the acute ROP lesion. Using a retinal probe or one specially designed, the cryotherapy lesions are applied confluently. The endpoint of cryotherapy is the appearance of whitening of the retina due to freezing. It is not usually necessary to open the conjunctiva unless the lesion is so posterior that the posterior section of the avascular zone cannot be reached.

In the absence of active ROP it is not necessary to retreat all skip areas. Ocular complications of cryotherapy include eyelid edema, lacerations and hemorrhage of the conjunctiva, and preretinal and vitreous hemorrhage.

Laser

A resurgence of interest in laser over the past decade has been facilitated by the introduction of portable diode and argon lasers delivered through an indirect ophthalmoscope. Had the clinical trial of treatment for ROP been delayed until after this development, this modality, rather than cryotherapy, may have been employed.[201] Portable indirect laser is now for most the treatment of choice.[202,205–212,216–220] A recent study reported a 10-year follow-up of 25 patients who participated in a randomized trial of laser versus cryotherapy for threshold ROP.[221] These investigators found best-corrected visual acuity of 20/66 in laser-treated eyes compared to 20/182 in cryo-treated eyes. In addition, eyes treated with cryotherapy were more likely to have retinal dragging. No large randomized trial comparing the outcomes after cryotherapy or laser treatment is likely to be undertaken due to the large sample needed for an equivalency study. Laser can be very accurately placed, is simpler to administer in experienced hands, and may be both easier to deliver and more

effective in zone 1 disease. Whether laser lesions should be confluent or one burn-width apart is still debated.[222] There are specific complications of laser. These include corneal, iris, and lens burn and the tunica vasculosa lentis may absorb energy. Cataract formation has been reported.[223] Retinal or vitreous hemorrhage may occur, but is probably not laser-specific. Evidence so far suggests that diode red (810 nm) may be preferable to argon green (514 nm) laser for ROP.[205] The former is more portable and requires less power. It causes less tissue destruction and as energy is less likely to be taken up by other ocular tissues, complications are less frequent (Figs 51.22–24).

Laser can also be applied by a transscleral probe, not dissimilar to the cryoprobe, to the external scleral surface, which induces retinal blanching as with transpupillary laser.[224,225]

Postoperative management

Postoperative eyedrops (steroid and antibiotic) are often instilled for a few days postoperatively. The response to treatment becomes visible by 6–7 days with the subsidence of plus disease, regression of the ROP lesion, and the appearance of ablative pigmented lesions. Should treatment fail to induce regression,

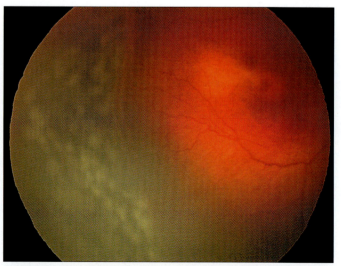

Fig. 51.22 Fresh laser lesions applied anterior to the ROP lesion.

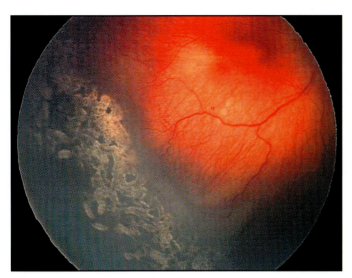

Fig. 51.23 Pigmented laser lesions in the other eye of baby in Figures 51.3 to 51.5. Taken 6 days after treatment and the ill-differentiated lesion is still visible.

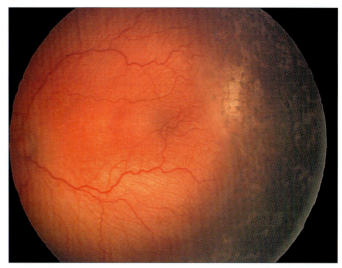

Fig. 51.24 Pigmentary response to laser delivered a few weeks previously.

retreatment should be considered within about 7–14 days. If left much later than this the fibrotic process will have set in and outcome will be compromised. Assessing whether ROP will resolve or require retreatment is one of the most difficult management problems.

Retinal detachment surgery

The management of stage 4 and 5 ROP is controversial. Around 67–70% of stage 4 and 40% stage 5 eyes can be surgically reattached but the visual outcome is unknown.[226] Recently, lens-sparing vitrectomy for partial retinal detachment have been advocated by some investigators,[227] while Hartnett used a variety of surgical procedures including scleral buckle and vitrectomy.[228] For older infants both "open sky"[229] and closed vitrectomy[230–233] approaches have been used with anatomical reattachment being achieved in 40–50% of cases. Infants who developed retinal detachment in the CRYO-ROP study were either managed conservatively (71 eyes) or by vitrectomy (58 eyes).[234] Reattachment was achieved in 28% of the former and none of the latter; only two eyes (both in the vitrectomy group) had any evidence of pattern vision, and that at the lowest measurable spatial frequency. A follow-up report in 1996 provided structural and functional results on the same cohort at age $5\frac{1}{2}$ years.[235] All except one of the 128 eyes in 98 children had vision limited to light perception or no light perception, regardless of whether a vitrectomy had been performed. In contrast, significantly better acuities were reported in a small number of infants following surgery for stage 5 ROP.[236,237] A series of eyes that had initially responded successfully to vitrectomy were reviewed[238]: retinas that were attached after surgery re-detached and the visual results were disappointing, although they concluded that "there is some evidence that vitrectomized eyes function better than non-vitrectomized eyes." With such dismal results surgical management cannot be recommended,[239] and it is critical that during any discussion parents are made aware of the difference between structural and functional success.

The situation for patients with regressed ROP who develop vitreoretinal complications in adult life is rather different as most eyes can be successfully treated.[240–242] With such a variable clinical picture the functional improvement in many cases is quite modest; however, the stability of the eye is improved.

Involving parents

The parents of a very preterm infant have much to cope with and they have a right to know what may befall their baby. Providing sensitive, balanced written information is essential to enable parents to be part of the decision-making process.[243] Information is required at several stages and must be individualized to meet the requirements of the baby. It is certainly important to discuss the possibility of ROP early during the baby's hospital stay even though serious disease may not develop until the child is nearing discharge. This discussion will eliminate the need to discuss surgical intervention at the first contact from the examining ophthalmologist.

Written information and counseling

This should be available at three levels: first, for all babies who are to be screened; second, for the parents of babies with ROP that might become severe; and third for the parents of the baby with end-stage disease. For the first group, a general description of ROP is required, which correctly emphasizes that, although ROP is a frequent occurrence, over 90% acute retinopathy resolves spontaneously without adverse sequelae. Generally, in the UK, the ophthalmologist does not personally counsel the parents of all babies who are screened. Of course he or she should be prepared to speak to any parent requiring more information. For the second group, when ROP is likely to become severe, further written information that emphasizes that treatment is available and may need to be considered should be supplied. At this stage the ophthalmologist should discuss the situation with parents, mindful of the fact that severe ROP occurs just when parents are beginning to relax for the first time since their baby was born. A member of the neonatal unit staff who knows the family should be present during any discussion so that post-interview queries can be dealt with. With severe ROP always keep parents fully and frequently informed.

Unfortunately not all eyes with ROP respond satisfactorily to treatment and blindness still occurs. Ophthalmologists should not lose contact with the family, for most accept that treatment carefully performed sometimes fails, but they cannot accept what is perceived as lack of interest or care.[13] There is still much to do and the ophthalmologist must ensure that the child gains early access to the services for the visually impaired. Registration as blind or partially sighted, if appropriate, is recommended as a positive act to ensure support, because in general terms the child not registered is less likely to receive adequate support. The need for liaison with the social and educational services cannot be overemphasized.

Summary of management for retinopathy of prematurity

In industrialized countries, infants at risk of developing severe ROP, i.e., less than 1501g birth weight and less than 32 weeks GA, should be screened according to recently developed protocols, and treatment for severe disease undertaken urgently using either cryotherapy or laser. The management of infants who develop stage 4 or 5 ROP is controversial, but at present treatment has not been shown to offer a significant functional benefit. All children who have progressed to stage 3 or more require prolonged follow-up as they are at risk of developing refractive errors, visual function deficits, and strabismus. The need for review of children who as infants developed mild retinopathy (stage 2 or less) is less well defined, as their ROP is unlikely to cause clinically significant problems.

OUTCOME

Being born early can affect the developing visual system by a number of mechanisms. These include:

(i) Removal of the fetus from an environment designed to promote development;

(ii) Exposure of immature tissues to an environment not encountered at any other time of life; and

(iii) Complications of preterm birth.

Clinical complications include neurological damage and retinopathy of prematurity, the former being considered elsewhere in this book. Teasing out the relative contributions of these contributing factors, especially differentiating between ROP and neurological problems is frequently not possible. There have been a number of reviews on preterm birth and visual system[176,244,245] and also on the neonatal environment.[246,247]

The visual pathway associations or complications of preterm birth have been reported a number of times;[248–250] however, relatively few include adequate data of the neonatal period.[251–261] To date only a few studies have prospectively studied infants in the neonatal period and compared the later findings with the presence and stage of acute ROP.

Preterm birth per se has a mild effect on visual functions so that median visual acuities and contrast sensitivity are both statistically significantly lower than those of control subjects while still falling within the normal range.[262–264] Most infants with ROP undergo complete resolution without adverse effects, and mild ROP (stages 1 and 2) has no additional adverse effect on visual function. Clearly severe ROP may impact acuity[192,259] and contrast sensitivity;[265] indeed the less than ideal response following cryotherapy generated the Early Treatment study. Color vision does not seem to be affected by preterm birth alone,[264] although the CRYO-ROP study noted an increased prevalence of blue-yellow deficits not related to ROP severity.[266] Visual field area measured at 10 or 11 years in children who had significant acute phase ROP is reduced regardless of whether the eyes underwent cryotherapy.[267,268]

The prevalence of strabismus is increased by preterm birth and by ROP stage (even mild ROP). The incidence of strabismus is raised from around 6% to over 30%,[250,251,254,256,257,259,269–272] and this rises with the severity of ROP.[123,273,274]

The direct consequences of ROP (Figs. 51.22–24) are more frequent in severe and posterior disease, but occasionally occur in mild acute ROP.[123] Retinal detachment can occur at any time of life, including after peripheral retinal ablation for severe ROP, although this is infrequent.[240,275] Large punched-out macular lesions are described as infrequent sequelae of severe ROP. When they develop is not well known but they have been observed during infancy. Originally thought to be the consequence of cryotherapy,[276] they are now known to occur in eyes that have not been treated.[277]

Anterior segment sequelae of severe ROP have been described.[197,278,279] Microcornea/microphthalmos may be the consequence of reduced growth during the acute phase or later shrinkage due to advanced cicatrization. Other changes are largely due to changes in the anterior vitreous causing anterior displacement of the iris-lens diaphragm, causing the frequent shallowing of the anterior chamber[123] and, if severe, the other complications of corneal opacity and cataract (Fig. 51.24).

Children who were born preterm have an increased prevalence of refractive errors, especially myopia.[123,264,273,280–284] Myopia is a consequence of low birth weight even in the absence of any ROP. The term "myopia of prematurity" has been coined to describe this state, in which the myopia is rather low and has the following characteristics: highly curved corneal curvature, shallow anterior chamber, thick lens, and an axial length shorter than expected for the degree of myopia.[262,264,283,285] Myopia is a well-known complication of severe ROP. In contrast to myopia of prematurity, which has its onset in school years, myopia associated with severe ROP has its onset in infancy with progression during the first year after birth but with relative stability thereafter, quite unlike most forms of myopia not associated with ROP.[281,285] There is no significant difference in myopia between eyes with severe ROP that were treated compared to those that were not.[286] Several studies report less myopia in eyes treated by laser than in those treated with cryotherapy.[222,287] This is of interest and merits further study although the possibility that eyes are treated with laser at an earlier stage than cryotherapy must be borne in mind.

REFERENCES

1. Terry TL. Extreme prematurity and fibroblastic overgrowth of persistent vascular sheath behind each crystalline lens I. Preliminary report. Am J Ophthalmol 1942; 25: 203–4.
2. Terry TL. Retrolental Fibroplasia in Premature Infants. Further studies on fibroblastic overgrowth of tunica vasculosa lentis. Arch Ophthalmol 1945; 33: 203–8.
3. Owens WC, Owens EU. Retrolental fibroplasia in premature infants. Trans Am Acad Ophthalmol Otolaryngol 1948; 53: 18–41.
4. Campbell K. Intensive oxygen therapy as a possible cause for retrolental fibroplasia. A clinical approach. Med J Austr 1951; 2: 48–50.
5. Ashton N, Ward B, Serpell G. Role of oxygen in the genesis of retrolental fibroplasia. A preliminary report. Br J Ophthalmol 1953; 37: 513–20.
6. Patz A. Oxygen studies in retrolental fibroplasia IV. Clinical and experimental observations. Am J Ophthalmol 1954; 38: 291–308.
7. Ashton N. Oxygen and retinal blood vessels. Trans Ophthalmol Soc UK 1980; 100: 359–62.
8. Lucey JL, Dangman B. A re-examination of the role of oxygen in retrolental fibroplasia. Pediatrics 1984; 73: 82–96.
9. Ben-Sira I, Nissenkorn I, Kremer I. Retinopathy of prematurity. Surv Ophthalmol 1988; 33: 1–16.
10. Weakley DR, Spencer R. Current concepts in retinopathy of prematurity. Early Hum Dev 1992; 30: 121–38.
11. Wheatley CM, Dickinson JL, Mackey DA, et al. Retinopathy of prematurity: recent advances in our understanding. Arch Dis Child 2002; 86: 696–700.
12. James LS, Lansman JT, editors. History of oxygen and retrolental fibroplasia. Pediatrics 1976; 57: 591–642.
13. Silverman WA. Retrolental Fibroplasia: a Modern Parable. New York: Grune & Stratton; 1980.
14. Flynn JT. Retinopathy of prematurity. Pediatr Clin North Am 1987; 34: 1487–516.
15. Simons BD, Flynn JT. Retinopathy of prematurity and associated factors. Int Ophthalmol Clin 1999; 39: 29–42.
16. Risau W. Mechanisms of angiogenesis. Nature 1997; 386: 671–4.
17. Provis JM. Development of the primate retinal vasculature. Prog Retinal Eye Res 2001; 20: 799–821.
18. Sellheyer K, Spitznas M. Morphology of the developing choroidal vasculature in the human fetus. Graefe's Arch Clin Exp Ophthalmol 1988; 226: 461–7.
19. Ashton N. Retinal angiogenesis in the human embryo. Br Med Bull 1970; 26: 103–6.
20. Keshet E. Preventing pathological regression of blood vessels. J Clin Invest 2003; 112: 27–9.
21. Hellström A, Peruzzi C, Ju M, et al. Low IGF-1 suppresses VEGF-survival signalling in retinal endothelial cells: direct correlation with clinical retinopathy of prematurity. Proc Natl Acad Sci USA 2001; 98: 5804–8.
22. Michaelson IC. The mode of development of the vascular system of the retina, with some observations on its significance for certain retinal diseases. Trans Ophthalmol Soc UK 1948; 68: 137–80.
23. Isenberg SJ. Macular development in the premature infant. Am J Ophthalmol 1986; 101: 74–80.
24. Editorial. Oxygen restriction and retinopathy of prematurity. Lancet 1992; 339: 961–3.
25. Editorial. Retinopathy of prematurity. Lancet 1991; 337: 83–4.
26. Prendiville A, Schulenburg WE. Clinical factors associated with retinopathy of prematurity. Eye 1988; 63: 522–7.
27. Darlow BA, Horwood LJ, Clemett RS. Retinopathy of prematurity: risk factors in a prospective population–based study. Paediatr Perinatal Epidemiol 1992; 6: 62–80.
28. Gallo JE, Jacobson L, Broberger U. Perinatal factors associated with retinopathy of prematurity. Acta Paediatr 1993; 82: 829–34.
29. Phelps DL. Retinopathy of prematurity. In: Isenberg SJ, editor. The Eye in Infancy. 2nd ed. St Louis: Mosby; 1994: 437–47.
30. McColm JR, Fleck BW. Retinopathy of prematurity: causation. Sem Neonatol 2001; 6: 453–60.
31. Kretzer FL, Hittner HM. Retinopathy of prematurity: clinical implications of retinal development. Arch Dis Child 1988; 63: 1151–67.
32. Pierce EA, Foley ED, Smith EH, et al. Regulation of vascular endothelial growth factor by oxygen in a model of retinopathy of prematurity. Arch Ophthalmol 1996; 114: 1219–28.
33. Smith LEH. Pathogenesis of retinopathy of prematurity. Acta Paediatr Suppl 2002; 437: 26–8.
34. Alon T, Hemo I, Itin A, et al. Vascular endothelial growth factor acts as a survival factor for newly formed retinal vessels and has implications for retinopathy of prematurity. Nature Medicine 1995; 1: 1024–8.
35. Shih SC, Ju M, Liu N, et al. Selective stimulation of VEGFR-1 prevents oxygen-induced retinal vascular degeneration in retinopathy of prematurity. J Clin Invest 2003; 112: 50–7.
36. D'Ercole AJ. ROP-forme fruste. J Perinatol 2002; 22: 257–8.
37. Sennlaub F, Chemtob S. VEGFR-1: a safe target for prophylaxis of retinopathy of prematurity. Ped Res 2004; 55: 1–2.
38. Brown DR, Milley JR, Ripepi UJ, et al. Retinopathy of prematurity. Risk factors in a five-year cohort of critically ill premature neonates. Am J Dis Child 1987; 141: 154–60.
39. Kinsey VE, Arnold HJ, Kalina RE, et al. PaO$_2$ levels and retrolental fibroplasia: a report of the co-operative study. Pediatrics 1977; 60: 655–68.
40. Flynn JT. Acute proliferative retrolental fibroplasia: multivariate risk analysis. Trans Am Ophthalmol Soc 1983; 81: 549–81.
41. Keith CG, Kitchen WH. Retinopathy of prematurity in extremely low birthweight infants. Med J Aust 1984; 141: 225–7.
42. Ng YK, Fielder AR, Shaw DE, et al. Epidemiology of retinopathy of prematurity. Lancet 1988; ii: 1235–8.
43. Fielder AR, Levene MI. Screening for retinopathy of prematurity. Arch Dis Child 1992; 67: 860–7.
44. Fielder AR, Shaw DE, Robinson J, et al. Natural history of retinopathy of prematurity: a prospective study. Eye 1992b; 6: 233–42.
45. Schaffer DB, Palmer EA, Plotsky DF, et al. on behalf of the Cryotherapy for Retinopathy of Prematurity Cooperative Group. Prognostic factors in the natural course of retinopathy of prematurity. Ophthalmology 1993; 100: 230–7.
46. Patz A, Hoeck LE, De La Cruz E. Studies on the effect of high oxygen administration in retrolental fibroplasia: a nursery observation. Am J Ophthalmol 1952; 35: 1248–52.
47. Lanman JT, Guy LP, Danus I. Retrolental fibroplasia and oxygen therapy. J Am Med Assoc 1954; 155: 223–6.
48. Kinsey VE, Twomey JT, Hamphill FM. Retrolental fibroplasia. Co-operative study of retrolental fibroplasia and the use of oxygen. Arch Ophthalmol 1956; 56: 481–529.
49. Avery ME, Oppenheimer EH. Recent increase in mortality from hyaline membrane disease. J Pediatr 1960; 57: 553–4.
50. McDonald AD. Cerebral palsy in children of very low birth weight. Arch Dis Child 1963; 38: 579–88.
51. Cross KW. Cost of preventing retrolental fibroplasia? Lancet 1973; ii: 954–6.
52. Flynn JT, Bancalari E, Bawol R, et al. Retinopathy of prematurity. A randomised, prospective trial of transcutaneous oxygen monitoring. Ophthalmology 1987b; 94: 630–8.
53. Flynn JT, Bancalari E, Snyder ES, et al. A cohort study of transcutaneous oxygen monitoring and the incidence and severity of retinopathy of prematurity. N Engl J Med 1992; 326: 1050–4.
54. Saito Y, Omoto T, Cho Y, et al. The progression of retinopathy of prematurity and fluctuation in blood gas tension. Graefe's Arch Clin Exp Ophthalmol 1993; 231: 151–6.
55. Cunningham S, Fleck BW, Elton RA, et al. Transcutaneous oxygen levels in retinopathy of prematurity. Lancet 1995; 346: 1464–5.
56. York JR, Landers S, Kirby RS, et al. Arterial oxygen fluctuation and retinopathy of prematurity in very-low-birth-weight infants. J Perinatology 2004; 24: 82–7.
57. Ng YK, Fielder AR, Levene MI, et al. Are severe retinopathy of prematurity and severe periventricular leucomalacia both ischaemic insults? Br J Ophthalmol 1989; 73: 111–14.
58. Ashton N, Henkind P. Experimental occlusion of retinal arterioles. Br J Ophthalmol 1965; 49: 225–34.
59. Fielder AR. Retinopathy of prematurity: aetiology. Clin Risk 1997; 3: 47–51.
60. Chan-Ling T, Gock B, Stone J. Supplemental oxygen therapy: basis for noninvasive treatment of retinopathy of prematurity. Invest Ophthalmol Vis Sci 1995; 36: 1215–30.

61. STOP-ROP Multicenter Study Group. Supplemental therapeutic oxygen for prethreshold retinopathy of prematurity (STOP-ROP), a randomized, controlled trial. I: primary outcomes. Pediatrics 2000; 105: 295–310.

62. Askie LM, Henderson-Smart DJ, Irwig L, et al. Oxygen-saturation targets and outcomes in extremely preterm infants. N Engl J Med 2003; 349: 959–67.

63. Tin W, Milligan DWA, Pennefather P, et al. Pulse oximetry, severe retinopathy of prematurity, and outcome at one year in babies of less than 28 weeks gestation. Arch Dis Child Fet Neonat Ed 2001; 84: F107–10.

64. Tin W, Wariyar U. Giving small babies oxygen: 50 years of uncertainty. Semin Neonatol 2002; 7: 361–7.

65. Chow LC, Wright KW, Sola A, the CSMC Oxygen Administration Study Group. Can changes in clinical practise decrease the incidence of severe retinopathy of prematurity in very low birth weight infants? Pediatrics 2003;111: 339–45.

66. Holmes JM, Zhang S, Leske DA, et al. Carbon dioxide-induced retinopathy in the neonatal rat. Curr Eye Res 1998; 17: 608–16.

67. Zhang S, Leske DA, Lanier WL, et al. Preretinal neovascularization associated with acetazolamide-induced systemic acidosis in the neonatal rat. Invest Ophthalmol Vis Sci 2001; 42: 1066–71.

68. Mariani G, Cifuentes J, Waldemar A, et al. Randomized trial of permissive hypercapnia in preterm infants. Pediatrics 1999; 104: 1082–8.

69. Gellen B, McIntosh N, McColm JR, et al. Is the partial pressure of carbon dioxide in the blood related to the development of retinopathy of prematurity? Br J Ophthalmol 2001; 85: 1044–5.

70. Higgins RD, Mendelsohn AL, DeFeo MJ, et al. Antenatal dexamethasone and decreased severity of retinopathy of prematurity. Arch Ophthalmol 1998; 116: 236–7.

71. Console V, Gagliardi L, De Giorgi A, et al. Retinopathy of prematurity and antenatal corticosteroids. The Italian ROP Study Group. Acta Biomed Ateneo Parmense. 1997; 68(Suppl 1): 75–9.

72. Cuculich PS, DeLozier KA, Mellen BG, et al. Postnatal dexamethasone treatment and retinopathy of prematurity in very-low-birth-weight neonates. Biol Neonate 2001; 79: 9–14.

73. Palmer EA, Flynn JT, Hardy RJ. The Cryotherapy for Retinopathy of Prematurity Cooperative Group. Incidence and early course of retinopathy of prematurity. Ophthalmology 1991; 98: 1628–40.

74. Saunders RA, Donahue ML, Christmann LM, et al. for the Cryotherapy for Retinopathy of Prematurity Cooperative Group. Racial variation in retinopathy of prematurity. Arch Ophthalmol 1997; 115: 604–8.

75. Tadesse M, Dhanireddy R, Mittal M, et al. Race, candida sepsis, and retinopathy of prematurity. Biol Neonate 2002; 81: 86–90.

76. Shastry BS, Pendergast SD, Hartzer MK, et al. Identification of missense mutations in the Norrie disease gene associated with advanced retinopathy of prematurity. Arch Ophthalmol. 1997; 115: 651–5.

77. Hiraoka M, Berinstein DM, Trese MT, et al. Insertion and deletion mutations in the dinucleotide repeat region of the Norrie disease gene in patients with advanced retinopathy of prematurity. J Hum Genet 2001; 46: 178–81.

78. Haider MZ, Devarajan LV, Al-Essa M, et al. A C597–a polymorphism in the Norrie disease gene is associated with advanced retinopathy of prematurity. J Biomed Sci 2002; 9: 365–70.

79. Dirnberger DR, Yoder BA, Gordon MC. Single versus repeated-course antenatal corticosteroids: outcomes in singleton and multiple-gestation pregnancies. Am J Perinatol 2001; 18: 267–7.

80. Blumenfeld LC, Siatkowski RM, Johnson RA, et al. Retinopathy of prematurity in multiple-gestation pregnancies. Am J Ophthalmol 1998; 125: 197–203.

81. Fellows RR, McGregor ML, Bremer DL, et al. Retinopathy of prematurity in discordant twins. J Pediatr Ophthalmol Strabismus 1995; 32: 86–8.

82. Frilling R, Rosen SD, Monos T, et al. Retinopathy of prematurity in mutiple-gestation, very low birth weight infants. J Pediatr Ophthalmol Strabismus 1997; 34: 96–100.

83. Phelps DL, Rosenbaum A. The role of tocopherol in oxygen-induced retinopathy: kitten model. Pediatrics 1977; 59: 998–1005.

84. Muller DPR. Vitamin E therapy in retinopathy of prematurity. Eye 1992; 6: 221–5.

85. Johnson AT, Kretzer JL, Hittner HM, et al. Development of the subretinal space in the preterm human eye: ultrastructural and immunocytochemical studies. J Comp Neurol 1985a; 232: 497–505.

86. Benaron DA, Bowen FW. Variation of initial serum bilirubin rise in newborn infants with type of illness. Lancet 1991; 338: 78–81.

87. Boynton BR, Boynton CA. Retinopathy of prematurity and bilirubin. N Engl J Med 1989; 321: 193.

88. Heyman E, Ohlsson A, Girschek P. Retinopathy of prematurity and bilirubin. N Engl J Med 1989; 320: 25.

89. Gaton DD, Gold J, Axer-Siegel R, et al. Evaluation of bilirubin as possible protective factor in the prevention of retinopathy of prematurity. Br J Ophthalmol 1991; 75: 532–4.

90. Johnson L, Bowen FW, Abbasi S, et al. Relationship of prolonged pharmacologic serum levels of vitamin E to incidence of sepsis and necrotising enterocolitis in infants with birth weights 1500 g or less. Pediatrics 1985; 75: 619–38.

91. Hittner HM, Godio LB, Rudolph AJ, et al. Retrolental fibroplasia: efficacy of vitamin E in a double-blind clinical study of preterm infants. N Engl J Med 1981; 305: 1365–71.

92. Finer NN, Grant G, Schindler RF, et al. Effect of intramuscular vitamin E on frequency and severity of retrolental fibroplasia: a controlled trial. Lancet 1982; i: 1087–91.

93. Phelps DL, Rosenbaum A, Isenberg SJ, et al. Tocopherol efficacy and safety for preventing retinopathy of prematurity: a randomised controlled double-masked trial. Pediatrics 1987; 79: 489–500.

94. Rosenbaum AL, Phelps DL, Isenberg SI, et al. Retinal haemorrhage in retinopathy of prematurity associated with tocopherol treatment. Ophthalmology 1985; 92: 1012–15.

95. Raju TN, Langenberg P, Bhutani V, et al. Vitamin E prophylaxis to reduce retinopathy of prematurity: A reappraisal of published trials. J Pediatr 1997; 131: 844–50.

96. Aranda JV, Clark TE, Maniello R, et al. Blood transfusions: a possible potentiating risk factor in retrolental fibroplasia. Pediatr Res 1975; 9: 362.

97. Bard H, Cornet A, Orquin J, et al. Retrolental fibroplasia and exchange transfusions. Pediatr Res 1975; 9: 362.

98. Clark C, Gibbs JAH, Maniello R, et al. Blood transfusions: a possible risk factor in retrolental fibroplasia. Acta Paediatr Scand 1981; 70: 535–9.

99. Allegaert K, de Coen K, Devlieger H, on behalf of the EpiBel Study. Threshold retinopathy at threshold of viability: the EpiBal study. Br J Ophthalmol 2004; 88; 239–42.

100. Brooks SE, Marcus DM, Gillis RN, et al. The effect of blood transfusion protocol on retinopathy of prematurity: a prospective, randomized study. Pediatrics 1999; 104: 514–8.

101. Long W, Corbet A, Cotton R, et al. A controlled trial of synthetic surfactant in infants weighing 1250 g or more with respiratory distress syndrome. N Engl J Med 1991; 325: 1696–703.

102. Rankin SJA, Tubman TRJ, Halliday HL, et al. Retinopathy of prematurity in surfactant treated infants. Br J Ophthalmol 1992; 76: 202–4.

103. Repka MX, Hardy RJ, Phelps DL, et al. Surfactant prophylaxis and retinopathy of prematurity. Arch Ophthalmol 1993; 111: 618–20.

104. Holmes JM, Cronin CM, Squires P, et al. Randomised clinical trial of surfactant prophylaxis in retinopathy of prematurity. J Pediatr Ophthalmol Strabismus 1994; 31: 189–91.

105. Axer-Siegel R, Snir M, Ma'ayan A, et al. Retinopathy of prematurity and surfactant treatment. J Pediatr Ophthalmol Strabismus 1996; 33: 171–4.

106. Gilbert CF, Canovas R, Kocksch de Canovas R, et al. Causes of blindness and severe visual impairment in children in Chile. Dev Med Child Neurol 1994; 36: 326–33.

107. Terry TL. Fibroblastic overgrowth of persistent tunica vasculosa lentis in premature infants. II: report of cases–clinical aspects. Arch Ophthalmol 1943; 29: 36–53.

108. Hepner WR, Krause AC, Davis ME. Retrolental fibroplasia and light. Pediatrics 1949; 3: 824–8.

109. Locke JC, Reese AB. Retrolental fibroplasia: the negative role of light, mydriatics and the ophthalmoscopic examination in its etiology. Arch Ophthalmol 1952; 48: 44–7.

110. Glass P, Avery GB, Kolinjavadi N, et al. Effect of bright light in the hospital nursery on the incidence of retinopathy of prematurity. N Engl J Med 1985; 313: 401–4.

111. Hommura S, Usuki Y, Takei K, et al. Ophthalmic care of very low birthweight infants. Report 4: clinical studies of the influence of light on the incidence of ROP. Nippon Gakkai Zasshi 1988; 92: 456–61.

112. Ackerman B, Sherwonit E, Williams J. Reduced incidental light exposure: effect on the development of retinopathy of prematurity in low birth weight infants. Pediatrics 1989; 83: 958–62.

113. Seiberth V, Linderkamp O, Knorz MC, et al. A controlled trial of light and retinopathy of prematurity. Am J Ophthalmol 1994; 118: 492–5.

114. Reynolds JD, Hardy RJ, Kennedy KA, et al. for the Light Reduction in Retinopathy of Prematurity (LIGHT-ROP) Cooperative Group. Lack of efficacy of light reduction in preventing retinopathy of prematurity. N Engl J Med 1998; 338: 1572-6.

115. Committee for the Classification of Retinopathy of Prematurity. The international classification of retinopathy of prematurity. Br J Ophthalmol 1984; 68: 690–7.

116. Committee for the Classification of Retinopathy of Prematurity II. The classification of retinal detachment. Arch Ophthalmol 1987; 105: 106–12.

117. Reese AB, King MJ, Owens WC. A classification of retrolental fibroplasia. Am J Ophthalmol 1953; 36: 1333–5.

118. Wallace DK, Kylstra JA, Chesnutt DA. Prognostic significance of vascular dilation and tortuosity insufficient for plus disease in retinopathy of prematurity. J AAPOS 2000; 4: 224–9.

119. Early Treatment for Retinopathy of Prematurity Cooperative Group. Revised indications for the treatment of retinopathy of prematurity. Arch Ophthalmol 2003; 121: 1684–96.

120. Repka MX, Palmer EA, Tung B, for the Cryotherapy for Retinopathy of Prematurity Cooperative Group. Involution of retinopathy of prematurity. Arch Ophthalmol 2000; 118: 645–9.

121. Flynn JT, O'Grady GE, Herrera J, et al. Retrolental fibroplasia I. Clinical observations. Arch Ophthalmol 1977; 95: 217–23.

122. Clemett R, Darlow B. Results of screening low-birth-weight infants for retinopathy of prematurity. Curr Op Ophthalmol 1999; 10: 155–63.

123. Darlow BA. Incidence of retinopathy of prematurity in New Zealand. Arch Dis Child 1988; 63: 1083–6.

124. Holmström G, el Azazi M, Jacobson L, et al. A population-based, prospective study of the development of ROP in prematurely born children in the Stockholm area of Sweden. Br J Ophthalmol 1993; 77: 417–23.

125. Cryotherapy for Retinopathy of Prematurity Cooperative Group. The natural ocular outcome of premature birth and retinopathy. Status at 1 year. Arch Ophthalmol 1994; 112: 903–12.

126. Bullard SR, Donahue SP, Feman SS, et al. The decreasing incidence and severity of retinopathy of prematurity. J AAPOS 1999; 3: 46–52.

127. Hussain N, Clive J, Bhandari V. Current incidence of retinopathy of prematurity, 1989–1997. Pediatrics 1999; 104: 1–8.

128. Rowlands E, Ionides ACW, Chin S, et al. Reduced incidence of retinopathy of prematurity. Br J Ophthalmol 2001; 85: 933–5.

129. Larsson E, Carle-Petrelius B, Cernerud G, et al. Incidence of ROP in two consecutive Swedish population based studies. Br J Ophthalmol 2002; 86: 1122–6.

130. O'Connor MT, Vohr BR, Tucker R, et al. Is retinopathy of prematurity increasing among infants less than 1250g birth weight? J Perinatol 2003; 23: 673–8.

131. Reynolds JD, Hardy RJ, Palmer EA. Incidence and severity of retinopathy of prematurity. J AAPOS 1999; 3: 321–2.

132. Vyas J, Field D, Draper ES, et al. Severe retinopathy of prematurity and its association with different rates of survival in infants of less than 1251 g birth weight. Arch Dis Child Fetal Neonat Ed 2000; 82: F145–9.

133. Cryotherapy for Retinopathy of Prematurity Cooperative Group. Multicenter trial of cryotherapy for retinopathy of prematurity: preliminary results. Arch Ophthalmol 1988; 106: 471–9.

134. Quinn GE. What do we do about ROP in larger birth weight babies? Editorial Br J Ophthalmol 2002; 86: 1072–3.

135. Gilbert C, Rahi J, Quinn GE. Visual impairment and blindness in children. In: Johnson GJ, Minassian DC, Weale RA, et al., editors. Epidemiology of Eye Disease. 2nd ed. London: Arnold; 2004: 260–86.

136. Patz A. Retrolental fibroplasia (retinopathy of prematurity). Trans Ophthalmol Soc NZ 1980; 32: 49–54.

137. Gibson DL, Sheps SB, Schechter MT, et al. Retinopathy of prematurity: a new epidemic? Pediatrics 1989; 83: 486–92.

138. Gibson DL, Sheps SB, Uh SH, et al. Retinopathy of prematurity-induced blindness: birth weight-specific survival and the new epidemic. Pediatrics 1990a; 86: 405–12.

139. Keith CG, Doyle LW. Retinopathy of prematurity in infants weighing 1000–1499 g at birth. J Paediatr Child Health 1995; 31: 134–6.

140. Rogers M. Vision impairment in Liverpool: prevalence and morbidity. Arch Dis Child 1996; 74: 299–303.

141. Rahi J, Dezateux C. Epidemiology of visual impairment in Britain. Arch Dis Child 1998; 78: 381–6.

142. Termote J, Schalif-Delfos NE, Donders ART, et al. The incidence of visually impaired children with retinopathy of prematurity and their concomitant disabilities. J AAPOS 2003; 7: 131–6.

143. Rahi J, Cable N, on behalf of the British Childhood Visual Impairment Study Group. Severe visual impairment and blindness in children in the UK. Lancet 2003; 362: 1359–65.

144. Gilbert C, Rahi J, Eckstein M, et al. Retinopathy of prematurity in middle-income countries. Lancet 1997; 350: 12–4.

145. Wood NS, Marlow N, Costeloe K, et al. Neurologic and developmental disability after extremely preterm birth. N Engl J Med 2000; 343: 378–84.

146. Fielder AR, Ng YK, Levene MI. Retinopathy of prematurity: age at onset. Arch Dis Child 1986; 61: 774–8.

147. Quinn GE, Johnson L, Abbasi S. Onset of retinopathy of prematurity as related to postnatal and postconceptual age. Br J Ophthalmol 1992b; 76: 284–8.

148. Noonan CP, Clark DI. Trends in the management of stage 3 retinopathy of prematurity. Br J Ophthalmol 1996; 80: 278–81.

149. Kivlin JD, Biglan AW, Gordon RA, et al. for the Cryotherapy for Retinopathy of Prematurity (CRYO-ROP) Cooperative Group. Early retinal vessel development and iris vessel dilatation as factors in retinopathy of prematurity. Arch Ophthalmol 1996; 114: 150–4.

150. Fielder AR, Robinson J, Shaw DE, et al. Light and retinopathy of prematurity: does retinal location offer a clue? Pediatrics 1992a; 89: 648–53.

151. Gallagher K, Moseley MJ, Tandon A, et al. Nasotemporal asymmetry of retinopathy of prematurity. Arch Ophthalmol 2003; 121: 1563–8.

152. Cryotherapy for Retinopathy of Prematurity Cooperative Group. Multicenter trial of cryotherapy for retinopathy of prematurity: 3–month outcome. Arch Ophthalmol 1990a; 108: 195–204.

153. Reynolds JD, Dobson V, Quinn GE, et al. on behalf of the CRYO-ROP and LIGHT-ROP Cooperative Groups. Evidence-based screening for retinopathy of prematurity: natural history data from CRYO-ROP and LIGHT-ROP Studies. Arch Ophthalmol 2002; 120: 1470–6.

154. Subhani M, Combs A, Weber P, et al. Screening for retinopathy of prematurity: the need for revision in extremely low birth weight infants. Pediatrics 2001; 107: 656–59.

155. Wallace DK, Jomier J, Aylward ST, et al. Computer-automated quantification of plus disease in retinopathy of prematurity. J AAPOS 2003; 7: 126–30.

156. Heneghan C, Flynn J, O'Keefe M, et al. Characterization of changes in blood vessel width and tortuosity in retinopathy of prematurity using image analysis. Med Image Anal 2002; 6: 407–9.

157. Swanson CR, Cocker KD, Parker KH, et al. Semi-automated computer analysis of retinal vessels in infants with acute-phase retinopathy of prematurity. Br J Ophthalmol 2003; 87: 1474–7.

158. Quinn GE, Dobson V, Repka MX, et al. for the Cryotherapy for Retinopathy of Prematurity Cooperative Group. Correlation of retinopathy of prematurity in fellow eyes in the cryotherapy for retinopathy of prematurity study. Arch Ophthalmol 1995; 113: 469–73.

159. Javitt J, Cas RD, Chiang Y-P. Cost-effectiveness of screening and cryotherapy for threshold retinopathy of prematurity. Pediatrics 1993; 91: 859–66.

160. Brown GC, Brown MM, Sharma S, et al. Cost-effectiveness of treatment for threshold retinopathy of prematurity. Pediatrics 1999; 104: e47.

161. Fledelius HC, Rosenberg T. Retinopathy of prematurity. Where to set the screening limits? Recommendations based on two Danish surveys. Acta Paediatr Scand 1990; 79: 906–10.

162. Report of a Joint Working Party of the Royal College of Ophthalmologists and British Association of Perinatal Medicine.

Retinopathy of prematurity: guidelines for screening and treatment. Early Hum Devel 1996; 46: 239–58.

163. Fielder AR, Reynolds JD. Retinopathy of prematurity: clinical aspects. Semin Neonatol 2001; 6: 461–75.

164. American Academy of Pediatrics, American Association for Pediatric Ophthalmology and Strabismus, American Academy of Ophthalmology. Screening Examination of Premature Infants for Retinopathy of Prematurity. Pediatrics 2001; 108: 809–11.

165. Fleck BW, Wright E, Dhillon B, et al. An audit of the 1995 Royal College of Ophthalmologists guidelines for screening for retinopathy of prematurity applied retrospectively in one regional neonatal intensive care unit. Eye 1995; 9(Suppl): 31–5.

166. Goble RR, Jones H, Fielder AR. Are we screening too many babies for retinopathy of prematurity? Eye 1997; 11: 509–14.

167. Hutchinson AK, Saunders RA, O'Neil JW, et al. Timing of initial screening examinations for retinopathy of prematurity. Arch Ophthalmol. 1998; 116: 608–12.

168. Wright K, Anderson ME, Walker E, et al. Should fewer premature infants be screened for retinopathy of prematurity in the managed care era? Pediatrics 1998; 102: 31–4.

169. Fledelius HC, Kjer B. Surveillance for retinopathy of prematurity in a Danish country. Epidemiological experience over 20 years. Acta Ophthalmol Scand 2004; 82: 38–41.

170. Trinavat A, Atchaneeyasakul LO, Udompunturak S. Applicability of American and British criteria for screening of the retinopathy of prematurity in Thailand. Jpn J Ophthalmol 2004; 48: 50–3.

171. Lee SK, Normand C, McMillan D, et al. For the Canadian Neonatal Network. Evidence for changing guidelines for routine screening for retinopathy of prematurity. Arch Pediatr Adolesc Med 2001; 155: 387–5.

172. Hutchinson AK, O'Neil JW, Morgan EN, et al. Retinopathy of prematurity in infants with birth weights greater than 1250 grams. J AAPOS 2003; 7: 190–4.

173. Aprahamian AD, Coats DK, Paysse EA, et al. Compliance with outpatient follow-up recommendations for infants at risk for retinopathy of prematurity. J AAPOS 2000; 4: 282–6.

174. Laws DE, Morton C, Weindling M, et al. Systemic effects of screening for retinopathy of prematurity. Br J Ophthalmol 1996; 80: 425–8.

175. Slevin M, Murphy JFA, O'Keefe M. Retinopathy of prematurity screening. Stress related responses, the role of nesting. Br J Ophthalmol 1997; 81: 762–4.

176. Bonthala S, Sparks JW, Musgrove KH, et al. Mydriatics slow gastric emptying in preterm infants. J Pediatr 2000; 137: 327–30.

177. Fielder AR, Moseley MJ, Ng YK. The immature visual system and premature birth. Br Med Bull 1988; 44: 1093–118.

178. Hittner HM, Hirsch NJ, Rudolph AJ. Assessment of gestational age by examination of the anterior vascular capsule of the lens. J Pediatr 1977; 91: 455–8.

179. Kushner BJ, Essner D, Cohen IJ, et al. Retrolental fibroplasia II. Pathologic correlation. Arch Ophthalmol 1977; 95: 29–38.

180. Schwartz SD, Harrison SA, Ferrone PJ, et al. Telemedical evaluation and management of retinopathy of prematurity using a fiberoptic digital fundus camera. Ophthalmology 2000; 107: 25–8.

181. Roth DB, Morales D, Feuer WJ, et al. Screening for retinopathy of prematurity employing the retcam 120: sensitivity and specificity. Arch Ophthalmol 2001; 119: 268–72.

182. Yen KG, Hess D, Burke B, et al. Telephotoscreening to detect retinopathy of prematurity: preliminary study of the optimum time to employ digital fundus camera imaging to detect ROP. J AAPOS 2002; 6: 64–70.

183. Sommer C, Gouillard C, Brugniart, et al. Retinopathy of prematurity screening and follow-up with Retcam 120: expertise of a team of neonatologists concerning 145 patients. Arch Pediatre 2003; 10: 694–9.

184. Ells A, Holmes JM, Astle WF, et al. Telemedicine approach to screening for severe retinopathy of prematurity: a pilot study. Ophthalmology 2003; 110: 2113–7.

185. Haines L, Fielder AR, Scrivener R, et al. Retinopathy of prematurity in the UK I: the organisation of services for screening and treatment. Eye 2002; 16: 33–8.

186. Saunders RA, Hutchinson AK. The future of screening for retinopathy of prematurity. J AAPOS 2002; 6: 61–3.

187. Saunders RA, Donahue ML, Berland JE, et al. Non-ophthalmologist screening for retinopathy of Prematurity. Br J Ophthalmol 2000; 84: 130–4.

188. Flynn JT, Tasman W, editors. Retinopathy of Prematurity. A Clinician's Guide. New York: Springer-Verlag; 1992.

189. Palmer EA. Treatment of ROP by peripheral retinal ablation. In: Isenberg SJ, editor. The Eye in Infancy. Chicago: Year Book Medical Publishers; 1994: 471–7.

190. Palmer EA, Biglan AW, Hardy RJ. Retinal ablative therapy for active retinopathy of prematurity: history, current status and prospects. In: Silverman WA, Flynn JT, editors. Contemporary Issues in Fetal Medicine and Neurology, Vol. 2. Retinopathy of Prematurity. Oxford: Blackwell Scientific; 1985: 207–28.

191. Fielder AR. Cryotherapy of Retinopathy of Prematurity. In: Davidson SI, Jay B, editors. Recent advances in ophthalmology. Edinburgh: Churchill Livingstone; 1992: 129–48. (Vol. 8.)

192. Cryotherapy for Retinopathy of Prematurity Cooperative Group. Multicenter trial of cryotherapy for retinopathy of prematurity: 1–year outcome. Arch Ophthalmol 1990b; 108: 1408–16.

193. Cryotherapy for Retinopathy of Prematurity Cooperative Group. Multicenter trial of cryotherapy for retinopathy of prematurity: ophthalmological outcome at 10 years. Arch Ophthalmol 2001a; 119: 1110–8.

194. Dobson V, Quinn GE, Biglan AW, et al. Acuity card assessment of visual function in the cryotherapy for retinopathy of prematurity trial. Invest Ophthalmol Vis Sci 1990; 31: 1702–8.

195. Cryotherapy for Retinopathy of Prematurity Cooperative Group. Multicenter trial of cryotherapy for retinopathy of prematurity: Snellen visual acuity and structural outcome at $5\frac{1}{2}$ years after randomization. Arch Ophthalmol 1996; 114: 417–24.

196. Summers G, Dale L, Phelps MD, et al. Ocular cosmesis in retinopathy of prematurity. Arch Ophthalmol 1992; 110: 1092–7.

197. Quinn GE, Dobson V, Barr CC, et al. Visual acuity of eyes after vitrectomy for ROP: follow-up at 5–1/2 years. Ophthalmology 1996; 103: 595–600.

198. Gilbert WS, Dobson V, Quinn GE, et al. on behalf of the Cryotherapy for Retinopathy of Prematurity Cooperative Group. The correlation of visual function with posterior retinal structure in severe retinopathy of prematurity. Arch Ophthalmol 1992; 110: 625–31.

199. Reynolds J, Dobson V, Quinn GE, et al. for the Cryotherapy for Retinopathy of Prematurity Cooperative Group. Prediction of visual function in eyes with mild to moderate posterior pole residua of retinopathy of prematurity. Arch Ophthalmol 1993; 111: 1050–6.

200. Fleming TN, Runge PE, Charles ST. Diode laser photocoagulation for prethreshold, posterior retinopathy of prematurity. Am J Ophthalmol 1992; 114: 589–92.

201. Tasman W. Threshold retinopathy of prematurity revisited. Arch Ophthalmol 1992; 110: 623–4.

202. Laser ROP Study Group. Laser therapy for retinopathy of prematurity. Arch Ophthalmol 1994; 112: 154–6.

203. Hardy RJ, Palmer EA, Dobson V, et al. for the Cryotherapy for Retinopathy of Prematurity Cooperative Group. Risk analysis of prethreshold retinopathy of prematurity. Arch Ophthalmol 2003; 121: 1697–701.

204. Schulenberg WE, Acheson JF. Cryosurgery for acute retinopathy of prematurity: factors associated with treatment success and failure. Eye 1992; 6: 215–20.

205. McNamara JA. Laser treatment for retinopathy of prematurity. Curr Opin Ophthalmol 1993; 4: 76–80.

206. Ling CS, Fleck BW, Wright E, et al. Diode laser treatment for retinopathy of prematurity: structural and functional outcome. Br J Ophthalmol 1995; 79: 637–41.

207. White JE, Repka MX. Randomized comparison of diode laser photocoagulation versus cryotherapy for threshold retinopathy of prematurity: 3-year outcome. J Pediatr Ophthalmol Strabismus 1997; 34: 83–7.

208. McGregor ML, Wherley AJ, Fellow RR, et al. A comparison of cryotherapy versus diode laser retinopexy in 100 consecutive infants treated for threshold retinopathy of prematurity. J AAPOS 1998; 2: 360–64.

209. Connolly BP, McNamara JA, Sharma S, et al. A comparison of laser photocoagulation with transscleral cryotherapy in the treatment of threshold retinopathy of prematurity. Ophthalmology 1998; 105: 1628–31.

210. Paysse EA, Lindsey JL, Coats DK, et al. Therapeutic outcomes of cryotherapy versus transpupillary diode laser photocoagulation for threshold retinopathy of prematurity. J AAPOS 1999; 3: 234–40.

211. Brooks SE, Johnson M, Wallace DK, et al. Treatment outcome in fellow eye after laser photocoagulation for retinopathy of prematurity. Am J Ophthalmol 1999; 127: 58–61.

212. Shalev B, Farr AK, Repka MX. Randomized comparison of diode laser photocoagulation versus cryotherapy for threshold retinopathy of prematurity: seven-year outcome. Am J Ophthalmol 2001; 132: 76–80.

213. Nissenkorn I, Axer-Siegel R, Kremer I, et al. Effect of partial cryoablation on retinopathy of prematurity. Br J Ophthalmol 1991; 75: 160–2.

214. Spencer R, Hutton W, Snyder W, et al. Limiting applications of cryotherapy for severe retinopathy of prematurity. Ophthalmic Surg 1992; 23: 766–9.

215. Brown GC, Tasman WS, Naidoff M, et al. Systemic complications associated with retinal cryoablation for retinopathy of prematurity. Ophthalmology 1989; 97: 855–8.

216. Landers MB, Toth CA, Semple C, et al. Treatment of retinopathy of prematurity with argon laser photocoagulation. Arch Ophthalmol 1992; 110: 44–7.

217. Capone A, Diaz-Rohena R, Sternberg P, et al. Diode-laser photocoagulation for zone 1 threshold retinopathy of prematurity. Am J Ophthalmol 1993; 116: 444–50.

218. Goggin M, O'Keefe M. Diode laser for retinopathy of prematurity–early outcome. Br J Ophthalmol 1993; 77: 559–62.

219. Hunter DG, Repka MX. Diode laser photocoagulation for threshold retinopathy of prematurity. A randomized study. Ophthalmology 1993; 100: 238–44.

220. Clark DI, Hero M. Indirect diode laser treatment for stage 3 retinopathy of prematurity. Eye 1994; 8: 423–6.

221. Ng EYJ, Connolly BP, McNamara JA, et al. A comparison of laser photocoagulation with cryotherapy for threshold retinopathy of prematurity at 10 years: Part 1. Visual function and structural outcome. Ophthalmology 2002; 109: 928–34.

222. Banach MJ, Ferrone PJ, Trese MT. A comparison of dense versus less dense diode laser photocoagulation patterns for threshold retinopathy of prematurity. Ophthalmology 2000; 107: 324–8.

223. Christiansen SP, Bradford JD. Cataract in infants treated with argon laser photocoagulation for threshold retinopathy of prematurity. Am J Ophthalmol 1995; 119: 175–80.

224. Seiberth V, Linderkamp O, Vardarli I. Transscleral vs transpupillary diode laser photocoagulation for the treatment of threshold retinopathy of prematurity. Arch Ophthalmol 1997; 115: 1270–5.

225. Davis AR, Jackson H, Trew D, et al. Transscleral diode laser in the treatment of retinopathy of prematurity. Eye 1999; 13: 571–6.

226. Trese M. Treatment of ROP by retinovitreous surgery. In: Isenberg SJ, editor. The Eye in Infancy. Chicago: Year Book Medical Publishers; 1994: 478–82.

227. Capone, A Jr, Trese MT. Lens-sparing vitreous surgery for tractional stage 4A retinopathy of prematurity retinal detachments. Ophthalmology 2001; 108: 2068–70.

228. Hartnett ME. Features associated with surgical outcome in patients with stages 4 and 5 retinopathy of prematurity. Retina 2003; 23: 322–9.

229. Tasman W, Borrone RN, Bolling J. Open sky vitrectomy for total retinal detachment in retinopathy of prematurity. Ophthalmology 1987; 94: 449–52.

230. Machemer R. Closed vitrectomy for severe retrolental fibroplasia in infants. Ophthalmology 1983; 90: 436–41.

231. Chong LP, Machemer R, de Juan E. Vitrectomy for advanced stages of retinopathy of prematurity. Am J Ophthalmol 1986; 102: 710–16.

232. Trese M. Visual results and prognostic factors for vision following surgery for stage V retinopathy of prematurity. Ophthalmology 1986; 93: 574–9.

233. Machemer R, de Juan E. Retinopathy of prematurity: approaches to surgical therapy. Aust NZ J Ophthalmol 1990; 18: 47–56.

234. Quinn GE, Dobson V, Barr CC, et al. Visual acuity in infants after vitrectomy for severe retinopathy of prematurity. Ophthalmology 1991; 98: 5–13.

235. Quinn GE, Dobson V, Hardy RJ, et al, for the CRYO-ROP Cooperative Group. Visual fields measured with double-arc perimetry in eyes with threshold retinopathy of prematurity (ROP) from the CRYO-ROP trial. Ophthalmol 1996; 103: 1432–7.

236. Katsumi O, Mehta MC, Matsui Y, et al. Development of vision in retinopathy of prematurity. Arch Ophthalmol 1991; 109: 1394–8.

237. Hirose T, Katsumi O, Mehta MC, et al. Vision in stage 5 retinopathy of prematurity after retinal reattachment by open-sky vitrectomy. Arch Ophthalmol 1993; 111: 345–9.

238. Seaber JH, Machemer R, Eliott D, et al. Long-term visual results of children after initially successful vitrectomy for stage V retinopathy of prematurity. Ophthalmology 1995; 102: 199–204.

239. Knight-Nanan DM, Algawi K, Bowell R, et al. Advanced cicatricial retinopathy of prematurity–outcome and complications. Br J Ophthalmol 1996; 80: 343–5.

240. Kaiser RS, Trese MT, Williams GA, et al. Adult retinopathy of prematurity: outcomes of rhegmatogenous retinal detachments and retinal tears. Ophthalmology 2001; 108: 1647–53.

241. Terasaki H, Hirose T. Late-onset retinal detachment associated with regressed retinopathy of prematurity. Jpn J Ophthalmol 2003; 47: 492–7.

242. Tufail A, Singh AJ, Haynes RJ, et al. Late onset vitreoretinal complications of regressed retinopathy of prematurity. Br J Ophthalmol 2004; 88: 243–6.

243. Harrison H. The principles for family-centered neonatal care. Pediatrics 1993; 92: 643–50.

244. Fielder AR, Foreman N, Moseley MJ, et al. Prematurity and visual development. In: Simons K, editor. Early Visual Development, Normal and Abnormal. New York: Oxford University Press; 1993: 485–504.

245. Birch EE, O'Connor AR. Preterm birth and visual development. Sem Neonatol 2001; 6: 467–97.

246. Robinson J, Fielder AR. Light and the neonatal eye. Behav Brain Res 1992; 49: 51–5.

247. Fielder AR, Moseley MJ. Environmental light and the preterm infant. Sem Perinatol 2000; 24: 291–8.

248. Fledelius HC. Prematurity and the eye. Ophthalmic follow-up of children of low and normal birthweight. Acta Ophthalmol 1976; 128(Suppl.): 1–245.

249. Hungerford J, Stewart A, Hope P. Ocular sequelae of preterm birth and their relation to ultrasound evidence of cerebral damage. Br J Ophthalmol 1986; 70: 463–8.

250. Burgess P, Johnson A. Ocular defects in infants of extremely low birth weight and low gestational age. Br J Ophthalmol 1991; 75: 84–7.

251. Keith CG, Kitchen WH. Ocular morbidity in infants of very low birth weight. Br J Ophthalmol 1983; 67: 302–5.

252. Nissenkorn I, Yassur Y, Mashkowski I, et al. Myopia in premature babies with and without retinopathy of prematurity. Br J Ophthalmol 1983; 67: 170–3.

253. Schaffer DB, Quinn GF, Johnson L. Sequelae of arrested mild retinopathy of prematurity. Arch Ophthalmol 1984; 102: 373–6.

254. Snir M, Nissenkorn I, Sherf I, et al. Visual acuity, strabismus, and amblyopia in premature babies with and without retinopathy of prematurity. Ann Ophthalmol 1988; 20: 256–8.

255. Gibson NA, Fielder AR, Trounce JQ, et al. Ophthalmic findings in infants of very low birthweight. Dev Med Child Neurol 1990; 32: 7–13.

256. Page JM, Schneeweiss S, Whyte HEA, et al. Ocular sequelae in premature infants. Pediatrics 1993; 92: 787–90.

257. Robinson R, O'Keefe M. Follow-up study on premature infants with and without retinopathy of prematurity. Br J Ophthalmol 1993;77: 91–4.

258. Holmström G, el Azazi M, Kugelberg U. Ophthalmological long term follow-up of preterm infants: a population based, prospective study of the refraction and its development. Br J Ophthalmol 1998; 82: 1265–71.

259. Holmström G, el Azazi M, Kugelberg U. Ophthalmological follow-up of preterm infants: a population based, prospective study of visual acuity and strabismus. Br J Ophthalmol 1999; 83: 143–50.

260. Dowdeswell HJ, Slater AM, Broomhall J, et al. Visual deficits in children born at less than 32 weeks' gestation with and without ocular pathology and cerebral damage. Br J Ophthalmol 1995; 79: 447–52.

261. Powls A, Botting N, Cooke RWI, et al. Visual impairment in very low birthweight children. Arch Dis Child Fetal Neonatal Ed 1997; 76: F82–7.

262. Fledelius HC. Ophthalmic changes from 10 to 18 years. A longitudinal study of sequels to low birthweight II. Visual acuity. Acta Ophthalmol 1981; 59: 64–70.

263. Sebris SL, Dobson V, Hartmann EE. Assessment and prediction of visual acuity in 3-4-year old children born prior to term. Hum Neurobiol 1984; 3: 87–92.

264. O'Connor AR, Stephenson T, Johnson A, et al. Long term ophthalmic outcome of low birth weight children with and without retinopathy of prematurity. Pediatrics 2002; 109: 12–8.

265. Cryotherapy for Retinopathy of Prematurity Cooperative Group. Contrast sensitivity at age 10 years in children who had threshold retinopathy of prematurity. Arch Ophthalmol 2001; 119: 1129–33.

266. Dobson V, Quinn GE, Abramov I, et al. Color vision measured with pseudoisochromatic plates at five-and-a-half years in eyes of children from the CRYO-ROP study. Invest Ophthalmol Vis Sci 1996; 37: 2467–74.

267. Cryotherapy for Retinopathy of Prematurity Cooperative Group. Effect of retinal ablative therapy for threshold retinopathy of prematurity. Results of Goldmann perimetry at the age of 10 years. Arch Ophthalmol 2001; 119: 1120–5.

268. Larsson E, Martin L, Holmström G. Peripheral and central visual fields in 11-year old children who had been born prematurely and at term. J Pediatr Ophthalmol Strabismus 2004; 41: 39–45.

269. McCormick AQ, Tredger EM, Dunn HG, et al. Ophthalmic disorders. In: Dunn HG, editor. Sequelae of Low Birthweight, the Vancouver Study, Clinics in Developmental Medicine No. 95/96. Oxford: MacKeith Press/Blackwell Scientific; 1986: 127–46.

270. Gallo JE, Lennerstrand G. A population-based study of ocular abnormalities in premature children aged 5 to 10 years. Am J Ophthalmol 1991; 111: 539–47.

271. McGinnity FG, Bryars JH. Controlled study of ocular morbidity in schoolchildren born preterm. Br J Ophthalmol 1992; 76: 520–4.

272. O'Connor AR, Stephenson TJ, Johnson A, et al. Strabismus in children of birth weight less than 1701g. Arch Ophthalmol 2002; 120: 767–71.

273. Laws D, Shaw DE, Robinson J, et al. Retinopathy of prematurity: a prospective study. Review at 6 months. Eye 1992; 6: 477–83.

274. Bremer DL, Palmer EA, Fellows RR, et al. for the Cryotherapy for Retinopathy of Prematurity Cooperative Group. Strabismus in premature infants in the first year of life. Arch Ophthalmol 1998; 116: 329–33.

275. Greven CM, Tasman W. Rhegmatogenous retinal detachment following cryotherapy in retinopathy of prematurity. Arch Ophthalmol 1989; 107: 1017–18.

276. Hindle NW. Cryotherapy for retinopathy of prematurity to prevent retrolental fibroplasia. Can J Ophthalmol 1982; 17: 207–12.

277. Williams JG, Trese MT. A macular lesion simulating an aberrant cryotherapy lesion in retinopathy of prematurity. Arch Ophthalmol 2000; 118: 438–9.

278. Hittner HM, Rhodes LM, McPherson AR. Anterior segment abnormalities in cicatricial retinopathy of prematurity. Ophthalmology 1979; 86: 803–16.

279. Kelly SP, Fielder AR. Microcornea associated with retinopathy of prematurity. Br J Ophthalmol 1987; 71: 201–3.

280. Gordon RA, Donzis PB. Myopia associated with retinopathy of prematurity. Ophthalmology 1986; 93: 1593–8.

281. Quinn GE, Dobson V, Repka MX, et al. on behalf of the Cryotherapy for Retinopathy of Prematurity Cooperative Group. Development of myopia in infants with birth weights less than 1251 g. Ophthalmology 1992; 99: 329–40.

282. Fledelius HC. Pre-term delivery and subsequent ocular development. 4 Oculometric–and other metric considerations. Acta Ophthalmol Scand 1996; 74: 301–5.

283. Fledelius HC. Pre-term delivery and subsequent ocular development. 3 Refraction. Myopia of prematurity. Acta Ophthalmol Scand 1996; 74: 297–300.

284. Larsson EK, Rydberg AC, Holmström GE. A population-based study of the refractive outcome in 10-year old preterm and full-term children. Arch Ophthalmol 2003; 121: 1430–6.

285. Quinn GE, Dobson V, Kivlin J, et al. Prevalence of myopia between three months and 5–1/2 years in preterm infants with and without retinopathy of prematurity. Ophthalmology 1998; 105: 1292–300.

286. Quinn GE, Dobson V, Siatkowski M, et al. for the Cryotherapy for Retinopathy of Prematurity Cooperative Group. Does cryotherapy affect refractive error? Results from treated versus control eyes in the cryotherapy for retinopathy of prematurity trial. Ophthalmology 2001; 108: 343–7.

287. Algawi K, Goggin M, O'Keefe M. Refractive outcome following diode laser versus cryotherapy with retinopathy of prematurity. Br J Ophthalmol 1994; 78: 612–14.

CHAPTER
52 Inherited Retinal Dystrophies

Michel Michaelides, Graham E Holder and Anthony T Moore

INTRODUCTION

The inherited retinal dystrophies are a clinically and genetically heterogeneous group of disorders of which many become symptomatic in childhood. Most occur as an isolated abnormality in an otherwise normal child but some dystrophies are associated with other systemic abnormalities (these are discussed in Chapter 53). Most dystrophies are progressive but others, notably stationary night-blindness, fundus albipunctatus, Oguchi disease and some cone dysfunction syndromes, are usually stationary.

Classification of childhood retinal dystrophies is problematic because of heterogeneity even amongst dystrophies sharing a common mode of inheritance; meaningful classification must await identification of the causative genetic mutations. However, these disorders can be usefully divided according to whether they (i) are stationary or progressive; and (ii) exhibit predominantly rod involvement or predominantly cone or central receptor disease. The dystrophies presenting at birth or in the first few months of life are considered separately, as they pose particular diagnostic problems.

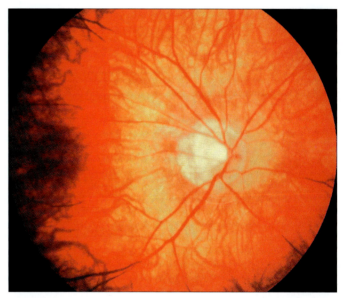

Fig. 52.1 X-linked congenital stationary night-blindness: tilted optic disc with myopic fundus.

STATIONARY RETINAL DYSTROPHIES

Stationary night-blindness

Congenital stationary night-blindness (CSNB)
Clinical findings
CSNB is characterized by night-blindness, variable visual loss and a normal fundus examination. It may be inherited as an autosomal dominant (AD), autosomal recessive (AR) or X-linked (XL) disorder.

The visual acuity is usually normal in the AD form[1] whereas mild central visual loss is common in the other two genetic subtypes. Other features that may be seen in XL and AR CSNB include moderate to high myopia, nystagmus, strabismus and paradoxical pupil responses.[2] Fundus examination is usually normal but some patients have pale or tilted optic discs (Fig. 52.1). Patients with AD CSNB usually present with symptomatic night-blindness, but in XL and AR CSNB, patients usually present in infancy with nystagmus, strabismus and reduced vision. Some affected individuals are not diagnosed until adulthood. The diagnosis is easily missed unless electroretinography (ERG) is performed.[2,3] XL CSNB is further subdivided into the *complete* and *incomplete* forms. This differentiation was originally made using electrophysiological criteria but has subsequently been shown to reflect genetically distinct disorders.[4-6]

Electrophysiology and psychophysics
Most patients show a monophasic dark adaptation curve although in some (predominantly those with AD CSNB and the incomplete form of XL CSNB) there is a recognizable rod component with a markedly elevated threshold.[7] Cone adaptation is also abnormal, as are other measures of cone function such as flicker fusion and photopic ERG.[8]

International recommendations for ERG are published by the International Society for Clinical Electrophysiology of Vision (ISCEV). Four main responses are defined; a rod-specific ERG and a maximal response performed under scotopic conditions, and two measures of cone function, a 30 Hz flicker ERG and a single flash photopic ERG. Both complete and incomplete CSNB show a negative or Schubert–Bornschein type of ERG such that the photoreceptor-derived a-wave in the maximal response is normal, but there is selective reduction in the inner nuclear derived b-wave, such that it is smaller than the a-wave. In complete CSNB there is no detectable rod-specific ERG and a profoundly negative maximal response. Cone ERGs show subtle abnormalities now known to reflect ON-pathway dysfunction (Fig. 52.2). There is a detectable rod-specific ERG in incomplete CSNB, and a profoundly negative maximal response. Cone ERGs are much more abnormal than in complete CSNB, reflecting involvement of both ON and OFF-pathways (Fig. 52.2).

In AR CSNB there is also usually ERG evidence of inner retinal dysfunction, and this may also occur in AD CSNB but in association with normal ISCEV cone ERGs. In other cases of AD CSNB, ERG rod responses are attenuated with normal cone responses, but the standard bright flash response does not have a negative waveform.

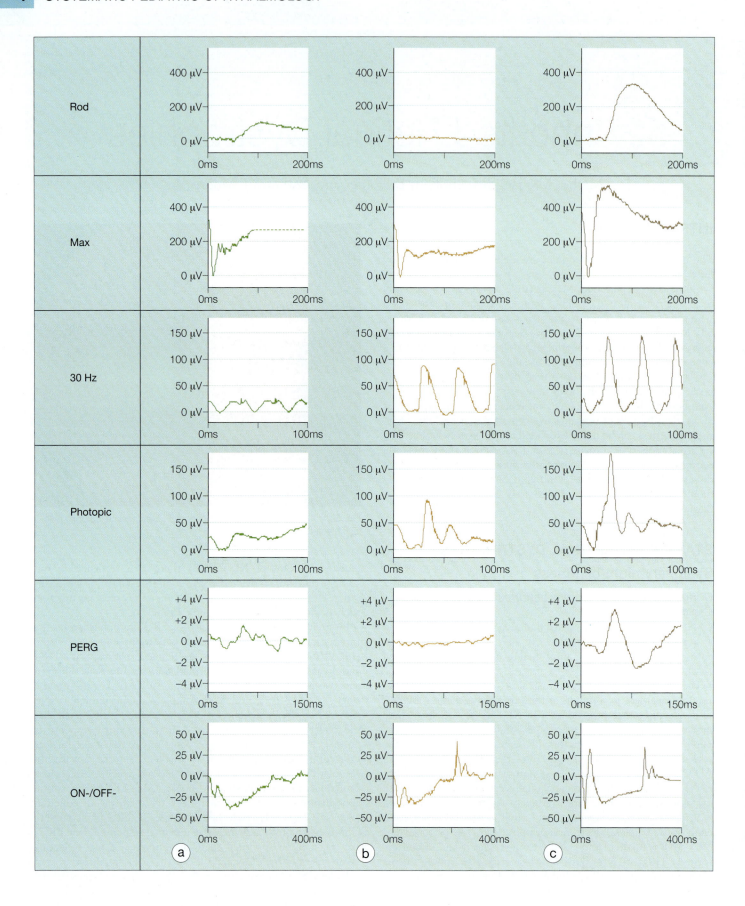

Molecular genetics and pathogenesis

Autosomal dominant CSNB

Mutations in the genes encoding three components of the rod phototransduction cascade have all been reported in association with the dominant form of stationary night-blindness; namely rhodopsin,[9,10] the α-subunit of rod transducin[11] and the rod cyclic guanosine monophosphate (cGMP) phosphodiesterase β-subunit (PDEβ).[12,13]

X-linked CSNB

The XL form of CSNB has been mapped to the short arm of the X chromosome to the region Xp11.4–11.23.[14] Two causative genes (*CACNA1F* and *NYX*) for XL CSNB have now been identified through positional cloning strategies. Incomplete CSNB is associated with mutation in *CACNA1F*, which encodes the retina-specific α_{1F}-subunit of the voltage-gated L-type calcium channel.[15–17] The expression of *CACNA1F* appears limited to the outer nuclear layer, inner nuclear layer, and ganglion cell layer. Most of the mutations are inactivating truncation sequence variants.[17,18] The loss of functional channels impairs the calcium flux into rod and cone photoreceptors required to sustain tonic neurotransmitter release from presynaptic terminals. This may result in inability to maintain the normal transmembrane potential of bipolar cells: the retina remains in a partially light-stimulated state, unable to respond to changes in light-levels.

Complete CSNB is associated with mutation in *NYX*, the gene encoding the leucine-rich proteoglycan nyctalopin.[17,19,20] Leucine-rich repeats may be important for protein interactions and most of the mutations occur within these repeats.[19] Nyctalopin is expressed in photoreceptor inner segments, outer and inner nuclear layers, and ganglion cells. Nyctalopin may guide and promote the formation and function of the ON-pathway within the retina.[19]

Several genotype-phenotype studies have been performed in individuals with either *CACNA1F* or *NYX* mutations. In a study of 66 male patients from 15 families, all with a common mutation in *CACNA1F* (L1056insC), there was considerable variability in the clinical expression of the incomplete CSNB phenotype.[21] At least one of the major features of CSNB (night-blindness, myopia and nystagmus) was absent in 72% of the patients. All the examined features varied widely, both between and within families, including refractive error which ranged from –18.25 spherical equivalent to +5.00, suggesting the presence of other genetic or environmental factors modifying the phenotype. Although most patients with XL CSNB have non-progressive disease, two brothers with a mutation in exon 4 of *CACNA1F* showed progressive decline in visual function and eventually had a nonrecordable rod and cone ERG.[22] Patients with complete CSNB (*NYX* mutations), are invariably myopic and have more pronounced night-blindness. Eighteen male patients with eight different *NYX* mutations have been assessed.[23] Patients with mutations changing structurally conserved residues tended to have a lower degree of myopia than patients with mutations of nonconserved residues; whilst visual acuity and 30 Hz flicker ERG recordings were similar in the two groups. The b:a amplitude ratio in the maximal response varied according to the identified mutation, with good agreement between different patients with the same genotype. Refractive error and the b:a amplitude ratio were highly concordant between the two eyes of an individual, suggesting that other genetic or environmental factors play a role in determining the phenotypic diversity seen in complete CSNB.

A third locus for XL CSNB has been mapped to Xp21,[24] to a region which also harbours the locus for a form of X-linked retinitis pigmentosa (RP3). Mutations in *CACNA1F* and *NYX* are likely to account for the majority of families with XL CSNB.[17]

Åland Island eye disease

Åland Island eye disease (AIED), an X-linked recessive disorder with similarities to incomplete CSNB, is characterized by reduced visual acuity, nystagmus, mild red-green dyschromatopsia and myopia.[25] Affected males may also show iris translucency, foveal hypoplasia and decreased fundus pigmentation. Nyctalopia is common. The clinical appearance may resemble X-linked ocular albinism (XLOA) but in XLOA color vision is usually normal and patients with AIED do not show the typical optic nerve fibre misrouting seen in albinism.[26]

The symptoms of night-blindness and the psychophysical and ERG changes seen in AIED are similar to those seen in the incomplete form of XL CSNB.[27] Both disorders map to the same region of Xp and it is likely that they are allelic.[28,29] However mutations in the *CACNA1F* gene have not yet been identified in AIED.[30]

Other related phenotypes

Patients with a contiguous gene syndrome, (glycerol kinase deficiency, congenital adrenal hypoplasia, Duchenne muscular dystrophy (DMD), and ocular abnormalities known as Oregon eye disease), associated with a deletion of Xp21, have some ocular features in common with affected males with Åland Island eye disease and have similar predominantly inner retinal ERG abnormalities. Furthermore, in DMD some affected males whose mutations are confined to the dystrophin gene at Xp21 have ERG abnormalities similar to those seen in CSNB. All of these multisystem disorders have a nonprogressive form of retinal dystrophy which predominantly affects the rod system.

Oguchi disease

Clinical findings

Oguchi disease is a rare form of stationary night-blindness in which there is a peculiar greyish or green-yellow discoloration of

Fig. 52.2 (*Facing page*) Congenital stationary night-blindness. Column (a) shows data from a patient with "incomplete" CSNB (iCSNB); the center column traces (b) are from a patient with "complete" CSNB (cCSNB); the traces in column (c) are from a representative normal subject. In iCSNB the rod ERG is mildly subnormal. The maximal response is electronegative, with a normal a-wave confirming normal photoreceptor function, but a profoundly reduced b-wave. The 30 Hz flicker ERG is markedly subnormal and clearly shows the delayed double peak usually found in iCSNB. The photopic single flash ERG shows marked reduction in the b:a ratio with simplification of the waveform and loss of the photopic oscillatory potentials, shown on ON/OFF-response recording (200 ms orange stimulus on a green background) to reflect involvement of both ON (depolarizing) and OFF (hyperpolarizing) cone bipolar cell pathways. The PERG is mildly subnormal in keeping with mild macular dysfunction. In cCSNB there is no detectable rod specific ERG and the profoundly electronegative maximal ERG confirms the site of the dysfunction to be post-phototransduction. The single flash photopic response shows a distinctive broadened a-wave and a sharply rising b-wave with a reduced b:a ratio and lack of photopic oscillatory potentials. This appearance indicates marked dysfunction of cone ON-bipolar cell pathways but preservation of the OFF-pathways. The profoundly negative ON-response, with preservation of the ON-a-wave and loss of the ON-b-wave, accompanied by a normal OFF-response supports this proposal. The somewhat broadened trough of the 30 Hz flicker ERG with a sharply rising peak is a manifestation of the same phenomenon. The PERG is almost undetectable. Overall, the findings in cCSNB are those of loss of ON-pathway function in both rod and cone systems.

the fundus, which reverts to normal on prolonged dark adaptation (Mizuo phenomenon). Although most cases have been reported from Japan it may occur in other races including Europeans[4] and African-Americans.[31] Oguchi disease is inherited as an autosomal recessive trait.

Most patients present with poor night vision. Visual acuity is usually normal or only mildly reduced and photopic visual fields and color vision are normal. The retina has a refractile grey-white appearance in the light-adapted state which reverts to normal after prolonged dark adaptation. Exposure to light then leads to the gradual reappearance of the abnormal discoloration in the majority of patients, which may take 10–20 minutes to reach its full effect. The abnormal appearance may be confined to the posterior pole or extend beyond the arcades.

Electrophysiology and psychophysics
Patients with Oguchi disease fall into two types according to the type of abnormality seen on dark adaptation:[7]

■ In **type 1** rod adaptation is markedly slowed; full recovery of sensitivity takes several hours and the absolute threshold is normal or only minimally elevated.

■ In **type 2** there is no recognizable rod adaptation; the abnormal retinal appearance is less marked and the Mizuo phenomenon may be absent.

Most patients with Oguchi disease have a "negative" maximal ERG, confirming the site of dysfunction to be post-phototransduction, as in XL CSNB. In contrast to fundus albipunctatus, the ERG remains abnormal even after prolonged dark adaptation.[6]

Molecular genetics and pathogenesis
A homozygous one base-pair deletion of nucleotide 1147 of the arrestin gene, has been reported in patients with Oguchi disease.[32,33] The mutation results in a truncated protein. Reduced activity of arrestin would be predicted to result in prolonged activation of transducin and rod phosphodiesterase on light exposure. Cyclic GMP levels would thereby be maintained at a low level in response to even dim light exposure and the outer segment cation channels would remain closed resulting in prolonged hyperpolarization of the rod. The rods would behave as if they were light adapted and would be unresponsive to light at low levels of illumination, explaining the psychophysical abnormalities seen in Oguchi disease.[32]

Null mutations in a second component of the rod phototransduction pathway, rhodopsin kinase (RK), have also been identified in Oguchi disease.[34] The key function, of both RK and arrestin, in the normal deactivation and recovery of the photoreceptor after exposure to light, is entirely consistent with the delayed recovery seen in Oguchi disease. The consequences of these reported RK mutations have been assessed by expression studies in COS7 cells of wild-type and human mutant RK. Markedly reduced mutant RK activity was demonstrated, thereby providing support to the pathogenicity of these mutations.[34,35]

Evidence from knock-out mice models suggest that patients with RK or arrestin mutations may be more susceptible to light-induced retinal damage; it may therefore be advisable to encourage patients to wear tinted spectacles thereby restricting excessive light exposure.[36,37]

Fundus albipunctatus
Clinical findings
This autosomal recessive form of stationary night-blindness has a characteristic fundus appearance with multiple white dots scattered throughout the retina. Patients either present with night-blindness or because the abnormal retinal appearance is noted on routine fundoscopy. The visual acuity is usually normal and the condition nonprogressive in the majority of affected individuals.

The deposits are discrete dull white lesions which lie at the level of the retinal pigment epithelium. They are most numerous in the mid-periphery and are usually absent at the macula; the optic discs and retinal vessels are normal. Fluorescein angiography shows multiple areas of hyperfluorescence which may not conform to the deposits seen clinically. The differential diagnosis is from other causes of flecked retina (Chapter 57).

Electrophysiology and psychophysics
Dark adaptation is severely delayed in fundus albipunctatus, reflecting abnormal regeneration of rhodopsin.[38] The rod–cone break is delayed and full rod adaptation may take several hours.[38] Rod ERGs are markedly abnormal, with the rod-specific ERG being undetectable under standard conditions, but becoming normal following prolonged dark adaptation (Fig. 52.3). To establish the diagnosis of fundus albipunctatus it is necessary to considerably exceed the ISCEV ERG Standard recommendations for dark adaptation.

There are two forms of fundus albipunctatus, the usual form in which cone ERGs are normal, and a second form described as fundus albipunctatus with cone dystrophy and negative ERG.[39]

Molecular genetics and pathogenesis
Mutations in *RDH5*, the gene encoding 11-*cis* retinol dehydrogenase, a component of the visual cycle, have been identified in fundus albipunctatus,[40] with recombinant mutant 11-*cis* retinol dehydrogenases having been demonstrated to have reduced activity compared with recombinant enzyme with wild-type sequence.[40] Fundus albipunctatus with or without cone dystrophy is caused by mutations in *RDH5*. The function of the protein product of *RDH5* is consistent with the delay in the regeneration of photopigments characteristic of the disorder.

Stationary cone disorders (cone dysfunction syndromes)

The cone dysfunction syndromes include congenital color vision disorders where there is normal visual acuity but defective color vision, and the various forms of cone dysfunction associated with reduced central vision and often nystagmus and photophobia (Table 52.1).[41]

Disorders of color vision with normal visual acuity
Color vision in humans is trichromatic; there are three classes of cone photoreceptor that contain visual pigments that are maximally sensitive at 560 nm (L-cones (red)), 535 nm (M-cones (green)) and 440 nm (S-cones (blue)). The genes for the protein component (opsin) of the red and green cone pigments have been identified on the long arm of the X chromosome, and the blue cone opsin gene on chromosome 7.[42,43] About 8% of men and 0.5% of women have a defect of the red-green system and these defects are associated with abnormalities of the red and green cone opsin genes. Tritanopia is an uncommon autosomal dominant disorder in which there is a specific deficiency of blue cone sensitivity associated with mutations of the blue cone opsin gene.[44]

This group of disorders, in which there is normal central vision, a normal eye examination but abnormal color vision will not be

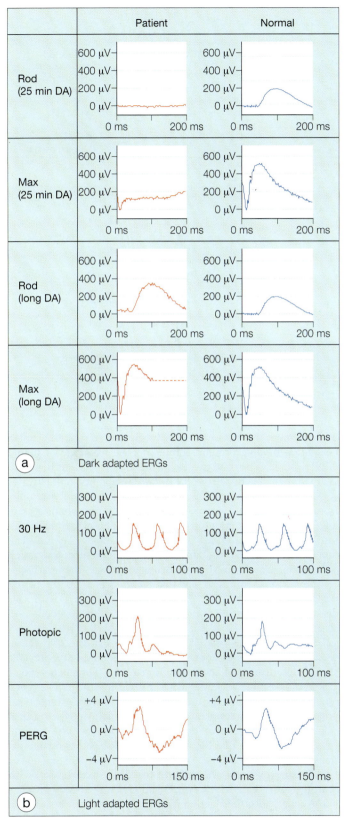

	Patient	Normal

Fig. 52.3 Fundus albipunctatus. (a) Dark adapted ERGs. (b) Light adapted ERGs. All ERGs under light adapted conditions fall within the normal range, including the 30 Hz flicker ERG, the single flash photopic ERG and the PERG. The rod-specific ERG is undetectable following a standard period of dark adaptation, and the maximal response is reduced and electronegative. However, following an extended period of dark adaptation both rod specific and maximal responses are completely normal in keeping with the delayed regeneration of rhodopsin that occurs in this disorder.

considered further. The clinical characteristics and the molecular pathology are reviewed in detail elsewhere.[45,46]

Achromatopsia

Achromatopsia refers to a genetically heterogeneous group of stationary retinal dystrophies in which there is an absence of functioning cones in the retina.[47] They are characterized by reduced central vision, poor color vision, photophobia and a normal fundus, and may occur in complete (typical) and incomplete (atypical) forms.

Complete achromatopsia (rod monochromatism)
Clinical and histopathological findings

This rare disorder is inherited as an autosomal recessive trait and results in impaired vision and complete color blindness. The incidence is approximately one in 30 000. The usual presentation is with reduced vision, nystagmus and marked photophobia in infancy. Parents often comment that vision is much better in dim illumination, and many say that, although there may be photophobia, the most significant symptom is that the vision is poorer in bright illumination (day-blindness). Pupil reactions are sluggish or may show pupillary constriction in the dark, the so-called paradoxical response.[48] High hyperopic refractive errors are common and fundus examination is normal. The nystagmus, although marked in infancy, may improve with age, as can the photophobia.

The visual acuity is usually about 6/60 and there is complete color blindness. Peripheral visual fields are normal but a small central scotoma can often be detected. Although histopathological studies have demonstrated cone-like structures in the retina,[49,50] psychophysical studies show that the achromat lacks cone vision.[47]

Electrophysiology and psychophysics

The dark adaptation curve is monophasic with no evidence of a cone contribution and spectral sensitivity studies show that rods mediate threshold under both photopic and scotopic conditions; there is no evidence of a Purkinje shift.[47] Electroretinography (Fig. 52.4) shows normal rod derived ERGs but no detectable cone-derived responses.[51,52]

Molecular genetics and pathogenesis

Complete achromatopsia is recessively inherited and genetically heterogeneous. Three achromatopsia genes have been identified, CNGA3, CNGB3, and GNAT2; all encoding components of the cone phototransduction cascade. However, the first potential locus reported followed the demonstration of maternal isodisomy of chromosome 14 (both copies of chromosome 14 were of maternal origin) in a 20-year-old woman with achromatopsia and multiple developmental abnormalities.[53] There has been no subsequent confirmation of a locus on chromosome 14.

CNGA3 and CNGB3, located at chromosome 2q11 and 8q21, respectively code for the α- and β-subunits of the cGMP-gated (CNG) cation channel in cone cells. In the dark, cGMP levels are high in cone photoreceptors, therefore enabling cGMP to bind to the α- and β-subunits of CNG channels, resulting in them adopting an open conformation and permitting an influx of cations, with consequent cone depolarization. When light is applied, activated photopigment initiates a cascade culminating in increased cGMP-phosphodiesterase activity, thereby lowering the concentration of cGMP in the photoreceptor which results in closure of CNG cation channels and consequent cone hyperpolarization.

Table 52.1 Summary of the cone dysfunction syndromes

Cone Dysfunction Syndrome	Alternative names	Mode of inheritance	Visual acuity	Refractive error	Nystagmus	Color vision	Fundi	Mutated gene(s) or chromosome locus
Complete achromatopsia	Rod monochromatism Typical achromatopsia	Autosomal recessive	6/36–6/60	Often hypermetropia	Present	Absent	Usually normal	CNGA3 CNGB3 GNAT2 Chromosome 14
Incomplete achromatopsia	Atypical achromatopsia	Autosomal recessive	6/24–6/60	Often hypermetropia	Present	Residual	Usually normal	CNGA3
Oligocone trichromacy	Oligocone syndrome	Autosomal recessive	6/12–6/24	Equal incidence of myopia and hypermetropia	Usually Absent	Normal	Normal	–
Cone monochromatism	–	Uncertain	6/6	–	Absent	Absent or markedly reduced	Normal	–
Blue cone monochromatism	X-linked atypical achromatopsia X-linked incomplete achromatopsia	X-linked	6/24–6/60	Often myopia	Present	Residual tritan discrimination	Usually normal or myopic	(i) Deletion of the LCR (ii) Single inactivated L/M hybrid gene
Bornholm eye disease	–	X-linked	6/9–6/18	Moderate to high myopia with astigmatism	Absent	Deuteranopia	Myopic	Xq28

More than 50 disease-causing mutations in *CNGA3* have been identified in patients with achromatopsia.[54–56] Mutations have been identified throughout the CNGA3 protein, including the five-transmembrane domains, the pore region and cGMP-binding site; with four mutations (Arg277Cys, Arg283Trp, Arg436Trp and Phe547Leu) accounting for approximately 40% of all mutant *CNGA3* alleles.[55] Moreover, subsequent analysis of the homologous *CNGA3* knockout-mouse model showed complete absence of physiologically measurable cone function, a decrease in the number of cones in the retina, and morphological abnormalities of the remaining cones.[57] By comparison, only approximately eight mutations have been identified in *CNGB3*;[56,58,59] the most frequent mutation is the 1 base-pair frameshift deletion, 1148delC (Thr383fs), which accounts for up to 84% of *CNGB3* mutant disease chromosomes.[56,59]

Currently there is far greater allelic heterogeneity of *CNGA3* mutants (over 50 mutations described) when compared to *CNGB3* (~8). It is known that CNGA3 subunits can form functional homomeric channels when expressed alone, whereas CNGB3 subunits alone do not appear to form functional channels.[60] It is therefore plausible that some *CNGB3* null mutations are not detected since sufficient channel function is possible solely with normal CNGA3 subunits, leading to a relatively normal phenotype.[41,56] The majority of *CNGA3* mutations identified to date are missense mutations, indicating that there is little tolerance for substitutions with respect to functional and structural integrity of the channel polypeptide. In contrast, the majority of *CNGB3* alterations are nonsense mutations. Approximately 25% of achromatopsia results from mutations of *CNGA3*[55] and 40–50% from mutations of *CNGB3*.[59]

Mutations within a third gene, *GNAT2*, located at 1p13, which encodes the α-subunit of cone transducin, have also been shown to cause achromatopsia.[61,62] In cone cells, light activated photopigment interacts with transducin, a three subunit guanine nucleotide binding protein, stimulating the exchange of bound GDP for GTP. The cone α-transducin subunit, which is bound to GTP, is then released from its β- and γ-subunits and activates cGMP-phosphodiesterase by removing the inhibitory γ-subunits from the active site of this enzyme. cGMP-phosphodiesterase lowers the concentration of cGMP in the photoreceptor which results in closure of cGMP-gated cation channels. The *GNAT2* mutations identified to date result in premature translation termination and in protein-truncation at the carboxy-terminus.[61,62] Mutations in this gene are thought to be responsible for less than 2% of patients affected with this disorder,[61] suggesting further genetic heterogeneity in achromatopsia.

The phenotype associated with mutations in the two cation channel protein genes appears to be in keeping with previous clinical descriptions of achromatopsia.[55,56,58,59] The phenotype of a large consanguineous family with *GNAT2* inactivation has been reported.[63] The findings of note were clinical evidence of progressive deterioration in older affected individuals, residual color vision, and relative preservation of S-cone ERGs in all subjects, suggesting that S-cones may express another distinct α-transducin.

The three genes described to date associated with achromatopsia, *CNGA3*, *CNGB3* and *GNAT2*, encode proteins in the cone phototransduction cascade. It is therefore reasonable to propose that further cone-specific intermediates involved in phototransduction represent potential candidates for disease.

Incomplete achromatopsia
Clinical findings
The presentation and clinical findings in infancy are similar to the complete form of achromatopsia, but the visual prognosis may be better. Visual acuity is often in the range 6/24–6/36 and there

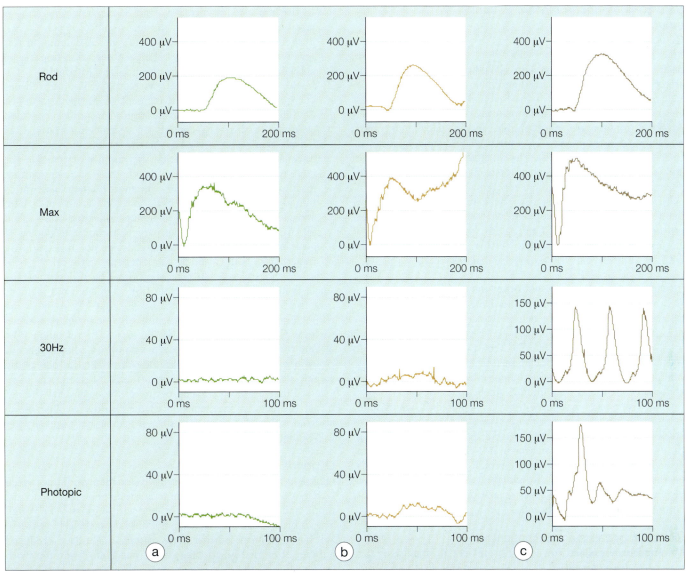

Fig. 52.4 Achromatopsia (rod monochromatism) and blue cone monochromatism (S-cone monochromatism). ERGs from a patient with rod monochromacy (a), a patient with S-cone monochromacy (b) and a representative normal (c). The rod specific and maximal ERGs show no definite abnormality in both of these cone dysfunction syndromes. The 30 Hz flicker ERG is undetectable in both, but the single flash photopic ERG is undetectable in rod monochromatism but small and delayed in S-cone monochromatism, typical of S-cone origins. Note that the scale for the photopic ERGs in the two patients differs from that in the normal subject better to illustrate the low amplitude photopic single flash response in the S-cone monochromat.

may be some residual color perception. This form is also inherited as an autosomal recessive trait. Three subtypes of incomplete achromatopsia have been demonstrated via color matching experiments:[64]
1. Color matches are governed by rods and M-cones (incomplete achromatopsia with protan luminosity).[65]
2. Color matches are governed by L- and M-cones.
3. Color matches mediated by rods, L-cones and S-cones (incomplete achromatopsia with deutan luminosity).[66,67]

Molecular genetics and pathogenesis

As in the complete form, mutations in *CNGA3*, have been identified in individuals with incomplete achromatopsia.[55] The nineteen mutations identified are all missense mutations, located throughout the channel polypeptide including the trans-membrane domains, ion pore and cGMP-binding region. Only three of these missense mutations, Arg427Cys, Arg563His, and

Thr565Met, were found exclusively in patients with incomplete achromatopsia.[55] Therefore in the majority of cases of incomplete achromatopsia, other factors may influence the phenotype, such as modifier genes or environmental factors. The missense variants identified in incomplete achromatopsia must be compatible with residual channel function since the phenotype is milder than in complete achromatopsia.

Mutations in *CNGB3* or *GNAT2* have not been reported in association with incomplete achromatopsia, despite mutant *CNGB3* alleles being identified twice as commonly as *CNGA3* variants as the cause of complete achromatopsia. However all *GNAT2* mutations to date, and the vast majority of *CNGB3* mutants, result in premature termination of translation, and thereby truncated and probably nonfunctional phototransduction proteins. Therefore an incomplete achromatopsia phenotype is unlikely to be compatible with these genotypes, which are predicted to encode mutant products lacking any residual function.

Blue cone monochromatism (S-cone monochromatism)
Clinical findings

Blue cone monochromatism (BCM) is an X-linked recessive disorder, affecting less than 1 in 100 000 individuals, in which affected males have normal rod and blue (S) cone function but lack red (L) and green (M) cone function. The clinical features are similar to complete achromatopsia but are less severe. Affected infants are photophobic and develop fine rapid nystagmus in early infancy. They are usually myopic, in contrast to achromatopsia (Fig. 52.5). The nystagmus reduces with time and is usually minimal by the late teens. There may be mild abnormalities on eye movement recording.[68]

BCM is generally accepted to be a stationary disorder but deterioration and the development of foveal pigmentary changes has been reported in one family with macular atrophy over a 12-year period.[69] There are two further reports of individuals with BCM displaying a progressive retinal degeneration.[70,71]

Electrophysiology and psychophysics

Achromatopsia (rod monochromatism) and BCM may be differentiated by the mode of inheritance, findings on psychophysical testing and electrophysiology. There is some preservation of the single flash photopic ERG in BCM (Fig. 52.4), and specialized spectral ERG techniques to measure S-cone ERGs can also be used.[72] Female carriers of X-linked BCM may have abnormal cone ERGs[73] and mild anomalies of color vision.[51]

Color vision tests that probe the tritan color confusion axis are necessary in order to distinguish between rod monochromatism and BCM. Blue cone monochromats display fewer errors along the vertical axis in the Farnsworth 100-Hue test (fewer tritan errors), and they may also display protan-like ordering patterns on the Farnsworth D-15.[74] In addition, the Berson plates have been claimed to provide a good separation of blue cone monochromats from rod monochromats.[75,76]

Molecular genetics and pathogenesis

Mutation analyses have proved highly efficient at establishing the molecular basis for BCM.[70,77] The mutations in the L- and M-pigment gene array causing BCM fall into two classes:

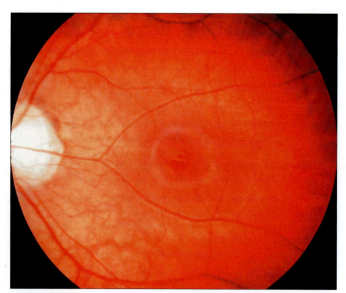

Fig. 52.5 Blue cone monochromatism: pale tilted optic disc with myopic fundus.

1. In the first class, a normal L- and M-pigment gene array is inactivated by a deletion in the locus control region (LCR), located upstream of the L-pigment gene. A deletion in this region abolishes transcription of all genes in the pigment gene array and therefore inactivates both L- and M-cones.
2. In the second class of mutations; the LCR is preserved but changes within the L- and M-pigment gene array lead to loss of functional pigment production. The most common genotype in this class consists of a single inactivated L/M hybrid gene. The first step in this second mechanism is unequal crossing over reducing the number of genes in the array to one, followed in the second step by a mutation that inactivates the remaining gene. The most frequent inactivating mutation is a thymine-to-cytosine transition at nucleotide 648, which results in a cysteine-to-arginine substitution at codon 203 (Cys203Arg), a mutation which disrupts the folding of cone opsin molecules.[78] BCM may also be due to Cys203Arg mutations in both L- and M-pigment genes in the array.[79]

A third molecular genetic mechanism has been described in a single family of BCM where exon 4 of an isolated red pigment gene had been deleted.[80] The data suggest that 40% of blue cone monochromat genotypes are a result of a one-step mutational pathway that leads to deletion of the LCR. The remaining 60% of blue cone monochromat genotypes comprise a heterogeneous group of multistep pathways. Studies have failed to detect the genetic alteration that would explain the BCM phenotype in all assessed individuals.[77,81] The structure of the opsin array did not reveal the genetic mechanism for the disorder in nine of 35 affected patients,[77] which may suggest genetic heterogeneity yet to be identified in BCM.

Oligocone trichromacy

Oligocone trichromacy is a rare cone dysfunction syndrome, which is characterized by reduced visual acuity, mild photophobia, normal fundi, and abnormal cone ERGs, but with normal color vision. The disorder was first described by Van Lith in 1973.[82]

It has been proposed that these patients might have a reduced number of normal functioning cones (oligocone syndrome) with preservation of the three cone types in the normal proportions, thereby permitting trichromacy.[82]

In a phenotype study of six patients with Oligocone syndrome, the findings included reduced visual acuity from infancy (6/12 to 6/24), mild photophobia, normal fundi and an absence of nystagmus.[83] Various color vision tests either revealed normal color vision or slightly elevated discrimination thresholds. The slightly elevated thresholds that were detected are compatible with a reduction in cone numbers. The cone ERG findings in these patients were poorly concordant. Five patients had absent or markedly reduced cone responses; the sixth showed more marked reduction in the cone b-wave than the a-wave, implying a predominantly inner-retinal abnormality in the cone system. These data suggest more than one disease mechanism and therefore more than one disease-causing gene.

Oligocone trichromacy is likely to be inherited as an autosomal recessive trait, but the molecular genetic basis of the disorder is unknown. Genes involved in retinal photoreceptor differentiation, when cone numbers are being determined, may represent good candidate genes.

Bornholm eye disease
Clinical findings

Bornholm eye disease (BED) is a rare X-linked disorder characterized by moderate to high myopia with astigmatism, impaired visual acuity, moderate optic nerve hypoplasia, thinning of the retinal pigment epithelium (RPE) in the posterior pole with visible choroidal vasculature, and abnormal cone ERG.[84] Affected members in this single family were all deuteranopes, with a stationary natural history. This disorder is therefore best characterized as an X-linked cone dysfunction syndrome with myopia and deuteranopia.

Molecular genetics and pathogenesis

Linkage analysis has mapped the locus to Xq28, in the same chromosomal region as the L/M opsin gene array.[85] Molecular genetic analysis of the opsin array may yet reveal mutations that account for both the cone dysfunction and the color vision phenotype. However, it is also possible that rearrangements within the opsin gene array may be found to account for the color vision findings, whilst the cone dysfunction component of the disorder may be ascribed to mutation within an adjacent but separate locus. The cone dystrophy that has been mapped to Xq27 (COD2) however, displays a progressive phenotype.[86]

PROGRESSIVE RETINAL DYSTROPHIES

Rod–cone dystrophies

The rod–cone dystrophies (often referred to as retinitis pigmentosa (RP)) are a clinically and genetically heterogeneous group of disorders in which there is progressive loss of rod and later cone photoreceptor function leading to severe visual impairment. RP usually occurs as an isolated retinal abnormality, but it may also be seen in association with systemic abnormalities; these syndromic disorders are addressed in Chapter 53.

Leber congenital amaurosis
Clinical findings

Leber congenital amaurosis (LCA) is a rod–cone dystrophy which presents at birth or the first few months of life with poor vision and nystagmus. It is usually inherited as an autosomal recessive trait, with affected individuals from the same family showing a similar phenotype.[87] Autosomal dominant inheritance has also been reported but is rare.[88] LCA is the most common inherited cause of severe visual impairment in children, accounting for 10–18% of children in institutions for the blind.[89]

The usual presentation is with severe visual impairment from birth or the first few months of life. Affected infants have roving eye movements or nystagmus and poor pupillary responses to light. Eye-poking, the "oculodigital" sign, is common (Fig. 52.6).

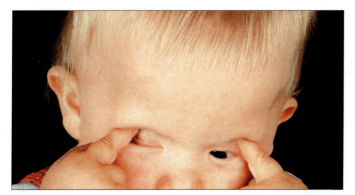

Fig. 52.6 Leber congenital amaurosis. Eye-poking, the "oculodigital sign" is very common but of unknown cause; it results in atrophy of orbital fat and enophthalmos.

Fundus examination is usually normal but a variety of abnormal fundus appearances may be present such as disc pallor, vessel attenuation or mild peripheral pigmentary retinopathy. Less commonly there may be optic disc edema or pseudopapilledema (Fig. 52.7), a flecked retina (Fig. 52.8), macular dysplasia (Fig. 52.9) or, rarely, nummular pigmentation. Affected infants often have high hyperopia, or less commonly high myopia, suggesting that the severe visual impairment may interfere with the process of emmetropization.

Although the majority of patients have normal fundi in infancy, most develop signs of a pigmentary retinopathy in later childhood with optic disc pallor and retinal arteriolar narrowing.[90] Rarely, yellow flecks may be seen in the equatorial fundus. Other late signs, which may be related to eye-poking, include enophthalmos, keratoconus and cataract. Eventual vision is in the region of 3/60 to perception of light: deterioration is demonstrable in some cases.[91]

Electrophysiology

The ERG is undetectable or severely abnormal in infants with LCA. It is important to distinguish the disorder from CSNB and achromatopsia, which may also present in infancy with nystagmus and poor vision. The visual evoked potential is usually absent but may be preserved in some infants despite an absent ERG and may indicate a better visual prognosis.

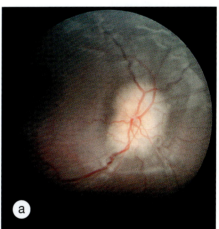

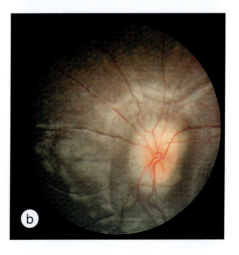

Fig. 52.7 Leber congenital amaurosis. (a, b) high hypermetropia and pseudopapilledema.

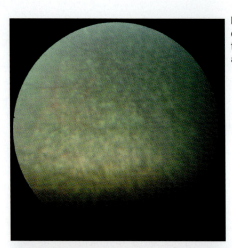

Fig. 52.8 Leber congenital amaurosis—flecked retina appearance.

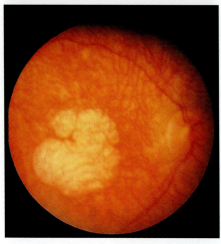

Fig. 52.9 Leber congenital amaurosis—macular dysplasia.

Non-ocular features

Most cases of LCA occur in otherwise normal infants and it may be preferable that the term LCA is confined to such children. However, a variety of associated systemic abnormalities including mental subnormality, neurological disorders, renal disease and hearing loss have been reported in association with a similar infantile retinal dystrophy.[91–94] It is still unclear whether most, if not all, of these complicated cases represent examples of other systemic disorders (Chapter 53).

Diagnosis

LCA should be suspected in any infant with poor vision, nystagmus, hypermetropia, sluggish pupil reactions and a normal fundus examination. The diagnosis is confirmed by ERG testing. Other inherited disorders such as the peroxisomal disorders or Joubert syndrome should be excluded if there are any unusual systemic features.

Molecular genetics and pathogenesis

Molecular genetic testing can now confirm and clarify the diagnosis in an increasing proportion of patients with LCA. To date, six genes have been identified that together account for approximately half of all LCA patients:

GUCY2D on 17p13.1[95,96]
RPE65 on 1p31[97,98]
CRX on 19q13.3[99,100]
AIPL1 on 17p13.1[101,102]
CRB1 on 1q31.3[103,104]
RPGRIP1 14q11[105]

These genes are expressed preferentially in the retina or the RPE. Their putative functions are quite diverse and include retinal photoreceptor development (*CRX*), photoreceptor cell structure (*CRB1*), phototransduction (*GUCY2D*), protein trafficking (*AIPL1*, *RPGRIP1*), and vitamin A metabolism (*RPE65*). Establishing a molecular diagnosis of LCA may facilitate advice about prognosis. Initial phenotype–genotype correlation studies have shown that patients with *RPE65* mutations have a better prognosis than those with *GUCY2D* mutations.[106] In addition, identification of disease-causing mutations in LCA patients allows improved genetic counseling, the potential for prenatal diagnosis and in the future may be used to select patients for gene-specific therapies.

Functional analysis has been performed of nine missense mutations in *GUCY2D*, the gene encoding photoreceptor-specific guanylyl cyclase (RETGC-1).[96] Mutants were expressed in COS7 cells and assayed for their ability to hydrolyze GTP into cGMP. All missense mutations lying in the catalytic domain showed a complete abolition of cyclase activity.[96] More than half the *GUCY2D* mutations identified in LCA are truncating mutations expected to result in a total abolition of RETGC-1 activity. A histopathological assessment of an eye from an 11-year-old with a known *GUCY2D* mutation has revealed rods and cones without outer segments in the macula and far retinal periphery.[107] Rods and cones were not identified in the mid-peripheral retina. The inner nuclear layer appeared normal in thickness throughout the retina, but ganglion cells were reduced in number. The finding of numerous photoreceptors at this age provides a potential target for treatments directed at improving vision.

Gene replacement therapy with subretinal injection of recombinant adeno-associated virus encoding an *RPE65* transgene in RPE65$^{-/-}$ dogs has provided promising results.[108,109] Marked improvements in visual behavior and ERGs occurred as early as 4 weeks after surgery in affected animals, with a gradual progressive improvement in ERG responses over time. Trials of gene therapy in patients with LCA due to mutations in *RPE65* are likely in the near future.

Retinitis pigmentosa

Retinitis pigmentosa (RP) is a term used for a genetically heterogeneous group of disorders characterized by night-blindness and visual field loss. ERGs are either undetectable or show the rod system to be more severely affected than the cone system, with dysfunction at the level of the photoreceptor. Dysfunction confined to the rod system is unusual but can occur. Onset is often in childhood and inheritance can be autosomal recessive (AR), autosomal dominant (AD) and X-linked (XL).

Clinical findings

Children with RP may present with night-blindness or with symptoms associated with extensive field loss or central retinal involvement. The age of onset is extremely variable. In some there may be no symptomatic night-blindness and the child is referred because of retinal abnormalities found on routine fundoscopy. When a parent or other close relative has RP, children may be referred early for investigation to exclude the disease.

In most cases the visual acuity is normal at presentation although later visual loss may occur as a result of posterior subcapsular cataract, macular edema or macular involvement. Early visual field changes are seen as small scotomata in the mid-peripheral retina and are more common in the upper visual field.

These field defects gradually coalesce to give the classical peripheral ring scotoma. Visual fields become very constricted in advanced disease, although there is often a small island of preserved field in the far temporal periphery. In sector RP, which commonly involves the lower nasal quadrant, bilateral upper temporal field loss may lead to unnecessary investigation to exclude a chiasmal lesion.

The appearance of the fundus in the early stages of RP is variable and in young children the changes may be subtle. The earliest change may be mild pigment epithelial atrophy in the mid-periphery often with small white dots at the level of the RPE (Fig. 52.10). Later, pigment deposition is seen in the equatorial retina and there may be arteriolar narrowing and optic disc pallor. Abnormal pigment may be lacking in some children (RP sine pigmento) and less commonly there may be multiple white deposits scattered throughout the retina (retinitis punctata albescens). The classical fundus appearance of optic disc pallor, retinal arteriolar attenuation and peripheral pigment epithelial atrophy and "bone corpuscle" pigmentation is seen in advanced disease (Figs 52.11, 52.12 and 52.13). Other changes include vitreous cells, posterior subcapsular cataract, optic disc drusen and macular edema. Occasionally, retinovascular changes similar to Coats disease are seen.

The retinal phenotype is similar in most forms of RP although there may be marked variation in severity between affected individuals. There are however some specific phenotypes that are seen more commonly with specific genetic mutations. AD sector RP is usually associated with mutations in the rhodopsin gene,[110] and RP with preserved para-arteriolar RPE, an uncommon AR form of RP (RP12), has been described in association with mutations in the *CRB1* gene.[111] Two early onset forms of AR RP caused by mutations in the *RLBP-1* gene are associated with multiple white deposits at the level of the RPE. These have been described in genetic isolates of North-Eastern Canada

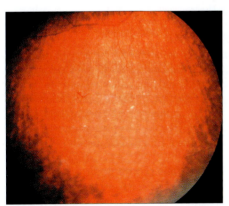

Fig. 52.10 Retinitis pigmentosa. Pigment epithelial atrophy in the mid-periphery with small white dots at the level of the RPE.

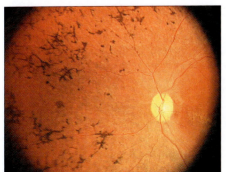

Fig. 52.11 Retinitis pigmentosa. "Bone spicule" formation and arteriolar narrowing.

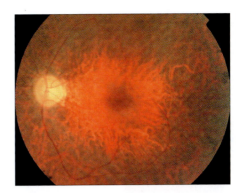

Fig. 52.12 Retinitis pigmentosa. Macular atrophy and arteriolar narrowing.

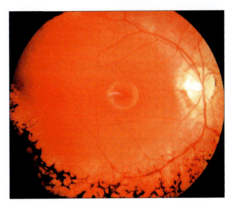

Fig. 52.13 Retinitis pigmentosa. Marked "bone spicule" formation encroaching on the posterior pole.

(Newfoundland rod–cone dystrophy) and northern Sweden (Bothnia dystrophy).[112,113]

Electrophysiology and psychophysics

The ERG in RP shows a rod–cone pattern of dysfunction such that the rod derived responses are more affected than the cone-derived responses. There is marked variation in severity related to the nature of the mutation, the inheritance pattern, and the age of the subject. The ERG may be undetectable in the late stages of RP, or small residual cone responses may be found. There is reduction in the amplitude of the rod a- and b-waves in mild disease or early RP and the rod-mediated b-wave implicit time may be prolonged. The 30 Hz cone flicker ERG is usually both delayed and reduced.

Although the EOG may be used in addition to the ERG in the assessment of patients with RP, it provides little further information and is difficult to perform in young children. In all types of RP there is a reduced or absent light rise, usually reflecting the severity of the rod ERG abnormality. The macula may be spared such that measures of central retinal function such as the PERG or multifocal ERG, may show minimal involvement despite almost complete loss of the conventional full-field ERG. PERG may also be helpful in demonstrating central retinal involvement prior to the development of visible abnormalities.

Psychophysical studies in all forms of RP show elevated rod and later cone thresholds[114,115] and in some patients the kinetics of dark adaptation is also abnormal.[110]

Sector retinitis pigmentosa

In sector RP, which is usually inherited as an autosomal dominant trait, the fundus abnormalities are confined to one sector of the fundus, usually the inferior retina (Fig. 52.14). Similar sectorial involvement may occasionally be seen in the female carriers of X-linked RP and can also occur as an early stage in more

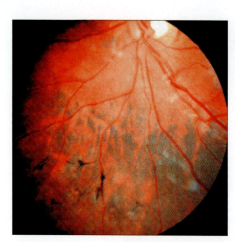

Fig. 52.14 Sector retinitis pigmentosa. Retinal pigmentary changes confined to the lower nasal quadrant.

generalized forms of RP. The term sector RP should be reserved for those forms of RP (usually autosomal dominant) where the fundoscopic abnormalities are confined to the inferior retina. The ERG in true sector RP may show no implicit time changes; the presence of marked implicit time shifts suggests a more generalized disorder. It is important in isolated cases to examine other family members as the disorder is often asymptomatic. Dominant sector RP is often associated with mutations of the rhodopsin gene.[110] Children with sector RP are usually asymptomatic and are referred when an abnormal fundus appearance is noted on routine fundoscopy or they are ascertained during family surveys.

Field loss on Goldmann perimetry is confined to one sector corresponding to the clinically involved retina. However, dark-adapted perimetry may show mild rod and cone threshold elevation in the apparently uninvolved retina indicating wide-spread disease.[110] Rod dark adaptation may be extremely delayed. The ERG is usually relatively well-preserved with mild or moderate reductions in both rod and cone amplitudes.[110] Disease progression is slow and confined to the clinically involved sector. The visual prognosis is excellent.

Autosomal dominant retinitis pigmentosa (adRP) with incomplete penetrance

Variability of expression is common in adRP but true incomplete penetrance is unusual. However, incomplete penetrance is a notable and common occurrence in some families, and there is some evidence that the disease in such families is of early onset and severe.[116,117] There is evidence for genetic heterogeneity in adRP with incomplete penetrance; linkage has been established to 7p[118] and 19q,[119] with mutations identified in the genes *RP9*[120] and *PRPF31*[121] respectively.

Genetic counseling in families showing incomplete penetrance may be problematic because of the high incidence of asymptomatic gene carriers, but molecular genetic diagnosis is now possible in some families.

X-linked retinitis pigmentosa

X-linked RP is a genetically heterogeneous, severe form of RP with early onset of night-blindness and progression to legal blindness by the 3rd to 4th decade. Most affected males show symptomatic night-blindness before the age of 10 years, are often myopic and show fundus abnormalities and ERG changes in early childhood (Fig. 52.15). Early onset myopia is common. If there is a family history of other affected males, the diagnosis is usually straightforward. Examination of close female relatives is helpful in the absence of a family history, as the recognition of the XL carrier state will confirm the diagnosis.

The carrier state for XL RP can be diagnosed with certainty in females who have affected sons or fathers and are therefore obligate gene carriers, or where they can be shown by molecular genetic testing to carry the causative mutation. In other female family members carrier detection depends upon recognition of the abnormal fundus appearance seen in the heterozygote or on the results of electrophysiological or psychophysical testing.

Fundus abnormalities are common in XL heterozygotes: a prominent 'tapetal' reflex may be seen at the posterior pole (Fig. 52.16) or mild pigment epithelial thinning and pigmentation may be present in the equatorial retina. Fluorescein angiography may help in confirming the peripheral pigment epithelial atrophy.

The ERG is usually abnormal in heterozygotes (Fig. 52.15). Delay in the 30 Hz flicker response is probably the most frequently found abnormality, but reduced rod amplitude may also occur. The proportion of obligate heterozygotes with abnormal ERG varies between series but most of these were performed before the introduction of standardized testing. Psychophysical testing can demonstrate elevated dark-adapted thresholds[122] and reduced rod flicker sensitivity[123] in XL heterozygotes.

XL carriers can therefore be identified in most cases using a combination of fundoscopy, electrophysiology and in selected cases psychophysics. Molecular genetic diagnosis is possible in many families and in future will be the method of choice for identification of heterozygotes.

The retinal dysfunction in some XL carriers appears to be progressive as older carriers may report symptoms of night-blindness and have detectable field loss and more extensive retinal pigmentation. Carrier females may be severely affected at a relatively young age in some pedigrees. In a large family with XL RP, the carrier female's phenotype varied from normal to a severe retinal dystrophy and blindness.[124] The severely affected females were shown to have skewed X inactivation with the X chromosome having the mutant allele active in most cells.

Unilateral retinitis pigmentosa

Fundus changes suggestive of unilateral RP have been described but have yet to be reported in families. Such cases are probably not genetically determined and may be related to retinal ischemia, inflammation or infection.[125] Some individuals with RP have an asymmetric fundus appearance at presentation so that one eye appears clinically unaffected, but psychophysical testing and ERG demonstrate abnormal function bilaterally.

Differential diagnosis of retinitis pigmentosa

Other disorders may be confused with RP either because there is symptomatic night-blindness or because a similar fundus appearance is present (Table 52.2, Fig. 52.17). The other inherited dystrophies can usually be differentiated from RP by the clinical findings and careful electrophysiological testing. Although history and examination may exclude many of the acquired causes of pigmentary retinopathy it is likely that some cases of apparently sporadic RP are due to acquired retinal or pigment epithelial disease.

Genetics of retinitis pigmentosa

RP may be inherited as an autosomal dominant, autosomal recessive or X-linked recessive disorder. There is genetic heterogeneity within these classes and it is particularly marked in autosomal recessive RP. The relative frequency of the different

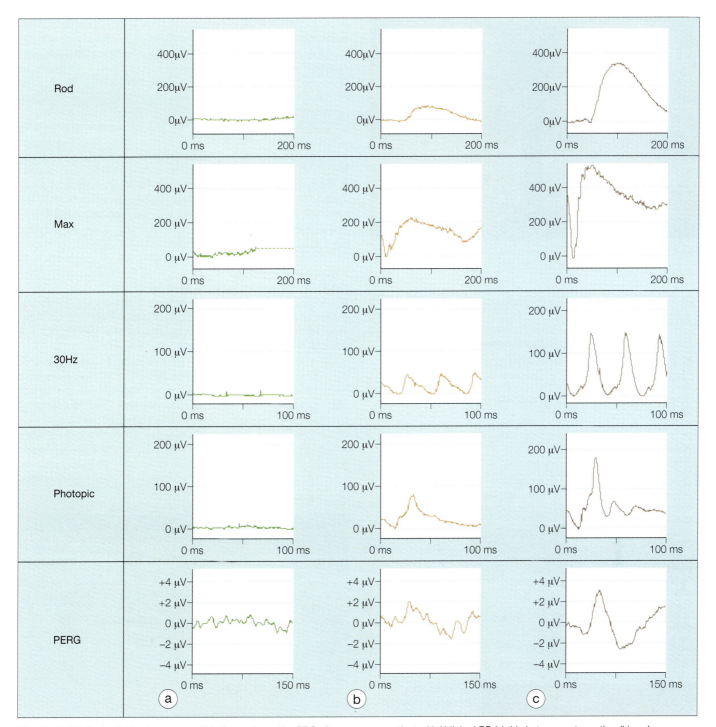

Fig. 52.15 X-linked retinitis pigmentosa. This figure shows the ERGs from a young patient with X-linked RP (a), his heterozygote mother (b) and a representative normal subject (c). There is only residual ERG activity detectable in the patient. The ERGs in his mother are mildly subnormal under all stimulus conditions, the subnormal a-wave of the maximal response demonstrating the abnormality to be at the level of the photoreceptor. ERG abnormalities are usually found in heterozygotes, and can vary from mild to severe.

modes of inheritance differs widely in the different series, but approximately 50% of patients have no family history of RP or evidence of parental consanguinity. It is unlikely that all such cases have autosomal recessive disease. Some males may have X-linked disease transmitted via asymptomatic female carriers; other cases may represent new autosomal dominant mutations or autosomal dominant disease in a family with reduced penetrance. It is also possible that some sporadic patients do not have genetic disease. Similar retinal dystrophies may also be seen with

mutations of mitochondrial DNA but there are usually other systemic abnormalities (Chapter 30).

Clinical experience shows that X-linked and autosomal recessive RP tend to have an earlier onset and are more severe than dominant disease. The clinical findings should be taken into account, particularly when counseling those patients with apparently sporadic disease. A severely affected female is more likely to have autosomal recessive disease whereas a severely affected male may have X-linked or autosomal recessive disease.

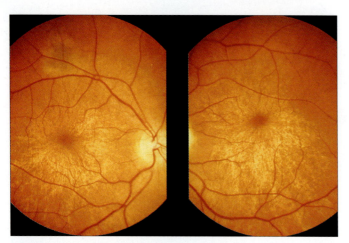

Fig. 52.16 X-linked RP carrier female showing the "tapetal reflex".

Table 52.3: Autosomal dominant retinitis pigmentosa (AD RP) with identified genes and known chromosomal loci

Pigmentary retinopathy	Night-blindness
Blunt trauma	**Genetic disorders**
Retained intraocular FB	Congenital stationary night–blindness
Congenital infection	Oguchi disease
Rubella	Fundus albipunctatus
Varicella	Choroideremia
Herpes simplex	Gyrate atrophy
Syphilis	Progressive cone–rod dystrophy
Acquired infection	
Measles	
Onchocerciasis	
Metabolic	**Acquired**
Cystinosis	Vitamin A deficiency
Oxallosis	Desferrioxamine toxicity
Drugs	
Phenothiazines	
Chloroquine	
Desferrioxamine	
Resolved retinal detachment	
Ophthalmic artery occlusion	
Other retinal dystrophies	
Cone–rod dystrophy	
Inherited vitreoretinal dystrophies	
Unknown etiology	
Paravenous retinochoroidal atrophy	

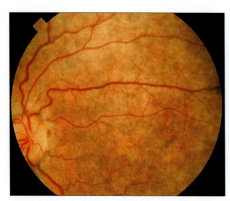

Fig. 52.17 Rubella retinopathy showing retinal pigment mottling. Retinal function is usually good and the ERG normal, whereas most retinal dystrophies with deafness have severely abnormal ERGs.

A significant number of patients with sporadic RP, however, have mild disease and a proportion of these probably have new autosomal dominant mutations. Prior to counseling it is important to examine other family members, especially the mothers of severely affected males who may show the fundus or electrophysiological abnormalities suggestive of an X-linked heterozygote.

Accurate genetic counseling hinges on identification of the causative mutations. Much progress has been made in recent years, and molecular genetic diagnosis is now possible in some forms of RP. To date, 39 loci have been implicated in non-syndromic RP, for which 30 genes are known; encoded proteins include components of the phototransduction cascade, proteins involved in vitamin A metabolism and cell–cell interaction, photoreceptor structural proteins and transcription factors, intracellular transport proteins and splicing factors.

Molecular genetics
Autosomal dominant retinitis pigmentosa
There is considerable genetic heterogeneity within autosomal dominant RP (adRP) (Table 52.3). Mutations in 13 genes have now been identified, with mutations in the rhodopsin gene (*RHO*)[126,127] being the commonest cause of RP.

Mutations of the rhodopsin gene account for about 25% of patients with adRP and more than 100 different mutations have been identified; there is considerable variation in the ocular phenotype seen with the different mutations.[141,115] Mutations of the rhodopsin gene have also been reported in dominant forms of CSNB[9,10] and autosomal recessive RP.[142] The phenotypic variability is more marked with mutations of the *RDS/peripherin* gene where the clinical picture may resemble retinitis pigmentosa, cone–rod dystrophy, a fleck retina syndrome or macular dystrophy

Table 52.3: Autosomal dominant retinitis pigmentosa (AD RP) with identified genes and known chromosomal loci

AD RP; OMIM number	Chromosome locus	Mutated gene	Reference
RP4 & RP5; 180380 & 180102	3q21–q24	*RHO*	126,127
RP7; 179605	6p21.1–cen	*RDS/peripherin*	129
ROM1 180721	11q13	*ROM1*	128
RP1; 603937	8p11–q13	*RP1*	130
RGR; 600342	10q23	*RGR*	131
RP27; 162080	14q11.1–q11.2	*NRL*	132
CRX; 602225	19q13.3	*CRX*	133
RP11; 606419	19q13.4	*PRPF31*	121
RP30; 607643	17q25	*FSCN2*	134
RP18 607301	1q21.2	*HPRP3*	135
RP10 146690	7q31.3–q32	*IMPDH1*	136
RP13 600059	17p13.3	*PRPF8*	137
RP9; 180104	7p14.2	*RP9*	120
RP17 600852	17q22	Not identified	138

(see Chapters 54, 57). Mutations of the *RDS/peripherin* gene account for about 5% of cases of autosomal dominant RP.[115]

An unusual form of RP (showing digenic inheritance), in which mutations of the *peripherin/RDS* gene and *ROM1* (rod outer segment protein 1) gene are present within the same family has been described.[128] Individuals with a mutation of one gene but not the other are clinically unaffected. Affected individuals are double heterozygotes with mutations of both the *ROM1* gene and the *peripherin/RDS* gene. Peripherin and *ROM1* are both located in rod and cone outer segments discs. In the photoreceptor outer segment, interaction of the two proteins is important for outer segment structure, and it appears that some mutations in the *peripherin/RDS* gene may be insufficient to cause significant photoreceptor disease unless accompanied by a defective ROM1 protein.

Splice factors have recently been identified as being associated with adRP, thereby establishing a new class of proteins involved in retinal dystrophy pathogenesis. Mutations in *PRPF31*,[121] *HPRP3*[135] and *PRPF8*,[137] have been identified. In a recent study of 150 families with adRP, approximately 5% were found to harbor mutations in one of these three pre-mRNA splicing-factor genes.[139] The functional consequences of two mutations, A194E and A216P, in *PRPF31* have been investigated.[140] Western blot analysis and immunofluorescence microscopy of mammalian cells transfected with *PRPF31* revealed that both mutations substantially hinder translocation of the protein into the nucleus; its site of action. It was suggested that an insufficiency in splicing function, may be disease-causing only under conditions of elevated splicing demand.[140] With the need to replenish disc proteins on a daily basis, such conditions will exist in rod photoreceptors, which may explain the paradox of isolated retinal disease caused by ubiquitously expressed splice-factor genes.

Since there are families that do not map to any of the currently known loci, more loci and genes remain to be identified. There have been several recent reviews.[115,143–145]

Autosomal recessive retinitis pigmentosa

Mutations in fourteen genes have been identified to date in autosomal recessive RP (arRP); with other genes and loci yet to be discovered (Table 52.4). Mutations in genes encoding many components of the rod phototransduction cascade have been identified including the rhodopsin gene,[142] the genes coding for the α-subunit[152] and the β-subunit[153] of the rod cGMP-phosphodiesterase, the genes for the α- and β-subunits of rod cGMP-gated cation channels[148,149] and also in *SAG*, encoding arrestin.[155] In addition, mutations in four genes coding for components of the visual cycle, involved in recycling vitamin A, have been implicated in arRP; namely *RPE65*[146], *ABCA4*[147], *LRAT*[150] and *RLBP1*.[154]

Recent reviews of the molecular genetics of arRP and phenotype correlations include the following references.[115,143–145]

X-linked retinitis pigmentosa

Mutations in two genes have been identified in X-linked RP, *RPGR* (RP3)[163,164] and *RP2* (RP2).[165,166] Three other loci have been reported: Xp22 (RP23),[167] Xp21.3–p21.2 (RP6),[168] and Xq26–27 (RP24).[169] Most families with XL RP have mutations in *RPGR*.

RPGR mutations are usually associated with typical rod–cone degeneration, but in a small number of patients, retinal dystrophy, deafness, and abnormalities in respiratory cilia have been noted.[170] The majority of mutations are predicted to result in

Table 52.4: Autosomal recessive retinitis pigmentosa (AR RP) with identified genes and known chromosomal loci

AR RP; OMIM number	Chromosome locus	Mutated gene	Reference
RHO; 180380	3q21-q24	*RHO*	142
RP20; 180069	1p31	*RPE65*	146
RP19; 601718	1p21-p13	*ABCA4*	147
RP12; 600105	1q31-q32.1	*CRB1*	111
CNGA1; 123825	4p12–cen	*CNGA1*	148
CNGB1; 600724	16q13	*CNGB1*	149
LRAT; 604863	4q31	*LRAT*	150
MERTK; 604705	2q14.1	*MERTK*	151
PDE6A; 180071	5q31.2-q34	*PDE6A*	152
PDE6B; 180072	4p16.3	*PDE6B*	153
RGR; 600342	10q23	*RGR*	131
RLBP1; 180090	15q26	*RLBP1*	154
Arrestin; 181031	2q37.1	*SAG*	155
RP14; 600132	6p21.3	*TULP1*	156
USH2A; 276901	1q41	*USH2A*	157
RP22; 602594	16p12.1–p12.3	Not identified	158
RP25; 602772	6q14-q21	Not identified	159
RP26; 608380	2q31-q33	*CERKL*	160
RP28; 606068	2p11–p16	Not identified	161
RP29	4q32–q34	Not identified	162

premature termination of translation. Exon ORF15 is a "hot spot" for mutation, at least in the British population; in a recent study, mutations in ORF15 were found to be responsible for 80% of cases of XL RP.[171] Most *RPGR* mutations are unique to single families, making meaningful phenotype–genotype correlations difficult. It has been suggested that RPGR may act as a regulator of a specific type of membrane transport or trafficking which is particularly active in the retina or RPE.[172]

Mutations in the retinitis pigmentosa protein gene *RP2* account for up to 15% of X-linked RP[170,173] RP2 is a novel protein of unknown function, which is targeted to the plasma membrane by dual N-terminal acyl-modification. Dual-acylated proteins are targeted to lipid rafts, suggesting a potential role for the protein in signal transduction.[174]

Management

Most forms of RP are not amenable to specific treatment. However in some systemic disorders the deterioration in retinal function may be slowed by dietary treatment (see Chapter 30). In one randomized controlled trial of vitamin A supplementation in RP there was a small effect on the rate of decline of the cone flicker ERG; the effect was however small and no beneficial effect was found on visual acuity or visual field loss.[175] This form of treatment has not gained widespread acceptance.

Despite the lack of effective treatment for RP, the ophthalmologist has an important role to play in the management both of the child and the whole family. Once the diagnosis is established, the parents and the child (if old enough) are given a full and sympathetic explanation; they can be reassured that most children complete their education at a normal school as central vision is preserved until late in the disease.

Parents are often concerned that other children may be at risk of developing the disease; they should be offered genetic counseling and it may be appropriate to examine other family members. It is also helpful to have available the addresses of patient self-help groups such as the British, American or other RP association (Chapter 31).

Practical help can also be given when there are visual difficulties. Many patients with RP have poor vision in bright sunlight and have problems in adapting from bright to dim illumination; tinted lenses may be helpful. Any significant refractive errors should be fully corrected. A trial of acetazolamide, orbital floor or systemic steroids should be given if there is macular edema. Low visual aids may be helpful in established edema or macular atrophy. Visual loss may also develop secondary to posterior subcapsular cataract, and although cataract surgery is often successfully performed in adults with RP, it is rarely necessary in childhood.

Prognosis

The prognosis in RP varies according to the type of disease and the causative genetic mutation. Ideally, prognosis should be inferred by the identification of the specific genetic mutation but widespread genetic testing is not yet available in clinical practice. Advice on prognosis therefore has to depend upon careful phenotyping to establish the diagnosis and a full family history to establish the mode of inheritance, and can be given with a greater degree of confidence once a more specific diagnosis has been established. It is also helpful to carry out a careful examination of all affected members to establish changes of disease severity with increasing age. Although intra-familial variability of disease expression may occur, the visual outcome of older affected family members serves as a good guide to the likely prognosis in children with retinal dystrophies.

In X-linked RP affected males are night-blind in early childhood, usually show extensive field loss by their teens and central visual loss in their twenties. By the fourth decade most have vision reduced to less than an ability to count fingers. Autosomal recessive RP is such a heterogeneous condition that accurate prognosis is difficult. The disease is usually of early onset and severe. Most patients have a severely constricted visual field by their teens and may have marked central visual loss by their late twenties. Some with recessive disease follow a more benign course.

The prognosis is better in autosomal dominant RP. Although night-blindness and field loss may develop in childhood, central vision may remain normal throughout life. Many patients maintain reasonable visual acuity until the fifth or sixth decade, although they may have extremely constricted visual fields. There is, however, wide variation even in RP caused by mutations at the same locus.[115] Severe, early onset forms are unusual.

True sector RP has the best prognosis of any form of the disease. Although there may be severe visual field loss (usually upper) corresponding to the involved retina, severe involvement of the macula is uncommon.

Paravenous retinochoroidal atrophy

This is a rare chorioretinal atrophy in which there is paravenous RPE atrophy and pigment clumping (Fig. 52.18). It is more common in males, most cases are sporadic and it is usually diagnosed on routine examination in asymptomatic patients. The ERG shows a spectrum of abnormalities and in contrast to most retinal dystrophies may show marked interocular asymmetry. Retinal function usually remains stable, but may show deterioration. It is uncertain whether this disorder has a genetic basis.[176] In one report the monozygotic twin of an affected adult was unaffected, suggesting that at least some cases are nongenetic.[177]

Acquired rod–cone dysfunction
Vitamin A deficiency

In developing countries vitamin A deficiency is usually caused by a combination of malnutrition and malabsorption associated with frequent gastrointestinal infection. In Europe and North America vitamin A deficiency is rare and usually seen in association with liver disease or malabsorption, although rarely an unusual diet may be the cause.

In early deficiency there is slowing of rod dark adaptation and later rod and cone thresholds are elevated.[178] Peripheral fields may be constricted and in some patients white dots at the level of the pigment epithelium are seen scattered throughout the peripheral retina. Rod ERGs are undetectable with cone responses well-preserved.

The ocular abnormalities are reversible with vitamin A supplementation if this is started early.[178] The recovery of retinal function is rapid and early diagnosis is important since vitamin A deficiency is treatable.

Desferrioxamine toxicity

Desferrioxamine is a chelating agent used in the treatment of iron storage disorders such as transfusion siderosis. Ocular side-effects

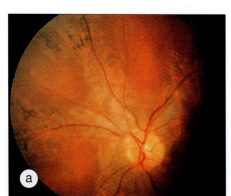

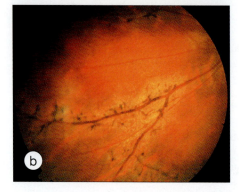

Fig. 52.18 Pigmented paravenous atrophy. (a, b) The veins are surrounded by a band of retinal pigment atrophy and clumping.

include cataract, optic neuropathy and retinal degeneration.[179] Patients with retinal toxicity develop night-blindness, peripheral field loss and a peripheral pigmentary retinopathy; dark adaptation is abnormal and the ERG shows reduced amplitude.[179] Some improvement occurs on stopping the drug.

Histological examination of the eyes of a patient with retinal toxicity showed that the RPE was predominantly affected.[180]

Isotretinoin toxicity

Isotretinoin (13-*cis*-retinoic acid) is an established treatment for acne vulgaris. It is known to have several severe potential adverse effects including liver toxicity and dysregulation of lipid metabolism, necessitating regular blood testing whilst on therapy. Ocular side-effects include photophobia, meibomian gland dysfunction, blepharoconjunctivitis, corneal opacities, keratitis, and decreased night vision.[181]

The mechanisms in human are unknown, but there is some evidence of slowed rhodopsin regeneration in rats receiving isotretinoin.[182]

Inherited chorioretinal dystrophies

Choroideremia
Clinical and histopathological findings

Choroideremia is an X-linked recessive disorder characterized by progressive atrophy of the RPE and choriocapillaris. Affected males usually present in early childhood with night-blindness and progressive field loss, but central vision is usually preserved until late in the disease. There is a slow rate of visual acuity loss and the prognosis for retention of central vision is generally good until the seventh decade.[183] There is, however, a wide variation in clinical expression.[184] Female carriers, although usually asymptomatic, are easily recognized by the characteristic appearance of the peripheral retina on fundoscopy with widespread fine RPE atrophy and granular pigment deposition in the mid-peripheral retina (Fig. 52.19). Cases associated with deafness, hypopituitarism and mental retardation probably represent a contiguous gene defect.[185]

Affected males usually present between the ages of 5 and 10 years with night-blindness. Mild myopia is common. The earliest fundus signs are fine pigment epithelial atrophy and pigmentation in the equatorial retina; at this stage the clinical appearance may be confused with RP. Focal areas of atrophy of the RPE and choriocapillaris develop as the disease progresses, which are particularly well demonstrated on fluorescein angiography or autofluorescence imaging (Figs 52.20 and 52.21).

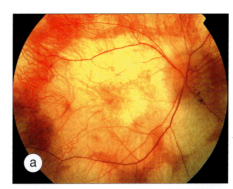

Fig. 52.20
Choroideremia. (a, b) Marked chorioretinal atrophy.

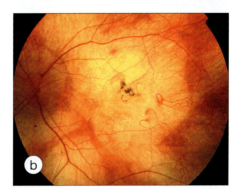

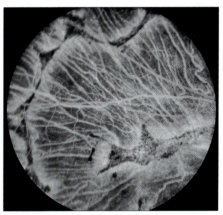

Fig. 52.21
Choroideremia. Fluorescein angiogram showing characteristic scalloped appearance given by the surviving retinal pigment epithelium and loss of the choriocapillaries.

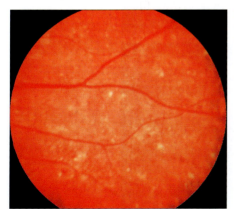

Fig. 52.19
Choroideremia carrier. Granular pigmented and depigmented areas in the peripheral retina.

These areas coalesce to give a widespread atrophic appearance throughout the equatorial retina. This later spreads to involve the peripheral and more posterior retina; the macula is spared until late in the disease.

Visual fields initially show small mid-peripheral scotomata corresponding to areas of atrophy. Marked constriction of the visual field develops with disease progression, but there is often a small preserved island of field in the far periphery.

Most eyes studied histopathologically have been from patients with advanced disease; there is however one report of the histological examination of the eyes of an 18-year-old male with early disease.[186] Marked degeneration of the outer retina was present with loss of RPE, Bruch's membrane and choriocapillaris. Biochemical studies showed reduced levels of interphotoreceptor retinal binding protein (IRBP) and increased levels of cAMP in the RPE and choroid.

Electrophysiology

The ERG is markedly abnormal at an early stage and may be undetectable. Rod and cone amplitudes are reduced in those with

ERG preservation. Implicit time changes are less prominent, but may be present later in the disease process.

Female heterozygotes

Most female carriers are asymptomatic, but the fundus appearance is characteristic. The EOG and ERG are usually normal. Some elderly heterozygotes may develop nyctalopia and show more extensive RPE atrophy with an abnormal ERG and elevated rod thresholds on psychophysical testing.[184] Molecular genetic diagnosis is now possible.

Molecular genetics and pathogenesis

The choroideremia gene (CHM) has been mapped to Xq21, with many different mutations in CHM having been identified.[187–189] The first intronic mutation remote from the exon–intron junctions has been reported in a recent mutation screening study of CHM, creating a strong acceptor splice site and leading to the inclusion of a cryptic exon into the CHM mRNA.[189] Intronic sequence is often not screened in inherited retinal dystrophy mutation investigations; this finding raises the possibility that a significant proportion of disease-causing variants are being missed.

CHM is widely expressed and the product of this gene, Rab escort protein (REP)-1, is involved in the post-translational lipid modification and subsequent membrane targeting of Rab proteins, small GTPases that play a key role in intracellular trafficking.[190]

Gyrate atrophy of the choroid and retina
See Chapter 53.

Cone and cone–rod dystrophies

The inherited cone dystrophies are a heterogeneous group of disorders characterized by variable photophobia, reduced central vision, abnormal color vision and abnormal cone ERGs. Autosomal recessive, autosomal dominant and X-linked recessive inheritance has been reported and there is heterogeneity even amongst these subtypes. The retinal dystrophy may be stationary or progressive; the stationary forms are discussed earlier in this chapter. The functional deficit is confined to the photopic system in some forms of cone dystrophy but in others, perhaps the majority, there is later evidence of rod dysfunction (cone–rod dystrophy). The distinction between cone and cone–rod dystrophies may be difficult, particularly during childhood and is dependent upon good electrophysiology. Most forms of cone and cone–rod dystrophy are seen in otherwise normal individuals; those associated with systemic abnormalities are discussed in Chapter 53.

Progressive cone dystrophy
Clinical findings

In contrast to the stationary cone disorder, achromatopsia, which presents in early infancy, the progressive cone dystrophies are not usually symptomatic until later childhood or early adult life.[51] The age of onset of visual loss and the rate of progression shows wide variability, but visual acuity usually deteriorates eventually to the level of 6/60 or to an ability to count fingers only. Photophobia is a prominent early symptom with progressive loss of central vision and color vision. Since all three classes of cone photoreceptor can be affected, the color vision defects seen are along all three color axes, often progressing to complete loss of color vision over time. Exceptions to this are cases where there is a predominant involvement of L-cones leading to a protan color

vision phenotype.[191,192] Autosomal dominant cone dystrophy pedigrees with early tritan color vision defects have also been reported.[193,194] Fine nystagmus is often seen even in older children. A small central scotoma is frequently detected on careful visual field testing but peripheral fields remain full.

Fundus examination may show a typical bull's eye maculopathy (Figs 52.22 and 52.23) (see Table 52.5 for the differential diagnoses of bull's eye maculopathies). However, in some cases there may only be minor macular pigment epithelial atrophy. The optic discs show a variable degree of temporal pallor. The retinal periphery is usually normal although rarely white flecks similar to those seen in fundus flavimaculatus may be seen.[51] Fluorescein angiography shows typical 'window' defects at the macula in the majority of cases and the so-called dark choroid sign is frequently seen.[195] A tapetal-like sheen which may change in appearance on dark adaptation (Mizuo–Nakamura phenomenon) may be seen in X-linked cone dystrophy.[196]

Electrophysiology and psychophysics

Electroretinography shows normal rod responses but substantially abnormal cone responses (Fig. 52.24). The 30 Hz flicker ERG is usually of increased implicit time but rarely, such as in the cone dystrophy related to GCAP1 mutation,[204] the

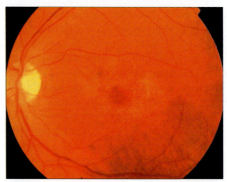

Fig. 52.22 Progressive cone dystrophy with bull's-eye maculopathy and temporal optic disc pallor.

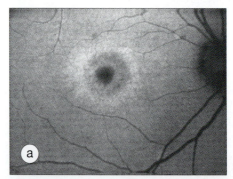

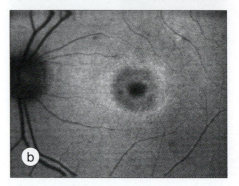

Fig. 52.23 Progressive cone dystrophy: autofluorescence (AF) images of bull's-eye maculopathy.

Table 52.5 Bull's eye maculopathy in childhood: differential diagnoses

Stargardt disease
Progressive cone dystrophy
Cone–rod dystrophy
Batten disease
Hallervorden–Spatz disease
Bardet–Biedl syndrome
Mucolipidosis IV
Fucosidosis
Drug toxicity (e.g. chloroquine)
Benign concentric macular dystrophy
Fenestrated sheen dystrophy

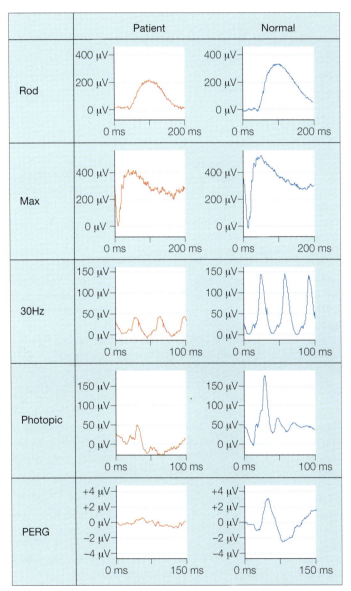

Fig. 52.24 Cone dystrophy. The rod specific and maximal (11.5 cd/m²) ERGs fall within the normal range. The 30 Hz flicker ERG is both delayed and reduced, typically present in most cone dystrophies. The photopic single flash ERG is markedly subnormal with particular reduction in the b-wave. The PERG is profoundly subnormal in keeping with marked macular involvement.

implicit time is normal and amplitude reduction is the only abnormality. A small subgroup of patients with cone dystrophy may show supernormal rod responses or rod responses within the normal range but with distinctive and specific abnormal characteristics.[197,198]

Dark adaptation studies show either a monophasic curve with no recognizable cone component, or a biphasic curve with elevated cone thresholds; rod-mediated thresholds are normal.[51] Spectral sensitivity studies show variable abnormalities of the photopic responses. In some families there is generalized depression of sensitivity across all wavelengths tested, whilst others show more specific functional deficits in the early stages of the disease. In advanced disease a typical rod sensitivity curve may be seen under both scotopic and photopic conditions.[51]

Obligate carriers of X-linked cone dystrophy may show evidence of cone dysfunction on electrophysiological or psychophysical testing.[191,196]

Progressive cone–rod dystrophy
Clinical findings
In this disorder affected patients develop the typical findings of a cone dystrophy in early life but later there is evidence of rod involvement with associated night-blindness. The age of onset is variable, but most present in the first two decades of life, with the retinal dystrophy either being isolated or associated with systemic abnormalities. Autosomal dominant, autosomal recessive and X-linked recessive inheritance have all been reported.

Fundus examination shows macular atrophy in the early stages, with peripheral RPE atrophy, retinal pigmentation, arteriolar attenuation and optic disc pallor in the late stages of the disease (Figs 52.25 and 52.26). A bull's-eye maculopathy may also be seen.[199]

Electrophysiology and psychophysics
Both rod and cone thresholds are elevated on psychophysical testing and the ERG shows reduced rod and cone amplitudes. Generalized abnormalities of rod and cone responses are seen with the cone ERGs being more abnormal than the rod ERGs. The 30 Hz cone flicker ERG implicit time is usually delayed. The maximal response a-wave is subnormal in keeping with rod photoreceptor involvement.

Molecular genetics of cone and cone–rod dystrophies
Most cases of progressive cone and cone–rod dystrophy are sporadic but autosomal dominant is the most common mode of inheritance in familial cases.[200] Most of the sporadic cases probably represent autosomal recessive inheritance. Well-documented families showing X-linked inheritance have also been reported.

Several loci and causative genes have been identified in the progressive cone dystrophies. XL cone dystrophies have been mapped to COD1 (Xp21–p11.1)[201] and COD2 (Xq27).[202] Mutations in *ABCA4*[203] and *CNGA3*[55] have been identified in autosomal recessive cone dystrophies, whilst *GCAP1* (*GUCA1A*) mutations have been reported in an autosomal dominant pedigree.[204]

In contrast, currently six genes have been associated with autosomal dominant cone–rod dystrophy:
CRX[206,207]
GUCY2D[209,210]
RIM1[211]
Peripherin/RDS[217]
GUCA1A[219]
AIPL1[221]

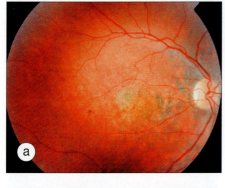
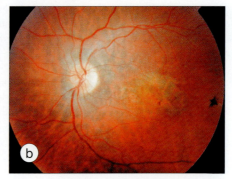

Fig. 52.25 Cone–rod dystrophy. (a, b) Bilateral macular atrophy. (c, d) Autofluorescence (AF) images showing decreased AF at the maculae corresponding to the atrophy seen ophthalmoscopically with an abnormal mottled appearance of the surrounding retina, with areas of relative increased and decreased AF.

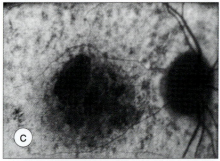
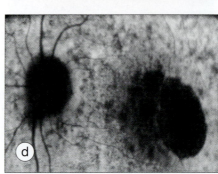

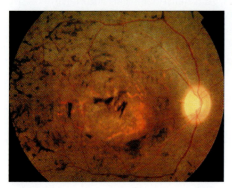

Fig. 52.26 Cone–rod dystrophy. End-stage disease with marked macular atrophy, retinal pigmentation and arteriolar narrowing.

Mutations in *ABCA4* have been shown to date to be the commonest cause of autosomal recessive cone–rod dystrophy.[203,208] *RPGRIP1* mutations have also been identified in autosomal recessive pedigrees,[218] whilst mutations in *RPGR*, the gene encoding the protein that interacts with RPGRIP1, have been associated with X-linked families.[214,215] The loci and genes identified in the cone–rod dystrophies are summarized in Table 52.6.

Goldmann–Favre disease and enhanced S-cone syndrome

Clinical findings and electrophysiology

Goldman–Favre is a rare autosomal recessive disorder characterized by gradual visual loss or night-blindness with ocular findings that include liquefaction of the vitreous, macular retinoschisis and peripheral retinal pigment epithelial atrophy and pigmentation. Peripheral retinoschisis and cataract may also occur. The retinal dystrophy is progressive resulting in extensive visual field loss and variable central visual loss. Fluorescein angiography may show evidence of peripheral capillary closure and vascular leakage.[222] ERG is markedly abnormal or undetectable. Studies of patients with the Goldmann–Favre syndrome using spectral ERG have demonstrated that S-cones are less affected than the mid-spectral cones.[223] This finding suggests that there is overlap between Goldmann–Favre syndrome and the enhanced S-cone syndrome (ESCS) where there are increased numbers of cones responsive to short wavelength light, nyctalopia and foveal schisis/cysts[224,225] (Fig. 52.27). Indeed some authorities believe that the Goldmann–Favre syndrome represents severe ESCS. Although the macular appearance may be similar, the vitreous changes, peripheral retinopathy, ERG abnormalities and mode of inheritance help differentiate this condition from X-linked juvenile retinoschisis and inherited forms of isolated foveal schisis.

The pigmentary deposition in ESCS is at the level of the RPE rather than intra-retinal, has a nummular appearance and tends to be mid-peripheral. Despite this characteristic appearance, patients are often mistaken for RP. The ERG in ESCS is diagnostic (Fig. 52.28). The responses to the same intensity flash under photopic and scotopic conditions are of similar waveform, being simplified and very delayed. In addition, the amplitude of the 30 Hz flicker ERG, which in a normal subject falls between that of the photopic single flash a- and b-waves, is usually of lower amplitude than the photopic a-wave.

Molecular genetics and pathogenesis

Mutations in *NR2E3* (encoding a transcription factor) have been identified in ESCS and Goldmann–Favre; the gene is believed to play a role in determining cone cell fate.[226,227] In ESCS there is evidence of a greater than normal number of S-cones, with mutation in *NR2E3* thought to cause disordered cone cell differentiation, possibly by encouraging default to the S-cone pathway and thereby altering the relative ratio of cone subtypes. A small number of cones co-express L/M- and S-opsins.[227]

CONCLUSIONS

Inherited retinal disorders are a common cause of childhood blindness and unfortunately most are not currently amenable to

Table 52.6 Cone–rod dystrophies (CORDs) with identified genes and known chromosomal loci

CORD; OMIM number	Mode of inheritance	Chromosome locus	Mutated gene	Reference
CORD1; 600624	Autosomal recessive	18q21.1–q21.3	Not identified	205
CORD2; 120970	Autosomal dominant	19q13.1–q13.2	CRX	206, 207
CORD3; 604116	Autosomal recessive	1p21–p13	ABCA4	208
CORD5 & CORD6; 600977 & 601777	Autosomal dominant	17p13–p12	GUCY2D	209, 210
CORD7; 603649	Autosomal dominant	6q14	RIM1	211
CORD8; 605549	Autosomal recessive	1q12–q24	Not identified	212
CORD	Autosomal recessive	8p11	Not identified	213
CORD; 304020	X-linked	Xp21.1–p11.3 (COD1)	RPGR	214, 215
CORD	X-linked	Xp11.4–q13.1 (COD4)	Not identified	216
CORD; 179605	Autosomal dominant	6p21.2–cen	Peripherin/RDS	217
CORD; 601691	Autosomal recessive	1p21–p13	ABCA4	203
CORD9; 608194	Autosomal recessive	14q11	RPGRIP1	218
CORD; 600053	Autosomal recessive	2q11	CNGA3	55
CORD; 600364	Autosomal dominant	6p21.1	GUCA1A	219
CORD; 604011	–	17q11.2	UNC119	220
CORD; 604392	Autosomal dominant	17p13.1	AIPL1	221

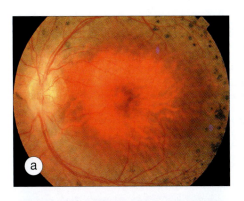
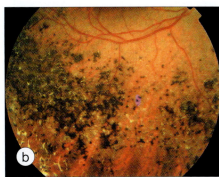
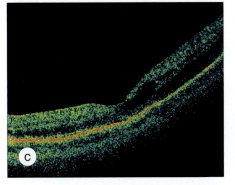
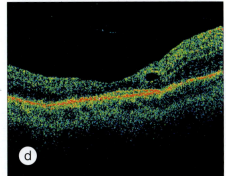

Fig. 52.27 Enhanced S-cone syndrome. (a, b) showing typical pigment clumps seen at the posterior pole and macular atrophy. (c, d) Optical coherence tomography images showing bilateral foveal cysts.

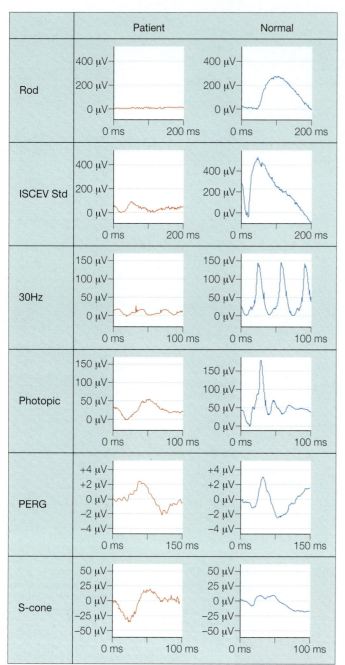

Fig. 52.28 Enhanced S-cone syndrome (ESCS). The rod-specific ERG is undetectable in keeping with the known absence of rods in this disorder. However, the two main diagnostic features are, firstly, the similarity in waveform between the photopic and scotopic ERG to the same stimulus, both of which show a simplified grossly delayed waveform, and, secondly, the amplitude of the grossly delayed 30 Hz flicker ERG being lower than that of the photopic a-wave. In a normal subject, the 30 Hz flicker ERG amplitude always falls between that of the photopic a-wave and the photopic b-wave. Note the profoundly delayed PERG, often present when the PERG is detectable in this disorder, and the increased sensitivity to short wavelength stimulation revealed by specific S-cone ERG recording (5 ms blue stimulus on a bright orange background). In a normal subject, the S-cone ERG consists of two components: a late S-cone specific component at ~50 ms and a L/M-cone component at ~30 ms. The earlier component is not present in the patient, and the later component is enhanced.

any form of treatment. Advances in molecular biology have led to the identification of many of the causative genetic mutations and it is likely that over the next few years the molecular pathology of most disorders will be known. This is the first stage in understanding the mechanisms that lead to photoreceptor cell death. Treatment strategies aimed at prolonging photoreceptor survival are currently being investigated in animal models, and include the use of exogenous growth factors,[228] gene therapy, and RPE or photoreceptor transplantation.[229] Gene therapy has recently been shown to have great potential.[108,109,230,231] Recent advances in stem cell biology are also now being applied to retinal disorders. Another approach, more applicable to those patients with minimal residual visual function, is the development of an artificial retina.[232] It is hoped that the success of some of these strategies in animal models will lead to human treatment trials in the near future. There is cautious optimism that treatment may at last become possible for some genetic retinal disease.

REFERENCES

1. Rosenberg T, Haim M, Piczenik Y, et al. Autosomal dominant stationary night-blindness. A large family rediscovered. Acta Ophthalmol 1991; 69: 694–703.
2. Price MJ, Judisch GF, Thompson HS. X-linked congenital stationary night-blindness with myopia and nystagmus without clinical complaints of nyctalopia. J Pediatr Ophthalmol Strabismus 1988; 25: 33–6.
3. Weleber RG, Tongue AC. Congenital stationary night-blindness presenting as Leber's congenital amaurosis. Arch Ophthalmol 1987; 105: 360–4.
4. Miyake Y, Yagasaki K, Horiguchi M, et al. Congenital stationary night-blindness with negative electroretinogram. Arch Ophthalmol 1986; 104: 1013–20.
5. Miyake Y, Horiguchi M, Terasaki H, et al. Scotopic threshold response in complete and incomplete types of congenital stationary night-blindness. Invest Ophthalmol Vis Sci 1994; 35: 3770–5.
6. Fishman GA, Birch DG, Holder GE, et al. Electrophysiologic Testing in Disorders of the Retina, Optic Nerve, and Visual Pathway. 2nd edn. Ophthalmology Monograph 2. San Francisco: The Foundation of the American Academy of Ophthalmology; 2001.
7. Krill AE. Congenital stationary night-blindness. In: Krill AE, ed. Hereditary Retinal and Choroidal Disease, Vol. II. London: Harper & Row; 1977: 391–417.
8. Krill AE, Martin D. Photopic abnormalities in congenital stationary night-blindness. Invest Ophthalmol Vis Sci 1971; 107: 625–36.
9. Sieving PA, Richards JE, Bingham EL, et al. Dominant congenital complete nyctalopia and Gly90Asp rhodopsin mutation. Invest Ophthalmol Vis Sci 1992; 33: 1397.
10. Dryja TP, Berson EL, Rao VR, et al. Heterozygous missense mutation in the rhodopsin gene as a cause of congenital stationary night-blindness. Nature Genet 1993; 4: 280–3.
11. Dryja TP, Hahn LB, Reboul T, et al. Missense mutation in the gene encoding the alpha subunit of rod transducin in the Nougaret form of congenital stationary night-blindness. Nat Genet 1996; 13: 358–60.
12. Gal A, Orth U, Baehr W, et al. Heterozygous missense mutation in the rod cGMP phosphodiesterase beta subunit gene in autosomal dominant stationary night-blindness. Nat Genet 1994; 7: 64–8.
13. Muradov KG, Granovsky AE, Artemyev NO. Mutation in rod PDE6 linked to congenital stationary night-blindness impairs the enzyme inhibition by its gamma-subunit. Biochemistry 2003; 42: 3305–10.
14. Musarella MA, Weleber RG, Murphey WH, et al. Assignment of the gene for complete X-linked congenital stationary night-blindness (CNSB1) to chromosome Xp11.3. Genomics 1989; 5: 727–37.
15. Bech-Hansen NT, Naylor MJ, Maybaum TA, et al. Loss-of-function mutations in a calcium-channel alpha1-subunit gene in Xp11.23 cause incomplete X-linked congenital stationary night-blindness. Nat Genet 1998; 19: 264–7.

16. Strom TM, Nyakatura G, Apfelstedt-Sylla E, et al. An L-type calcium-channel gene mutated in incomplete X-linked congenital stationary night-blindness. Nat Genet 1998; 19: 260–3.

17. Zito I, Allen LE, Patel RJ, et al. Mutations in the CACNA1F and NYX genes in British CSNBX families. Hum Mutat 2003; 21: 169.

18. Boycott KM, Maybaum TA, Naylor MJ, et al. A summary of 20 CACNA1F mutations identified in 36 families with incomplete X-linked congenital stationary night-blindness, and characterization of splice variants. Hum Genet 2001; 108: 91–7.

19. Bech-Hansen NT, Naylor MJ, Maybaum TA, et al. Mutations in NYX, encoding the leucine-rich proteoglycan nyctalopin, cause X-linked complete congenital stationary night-blindness. Nat Genet 2000; 26: 319–23.

20. Pusch CM, Zeitz C, Brandau O, et al. The complete form of X-linked congenital stationary night-blindness is caused by mutations in a gene encoding a leucine-rich repeat protein. Nat Genet 2000; 26: 324–7.

21. Boycott KM, Pearce WG, Bech-Hansen NT. Clinical variability among patients with incomplete X-linked congenital stationary night-blindness and a founder mutation in CACNA1F. Can J Ophthalmol 2000; 35: 204–13.

22. Nakamura M, Ito S, Piao CH, et al. Retinal and optic disc atrophy associated with a CACNA1F mutation in a Japanese family. Arch Ophthalmol 2003; 121: 1028–33.

23. Jacobi FK, Andreasson S, Langrova H, et al. Phenotypic expression of the complete type of X-linked congenital stationary night-blindness in patients with different mutations in the NYX gene. Graefes Arch Clin Exp Ophthalmol 2002; 240: 822–8.

24. Bergen AA, ten Brink JB, Riemslag F, et al. Localization of a novel X-linked congenital stationary night-blindness locus: close linkage to the RP3 type retinitis pigmentosa gene region. Hum Mol Genet 1995; 4: 931–5.

25. Forsius H, Eriksson AW. Ein neues augensyndrom mit X-chromosomaler transmission. Klin Monatsbl Augenheilkd 1964; 144: 447–57.

26. van Dorp DB, Eriksson AW, Delleman JW, et al. Aland eye disease—no albino misrouting. Clin Genet 1985; 28: 526–31.

27. Hawksworth NR, Headland S, Good P, et al. Åland eye disease: clinical and electrophysiological studies of a Welsh family. Br J Ophthalmol 1995; 79: 424–30.

28. Glass IA, Good P, Coleman MP, et al. Genetic mapping of cone and rod dysfunction (Åland eye disease) to the proximal short arm of the human X chromosome. J Med Genet 1993; 30: 1044–50.

29. Aldred MA, Kry KL, Sharp DM, et al. Linkage analysis in X-linked congenital stationary night-blindness. Genomics 1992; 14: 99–104.

30. Wutz K, Sauer C, Zrenner E, et al. Thirty distinct CACNA1F mutations in 33 families with incomplete type of XLCSNB and Cacna1f expression profiling in mouse retina. Eur J Hum Genet 2002; 10: 449–56.

31. Winn S, Tasman JW, Spaeth G, et al. Ogouchi's disease in negroes. Arch Ophthalmol 1968; 81: 501–7.

32. Fuchs S, Nakazawa M, Maw M, et al. A homozygous 1 base pair deletion in the arrestin gene is a frequent cause of Ogouchi's disease in Japanese. Nature Genet 1995; 10: 360–2.

33. Yoshii M, Murakami A, Akeo K, et al. Visual function and gene analysis in a family with Oguchi's disease. Ophthalmic Res 1998; 30: 394–401.

34. Yamamoto S, Sippel KC, Berson EL, et al. Defects in the rhodopsin kinase gene in the Oguchi form of stationary night-blindness. Nat Genet 1997; 15: 175–8.

35. Khani SC, Nielsen L, Vogt TM. Biochemical evidence for pathogenicity of rhodopsin kinase mutations correlated with the Oguchi form of congenital stationary night-blindness. Proc Natl Acad Sci USA 1998; 95: 2824–7.

36. Chen J, Simon MI, Matthes MT, et al. Increased susceptibility to light damage in an arrestin knockout mouse model of Oguchi disease (stationary night-blindness). Invest Ophthalmol Vis Sci 1999; 40: 2978–82.

37. Chen CK, Burns ME, Spencer M, et al. Abnormal photoresponses and light-induced apoptosis in rods lacking rhodopsin kinase. Proc Natl Acad Sci USA 1999; 96: 3718–22.

38. Carr RE, Rupps H, Siegel IM. Visual pigment kinetics and adaptation in fundus albipunctatus. Doc Ophthalmol Proc Ser 1974; 4: 193–204.

39. Miyake Y, Shiroyama N, Sugita S, Horiguchi M, Yagasaki K. Fundus albipunctatus associated with cone dystrophy. Br J Ophthalmol 1992; 76: 375–9.

40. Yamamoto H, Simon A, Eriksson U, et al. Mutations in the gene encoding 11-cis retinol dehydrogenase cause delayed dark adaptation and fundus albipunctatus. Nat Genet 1999; 22: 188–91.

41. Michaelides M, Hunt DM, Moore AT. The cone dysfunction syndromes. Br J Ophthalmol 2004; 88: 291–7.

42. Nathans J, Piantadida TP, Eddy RI, et al. Molecular genetics of inherited variation in human color vision. Science 1986; 232: 203–10.

43. Nathans J, Thomas D, Hogness DS. Molecular genetics of human vision: the genes encoding blue, green, and red pigments. Science 1986; 232: 193–203.

44. Weitz CJ, Miyake Y, Shinzato K. Human tritanopia associated with two amino acid substitutions in the blue sensitive opsin. Am J Hum Genet 1992; 50: 498–507.

45. Krill AE. Congenital color vision defects. In: Krill AE, ed. Hereditary Retinal and Choroidal Disease, Vol II. London: Harper & Row; 1977: 355–90.

46. Neitz M, Neitz J. Molecular genetics of color vision and color vision defects. Arch Ophthalmol 2000; 118: 691–700.

47. Sharpe LT, van Norrend D, Nordby K. Pigment regeneration, visual adaptation and spectral sensitivity in the achromat. Clin Vis Sci 1988; 3: 9–17.

48. Price MJ, Thompson HS, Judisch FG, et al. Pupillary constriction to darkness. Br J Ophthalmol 1985; 69: 205–11.

49. Falls HF, Wolter JR, Alpern M. Typical total monochromacy. Arch Ophthalmol 1965; 74: 610–16.

50. Glickstein M, Heath GG. Receptors in the monochromat eye. Vision Res 1975; 15: 633–6.

51. Krill AE. Cone degenerations. In: Krill AE, ed. Hereditary Retinal and Choroidal Disease, Vol II. London: Harper & Row; 1977: 335–90.

52. Andreasson S, Tornquist K. Electroretinograms in patients with achromatopsia. Acta Ophthalmologica 1991; 69: 711–16.

53. Pentao L, Lewis RA, Ledbetter DH, et al. Maternal uniparental isodisomy of chromosome 14: association with autosomal recessive rod monochromacy. Am J Hum Genet 1992; 50: 690–9.

54. Kohl S, Marx T, Giddings I, et al. Total color-blindness is caused by mutations in the gene encoding the alpha-subunit of the cone photoreceptor cGMP-gated cation channel. Nat Genet 1998; 19: 257–9.

55. Wissinger B, Gamer D, Jägle H, et al. CNGA3 mutations in hereditary cone photoreceptor disorders. Am J Hum Genet 2001; 69: 722–37.

56. Johnson S, Michaelides M, Aligianis IA, et al. Achromatopsia caused by novel mutations in both CNGA3 and CNGB3. J Med Genet 2004; 41: e20.

57. Biel M, Seeliger M, Pfeifer A, et al. Selective loss of cone function in mice lacking the cyclic nucleotide-gated channel CNG3. Proc Natl Acad Sci USA 1999; 96: 7553–7.

58. Sundin OH, Yang J-M, Li Y, et al. Genetic basis of total color-blindness among the Pingelapese islanders. Nat Genet 2000; 25: 289–93.

59. Kohl S, Baumann B, Broghammer M, et al. Mutations in the CNGB3 gene encoding the beta-subunit of the cone photoreceptor cGMP-gated channel are responsible for achromatopsia (ACHM3) linked to chromosome 8q21. Hum Mol Genet 2000; 9: 2107–16.

60. Finn JT, Krautwurst D, Schroeder JE, et al. Functional co-assembly among subunits of cyclic-nucleotide-activated, nonselective cation channels, and across species from nematode to human. Biophys J 1998; 74: 1333–45.

61. Kohl S, Baumann B, Rosenberg T, et al. Mutations in the cone photoreceptor G-protein alpha-subunit gene GNAT2 in patients with achromatopsia. Am J Hum Genet 2002; 71: 422–5.

62. Aligianis IA, Forshew T, Johnson S, et al. Mapping of a novel locus for achromatopsia (ACHM4) to 1p and identification of a germline mutation in the α-subunit of cone transducin (GNAT2). J Med Genet 2002; 39: 656–60.

63. Michaelides M, Aligianis A, Holder GE, et al. Cone dystrophy phenotype associated with a frameshift mutation (M280fsX291) in the α-subunit of cone-specific transducin (GNAT2). Br J Ophthalmol 2003; 87: 1317–20.

64. Pokorny J, Smith VC, Pinckers AJ, et al. Classification of complete and incomplete autosomal recessive achromatopsia. Graefes Arch Clin Exp Ophthalmol 1982; 219: 121–30.

65. Smith VC, Pokorny J, Newell FW. Autosomal recessive incomplete achromatopsia with protan luminosity function. Ophthalmologica 1978; 177: 197–207.

66. Smith VC, Pokorny J, Newell FW. Autosomal recessive incomplete achromatopsia with deutan luminosity. Am J Ophthalmol 1979; 87: 93–402.

67. van Norren D, de Vries-de Mol EC. A case of incomplete achromatopsia of the deutan type. Doc Ophthalmol 1981; 51: 365–72.

68. Gottlob I. Eye movement abnormalities in carriers of blue cone monochromatism. Invest Ophthalmol Vis Sci 1994; 35: 3556–60.

69. Fleischman JA, O'Donnell FE Jr. Congenital X-linked incomplete achromatopsia. Evidence for slow progression, carrier fundus findings, and possible genetic linkage with glucose-6-phosphate dehydrogenase locus. Arch Ophthalmol 1981; 99: 468–72.

70. Nathans J, Davenport CM, Maumenee IH, et al. Molecular genetics of human blue cone monochromacy. Science 1989; 245: 831–8.

71. Ayyagari R, Kakuk LE, Coats EL, et al. Bilateral macular atrophy in blue cone monochromacy (BCM) with loss of the locus control region (LCR) and part of the red pigment gene. Mol Vis 1999; 5: 13–18.

72. Gouras P, MacKay CJ. Electroretinographic responses of the short-wavelength-sensitive cones. Invest Ophthalmol Vis Sci 1990; 31: 1203–9.

73. Berson EL, Sandberg MA, Maguire A. Electroretinogram in carriers of blue cone monochromatism. Am J Ophthalmol 1986; 102: 254–61.

74. Weis AH, Biersdorf WR. Blue cone monochromatism. J Pediatr Ophthalmol Strabismus 1989; 26: 218–23.

75. Berson EL, Sandberg MA, Rosner B, et al. Color plates to help identify patients with blue cone monochromatism. Am J Ophthalmol 1983; 95: 741–7.

76. Haegerstrom-Portnoy G, Schneck ME, Verdon WA, et al. Clinical vision characteristics of the congenital achromatopsias. II. Color vision. Optom Vis Sci 1996; 73: 457–65.

77. Nathans J, Maumenee IH, Zrenner E, et al. Genetic heterogeneity among blue-cone monochromats. Am J Hum Genet 1993; 53: 987–1000.

78. Kazmi MA, Sakmar TP, Ostrer H. Mutation of a conserved cysteine in the X-linked cone opsins causes color vision deficiencies by disrupting protein folding and stability. Invest Ophthalmol Vis Sci 1997; 38: 1074–81.

79. Reyniers E, Van Thienen MN, Meire F, et al. Gene conversion between red and defective green opsin gene in blue cone monochromacy. Genomics 1995; 29: 323–8.

80. Ladekjaer-Mikkelsen AS, Rosenberg T, Jorgensen AL. A new mechanism in blue cone monochromatism. Hum Genet 1996; 98: 403–8.

81. Ayyagari R, Kakuk LE, Bingham EL, et al. Spectrum of color gene deletions and phenotype in patients with blue cone monochromacy. Hum Genet 2000; 107: 75–82.

82. van Lith GHM. General cone dysfunction without achromatopsia. In: Pearlman JT, ed. 10th ISCERG Symposium. Doc Ophthalmol Proc Ser 1973; 2: 175–80.

83. Michaelides M, Holder GE, Radshaw K, et al. Oligocone trichromacy—a rare and unusual cone dysfunction syndrome. Br J Ophthalmol 2004; 88: 497–500.

84. Haim M, Fledelius HC, Skarsholm D. X-linked myopia in a Danish family. Acta Ophthalmol 1988; 66: 450–6.

85. Schwartz M, Haim M, Skarsholm D. X-linked myopia: Bornholm eye disease. Linkage to DNA markers on the distal part of Xq. Clin Genet 1990; 38: 281–6.

86. Bergen AA, Pinckers AJ. Localization of a novel X-linked progressive cone dystrophy gene to Xq27: evidence for genetic heterogeneity. Am J Hum Genet 1997; 60: 1468–73.

87. Lambert SR, Sherman S, Taylor D, et al. Concordance and recessive inheritance of Leber's congenital amaurosis. Am J Med Genet 1993; 46: 275–7.

88. Sorsby A, Williams CF. Retinal aplasia as a clinical entity. Br Med J 1960; 1: 293–7.

89. Schappert-Kimmijser J, Henkes HE, van den Bosch J. Amaurosis congenita (Leber). Arch Ophthalmol 1959; 61: 211–18.

90. Sullivan TJ, Lambert SR, Buncic JR, et al. The optic disc in Leber's congenital amaurosis. J Pediatr Ophthalmol Strabismus 1992; 29: 246–9.

91. Lambert SR, Kriss A, Taylor D, et al. Leber's congenital amaurosis: a follow-up diagnostic reappraisal of 75 patients. Am J Ophthalmol 1989; 107: 624–31.

92. Vaizey MJ, Sanders MD, Wybar KC, et al. Neurological abnormalities in congenital amaurosis of Leber. Review of 30 cases. Arch Dis Child 1977; 52: 399–402.

93. Moore AT, Taylor DS. A syndrome of congenital retinal dystrophy and saccade palsy–a subset of Leber's amaurosis. Br J Ophthalmol 1984; 68: 421–31.

94. Nickel B, Hoyt CS. Leber's congenital amaurosis. Is mental retardation a frequently associated defect? Arch Ophthalmol 1982; 100: 1089–92.

95. Perrault I, Rozet JM, Calvas P, et al. Retinal-specific guanylate cyclase gene mutations in Leber's congenital amaurosis. Nat Genet 1996; 14: 461–4.

96. Rozet JM, Perrault I, Gerber S, et al. Complete abolition of the retinal-specific guanylyl cyclase (retGC-1) catalytic ability consistently leads to Leber congenital amaurosis (LCA). Invest Ophthalmol Vis Sci 2001; 42: 1190–2.

97. Marlhens F, Bareil C, Griffoin JM, et al. Mutations in RPE65 cause Leber's congenital amaurosis. Nat Genet 1997; 17: 139–41.

98. Gu SM, Thompson DA, Srikumari CR, et al. Mutations in RPE65 cause autosomal recessive childhood-onset severe retinal dystrophy. Nat Genet 1997; 17: 194–7.

99. Freund CL, Wang QL, Chen S, et al. De novo mutations in the CRX homeobox gene associated with Leber congenital amaurosis. Nat Genet 1998; 18: 311–2.

100. Jacobson SG, Cideciyan AV, Huang Y, et al. Retinal degenerations with truncation mutations in the cone–rod homeobox (CRX) gene. Invest Ophthalmol Vis Sci 1998; 39: 2417–26.

101. Sohocki MM, Bowne SJ, Sullivan LS, et al. Mutations in a new photoreceptor–pineal gene on 17p cause Leber congenital amaurosis. Nat Genet 2000; 24: 79–83.

102. Damji KF, Sohocki MM, Khan R, et al. Leber's congenital amaurosis with anterior keratoconus in Pakistani families is caused by the Trp278X mutation in the AIPL1 gene on 17p. Can J Ophthalmol 2001; 36: 252–9.

103. Lotery AJ, Jacobson SG, Fishman GA, et al. Mutations in the CRB1 gene cause Leber congenital amaurosis. Arch Ophthalmol 2001; 119: 415–20.

104. den Hollander AI, Heckenlively JR, van den Born LI, et al. Leber congenital amaurosis and retinitis pigmentosa with Coats-like exudative vasculopathy are associated with mutations in the crumbs homologue 1 (CRB1) gene. Am J Hum Genet 2001; 69: 198–203.

105. Dryja TP, Adams SM, Grimsby JL, et al. Null RPGRIP1 alleles in patients with Leber congenital amaurosis. Am J Hum Genet 2001; 68: 1295–8.

106. Cremers FP, van den Hurk JA, den Hollander AI. Molecular genetics of Leber congenital amaurosis. Hum Mol Genet 2002; 11: 1169–76.

107. Milam AH, Barakat MR, Gupta N, et al. Clinicopathologic effects of mutant GUCY2D in Leber congenital amaurosis. Ophthalmology 2003; 110: 549–58.

108. Acland GM, Aguirre GD, Ray J, et al. Gene therapy restores vision in a canine model of childhood blindness. Nat Genet 2001; 28: 92–5.

109. Narfstrom K, Katz ML, Ford M, et al. In vivo gene therapy in young and adult RPE65$^{-/-}$ dogs produces long-term visual improvement. J Hered 2003; 94: 31–7.

110. Moore AT, Fitzke FW, Kemp CM, et al. Abnormal dark adaptation kinetics in autosomal dominant sector retinitis pigmentosa due to a rod opsin mutation. Br J Ophthalmol 1992; 76: 465–9.

111. den Hollander AI, ten Brink JB, de Kok YJ, et al. Mutations in a human homologue of Drosophila crumbs cause retinitis pigmentosa (RP12). Nat Genet 1999; 23: 217–21.

112. Eichers ER, Green JS, Stockton DW, et al. Newfoundland rod–cone dystrophy, an early-onset retinal dystrophy, is caused by splice-junction mutations in RLBP1. Am J Hum Genet 2002; 70: 955–64.

6666

113. Burstedt MS, Sandgren O, Holmgren G, et al. Bothnia dystrophy caused by mutations in the cellular retinaldehyde-binding protein gene (RLBP1) on chromosome 15q26. Invest Ophthalmol Vis Sci 1999; 40: 995–1000.

114. Massof RW, Finkelstein D. Two forms of autosomal dominant primary retinitis pigmentosa. Doc Ophthalmol 1981; 51: 289–346.

115. Bird AC. Retinal photoreceptor dystrophies. Am J Ophthalmol 1995; 118: 543–62.

116. Evans K, Moore AT, Jubb C, et al. Bimodal expressivity in autosomal dominant retinitis pigmentosa genetically linked to chromosome 19q. Br J Ophthalmol 1995; 99: 841–6.

117. Kim RY, Fitzke FW, Moore AT, et al. Autosomal dominant retinitis pigmentosa mapping to chromosome 7p exhibits variable expression. Br J Ophthalmol 1995; 79: 23–7.

118. Inglehearn CF, Carter SA, Keen TJ, et al. A new locus for autosomal dominant retinitis pigmentosa on chromosome 7p. Nat Genet 1993; 4: 51–3.

119. al Maghtheh M, Inglehearn CF, Keen TJ, et al. Identification of a sixth locus for autosomal dominant retinitis pigmentosa on chromosome 19. Hum Mol Genet 1994; 3: 351–4.

120. Keen TJ, Hims MM, McKie AB, et al. Mutations in a protein target of the Pim-1 kinase associated with the RP9 form of autosomal dominant retinitis pigmentosa. Eur J Hum Genet 2002; 10: 245–9.

121. Vithana EN, Abu-Safieh L, Allen MJ, et al. A human homolog of yeast pre-mRNA splicing gene, PRPF31, underlies autosomal dominant retinitis pigmentosa on chromosome 19q13.4 (RP11). Mol Cell 2001; 8: 375–81.

122. Bird AC. X-linked retinitis pigmentosa. Br J Ophthalmol 1975; 59: 177–99.

123. Ernst W, Clover G, Faulkner DJ. X-linked retinitis pigmentosa: reduced rod flicker sensitivity in heterozygous females. Invest Ophthalmol Vis Sci 1981; 20: 812–16.

124. Friedrich U, Warburg M, Jorgensen AL. X-inactivation pattern in carriers of X-linked retinitis pigmentosa: a valuable means of prognostic evaluation. Hum Genet 1993; 92: 359–63.

125. Carr RE, Siegel IM. Unilateral retinitis pigmentosa. Arch Ophthalmol 1973; 90: 21–6.

126. Dryja TP, McGee TI, Hahn LB, et al. Mutations within the rhodopsin gene in patients with autosomal dominant retinitis pigmentosa. New Eng J Med 1990; 323: 1302–7.

127. Farrar GJ, Findlay JBC, Kumar-Singh R, et al. Autosomal dominant retinitis pigmentosa: a novel mutation in the rhodopsin gene in the original 3q linked family. Hum Mol Genet 1992; 1: 769–71.

128. Kajiwara K, Berson EL, Dryja TP. Digenic retinitis pigmentosa due to mutations at the unlinked peripherin/RDS and ROM1 loci. Science 1994; 264: 1604–8.

129. Kajiwara K, Hahn LB, Mukai S, et al. Mutations in the human retinal degeneration slow gene in autosomal dominant retinitis pigmentosa. Nature 1991; 354: 480–3.

130. Pierce EA, Quinn T, Meehan T, et al. Mutations in a gene encoding a new oxygen-regulated photoreceptor protein cause dominant retinitis pigmentosa. Nat Genet 1999; 22: 248–54.

131. Morimura H, Saindelle-Ribeaudeau F, Berson EL, et al. Mutations in RGR, encoding a light-sensitive opsin homologue, in patients with retinitis pigmentosa. Nat Genet 1999; 23: 393–4.

132. Bessant DA, Payne AM, Mitton KP, et al. A mutation in NRL is associated with autosomal dominant retinitis pigmentosa. Nat Genet 1999; 21: 355–6.

133. Sohocki MM, Sullivan LS, Mintz-Hittner HA, et al. A range of clinical phenotypes associated with mutations in CRX, a photoreceptor transcription-factor gene. Am J Hum Genet 1998; 63: 1307–15.

134. Wada Y, Abe T, Takeshita T, et al. Mutation of human retinal fascin gene (FSCN2) causes autosomal dominant retinitis pigmentosa. Invest Ophthal Vis Sci 2001; 42: 2395–400.

135. Chakarova CF, Hims MM, Bolz H, et al. Mutations in HPRP3, a third member of pre-mRNA splicing factor genes, implicated in autosomal dominant retinitis pigmentosa. Hum Mol Genet 2002; 11: 87–92.

136. Bowne SJ, Sullivan LS, Blanton SH, et al. Mutations in the inosine monophosphate dehydrogenase 1 gene (IMPDH1) cause the RP10 form of autosomal dominant retinitis pigmentosa. Hum Mol Genet 2002; 11: 559–68.

137. McKie AB, McHale JC, Keen TJ, et al. Mutations in the pre-mRNA splicing factor gene PRPF8 in autosomal dominant retinitis pigmentosa (RP13). Hum Mol Genet 2001; 10: 1555–62.

138. Bardien S, Ebenezer N, Greenberg J, et al. An eighth locus for autosomal dominant retinitis pigmentosa is linked to chromosome 17q. Hum Mol Genet 1995; 4: 1459–62.

139. Martinez-Gimeno M, Gamundi MJ, Hernan I, et al. Mutations in the pre-mRNA splicing-factor genes PRPF3, PRPF8, and PRPF31 in Spanish families with autosomal dominant retinitis pigmentosa. Invest Ophthalmol Vis Sci 2003; 44: 2171–7.

140. Deery EC, Vithana EN, Newbold RJ, et al. Disease mechanism for retinitis pigmentosa (RP11) caused by mutations in the splicing factor gene PRPF31. Hum Mol Genet 2002; 11: 3209–19.

141. al Maghtheh M, Gregory CY, Inglehearn CF, et al. Rhodopsin mutations in autosomal dominant retinitis pigmentosa. Hum Mutat 1993; 2: 249–55.

142. Rosenfeld PJ, Cowley GS, McGee TL, et al. A null mutation in the rhodopsin gene causes rod photoreceptor dysfunction and autosomal recessive retinitis pigmentosa. Nat Genet 1992; 1: 209–13.

143. Dryja TP, Li T. Molecular genetics of retinitis pigmentosa. Hum Mol Genet 1995; 4: 1739–43.

144. Hims MM, Diager SP, Inglehearn CF. Retinitis pigmentosa: genes, proteins and prospects. Dev Ophthalmol 2003; 37: 109–25.

145. Wang Q, Chen Q, Zhao K, et al. Update on the molecular genetics of retinitis pigmentosa. Ophthalmic Genet 2001; 22: 133–54.

146. Morimura H, Fishman GA, Grover SA, et al. Mutations in the RPE65 gene in patients with autosomal recessive retinitis pigmentosa or Leber congenital amaurosis. Proc Natl Acad Sci USA 1998; 95: 3088–93.

147. Martinez-Mir A, Paloma E, Allikmets R, et al. Retinitis pigmentosa caused by a homozygous mutation in the Stargardt disease gene ABCR. Nat Genet 1998; 18: 11–12.

148. Dryja TP, Finn JT, Peng Y-W, et al. Mutations in the gene encoding the alpha subunit of the rod cGMP-gated channel in autosomal recessive retinitis pigmentosa. Proc Natl Acad Sci USA 1995; 92: 10177–81.

149. Bareil C, Hamel CP, Delague V, et al. Segregation of a mutation in CNGB1 encoding the beta-subunit of the rod cGMP-gated channel in a family with autosomal recessive retinitis pigmentosa. Hum Genet 2001; 108: 328–34.

150. Ruiz A, Kuehn MH, Andorf JL, et al. Genomic organization and mutation analysis of the gene encoding lecithin retinol acyltransferase in human retinal pigment epithelium. Invest Ophthalmol Vis Sci 2001; 42: 31–7.

151. Gal A, Li Y, Thompson DA, et al. Mutations in MERTK, the human orthologue of the RCS rat retinal dystrophy gene, cause retinitis pigmentosa. Nat Genet 2000; 26: 270–1.

152. Huang SH, Pittler SJ, Huang X, et al. Autosomal recessive retinitis pigmentosa caused by mutations in the alpha subunit of rod cGMP phosphodiesterase. Nat Genet 1995; 11: 468–71.

153. McLaughlin ME, Sandberg MA, Berson EL, Dryja TP. Recessive mutations in the gene encoding the beta-subunit of rod phosphodiesterase in patients with retinitis pigmentosa. Nat Genet 1993; 4: 130–4.

154. Maw MA, Kennedy B, Knight A, et al. Mutation of the gene encoding cellular retinaldehyde-binding protein in autosomal recessive retinitis pigmentosa. Nat Genet 1997; 17: 198–200.

155. Nakazawa M, Wada Y, Tamai M. Arrestin gene mutations in autosomal recessive retinitis pigmentosa. Arch Ophthalmol 1998; 116: 498–501.

156. Banerjee P, Kleyn PW, Knowles JA, et al. TULP1 mutation in two extended Dominican kindreds with autosomal recessive retinitis pigmentosa. Nat Genet 1998; 18: 177–9.

157. Rivolta C, Sweklo EA, Berson EL, et al. Missense mutation in the USH2A gene: association with recessive retinitis pigmentosa without hearing loss. Am J Hum Genet 2000; 66: 1975–8.

158. Finckh U, Xu S, Kumaramanickavel G, et al. Homozygosity mapping of autosomal recessive retinitis pigmentosa locus (RP22) on chromosome 16p12.1-p12.3. Genomics 1998; 48: 341–5.

159. Ruiz A, Borrego S, Marcos I, et al. A major locus for autosomal recessive retinitis pigmentosa on 6q, determined by homozygosity mapping of chromosomal regions that contain gamma-aminobutyric acid-receptor clusters. Am J Hum Genet 1998; 62: 1452–9.

160. Bayes M, Goldaracena B, Martinez-Mir A, et al. A new autosomal recessive retinitis pigmentosa locus maps on chromosome 2q31–q33. J Med Genet 1998; 35: 141–5.

161. Gu S, Kumaramanickavel G, Srikumari CR, et al. Autosomal recessive retinitis pigmentosa locus RP28 maps between D2S1337 and D2S286 on chromosome 2p11–p15 in an Indian family. J Med Genet 1999; 36: 705–7.

162. Hameed A, Khaliq S, Ismail M, et al. A new locus for autosomal recessive RP (RP29) mapping to chromosome 4q32–q34 in a Pakistani family. Invest Ophthalmol Vis Sci 2001; 42: 1436–8.

163. Meindl A, Dry K, Herrmann K, et al. A gene (RPGR) with homology to the RCC1 guanine nucleotide exchange factor is mutated in X-linked retinitis pigmentosa (RP3). Nat Genet 1996; 13: 35–42.

164. Roepman R, van Duijnhoven G, Rosenberg T, et al. Positional cloning of the gene for X-linked retinitis pigmentosa 3: homology with the guanine-nucleotide-exchange factor RCC1. Hum Mol Genet 1996; 5: 1035–41.

165. Schwahn U, Lenzner S, Dong J, et al. Positional cloning of the gene for X-linked retinitis pigmentosa 2. Nat Genet 1998; 19: 327–32.

166. Schwahn U, Paland N, Techritz S, et al. Mutations in the X-linked RP2 gene cause intracellular misrouting and loss of the protein. Hum Mol Genet 2001; 10: 1177–83.

167. Hardcastle AJ, Thiselton DL, Zito H, et al. Evidence for a new locus for X-linked retinitis pigmentosa (RP23). Invest Ophthalmol Vis Sci 2000; 41: 2080–6.

168. Ott J, Bhattacharya S, Chen JD, et al. Localizing multiple X chromosome-linked retinitis pigmentosa loci using multilocus homogeneity tests. Proc Natl Acad Sci USA 1990; 87: 701–4.

169. Gieser L, Fujita R, Göring HHH, et al. A novel locus (RP24) for X-linked retinitis pigmentosa maps to Xq26–q27. Am J Hum Genet 1998; 63: 1439–47.

170. Zito I, Downes SM, Patel RJ, et al. RPGR mutation associated with retinitis pigmentosa, impaired hearing, and sinorespiratory infections. J Med Genet 2003; 40: 609–15.

171. Vervoort R, Wright AF. Mutations of RPGR in X-linked retinitis pigmentosa (RP3). Hum Mutat 2002; 19: 486–500.

172. Linari M, Ueffing M, Manson F, et al. The retinitis pigmentosa GTPase regulator, RPGR, interacts with the delta subunit of rod cyclic GMP phosphodiesterase. Proc Natl Acad Sci USA 1999; 96: 1315–20.

173. Teague PW, Aldred MA, Jay M, et al. Heterogeneity analysis in 40 X-linked retinitis pigmentosa families. Am J Med Genet 1994; 55: 105–11.

174. Chapple JP, Grayson C, Hardcastle AJ, et al. Organization on the plasma membrane of the retinitis pigmentosa protein RP2: investigation of association with detergent-resistant membranes and polarized sorting. Biochem J 2003; 372: 427–33.

175. Berson EL, Rosner B, Sandberg MA, et al. A randomized trial of vitamin A and vitamin E supplementation for retinitis pigmentosa. Arch Ophthalmol 1993; 111: 761–72.

176. Traboulsi EI, Maumenee IH. Hereditary pigmented paravenous chorioretinal atrophy. Arch Ophthalmol 1986; 104: 1636–40.

177. Small K, Anderson WB. Pigmented paravenous retinochoroidal atrophy: discordant expression in monozygotic twins. Arch Ophthalmol 1991; 109: 1408–10.

178. Walt RP, Kemp CM, Lyness L, et al. Vitamin A treatment for night-blindness in primary biliary cirrhosis. Br Med J 1984; 288: 1030–1.

179. Lakhampal V, Schockett SS, Jiji R. Desferrioxamine (Desferol) induced toxic retinal pigmentary degeneration and presumed optic neuropathy. Ophthalmology 1984; 91: 443–51.

180. Rahi AH, Hungerford JL, Ahmed AI. Ocular toxicity of desferrioxamine: light microscopic, histochemical, and ultrastructural findings. Br J Ophthalmol 1986; 70: 373–81.

181. Fraunfelder FT, Fraunfelder FW, Edwards R. Ocular side effects possibly associated with isotretinoin usage. Am J Ophthalmol 2001; 132: 299–305.

182. Sieving PA, Chaudhry P, Kondo M, et al. Inhibition of the visual cycle in vivo by 13-cis-retinoic acid protects from light damage and provides a mechanism for night-blindness in isotretinoin therapy. Proc Natl Acad Sci USA 2001; 98: 1835–40.

183. Roberts MF, Fishman GA, Roberts DK, et al. Retrospective, longitudinal, and cross sectional study of visual acuity impairment in choroideraemia. Br J Ophthalmol 2002; 86: 658–62.

184. Karna J. Choroideremia: a clinical and genetic study of 84 Finnish patients and 126 female carriers. Acta Ophthalmol 1986; 176(Suppl.): 1–68.

185. Rosenberg T, Niebatir E, Yang MM. Choroideremia, congenital deafness and mental retardation in a family with an X-chromosomal deletion. Ophthalmol Paediatr Genet 1987; 8: 139–43.

186. Rodrigues MM, Ballintine EJ, Wiggert B, et al. Choroideremia: a clinical electron microscopic and biochemical report. Ophthalmology 1984; 91: 873–83.

187. Cremers PM, van der Pol DJ, van Kerkhof LP, et al. Cloning of a gene that is rearranged in patients with choroideremia. Nature 1990; 347: 674–7.

188. Schwartz M, Rosenberg T, van der Hurk JA, et al. Identification of mutations in Danish choroideremia families. Hum Mutat 1993; 2: 43–7.

189. van den Hurk JA, van de Pol DJ, Wissinger B, et al. Novel types of mutation in the choroideremia (CHM) gene: a full-length L1 insertion and an intronic mutation activating a cryptic exon. Hum Genet 2003; 113: 268–75.

190. Seabra MC, Mules EH, Hume AN. Rab GTPases, intracellular traffic and disease. Trends Mol Med 2002; 8: 23–30.

191. Reichel E, Bruce AM, Sandberg MA, et al. An electroretinographic and molecular genetic study of X-linked cone degeneration. Am J Ophthalmol 1989; 108: 540–7.

192. Kellner U, Sadowski B, Zrenner E, et al. Selective cone dystrophy with protan genotype. Invest Ophthalmol Vis Sci 1995; 36: 2381–7.

193. Went LN, van Schooneveld MJ, Oosterhuis JA. Late onset dominant cone dystrophy with early blue cone involvement. J Med Genet 1992; 29: 295–8.

194. Bresnick GH, Smith VC, Pokorny J. Autosomal dominantly inherited macular dystrophy with preferential short-wavelength sensitive cone involvement. Am J Ophthalmol 1989; 108: 265–76.

195. Uliss A, Moore AT, Bird AC. The dark choroid in posterior retinal dystrophies. Ophthalmology 1987; 94: 1423–8.

196. Jacobson DM, Thompson S, Bartley JA. X-linked progressive cone dystrophy. Clinical characteristics of affected males and female carriers. Ophthalmology 1989; 96: 885–95.

197. Gouras P, Eggers HM, Mackay C. Cone dystrophy, nyctalopia and supernormal rod responses. A new retinal degeneration. Arch Ophthalmol 1983; 101: 718–24.

198. Alexander KR, Fishman GA. Supernormal scotopic ERG in cone dystrophy. Br J Ophthalmol 1984; 68: 69–78.

199. Kurz-Levin M, Halfyard AS, Bunce C, et al. Clinical variations in assessment of Bull's eye maculopathy. Arch Ophthalmol 2002; 120: 567–75.

200. Krill AE, Deutman AF. Dominant macular degeneration. The cone dystrophies. Am J Ophthalmol 1972; 73: 352–9.

201. Meire FM, Bergen AA, De Rouck A, et al. X-linked progressive cone dystrophy. Localisation of the gene locus to Xp21–p11.1 by linkage analysis. Br J Ophthalmol 1994; 78: 103–8.

202. Bergen AA, Pinckers AJ. Localisation of a novel X-linked progressive cone dystrophy gene to Xq27: evidence for genetic heterogeneity. Am J Hum Genet 1997; 60: 1468–73.

203. Maugeri A, Klevering BJ, Rohrschneider K, et al. Mutations in the ABCA4 (ABCR) gene are the major cause of autosomal recessive cone–rod dystrophy. Am J Hum Genet 2000; 67: 960–6.

204. Payne AM, Downes SM, Bessant DA, et al. A mutation in guanylate cyclase activator 1A (GUCA1A) in autosomal dominant cone dystrophy mapping to a new locus on chromosome 6p21.1. Hum Mol Genet 1998; 7: 273–7.

205. Warburg M, Sjo O, Tranebjaerg L, et al. Deletion mapping of a retinal cone–rod dystrophy:assignment to 18q211. Am J Med Genet 1991; 39: 288–93.

206. Evans K, Fryer A, Inglehearn C, et al. Genetic linkage of cone–rod retinal dystrophy to chromosome 19q and evidence for segregation distortion. Nat Genet 1994; 6: 210–3.

207. Freund CL, Gregory-Evans CY, Furukawa T, et al. Cone–rod dystrophy due to mutations in a novel photoreceptor-specific homeobox gene (CRX) essential for maintenance of the photoreceptor. Cell 1997; 91: 543–53.

208. Cremers FP, van de Pol DJ, van Driel M, et al. Autosomal recessive retinitis pigmentosa and cone–rod dystrophy caused by splice site mutations in the Stargardt's disease gene ABCR. Hum Mol Genet 1998; 7: 355–62.

209. Kelsell RE, Gregory-Evans K, Payne AM, et al. Mutations in the retinal guanylate cyclase (RETGC-1) gene in dominant cone–rod dystrophy. Hum Mol Genet 1998; 7: 1179–84.

210. Udar N, Yelchits S, Chalukya M, et al. Identification of GUCY2D gene mutations in CORD5 families and evidence of incomplete penetrance. Hum Mutat 2003; 21: 170–1.

211. Johnson S, Halford S, Morris AG, et al. Genomic organisation and alternative splicing of human RIM1, a gene implicated in autosomal dominant cone–rod dystrophy (CORD7). Genomics 2003; 81: 304–14.

212. Khaliq S, Hameed A, Ismail M, et al. Novel locus for autosomal recessive cone–rod dystrophy CORD8 mapping to chromosome 1q12–q24. Invest Ophthalmol Vis Sci 2000; 41: 3709–12.

213. Danciger M, Hendrickson J, Lyon J, et al. CORD9 a new locus for arCRD: mapping to 8p11, estimation of frequency, evaluation of a candidate gene. Invest Ophthalmol Vis Sci 2001; 42: 2458–65.

214. Demirci FY, Rigatti BW, Wen G, et al. X-linked cone–rod dystrophy (locus COD1): identification of mutations in RPGR exon ORF15. Am J Hum Genet 2002; 70: 1049–53.

215. Mears AJ, Hiriyanna S, Vervoort R, et al. Remapping of the RP15 locus for X-linked cone–rod degeneration to Xp11.4–p21.1, and identification of a de novo insertion in the RPGR exon ORF15. Am J Hum Genet 2000; 67: 1000–3.

216. Jalkanen R, Demirci FY, Tyynismaa H, et al. A new genetic locus for X linked progressive cone–rod dystrophy. J Med Genet 2003; 40: 418–23.

217. Nakazawa M, Kikawa E, Chida Y, et al. Autosomal dominant cone–rod dystrophy associated with mutations in codon 244 (Asn244His) and codon 184 (Tyr184Ser) of the peripherin/RDS gene. Arch Ophthalmol 1996; 114: 72–8.

218. Hameed A, Abid A, Aziz A, et al. Evidence of RPGRIP1 gene mutations associated with recessive cone–rod dystrophy. J Med Genet 2003; 40: 616–9.

219. Downes SM, Holder GE, Fitzke FW, et al. Autosomal dominant cone and cone–rod dystrophy with mutations in the guanylate cyclase activator 1A gene-encoding guanylate cyclase activating protein-1. Arch Ophthalmol 2001; 119: 96–105.

220. Kobayashi A, Higashide T, Hamasaki D, et al. HRG4 (UNC119) mutation found in cone–rod dystrophy causes retinal degeneration in a transgenic model. Invest Ophthalmol Vis Sci 2000; 41: 3268–77.

221. Sohocki MM, Perrault I, Leroy BP, et al. Prevalence of AIPL1 mutations in inherited retinal degenerative disease. Mol Genet Metab 2000; 70: 142–50.

222. Fishman GA, Jampol LM, Goldberg MF. Diagnostic features of the Favre-Goldmann syndrome. Br J Ophthalmol 1976; 60: 345–53.

223. Jacobsen SG, Roman AJ, Roman MI, et al. Relatively enhanced S cone function in the Goldmann-Favre syndrome. Am J Ophthalmol 1991; 111: 446–53.

224. Jacobson SG, Marmor MF, Kemp CM, et al. SWS (blue) cone hypersensitivity in a newly identified retinal degeneration. Invest Ophthalmol Vis Sci 1990; 31: 827–38.

225. Marmor MF, Jacobson SG, Foerster MH, et al. Diagnostic clinical findings of a new syndrome with night-blindness, maculopathy, and enhanced S cone sensitivity. Am J Ophthalmol 1990; 110: 124–34.

226. Haider NB, Jacobson SG, Cideciyan AV, et al. Mutation of a nuclear receptor gene, NR2E3, causes enhanced S cone syndrome, a disorder of retinal cell fate. Nat Genet 2000; 24: 127–31.

227. Milam AH, Rose L, Cideciyan AV, et al. The nuclear receptor NR2E3 plays a role in human retinal photoreceptor differentiation and degeneration. Proc Natl Acad Sci USA 2002; 99: 473–8.

228. Tao W, Wen R, Goddard MB, et al. Encapsulated cell-based delivery of CNTF reduces photoreceptor degeneration in animal models of retinitis pigmentosa. Invest Ophthalmol Vis Sci 2002; 43: 3292–8.

229. Lund RD, Ono SJ, Keegan DJ, et al. Retinal transplantation: progress and problems in clinical application. J Leukoc Biol 2003; 74: 151–60.

230. Ali RR, Sarra GM, Stephens C, et al. Restoration of photoreceptor ultrastructure and function in retinal degeneration slow mice by gene therapy. Nat Genet 2000; 25: 306–10.

231. Dejneka NS, Rex TS, Bennett J. Gene therapy and animal models for retinal disease. Dev Ophthalmol 2003; 37: 188–98.

232. Lakhanpal RR, Yanai D, Weiland JD, et al. Advances in the development of visual prostheses. Curr Opin Ophthalmol 2003; 14: 122–7.

CHAPTER 53 Retinal Dystrophies with Systemic Associations

Isabelle M Russell-Eggitt and Andrew A M Morris

RETINAL DYSTROPHIES ASSOCIATED WITH PREDOMINANTLY NEUROLOGICAL ABNORMALITIES

This chapter discusses retinal dystrophies associated with systemic disorders. Dystrophy literally means a "nutritional failure". In this context this is a failure at the cellular level of enzymes and other proteins necessary for normal growth and health of retinal cells. Isolated retinal dystrophies and retinal dysplasia are covered in Chapters 49 and 52.

RETINAL DYSTROPHY: THE INFANT WITH AN ABNORMAL ERG, "QUICK GUIDE TO DIAGNOSIS"

History
Family history (and family examination)
Breathing irregularity, e.g. Joubert, heart failure of Alström
Developmental concern
Hearing concern
General examination
Look at the whole baby
- Dysmorphism, e.g. Zellweger: refer to genetics, search on features on syndrome database
- Pick up the baby: floppy?
- Weight above 90th centile, e.g. Bardet–Biedl, Alström, Cohen
Development: if impaired on milestones corrected for vision impairment investigate
Hair
- Brittle, e.g. trichothiodystrophy, uncombable hair-pigmentary retinal dystrophy-dental anomalies-brachydactyly
- Fine, e.g. Sensenbrenner, hypotrichosis: juvenile macular dystrophy, ectodermal dysplasia–ectrodactyly–macular dystrophy
- Premature greying, e.g. Werner syndrome
Skin
- Photosensitivity, e.g. Cockayne, trichothiodystrophy
- Acanthosis nigricans, e.g. Alström
- Recurrent infections, e.g. Cohen
- Tight atrophic, e.g. Werner
- Ichthyosis/dry scaly, e.g. trichothiodystrophy, Refsum disease, Sjögren–Larsson syndrome
Teeth
- Missing, e.g. BBS4, Sensenbrenner
- Small widely spaced, e.g. EEC
Skeletal
- Stubby fingers X-ray for cone-shaped epiphyses, e.g. Mainzer–Saldino
- Polydactyly, e.g. Bardet–Biedl, Jeune, Joubert

- Malformed chest: Jeune, Sensenbrenner
- Chondrodysplasia punctata: peroxisomal disorders
Heart
- Infantile heart failure, e.g. Alström, mitochondrial disorders
Eye examination
Chorioretinal coloboma, e.g. Joubert, Cohen syndromes
Macula
- "Coloboma", e.g. cobalamin (cbl) C disease, idiopathic infantile hypercalciuria
- "Bull's eye", e.g. Hallervorden–Spatz, Cohen syndrome
- Flecks or glistening bodies, e.g. olivopontocerebellar atrophy, gyrate atrophy, Sjögren–Larsson, primary hyperoxaluria type 1, Hallervorden–Spatz
Refraction
- Myopia, e.g. Cohen, gyrate atrophy, LCHADD, Sensenbrenner, congenital disorders of glycosylation
Ocular electrophysiology
- Cone or cone-rod pattern of dysfunction, e.g. some BBS, Alström
Hearing tests
- It is important to screen for hearing defect in all children with severe vision impairment
Blood tests
- Full blood count, e.g. neutropenia in Cohen syndrome, anemia in Cbl C disease
- Very long chain fatty acid and phytanic acid levels
- Acylcarnitines, e.g. LCHADD
Urine tests
- Routine analysis for red blood cells and protein, e.g. Bardet–Biedl, Joubert
- Organic and amino acids, e.g. CblCdisease, L-2-hydroxyglutaric aciduria
MRI
- Olivopontocerebellar anomaly, e.g. congenital disorders of glycosylation, Joubert
EEG
- Seizures, e.g. infantile Refsum, L-2-hydroxyglutaric aciduria, Sjögren–Larsson syndrome, multiple sulfatase deficiency, Hirabayashi
Renal ultrasound: a renal ultrasound should be performed on all children with severe early onset combined rod and cone retinal dystrophy
- Cystic kidneys, e.g. Leber Amaurosis, Joubert, Mainzer–Saldino syndromes
Skin biopsy
- Fibroblast culture for DNA tests, e.g. Cockayne
Genetic tests, chromosomes, gene screening
- Organelle diseases
- Retinal dystrophies associated with predominantly neurological abnormalities
- Mitochondrial disorders

ORGANELLE DISEASES AND MITOCHONDRIAL DISORDERS

Mitochondrial biochemistry and genetics are considered in Chapter 65. Retinal dystrophy occurs in many patients with respiratory chain defects but has been best documented in patients with mitochondrial DNA (mtDNA) deletions and certain mtDNA point mutations. Most mtDNA mutations are heteroplasmic, i.e. they only affect a proportion of copies of mtDNA. Clinical syndromes can usually be caused by several different mutations and, conversely, the same mutation can present in different ways depending on the level of heteroplasmy. The level of heteroplasmy is generally lower in blood than muscle and mtDNA deletions, for example, are often only detectable in muscle.

Kearns–Sayre syndrome (KSS)

KSS is characterized by progressive external ophthalmoplegia and retinal dystrophy with onset before 20 years of age. Ptosis is the commonest complaint, patients seldom suffer diplopia even when there is severe strabismus. Other features may include cerebellar ataxia, progressive hearing loss, dementia, a high CSF protein, heart block, cardiomyopathy, renal tubular disorders and endocrine abnormalities. At least 80% of patients have heteroplasmic mtDNA deletions or duplications: the "common" 4.9 kb deletion is found in 50%. Studies on muscle biopsies generally show that a proportion of fibers have cytochrome-c-oxidase deficiency and there may also be "ragged red fibers". Recurrence risks are low where the child has an mtDNA deletion, but studies may be undertaken on the mother if further reassurance is required.

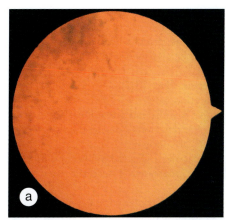

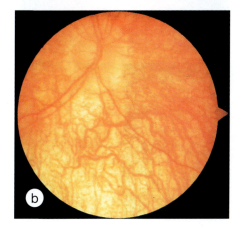

Fig. 53.1 Mitochondrial cytopathy. (a) "Salt and pepper" pigmentation in the retinal dystrophy associated with mitochondrial cytopathy. (b) RPE atrophy and arteriolar thinning in mitochondrial cytopathy.

Ophthalmic features:

Progressive external ophthalmoplegia (CPEO) and ptosis.

Retinal dystrophy. Most patients retain good visual function with mild but probably progressive cone-rod dystrophy and a "salt and pepper" appearance (Fig. 53.1), with regions of increased and decreased pigmentation particularly in the equatorial fundus.[1] Other cases develop severe receptor loss, blindness and no recordable electroretinogram (ERG): these may either have a typical retinitis pigmentosa fundus or severe retinal pigment epithelial atrophy which may mimic choroideremia.[2]

Corneal clouding. Rarely KSS may present with corneal clouding associated with either congenital glaucoma or corneal dystrophy.[3] Structural changes in endothelium and Descemet's membrane have been reported or the corneal edema may be due to reduced pump action of corneal mitochondria.[4] Rarely corneal changes may precede systemic signs by several years.[4]

Optic neuritis.

Macular dystrophy. A single case with a vitelliform macular dystrophy.

MtDNA point mutations

Retinal dystrophy is common in patients with the 8993T>G and 8993T>C mtDNA point mutations. Some patients have a peripheral "salt and pepper" retinopathy, which may be asymptomatic. Others have a "bone spicule" appearance with loss of peripheral and night-vision. Later some patients develop optic atrophy or maculopathy with severe visual loss.[5,6] These patients may also suffer neurological problems, the severity depending on the level of heteroplasmy. Patients with >90% mutant mtDNA often present with a childhood neurodegenerative disorder called **Leigh syndrome** (see Chapter 65). Patients with a slightly lower level of mutant mtDNA may present with **NARP syndrome** (**N**eurogenic weakness, **A**taxia and **R**etinitis **P**igmentosa).[7]

The 3243A>G mtDNA mutation is also associated with a range of clinical presentations, depending on the level of heteroplasmy. High mutant mtDNA levels are associated with **M**yopathy, **E**ncephalopathy, **L**actic **A**cidosis and **S**troke-like episodes, which may lead to visual field defects (MELAS syndrome). Patients with lower levels of the mutation may present with diabetes and deafness, cardiomyopathy or progressive external ophthalmoplegia. A number of patients have a retinal dystrophy with a "salt and pepper" appearance. Macular pattern dystrophy is common in older patients.[8]

Long-chain 3-hydroxyacyl-CoA dehydrogenase deficiency (LCHADD)

This is a rare disorder of mitochondrial fatty acid oxidation. LCHADD usually presents in infancy with acute hypoketotic hypoglycemia, encephalopathy, liver disease, cardiomyopathy and, sometimes, rhabdomyolysis.[9] The diagnosis is usually made by analysis of blood acylcarnitines or urine organic acids; it can be confirmed by measuring enzyme activity or by finding the common gene mutation. Patients who survive the presenting episode are treated with a low-fat diet, supplements of medium-chain triglyceride and avoidance of fasting. Unfortunately, this does not prevent the long-term complications, pigmentary retinopathy and peripheral neuropathy.

Ophthalmic features:
Retinal dystrophy. This has a variable age of onset and severity,[10] it is progressive with symptoms of night-blindness from 2 years of age. The retinopathy may be classified into four stages:

- Stage 1: normal fundus.
- Stage 2 pigment dispersion (Fig. 53.2).
- Stage 3 central chorioretinopathy.
- Stage 4 with progressive myopia and posterior staphyloma.

ERGs are initially normal, but deteriorate during the first decade. VEPs to a flash stimulus are normal.

Cataract. Flake-like lens opacities[10] (Fig. 53.3a) occur with stage 4 chorioretinal disease. Progressive cataract occurs[11] (Fig. 53.3b).

The variability of the severity of ocular complications makes it difficult to test the effectiveness of therapeutic options on the ophthalmic complications.

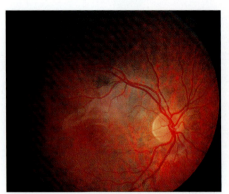

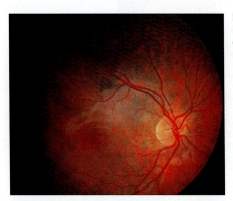

Fig. 53.2 LCHADD. Mild pigmentary disturbance at the macula.

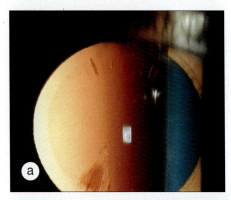

Fig. 53.3 LCHADD. (a) "Flake" lens opacities. (b) Progressive lens opacities.

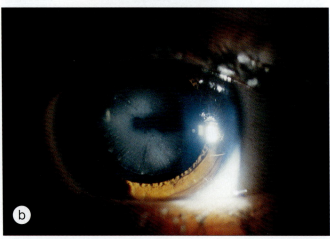

PEROXISOMAL DISORDERS

Peroxisomal biogenesis disorders

These disorders are caused by impaired import of proteins into the peroxisomal matrix or the peroxisomal membrane; Chapter 65. Two clinical patterns can be distinguished, for each there is a wide range of severity:

Zellweger spectrum (80%)

Patients with Zellweger syndrome are dysmorphic with multiple congenital anomalies and severe neurodevelopmental problems; most die within a few months of birth. "Neonatal adreno-leukodystrophy" and "infantile Refsum syndrome" refer to milder phenotypes within the Zellweger spectrum. Patients present in infancy or early childhood with mild dysmorphism, hypotonia, mental retardation, seizures, sensorineural hearing loss and retinal dystrophy. Peroxisomal biogenesis disorders are caused by mutations in the peroxin genes, 15 of which have now been identified. Defects of *PEX1* are the commonest cause of the Zellweger spectrum.[12] The most mildly affected patients show mosaicism. Neonatal adrenoleukodystrophy is unrelated to X-linked adrenoleukodystrophy and infantile Refsum syndrome is unrelated to classical Refsum disease.

Ophthalmic features:
Retinal dystrophy.

- **Zellweger syndrome.** Patients generally have hypopigmentation of the retina, sometimes accompanied by pigment clumping in the mid-periphery. The ERG is absent or severely abnormal. Histopathology shows photoreceptor degeneration, ganglion cell loss, gliosis of the nerve fiber layer and optic nerve, and optic atrophy.
- **Infantile Refsum disease** and **neonatal adrenoleukodystrophy.** In patients who survive beyond a year or two, pigmentary retinopathy is almost universal; it is even seen with peroxisomal mosaicism.[13] There is granular depigmentation at the posterior pole and retinal edema may be an early feature. Later there is vascular attenuation, with depigmentation of the macula and coarse black pigment clumps in the mid and far periphery. Patients are night-blind and suffer progressive loss of peripheral vision that often progresses to complete blindness. In advanced cases, the ERG rod- and cone-mediated responses are equally affected, later completely extinguished. Histopathology shows photoreceptor degeneration and atrophy of the nerve fiber layer.[14] The pathogenesis of the retinopathy is uncertain but deficiency of peroxisomal docosahexanoic acid (DHA) may play a role: it is present at high concentrations in the normal retina. DHA treatment may improve the retinal outcome in Zellweger spectrum patients.[15]

Corneal clouding. Patients with Zellweger syndrome sometimes have malformations of the eye and often have corneal clouding, glaucoma or cataracts.

Cataract. Cataracts occur in about 10% of cases.

Rhizomelic chondrodysplasia punctata (20%)

See Chapter 65.

Classical Refsum disease

The cardinal features:

1. Retinitis pigmentosa. Night-blindness is usually the first symptom and may start before 10 years of age. Retinal pigmentation appears as "bone spicules", "salt and pepper" or

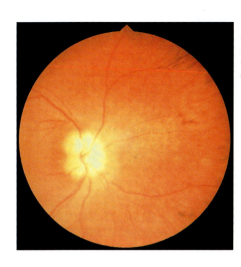

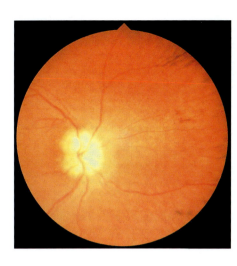

Fig. 53.4 "Bone spicule" pigmentation and a pale swollen optic disc in Refsum disease.

fine granules (Fig. 53.4). Retinal pathology shows loss of photoreceptors and ganglion cells and thinning of the inner nuclear layer.
2. Cerebellar ataxia.
3. Peripheral neuropathy (especially legs).

Less constant features:
1. Other ophthalmological complications include cataracts, vitreous opacities, optic atrophy and impaired pupil reactions but these are all rare during childhood.
2. Deafness.
3. Anosmia.
4. Ichthyosis.
5. Cardiomyopathy.

Refsum syndrome is inherited as an autosomal recessive trait and is usually caused by deficiency of the peroxisomal enzyme, phytanoyl-CoA hydroxylase[16] encoded by the *PHYH* gene.[17] A few patients with Refsum syndrome have mutations in the *PEX7* gene,[18] which is usually associated with rhizomelic chondrodysplasia punctata type 1.

Accumulation of phytanic acid in blood and tissues causes cell damage. Phytanic acid is not synthesized in man and its concentration can be lowered by dietary restriction of dairy products and ruminant meat or fat. This may reduce the rate of further neurological deterioration in classical Refsum disease and the peripheral neuropathy usually improves but the retinal degeneration remains unchanged.

Primary hyperoxaluria type 1 (PH 1)

See Chapter 57.

PH1 is an autosomal recessive disorder caused by deficiency of the peroxisomal enzyme, alanine-glyoxylate aminotransferase which is encoded by the *AGXT* gene on chromosome 2q37.3. High urinary excretion of calcium oxalate leads to stone formation and nephrocalcinosis. The median age of presentation with renal dysfunction is 5 years. As renal function deteriorates, calcium oxalate is deposited elsewhere with bone pain, livedo reticularis and heart block.

Ophthalmic features:

Retinopathy. Oxalate crystals are deposited in the retinal pigment epithelium, at the posterior pole appearing as minute yellow or white flecks.[19] Visual impairment tends to be relatively

mild unless complicated by subretinal neovascularization at the macula[20] or a subretinal fibrosis at the macula ("white geographic maculopathy") which can occur as young as 4 years of age in spite of successful combined liver/renal transplantation. Reaction of the epithelial cells to the crystals may be the cause of subretinal black ringlets, which may coalesce to form a large black geographical lesion ("black geographic maculopathy").

Optic neuropathy. A few patients have optic atrophy associated with more severe loss of acuity.

LYSOSOMAL DISORDERS

Nephropathic cystinosis

This is a rare autosomal recessive disorder of lysosomal cystine transport. Cystine crystals accumulate in lysosomes of most tissues. The defective gene (*CTNS*) encodes a transmembrane protein.[21] The infantile form presents as growth retardation and renal failure. Most children require renal transplantation by the second decade.

Ophthalmic features:

Crystal deposits. All tissues of the eye including the conjunctiva and the lens may have crystal deposits but the most visually disabling are those in the cornea and retina. Most patients have a visual acuity of 20/40 or better.[22]

Corneal crystals (Chapter 29) are needle shaped and develop initially in the superficial peripheral cornea progressing deeper and centrally. Photophobia and discomfort is usually not symptomatic until the second decade. Topical lubricants and sunglasses are helpful. Oral cysteamine does not reduce corneal crystals but topical may be effective in reducing number of crystals and photophobia.[22]

Retinopathy may occur within the first few years of life, but usually asymptomatic before the second decade. There is patchy depigmentation initially of the peripheral retina and later macular involvement is associated with vision loss. Early in the disease the ERG is normal.

Multiple sulphatase deficiency (MSD)

See page 567.

Neuronal ceroid lipofuscinoses and other lysosomal disorders

See Chapter 65.

NON-ORGANELLE DISEASES

Hallervorden–Spatz syndrome

This is an autosomal recessive disorder characterized by dystonia, spastic quadriparesis, dystonia, parkinsonism, and iron accumulation in the brain. Many patients with this disease have mutations in the gene encoding pantothenate kinase 2 (*PANK2*).[23] Mutations in this gene also cause the syndrome previously known as **H**ypoprebetalipoproteinemia, **A**canthocytosis, **R**etinitis pigmentosa, and **P**allidal degeneration (HARP) syndrome.[24]

Ophthalmic features:

Retinal dystrophy. The retina has early flecks and later bone-spicule formation and "bull's-eye" annular maculopathy (Fig. 53.5). "Bone spicules" can be found as early as 7 years of age in a child with severe progressive neurological handicap.

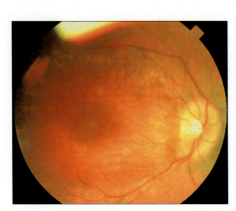

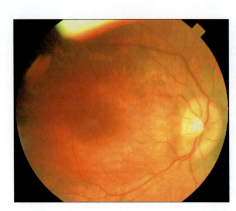

Fig. 53.5
Hallervorden–Spatz syndrome. Annular maculopathy.

Ocular histopathological findings[25] include degeneration of photoreceptors and RPE, marked thinning of the outer nuclear and outer plexiform layers, retinal gliosis, narrowing and obliteration of blood vessels with a perivascular cuffing of pigment cells.

Cerebellar ataxia with pigmentary macular dystrophy (spinocerebellar ataxia type 7)

Cerebellar ataxia associated with visual failure secondary to a pigmentary macular dystrophy inherited as an autosomal dominant and may be more severe in infants born to affected fathers (anticipation).[26] Diagnosis is confirmed by the demonstration of an expansion of a CAG repeat in the coding region of the gene on chromosome 3p. The presenting symptom is usually ataxia, sometimes with visual failure.

Ophthalmic features:

Retinal dystrophy. The macular abnormalities are often subtle (Fig. 53.6) in early cases, even in some with moderately reduced visual acuity.[27] Age of onset and clinical course is very variable even within pedigrees. The infantile onset phenotype is rapidly progressive.

Eye movement abnormalities. Other neurological features include pyramidal tract signs and supranuclear ophthalmoplegia with progressive saccadic palsy.

L-2-hydroxyglutaric aciduria

This is a rare disorder with increased urinary, plasma and CSF concentrations of L-2-hydroxyglutarate, neurodevelopmental regression, seizures, and cerebellar ataxia. The CSF concentration of L-2-hydroxyglutarate is around five times its plasma concentration. MRI findings are characteristic and include cerebellar atrophy, increased T2-weighted signal in the subcortical white matter, dentate nucleus and basal ganglia.[28]

Ophthalmic feature:

Retinal dystrophy. Pigmentary retinopathy with reduced ERG has been reported.

Osteopetrosis

Osteopetrosis is genetically heterogeneous.[29] The autosomal recessive forms have earlier onset and are characterized by osteopetrosis and cerebral calcification with developmental delay, anemia and loss of vision and hearing. One type is caused by deficiency of carbonic anhydrase II and is associated with renal tubular acidosis which is rare in other forms of osteopetrosis.[30] Malignant osteopetrosis (MOP) is an aggressive variant associated with early infant death.

Patients with mutations in one allele of the chloride channel gene *CLCN7* have a milder autosomal dominant phenotype.

Ophthalmic features:

Optic atrophy. Visual loss occurs because of optic nerve compromise (see Chapter 61) and more rarely retinal dysfunction which may be a part of a primary neurodegeneration.[31] Treatment is with optic canal decompression or bone marrow transplantation (BMT). There is controversy as to whether vision loss is reversible, but vision may be preserved with early treatment.[32] Blindness due to optic atrophy occured in 5/35 cases in one series of carbonic anhydrase II type osteopetrosis.[33]

Retinal dystrophy. ERG changes indicating loss of both rod and cone function are only detected in the minority of patients[31] and this may be unique to the CLCN7 type of osteopetrosis. These children may have a normal fundus appearance or abnormal retinal pigmentation (Fig. 53.7). The retinal degeneration is usually progressive and may be associated with congenital stationery night-blindness.[34]

Lacrimal symptoms. The lacrimal drainage system also becomes blocked leading to dacryocystitis and dacryocystorhinostomy is difficult due to bone thickness and the ostium commonly closes over with a relapse of symptoms.

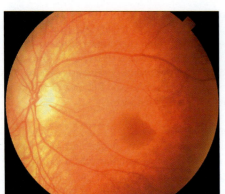

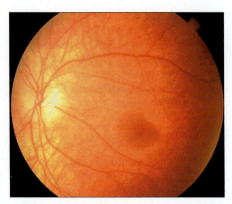

Fig. 53.6
Spinocerebellar ataxia. Early retinal dystrophy with macular pigmentation.

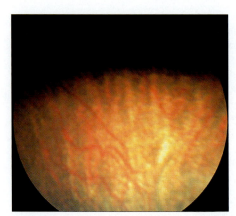

Fig. 53.7
Osteopetrosis. Peripheral retinal mottling associated with an abnormal ERG.

Usher syndrome

Usher syndrome (USH) is genetically heterogeneous: it is characterized by sensorineural deafness and progressive pigmentary retinopathy with or without a vestibular abnormality.[35,36]

USH1

Congenital severe to profound sensorineural hearing loss and abnormal vestibular dysfunction which causes delayed developmental motor milestones for sitting and walking. Psychological problems and developmental delay occur in some cases. USH1 genes are expressed in the stereocilia of the cochlea and in the retinal photoreceptors or retinal pigment epithelium[37] Genes identified include *MYO7A* (encoding myosin 7A, causes both USH1B and nonsyndromic deafness,[38] *USH1C* (encoding harmonin,[39]), *CDH23* (USH1D, encoding cadherin 23[40] may be modified by other genes[41] and missense mutations may be associated with nonsyndromic deafness,[42] *PCDH15* (encoding protocadherin 15,[43] USH1F), *USH1G* (encoding SANS[44]). USH1C is deleted in a contiguous gene syndrome characterized by severe hyperinsulinism, profound congenital sensorineural deafness, enteropathy and renal tubular dysfunction.[45]

USH2

Congenital mild to severe sensorineural hearing loss and normal vestibular function. The USH2 phenotype is caused by defects of extracellular matrix or cell surface receptor proteins. USH 2A encodes usherin.[46]

USH3

Progressive hearing loss and progressive deterioration of vestibular function. USH3 may be due to synaptic disturbances. USH3A encodes clarin 1,[47] and USH3.[47]

Ophthalmic features:

Retinal dystrophy. There is a wide variation in the presentation of the retinal dystrophy.[48] Early in the disease the RPE often appears mottled sometimes with retinal edema and a macula hole. Later, "bone spicules" appear especially in the retinal periphery. In USH1 the ERG may be abnormal in the first year yet may still be normal as late as the 9th year.

Generally, USH2 and 3 mostly are not symptomatic in the first decade and initially have a normal fundus appearance. Many patients retain good acuity in spite of constricted visual fields. The electroretinogram (ERG) may initially be normal; however ERG changes may be detected in presymptomatic young children. During the second decade, night-blindness and loss of peripheral vision become evident and inexorably progress. Flicker ERG characteristics differ between USH1 and USH2 phenotypes.[49]

Fuchs heterochromic cyclitis may rarely be associated with Usher syndrome.[50]

Posterior subcapsular cataracts are common by the third decade as they are in many other retinal degenerations.

Hallgren syndrome

Hallgren described congenital sensorineural hearing loss, pigmentary retinopathy, nystagmus, cataracts and ataxia, 25% are mentally retarded and there is an increased incidence of psychotic episodes. This may be a type of Usher type 1 that is rare outside Scandinavia.[51]

SYNDROMES ASSOCIATED WITH OBESITY

Alström syndrome

Alström syndrome (AS) is a rare autosomal recessive multi-organ degenerative disorder characterized by severe early onset cone-rod retinal dystrophy, obesity, progressive sensorineural hearing impairment, dilated cardiomyopathy, insulin resistance, and developmental delay.[52] It is variable in expression even between siblings. The *ALMS1* gene (2p13) has been identified and is thought to be responsible for all cases of ALMS.[53]

Children usually become truncally obese during their first year. Many develop cardiac failure as a result of dilated cardiomyopathy[54] presenting in infancy or in the second decade. The retinal dystrophy is initially cone-rod as distinct from the rod-cone presentation in Bardet-Biedl syndrome (BBS). Glue ear is frequent. Sensorineural hearing loss presents in the first decade in up to 70%; it may progress to the moderately severe range (40–70 db) by the end of the first to second decade. Insulin resistant type 2 diabetes mellitus often presents in the second decade and is accompanied by acanthosis nigricans. Other endocrine and metabolic abnormalities include hypothyroidism, diabetes insipidus, growth hormone deficiency, hyperuricemia, hyperlipidemia, hypothyroidism and hypogonadotrophic hypogonadism. Urological disorders of varying severity, characterized by detrusor-urethral dyssynergia, presents in females in the second decade. Hepatic and renal dysfunction present in the second decade. Delay in receptive and expressive language skills has been described, but this may partially be a result of the severe sensory deficits. The majority of patients are of normal intelligence.

Ophthalmic features:

Retinal dystrophy. Most cases present soon after birth with vision failure, photophobia and nystagmus due to severe retinal dystrophy affecting both rods and cones, rarely as late as 15 months. The photoreceptors are abnormal in structure and function with some residual function of rod receptors and the lack of development of foveal region. In the majority of cases there is useful vision early in life. Comfort and functional vision is optimized if prescription dark glasses are given to utilize rod vision. Visual acuity is 6/60 or less by age ten years with increasing constriction of visual fields and no light perception by age 20 years.[55] In the first decade, retinal changes are subtle with mild narrowing of the retinal vessels and optic disc pallor (Fig. 53.8). Later, chorioretinal atrophy and pigmentary clumping occur. Vision progressively deteriorates to lack of light perception in the second decade.

Cataracts. Posterior subcapsular cataracts are common by the second decade. They are secondary to the retinal degeneration and removal is not usually helpful.

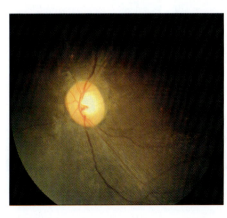

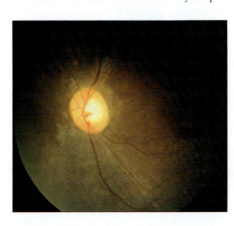

Fig. 53.8 Alström syndrome. Narrowed arterioles and optic disc pallor associated with a severely abnormal ERG.

Bardet–Biedl syndrome

The Bardet–Biedl (BBS) phenotype of pigmentary retinopathy, truncal obesity, polydactyly (Fig. 53.9), renal malformations and hypogenitalism in males.

Additional features include hypertension, diabetes mellitus congenital heart disease, small or missing teeth.[56] BBS4 is associated with early-onset morbid obesity, while BBS2 appears to present the "leanest" end of BBS. Sensorineural hearing loss is reported in less than 5% of BBS cases.

BBS1 is the commonest form of BBS and is inherited as an autosomal recessive trait with both alleles of the gene having to be mutant for the disorder to be manifest.[57] However in some cases of BBS1, but more often in other BBS genotypes, there may be a more complex inheritance pattern and intrafamilial variability[58]; in some families three mutations at two loci are required for BBS phenotype to manifest.[59] Some published reviews include other conditions such as Alström syndrome.

Ophthalmic features:

Retinal dystrophy. The onset of the progressive retinal dystrophy (Fig. 53.10) is in the first decade; it usually affects rods more than cones but both types of receptors rapidly become involved. Abnormality in the ERG may precede pigmentary changes in the retina. In BBS4 an early onset and severe

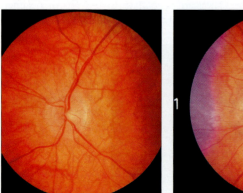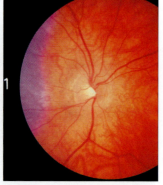

Fig. 53.9 Bardet–Biedl syndrome. Postaxial polydactyly; in this case the extra digit had been removed in infancy leaving minimal signs.

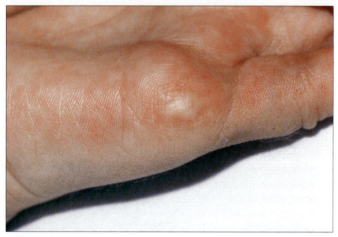

Fig. 53.10 Bardet–Biedl syndrome. Normal fundus (myopic). The ERG was abnormal, however.

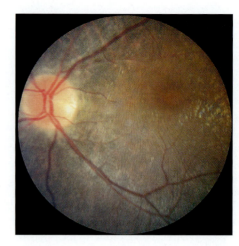

Fig. 53.11 Bardet–Biedl syndrome. Severe retinal dystrophy with a "shot-silk" appearance. The ERG was very attenuated.

retinal dystrophy (Fig. 53.11) occurs with a characteristic fundus appearance.[56]

Nystagmus. Many patients with BBS and retinal dystrophy do not have nystagmus. This helps to distinguish BBS from Alström syndrome. Some do have strabismus and nystagmus which may even present as spasmus nutans.[60]

Ocular motor apraxia (saccade initiation failure) has been reported in BBS.

Blepharospasm has been reported in one case.[61]

McKusick–Kaufman syndrome

McKusick–Kaufman syndrome (MKKS) is a rare autosomal recessive disease with features in common with Bardet–Biedl syndrome including, in a minority of cases, a retinal dystrophy. There have been various reports of patients with Bardet–Biedl syndrome with mutations in the MKKS gene which is responsible for Kaufman–McKusick syndrome.[62] Homozygosity for null mutation may cause the BBS phenotype, but hypomorphic alleles cause the MKKS phenotype.[63] However no evidence of digenic inheritance with interaction of MKKS and BBS2 has been found.[62]

The distinguishing features of MKKS are vaginal atresia or an imperforate hymen that presents as congenital abdominal swelling with hydrometrocolpos. Additional features may include an imperforate anus, a urogenital sinus, malrotation of the gut, esophageal atresia, Hirschsprung disease, choanal atresia, pituitary dysplasia, vertebral anomalies, laryngeal stenosis and congenital heart disease.[64]

Cohen syndrome

This is a rare autosomal recessively inherited condition with facial dysmorphism, microcephaly, developmental delay, hypotonia, obesity, episodic neutropenia, long tapered fingers, joint laxity, myopia and a progressive retinal dystrophy.[65,66] Most reports come from Finland which may reflect a founder effect with under-recognition and under reporting elsewhere. The COH1 gene mapped to 8q22–23 has recently been characterized; it encodes a putative transmembrane protein of 4022 amino acids. It may have a role in vesicle-mediated sorting and transport of proteins within the cell.[67] The facial features are downward slanting "wave-shaped" palpebral fissures, prominent beak-shaped nose, short upturned philtrum and open mouth with downturned corners. Commonly there is a history of neonatal hypotonia with poor feeding and delay in motor milestones; speech

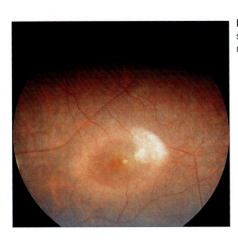

Fig. 53.12 Cohen syndrome. "Bulls-eye" maculopathy.

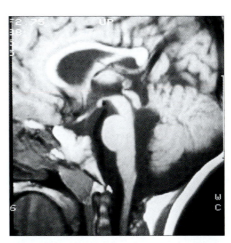

Fig. 53.13 Joubert syndrome. Cerebellar vermis hypoplasia.

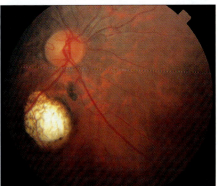

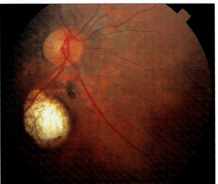

Fig. 53.14 Joubert syndrome. Chorioretinal coloboma. The ERG was also abnormal.

delay, and stridor secondary to laryngomalacia. Truncal obesity is common but not invariable by 5 years of age as is microcephaly although head circumference may be normal at birth. Neutropenia may result in frequent skin and dental infections. MRI may show a relatively large corpus callosum.

Ophthalmic features:

Myopia. The onset of myopia is usually under 5 years of age and exceeds 7 diopters by the second decade: is thought to be mainly due to high corneal and lenticular power super-imposed on variable axial myopia.[68]

Retinal dystrophy. The macula may develop a "bull's eye" appearance (Fig. 53.12) in the first decade and the retinal pigment epithelium may appear thin especially around the optic disc with mottled retinal pigmentation, narrowing of the retinal vessels and optic disc pallor. The first symptoms are of myopia and night-blindness. There is reduced acuity, visual field, night-blindness, generalized pigmentary retinopathy with bone spicules or lacunar RPE atrophy in the mid-periphery by the second decade. Although the myopia and retinal dystrophy are progressive, acuity of 6/18 may be maintained into the third decade. Microphthalmos and retinochoroidal coloboma are rare features.[69,70]

SYNDROMES ASSOCIATED WITH RENAL AND/OR SKELETAL DISORDER

Skeletal dysplasia in a child with a retinal dystrophy may be a sign of asymptomatic renal or hepatic disease.

Joubert syndrome

Joubert syndrome (JS) is an autosomal recessive disorder characterized by early episodic tachypnea and apnea, abnormal eye movements, developmental delay, ataxia, cerebellar vermis hypoplasia and hypotonia.[71] The cerebellar hypoplasia (Fig. 53.13) is often associated with a more complex brainstem malformation with the "molar tooth sign" on magnetic resonance imaging. Other reported associations include occipital encephalocele, Dandy–Walker malformation, polydactyly, dysmorphic facies, facial palsy, soft-tissue tumors of the tongue, cystic kidneys, congenital hepatic fibrosis, duodenal atresia, retinal dystrophy and ocular colobomas. Some cases have a phenotype that straddles two syndromes. There is overlap of clinical features with Bardet–Biedl and Senior–Loken syndromes.[72]

Joubert syndrome is likely to be genetically heterogenous, it may be subdivided into those with (A) or without (B) retinal dystrophy[73] and renal involvement may occur only in the latter. Families with the JS type B phenotype show linkage to chromosome 11p12-q13.3.[74]

Ophthalmic features:

Retinal dystrophy. An early onset retinal dystrophy affecting both rod and cones has been reported in JS and there is evidence of slow deterioration in many cases. Early in childhood there is often preservation of the flash VEP in spite of an attenuated or unrecordable electroretinogram.[75] The fundus may be normal or have mottled pigmentation especially at the macula.

Eye movement disorders. Intermittent saccadic failure, nystagmus, strabismus and ocular motor palsies are all reported in JS.

Chorioretinal coloboma. Chorioretinal coloboma (Fig. 53.14) has been reported in association with JS[76] and may co-exist with a progressive retinal dystrophy.

Coloboma with abnormal ERG

Macula "coloboma"

A congenital and usually bilateral defect of the macula that is not associated with intrauterine infection is often referred to as a macula "coloboma". However the defect is not along the fetal fissure and more correctly should be termed a macula dysplasia. Macula dysplasia has been reported in siblings and in two or more generations. The abnormality of the retina is often widespread and dysplasia of the macula can be a phenotype of various different genetic types of Leber Congenital Amaurosis (LCA). A dysplastic macula is a feature of various metabolic disorders including Cobalamin C deficiency (see below), idiopathic infantile hypercalcuria[77] and in association with polydactyly,[78] brachydactyly[79] and other skeletal abnormalities.[80] A similar macula appearance has been reported as a complication of cryotherapy for retinopathy of prematurity.[81]

Senior–Loken syndrome

Senior–Loken syndrome (SLS) is a genetically heterogeneous autosomal recessive disorder characterized by juvenile nephronophthisis and retinal dystrophy. The SLS phenotype is associated with homozygous mutations in the *NPH1* (the main nephronophthisis gene) and in the *NPHP4* gene. *NPHP3* is another candidate gene. End stage renal failure usually occurs by 20 years of age, but rarely may be delayed until the fourth or fifth decade.[82] Other features include short stature, kyphoscoliosis, short metacarpals, cerebellar hypoplasia, cutis laxa and sensorineural hearing loss. Patients with SLS may present with anemia as the presenting sign of renal failure in the first decade.[83] The family may not be aware of the vision failure due to an associated retinal dystrophy especially if there is mental retardation.

Ophthalmic features:
Retinal dystrophy. There is very variable age of onset of the retinal dystrophy (Fig. 53.15) with some cases presenting with a severe infantile onset with nystagmus and others with more insidious onset. ERG abnormalities have been reported in some asymptomatic heterozygotes.
Cataracts. Cataract surgery in Senior–Loken syndrome may be beneficial despite severe retinopathy.[84]

Hirabayashi syndrome

A single case with developmental arrest, early-onset seizures, retinal pigmentary degeneration, progressive central nervous symptoms and peripheral neuropathy, associated with progressive renal dysfunction, anemia and nephrotic syndrome.[85]

Mainzer–Saldino syndrome

This is a heterogeneous disorder characterized by the association of juvenile nephronophthisis, cerebellar ataxia, cone-shaped epiphyses of the hands and feet with "stubby" fingers and an early onset severe retinal dystrophy.[86]

Ophthalmic features:
Panretinal atrophy, increased retinal reflex with wrinkled

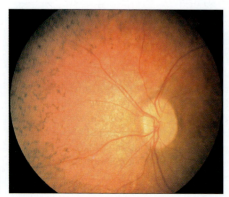

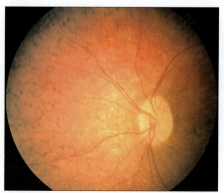

Fig. 53.15 Senior–Loken syndrome with "bone-spicule" retinal dystrophy.

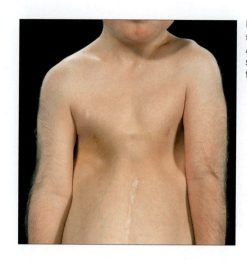

Fig. 53.16 Jeune syndrome. Asphyxiating dystrophy showing the severe thoracic dysplasia.

appearance and few scattered pigmentary deposits or yellow flecks at equator, narrow vessels, temporal disc pallor, and the ERG was unrecordable.

Jeune syndrome

Asphyxiating thoracic dystrophy (ATD), or Jeune syndrome, is a multisystem autosomal recessive disorder with a characteristic skeletal dysplasia with respiratory insufficiency related to the abnormally small thorax (Fig. 53.16) and variable renal, hepatic, pancreatic abnormalities. Growth retardation and chronic renal insufficiency due to nephronophthisis may occur in patients who survive the respiratory failure. Other clinical manifestations include cystic lesions of the pancreas, Hirschsprung disease,[87] polydactyly.[88] It maps to 15q13.[89]

Ophthalmic features:
They may present with nystagmus, unrecordable ERG and poor vision in infancy[90] or later with night-blindness.[88] There is a variable fundus appearance with pigment clumping, retinal arteriolar narrowing and RPE atrophy in the mid-periphery.

Sensenbrenner syndrome

Sensenbrenner syndrome or cranioectodermal dysplasia is a rare autosomal recessive condition with dolichocephaly due to sagittal craniostenosis, narrow thorax, short limbs, short fingers, sparse, slow-growing, fine hair, small and absent or unusually shaped teeth. Additional features include chronic renal failure, congenital heart defects, osteoporosis and retinal dystrophy.[91]

Ophthalmic features:
The retinal dystrophy may present in infancy with poor vision and nystagmus or at about 5 years of age with nyctalopia.

SYNDROMES WITH ABNORMALITY OF HAIR AND/OR SKIN

Cockayne syndrome

Cockayne syndrome (CS) is a heterogenous group of DNA repair disorders whose classification is based upon complementation groups CS-A (ERCC8 mutation CKN1 chromosome 5) and CS-B (80% cases) (ERCC6 mutation chromosome 10), XPD and XPG.

are normal, indicating that there is no generalized retinal dysfunction. The only significant differences between this phenotype and MCDR1 is that in MCDR3 color vision is abnormal in the majority of affected individuals, and there was evidence of disease progression, albeit in a single case.

Molecular genetics
Genetic linkage analysis established linkage to chromosome 5p13.1–p15.33, and excluded linkage to the MCDR1 locus.

North Carolina-like macular dystrophy and progressive sensorineural hearing loss

Clinical and electrophysiological findings
The second family is characterized by a nonprogressive MCDR1-like macular dystrophy in association with progressive sensorineural hearing loss.[36] The EOG and full-field ERG are normal. Progressive sensorineural deafness is present in all affected individuals over the age of 20 years.

Molecular genetics
Genotyping excluded linkage to the MCDR1 locus and established linkage to chromosome 14q.

Progressive bifocal chorioretinal atrophy (PBCRA)

Clinical and histological findings
PBCRA is an early-onset autosomal dominant disorder characterized by nystagmus, myopia, poor vision, and slow progression. A large atrophic macular lesion and nasal subretinal deposits are present soon after birth (Fig. 54.11). An atrophic area nasal to the optic nerve head appears in the second decade of life, and enlarges progressively. Marked photopsia in early/middle age and retinal detachment extending from the posterior pole are recognized complications. FFA and indocyanine green angiography

(IGA) demonstrate a large circumscribed area of macular choroidal atrophy with staining of deposits in the peripheral retina.

Electrophysiology
Both ERG and EOG are abnormal, reflecting widespread abnormality of photoreceptors and RPE.

Molecular genetics and pathogenesis
PBCRA has been linked to 6q14-q16.2.[37] The PBCRA disease interval overlaps with the established MCDR1 interval. These two autosomal dominant macular dystrophies have some phenotypic similarities, and both are thought to result from a failure of normal macular development. However, PBCRA differs significantly from MCDR1 in several important ways, including slow progression, abnormal color vision, extensive nasal as well as macular atrophy, and abnormal ERG and EOG. Therefore, if allelic, it is likely that different mutations are involved; alternatively they might be caused by mutations in adjacent genes.

Central areolar choroidal dystrophy (CACD)

Clinical and histological findings
CACD is characterized by bilateral, symmetrical, subtle mottling of the RPE at the macula in the second decade. The mottling progresses to atrophy of the RPE and choriocapillaris. The round or oval macular lesion is well demarcated. CACD has been divided into four stages:[38]

Stage I: Slight parafoveal changes of the RPE;
Stage II: RPE mottling encircling the fovea;
Stage III: Additional atrophy of the choriocapillaris without central involvement; and
Stage IV: Same as stage III but with central involvement.

Color vision is abnormal and central scotomata are present with normal peripheral visual fields. FFA and IGA reveal RPE atrophy and various degrees of choriocapillaris loss.

Electrophysiology
Full-field ERGs are normal in the early stages, but may become abnormal in advanced stages.

Molecular genetics and pathogenesis
An Arg142Trp mutation in *peripherin/RDS* has been implicated as one cause of this rare autosomal dominant macular dystrophy.[39] Sporadic cases of CACD have also been described but no mutations have been found in *peripherin/RDS* suggestive of further genetic heterogeneity. A locus at 17p13 has also been identified by a genome-wide linkage search.[40]

X-LINKED INHERITANCE

X-linked juvenile retinoschisis (XLRS)
(see Chapter 49)

XLRS is a vitreoretinal degeneration that presents either in an infant with nystagmus (when there are large congenital cystic schisis cavities)[41] or more commonly in childhood with mild loss of central vision. The characteristic fundus abnormality is a cystic spokewheel-like maculopathy (foveal schisis) in affected males (Fig. 54.12). However, recent studies suggest that only about two-thirds of males show the typical foveal schisis.[42] About 50% of affected males show additional peripheral retinal changes. The finding of a typical negative wave ERG in response to the standard bright flash stimulus is helpful in confirming the

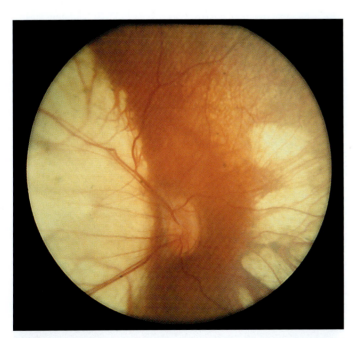

Fig. 54.11 Progressive bifocal chorioretinal atrophy. Large oval areas of atrophy extending nasal and temporal to the optic disc. (Prof. A.C. Bird's patient.)

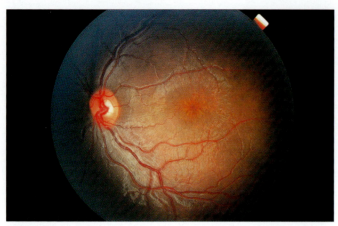

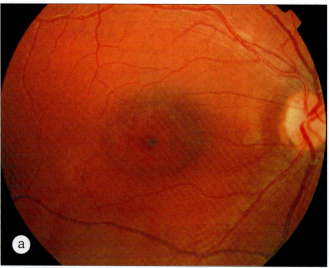

Fig. 54.12 X-linked juvenile retinoschisis. Characteristic fundus abnormality of a cystic spokewheel-like maculopathy (foveal schisis).

diagnosis. Molecular genetic testing is now possible. XLRS is discussed in detail in Chapter 49.

FOVEAL HYPOPLASIA

This disorder is characterized by reduced vision, normal color vision, nystagmus, and a poorly developed macula and fovea; there is no readily recognized foveola or luteal pigment, and blood vessels may cross the presumed macular region. Foveal hypoplasia is seen in aniridia and in albinism; it may also be seen as an isolated abnormality.[43,44] Most cases are sporadic, but one dominant pedigree has been reported.[44]

BULL'S EYE MACULOPATHY

The term "bull's-eye" maculopathy (BEM) was first introduced to describe the characteristic appearance of chloroquine retinopathy. Bull's-eye lesions have since been reported in cone dystrophy and cone–rod dystrophy,[45] rod–cone dystrophy,[46] and benign concentric annular dystrophy[47] and fenestrated sheen

macular dystrophy.[48] In addition, BEM is a frequent finding in neurodegenerative disorders, especially Batten disease, Hallervorden–Spatz disease, and olivopontocerebellar atrophy.

The pathogenesis of BEM is poorly understood. The characteristic appearance in which there is annular RPE atrophy and central sparing may correspond to the pattern of lipofuscin accumulation in the RPE, which in healthy individuals is highest at the posterior pole and shows a depression at the fovea (Figs. 54.13a, 54.13b). The initially spared center usually becomes involved as the disease advances. It is evident that BEM is not a discrete macular disorder but describes a recognizable retinal phenotype that may be seen in a wide variety of macular dystrophies at an early stage of their evolution.

MANAGEMENT

There is currently no established treatment for any of the inherited macular dystrophies. Nevertheless, it is important that the correct diagnosis is made, in order to be able to provide accurate information on prognosis and to be able to offer informed genetic counseling. Prenatal diagnosis is possible when the mutation(s) causing disease in the family is known.

Although there is no specific treatment available for this group of disorders, the provision of the best refractive correction, appropriate low-vision aids, and educational support is very important. Photophobia may be a prominent symptom in the inherited macular dystrophies, and therefore tinted spectacles or contact lenses may help, improving comfort and vision.

Our improved knowledge of the pathogenesis of the inherited macular dystrophies and the underlying molecular genetics has helped to improve genetic counseling. To this end, accurate genotype–phenotype correlation, where applicable, will allow a more informed prediction of disease progression and prognosis.

CONCLUSIONS

The inherited macular dystrophies are a clinically and genetically heterogeneous group of disorders. Their phenotypes have now some forms of dominantly inherited macular dystrophy, including

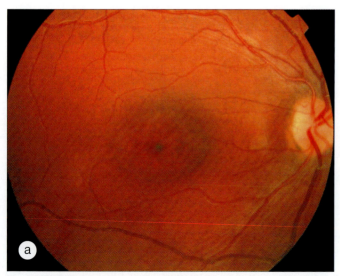

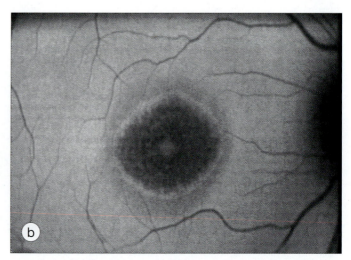

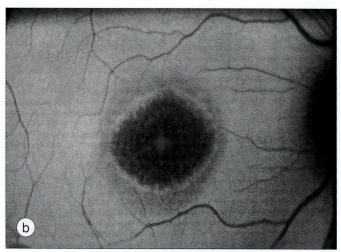

Fig. 54.13 Bull's-eye maculopathy (BEM). (a) Characteristic ophthalmoscopic appearance in which there is annular RPE atrophy and central sparing. (b) Typical autofluorescence image of BEM.

been well characterized, and many causative genes have been identified. Establishing the diagnosis at an early stage can be helpful in enabling accurate prognosis and effective genetic counseling. At the present time there is no effective treatment for these early-onset inherited macular dystrophies.

Although in some inherited macular dystrophies, the disease appears to be confined to the macular region, in the majority of disorders, there is electrophysiological, psychophysical, or histological evidence of widespread retinal dysfunction. Indeed

in the case of autosomal recessive STGD the presence of widespread full-field ERG abnormalities can be used as an accurate indicator of a worse prognosis.

Improved knowledge of the mechanisms of inherited macular dystrophy and the underlying molecular genetics has not only raised the potential for future development of rational therapeutic regimens but has also helped to refine diagnosis, disease-classification and prognosis, and improved genetic counseling.

REFERENCES

1. von Rückmann A, Fitzke FW, Bird AC. In vivo fundus autofluorescence in macular dystrophies. Arch Ophthalmol 1997; 115: 609–15.
2. Lois N, Holder GE, Bunce C, et al. Phenotypic subtypes of Stargardt macular dystrophy-fundus flavimaculatus. Arch Ophthalmol 2001; 119: 359–69.
3. Eagle RC, Lucier AC, Bernardino VB, et al. Retinal pigment epithelial abnormalities in fundus flavimaculatus: a light and electron microscopic study. Ophthalmology 1980; 87: 1189–200.
4. Allikmets R, Singh N, Sun H, et al. A photoreceptor cell-specific ATP-binding transporter gene (ABCR) is mutated in recessive Stargardt macular dystrophy. Nat Genet 1997; 15: 236–46.
5. Weng J, Mata NL, Azarian SM, et al. Insights into the function of Rim protein in photoreceptors and etiology of Stargardt's disease from the phenotype in ABCR knockout mice. Cell 1999; 98: 13–23.
6. Sun H, Smallwood PM, Nathans J, et al. Biochemical defects in ABCR protein variants associated with human retinopathies. Nat Genet 2000; 26: 242–6.
7. Gerth C, Andrassi-Darida M, Bock M, et al. Phenotypes of 16 Stargardt macular dystrophy/fundus flavimaculatus patients with known ABCA4 mutations and evaluation of genotype-phenotype correlation. Graefes Arch Clin Exp Ophthalmol 2002; 240: 628–38.
8. Sparrow JR, Vollmer-Snarr HR, Zhou J, et al. A2E-epoxides damage DNA in retinal pigment epithelial cells. Vitamin E and other antioxidants inhibit A2E-epoxide formation. J Biol Chem 2003; 278: 18207–13.
9. Radu RA, Mata NL, Nusinowitz S, et al. Treatment with isotretinoin inhibits lipofuscin accumulation in a mouse model of recessive Stargardt's macular degeneration. Proc Natl Acad Sci USA 2003; 100: 4742–7.
10. Donoso LA, Edwards AO, Frost A, et al. Autosomal dominant Stargardt-like macular dystrophy. Surv Ophthalmol 2001; 46: 149–63.
11. Lopez PF, Maumenee IH, de la Cruz Z, et al. Autosomal-dominant fundus flavimaculatus. Clinicopathologic correlation. Ophthalmology 1990; 97: 798–809.
12. Zhang K, Kniazeva M, Han M, et al. A 5-bp deletion in ELOVL4 is associated with two related forms of autosomal dominant macular dystrophy. Nat Genet 2001; 27: 89–93.
13. Maw MA, Corbeil D, Koch J, et al. A frameshift mutation in prominin (mouse)-like 1 causes human retinal degeneration. Hum Mol Genet 2000; 9: 27–34.
14. Michaelides M, Johnson S, Poulson A, et al. An autosomal dominant bull's-eye macular dystrophy (MCDR2) that maps to the short arm of chromosome 4. Invest Ophthalmol Vis Sci 2003; 44: 1657–62.
15. Mohler CW, Fine SL. Long-term evaluation of patients with Best's vitelliform dystrophy. Ophthalmology 1981; 88: 688–92.
16. Petrukhin K, Koisti MJ, Bakall B, et al. Identification of the gene responsible for Best macular dystrophy. Nat Genet 1998; 19: 241–7.
17. Weber BH, Walker D, Muller B. Molecular evidence for non-penetrance in Best's disease. J Med Genet 1994; 31: 388–92.
18. Sun H, Tsunenari T, Yau KW, et al. The vitelliform macular dystrophy protein defines a new family of chloride channels. Proc Natl Acad Sci USA 2002; 99: 4008–13.
19. Pianta MJ, Aleman TS, Cideciyan AV, et al. In vivo micropathology of Best macular dystrophy with optical coherence tomography. Exp Eye Res 2003; 76: 203–11.
20. Deutman AF, van Blommestein JD, Henkes HE, et al. Butterfly-shaped pigment dystrophy of the fovea. Arch Ophthalmol 1970; 83: 558–69.
21. Deutman AF, Rumke AM. Reticular dystrophy of the retinal pigment epithelium. Dystrophia reticularis laminae pigmentosa retinae of H. Sjogren. Arch Ophthalmol 1969; 82: 4–9.
22. Kingham JD, Fenzl RE, Willerson D, et al. Reticular dystrophy of the retinal pigment epithelium. A clinical and electrophysiologic study of three generations. Arch Ophthalmol 1978; 96: 1177–84.
23. Slezak H, Hommer K. Fundus pulverulentus. Albrecht von Graefes Arch Klin Exp Ophthalmol 1969; 178: 176–82.
24. Nichols BE, Drack AV, Vandenburgh K, et al. A 2 base pair deletion in the RDS gene associated with butterfly-shaped pigment dystrophy of the fovea. Hum Mol Genet 1993; 2: 601–3.
25. van Lith-Verhoeven JJ, Cremers FP, van den Helm B, et al. Genetic heterogeneity of butterfly-shaped pigment dystrophy of the fovea. Mol Vis 2003; 9: 138–43.
26. Downes SM, Fitzke FW, Holder GE, et al. Clinical features of codon 172 RDS macular dystrophy: similar phenotype in 12 families. Arch Ophthalmol 1999; 117: 1373–83.
27. Weleber RG, Carr RE, Murphy WH, et al. Phenotypic variation including retinitis pigmentosa, pattern dystrophy, and fundus flavimaculatus in a single family with a deletion of codon 153 or 154 of the peripherin/RDS gene. Arch Ophthalmol 1993; 111: 1531–42.
28. Ali RR, Sarra GM, Stephens C, et al. Restoration of photoreceptor ultrastructure and function in retinal degeneration slow mice by gene therapy. Nat Genet 2000; 25: 306–10.
29. Small KW, Voo I, Flannery J, et al. North Carolina macular dystrophy: clinicopathologic correlation. Trans Am Ophthalmol Soc 2001; 99: 233–7.
30. Small KW, Udar N, Yelchits S, et al. North Carolina macular dystrophy (MCDR1) locus: a fine resolution genetic map and haplotype analysis. Mol Vis 1999; 5: 38–42.
31. Reichel MB, Kelsell RE, Fan J, et al. Phenotype of a British North Carolina macular dystrophy family linked to chromosome 6q. Br J Ophthalmol 1998; 82: 1162–8.
32. Stefko ST, Zhang K, Gorin MB, et al. Clinical spectrum of chromosome 6-linked autosomal dominant drusen and macular degeneration. Am J Ophthalmol 2000; 130: 203–8.
33. Kniazeva M, Traboulsi EI, Yu Z, et al. A new locus for dominant drusen and macular degeneration maps to chromosome 6q14. Am J Ophthalmol 2000; 130: 197–202.
34. Griesinger IB, Sieving PA, Ayyagari R. Autosomal dominant macular atrophy at 6q14 excludes CORD7 and MCDR1/PBCRA loci. Invest Ophthalmol Vis Sci 2000; 41: 248–55.
35. Michaelides M, Johnson S, Tekriwal AK, et al. An early-onset autosomal dominant macular dystrophy (MCDR3) resembling North Carolina macular dystrophy maps to chromosome 5. Invest Ophthalmol Vis Sci 2003; 44: 2178–83.
36. Francis PJ, Johnson S, Edmunds B, et al. Genetic linkage analysis of a novel syndrome comprising North Carolina-like macular dystrophy and progressive sensorineural hearing loss. Br J Ophthalmol 2003; 87: 893–8.
37. Kelsell RE, Godley BF, Evans K, et al. Localization of the gene for progressive bifocal chorioretinal atrophy (PBCRA) to chromosome 6q. Hum Mol Genet 1995; 4: 1653–6.
38. Hoyng CB, Deutman AF. The development of central areolar choroidal dystrophy. Graefes Arch Clin Exp Ophthalmol 1996; 234: 87–93.
39. Hoyng CB, Heutink P, Testers L, et al. Autosomal dominant central areolar choroidal dystrophy caused by a mutation in codon 142 in the peripherin/RDS gene. Am J Ophthalmol 1996; 121: 623–9.
40. Hughes AE, Lotery AJ, Silvestri G. Fine localisation of the gene for central areolar choroidal dystrophy on chromosome 17p. J Med Genet 1998; 35: 770–2.

41. George ND, Yates JR, Bradshaw K, et al. Infantile presentation of X linked retinoschisis. Br J Ophthalmol 1995; 79: 653–7.

42. George ND, Yates JR, Moore AT. Clinical features in affected males with X-linked retinoschisis. Arch Ophthalmol 1996; 114: 274–80.

43. Curran RE, Robb RM. Isolated foveal hypoplasia. Arch Ophthalmol 1976; 94: 48–50.

44. O'Donnell FE Jr, Pappas HR. Autosomal dominant foveal hypoplasia and presenile cataracts. A new syndrome. Arch Ophthalmol 1982; 100: 279–81.

45. Krill AE, Deutman AF, Fishman M. The cone degenerations. Doc Ophthalmol 1973; 35: 1–80.

46. Fishman GA, Fishman M, Maggiano J. Macular lesions associated with retinitis pigmentosa. Arch Ophthalmol 1977; 95: 798–803.

47. Deutman AF. Benign concentric annular macular dystrophy. Am J Ophthalmol 1974; 78: 384–96.

48. O'Donnell FE, Welch RB. Fenestrated sheen macular dystrophy. A new autosomal dominant maculopathy. Arch Ophthalmol 1979; 97: 1292–6.

Congenital Hamartomatous Lesions of the Retina and Retinal Pigment Epithelium

CHAPTER 55

Graeme C M Black

CONGENITAL HYPERTROPHY OF THE RETINAL PIGMENT EPITHELIUM

Congenital hypertrophy of the retinal pigment epithelium (CHRPE) is a discrete, usually slightly raised, pigmented lesion of the fundus.[1] Such lesions are congenital and in the majority of cases do not cause clinical problems. At the cellular level the lesions are composed of a layer of hypertrophic RPE cells with atrophic photoreceptors above.[2,3] They are strongly pigmented (Fig. 55.1) and often have a surrounding area of depigmentation and discrete areas of depigmentation within.[1] Fluorescein angiography demonstrates masking of the choroidal fluorescence in areas of pigmentation. While occasionally CHRPEs have been shown to grow slowly with time, the majority are static. Secondary retinovascular changes may occur over CHRPEs[4] and a very small number of reports describe late, associated, malignant change.[5]

CHRPEs and adenomatous polyposis of the colon (APC)

In the majority of cases, CHRPEs have neither visual nor health implications. However many bilateral cases have been described in association with adenomatous polyposis of the colon (APC) or familial adenomatous polyposis (FAP).[6,7]

Adenomatous polyposis of the colon (APC) is an uncommon, autosomal dominant, monogenic disorder that predisposes to malignancy. Its prevalence is estimated to be around three in 100 000.[8] That subset of APC patients who have Gardner syndrome, that is APC with extracolonic manifestations, e.g. osteomas and CHRPEs,[9] are now known to have an identical condition. Turcot syndrome describes the co-occurrence of FAP

with primary brain (medulloblastoma) tumor.[10] Both conditions map to the same gene and may be caused by identical mutations.[11]

The majority of affected individuals with APC develop adenomatous colorectal polyps between the second and fourth decades.[12] Malignant transformation of the polyps is high, of the order of 90% by age 50 years. Identification of gene carriers is important for management as tumor surveillance by means of colonoscopy begins from around the age of 12 years. This is effective in detecting premalignant or early malignant lesions and may ultimately lead to elective colectomy. Polyps may also develop in the upper GI tract including stomach, small bowel and duodenal polyps. The last are associated with a significant risk of malignant transformation. Around 10% of patients develop desmoid tumors which are benign and locally invasive fibrous tissue tumors. Osteomas of the mandible are recognized with dental anomalies including missing or supernumerary teeth are also common.[13]

Multiple, (more than three) bilateral CHRPE are a highly specific and sensitive marker of APC. The lesions are congenital[14] and while they may be may be ovoid or pisciform in shape and may be surrounded by a palish grey halo they are often atypical. They may vary in size, from dot-like lesions to CHRPEs of multiple disc diameters, and position.[7,15]

Ophthalmic examination for CHRPEs can be useful as a clinical marker for a genetic mutation in at-risk individuals.[7,8] CHRPEs are not seen in all individuals with the APC phenotype and, when present suggest the presence of a mutation between codons 463–1387. In families where they are present it is very rare for a mutation carrier not to have CHRPEs.[16,17] In many cases this has been superseded by molecular genetic testing in many families where a gene mutation is known. Mutations in the *APC* gene are found in around 85% of families,[18] the overwhelming majority resulting in premature protein truncation.

CONGENITAL GROUPED PIGMENTATION OF THE RPE

Congenital grouped pigmentation of the RPE or "bear track" pigmentation is an uncommon condition which may be misdiagnosed as being related to APC. Here, there are numerous, pigmented lesions (Fig. 55.2) which resemble animal footprints (bear tracks).[1] Like CHRPEs they show masking of choroidal fluorescence on angiography. Histopathology suggests that CHRPE and congenital grouped pigmentation may be different expressions of a similar process, with the former being focal and the latter multifocal.[19] Congenital grouped pigmentation of the RPE may be bilateral or, in unilateral cases may be confined to one sector of the fundus. While familial cases have been reported

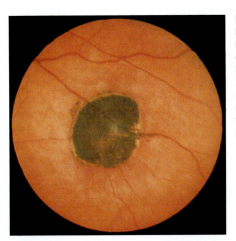

Fig. 55.1 Congenital hypertrophy of the retinal pigment epithelium (CHRPE). Slightly raised jet black lesion in the midperiphery with an associated small visual field defect (Professor AC Bird's patient.)

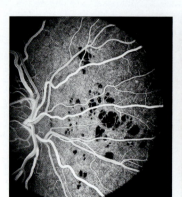
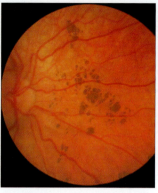

Fig. 55.2 Congenital grouped pigmentation ("bear track"). Unilateral, multiple brown patches in the retinal pigment epithelium of no functional significance. Fluorescein angiography shows masking of the underlying choroidal fluorescence (Professor AC Bird's patient.)

they are rarely seen.[20] Patients are asymptomatic and have normal EOGs and ERGs. There is no association between congenital grouped pigmentation of the RPE and APC.[21]

ASTROCYTIC HAMARTOMA

Astrocytic hamartoma is the classic ocular lesion of tuberous sclerosis. It has also been reported as an isolated finding (Fig. 55.3),[22,23] in association with neurofibromatosis type 1[24] and retinitis pigmentosa.[25] Histologically astrocytic hamartomas contain several glial cell types including those that stain positively for glial fibrillary acidic protein.[26]

Tuberous sclerosis complex (TSC) is a variable, autosomal dominant, disorder described in Chapter 69.

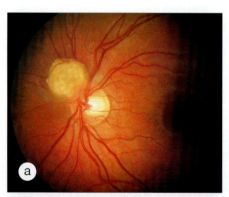

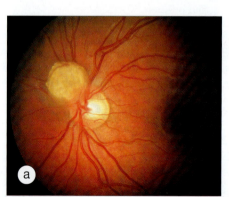

Fig. 55.3 Astrocytic hamartoma. (a) Peripapillary hamartoma in a patient who did not have tuberous sclerosis. The acuity was 6/6 and the lesion was discovered at an examination for myopia. (b). Same patient as (a) showing the calcification in the hamartoma on CT scan.

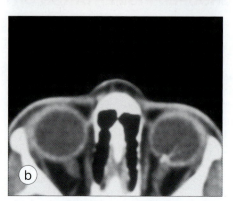

The manifestations of TSC in the eye are common and in most cases do not cause symptoms. The classical retinal hamartomas include (i) flat, smooth, noncalcified translucent lesions; (ii) classical elevated, multinodular hamartoma or "mulberry tumors" which are usually found at or close to the optic disc[27] (iii) a transitional type with features of the two, being calcified centrally but translucent in its periphery. Progression from flat, noncalcified lesions to elevated calcified lesions may occur.[28]

The majority of astrocytic hamartomas are static lesions. However they can undergo necrosis leading to vitreous seeding vitreous hemorrhage,[29] retinal detachment[30] or necrotizing retinochoroiditis[31] and rarely may behave in a locally invasive fashion.[26] Occasionally, in particular in sporadic cases, an astrocytic hamartoma will be mistaken for a retinoblastoma.[32]

TSC is a genetically heterogenous condition which may be caused by mutations in two genes, *TSC1* on chromosome 9q34 which encodes the hamartin protein and *TSC2* on chromosome 16p13 which encodes tuberin.[33] Mutation testing is now available but only identifies mutations in around three quarters of cases;[34] ophthalmic examination therefore remains an important adjunct to diagnosis. Both hamartin and tuberin are thought to act as tumor suppressor genes which have been shown to form heterodimers and are believed to regulate cell cycle and cell proliferation.[35]

CAPILLARY HAEMANGIOMA

Capillary hemangiomas (more correctly, hemangioblastomas) are found as an isolated finding or as part of the multisystemic manifestations of von Hippel–Lindau disease (Chapter 69), which must be excluded in all cases.[36] While they may be solitary in VHL they are more often multiple. Symptoms are rare before the age of 5 years at which age annual screening should begin since treatment can successfully preserve vision.[37,38] Those presenting with symptoms (commonly blurring of vision) are at greatest risk while the majority of those who lose vision do so before the age of 30 years.[36,39]

The majority of hemangiomas are seen in the periphery of the fundus where they are usually well circumscribed, growing inwards from the outer retina (endophytic) and, in the case of larger tumors, associated with large feeder and draining vessels. Angiomas are most commonly present anterior to the equator and are most frequent in the superotemporal quadrant.[38,40] Smaller hemangiomas may not have obvious feeder vessels and can be difficult to detect on ophthalmoscopy although they will be readily visible as hyperfluorescent lesions on fluorescein angiography. Juxtapapillary hemangiomas may be endophytic or exophytic[41] and are seen in 10–15% of eyes from VHL gene carriers.

Retinal hemangiomas cause a variety of complications including exudation, tractional retinal detachment, neovascularization and in late stages, neovascular glaucoma and phthisis bulbi. The exophytic tumors close to the disc may simulate papilledema and may result in juxtapapillary exudation or exudative detachment.

Hemangioblastomas of the retina and nervous system are indistinguishable histologically and are characterized by a high degree of vascularization with a dense network of capillaries. Vascularization is induced by overexpression of vascular endothelial growth factor (VEGF). The mixed cellular populations of the tumors include vascular endothelial and pericyte cells as well as intervascular, or stromal, cells of uncertain cellular origin.[42]

Treatment depends on the size, position and nature of the lesion. The majority of small peripheral lesions may, in the presence of clear media, be treated by laser photocoagulation which can be applied to the feeder vessels, to the tumor itself, or both. This is most effective for smaller tumors (<1.5 mm in diameter) but, when applied over several sessions, has been shown to be effective for tumors up to 3 mm. Cryotherapy is valuable in particular for anterior lesions, situations where laser uptake may be reduced, (for example in the presence of subretinal fluid) and for larger tumors (>3 mm in diameter). Larger tumors (>4 mm diameter) may not be effectively managed with either photocoagulation or cryotherapy; here other treatment modalities may be considered including both external beam and plaque radiotherapy.[43,44]

The use of photodynamic therapy for retinal hemangiomas has been reported to be successful[45] although there is currently only limited experience of its use. For the future it is possible that novel, targeted therapies will be developed; for example recent reports describe the use of VEGF inhibitors (VEGF is highly expressed in the tumors) in a small number of cases with variable results.[46,47]

Juxtapapillary hemangiomas in particular present a therapeutic challenge due to the risk of damage to the optic nerve and/or nerve fiber layer.[48] In many cases these can remain stable over long periods suggesting that observation is a reasonable first-line approach to management. Where there are symptoms or evidence of progression, laser photocoagulation may be effective especially when used in multiple treatments at low energy although plaque radiotherapy and photodynamic therapy have all be used.[49]

The VHL gene is located at chromosome 3p25–p26 and encodes a ubiquitous 213 amino acid protein (Chapter 69), mutations are found in almost all patients. It is a tumor suppressor gene requiring loss of both alleles for tumorigenesis.

FAMILIAL RETINAL ARTERIOLAR TORTUOSITY

Familial retinal arteriolar tortuosity is a rare autosomal dominant condition in which retinal arteriolar tortuosity develops, in particular at the posterior pole, during childhood or early adulthood and may progress with age.[50] No leakage is seen on fluorescein angiography and the major retinal vasculature and venous system are both normal. Intra- and preretinal hemor-

rhages may develop both spontaneously or after exertion but resolve without complication or loss of vision. There are no systemic associations

CONGENITAL RETINAL MACROVESSEL

In this uncommon disorder a large retinal vessel, usually a vein, runs from the disc towards the macular region to supply the retina both above and below the horizontal raphe.[51] Fluorescein angiography often shows arteriovenous communications and areas of capillary nonperfusion. It can be divided into three groups,[51] depending upon the extent of the arteriovenous anastomosis:

1. There is a small arteriovenous anastomosis which occurs across a capillary complex; although venous pressure is raised it is well-compensated and vision remains good.
2. There is direct arteriolar venous communication and high flow between the arterial and venous sides of the circulation (Fig. 55.4). This leads to secondaries such as arteriolar and venous dilatation and capillary nonperfusion in neighboring vessels.
3. This consists of patients with complex large vessel anastomoses. Many vessels is in the fundus may be widely dilated and vision is often poor.

The vascular abnormalities are thought to be congenital and are usually nonprogressive. They may rarely give rise to ocular complications including retinal, subhyaloid and vitreous hemorrhage, venous occlusion, retinal neovascularization and neovascular glaucoma.[52,53] Treatment is not usually necessary but retinal neovascularization or rubeotic glaucoma may respond to panretinal photocoagulation.[53]

The retinal arteriovenous malformations may be associated with similar facial and intracranial vascular malformations. In Wyburn–Mason syndrome similar vascular malformations in the midbrain and cerebrum (Fig. 55.4).

INHERITED RETINAL VENOUS BEADING

In this dominantly inherited disorder, affected individuals have prominent segmental venous beading.[54,55] Conjunctival venous anomalies are present in some family members and occasionally renal disease and hearing loss. Although all affected

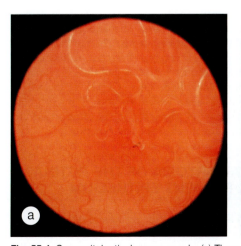

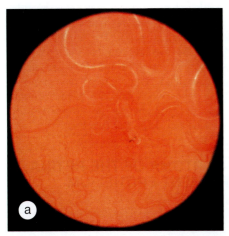
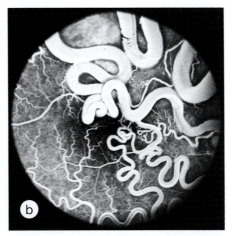
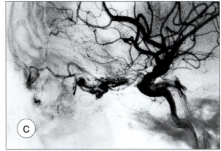

Fig. 55.4 Congenital retinal macrovessels. (a) There are multiple very large anastomotic vessels in the right fundus: the acuity was 6/18. (b) The fluorescein angiogram showed no leakage. (c) Carotid angiogram showing cerebral vascular malformation.

individuals show the typical segmental venous abnormality there is wide range of clinical expression. Microvascular abnormalities including arteriolar narrowing, capillary closure, vascular leakage, microaneurysm formation and retinal neovascularization are evident in some individuals. Visual loss may occur as a result of macular edema or exudates, venous occlusion or vitreous hemorrhage. The underlying cause of the vascular abnormality is not known.

FAMILIAL RETINAL ARTERIAL MACROANEURYSMS

Three pairs of siblings from three families have been described[56] with multiple retinal arterial macroaneurysms. All affected individuals had symptoms in childhood and had an aneurysm formation with beading along the major retinal arteries. There was recurrent hemorrhaging, which often resorbed spontaneously, and leakage from the macroaneurysms.

CAVERNOUS HEMANGIOMA

Retinal cavernous hemangioma is an uncommon vascular hamartomatous lesion of the retina involving the optic nerve head or peripheral retina. Retinal cavernous hemangiomas are usually asymptomatic and while reported in childhood, most are seen in adults and are said to be commoner in females. They are usually unilateral and most are sporadic. A cavernous hemangioma is often visible as a cluster of grape-like vascular dilatations (Fig. 55.5) near a retinal vein (which may be dilated) and which is often associated with fibrous tissue and superficial hemorrhage. The absence of dilated feeder vessels helps in differentiating from a capillary hemangioma.[57,58] On fluorescein angiography the

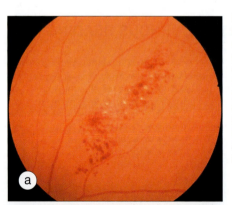

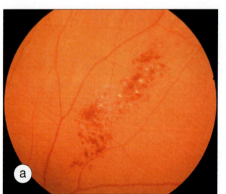

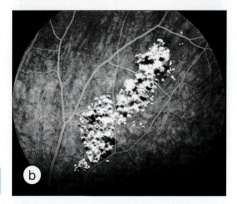

Fig. 55.5 Cavernous hemangioma of the retina. (a) There is a grape-like cluster of aneurysmal dilatations in the superior retina. (b) Fluorescein angiogram of the same patient showing slow flow and pooling. (Mr Anthony Moore's patient.)

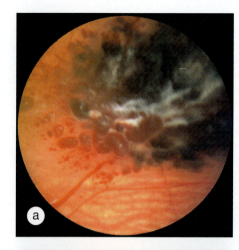

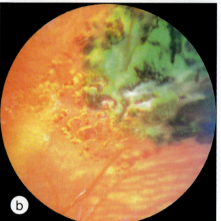

Fig. 55.6 Cavernous hemangioma of the retina. (a) This 11-month-old child presented with a strabismus, but with patching the eye acuity remained at 6/18. The grape-like cluster of abnormal vessels was adjacent to the macula and regressed over 3 years. (b) Photograph taken a few minutes after fluorescein injection. The pooling of fluorescein occurs due to the very slow blood flow. No leakage occurred.

lesions fill slowly and incompletely without leakage or arteriovenous shunting (Figs 55.5 and 55.6). Histologically cavernous hemangiomas comprise normal-looking vascular tissue.[58] Where a lesion is distant from the macula vision is usually good, when near it may be reduced.[59] Treatment is seldom necessary except in rare instances of recurrent vitreous hemorrhage where both cryotherapy or photocoagulation may be used.[60]

In a small number of cases an individual may have multiple vascular malformations. Such vascular malformations included cavernous hemangiomas of the brain or spinal cord or cutaneous vascular malformations.[61] In some cases there may be a relevant family history including others with similar vascular abnormalities, seizures, cutaneous vascular lesions, recognized intracranial hemorrhage, or sudden unexplained death. The familial cases of cavernous hemangiomas (CCM cerebral cavernous malformations) are now recognized as a distinct condition and three genetic loci (CCM1-3) have been identified. One, CCM1 is caused by mutation of the KRIT1 gene which encodes a microtubule-associated protein that is thought to be important for determination of endothelial cell shape and function.[62,63]

COMBINED HAMARTOMA OF THE RETINA AND RETINAL PIGMENT EPITHELIUM

The term combined hamartoma of the retina and retinal pigment epithelium describes a group of hamartomatous lesions involving the RPE, retina, retinal vasculature and overlying vitreous (Figs 55.7 and 55.8).[64] They may be juxtapapillary or extrapapillary,

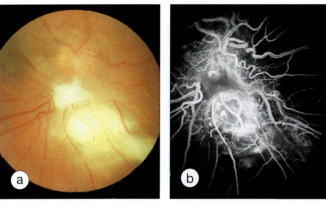

Fig. 55.7 Combined hamartoma of the retina and retinal pigment epithelium. (a) Elevated peripapillary lesion with retinal traction and exudative detachment. (b) The fluorescein angiogram of the same patient shows marked vascular tortuosity and distortion. (Professor AC Bird's patient.)

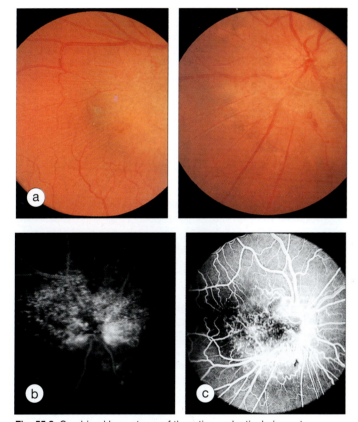

Fig. 55.8 Combined hamartoma of the retina and retinal pigment epithelium. (a) This patient has a marked elevation of the optic disc with radial retinal traction, wrinkled internal limiting membrane and retinal pigment epithelium changes around the disc. (b) Fluorescein angiogram showing the capillary beading and (c) late leakage. (Professor AC Bird's patient.)

the latter affecting either the macular or peripheral retina.[65,66] The most common site is in the juxtapapillary region where the lesions are elevated, pigmented and associated with intraretinal gliosis and distortion of the retinal vessels. Fluorescein angiography shows capillary dilation within the lesions, vessel

tortuosity with some leakage and blockage of the choroidal fluorescence. Extrapapillary lesions may result in visual reduction as a result of contraction of the glial component.

Most cases are unilateral and sporadic. However bilateral cases are described[67] and in particular are seen in association with a number of inherited diseases:

Neurofibromatosis type 2 (NF2).[68,69]
Neurofibromatosis type 1 (NF1).[70,71]
Basal cell nevus (Gorlin) syndrome.[72]

Presentation (amblyopia, strabismus or reduction in vision) usually suggests a congenital lesion while the clinical findings (reduced visual acuity, field defect or afferent pupil defect) depend upon the extent of disc and macular involvement or the degree of macular distortion. Apart from management of amblyopia, management is usually conservative as, in the majority of cases, combined hamartomas remain stable. The lesions may show some increase in size with time while the presence of contractile glial elements within the lesions may give rise to changes with time and to a reduction in visual acuity[73] and may require intervention.[74,75] Occasionally vitreous hemorrhage, which may be recurrent, is described.[76]

The lesions may simulate ocular tumors such as melanoma or retinoblastoma and have occasionally resulted in enucleation. In these, rare cases, histopathology, shows abundant glial tissue, capillary hyperplasia and pigment epithelial proliferation with a variable distribution of the tissue types throughout the lesion.[64,65]

COATS DISEASE

Coats disease of the retina is a form of retinal telangiectasia characterized by a defect of retinal vascular development which results in vessel leakage, subretinal exudation and retinal detachment. Described by Coats,[77] the condition in its classical form is almost invariably seen in males and is unlike other forms of retinal telangiectasis, such as idiopathic juxtafoveal telangiectasis as it is unilateral. The condition usually presents during the first decade of life with unilateral visual loss, strabismus or rarely, leukocoria or ocular pain. The condition may simulate retinoblastoma which may be a common referral diagnosis.

Fundus examination demonstrates retinal telangiectasia with aneurysm formation (Fig. 55.9), which is most often seen in the temporal retina but which may affect any quadrant. The subretinal exudation may be more far-reaching than the telangiectasia (Fig. 55.10). On retinal fluorescein angiography, areas of capillary nonperfusion and dilatation together with fusiform aneurysms are observed. Leakage from the vessels may be observed.

Where eyes with Coats disease have been enucleated they show aneurysmal dilatation of small vessels, and a subretinal exudate characterized by lipid-laden macrophages and cholesterol crystals. The majority of cases show progression with time, leading to total retinal detachment, neovascular glaucoma and phthisis bulbi. The extent and severity of detachment has been observed to be more severe in those diagnosed at a younger age.

Treatment with either cryotherapy or photocoagulation may slow the progression of the disease and in some cases may result in improvement of vision with reduction in the exudate. Treatment depends on disease severity. The most widely used modalities, cryotherapy or laser photocoagulation, are most effective if the retinal telangiectasias is limited and the associated detachment mild.[78,79] Cryotherapy is best for small, anterior lesions while photocoagulation may be used for macular edema and exudation.[80] In severe cases where cryotherapy and laser are

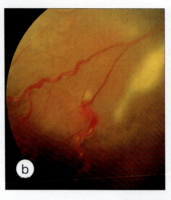
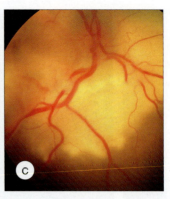

Fig. 55.9 Coats disease. (a) Beading and aneurysmal dilatation of the retinal arterioles in the upper temporal quadrant of this 8-year-old boy. There is a localized retinal detachment. (b) Large aneurysmal dilatation of a peripheral vessel and dilatation and tortuosity of the adjacent vessel. (c) Exudative retinal detachment with subretinal solid exudate.

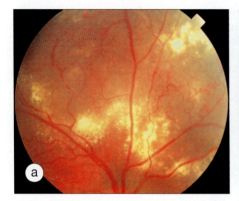
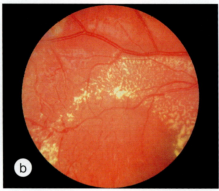

Fig. 55.10 Coats disease. (a) In the superior fundus a number of dilated and telangiectatic retinal vessels can be seen. There is a serous retinal detachment and subretinal exudates. (b) In the inferior and temporal fundus of this child with Coats disease a number of dilatations of the retinal vessels can be seen. There has been a serous retinal detachment which has now reabsorbed leaving a ring of subretinal exudates.

ineffective, vitrectomy has been attempted with success in some cases.

Coats disease is idiopathic. However, the observations that the condition is often unilateral, segmental and found in males are consistent with the suggestion that this represents a mosaic phenotype. It has been demonstrated that somatic mutation of *NDP*, the gene mutated in Norrie disease (See Chapter 49) can cause Coats disease. In this case it is presumed that a mutation occurs within cells of neuroectodermal origin at a stage of development that results in a segment of the retina carrying the mutant allele.[81]

Coats disease has been described in a number of systemic diseases:

- **Retinitis pigmentosa**. In one study this was in particular associated with mutations in the *CRB1* mutations in patients with both RP and with RP with preserved para-arteriolar retinal pigment epithelium (PPRPE) phenotype[82] which suggested that patients with PRPE should be checked regularly for a Coats-like complication.
- **Cranial, cutaneous and systemic conditions.** Coats disease has been reported in association with a number of inherited and also extraocular conditions. A number of children have

been described with Coats disease in association with what is presumed to be an autosomal recessive condition characterized by intracerebral calcification, cerebral microangiopathy, sparse hair, dystrophic nails, intrauterine growth retardation and bone marrow involvement and postnatal growth failure.[83–85]

- **Plasminogen deficiency type 1**.[86]
- **Cornelia de Lange syndrome**.[87]
- **Hallerman-Streiff syndrome**.[88]
- **Senior Loken syndrome**.[89]
- **Multiple glomus tumors**.[90]
- **Factoscapulohumeral muscular dystrophy.**
Retinal microvasculopathy including tortuosity and aneurysm formation with Coats' disease has been described in association with facioscapulohumeral muscular dystrophy a rare autosomal dominant condition that is also associated with hearing loss.[91] The microvascular changes include retinal telangiectasis and microaneurysm formation, capillary closure and vascular leakage. In larger studies microvascular abnormalities were present in half to two-thirds of affected individuals and may been seen in childhood and may even precede the muscle disease.[92]

REFERENCES

1. Gass JD. Focal congenital anomalies of the retinal pigment epithelium. Eye 1989; 3: 1–18.

2. Parker JA, Kalnins VI, Deck JH, et al. Histopathological features of congenital fundus lesions in familial adenomatous polyposis. Can J Ophthalmol 1990; 25: 159–63.

3. Traboulsi EI, Murphy SF, de la Cruz ZC, et al. A clinicopathologic study of the eyes in familial adenomatous polyposis with extracolonic manifestations (Gardner's syndrome). Am J Ophthalmol 1990; 110: 550–61.

4. Cohen SY, Quentel G, Guiberteau B, et al. Retinal vascular changes in congenital hypertrophy of the retinal pigment epithelium. Ophthalmology 1993; 100: 471–4.

5. Shields JA, Shields CL, Eagle RC Jr, et al. Adenocarcinoma arising from congenital hypertrophy of retinal pigment epithelium. Arch Ophthalmol 2001; 119: 597–602.

6. Blair NP, Trempe CL. Hypertrophy of the retinal pigment epithelium associated with Gardner's syndrome. Am J Ophthalmol 1980; 90: 661–7.

7. Moore AT, Maher ER, Koch DJ, et al. Incidence and significance of congenital hypertrophy of the retinal pigment epithelium (CHRPE) in familial adenomatous polyposis coli (FAPC). Ophthalmic Paediatr Genet 1992; 13: 67–71.

8. Burn J, Chapman P, Delhanty J, et al. The UK Northern region genetic register for familial adenomatous polyposis coli: use of age of onset, congenital hypertrophy of the retinal pigment epithelium, and DNA markers in risk calculations. J Med Genet 1991; 28: 289–96.

9. Gardner EJ. Follow-up study of a family group exhibiting dominant inheritance for a syndrome including intestinal polyps, osteomas, fibromas and epidermal cysts. Am J Hum Genet 1962; 14: 376–90.

10. Turcot J, Despres JP, St. Pierre F. Malignant tumors of the central nervous system associated with familial polyposis of the colon: report of two cases. Dis Colon Rectum 1959; 2: 465–468.

11. Nishisho I, Nakamura Y, Miyoshi Y, et al. Mutations of chromosome 5q21 genes in FAP and colorectal cancer patients. Science. 1991; 253: 665–9.

12. Petersen GM, Slack J, Nakamura Y. Screening guidelines and premorbid diagnosis of familial adenomatous polyposis using linkage. Gastroenterology 1991; 100: 1658–64.

13. Thakker N, Davies R, Horner K, et al. The dental phenotype in familial adenomatous polyposis: diagnostic application of a weighted scoring system for changes on dental panoramic radiographs. J Med Genet 1995; 32: 458–64.

14. Aiello LP, Traboulsi EI. Pigmented fundus lesions in a preterm infant with familial adenomatous polyposis. Arch Ophthalmol 1993; 111: 302–3.

15. Tiret A, Taiel-Sartral M, Tiret E, et al. Diagnostic value of fundus examination in familial adenomatous polyposis. Br J Ophthalmol 1997; 81: 755–8.

16. Wallis YL, Macdonald F, Hulten M, et al. Genotype-phenotype correlation between position of constitutional APC gene mutation and CHRPE expression in familial adenomatous polyposis. Hum Genet 1994; 94: 543–8.

17. Davies DR, Armstrong JG, Thakker N, et al. Severe Gardner syndrome in families with mutations restricted to a specific region of the APC gene. Am J Hum Genet 1995; 57: 1151–8.

18. Ballhausen WG. Genetic testing for familial adenomatous polyposis. Ann NY Acad Sci 2000; 910: 36–47; discussion 47–9.

10. Regillo CD, Eagle RC Jr, Shields JA, et al. Histopathologic findings in congenital grouped pigmentation of the retina. Ophthalmology 1993; 100: 400–5.

20. Renardel de Lavalette VW, Cruysberg JR, Deutman AF. Familial congenital grouped pigmentation of the retina. Am J Ophthalmol 1991; 112: 406–9.

21. Shields JA, Shields CL, Shah PG, et al. Lack of association among typical congenital hypertrophy of the retinal pigment epithelium, adenomatous polyposis, and Gardner syndrome. Ophthalmology 1992; 99: 1709–13.

22. Ramsay RC, Kinyoun JL, Hill CW, et al. Retinal astrocytoma. Am J Ophthalmol 1979; 88: 32–6.

23. Arnold AC, Hepler RS, Yee RW, et al. Solitary retinal astrocytoma. Surv Ophthalmol 1985; 30: 173–81.

24. Destro M, D'Amico DJ, Gragoudas ES, et al. Retinal manifestations of neurofibromatosis. Diagnosis and management. Arch Ophthalmol 1991; 109: 662–6.

25. Bec P, Mathis A, Adam P, et al. Retinitis pigmentosa associated with astrocytic hamartomas of the optic disc. Ophthalmologica 1984; 189: 135–8.

26. Milot J, Michaud J, Lemieux N, et al. Persistent hyperplastic primary vitreous with retinal tumor in tuberous sclerosis: report of a case including tumoral immunohistochemistry and cytogenetic analyses. Ophthalmology 1999; 106: 630–4.

27. Rowley SA, O'Callaghan FJ, Osborne JP. Ophthalmic manifestations of tuberous sclerosis: a population based study. Br J Ophthalmol 2001; 85: 420–3.

28. Robertson DM. Ophthalmic findings. In: Gomez MR, ed. Tuberous Sclerosis Complex. 3rd edn. New York: Oxford University Press, 1999: 145–59.

29. Atkinson A, Sanders MD, Wong V. Vitreous haemorrhage in tuberous sclerosis. Report of two cases. Br J Ophthalmol 1973; 57: 773–9.

30. Bloom SM, Mahl CF. Photocoagulation for serous detachment of the macula secondary to retinal astrocytoma. Retina 1991; 11: 416–22.

31. Coppeto JR, Lubin JR, Albert DM. Astrocytic hamartoma in tuberous sclerosis mimicking necrotizing retinochoroiditis. J Pediatr Ophthalmol Strabismus 1982; 19: 306–13.

32. Robertson DM. Ophthalmic manifestations of tuberous sclerosis. Ann NY Acad Sci 1991; 615: 17–25.

33. Sampson JR. TSC1 and TSC2: genes that are mutated in the human genetic disorder tuberous sclerosis. Biochem Soc Trans 2003; 31: 592–6.

34. Jones AC, Shyamsundar MM, Thomas MW, et al. Comprehensive mutation analysis of TSC1 and TSC2-and phenotypic correlations in 150 families with tuberous sclerosis. Am J Hum Genet 1999; 64: 1305–15.

35. Rosner M, Hofer K, Kubista M, et al. Cell size regulation by the human TSC tumor suppressor proteins depends on PI3K and FKBP38. Oncogene 2003; 22: 4786–98.

36. Webster AR, Maher ER, Moore AT. Clinical characteristics of ocular angiomatosis in von Hippel-Lindau disease and correlation with germline mutation. Arch Ophthalmol 1999; 117: 371–8.

37. Moore AT, Maher ER, Rosen P, et al. Ophthalmological screening for von Hippel-Lindau disease. Eye 1991; 5: 723–8.

38. Schmidt D, Natt E, Neumann HP. Long-term results of laser treatment for retinal angiomatosis in von Hippel-Lindau disease. Eur J Med Res 2000; 5: 47–58.

39. Dollfus H, Massin P, Taupin P, et al. Retinal hemangioblastoma in von Hippel-Lindau disease: a clinical and molecular study. Invest Ophthalmol Vis Sci 2002; 43: 3067–74.

40. Webster AR, Maher ER, Bird AC, et al. A clinical and molecular genetic analysis of solitary ocular angioma. Ophthalmology 1999; 106: 623–9.

41. Gass JD, Braunstein R. Sessile and exophytic capillary angiomas of the juxtapapillary retina and optic nerve head. Arch Ophthalmol 1980; 98: 1790–7.

42. Joussen AM, Kirchhof B. Solitary peripapillary hemangioblastoma. A histopathological case report. Acta Ophthalmol Scand 2001; 79: 83–7.

43. Palmer JD, Gragoudas ES. Advances in treatment of retinal angiomas. Int Ophthalmol Clin 1997; 37: 159–70.

44. Kreusel KM, Bornfeld N, Lommatzsch A, et al. Ruthenium-106 brachytherapy for peripheral retinal capillary hemangioma. Ophthalmology 1998; 105: 1386–92.

45. Atebara NH. Retinal capillary hemangioma treated with verteporfin photodynamic therapy. Am J Ophthalmol 2002; 134: 788–90.

46. Aiello LP, George DJ, Cahill MT, et al. Rapid and durable recovery of visual function in a patient with von Hippel-Lindau syndrome after systemic therapy with vascular endothelial growth factor receptor inhibitor su5416. Ophthalmology 2002; 109: 1745–51.

47. Girmens JF, Erginay A, Massin P, et al. Treatment of von Hippel-Lindau retinal hemangioblastoma by the vascular endothelial growth factor receptor inhibitor SU5416 is more effective for associated macular edema than for hemangioblastomas. Am J Ophthalmol 2003; 136: 194–6.

48. McDonald HR. Diagnostic and therapeutic challenges. Juxtapapillary retina capillary hemangioma. Retina 2003; 23: 86–91.

49. Schmidt-Erfurth UM, Kusserow C, Barbazetto IA, et al. Benefits and complications of photodynamic therapy of papillary capillary hemangiomas. Ophthalmology 2002; 109: 1256–66.

50. Sutter FK, Helbig H. Familial retinal arteriolar tortuosity: a review. Surv Ophthalmol 2003; 48: 245–55.

51. Archer DB, Deutman A, Ernest JT, et al. Arteriovenous communications of the retina. Am J Ophthalmol 1973; 75: 224–41.

52. Mansour AM, Wells CG, Jampol LM, et al. Ocular complications of arteriovenous communications of the retina. Arch Ophthalmol 1989; 107: 232–6.

53. Schatz H, Chang LF, Ober RR, et al. Central retinal vein occlusion associated with retinal arteriovenous malformation. Ophthalmology 1993; 100: 24–30.

54. Stewart MW, Gitter KA. Inherited retinal venous beading. Am J Ophthalmol 1988; 106: 675–81.

55. Piquet B, Gross-Jendroska M, Holz FG, et al. Inherited venous beading. Eye 1994; 8: 84–8.

56. Dhindsa HS, Abboud EB. Familial retinal arterial macroaneurysms. Retina 2002; 22: 607–15.

57. Bottoni F, Canevini MP, Canger R, et al. Twin vessels in familial retinal cavernous hemangioma. Am J Ophthalmol 1990; 109: 285–9.

58. Messmer E, Laqua H, Wessing A, et al. Nine cases of cavernous hemangioma of the retina. Am J Ophthalmol 1983; 95: 383–90.

59. Naftchi S, la Cour M. A case of central visual loss in a child due to macular cavernous haemangioma of the retina. Acta Ophthalmol Scand 2002; 80: 550–2.

60. Brown GC, Shields JA. Tumors of the optic nerve head. Surv Ophthalmol 1985; 29: 239–64.

61. Sarraf D, Payne AM, Kitchen ND, et al. Familial cavernous hemangioma: an expanding ocular spectrum. Arch Ophthalmol 2000; 118: 969–73.

62. Couteulx SL, Brezin AP, Fontaine B, et al. A novel KRIT1/CCM1 truncating mutation in a patient with cerebral and retinal cavernous angiomas. Arch Ophthalmol 2002; 120: 217–8.

63. Gunel M, Laurans MS, Shin D, et al. KRIT1, a gene mutated in cerebral cavernous malformation, encodes a microtubule-associated protein. Proc Natl Acad Sci USA 2002; 99: 10677–82.

64. Gass JD. An unusual hamartoma of the pigment epithelium and retina simulating choroidal melanoma and retinoblastoma. Trans Am Ophthalmol Soc 1973; 71: 171–83; discussions 184–5.

65. Cosgrove JM, Sharp DM, Bird AC. Combined hamartoma of the retina and retinal pigment epithelium: the clinical spectrum. Trans Ophthalmol Soc UK 1986; 105: 106–13.

66. Wiechens B, Amm M. Macular combined malformation (hamartoma) of the retina and retinal pigment epithelium Ophthalmologe 1996; 93: 724–8.

67. Blumenthal EZ, Papamichael G, Merin S. Combined hamartoma of the retina and retinal pigment epithelium: a bilateral presentation. Retina 1998; 18: 557–9.

68. Sivalingam A, Augsburger J, Perilongo G, et al. Combined hamartoma of the retina and retinal pigment epithelium in a patient with neurofibromatosis type 2. J Pediatr Ophthalmol Strabismus 1991; 28: 320–2.

69. Bouzas EA, Parry DM, Eldridge R, et al. Familial occurrence of combined pigment epithelial and retinal hamartomas associated with neurofibromatosis 2. Retina 1992; 12: 103–7.

70. Tsai P, O'Brien JM. Combined hamartoma of the retina and retinal pigment epithelium as the presenting sign of neurofibromatosis-1. Ophthal Surg Lasers 2000; 31: 145–7.

71. Vianna RN, Pacheco DF, Vasconcelos MM, et al. Combined hamartoma of the retina and retinal pigment epithelium associated with neurofibromatosis type-1. Int Ophthalmol 2001; 24: 63–6.

72. De Potter P, Stanescu D, Caspers-Velu L, et al. Photo essay: combined hamartoma of the retina and retinal pigment epithelium in Gorlin syndrome. Arch Ophthalmol 2000; 118: 1004–5.

73. Mason JO 3rd, Kleiner R. Combined hamartoma of the retina and retinal pigment epithelium associated with epiretinal membrane and macular hole. Retina 1997; 17: 160–2.

74. McDonald HR, Abrams GW, Burke JM, et al. Clinicopathologic results of vitreous surgery for epiretinal membranes in patients with combined retinal and retinal pigment epithelial hamartomas. Am J Ophthalmol 1985; 100: 806–13.

75. Sappenfield DL, Gitter KA. Surgical intervention for combined retinal-retinal pigment epithelial hamartoma. Retina 1990; 10: 119–24.

76. Moschos M, Ladas ID, Zafirakis PK, et al. Recurrent vitreous hemorrhages due to combined pigment epithelial and retinal hamartoma: natural course and indocyanine green angiographic findings. Ophthalmologica 2001; 215: 66–9.

77. Coats G. Forms of retinal disease with massive exudation. R Lon Ophthalmic Hosp Rev 1908; 17: 440–525.

78. Silodor SW, Augsburger JJ, Shields JA, et al. Natural history and management of advanced Coats' disease. Ophthalmic Surg 1988; 19: 89–93.

79. Jones JH, Kroll AJ, Lou PL, et al. Coats' Disease. Int Ophthalmol Clin 2001; 41: 189–98.

80. Tarkkanen A, Laatikainen L. Coats' disease: clinical, angiographic, histopathological findings and clinical management. Br J Ophthalmol 1983; 67: 766–76.

81. Black GC, Perveen R, Bonshek R, et al. Coats' disease of the retina (unilateral retinal telangiectasis) caused by somatic mutation in the NDP gene: a role for norrin in retinal angiogenesis. Hum Mol Genet 1999; 8: 2031–5.

82. den Hollander AL, Heckenlively JR, van den Bornli, et al. Laber congenital amaurosis and retinitis pigmentosa with Coats-like exudative vasculopathy are associated with mutations in the crumbs homologue (CRBI) gene. Am J Hum Genet 2001; 69: 198–203.

83. Gayatri NA, Hughes MI, Lloyd IC, et al. Association of the congenital bone marrow failure syndromes with retinopathy, intracerebral calcification and progressive neurological impairment. Eur J Paediatr Neurol 2002; 6: 125–128.

84. Kajtár P, Mehés K. Bilateral Coats' retinopathy associated with aplastic anaemia and mild dyskeratotic signs. Am J Med Genet 1994; 49: 374–377.

85. Tolmie JL, Browne BH, McGettrick PM, et al. A familial syndrome with Coats' reaction, retinal angiomas, hair and nail defects and intracranial calcification. Eye 1988; 2: 297–303.

86. Patrassi GM, Sartori MT, Piermarocchi S, et al. Unusual thrombotic-like retinopathy (Coats' disease) associated with congenital plasminogen deficiency type I. J Intern Med 1993; 234: 619–23.

87. Folk JC, Genovese FN, Biglan AW. Coats' disease in a patient with Cornelia de Lange syndrome. Am J Ophthalmol 1981; 91: 607–10.

88. Newell SW, Hall BD, Anderson CW, et al. Hallermann-Streiff syndrome with Coats disease. J Pediatr Ophthalmol Strabismus 1994; 31: 123–5.

89. Schuman JS, Lieberman KV, Friedman AH, et al. Senior-Loken syndrome (familial renal-retinal dystrophy) and Coats' disease. Am J Ophthalmol 1985; 100: 822–7.

90. Bhushan M, Kumar S, Griffiths CE. Multiple glomus tumors, Coats' disease and basic fibroblast growth factor. Br J Dermatol 1997; 137: 454–6.

91. Gurwin EB, Fitzsimons RB, Sehmi KS, et al. Retinal telangiectasis in facioscapulohumeral muscular dystrophy with deafness. Arch Ophthalmol 1985; 103: 1695–700.

92. Padberg GW, Brouwer OF, de Keizer RJ, et al. On the significance of retinal vascular disease and hearing loss in facioscapulohumeral muscular dystrophy. Muscle Nerve 1995; 2: S73–80.

Retinal Detachment in Childhood

CHAPTER 56

Martin P Snead

Retinal detachment is uncommon in childhood and frequently presents late with advanced or second eye involvement at the time of diagnosis (Table 56.1). Several inherited disorders associated with an increased risk of retinal detachment and detachment complicating preexisting developmental abnormalities are particularly difficult to repair. In addition retinoblastoma or other tumors may give rise to a "solid" detachment. Congenital retinal detachment, or so-called congenital nonattachment of the retina, is now recognized as part of the spectrum of vitreoretinal dysplasia, which may have a variety of causes (see Chapter 49).

RHEGMATOGENOUS RETINAL DETACHMENT

Most cases of rhegmatogenous retinal detachment in children are related to genetic, developmental, or traumatic causes.

Traumatic retinal detachment

Traumatic retinal detachment is seen most commonly in older children and is usually caused by blunt trauma where retinal tears may be found in approximately 2–5%.[1] Penetrating injuries and retained intraocular foreign bodies are less frequent causes[2,3] but are associated with severe proliferative vitreoretinopathy (PVR).

Blunt ocular trauma

Retinal detachment due to blunt trauma is most commonly caused by a disinsertion at the ora serrata and usually occurs in older children. Sudden anteroposterior compression is associated with a corresponding coronal expansion and retinal avulsion injury

characterized by an accompanying festoon of nonpigmented pars plana epithelium (Fig. 56.1). The preponderance for superior quadrant involvement is greater than the usual lower temporal quadrant involvement in nontraumatic dialysis.[4,5] Although the disinsertion may exceed 90° of the circumference and superficially resemble a giant retinal tear, the vitreous gel characteristically remains attached to the posterior flap so that independent mobility is not a feature, and dialyses respond well to conventional scleral buckling techniques. Further distinguishing features are the absence of radial extensions, which frequently occur at the apices

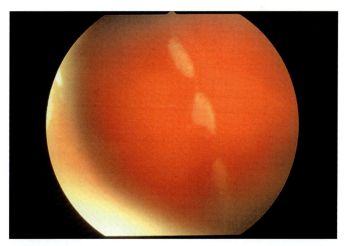

Fig. 56.1 A traumatic dialysis is characterized by an avulsed festoon of nonpigmented pars planar epithelium.

Table 56.1 The "Cambridge Guide" to the features associated with the 7 common varieties of primary retinal break in rhegmatogenous retinal detachment

Break type	PHM status	Vitreous architecture	Sex	Typical age group (yr)	Refractive error	Fellow eye involvement/pathology
Nontraumatic dialysis	On	Normal	M > F	8–20	Emmetropic/hypermetropic	5–15%
Giant retinal tear	Off	Check for anomaly	M = F	5–50	Moderate/high myopia	Variable up to 80%
Horseshoe tear	Off	Usually syneretic	M = F	45–65	Moderate/high myopia	10%
Round retinal hole	On	Usually normal	F > M	20–40	Moderate myopia	50%
Macular hole	Off	Syneretic	M = F	45–65	High myopia	Rare
Reticular schisis	On	Normal	M > F	70+	Hypermetropic	80%
X-linked retinoschisis	On	Normal, may have hemorrhage	M	10–20	Emmetropic	100%

Pediatric groups are in bold. PHM = posterior hyaloid membrane. "Macular hole" refers to macular hole associated with retinal detachment as distinct from isolated "idiopathic" macular hole. Note the importance of vitreous examination and PHM status.

of giant retinal tears and the normal compact healthy vitreous gel architecture. Giant tears in childhood are typically associated with abnormal gel and inherited vitreoretinopathies (see below). Subretinal fluid recruitment in dialyses is typically slow so that unless the ora serrata is routinely inspected after blunt trauma, the diagnosis may be delayed by several weeks until macular involvement ensues.[3]

Ragged impact necrosis breaks account for about one-fifth of retinal breaks seen in blunt trauma.[3] Retinal vessel and retinal pigment epithelial disruption may be confirmed on fundus fluorescein angiography: the retinal detachment usually presents within 6 weeks.[3] These breaks are often large, postequatorial, and irregular, making closure by conventional scleral buckling problematic so that an internal approach is often preferred. Giant retinal tears account for a minority of retinal breaks due to blunt trauma.[4] They respond well to vitrectomy and internal tamponade although the visual prognosis is often limited by associated ocular damage.[6]

Penetrating ocular trauma

Penetrating injury is an uncommon cause of detachment in childhood and may rarely follow inadvertent perforation of the globe at strabismus surgery. More common causes include accidental scissors, knife, pencil, or other sharp penetrating injuries. Intraocular foreign bodies are rarely seen although penetrating injuries from air-gun pellets are typically seen in older children and adolescents and have a poor prognosis because of the associated collateral damage and severe PVR.

Retinal perforation or incarceration from penetrating trauma rarely causes acute rhegmatogenous retinal detachment. The associated corneoscleral wound provides access for extrinsic fibroblasts so that the more common sequel is late retinal detachment complicated by combined tractional and rhegmatogenous components.[6] Vitrectomy and internal tamponade with or without relieving retinectomy may be required. A dialysis may also develop following penetrating trauma with vitreous loss when it tends to occur on the opposite side of the eye to the penetrating wound.

Nontraumatic retinal dialysis

Nontraumatic retinal dialysis accounts for approximately 10% of all juvenile retinal detachment[2,4] and in 97% of cases affects the inferotemporal quadrant.[2] It is important to examine the entire retinal periphery as occasionally two or more separate dialyses are found within the same eye. There is a 2/3 male propensity[2] and the majority of patients are hypermetropic or emmetropic (see Table 56.1).[4,5,7] Detachments associated with dialyses progress slowly and characteristically present either as an incidental finding or when the macula becomes detached.[8] They can be managed routinely with conventional buckling techniques, and the use of a small (typically 3 mm) circumferential sponge reduces the likelihood of postoperative motility problems to a minimum. Although the anatomical success rate of surgery is high, visual recovery may remain poor if there has been chronic macular involvement. Familial dialyses are rare but consideration should be given to sibling examination because (i) the patients are asymptomatic and (ii) visual recovery once macular involvement has occurred may be poor. Examination of the fellow eye under anesthesia is also important as retinal dialysis may be bilateral and oral abnormalities, in the form of a "frill" or flat dialysis, are found in the fellow eye in up to 30% of cases (Fig. 56.2).

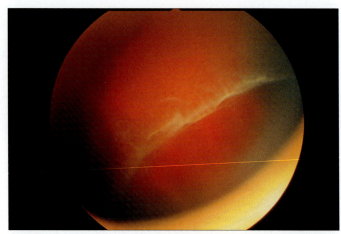

Fig. 56.2 Nontraumatic dialysis. Note the characteristic bridges spanning the retraction and the cystic change in the border of the dialysis, which is continuous with the frill at the ora serrata.

RETINAL DETACHMENT COMPLICATING DEVELOPMENTAL ABNORMALITIES

Ocular colobomas

Eyes with ocular colobomas are at a significantly increased risk of detachment and account for approximately 0.5% of pediatric retinal detachments;[9,10] giant retinal tears are seen in association with lens colobomas;[11] and rhegmatogenous detachment may develop in eyes with choroidal coloboma, when small retinal breaks may be found in the hypoplastic retina overlying the coloboma. Assessment of vision can be difficult and the diagnosis of detachment can be further impaired by nystagmus, microphthalmos, and cataract. The intercalary membrane stretched across the coloboma cavity can simulate retina on ultrasound examination so that care should be exercised to assess any mobility on dynamic examination. Histopathological studies demonstrate the intercalary membrane to consist of hypoplastic inner retina with reversal and duplication of outer neuroblastic layers at the coloboma margin.[12] This marginal duplication has been proposed as a "locus minoris resistentiae" providing adhesion. Both retinal pigment epithelium and Müller cells are vestigial or absent within the coloboma so that effective retinopexy is impossible unless applied outside the margin.

Where retinal breaks occur away from the colobomatous area they may be managed by conventional buckling techniques provided the sclera is of sufficient quality for suturing (Fig. 56.3a) and the break can be adequately closed. More usually, the retinal break overlies the colobomatous area so that identification and closure with adequate retinopexy may be impossible without internal tamponade. Retinal breaks over a coloboma are often small and may be multiple and their localization can be aided preoperatively by the identification of "schlieren" during internal drainage. Argon laser photocoagulation may be applied around the border of the colobomatous area and where this includes the papillomacular bundle this may be applied prior to retinal reattachment to minimize associated thermal damage to the nerve fiber layer.

Maintenance of tamponade throughout the maturation of the retinopexy can be compromised by the abnormal configuration of the colobomatous globe (Fig. 56.3b). Redetachment may occur in up to 30% of cases,[13] so that permanent internal tamponade may be required.

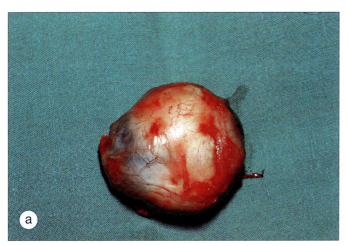
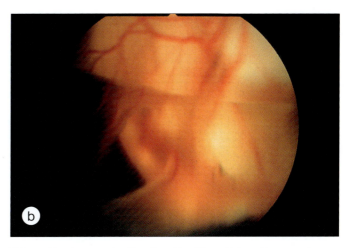

Fig. 56.3 Rhegmatogenous retinal detachment complicating ocular coloboma. (a) A combined approach with external buckle and internal tamponade may be required but care should be exercised with scleral buckling because of associated scleral ectasia as in this enucleated eye. (b) Even with internal tamponade effective break closure can be compromised by the abnormal configuration of the globe.

Spontaneous reattachment of the retina has been occasionally reported in retinal detachment associated with the morning glory anomaly (see Chapter 59) and optic nerve coloboma.

Optic disc pits and serous macular detachment

The association of serous macular detachment and optic disc pits and coloboma is well recognized and similar findings with the morning glory disc abnormality indicate that these two conditions are variations of the same basic abnormality (Fig. 56.4). The vitreous is characteristically attached,[14,15] and it has been suggested that up to 45% of optic disc pits may be complicated by serous retinal detachment.[16,17] Although spontaneous resolution has been reported in some cases,[18] the visual prognosis is poor if the detachment persists beyond 6 months.[17]

Photocoagulation alone has met with mixed success. In some series no patients were successfully reattached with laser alone,[14] and in others[16] the limited success must be balanced against the only long-term natural history study, which showed eventual spontaneous reattachment in 25% of cases.[17] The combination of argon laser photocoagulation with internal tamponade either with or without vitrectomy appears to offer greater chance of successful retinal reattachment albeit at greater risk of operative morbidity.[14–16,19]

Retinal detachment may also occur in eyes with anterior or posterior persistent hyperplastic primary vitreous (see Chapter 47). Other ocular abnormalities associated with an increased risk of retinal detachment include congenital cataract, congenital glaucoma, and retinopathy of prematurity (see Chapter 51).

Familial retinal detachment

Retinal detachment may be seen in a variety of inherited systemic disorders in which there is ocular involvement. In most cases there is associated high myopia, although in some conditions, for example incontinentia pigmenti and familial exudative vitreoretinopathy (FEVR), there is an underlying retinovascular abnormality. Infrequently a true detachment may complicate juvenile X-linked retinoschisis.[2,20]

High myopia and retinal detachment is seen in Marfan syndrome, Ehlers–Danlos syndrome, Smith–Magenis syndrome, the Stickler syndromes (both with and without systemic involvement), Kniest syndrome, and spondyloepiphyseal dysplasia congenita and in association with midfacial clefting syndromes and the EEC syndrome. The detachments are often complex and frequently with associated giant retinal tear.

Genetics of rhegmatogenous retinal detachment

Stickler syndrome is the commonest inherited cause of rhegmatogenous retinal detachment in childhood. It forms part of the spectrum of type II/XI collagenopathies, which also includes the more severe Kniest dysplasia (MIM 156550 (see Online Mendelian Inheritance in Man: http://www4.ncbi. nlm.nih.gov/PubMed/)), spondyloepiphyseal dysplasia congenita (SEDC, MIM183900), and spondyloepimetaphyseal dysplasia (Strudwick type, MIM 184250).

In contrast to the more severe disproportionate stature syndromes that result mainly from dominant negative mutations (Table 56.2), the majority of patients with Stickler syndrome have premature termination mutations in the gene for type II collagen. This results in haploinsufficiency, exhibiting a characteristic membranous vitreoretinal phenotype[21] (Fig. 56.5a).

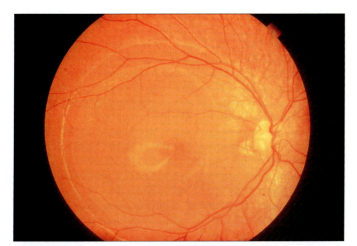

Fig. 56.4 Serous macular detachment linked to an optic disc pit in a 10-year-old boy. (Image courtesy of Mr Paul Jacobs.)

Table 56.2 Summary of molecular genetics of chondrodysplasias and phenotype in relation to rhegmatogenous retinal detachment

Collagen	Gene	Locus	Mutation	Phenotype	Clinical features	MIM
Type II	COL2A1	12q13.2	Haploinsufficiency	Type 1 Stickler	Normal stature, membranous vitreous anomaly, skeletal and aural features	108300
			Exon 2	"Ocular only" type 1 Stickler syndrome	Membranous vitreous anomaly, little or no systemic features	108300
			Dominant negative	Kniest dysplasia	Short stature, flat face, large head, knobbly fingers	156550
		12q13.11–13.2	Dominant negative	SEDC	Short trunk, disproportionate proximal limb shortening	183900
			C-Propeptide	VPED	Normal stature, developmental phalangeal epiphyseal dysplasia	Not assigned
Type XI	COL11A1	1p21	Haploinsufficiency	*Unreported*		
			Dominant negative	Type 2 Stickler syndrome	Normal stature, beaded vitreous anomaly, skeletal and aural features	604841
	COL11A2	6p21.3	Recessive, dual haploinsufficiency	OSMED	Cleft, arthropathy	215150
	COL11A2	6p21.3	Dominant negative	No ocular involvement	Deafness, arthropathy, normal vitreous	184840

MIM = Mendelian inheritance in man.

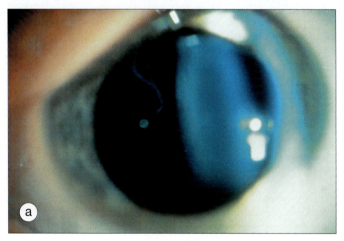 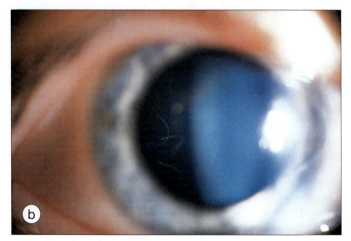

Fig. 56.5 Vitreous phenotypes. (a) Type 1 Stickler syndrome (membranous phenotype). (b) Type 2 Stickler syndrome (beaded phenotype)

Pedigrees with a different vitreous phenotype have mutations in the gene *COL11A1* encoding type XI collagen[22–24] and are now known as type II Stickler (STL2) syndrome (Fig. 56.5b). Other families exhibit neither of these two vitreoretinal phenotypes or linkage to known loci so there is further locus heterogeneity to be resolved. Exon 2 of the *COL2A1* gene is principally expressed in the eye and spliced out of cartilage so that it should be remembered that mutations in this exon result in a predominantly ocular form of Stickler syndrome with minimal or absent systemic involvement.[25]

Dominant rhegmatogenous retinal detachment (DRRD)

Recent work has identified a number of novel missense mutations in *COL2A1*. One of these, an Arg to Cys mutation,[25] resulted in the membranous vitreous phenotype as seen in cases of type 1 Stickler syndrome, but others have resulted in vitreous phenotypes similar to those seen in isolated cases of rhegmatogenous detachment rather than those seen in Stickler syndrome. A family with a novel L467F mutation exhibited an extremely high incidence of retinal detachment, with systemic features virtually absent in all affected individuals, suggesting "dominant rhegmatogenous retinal detachment" (DRRD) as a more appropriate description for this subtype.[26,27] Families such as these are one indication that there is also a genetic component to the risk of isolated retinal detachment. A proportion of cases of RRD have significant pathology in the fellow eye and will later develop bilateral detachment. Some of these also have other family members with bilateral retinal detachment. The mode of inheritance in these cases is unclear as they may have specific dominant mutations, or alternatively inherit a specific set of gene alleles that predispose to retinal detachment.

Marfan syndrome

Marfan syndrome is a dominantly inherited disorder of fibrillin production with a prevalence of approximately 1 in 20,000.[28] The fibrillins are high-molecular-weight extracellular glycoproteins, and mutations in the fibrillin gene on chromosome 15 (*FBN1*) cause Marfan syndrome and dominant ectopia lentis. Mutations in a second fibrillin gene on chromosome 5 are responsible for congenital contractural arachnodactyly.[28] Recent work has confirmed fibrillin to be widespread in lens capsule, iris, ciliary body, and sclera.[29]

The association of rhegmatogenous retinal detachment with Marfan syndrome is well recognized and has been reported in 8–50% of cases;[30] approximately 75% of these occur before 20 years of age.[30] Although there is a significant association with myopia, this is characteristically developmental, and no case of myopia was found under 3 years of age in one large series.[30] This is in contrast to the congenital nonprogressive myopia found in type 1 Stickler syndrome. In Marfan syndrome the pupils characteristically dilate poorly because of a structural iris abnormality,[29] and when combined with lens subluxation and weak scleral architecture the repair of retinal detachment in Marfan syndrome patients can provide a formidable surgical challenge. Pars plana lensectomy and internal tamponade are often required and appropriate equipment for such procedures should always be available when managing these patients.

The Stickler syndromes

The Stickler syndromes (hereditary arthro-ophthalmopathy, McKusick Nos. 108300, 604841, 184840) are dominantly inherited disorder of collagen connective tissue and the commonest inherited cause of rhegmatogenous retinal detachment in childhood. Other variable features include cleft palate, deafness, and arthropathy. Ophthalmic complications are severe, particularly congenital myopia and the risk of giant retinal tear (GRT), which is commonly bilateral and a frequent cause of blindness.

The diagnosis should be considered in:
1. Neonates with Pierre–Robin sequence or midline cleft;
2. Infants with spondyloepiphyseal dysplasia associated with myopia or deafness;
3. Patients with a family history of rhegmatogenous retinal detachment; and
4. Sporadic cases of retinal detachment associated with joint hypermobility, midline clefting, or deafness.

Type 1 Stickler syndrome (STL1; MIM 108300)

Pedigrees expressing the type 1 (membranous) phenotype show linkage to the gene-encoding type II collagen (*COL2A1*). The vitreous phenotype, "empty vitreous," is a pathognomonic hallmark for the ophthalmologist given the variability of facial and systemic features. Mutation screening thus far has shown a high propensity for stop mutations, and in this respect type 1 Stickler syndrome appears unique among the inherited fibrillar collagen disorders. The myopia is typically congenital and of high degree although some patients also exhibit cornea plana and are not refractively myopic despite increased axial length.

Classically, patients show a flat midface with a depressed nasal bridge, reduced nasal protrusion, anteverted nares, and micrognathia (Figs. 56.6a, 56.6b). These findings are usually most evident in childhood and with increasing age often become less distinctive. Facial features are so variable that in isolation they are unreliable for making a diagnosis. Many patients have some evidence of midline clefting ranging from the extreme of the

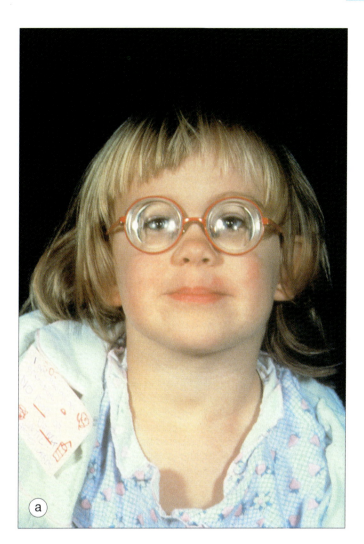
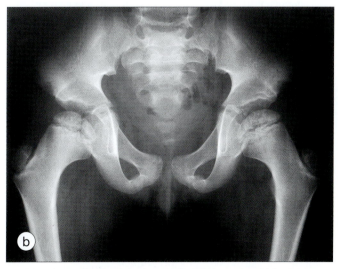

Fig. 56.6 Type 1 Stickler syndrome. (a) Facial phenotype. (b) Radiology: there is wide phenotypic variation in the radiological appearances. In this patient there is mild platyspondyly with irregular end plates, and in the pelvis, there is some widening of the metaphyses and irregularity of the weight-bearing surface of the femoral epiphyses with a moderate degree of coxa vara on the left (radiology courtesy of Dr Philip Bearcroft).

Pierre–Robin sequence, through clefting of the hard/soft palate, to the mildest manifestation of bifid uvula. It is important to remember to examine for subtle evidence of midline clefting as this is easily overlooked.

Patients with Stickler syndrome may suffer hearing difficulties for two reasons. Firstly, the association with cleft and high-arched palate leads to an increased incidence of serous otitis media, causing a conductive hearing deficit that may be remedial. In some patients a mild conductive element persists because of ossicle defects. Secondly, there can be an associated sensorineural defect. Stickler syndrome patients typically show high-tone sensorineural hearing loss, and in many patients this may be so subtle that they are unaware of the deficit. Baseline audiometry therefore has an important diagnostic role to reveal subtle asymptomatic high-tone loss.

Children with Stickler syndrome classically exhibit joint hypermobility and the diagnosis should be considered in hypermobile patients who are myopic. Joint mobility can be assessed objectively using the Beighton scoring system to allow comparison with an age, sex, and race matched population. With increasing age, the hypermobility reduces or is lost completely, and a degenerative arthropathy of variable severity may develop by the third or fourth decade. Typical radiological changes show irregularity of articular contour and loss of joint space. By middle age some patients require joint replacement surgery for hips or knees.

Slender extremities, long fingers, and normal height characterize the body habitus. Mild spondyloepiphyseal dysplasia is often apparent radiologically. Early reports of increased mitral valve prolapse have not been substantiated by recent studies.[31]

Once the diagnosis of Stickler syndrome has been established, a coordinated multidisciplinary approach is desirable, comprising the following:

1. Ophthalmological assessment with refraction and correction of myopic/astigmatic error. The quality of best-corrected vision may be improved with contact lens rather than spectacle correction. Many centers are now offering prophylactic retinopexy to reduce the risk of retinal detachment and because of the risk of detachment, all patients require long-term follow-up and should be advised that if they see new floaters or shadows in their vision they should seek urgent ophthalmological assessment.

2. Maxillofacial assessment as to whether midline clefting is present.

3. Hearing assessment and management of combined conductive and sensorineural deafness if present.

4. Educational assessment. Although intelligence is normal, patients of school age may face considerable educational difficulties because of combined visual, auditory, and speech impairment. Educational authorities may need to be notified of a child's special needs. Patient support and public education has been helped substantially by the formation of the Stickler Syndrome Group (http://www.stickler.org.uk).

Stickler syndrome shows autosomal dominant inheritance but with wide variation in expression so that the disease status of mildly affected relatives may only become apparent on careful slit-lamp examination of the vitreous. The pediatric ophthalmologist should remember to examine parents and other adult siblings so that affected members of the family are identified and assessed for prophylaxis against retinal detachment and offered genetic advice.

Type 2 Stickler syndrome (STL2; MIM 604841)

In a minority of pedigrees there is a different phenotype with sparse and irregularly thickened bundles of fibers throughout the vitreous cavity (type 2 vitreous phenotype Fig. 56.5b) and linkage to COL2A1 can be excluded. Mutations in the gene encoding the 1 chain of type XI collagen (COL11A1) on chromosome 1p21 have so far been found in 7 families and these are, to date, the only mutations associated with the type 2 vitreous phenotype. These pedigrees have a similarly high risk of detachment and giant retinal tear but appear to have a greater propensity for sensorineural deafness than the STL1 families.

Type 3 Stickler syndrome (STL3; MIM 184840)

The other polypeptide chain (α2) of type XI collagen is not expressed in the vitreous so that mutations in its encoding gene (COL11A2) produce syndromes with the systemic features of Stickler syndrome but without eye involvement. These include nonsyndromic hearing loss, Weissenbacher–Zweymüller syndrome, and otospondyloepimetaphyseal dysplasia (OSMED).

"Ocular only" Stickler syndrome

Of the Stickler syndrome pedigrees exhibiting the type 1 vitreous phenotype, a subgroup characterized as a predominantly "ocular only" disorder without systemic skeletal or auditory involvement has also been identified. It is possible that in the past some of these pedigrees may have been confused with another inherited vitreoretinopathy, Wagner syndrome (MIM 143200). However, although Wagner syndrome also appears to be a purely ocular vitreoretinopathy without systemic manifestations, it has distinct clinical differences from Stickler syndrome and is now clearly linked to a separate locus. The term "Wagner–Stickler" syndrome is therefore confusing and should be abandoned. Type II procollagen exists in two alternatively spliced forms. A short form, which is expressed in cartilage, has exon 2 spliced out, resulting in a molecule with a smaller N-propeptide (αIIb). The short form also functions as a third α(XI) chain in cartilage. It coassembles with products of the COL11A1 and COL11A2 genes, to form a α1(XI)-α2(XI)-α1(IIb) heterotrimer. Mutations in exon 2 of the COL2A1 gene therefore result in a "pure" ocular variant of this disorder although these patients are also at high risk of retinal detachment. This has important implications for counseling patients with regard to the development of systemic complications and emphasizes the importance of the ophthalmic examination in the differential diagnosis of Stickler syndrome from Wagner vitreoretinopathy and also the need to consider the diagnosis of the Stickler syndromes in sporadic giant tear.

Kniest syndrome (MIM 156550)

Kniest syndrome is an autosomal dominant disorder that shares many similarities with Stickler syndrome. Mutations are found in the same gene as for type 1 Stickler syndrome (COL2A1), but result in dominant-negative effects rather than haploinsufficiency with consequently more severe arthropathy. It typically presents at birth with shortened trunk and limbs, congenital megalophthalmos, and flattened nasal bridge (Figs. 56.7a, 56.7b). The joints are often large at birth and the fingers long and knobbly.[32] Motor milestones can be delayed because of joint deformities, and muscle atrophy may result from disuse. Both conductive and sensorineural hearing loss may be present as with the Stickler syndromes. The intellect is normal, and myopia, retinal detachment, and giant retinal tear are the major ophthalmic complications.

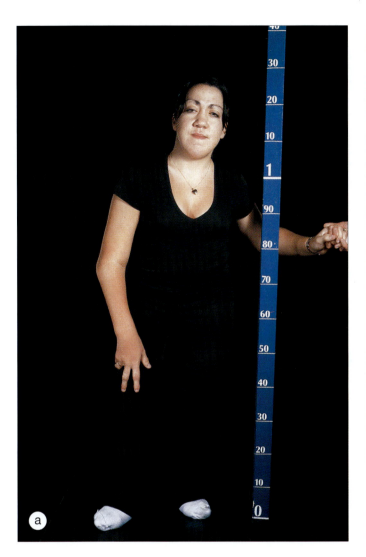

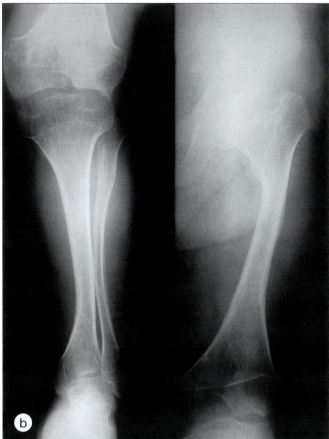

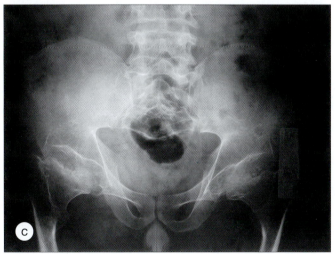

Fig. 56.7 Kniest dysplasia. (a) Severe short stature is present from birth, and the face is usually flat with the head disproportionally large. Note the typical phalangeal changes. The capital epiphyses are irregular, and the metaphyses are wide. Patients with Kniest dysplasia often exhibit severe but variable platyspondyly. The shortening of the limbs is exemplified and note that the epiphyses are wide and irregular, but the metaphyses are also involved with splaying, a feature not seen in spondyloepiphyseal dysplasia (b,c) (radiology courtesy of Dr Philip Bearcroft).

Spondyloepiphyseal dysplasia congenita (SEDC; MIM 183900)

SEDC presents at birth with shortening of the trunk and to a lesser extent the extremities. It is inherited as an autosomal dominant disorder and characteristically results from dominant-negative mutations in the gene for type II collagen (*COL2A1*). Patients classically develop a barrel-shaped chest associated with an exaggerated lumbar lordosis, which may compromise respiratory function.[32] Odontoid hypoplasia may be present, predisposing to cervicomedullary instability, and imaging of the cervical spine should be considered prior to general anesthesia. The limb

shortening is disproportionate, affecting mainly the proximal limbs with hands and feet appearing relatively normal (Figs. 56.8a, 56.8b). Myopia, retinal detachment, and giant retinal tear are the major ophthalmic complications, and as with the other type II collagenopathies, both conductive and sensorineural hearing loss may be present.

Spondyloepimetaphyseal dysplasia (Strudwick type; MIM 184250)

SEMD also forms part of the clinical spectrum of dominantly inherited type II collagenopathies. The features include severe

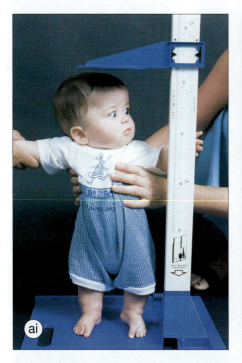
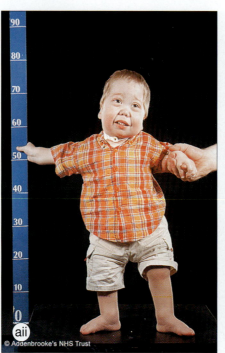
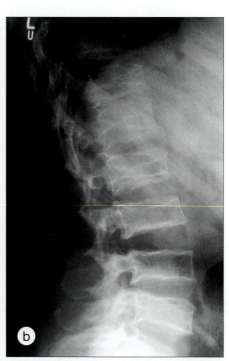

Fig. 56.8 (a) Congenital spondyloepiphyseal dysplasia and (b) radiology. In the spine, the vertebral bodies show flattening (platyspondyly) with irregular end plates. Clinically the patients are small with a short trunk, and commonly a marked lordosis. Onset is at birth, but severe short stature may not be obvious until 2–3 years (radiology courtesy of Dr Philip Bearcroft).

dwarfism, superficially resembling the Morquio syndrome, pectus carinatum, and scoliosis, which are usually marked.[32] Cleft palate and retinal detachment are frequently associated, as with SEDC. Disproportionately short limbs and delayed epiphyseal maturation are present at birth. Radiologically the disorder is indistinguishable from SEDC during infancy but a characteristic mottled appearance created by alternating zones of osteosclerosis and osteopenia develops during early childhood.[32]

Other connective tissue dysplasias

Vitreoretinopathy associated with phalangeal epiphyseal dysplasia (VPED)

Richards et al. reported a large family with dominantly inherited rhegmatogenous retinal detachment, premature arthropathy, and development of phalangeal epiphyseal dysplasia, resulting in brachydactyly.[33] The phenotype appears distinct from other type II collagenopathies but sequencing identified a novel mutation in the C-propeptide region of *COL2A1*. The glycine to aspartic acid change occurred in a region highly conserved in all fibrillar collagen molecules.

Ehlers–Danlos syndrome

The Ehlers–Danlos syndromes (EDS) are a clinically and genetically heterogeneous group of connective tissue disorders affecting mainly skin, joints, and ligaments, but in some cases also arteries and the gastrointestinal tract.[34] In common with both Stickler and Marfan syndromes, joint laxity is a prominent feature, but associated with hyperelasticity of the skin and tissue fragility. The classification is complex and regularly revised as underlying primary defects are defined. Subclassification is made on clinical grounds and substantiated by consideration of the most likely inheritance pattern and biochemical and molecular genetic analysis when possible. Ophthalmic manifestations include

dermatochalasis, myopia, and corneal abnormalities (keratoconus, microcornea, megalocornea), but retinal detachment is typically associated with type VI (kyphoscoliotic, lysyl hydroxylase deficiency; MIM 225400) where ectopia lentis, scleromalacia, and Marfanoid habitus may also feature. EDS VI is rare and inheritance is autosomal recessive.[34]

Wagner vitreoretinopathy

Wagner described a new ocular disease in a three-generation pedigree from the Kanton of Zurich with 13 affected individuals. It featured autosomal dominant inheritance, low myopia (3.00 diopters or less), fluid vitreous, cortical cataract, and inconstant and variably affected dark adaptation. No affected individual suffered a retinal detachment. The cardinal features noted were the complete absence of the normal vitreal scaffolding and preretinal, equatorial, and avascular grayish-white membranes. Clear lenses in childhood developed anterior and posterior cortical opacities in puberty and cataracta complicata during the fourth decade. Rhegmatogenous retinal detachment was not originally reported but has since been noted in a minority of individuals. Frequent reference to the "Wagner–Stickler" syndrome or "Wagner syndrome with arthropathy" implies phenotypic variation of the same basic underlying disorder. However, it has recently been shown that families with Stickler syndrome and a nonocular variant have mutations in the genes *COL2A1*, *COL11A1*, and *COL11A2*, whereas several families with Wagner syndrome (WGN1) including the original family have been linked to a separate locus at 5q14.3.[35]

X-linked retinoschisis

X-linked retinoschisis is an uncommon cause of retinal detachment in childhood accounting for 2.5–5% of all pediatric retinal

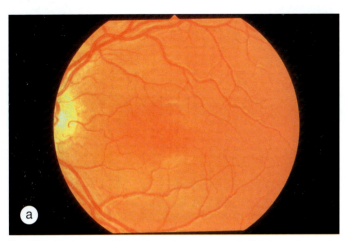

Fig. 56.9 (a) Foveal and (b) peripheral appearances in X-linked retinoschisis.

detachments.[2,9] The incidence of retinal detachment varies in the different series but it may occur in up to 16% of affected males.[36] Vitreous hemorrhage is another cause of visual loss. Peripheral retinoschisis is found in approximately 50% of cases (Figs. 56.9a, 56.9b) and can be complicated by retinal detachment by various mechanisms. A full-thickness retinal break occurring *de novo* or a communication between outer and inner leaf defects in the schisis wall may lead to rhegmatogenous retinal detachment. Full-thickness breaks may be managed effectively by scleral buckling procedures provided complete break closure can be satisfactorily achieved. Where communication exists between inner and outer leaf breaks an internal approach may be required to effect and maintain closure.

Occasionally X-linked retinoschisis can be complicated by cyst formation, which may develop hemorrhaging into the cavity[36] or even be so bullous as to obscure the visual axis. There is some evidence that spontaneous resolution can occur,[36] but prolonged delay may compromise the visual prognosis so that some authors have advocated surgical drainage and deroofing of the cyst by internal means.

Prophylaxis in rhegmatogenous retinal detachment

In contrast to most other pediatric blinding retinal disorders, blindness through retinal detachment is in most cases potentially avoidable if a rationale for the prediction and prevention of retinal detachment could be developed. This goal has been frustrated by a lack of understanding of the factors influencing retinal detachment even in high-risk groups, which are only now beginning to be unraveled.

Factors traditionally associated with retinal detachment include refractive error, a positive family history, visible lattice retinopathy, and fellow eye involvement, but the nature of these associations is poorly understood. The prevalence of myopia varies enormously and even in Stickler syndrome up to 20% of patients may exhibit no significant refractive error. Many patients with retinal detachment exhibit none of the accepted risk features such as lattice retinopathy, and in those that do retinal tear formation frequently occurs remote from such areas so that the associations with habitually accepted risk factors require refinement.

Although the systemic features are widespread, the sight-threatening complications are perhaps the most conspicuous and

serious manifestations, particularly the risk of giant retinal tear (GRT), which is frequently bilateral and a frequent cause of blindness. The rationale for offering prophylaxis in such high-risk cases is to prevent progression of GRT to detachment by applying treatment at the post-oral retina at the site of giant tear development (Fig. 56.10, Figs. 56.11a, 56.11b).

TRACTIONAL RETINAL DETACHMENT

Traction on the retina leading to detachment is rare in childhood; it may complicate primary retinovascular disease such as retinopathy of prematurity, FEVR, the inherited vitreoretinal degenerations (see Chapter 49), or incontinentia pigmenti, or may develop following penetrating trauma, or intraocular inflammation associated with, for example, ocular toxocariasis. Such traction may lead to retinal detachment directly or cause retinal breaks and subsequent rhegmatogenous detachment. Proliferative vitreoretinopathy (PVR) may also complicate unsuccessful rhegmatogenous detachment repair, and extensive vitreoretinal fibrosis is a common result of failed reattachment surgery.

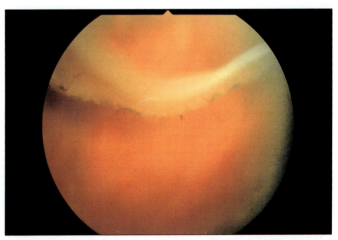

Fig. 56.10 Unsuccessful prophylaxis: laser applied too posteriorly to prevent giant tear initiation and progression. Only eye with type 1 Stickler syndrome; fellow eye became blind following detachment.

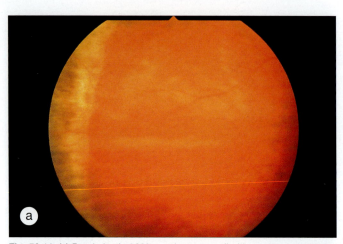 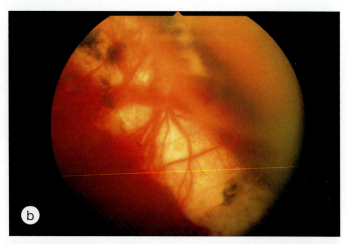

Fig. 56.11 (a) Prophylactic 360° cryotherapy applied in contiguous ribbon to prevent giant tear progression from pars plana. (b) Effective prophylaxis: this giant tear occurred 2 years after prophylaxis. Retinal detachment did not ensue.

Retinopathy of prematurity

Retinopathy of prematurity accounts for approximately 2% of all pediatric retinal detachments.[9] These may be broadly classified into those with early (within 1 year) and late (after 1 year) presentation.

The incidence of early retinal detachment following advanced retinopathy of prematurity has been substantially reduced by better screening and prophylactic cryotherapy (see Chapter 51). However, the visual results following vitreoretinal surgery for those that do progress to retinal detachment have been very disappointing. The major and often multiple surgical challenges posed (the redetachment rate is high) need to be carefully weighed against a partial and spontaneous retinal reattachment in perhaps 10% of cases.

The prognosis for retinal reattachment and the visual outcome are more favorable in eyes that have not progressed to stage 5. Lens-sparing techniques have been advocated for pathology confined posterior to the equator.[37] Preservation of the crystalline lens with surgical access to the vitreous base in the neonatal eye requires adequate visualization of the pars plicata facilitated by use of the operating indirect ophthalmoscope or wide-angle viewing systems.

Late retinal detachment following treated or untreated retinopathy of prematurity is a well-recognized phenomenon. Detachments are most commonly rhegmatogenous but may be tractional or a combination of the two. Presentation may be late and although reattachment is frequently possible with vitreoretinal surgery the prognosis relates more to the preexisting visual potential prior to retinal detachment.

Incontinentia pigmenti

Incontinentia pigmenti is an X-linked dominantly inherited disorder causing death in males and dermatological, dental, central nervous system, and ocular abnormalities in females. Ocular abnormalities occur in approximately one-third of patients, usually within the first year of life[38] and consist mainly of vascular abnormalities with abnormal peripheral perfusion and retinal pigment epithelial defects together with an isolated report of foveal hypoplasia.[39] The affected eye is often microphthalmic and complications can arise from late tractional retinal detachment. Limited success has been achieved using complex vitreoretinal techniques and attention has been focused on prophylaxis. Although prophylactic cryotherapy to the peripheral avascular retina has been reported to arrest vascular proliferation and thereby prevent late tractional detachment this has not been universally successful and direct vessel ablation has been suggested.[40]

Congenital falciform folds

An association between congenital falciform retinal folds and retinal detachment has been described.[41] These eyes are often microphthalmic and histology shows malformative retinal rosettes, persistent hyperplastic primary vitreous and occasionally vascular proliferation. It has been postulated that a retinal fold devoid of the influence of retinal pigment epithelium fails to acquire the potential for secreting secondary vitreous.[41] These cases are rare. If retrolental adhesion is minor then it may be possible to establish a surgical plane so that retinal reattachment can be achieved, but the visual prognosis remains poor.

Exudative retinal detachment

Exudative detachment although uncommon has a wide variety of causes in childhood, including Coats disease, retinoblastoma, retinopathy of prematurity, ocular toxocariasis, choroidal hemangioma, capillary hemangioma, posterior scleritis, and Harada's disease. If there is doubt about the diagnosis computed tomographic (CT) scan or ultrasound and a careful examination under anesthetic (EUA) should be performed to rule out retinoblastoma. Treatment is usually directed at the underlying cause, for example, laser photocoagulation of Coats disease or retinal hemangiomas.

REFERENCES

1. Eagling EM. Ocular damage after blunt trauma to the eye: its relationship to the nature of the injury. Br J Ophthalmol 1974; 58: 126–40.
2. Verdaguer J. Juvenile retinal detachment. Arch Ophthalmol 1982; 93: 145–56.
3. Johnson PB. Traumatic retinal detachment. Br J Ophthalmol 1991; 75: 18–21.
4. Hagler WS. Retinal dialysis: a statistical and genetic study to determine pathogenic factors. Trans Am Ophthalmol Soc 1980; 78: 686–733.
5. Ross WH. Retinal dialysis: lack of evidence for a genetic cause. Can J Ophthalmol 1991; 26: 309–12.
6. Aylward GW, Cooling RJ, Leaver PK. Trauma-induced retinal detachment associated with giant retinal tears. Retina 1993; 13: 136–41.
7. Scott JD. Retinal dialysis. Trans Ophthalmol Soc UK 1977; 97: 33–5.
8. Chignell AH. Retinal dialysis. Br J Ophthalmol 1973; 57: 572–7.
9. Daniel R, Kanski JJ, Glasspool MG. Retinal detachment in children. Trans Ophthalmol Soc UK 1974; 94: 5–34.
10. McDonald HR, Lewis H, Brown G, et al. Vitreous surgery for retinal detachment associated with choroidal coloboma. Arch Ophthalmol 1991; 109: 1399–402.
11. Hovland KR, Schepens CL, Freeman HM. Developmental giant retinal tears associated with lens coloboma. Arch Ophthalmol 1968; 80: 325–31.
12. Schubert HD. Schisis-like rhegmatogenous retinal detachment associated with choroidal colobomas. Graefe's Arch Clin Exp Ophthalmol 1995; 233: 74–9.
13. Gopal L, Kini MM, Badrinath SS, et al. Management of retinal detachment with choroidal coloboma. Ophthalmology 1991; 98: 1622–7.
14. Bonnet M. Serous macular detachment associated with optic nerve pits. Graefe's Arch Clin Exp Ophthalmol 1991; 229: 526–32.
15. Snead MP, James N, Jacobs PM. Vitrectomy, argon laser, and gas tamponade for serous retinal detachment associated with an optic disc pit. Br J Ophthalmol 1991; 75: 381–2.
16. Cox MS, Witherspoon CD, Morris RE, et al. Evolving techniques in the treatment of macular detachment caused by optic nerve pits. Ophthalmology 1988; 95: 889–96.
17 Sobol WM, Blodi CF, Folk JC, et al. Long-term visual outcome in patients with optic nerve pit and serous retinal detachment of the macula. Ophthalmology 1990; 97: 1539–42.
18. Sugar HS. Congenital pits in the optic disc and their equivalents (congenital colobomas and coloboma-like excavations) associated with submacular fluid. Am J Ophthalmol 1967; 63: 298–307.
19. Lincoff H, Yannuzzi L, Singerman L, et al. Improvement in visual function after displacement of the retinal elevations emanating from optic pits. Arch Ophthalmol 1993; 111: 1071–9.
20. George ND, Yates JR, Moore AT. Clinical features in affected males with X-linked retinoschisis. Arch Ophthalmol 1996; 114: 274–80.
21. Snead MP, Payne SJ, Barton DE, et al. Stickler syndrome: correlation between vitreo-retinal phenotypes and linkage to COL 2A1. Eye 1994; 8: 609–14.
22. Richards AJ, Yates JR, Williams R, et al. A family with Stickler syndrome type 2 has a mutation in the COL11A1 gene resulting in the substitution of glycine 97 by valine in alpha 1 (XI) collagen. Hum Mol Genet 1996; 5: 1339–43

23. Martin S, Richards AJ, Yates JR, et al. Stickler syndrome: further mutations in COL11A1 and evidence for additional locus heterogeneity. Eur J Hum Genet 1999; 7: 807–14
24. Snead MP, Yates JR. Clinical and molecular genetics of Stickler syndrome. J Med Genet 1999; 5: 353–9.
25. Richards AJ, Martin S, Yates JR, et al. COL2A1 exon 2 mutations: relevance to the Stickler and Wagner syndromes. Br J Ophthalmol 2000; 84: 364–71.
26. Richards AJ, Baguley DM, Yates JR, et al. Variations in the vitreous phenotype of Stickler syndrome can be caused by different amino acid substitutions in the X position of the type II collagen Gly-X-Y triple helix. Am J Hum Genet 2000; 67: 1083–94.
27. Richards AJ, Scott JD, Snead MP. Molecular genetics of rhegmatogenous retinal detachment. Eye 2002; 16: 88–92.
28. Pyeritz RE, Dietz HC. The Marfan syndrome and other microfibrillar disorders. In: Royce PM, Steinmann B, editors. Connective tissue and its heritable disorders. 2nd ed. New York: Wiley-Liss; 2002: 585–626.
29. Wheatley HM, Traboulsi EI, Flowers BE, et al. Immunohistochemical localisation of fibrillin in human ocular tissues. Relevance to the Marfan syndrome. Arch Ophthalmol 1995; 113: 103–9.
30 Maumenee IH. The eye in Marfan syndrome. Trans Am Ophthalmol Soc 1981; 79: 684–733.
31 Ahmad N, Richards AJ, Murfett HC, et al. Mitral valve prolapse in Stickler syndrome. Am J Med Genet 2003; 116A: 234–7.
32. Horton WA, Hecht JT. Chondrodysplasias: disorders of cartilage matrix proteins. In: Royce PM, Steinmann B, editors. Connective tissue and its heritable disorders. 2nd ed. New York: Wiley-Liss; 2002: 909–37.
33. Richards AJ, Morgan J, Bearcroft PW, et al. Vitreoretinopathy with phalangeal epiphyseal dysplasia, a type II collagenopathy resulting from a novel mutation in the C-propeptide region of the molecule. J Med Genet 2002; 39: 661–5.
34. Steinmann B, Royce PM, Superti-Furga A. The Ehlers-Danlos syndrome. In: Royce PM, Steinmann B, editors. Connective tissue and its heritable disorders. 2nd ed. New York: Wiley-Liss; 2002: 431–524.
35. Brown, DM, Graemiger RA, Hergersberg M, et al. Genetic linkage of Wagner disease and erosive vitreoretinopathy to chromosome 5q13–14. Arch Ophthalmol 1995; 113: 671–5.
36. George ND, Yates JR, Bradshaw K, et al. Infantile presentation of X-linked retinoschisis. Br J Ophthalmol 1995; 79: 653–7.
37. Capone A, Trese MT. Lens-sparing vitreous surgery for tractional stage 4A retinopathy of prematurity retinal detachments. Ophthalmology 2001; 108: 2068–70.
38. Catalano RA. Incontinentia pigmenti. Am J Ophthalmol 1990; 110: 696–700.
39. Goldberg MF, Custis PH. Retinal and other manifestations in nine cases of incontinentia pigmenti (Bloch-Sulzberger syndrome). Inv Ophthalmol Vis Sci 1992; 33: 1084.
40. Catalano RA, Lopatynsky M, Tasman WS. Treatment of proliferative retinopathy associated with incontinentia pigmenti. Am J Ophthalmol 1990; 110: 701–2.
41. Warburg M. Retinal malformations. Doyne Memorial lecture 1979. Retinal malformations: aetiological heterogeneity and morphological similarity in congenital retinal non-attachment and falciform folds. Trans Ophthalmol Soc UK 1979; 99: 272–83.

CHAPTER
57 Flecked Retinal Disorders

Peter J Francis and Anthony T Moore

The flecked retinal disorders comprise a heterogeneous group of conditions in which there are multiple white or yellow "flecks" or crystalline deposits scattered throughout the retina. They may be inherited or acquired and are associated with variable retinal dysfunction. We review the differential diagnosis of the flecked retina in childhood, although some disorders predominantly seen in adults are included for completeness. Some of these disorders are considered in Chapters 52–55 and 58.

CLINICAL EVALUATION

When a flecked retina appearance is noted on ophthalmoscopy, a full history, careful clinical evaluation and electrophysiological testing can provide clues to the etiology. It is important to enquire about visual symptoms such as blurred vision, night or day vision difficulty, to obtain a full family history and to enquire about current or previous systemic drug administration. Careful note should be taken of other medical disorders particularly those associated with malabsorption as vitamin A deficiency may be seen in association with fat malabsorptive conditions such as cystic fibrosis.[1] Recognition is important, as treatment will reverse visual loss.

In examining the eye, it is important to document the distribution of the retinal deposits, their depth in the retina (sensory retina or RPE) and the whether the flecks are crystalline in nature. All of these factors can prove useful in identifying the cause. Investigations useful in identifying the specific retinal disorder include visual field testing, electroretinography, psychophysical evaluations such as dark adaptometry and fundus imaging including color photography, fluorescein angiography and autofluorescence imaging.[2]

PATHOGENESIS OF FLECK RETINA DISORDERS

It is not known how generalized genetic and metabolic defects can produce apparently discrete accumulations of reflective material in the retina and localized areas of retinal pigment epithelial and photoreceptor dysfunction. It is tempting to speculate that variations in the distribution[3] and metabolic activity of photoreceptor subtypes[4] or Müller cells,[5,6] differences in the morphology and density[7] of retinal pigment epithelial cells and their metabolic relationships with photoreceptors[8] may play a role .

INHERITED FLECKED RETINA SYNDROMES

Stargardt disease (STGD) and fundus flavimaculatus (FFM)

See Chapters 52 and 54.

This disorder is an autosomal recessive retinal dystrophy caused by mutations in the *ABCA4* gene.[9] It is characterized by the presence of yellow-white "fish-tail" shaped flecks at the level of the retinal pigment epithelium (RPE) scattered throughout the posterior pole and peripheral retina (Fig. 57.1).[10] There is macular atrophy and the main presentation is with poor acuity. Some patients have minimal or no macular involvement at presentation have good visual acuity and may be diagnosed

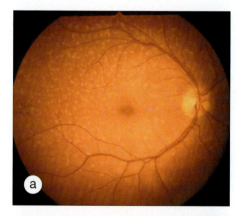

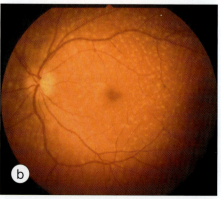

Fig. 57.1 Stargardt disease. Right (a) and left (b) fundus photograph of a patient with Stargardt disease. There are multiple flecks at the level of the retinal pigment epithelium and some mild macular atrophy.

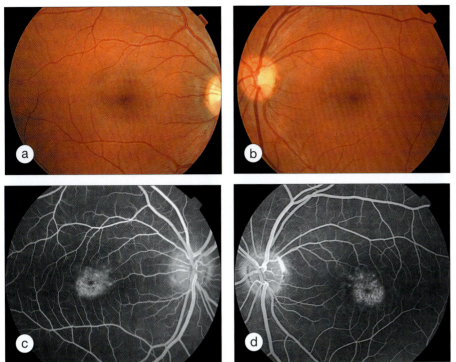

Fig. 57.2 Stargardt disease. Fundus photograph of the right (a) and left (b) eyes showing mild macular atrophy with white flecks at the level of the RPE. The corresponding fluorescein angiogram (c and d) shows a dark choroid except in the central macula where there is hyperfluorescence secondary to RPE atrophy.

as having fundus flavimaculatus (FFM) but both STGD and FFM form parts of the same disorder with mutation of the same gene. Patients rarely complain, at presentation, of poor night vision or field constriction despite delayed dark adaptation on psychophysical testing.[11] Electrophysiological testing shows an abnormal pattern electroretinogram but the full field electroretinography and electroculogram are often normal in the early stages. Electrophysiological testing may be helpful in predicting the visual prognosis.[12] On fluorescein angiography, a "dark choroid" is seen,[13,14] but not universally (Fig. 57.2). The dark choroid is thought to be due to the presence of an abnormal absorbing material at the level of the RPE masking the underlying choroidal fluorescence. Early in the disease, the individual flecks mask the underlying choroidal fluorescence but later the flecks hyperfluoresce due to atrophy of the underlying RPE.

Histopathological examinations of donor eyes from patients with STGD[15] have demonstrated accumulation of lipofuscin throughout the RPE. Autofluorescence imaging is useful in the diagnosis of STGD and FFM (Fig. 57.3).[16]

Dominant Stargardt disease

See Chapters 52 and 54.

A number of families with a fundus appearance similar to Stargardt disease show autosomal dominant inheritance.[17,18] The usual presentation is with progressive central visual loss in the first or second decade of life that may precede ophthalmoscopic abnormalities. Initially, there are subtle RPE abnormalities and temporal pallor of the optic disc; later there is macular atrophy often with yellowish fundus flecks. A "dark" choroid is uncommon. Electrophysiology is usually normal until late in the disease process.[19]

Most families show linkage to chromosome 6q[20] and genealogical and molecular evidence points towards a founder ancestor.[19] In one large family a deletion in the gene, *ELOVL4*, a component of the mammalian fatty acid elongation system, has been identified.[17]

Other dominant Stargardt families map to 4p,[21] and 13q.[22] A mutation of the peripherin/RDS gene has been reported in a

family with a dominantly inherited retinal dystrophy with a very variable phenotype with a FFM fundus appearance.[23]

Kandori flecked retina syndrome

This is a rare[24–26] autosomal recessive stationary dystrophy characterized by onset in childhood, mild slowing of dark adap-

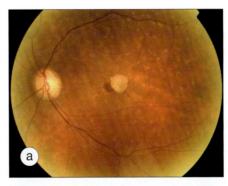

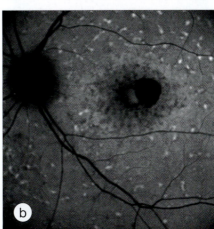

Fig. 57.3 Stargardt disease. (a) Fundus photography in a patient with Stargardt disease. (b) Autofluorescence imaging: areas of RPE atrophy are hypofluorescent but in other areas there are areas of increased fluorescence which reflect accumulation of lipofuscin in the RPE. This appearance is characteristic of Stargardt disease.

tation, normal vision and visual fields. Fundus examination reveals distinctive mid-peripheral deposition of yellow flecks at the level of the RPE that spare the macula and are hypofluorescent on angiography. The ERG and EOG are normal and the results of psychophysical testing are similar to those in fundus albipunctatus.

Benign flecked retina syndrome

Aish and Dajani[27] described a flecked retina syndrome in seven out of ten siblings born to consanguineous parents. The visual acuity, peripheral visual fields and dark adaptation were all normal. The flecks, first seen in infancy, were discrete white-yellow lesions at the level of the RPE and were scattered throughout the fundus. Fluorescein angiography showed multiple areas of hyperfluorescence that did not correlate with the flecks. Although there are many similarities to fundus flavimaculatus the lack of macular involvement in all of the seven affected siblings and the good visual prognosis suggest that this represents different disorder.

Fundus albipunctatus

Fundus albipunctatus (FA) is a rare autosomal recessive condition characterized by widespread numerous small yellow-white punctate lesions at the level of the RPE (Fig. 57.4).[28,29] The prominence and number of these lesions appear to change with age.[30–32] Individuals complain of night-blindness from a young age and delayed dark adaptation following exposure to bright light. Acuity is usually normal as are visual fields and this combination helps to differentiate FA from other fleck retina syndromes.

Dark adaptometry reveals elevated rod and cone final thresholds and prolonged recovery of rod and cone sensitivity. Rod and cone electroretinogram (ERG) responses are subnormal when recorded following routine dark adaptation but reach normal or near normal levels following extended dark adaptation.[29,30,33]

A gene for FA (*RDH5*) has now been cloned and encodes 11-*cis*-retinol dehydrogenase.[34] The enzyme catalyses the dehydrogenation of 11-*cis*-retinol to 11-*cis*-retinal in the RPE which is then transported to the photoreceptors for use as the chromophore in rhodopsin and the cone opsins.[35] Defects in RDH5 are thought therefore to result in delayed photopigment regeneration which would account for the prolongation of dark adaptation seen in patients with fundus albipunctatus. In bright light, the demand for regenerated cone opsins outstrips supply with resultant hemeralopia.[34]

Traditionally, FA has been considered a type of congenital stationary night-blindness, but it is clear that some older individuals, who have RDH5 mutations, develop poor acuity as a result of a progressive cone dystrophy.[36–38] Miyake *et al.*[28] have described five unrelated individuals with a fundal appearance similar to FA, poor color vision since childhood, a bull's eye maculopathy and electrophysiological evidence of a cone dystrophy.

Retinitis punctata albescens, Bothnia and Newfoundland retinal dystrophies

Some patients with retinitis pigmentosa (RP) have multiple white dots throughout the retina rather than the usual pigment deposition; such patients are described as having retinitis punctata albescens (Fig. 57.5). It is doubtful whether this phenotype represents a unique subtype of the condition as it may be seen in patients from families where other relatives have the classical fundus appearance of RP.[39] The retinal appearance in patients with these white deposits may later evolve to give rise to the more classical pigmentary retinopathy. Clinically, retinitis punctata albescens can be distinguished from fundus albipunctatus by the progressive field loss and differences in ERG testing.[39]

Mutations in peripherin/RDS,[40] cellular retinal binding protein-1 (RLBP-1)[41] and the rhodopsin gene[42] have all been described in association with a retinitis punctata albescens phenotype.

Two early onset forms of autosomal recessive retinitis pigmentosa with multiple white deposits at the level of the RPE have been described, both of which have high prevalence in the genetic isolates of north-eastern Canada (Newfoundland rod-cone dystrophy) and northern Sweden (Bothnia dystrophy). In both instances, mutations in the gene encoding RLBP-1 have been described.[43–45]

Enhanced S cone syndrome (ESCS)

See Chapter 52.

ESCS is unique among retinal dystrophies since although there is retinal degeneration resulting in visual loss, there is gain of function in a subset of photoreceptors, the S cones. The abnormalities may be minimal (ESCS) or severe (Goldmann–Favre syndrome) and comprise cystic changes at the fovea, vitreous degeneration (veils and opacities), peripheral retinoschisis and cataract. In addition, mid-peripheral deep retinal flecks can be seen together with pigmentary changes.[46] ESCS can be distinguished by a characteristic electrophysiological pattern. Rod and L/M cone responses are reduced. However, S cone-mediated sensitivities are typically 30 times higher than in normal individuals.[47] ESCS is caused by mutations in the *NR2E3* gene.[48]

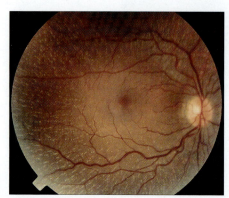

Fig. 57.4 Wide angle view of fundus albipunctatus.

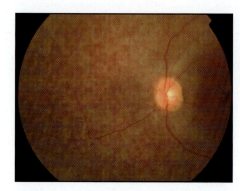

Fig. 57.5 Fundus photograph of 16-year-old boy with autosomal recessive rod cone dystrophy. There are multiple white deposits at the level of the RPE. The ERG is unrecordable.

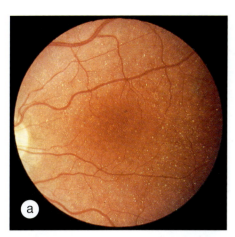

Fig. 57.8 Bietti crystalline retinal dystrophy. (a) There are numerous crystals at the posterior pole. (b) The fluorescein angiogram shows choroidal and retinal pigment atrophy.

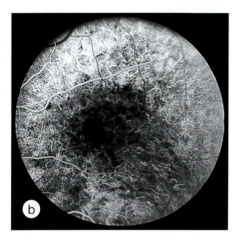

Bietti crystalline retinopathy[89]: sequencing of the XLRS gene (*RS1*) demonstrated that the grandfather and grandson were hemizygous and the daughter heterozygous for the same mutation. The finding is strongly suggestive that this genetic defect was causative of both retinal pathologies indicating that RS1 should be considered a candidate gene for Bietti crystalline dystrophy.

Autosomal dominant crystalline retinopathy

A large family had some individuals with retinal findings compatible with Bietti dystrophy.[90] There were no corneal deposits. The onset was in the mid-teens and the inheritance was autosomal dominant (with incomplete penetrance and variable expressivity). For these reasons, the authors and others[91] felt this was a distinct syndrome.

Primary hereditary oxalosis

Primary hereditary oxalosis is a rare autosomal recessive disorder of glyoxylate metabolism resulting in increased serum and urinary levels of oxalate. As serum levels rise, calcium precipitates with oxalate to form insoluble crystals which are then deposited in many tissues. Renal involvement leading to chronic renal failure is major cause of premature death.

Two different types of the disorder have been described with a specific enzyme deficiency. In type 1 hyperoxaluria, mutations in the AGXT gene resulting defective a-ketoglutarate: glyoxalate carboligase activity resulting in excessive oxalate formation in the liver. In type 2 disease, a deficiency in D-glyceric dehydrogenase likewise results in increased oxalate synthesis.[92,93] The ocular abnormalities are confined to type 1 disease.[94,95]

Hereditary oxalosis usually presents in early childhood and affected children may show multiple yellow crystals deposited at the level of the RPE more numerously at the posterior pole (Fig. 57.9). Over time, hyperplasia of the RPE results in a ring of hyperpigmentation around the macula. Angiography in one case showed masking of fluorescence over this area with surrounding hyperfluorescence presumably related to the crystal deposition. Retinal oxalate crystal deposition may also occur in secondary hyperoxaluria resulting from methoxyflurane anesthesia.[94–96]

Histological examination of tissue from corneal and conjunctival biopsies from affected patients has shown lipid noncholesterol inclusions[82,86] suggesting a defect in lipid-binding proteins or one or more enzymes active in fatty acid elongation and desaturation.[87]

A gene for Bietti crystalline dystrophy lies on chromosome 4q35.[88] A male infant was described with juvenile retinoschisis (XLRS) whose maternal grandfather had been diagnosed with

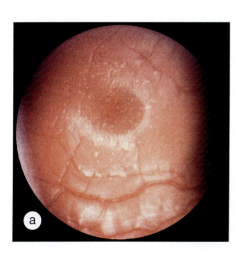

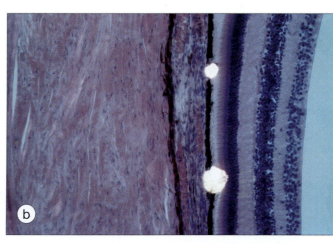

Fig. 57.9 Oxalosis type 1. (a) Fundus photograph showing the flecks predominantly at the macula. (b). Crystal deposition at the level of the retinal pigment epithelium. (Professor A. Fielder's patient.)

Sjögren–Larsson syndrome

Sjögren–Larsson syndrome (SLS)[97] is an autosomal recessively inherited neurocutaneous disorder of childhood caused by defects in the gene for the microsomal enzyme fatty aldehyde dehydrogenase (*FALDH* on chromosome 17[98]). Affected individuals show the classical triad of congenital ichthyosis, mental retardation and spastic diplegia.[97] Most patients are born preterm and all have yellow-white glistening deposits in their retinae distributed around the macula and paramacular areas (Fig. 57.10).[99,100] Fluorescein angiography shows patchy hyperfluorescence at the macula due to pigment epithelial atrophy. The ERG and EOG are normal.[99,100]

Histopathological examination of the eyes from one case showed increased lipofuscin levels in the pigment epithelium in the macular area but no evidence of any other retinal or subretinal deposits.[101]

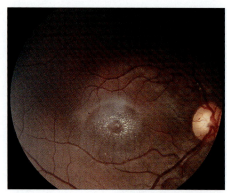

Fig. 57.10
Sjögren–Larssen syndrome. Crystal-like particles at the macula.

REFERENCES

1. Sommer A. Vitamin A: its effect on childhood sight and life. Nutr Rev 1994; 52: S60–6.
2. von Ruckmann Av, Fitzke F, Bird A. In vivo fundus auto-fluorescence in macular dystrophies. Arch Ophthalmol 1997; 115: 609–15.
3. Ahnelt PK, Kolb H, Pflug R. Identification of a subtype of cone photoreceptor, likely to be blue sensitive, in the human retina. J Comp Neurol 1987; 255: 18–34.
4. Mata N, Radu R, Clemmons R, et al. Isomerisation and oxidation of vitamin A in cone dominant retinas: a novel pathway for visual-pigment regeneration in daylight. Neuron 2002; 36: 69–80.
5. Li Q, Puro DG. Diabetes-induced dysfunction of the glutamate transporter in retinal Muller cells. Invest Ophthalmol Vis Sci 2002; 43: 3109–16.
6. Chao TI, Grosche J, Friedrich KJ, et al. Comparative studies on mammalian Muller (retinal glial) cells. J Neurocytol 1997; 26: 439–54.
7. Snodderly DM, Sandstrom M, Leung IY, et al. Retinal pigment epithelial cell distribution in retinol deficiency in central retina of monkeys. Invest Ophthalmol Vis Sci 2002; 43: 2815–8.
8. Wikler KC, Williams RW, Rakic P. Photoreceptor mosaic: number and distribution of rods and cones in the rhesus monkey retina. J Comp Neurol 1990; 297: 499–508.
9. Koenekoop RK. The gene for Stargardt disease, ABCA4, is a major retinal gene: a mini-review. Ophthalmic Genet 2003; 24: 75–80.
10. Zhang K, Nguyen TH, Crandall A, et al. Genetic and molecular studies of macular dystrophies: recent developments. Surv Ophthalmol 1995; 40: 51–61.
11. Fishman GA, Farbman JS, Alexander KR. Delayed rod dark adaptation in patients with Stargardt's disease. Ophthalmology 1991; 98: 957–62.
12. Lois N, Holder G, Bunce C, et al. Phenotypic subtypes of Stargardt macular dystrophy-fundus flavimaculatus. Arch Ophthalmol 2001; 119: 359–69.
13. Bonnin P, Passot M, Tricolaire-Cotten M. Le signe du silence choroidien dans les degenerescences tapeto-retienes posteriorieures. Doc Ophthalmol Proc Ser 1976; 9: 461–3.
14. Uliss AE, Moore AT, Bird AC. The dark choroid in posterior retinal dystrophies. Ophthalmology 1987; 94: 1423–7.
15. Birnbach CD, Jarvelainen M, Possin DE, et al. Histopathology and immunocytochemistry of the neurosensory retina in fundus flavimaculatus. Ophthalmology 1994; 101: 1211–9.
16. Lois N, Holder GE, Fitzke FW, et al. Intrafamilial variation of phenotype in Stargardt macular dystrophy-fundus flavimaculatus. Invest Ophthalmol Vis Sci 1999; 40: 2668–75.
17. Edwards AO, Donoso LA, Ritter R, 3rd. A novel gene for auto-somal dominant Stargardt-like macular dystrophy with homology to the SUR4 protein family. Invest Ophthalmol Vis Sci 2001; 42: 2652–63.
18. Lagali PS, MacDonald IM, Griesinger IB, et al. Autosomal dominant Stargardt-like macular dystrophy segregating in a large Canadian family. Can J Ophthalmol 2000; 35: 315–24.
19. Donoso LA, Edwards AO, Frost A, et al. Autosomal dominant Stargardt-like macular dystrophy. Surv Ophthalmol 2001; 46: 149–63.
20. Stone EM, Nichols BE, Kimura AE, et al. Clinical features of a Stargardt-like dominant progressive macular dystrophy with genetic linkage to chromosome 6q. Arch Ophthalmol 1994; 112: 765–72.
21. Kniazeva M, Chiang MF, Morgan B, et al. A new locus for autosomal dominant Stargardt-like disease maps to chromosome 4. Am J Hum Genet 1999; 64: 1394–9.
22. Zhang K, Bither PP, Park R, et al. A dominant Stargardt's macular dystrophy locus maps to chromosome 13q34. Arch Ophthalmol 1994; 112: 759–64.
23. Weleber RG, Carr RE, Murphey WH, et al. Phenotypic variation including retinitis pigmentosa, pattern dystrophy, and fundus flavimaculatus in a single family with a deletion of codon 153 or 154 of the peripherin/RDS gene. Arch Ophthalmol 1993; 111: 1531–42.
24. Kandori F, Tamai A, Kurimoto S, et al. Fleck retina. Am J Ophthalmol 1972; 73: 673–85.
25. Kandori F, Setogawa T, Tamai A. Electroretinographical studies on "fleck retina with congenital nonprogressive nightblindness". Yonago Acta Med 1966; 10: 98–108.
26. Kandori F, Kurimoto S, Fukunaga K, et al. Studies on fluorescein fundus photography in cases of "fleck retina with congenital nonprogressive nightblindness". Nippon Ganka Gakkai Zasshi 1968; 72: 1253–9.
27. Sabel Aish SF, Dajani B. Benign familial flecked retina. Br J Ophthalmol 1980; 64: 652–9.
28. Miyake Y, Shiroyama N, Sugita S, et al. Fundus albipunctatus associated with cone dystrophy. Br J Ophthalmol 1992; 76: 375–9.
29. Marmor MF. Fundus albipunctatus: a clinical study of the fundus lesions, the physiologic deficit, and the vitamin A metabolism. Doc Ophthalmol 1977; 43: 277–302.
30. Carr RE, Margolis S, Siegel IM. Fluorescein angiography and vitamin A and oxalate levels in fundus albipunctatus. Am J Ophthalmol 1976; 82: 549–58.
31. Dryja TP. Molecular genetics of Oguchi disease, fundus albipunctatus, and other forms of stationary night blindness: LVII Edward Jackson Memorial Lecture. Am J Ophthalmol 2000; 130: 547–63.
32. Marmor MF. Long-term follow-up of the physiologic abnormalities and fundus changes in fundus albipunctatus. Ophthalmology 1990; 97: 380–4.
33. Miyake Y, Asano T, Sakai T, et al. ERG and EOG in retinitis punctata albescens. Nippon Ganka Gakkai Zasshi 1972; 76: 247–56.
34. Yamamoto H, Simon A, Eriksson U, et al. Mutations in the gene encoding 11-cis retinol dehydrogenase cause delayed dark adaptation and fundus albipunctatus. Nat Genet 1999; 22: 188–91.

35. Gonzalez-Fernandez F, Kurz D, Bao Y, et al. 11-cis retinol dehydrogenase mutations as a major cause of the congenital night-blindness disorder known as fundus albipunctatus. Mol Vis 1999; 5: 41.
36. Wada Y, Abe T, Sato H, et al. A novel Gly35Ser mutation in the RDH5 gene in a Japanese family with fundus albipunctatus associated with cone dystrophy. Arch Ophthalmol 2001; 119: 1059–63.
37. Nakamura M, Hotta Y, Tanikawa A, et al. A high association with cone dystrophy in Fundus albipunctatus caused by mutations of the RDH5 gene. Invest Ophthalmol Vis Sci 2000; 41: 3925–32.
38. Liden M, Romert A, Tryggvason K, et al. Biochemical defects in 11–cis-retinol dehydrogenase mutants associated with fundus albipunctatus. J Biol Chem 2001; 276: 49251–7.
39. Katsanis N, Shroyer NF, Lewis RA, et al. Fundus albipunctatus and retinitis punctata albescens in a pedigree with an R150Q mutation in RLBP1. Clin Genet 2001; 59: 424-9.
40. Kajiwara K, Sandberg MA, Berson EL, et al. A null mutation in the human peripherin/RDS gene in a family with autosomal dominant retinitis punctata albescens. Nat Genet 1993; 3: 208–12.
41. Morimura H, Berson EL, Dryja TP. Recessive mutations in the RLBP1 gene encoding cellular retinaldehyde-binding protein in a form of retinitis punctata albescens. Invest Ophthalmol Vis Sci 1999; 40: 1000–4.
42. Souied E, Soubrane G, Benlian P, et al. Retinitis punctata albescens associated with the Arg135Trp mutation in the rhodopsin gene. Am J Ophthalmol 1996; 121: 19–25.
43. Burstedt MS, Sandgren O, Holmgren G, et al. Bothnia dystrophy caused by mutations in the cellular retinaldehyde-binding protein gene (RLBP1) on chromosome 15q26. Invest Ophthalmol Vis Sci 1999; 40: 995–1000.
44. Burstedt MS, Forsman-Semb K, Golovleva I, et al. Ocular phenotype of Bothnia dystrophy, an autosomal recessive retinitis pigmentosa associated with an R234W mutation in the RLBP1 gene. Arch Ophthalmol 2001; 119: 260–7.
45. Eichers ER, Green JS, Stockton DW, et al. Newfoundland rod-cone dystrophy, an early-onset retinal dystrophy, is caused by splice-junction mutations in RLBP1. Am J Hum Genet 2002; 70: 955–64.
46. Marmor MF, Jacobsen SG, Foerster MH, et al. Diagnostic clinical findings of a new syndrome with night-blindness, maculopathy and enhanced S cone sensitivity. Am J Ophthalmol 1990; 110: 124–34.
47. Jacobson SG, Marmor MF, Kemp CM, et al. SWS (blue) cone hypersensitivity in a newly identified retinal degeneration. Invest Ophthalmol and Vis Sci 1990; 31: 827–38.
48. Haider NB, Jacobson SG, Cideciyan AV, et al. Mutation in a nuclear receptor gene, NR2E3, causes enhanced S cone syndrome, a disorder of retinal cell fate. Nat Genet 2000; 24: 127–31.
49. Stone EM, Lotery AJ, Munier FL, et al. A single EFEMP1 mutation associated with both Malattia Leventinese and Doyne honeycomb retinal dystrophy. Nat Genet 1999; 22: 199–202.
50. Krill AE, Klein BA. Flecked retina syndrome. Arch Ophthalmol 1965; 74: 496–508.
51. Small K, Killian J, McLean. North Carolina dominant progressive foveal dystrophy: how progressive is it? Br J Ophthalmol 1990; 75: 401–6.
52. Small K, Hermsen V, Gurney N, et al. North Carolina macular dystrophy and central areolar pigment epithelial dystrophy. Arch Ophthalmol 1992; 110: 515–8.
53. Reichel MB, Kelsell RE, Fan J, et al. Phenotype of a British North Carolina macular dystropy family linked to chromosome 6q. Br J Ophthalmol 1998; 82: 1162–8.
54. Small KW, Weber JL, Roses A, et al. North Carolina macular dystrophy is assigned to chromosome 6. Genomics 1992; 13: 681–5.
55. Michaelides M, Johnson S, Tekriwal AK, et al. An early-onset autosomal dominant macular dystrophy (MCDR3) resembling North Carolina macular dystrophy maps to chromosome 5. Invest Ophthalmol Vis Sci 2003; 44: 2178–83.
56. Francis PJ, Johnson S, Edmunds B, et al. Genetic linkage analysis of a novel syndrome comprising North Carolina-like macular dystrophy and progressive sensorineural hearing loss. Br J Ophthalmol 2003; 87: 893–8.
57. Holz FG, Evans K, Gregory CY, et al. Autosomal dominant macular dystrophy simulating North Carolina macular dystrophy. Arch Ophthalmol 1995; 113: 178–84.
58. Scholl HP, Zrenner E. Electrophysiology in the investigation of acquired retinal disorders. Surv Ophthalmol 2000; 45: 29–47.
59. Kemp CM, Jacobson SG, Faulkner DJ, et al. Visual function and rhodopsin levels in humans with vitamin A deficiency. Exp Eye Res 1988; 46: 185–97.
60. Dieckert JP, White M, Christmann L, et al. Angioid streaks associated with abetalipoproteinemia. Am J Ophthalmol 1989; 21: 173–9.
61. Lloyd JK. Disorders of the serum lipoproteins. I. Lipoprotein deficiency states. Arch Dis Child 1968; 43: 393–403.
62. Cogan DG, Rodrigues M, Chu F, et al. Ocular abnormalities in abetalipoproteinemia: a clinicopathologic correlation. Ophthalmology 1984; 91: 991–8.
63. Kashtan CE. Alport syndromes: phenotypic heterogeneity of progressive hereditary nephritis. Pediatr Nephrol 2000; 14: 502–12.
64. Colville D, Savige J, Branley P, et al. Ocular abnormalities in thin basement membrane disease. Br J Ophthalmol 1997; 81: 373–7.
65. Colville D, Savige J, Morfis M, et al. Ocular manifestations of autosomal recessive Alport syndrome. Ophthalmic Genet 1997; 18: 119–28.
66. Raines MF, Duvall-Young J, Short CD. Fundus changes in mesangiocapillary glomerulonephritis type II: vitreous fluorophotometry. Br J Ophthalmol 1989; 73: 907–10.
67. Duvall-Young J, Short CD, Raines MF, et al. Fundus changes in mesangiocapillary glomerulonephritis type II: clinical and fluorescein angiographic findings. Br J Ophthalmol 1989; 73: 900–6.
68. O'Brien C, Duvall-Young J, Brown M, et al. Electrophysiology of type II mesangiocapillary glomerulonephritis with associated fundus abnormalities. Br J Ophthalmol 1993; 77: 778–80.
69. Innis JW, Sieving PA, McMillan P, et al. Apparently new syndrome of sensorineural hearing loss, retinal pigment epithelium lesions, and discolored teeth. Am J Med Genet 1998; 75: 13–7.
70. Eustis HS, Curry T, Superneau D. Peroxisomal bifunctional enzyme complex deficiency with associated retinal findings. J Pediatr Ophthalmol Strabismus 1995; 32: 125–7.
71. Al-Hazzaa S, Ozand P. Peroxisomal bifunctional enzyme deficiency with associated retinal findings. Ophthalmic Genet 1997; 18: 93–9.
72. Traboulsi EI. Fleck retina in Kjellin's syndrome. Am J Ophthalmol 1985; 99: 738–9.
73. Frisch IB, Haag P, Steffen H, et al. Kjellin's syndrome: fundus autofluorescence, angiographic, and electrophysiologic findings. Ophthalmology 2002; 109: 1484–91.
74. Ono K, Suzuki Y, Fujii I, et al. A case of ring chromosome E17: 46, XX, r17 (p13 yields q25) (author's transl). Jinrui Idengaku Zasshi 1974; 19: 235–42.
75. Gass JD, Taney BS. Flecked retina associated with cafe au lait spots, microcephaly, epilepsy, short stature, and ring 17 chromosome. Arch Ophthalmol 1994;112:738–9.
76. Charles SJ, Moore AT, Davison BC, et al. Flecked retina associated with ring 17 chromosome. Br J Ophthalmol 1991; 75: 125–7.
77. Protzko EE, Schatz H, Raymond W, et al. Bread crumb-flecked retinopathy. Retina 1992; 12: 21–3.
78. Hotta Y, Nakamura M, Okamoto Y, et al. Different mutation of the XLRS1 gene causes juvenile retinoschisis with retinal white flecks. Br J Ophthalmol 2001; 85: 238–9.
79. Hayasaka S, Kiyosawa M, Katsumata S, et al. Clinical and retinal changes in myotonic dystrophy. Arch Ophthalmol 1984; 102: 88–93.
80. Singerman LJ, Berkow JW, Patz A. Dominant slowly progressive macular dystrophy. Am J Ophthalmol 1977; 83: 680–93.
81. Bietti G. Ueber familiares Vorkommen von Retinitis pigmentosa albescens (verbinden mit Dystrophia marginalis crystillinea corneae) Glizern des Glaskverpers und anderen degenerativen Augenveranderungen. Klin Monatsbl Augenheilkd 1937; 99: 737–56.
82. Wilson DJ, Weleber RG, Klein ML, et al. Bietti's crystalline dystrophy. A clinicopathologic correlative study. Arch Ophthalmol 1989; 107: 213–21.
83. Bernauer W, Daicker B. Bietti's corneal-retinal dystrophy. A 16-year progression. Retina 1992; 12: 18–20.
84. Fujiwara H, Nishikion T, Kano M. Two cases of crystalline retinopathy. Jpn J Ophthalmol 1982; 36: 301–6.

613

85. Grizzard WS, Deutman AF, Nijhuis F. Crystalline retinopathy. Am J Ophthalmol 1978; 86: 81–8.

86. Kaiser-Kupfer MI, Chan CC, Markello TC. Clinical biochemical and pathologic correlations in Bietti's crystalline dystrophy. Am J Ophthalmol 1994; 118: 569–82.

87. Lee J, Jiao X, Hejtmancik JF, et al. Identification, isolation, and characterization of a 32-kDa fatty acid-binding protein missing from lymphocytes in humans with Bietti crystalline dystrophy (BCD). Mol Genet Metab 1998; 65: 143–54.

88. Jiao X, Munier FL, Iwata F, et al. Genetic linkage of Bietti crystallin corneoretinal dystrophy to chromosome 4q35. Am J Hum Genet 2000; 67: 1309–13.

89. Weinberg DV, Sieving PA, Bingham EL, et al. Bietti crystalline retinopathy and juvenile retinoschisis in a family with a novel RS1 mutation. Arch Ophthalmol 2001; 119: 1719–21.

90. Richards BW, Brodstein DE, Nussbaum JJ, et al. Autosomal dominant crystalline dystrophy. Ophthalmology 1991; 98: 658–65.

91. Miyauchi O, Murayama K, Adachi-Usami E. A family with crystalline retinopathy demonstrating an autosomal dominant inheritance pattern. Retina 1999; 19: 573–4.

92. Milosevic D, Rinat C, Batinic D, et al. Genetic analysis – a diagnostic tool for primary oxaluria type 1. Pediatr Nephrol 2002; 17: 896–8.

93. Rumsby G. Biochemical and genetic diagnosis of the primary hyperoxalurias: a review. Mol Urol 2000; 4: 349–54.

94. Zak TA, Buncic R. Primary hereditary oxalosis retinopathy. Arch Ophthalmol 1983; 101: 78–80.

95. Fielder AR, Garner A, Chambers T. Ophthalmic manifestations of primary oxalosis. Br J Ophthalmol 1980; 64: 782–8.

96. Meredith TA, Wright J, Gammon J, et al. Ocular involvement in primary hyperoxaluria. Arch Ophthalmol 1984; 102: 584–7.

97. Sjogren T, Larsson T. Oligophrenia in combination with congenital ichthyosis and spastic disorders. Acta Psychiatr Scand 1957; 32: 1–113.

98. Pigg M, Jagell S, Sillen A, et al. The Sjogren-Larsson syndrome gene is close to D17S805 as determined by linkage analysis and allelic association. Nat Genet 1994; 8: 361–4.

99. Jagell S, Gustavson KH, Holmgren G. Sjogren-Larsson syndrome in Sweden. A clinical, genetic and epidemiological study. Clin Genet 1981; 19: 233–56.

100. Gilbert WR, Jr, Smith JL, Nyhan WL. The Sjogren-Larsson syndrome. Arch Ophthalmol 1968; 80: 308–16.

101. Nilsson SE, Jagell S. Lipofuscin and melanin content of the retinal pigment epithelium in a case of Sjogren-Larsson syndrome. Br J Ophthalmol 1987; 71: 224–6.

CHAPTER 58 Miscellaneous Retinal Disorders

David A Hollander and Robert B Bhisitkul

DIABETIC RETINOPATHY

Diabetic retinopathy, while uncommon in children, is strongly correlated with duration of diabetes and overall glycemic control (percentage of glycosylated hemoglobin). The prevalence of diabetic retinopathy rises steadily following puberty, with a 4.8 times greater risk of postpubescent adolescents developing retinopathy relative to pubescent or pre-pubescent children with the same duration of diabetes.[1] Studies in the past discounted the influence of the duration of diabetes prior to puberty,[2] yet recent reports have suggested that the number of years of systemic illness prior to puberty do have a significant impact on the prevalence and complications of diabetic retinopathy.[3–5] The progression of diabetic retinopathy associated with puberty is likely a combination of metabolic changes as well as decreased patient compliance.

Until recently, pediatric diabetes was almost exclusively the type 1 insulin-dependent form. With increasing obesity in the pediatric population however, type 2 diabetes and insulin resistance now represents an emerging epidemic in children and adolescents, comprising 8–45% of all juvenile diabetes.[6] Initial screening of pediatric diabetic patients by an ophthalmologist between 3–5 years following diagnosis remains critical. Early retinopathy in children is best detected by fluorescein angiography, as over 50% of juvenile diabetic patients negative by ophthalmoscopy may have angiographic findings, most commonly microaneurysms.[7] The Diabetes Control and Complications Trial (DCCT) demonstrated in its pediatric cohort (ages 13–17 years) that intensive insulin therapy delayed the onset and reduced the progression of diabetic retinopathy.[8] Insulin therapy however, must be specifically tailored to the patient in order to avoid hypoglycemic events, episodes more common in young children whose eating and exercise behaviors are highly variable.[9]

Retinopathy is slowly progressive, affecting between 5–44% of insulin dependent diabetic children after five years of systemic disease and nearly 100% of patients within 20 years.[10–12] Longitudinal studies have demonstrated clinically significant macular edema after seven years of systemic disease, with a linear yearly cumulative risk as high as 6.7% between 10 and 20 years of duration.[13] Proliferative diabetic retinopathy (Fig. 58.1), though extremely rare in the pediatric population, has been observed in children as young as 13 years old with an 8 year history of diabetes.[14]

SICKLE CELL RETINOPATHY

Ocular manifestations of sickle cell disease are most commonly seen in hemoglobin SC disease, homozygous sickle cell (SS) disease, sickle cell thalassemia (S-Thal), and heterozygous sickle

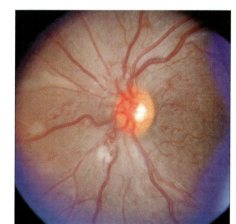

Fig. 58.1 Diabetic retinopathy. Proliferative diabetic retinopathy in a young adult. Neovascularization of the disc is present, in addition to multiple cotton-wool spots and intraretinal hemorrhages.

cell trait (AS). Sickle hemoglobinopathies occur secondary to point mutations in the hemoglobin gene. Under conditions of hypoxia, dehydration, acidosis, and hyperviscosity, the abnormal hemoglobins tend to polymerize, resulting in sickled erythrocytes.[15] Sickled erythrocytes are less pliable and cannot easily migrate through small diameter capillaries or pores of the trabecular meshwork.

The earliest ocular complication of sickle cell disease is peripheral retinal arteriolar occlusion resulting from intravascular sickling and thrombosis.[16] Retinal nonperfusion initiates a complex cascade of vascular remodeling at the junction of perfused and nonperfused retina. Arteriovenous anastomoses may develop, which eventually give rise to classic sea fan proliferative retinopathy (Fig. 58. 2), most commonly seen in SC and S-Thal disease.[17–19] Classic intraretinal salmon patch hemorrhages are often observed, which upon resorption may result in refractile spots of hemosiderin deposition beneath the internal limiting membrane. Black sunburst lesions, likely the sequela of subretinal hemorrhage, are focal areas of retinal pigment epithelial hypertrophy and hyperplasia.[20] Additional

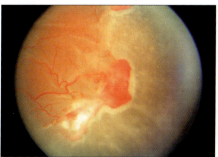

Fig. 58.2 Sickle cell retinopathy. Proliferative sickle cell retinopathy in a young male with hemoglobin SC disease. Proliferative retinopathy is seen at the border of perfused and nonperfused retina. The patient subsequently developed a tractional retinal detachment.

615

ophthalmic manifestations include conjunctival microvascular segmentation (comma sign), iris atrophy,[21] synechia, angioid streaks,[22] transient red spots on the optic disc,[23] venous tortuosity,[24] as well as branch and central retinal artery occlusions.[25]

Vascular remodeling begins early, with longitudinal studies demonstrating peripheral vascular closure in 50% of children with SS and SC disease at age 6, and vascular changes in up to 90% of children by age 12.[26] Though proliferative retinopathy is rare in children, angiographic evidence of neovascularization was found in five (8%) males and two (3%) females in a series of 199 patients below 20 years of age with SC, SS and S-Thal disease.[27] Vision loss in children may also occur secondary to occlusions in terminal arterioles near the foveal avascular zone[28-30] or central retinal artery occlusions, exacerbated by raised intraocular pressure.

Proliferative sickle cell retinopathy may lead to vitreous hemorrhage, tractional and rhegmatogenous retinal detachments, but more frequently, undergoes spontaneous regression.[31-32] Suggested mechanisms for autoinfarction include feeder arteriolar occlusion, capillary occlusion, or hemodynamic alterations induced by vitreous traction.[33-34] Progression of lesions in both SC and SS disease is most likely to take place in patients between 20 and 39 years of age.[32] Peripheral scatter photocoagulation may be utilized to induce regression and reduce the risk of vitreous hemorrhage.[35] Careful monitoring of the delicate balance of regression and progression is critical, as neither spontaneous regression nor scatter photocoagulation prevents the development of new proliferative lesions. In the event of retinal detachment, caution should be taken to minimize the risk of anterior segment ischemia as reported with encircling scleral buckles.[36]

Traumatic hyphema in children with sickle cell hemoglobinopathies poses an increased risk of complications, including raised intraocular pressure as a result of aqueous outflow obstruction by sickled erythrocytes.[37-38] Even mild elevations in intraocular pressure may produce sludging in the vascular supply to the optic nerve and retina, leading to central retinal artery occlusion or optic atrophy.[39] Therefore surgical intervention or antifibrinolytic therapy with aminocaproic acid may be necessary in certain cases. Additionally, there is an increased risk of rebleeding after the initial hyphema in pediatric sickle cell patients.[40]

RADIATION RETINOPATHY

Radiation retinopathy, first reported by Stallard and Moore in the 1930s,[41-42] continues to be seen in children secondary to both focal plaque (brachytherapy) and external beam treatments for retinoblastoma and orbital tumors.[43-44] The total dose and the fraction size of radiation are the key elements predisposing to radiation retinopathy, with retinal vascular damage occurring at lower doses with external beam than plaque therapy.[43] The threshold for retinopathy is typically at a total dose of 3000–3500 cGy with external beam radiotherapy, but retinopathy has been reported with as little as 1500 total cGy.[43,45] Radiation retinopathy most commonly develops between 6 months and 3 years following treatment, though retinal changes have been observed as early as 1 month following both plaque and external beam modalities.[46-48]

Radiation induces a cascade of changes in the retinal vascular architecture, predominantly in the macula, which lead to vascular nonperfusion, incompetence, and proliferation. Early histological studies have demonstrated a preferential loss of vascular endothelial cells with a relative sparing of the pericytes, a distinct contrast to the early loss of pericytes in diabetic retinopathy.[46] Progressive endothelial cell loss results in capillary occlusion as well as irregular dilatations, telangiectasias, and microaneurysms of the neighboring capillary bed.[49] Vascular changes are more common on the arterial side, likely the result of a greater number of free radicals promoted by the higher oxygen tension. Additional posterior segment findings may include arteriolar narrowing and sheathing, intraretinal hemorrhages, cotton-wool spots, lipid exudates, macular edema, retinal pigment epithelial atrophy, optic neuropathy, and proliferative retinopathy.

Retinoblastoma is relatively radiosensitive, and therefore plaque and external beam radiotherapy are often necessary treatment modalities, despite the risks of radiation retinopathy. In a retrospective study of 141 retinoblastoma patients treated with plaque therapy, a maculopathy was seen in 25% and proliferative retinopathy was seen in 15% of treated eyes at 5 years.[44] In children treated with external beam radiotherapy for retinoblastoma, radiation retinopathy was observed in 23% of 44 treated eyes.[50] More severe and extensive radiation retinopathy is associated with diabetes mellitus and the administration of chemotherapeutic agents.[43,51-52] Efforts to reduce the total dose and increase the fractionation may help reduce the complications of radiotherapy.

BONE MARROW TRANSPLANT RETINOPATHY

An ischemic retinopathy, similar to that observed with radiotherapy, is seen in children and adults receiving bone marrow transplantation (BMT) for hematological malignancies and aplastic anemia. The retinal manifestations typically include capillary nonperfusion, cotton-wool spots, and intraretinal hemorrhages (Fig. 58.3).[53] The vasculopathy generally develops within 6 months of BMT, with histological changes resembling those of early radiation retinopathy.[53-54] While the majority of ocular complications associated with BMT are anterior segment related, namely cataract and dry eye, the incidence of posterior segment changes, most notably ischemic retinopathy and disc swelling, ranges from 6.9–13.5%.[53,55-58] The vast majority of the retinopathy resolves,[59] with rare reports of proliferative retinopathy associated with BMT.[60] Additional posterior segment complications include vitreous hemorrhage secondary to

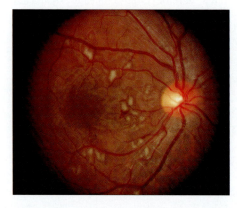

Fig. 58.3 Bone marrow transplant retinopathy. Multiple cotton-wool spots and a small perifoveal hemorrhage occurring three months after bone marrow transplant.

thrombocytopenia, opportunistic infections,[55,58] and progressive outer retinal necrosis.[61] In a retrospective study of 104 consecutive pediatric patients undergoing bone marrow transplantation, 95.7% of eyes retained visual acuity of 20/40 or better, with poor visual outcomes associated with cytomegalovirus retinitis, a presumed submacular *Nocardia* abscess, corneal ulcers secondary to dry eye syndrome, and cataracts.[58]

The pathogenesis of the retinopathy in BMT patients remains unclear, confounded by the conditioning regimens prior to transplantation which typically involve total body radiation and chemotherapy, as well as the administration of agents following transplantation designed to suppress graft-versus-host disease. The chemotherapeutic agents may be directly toxic to the retinal vasculature, potentially increasing the susceptibility to retinopathy, as retinopathy develops with relatively low doses of total radiation[58–59] as well as in its absence.[62] Both cyclosporin A and campath-1G, suppressors of T-cell function which alone do not cause a retinopathy,[63] may similarly lower the threshold for radiation induced retinal ischemia.[53–54]

RETINAL VASCULITIS

Retinal vasculitis may occur secondary to a systemic disease or an infectious agent, or simply as an isolated retinal etiology. Posterior segment manifestations include vascular sheathing, intraretinal hemorrhages, retinal exudates, vitritis, as well as macular edema. Both vascular incompetence and ischemia may be seen on fluorescein angiography, in which vessel staining or leakage are common findings. Nonperfusion may produce cotton-wool spots (Fig. 58.4), intraretinal whitening, and proliferative retinopathy. Clinical fundus features are often nonspecific, and other ocular or systemic features may aid in the diagnosis of the underlying etiology.

The most common causes of retinal vasculitis in the pediatric population are listed in Table 58.1, and may include collagen vascular disorders,[64] Behçet disease,[65] Eales disease,[66] acquired toxoplasmosis,[67] multiple sclerosis,[68] human immunodeficiency virus (HIV), Human T-cell lymphotropic virus type-1 (HTLV-1),[69] common variable immunodeficiency syndrome,[70] Henoch–Schönlein purpura,[71] and the syndrome of idiopathic vasculitis, aneurysms and neuroretinitis.[72] Treatment is tailored to the underlying etiology and retinal pathology.

Table 58.1 Conditions associated with retinal vasculitis in children and adolescents

Idiopathic
Eales disease
System lupus erythematous (SLE) and other collagen vascular diseases
Sarcoidosis
Behçet disease
Human immunodeficiency virus (HIV) and acquired immunodeficiency syndrome (AIDS)
Common variable immunodeficiency
Human T-cell lymphotropic virus type 1 (HTLV-1)
Acute retinal necrosis
Toxoplasmosis
Pars planitis
Multiple sclerosis
Takayasu arteritis
Henoch–Schönlein purpura
Inflammatory bowel disease
Idiopathic retinal vasculitis, aneurysms, and neuroretinitis syndrome (IRVAN)

FROSTED BRANCH ANGIITIS

Frosted branch angiitis, first described in Japan, is a syndrome of acute, often bilateral vision loss in otherwise healthy patients, commonly children and young adults.[73] Fundus examination reveals thick inflammatory sheathing surrounding the veins (and arteries to a lesser extent), extending from the optic nerve to the periphery (Fig. 58.5). The visual acuity is often reduced to counting fingers, but may be relatively unaffected in mild cases.[74] Intraretinal hemorrhages, serous macular detachment, optic disc swelling, conjunctival injection, anterior uveitis and vitreous inflammation may also be present.[75–76] Fluorescein angiography demonstrates late staining and leakage from the veins without any evidence of stasis or occlusion.

Systemic corticosteroids remain the mainstay of treatment, with prompt resolution of perivascular infiltrates and recovery of vision in the majority of cases.[73,75–77] Isolated case reports have demonstrated a similar recovery with topical or subconjunctival steroids alone.[74,78–79] Visual recovery however, may be limited by macular scarring, branch retinal vein occlusions and diffuse retinal fibrosis.[75,80] Despite visual recovery, persistent visual field constriction and depressed electroretinogram (ERG) amplitudes may persist.[81]

The origin of frosted branch angiitis remains uncertain, though the efficacy of corticosteroid therapy suggests an underlying immune response. Frosted branch appearances have been described in patients with lymphoma and leukemia, likely the result of malignant vascular infiltration.[82] Frosted branch-like

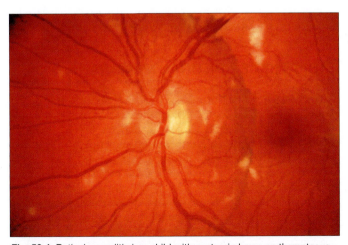

Fig. 58.4 Retinal vasculitis in a child with systemic lupus erythematosus. Shows multiple cotton-wool spots.

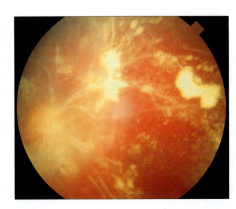

Fig. 58.5 Frosted branch angiitis. Unilateral frosted branch angiitis, in a 10-year-old girl, of no known cause. Sheathed retinal vessels, and subretinal exudates.

appearances have also been associated with cytomegalovirus (CMV) retinitis in immunosuppressed patients,[83–86] as well as with autoimmune diseases such as systemic lupus erythematosus[87] and Crohn disease.[88]

ANGIOID STREAKS

Angioid streaks are irregular linear streaks of variable pigmentation which may radiate in all directions from the peripapillary retina (Fig. 58.6). The streaks taper as they approach the optic disc, producing a circumferential peripapillary ring. The lesions are typically bilateral and vary in coloration depending on the pigmentation of the fundus. Angioid streaks are not seen at birth and only rarely have been observed in children, with earliest observations at 8 years of age.[89–91] Angioid streaks have been noted to increase in length and width over time. The incidence of angioid streaks increases with age, especially in the sickle hemoglobinopathies in which angioid streaks are typically observed only after the age of 25 years.[22,92]

The term angioid streak was originally coined by Knapp in 1892, reflecting the prevailing notion of the time that this fundus abnormality had a vascular etiology.[93] Subsequent clinical and histopathological studies have demonstrated that the streaks represent localized breaks at the level of Bruch's membrane.[94] Indocyanine green has proven to be a useful diagnostic tool in identifying angioid streaks and their associated ocular pathology.[95]

Angioid streaks, in up to 50% of cases, are associated with a systemic condition (Table 58.2), most commonly pseudoxanthoma

Table 58.2 Conditions associated with angioid streaks
Hematologic Sickle cell anemia Beta-thalassemia Beta-thalassemia major and intermedia Sickle cell beta-thalassemia Spherocytosis Abetalipoproteinemia
Endocrine Paget's disease of bone Hyperparathyroidism Hyperphosphatemia Acromegaly
Miscellaneous Pseudoxanthoma elasticum (PXE) Ehlers–Danlos syndrome Lead poisoning
Rare reports Familial polyposis Diabetes mellitus Sturge–Weber syndrome Facial angiomatosis Myopia Neurofibromatosis Senile elastosis Tuberous sclerosis

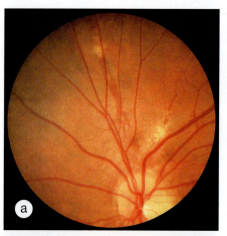

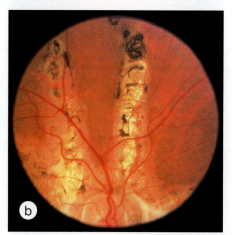

Fig. 58.6 Angioid streaks. (a) Angioid streak above the left optic disc in a 10-year-old girl with abetalipoproteinemia. (b) Marked angioid streaks in an adult with PXE. They taper away from the optic disc where they have formed a confluent ring around the disc. Neovascularization and hemorrhage occur at the margins of the streaks.

elasticum (PXE) (Fig. 58.7), Paget disease of bone, and sickle hemoglobinopathies.[96] Extensive calcification of Bruch's membrane has been demonstrated in cases of Paget disease and PXE, potentially rendering Bruch's membrane more brittle and subject to breaks. In hereditary spherocytosis, iron deposition may similarly predispose Bruch's membrane to breaks.[97] The distribution of angioid streaks may represent the effects of biomechanical forces and the traction exerted by the extraocular muscles.[98–99]

Choroidal neovascularization, though a rare phenomenon in children, may develop secondary to the breaks in Bruch's membrane, resulting in serous detachments, subretinal hemorrhage, and disciform scarring. Fundus precursors to angioid streaks may be seen in children with PXE, and include a peau d'orange pigment speckling in the posterior pole (Fig. 58.7), as well as peripheral salmon spots, yellow deposits in the retinal pigment epithelium.[89] Additionally, subretinal hemorrhages following blunt ocular trauma, has been observed in eyes with angioid streaks.[100] Identifying angioid streaks necessitates a diagnostic work-up for an underlying systemic disorder as well as close follow-up for potential ocular complications.

IDIOPATHIC EPIRETINAL MEMBRANE

Epiretinal membrane formation (macular pucker, premacular gliosis, premacular fibrosis, cellophane maculopathy) in young adults is often associated with an underlying etiology such as ocular trauma, posterior segment inflammation,[101] combined hamartoma of the RPE and retina,[102] Coats disease,[103] and neurofibromatosis type II.[104] Unlike in the adult population, idiopathic epiretinal membrane (Fig. 58.8) is rare in children and adolescents.[105] Histopathological studies have demonstrated that epiretinal membranes predominantly consist of glial and retinal pigment epithelial cells, with a greater proportion of myofibroblasts and collagen formation observed in the epiretinal membranes of adolescents than in those of the elderly.[106–107]

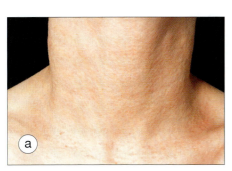
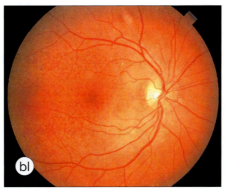
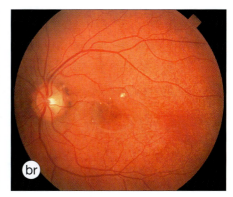

Fig. 58.7 Pseudoxanthoma elasticum. (a) The skin lesions of PXE consist of small, yellowish bumps in rows or a lacy pattern, which may join to make large patches. The skin is soft, lax and slightly wrinkled or pebbly in appearance, which has been described as cobblestoned. The neck is often affected. (b). A 14-year-old child with PXE. "Peau d'orange" pigment speckling in the RPE at the posterior pole, yellow deposits in the RPE in both eyes and angioid streaks at 12 and 6 o'clock in the right eye and 3 o'clock in the left.

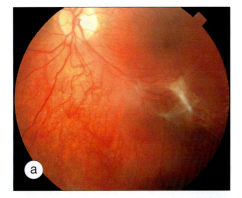
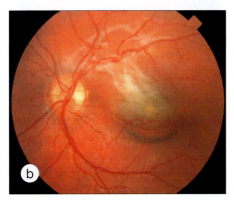

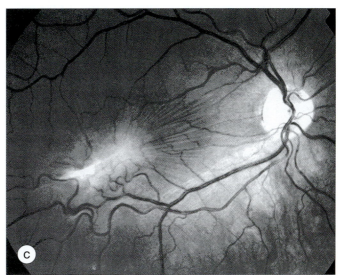

Fig. 58.8 Epiretinal membranes. (a) Preretinal fibrosis in a child with neurofibromatosis type 2. It is distorting the inferior vascular arcade and puckering the macula. (b) Macular epiretinal membrane causing traction on the superior and inferior arcades and a subretinal disturbance. (c) Idiopathic epiretinal membrane in 15-year-old leading to retinal folds and macular distortion. (Photo courtesy of Prof. Alain Gaudric, from Benhamou N, Massin P, Spolaore R, et al. Surgical Management of Epiretinal Membrane in Young Patients. Am J Ophthalmol 2002; 133: 358–364.

The etiology of idiopathic epiretinal formation in young adults remains unknown, with cases of epiretinal membranes in both the presence and absence of an attached posterior vitreous.[107–108] The congenital persistence of primary vitreous has been proposed, supported by reports of epiretinal membranes in young patients with both a Mittendorf dot and a Bergmeister papilla.[109–110] In contrast, epiretinal membrane formation in young adults may be an acquired abnormality, with reported cases of epiretinal membrane in eyes with previous normal funduscopic examinations.[111]

Many young adults with epiretinal membranes can be followed conservatively without surgical intervention.[111–113] Surgical studies have demonstrated that epiretinal membranes in young adults tend to be thicker, more adherent, and associated with a higher recurrence rate than in adults.[107–108] Spontaneous peeling of idiopathic epiretinal membrane in young patients, even in the absence of a posterior vitreous detachment, has been

reported.[114–115] Banach et al. demonstrated that patients with a visual acuity of 20/50 or better have favorable outcomes with observation alone, while those with 20/60 vision or worse had significant improvement following vitrectomy and membrane peeling.[116]

LIPEMIA RETINALIS

Lipemia retinalis, first described by Heyl in 1880, is a rare ocular manifestation of hypertrigylceridemia.[117] With serum triglycerides levels greater than 1000–2500 mg/dl (normal <200 mg/dl), the retinal arteries and veins may appear uniform creamy white in color, distinguishable only by vessel caliber.[118–119] Earliest fundus changes are seen in the periphery, with posterior involvement correlating with progressively higher triglyceride levels.[118] The

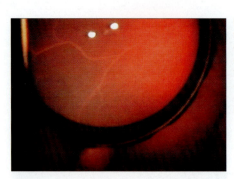

Fig. 58.9 Lipemia retinalis. Indirect ophthalmoscopic view of the retinal vessels, which stand out pale against the background, in a child with hyperchylomicronemia.

Table 58.3 Associations with CNV in children and adolescents

Inflammatory/infectious
Presumed ocular histoplasmosis syndrome
Toxocara canis
Toxoplasmosis
Rubella retinopathy
Chronic uveitis
Trauma
Choroidal rupture
Inherited retinal disorders
Best vitelliform macular dystrophy
Choroideremia
Fundus flavimaculatus
Miscellaneous
Congenital optic pits
Optic nerve head drusen
Angioid streaks
Myopia
Choroidal osteoma
Choroidal hemangioma
Combined retinal pigment epithelium: retinal hamartomas
Photocoagulation
Idiopathic

background fundus may also appear lightened or salmon colored as a result of elevated triglycerides in the choroidal circulation.

Lipemia retinalis may occur in neonates[120] and children[121] as a result of a primary familial lipid disorder (hyperlipoproteinemias types I, III, IV, and V) in chylomicrons (Fig. 58.9) and very low-density lipoproteins (VLDL), the lipoproteins which transport triglycerides, or as an acquired abnormality. Secondary hyperlipidemia has been associated with diabetes mellitus,[121] biliary obstruction, nephrotic syndrome, pancreatitis, hypothyroidism, alcoholism, medications (estrogens, β-blockers, protease inhibitors) and acquired immunodeficiency syndrome.[122]

Visual acuity typically remains unaffected, though retinal vein sludging secondary to hyperchylomicronemia has been demonstrated,[123] and a significant lipid exudative response has been observed following vein occlusion.[124] Recognition of lipemia retinalis may facilitate the earlier detection and treatment of hyperlipidemia in order to prevent complications such as pancreatitis and accelerated atherosclerosis. Treating the underlying systemic condition may simply require instituting insulin therapy or thyroid supplementation,[121] or discontinuing particular medications. Dietary modifications alone, including fat restriction[125] and the use medium-chain triglyceride (MCT) milk for neonates,[126] are often sufficient to reverse the ocular findings.

CYSTOID MACULAR EDEMA

Cystoid macular edema (CME) may be observed in children secondary to chronic ocular inflammation,[127] retinitis pigmentosa,[128] diabetes,[13] radiation,[46] Coats disease,[103] Letterer–Siwe disease,[129] retinoschisis,[130] an autosomal dominant hereditary dystrophy,[131] and following cataract extraction.[132] While Hoyt and Nickel observed cystoid macular edema in 10 of 27 eyes (37%) which underwent lensectomy and anterior vitrectomy,[132] a much lower incidence (0–4%) has been reported by others.[133–137] Explanations for the lower incidence of postoperative CME in children than adults include a healthier vitreous body and vasculature, a lack of systemic disease, and possible differences in prostaglandin physiology.[137] Different surgical techniques have not been shown to pose any additional risk for developing postoperative CME in children.[135,138]

CHOROIDAL NEOVASCULARIZATION

Choroidal neovascularization (CNV) is rare in children and adolescents, but is most commonly associated with intraocular inflammation and infection.[139] Patients may be asymptomatic or complain of metamorphopsia and blurring of vision. Fundus findings may include a deep greyish membrane, subretinal or intraretinal hemorrhage, and pigmentary changes, most commonly in the macula or peripapillary region.[140] Reported associations in the pediatric population, listed in Table 58.3, include congenital toxoplasmosis,[141–142] presumed ocular histoplasmosis syndrome,[143] congenital rubella (Fig. 58.10),[144] Best disease,[145] optic nerve head drusen,[146] traumatic choroidal rupture,[147] and choroidal coloboma.[148]

The natural history of CNV in children has a more favorable prognosis than that in adults with age related macular degeneration (ARMD). Goshorn et al. reported spontaneous involution of CNV in 11 of 19 (58%) untreated eyes in a pediatric population, in which nine patients achieved visual acuity better than or equal to 20/50.[139] Various modalities have been employed successfully in selected cases including laser photocoagulation,[140] photodynamic therapy with verteporfin,[149] and submacular surgery.[150–151]

CHRONIC GRANULOMATOUS DISEASE

Chronic granulomatous disease (CGD) is a group of rare, inherited disorders of the immune system that are caused by

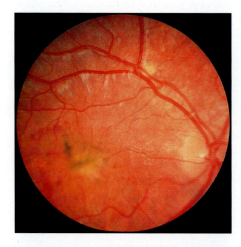

Fig. 58.10 Choroidal neovascularization. This 7-year-old with congenital rubella had a congenital cataract in the left eye and noted a reduction in the vision in the right eye. Background pigment mottling is present as well a serous detachment and a disciform lesion. The acuity fell to 6/60 but recovered to 6/12 over 4 months.

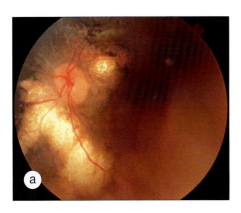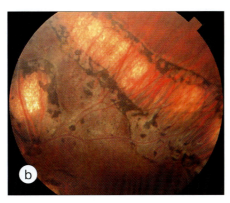

Fig. 58.11 Chronic granulomatous disease. (a) Chorioretinal atrophy and pigment clumping in the retinal arcades. (b). Linear peripheral chorioretinal atrophy and pigment clumping.

defects in phagocytes giving rise to often severe recurrent bacterial and fungal infections and chronic inflammatory conditions such as gingivitis, lymphadenopathy, or granulomas. Two-thirds of people with CGD inherit the disease as an X-linked trait, one third are thought to be autosomal recessive.

The eye is frequently affected with chorioretinal lesions in about a quarter or more of patients.[152] The chorioretinal lesions include RPE atrophy or pigment clumping (Fig. 58.11) and chorioretinal atrophy, neovascular membrane, and macular edema.[153]

REFERENCES

1. Murphy RP, Nanda M, Plotnick L, Enger C, Vitale S, Patz A. The relationship of puberty to diabetic retinopathy. Arch Ophthalmol 1990; 108: 215–8.
2. Kostraba JN, Dorman JS, Orchard TJ, et al. Contribution of diabetes duration before puberty to development of microvascular complications in IDDM subjects. Diabetes Care 1989; 12: 686–93.
3. McNally PG, Raymond NT, Swift PG, Hearnshaw JR, Burden AC. Does the prepubertal duration of diabetes influence the onset of microvascular complications? Diabetic Med 1993; 10: 906–8.
4. Flack A, Kaar ML, Laatikainen L. A prospective, longitudinal study examining the development of retinopathy in children with diabetes. Acta Paediatr 1996; 85: 313–9.
5. Donaghue KC, Fung AT, Hing S, et al. The effect of prepubertal diabetes duration on diabetes. Microvascular complications in early and late adolescence. Diabetes Care 1997; 20: 77–80.
6. Aye T, Levitsky LL. Type 2 diabetes: an epidemic disease in childhood. Curr Opin Pediatr 2003; 15: 411–5.
7. Brooser G, Barta L, Anda L, Molnar M. Early diagnosis of microangiopathy in infantile diabetes. Klin Monatsbl Augenheilkd 1975; 166: 233–6.
8. DCCT Research Group. Effect of intensive diabetes treatment on the development and progression of long-term complications in adolescents with insulin-dependent diabetes mellitus: Diabetes Control and Complications Trial. J Pediatr 1994; 125: 177–88.
9. Geffner ME. Reviewing the Diabetes Control and Complications Trial: one member of the 'control panel' speaks. J Pediatr 1994; 125: 228–9.
10. Burger W, Hovener G, Dusterhus R, Hartmann R, Weber B. Prevalence and development of retinopathy in children and adolescents with type 1 (insulin-dependent) diabetes mellitus. A longitudinal study. Diabetologia 1986; 29: 17–22.
11. Kokkonen J, Laatikainen L, van Dickhoff K, et al. Ocular complications in young adults with insulin-dependent diabetes mellitus since childhood. Acta Paediatr 1994; 83: 273–8.
12. Ben Hamouda H, Messaoud R, Grira S, et al. Prevalence and risk factors of diabetic retinopathy in children and young adults. J Fr Ophthalmol 2001; 24: 367–70.
13. Vitale S, Maguire MG, Murphy RP, et al. Clinically significant macular edema in type 1 diabetes. Incidence and risk factors. Ophthalmology 1995; 102: 1170–6.
14. Kimmel AS, Magargal LE, Annesley WH Jr, Donoso LA. Diabetic retinopathy under age 20. A review of 71 cases. Ophthalmology 1985; 92: 1047–50.
15. Dean J, Schechter AN. Sickle-cell anemia: molecular and cellular basis of therapeutic approaches. N Eng J Med 1978; 299: 863–70.
16. Goldberg MF. Classification and pathogenesis of proliferative sickle retinopathy. Am J Ophthalmol 1971; 71: 649–65.
17. Raichand M, Goldberg MF, Nagpal KC, Goldbaum MH, Asdourian GK. Evolution of neovascularization in sickle cell retinopathy. A prospective fluorescein angiographic study. Arch Ophthalmol 1977; 95: 1543–52.
18. Fox PD, Dunn DT, Morris JS, Serjeant GR. Risk factors for proliferative sickle retinopathy. Br J Ophthalmol 1990; 74: 172–6.
19. Kent D, Arya R, Aclimandos WA, Bellingham AJ, Bird AC. Screening for ophthalmic manifestations of sickle cell disease in the United Kingdom. Eye 1994; 8: 618–22.
20. Asdourian G, Nagpal KC, Goldbaum M, Patrianakos D, Goldberg MF, Rabb M. Evolution of the retinal black sunburst in sickling hemoglobinopathies. Br J Ophthalmol 1975; 59: 710–6.
21. Acheson RW, Ford SM, Maude GH, Lyness RW, Serjeant GR. Iris atrophy in sickle cell disease. Br J Ophthalmol 1986; 70: 516–21.
22. Nagpal KC, Asdourian G, Goldbaum M, Apple D, Goldberg MF. Angioid streaks and sickle haemoglobinopathies. Br J Ophthalmol 1976; 60: 31–4.
23. Goldbaum MH, Jampol LM, Goldberg MF. The disc sign in sickling hemoglobinopathies. Arch Ophthalmol 1978; 96: 1597–600.
24. Welch RB, Goldberg MF. Sickle-cell hemoglobin and its relation to fundus abnormality. Arch Ophthalmol 1966; 75: 353–62.
25. Fine LC, Petrovic' V, Irvine AR, Bhisitkul RB. Spontaneous central retinal artery occlusion in hemoglobin sickle cell disease. Am J Ophthalmol 2000; 129: 680–1.
26. Talbot JF, Bird AC, Maude GH, Acheson RW, Moriarty BJ, Serjeant GR. Sickle cell retinopathy in Jamaican children: further observations from a cohort study. Br J Ophthalmol 1988; 72: 727–32.
27. Kimmel AS, Magargal LE, Maizel R, Robb-Doyle E. Proliferative sickle cell retinopathy under age 20: a review. Ophthalmic Surg 1987; 18: 126–8.
28. Knapp JW. Isolated macular infarction in sickle cell (SS) disease. Am J Ophthalmol 1972; 73: 857–9.
29. Merritt JC, Risco JM, Pantell JP. Bilateral macular infarction in SS disease. Pediatr Ophthalmol Strabismus 1982; 19: 275–8.
30. Al-Abdulla NA, Haddock TA, Kerrison JB, Goldberg MF. Sickle cell disease presenting with extensive peri-macular arteriolar occlusions in a nine-year-old boy. Am J Ophthalmol 2001; 131: 275–6.
31. Condon PI, Serjeant GR. Behaviour of untreated proliferative sickle retinopathy. Br J Ophthalmol 1980; 64: 404–11.
32. Fox PD, Vessey SJ, Forshaw ML, Serjeant GR. Influence of genotype on the natural history of untreated proliferative sickle retinopathy – an angiographic study. Br J Ophthalmol 1991; 75: 229–31.
33. Nagpal KC, Patrianakos D, Asdourian GK, Goldberg MF, Rabb M, Jampol L. Spontaneous regression (autoinfarction) of proliferative sickle retinopathy. Am J Ophthalmol 1975; 80: 885–92.
34. McLeod DS, Merges C, Fukushima A, Goldberg MF, Lutty GA.

Histopathologic features of neovascularization in sickle cell retinopathy. Am J Ophthalmol 1997; 124: 455–72.

35. Farber MD, Jampol LM, Fox P, et al. A randomized clinical trial of scatter photocoagulation of proliferative sickle cell retinopathy. Arch Ophthalmol 1991; 109: 363–7.

36. Ryan SJ, Goldberg MF. Anterior segment ischemia following scleral buckling in sickle cell hemoglobinopathy. Am J Ophthalmol 1971; 72: 35–50.

37. Michelson PE, Pfaffenbach D. Retinal artery occlusion following ocular trauma in youths with sickle-trait hemoglobinopathy. Am J Ophthalmol 1972; 74: 494–7.

38. Lai JC, Fekrat S, Barron Y, Goldberg MF. Traumatic hyphema in children: risk factors for complications. Arch Ophthalmol 2001; 119: 64–70.

39. Goldberg MF. Sickled erythrocytes, hyphema, and secondary glaucoma: I. The diagnosis and treatment of sickled erythrocytes in human hyphemas. Ophthalmic Surg 1979; 10: 17–31.

40. Nasrullah A, Kerr NC. Sickle cell trait as a risk factor for secondary hemorrhage in children with traumatic hyphema. Am J Ophthalmol 1997; 123: 783–90.

41. Stallard HB. Radiant energy as (a) a pathogenic and (b) a therapeutic agent in ophthalmic disorders. Br J Ophthalmol Monogr 1933; 6(Suppl): 1–126.

42. Moore RF. The value of radium in intraocular lesions. Trans Ophthalmol Soc UK 1935; 55: 3–26.

43. Brown GC, Shields JA, Sanborn G, Augsburger JJ, Savino PJ, Schatz NJ. Radiation retinopathy. Ophthalmology 1982; 89: 1494–501.

44. Shields CL, Shields JA, Cater J, Othmane I, Singh AD, Micaily B. Plaque radiotherapy for retinoblastoma: long-term tumor control and treatment complications in 208 tumors. Ophthalmology 2001; 108: 2116–21.

45. Perrers-Taylor M, Brinkley D, Reynolds T. Choroido-retinal damage as a complication of radiotherapy. Acta Radiol Ther Phys Biol 1965; 3: 431–40.

46. Archer DB. Doyne lecture. Responses of retinal and choroidal vessels to ionising radiation. Eye 1993; 7: 1–13.

47. Wara WM, Irvine AR, Neger RE, Howes EL Jr, Phillips TL. Radiation retinopathy. Int J Radiat Oncol Biol Phys 1979; 5: 81–3.

48. Ehlers N, Kaae S. Effects of ionizing radiation on retinoblastoma and on the normal ocular fundus in infants. A photographic and fluorescein angiographic study. Acta Ophthalmol (Copenh) 1987; 65(Suppl 181): 1–84.

49. Hayreh SS. Post-radiation retinopathy. A fluorescence fundus angiographic study. Br J Ophthalmol 1970; 54: 705–14.

50. Coucke PA, Schmid C, Balmer A, Mirimanoff RO, Thames HD. Hypofractionation in retinoblastoma: an increased risk of retinopathy. Radiother Oncol 1993; 28: 157–61.

51. Amoaku WM, Archer DB. Cephalic radiation and retinal vasculopathy. Eye 1990; 4: 195–203.

52. Gragoudas ES, Li W, Lane AM, Munzenrider J, Egan KM. Risk factors for radiation maculopathy and papillopathy after intraocular irradiation. Ophthalmology 1999; 1571–7.

53. Bernauer W, Gratwohl A, Keller A, Daicker B. Microvasculopathy in the ocular fundus after bone marrow transplantation. Ann Intern Med 1991; 115: 925–30.

54. Webster AR, Anderson JR, Richards EM, Moore AT. Ischaemic retinopathy occurring in patients receiving bone marrow allografts and campath-1G: a clinicopathological study. Br J Ophthalmol 1995; 79: 687–91.

55. Coskuncan NM, Jabs DA, Dunn JP, et al. The eye in bone marrow transplantation. VI. Retinal complications. Arch Ophthalmol 1994; 112: 372–9.

56. De Marco R, Dassio DA, Vittone P. A retrospective study of ocular side effects in children undergoing bone marrow transplantation. Eur J Ophthalmol 1996; 6: 436–9.

57. Ng JS, Lam DS, Li CK, et al. Ocular complications of pediatric bone marrow transplantation. Ophthalmology 1999; 106: 160–4.

58. Suh DW, Ruttum MS, Stuckenschneider BJ, Mieler WF, Kivlin JD. Ocular findings after bone marrow transplantation in a pediatric population. Ophthalmology 1999; 106: 1564–70.

59. Lopez PF, Sternberg P Jr, Dabbs CK, Vogler WR, Crocker I, Kalin NS. Bone marrow transplant retinopathy. Am J Ophthalmol 1991; 112: 635–46.

60. Gomez-Ulla F, Rodriguez-Cid MJ, Gomez-Torreiro M, Abelenda D. Bone marrow transplantation retinopathy. Int Ophthalmol 2001; 24: 33–5.

61. Lewis JM, Nagae Y, Tano Y. Progressive outer retinal necrosis after bone marrow transplantation. Am J Ophthalmol 1996; 122: 892–5.

62. Cunningham ET Jr, Irvine AR, Rugo HS. Bone marrow transplantation retinopathy in the absence of radiation therapy. Am J Ophthalmol 1996; 122: 268–70.

63. Oechslin M, Thiel G, Landmann J, Gloor B. Cotton-wool exudates not observed in recipients of renal transplants treated with cyclosporine. Transplantation 1986; 41: 60–2.

64. Brissaud P, Laroche L, Krulik M, et al. Retinal vasculitis in lupic disease. Rev Med Interne 1985; 6: 36–40.

65. Atmaca LS. Fundus changes associated with Behcet's disease. Graefes Arch Clin Exp Ophthalmol 1989; 227: 340–4.

66. Elliot AJ. 30-year observation of patients with Eale's disease. Am J Ophthalmol 1975; 80: 404–8.

67. Holland GN, Muccioli C, Silveira C, Weisz JM, Belfort R Jr, O'Connor GR. Intraocular inflammatory reactions without focal necrotizing retinochoroiditis in patients with acquired systemic toxoplasmosis. Am J Ophthalmol 1999; 128: 413–20.

68. Kerrison JB, Flynn T, Green WR. Retinal pathologic changes in multiple sclerosis. Retina 1994; 14: 445–451.

69. Nakao K, Ohba N. Human T-cell lymphotropic virus type 1-associated retinal vasculitis in children. Retina 2003; 23: 197–201.

70. van Meurs JC, Lightman S, de Waard PW, et al. Retinal vasculitis occurring with common variable immunodeficiency syndrome. Am J Ophthalmol 2000; 129: 269–70.

71. Chen CL, Chiou YH, Wu CY, Lai PH, Chung HM. Cerebral vasculitis in Henoch-Schonlein purpura: a case report with sequential magnetic resonance imaging changes and treated with plasmapheresis alone. Pediatr Nephrol 2000; 15: 276–8.

72. Chang TS, Aylward GW, Davis JL, et al. Idiopathic retinal vasculitis, aneurysms, and neuro-retinitis. Retinal Vasculitis Study. Ophthalmology 1995; 103: 1089–97.

73. Ito Y, Nakano M, Kyu N, Takeuchi M. Frosted branch angiitis in a child. Jpn J Clin Ophthalmol 1976; 30: 797–803.

74. Browning DJ. Mild frosted branch periphlebitis. Am J Ophthalmol 1992; 114: 505–506.

75. Kleiner RC, Kaplan HJ, Shakin JL, Yannuzzi LA, Crosswell HH Jr, McLean WC Jr. Acute frosted retinal periphlebitis. Am J Ophthalmol 1988; 106: 27–34.

76. Sugin SL, Henderly DE, Friedman SM, Jampol LM, Doyle JW. Unilateral frosted branch angiitis. Am J Ophthalmol 1991; 111: 682–5.

77. Sakanishi Y, Kanagami S, Ohara K. Frosted retinal angiitis in children. Jpn J Clin Ophthalmol 1984; 38: 803–7.

78. Vander JF, Masciulli L. Unilateral frosted branch angiitis. Am J Ophthalmol 1991; 112: 477–8.

79. Hamed LM, Fang EN, Fanous MM, Mames R, Friedman S. Frosted branch angiitis: the role of systemic corticosteroids. J Pediatr Ophthalmol Strabismus 1992; 29: 312–3.

80. Atmaca LS, Gunduz K. Acute frosted retinal periphlebitis. Acta Ophthalmol (Copenh) 1993; 71: 856–9.

81. Watanabe Y, Takeda N, Adachi-Usami E. A case of frosted branch angiitis. Br J Ophthalmol 1987; 71: 553–8.

82. Kim TS, Duker JS, Hedges TR 3rd. Retinal angiopathy resembling unilateral frosted branch angiitis in a patient with relapsing acute lymphoblastic leukemia. Am J Ophthalmol 1994; 117: 806–8.

83. Rabb MF, Jampol LM, Fish RH, Campo RV, Sobol WM, Becker NM. Retinal periphlebitis in patients with acquired immunodeficiency syndrome with cytomegalovirus retinitis mimics acute frosted retinal periphlebitis. Arch Ophthalmol 1992; 110: 1257–60.

84. Secchi AG, Tognon MS, Turrini B, Carniel G. Acute frosted retinal periphlebitis associated with cytomegalovirus retinitis. Retina 1992; 12: 245–7.

85. Mansour AM, Li HK. Frosted retinal periphlebitis in the acquired immunodeficiency syndrome. Ophthalmologica 1993; 207: 182–6.

86. Cortina P, Diaz M, Espana E, Almenar L, Lopez-Aldeguer J. Acute frosted retinal periphlebitis associated with cytomegalovirus retinitis in a heart transplant patient. Retina 1994; 14: 463–4.

87. Quillen DA, Stathopoulos NA, Blankenship GW, Ferriss JA. Lupus associated frosted branch periphlebitis and exudative maculopathy. Retina 1997; 17: 449–51.

88. Sykes SO, Horton JC. Steroid-responsive retinal vasculitis with a frosted branch appearance in Crohns disease. Retina 1997; 17: 451–54.

89. Krill AE, Klien BA, Archer DB. Precursors of angioid streaks. Am J Ophthalmol 1973; 76: 875–9.

90. Gomolin JE. Development of angioid streaks in association with pseudoxanthoma elasticum. Can J Ophthalmol 1992; 27: 30–1.

91. Mansour AM, Ansari NH, Shields JA, Annesley WH Jr, Cronin CM, Stock EL. Evolution of angioid streaks. Ophthalmologica 1993; 207: 57–61.

92. Condon PI, Serjeant GR. Ocular findings in hemoglobin SC disease in Jamaica. Am J Ophthalmol 1972; 74: 921–31.

93. Knapp H. On the formation of dark angioid streaks as an unusual metamorphosis of retinal hemorrhage. Arch Ophthalmol 1892; 21: 289–92.

94. Klien BA. Angioid streaks: A clinical and histopathological study. Am J Ophthalmol 1947; 30: 955–68.

95. Quaranta M, Cohen SY, Krott R, Sterkers M, Soubrane G, Coscas GJ. Indocyanine green videoangiography of angioid streaks. Am J Ophthalmol 1995; 119: 136–42.

95. Clarkson JG, Altman RD. Angioid streaks. Surv Ophthalmol 1982; 26: 235–46.

97. McLane NJ, Grizzard WS, Kousseff BG, Hartmann RC, Sever RJ. Angioid streaks associated with hereditary spherocytosis. Am J Ophthalmol 1984; 97: 444–9.

98. Adelung JC. Zur genese der angioid streaks (Knapp). Klin Monatsbl Augenheilkd 1951; 119: 241–50.

99. Pruett RC, Weiter JJ, Goldstein RB. Myopic cracks, angioid streaks, and traumatic tears in Bruch's membrane. Am J Ophthalmol 1987; 103: 537–43.

100. Pandolfo A, Verrastro G, Piccolino FC. Retinal hemorrhages following indirect ocular trauma in a patient with angioid streaks. Retina 2002; 22: 830–1.

101. Small KW, McCuen BW 2nd, de Juan E Jr, Machemer R. Surgical management of retinal traction caused by toxocariasis. Am J Ophthalmol 1989; 108: 10–14.

102. Schachat AP, Shields JA, Fine SL, et al. Combined hamartomas of the retina and retinal pigment epithelium. Ophthalmology 1984; 91: 1609–15.

103. Wolfensberger TJ, Holz FG, Gregor ZJ. Juvenile coats disease associated with epiretinal membrane formation. Retina 1995; 15: 261–3.

104. Meyers SM, Gutman FA, Kaye LD, Rothner AD. Retinal changes associated with neurofibromatosis 2. Trans Am Ophthal Soc 1995; 93: 245–52.

105. Appiah AP, Hirose T, Kado M. A review of 324 cases of idiopathic premacular gliosis. Am J Ophthalmol 1988; 106: 533–5.

106. Smiddy WE, Maguire AM, Green WR, et al. Idiopathic epiretinal membranes. Ultrastructural characteristics and clinicopathologic correlation. Ophthalmology 1989; 96: 811–20.

107. Smiddy WE, Michels RG, Gilbert HD, Green WR. Clinico-pathologic study of idiopathic macular pucker in children and young adults. Retina 1992; 12: 232–6.

108. Benhamou N, Massin P, Spolaore R, Paques M, Gaudric A. Surgical management of epiretinal membrane in young patients. Am J Ophthalmol 2002; 133: 358–64.

109. Wise GN. Congenital preretinal macular fibrosis. Am J Ophthalmol 1975; 79: 363–5.

110. Webster AR, Jordan K. Epiretinal membranes presenting in two young adults with evidence of persistent primary vitreous. Eye 1994; 8: 706–8.

111. Barr CC, Michels RG. Idiopathic nonvascularized epiretinal membranes in young patients: report of six cases. Ann Ophthalmol 1982; 14: 335–41.

112. Laatikainen L, Punnonen E. 'Idiopathic' preretinal macular fibrosis in young individuals. Int Ophthalmol 1987; 10: 11–14.

113. Kimmel AS, Weingeist TA, Blodi CF, Wells KK. Idiopathic premacular gliosis in children and adolescents. Am J Ophthalmol 1989; 108: 578–81.

114. Mulligan TG, Daily MJ. Spontaneous peeling of an idiopathic epiretinal membrane in a young patient. Arch Ophthalmol 1992; 110: 1367–8.

115. Desatnik H, Treister G, Moisseiev J. Spontaneous separation of an idiopathic macular pucker in a young girl. Am J Ophthalmol 1999; 127: 729–31.

116. Banach MJ, Hassan TS, Cox MS, et al. Clinical course and surgical treatment of macular epiretinal membranes in young subjects. Ophthalmology 2001; 108: 23–6.

117. Heyl AG. Intraocular lipemia. Trans Am Ophthalmol Soc 1880; 3: 55.

118. Vinger PF, Sachs BA. Ocular manifestations of hyperlipoproteinemia. Am J Ophthalmol 1970; 70: 563–73.

119. Schaefer EJ, Levy RI. Pathogenesis and management of lipoprotein disorders. N Engl J Med 1985; 312: 1300–10.

120. Ozdemir M, Bay A, Yasar T, Cinal A. A newborn with lipemia retinalis. Ophthalmic Surg Lasers Imaging 2003; 34: 221–2.

121. Martinez KR, Cibis GW, Tauber JT. Lipemia retinalis. Arch Ophthalmol 1992; 110: 1171.

122. Eng KT, Liu ES, Silverman MS, Berger AR. Lipemia retinalis in acquired immunodeficiency syndrome treated with protease inhibitors. Arch Ophthalmol 2000; 118: 425–6.

123. Chazan BI, Ferguson BD, Castelli WP, Touborg JN, Balodimos MC, Rutstein DD. Lipemia retinalis: microcirculatory changes and lipid studies in a family. Metabolism 1969; 18: 978–85.

124. Nagra PK, Ho AC, Dugan JD Jr. Lipemia retinalis associated with branch retinal vein occlusion. Am J Ophthalmol 2003; 135: 539–42.

125. Ram J, Pandav SS, Jain S, Arora S, Gupta A, Sharma A. Reversal of lipaemia retinalis with dietary control. Eye 1993; 7: 763–5.

126. Ikesugi K, Doi M, Nishi A, Uji Y. Lipemia retinalis of prematurity. Arch Ophthalmol 1996; 114: 1283–4.

127. Smith RE, Godfrey WA, Kimura SJ. Complications of chronic cyclitis. Am J Ophthalmol 1976; 82: 277–82.

128. Fetkenhour CL, Choromokos E, Weinstein J, Shoch D. Cystoid macular edema in retinitis pigmentosa. Trans Am Acad Ophthalmol Otolaryngol 1977; 83: OP515–21.

129. Angell LK, Burton TC. Posterior choroidal involvement in Letterer-Siwe disease. J Pediatr Ophthalmol Strabismus 1978; 15: 79–81.

130. Trese MT, Foos RY. Infantile cystoid maculopathy. Br J Ophthalmol 1980; 64: 206–10.

131. Deutman AF, Pinckers AJ, Aan de Kerk AL. Dominantly inherited cystoid macular edema. Am J Ophthalmol 1976; 82: 540–8.

132. Hoyt CS, Nickel B. Aphakic cystoid macular edema: occurrence in infants and children after transpupillary lensectomy and anterior vitrectomy. Arch Ophthalmol 1982; 100: 746–9.

133. Poer DV, Helveston EM, Ellis FD. Aphakic cystoid macular edema in children. Arch Ophthalmol 1981; 99: 249–52.

134. Gilbard SM, Peyman GA, Goldberg MF. Evaluation for cystoid maculopathy after pars plicata lensectomy-vitrectomy for congenital cataracts. Ophthalmology 1983; 90: 1201–6.

135. Pinchoff BS, Ellis FD, Helveston EM, Sato SE. Cystoid macular edema in pediatric aphakia. J Pediatr Ophthalmol Strabismus 1988; 25: 240–3.

136. Green BF, Morin JD, Brent HP. Pars plicata lensectomy/vitrectomy for developmental cataract extraction: surgical results. J Pediatr Ophthalmol Strabismus 1990; 27: 229–32.

137. Rao SK, Ravishankar K, Sitalakshmi G, Ng JS, Yu C, Lam DS. Cystoid macular edema after pediatric intraocular lens implantation: fluorescein angioscopy results and literature review. J Cataract Refract Surg 2001; 27: 432–6.

138. Ahmadieh H, Javadi MA, Ahmady M, et al. Primary capsulectomy, anterior vitrectomy, lensectomy, and posterior chamber lens implantation in children: limbal versus pars plana. J Cataract Refract Surg 1999; 25: 768–75.

139. Goshorn EB, Hoover DL, Eller AW, Friberg TR, Jarrett WH 2nd, Sorr EM. Subretinal neovascularization in children and adolescents. J Pediatr Ophthalmol Strabismus 1995; 32: 178–82.

140. Wilson ME, Mazur DO. Choroidal neovascularization in children: report of five cases and literature review. J Pediatr Ophthalmol Strabismus 1988; 25: 23–9.

141. Fine SL, Owens SL, Haller JA, Knox DL, Patz A. Choroidal neovascularization as a late complication of ocular toxoplasmosis. Am J Ophthalmol 1981; 91: 318–22.

142. Cotliar AM, Friedman AH. Subretinal neovascularisation in ocular toxoplasmosis. Br J Ophthalmol 1982; 66: 524–9.

143. Gutman FA. The natural course of active choroidal lesions in the presumed ocular histoplasmosis syndrome. Trans Am Ophthalmol Soc 1979; 77: 515–41.

144. Deutman AF, Grizzard WS. Rubella retinopathy and subretinal neovascularization. Am J Ophthalmol 1978; 85: 82–7.

145. Jain K, Shafiq AE, Devenyi RG. Surgical outcome for removal of subfoveal choroidal neovascular membranes in children. Retina 2002; 22: 412–7.

146. Brown SM, Del Monte MA. Choroidal neovascular membrane associated with optic nerve head drusen in a child. Am J Ophthalmol 1996; 121: 215–7.

147. Hilton GF. Late serosanguineous detachment of the macula after traumatic choroidal rupture. Am J Ophthalmol 1975; 79: 997–1000.

148. Shaikh S, Trese M. Infantile choroidal neovascularization associated with choroidal coloboma. Retina 2003; 23: 585–6.

149. Mimouni KF, Bressler SB, Bressler NM. Photodynamic therapy with verteporfin for subfoveal choroidal neovascularization in children. Am J Ophthalmol 2003; 135: 900–2.

150. Sears J, Capone A Jr, Aaberg T Sr, et al. Surgical management of subfoveal neovascularization in children. Ophthalmology 1999; 106: 920–4.

151. Uemura A, Thomas MA. Visual outcome after surgical removal of choroidal neovascularization in pediatric patients. Arch Ophthalmol 2000; 118: 1373–8.

152. Goldblatt D, Butcher J, Thrasher AJ, et al. Chorioretinal lesions in patients and carriers of chronic granulomatous disease. J Pediatr 1999; 134: 780–3.

153. Kim SJ, Kim JG, Yu YS. Chorioretinal lesions in patients with chronic granulomatous disease. Retina 2003; 23: 360–5.

Congenital Optic Disc Anomalies

Michael C Brodsky

INTRODUCTION

A comprehensive evaluation of congenital anomalies of the optic disc needs an understanding of the ophthalmoscopic features, associated findings, pathogenesis, and ancillary studies for each anomaly.[1] New ocular and systemic associations have emerged and theories of pathogenesis for many optic disc anomalies have been revised. Our ability to subclassify different forms of excavated optic disc anomalies that were previously lumped together as colobomatous defects has further refined our ability to predict associated central nervous system (CNS) anomalies based solely on the appearance of the optic disc. The widespread application of high-resolution neuroimaging has refined our ability to predict subtle neurodevelopmental and endocrinological associations of CNS anomalies.[1]

Four general concepts are helpful in the management of congenital optic disc anomalies:

1. Children with bilateral optic disc anomalies generally present in infancy with poor vision and nystagmus; those with unilateral optic disc anomalies present during their preschool years with sensory esotropia.
2. CNS malformations are common in patients with malformed optic discs.
   - Small discs are associated with malformations involving the cerebral hemispheres, pituitary infundibulum and midline intracranial structures (e.g. septum pellucidum, corpus callosum).
   - Large optic discs of the morning glory configuration are associated with the transsphenoidal form of basal encephalocele.
   - Colobomatous optic discs are associated with systemic anomalies in a variety of syndromes.[1]
3. Any structural ocular abnormality that reduces visual acuity in infancy may lead to superimposed amblyopia.[2] A trial of occlusion therapy may be warranted in patients with asymmetrical optic disc anomalies and decreased vision.
4. The finding of a discrete V- or tongue-shaped zone of infrapapillary retinochoroidal depigmentation in an eye with an anomalous optic disc should prompt a search for a transsphenoidal encephalocele.[3]

OPTIC NERVE HYPOPLASIA

Optic nerve hypoplasia is an anomaly that, until recently, escaped scrutiny.[1] Optic nerve hypoplasia is now unquestionably the most common optic disc anomaly encountered in ophthalmologic practice.[1] This dramatic increase reflects a greater recognition by clinicians. Many cases of optic nerve hypoplasia that previously went unrecognized or were misconstrued as congenital optic atrophy are now correctly diagnosed. In addition, parental drug and alcohol abuse, which have become more widespread in recent years, may also contribute to an increasing prevalence of optic nerve hypoplasia.[1,4] Teratogenic agents factors and systemic disorders that have been associated with optic nerve hypoplasia are summarized in Table 59.1.

Optic nerve hypoplasia is now the most common optic disc anomaly encountered in ophthalmologic practice. Ophthalmoscopically, it appears as an abnormally small optic nerve head, that may appear gray or pale in color, and is often surrounded by a yellowish mottled peripapillary halo, bordered by a ring of increased or decreased pigmentation ("double-ring" sign) (Fig. 59.1).[4] The major retinal veins are often tortuous.[5] When nystagmus precludes accurate assessment of the optic disc size, this selective venous tortuosity provides an important clue to the diagnosis.

Histopathologically, optic nerve hypoplasia is characterized by a subnormal number of optic nerve axons with normal mesodermal elements and glial supporting tissue.[6,7] The double-ring sign has been found histopathologically to consist of a normal junction between the sclera and lamina cribrosa, which corresponds to the outer ring, and an abnormal extension of retina and pigment epithelium over the outer portion of the lamina cribrosa, which corresponds to the inner ring.[6,7]

Table 59.1 Systemic and teratogenic associations with optic nerve hypoplasia

Systemic associations	Teratogenic agents
Albinism	Dilantin
Aniridia	Quinine
Duane syndrome	PCP
Median facial cleft syndrome	LSD
Klippel–Trénauney–Weber syndrome	Alcohol
Goldenhar syndrome	Maternal diabetes
Linear sebaceous nevus syndrome	
Meckel syndrome	
Hemifacial atrophy	
Blepharophimosis	
Osteogenesis imperfecta	
Chondrodysplasia punctata	
Aicardi syndrome	
Apert syndrome	
Trisomy 18	
Potter syndrome	
Chromosome 13q-	
Neonatal isoimmune thrombocytopenia	
Fetal alcohol syndrome	
Dandy–Walker syndrome	
Delleman syndrome	
Frontonasal dysplasia	
Kallmann syndrome	
Congenital retinal arterial malformations	

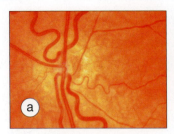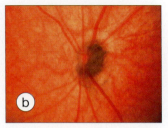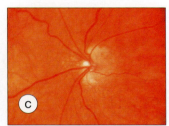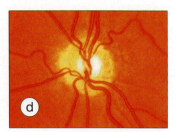

Fig. 59.1 Variants of optic nerve hypoplasia. (a) Double ring-sign. (b) With congenital optic disc pigmentation. (c) With choroid and RPE eclipsing temporal disc. (d) Double-ring sign simulating normal disc despite vision of NLP. (With permission from the American Medical Association.)

Visual acuity in optic nerve hypoplasia ranges from 20/20 to no light perception; affected eyes show localized visual field defects, often combined with a generalized constriction.[8] Since visual acuity is determined primarily by the integrity of the papillo-macular nerve fiber bundle, it does not necessarily correlate with the overall size of the disc. The strong association of astigmatism with optic nerve hypoplasia warrants careful attention to correction of refractive errors.[9]

Amblyopic eyes have smaller optic discs and smaller axial lengths compared to fellow eyes, which suggested that vision impairment in presumed amblyopia may be caused by optic nerve hypoplasia with relative microphthalmos.[10] This might be due to amblyopia by being correlated with hyperopia and anisometropia rather than being the cause of the decreased vision,[11] but when axial length was factored into the calculation, the optic disc areas of eyes with hyperopic strabismus with and without amblyopia were significantly reduced compared with hyperopic eyes without amblyopia or esotropia.[12]

Except when amblyopia develops in one eye, visual acuity usually remains stable throughout life. However, mild optic nerve hypoplasia occurs in children with congenital suprasellar tumors, which could slowly enlarge to produce the confusing diagnostic picture of acquired visual loss in the child with optic nerve hypoplasia.[13]

Optic nerve hypoplasia is often associated with a wide variety of CNS abnormalities. Septo-optic dysplasia (de Morsier syndrome) refers to the constellation of small anterior visual pathways, absence of the septum pellucidum, and thinning or agenesis of the corpus callosum;[14] it may be associated with pituitary dwarfism[15] from a pituitary hormone defect. Growth hormone deficiency is the most common, followed by thyrotropin, corticotropin, and antidiuretic hormone (Fig. 59.2).[1,16] Hypothyroidism, panhypopituitarism, diabetes insipidus, and hyperprolactinemia may also occur.[17–19] Growth hormone deficiency may be clinically inapparent within the first 3 to 4 years of life because high prolactin levels may stimulate normal growth over this period.[20] Puberty may be precocious or delayed in children with hypopituitarism.[21] Subclinical hypopituitarism can manifest as acute adrenal insufficiency following general anesthesia and suggests that it may be prudent to treat

children who have optic nerve hypoplasia with perioperative corticosteroids.[22]

In an infant with optic nerve hypoplasia, a history of neonatal jaundice suggests congenital hypothyroidism, while neonatal hypoglycemia or seizures suggests congenital panhypopituitarism.[4] A serum thyroxine level in infants with optic nerve hypoplasia may diagnose neonatal hypothyroidism. Because of inherent difficulties in measuring normal physiologic growth hormone levels, which vary diurnally, most patients with optic nerve hypoplasia are followed clinically and only investigated biochemically if growth is subnormal. However, when MRI shows posterior pituitary ectopia, or when a clinical history of neonatal jaundice or neonatal hypoglycemia is obtained, anterior pituitary hormone deficiency is probable, and more extensive endocrinologic testing becomes mandatory.[23]

Children with septo-optic dysplasia and corticotropin deficiency are at risk for sudden death during febrile illness,[24] which may be caused by an impaired ability to increase corticotropin secretion to maintain blood pressure and blood sugar in response to the stress of infection. They may have co-existent diabetes insipidus that contributes to dehydration during illness and hastens the development of shock. Some also have hypothalamic thermoregulatory disturbances signaled by episodes of hypothermia during well periods and high fevers during illnesses with life-threatening hyperthermia; they have usually had multiple hospital admissions for viral illnesses which can precipitate hypoglycemia, dehydration, hypotension, or fever of unknown origin.[24] Because corticotropin deficiency represents the pre-eminent threat to life in children with septo-optic dysplasia, a complete anterior pituitary hormone evaluation, including provocative serum cortisol testing and assessment for diabetes insipidus, should be performed in children who have clinical symptoms (history of hypoglycemia, dehydration, or hypothermia) or neuroimaging signs (absent pituitary infundibulum with or without posterior pituitary ectopia) of pituitary hormone deficiency.

Magnetic resonance imaging is best for delineating associated CNS malformations in patients with optic nerve hypoplasia.[25] MRI provides high-contrast resolution and multiplanar imaging capability, allowing the anterior visual pathways to be visualized as distinct, well-defined structures.[25] In optic nerve hypoplasia, coronal and sagittal Tl-weighted MR images shows thinning and attenuation of the corresponding prechiasmatic intracranial optic nerve (Fig. 59.3). Coronal TI-weighted MR imaging in bilateral optic nerve hypoplasia shows diffuse thinning of the optic chiasm in bilateral optic nerve hypoplasia and focal thinning or absence of the side of the chiasm corresponding to the hypoplastic nerve in unilateral optic nerve hypoplasia.[25] Then MR imaging shows a decrease in intracranial optic nerve size accompanied by other

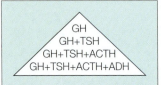

Fig. 59.2 Pyramid of pituitary hormone deficiencies in optic nerve hypoplasia.

features of septo-optic dysplasia, a presumptive diagnosis of optic nerve hypoplasia can be made.[25]

Because MRI often shows structural abnormalities involving the cerebral hemispheres and the pituitary infundibulum, septo-optic dysplasia cannot be considered a single condition.[26] Cerebral hemispheric abnormalities, are evident in approximately 45% of patients with optic nerve hypoplasia (Fig. 59.4). They may consist of hemispheric migration anomalies (e.g. schizencephaly, cortical heterotopia), intrauterine or perinatal hemispheric injury (e.g. periventricular leukomalacia, encephalomalacia).[26] Evidence of perinatal injury to the pituitary infundibulum (seen on MR imaging as posterior pituitary ectopia) is found in approximately 15% of patients with optic nerve hypoplasia.[26] Normally, the posterior pituitary gland appears bright on TI-weighted images, because of the composition of the vesicles within it.[23,26] In posterior pituitary ectopia, MRI demonstrates absence of the normal posterior pituitary bright spot, absence of the pituitary infundibulum, and an ectopic posterior pituitary bright spot where the upper infundibulum is normally located (Fig. 59.5).[23,26]

In optic nerve hypoplasia, posterior pituitary ectopia is virtually pathognomonic of anterior pituitary hormone deficiency, whereas cerebral hemispheric abnormalities are highly predictive of neurodevelopmental deficits.[26] Absence of the septum pellucidum alone does not portend neurodevelopmental deficits or pituitary hormone deficiency.[27] Thinning or agenesis of the corpus callosum predicts neurodevelopmental problems by virtue of its

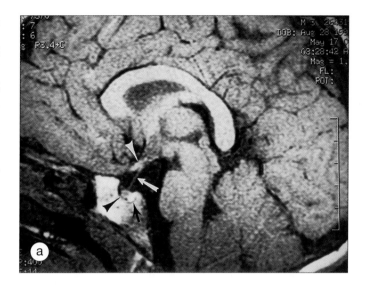

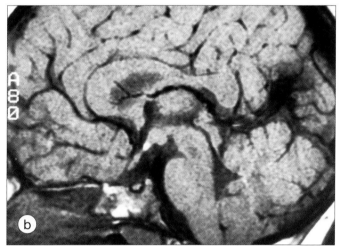

Fig. 59.5 Posterior pituitary ectopia. (a) Normal pituitary infundibulum, and posterior pituitary gland. (b) Absence of the pituitary infundibulum, absence of posterior pituitary gland, with ectopic posterior pituitary gland adjacent to optic chiasm. (With permission from the American Medical Association.)

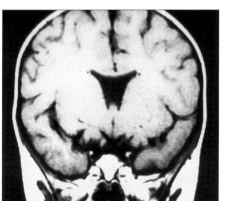

Fig. 59.3 Optic nerve hypoplasia. Coronal MR image showing absence of the septum pellucidum, normal right optic nerve, and hypoplasia of the left optic nerve.

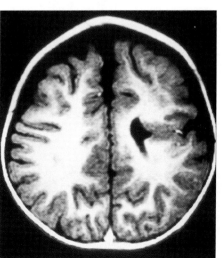

Fig. 59.4 Schizencephaly involving the left cerebral hemisphere. (With permission from the American Medical Association.)

frequent association with cerebral hemispheric abnormalities. The finding of unilateral optic nerve hypoplasia does not preclude co-existent intracranial malformations.[26] Therefore, MRI can be used to provide wide prognostic information in the infant or young child with optic nerve hypoplasia.[26]

Segmental optic nerve hypoplasia

Some forms of optic nerve hypoplasia are segmental.[28] A pathognomonic "superior segmental optic hypoplasia" (SSOH) with an inferior visual field defect occurs rarely in children of insulin-dependent diabetic mothers (Fig. 59.6).[29,30] Despite the multiple teratogenic effects of maternal diabetes early in the first trimester, SSOH is usually an isolated anomaly.[31] The incidence of SSOH has been estimated at approximately 8%. The inferior visual field defects in superior segmental optic hypoplasia differ from typical nerve fiber bundle defects and a regional impairment in retinal development may play a role in the pathogenesis.[30]

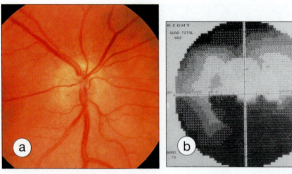

Fig. 59.6 Superior segmental optic hypoplasia. (a) Right optic disc shows superior entrance of central retinal vessels, relative pallor, superior peripapillary crescent, and selective loss of superior nerve fiber layer. (b) Corresponding visual field showing characteristic inferior loss. (With permission from Survey of Ophthalmology.)

SSOH has also been documented in patients whose mothers were not diabetic; it therefore is not pathognomonic for maternal diabetes.[32] The mechanism by which insulin-dependent diabetes mellitus selectively interferes with the early gestational development of superior retinal ganglion cells or their axons remains elusive.[33] Mice lacking EphB receptor guidance proteins exhibit specific guidance defects in axons originating from the dorsal or superior part of the retina[34] which may eventually explain this segmental hypoplasia.[34]

Congenital lesions involving the retina, optic nerve, chiasm, tract, or retrogeniculate pathways are associated with segmental hypoplasia of the corresponding portions of each optic nerve (Fig. 59.7).[28] Chiasmal hypoplasia produces focal loss of the nasal and temporal nerve fiber layer with hypoplasia of corresponding portions of the optic nerve (Fig. 59.7). The term "homonymous

hemioptic hypoplasia" describes an asymmetrical form of segmental optic nerve hypoplasia seen in patients with unilateral congenital lesions involving the postchiasmal afferent visual pathways.[35] The nasal and temporal aspects of the optic disc contralateral to the hemispheric lesion show segmental hypoplasia and loss of the corresponding nerve fiber layer. There may be a central band of horizontal pallor across the disc. The ipsilateral optic disc may range from normal in size to frankly hypoplastic.[28] Homonymous hemioptic hypoplasia in retrogeniculate lesions results from transsynaptic degeneration of the optic tract that is usually seen in congenital hemispheric lesions.[28,35]

Periventricular leukomalacia (PVL) produces another form of segmental optic nerve hypoplasia. PVL produces a form of bilateral optic nerve hypoplasia characterized by an abnormally large optic cup and a thin neuroretinal rim contained within a normal-sized optic disc (Fig. 59.8).[36] This may be due to intrauterine injury to the optic radiations with retrograde trans-

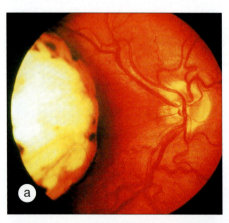

Fig. 59.7 Segmental optic nerve hypoplasia. (a) Macular "coloboma" produces selective temporal nerve fiber loss and corresponding temporal hypoplasia of the optic disc. (b) Segmental "band" hypoplasia in a patient with chiasmal hypoplasia. Note normal superior and inferior nerve fiber layers and absence of nasal and temporal nerve fiber layers bilaterally. (From Novakovic et al. Localizing patterns of optic nerve hypoplasia-retina to occipital lobe. Br J Ophthalmol 1988; 72: 176–82.)

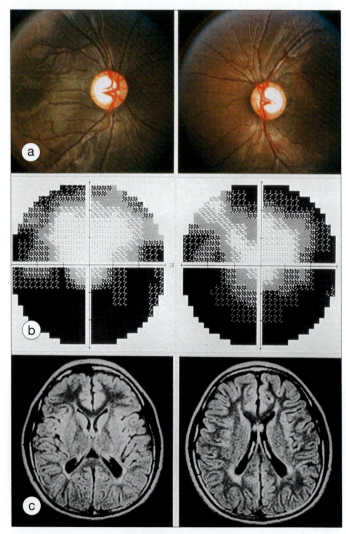

Fig. 59.8 Periventricular leukomalacia. (a) Enlarged optic cups with greater thinning of superior than inferior neuroretinal rim. (b) Characteristic inferior visual field defects. (c) MR imaging showing causative lesions involving optic radiations. (With permission from the American Medical Association.)

synaptic degeneration of retinogeniculate axons after the scleral canals had established normal diameters. It is not associated with endocrinologic deficiency. The large optic cups can simulate glaucoma, but the history of prematurity; normal intraocular pressure; and characteristic symmetrical inferior visual field defects all serve to distinguish PVL from glaucomatous optic atrophy.[37] The selective inferior visual field loss suggests that this may be a new form of segmental optic nerve hypoplasia, although some believe that it is a prenatal form of optic atrophy because of its normal optic disc diameter.[37]

At least two distinct mechanisms appear to be operative in the embryogenesis of optic nerve hypoplasia. Optic nerve hypoplasia was attributed to a primary failure of retinal ganglion cell differentiation at the 13–15 mm stage of embryonic life (4–6 weeks of gestation).[38] A deficiency of axon guidance molecules at the optic disc can lead to optic nerve hypoplasia. Netrin-1 is an axon guidance molecule that is expressed by neuroepithelial cells at the developing optic nerve head. Retinal ganglion cells *in vitro* respond to netrin-1 as a guidance molecule. Mice with a targeted deletion of the netrin-1 gene exhibit pathfinding errors at the optic disc, where retinal ganglion cells fail to exit into the optic nerve, and they exhibit optic nerve hypoplasia.[39–41] The lack of netrin-1 function also results in abnormalities in other parts of the CNS, such as agenesis of the corpus callosum, and cell migration and axonal guidance defects in the hypothalamus.[40] However, the timing of co-existent CNS injuries suggests that some cases of optic nerve hypoplasia may result from intrauterine destruction of a normally developed structure (i.e. an encephaloclastic event), whereas others represent a primary failure of axons to develop.[16] In human fetuses, Provis et al. found a peak of 3.7 million optic axons at 16–17 weeks of gestation, with a subsequent decline to 1.1 million axons by the 31st gestational week.[43] This massive normal loss of supernumerary axons, termed "apoptosis", may serve to establish the correct topography of the visual pathways.[4] Toxins or associated CNS injury could augment the usual processes by which superfluous axons are eliminated from the developing visual pathways.[4,16,26] The common association of optic nerve hypoplasia with periventricular leukomalacia,[26] which clearly cannot be reconciled with a deficiency of axon guidance molecules at the optic disc, demonstrates the importance of retrograde transsynaptic degeneration in the development of some forms of optic nerve hypoplasia.[36,37]

Cases of optic nerve hypoplasia in siblings.[44,45] are rare, and parents of a child with optic nerve hypoplasia can reasonably be assured that subsequent siblings are at little additional risk. While genetic mutations in the human netrin-1 and DCC genes have not been described, homozygous mutations in the *Hesx1* gene has been identified in two siblings with optic nerve hypoplasia, absence of the corpus callosum, and hypoplasia of the pituitary gland.[46] Five additional mutations in *Hesx1* have recently been observed in children with sporadic pituitary disease and septo-optic dysplasia.[47] Mutations have clustered in the DNA-binding region of the protein consistent with a presumed loss in protein function. Formal examination of homeobox genes with expression patterns similar to *Hesx1*, such as *Six3* and *Six6*, may yield additional genes responsible for both sporadic and familial septo-optic dysplasia.[48] Optic nerve hypoplasia may accompany other ocular malformations in patients with mutations in the PAX6 gene.[49]

Excavated optic disc anomalies

Excavated optic disc anomalies include optic disc coloboma, morning glory disc anomaly, peripapillary staphyloma, megalopapilla, and optic pit. Recently, two new excavated optic disc anomalies

have been associated with periventricular leukomalacia and the "vacant optic disc" associated with papillorenal syndrome.

Morning glory disc anomaly

In the morning glory disc anomaly and peripapillary staphyloma, an excavation of the posterior globe surrounds and incorporates the optic disc, while in the other conditions, the excavation is contained within the optic disc. The terms morning glory disc, optic disc coloboma, and peripapillary staphyloma are often confused in the literature, which has propagated confusion regarding their diagnostic criteria, associated systemic findings, and pathogenesis.[50] It is now clear that optic disc colobomas, morning glory optic discs, and peripapillary staphylomas are distinct anomalies, each with its own specific embryological origin, and not simply clinical variants along a broad phenotypic spectrum.[50]

The morning glory disc anomaly is a congenital, funnel-shaped excavation of the posterior fundus that incorporates the optic disc[50] which resembles a morning glory flower.[51] Ophthalmoscopically, the disc is markedly enlarged, it is orange or pink and it may appear to be recessed or elevated centrally within the confines of a funnel-shaped peripapillary excavation (Fig. 59.9).[50] Wide annulus of chorioretinal pigmentary disturbance surrounds the disc.[50] A white tuft of glial tissue overlies the central portion of the disc. The blood vessels appear increased in number and often arise from the periphery of the disc.[50] They often curve abruptly as they emanate from the disc and then run an abnormally straight course over the peripapillary retina. It is often difficult to distinguish arterioles from venules. Close inspection occasionally reveals the presence of small peripapillary arteriovenous communications.[52] The macula may be incorporated

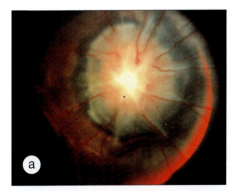
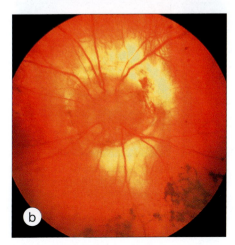

Fig. 59.9 Morning glory disc anomaly. (a) Without transsphenoidal encephalocele. (From Pollock S. The morning glory disc anomaly: Contractile movement, classification, and embryogenesis. Doc Ophthalmol 1987;65:439–60, with permission.) (b) With V-shaped infrapapillary depigmentation signifying transsphenoidal encephalocele. (With permission from the American Medical Association.)

into the excavation ("macular capture").[53] Neuroimaging shows a funnel-shaped enlargement of the distal optic nerve at its junction with the globe.[1]

The morning glory disc anomaly is usually unilateral, but several bilateral cases have been reported.[50,53] Visual acuity usually ranges from 20/200 to finger counting in the morning glory disc anomaly, but cases with 20/20 vision as well as no light perception have been reported. Amblyopia may contribute to visual loss in unilateral cases,[2] and a trial of occlusion therapy is warranted in small children. Unlike optic disc colobomas that have no racial or gender predilection, morning glory discs are conspicuously more common in females and rare in black people.

The morning glory disc anomaly is associated with a transsphenoidal basal encephalocele.[53–55] It may be accompanied by a V- or tongue-shaped zone of infrapapillary depigmentation, which can be a clinical sign of transsphenoidal encephalocele (Fig. 59.9).[3] Transsphenoidal encephalocele is a rare midline congenital malformation in which a meningeal pouch, often containing the chiasm and adjacent hypothalamus, protrudes inferiorly through a defect in the sphenoid bone (Fig. 59.10). Children with this occult basal meningocele have a wide head, a flat nose, mild hypertelorism, a midline notch in the upper lip, and sometimes a midline cleft in the soft palate (Fig. 59.11). The meningocele protrudes into the nasopharynx, where it may obstruct the airway. Symptoms in infancy may include rhinorrhea, nasal obstruction, mouth breathing, or snoring,[56,57] and may be overlooked unless the morning glory disc anomaly or the facial configuration is recognized. A transsphenoidal encephalocele may appear clinically as a pulsatile posterior nasal mass or as a "nasal polyp" high in the nose; surgical biopsy or excision can have lethal consequences.[56] Associated brain malformations include agenesis of the corpus callosum and posterior dilatation of the lateral ventricles. Absence of the chiasm is seen in approximately one-third of patients at surgery or autopsy. Most of the affected children have no overt intellectual or neurological deficits, but panhypopituitarism is common.[56] Surgery for transsphenoidal encephalocele is considered by many authorities to be contraindicated, since herniated brain tissue may include vital structures.[1,3]

The morning glory disc anomaly can be associated with hypoplasia of the ipsilateral intracranial vasculature.[58] With MR angiography, there are reports of ipsilateral intracranial vascular dysgenesis (with or without Moyamoya syndrome), in patients with morning glory disc anomaly (Fig. 59.12).[58–60] The co-existence of these intracranial vascular anomalies suggests that

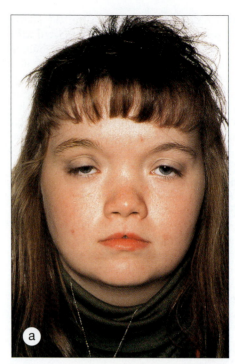

Fig. 59.11 Midfacial anomalies associated with transsphenoidal encephalocele. (a) Facial photograph showing hypertelorism, flat nasal bridge, widened bitemporal diameter. (b) Closer photograph showing midline cleft in the upper lip. (With permission from the American Medical Association.)

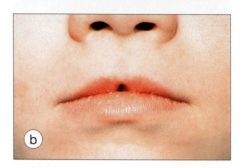

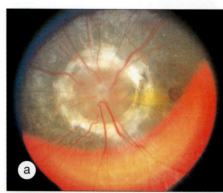

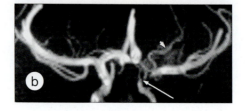

Fig. 59.12 Morning glory disc anomaly (a) with moyamoya syndrome. Note hypoplasia of left internal carotid artery (b) (large arrow) with moyamoya vessels (small arrow). (With permission from the American Medical Association.)

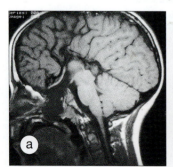
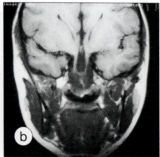

Fig. 59.10 MR imaging of transsphenoidal encephalocele. (a) Sagittal image showing encephalocele extending down through the sphenoid bone into the nasopharynx. (b) Coronal image showing third ventricle and chiasm extending inferiorly into the encephalocele. (From Barkovich AJ. Pediatric Neuroimaging. Vol 1, Raven Press, New York, 1990, p 89, with permission.)

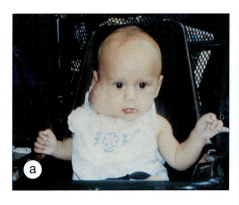
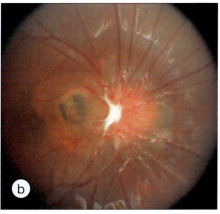
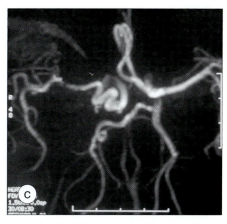

Fig. 59.13 PHACE syndrome. (a) Orofacial hemangioma (b) morning glory disc anomaly and (c) tortuous supraclinoid right internal carotid artery with hypoplasia of the ipsilateral middle cerebral artery on MR angiography. (Kniestedt C, Landau K, Brodsky MC et al. Infantile orofacial hemangioma with ipsilateral peripapillary excavation in girls: a variant of PHACE syndrome. Arch Ophthalmol. 2004 Mar; 122: 413–415, with permission from the American Medical Association.)

the morning glory disc anomaly results from a primary vascular dysgenesis in the context of a regional mesodermal dysgenesis.[61]

With rare exceptions, the morning glory disc anomaly is not part of a genetic disorder,[1,50] but it has been associated with ipsilateral orofacial hemangioma.[62] This association may fall within the spectrum of the PHACE syndrome (posterior fossa malformations, large facial hemangiomas, arterial anomalies, cardiac anomalies and aortic coarctation, and eye anomalies), which occurs only in girls.[63] Ipsilateral intracranial vascular dysgenesis in such patients (Fig. 59.13) support this.[64] Atypical morning glory disc anomalies have also rarely been reported in patients with neurofibromatosis 2.[65]

Serous retinal detachments may develop in 26–38% of eyes with morning glory optic disk anomalies;[50] they typically originate in the peripapillary area and extend through the posterior pole, occasionally progressing to total detachments. Although retinal tears are rarely evident, several reports have identified small retinal tears adjacent to the optic nerve in patients with morning glory disc-associated retinal detachments.[66] Subretinal neovascularization may occasionally develop within the circumferential zone of pigmentary disturbance adjacent to a morning glory disc.[67] Contractile movements occur in morning glory optic discs,[50] perhaps due to fluctuations in subretinal fluid volume altering the degree of retinal separation within the confines of the excavation.[50] One patient had episodes of amaurosis with transient dilation of the retinal veins in an eye with a morning glory disc.[68]

The embryological defect leading to the morning glory disc anomaly is widely disputed.[69] Histopathological reports have lacked clinical confirmation.[1] It may result from defective closure of the fetal fissure and is but one phenotypic form of a colobomatous (i.e. embryonic fissure-related) defect.[69,70] The central glial tuft, vascular anomalies, and a scleral defect, together with the histological findings of adipose tissue and smooth muscle within the peripapillary sclera perhaps signify a primary mesenchymal abnormality. The midfacial anomalies in some patients further support a primary mesenchymal defect, since most of the cranial structures are derived from mesenchyme.[69] The basic defect may be mesodermal, but some features may result from a dynamic disturbance between the relative growth of mesoderm and ectoderm.[61]

The symmetry of the fundus excavation with respect to the disc implicates an anomalous funnel-shaped enlargement of the distal optic stalk at its junction with the primitive optic vesicle, as the primary embryological defect.[50] According to this hypothesis, the glial and vascular abnormalities that characterize the morning glory disc anomaly would be explainable as the secondary effects of a primary neuroectodermal dysgenesis on the formation of mesodermal elements that arise later in embryogenesis.[50]

Optic disc coloboma

The term *coloboma*, of Greek derivation, means curtailed or mutilated.[72] In optic disc coloboma, a sharply delimited, glistening white, bowl-shaped excavation occupies an enlarged optic disc (Fig. 59.14). The excavation is decentered inferiorly, reflecting the position of the embryonic fissure relative to the primitive epithelial papilla.[50] The inferior neuroretinal rim is thin or absent while the superior neuroretinal rim is relatively spared. Rarely, the entire disc may appear excavated; however, the colobomatous nature of the defect can still be appreciated ophthalmoscopically since the excavation is deeper inferiorly.[50] The defect may extend further inferiorly to involve the adjacent choroid and retina, in which case microphthalmia is frequently present.[74] Iris and ciliary colobomas often co-exist. Axial CT scanning shows a crater like excavation of the posterior globe at its junction with the optic nerve.[70]

Visual acuity, which depends primarily upon the integrity of the papillomacular bundle, may be variably decreased and is difficult to predict from the appearance of the disc.[1] Unlike the

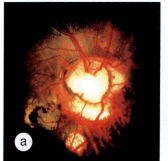
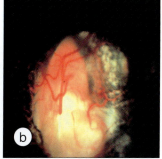

Fig. 59.14 Variants of optic disc coloboma. (Courtesy of William F. Hoyt, MD.)

morning glory disc anomaly, which is usually unilateral, optic disc colobomas occur unilaterally or bilaterally with approximately equal frequency.[50] Optic disc colobomas may arise sporadically or be inherited in an autosomal dominant fashion. Ocular colobomas may be accompanied by multiple systemic abnormalities in myriad conditions including, the CHARGE association,[73] Walker–Warburg syndrome, Goltz focal dermal hypoplasia, Aicardi syndrome, Goldenhar sequence, and linear sebaceous nevus syndrome.[1] Rarely, large orbital cysts can occur in conjunction with atypical excavations of the disc, which are probably colobomatous in nature.[74,75] The cyst may communicate with the excavation.[75,76] Histopathological examination has demonstrated intrascleral smooth muscle strands oriented concentrically around the distal optic nerve,[77] which may account for the contractility of the optic disc seen in rare cases of optic disc coloboma.[78]

Eyes with isolated optic disc colobomas are prone to develop serous macular detachments (in contrast to the rhegmatogenous retinal detachments that complicate retinochoroidal colobomas)[79,80] perhaps from diffusion of retrobulbar fluid into the subretinal space.[80] Treatments have included patches, bedrest, corticosteroids, vitrectomy, scleral buckling procedures, gas–fluid exchange, and photocoagulation.[81,82] Spontaneous reattachment may occur.[82]

Coronal T1-weighted MR imaging confirms that the intracranial portion of the optic nerve is reduced in size.[82] Many uncategorizable dysplastic optic discs are indiscriminately labeled as optic disc colobomas. This complicates the nosology of coloboma-associated genetic disorders. It is therefore crucial that the diagnosis of optic disc coloboma be reserved for discs that show an inferiorly decentered, white-colored excavation with minimal peripapillary pigmentary changes.[1,50] For example, the purported association between optic disc coloboma and basal encephaloceles deeply entrenched in the literature; there are, however, only two photographically documented cases.[84,85] In striking contrast to the numerous well-documented reports of morning glory optic discs occurring in conjunction with basal encephaloceles, cases of optic disc coloboma with basal encephalocele are conspicuous by their absence.

Von Szily stated that "all the true morphological malformations of the optic disc, including true colobomas ... are only different manifestations of the same developmental anomaly, namely, a different form and degree of malformation of the primitive or epithelial optic papilla".[86] Although the phenotypic profiles of optic disc coloboma and the morning glory disc anomaly may occasionally overlap, the ophthalmoscopic features of optic disc coloboma (Table 59.2) are most consistent with a primary structural dysgenesis involving the proximal embryonic fissure, as opposed to an anomalous dilatation confined to the distal optic stalk in the morning glory disc anomaly.[50] The differences in associated ocular and systemic findings between the two anomalies (Table 59.3) lend further credence to this hypothesis.[1]

"Hybrid" anomalous optic discs with features of the morning glory disc anomaly and optic disc coloboma are occasionally seen. These anomalies could easily represent instances of early embryonic injury involving both the proximal embryonic fissure and the distal optic stalk. They should not obscure the fact that colobomatous and morning glory optic discs are distinct anomalies in the great majority of cases.

Peripapillary staphyloma

Peripapillary staphyloma is an extremely rare, usually unilateral anomaly, in which a deep fundus excavation surrounds the optic

Table 59.2 Ophthalmoscopic findings that distinguish the morning glory disc anomaly from optic disc coloboma

Morning glory disc	Optic disc coloboma
Optic disc lies within the excavation	Excavation lies within the optic disc
Symmetrical defect (disc lies centrally within the excavation)	Asymmetrical defect (excavation lies inferiorly within the disc
Central glial tuft	No central glial tuft
Severe peripapillary	Minimal peripapillary
Pigmentary disturbance	Pigmentary disturbance
Anomalous retinal vasculature	Normal retinal vasculature

Table 59.3 Associated ocular and systemic findings that distinguish the morning glory disc from isolated optic disc coloboma

Morning glory disc	Optic disc coloboma
More common in females; rare in blacks	No sex or racial preference
Rarely familial	Often familial
Rarely bilateral	Often bilateral
No iris, ciliary, or retinal colobomas	Iris, ciliary, and retinal colobomas common
Rarely associated with multisystem genetic disorders	Often associated with multisystem genetic disorders
Basal encephalocele common	Basal encephalocele rare

disc.[87,88] The disc is seen at the bottom of the excavated defect and may appear normal or show temporal pallor (Fig. 59.15).[88] The walls and margin of the defect may show atrophic pigmentary changes is the retinal pigment epithelium (RPE) and choroid.[88] There is no central glial tuft overlying the disc, and the retinal vascular pattern remains normal, apart from reflecting the essential contour of the lesion. The staphylomatous excavation in peripapillary staphyloma is also notably deeper than that seen in the morning glory disc anomaly. Several cases of contractile peripapillary staphyloma have been documented,[89–91] sometimes with transient visual obscurations.[92]

Visual acuity is usually reduced, but cases with normal acuity have also been reported.[93] Affected eyes are usually emmetropic or slightly myopic.[87] Eyes with decreased vision frequently have centrocecal scotomas.[87] Although peripapillary staphyloma is clinically and embryologically distinct from morning glory disc

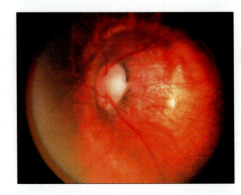

Fig. 59.15 Peripapillary staphyloma. (With permission from Lippincott).

anomaly, these conditions are frequently transposed in the literature. Although peripapillary staphyloma is usually unassociated with systemic or intracranial disease, it has been reported in association with transsphenoidal encephalocele,[94] PHACE syndrome,[63,95] linear nevus sebaceous syndrome, and 18q- syndrome.[96]

The relatively normal appearance of the optic disc and retinal vessels in peripapillary staphyloma suggest that the development of these structures is complete prior to the onset of the staphylomatous process.[50] The clinical features of peripapillary staphyloma are consistent with diminished peripapillary structural support, perhaps resulting from incomplete differentiation of sclera from posterior neural crest cells in the fifth month of gestation. Staphyloma formation presumably occurs when establishment of normal intraocular pressure leads to herniation of unsupported ocular tissues through the defect.[50] Thus, peripapillary staphyloma and the morning glory disc anomaly appear to be pathogenetically distinct both in the timing of the insult (five months gestation versus four weeks gestation) as well as the embryological site of structural dysgenesis (posterior sclera versus distal optic stalk).

Megalopapilla

Megalopapilla[97] has become a generic term for an abnormally large optic disc that lacks the inferior excavation of optic disc coloboma or the features of the morning glory disc anomaly.

Megalopapilla comprises two phenotypic variants:

1. The optic disc is greater than 2.1 mm in diameter and retains an otherwise normal configuration.[87,97] This relatively common form is usually bilateral and often associated with a large cup-to-disc ratio, which raises the diagnostic consideration of glaucoma (Fig. 59.16).[1] The optic cup is usually round or horizontally oval with no vertical notching or encroachment, in contradistinction to glaucomatous optic atrophy. Because the axons are spread over a larger surface area, the neuroretinal rim may also appear pale, mimicking optic atrophy.[98]

2. A unilateral form of megalopapilla is occasionally seen in which the normal optic cup is replaced by a grossly anomalous noninferior excavation that obliterates the adjacent neuroretinal rim. It is distinct from coloboma. Cilioretinal arteries are more common in megalopapilla.[99] A high prevalence of megalopapilla has been observed in natives of the Marshall Islands.[100]

Two reports have documented large optic discs in patients with optic nerve hypoplasia associated with a congenital homonymous hemianopia.[101,102] This rare combination of findings suggests that a prenatal loss of optic nerve axons leading to optic nerve hypoplasia may not always alter the genetically predetermined size of the scleral canals.[102]

Visual acuity is usually normal but may be mildly decreased. Visual fields are usually normal, except for an enlarged blind spot, ruling out normal tension glaucoma or compressive optic atrophy. Colobomatous discs are distinguished from megalopapilla by their predominant excavation of the inferior optic disc. The differential diagnosis of megalopapilla includes orbital optic glioma, which in children can cause progressive enlargement of a previously normal-sized optic disc.[103]

Most cases of megalopapilla may represent a statistical variant of normal. However, it is likely that megalopapilla can result from altered optic axonal migration early in embryogenesis, as evidenced by a report of megalopapilla in a child with basal encephalocoele.[54] The rarity of this association, however, suggests that neuroimaging is unwarranted unless midfacial anomalies co-exist.

Optic pit

An optic pit is a round or oval, gray, white, or yellowish depression in the optic disc (Fig. 59.17). Optic pits commonly involve the temporal optic disc but may be situated in any sector.[104] Temporally located pits are often accompanied by adjacent peripapillary pigment epithelial changes. One or two cilioretinal arteries are seen to emerge from the bottom or the margin of the pit in greater than 50% of cases.[87,105] Although optic pits are typically unilateral, bilateral pits are seen in 15% of cases.[87] Histologically, optic pits consist of herniations of dysplastic retina into a collagen-lined pocket extending posteriorly, often into the subarachnoid space, through a defect in the lamina cribrosa.[87] Reports of familial optic pits suggest an autosomal dominant mode of transmission.[106–108]

In unilateral cases, the involved disc is slightly larger than the normal disc.[87] Visual acuity is typically normal in the absence of subretinal fluid. Although visual field defects are variable and often correlate poorly with the location of the pit, the most common defect appears to be a para-central arcuate scotoma connected to an enlarged blind spot.[104] Optic pits rarely portend additional CNS malformations.[109] Acquired depressions in the optic disc, indistinguishable from optic pits, have been documented in normal-tension glaucoma.[110]

Serous macular elevations have been estimated to develop in 25–75% of eyes with optic pits.[104] Optic pit-associated maculopathy generally becomes symptomatic in the third and fourth decade of life. Vitreous traction on the margins of the pit and

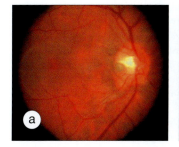
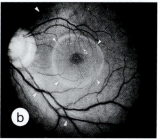

Fig. 59.17 Optic pit. (a) Inferotemporal olive-colored optic pit with associated retinoschisis cavity (corresponding to large area of horizontal striations, outer layer hole, and serous macular detachment. (b) Black and white photograph demonstrating an inner-layer separation (delimited by large arrowheads), macular hole (open arrowhead, and an outer-layer sensory detachment (delimited by small arrowheads). (From Lincoff H, Lopez R, Kreissig I, et al. Retinoschisis associated with optic pits. Arch Ophthalmol 1988; 106: 61–7, with permission. Copyright 1988, American Medical Association. Photographs courtesy of Harvey Lincoff, MD.)

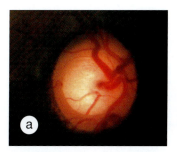
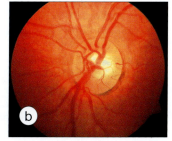

Fig. 59.16 Two cases of megalopapilla. The left figure illustrates pseudoglaucomatous cupping.

tractional changes in the roof of the pit may be the inciting events that ultimately lead to late-onset macular detachment.[105]

Until recently, all optic pit-associated macular elevations were thought to represent serous detachments, but careful stereoscopic examination of the macula in conjunction with kinetic perimetry[111] demonstrates the following progression of events:

1. A schisis-like inner-layer retinal separation initially forms in direct communication with the optic pit, which produces a mild, relative, centrocecal scotoma.
2. An outer-layer macular hole develops beneath the boundaries of the inner-layer separation and produces a dense central scotoma.
3. An outer-layer retinal detachment develops around the macular hole (presumably from influx of fluid from the inner-layer separation). This outer-layer detachment ophthalmoscopically resembles an RPE detachment but fails to hyperfluoresce on fluorescein angiography.
4. The outer-layer detachment may eventually enlarge and obliterate the inner-layer separation. At this stage, it is no longer ophthalmoscopically or histopathologically distinguishable from a primary serous macular detachment.

Fig. 59.17 depicts the retinal findings that can be observed in the evolution of an optic pit-associated macular detachment. The histopathological finding of a sensory macular detachment in eyes with optic pits presumably represents the endstage, but whether this sequence of events leads to all optic pit-associated macular detachments is unclear.

The risk of optic pit-associated macular detachment is greater in eyes with large optic pits and in eyes with temporally located pits.[104] Perhaps because of age-related differences in vitreopapillary traction, optic pit-associated serous maculopathy in children may have a tendency toward spontaneous resolution.[112,113]

Spontaneous reattachment is seen in approximately 25% of cases.[104,114] Early reports of spontaneous resolution of most optic pit-associated macular detachments with good visual recovery[115] differ from the experience of subsequent investigators who have noted permanent visual loss in untreated patients, even when spontaneous reattachment occurs.[114,116] Bedrest and bilateral patching have led to retinal reattachment in some patients, presumably by decreasing vitreous traction.[80,117] Laser photocoagulation to block the flow of fluid from the pit to the macula has been largely unsuccessful, perhaps due to the inability of laser photocoagulation to seal a retinoschisis cavity.[111,118] Vitrectomy with internal gas tamponade laser photocoagulation has produced long-term improvement in acuity.[80,111,117] Although the aim of this treatment is to compress the retina at the edge of the disc to enhance the effect of laser treatment, internal gas tamponade may function to mechanically displace subretinal fluid away from the macula, allowing a shallow, inner-layer separation to persist, which is associated with a mild scotoma and relatively good visual acuity and laser photocoagulation probably does not contribute to the success of this procedure.[118]

The source of intraretinal fluid in eyes with optic pits is controversial.[86] Possible sources include:

■ Vitreous cavity via the pit.
■ The subarachnoid space.
■ Blood vessels at the base of the pit.
■ The orbital space surrounding the dura.

Although fluorescein angiography shows early hypofluorescence of the pit followed in many cases by late hyperfluorescent staining, optic pits do not generally leak fluorescein, and there is no extension of fluorescein into the subretinal space toward the macula.[104] The finding of late hyperfluorescent staining correlates strongly with cilioretinal arteries emerging from the pit.[105] Slit-lamp biomicroscopy often reveals a thin membrane overlying the pit[104] or a persistent Cloquet's canal terminating at the margin of the pit.[119] Although active flow of fluid from the vitreous cavity through the pit to the subretinal space has been demonstrated in collie dogs, this mechanism has never been conclusively demonstrated in humans.[120]

Although the pathogenesis of optic pits is unclear, the great majority of authors view them as the mildest variant of optic disc colobomas.[1] But:

1. Optic pits are usually unilateral, sporadic, and unassociated with systemic anomalies. Colobomas are bilateral as often as unilateral, commonly autosomal dominant, and may be associated with a variety of multisystem disorders.
2. It is rare for optic pits to co-exist with iris or retinochoroidal colobomas.
3. Optic pits usually occur in locations unrelated to the embryonic fissure.

Papillorenal (renal–coloboma) syndrome ("the vacant optic disc")

The papillorenal syndrome, previously known as renal–coloboma syndrome, was first described by Rieger.[121] It is a rare autosomal dominant disorder consisting of bilateral optic disc anomalies associated with hypoplastic kidneys.[122] Associated retinal detachments were described, as was renal failure. There are sometimes mutations in the PAX2 gene, in affected families.[123,124]

Renal abnormalities may include hypoplasia, variable proteinuria, vesiculoureteral reflux, recurrent pyelonephritis, microhematuria, echogenicity on ultrasound, or high resistance to blood flow on Doppler ultrasound.

The papillorenal syndrome is characterized by a distinct optic disc malformation.[122] In this syndrome, the excavated optic disc is normal in size, and may be surrounded by variable pigmentary disturbance.[122] Unlike colobomatous defects, the excavation is centrally positioned (Fig. 59.18). According to Parsa et al., the defining feature is the multiple cilioretinal vessels which emanate from the periphery of the disc, and variable attenuation or atrophy of the central retinal vessels (Fig. 59.18).[122] Color Doppler imaging has confirmed the absence of central retinal circulation in patients with papillorenal syndrome.[122] Visual acuity is usually good but may be severely diminished secondary to choroidal and retinal hypoplasia and, in some cases, to later-onset serous retinal detachments.[122,125] Peripheral visual field defects corresponding to areas of retinal hypoplasia are often present. The central optic disc excavation and peripheral field defects can simulate coloboma as well as normal tension glaucoma. Follow-up examination has shown renal disease in some patients who were originally reported as having isolated familial autosomal dominant "coloboma".[126,127]

This malformation is attributed to a primary deficiency in angiogenesis involved in vascular development.[122] There is a failure of the hyaloid system to convert to normal central retinal vessels analogous to an evolutionary regression to a feline pattern of circulation.[122] Many patients with papillorenal syndrome have no detectable mutations in the PAX2 gene.[122,125]

Congenital tilted disc syndrome

The tilted disc syndrome is a nonhereditary bilateral condition in which the superotemporal optic disc is elevated and the inferonasal disc is posteriorly displaced, resulting in an oval-appearing optic

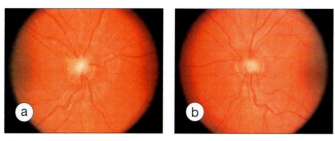

Fig. 59.18 Papillorenal syndrome. This 9-year-old girl with chronic renal failure secondary to interstitial fibrosis had vacant optic discs with an exclusive cilioretinal circulation. (Photographs courtesy of Erika M. Levin, MD.)

disc, with its long axis obliquely oriented (Fig. 59.19).[1] This configuration is accompanied by situs inversus of the retinal vessels, congenital inferonasal conus, thinning of the inferonasal RPE and choroid, and bitemporal hemianopia.[128] The anomalous optic disc appearance is secondary to a posterior ectasia of the inferonasal fundus and optic disc. Because of the regional fundus ectasia, affected patients have myopic astigmatism, with the plus axis oriented parallel to the ectasia. Corneal topography studies

indicate that an irregular corneal curvature contributes to the associated astigmatism.[129] The cause of the condition is unknown, but the inferonasal or inferior location of the excavation is vaguely suggestive of a relationship to retinochoroidal coloboma.[130]

Familiarity with the tilted disc syndrome is crucial for the ophthalmologist, since affected patients may present with bitemporal hemianopia or optic disc elevation that simulates papilledema.[1,130] The bitemporal hemianopia in affected patients, which is typically incomplete and confined primarily to the superior quadrants, represents a refractive scotoma, secondary to regional myopia localized to the inferonasal retina. Unlike the visual field loss from chiasmal lesions, the field defects seen in the tilted disc syndrome fail to respect the vertical meridian on kinetic perimetry. Furthermore, the superotemporal depression is selectively confined to the midsize isopter, while the large and small isopters remain fairly normal, due to the marked ectasia of the mid-peripheral fundus. Repeat perimetry after addition of a −4.00 lens often eliminates the visual field abnormality, confirming the refractive nature of the defect. In some cases, retinal sensitivity may be decreased in the area of the ectasia, and the defect persists to some degree despite appropriate refractive correction.[128]

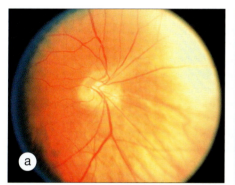
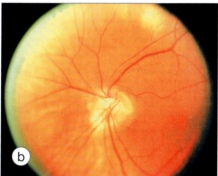
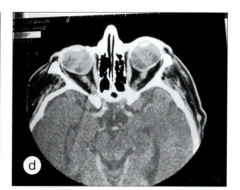

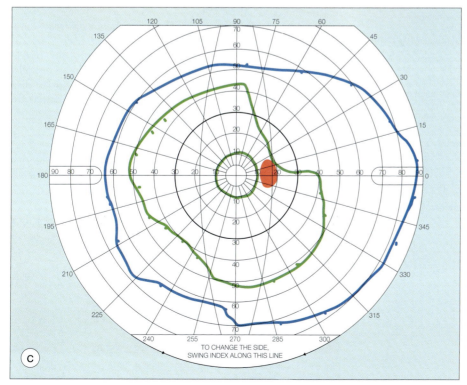

Fig. 59.19 Congenital tilted disc syndrome. (a) Right optic disc. (b) Left optic disc. (c) Right visual field showing superotemporal defect confined to the mid-peripheral isopter that does not respect the vertical meridian. (d) CT scan showing increased curvature of the posterior sclera nasally and flattening of the posterior sclera temporally nasally. (With permission from Survey of Ophthalmology).

The tilted disc syndrome has been associated with true bitemporal hemianopia in several patients who were found to harbor a congenital suprasellar tumor. These seemingly disparate findings may reflect the disruptive effect of the suprasellar tumor on optic axonal migration during embryogenesis.[13] This makes neuroimaging mandatory in any patient with a tilted disc syndrome whose bitemporal hemianopia either respects the vertical meridian or fails to preferentially involve the mid-peripheral isopter on kinetic perimetry.[131,132] Tilted discs without retinal ectasia occur in patients with transsphenoidal encephalocele.[3] The tilted disc syndrome has also been reported in patients with X-linked congenital stationary night blindness.[84,86–133] In eyes with tilted discs or the full tilted disc syndrome, anomalies at the junction of the staphyloma or at the junction of between peripapillary retina and the altered disc margin may cause serous macular detachments.[134–136]

Optic disc dysplasia

The term "optic disc dysplasia" should be viewed not as a diagnosis but as a descriptive term that connotes a markedly deformed optic disc that fails to conform to any recognizable diagnostic category (Fig. 59.20). The distinction between an uncategorizable "anomalous" disc and a "dysplastic" disc is arbitrary and based upon the severity of the lesion. In the past, the term optic disc dysplasia has been applied to cases that are now recognizable as the morning glory disc anomaly.[53,137] Conversely, many dysplastic optic discs have been indiscriminately labeled as optic disc colobomas.[1] It is likely that additional variants of optic disc dysplasia will be recognized and identified as distinct anomalies.

Dysplastic optic discs can occur in association with transsphenoidal encephalocele.[3] A discrete infrapapillary zone of V- or tongue-shaped retinochoroidal depigmentation has been described in five patients with anomalous optic discs and transsphenoidal encephalocele (Fig. 59.20). These juxtapapillary defects differ from retinochoroidal colobomas, which widen inferiorly and are not associated with basal encephalocele and there is minimal scleral excavation and no visible disruption in the integrity of the overlying retina. In patients with anomalous optic discs, the finding of this V- or tongue-shaped infrapapillary retinochoroidal anomaly should prompt neuroimaging for transsphenoidal encephalocele.[3]

Congenital optic disc pigmentation

Congenital optic disc pigmentation is a condition in which melanin deposition anterior to or within the lamina cribrosa imparts a gray appearance to the optic disc (Fig. 59.21).[138] True congenital optic disc pigmentation is extremely rare, but it has been described in a child with an interstitial deletion of chromosome 17 and in Aicardi syndrome.[138] Congenital optic disc pigmentation is compatible with good visual acuity but may be associated with co-existent optic disc anomalies that decrease vision.[138] In developing mice and rats, a transient zone of melanin in the distal developing optic stalk influences migration of the earliest optic nerve axons.[139] The effects of abnormal pigment deposition on optic nerve embryogenesis could explain the frequent co-existence of congenital optic disc pigmentation with other anomalies, particularly optic nerve hypoplasia.

The great majority of patients with gray optic discs do not have congenital optic disc pigmentation. Some optic discs of infants with delayed visual maturation and albinism may have a diffuse gray tint when viewed ophthalmoscopically which often disappears within the first year of life without visible pigment migration. Beauvieux observed gray optic discs in premature and in albino infants who were apparently blind but who later developed good vision.[140,141] He attributed the gray appearance of these neonatal discs to delayed optic nerve myelination with preservation of the "embryonic tint". Gray optic discs may also be seen in normal neonates and are therefore a nonspecific finding of little diagnostic value, except in delayed visual maturation or albinism.

Despite their fundamental differences, "optically gray optic discs" and congenital optic disc pigmentation have unfortunately been lumped together in many reference books. These two conditions can usually be distinguished ophthalmoscopically, since melanin deposition in true congenital optic disc pigmentation is often discrete, irregular, and granular in appearance.[20]

Aicardi syndrome

Aicardi syndrome is a cerebroretinal disorder of unknown etiology. Its salient clinical features are infantile spasms, agenesis

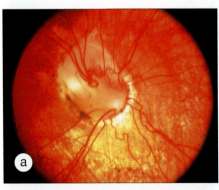
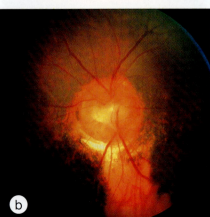

Fig. 59.20 Optic disc dysplasia with and without transsphenoidal encephalocele. (a) Without transsphenoidal encephalocele. (b) With tongue-shaped infrapapillary depigmentation signifying transsphenoidal encephalocele. (From Brodsky MC, Baker RS, Hamed LF. Pediatric Neuro-ophthalmology. Springer Verlag 1996, with permission © 1996 Springer Verlag.)

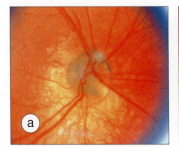
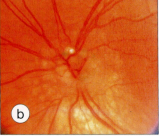

Fig. 59.21 Congenital optic disc pigmentation. (With permission from Survey of Ophthalmology.)

of the corpus callosum, a characteristic electroencephalographic pattern termed hypsarrhythmia, and a pathognomonic optic disc appearance consisting of multiple depigmented "chorioretinal lacunae" clustered around the disc (Fig. 59.22).[142,143] Histologically, chorioretinal lacunae consist of well-circumscribed, full-thickness defects limited to the RPE and choroid. The overlying retina remains intact but is often histologically abnormal.[143]

Congenital optic disc anomalies, including optic disc coloboma, optic nerve hypoplasia, and congenital optic disc pigmentation, may accompany chorioretinal lacunae.[143,144] Other ocular abnormalities include microphthalmos, retrobulbar cyst, pseudoglioma, retinal detachment, macular scars, cataract, pupillary membranes, iris synechiae, and iris colobomas.[142,144] The most common systemic findings associated with Aicardi syndrome are vertebral malformations (e.g. fused vertebrae, scoliosis, spina bifida) and costal malformations (e.g. absent ribs, fused or bifurcated ribs).[142-144] Other systemic associations include muscular hypotonia, microcephaly, dysmorphic facies, and auricular anomalies. Severe mental retardation is almost invariable.[142,143] Choroid plexus papilloma and Aicardi syndrome has been documented in five patients.[145]

Central nervous system anomalies in Aicardi syndrome include agenesis of the corpus callosum, cortical migration anomalies (e.g. pachygyria, polymicrogyria, cortical heterotopias), and multiple structural CNS malformations (e.g. cerebral hemispheric asymmetry, Dandy–Walker variant, colpocephaly, midline arachnoid cysts) (Fig. 59.22).[143] An overlap between Aicardi syndrome and septo-optic dysplasia has been recognized in several patients.[143]

Aicardi syndrome may result from an X-linked mutational event that is lethal in males.[144,146] Parents should therefore be asked about a previous history of miscarriages. All cases of Aicardi syndrome probably represent fresh mutations since cases of affected siblings have rarely been reported,[144] but a report of Aicardi syndrome in two sisters indicates that parental gonadal mosaicism for the mutation may be an additional mechanism of inheritance.[147] Although early infectious CNS insults can lead to severe CNS anomalies, tests for infective agents have been consistently negative. No teratogenic drug or other toxin has yet been associated with Aicardi syndrome.[143] Based on the pattern of cerebroretinal malformations, an insult to the CNS might take place between the fourth and eighth week of gestation.[144]

The neurodevelopmental prognosis of Aicardi syndrome is poor, with most children having intractable seizures, and 91% attaining milestones no higher than 12 months.[148] Based on the associated intraocular malformations such as microphthalmos, persistent pupillary membrane, persistent hyperplastic primary vitreous, vascular loops on the optic disc, and epiretinal glial tissue,[149] persistence of fetal vasculature between gestational weeks 9 and 12 may provide a unifying hypothesis for the embryogenesis of Aicardi syndrome.

Doubling of the optic disc

Doubling of the optic disc is a rare anomaly in which two discs appear to be in close proximity to one another.[150] This ophthalmoscopic finding is presumed to result from a duplication or separation of the distal optic nerve into two fasciculi.[150] Most reports describe a "main" disc and a "satellite" disc, each with its own vascular system (Fig. 59.23). It is usually unilateral and associated with decreased vision in the involved eye.[150]

The majority of clinical reports antedate the era of high resolution neuroimaging and have relied upon the roentgenographic demonstration of two optic nerves in the same orbit, results of fluorescein angiography, synchronous pulsations of each major disc artery, dual blind spots, and angioscotomas to provide indirect evidence of optic nerve diastasis.[150] In some cases, an apparent doubling of the optic disc results from a focal, juxtapapillary retinochoroidal coloboma that displays an abnormal vascular anastomosis with the optic disc.[150]

Separation of the optic nerve into two or more is rare in humans but common in lower vertebrates.[150] However, separation of various portions of an intracranial or orbital optic nerve has been documented in a handful of autopsy cases.[151-154] MRI should confirm optic nerve diastasis in doubling of the optic disc.

Optic nerve aplasia

Optic nerve aplasia is a rare nonhereditary malformation, which is usually seen in a unilaterally malformed eye of an otherwise healthy person.[155] The term optic nerve aplasia denotes complete absence of the optic nerve and disc, retinal ganglion and nerve

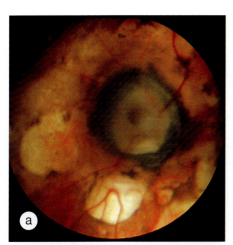
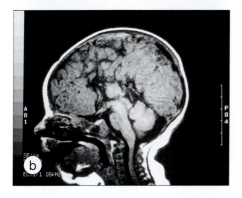

Fig. 59.22 Aicardi syndrome. (a) Peripapillary chorioretinal lacunae are clustered around the optic disc. (With permission from Williams and Wilkins). (b) MR imaging shows agenesis of the corpus callosum. (From Brodsky MC, Baker RS, Hamed LF. Pediatric Neuro-ophthalmology, Springer Verlag 1996, with permission © 1996 Springer Verlag.)

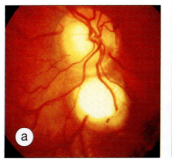
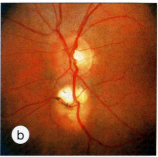

Fig. 59.23 "Doubling of the optic disc" produced by infrapapillary chorioretinal coloboma. ((a) Left figure courtesy of Klara Landau, MD, (b) figure courtesy of Anthony C. Arnold MD.)

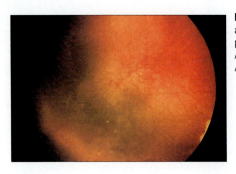

Fig. 59.24 Optic nerve aplasia. (With permission from American Medical Association.)

fiber layers, and optic nerve vessels.[156] Histopathological examination usually demonstrates a vestigial dural sheath entering the sclera in its normal position, as well as retinal dysplasia with rosette formation (Fig. 59.24).[155] Some early reports of optic nerve aplasia actually described patients with severe hypoplasia at a time when the latter entity was not clearly recognized.[156,157]

Ophthalmoscopically, optic nerve aplasia may take on any of the following appearances[158]:

■ Absence of a normally defined optic nerve head or papilla without central blood vessels and with an absence of macular differentiation.
■ A whitish area corresponding to the optic disc, without central vessels or macular differentiation.
■ A deep avascular cavity in the site corresponding to the optic disc, surrounded by a whitish annulus.

Optic nerve aplasia is fundamentally distinct from optic nerve hypoplasia; it is unilateral, and frequently associated with malformations confined to the involved eye (microphthalmia, malformations in the anterior chamber angle, hypoplasia or segmental aplasia of the iris, cataracts, persistent hyperplastic primary vitreous, colobomas, and retinal dysplasia), as opposed to the brain.[158–161] The pathogenesis is unknown. When it occurs bilaterally, it is usually associated with other CNS malformations.[162–164]

One patient with unilateral anophthalmos had optic nerve aplasia associated with a congenital giant suprasellar aneurysm.[165] The remaining optic nerve was identified at craniotomy as passing posteriorly as a single cord to form an optic tract with no adjoining chiasm. It was speculated that the absent optic nerve and chiasm may have formed initially and then degenerated in a retrograde fashion. Necropsy findings from a patient with a Hallerman–Streiff-like syndrome and left optic nerve hypoplasia showed normal geniculate bodies and optic tracts with only a single nerve that emerged anteriorly from a chiasm that deviated to the right.[166] In another patient with unilateral optic nerve aplasia and microphthalmos, MR imaging disclosed optic nerve aplasia and hemichiasmal hypoplasia on the affected side.[156] Visual evoked cortical responses demonstrated increased signals over the occipital lobe contralateral to the intact optic nerve, suggesting chiasmal misdirection of axons from the temporal retina of the normal eye, as seen in albinos. The authors speculated that this abnormal decussation may represent an atavistic form of neuronal reorganization.[156]

Myelinated (medullated) nerve fibers

Myelination of the afferent visual pathways begins at the lateral geniculate body at 5 months of age and terminates at the lamina cribrosa at term or shortly thereafter.[167] Oligodendrocytes, responsible for myelination of the CNS, are not normally present in the human retina.[167] Histological studies have confirmed the presence of presumed oligodendrocytes and myelin in areas of myelinated nerve fibers and their absence in other areas.[168] Myelinated retinal nerve fibers have been found in approximately 1% of eyes examined at autopsy and in 0.3–0.6% of routine ophthalmic patients.[167]

Ophthalmoscopically, myelinated nerve fibers usually appear as white striated patches at the upper and lower poles of the disc (Fig. 59.25). In this location, they may simulate papilledema, both by elevating the involved portions of the disc and by obscuring the disc margin and the underlying retinal vessels.[167,169] Distally, they have an irregular fan-shaped appearance that facilitates their recognition. Small slits or patches of normal-appearing fundus color are occasionally visible within an area of myelination.[167] Myelinated nerve fibers are bilateral in 17–20% of cases, and clinically, they are discontinuous with the optic nerve head in 19%. Isolated patches of myelinated nerve fibers in the peripheral retina are rarely found nasal to the optic disc.[169]

The pathogenesis of myelinated nerve fibers remains largely speculative,[169] but animals with little or no evidence of a lamina cribrosa tend to have deep physiological cups and extensive myelination of retinal nerve fibers, while animals with a well-developed lamina cribrosa tend to show fairly flat nerve heads and no myelination of retinal nerve fibers. This suggests several mechanisms[169]:

1. A defect in the lamina cribrosa may allow oligodendrocytes to gain access to the retina and produce myelin there.
2. There may be fewer axons relative to the size of the scleral canal, producing enough room for myelination to proceed into the eye. In eyes with remote, isolated peripheral patches of myelinated nerve fibers, an anomaly in the formation or timing of formation of the lamina cribrosa permits access of oligodendrocytes to the retina. These cells then migrate through the nerve fiber layer until they find a region of relatively low nerve fiber layer density, where they proceed to myelinate some axons.
3. Late development of the lamina cribrosa may allow oligodendrocytes to migrate into the eye. The sclera begins to

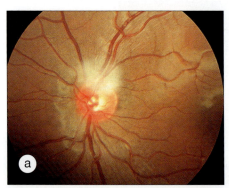

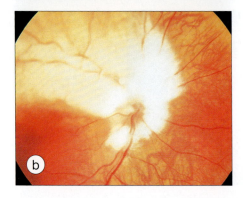

Fig. 59.25 Myelinated nerve fibers.

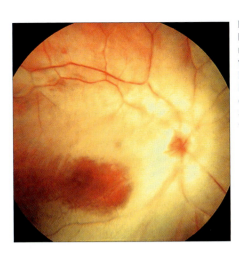

Fig. 59.26 Unilateral high myopia with myelinated nerve fibers. (From Brodsky MC, Baker RS, Hamed LF. Pediatric Neuro-ophthalmology. Springer Verlag 1996, with permission © 1996 Springer Verlag.)

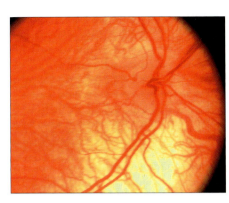

Fig. 59.27 Albinotic optic disc (Pollock's sign). (From Brodsky MC, Baker RS, Hamed LF. Pediatric Neuro-ophthalmology. Springer Verlag 1996, with permission © 1996 Springer Verlag.)

consolidate in the limbal region, then proceeds posteriorly toward the lamina cribrosa.

Extensive unilateral (or rarely bilateral) myelination of nerve fibers can be associated with high myopia and severe refractory amblyopia[170] (Fig. 59.26). In such patients, myelin envelops most or all of the circumference of the disc. Additionally, the macular region (although unmyelinated) usually appears abnormal, showing a dulled reflex or pigment dispersion.[171] The appearance of the macula may be the best direct correlate of response to occlusion therapy.[171]

Myelinated nerve fibers occur in association with the Gorlin (multiple basal cell nevi) syndrome,[172] and an autosomal dominant vitreoretinopathy characterized by congenitally poor vision, bilateral extensive myelination of the retinal nerve fiber layer, severe vitreal degeneration, high myopia, a retinal dystrophy with night-blindness, reduction of the electroretinographic responses, and limb deformities.[173]

Myelinated nerve fibers may also be inherited in an autosomal dominant fashion.[174] Isolated cases of myelinated nerve fibers have also been described in association with abnormal length of the optic nerve (oxycephaly),[175] effects in the lamina cribrosa (tilted disc),[176] anterior segment dysgenesis,[169] and NF-2.[177] Although myelinated nerve fibers are purported to be associated with neurofibromatosis,[177] many authorities feel that this association is questionable.[167]

Rarely, areas of myelinated nerve fibers may be acquired after infancy and even in adulthood.[178,179] Trauma to the eye (a blow to the eye in one patient and an optic nerve sheath fenestration in the other) seems to be a common denominator in these cases. Perhaps there is sufficient damage to the lamina cribrosa to permit oligodendrocytes to enter the retina.[169] Myelinated nerve fibers have also disappeared as a result of tabetic optic atrophy, pituitary tumor, glaucoma, central retinal artery occlusion, and optic neuritis.[167]

The optic disc in albinism

The optic discs of albinos have a number of distinct ophthalmoscopic appearances. They often have a diffuse gray tint when viewed within the first few years of life. This discoloration must be related to optical effects resulting from surrounding chorioretinal depigmentation since it is no longer evident in older children and adults.

Five ophthalmoscopic findings characterize albino optic discs[180]:

1. Small disc diameter.
2. Absence of the physiological cup.
3. Oval shape with long axis oriented obliquely.
4. Origin of the retinal vessels from the temporal aspect of the disc.
5. Abnormal course of retinal vessels consisting of initial nasal deflection followed by abrupt divergence and reversal of direction to form the temporal vascular arcades (Fig. 59.27). The purported association between albinism and optic nerve hypoplasia is dubious.[181]

PSEUDOPAPILLEDEMA

Anomalous elevation of the optic disc is a primary diagnostic consideration in the child referred for papilledema.[182] Buried drusen within the optic disc is the most common form of pseudo-papilledema in childhood and must be distinguished from other causes of pseudopapilledema, such as hyperopia, myelinated nerve fibers, epipapillary glial tissue, and hyaloid traction on the disc.[183]

Optic disc drusen

The word *drusen*, of Germanic derivation, originally meant tumor, swelling, or tumescence.[184] The word was used in the mining industry approximately 500 years ago to indicate a crystal-filled space in a rock.[184] Other terms such as *hyaline* bodies and *colloid* bodies are occasionally used to describe drusen of the optic disc.[185]

The fact that drusen may closely simulate papilledema, that they are associated with visual field defects, and that they may occasionally show solitary hemorrhages often serves to complicate the diagnostic picture and impart a sense of urgency to the diagnosis.[186] If buried drusen go unrecognized, the elevated optic discs may precipitate inappropriate diagnostic studies.[187]

The conceptual problem that persists in understanding the evolution of disc drusen comes from viewing drusen as the cause rather than the effect of an underlying configurational anomaly of the disc. This tendency carries over into our analysis of associated complications (e.g. the lack of correspondence between visual field abnormalities with the position of visible drusen on the disc has puzzled many). The time course of evolution of optic disc drusen and the histopathological findings suggest that disc drusen result from axonal degeneration, rather than encroaching upon adjacent axons to cause their degeneration. Disc drusen signify a chronic, low-grade optic neuropathy measured over decades.

Lorentzen examined 3200 routine cases from an ophthalmological practice in Denmark and found that 11 had drusen of the optic disc (a prevalence of 0.34%).[184] This prevalence increased by a factor of 10 in family members of patients with disc drusen. Friedman et al. examined 737 cadavers and found disc drusen in 15.[185] The drusen are often minute and situated deep within the optic nerve tissue.[188] Familial drusen are transmitted as an autosomal dominant trait.[189-191] Disc drusen are rare in African-Americans.[187] The early notion that disc drusen are associated with hyperopia has not been substantiated.[187,191,193] Visible disc drusen are bilateral in approximately two-thirds of cases, whereas buried drusen are bilateral in 86% of cases.[187] Clumsiness, learning disabilities, and neurological problems were found in children with drusen,[194] but subsequent studies have failed to substantiate this.

Ophthalmoscopic appearance in children

Most childhood cases present initially with pseudopapilledema secondary to buried drusen (Fig. 59.28). The disc is elevated, and its margins are blurred or obscured.[185] The elevated disc may have a gray or a yellow-white discoloration. Disc drusen tend to become more conspicuous with age.[195] Discrete hyaline bodies are first noted at a mean age of 12.1 years[196]; in older children, there is often a scalloped contour to the disc margins, due to partially buried drusen protruding from the edge of the disc into the peripapillary retina.[185]

Buried drusen are most visible at the margin of the disc, where they impart an irregular lumpy-bumpy contour (Fig. 59.28). Exposed drusen are more frequent on the nasal side of the optic disc. Surface drusen appear as yellowish, globular, translucent bodies on the optic disc, often in larger or smaller conglomerations[184] (Fig. 59.29). They may occur singularly, in grapelike clusters, or as fused conglomerations, varying in size from small dots to several vein widths in diameter.[185] By direct illumination, the central portion of each shines uniformly, while the border may appear as a glistening ring. With indirect illumination from light focused on the peripapillary retina, the druse shines uniformly, except for a brighter, semicircular marginal zone on the side opposite from the spot of light ("inverse shading"). In addition to the small size of the optic disc and the absence of a physiological cup, the disc vasculature is anomalous. The major retinal vessels are increased in number and often tortuous (Fig. 59.28). They tend to branch early and may trifurcate or quadrificate. The prevalence of cilioretinal arteries is also increased, with estimates ranging from 24.1%[193] to 43%.[194] Peripapillary atrophy or pigment epithelial derangement occurs in a third of eyes.[193] Retinal venous loops or anomalous retinociliary shunt vessels are occasionally seen.

Distinguishing buried disc drusen from papilledema

The distinction between pseudopapilledema associated with buried drusen from papilledema (or other forms of optic disc edema) can at times be difficult, but there are several clinical signs that serve to distinguish these two conditions (Table 59.4).[182] In papilledema, the swelling extends into the peripapillary retina and obscures the peripapillary retinal vasculature. In pseudopapilledema, there is a discrete, sometimes grayish or straw-colored elevation of the disc without obscuration of vessels or opacification of peripapillary retina. There is a graying or muddying of the peripapillary nerve fiber layer that occurs with swelling of the optic disc from papilledema or other causes.[197] In pseudopapilledema associated with buried drusen, light reflexes of the peripapillary nerve fiber layer appear sharp, and the elevated disc is often haloed by a crescentic peripapillary

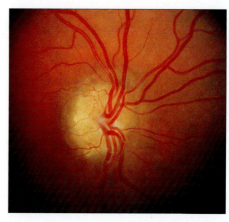

Fig. 59.29 Visible disc drusen. (From Brodsky MC, Baker RS, Hamed LF. Pediatric Neuro-ophthalmology. Springer Verlag 1996, with permission © 1996 Springer Verlag.)

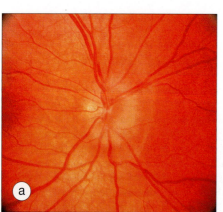
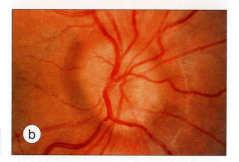

Fig. 59.28 (a) Pseudopapilledema with buried disc drusen. (b) Note cupless discs with elevation confined to the disc, increased retinal vessels that overlie the disc without obscuration, and clear circumpapillary light reflex from the internal limiting membrane.

Table 59.4 Ophthalmoscopic features useful in differentiating optic disc edema from pseudopapilledema associated with buried drusen	
Optic disc edema	Pseudopapilledema with buried drusen
Disc vasculature obscured at disc margins	Disc vasculature remains visible at disc margins
Elevation extends into peripapillary retina	Elevation confined to optic disc
Graying and muddying of peripapillary nerve fiber layer	Sharp peripapillary nerve fiber
Venous congestion	No venous congestion
+/- Exudates	No exudates
Loss of optic cup only in moderate to severe disc edema	Small cupless disc
Normal configuration of disc vasculature despite venous congestion	Increased major retinal vessels with early branching
No circumpapillary light reflex	Crescentic circumpapillary light reflex
Absence of spontaneous venous pulsations	Spontaneous venous pulsations may be present or absent

ring of light that reflects from the concave internal limiting membrane surrounding the elevation (Fig. 59.28). This crescentic light reflex is absent in papilledema, due to diffraction of light from distended peripapillary axons.[194,197] Single splinter or subretinal optic disc hemorrhages are occasionally seen with disc drusen, but exudates, cotton-wool spots, hyperemia, and venous congestion are conspicuously absent.[198]

Fluorescein angiography

Discs with ophthalmoscopically prominent drusen (Fig. 59.29) may exhibit autofluorescence in the preinjection phase.[185] This is followed by a true nodular hyperfluorescence corresponding to the location of the drusen. Hyperfluorescence, which typically is mild, begins in the arteriovenous phase and continues into the late phases. The superficial disc capillary network may show prominence in areas overlying buried drusen.[185] The late phases may be characterized by some minimal blurring of the drusen that may either fade or maintain fluorescence (staining). Unlike papilledema, however, there is no visible leakage along the major vessels.[186,192] Venous anomalies (venous stasis, venous convolutions, and retinociliary venous communications) and staining of the peripapillary vein walls are occasionally seen.[199]

Neuroimaging of pseudopapilledema

The distinction between papilledema and pseudopapilledema with buried drusen has been aided by CT scanning and ultrasonography which shows calcifications within the elevated optic disc (Fig. 59.30).[200–203] It is not uncommon to see a child referred for possible papilledema arrive for consultation with the "negative" CT scan in hand, only to find undetected calcification of the optic discs upon review of the scan. B-scan ultrasonography appears to be superior to either CT scanning or photography to look for autofluorescence in the detection of disc drusen.[203]

Histopathology

Optic disc drusen are situated anterior to the lamina cribrosa; they occur nowhere else in the brain. They consist of homogenous, globular concretions, often collected in larger, multilobulated agglomerations. Individual druse usually exhibit a concentrically laminated structure, which is not encapsulated and contains no cells or cellular debris.[184] Drusen are often most concentrated within the nasal portion of the disc. The optic disc axons are atrophic adjacent to large accumulations of drusen.[184,204,205] Drusen take up calcium salts and must be decalcified before being cut into sections for histological study.[184]

Pathogenesis

The primary developmental expression of the genetic trait for drusen may be a smaller-than-normal scleral canal.[206,207] The peripapillary sclera forms after the optic stalks are complete.[207] Mesenchymal elements from the sclera then invade the glial framework of the primitive lamina, reinforcing it with collagen.[207] An abnormal encroachment of sclera, Bruch's membrane, or both upon the developing optic stalk would narrow the exit space of optic axons from the eye. The absence of a central cup in affected eyes is consistent with the existence of axonal crowding. Drusen are often first detected clinically and histopathologically at the margins of the optic disc, which raises the possibility that the rigid edge of the scleral canal may be an

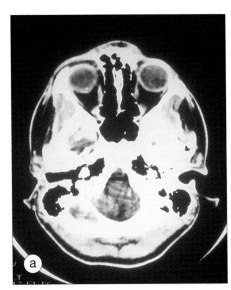

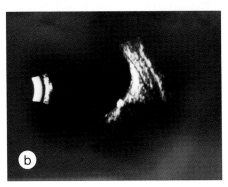

Fig. 59.30 Ancillary studies showing calcifications in patients with pseudopapilledema and buried disc drusen. (a) CT scan. (Courtesy of Stephen C. Pollock, MD.) (b) B-scan ultrasonography. (Courtesy of Laurie Barber, MD.) (From Brodsky MC, Baker RS, Hamed LF. Pediatric Neuro-ophthalmology. Springer Verlag 1996, with permission © 1996 Springer Verlag.)

aggravating factor in producing a relative mechanical interruption of axonal transport.[208–212] The lower prevalence of optic disc drusen in African-Americans, who have a larger disc area with less potential for axonal crowding, is consistent with the notion of axonal crowding as a fundamental anatomical substrate for formation of disc drusen.[206]

Ocular complications and associated systemic conditions

Despite the gradual attrition of optic axons that occurs throughout life, most patients with pseudopapilledema remain asymptomatic. Nevertheless, most develop visual field defects (measurable in 71–87% of eyes).[181] Other rare but recognized defects include superficial and deep hemorrhages in or adjacent to the disc peripapillary subretinal neovascularization, ischemic optic neuropathy, peripapillary central serous choroidopathy, and acute loss of central acuity.[181]

Associated systemic conditions

Systemic disorders associated with pseudopapilledema include Down syndrome, Alagille syndrome, Denny syndrome, Weber hereditary optic neuropathy, mucopolysaccharidosis, linear sebaceous nevus syndrome, orbital hypotelorism and trisomy 13q-.[181] Systemic disorders associated with visible optic disc drusen include retinitis pigmentosa, pseudoxanthoma elasticum, megalencephaly, migraine headaches and pigmented paravenous retinochoroidal atrophy.[181]

REFERENCES

1. Brodsky MC. Congenital optic disk anomalies. Surv Ophthalmol 1994; 39: 89–112.

2. Kushner BJ. Functional amblyopia associated with abnormalities of the optic nerve. Arch Ophthalmol 1985; 102: 683–5.

3. Brodsky MC, Hoyt WF, Hoyt CS, et al. Atypical retinochoroidal coloboma in patients with dysplastic optic discs and transsphenoidal encephalocele. Arch Ophthalmol 1995; 113: 624–8.

4. Lambert SR, Hoyt CS, Narahara MH. Optic nerve hypoplasia. Surv Ophthalmol 1987; 32: 1–9.

5. Hellström A, Wiklund L-M, Svensson E, et al. Optic nerve hypoplasia with isolated tortuosity of the retinal veins. Arch Ophthalmol 1999; 117: 880–4.

6. Mosier MA, Lieberman MF, Green WR, et al. Hypoplasia of the optic nerve. Arch Ophthalmol 1978; 96: 1437–42.

7. Hotchkiss ML, Green WR. Optic nerve aplasia and hypoplasia. J Pediatr Ophthalmol Strabismus 1979; 16: 225–40.

8. Frisen L, Holmegaard L. Spectrum of optic nerve hypoplasia. Br J Ophthalmol 1975; 62: 7–15.

9. Zeki SM. Optic nerve hypoplasia and astigmatism: a new association. Br J Ophthalmol 1990; 74: 297–9.

10. Lempert P. Optic nerve hypoplasia and small eyes in presumed amblyopia. J AAPOS 2000; 4: 258–66.

11. Archer SM. Amblyopia? J AAPOS 2000; 4: 257.

12. Lempert P. Axial length-disc area ratio in esotropic amblyopia. Arch Ophthalmol 2003; 121: 821–4.

13. Taylor D. Congenital tumors of the anterior visual system with dysplasia of the optic discs. Br J Ophthalmol 1982; 66: 455–63.

14. de Morsier G. Études sur les dysraphies crânioencéphaliques. III. agénésis du septum lucidum avec malformation du tractus optique. La dysplasie septo-optique. Schweiz Arch Neurol Psychiatr 1956; 77: 267–92.

15. Hoyt WF, Kaplan SL, Grumbach MM, et al. Septo-optic dysplasia and pituitary dwarfism. Lancet 1970; 2: 893–4.

16. Skarf B, Hoyt CS. Optic nerve hypoplasia in children. Association with anomalies of the endocrine and CNS. Arch Ophthalmol 1984; 102: 255–8.

17. Arslanian SA, Rothfus WE, Foley TP, et al. Hormonal, metabolic, and neuroradiologic abnormalities associated with septo-optic dysplasia. Acta Endocrinol 1984; 139: 249–54.

18. Izenberg N, Rosenblum M, Parks JS. The endocrine spectrum of septo-optic dysplasia. Clin Pediatr 1984; 23: 632–6.

19. Margalith D, Tze WJ, Jan JE. Congenital optic nerve hypoplasia with hypothalamic-pituitary dysplasia. A review of 16 cases. Am J Dis Child 1985; 139: 361–6.

20. Costin G, Murphree AL. Hypothalamic pituitary dysfunction in children with optic nerve hypoplasia. Am J Dis Child 1985; 143: 249–54.

21. Hanna ME, Mandel SH, LaFranchi SH. Puberty in the syndrome of septo–optic dysplasia. Am J Dis Child 1989; 143: 186–9.

22. Sherlock DA, McNicol LR. Anaesthesia and septo-optic dysplasia. Anaesthesia 1987; 42: 1302–5.

23. Phillips PH, Spear C, Brodsky MC. Magnetic resonance diagnosis of congenital hypopituitarism in children with optic nerve hypoplasia. J AAPOS 2001; 5: 275–80.

24. Brodsky MC, Conte FA, Taylor D, et al. Sudden death in septo-optic dysplasia. Report of five cases. Arch Ophthalmol 1997; 15: 66–70.

25. Brodsky MC, Glasier CM, Pollock SC, et al. Optic nerve hypoplasia: identification by magnetic resonance imaging. Arch Ophthalmol 1990; 108: 562–7.

26. Brodsky MC, Glasier CM. Optic nerve hypoplasia: clinical significance of associated central nervous system abnormalities on magnetic resonance imaging. Arch Ophthalmol 1993; 111: 66–74.

27. Williams J, Brodsky MC, Griebel M, et al. Septo-optic dysplasia: clinical significance of an absent septum pellucidum. Dev Med Child Neurol 1993; 35: 490–501.

28. Novakovic P, Taylor DS, Hoyt WF. Localizing patterns of optic nerve hypoplasia-retina to occipital lobe. Br J Ophthalmol 1988; 72: 176–82.

29. Petersen RA, Walton DS. Optic nerve hypoplasia with good visual acuity and visual field defects: a study of children of diabetic mothers. Arch Ophthalmol 1977; 95: 254–8.

30. Kim RY, Hoyt WF, Lessell S, et al. Superior segmental optic hypoplasia: a sign of maternal diabetes. Arch Ophthalmol 1989; 107: 1312–5.

31. Landau K, Bajka JD, Kirchschlager BM. Topless optic disks in children of mothers with type I diabetes mellitus. Am J Ophthalmol 1998; 125: 605–11.

32. Hashimoto M, Ohtsuka K, Nakagawa T, et al. Topless optic disk syndrome without maternal diabetes mellitus. Am J Ophthalmol 1999; 128: 111–2.

33. Brodsky MC, Schroeder GT, Ford R. Superior segmental optic hypoplasia in identical twins. J Clin Neuro-ophthalmol 1993; 13: 152–4.

34. Birgbauer E, Cowan CA, Sretavan DW, et al. Kinase independent function of EphB receptors in retinal axon pathfinding to the optic disc from dorsal but not ventral retina. Development 2000; 127: 1231–41.

35. Hoyt WF, Rios-Montenegro EN, Behrens MM, et al. Homonymous hemioptic hypoplasia: funduscopic features in standard and red-free illumination in three patients with congenital hemiplegia. Br J Ophthalmol 1972; 56: 537–45.

36. Jacobson L, Hellström A, Flodmark O. Large cups in normal-sized optic discs. Arch Ophthalmol 1997; 115: 1263–9.

37. Brodsky MC. Periventricular leukomalacia: an intracranial cause of pseudoglaucomatous cupping. Arch Ophthalmol 2001; 119: 626–7.

38. Scheie HG, Adler FH. Aplasia of the optic nerve. Arch Ophthalmol 1941; 26: 61–70.

39. Deiner MS, Kennedy TE, Fazeli A, et al. Netrin-1 and DCC mediate axon guidance locally at the optic disc: loss of function leads to optic nerve hypoplasia. Neuron 1997; 19: 575–589.

40. Oster SF, Sretavan DW. Connecting the eye to the brain: the molecular basis of ganglion cell axon guidance. Br J Ophthalmol 2003; 87: 639–45.

41. Deiner MS, Kennedy TE, Fazeli A, et al. Netrin-1 and DCC mediate axon guidance locally at the optic disc: loss of function leads to optic nerve hypoplasia. Neuron 1997; 19: 575–89

42. Deiner MS, Sretavan DW. Altered midline axon pathways and ectopic neurons in the developing hypothalamus of netrin-1 and DCC deficient mice. J Neurosci 1999; 19: 9900–12.

43. Provis JM, Van Driel D, Billson FA, et al. Human fetal optic nerve: overproduction and elimination of retinal axons during development. J Comp Neurol 1985; 238: 92–100.

44. Hackenbruch Y, Meerhoff E, Besio R, et al. Familial bilateral optic nerve hypoplasia. Am J Ophthalmol 1975; 79: 314–20.

45. Brenner JD, Preslan MW, Gratz E, et al. Septo-optic dysplasia in two siblings. Am J Ophthalmol 1990; 109: 632–9.

46. Dattani M, Martinez-Barbera JP, Thomas PQ, et al. Mutations in the homeobox gene HESX/Hesx1 associated with septo-optic dysplasia in human and mouse. Nat Genet 1998; 19: 125–33.

47. Dattani M, Martinez-Barbera JP, Thomas PQ, et al. Molecular genetics of septo-optic dysplasia. Horm Res 1000; 53: Suppl 1, 26–33.

48. Bennett JL. Developmental neurogenetics and neuro-ophthalmology. J Neuro-ophthalmol 2003; 22: 286–93.

49. Azuma N, Yamaguchi Y, Handa H, et al. Mutations of the PAX6 gene detected in patients with a variety of optic nerve malformations. Am J Hum Genet 2003; 72: 1565–70.

50. Pollock S. The morning glory disc anomaly: contractile movement, classification, and embryogenesis. Docum Ophthalmol 1987; 65: 439–60.

51. Kindler P. Morning glory syndrome: unusual congenital optic disk anomaly. Am J Ophthalmol 1970; 69: 376–84.

52. Brodsky MC, Wilson RS. Retinal arteriovenous communications in the morning glory disc anomaly. Arch Ophthalmol 1995; 115: 410–11.

53. Beyer WB, Quencer RM, Osher RH. Morning glory syndrome: a functional analysis including fluorescein angiography, ultra-sonography, and computerized tomography. Ophthalmology 1982; 89. 1362–4.

54. Goldhammer Y, Smith JL. Optic nerve anomalies in basal encephalocele. Arch Ophthalmol 1975; 93: 115–8.

55. Koenig SP, Naidich TP, Lissner G. The morning glory syndrome associated with sphenoidal encephalocele. Ophthalmology 1982; 89: 1368–72.

56. Pollack JA, Newton TH, Hoyt WF. Transsphenoidal and

transethmoidal encephalocele: a review of clinical and roentgen features in 8 cases. Radiology 1968; 90: 442–53.

57. Yokota A, Matsukado Y, Fuwa I, et al. Anterior basal encephalocele of the neonatal and infantile period. Neurosurgery 1986; 19: 468–78.

58. Hansen MR, Price RL, Rothner AD, et al. Developmental anomalies of the optic disc and carotid circulation: A new association. J Clin Neuro-ophthalmol 1985; 5: 3–8.

59. Massaro M, Thorarensen O, Liu GT, et al. Morning glory disc anomaly and moyamoya vessels. Arch Ophthalmol 1998; 116: 253–4.

60. Bakri SJ, Skier D, Masaryk T, et al. Ocular malformations, moyamoya disease, and midline cranial defects. A distinct syndrome. Am J Ophthalmol 1999; 127: 356–7.

61. Dempster AG, Lee WR, Forrester JV, et al. The "morning glory syndrome". A mesodermal defect? Ophthalmologica 1983; 187: 222–30.

62. Holmström G, Taylor D. Capillary haemangiomas in association with morning glory disc anomaly. Acta Ophthalmol Scand 1998; 76: 613–6.

63. Metry DW, Dowd CF, Barkovich AJ, et al. The many faces of PHACE syndrome. J Pediatr 2001; 139: 117–23.

64. Kniestedt C, Brodsky MC, North P, et al. Infantile orofacial hemangioma with ipsilateral peripapillary excavation in girls. A variant of the PHACE syndrome. Arch Ophthalmol 2004 (in press).

65. Brodsky MC, Landau K, Wilson RS, et al. Morning glory disc anomaly in neurofibromatosis type 2. Arch Ophthalmol 1999; 117: 839–41.

66. Harris MJ, De Bustros S, Michels RG, et al. Treatment of combined traction–rhegmatogenous retinal detachment in the morning glory syndrome. Retina 1984; 4: 249–52.

67. Sobol WM, Bratton AR, Rivers MB, et al. Morning glory disk syndrome associated with subretinal neovascularization. Am J Ophthalmol 1990; 110: 93–4.

68. Graether JM. Transient amaurosis in one eye with simultaneous dilatation of retinal veins. Arch Ophthalmol 1963; 70: 342–5.

69. Traboulsi EI, O'Neill JF. The spectrum in the morphology of the so-called "morning glory disc anomaly: J Ped Ophthalmol Strabismus 1988; 25: 93–8.

70. Gardner TW, Zaparackas ZG, Naidich TP. Congenital optic nerve colobomas: CT demonstration. J Comput Assist Tomogr 1984; 8: 95–102.

71. Mafee MF, Jampol LM, Langer BG, et al. Computed tomography of optic nerve colobomas, morning glory disc anomaly, and colobomatous cyst. Radiol Clin of North Am 1987; 25: 693–9.

72. Mann I. Developmental Abnormalities of the Eye. Philadelphia: JB Lippincott; 1957: 74–91.

73. Pagon RA. Ocular coloboma. Surv Ophthalmol 1981; 25: 223–36.

74. Francois J. Colobomatous malformations of the ocular globe. Int Ophthalmol Clin 1968; 8: 797–816.

75. Calhoun FP. Bilateral coloboma of the optic nerve associated with holes in the disc and a cyst of the optic nerve sheath. Arch Ophthalmol 1930; 3: 71–9.

76. Slamovits TL, Kimball GP, Friberg TR, et al. Bilateral optic disc colobomas with orbital cysts and hypoplastic optic nerves and chiasm. J Clin Neuro-ophthalmol 1989; 9: 172–7.

77. Font RL, Zimmerman LE. Intrascleral smooth muscle in coloboma of the optic disc. Am J Ophthalmol 1971; 72: 452–7.

78. Willis R, Zimmerman LE, O'Grady R, et al. Heterotopic adipose tissue and smooth muscle in the optic disc, association with isolated colobomas. Arch Ophthalmol 1972; 88: 139–46.

79. Foster JA, Lam S. Contractile optic disc coloboma. Arch Ophthalmol 1991; 109: 472–3.

80. Lin CC, Tso MO, Vygantas CM. Coloboma of the optic nerve associated with serous maculopathy: a clinicopathologic correlative study. Arch Ophthalmol 1984; 1651–4.

81. Schatz H, McDonald HR. Treatment of sensory retinal detachment associated with optic nerve pit or coloboma. Ophthalmology 1988; 95: 178–86.

82. Bochow TW, Olk RJ, Knupp JA, et al. Spontaneous reattachment of a total retinal detachment in an infant with microphthalmos and an optic nerve coloboma. Am J Ophthalmol 1991; 112: 347–9.

83. Brodsky MC. Magnetic resonance imaging of colobomatous optic hypoplasia. Br J Ophthalmol 1999; 83: 755–6.

84. Corbett JJ, Savino PJ, Schatz NJ, et al. Cavitary developmental defects of the optic disc: visual loss associated with optic pits and colobomas. Arch Neurol 1980; 37: 210–3.

85. Streletz LJ, Schatz NJ. Transsphenoidal encephalocele associated with colobomas of the optic disc and hypopituitary dwarfism. In Smith JL, Glaser JS, ed. Neuroophthalmology Symposium of the University of Miami and the Bascom Palmer Eye Institute. St Louis, MO: CV Mosby; 1973: 78–86.

86. von Szily A. Die Obntogenese der idiopathiachen (erbbildlichen Spaltbildungen des Auges des Mikrophthalmus und der Orbitalcysten). Z Anat Entwicklungsgesch 1924; 74: 1–230.

87. Brown G, Tasman W. Congenital Anomalies of the Optic Disc. New York, NY: Grune & Stratton; 1983: 31–215.

88. Singh D, Verma A. Bilateral peripapillary staphyloma (ectasia). Ind J Ophthalmol 1978; 25: 50–1.

89. Wise JB, Maclean AL, Gass JD. Contractile peripapillary staphyloma. Arch Ophthalmol 1966; 75: 626–30.

90. Konstas P, Katikos G, Vatakas LC. Contractile peripapillary staphyloma. Ophthalmologica 1971; 172: 379–81.

91. Kral K, Svarc D. Contractile peripapillary staphyloma. Am J Ophthalmol 1971; 71: 1090–2.

92. Seybold ME, Rosen PN. Peripapillary staphyloma. Ann Ophthalmol 1977; 9: 139–41.

93. Caldwell JBH, Sears ML, Gilman M. Bilateral peripapillary staphyloma with normal vision. Am J Ophthalmol 1971; 71: 423–5.

94. Hodgkins P, Lees M, Lawson J, et al. Optic disc anomalies and frontonasal dysplasia. Br J Ophthalmol 1998; 82: 290–3.

95. Kiratli H, Bozkurt B, Mocan C. Peripapillary staphyloma associated with orofacial capillary hemangioma. Ophthal Genet 2001; 22: 249–53.

96. Izquierdo NJ, Maumenee IH, Traboulsi EI. Anterior segment malformations in 18q- (de Grouchy) syndrome. Ophthal Pediatr Genet 1993; 14: 91–4.

97. Franceschetti A, Bock RH. Megalopapilla: a new congenital anomaly. Am J Ophthalmol 1950; 33: 227–35.

98. Bynke H, Holmdahl G. Megalopapilla: a differential diagnosis in suspected optic atrophy. Neuro-ophthalmology 1981; 2: 53–7.

99. Jonas JB, Koniszewski G, Naumann GO. Pseudoglaucomatous physiologic optic cups. Am J Ophthalmol 1989; 107: 137–44.

100. Maisel JM, Pearlstein CS, Adams WH, et al. Large optic discs in the Marshallese population. Am J Ophthalmol 1989; 107: 145–50.

101. Manor RS, Kesler A. Optic nerve hypoplasia, big discs, large cupping, and vascular malformation embolized: a 22 year follow-up. Arch Ophthalmol 1993; 111: 901–2.

102. Ragge N, Hoyt WF, Lambert SR. Big discs with optic nerve hypoplasia. J Clin Neuro-ophthalmol 1991; 11: 137.

103. Grimson BS, Perry DD. Enlargement of the optic disk in childhood optic nerve tumors. Am J Ophthalmol 1984; 97: 627–31.

104. Brown GC, Shields JA, Goldberg RE. Congenital pits of the optic nerve head. II. Clinical studies in humans. Ophthalmology 1980; 87: 51–65.

105. Theodossiadis GP, Kollia AK, Theodossiadis PG. Cilioretinal arteries in conjunction with a pit of the optic disc. Ophthalmologica 1992; 204; 115–21.

106. Stefko ST, Campochiaro P, Wang P, et al. Dominant inheritance of optic pits. Am J Ophthalmol 1997; 124: 112–3.

107. Ragge NK. Dominant inheritance of optic pits. Am J Ophthalmol 1998; 125: 124–5.

108. Jonas JB, Freisler KA. Bilateral congenital optic nerve head pits in monozygotic twins. Am J Ophthalmol 1997; 844–5.

109. Van Nouhuys JM, Bruyn GW. Nasopharyngeal transssphenoidal encephalocele, craterlike hole in the optic disc and agenesis of the corpus callosum: pneumoencephalographic visualization in a case. Psychiatr Neurol Neurochir 1964; 67: 243–58.

110. Javitt JC, Spaeth GL, Katz LJ, et al. Acquired pits of the optic nerve. Ophthalmology 1990; 97: 1038–44.

111. Lincoff H, Lopez R, Kreissig I, et al. Retinoschisis associated with optic nerve pits. Arch Ophthalmol 1988; 106: 61–7.

112. Yuen CH, Kaye SB. Spontaneous resolution of serous maculopathy associated with optic disc pit in a child: a case report. J AAPOS 2002; 6: 330–1.

113. Brodsky MC. Congenital optic pit with serous maculopathy in childhood. J AAPOS 2003; 7: 150.

114. Sobol WM, Blodi CF, Folk JC, et al. Long-term visual outcome in patients with optic nerve pit and serous retinal detachment of the macula. Ophthalmology 1990; 97: 1539–42.

115. Sugar HS. Congenital pits of the optic disc and their equivalents (congenital colobomas and colobomalike excavations) associated with submacular fluid. Am J Ophthalmol 1967; 63: 298–307.

116. Gass JD. Serous detachment of the macula: secondary to congenital pit of the optic nervehead. Am J Ophthalmol 1969; 67: 821–41.

117. Cox MS, Witherspoon CD, Morris RE, et al. Evolving techniques in treatment of macular detachment caused by optic nerve pits. Ophthalmology 1988; 95: 889–96.

118. Lincoff H, Yannuzzi L, Singerman L, et al. Improvement in visual function after displacement of the retinal elevation emanating from optic pits. Arch Ophthalmol 1993; 111: 1071–9.

119. Akiba J, Kakehashi A, Hikichi T, et al. Vitreous findings of optic nerve pits and serous macular detachment. Am J Ophthalmol 1993; 116: 38–41.

120. Brown GC, Shields JA, Patty BE, et al. Congenital pits of the optic nerve head. I. experimental studies in collie dogs. Arch Ophthalmol 1979; 97: 1341–4.

121. Rieger G. Zum Krankheitsbild der Handmannschen Sehnerven-anomalie: "Windenblüten"-("Morning Glory"-) Syndrom? Klin Monatsbl Augenheilkd 1977; 697–706.

122. Parsa CF, Silva ED, Sundin OH, et al. Redevining papillorenal syndrome: An underdiagnosed cause of ocular and renal morbidity. Ophthalmology 2001; 108: 738–49.

123. Sanyanusin P, Schimmenti LA, McNoe A, et al. Mutation of the PAX2 gene in a family with optic nerve colobomas, renal anomalies, and vesiculoureteral reflux. Nat Genet 1995; 9: 358–64.

124. Schimmenti LA, Cunliffe HE, McNoe LA, et al. Further delineation of renal-coloboma syndrome in patients with extreme variability of phenotype and identical PAX2 mutations. Am H Hum Genet 1997; 60: 869–78.

125. Dureau P, Attie-Bitach T, Salomon R, et al. Renal-coloboma syndrome. Ophthalmology 2001; 108: 1912–16.

126. Savell J, Cook JR. Optic nerve colobomas of autosomal dominant heredity. Arch Ophthalmol 1979; 94: 395–400.

127. Parsa CF, Attie-Bitach T, Salomon R, et al. Papillorenal ("renal-coloboma") syndrome. Am J Ophthalmol 2002; 134: 301–2.

128. Young SE, Walsh FB, Knox DL. The tilted disc syndrome. Am J Ophthalmol 1976; 82: 16–23.

129. Banu B, Murat I, Gedik S, et al. Topographical analysis of corneal astigmatism in patients with tilted disc syndrome. Cornea 2002; 21: 458–62.

130. Apple DJ, Rabb MF, Walsh PM. Congenital anomalies of the optic disc. Surv Ophthalmol 1982; 27: 3–41.

131. Keane JR. Suprasellar tumors and incidental optic disc anomalies: diagnostic problems in two patients with hemianopic temporal scotomas. Arch Ophthalmol 1977; 95: 2189–93.

132. Osher RH, Schatz NJ. A sinister association of the congenital tilted disc syndrome with chiasmal compression. In: Smith JL, ed. Neuro-Ophthalmology Focus 1980. New York, NY: Masson; 1979: 117–23.

133. Hittner HM, Borda RP, Justice J. X-linked recessive congenital stationary night blindness, myopia, and tilted discs. J Pediatr Ophthalmol Strabismus 1981; 18: 15–20.

134. Cohen SY, Quentel G, Guiberteau B, et al. Macular serous retinal detachment caused by subretinal leakage in tilted disc syndrome. Ophthalmology 1998; 105; 1831–4.

135. Tosti G. Serous macular detachment and tilted disc syndrome. Ophthalmology 1999; 106: 1453–4.

136. Brodsky MC. Central serous papillopathy. Br J Ophthalmol 1999; 83: 878.

137. Handmann M. Erbliche, vermutlich angeborene zentrale gliose entartung des sehnerven mit besonderer beteilgung der zentralgefasse. Klin Monatsbl Augenheilkd 1929; 83: 145.

138. Brodsky MC, Buckley EG, Rosell-McConkie A. The case of the gray optic disc! Surv Ophthalmol 1989; 33: 367–72.

139. Silver J, Sapiro J. Axonal guidance during development of the optic nerve: the role of pigmented epithelia and other factors. J Comput Neurol 1981; 202: 521–38.

140. Beauvieux J. La pseudo-atrophie optique dés nouveau-nes (dysgénésie myélinique des voies optiques). Ann Ocul (Paris) 1926; 163: 881–921.

141. Beauvieux J. La cécité apparente chez le nouveau-né: la pseudoatrophie grise du nerf optique. Arch Ophtalmol 1947; 7: 241–9.

142. Hoyt CS, Billson F, Ouvrier R, et al. Ocular features of Aicardi's syndrome. Arch Ophthalmol 1978; 96: 291–5.

143. Carney SH, Brodsky MC, Good WV, et al. Aicardi syndrome: more than meets the eye. Surv Ophthalmol 1993; 37: 419–24.

144. Chevrie JJ, Aicardi J. The Aicardi syndrome. In: Pedley TA, Meldrum BS, eds. Recent Advances in Epilepsy. New York, NY: Churchill Livingstone; 1986; 189–210.

145. Tagawa T, Mimaki T, Ono J, et al. Aicardi syndrome associated with an embryonal carcinoma. Pediatr Neurol 1989; 5: 45–57.

146. Neidich JA, Nussbaum RL, Packer RJ, et al. Heterogeneity of clinical severity and molecular lesions in Aicardi syndrome. J Pediatr 1990; 116: 911–17.

147. Molina JA, Mateos F, Merino M, et al. Aicardi syndrome in two sisters. J Pediatr 1989; 115: 282–3.

148. Rosser TL, Acosta MT, Packer RJ. Aicardi syndrome: spectrum of disease and long-term prognosis in 77 females. Pediatr Neurol 2002; 77: 343–6.

149. Ganesh A, Mitra S, Koul RL, et al. The full spectrum of persistent fetal vasculature in Aicardi syndrome: an integrated interpretation of ocular malformations. Br J Ophthalmol 2000; 84: 227–8.

150. Donoso LA, Magargal LE, Eiferman RA, et al. Ocular anomalies simulating double optic disc. Can J Ophthalmol 1981; 16: 84–7.

151. Snead CM. Congenital division of the optic nerve at the base of the skull. Arch Ophthalmol 1915; 44: 418–20.

152. Fuchs E. Über den anatomischen Befun einiger angeborener Anomalien der Netzhaut und des Sehnerven. Albrech von Graefes Arch Opthalmol 1917; 93: 1.

153. Slade HW, Weekley RD. Diastasis of the optic nerve. J Neurosurg 1957; 14: 571–4.

154. Collier M. Communications sur le sujet du rapport les doubles papilles optiques. Bull Soc Ophtalmol Fr 1958; 71: 328–52.

155. Weiter JJ, McLean IW, Zimmerman LE. Aplasia of the optic nerve and disk. Am J Ophthalmol 1977; 83: 569–76.

156. Margo CE, Hamed LM, McCarty J. Congenital optic tract syndrome. Arch Ophthalmol 1992; 110: 1610–13.

157. Little LE, Whitmore PV, Wells TW Jr. Aplasia of the optic nerve. J Pediatr Ophthalmol 1976; 13: 84–8.

158. Blanco R, Salvador F, Galan A, et al. Optic nerve aplasia: report of three cases. J Pediatr Ophthalmol Strabismus 1992; 29: 228–31.

159. Ginsberg J, Bove KE, Cuesta MG. Aplasia of the optic nerve with aniridia. Ann Ophthalmol 1980; 12: 433–9.

160. Howard MA, Thompson JT, Howard RO. Aplasia of the optic nerve. Trans Am Ophthalmol Soc 1993; 91: 276–81.

161. Recupero SM, Lepore GF, Plateroti R, et al. Optic nerve aplasia associated with macular "atypical coloboma". Acta Ophthalmol 1994; 72: 768–79.

162. Barry DR. Aplasia of the optic nerves. Int Ophthalmol 1985; 7: 235–42.

163. Storm RL, PeBenito R. Bilateral optic nerve aplasia associated with hydroencephaly. Ann Ophthalmol 1984; 16: 988–92.

164. Yanoff M, Rorke LB, Allman MI. Bilateral optic system aplasia with relatively normal eyes. Arch Ophthalmol 1978; 96: 97–101.

165. Hoff J, Winestock D, Hoyt WF. Giant suprasellar aneurysm associated with optic stalk agenesis and unilateral anophthalmos. J Neurosurg 1975; 43: 495–8.

166. Hotchkiss ML, Green WR. Optic nerve aplasia and hypoplasia. J Pediatr Ophthalmol Strabismus 1979; 16: 225–40.

167. Miller NR. Walsh and Hoyt's Clinical Neuro-Ophthalmology. 4th edn. Baltimore, MD: Williams and Wilkins; 1982: 343–69.

168. Straatsma BR, Foos FY, Heckenlively JR, et al. Myelinated retinal nerve fibers. Am J Ophthalmol 1981; 91: 25–38.

169. Williams TD. Medullated retinal nerve fibers: speculations on their cause and presentation of cases. Am J Optom Physiol Opt 1986; 63: 142–51.

170. Ellis GS, Frey T, Gouterman RZ. Myelinated nerve fibers, axial myopia, and refractory amblyopia: an organic disease. J Pediatr Ophthalmol Strabismus 1987; 24: 111–19.

171. Hittner HM, Kretzer FL, Antoszyk JH, et al. Variable expressivity of autosomal dominant anterior segment mesenchymal dysgenesis in six generations. Am J Ophthalmol 1982; 93: 57–70.

172. De Jong, PT, Bistervels B, Cosgrove J, et al. Medullated nerve fibers: a sign of multiple basal cell nevi (Gorlin's syndrome). Arch Ophthalmol 1985; 103: 1833–6.

173. Traboulsi EI, Lim JI, Pyeritz R, et al. A new syndrome of myelinated nerve fibers, vitreoretinopathy and skeletal malformations. Arch Ophthalmol 193; 111: 1543–5.

174. Francois J. Myelinated nerve fibers. In: Heredity in Ophthalmology. St Louis, MO, C.V. Mosby; 1961: 767–8.

175. Bertelsen TI. The premature synostosis of the cranial sutures. Acta Ophthalmol 1958; 51 (suppl): 62–92.

176. Cockburn DM. Tilted disc and medullated nerve fibers. Am J Optom Physiol Opt 1982; 59: 760–1.

177. Goldsmith J. Neurofibromatosis associated with tumors of the optic papilla. Arch Ophthalmol 1949; 41: 718–29.

178. Aaby AA, Kushner BJ. Acquired and progressive myelinated nerve fibers. Arch Ophthalmol 1985; 103: 542–4.

179. Baarsma GS. Acquired medullated nerve fibers. Br J Ophthalmol 1980; 64: 651.

180. Schatz MP, Pollock SC. Optic disc morphology in albinism. Presented as a poster at the North American Neuro-Ophthalmology Society, Durango, CO, February 27–March 3, 1994.

181. Brodsky MC, Baker RS, Hamed LM. Pediatric Neuro-Ophthalmology. Springer Verlag, New York; 1996: 42–124.

182. Hoyt WF, Beeston D. The Ocular Fundus in Neurologic Disease. St Louis, MO: CV Mosby; 1966.

183. Savino PJ, Glaser JS, Rosenberg MA. A clinical analysis of pseudopapilledema. II. Visual field defects. Arch Ophthalmol 1979; 97: 71–5

184. Lorentzen SE. Drusen of the optic disk. Dan Med Bull 1967; 14: 293–8

185. Friedman AH, Beckerman B, Gold DH, et al. Drusen of the optic disc. Surv Ophthalmol 1977; 21: 375–90

186. Sanders MD, Ffytche TJ. Flourescein angiography in the diagnosis of drusen of the disc. Trans Ophthalmol Soc UK 1967; 87: 457–68

187. Rosenberg MA, Savino PJ, Glaser JS. A clinical analysis of pseudopapilledema: I: population, laterality, acuity, refractive error, ophthalmoscopic characteristics, and coincident disease. Arch Ophthalmol 1979; 97: 65–70.

188. Friedman AH, Gartner S, Modi SS. Drusen of the optic disc. A retrospective study in cadaver eyes. Br J Ophthalmol 1975; 59: 413–521

189. Francois J. L'hérédité en ophtalmologie. Paris: Masson; 1958: 509–602.

190. Lorentzen SE. Drusen of the optic disk, an irregular dominant hereditary affectation. Arch Ophthalmol 1961; 39: 626–43.

191. Hoyt WF, Pont ME. Pseudopapilledema. Anomalous elevation of optic disk. Pitfalls in diagnosis and management. JAMA 1962; 181: 191–6.

192. Singleton EM, Kinsbourne M, Anderson WB. Familial pseudopapilledema. South Med J 1973; 66: 796–802.

193. Mustonen E. Pseudopapilloedema with and without verified optic disc drusen. A clinical analysis II: visual fields. Acta Ophthalmol 1983; 61: 1057–66.

194. Erkkila H. Optic disc drusen in children. Acta Ophthalmol 1977; 129 (suppl): 7–44.

195. Miller NR. Appearance of optic disc drusen in a patient with anomalous elevation of the optic disc. Arch Ophthalmol 1986; 104: 794–5.

196. Hoover DL, Robb RM, Petersen RA. Optic disc drusen in children. J Pediatr Ophthalmol Strabismus 1988; 25: 191–5.

197. Hoyt WF, Knight CL. Comparison of congenital disc blurring and incipient papilledema in red-free light-a photographic study. Invest Ophthalmol 1973; 12: 241–7.

198. Hitchings RA, Corbett JJ, Winkleman J, et al. Hemorrhages with optic nerve drusen. Arch Neurol 1976; 33: 675–7.

199. Karel I, Otradovec J, Peleska M. Fluorescein angiography in circulatory disturbances in drusen of the optic disc. Ophthalmologica 1972; 164: 449–62.

200. Bec P, Adam P, Mathis A, et al. Optic nerve head drusen: high resolution computed tomographic approach. Arch Ophthalmol 1984; 102: 680–2.

201. Frisen L, Scholdstrom G, Svendsen P. Drusen in the optic nerve head: verification by computed tomography. Arch Ophthalmol 1978; 96: 1611–14.

202. Boldt HC, Byrne SF, DiBernardo C. Echographic evaluation of optic disc drusen. J Clin Neuro-ophthalmol 1991; 11: 85–91.

203. Kurz-Levin M, Landau K. A comparison of imaging techniques for diagnosing drusen of the optic nerve head. Arch Ophthalmol 1999; 117: 1045–9.

204. Boyce SW, Platia EV, Green WR. Drusen of the optic nerve head. Ann Ophthalmol 1978; 10: 695–704.

205. Friedman DH, Henkind P, Gartner S. Drusen of the optic disc: a histopathological study. Trans Ophthalmol Soc UK 1975; 95: 4–9.

206. Mansour AM, Hamed LM. Racial variation of optic nerve disease. Neuro-ophthalmology 1991; 11: 319–23.

207. Mullie MA, Sanders MD. Scleral canal size and optic nerve head drusen. Am J Ophthalmol 1985; 99: 356–9.

208. Spencer WH. Drusen of the optic disc and aberrant axoplasmic transport. Am J Ophthalmol 1978; 85; 1–12.

209. Seitz R, Kersting G. Die drusen der sehnervenpapille und des pigmentphitels. Klin Monatsbl Augenheilkd 1962; 140: 75–88.

210. Seitz R. Die intraocular drusen. Klin Montasbl Augenheilkd 1968; 152: 203.

211. Sacks JG, O'Grady RB, Choromokos E, et al. The pathogenesis of optic nerve drusen. A hypothesis. Arch Ophthalmol 1977; 95: 425–8.

212. Tso MO. Pathology and pathogenesis of drusen of the optic nervehead. Ophthalmology 1981; 88: 1066–80.

CHAPTER 60 Hereditary Optic Neuropathies

Valérie Biousse and Nancy J Newman

The hereditary optic neuropathies comprise a group of disorders in which the cause of optic nerve dysfunction appears to be hereditary based on familial expression or genetic analysis. Clinical variability, both within and among families with the same disease, often makes recognition and classification difficult.[1] Inherited optic neuropathies are often classified by pattern of transmission. The most common patterns of inheritance include autosomal dominant, autosomal recessive, and maternal (mitochondrial). The same genetic defect may not be responsible for all pedigrees with optic neuropathy inherited in a similar fashion. Similarly, different genetic defects may cause identical or similar phenotypes–some inherited in the same manner, others not. Alternatively, the same genetic defect may result in different clinical expression, although the pattern of inheritance should be consistent. Also, single cases are often presumed or proven to be caused by inherited genetic defects, making the pattern of familial transmission unavailable as an aid in classification.[1]

The inherited optic neuropathies typically manifest as symmetric, bilateral, painless, central visual loss (Table 60.1). In many of these disorders, the papillomacular nerve fiber bundle is affected, with resultant central or cecocentral scotomas. The exact location of initial pathology along the ganglion cell and its axon, and the pathophysiologic mechanisms of optic nerve injury remain unknown.

Optic nerve damage is usually permanent and, in many diseases, may be progressive. Once optic atrophy is observed, substantial nerve injury has already occurred.[1]

In some of the hereditary optic neuropathies, optic nerve dysfunction is typically isolated. In others, various neurologic and systemic abnormalities are regularly observed. Furthermore, inherited diseases with primarily neurologic or systemic manifestations, such as the multisystem degenerations, can include optic atrophy. In this chapter the hereditary optic neuropathies are arbitrarily classified into three major groups:

1. Those that occur primarily without associated neurologic or systemic signs;

2. Those that frequently have associated neurologic or systemic signs; and

3. Those in which the optic neuropathy is secondary in the overall disease process.

As more specific genetic defects are discovered, our concept of the phenotypes of these disorders will likely change, as will our classification.

MONOSYMPTOMATIC HEREDITARY OPTIC NEUROPATHIES

Leber hereditary optic neuropathy (LHON)

LHON is one of the first diseases to be etiologically linked to specific mitochondrial DNA (mtDNA) defects.[2] It is the most common mitochondrial disease with bilateral optic atrophy.[3,4] LHON is expressed predominantly in males of the lineage, but the greater susceptibility of males to visual loss in LHON remains unexplained. Age of onset typically occurs between 15 and 35, but may range from 1 to 80 years. Variability is seen even among members of the same pedigree.[1,5] Visual loss is painless, central, and occurs in one eye weeks to months before second eye involvement. Vision worsens in each eye over weeks or months, and often deteriorates to acuities of 20/200 or worse. Color vision is affected early and severely, and visual fields typically show central or cecocentral defects. Funduscopic abnormalities may be seen in patients with LHON and in their asymptomatic maternal relatives. Especially during the acute phase of visual loss, there may be hyperemia of the optic nerve head, dilation and tortuosity of vessels, hemorrhages, circumpapillary telangiectatic microangiopathy, or circumpapillary nerve fiber layer swelling (pseudoedema) (Fig. 60.1). Eventually, the only fundus findings will be optic atrophy with nerve fiber layer dropout, especially in the papillomacular bundle. There may be nonglaucomatous cupping of the disc and arterial attenuation.[1,5] In most LHON patients, visual loss is the only manifestation of the disease. Some

Table 60.1 Monosymptomatic hereditary optic neuropathies–characteristics and genetic defects

	Age of onset (years)	Other signs	First sign	Pattern of inheritance	Genetic defect
Leber's optic neuropathy	15–35	Heart block "Leber's plus"	Visual loss	Maternal	Mitochondrial DNA point mutations Primary mutations (11778, 3460, 14484)
Dominant optic atrophy (Kjer)	4–6	None	Visual loss	Autosomal dominant	Chromosomes 3q and 18 q
Congenital recessive optic atrophy	Birth–4	None	Visual loss	Autosomal recessive	?
Apparent sex-linked optic atrophy	Early childhood	? Retinopathy	Visual loss	X-linked recessive	Xp11.4–11.2

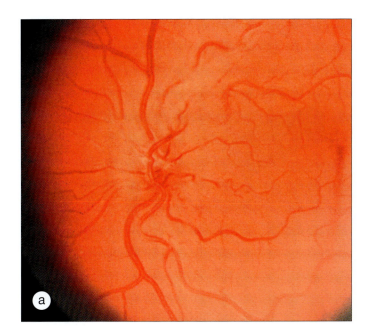

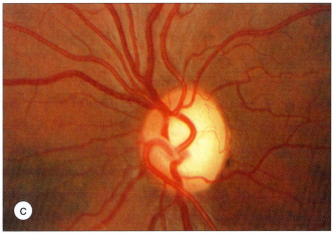

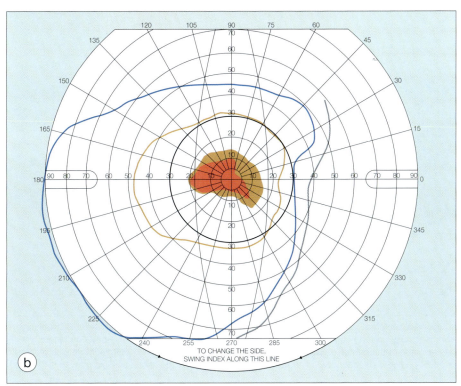

Fig. 60.1 Leber hereditary optic neuropathy.
(a) Left fundus at the time of visual loss showing
mild hyperemia of the optic discs with
peripapillary telangiectasias. (b) Goldmann visual
field demonstrating a central scotoma in the left
eye. (c) Left optic disc pallor with cupping
5 months after visual loss in a patient with Leber's
hereditary optic neuropathy.

pedigrees have family members with associated cardiac conduction abnormalities, especially preexcitation syndromes.[1-5] Minor neurologic and skeletal abnormalities have been reported in some patients, as has like disease.[1,6]

Ancillary tests in LHON are of limited clinical value. Fluorescein angiography may help distinguish the LHON optic disc from true disc edema. Electrocardiograms may show cardiac conduction abnormalities. Visually evoked responses are predictably abnormal when there is visual loss. Standard flash electroretinograms are typically normal. Electroencephalograms, cerebrospinal fluid, and brain CT and MRI are generally unremarkable. MRI has shown optic nerve enhancement acutely in rarely affected LHON

patients and bright T2 lesions in the late phases.[1] Phosphorus-31 magnetic resonance spectroscopy has suggested impaired mitochondrial metabolism within several LHON patients' limb muscles and occipital lobes.[1] Deficiency in respiratory chain complex I function has been demonstrated in muscle and blood samples of some LHON patients.[1]

LHON pedigrees follow a maternal inheritance pattern, and the disease has been linked to point mutations in the mtDNA[1,2,7,8] (Fig. 60.2). Three point mutations in the mtDNA, known as the "primary LHON mutations," are believed to cause 90–95% of cases of LHON worldwide. They are located at mtDNA nucleotide positions 11778 (69% of cases), 3460 (13% of cases),

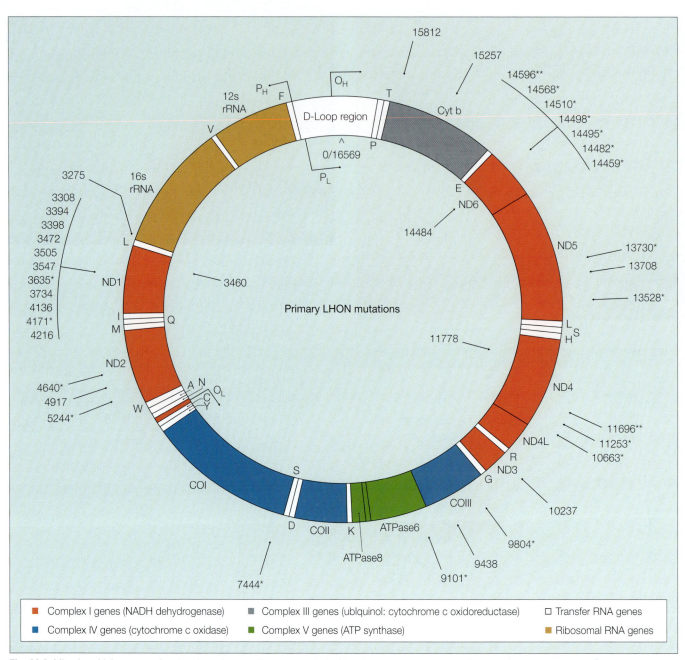

Fig. 60.2 Mitochondrial genome showing the point mutations associated with Leber's optic neuropathy. Over 90% of all cases of LHON are associated with the three primary mutations located inside the genome (circle), and the other mutations are shown outside the genome. These other mutations vary markedly in their prevalence, degree of evolutionary conservation of the encoded amino acids altered, and frequency among controls. Mutations marked * may be primary, but they each account for only one or a few pedigrees worldwide. Mutations marked ** are primary mutations associated with LHON and dystonia. (Adapted from Newman.)[10]

and 14484 (14% of cases)[1,2,7–10] (Fig. 60.2). Other point mutations have been found with a greater frequency in LHON patients than controls, but caution must be taken in assuming a causal significance for these secondary mutations. Some may truly be primary mutations but account for only a few pedigrees worldwide.[1,2,5–10] Others' pathogenic significance remains unclear.[1,10] Screening for LHON in a patient with visual loss should begin with the three primary mutations. In those primary mutation-negative patients in whom suspicion remains high, testing for the other mtDNA mutations associated with LHON is srobably warranted, especially for those mutations deemed likely to be causal in a few pedigrees.[1,9,10] Alternatively, since the majority of these other mtDNA mutations reside in genes

encoding subunits of complex I, complete sequencing of complex I, perhaps beginning with the so-called "hot spot" *ND6* gene,[10] might also be considered. Finally, sequencing the entire mitochondrial genome is possible, although labor intensive. This should be performed only in those cases of high suspicion, and interpreted by someone versed in the complexities of mitochondrial genetics.[1,10]

Among the primary mutations, the LHON clinical phenotype is remarkably similar. The only consistent differentiating feature is the better prognosis for visual outcome in those patients with the 14484 mutation.[11] Up to 60% of patients with the 14484 mutation will have some degree of visual improvement compared to only 5% of patients with the 11778 mutation.[1,11] Patients with the 3460 mutation may have a better chance of visual recovery than those with the 11778 mutation, but the numbers of patients are too small for meaningful analysis.[1,11] Patients with a younger age of onset of visual loss, especially less than 15 years, have a much better visual prognosis.[1,11]

The genetic defects, however, cannot fully explain the determinants of expression in this disease. The presence of a mtDNA mutation is necessary for phenotypic expression, but it is not sufficient.[1,7,10,12] The presence of heteroplasmy (the co-existence of both mutant and normal mtDNA) may be a factor in expression.[1,7,10,12] In heteroplasmic pedigrees, individuals with a greater amount of mutant mtDNA may be at higher risk for visual loss. However, many individuals with 100% mutant mtDNA never suffer visual loss.[1,7,10,12] The interaction of genetic, mitochondrial or nuclear, and environmental factors may complicate the issue of assigning a pathogenic role to individual mtDNA mutations.[10] Other mitochondrial or nuclear DNA factors may modify expression of the disease, including X-linkage. Various environmental triggers for the development of visual loss in LHON have been suggested.[1,2,10,13] Systemic illnesses, nutritional deficiencies, head trauma, or toxins that stress the organism's mitochondrial energy production might be detrimental to those individuals already genetically at risk for mitochondrial energy deficiency. However, a large recent case-control study showed no association between tobacco or alcohol consumption and visual loss among individuals harboring LHON primary mutations.[13]

The pathophysiology of LHON remains unknown.[10] It may involve abnormal oxidative phosphorylation and deficient generation of ATP, either directly or indirectly related to free radical production, resulting in irreversible damage to the ganglion cells and their axons.[1,7,10,12] The reason these mechanisms result in selective damage to the optic nerve remains uncertain.[10,14] Histochemical studies of the optic nerve in animals have shown a high degree of mitochondrial respiratory activity within the unmyelinated, prelaminar portion of the optic nerve, suggesting a particular high requirement for mitochondrial function in this region.[1,14] Of great interest is the recent identification of a genetically-induced mouse model of complex I deficiency that shows the histopathological features of optic nerve degeneration seen in LHON patients.[15,16] Further development of mouse models for mitochondrial diseases should better facilitate the understanding of the pathogenesis of human mitochondrial disorders.[17]

Therapies tried in the treatment of LHON include coenzyme Q_{10}, idebenone, L-carnitine, succinate, dichloroacetate, vitamin K_1, vitamin K_3, vitamin C, thiamine, vitamin B_2, and vitamin E.[1] However, irreversible damage makes optic atrophy unlikely candidates for a good response to any therapy. Avoiding agents that might stress mitochondrial energy production is a nonspecific recommendation with no proven benefit. However, the authors suggest that their patients avoid tobacco, cyanide-containing products, excessive alcohol, and environmental toxins. Symptomatic therapies include pacemakers in the patient with heart block or serious cardiac conduction defects and low-vision aids for the patient with severe visual loss. As the specific genetic and biochemical abnormalities are better defined, more directed therapies may be created to replace or bypass the genetic or metabolic deficiencies in patients with the disease and in their relatives at risk. A promising form of gene therapy known as allotypic expression may play a future role in the therapy of LHON and other mitochondrial diseases.[16] Meanwhile, one should not underestimate the importance of informed genetic counseling among family members.[18]

Dominant optic atrophy

Autosomal dominant ("Kjer type") optic atrophy is the most common of the hereditary optic neuropathies, with an estimated disease prevalence in the range of 1:50 000 or as high as 1:10 000 in Denmark.[1,19]

Although it is difficult for patients to identify a precise onset of reduced vision, the majority of affected patients date the onset of visual symptoms between 4 and 6 years of age. Rarely, severely affected individuals are noted to have visual difficulties and sensory nystagmus prior to beginning schooling. Many patients are unaware of a visual problem and are discovered to have optic atrophy as a direct consequence of examination of other affected family members. These phenomena attest to the usually imperceptible onset in childhood, mild degree of visual dysfunction, absence of night-blindness, and absence of substantial or dramatic progression.[1,19] Visual acuity is usually reduced to the same mild extent in both eyes. Acuities range from 20/20 to 20/800, with only about 15% of patients with vision of 20/200 or worse. Hand motion or light perception vision is extremely rare. There is considerable interfamilial and intrafamilial variation in acuities. Although blue-yellow defects are classic in patients with dominant optic atrophy, a mixed color deficit is most common. There is no correlation between the severity of the dyschromatopsia and the visual acuity. Visual fields in patients with dominant optic atrophy characteristically show central, para-central, or cecocentral scotomas. Rarely, a visual field pattern with bitemporal depression may be seen, mimicking the field defects of chiasmal compression. The optic atrophy in patients with dominantly inherited optic neuropathy may be subtle, temporal only, or involve the entire disc (Fig. 60.3). The most characteristic change is a translucent pallor with the absence of fine superficial capillaries of the temporal aspect of the disc, and a peculiar triangular excavation of the temporal portion of the disc. Other ophthalmoscopic findings reported in these patients include peripapillary atrophy, absent foveal reflex, mild macular pigmentary changes, arterial attenuation, and nonglaucomatous cupping.[1,19] Although there are dominantly inherited syndromes of optic atrophy associated with neurologic dysfunction (see below), most of the patients with the syndrome of autosomal dominant optic atrophy have no additional neurologic deficits. Mild hearing loss has been reported in some families.[1]

Dominant optic atrophy is believed to be a primary degeneration of the retinal ganglion cells. The predominant gene is localized on the long arm of chromosome 3 3q28–q29.[1,20] This nuclear gene (called OPA1) is widely expressed and is most abundant in the retina. It encodes a dynamin-related protein localized to the mitochondria, suggesting a role for mitochondria in retinal ganglion cell pathophysiology.[1,20] Kerrison et al. recently identified a second locus for dominant optic atrophy on chromosome 18q, thereby demonstrating genetic heterogeneity.[21] Interestingly, linkage analysis of patients with normal tension glaucoma has shown an association with polymorphisms of the OPA1 gene.[22]

Congenital recessive optic atrophy

This form of optic atrophy is present at birth or develops at an early age and is usually discovered before the patient is 3 or 4 years of age. It is presumed to have autosomal recessive transmission and there is often consanguinity between parents. The visual acuity is so severely affected that the patient may be completely blind with sensory nystagmus. The visual fields show variable constriction, and there are often paracentral scotomas. The optic discs are

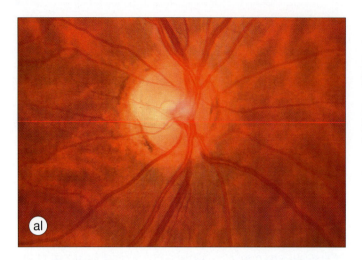

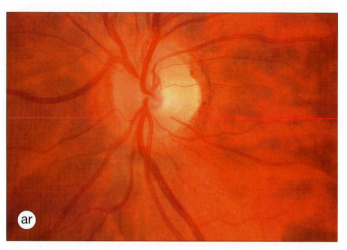

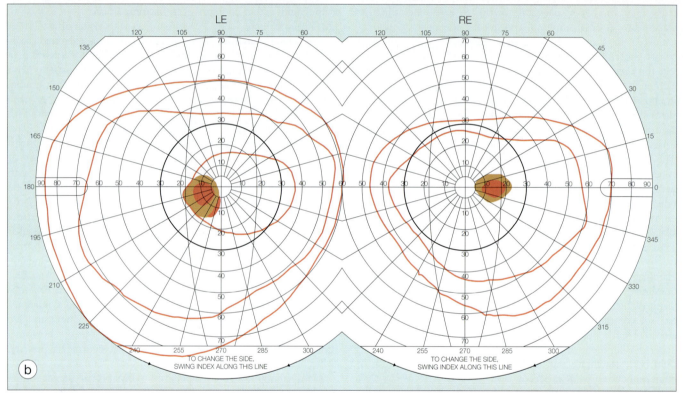

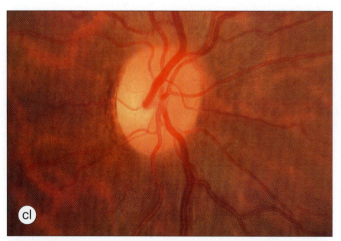

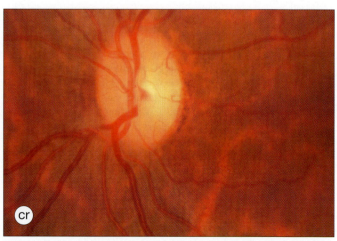

Fig. 60.3 Dominant optic atrophy. (a) Funduscopy showing bilateral temporal pallor with excavated appearance. (b) Goldmann visual field showing bilateral cecocentral scotomas (depression). Dominant optic atrophy. (c) Funduscopy of the above patient's mother who is asymptomatic. Note the temporal pallor of both optic discs.

completely atrophic and often deeply cupped. By funduscopic appearance alone, it is difficult to differentiate this entity from infantile tapetoretinal degeneration, making electroretinography important. This form of optic atrophy is extremely rare.[1]

Apparent sex-linked optic atrophy

Pedigrees with optic atrophy inherited in a documented sex-linked fashion are extremely rare. In the few cases described, neurologic and even retinal abnormalities were often present, making the designation of this disorder as a distinct sex-linked optic atrophy problematic.[1]

HEREDITARY OPTIC ATROPHY WITH OTHER NEUROLOGIC OR SYSTEMIC SIGNS
(see Table 60.2)

Autosomal dominant progressive optic atrophy and deafness

Several pedigrees with presumed autosomal dominant optic atrophy and hearing loss have been described. In all of the cases,

there were no systemic or neurologic abnormalities except for sensorineural hearing loss. The hearing loss in these pedigrees may be severe at birth with few patients developing speech. Although visual dysfunction may be present at an early age, most of the patients had normal acuity until their third decade. In most cases, visual loss remains better than 20/200. In one Turkish family, linkage analysis excluded the two known genes associated with autosomal dominant optic atrophy.[1]

Autosomal dominant progressive optic atrophy with progressive hearing loss and ataxia

In this rare syndrome, progressive bilateral optic atrophy and hearing loss are associated with ataxia and limb weakness. The onset of visual loss is between $2\frac{1}{2}$ and 9 years of age. The hearing loss is only moderate and slowly progressive. The acronym CAPOS (cerebellar ataxia, areflexia, pes cavus, and sensorineural deafness) has been suggested.[1]

Table 60.2 Hereditary optic atrophy with other neurologic or systemic signs–characteristics and genetic defects

	Age of onset (years)	Other signs	First sign	Pattern of inheritance	Genetic defect
Autosomal dominant progressive optic atrophy and deafness	Birth	Hearing loss	Hearing loss 3rd decade visual loss	Autosomal dominant	?
Autosomal dominant progressive optic atrophy with progressive hearing loss and ataxia	2.5–9	Hearing loss Ataxia	Visual loss	Autosomal dominant	?
Hereditary optic atrophy with progressive hearing loss and polyneuropathy	1st decade	Hearing loss Polyneuropathy	Visual loss	?	?
Opticocochleodendate degeneration	Infancy	Hearing loss Spastic quadriplegia Mental retardation Death in childhood	Visual loss	Autosomal recessive	?
Sex-linked recessive optic atrophy, ataxia, deafness, tetraplegia, and areflexia	Infancy	Hearing loss Flaccid tetraplegia Areflexia	Tetraplegia	X-linked	?
Opticoacoustic nerve atrophy with dementia	Infancy	Hearing loss Dementia in adulthood	Hearing loss Visual loss 3rd decade	? X-linked	? Mitochondrial disease
Wolfram/DIDMOAD syndrome	1st–2nd decade	Diabetes insipidus Diabetes mellitus Hearing loss Urinary tract atonia	Diabetes mellitus	Autosomal recessive ? Maternal	Chromosome 4p ? Nuclear or mitochondrial genome
Dominant optic atrophy, deafness, ophthalmoplegia, and myopathy	1st decade	Hearing loss Ophthalmoplegia Myopathy	Visual loss	Autosomal dominant	? Mitochondrial disease
PEHO syndrome	First 6 months	Encephalopathy Hypsarrhythmia	Encephalopathy Optic atrophy at 1–2 y	Autosomal recessive	?
Behr syndrome	<10	Spastic paraparesis Ataxia Mental retardation Pes cavus	Visual loss	Autosomal recessive	?

PEHO: Progressive encephalopathy with Edema, Hypsarrhythmia, and Optic atrophy
DIDMOAD: Diabetes Insipidus, Diabetes Mellitus, Optic Atrophy, and Deafness

Hereditary optic atrophy with progressive hearing loss and polyneuropathy

Several pedigrees in which progressive optic atrophy is accompanied by sensorineural deafness and symptomatic or asymptomatic polyneuropathy have been described. The affected individuals vary in the extent of visual and neurologic impairment, and different modes of inheritance, including autosomal dominant, autosomal recessive, and X-linked recessive, have been proposed.[1]

Autosomal recessive optic atrophy with progressive hearing loss, spastic quadriplegia, mental deterioration, and death (opticocochleodentate degeneration)

In this autosomal recessive syndrome, severe optic atrophy begins in infancy and is associated with progressive hearing loss. Progressive spastic quadriplegia and progressive mental deterioration result in death in childhood. All patients have a selective, systematized degeneration of the optic, cochlear, dentate, and medial lemniscal systems without involvement of the basal ganglia.[1]

Sex-linked recessive optic atrophy, ataxia, deafness, tetraplegia, and areflexia

Affected family members of a single Dutch family had optic atrophy, ataxia, deafness, flaccid tetraplegia, and areflexia. The course was generally progressive to death. It followed an X-linked recessive inheritance pattern.[1]

Opticoacoustic nerve atrophy with dementia

This very rare syndrome is characterized by severe sensorineural hearing loss with onset in infancy, followed by progressive optic atrophy in the second or third decade and progressive dementia in adulthood. An X-linked recessive inheritance has been proposed, but mitochondrial inheritance is also possible.[1]

Progressive optic atrophy with juvenile diabetes mellitus, diabetes insipidus, and hearing loss (Wolfram syndrome, DIDMOAD)

The hallmark of this syndrome is the association of juvenile diabetes mellitus and progressive visual loss with optic atrophy, almost always associated with diabetes insipidus, neurosensory hearing loss, or both (hence, the eponym DIDMOAD for diabetes insipidus, diabetes mellitus, optic atrophy, and deafness).[1,23] Diabetes mellitus usually develops within the first or second decade of life and usually precedes the development of optic atrophy. In several cases, however, visual loss with optic atrophy is the first sign of the syndrome. In the early stages, visual acuity may be normal despite mild dyschromatopsia and optic atrophy. In later stages, visual loss becomes severe. Visual fields have shown both generalized constriction and central scotomas. Optic atrophy is uniformly severe (Fig. 60.4), and there may be mild to moderate cupping of the disc. Both hearing loss and diabetes insipidus begin in the first or second decade of life and may be quite severe. Atonia of the efferent urinary tract is present in half of patients and is associated with recurrent urinary tract infections, neurogenic incontinence, and even fatal complications. Other systemic and neurologic abnormalities

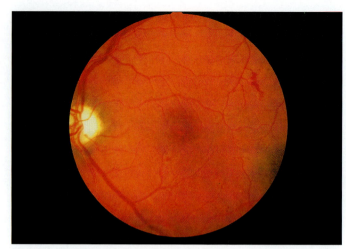

Fig. 60.4 DIDMOAD The optic disc is atrophic and there is retinal hemorrhage associated with the diabetes mellitus.

include ataxia, axial rigidity, seizures, startle myoclonus, tremor, gastrointestinal dysmotility, vestibular malfunction, central apnea, neurogenic upper airway collapse, ptosis, cataracts, pigmentary retinopathy, iritis, lacrimal hyposecretion, Adie's pupil, ophthalmoplegia, convergence insufficiency, vertical gaze palsy, nystagmus, mental retardation, psychiatric abnormalities, short stature, primary gonadal atrophy, other endocrine abnormalities, anosmia, megaloblastic and sideroblastic anemia, abnormal electroretinography, and elevated CSF protein. Neuroimaging and pathology in some patients reveal widespread atrophic changes and suggest a diffuse neurodegenerative disorder, with particular involvement of the midbrain and pons.

Many of the associated abnormalities reported in Wolfram syndrome are commonly encountered in patients with presumed mitochondrial diseases, especially those patients with the chronic progressive external ophthalmoplegia syndromes. This has led to speculation that the Wolfram phenotype may be nonspecific and reflect a wide variety of underlying genetic defects in either the nuclear or mitochondrial genomes. Indeed, most cases of Wolfram have been classified as sporadic or recessively inherited, the latter usually concluded from sibling expression (which is now known to also occur from maternal transmission). Linkage analysis in several families suggests localization of a Wolfram gene to the short arm of chromosome 4. The gene responsible at this locus has been designated *WFS1*, in which multiple point mutations and deletions have been identified. When the syndrome is accompanied by anemia, treatment with thiamine may ameliorate the anemia and decrease the insulin requirement.[1,23]

Dominant optic atrophy, deafness, ophthalmoplegia, and myopathy

This is a rare syndrome characterized by optic atrophy, deafness, ptosis, ophthalmoplegia, dystaxia, and myopathy. The visual loss occurs in the first decade and progresses to the 20/30 to 20/400 range. The electroretinogram is abnormal, although retinal pigmentary changes are absent. Hearing loss is sensorineural and progressive, with onset in the first or second decade. Ophthalmoplegia and myopathy occur in midlife. Male-to-male transmission confirms autosomal dominant inheritance, but this disorder may represent a mitochondrial disease secondary to a nuclear genetic abnormality.[1]

Progressive encephalopathy with edema, hypsarrhythmia, and optic atrophy (PEHO syndrome)

Several families have been described with a progressive encephalopathy with onset in the first 6 months of life, followed by severe hypotonia, convulsions with hypsarrhythmia, profound mental deterioration, hyperreflexia, transient or persistent facial and body edema, and optic atrophy. Optic atrophy is usually noted by the first or second year of life and nystagmus is common. A metabolic defect has yet to be determined and an autosomal recessive mode of inheritance is likely.[1] This could be considered a form of Behr syndrome, which likely represents a heterogeneous group of disorders (see next section).

Complicated hereditary infantile optic atrophy (Behr syndrome)

In this heredofamilial syndrome, optic atrophy beginning in early childhood is associated with variable pyramidal tract signs, ataxia, mental retardation, urinary incontinence, and pes cavus. Both sexes are affected and the syndrome is usually inherited as an autosomal recessive trait. Visual loss usually manifests before age 10 years, is moderate to severe, and is frequently accompanied by nystagmus. In most cases, the abnormalities do not progress after childhood. Neuroimaging may demonstrate diffuse symmetric white matter abnormalities. Clinical findings in some patients with Behr syndrome may be similar to those in cases of hereditary ataxia. Behr syndrome is likely heterogeneous, reflecting different etiologic and genetic factors.[1]

OPTIC NEUROPATHY AS A MANIFESTATION OF HEREDITARY DEGENERATIVE OR DEVELOPMENTAL DISEASES (see Table 60.3)

Hereditary ataxias

The hereditary ataxias comprise a group of chronic progressive neurodegenerative conditions involving the cerebellum and its connections, and are sometimes associated with optic atrophy. A genomic classification by chromosomal location is available for many of these disorders and the abnormal gene products involved are under investigation.[1,24–26]

Friedreich ataxia is inherited in an autosomal recessive manner, and the gene defect has been localized to the proximal long arm of the ninth chromosome (9q13–q21). The majority of cases are homozygous for a GAA trinucleotide expansion in a gene designated *FRDA/X25* that codes for a protein called frataxin, which regulates iron levels in the mitochondria.[1,26] The disease usually begins during the second decade of life and includes progressive ataxia, dysarthria, loss of joint position and vibratory sensation, absent lower extremity tendon reflexes, and extensor

Table 60.3 Optic neuropathy as manifestation of hereditary degenerative or developmental diseases–characteristics and genetic defects

	Age of onset (years)	Other signs	First sign	Pattern of inheritance	Genetic defect
Hereditary ataxias					
Friedreich's ataxia	8–15	Ataxia Loss of vibratory sensation Extensor plantar response	Ataxia	Autosomal recessive	Chromosome 9q
Spinocerebellar ataxias	2nd decade	Ataxia ophthalmoplegia Basal ganglia symptoms	Ataxia	Autosomal dominant	Variable depending on the type of SCA
Hereditary polyneuropathies					
Charcot-Marie-Tooth disease	1st and 2nd decade	Polyneuropathy	Polyneuropathy	Mendelian	Variable depending on the type of CMT ?
Familial dysautonomia (Riley-Day syndrome)	2nd decade	Polyneuropathy with autonomic dysfunction	Polyneuropathy	Autosomal recessive	
Storage diseases and cerebral degenerations of childhood (see Table 60.4)					
Mitochondrial diseases of childhood Leigh syndrome	2mo–6y	Ataxia Encephalopathy Seizures Polyneuropathy Retinopathy	Encephalopathy	Maternal Autosomal recessive X-linked	MtDNA point mutations (especially 8993T-C) ? ?
MELAS syndrome	1st or 2nd decade	Headaches Stroke-like episodes Seizures Lactic acidosis	Neurologic	Maternal	MtDNA point mutations (especially 3243A-G)
MERFF syndrome	1st or 2nd decade	Myoclonus Seizures Myopathy Ataxia Dementia	Neurologic	Maternal	MtDNA point mutations (8344A-G)
CPEO/KSS syndrome	1st or 2nd decade	Myopathy Ophthalmoplegia Ptosis	Ophthalmoplegia	Maternal	MtDNA rearrangements (especially deletions)

CPEO: Chronic progressive external ophthalmoplegia.
KSS: Kearns-Sayre syndrome.
MELAS: Mitochondrial myopathy, encephalopathy, lactic acidosis, and stroke-like episodes.
MERFF: Myoclonic epilepsy and ragged red fibers.

Table 60.4 Familial-storage diseases and cerebral degenerations of childhood associated with optic neuropathies

Mucopolysaccharidoses (MPS IH, IS, IHS, IIA, IIB, IIIA, IIIB, IV, VI)
Lipidoses (infantile and juvenile GM1-1 and GM1-2, GM2, infantile Niemann-Pick disease)
Metachromatic leukodystrophy
Krabbe's disease
Adrenoleukodystrophy
Zellweger syndrome
Pelizaeus-Merzbacher disease
Infantile neuroaxonal dystrophy
Hallervorden-Spatz disease
Menkes syndrome
Canavan's disease
Cockayne syndrome
COFS
Allgrove syndrome ("4A")
Smith-Lemli-Opitz syndrome
GAPO syndrome
Cerebral palsy

MPS IH: Hurler; MPS IS: Sheie; MPS HIS: Hurler-Sheie; MPS IIA and IIB: Hunter; MPS IIIA and IIIB: Sanfilippo; MPS IV: Morquio; MPS VI: Maroteaux-Lamy.
GM1-Gangliosidoses: GM1-1 and GM1-2.
GM2-Gangliosidoses: Tay-Sachs disease, Sandhoff disease, late infantile, juvenile and adult GM2-Gangliosidose
COFS: Cerebro-oculo-facio-skeletal syndrome
"4A": Alacrine, achalasia, autonomic disturbance, and ACTH insensitivity.
GAPO: Growth retardation, alopecia, pseudoanodontia, and optic atrophy.

plantar responses. Scoliosis, foot deformity, diabetes mellitus, and cardiac disease are common. Other manifestations include pes cavus, distal wasting, deafness, nystagmus, eye movement abnormalities consistent with abnormal cerebellar function, and optic atrophy. The course is progressive, with most patients unable to walk within 15 years of onset, and death from infectious or cardiac causes usually in the fourth or fifth decade. A later-onset, more slowly progressive form has also been described. Optic atrophy is present in up to 50% of cases of Friedreich ataxia, although severe visual loss is uncommon. A condition resembling Friedreich ataxia associated with decreased vitamin E levels has been localized to chromosome 8. Vitamin E supplementation of these patients may be efficacious early in the course of the disease.[1]

The spinocerebellar ataxias, previously called olivopontocerebellar atrophy (OPCA) and autosomal dominant cerebellar ataxia, include a group of hereditary ataxic disorders in which the ataxia is related more to degeneration of the cerebellum than rather than the spinal cord.[1,25,26] As of 2003, there were at least 23 different genetic loci for SCAs (SCA1 to SCA17). The combination of SCA1 (chromosome 6p), SCA2 (chromosome 12q), SCA3 (chromosome 14q), SCA6 (chromosome 19p), and SCA7 (chromosome 3p) comprises approximately 80% of the autosomal dominant ataxias.[1,26] Many of the SCAs are caused by mutations involving the expansion of a CAG trinucleotide repeat in the protein-coding sequences of specific genes. As with other diseases that involve abnormal repeats, the expanded regions can become larger with each successive generation, resulting in a younger age of onset in each generation, so-called anticipation.[1] Clinically, the SCAs are characterized by signs and symptoms attributable to cerebellar degeneration and sometimes other neurologic dysfunction secondary to neuronal loss. Loss of vision is usually mild but may be a prominent symptom, occurring in association with constricted visual fields and diffuse optic atrophy. However, it is not clear in some cases whether the primary process is retinal with secondary optic atrophy or

primarily involving the optic nerve. SCA7 is specifically associated with retinal degeneration.

Hereditary polyneuropathies

Charcot-Marie-Tooth disease (CMT) encompasses a group of heredofamilial disorders characterized by progressive muscular weakness and atrophy that begins during the first two decades of life.[1] This group of hereditary polyneuropathies accounts for 90% of all hereditary neuropathies, with the prevalence in the United States being about 40 per 100 000. Most forms of CMT begin between the ages of 2 and 15 years, and the first signs may be pes cavus, foot deformities, or scoliosis. There is slowly progressive weakness and wasting, first of the feet and legs, and then of the hands. Motor symptoms predominate over sensory abnormalities. As of 2002, causative mutations for the hereditary peripheral neuropathies have been identified in 17 different genes.[1] Numerous patients with CMT and optic atrophy have been reported. Associated visual loss, if present, is usually mild. However, taking into account both electrophysiologic and clinical data, up to 75% of patients with CMT have some afferent visual pathway dysfunction, demonstrating that subclinical optic neuropathy may occur in a high proportion of patients with CMT. Pedigrees specifically designated CMT type 6 show a regular association of CMT and optic atrophy. This type of CMT is as yet genetically unspecified and may prove genetically heterogeneous.[1]

Familial dysautonomia (Riley-Day syndrome) is an autosomal recessive disease that almost exclusively affects Ashkenazi Jews. Abnormalities of the peripheral nervous system cause the clinical manifestations of sensory and autonomic dysfunction. Optic atrophy is very common in patients with familial dysautonomia, usually noted after the first decade of life. However, in most cases, early mortality from the disease probably precludes the later development of optic atrophy.[1]

Hereditary spastic paraplegias

The hereditary spastic paraplegias (Strumpell-Lorrain disease) are autosomal dominant disorders characterized by progressive spasticity of the lower limbs and pathological reflexes with degeneration or demyelination of the corticospinal system and of the spinocerebellar system. Optic neuropathies with visual acuities ranging from 20/20 to 20/200 have been reported in a small number of patients with this disease.[1]

Hereditary muscular dystrophies

Myotonic dystrophy is a relatively common autosomal dominant disorder with a prevalence of 1 in 20 000, characterized by progressive myopathy, ptosis, cataracts, cardiomyopathy with conduction defects, frontal balding, bifacial weakness, and diabetes mellitus. Less common ophthalmic manifestations include external ophthalmoplegia, pigmentary retinopathy, and optic atrophy.[1,26] Most patients with myotonic dystrophy have an expansion of a CTG repeat in a protein kinase gene on chromosome 19q13.3.

Storage diseases and cerebral degenerations of childhood

About 100 inherited metabolic diseases with ocular manifestations have been described and some are detailed in Chapter 65 (see also Table 60.4).

Children with cerebral palsy have a higher prevalence of ocular defects than normal children. In one study, optic atrophy was found in 10% of children with cerebral palsy. The etiology for the atrophy in these patients was not explained, nor were the clinical characteristics of the patients elucidated.[1]

Mitochondrial disorders

The subacute necrotizing encephalomyelopathy of Leigh results from multiple different biochemical defects that all impair cerebral oxidative metabolism.[1,3,4] This disorder may be inherited in an autosomal recessive, X-linked, or maternal pattern, depending on the genetic defect. The onset of symptoms is typically between the ages of 2 months and 6 years, and consists of progressive deterioration of brainstem functions, ataxia, seizures, peripheral neuropathy, intellectual deterioration, impaired hearing, and poor vision. Visual loss may be secondary to optic atrophy or retinal degeneration. The syndrome of Leigh is likely a nonspecific phenotypic response to certain abnormalities of mitochondrial energy production.[1,3,4]

Other presumed mitochondrial disorders of both nuclear and mitochondrial genomic origins may manifest optic atrophy as a secondary clinical feature, often a variable manifestation of the disease.[1,3,4] Examples include cases of MERRF, MELAS, and chronic progressive external ophthalmoplegia, both with and without the full Kearns-Sayre phenotype. The other, more constant, phenotypic characteristics of all of these mitochondrial disorders distinguish them from diseases such as Leber optic neuropathy in which visual loss from optic nerve dysfunction is the primary manifestation of the disorder.[1,3,4]

ACKNOWLEDGMENTS

This study was supported in part by a departmental grant (Department of Ophthalmology) from Research to Prevent Blindness, Inc., New York, NY, and by Core Grant P30-EY06360 (Department of Ophthalmology) from the National Institutes of Health, Bethesda, MD. Dr Newman is a recipient of a Research to Prevent Blindness Lew R. Wasserman Merit Award.

REFERENCES

1. Newman NJ. Hereditary optic neuropathies. In: Miller NR, Newman NJ, Biousse V, et al. editors. Walsh and Hoyt's Clinical Neuro-ophthalmology. 6th ed. Baltimore, MD: Williams & Wilkins. In press.
2. Wallace DC, Singh G, Lott MT, et al. Mitochondrial DNA mutation associated with Leber's hereditary optic neuropathy. Science 1988; 242: 1427–30.
3. Phillips PH, Newman NJ. Mitochondrial diseases in pediatric ophthalmology. J AAPOS 1997; 1: 115–22.
4. Biousse V, Newman NJ. The neuro-ophthalmology of mitochondrial diseases. Sem Neurol 2001; 21: 275–91.
5. Man PY, Turnbull DM, Chinnery PF. Leber hereditary optic neuropathy. J Med Genet 2002; 39: 162–9.
6. Bhatti MT, Newman NJ. A multiple sclerosis-like illness in a man harboring the mtDNA 14484 mutation. J Neuro-ophthalmol 1999; 19: 28–33.
7. Brown MD. The enigmatic relationship between mitochondrial dysfunction and Leber's hereditary optic neuropathy. J Neurol Sci 1999; 165: 1–5.
8. Huopenen K. Leber hereditary optic neuropathy: clinical and molecular genetic findings. Neurogenetics 2001; 3: 119–25.
9. Chinnery PF, Howell N, Andrews RM, et al. Mitochondrial DNA analysis; polymorphisms and pathogenicity. J Med Genet 1999; 36: 505–10.
10. Newman NJ. From genotype to phenotype in Leber's hereditary optic neuropathy: still more questions than answers. J Neuro-ophthalmol 2002; 22: 257–61.
11. Nakamura M, Yamamoto M. Variable pattern of visual recovery of Leber's hereditary optic neuropathy. Br J Ophthalmol 2000; 84: 534–5.
12. Went LN. Leber hereditary optic neuropathy (LHON): a mitochondrial disease with unresolved complexities. Cytogenet Cell Genet 1999; 86: 153–6.
13. Kerrison JB, Miller NR, Hsu FC, et al. A case-control study of tobacco and alcohol consumption in Leber's hereditary optic neuropathy. Am J Ophthalmol 2000; 130: 803–12.

14. Bristow EA, Griffiths PG, Andrews RM, et al. The distribution of mitochondrial activity in relation to optic nerve structure. Arch Ophthalmol 2002; 120: 791–6.
15. Qi X, Lewin A, Hauswirth WW, et al. Suppression of complex I expression induces optic neuropathy. Ann Neurol 2003; 53: 198–205.
16. Guy J, Qi X, Pallotti F, et al. Rescue of a mitochondrial deficiency causing LHON. Ann Neurol 2003; 52: 534–42.
17. Biousse V, Pardue MT, Wallace DC, et al. The eyes of mito-mouse. Mouse models of mitochondrial disease. J Neuro-ophthalmol 2002; 22: 279–85.
18. Huoponen K, Puomila A, Savontaus ML, et al. Genetic counseling in Leber's hereditary optic neuropathy (LHON). Acta Ophthalmol Scand 2002; 80: 38–43.
19. Votruba M, Fitzke FW, Holder GE, et al. Clinical features in affected individuals from 21 pedigrees with dominant optic atrophy. Arch Ophthalmol 1998; 116: 351–8.
20. Delettre C, Lenaers G, Pelloquin L, et al. OPA1 (Kjer type) dominant optic atrophy: a novel mitochondrial disease. Mol Genet Metab 2002; 75: 97–107.
21. Kerrison JB, Arnould VJ, Ferraz Sallum JM, et al. Genetic heterogeneity of dominant optic atrophy, Kjer type: identification of a second locus on chromosome 18q12.2–12.3. Arch Ophthalmol 1999; 117: 805–10.
22. Aung T, Ocaka L, Poinoosawmy D, et al. The phenotype of normal tension glaucoma patients with and without OPA1 polymorphisms. Br J Ophthalmol 2003; 87: 149–52.
23. Barrett TG, Bundey SE, Macleod AF. Neurodegeneration and diabetes: UK nationwide survey of (Wolfram) DIDMOAD syndrome. Lancet 1995; 346: 1458–63.
24. Klockgether T, Wullner U, Spauschus A, et al. The molecular biology of the autosomal dominant cerebellar ataxias. Mov Disord 2000; 15: 604–12.
25. Abe T, Abe K, Aoki M, et al. Ocular changes in patients with spinocerebellar degeneration and repeated trinucleotide expansion of spinocerebellar ataxia type 1 gene. Arch Ophthalmol 1997; 115: 231–6.
26. Lynch Dr, Farmer JF. Practical approaches to neurogenetic disease. J Neuro-ophthalmol 2002; 22: 297–304.

CHAPTER 61 Other Optic Neuropathies

Creig S Hoyt

Childhood optic neuritis

Childhood optic neuritis is rare, but significant because of its presentation and the importance of the differential diagnosis. It probably occurs throughout childhood, but is rarely recognized in toddlers because any visual defect has to be very profound, and bilateral before the child is obviously abnormal to the parents. The most frequent age at presentation is 7 years; it probably occurs with equal sex distribution.[1] It is often bilateral.

The onset may be sudden, but it may develop over a few days with increasing visual difficulty. Smaller children often do not present until they are profoundly affected (Fig. 61.1) with some children saying they want lights put on in bright daylight, or that their parents have woken them in the night. Others have ataxia, actually due to blindness. The loss of acuity and color vision is usually profound; there is a central scotoma or diffuse visual field loss (Fig. 61.2). There is an afferent pupil defect that may be apparent to the parents, if the optic neuritis is bilateral and

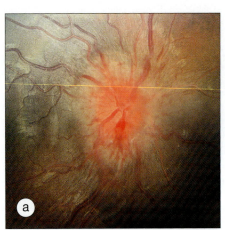
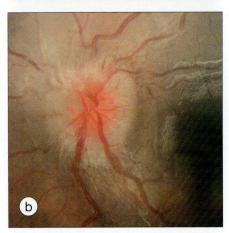

Fig. 61.1 Bilateral optic neuritis. The severely swollen right (a) and left (b) eye of a seven-year-old girl with bilateral optic neuritis. When she presented she was blind; after six weeks her acuities were 0.3 light, 0.4 left.

severe, as dilated pupils even in bright light. The optic discs are swollen in the majority,[1,2] (Fig. 61.3) marked in 53%.[2] Hemorrhages around the disc are rare and exudates unusual (Figs 61.4, 61.5). Fluorescein angiography of the discs in the acute phase shows dilated capillaries and leakage. When the optic disc is not swollen it is known as retrobulbar neuritis; if it is, it may be called papillitis.

The visual prognosis is excellent,[1-5] often with residual optic atrophy. High-dose systemic steroids sometimes bring about a dramatic and rapid visual improvement,[6] but long-term efficacy is unproven. Patients usually improve in days without treatment, and the steroids may just speed the improvement, most useful when the child is blind.

Unlike adults, the systemic prognosis is also good. Eighty per cent of children in one series had no subsequent neurological signs and no recurrence of optic neuritis.[2] Other series have reported a higher incidence of neurological problems, including multiple sclerosis,[7,8] varying with selection of the patients.

Patients with suspected optic neuritis should preferably be managed jointly with a neurologist, and further investigations should include neuroimaging especially MRI scanning, cerebrospinal fluid studies, sinus X-ray, hematology and studies for infectious diseases. MRI studies reflect not only the expected inflammatory changes in the optic nerves but have also shown acute disseminated encephalomyelitis (ADEM). Visual evoked responses are always abnormal in the acute stage but, different from adults, pattern responses are often normal on follow-up.[2]

The etiology of childhood optic neuritis may be different from adults, more frequently an infectious or parainfectious syndrome.[1]

Neuroretinitis

The symptoms are similar to optic neuritis; the difference is in the finding of a macular star, which is a collection of para-foveal intraretinal lipids, determined by the macular anatomy. It seems likely that the star is due to a serous exudate from the optic disc (Fig. 61.6). Perhaps it is similar to childhood optic neuritis, but a different part of the neuron is affected.[2] The prognosis is good.[9,10] Neuroretinitis occurs with toxoplasmosis and varicella-zoster, but cat scratch disease (*Bartonella henselae*) is a common cause[12] and may be treated with antibiotics.

Optic neuritis in infectious diseases

Exanthemas

Optic neuritis in childhood may be preceded by a nonspecific illness or an exanthem, chickenpox being the most common.[13] Visual symptoms usually follow the rash by a few days, with profound visual loss, but good recovery despite residual optic atrophy.[14] Varicella may also cause central retinal artery occlusion.[15]

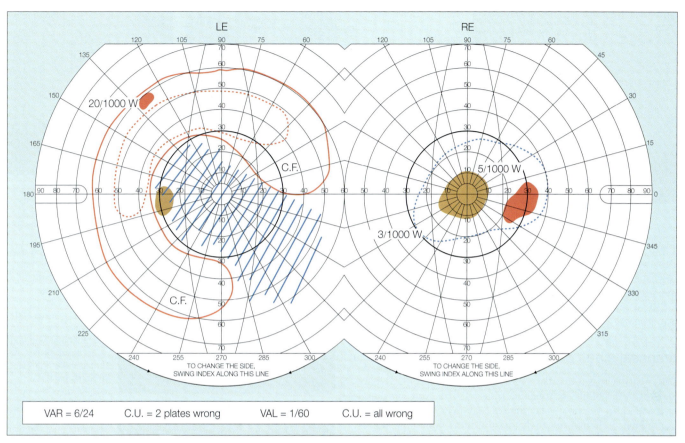

| VAR = 6/24 | C.U. = 2 plates wrong | VAL = 1/60 | C.U. = all wrong |

Fig. 61.2 Optic neuritis in a 7-year-old boy. Sudden onset of visual loss to 6/24 acuity right eye, 1/60 left eye, central scotomas and color vision loss.

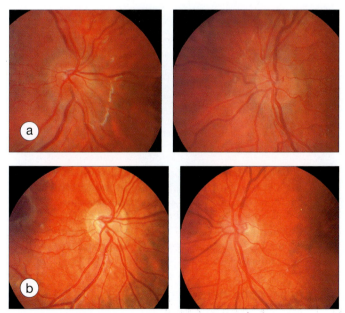

Fig. 61.3 Bilateral optic neuritis. (a) Bilaterally swollen optic discs. (b) Normal optic discs 2 months later. Complete visual recovery. Same patient as Fig. 61.2.

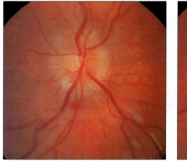

Fig. 61.4 Bilateral optic neuritis with swollen optic discs and a few peripapillary nerve fiber hemorrhages.

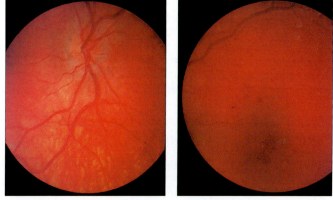

Fig. 61.5 Unilateral optic neuritis with paramacular preretinal hemorrhage.

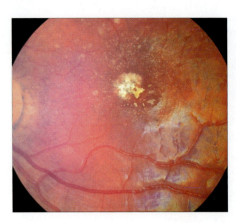

Fig. 61.6 Optic neuritis with remains of macular "star"—the acuity is 6/9. There are similarities between childhood optic neuritis and neuroretinitis.

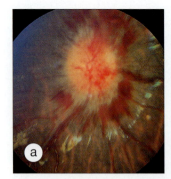
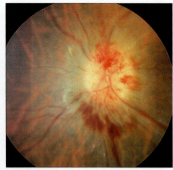

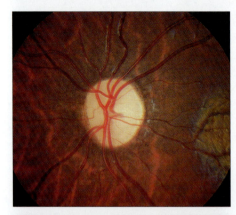

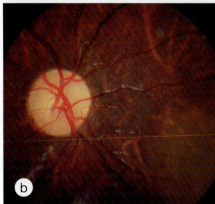

Fig. 61.7 Acute optic neuropathy. (a) Acute optic neuropathy in a child with treated neuroblastoma on no therapy for 6 months. There was a bilateral central scotoma, acuities of 1/60 right eye, 4/60 left eye and color vision loss. The cerebrospinal fluid and neuroradiological studies were normal. (b) Same patient 3 months later. The optic neuropathy settled on corticosteroid treatment only and the acuity (despite the obvious optic atrophy) has remained normal for 10 years.

Optic neuritis may follow rubella, measles, mumps or other vaccination.[16,17] Optic neuritis and encephalitis with a good prognosis have been described Epstein–Barr virus infection.[18] Optic nerve dysfunction in Lyme borreliosis may be due to optic neuritis or elevated intracranial pressure.[19] Papillitis with toxoplasmosis may not have marked visual loss or chorioretinitis.

Paranasal sinus disease

Optic neuritis or a chiasmal syndrome (see Chapter 62) may occur with ethmoiditis or sphenoid sinusitis. The optic canal and nerve are close to, or in the sinuses and may be affected by compression, ischemia or "toxic" local effects. Sinus imaging is indicated in all cases of childhood optic neuritis even without clinical sinusitis. Antibiotic treatment may be accompanied by systemic steroids.

Optic neuropathy of malnutrition

It has long been known that patients on near-starvation diets are liable to an optic neuropathy and children on a ketogenic diet may have a thiamine-reversible optic neuropathy.[20]

Malnutrition optic neuropathy may occur in a child from a developing country or from the less privileged sectors of developed countries on an unusual diet, or with gut diseases.

Optic neuropathy in leukemia and systemic neoplasms

Optic nerve involvement in leukemia is serious and sometimes a preterminal event.[21] Optic nerve compression, sometimes bilateral, also occurs in Langerhans cell histiocytosis, neuroblastoma, leukemias and non-Hodgkin lymphoma.[22] Patients with clinical optic neuritis may rarely have tumour compression with temporary steroid responsiveness[23.] It may rarely occur as a remote effect of tumors.

Neuroblastoma may present with acute visual loss which demands rapid action to prevent blindness[22] (Fig. 61.7).

Radiation optic neuropathy and encephalopathy occur weeks after the treatment.[24,25]

Compressive optic neuropathy

Optic atrophy from compression occurs from trauma, neoplasm, bone disease (Fig. 61.8), orbital tumors and infections. In osteopetrosis there may be early narrowing of the optic canal; poor vision may be the presenting sign in these infants (see

Chapter 53). Decompression of the optic canal may prevent visual loss and may be indicated before or during bone marrow transplantation, the effects of which may take time.[27] Neurophysiological studies are helpful to detect a retinal dystrophy and visual evoked potentials (VEPs) can be used to monitor progress (see Chapter 11).[28] Eye-poking may explain transient optic disc swelling in patients with Down syndrome[29] (Fig. 61.9).

Traumatic optic neuropathy

Soft tissue trauma

Blunt orbital trauma (Fig. 61.10) may cause a functional optic nerve transection if the optic nerve is compressed at the orbital apex or if there is an orbital hematoma. Optic atrophy takes several weeks to appear.

Skull fracture

Fractures of the sphenoid bone resulting from frontal trauma may cause a sudden blindness in one or, rarely, both eyes. It is often discovered too late for treatment, either because it is

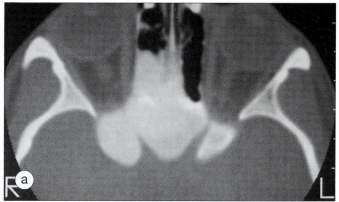

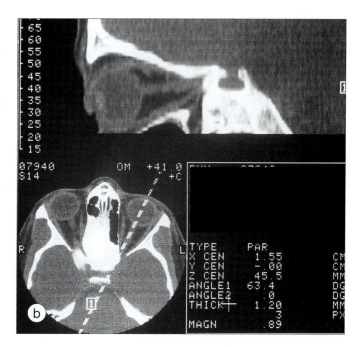

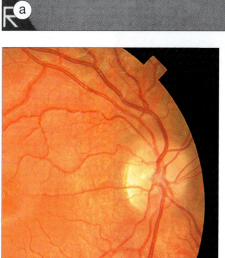

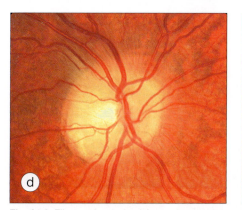

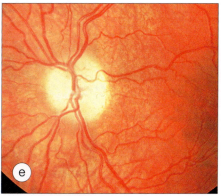

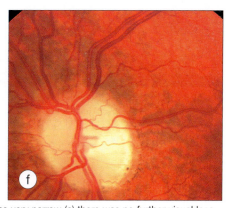

Fig. 61.8 Fibrous dysplasia giving a chronic compressive optic neuropathy. Although the optic canal was very narrow (a) there was no further visual loss after the age of 14 years (b). (c) In the right eye the acuity was 6/9. (d) The same patient's right eye 5 years later. (e) In the left eye the acuity was 6/60 after optic canal decompression; five years later (f), the acuity was unchanged.

unilateral or the relative afferent pupil defect is difficult to detect, because the child is restless. In bilateral cases, the other effects of trauma, including lid swelling, are the overwhelming signs. If detected early high-dose systemic steroids and optic canal decompression may help.[30,31] Surgery is not universally effective but, with neuroimaging, the site of the injury is more readily identified and the best transcranial or extracranial approach may be selected.[31] Recovery may be prolonged.[32] Poor prognostic signs for visual recovery include age of patient, loss of consciousness, blood in the ethmoids, and no visual recovery after systemic steroid administration.[33]

Ischemic optic neuropathy

Ischemic optic neuropathy results from hypertension[34] (Fig. 61.11), vasculitis in polyarteritis nodosa, systemic lupus or primary Sjögren syndrome,[35] in anomalous optic discs in profoundly anemic patients[36] and dialysis.[37]

Toxic optic neuropathy

In any child presenting with an unexplained optic neuropathy (acuity and color vision loss and a central scotoma), a careful history of toxic intake must be taken.

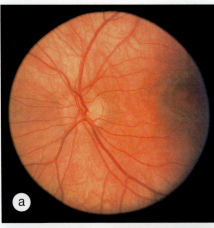

Fig. 61.10 Traumatic optic neuropathy. (a) Right optic disc 4 hours after the eye was blinded by a billiards cue being accidentally thrust into the orbit of a 10-year-old boy. (b) Same patient 6 weeks later at the first appearance of optic atrophy.

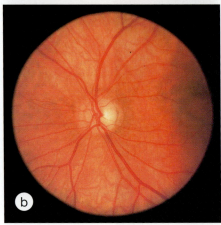

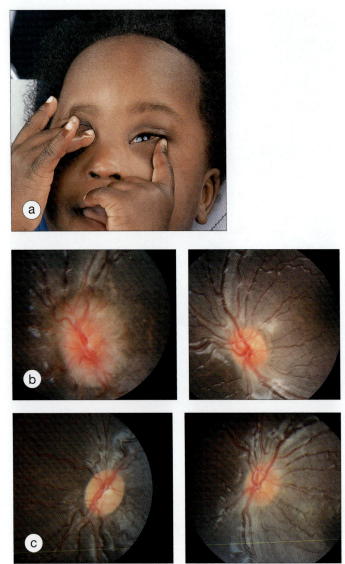

Fig. 61.9 Eye poking. (a) Child with severe Down syndrome who relentlessly poked both eyes, mostly the right eye. (b) Right optic disc edema. (c) After 2 weeks of using elbow restraints to stop the eye-poking, the optic disc edema had resolved.

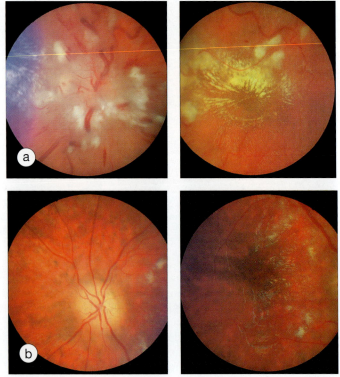

Fig. 61.11 Ischemic optic neuropathy. (a) Optic neuropathy in malignant hypertension in an 11-year-old boy with reflux nephropathy. The vision had suddenly dropped associated with a gut hemorrhage: this was the presenting symptom. (b) Same patient showing the profound optic atrophy that subsequently occurred.

Antituberculous drugs
Ethambutol, streptomycin, and isoniazid have a direct effect on optic nerve neurons and retinal ganglion cells.[38] Their continued use in tuberculous meningitis of the chiasm and optic nerves calls for fine judgment (Fig. 61.12).

Desferrioxamine
High-dose desferrioxamine given for refractory anemia may cause a partially reversible optic neuropathy or retinal pigmentation[39] that presents with night-blindness. Screening of acuity, color vision and visual fields is indicated in at-risk patients.

Cardiac drugs
Amiodarone causes largely asymptomatic cornea verticillata[40] and symptomatic[41] retinal changes that are unusual but usually. A papillopathy with decreased visual acuity and field loss has been described.[42] Digitalis and propranolol[43] may cause an optic neuropathy.

Hydroxyquinolines
Iodochlorhydroxyquin (dioquinol), an antidiarrheal, and diiodohydroxyquin (iodoquinol) may give optic atrophy; the former in the form of subacute myelo-optic neuropathy (SMON)[44] and the latter as chronic optic atrophy.[45]

Antibiotics
Chloramphenicol and sulphonamides (and their derivatives, tolbutamide and chlorpropamide) may cause a reversible optic neuropathy.

Antineoplastic agents
Carmustine (BCNU) and vincristine both give an optic neuropathy.[46]

Anti-inflammatory agents
A toxic optic neuropathy has been associated with the use of the tumor necrosis factor alpha antagonist, infliximab.[47]

Others
Heavy metals, lead in particular, methanol, hexachlorophene and solvents (carbon tetrachloride, carbon disulphide, trichlorethylene or toluene) should also be suspected in undiagnosed optic neuropathy.

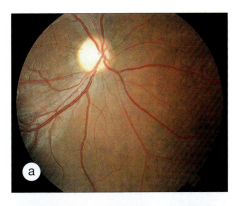

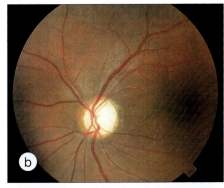

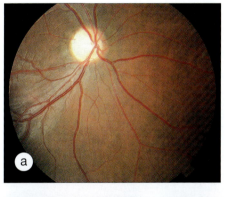 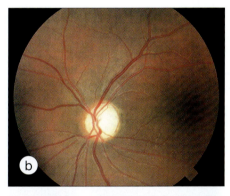
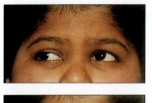 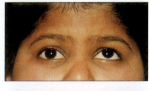 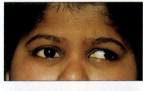
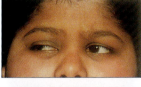 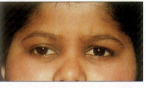 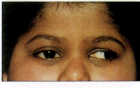
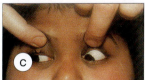 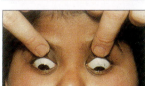 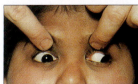

Fig. 61.12 A patient with tuberculosis meningitis. (a and b) Bilateral optic neuropathy. The organism was only sensitive to ethambutol which may cause a toxic optic neuropathy. (c) A partial right third nerve palsy in the same patient.

REFERENCES

1. Franco AF, Cabrera D, Carrizosa J, et al. Clinical characteristics of optical neuritis in childhood. Rev Neurol 2003; 36: 208–11.
2. Taylor D, Cuendet F. Optic neuritis in childhood. In: Hess RF, Plant GT, eds. Optic Neuritis. Cambridge: Cambridge University Press; 1986: 73–85.
3. Heirons R, Lyle TK. Bilateral retrobulbar neuritis. Brain 1959; 82: 56–67.
4. Kennedy C, Carroll FD. Optic neuritis in children. Arch Ophthalmol 1960; 63: 747–55.
5. Meadows SP. Retrobulbar and optic neuritis in childhood and adolescence. Trans Ophthalmol Soc UK 1969; 89: 603–38.
6. Farris BK, Pickard DJ. Bilateral post-infectious optic neuritis and intravenous steroid therapy in children. Ophthalmology 1990; 97: 339–45.
7. Kennedy C, Carter W. Relation of optic neuritis to multiple sclerosis in children. Pediatrics 1961; 28: 377–87.
8. Parkin PJ, Heirons R, McDonald WI. Bilateral optic neuritis. A long-term follow-up. Brain 1984; 107: 951–64.
9. Maitland CG, Miller NR. Neuroretinitis. Arch Ophthalmol 1984; 102: 1146–50.
10. Dreyer RF, Hopen G, Gass JDM, et al. Leber's idiopathic stellate neuroretinitis. Arch Ophthalmol 1984; 102: 1140–5.
11. De Schryver I, Stevens AM, Vereecke G, et al. Cat scratch disease in patients with stellate neuroretinitis. Bull Soc Belge Opthalmol 2002; 286: 41–6.
12. McDonald HR. Diagnostic and therapeutic challenges. Diffuse unilateral subacute neuroretinitis. Retina 2003; 23: 92–6.
13. Purvin V, Hrisomalos N, Dunn N. Varicella optic neuritis. Neurology 1988; 38: 501.
14. Sellost RG, Selhorst JB, Harbison EC. Parainfectious optic neuritis. Arch Neurol 1983; 40: 347–50.
15. Friedburg MA, Miale AJ. Monocular blindness from central retinal artery occlusion associated with chickenpox (letter). Am J Ophthalmol 1994; 117: 117–18.
16. Kazarian EL, Gager WE. Optic neuritis complicating measles, mumps and rubella vaccination. Am J Ophthalmol 1979; 86: 544–7.
17. Kline LB, Margulies SL, Oh SJ. Optic neuritis and myelitis following rubella vaccination. Arch Neurol 1982; 39: 443–5.
18. Straussberg R, Amir J, Cohen H, et al. Epstein-Barr virus infection associated with encephalitis and optic neuritis. J Pediatr Ophthalmol Strabismus 1993; 30: 262–3.
19. Rothermal H, Hedges TR III, Steere AC. Optic neuropathy in children with lyme disease. Pediatrics 2001; 108: 477–81.
20. Hoyt CS, Billson FA. Optic neuropathy in ketogenic diet. Br J Ophthalmol 1979a; 63: 191–4.
21. Rosenthal AR. Ocular manifestations of leukemia: A review. Opthalmology 1983; 90: 899–905.
22. Manschot WA. Transverse ischaemic optic nerve necrosis in neuroblastoma. Arch Ophthalmol 1969; 89: 707–9.
23. Hirst LW, Miller NR, Kumar AJ, et al. Medulloblastoma causing a corticosteroid-responsive optic neuropathy. Am J Ophthalmol 1980; 89: 437–41.
24. Oliff A, Bleyer WA, Poplack DG. Acute encephalopathy after initiation of cranial irradiation for meningeal leukaemia. Lancet 1978; ii: 13.
25. Brown GC, Shields JA, Sanborn G, et al. Radiation optic neuropathy. J Am Acad Ophthalmol 1982; 89: 1489–93.
26. Ainsworth J, Bryce I, Dudgeon J. Visual loss in infantile osteopetrosis. J Pediatr Ophthalmol Strabismus 1993; 30: 201–3.
27. Haines SJ, Erickson DL, Wirtschafter JD. Optic nerve decompression for osteopetrosis in early childhood. Neurosurgery 1988; 23: 470–5.
28. Hoyt CS, Billson FA. Visual loss in osteopetrosis. Am J Dis Child 1979b; 133: 955–8.
29. Catalano R, Simon JW. Optic disc elevation in Down's syndrome. Am J Ophthalmol 1990; 110: 28–32.
30. Seiff SR. High dose corticosteroids for treatment of vision loss due to indirect injury to the optic nerve. Ophthalmic Surg 1990; 21: 389–95.
31. Levin LA, Baker RS. Management of traumatic optic neuropathy. J Neurophthalmol 2003; 23: 72–5.
32. Feist RM, Kline LB, Morris RE, et al. Recovery of vision after presumed direct optic nerve injury. J Am Acad Ophthalmol 1987; 94: 1567–70.
33. Canta A, Ferrigno L, Salvo M, et al. Visual prognosis after indirect traumatic optic neuropathy. JNNP 2003; 74: 246–8.
34. Taylor D, Ramsay J, Day S, et al. Infarction of the optic nerve head in children with accelerated hypertension. Br J Ophthalmol 1981; 65: 152–60.
35. Berman JL, Kashii S, Trachtman M, et al. Optic neuropathy and central nervous system disease secondary to Sjögren's syndrome in a child. Ophthalmology 1990; 97: 1606–10.
36. Burde R. Optic disc risk factors for non-arteritic anterior ischaemic optic neuropathy. Am J Ophthalmol 1993; 116: 759–64.
37. Chutorian AM, Winterkorn JM, Geffner A. Anterior ischemic optic neuropathy in children. Pediatr Neurol 2002; 26: 358–64.
38. Heng JE, Vorwerk CK, Lessel E. Ethambutol is toxic to retinal ganglion cells via an excitotoxic. Invest Ophthalmol Vis Sci 1999; 40: 190–6.
39. Lakhanpal V, Schocket SS, Jiji R. Desferoxiamine-induced toxic retinal pigmentary degeneration and presumed optic neuropathy. Ophthalmology 1984; 91: 443–51.
40. Orlando RG, Dangel ME, School SF. Clinical experience and grading of amiodarone keratopathy. Ophthalmology 1984; 91: 1184–8.
41. Ingram DV, Jaggarao NSV, Chamberlain DA. Ocular changes resulting from therapy with amiodarone. Br J Ophthalmol 1982; 66: 676–80.
42. Nagra PK, Foroozan R, Savino PJ. Amiodarone induced optic neuropathy. Br J Ophthalmol 2003; 4: 420–2.
43. Parrish DO, Todorov AB. Transient bilateral visual reduction and mydriasis after propranolol treatment. Ann Neurol 1981; 10: 583.
44. Oakley GP. The neurotoxicity of the halogenated hydroxyquinolines. J Am Med Assoc 1973; 225: 395–8.
45. Behrens MM. Optic atrophy in children after di-iodohydroxyquin therapy. J Am Med Assoc 1974; 228: 693–4.
46. Fraunfelder FT, Meyer SM. Ocular toxicity of antineoplastic agents. Ophthalmology 1983; 90: 1–3.
47. ten Tusscher MP, Jacobs PJ, Busch MJ. Bilateral toxic optic neuropathy and the use of infliximab BMJ 2003; 326: 579.

CHAPTER
62 Chiasmal Defects

Michael C Brodsky

THE OPTIC CHIASM

Introduction

The chiasm is so named because it is shaped like the Greek letter chi.[1] Over 2 million nerve fibers pass through it: most are visual but some nonvisual fibers project from the optic chiasm to hypothalamic nuclei, forming the retinohypothalamic tract that subserves circadian rhythms through its central connections with the suprachiasmatic nucleus.[2] The ratio of crossed to uncrossed fibers in the human chiasm is about 53:47.[3]

The optic chiasm is important for binocular vision. To establish fusion, it is necessary to have overlapping visual fields, congruence of corresponding retinal elements, and extraocular muscles to maintain alignment of the visual axes.[4] Decreased stereoacuity is present in the majority of patients with chiasmal lesions, even when no visual field abnormalities are detectable.[4]

Evolutionary considerations

The chiasm provides the major route for the juxtaposition of corresponding parts of the visual field in each eye and single binocular vision in humans depends on the balance between crossed and uncrossed fibers. During the evolution of single binocular vision, all messages from the right half of the visual field (most from the right eye but some from the left eye) reach the left side of the brain. In lateral-eyed animals, optic fibers from each eye decussate entirely to the contralateral hemisphere. Generally, the percentage of uncrossed fibers increases as the orbits rotate anteriorly and the frontal field of single binocular vision increases.[5] Throughout evolution, the stake of the left brain in the right visual field remains absolute.[6] The reason that our visual system is crossed is an issue of some debate, and the interested reader is referred to fascinating evolutionary analyses by Polyak[5] and Linksz (Fig. 62.1).[6]

In humans, there is more retina nasal to the fovea than temporally so that the right eye covers more right visual field (some exclusively) than left visual field. The primordial nasal retinal halves are concerned with a phylogenetically older "panoramic" function in that each covers half of the visual field and their fibers cross. The temporal retinal halves of each eye have entered into a phylogenetically younger "binocular" function. By placing a hand in front of the nose (to block the temporal retinas) and viewing the world, we can appreciate the fact that our panoramic appreciation of the world is unaltered, despite the loss of binocularity.

Our foveas are placed where nasal (panoramic) and temporal (binocularity providing) retinas meet.[6] This arrangement allows human vision to subserve its elemental functions:

1. Exploration (mobility).
2. Detail (foveas).
3. Stereopsis (binocularity).[6]

Exploration of the surround is a primordial panoramic function that concerns the nasal retinal halves, while binocular vision, stereopsis, and convergence concern the temporal retinal halves. The latter are newer, less essential, easily lost, often missing and not missed functions.[6]

Anatomy

The optic nerves, chiasm and optic tracts extend posteriorly and upwards from the optic canals at about 45°. The anatomical relationships are not significantly different from those in the adult.[7] The chiasm lies in the suprasellar cistern, above the diaphragma sellae from which it is separated by several millimeters by its oblique course. The anterior cerebral arteries and the anterior communicating arteries lie anteriorly and above the chiasm and optic nerves. The carotid arteries lie laterally with the posterior communicating artery passing underneath the optic tracts. The chiasm lies in the floor of the anterior end of the third ventricle which is above it (expansion of the third ventricle in hydrocephalus is a potent cause of visual damage from chiasmal compression). Posteriorly lies the hypothalamus and the pituitary stalk, the tuber cinereum and the mamillary bodies. The optic nerves emerge from the optic canals where they are fixed; the length of the intracranial portion of the optic nerve varies so that the position of the chiasm in relation to the tuberculum sellae and other structures is different; when the optic nerves are short the chiasm is said to be prefixed, when long it is said to be postfixed. The time-honored Willebrand's knee is an artifact of enucleation in mice.[8]

Embryology

In humans, the chiasm appears within the first month of life,[9] its precursor appears as a thickening of the floor of the forebrain between the optic stalks at the junction of the telencephalon and the diencephalon. Retinal ganglion cells grow down the optic stalks and enter the floor of the third ventricle where they decussate to form the optic chiasm. The highly specific pattern of axon crossing is fundamental to visual processing; its formation occurs in two phases.[10] As the first retinal axons meet in the midline at the ventral diencephalon they form an X-shaped chiasm; subsequent axons grow into either the ipsilateral or contralateral optic tract.[11]

Each axon is tipped by a morphological specialization called a growth cone which allows the axon to sense and respond to signals in the embryonic brain environment.[12] Neuronal and glial cell populations in the developing ventral hypothalamus provide guidance information to ingrowing RGC axons.

Early generated neurons and radial glial cells present locally in the ventral diencephalon where the chiasm will be formed, may

663

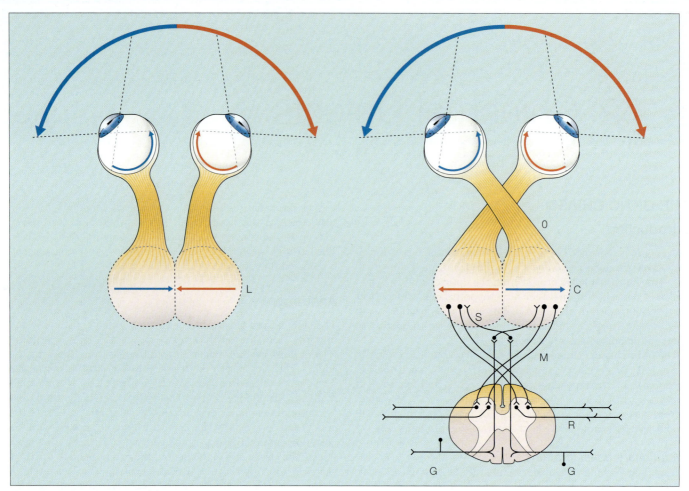

Fig. 62.1 Ramón y Cajal's original diagram of the hypothetical uncrossed chiasm. He believed this arrangement was never found in nature (left). On the right is the completely crossed chiasm in lateral-eyed animals. (With permission from Polyak S. The Vertebrate Visual System. Edited by Heinrich Kluver. © 1957 University of Chicago Press.)

serve a role in retinal ganglion cell axon guidance during chiasm formation. Growth associated proteins in retinal growth cones enable RGC axons to progress from the optic chiasm to enter the optic tract and perform pathfinding tasks. In the mouse, the presence of early-generated neurons at the site of the future chiasm is required for the formation of the optic chiasm by retinal ganglion cell axons. A growth associated protein essential for chiasm formation has also been identified.[13] At first there is a substantial overproduction of neurones which later die back by apoptosis.[14] The chiasm reaches its definitive form by the fourth month of gestation.

Signs and symptoms

While pituitary tumors are most common in adults, developmental defects and suprasellar tumors are most common in children (Table 62.1). While most chiasmal syndromes result from neoplastic disorders, developmental derangements, radiation injury, inflammation, infection, demyelination, intoxication, infarction, transection, or hypoplasia are also well-recognized.[15] Dominant optic atrophy may be associated with a bitemporal hemianopia that simulates a hereditary chiasmal disorder.[15]

In young children, chiasmal disease often presents late, particularly if the process is chronic, because the child compensates well and is not suspected of having poor vision until there is a substantial and bilateral visual defect. It is often only when the last

remaining vision of the second eye to be affected finally deteriorates to nil that the small child will be noticed to have poor vision by the parents.

The hallmark of chiasmal disease is a bitemporal hemianopia. An initial clue to this visual field defect is the child's consistent omission of letters at the beginning or end of the line corresponding to the temporal visual field during monocular acuity testing. Even if formal visual field testing is not possible, it is still vital to carry out visual field testing by turning the test into a game (see Chapter 10). Lesions from below, usually from the pituitary gland, the surrounding bone or sometimes from the pituitary stalk, for instance craniopharyngiomas, have to grow large before signs of chiasmal compression appear. Inferior lesions compress the

Table 62.1 Signs and symptoms of chiasmal disease
Loss of stereopsis
Postfixational blindness
Loss of motor fusion
Hemifield slide
Bitemporal hemianopia
Band atrophy
See-saw nystagmus
Spasmus nutans

lower nasal fibers first and tend to give an upper bitemporal field defect. Similarly lesions from above tend to cause an inferior defect. By the time a compressive lesion has caused defects there is usually gross thinning of the chiasm and the pattern of appearance of the field defects is not usually clear-cut.

In a child in whom acuity can be measured, there is often an acuity defect. Chiasm splitting lesions, such as trauma, do not affect acuity greatly because the nasal field and the nasal half of the fovea is not affected, but usually there is involvement of the optic nerve or widespread involvement of both crossed and uncrossed fibers in the chiasm which gives rise to the acuity defect. Most frequently, one eye has a very severe acuity defect and the other is relatively spared, except for a field defect. In very chronic lesions, there is often a most impressive preservation of a high level of acuity in the face of funduscopic evidence of a profound loss of neurons.

With widespread abnormalities or optic nerve involvement there is a significant color vision defect. This is best tested for by pseudoisochromatic plates, though in the small child it is often difficult and only gross color vision defects are detectable. Stereopsis has been elicited in a patient with complete chiasmal transection by haploscopic stimulation of the intact temporal retinas.[16] While this shows that patients with chiasmal transection retain the sensory capacity for stereopsis, the absence of motor fusion may preclude stereopsis under real world viewing conditions.[17]

Children with chiasmal disease may present with nystagmus, if the onset is early in their life. The classic form of nystagmus is known as see-saw nystagmus. Most patients, however, have a less clear-cut abnormality with a compound nystagmus with vertical, horizontal and rotary components (see Chapter 73). The presence of this sort of nystagmus in a child demands appropriate investigations.

Optic atrophy frequently occurs when there is substantial loss of neurons in the chiasm. Although often there is a generalized loss of neurons, sometimes there may be a characteristic pattern due to the loss of the fibers subserving the defunct temporal fields and the relative preservation of those fibers which subserve the intact nasal field (Fig. 62.2). These, because of the temporal retinal location of their ganglion cells, have to arch over the macula and are inserted into the upper and lower quadrants of the optic disc. In cases of developmental chiasmal defects and tumors there are often optic disc defects (Figs 62.3, 62.4), for instance hypoplasia or coloboma, and the presence of one of these defects should alert the practitioner to the possibility of a chiasmal defect.[18,19] Papilledema occurring in these optic discs may reflect the anomaly and the bitemporal hemianopia, occurring predominantly in the superior and inferior poles (Fig. 62.2c).

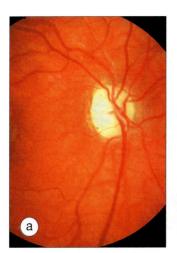
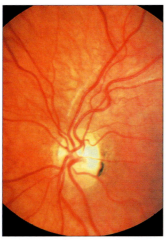
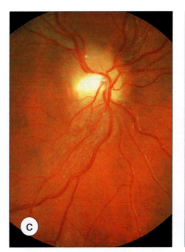
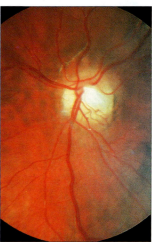
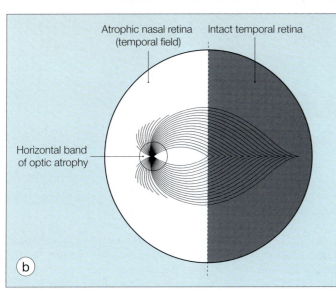

Fig. 62.2 Craniopharyngioma. (a) The right eye has bare perception of hand movements but the left has an absolute temporal hemianopia, normal color vision and 6/5 acuity. The left optic disc shows band atrophy-there is all-round loss of the nerve fibers that subserve the defunct temporal visual field but preservation of those that subserve the intact nasal field which are inserted into the upper and lower segments of the disc. (b) The origin of the band of atrophy is due to the fact that the horizontal band or bow-tie area is the visible area of atrophy where temporal field fibers alone are inserted into the disc. (c) Craniopharyngioma showing bilobed papilledema during a period of raised intracranial pressure. Since papilledema occurs only when the retinal ganglion cell axons are swollen and only the superior and inferior (nasal field) axons survive in chiasmal compression, the papilledema occurs only in the upper and lower poles giving bilobed or "twin peaks" papilledema.

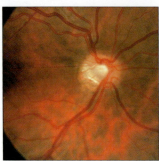
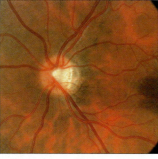

Fig. 62.3 Craniopharyngioma. Bilateral segmental hypoplasia or "tilted" optic disc. Bitemporal hemianopia with 6/5 acuity right eye (–4.0) and 6/4 left eye (–4.50).

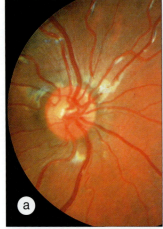
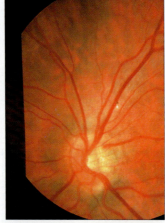
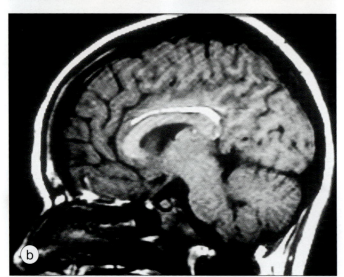

Fig. 62.4 Midline facial defect. (a) Dysplastic tilted left optic disc in a patient with a midline facial defect. (b) MRI of corpus callosum lipoma in a patient with a midline facial defect.

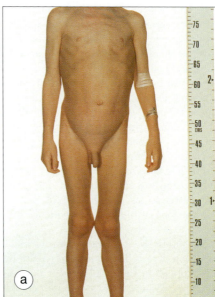
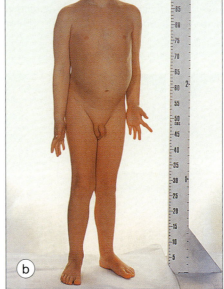
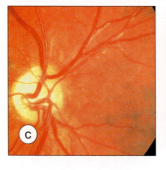
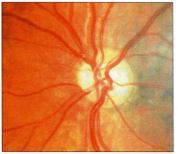

Fig. 62.5 Chiasmal glioma. (a) This boy presented with poor vision and recent weight loss. Photograph on 12 February 1973. (b) Photograph on 31 January 1974 showing rapid growth in weight and height. Weight and growth rate fluctuation are common in chiasmal glioma. (c) Bilateral band atrophy. (Same patient a–c.)

Because of the proximity of the hypothalamus and pituitary gland, endocrine and growth defects may occur. Some infants with hypothalamus-involving tumors have a combination of emaciation with loss of subcutaneous fat (Fig. 62.5), accelerated growth in length relative to weight (Fig. 62.6) and personality changes with euphoria and hyperactivity: a condition known as Russell diencephalic syndrome of infancy. The pediatric ophthal-mologist must examine and measure the infant's general body habitus and inquire about normal weight gain.

In older children there may be visual complaints that often sound rather nonorganic. The patient with bitemporal hemianopia experiences a unique sensorimotor disability known as the hemifield slide phenomenon (Fig. 62.7). Since only the nasal portion of each visual field is functioning fully, corresponding

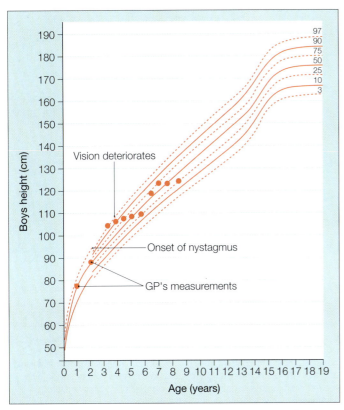

Fig. 62.6 Height growth record of a child with chiasmal glioma showing height growth rate fluctuation. Pediatric ophthalmology clinics need to have these charts available.

retinal points between the two eyes no longer exist. Sensory fusion becomes impossible, and motor fusion cannot maintain alignment. A previous heterophoria becomes a manifest deviation. If the child has an esophoria or intermittent esotropia, when the eyes drift in, letters or words appear deleted. When the eyes drift out, letters or words appear duplicated. A vertical hemifield slide causes the child to lose track of which line of text they are reading. Parents report that the child frequently misreads printed text. These children do not complain of diplopia (i.e. two separate images that appear subjectively abnormal) but rather a duplication of the middle of words or objects. Interestingly, the hemifield slide phenomenon does not require a complete bitemporal hemianopia and can occur as the initial symptom of a central bitemporal defect.[20] Neuro-ophthalmologic signs and symptoms of chiasmal disease are summarized in Table 62.2.

Further investigations

Clinical suspicion of an underlying chiasmal pathology, and the subsequent clinical evaluation are the vital starting points in the investigation; the further investigations consist of endocrine studies, neurophysiological evaluation (see Chapter 11) and neuroimaging (see Chapter 13). Neurophysiological studies are totally risk-free and inexpensive; their main role is in detection of a crossover defect in a child (particularly a preverbal child) with a nonspecific defect and in the quantitative and qualitative assessment of the visual defect, including serial studies to detect progression.

Magnetic resonance imaging (MRI)[21,22] provides exquisite neuro-anatomical detail of the chiasm and surrounding structures, but it obviously cannot assess function. Computed tomography

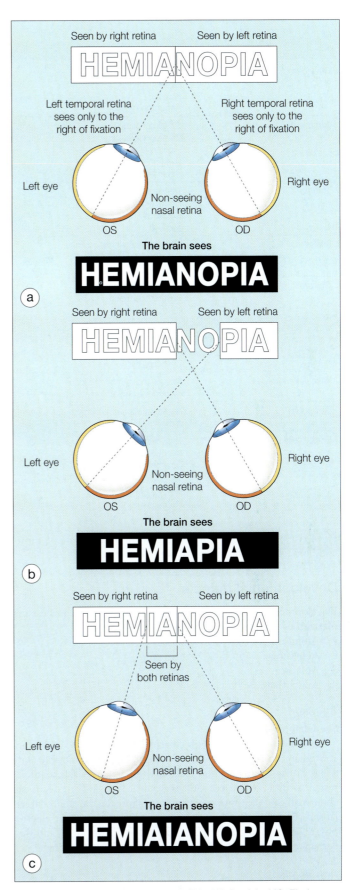

Fig. 62.7 Hemifield slide phenomenon. (Fritz KJ, Brodsky MC. Elusive neuro-ophthalmic reading impairment. American Orthoptic Journal 1992; 42: 159–164. Reprinted by permission of The University of Wisconsin Press.)

Table 62.2 Chiasmal diseases in children

Developmental defects	Albinism Achiasmia Aplasia Anophthalmia
Tumors	Chiasmal glioma Craniopharyngioma Pituitary adenoma Dysgerminoma Retinoblastoma ("trilateral")
Trauma	Transection Hematoma Contusion Traction
Infiltration	Langerhans cell histiocytosis Sarcoidosis Juvenile xanthogranuloma
Chiasmal neuritis	Postviral Postimmunization Multiple sclerosis
Optochiasmatic arachnoiditis	Tuberculosis Neurosyphilis Fungal Cysticercosis
Vascular anomalies	Arteriovenous malformation Cavernous angioma
Radiation	Acute visual loss months to years after radiation
Empty sella	Third ventricular distension secondary to aqueductal stenosis Downward traction on chiasm secondary to surgical scarring on pituitary apoplexy

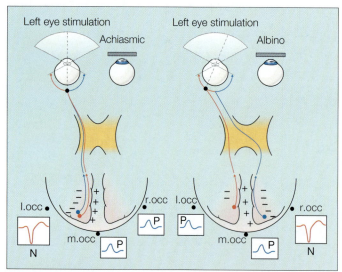

Fig. 62.8 Schematic comparing the visual pathway and VEP distribution in albino and achiasmic patients for flash stimulation of the left eye. Stimulation of the right eye produces the mirror image distribution for either condition. In the achiasmic subject, all the visual fibers from the left eye project to the left occipital cortex, and at 80–100 milliseconds, a positivity is recorded over the right scalp and a negativity over the left. In contrast, most of the fibers from one eye cross at the chiasm in albinism, and the VEP distribution is the opposite, with a positivity recorded over the left scalp, and a negativity over the right. (Courtesy of Dr Dorothy Thompson.)

(CT) scanning may provide important information about tumor and bony changes involving the parasellar area.

Developmental defects

Developmental derangements of the optic chiasm can be summarized by the four A's of chiasmal misdirection:

1. Albinism.
2. Achiasmia.
3. Aplasia.
4. Anophthalmia.

Albinism
See Chapter 45.

Anomalous decussation of chiasmal projections was demonstrated in albino animals over 30 years ago.[23] Retinogeniculate axons arising from ganglion cells in the portion of the temporal retina within 20 degrees of the vertical meridian decussate abnormally in the optic chiasm to synapse in the contralateral lateral geniculate nucleus.[23–25] This results in consistent electrophysiological changes[27,28] (Fig. 62.8) (see Chapters 11 and 45). Perhaps pigmentation of the optic stalk directs axon routing.[26]

Achiasmia
Belgian sheep dogs with achiasmia have a combination of congenital nystagmus and see-saw nystagmus.[29,30] Two unrelated girls had achiasmia with normal visual fields and no stereoacuity.[31] Eye movement recordings showed congenital

nystagmus in the horizontal plane and see-saw nystagmus in the vertical and torsional planes. MR imaging showed absence of the chiasm with each optic nerve projecting entirely to the ipsilateral hemisphere. The polarity of the VEP distribution across the occiput was the reverse of the crossed asymmetry that has been described in albinism (Fig. 62.8).[32]

The achiasmia may be complete (Fig. 62.9) or partial (Fig. 62.10), patients with bilateral optic nerve hypoplasia invariably have chiasmal hypoplasia, while those with unilateral optic nerve hypoplasia have selective hypoplasia of the ipsilateral side of the chiasm.[33] Rare patients with isolated chiasmal hypoplasia can have a segmental form of optic nerve hypoplasia that is confined to the nasal and temporal sectors of the optic discs.[34,35] Chiasmal anomalies, as evidenced by clinical findings or by abnormalities on neuroimaging have been described in patients with midline defects, for instance septo-optic dysplasia, or midfacial defects, or basal encephaloceles. The chiasm may be abnormal in the various midline facial and skull clefting syndromes that are associated with hypertelorism and encephalocele.[36,37]

Aplasia and anophthalmia
Unilateral anophthalmos or optic nerve aplasia produces an asymmetrical chiasm,[38] while bilateral anophthalmia or optic nerve aplasia is usually associated with absence of optic nerves, chiasm and lateral geniculate bodies[39–41]: some cases show remnants of the optic nerve and chiasm.[42] Bilateral optic nerve aplasia is also associated with an absent chiasm. In mice, prenatal removal of one eye produces a preponderance in crossed fibers from the other eye, whereas, in several animal species, postnatal removal of one eye produces an increase in the surviving uncrossed component.[25] Patients with unilateral optic nerve aplasia may show crossed hemispheric VEP asymmetry.[38]

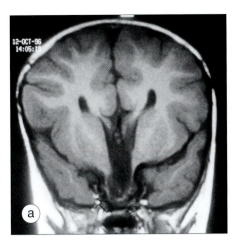
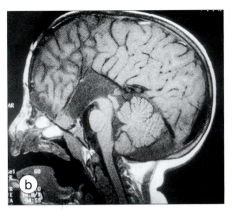
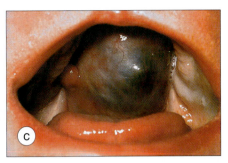

Fig. 62.9 Achiasmia in a child who presented with a cleft lip and palate, see-saw nystagmus. (a) Coronal MRI and (b) saggital MRI showing a large encephalocele completely dividing the chiasm. (Photographs courtesy of Dr Dorothy Thompson.) (c) The encephalocele protruding through the hard palate.

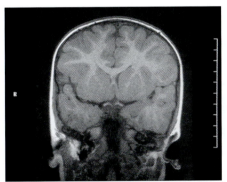

Fig. 62.10 Chiasmal hypoplasia. The chiasm is divided into two halves which are joined by a fragment of tissue. Electrophysiologically the patient was achiasmic. (Photograph courtesy of Dr Dorothy Thompson.)

Trauma

Occasionally, following closed head trauma, the child develops an absolute bitemporal hemianopia and poor acuity and color vision if there is also damage to the noncrossing fibers or optic nerve.[43] Other defects result from damage to surrounding structures which may lead to diabetes insipidus, anosmia, cerebrospinal fluid rhinorrhea, growth defects and mood changes. Traumatic enucleations can produce tractional injury to the optic chiasm and a temporal hemianopic defect in the other eye.[44]

Tumors

Chiasmal glioma

Chiasmal glioma, optic nerve glioma and hypothalamic glioma are closely related tumors, often one indistinguishable from the other and showing common histopathological features and clinical behavior. All occur with increased frequency in neurofibromatosis (NF), and up to one-half of patients with chiasmal or optic glioma have this disease.[45] It may occur in association with the Beckwith–Wiedemann syndrome of macrosomia, macroglossia, encephalocele, hemihypertrophy, hepatomegaly and advanced bone age.[46]

Children with chiasmal glioma present in a variety of ways. Infants with large chiasmal-hypothalamic glioma can present with Russell diencephalic syndrome. The main features of this condition are emaciation despite a normal or only slightly diminished caloric intake, alert appearance, hyperkinesis or increased vigor, euphoria, skin pallor, irritability, and normal

or accelerated linear growth (Fig. 62.5). These infants usually have large chiasmal gliomas and, in this specific setting, radiation therapy can induce dramatic tumor shrinkage and long-term regression of clinical abnormalities.[47,48]

Small children often present with a compound nystagmus and typically this is see-saw in nature (see Chapter 73). Any child with a compound nystagmus with rotary, vertical and horizontal elements should be suspected of having a chiasmal lesion.[49] Visual loss is often profound before it is noticed by parents of young children, but in older children the visual defect may be noticed by the child himself or detected by preschool or school visual testing. Some optic gliomas may be large but without gross visual defect.[50] Chiasmal glioma may reveal itself by its effects on growth and development. An unusual presentation is that of head bobble–the bobble-headed doll syndrome–this is usually an indication that the child also has hydrocephalus.

The diagnosis can be made easier by visual field testing or by visual field analysis on visual evoked cortical potential testing. Plain X-rays are seldom used now but the classical finding is an expanded and pear-shaped sella turcica (Fig. 62.11), with chronic bone changes and without calcification. Often one or both optic foramina are enlarged, especially if there is an optic nerve component to the tumor. CT scanning shows three diagnostic patterns (Fig. 62.12).[51]

1. A tube-like thickening of optic nerve and chiasm.
2. A suprasellar tumor with contiguous optic nerve expansion.
3. A suprasellar tumor with optic tract involvement.

Cystic or "globular" suprasellar tumors are not characteristic and may require histological confirmation. CT scanning demonstrated growth in three out of 22 cases and all were globular types.[51] MRI scanning better delineates the extent and nature of the tumor.[52] CT and MRI scanning will both show whether there is hydrocephalus. Tumors may evolve in areas thought to be normal on initial CT and even MRI scans.[53]

The histopathological nature of optic gliomas has long been the subject of a discussion that is important because of its relevance to treatment. Optic gliomas are benign tumors that are generally thought of as being hamartomas.[54]

They undergo enlargement by an accumulation of mucosubstance, by local invasion, by induction of hyperplasia in adjacent glial cells, or by growth of cell "rests" already present in adjacent optic nerve or chiasm.[55] Malignant gliomas do occur but are very rare and mainly in adults. Meningeal spread in children,

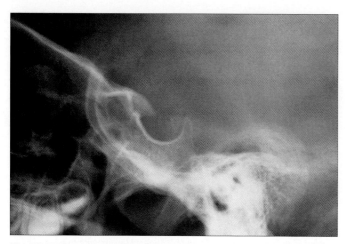

Fig. 62.11 Expanded pituitary fossa shown on plain X-ray with some calcification due to a craniopharyngioma.

however, is not unknown[56,57] and spread through a ventriculo-peritoneal shunt has been recorded.[58]

The clinical course of 36 optic gliomas, 29 of which were chiasmal were reviewed[54]: some were reviewed in 1971[59] and in

1986.[45] The 1971 follow-up showed a very stable course but the later follow-up showed that 57% of the 29 patients with chiasmal gliomas were dead, although only 18% from the direct effects of the glioma. The patients were more at risk from other tumors, thus reflecting the high proportion of patients who had neurofibromatosis Type I. Twelve survivors had not had radiation therapy whereas 11 of 16 patients who died had.[45]

Although early studies reported that the presence of NF had no influence on the prognosis of optic pathway glioma, it is now accepted that NF acts as a protective factor, both visually and neurologically.[60–62] In one large study, the most common site of visual pathway involvement in neurofibromatosis was the orbital optic nerve (66%) followed by the chiasm (62%). This contrasted to patients without NF in which the chiasm was the most common site of involvement (91%) and the orbital optic nerves were involved in only 32%. Extension beyond the optic pathway at diagnosis was uncommon in the NF group (2%) but frequent in the non-NF group (68%). In the NF group, the tumor was smaller and the original shape of the optic pathways was preserved (91% vs. 27% in the non-NF group). The presence of a cystic tumor component was significantly more common in non-NF patients 66% vs. 9% in the NF group). During follow-up, the tumors in half the NF patients remained stable, in contrast to 5% of the non-NF group.

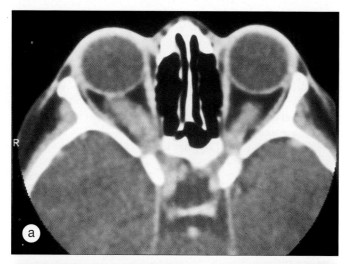

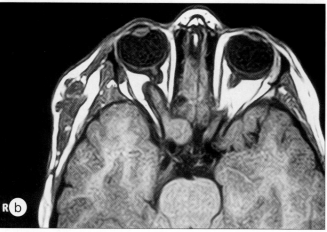

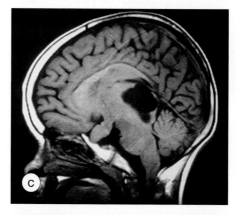

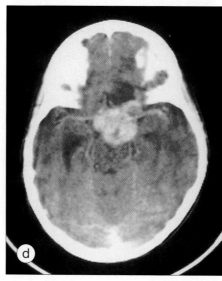

Fig. 62.12 Chiasmal glioma. (a) CT scan of bilateral optic nerve gliomas extending to the chiasm. (b) MRI scan of left optic nerve glioma extending to the chiasm and kinking the intra-orbital optic nerve. (Courtesy of Dr Kling Chong, Great Ormond Street Hospital, London and Dr Bob Zimmerman of the Children's Hospital, Philadelphia). (c) Saggital MRI of an optic nerve and chiasmal glioma. (d) CT scan with contrast of a cystic chiasmal glioma.

Hydrocephalus as a presenting symptom was found only in the non-NF group.

In children with neurofibromatosis and optic pathway gliomas, the likelihood of visual loss is dependent on the extent and location of the tumor and is particularly associated with involvement of postchiasmal structures.[63] The biological behavior of optic gliomas determines the way in which individual patients should be managed. For example, we now know that complete spontaneous regression can occur in both NF and non-NF-associated gliomas.[64] Similarly, spontaneous visual improvement can also take place in the absence of MRI changes.[65] Many authors have reported at least reasonable long-term prognosis that does not seem to be improved by treatment.[66,67,45] and although radiotherapy may decrease the size of the tumor[51] and some say improve the vision of treated patients[68–72] its use should be avoided except in infants with Russell diencephalic syndrome, because of its serious side-effects, especially in young children.[73–75] Chemotherapy[56,76,77] is as yet of uncertain benefit but with newer agents the outlook is promising and may allow deferment of damaging radiotherapy in the particularly susceptible younger child.[77]

Surgery is not indicated except to treat obstructive hydrocephalus in patients with large chiasmal/hypothalamic gliomas[78] or if there is a cystic tumor with serious doubts about the possibility of alternative pathology when biopsy and cyst aspiration may be indicated.

Follow-up after diagnosis usually involves periodic review of the visual fields, acuity, color vision and optic discs, neuro-physiological studies where available and CT or MRI scanning, the frequency needed being judged on the apparent clinical course of the disease.

Craniopharyngioma

These cystic tumors grow slowly and do not usually present until the child is 3 or 4 years old or later but they may present even in old age. Because of its origin from the pituitary stalk the tumor tends to compress the chiasm in any direction but classically from behind and above. Hypothalamic disturbances are frequent and the loss of vision may be profound. Young children tend to develop symptoms of hypothalamic disturbance or hydro-cephalus, whilst older children (first decade) are more likely to present with visual disturbance, strabismus or nystagmus (Figs 62.11 and 62.13). The diagnosis is made by CT or MRI scanning (Fig. 62.13). Calcification occurs in virtually every case in child-hood and the tumors are often cystic. Pre- and postoperative endocrine assessment and management is essential. The tumors are usually treated by surgery with or without radiotherapy; total removal is sometimes possible.

Pituitary adenomas

Pituitary tumors are relatively uncommon in childhood. Most pediatric cases present in adolescence.[79] When pituitary adenomas present in the pubertal period, they may be more likely to show extrasellar extension and hemorrhage.[79,80] Children with macroadenomas may also develop pituitary apoplexy, characterized by sudden headache, visual deterioration, ophthalmoplegia, depressed consciousness consequent to hemor-rhage into the tumor.[81,82]

Dysgerminoma

The clinical clue to the presence of a dysgerminoma is when diabetes insipidus is a symptom at presentation together with chiasmal defects, including acuity and visual field loss and hypo-

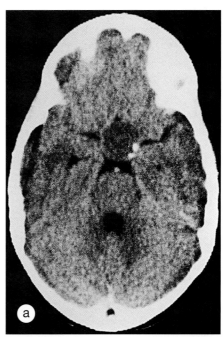
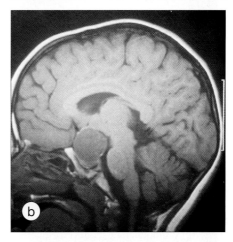
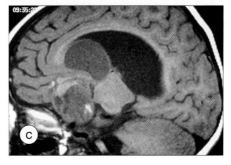

Fig. 62.13
Craniopharyngioma. (a) CT scan of a small cystic craniopharyngioma with calcification in its wall. (b) Saggital MRI of small craniopharyngioma. (c) MRI scan of a large cystic craniopharyngioma with calcification in its wall. There is hydrocephalus.

thalamic or pituitary disturbances.[83,84] The tumors are often not large[85] and occur in older children or young adults.[86]

Other chiasmal tumors

Trilateral retinoblastoma describes the association of bilateral retinoblastomas and ectopic intracranial primitive neuroectodermal tumor. While these midline intracranial tumors most commonly occur in the pineal region, it is important to remember that they can also occur in the suprasellar area and involve the chiasm.[87] These suprasellar tumors can present before the diagnosis of ocular retinoblastoma.[88]

Other rare tumors, such as metastatic neuroblastoma, arachnoid cysts, choristomas[89] such as ependymomas, epidermoid tumors, leukemic deposits, ectopic pinealomas, teratomas can occur.[90]

Granulomas and chronic inflammatory disorders

The chiasm and surrounding structures may be involved in abnormalities of the skull base as Langerhans cell histiocytosis (see Chapter 38). A variant of this condition tends to present with diabetes insipidus and visual defects. Sarcoidosis, juvenile xanthogranulomas and pseudotumors similar to those found in adults with the Tolosa–Hunt syndrome may also affect the chiasmal area.

Sphenoid sinus disease

In children whose sinuses have developed, a chiasmal syndrome or even rapid blindness may result from the formation and expansion of a mucocele,[91] even in the absence of symptomatic sinus disease.[92]

Chiasmal neuritis

Chiasmal neuritis is characterized by a chiasmal syndrome with visual loss and bitemporal hemianopia.[93] Most cases are been associated with demyelinating disease,[93] although Purvin et al. described a 13-year-old boy with infectious mononucleosis and chiasmal neuritis.[94] MR imaging shows swelling and enhancement of the chiasm.[93]

Optochiasmatic arachnoiditis

In rare cases, optochiasmatic arachnoiditis, characterized by localized thickening of the arachnoid at the base of the brain, may surround the optic nerves and chiasm, and compress these visual structures or their vascular supply. Tuberculous meningitis, hydatid disease and cysticercosis together with fungal disorders (especially in debilitated, immunodeficient children) may all affect the suprasellar cistern with damage to the chiasm and surrounding structures. Historically, this diagnosis has been assigned to patients with active infection, head trauma, or demyelinating disease (chiasmal optic neuritis).[95–97] Although the diagnosis has come to imply that surgical lysis of intracranial adhesions may be necessary to restore vision, the efficacy of surgical treatment remains unproven. Corticosteroids and cytotoxic agents are reportedly effective in some instances.[98] Modern neuroimaging seems to have rendered the diagnosis of optochiasmatic arachnoiditis an anachronism.

Third ventricle distention

In hydrocephalic patients, distention of the third ventricle may cause chiasmal damage and bitemporal or more widespread visual field defects,[99] with sometimes profound vision loss due to stretching or compression of the optic nerves and chiasm, to which may be added cortical blindness from posterior cerebral artery stretching and distortion (see empty sella). A unilateral visual defect has been described due to compression of one optic nerve against the internal carotid artery.[100]

Vascular malformations

Aneurysm is an extremely rare cause of chiasmal defects in children[101,102] and does not produce specific symptoms or signs. In children symptomatic intracranial aneurysms are sometimes large and may be associated with polycystic kidneys, coarctation of the aorta, and Marfan and Ehlers–Danlos syndromes.

Multiple aneurysms (usually small) may also occur in "mycotic" aneurysms with subacute bacterial endocarditis and moya moya disease[103–105]: these mostly affect cerebral hemispheres.

Arteriovenous or cavernous malformations localized to the chiasm may hemorrhage to produce the sudden-onset chiasmal visual deficit accompanied by headache (termed *chiasmal apoplexy*).[106]

Radionecrosis

Radiation injury to the optic chiasm is an uncommon but serious complication of radiation treatment of intracranial and paranasal sinus neoplasms. When vision becomes impaired, enhancement of the chiasm after gadolinium injection is a consistent finding. Chiasmal enlargement may also be present, and these neuro-imaging abnormalities may antedate the visual loss by several months.[107]

The pathogenesis involves damage to the capillary beds. The risk of radionecrosis appears to be increased by the concomitant use of chemotherapy.

Empty sella syndrome

Empty sella syndrome is an anatomic condition in which subarachnoid space extends into the sella turcica, and the pituitary gland is flattened against the sellar floor or walls.[108,109] Chiasmal visual field defects occasionally occur and the sella may be enlarged.[109,110] Empty sella with chiasmal prolapse can be caused either by a distended third ventricle pushing the chiasm down into the sella, or by scarring and contracture pulling the chiasm into the sella. While communicating hydrocephalus produces diffuse ventricular enlargement, aqueductal stenosis is particularly prone to produce ballooning of the third ventricle with downward herniation of the chiasm.[111] Pituitary apoplexy or sellar surgery can produce adhesions and cause downward traction of the chiasm into the sella.[110] Although pseudotumor cerebri is undoubtedly the most common cause of empty sella,[109] the empty sella that accompanies pseudotumor cerebri is never associated with chiasmal prolapse. Since patients can have empty sella syndrome with normal vision, the diagnosis of empty sella with visual loss should prompt a careful search for ocular causes.[110]

REFERENCES

1. Slamovits TL. In: Walsh and Hoyt's Clinical Neuro-Ophthalmology. Miller NR and Newman NJ, eds. Anatomy and Physiology of the Optic Chiasm. 5th edn. Baltimore, Maryland: Williams & Wilkins; 1998: 85–100.

2. Lubkin V, Beizai P, Sadun AA. The eye as metronome of the body. Surv Ophthalmol 2002; 47: 17–26.

3. Kupfer C, Chumbley L, Downer JC. Quantitative histology of optic nerve, optic tract and lateral geniculate nucleus of man. J Anat 1967; 101: 393–401.

4. Hirai T, Ito Y, Arai M, et al. Loss of stereopsis with optic chiasmal lesions and stereoscopic tests as a differential test. Ophthalmology 2002; 109: 1692–702.

5. Polyak S. The Vertebrate Visual System. Chicago: University of Chicago Press; 1957: 779–89.

6. Linksz A. On Writing, Reading and Dyslexia. New York: Grune and Stratton; 1973.

7. Hoyt WF. Correlative functional anatomy of the optic chiasm. Clin Neurosurg 1970; 17: 189–208.

8. Horton JC. Willebrand's knee of the primate optic chiasm is an artefact of monocular enucleation. Trans Am Ophthalmol Soc 1997; 95: 579–609.

9. Barber AN, Ronstrom GN, Muelling RH. Development of the visual pathway; optic chiasm. Arch Ophthalmol 1954; 52: 447–56.

10. Sretavan DW, Reichardt LF. Time-lapse video analysis of retinal ganglion cell axon pathfinding at the mammalian optic chiasm: growth cone guidance using intrinsic chiasm cues. Neuron 1993; 10: 761–77.

11. Guillery RW, Mason CA, Taylor JS. Developmental determinants of the mammalian optic chiasm. J Neurosci 1995; 15: 4727–37.

12. Sretavan DW, Pure E, Siegel MW, et al. Disruption of retinal axon ingrowth by ablation of embryonic mouse optic chiasm neurons. Science 1995; 269: 98–101.

13. Mason CA, Sretavan DW. Glia, neurons, and axon pathfinding during optic chiasm development. Curr Opin Neurobiol 1997; 7: 647–53.

14. Provis JM, van Driel P, Billson FA, et al. Human fetal optic nerve: overproduction and elimination of retinal axons during development. J Comp Neurol 1985; 238: 92–100.

15. Pomeranz HD, Lessell S. A hereditary chiasmal optic neuropathy. Arch Ophthalmol 1999; 117: 128–31.

16. Blakemore C. Binocular depth perception and the optic chiasm. Vision Res 1970; 10: 43–7.

17. Fisher NF. The optic chiasm and the corpus callosum: their relationship to binocular vision in humans. J Pediatr Ophthalmol Strabismus 1986; 23: 126–31.

18. Taylor D. Congenital tumors of the anterior visual system with dysplasia of the optic discs. Br J Ophthalmol 1982; 66: 455–63.

19. Zeki SM, Hollman AS, Dutton GN. Neuroradiological features of patients with optic nerve hypoplasia. J Pediatr Ophthalmol Strabismus 1992; 29: 107–12.

20. Nachtigaller H, Hoyt WF. Storungen des Seheindruckes bei bitemporaler Hemianopsie und verscheibung der sehachsen. Klin Monatsbsbl Augenheilkd 1970; 156: 821–36.

21. Hupp SL, Kline LB. Magnetic resonance imaging of the optic chiasm. Surv Ophthalmol 1991; 36: 207–16.

22. Tang RA, Kramer LA, Schiffman J, et al. Chiasmal trauma: clinical and imaging considerations. Surv Ophthalmol 1994; 38: 381–83.

23. Guillery RW, Kaas JH. A study of normal and congenitally abnormal retinogeniculate projections in cats. J Comp Neurol 1971; 143: 73–100.

24. Shatz C. A comparison of visual pathways in Boston and Midwestern Siamese cats. J Comp Neurol 1977; 171: 205–28.

25. Guillery RW. Why do albinos and other hypopigmented mutants lack normal binocular vision, and what else is abnormal in their central visual pathways? Eye 1996; 10: 217–21.

26. Silver J, Sapiro J. Axonal guidance during development of the optic nerve: the role of pigmented epithelia and other factors. J Comp Neurol 1981; 202: 521–38.

27. Creel D, Witkop CJ Jr, King RA. Asymmetric visually evoked potentials in human albinos: evidence for visual system anomalies. Invest Ophthalmol 1974; 13: 430–40.

28. Apkarian P. Chiasmal crossing defects in disorders of binocular vision. Eye 1996; 10: 222–32.

29. Williams RW, Hogan D, Garraghty PE. Target recognition and visual maps in the thalamus of achiasmatic dogs. Nature 1994; 367: 637–9.

30. Dell'Osso LF, Williams RW, Jacobs JB, et al. The congenital and see-saw nystagmus in the prototypical achiasmia of canines: comparison to the human achiasmatic prototype. Vision Res 1998; 38: 1629–41.

31. Apkarian P, Bour LJ, Barth PG, et al. Non-decussating retinal-fugal fiber syndrome. An inborn achiasmatic malformation associated with visuotopic misrouting, visual evoked potential ipsilateral asymmetry and nystagmus. Brain 1995; 118: 1195–216.

32. Apkarian P, Bour L, Barth PG. A unique achiasmatic anomaly detected in non-albinos with misrouted retino-fugal projections. Eur J Neurosci 1994; 6: 501–7.

33. Brodsky MC, Glasier CM, Pollock SP. Optic nerve hypoplasia: identification by magnetic resonance imaging. Arch Ophthalmol 1990; 108: 562–67.

34. Taylor D. Chiasmal disease in young children. In:Wybar KC, Taylor D, eds. Paediatric Ophthalmology: Current Aspects. New York: Dekker; 1983: 255–65.

35. Novakovic P, Taylor DS, Hoyt WF. Localizing patterns of optic nerve hypoplasia – retina to occipital lobe. Br J Ophthalmol 1998; 72: 176–82.

36. Leitch RJ, Thompson D, Harris CM, et al. Achiasmia in a case of midline craniofacial cleft with seesaw nystagmus. Br J Ophthalmol 1996; 80: 1023–4.

37. Thompson DA, Kriss A, Chong K, et al. Visual-evoked potential evidence of chiasmal hypoplasia. Ophthalmology 1999; 106: 2354–61.

38. Margo CE, Hamed LM, Fang LE, et al. Optic nerve aplasia. Arch Ophthalmol 1992; 110: 1610–3.

39. Recordon E, Griffiths GM. A case of primary bilateral anophthalmia. Br J Ophthalmol 1936; 22: 353–61.

40. Haberland C, Perou M. Primary bilateral anophthalmia. J Neuropathol Exp Neurol 1969; 28: 337–51.

41. Penner H, Schlack HG. Anophthalmie und begleitende fehlbidungen. Klin Pediatr 1976; 188: 320–7.

42. Calgianut B, Theiler K. Zur aplaise der sehnerven. Graefe's Arch Klin Exp Ophthalmol 1976; 200: 93–8.

43. Heinz GW, Nunery WR, Grossman CB: Traumatic chiasmal syndrome associated with midline basilar skull fractures. Am J Ophthalmol 1994; 117: 90–6.

44. Parmar B, Edmunds B, Plant G. Traumatic enucleation with chiasmal damage: magnetic resonance image findings and response to steroids. Br J Ophthalmol 2002; 86: 1317–8.

45. Imes RK, Hoyt WF. Childhood chiasmal gliomas: update on the fate of patients in the 1969 San Francisco study. Br J Ophthalmol 1986; 70: 179–82.

46. Weinstein JM, Backonja M, Houston LW, et al. Optic glioma associated with the Beckwith-Wiedemann syndrome. Pediatr Neurol 1986; 2: 308–10.

47. Russell A. A diencephalic syndrome of emaciation in infancy and childhood. Arch Dis Child 1951; 26: 274–9.

48. Burr IM, Slonim AE, Danish RK, et al. Diencephalic syndrome revisited. J Pediatr 1976; 88: 439–44.

49. Schulman JA, Shults WT, Jones JM Jr. Monocular vertical nystagmus as an initial sign of chiasmal glioma. Am J Ophthalmol 1979; 87: 87–90.

50. Goodman SJ, Rosenbaum AL, Hasso A, et al. Large optic nerve glioma with normal vision. Arch Ophthalmol 1975; 93: 991–5.

51. Fletcher WA, Imes RK, Hoyt WF. Chiasmal gliomas: appearance and long-term changes demonstrated by computerized tomography. J Neurosurg 1986; 65: 154–9.

52. Holman RE, Grimson BS, Drayer BP, et al. Magnetic resonance imaging of optic gliomas. Am J Ophthalmol 1985; 100: 596–601.

53. Listernick R, Charrow J, Greenwald M. Emergence of optic pathway gliomas in children with neurofibromatosis type 1 after normal neuroimaging results. J Pediatr 1992; 121: 584–7.

54. Hoyt WF, Baghdassarian SA. Optic glioma of childhood. Br J Ophthalmol 1969; 53: 793–8.

55. Anderson DR, Spencer WH. Ultrastructural and histochemical observations of optic nerve gliomas. Arch Ophthalmol 1970; 83: 324–35.

56. Civitello LA, Packer RJ, Rorke LB, et al. Leptomeningeal dissemination of low grade gliomas in childhood. Neurology 1988; 38: 562–6.

57. Bruggers CS, Friedman HS, Phillips PC, et al. Leptomeningeal dissemination of optic pathway gliomas in three children. Am J Ophthalmol 1991; 111: 719–23.

58. Trigg ME, Swanson JD, Letellier MA. Metastasis of an optic glioma through a ventriculoperitoneal shunt. Cancer 1983; 52: 599–601.

59. Glaser JS, Hoyt WF, Corbett J. Visual morbidity with chiasmal glioma. Long-term studies of visual fields in untreated and irradiated cases. Arch Ophthalmol 1971; 85: 3–12.

60. Listernick R, Charrow J, Greenwald M, et al. Natural history of optic pathway tumors in children with neurofibromatosis type 1: a longitudinal study. J Pediatr 1994; 125: 63–6.

61. Kornreich L, Blaser S, Schwarz M, et al. Optic pathway glioma: correlation of imaging findings with the presence of neurofibromatosis. Am J Neuroradiol 2001; 22: 1963–9.

62. Tow SL, Chandela S, Miller NR, et al. Long-term outcome in children with gliomas of the anterior visual pathway. Pediatr Neurol 2003; 28: 262–70.

63. Balcer LJ, Liu GT, Heller G, et al. Visual loss in children with neurofibromatosis type 1 and optic pathway gliomas: relation to tumor location by magnetic resonance imaging. Am J Ophthalmol 2001; 131: 442–5.

64. Parsa CF, Hoyt CS, Lesser RL, et al. Spontaneous regression of optic gliomas. Arch Ophthalmol 2001; 119: 516–29.

65. Liu GT, Lessell S. Spontaneous visual improvement in chiasmal gliomas. Am J Ophthalmol 1992; 114: 193–201.

66. Borit A, Richardson EP, Jr. The biological and clinical behavior of pilocytic astrocytomas of the optic pathways. Brain 1982; 105: 161–87.

67. Rush JA, Younge BR, Campbell RJ, et al. Optic glioma: long-term follow-up of 85 histopathologically verified cases. Ophthalmology 1982; 89: 1213–9.

68. Roberson C, Till K. Hypothalamic gliomas in children. J Neurol Neurosurg Psychiatr 1974; 30: 1047–52.

69. Brand WN, Hoover SV. Optic glioma in children. Review of 16 cases given megavoltage radiation therapy. Childs Brain 1979; 5: 459–66.

70. MacCarty CS, Boyd AS Jr., Childs DS Jr. Tumors of the optic nerve and optic chiasm. J Neurosurg 1970; 33: 439–44.

71. Flickinger JC, Torres C, Deutsch M. Management of low grade gliomas of the optic nerve and chiasm. Cancer 1988; 61: 635–42.

72. Kovalic JJ, Grigsby PW, Shepard MJ, et al. Radiation therapy for gliomas of the optic nerve and chiasm. Int J Radiation Oncol Biol Phys 1990; 18: 927–32.

73. Weiss L, Sagerman RH, King GA, et al. Controversy in the management of optic nerve glioma. Cancer 1987; 59: 1000–4.

74. Pierce SM, Barnes PD, Loeffler JS, et al. Definitive radiation therapy in the management of symptomatic patients with optic glioma. Cancer 1990; 65: 45–52.

75. Jenkin D, Angyalfi S, Becker L, et al. Optic glioma in children: surveillance, resection or irradiation. Int J Radiation Oncol Biol Phys 1993; 25: 215–25.

76. Packer RJ, Sutton LN, Bilaniuk LT, et al. Treatment of chiasmatic-hypothalamic gliomas of childhood with chemotherapy. An update. Ann Neurol 1988; 23: 79–85.

77. Petronio J, Edwards MS, Prados M, et al. Management of chiasmal and hypothalamic gliomas of infancy and childhood with chemotherapy. J Neurosurg 1991; 74: 701–8.

78. Housepian EM, Chi TL. Neurofibromatosis and optic pathways gliomas. J Neurooncol 1993; 15: 51–5.

79. Poussaint TY, Barnes PD, Anthony DC, et al. Hemorrhagic pituitary adenomas of adolescence. Am J Neuroradiol 1996; 17: 1907–12.

80. Lee AG, Sforza PD, Fard AK, et al. Pituitary adenoma in children. J Neuro-ophthalmol 1998; 18: 102–105.

81. Sugita S, Hirohata M, Tokutomi T, et al. A case of pituitary apoplexy in a child. Surg Neurol 1995; 43: 154–7.

82. Shah SA, Pereira JK, Becker CJ, et al. Pituitary apoplexy in adolescence. Pediatr Radiol (Suppl 1) 1995; 25: S26–S27.

83. Jennings MT, Gelman R, Hochberg F. Intracranial germ-cell tumors: natural history and pathogenesis. J Neurosurg 1985; 63: 155–67.

84. Bowman CB, Farris BK. Primary chiasmal germinoma: a case report and review of the literature. J Clin Neuro-ophthalmol 1990; 10: 9–17.

85. Takeuchi J, Handa H, Nagatal I. Suprasellar germinoma. J Neurosurg 1978; 49: 418.

86. Camins MB, Mount LA. Primary suprasellar atypical teratoma. Brain 1974; 97: 447–56.

87. Chang YW, Yoon H-K, Shin H-J, et al. Suprasellar retinoblastoma in a 5-month-old girl. Pediatr Radiol 2002; 32: 869–71.

88. DePotter P, Shields CL, Shields JA. Clinical variations of trilateral retinoblastoma. A report of 13 cases. J Pediatr Ophthalmol Strabismus 1994; 31: 26–31.

89. Kazim M, Kennerdell J, Maroon J, et al. Choristoma of the optic nerve and chiasm. Arch Ophthalmol 1992; 110: 236–8.

90. Till K. Paediatric Neurosurgery for Paediatricians and Neurosurgeons. Oxford: Blackwell Scientific Publications; 1975.

91. Goodwin J, Glaser JS. Chiasmal syndrome in sphenoid sinus mucocoele. Ann Neurol 1978; 4: 440–4.

92. Casteels I, De Loof E, Brock P, et al. Sudden blindness in a child: presenting symptoms of a sphenoid sinus mucocoele. Br J Ophthalmol 1992; 76: 502–4.

93. Newman NJ, Lessell S, Winterkorn JM. Optic chiasmal neuritis. Neurology 1991; 41: 1203–10.

94. Purvin V, Herr GJ, De Myer W. Chiasmal neuritis as a complication of Epstein-Barr infection. Arch Neurol 1988; 45: 458–60.

95. Bell RA, Robertson DM, Rosen DA, et al. Optochiasmiatic arachnoiditis in multiple sclerosis. Arch Ophthalmol 1975; 93: 191–3.

96. Navarro IM, Peralta VH, Leon JA, et al. Tuberculous optochiasmatic arachnoiditis. Neurosurg 1981; 9: 654–60.

97. Takahashi T, Isayama Y. Chiasmal meningitis. Neuro-ophthalmol 1980; 1: 19.

98. Marus AO, Demakas JJ, Ross A, et al. Optochiasmatic arachnoiditis with treatment by surgical lysis of adhesions, corticosteroids, and cyclophosphamide. Report of a case. Neurosurgery 1986; 19: 101–3.

99. Sinclair AH, Doff NM. Hydrocephalus-simulating tumor in the production of chiasmal and other parahypophyseal lesions. Trans Ophthalmol Soc UK 1931; 51: 232–41.

100. Calogero JA, Alexander E. Unilateral amaurosis in a hydrocephalic child with an obstructed shunt. J Neurosurg 1971; 34: 236–8.

101. Roche JL, Choux M, Czorny A, et al. L'aneurysme artériel intracranien chez l'enfant: étude cooperative. À propos de 43 observations. Neurochirurgie 1988; 34: 243–51.

102. Meyer FB, Sundt TM, Fode NC, et al. Cerebral aneurysms in childhood and adolescence. J Neurosurg 1989; 70: 420–5.

103. Schoenberg BS, Mellinger JF, Schoenberg DG. Moya-moya disease in children. South Med J 1978; 71: 237–41.

104. Waga S, Tochio H. Intracranial aneurysm association with moyamoya disease. Surg Neurol 1985; 23: 237–43.

105. Noda S, Hayasaka S, Setogawa T, et al Ocular symptoms of moya moya disease. Am J Ophthalmol 1987; 103: 812–7.

106. Maitland CG, Abiko S, Hoyt WF, et al. Chiasmal apoplexy: report of four cases. J Neurosurg 1982; 56: 118–22.

107. Lessell S. Magnetic resonance imaging signs may antedate visual loss in chiasmal radiation injury. Arch Ophthalmol 2003; 121: 287–8.

108. Jaffer KA, Obbens EA, El Gammal TA. Empty sella: review of 79 cases. South Med J 1979; 72: 294–6.

109. Pollock SC, Bromberg BS. Visual loss in a patient with primary empty sella. Arch Ophthalmol 1987; 105: 1487–8.

110. McFadzean RM. The empty sella syndrome. A review of 14 cases. Trans Ophthalmol Soc UK 1983; 103: 537–42.

111. Osher RH, Corbett JJ, Schatz NJ, et al. Neuro-ophthalmological complications of enlargement of the third ventricle. Br J Ophthalmol 1978; 62: 536–42.

CHAPTER
63

Hydrocephalus, Brain Anomalies and Cortical Visual Impairment

Creig S Hoyt

HYDROCEPHALUS

A precise, all-inclusive, definition of "hydrocephalus" is difficult to articulate. A working definition can be put forth however: Hydrocephalus is a disorder characterized by an imbalance of cerebrospinal fluid formation and absorption: the result is an excess of cerebrospinal fluid (CSF) accumulating within the central nervous system causing an elevation in intracranial pressure. This, in turn, exerts a pressure on the brain substance itself. Hydrocephalus can exist in the presence of normal sized cerebral ventricles although in most cases they are enlarged. The degree of dilatation of the cerebrospinal fluid pathways and the amount of damage done to the brain depends upon both the extent and etiology of the hydrocephalus. The age of the patient at the time when the hydrocephalus develops is also critical.[1] A number of important ocular consequences of hydrocephalus are relatively common.

The formation of CSF and its pathways

The embryology of the neural tube is essential in considering hydrocephalus. Closure of the neural tube occurs at about 28 postconceptual days. Constriction of portions of the central lumen of the neural tube are accompanied by expansion of other portions that form the basic ventricular system. During the second gestational month the fourth ventricle is formed by mesenchymal invagination. This is followed by a similar process that produces the lateral and third ventricles. The choroid plexuses form within these invaginations and initially are quite large, filling up to 75% of the ventricular lumen during the third month of gestation. Gradually, the size of the choroid plexuses relative to lateral ventricles diminish.

The cerebrospinal fluid (CSF) pathway appears as the result of a degeneration of the primitive mesenchyme of the developing brain.[2] Circulating cerebrospinal fluid probably is not detectable until the ninth or tenth gestational week at which time the fourth ventricular foramen outflow develops.[3]

CSF flows from the cerebral ventricles through the ventricular foramen and into the subarachnoid spaces, ultimately to be absorbed in the venous system.[4,5] This notion of bulk flow of cerebrospinal fluid within the ventricular system is challenged by other authorities who believe it is nearly entirely pulsatile with few cerebrospinal fluid molecules actually circulating.

Theories of hydrocephalus

All of the several theories of the development of hydrocephalus are founded on the notion that an imbalance between cerebrospinal fluid production and absorption is essential. The rate of cerebrospinal fluid production is relatively constant within the brain, and with the exception of choroid plexus papillomas, overproduction of the cerebrospinal fluid is rare. Excess cerebrospinal fluid does not seem to be a major cause of hydrocephalus. Rather, it appears to be the result of impaired absorption of cerebrospinal fluid. This diminished absorption may result from blockage of CSF flow within the ventricular system itself or through the cisterna magna, the basilar systems or over the cerebral convexities. Diminished absorption may also take place at the level of the arachnoid villa or lymphatic channels associated with cranial nerves, spinal nerves and the adventia of cerebral vessels.[5,6]

The pathophysiology of brain damage

Mild increases in intracranial pressure may be compensated for by absorption of cerebrospinal fluid through the arachnoid membrane, the cisterna of the choroid plexus or even by passing through the extracellular space of the cortical mantle to reach the surface of the brain.[6] This situation is referred to as compensated hydrocephalus.

Damage to the brain may come about in several ways. Obstructive changes in small blood vessels especially in the periventricular white matter of hydrocephalic patients results in neuronal and astrocytic swelling in the deep gray matter and atrophic changes in the white matter of the cerebral hemispheres.[7] This reduction in blood flow in the periventricular area can be measured by positron emission tomography.[8] Additional damage is done to the cilia normally covering the ependymal surface of the ventricular walls, which may completely disappear in chronic hydrocephalus.[9] In addition, ependymal cells in the walls of the ventricle stretch and degenerate. Fibrosis of the choroid plexus may ultimately occur.

Systemic results of hydrocephalus

By far, the most important and consistent associated abnormality in the childhood with hydrocephalus is an excessive rate of head growth. It is the growth that should be emphasized. A large head circumference percentile by itself should not be concerning. However, serial circumference measurements of a child's head that demonstrates excessive rate of head growth across percentiles should always raise suspicions of hydrocephalus. Head growth associated with hydrocephalus is more dramatic in the younger, more distensible brain and the not-yet-fused sutures of the skull of the young infant.

Hydrocephalus is now often detected prenatally by ultrasonography. Intrauterine hydrocephalus carries a poor prognosis because of the frequently associated malformations of the central nervous system and elsewhere that are found in the majority of these infants[10] (Fig. 63.1). Even if treated, hydrocephalus in this

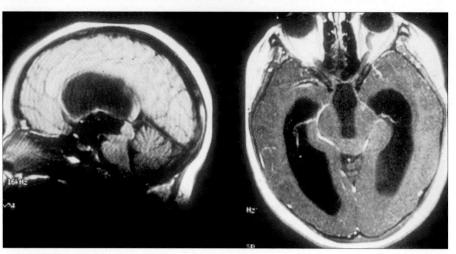

Fig. 63.1 Agenesis of the corpus callosum and hydrocephalus in a patient with septo-optic dysplasia.

group has a poor prognosis for normal development. The average life expectancy is a few years.

In contrast, hydrocephalus detected even in early infancy has a better prognosis for development and survival.[7] The Chiari formation, aqueductal stenosis, and aqueductal gliosis account for at least 3/4 of the hydrocephalus seen in infancy[7] (Fig. 63.2). Other relatively common causes of hydrocephalus in infancy including uterine perinatal and neonatal infection as well as perinatal–neonatal hemorrhage.

In addition to the enlargement of the skull associated with hydrocephalus, spasticity of the lower extremities is relatively common. The axons subserving motor function in the lower extremities must travel around the dilated ventricles and have a longer distance to travel than those that supply the upper extremities. Stretching and distortion of these fibers resulted in weakness and spasticity in the lower extremities.[7]

Hydrocephalus in the child of greater than 2 years of age may present with focal neurologic deficits that reflect the primary lesion or cause of the hydrocephalus. As the child gets older, the most common cause of hydrocephalus shifts from congenital anomalies of the central nervous system to tumors of the posterior fossa and obstruction of the aqueduct.[7]

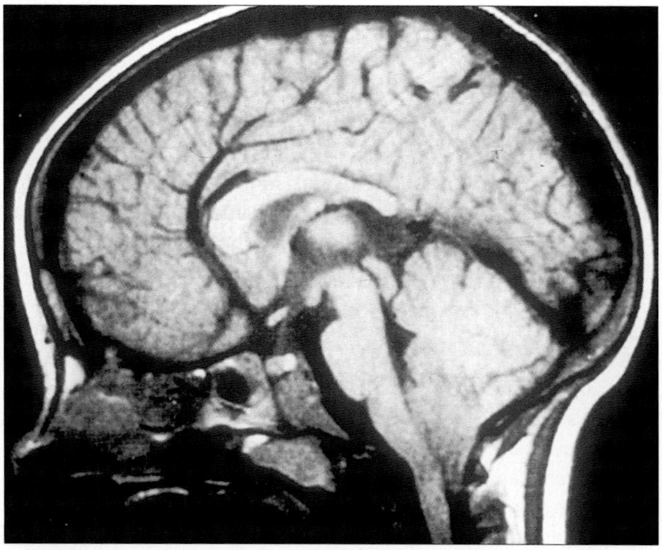

In most patients of any age group, increased intracranial pressure is often accompanied by an early morning headache that improves with an upright posture but may be aggravated by straining. Hypothalamic–pituitary dysfunction may occur, resulting in a wide range of endocrine abnormalities. A complex of perceptual and motor deficits including visual, spacial and visual attentional disorders may result from stretching of axons within the frontal, parietal and occipital globes.[7]

Ocular complications of hydrocephalus

A wide range of ocular motor, sensory and optic nerve pathway changes may be associated with elevated intracranial pressure in hydrocephalus. Disturbances of ocular motility such as acquired comitant and incomitant strabismus, nystagmus, gaze palsies, and unusual abnormalities of eye movement including the bobble-headed doll syndrome may all be associated with elevated intracranial pressure. Pupillary abnormalities may include a light-near dissociation phenomena as well as an afferent pupillary defect. Disorders of the anterior visual pathway may be manifested as papilledema, optic atrophy, optociliary shunt vessels, and chiasmal and/or optic tract visual field abnormalities. Cortical disabilities associated with hydrocephalus include cortical visual impairment, visual attention and visual spatial disorders. Visual field loss may result from involvement of the optic radiations and/or primary visual cortex. Although these ocular abnormalities can be directly associated with the elevated intracranial pressure and usually the associated ventricular enlargement treatment of the elevated intracranial pressure does not always reverse these abnormalities.

Optic nerve

Papilledema

The term papilledema is usually restricted by most authorities to optic nerve head swelling specifically associated with elevated intracranial pressure. It is a frequent finding in the child with hydrocephalus although less so in the infant with an incompletely fused skull.[11] However one suspects that papilledema is more frequent even in infants than generally recognized since evaluation of the disc by ophthalmoscopy photography and even retinal imaging instrumentation is difficult in this age group. In

Fig. 63.2 Cerebellar tonsil inferior displacement in Arnold Chiari type II malformation.

older more co-operative children hydrocephalus is frequently associated with dramatic degrees of disc elevation, hemorrhage, exudate, and even macular changes.

Optic atrophy

Optic atrophy is common in all forms of hydrocephalus and is a major cause of visual morbidity.[11,12] However, one should be cautious in trying to predict the degree of visual disability in a child with optic atrophy based on the appearance of the optic nerve alone. It is striking how often profound optic atrophy is seen in hydrocephalic children with relatively good visual function. However these very children may be especially vulnerable to dramatic and catastrophic visual loss as the result of sudden shunt failure or with episodic elevation in intracranial pressure. Children with hydrocephalus who have significant optic atrophy have a higher incidence of visual impairment and associated severe neurologic deficits than those with normal appearing optic nerves.[12]

The mechanism for optic nerve damage in hydrocephalus is multifaceted. Long-standing papilledema may result in post-papilledema optic atrophy with significant visual loss which is almost always bilateral although often asymmetric in its appearance.[11] The optic nerve may also be damaged as a result of the dilation of the ventricles especially the third ventricle which may compress the chiasm directly or the adjacent arterial supply of it. Third ventricular compression of the vascular supply of the optic tracts may also occur resulting ultimately in the appearance of optic atrophy.[13] Elevation of intracranial pressure may result in arterial compression and ischemia of the optic nerve itself. It remains controversial whether retrograde transsynaptic neuronal degeneration through the lateral geniculate body from the optic radiations and/or visual cortex accounts for some of the optic atrophy seen in infants with elevated intracranial pressure. However the well-recognized and frequent disc problems associated with periventricular leukomalacia lends weight to the argument that transsynaptic neuronal degeneration may occur in the human infant.[14]

Chiasmal disorders

Typical bitemporal visual field defects can be seen in patients with hydrocephalus and no intrinsic chiasmal lesion nor any other extrinsic compressive pathology. The close anatomical relationship between the third ventricle and the optic chiasm is easily distorted when the third ventricle is enlarged. In most cases where third ventricle enlargement compromises chiasmal function some degree of aqueductal stenosis can be found. These patients usually have other ocular manifestations associated with the chiasmal defects especially signs of dorsal midbrain dysfunction.[13]

Posterior visual pathway disorders

Bilateral visual loss or homonymous hemianopic field defects may result from damage to the visual cortex in the patient with hydrocephalus.[15] This is usually attributed to posterior cerebral artery circulation compromise thought to result from bilateral compression of these vessels on the tentorial edge as the result of rostral–caudal deterioration as movement of the intracranial contents through the foreman magnum attempts to spontaneously decompress the hydrocephalic brain. As previously stated however, some of the visual loss experienced in the posterior visual pathways probably comes about as the result of periventricular white matter loss resulting from compression of small intrinsic blood vessels.[7] Some authorities assert that posterior visual pathway damage occurs more commonly after shunt failure than as a primary result of hydrocephalus. One also occasionally sees children in whom partial visual field loss associated with raised intracranial pressure was detected preshunt implantation and deterioration or total blindness occurs despite successful shunt implantation.[12] The precise mechanism for the paradoxical deterioration in visual function following successful shunt placement is not completely understood. It may result from ischemic changes that occur with the decompression of the ventricular system. Protracted visual recovery following shunt surgery can also be seen with improved visual function being recorded over several weeks or months. The mechanism for this phenomenon is also incompletely understood.

Ocular motor defects

A wide range of ocular motor abnormalities are seen in association with hydrocephalus and/or its associated central nervous system disorder.

Strabismus

Strabismus in many forms is by far the most common ocular complication of hydrocephalus occurring in the majority of patients. Although most of these patients have horizontal forms of strabismus, vertical and combined forms of strabismus, as well as skew deviation may be seen.[12]

It is well-recognized that unilateral or bilateral sixth nerve palsies frequently accompany hydrocephalus. This results in an incomitant esotropia in most cases although divergence paralysis, defined as a comitant esotropia larger at distance than at near may represent a subclinical bilateral sixth nerve palsy in some circumstances.[16] Comitant esotropia is actually more common in patients with hydrocephalus than incomitant strabismus.[17] In infants under the age of one, this comitant esotropia may be indistinguishable from typical infantile esotropia and be associated with all of the accompanying ocular motor disorders seen in infantile esotropia (dissociative vertical deviation, inferior oblique overaction, and latent nystagmus).[18] In the older child an acquired comitant esotropia may be seen as the sign of either the onset of hydrocephalus or shunt failure.[19] Of particular note is the frequency with which A pattern esotropia is seen in association with hydrocephalus.[20] This seems to be specifically related to certain associated central nervous system pathologies including spina bifida, meningocele,[21] Chiari 1 malformation,[22] and other low brainstem anomalies.[23] It is not seen in association with disorders of the aqueduct.

Much less frequently unilateral or even bilateral fourth nerve palsies may occur in association with hydrocephalus.[24] This appears to result from compression of the trochlear nerve by the tentorial margin. The fourth nerve is especially vulnerable because of its decussation within the anterior medullary vellum where the two trochlear nerves interdigitate and can be compressed easily by tumor, by a dilated aqueduct or affected by downward pressure from an enlarged third ventricle. Unequivocally acquired non-traumatic bilateral fourth nerve palsies should raise the concern of undetected hydrocephalus in children.[24]

Third nerve palsies are distinctly unusual as a result of hydrocephalus. When they occur they are often the sign of fatal rostral-caudal deterioration in uncontrolled raised intracranial pressure.

Exotropia does occur occasionally in the hydrocephalic child although in most circumstances this is probably sensory in origin as the result of unilateral or asymmetric visual loss related to optic atrophy.[12]

Supranuclear ocular motor disturbances

In young infants with hydrocephalus the so called "setting sun" sign with bilateral upper lid refraction and forceful downward deviation of the eyes is associated with a supranuclear up gaze palsy that effects both saccades and pursuits.[25] This is a poor prognostic sign and is often accompanied by severe optic atrophy and visual loss. It is almost always accompanied by severe obstructive hydrocephalus especially aqueductal stenosis. It must be distinguished from the transient downward deviation seen in otherwise healthy neonates in which the downward deviation is not accompanied by an upgaze palsy. In older children with hydrocephalus a dorsal midbrain syndrome usually in association with aqueductal stenosis results from dilation of the third ventricle or enlargement of suprapineal recess with resulting pressure on the posterior commissure and its surrounding area. This dorsal midbrain syndrome usually consists of a supranuclear upgaze palsy, gaze paretic up-beating nystagmus, light–near dissociation of the pupillary reflexes and other forms of nystagmus. Convergence retraction nystagmus may be seen in severe cases. A variant of convergence retraction nystagmus has been termed V-pattern pretectal pseudo bobbing and consists of arrhythmic, repetitive, fast downward and inward movements of the eye.

Another rare abnormality seen in hydrocephalus is the bobble-headed doll syndrome. In this condition flexion–extension movements of the head and neck on the trunk are seen. The condition is almost invariably associated with an enlarged third ventricle associated with an intracranial tumor and usually resolves after successful shunt surgery.

Nystagmus

Several different forms of nystagmus may occur in hydrocephalus.[12] The idiopathic congenital nystagmus syndrome is frequently seen as the result of early bilateral significant optic atrophy and associated visual loss. Gaze paretic nystagmus may be seen in association with vertical gaze palsies or sixth nerve palsies. Children with hydrocephalus and associated specific and other associated specific intracranial pathology may show very unique forms of nystagmus that are highly diagnostic. For example, acquired downbeat nystagmus especially in the presence of an A pattern esotropia is highly suggestive of the Chiari 1 malformation and may be associated with hydrocephalus.[22]

Radiologic diagnosis of hydrocephalus

The prenatal diagnosis of hydrocephalus is made almost exclusively using ultrasonography. The postnatal diagnosis of hydrocephalus can be made clinically together with ultrasound, and CT or MR imaging. Using any of these techniques hydrocephalus is suspected when the ventricles are enlarged in the absence of significant white matter atrophy. This differentiation is not always as easy as it sounds (Fig. 63.3). The most reliable signs to differentiate hydrocephalus from ex vacuo ventricular enlargement of white matter are enlargement of anterior and posterior recesses of the third ventricle and commensurate dilation of the temporal horns. While radiographic techniques can usually detect enlargement of the ventricles, often direct measurement of the intracranial pressure is usually a necessary part of the diagnostic evaluation.

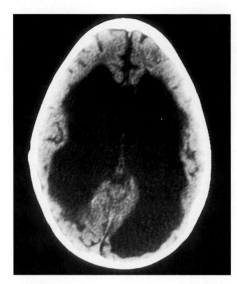

Fig. 63.3 Cortical atrophy with ex-vacuo dilation of ventricles following perinatal hypoxic ischemic encephalopathy.

Treatment

Untreated hydrocephalus inevitably leads to tissue damage and hemispheric atrophy. White matter is disproportionately damaged more than the gray matter in almost all cases. Hydrocephalus is treated by placement of some type of ventricular shunting device either ventriculoperitoneal or ventriculoatrial. Early diagnosis with prompt surgery is essential in order to minimize permanent neurologic and ophthalmic consequences. Early treatment can result in complete regression of ventricular dilatation with no apparent residual neurologic deficits. Neurologic recovery following shunting can be dramatic and occur over a short period of time. However, in the case of children with cortical visual impairment associated with hydrocephalus visual recovery following shunt revision or placement may take weeks to months.[25] Despite effective treatment, a significant percentage of hydrocephalic children will continue to perform below average in various neurologic, visual and intellectual tests.

Advice to the parents

Most causes of hydrocephalus should be viewed as chronic disorders. Many children will require multiple shunt replacements in their childhood in order to maintain normal intracranial pressure. Timely detection of shunt failure is an important part of the management of these children. In many cases, changes in the ocular status of these children may be the first sign of shunt failure or elevation of intracranial pressure. Decrease in vision, acute onset of strabismus, deterioration of previously well-controlled strabismus in the presence of other unusual eye movements may be the first sign that something is amiss. Children with hydrocephalus require periodic ophthalmic re-evaluation and parents should be urged to seek ophthalmic consultation when any new and unusual changes occur in the child's visual function.

BRAIN PROBLEMS: CONGENITAL AND ACQUIRED

A wide range of congenital and acquired disorders of the central nervous system are important in dealing with children's visual problems. Many of the central nervous system disorders impinge directly upon important and vital visual structures. Others do not but are associated with structural eye defects.

Developmental and structural defects

Cephalocele

Most congenital abnormalities of the central nervous system that effect the visual pathways are best understood in the context of the developmental stage in which they occur. During the first month of embryogenesis, a neural plate is formed which invaginates into the neural groove and then fuses into a neural tube. Classic teaching holds that a disturbance in the closure of the neural groove may result in a cephalocele.[26] Others argue that cephaloceles are the result of a postneurulation event in which brain tissue herniates through a defect in the mesenchyme that will become cranium and dura.[27] In any case "cephalocele" refers to a defect in the skull and dura with extracranial extension of intracranial structures. These are classified by the location of the bone defect through which they pass. Three of the major four types of cephaloceles are important to ophthalmologists. Occipital cephaloceles are the most common in white populations of Europe and North America.[28] In these defects the occipital cortex and portions of the occipital horn of the lateral ventricle herniate into the sack. Severe visual defects are associated both with this anomaly and the consequences of its surgical correction. Frontal-ethmoidal cephaloceles are the most common in South East Asia.[30] These do not usually impinge upon the visual system but ipsilateral optic disc dysplasia is frequently associated with them. Nasal pharyngeal cephaloceles are uncommon. Because of their occult nature they are important. Visual function is almost always affected as a result of the optic chiasm being stretched as it extends into the sack of the defect.[31]

Holoprosencephaly

During the second month of gestation the forebrain or prosencephalon is cleaved transversely into the telencephalon and diencephalon and sagittally into cerebral hemispheres and lateral ventricles. Failure of differentiation and cleaving of the prosencephalon result in a group of disorders referred to as holoprosencephalies.[32] The embryogenesis of this disorder is incompletely understood but is thought to result from a deficient or defective cranial mesenchyme with subsequent lack of induction and differentiation of basal midline structures. It is caused by both teratogens and genetic factors.[33] The most common recognized teratogenic cause is diabetes. A variety of associated central nervous system anomalies may accompany it, especially corpus callosum dysgenesis. Not surprisingly therefore optic nerve hypoplasia is commonly associated with holoprosencephaly.[34]

Neuronal migration anomalies

Between the second and fourth gestational months, the neurons in the ventricular and subventricular zones proliferate and then migrate to the cortical plates. While neurons early in embryogenesis migrate relatively short distances, neurons later in development often migrate long distances across the intermediate zones. Their migration may be facilitated by radial glial cells which appear to serve as guidelines. The neurons arriving first in the cortical mantle assume the deepest locations while neurons arriving later assume a more superficial location.[35]

Aberrations in normal neuronal migration result in a variety of neural abnormalities. Lissencephaly (smooth brain) occurs when neurons end their migration in the intermediate zone resulting in an absence of cortical gyri. There are two major subtypes of lissencephaly–"classical" and "cobblestone". Ophthalmologists have a special interest in "cobblestone" lissencephaly which results from an overmigration of neurons. "Cobblestone" lissencephaly is associated with at least three disorders in which congenital muscular dystrophies, central nervous system anomalies and eye abnormalities are associated.[36] These are:

1. Fukuyama type congenital muscular dystrophy, an autosomal recessive condition prevalent in Japan.
2. Walker–Warburg syndrome in which patients have "cobblestone" lissencephaly, congenital hydrocephalus, severe congenital muscular hypotonia and severe congenital eye malformations.
3. Muscle–eye brain disease which has been primarily described in Finland.[37] In this latter syndrome patients are hypotonic and have poor visual function as the result of a retinal dystrophy. On pathologic examination the cerebral cortex of patients with muscle–eye brain disease show abnormal convolutions with a granular ("cobblestone") surface to the cerebral cortex although the cortical defect in this syndrome seems to be less severe than in the two previously described.

Pachygyria is related to lissencephaly but develops when neuronal migration is disturbed at a later stage. It is characterized by reduced numbers of gyri, abnormally thick cortex and fewer cortical neurons than normal. Incomplete lissencephaly, in which areas of pachygyria are present together with areas of agyria or areas of normal brain is much more common than complete lissencephaly.[35]

Polymicrogyria is a malformation of cortical development in which the neurons reach the cortex but distribute abnormally resulting in the formation of multiple small gyri (Fig. 63.4). Although its effect on neurologic function is less severe than the disorders of neuronal migration described above polymicrogyria accounts for at least some of the cases of congenital homonomous hemianopia.[38] In these patients the polymicrogyria may be limited to just one occipital cortex area. Polymicrogyria, as well as neuronal ectopias and dysplasias have been found in the inferior frontal and superior temporal regions of the left hemisphere in dyslexic subjects.[39]

The fetal brain responds differently to injuries compared to the neonatal or adult brain. Injuries to the brain during fetal development cause total dissolution of the affected parenchyma, often with well circumscribed borders. Insults early in fetal development may result in loss of portions of the brain. Schizencephaly, sometimes called "agenetic porencephaly" is a term used to describe gray matter lined clefts that extend through the entire hemisphere from the ependymal lining of the lateral ventricles to the pial covering of the cortex (Fig. 63.5). Schizencephaly seems to result from both genetic and acquired causes.[40] Porencephaly is usually used to describe focal cavities with smooth walls and minimal surrounding glial reaction in the brain (Fig. 63.6). It is obvious that schizencephaly and porencephaly are essentially synonymous in describing an anomaly that results from destruction of a portion of the germinal matrix and surrounding brain before the hemispheres are fully formed. Hydranencephaly is a condition in which most of the brain mantle has been damaged, liquefied and resorbed. In a sense it can be seen as porencephaly of the entire cerebrum. The cerebral hemispheres are largely replaced by thin walled sacks containing cerebral spinal fluid. It is sometimes difficult to differentiate hydranencephaly from severe hydrocephalus.

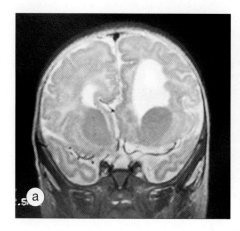

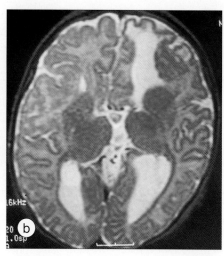

Fig. 63.4 Polymicrogyria. (a & b) Agenesis of the corpus callosum and ectopic gray matter in a patient with Aicardis syndrome.

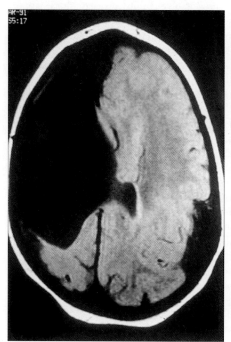

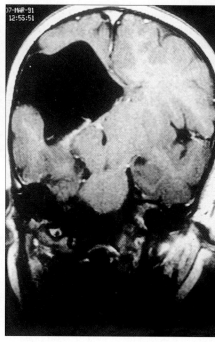

Fig. 63.5 Schizencephaly in a patient with prenatal infarction.

Developmental disorders of the corpus callosum are relatively common and important to ophthalmologists because of their frequent association with optic disc anomalies[34] (Fig. 63.7a, b). When agenesis of the corpus callosum is accompanied by agenesis of the cingulum the posterior portions of the lateral ventricles expand resulting in dilation of the trigons and occipital horns of the lateral ventricles. This condition is known as colpocephaly. Not surprisingly optic disc hypoplasia frequently accompanies it.

Congenital vascular anomalies may occur in the occipital lobes resulting in hemianopias or other more subtle field defects. These anomalies may be part of a more widespread vascular disorder such as the Sturge–Weber or Wyburn–Mason syndrome or may occur as isolated arteriovenous malformations. They are often calcified.

Congenital tumors of the occipital lobes are uncommon.

Congenital lesions of the geniculostriate pathway may result in transsynaptic degeneration of the ipsilateral temporal hemiretina which causes thinning of the arcuate nerve fiber bundles inferiorly and superiorly. Transsynaptic degeneration of the nasal hemiretina contralateral to the lesion produces a horizontal band

of optic disc atrophy. It is usually thought that an isolated defect of the geniculostriate pathway associated with either optic nerve atrophy or hypoplasia implies a prenatal injury. Some argue that the frequent optic disc anomaly seen in periventricular leukomalacia argues against this rule.[14]

Congenital homonomous hemianopia often remains undetected until early adulthood. It frequently occurs secondary to periventricular leukomalacia, but on occasion may occur secondary to lesions of the optic tracts. Congenital optic tract lesions are also usually associated with congenital nystagmus, which can help to distinguish them from lesions of the geniculostriate pathway. Patients with congenital homonomous hemianopia may show an afferent pupillary defect on the side contralateral to the cerebral lesion. This has been attributed to the transsynaptic degeneration of the pupillomotor fibers. Thus, it would appear that the pupillomotor fibers which do not synapse at the lateral geniculate body but at the pretectal area may also be susceptible to transsynaptic degeneration. Generally patients with congenital hemianopia cope better with their defect than those who acquire

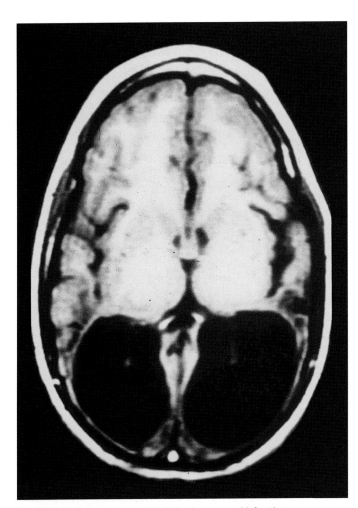

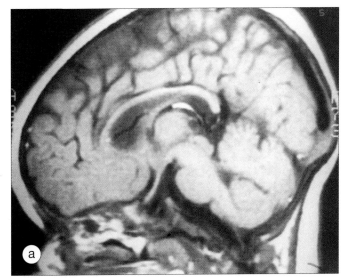

Fig. 63.6 Occipital porencephaly following prenatal infarction.

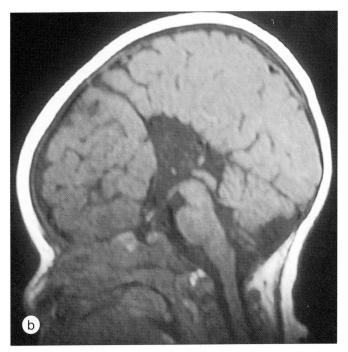

Fig. 63.7 Septo-optic dysplasia. (a) Hypoplasia of corpus callosum in septo-optic dysplasia. (b) Agenesis of corpus callosum in patient with septo-optic dysplasia.

similar field defects later in life. A complete understanding of the mechanism of compensation for this is not yet known. However at least in part some of the compensation appears to be a unique saccadic strategy for fixating an eccentric target in which the patient produces a single large saccadic movement into the blind field that overshoots the intended visual target.

CORTICAL VISUAL IMPAIRMENT

The term "cortical blindness" is used to refer to the patient who has been rendered blind by bilateral damage to the occipital cortex. It is a term introduced as the result of studies of adult patients.[41] Cortical blindness is defined clinically as a bilateral loss of vision with normal pupillary responses and an eye examination, which shows no abnormalities.[42] In adults, this is considered to be an infrequent event and usually the result of arterial circulatory disease.

For several reasons, the term "cortical blindness" does not seem appropriate to describe the clinical conditions responsible for visual loss due to damage to the occipital cortex and its associated structures in children.[42] First and foremost, total absence of sight in children due to a bilateral disturbance of the optic radiations and/or calcarine cortex is extremely rare.[42,43] Moreover, unlike the case in adults, significant visual recovery can be documented in a large proportion of the children with visual

loss due to calcarine cortex injury. Roland and associates studied 30 children with visual loss due to occipital cortex injury and documented some degree of visual recovery in 50%.[44] In a study of 19 babies with perinatal hypoxic-ischemic insults, 16 could be documented to have improved visual function over a 3–7 year follow-up.[45] In a series of 170 children with visual loss due to optic radiation and/or visual cortex damage from a number of different causes,[46] 60% of children showed some visual recovery. For these reasons, the term, "cortical visual impairment" was introduced to emphasize the visual potential in these neurologically damaged children.[42]

The term "cortical visual impairment" is unfortunately equally misleading in describing many of these children. It fails to accurately describe the group of children with visual impairment resulting from primarily deep subcortical white matter insults (periventricular leukomalacia). For this reason, the term "cerebral visual impairment" has been suggested as a replacement for "cortical visual impairment." This problem surrounding a precise terminology to describe children with visual impairment due to neurologic disease has been compounded by some who would use the term "cortical visual impairment" to describe children with ocular motor apraxia, saccadic paralysis, visual inattention, etc.[47]

In the past most cases of CVI were due to meningitis and/or encephalitis or hydrocephalus. The most common organism responsible for meningitis and cortical visual impairment is *H. influenzae*.[48] The onset of neurological visual loss associated with meningitis may be late and usually occurs after the child has recovered from the acute infection. Thrombophlebitis[48] and arterial occlusion play a prominent role in the pathophysiology of cortical visual impairment associated with meningitis. Encephalitis, especially the cases due to neonatal herpes simplex infection, may cause cerebral visual impairment.[49]

Hydrocephalus can cause acute and chronic cortical visual impairment.[50] With significant dilation of the ventricles and the resulting distention of the posterior cortex occlusion of the posterior cerebral arteries and resulting occipital cortex infarction may occur.[51] However, most cases of cortical visual impairment associated with hydrocephalus are not associated with infarction of the occipital cortex but simply dilation of the ventricles. Long-term shunt malfunction can cause permanent cortical visual impairment.[52] Ironically, cortical visual impairment may occur following a successful shunt procedure, presumably due to too rapid correction of the elevated intracranial pressure.[53]

Cortical visual impairment may occur secondary to a variety of other causes including hypoglycemia, hemodialysis, cisplatin therapy, seizures, cerebral arteriography, malaria, inflammatory and neurodegenerative disorders[43] (Fig. 63.8). Trauma may produce either a transient or a permanent form of cortical visual impairment. It is a tragedy that "nonaccidental" trauma is increasingly seen as a significant cause of cortical visual impairment in all societies.

However, a single cause accounts for the overwhelming majority of cases of cortical visual impairment in children—perinatal hypoxic-ischemia.[46,54] With advances in perinatal care has come increased survival rates for children with hypoxic-ischemic insults.[55] Indeed, the increasing prevalence of cortical visual impairment in many ways parallels the resurgence of retinopathy of prematurity as a cause of visual impairment in children in developed countries.[46]

Cortical visual impairment is now clearly the single greatest cause of visual impairment in young children in developed countries.[56,57] Cortical visual impairment places a major burden on ophthalmological and educational services in these countries. Moreover, cortical visual impairment is rarely an isolated defect as the vast majority of affected patients have associated neurological or ophthalmological defects.

In one study, 75% of the children had associated neurological deficits, many of which require ongoing management and some of which interfered with visual function (for example, seizures and anticonvulsant therapy).[46] Over 50% of the patients with cortical visual impairment had seizures. A significant number of these patients are afflicted with cerebral palsy or other motor deficits: over 40% had significant neurological deficits affecting mobility. In one study, 53% of the patients with cortical visual impairment had cerebral palsy.[55] One hundred percent of congenital and 88% of acquired cortical visual impairment patients were found to have associated neurological abnormalities.[58] The results of these

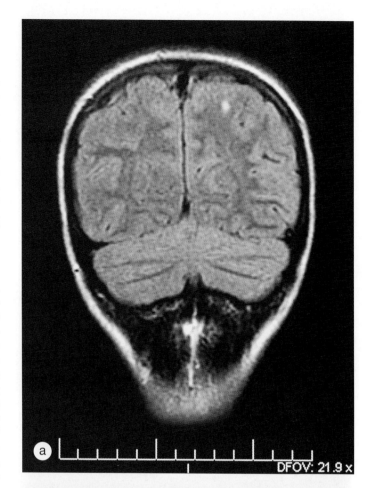

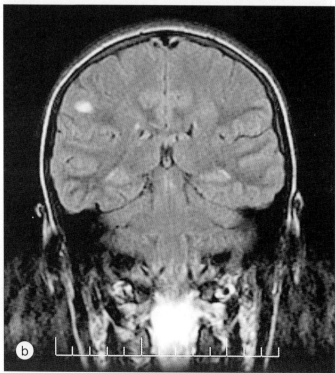

Fig. 63.8 Acute disseminated encephalomyelopathy (ADEM). (a & b) 12-year-old with white matter enhancement in ADEM.

can be seen by visiting any residential blind school in the developed world where the vast majority of students are now multiply handicapped and the teaching strategies developed for children with visual impairment due to isolated ocular disease are found not to be appropriate or effective for these children with cortical visual impairment.[59]

The premature infant

Several types of brain injury may occur in premature infants due to a mild to moderate episode of hypoxia and hypoperfusion. These included periventricular leukomalacia, periventricular hemorrhagic infarction, germinal matrix hemorrhage, intraventricular hemorrhage, and cerebellar infarction. However, I will limit this discussion to injury of the periventricular white matter–the most common site of brain injury related to hypoxia-hypoperfusion in premature infants. The corticospinal tracts run through the periventricular region and for this reason, impaired motor function is the most common sequela of periventricular white matter injury. Spastic diplegia, weakness of the lower extremities, is the most common neurologic disability in premature infants with an incidence of 5–15%.[60] Visual impairment is quite common in premature children with spastic diplegia, with the incidence as high as 70%.[61] These children almost invariably have some form of periventricular leukomalacia.

CT and MRI studies of these patients may demonstrate:
1. Ventriculomegaly with an irregular outline of the body and trigone of the lateral ventricles.
2. Reduced volume of periventricular white matter.
3. Deep, prominent sulci that abut or nearly abut the ventricles with little or no interposed white matter.[62]

In addition, MRI will show increased signal intensity in the area of the periventricular white matter and delayed myelination.[63] It is especially important to note that sagittal MRI may reveal thinning of the corpus callosum due to degeneration of the transcallosal fibers.[64]

An entirely different pattern of brain injury is seen in premature infants who have suffered a profound hypotensive event or cardiopulmonary arrest. Injury is concentrated in the deep gray matter and brainstem nuclei, although some periventricular damage may occur as well.[65] The brainstem, cerebellum, and thalami are predominately injured: An MRI performed several months after injury will reveal small thalami, brainstem, and cerebellum, often accompanied by reduced cerebral white matter. The survival rates for this group is poor but if they survive, they may present with athetosis in addition to quadriparesis, severe seizure disorder, and mental retardation.[44]

Because of improved survival rates of very premature infants,[66] periventricular leukomalacia is seen with increasing frequency as a cause of cortical visual impairment.[67] In contrast, the incidence of encephalopathy secondary to hypoxic-ischemic injury in term infants appeared to be decreasing.[68] Nevertheless, 10–15% of cerebral palsy is secondary to perinatal hypoxic-ischemic injury in term infants.[69]

The full-term infant

The primary injury in term infants who suffer a mild to moderate hypoxic-hypoperfusion event occurs at the watershed areas, the regions between the middle and posterior cerebral arteries and between the anterior and middle cerebral arteries. The results in discrete, often cystic infarctions in the boundary zones between the major vascular territories (Fig. 63.9). Thus, infarction is most

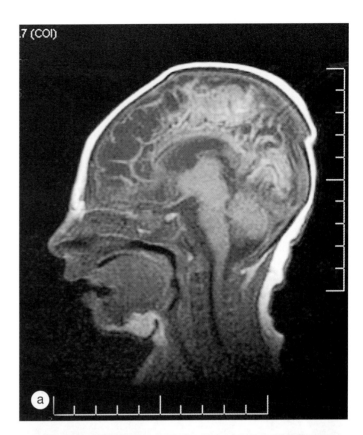

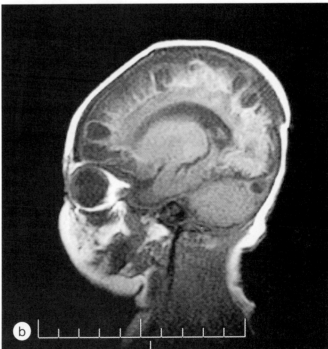

Fig. 63.9 Cystic encephalomalacia. (a & b) Cystic encephalomalacia in a 3-week-old girl following meconium aspiration.

likely to occur in the frontal and the parieto-occipital regions. After the child has recovered from the acute hypoxic-ischemic insult, MRI studies may reveal: (i) Cortical thinning and diminution of the underlying white matter in the area of infarction; (ii) ex-vacuo dilation of the lateral ventricles; (iii) the development of a gyral anomaly, ulegyria, due to the pattern of shrinking cortex; (iv) wedge-shape infarction in the watershed zones[70] (Fig. 63.10).

A distinctly different pattern of brain injury is seen in term infants who suffer a profound hypoxic-hypoperfusion event or cardiocirculatory arrest. Most of these children do not however survive.[71] Injury occurs primarily in the lateral thalami, posterior putamina, hippocampus, and corticospinal tracts.[72] It is essential to know that many of these children will also show significant injury to the lateral geniculate bodies and the optic radiations. The cortex is usually spared except for the peri-Rolandic gyri.[72]

Visual recovery in CVI

There are several possible reasons why infants with some forms of cortical visual impairment seem to improve over time. One may be simply that the normal maturation of visual systems that occurs in normal infants allows residual visual potential in these brain damage children to become apparent over time.[73] Another is that the damage to the visual cortex and/or optic radiations is usually incomplete in these children. Thus, residual visual function can be attributed to the residual intact functioning visual cortex and radiations. Yet, most investigators who study these children seem to believe that some unique mechanism of plasticity of the brain in infants is an important factor in the apparent visual recovery that occurs in many of these children.[43]

In cats, there are pronounced functional and anatomical differences between animals who experienced visual cortex ablation as neonates and those who undergo it as adults. Neonatal lesions of the primary visual cortex in cats lead to significant changes in the organization of visual pathways including severe retrograde degeneration of retinal ganglion cells. If kittens undergo visual cortex ablation (up to the age of 2 weeks), there will be a 78% loss of retinal ganglion cells of the x/beta class, whereas visual cortex ablation in adult cat results in only a 22% loss of x/beta cells.[74]

At the cortex level, most of the adaptive changes seem to take place in the posteromedial lateral suprasylvian (PMLS) cortex. Anatomical studies with both anterograde and retrograde tracing methods reveal an increased projection from the retina through the thalamus to the posteromedial lateral suprasylvian extrastriate visual areas of cortex in the damaged hemisphere of cats with a neonatal visual cortex ablation.[75] No such enhanced projections are seen in cats who undergo visual cortex ablation as adults. Single-cell neurophysiological studies indicate that physiological compensation is present in the posteromedial lateral suprasylvian cortex and these cells developed normal receptive field properties.[76] However, these cells in the posteromedial lateral suprasylvian cortex do not acquire the response properties of the striate neurons that were damaged (high spatial frequency tuning and low contrast threshold).[76,77] Nevertheless, the data in experimental animals seem clear. An incomplete, but nonetheless impressive compensation takes place primarily in the posteromedial lateral suprasylvian cortex of cats who undergo visual cortex ablation as neonates. No comparable compensation occurs in animals who undergo ablation as adults. Whether other areas of the cortex are also important in the visual recovery of infant cats with visual cortex ablation remains unclear.

Almost nothing is known about the underlying neuroanatomical substrates responsible for recovery from visual cortex damage in adult or neonatal experimental primates. Rodman and co-workers demonstrated in adult macaques that after ablation of the visual cortex, neurons in the area MT of the peristriate cortex still respond appropriately albeit less robustly and they retain direction selectivity. This would suggest that at least motion detection can be processed without striate cortex via pathways of the extrageniculostriate system from the thalamus directly to area MT.[78] Whether this explains the Riddoch phenomenon in man has yet to be determined. The compensatory nature of the posteromedial lateral suprasylvian cortex has been conclusively demonstrated in cats but the possibility that it plays a similar compensatory role in primates who undergo comparable neonatal visual cortex damage has recently been challenged.[79]

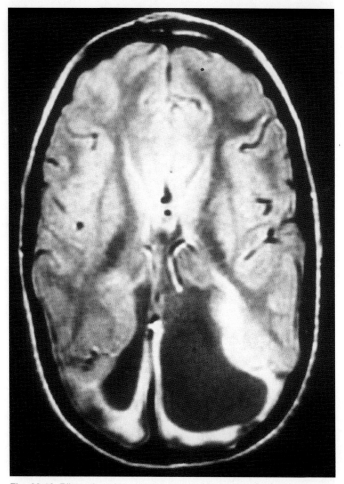

Fig. 63.10 Bilateral wedge-shaped occipital "watershed" infarctions.

REFERENCES

1. Barkovitch AJ. Pediatric Neuro Imaging. Philadelphia: Lippincott Williams and Wilkins; 2000: 581–94.
2. Osaka K, Handa R, Matsumoto S, et al. Development of the cerebrospinal fluid pathway in the normal and abnormal human embryo. Child's Brain 1980; 60: 26–38.
3. Dooling EC, Chi Je G, Jilles FH. Ependymal changes in the human fetal brain. Ann Neurol 1977; 1: 535–7.
4. McComb JG. Recent research into the nature of cerebrospinal fluid formation and absorption. J Neurosurg 1983; 59: 369–83.
5. McComb JG. Cerebrospinal fluid physiology of the developing fetus. AJNR Am J Neuroradiol 1992; 13: 595–9.
6. Milhorat TH. Classifications of the cerebral edemas with reference to hydrocephalus and pseudotumor cerebri. Childs Nerv Syst 1992; 8: 301–6.
7. Milhorat TH. Hydrocephaly. In: Myrianthopoulos NC, ed. Malformations of the Central Nervous System. New York: Elsevier; 1987: 285–300.
8. Shirane R, Sako S, Sako K, et al. Cerebral blood flow and oxygen metabolism in infants with hydrocephalus. Childs Nerv Syst 1992; 8: 118–23.
9. Hill A, Volpe JJ. Decrease in pulsatile flow in the anterior cerebral arteries in infantile hydrocephalus. Pediatrics 1982; 69: 4–10.
10. Rosseau GL, McCullough DC, Joseph AL. Current prognosis in fetal ventriculomegaly. J Neurosurg 1992; 77: 551–5.
11. Ghose S. Optic nerve changes in hydrocephalus. Trans Ophthalmol Soc UK 1983; 103: 217–20.
12. Gaston H. Ophthalmic complications of spina bifidi-hydrocephalus. Eye 1991; 5: 279–90.
13. Osher RH, Corbett JJ, Schatz NJ, et al. Neuro-ophthalmological complications of enlargement of the third ventricle. Br J Ophthalmol 1978; 62: 536–42.
14. Jacobson LK, Dutton GN. Periventricular leukomalacia: an important cause of visual and ocular motility dysfunction in children. Surv Ophthalmol 2000; 45: 1–13.
15. Smith JL, Walsh TJ, Shipley T. Cortical blindness in congenital hydrocephalus. Am J Ophthalmol 1966; 62: 251–7.
16. Hogg JE, Schoenberg PX. Paralysis of divergence in an adult with aqueduct stenosis. Arch Neurol 1979; 36: 511–2.
17. Harcourt RB. Ophthalmic complications of meningomyelocele and hydrocephalus in children. Br J Ophthalmol 1968; 52: 670–8.
18. Charles SJ, Moore AT. Infantile esotropia in normal infants and those with neuro developmental disorders. Eye 1992; 6: 603–6.
19. Vollrath-Junger C, Lange J. Akuten Strabismus Convergens bei erhohtem Hirnvruck. Monatsbl Augenheilkd 1987; 190: 359–63.
20. Hoyt CS, Good WV. Acute onset concomitant esotropia. When is it a sign of serious neurological disease? Br J Ophthalmol 1995; 79: 498–502.
21. Biglan AW. Ophthalmological complications of meningomyelocele: a longitudinal study. Trans Am Ophthalmol Soc 1990; 88: 389–462.
22. Paseo M, Shults WT, Talbot T, et al. Acquired esotropia. A manifestation of Chiari one malformation. J Clin Neuro-ophthalmol 1984; 4: 151–4.
23. Akman A, Dayanir V, Sanac A, et al. Acquired esotropia as presenting sign of cranio-cervical junctional anomalies. Neuro-ophthalmology 1995; 15: 311–4.
24. Guy JR, Freedman WF, Nickle JP. Bilateral trochlear nerve paresis in hydrocephalus. J Clin Neuro-ophthalmol 1989; 9: 105–11.
25. Lorber J. Recovery of vision following prolonged blindness in children with hydrocephalus or following pyogenic meningitis. Clin Pediatr 1967; 6: 699–703.
26. Van Allen M, Kalousek D, Chernoff G, et al. Evidence for multisite closure of the neural tube in humans. Am J Med Genet 1993; 47: 723–43.
27. Gluckman TJ, George TM, McLone DJ. Postneurulation rapid brain growth represents a critical time for encephalocele formation: a chick model. Pediatr Neurosurg 1996; 25: 130–6.
28. Naidich TP, Altman MR, Braffman BH, et al. Cephaloceles and related malformations. AJNR Am J Neuroradiol 1992; 13: 655–90.
29. Martinez-Lage JF, Poza M, Sola J, et al. The child with a cephalocele: ideology, neuroimaging, and outcome. Childs Nerv Syst 1996; 12: 540–50.
30. Sewanwela C, Sukabote C, Sewanwela N. Frontoethmoidal encephalomeningocele. Surgery 1971; 69: 617–25.
31. Yokata A, Matsukabo Y, Fuwa I, et al. Anterior basal encephalocele of the neonate and infant. Neurosurgery 1986; 19: 468–78.
32. Muller F, O'Rahilly R. Mediobasal prosencephalic defects including holoprosencephaly. Am J Anat 1989; 185: 391–414.
33. Roessler E, Meunke M. Holoprosencephaly: a paradigm for the complex genetics of brain development. J Inherit Metab Bis 1998; 21: 481–97.
34. Lambert SR, Hoyt CS, Narahara NH. Optic nerve hypoplasia. Surv Ophthalmol 1987; 32: 1–9.
35. Barkovich AJ, Gressens P, Ebrard P. Formation, maturation and disorders of brain neocortex AJNR. Am J Neuroradiol 1992; 13: 423–46.
36. Voit T. Congenital muscular dystrophies. Brain Dev 1998; 20: 55–8.
37. Haltia M, Leivo I, Somer H, et al. Muscle-eye-brain disease: a neuropathological study. Ann Neurol 1997; 41: 173–80.
38. Tychsen L, Hoyt WF. Occipital lobe dysplasia. Magnetic resonance findings in two cases of isolated congenital hemianopia. Arch Ophthalmol 1985; 103: 680–2.
39. Galaburda AM, Sherman GF, Rosen GD, et al. Developmental dyslexia: four consecutive patients with cortical anomalies. Ann Neurol 1985; 8: 222–3.
40. Granata P, Farina L, Faiella A, et al. Familial schizencephaly associated with EMX2 mutation. Neurology 1997; 48: 1403–6.
41. Girkin CA, Miller NR. Central disorders of vision in humans. Surv Ophthalmol 2001; 45: 379–405.
42. Jan JE, Groenveld M, Sykanda AM, et al. Behavioral characteristics of children with permanent cortical visual impairment. Dev Med Child Neurol 1987; 29: 571–6.
43. Good WV, Jan JE, deSa L, et al. Cortical visual impairment in children. Surv Ophthalmol 1994; 38: 351–64.
44. Roland EH, Jan JE, Hill A, et al. Cortical visual impairment following birth asphyxia. Pediatr Neurol 1986; 2: 133–7.
45. Casteels I, Demaerel P, Spileers W, et al. Cortical visual impairment following perinatal hypoxia: clinicoradiologic correlation using magnetic resonance imaging. J Pediatr Ophthalmol 1997; 34: 297–305.
46. Huo R, Burden S, Hoyt CS, et al. Chronic cortical visual impairment in children: etiology, prognosis, and associated neurological deficits. Br J Ophthalmol 1999; 83: 670–5.
47. Weiss AH, Kelly JP, Phillips JO. The infant who is visually unresponsive on a cortical basis. Ophthalmology 2001; 108: 2076–87.
48. Ackroyd RS. Cortical blindness following bacterial meningitis: case report with reassessment of prognosis and etiology. Dev Med Child Neurol 1984; 26: 227–30.
49. Tepperberg J, Nussbaum D, Feldman F. Cortical blindness following meningitis due to Haemophilus influenzae type B. J Pediatr 1977; 91: 434–6.
50. Lorber J. Recovery of vision following prolonged blindness in children with hydrocephalus or following pyogenic meningitis. Clin Pediatr 1967; 6: 699–703.
51. Connolly MB, Jan JE, Cochrane DD. Rapid recovery from cortical visual impairment following correction of prolonged shunt malfunction in congenital hydrocephalus. Arch Neurol 1991; 48: 956–7.
52. Arroyo HA, Jan JE, McCormick AQ, et al. Permanent visual loss after shunt malfunction. Neurology 1985; 35: 25–9.
53. Corbett JJ. Neuro-ophthalmologic complications of hydrocephalus and shunting procedures. Sem Neurol 1986; 6: 111–23.
54. Flodmark O, Jan JE, Wong PK. Computed tomography of the brains of children with cortical visual impairment. Dev Med Child Neurol 1990; 32: 611–20.
55. Rogers M. Vision impairment in Liverpool: prevalence and morbidity. Arch Dis Child 1996; 74: 299–303.
56. Rosenberg T, Flage T, Hansen E. Incidence of registered visual impairment in the Nordic child population. Br J Ophthalmol 1996; 80: 49–53.
57. Dutton G, Ballantyne J, Boyd G, et al. Cortical visual impairment. Eye 1996; 10: 291–2.
58. Wong VN. Cortical blindness in children: a study of etiology and prognosis. Pediatr Neurol 1991; 7: 178–85.
59. Morse M. Argumented assessment procedures for children who have severe and multiple handicaps in addition to sensory impairments. J Vis Impair Blind 1992; 86: 73–7.

60. Weisglas-Kuper N, Baerts W, Fetter W. Minor neurological dysfunction and quality of movement in relation to neonatal cerebral damage and subsequent development. Dev Med Child Neurol 1994; 36: 727–35.

61. Schenk-Rootlieb AJ, van Nieuwenhuizen O, van der Graaf Y, et al. The prevalence of cerebral disturbance in children with cerebral palsy. Dev Med Child Neurol 1992; 34: 473–80.

62. Flodmark O, Roland EH, Hill A, et al. Periventricular leukomalacia: radiologic diagnosis. Radiology 1987; 162: 119–24.

63. Baker LL, Stevenson DK, Enzmann DR. End-stage periventricular leukomalacia: MR evaluation. Radiology 1988; 168: 809–15.

64. Mercuri E, Jongmans N, Henderson S. Evaluation of the corpus callosum in clumsy children born prematurely: a functional and morphological study. Neuropediatrics 1996; 27: 317–22.

65. Barkovich AJ. MR and CT evaluation of the profound neonatal and infantile asphyxia. Am J Neuroradiol 1992; 13: 959–72.

66 Tin W, Wariyar U, Hey E. Changing prognosis for babies of the less than 28 weeks gestation in the north of England between 1983–1984. Northern Neonatal Network. BMJ 1997; 314: 107–11.

67. Emslie HC, Wardle SP, Sims DG, et al. Increased survival and deteriorating developmental outcome in 23–25 weeks gestation infants. 1990–1994 compared with 1984–1989. Arch Dis Child Fetal Neonatal Ed 1998; 78: 99–104.

68. Hull J, Dodd KL. Falling incidence of hypoxic-ischemic encephalopathy in term infants. Br J Obstet Gynecol 1992; 99: 386–91.

69. Nelson K, Ellenberg J. Antecedents of cerebral palsy: multivariate analysis of risk. N Eng J Med 1986; 315: 81–6.

70. Johnson MA, Pennock JM, Bydder GM. Serial MR imaging in neonatal cerebral injury. Am J Roentgenol 1987; 8: 83–92.

71. Schneider H, Ballowitz L, Schachinger H. Anoxic encephalopathy with predominant involvement of basal ganglia, brainstem and spinal cord in the perinatal period. Acta Neuropathol 1975; 32: 287–98.

72. Mercuri E, Atkinson J, Braddick O. Visual function in full-term infants with hypoxic-ischemic encephalopathy. Neuropediatrics 1997; 28: 155–61.

73. Hoyt CS, Nickel BL, Billson FA. Ophthalmological examination of the infant: developmental aspects. Surv Ophthalmol 1982; 26: 177–89.

74. Tong L, Spear PD, Kalil RE, et al. Loss of retinal X cells in cats with neonatal or adult visual cortex damage. Science 1982; 217: 72–5.

75. Spear PD, Tong L, McCall MA. Functional influence of areas 17, 18, and 19 on lateral suprasylvian cortex in kittens and adult cats: implications for compensation following early visual cortex damage. Brain Res 1988; 447: 79–91.

76. Guido W, Spear PD, Tong L. How complete is physiological compensation in extrastriate cortex after visual cortex damage in kittens? Exp Brain Res 1992; 91: 455–66.

77. Spear PD. Plasticity following neonatal visual cortex damage in cats. Can J Physiol Pharmacol 1995; 73: 1389–97.

78. Rodman HR, Gross, CG, Albright TD. Afferent basis of visual response properties in area MT of the macaque. I. Effects of striate cortex removal. J Neurosci 1989; 9: 2033–50.

79. Sorenson KM, Rodman HR. A transient geniculo-striate pathway in macaques? Implications for blindsight. Neuroreport 1999; 10: 3295–9.

CHAPTER
64 Nonorganic Visual Disorders

William V Good

What can cause otherwise well children to have symptoms, the reality of which cannot be doubted, without evidence of organic disease and why is the visual system so often chosen as the site for these manifestations?

DEFINITIONS

The American Psychiatric Association periodically revises and reclassifies diagnostic categories of psychiatric disease, basing revised diagnoses on evidence-based findings. The Diagnostic and Statistical Manual (now IV-SR) of the American Psychiatric Association not only provides guidelines for diagnostic categorization, but also other diagnostic axes for severity of symptoms and other features. The design of the DSM IV is such that inexperienced health care providers may be able to use it.[1] In this chapter diagnostic categories for nonorganic visual function are simplified so that the nonpsychiatrist might be able to consider appropriate dispositions and management of children with suspected "functional" disorders.

The concept of hysteria in the eyes of the public has achieved such a distorted and variable meaning that its use has been criticized and the American Pediatric Association's classification now does not use the term. In practice, however, clinicians use the terms "hysteria", "functional" and "psychogenic" rather loosely.[2] Many clinical subdivisions that were included in the catch-all term "hysteria" are used instead, including malingering, conversion disorder, Münchausen, and somatization disorder. The most enigmatic of these is conversion disorder, described by Marsden[3] as a loss or distortion of neurological function not fully explained by organic disease. In this chapter, the term "functional visual loss" is used to describe any visual deficit that cannot be explained by physical findings. The term encompasses the many causes of nonorganic visual loss.

Conversion disorder

Freud, nurtured by Charcot, developed the forerunner of the conversion theory. He believed that the patient had an internal conflict (usually sexual) of which he was unaware, which became converted into a symptom as a means of expression after a process of dissociation, which is a mental mechanism whereby underlying feelings and the symptoms are separated. Conversion disorder can be distinguished from other psychiatric disorders mimicking organic loss by its absence of conscious, or intentional desire to trick the doctor (or parent). The child with conversion disorder develops nonorganic loss due to unconscious problems–mental disturbances outside of the child's awareness. Often such children have a history of having had previous conversion reactions, not necessarily involving the visual system (e.g. nonorganic loss of motor function).

Mersky[4] made a useful clinical definition of conversion symptoms:
1. They correspond to an idea in the mind of the patient concerning physical or sensory changes or psychological dysfunction.
2. They are definable, if somatic, in terms of positive evidence and, if psychological, by techniques of clinical examination.
3. They are related to emotional conflict.

Three terms are commonly applied to this situation: one is hysterical visual loss and the others are functional and nonorganic visual loss. The latter two are used rather loosely to describe the same phenomenon, implying that the impairment is the result of a disorder of function rather than structure and is therefore restorable.[5]

Conversion disorders are rare under 6 years old, and the sex ratio is equal up to 10 years, then females outnumber males by 3:1. Family disharmony is common and incestuous relationships should be borne in mind as an underlying cause.[6]

Münchausen syndrome

Some children intentionally develop loss of visual function. Patients with self-inflicted injuries have ocular *Münchausen syndrome*.[7] When their injuries are intentionally inflicted by adult caregivers, these children have Münchausen by proxy (Chapter 71). This latter condition indicates serious psychopathology on the part of the caregiver, who is frequently a health care professional. Simple Münchausen syndrome is also a sign of significant psychopathology on the part of the child. Ophthalmologists will do well to remember that certain diseases will result in self-abuse, including Lesch–Nyhan syndrome, and, occasionally, Riley–Day syndrome.[8]

Malingering

Malingerers are those who intentionally feign loss of function, often for secondary gain, i.e. they hope to achieve some tangible goal by feigning illness. Examples include faking illness to miss school, or to obtain a pair of glasses because a friend has glasses. The malingering child seems to be very different from the adult malingerer. He is usually a normal child, usually not from a very disturbed background (although serious underlying social problems may co-exist), and he does not usually have any eye or psychiatric disease.

Depression

Some children develop somatic complaints in response to depression. However, children and adolescents who are depressed do not always experience depressive feelings. Therefore, questions that can elicit signs of depression should be raised, when depression is suspected. For example, depressed children may have sleep and eating disturbances, and may have suicidal ideation. Their peer relationships may have suffered in the preceding few months, and they may appear irritable.

ASSOCIATION WITH ORGANIC DISEASE

Nonorganic symptoms are common amongst children referred to a pediatric ophthalmology service,[9] and their prompt and correct diagnosis, with appropriate management, saves the doctor, the child and the parents much heartache and time and saves the discomfort and risk of unnecessary investigations.

The fear of missing organic disease means that doctors have become more cautious about diagnosing hysteria. Several conditions previously regarded as hysterical are now thought to have an organic basis including spasmodic torticollis, blepharospasm, and writer's cramp; there may be some more to come. Nevertheless, there is a nucleus of patients for whom no diagnosis, other than hysteria, seems right.[10]

In psychiatry, it is well-recognized that the presence of organic disease may be associated with nonorganic disease, with the classic situation being the occurrence of pseudoseizures in epileptics.[11] The same may well be true of ocular hysterics, but in childhood the symptoms usually occur free of organic disease, or psychiatric disease.[12] Exceptions to this rule have recently been noted. Ocular tics have come into question as occasionally associated with, or caused by, real organic disease.[13] Nevertheless, the vast majority of children with tics involving musculature around the eyes are afflicted with nonorganic problems.

CLINICAL PRESENTATION AND SYMPTOMS

The child with a nonorganic ocular defect is aged between 6 and 16 years, most frequently 10 years old ; girls are more frequently affected than boys.[14] There may be a family history of illness or of eye disease, such as retinitis pigmentosa.[15] The symptoms seem to come on gradually in most cases, often the first problem being a marginal failure at a school eye test. Subsequent examinations by optometrists or ophthalmologists reveal varying degrees of acuity and visual field loss, often worsening as time goes on, but rarely to the extent that the child becomes bilaterally blind. The remarkable thing is how little most children are inconvenienced by an apparently marked visual loss. Repeated objective examinations and further examinations, including neurophysiology and radiology, are all normal. The condition is usually bilateral,[14] the most common complaints are of "just not seeing", blurred vision, or distorted or small images; occasionally symptomatic visual field defects are described, such as "tunnel vision" which is the most common, and hemianopias are occasionally encountered.[16] Central scotomas are rare and should make one think of associated organic disease. Nonocular defects occasionally also occur, including spasm of the near reflex, headaches, voluntary nystagmus,[12] and eye movement tics[17]; horizontal gaze paresis has occurred in an adult,[18] contraversive eye deviation[19] and accommodation paralysis has also been described.

Psychological background

Enquiry into the background, looking for the underlying stress that produces the symptoms, should center on two main areas:

(i) The home and family

Conflict between children, sibling rivalry, the child who needs more attention, an unhappy marriage, overcrowding, sexual

abuse[20] or harassment by relatives or others, or conflict with neighbors and their children may all be predisposing factors.

(ii) The school

In the school it is the slow child who is being overstretched, or the bright child who is being understretched who may produce visual symptoms, but unsympathetic or aggressive teachers, teasing or bullying, sexual or nonsexual harassment or abuse[20] are all factors to look for as predisposing to nonorganic visual loss. It is of utmost importance to enlist the help of the parents, and to tell them explicitly of the possible underlying problems so that they can best help their own child, because it is by relieving underlying factors that the symptoms are best treated.

DETECTION OF FUNCTIONAL OCULAR DISORDERS IN CHILDREN

It is of crucial importance that the diagnosis is made positively, with the clear demonstration of signs that are widely outside the bounds of physiological possibility. Marginal anomalies should be treated with the greatest of caution.

There are certain situations that are particularly suggestive of hysteria:

- A severe functional defect in the presence of a normal physical examination and especially when there is a severe unilateral defect with normal pupil reactions and no refractive error.
- The sudden onset of a disorder related to an emotionally significant event or situation.
- Step-like deterioration, with the patient's acuity becoming one or two lines worse on each examination but with no objective abnormalities.
- The ability of a patient to achieve a better acuity or better visual fields with coaxing or cajoling.
- A monotonous and excessively slow reading of all the letters on a letter chart, regardless of whether they are large or small.
- A single symptom is most frequent in hysterics whereas psychoneurotic patients will tend to have numerous symptoms. Children rarely have substantial ocular complaints.
- A previous history of hysterical manifestations, ocular or nonocular, is a recognized predisposing factor to further hysterical disorders.
- The occurrence of visual problems in other members of the family, especially if serious.

Bilateral total blindness

Although unusual, this severe disturbance is usually easy to detect as being nonorganic.

1. Direct threat or throwing a ball on a string at the patient while the eyes are open invariably produces a blink (Fig. 64.1). By asking the patient to close his eyes, the string can be concealed before the ball is thrown, making the test more effective.
2. When facing a mirror a patient will involuntarily move his eyes when the mirror is rotated about a vertical axis running through the center of the mirror. The velocity of the eye movement is proportional to the velocity of rotation of the mirror and the only way in which the patient can inhibit the eye movement is by "looking through" the mirror, usually easily detected by a change in convergence of the eyes and an associated pupil reaction (Fig. 64.2).

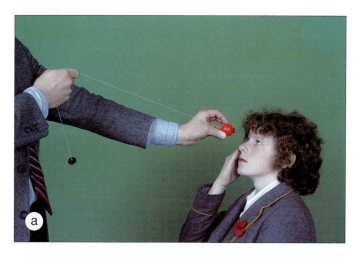

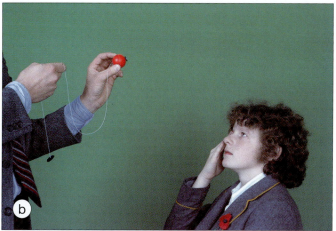

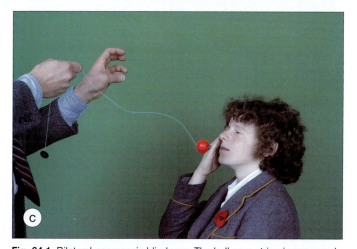

Fig. 64.1 Bilateral nonorganic blindness. The ball on a string is measured for distance (a), withdrawn (b) and then thrown at the child, eliciting a blink if she is indeed sighted (c).

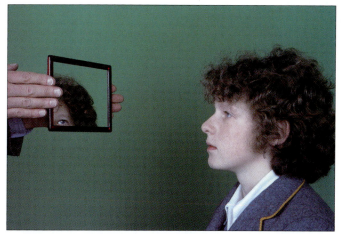

Fig. 64.2 Bilateral nonorganic blindness. When a blind person looks at a mirror, no movement takes place when the mirror is rotated. The sighted person's eyes will move as the mirror rotates although he feels he is looking straight ahead.

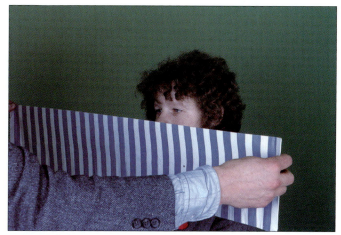

Fig. 64.3 Bilateral nonorganic blindness. As long as the patient does not "look through" the tape, the patient's eyes will move with the OKN tape.

3. An optokinetic drum or tape, subtending a large angle at the eye, can be held in front of the patient and the drum rotated to elicit visual evoked movement (Fig. 64.3). It is possible for the patient to look through the tape or drum giving the impression that he is not seeing it. If a large drum, in which the patient sits, is available (some eye movement laboratories have these), this provides whole field stimulation and an irresistible source of visual evoked eye movement. Some workers[21] have found the Catford drum[22] is a useful test in functional visual loss but this is not a universal experience since it is very easy to avoid fixation of the target of this machine.

4. Another occasionally useful device is to hold up a cartoon or joke on a card in order to obtain a reaction. This is considerably less effective than the adult equivalent (holding up a pornographic photograph) but may help if the child's emotional state and the joke are appropriate.

5. A 5 or 25 diopter prism placed base out in front of a seeing eye will normally induce an appropriate, and totally involuntary, fusional movement (Fig. 64.4). This will not occur in severe visual defect.

Unilateral blindness

The same test as described in the previous section can be used by covering the normal eye. In addition there are several subtle tests that can be applied.

1. A dexterous refractionist can usually manage to confuse the patient into reading with the "blind" eye while he thinks that he is using his good eye. Putting a high plus lens or rotating two cylinders (Fig. 64.5) from a cancelling to an additive

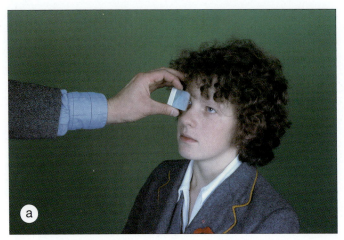
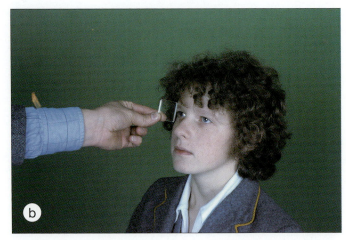

Fig. 64.4 Bilateral nonorganic blindness. A 25 diopter prism (a) elicits a movement even with only peripheral vision. A 4 diopter prism (b) requires central vision to elicit a movement.

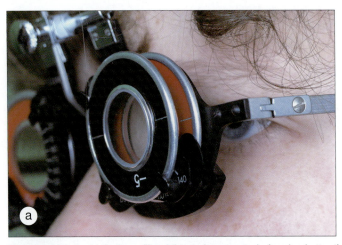
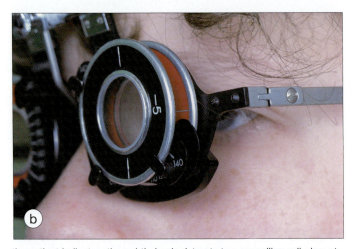

Fig. 64.5 Unilateral blindness. The right eye is suspected of seeing better than the patient indicates; the ophthalmologist puts two cancelling cylinders at the same axis in front of the left eye (a), obscures the patient's view of the test type by moving across him, switches the lenses to add to each other (b) and occlude the left eye and as he moves away from the patient urges him to read quickly. The left eye is obscured by the lens combination and the right is forced to be used; the patient does not usually detect the change to being forced to use the right eye.

position to occlude the good eye causes the patient to unsuspectingly read down the chart to a normal level. Polaroid lenses or Polaroid projection devices can also be used to trick the patient into reading with the affected eye.

2. Worth's dots, in which four illuminated spots, two green, one white and one red, are viewed by the patient wearing a red goggle over the right eye and a green over the left (Fig. 64.6). A normal person will see two spots with the right eye (the red and the white appear red) through the red filter and three with the left eye (two green and one white all appearing green through the green filter). With both eyes open the patient sees four dots if he is able to fuse the two white dots. If there is a latent or manifest strabismus without suppressions he sees five dots. If the patient sees more than three green or two red he must be using both eyes.

3. Various tests of stereoacuity are available but the one most useful for this purpose is the Frisby stereotest[23] since this does not require the use of Polaroid or red/green glasses to achieve dissociation of the eyes. While the plate shown is held steadily (movement induces parallax and detection of the target) the patient is invited to point out the square containing a circle. It requires quite a high degree of binocular vision to achieve this.

4. Either a horizontal prism, as described in the previous section, or a vertical prism may be placed in front of the apparently defective eye. The vertical prism, if over 5 diopters

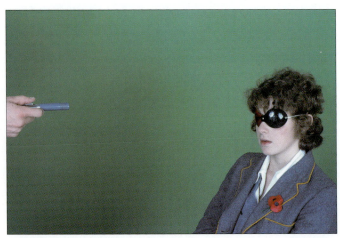

Fig. 64.6 Worth's four dot test being used to detect nonorganic unilateral visual defect. (See text).

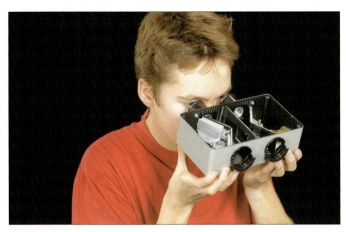

Fig. 64.7 The pseudoscope. This is a system of mirrors arranged to be used in a device similar to a pair of binoculars. The patient obscures what he or she thinks is (say) the left aperture, but is actually obscuring the right eye. The apparatus is seen here with the lid removed.

in power, usually invokes diplopia and the patient may report this or terminate the examination.

5. It is in this group that pupil reactions are most useful; if one eye is blind and the other is normal there is always a relative afferent pupil defect.

6. Bar reading is a commonly used technique in orthoptics. To read with a bar placed in an appropriate position between the reading matter and the patient's eyes requires both eyes to work simultaneously in order to read a complete line.

7. A pseudoscope (Fig. 64.7) is a device in which a system of mirrors in a box is used to confuse the observer as to which eye he is using. When the patient thinks he is covering one eye he is in fact covering the other. The device is fitted with lens holders to enable refraction to be carried out.

Unilateral partial acuity loss

In this group the same tests that are used for unilateral complete visual loss are applicable. The results, however, are often less easy to interpret. Pupil reactions are rarely helpful and since there are no clear norms for the correlation between acuity and stereoacuity, the stereoacuity tests are difficult to interpret. The pseudoscope and the confusion-refraction test are most useful in this situation.

Bilateral partial acuity loss

This group is the most difficult to diagnose as nonorganic but they nearly always have associated functional field defects that can establish the diagnosis.

1. The finding of an acuity that greatly varies in terms of the angle subtended, at different distances is an indicator of the hysterical defect. The patient may sometimes, by the use of a second chart with different sized figures or a mirror placed so as to hide the increased distance between the patient and the chart, be induced to read letters of a size that he was not previously able to read. Similarly, near vision testers, using Snellen near equivalent letters, may show a disparity.

2. A severe bilateral loss of acuity due to organic disease is not compatible with a high level of stereoacuity.

3. Similarly it is unusual for a patient to make fusional movement when a 5 diopter prism is placed base out in front of the other eye, if that eye has organically reduced acuity.

Visual field defects

In children, the most common functional presentation is one in which acuity is abnormal, but visual fields are normal. But when having their visual fields tested, even normals may apparently perform in a nonorganic manner if the examination is not carefully conducted. Abnormal fields are often associated with an apparently reduced acuity in functional visual loss, or sometimes with other symptoms including reading disability.[24]

Tunnel vision is the most common of hysterical field defects.[25] In tunnel vision the size of the field is the same at all distances; usually the field is also small. Purely constricted fields, for instance in retinitis pigmentosa, are conical becoming larger as the patient moves away from the testing screen. The defect is always gross; there is an apparently dense defect involving the whole visual field only a few degrees away from the fixation point and this is the same size whether tested at 1, 2 or more meters away from the screen.

The defect, characterized by the piling of isopters, is usually "sharp-edged" so that both large and small targets are perceived at the same point which is often remarkably constant. This "piling up" of the isopters may occur even in the face of gross changes in the contrast between the brightness of the background and the target; a distinctly unphysiological effect!

The absolute nature of the defect may make it easier to detect as being functional.

1. In a confrontation technique, if the patient alternates fixation between the examiner's eye and a fixation point on a stick held by the examiner, and at a time when he is fixing the examiner's eye, the fixation point is moved (Fig. 64.8). If the patient has organic disease with constricted fields, he will have difficulty in relocating the spot, whereas a hysteric will find it accurately.

2. On parting, the examiner fixes the patient in the eye and, without speaking, raises his hand from the elbow as though to shake hands. Given the variations of social backgrounds, most patients with organically constricted fields do not see the examiner's hand, while the hysteric will.

Using large targets, one may obtain a square visual field, the target when moved inwards from one direction being detected in areas previously blind.

On successive testing the field may become smaller. If the target is moved inwards as though around a clockface the target becomes detectable at an ever decreasing distance from fixation giving rise to "spiraling".

A binasal field defect is rare and may be a functional phenomenon.[26] Pilley and Thompson pointed out that with a binasal hemianopia, if the patient fixes the examiner, there is a blind area between the two which is wedge-shaped, with a base between the patient's eyes and the apex at the examiner's nose. In organic disease targets that were not visible in this wedge are visible and the functional patient therefore may see them. Functional binasal defects are usually clear-cut, organic ones are not.

In the very rare bitemporal functional visual field defect there is a wedge of blindness extending away from the fixation point. Therefore, if the patient fixes the examiner's nose and then fixes a point between the examiner's nose and himself, if the bitemporal hemianopia is complete there will be a loss or blurring of the central features of the examiner's face. Obviously this does not occur in hysterical amblyopia.

De Schweinitz[27] stressed the importance of inverted color fields in functional visual loss. In this, the red targets are detected more peripherally than the blue targets of identical size and

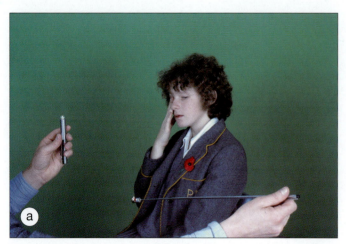
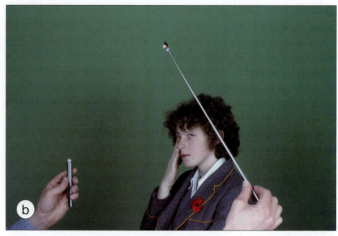

Fig. 64.8 Visual field defects. The patient, who has been shown to have very constricted visual fields, looks accurately between the light and the mobile target which moves in the apparently blind part of the visual field.

brightness, whereas the reverse is normal. This is not a test frequently done today but may be a useful adjunct.

Lastly it must be emphasized that an examiner skilled in testing for functional loss should not let his enthusiasm for testing to allow him either to overlook co-existing organic disease, or to encourage the patient to give apparently hysterical results when none are normally present, and do not forget that Eames[25] demonstrated tunnel vision in 9% of 193 normal schoolchildren! The visual field testing is best done with a tangent screen but defects can be detected even using automated perimetry.[28]

CONFIRMATORY STUDIES

It is easy to diagnose the condition too late and over-investigate.[29] Once the clinician has made a positive diagnosis of nonorganic visual loss and has not found evidence of any disease, there remains little to do from the point of view of diagnosis and one can easily argue that the more one investigates the child the more stress one creates and the more one reinforces his underlying problem. If there is any doubt in the mind of the doctor, parent or the older child, about the possibility of organic disease, detailed neurophysiological studies, including an electroretinogram and pattern visually evoked responses may be very reassuring and may inspire sufficient confidence to base the treatment only on reassurance. Hysterical symptoms may also occur in brain disorders such as Batten disease or adrenoleukodystrophy, many of which are accompanied by neurophysiological changes. So these are useful confirmatory studies in many cases and are risk-free. Further investigations such as a computed tomography or magnetic resonance imaging are not completely risk-free and are therefore only indicated if the neurophysiological tests are abnormal or if there is real doubt in the doctor's mind.

MANAGEMENT

The most important thing is to try to find the underlying cause and this is possible in most cases; appropriate and sensitive modification of these underlying predisposing factors will abolish the symptom. It is useful to demonstrate the nonorganic nature of the defect to the parents and to reassure them strongly that it is such a common problem that it could almost be regarded as a

"normal stress reaction". There is a very strong need to discuss the condition in full with both child and parents, in language appropriate to both; it is this that makes most pediatric ophthalmologists' hearts fall when they make the diagnosis in the middle of a busy clinic! The contributions of a psychiatrist or psychologist may be helpful in refractory cases, but it is probably preferable to avoid involvement with too many professionals, because this may tend to reinforce the problem.

The ophthalmologist should maintain a dispassionate approach to the functional patient. Countertransference problems (doctors' emotional reactions to patients) can be complex, with anger at the patient for "wasting the doctor's time" a common feature.

PITFALLS IN DIAGNOSIS OF FUNCTIONAL VISUAL LOSS

A few caveats and pitfalls in the diagnosis of functional visual loss should be mentioned. When children first present with a visual complaint caused by chiasmal tumor, they may not have any observable optic atrophy, and responses to visual field examination may be variable. Multiple sclerosis causes variable neurological findings and should be suspected when the history supports the diagnosis. Positive historical findings of symptoms worsening with exercise, for example, may help to rule in the need for a work-up. Similarly, loss of neurological function due to two noncontiguous brain abnormalities (two problems separated in space) is suggestive of multiple sclerosis.

PROGNOSIS

The prognosis is good[12] and strong reassurance with minimal follow-up is usually indicated. Psychiatric help may be useful in certain cases and it is likely that "integrative" and family therapy may improve the prognosis.[30] Good prognostic factors are younger age, treatment compliance, early intervention, healthy family functioning, lack of psychopathology, insight and acceptance by the family of the psychological natures of the illness.[30] If there is any indication of an underlying psychiatric disorder, or of a more widespread psychoneurosis, for instance if the patient has recurrent episodes especially affecting more than one system, the psychiatrist's expert help is mandatory.

REFERENCES

1. Yutzy SH, Cloninger CR, Guze SB, et al. DSM-IV field trial: testing a new proposal for somatization disorder. Am J Psychiatr 1995; 152: 97–101.
2. Mace CJ, Trimble MR. 'Hysteria', 'functional' or 'psychogenic'? A survey of British neurologist's preferences. J Roy Soc Med 1991; 84: 471–6.
3. Marsden CD. Hysteria: a neurologist's view. Psychol Med 1986; 149: 28–37.
4. Mersky H. Disorders of conscious awareness: hysterical phenomena. Br J Hosp Med 1986; 19: 305–9.
5. Thompson SH. Functional visual loss. Am J Ophthalmol 1985: 100: 209–13.
6. Editorial. Neurological conversion disorders in childhood. Lancet 1991; 337: 889–90.
7. Rosenberg PN, Krohel GB, Webb RM, et al. Ocular Münchausen's syndrome. Ophthalmology 1986; 93: 1120–4.
8. Robey KL, Reck JF, Giacomini KD, et al. Modes and patterns of self-mutilation in persons with Lesch-Nyhan disease. Dev Med Child Neurol 2003; 45: 167–71.
9. Schlaegel TF Jr, Quilala FV. Hysterical amblyopia; statistical analysis of 42 cases found in a survey of 800 unselected eye patients at a state medical center. Arch Ophthalmol 1955; 54: 875–84.
10. Lloyd GG. Hysteria: a case for conservation. Br Med J 1986; 293: 1255–6.
11. Fenton GW. Epilepsy and hysteria. Br J Psychiatr 1986; 149: 28–37.
12. Catalano RA, Simon JW, Krohel GB, et al. Functional visual loss in children. J Am Acad Ophthalmol 1986; 93: 385–91.
13. Coats DK, Paysse EA, Kim DS. Excessive blinking in childhood: a prospective evaluation of 99 children. Ophthalmology 2001; 108: 1556–1561.
14. Yasuna ER. Hysterical amblyopia in children and young adults. Arch Ophthalmol 1951; 45: 70–6.
15. Holden R, Duvall-Young J. Functional visual deficit in children with a family history of retinitis pigmentosa. J Pediatr Ophthalmol Strabismus 1994; 31: 323–4.
16. Keane JR. Hysterical hemianopia. Arch Ophthamol 1979; 97: 865–6.
17. Shawkat F, Harris C, Jacobs M, et al. Eye movement tics. Br J Ophthalmol 1992; 76: 697–9.
18. Troost TB, Troost GE. Functional paralysis of horizontal gaze. Neurology 1979; 29: 82–5.
19. Armon C. The alternating eye deviation sign. Neurology 1991; 41: 1845.
20. Roelofs K, Keijsers GP, Hoogduin KA, et al. Childhood abuse in patients with conversion disorder. Am J Psychiatr 2002; 159: 1908–13.
21. Aichner H, Rubi E. Objective Seh Scharf Bentimmung bei Kleinstkmodern. Klin Monatbsbl Augenheilkd 1976; 169: 255–9.
22. Catford GV, Oliver A. A method of visual acuity detection. Proceedings of the Second International Orthoptic Congress, Amsterdam. Excerpta Med 1971; 183–20.
23. Hinchcliff H. Clinical evaluation of stereopsis. Br Orthopt J 1978; 35: 46–50.
24. Leary PM, Van Selm JL. Tunnel vision presenting as reading disability. J Roy Soc Med 1987; 80: 585–7.
25. Eames TH. A study of tubular and spiral central fields. Am J Ophthalmol 1947; 30: 610–11.
26. Pilley SJH, Thompson HS. Binasal field loss and prefixation blindness. In: Glaser J, Smith JL, eds. Neuro-ophthalmology, Vol. 8. St Louis: CV Mosby; 1975: 277–84.
27. De Schweinitz GW. Neuroses and psychoses. In: Posey WC, Spiller WG, eds. The Eye and the Nervous System. Philadelphia: Lippincott; 1906: 614–96.
28. Smith TJ, Baker RS. Perimetric findings in functional disorders using automated techniques. J Am Acad Ophthalmol 1987; 94: 1562–7.
29. Leary PM. Conversion disorder in childhood: diagnosed too late, investigated too much? J R Soc Med 2003; 96: 436–8.
30. Turgay A. Treatment outcome for children and adolescents with conversion disorder. Can J Psychiatr 1990; 35: 585–9.

CHAPTER 65 Inborn Errors of Metabolism and the Eye

Maureen Cleary, Andrew Morris and David Taylor

Relatively few inherited metabolic diseases present with eye disease, but many are associated with ophthalmological complications. Ophthalmologists may provide diagnostic clues, and monitor or treat complications in diagnosed patients. Further information can be found in the major texts.[1,2]

Most of the diseases described here are autosomal recessive and rare, many having an incidence of approximately 1:100 000. Prenatal diagnosis is now possible, using biochemical or molecular techniques, for the majority of inborn errors, apart from most mitochondrial disorders.

Inborn errors of metabolism are sometimes classified into diseases affecting organelles (such as lysosomes, mitochondria and peroxisomes) and other diseases, most of which involve relatively small molecules.

LYSOSOMAL DISORDERS

Lysosomes are membrane-bound intracellular organelles containing hydrolytic enzymes at acidic pH whose main function is the degradation of complex macromolecules. The 30 or so lysosomal storage disorders are due to an enzyme deficiency resulting in abnormal storage in the lysosomes: all are autosomal recessive, except Fabry and Hunter diseases which are X-linked.

Their clinical spectrum is wide, ranging from prenatal hydrops fetalis to mild disease in adulthood. Suggestive signs include coarsening of facial features, neurological deterioration and hepatosplenomegaly, a characteristic skeletal dysplasia (dysostosis multiplex) with a large skull, spinal deformities and short, thick tubular bones. Hepatosplenomegaly is frequent but the clinical picture is often dominated by neurodevelopmental regression.

Diagnosis relies on measurement of enzyme activity in leukocytes or fibroblasts for all cases.

Other helpful investigations are:
1. Urinary mucopolysaccharides and oligosaccharides (MPS, ML, mannosidosis, sialidosis).
2. Vacuolated cells in peripheral blood smear (GM1 gangliosidosis, Niemann–Pick Disease).
3. Foamy cells on bone marrow aspirate (GM1 gangliosidosis, Niemann–Pick, Gaucher).
4. Dysostosis multiplex on skeletal survey (MPS, GM1 gangliosidosis, ML).

Prenatal diagnosis is possible for the whole group.

They are chronic, progressive diseases previously regarded as untreatable, but many now have treatment options.[3] Bone marrow transplantation is effective in some, the donor marrow providing the deficient enzyme.[4] Also, the enzymes are targeted to the lysosome by mannose-6 phosphate enabling enzyme replacement therapy for several diseases. Enzyme injected intravenously migrates to the lysosomes in affected tissues, but not across the blood–brain barrier and they will not therefore treat the neurological disease. "Substrate deprivation therapy"[5,6] reduces the stored lysosomal compound by blocking an earlier step in the pathway even across the blood–brain barrier. These new treatments may alter the outcome of these disorders, and modify their effects on the eye.

Depending on the primary storage product, the disorders may be divided into four major groups:

Sphingolipidoses

Sphingolipids are complex membrane lipids composed of sphingosine and a long-chain fatty acid. Since these intricate molecules form an integral part of cerebral membranes, the sphingolipidoses, in which catabolism is deranged, are often associated with relentless neurodegeneration. There are many effects on the eye, but the ophthalmological hallmark of the neurodegenerative subgroup of sphingolipidoses is the cherry-red spot.

There is a wide range of severity and many presentations in most of the sphingolipidoses.

GM2 gangliosidosis
(i)   Tay–Sachs disease.
(ii) Sandhoff disease.
Two variants where the enzyme is present but there is either:
(iii) Altered substrate specificity.
(iv) Activator protein deficiency.

These are severe neurodegenerative disorders. A cherry-red spot is the typical eye finding (Table 65.1)

Tay–Sachs (hexosaminidase A deficiency) usually presents in infancy with an exaggerated startle response. Early milestones are lost by the first birthday. Loss of visual attentiveness occurs early. Progressive neurological deterioration occurs with spasticity, feeding difficulties and seizures. Macrocephaly is common and death usually occurs by 2–4 years. It is autosomal recessive and the gene has been mapped to 15q23-q24.[7]

Table 65.1 Diseases with a cherry-red spot

GM2 Gangliosidoses
   GM2 type 1 Tay–Sachs disease
   GM2 type 2 Sandhoff disease
   GM2 type 3
Metachromatic leukodystrophy, Niemann–Pick disease types A & B
GM1 gangliosidosis
Sialidosis types 1 & 2
Mucolipidosis III
Farber disease

Sandhoff disease (hexosaminidase A and B deficiency) follows a similar pattern. The gene for hexosaminidase B has been localized to 5q31-qter.[8]

Both disorders also have a later-onset variety; ataxia and dementia begin in the second year of life and the disease follows a more attenuated form. The neurological picture differs in the adult-onset type, and may include psychosis, dystonia and cerebellar ataxia in addition to a supranuclear ophthalmoplegia; a cherry-red spot is less common.

Ophthalmoscopy at an early stage reveals the cherry-red spot, due to GM2 ganglioside accumulation in the retinal ganglion cells. The absence of ganglion cells at the fovea gives rise to the red spot surrounded by white diseased cells. As the ganglion cells die the cherry-red spot fades and optic atrophy becomes apparent. The electroretinogram (ERG) is normal or large[9] but the visual evoked response (VER) extinguished.[10] There is no treatment.

Metachromatic leukodystrophy (arylsulfatase deficiency)

In metachromatic leukodystrophy (MLD), variable presentations in infancy, childhood, adolescence and adulthood are recognized. Classically, a previously normal child develops problems when they learn to walk, the gait deteriorates with spasticity and reflexes are lost due to peripheral neuropathy; death usually occurs by 6 years of age. MRI shows central demyelination and cerebellar atrophy.

The juvenile form runs a slower course, and the ataxia and spasticity usually begin after age seven years, with behavioral difficulties. Bulbar dysfunction leads to speech difficulties and feeding problems. In the adult with MLD, psychiatric symptoms predominate.

The disease arises from accumulation of sulphatide, a constituent of myelin. The diagnosis is made by measuring the enzyme arylsulfatase. There is a "pseudo-deficiency" state where there is sufficient enzyme activity to avoid the clinical picture of MLD. No effective treatment exists, but bone marrow transplant may prevent deterioration early in the disease.[11]

Optic atrophy occurs in one-third of cases. It may be caused optic nerve axon involvement or by retinal ganglion cell degeneration, rarely with a cherry-red spot.

Krabbe disease (galactocerebrosidase deficiency)

This is a severe neurodegenerative disorder with infantile, childhood and late onset forms. The early onset form develops symptoms in the first few months with irritability, poor feeding and progresses quickly to spasticity and a vegetative state. There is no treatment but in patients diagnosed very early in the course of their disease, BMT may have a role.[12]

Visual impairment is common due to optic atrophy or cortical blindness. The rapid neurodegeneration, however, overshadows this complication.

GM1 gangliosidosis

Infantile GM1 gangliosidosis causes hypotonia from birth. By six months, developmental delay and a coarse appearance with puffy skin, maxillary hyperplasia, hypertrophied gums and macroglossia develop. Affected children have dysostosis multiplex and about half have a cherry-red spot, occasionally retinal hemorrhages and corneal clouding. Rapid neurological deterioration is usual with seizures and swallowing difficulties and death by about two years. There is no curative treatment. Juvenile and adult forms are recognized in which there is neurological deterioration but no physical changes.

Niemann–Pick disease

Disorders in which there is storage of sphingomyelin were previously termed Niemann–Pick disease types A, B, C, and D. These terms are still used despite only types A and B being due to sphingomyelinase deficiency; in types C and D, sphingomyelin accumulates in the spleen and liver due to disorders of cholesterol uptake.

Niemann–Pick disease types A and B (sphingomyelinase deficiency)

Niemann–Pick type A presents in infancy with nonspecific symptoms: failure to thrive, feeding difficulties and respiratory infections. Hepatomegaly (Fig. 65.1) is prominent and, in contrast to infantile Gaucher, is more marked than splenomegaly. Neurological degeneration starts around 18 months with loss of vision and floppiness evolving to spasticity. Death usually occurs around three years. Cherry-red spots (Fig. 65.2) lead on to retinal ganglion cell degeneration and optic atrophy; there may be a brown discoloration of the anterior lens capsule, but minimal corneal opacification.[13]

Niemann–Pick disease type B is less severe and presents later in childhood with hepatosplenomegaly. Usually there are no neurological symptoms, but patients may have ataxia but are of normal intelligence. Clinical problems include hypersplenism arising from massive splenic enlargement, cirrhosis of the liver and pulmonary infiltration. Eye abnormalities include periorbital fullness, macular granular deposits and cherry-red spot.[14]

Both are autosomal recessive and more prevalent in the Ashkenazi Jewish population. There is no treatment for type A, but type B may be amenable to bone marrow transplantation.[15] Enzyme replacement has shown positive results in the mouse model with human trials underway. The finding of lipid-laden histiocytes (Fig. 65.3a) on bone marrow examination may be helpful in diagnosis.

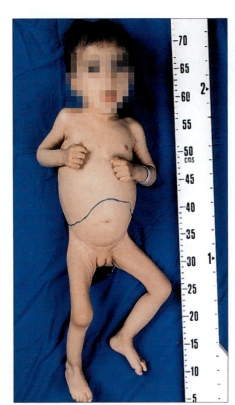

Fig. 65.1 An infant with Niemann-Pick type A showing the hepatomegaly and spastic posture.

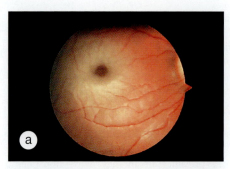

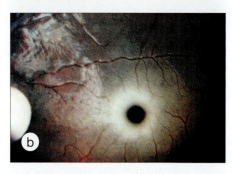

Fig. 65.2 (a) Cherry-red spot in a patient with Niemann-Pick type A: the spot is brownish because of dark pigmentation. (b) Cherry-red spot in a black infant with Niemann-Pick type A. (Professor C S Hoyt's patient.)

Niemann–Pick types C and D (NPC/NPD)

Types C and D are due to impaired intracellular transport of cholesterol[16] as a result of mutations in the NPC1 gene. Whilst type C is seen world-wide, type D is seen only in Nova Scotia.[17]

Type C has variable presentations:
1. Neonatal transient cholestatic liver disease.
2. Neonatal liver disease, rapidly progressive resulting in death.

3. Childhood detection of isolated splenomegaly.[18]
4. Onset of neurological problems.

Neurological progression occurs in late childhood with the development of seizures, dystonia, cerebellar ataxia and dementia with death by the second decade.

Currently there is no effective therapy for either types but a trial of substrate deprivation for type C where synthesis of metabolites is blocked is underway.

Early-onset supranuclear palsy (Fig. 65.3b) is characteristic of this disorder,[19] with loss of voluntary vertical saccades (rapid eye movements) and fast phases of optokinetic nystagmus, especially downwards; there are preserved doll's eye movements. There may be vertical pursuit and horizontal supranuclear eye movement defects or a supranuclear disorder of convergence. It has been suggested that there are separate feedback loops for horizontal and vertical burst neurons and that NPC usually selectively affects vertical burst neurons.[20] Head thrusts may compensate for the saccade disorder.

A faint cherry-red spot due to opalescence of the perifoveal retina has been observed and histologically, membranous inclusions are found in many tissues.[21]

Gaucher disease (glucocerebrosidase deficiency)

Gaucher disease arises from deficiency of glucocerebrosidase, which cleaves glucose from glucosyl ceramide. There are three subtypes depending on severity of the enzyme deficiency; only 2 and 3 have brain involvement.

Type 1

This is more common in Ashkenazi Jews, with storage in the liver, spleen and bones causing hepatosplenomegaly, anemia, thrombocytopenia and leucopenia. Splenic infarctions cause abdominal

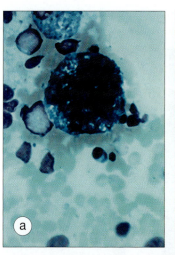

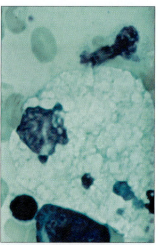

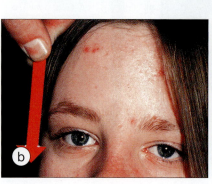

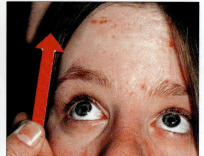

Fig. 65.3 (a) Niemann-Pick type B showing foamy macrophages (right) and sea-blue histiocytes (left). (b) Downgaze palsy in child with Niemann-Pick type C. The arrow denotes the direction that the child is being told to look. Horizontal and upgaze were normal (Mr M.D.Sanders patient).

pain and the lungs may become infiltrated. In a minority, the bones develop the typical Erlenmeyer deformity. Infarction of long bones may cause severe pain, and osteopenia is common. Dark brown-yellow pingueculae occur in the nasal bulbar conjunctivae which are characterized by numerous Gaucher cells on histological examination. Macular degeneration has been described.

Type 2

Hepatosplenomegaly is present within the first six months of life and neurological involvement is severe with feeding problems, spasticity and regression. Involvement of the bulbar centers is characteristic and this, with the eye findings of a strabismus and the severe spasticity gives the clinical triad of opisthotonus, trismus and strabismus (Fig. 65.4). The typical ophthalmological finding is horizontal gaze palsy.

Type 3 (Norbottnian)

Intermittent strabismus and vertical gaze palsy are early findings,[22] and there is often massive splenomegaly. Progression may be very gradual.

Bone marrow examination may show Gaucher cells, reticuloendothelial cells with displaced nuclei and a "crumpled paper"-like cytoplasm. The enzyme chitotriosidase (a marker of macrophage activity) is markedly elevated, but final diagnosis is made with enzyme testing in leukocytes or fibroblasts.

There is no effective treatment for type 2 Gaucher. Bone marrow transplant halts progression in type 1. Enzyme replacement with glucocerebrosidase is very effective in type 1 and helps the systemic problems of type 3, possibly halting neurological progression.

Glycoprotein disorders

This group clinically has similarities to the mucopolysaccharidoses, but urinary MPS pattern is normal.

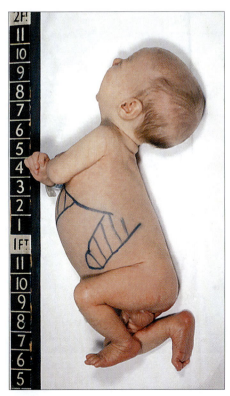

Fig. 65.4 Gaucher Type 2 showing splenomegaly, hepatomegaly and opisthotonic posturing.

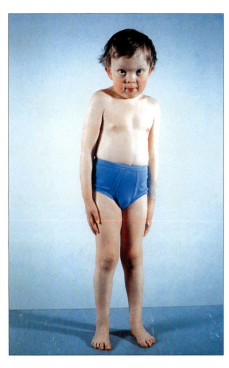

Fig. 65.5 A child with Mannosidosis showing the mild coarsening of the features. When older there was an increase in the facial coarsening. (Patient of Dr J.E. Wraith, Manchester Children's Hospital).

α-Mannosidosis (α-mannosidase deficiency)

There is mild facial coarsening (Fig 65.5), skeletal abnormalities, a variable degree of learning difficulty and, frequently, deafness. Corneal opacity is not usually marked and spoke-like cataract is more frequent. The spokes are posterior cortical, composed of multiple discrete clear round vacuoles lying at different depths in the lens, best seen by slit-lamp retroillumination.[23] MRI findings suggest demyelination and there is cerebellar atrophy and a thick calvarium.[24] There is no specific treatment.

Fucosidosis

Typically, it is a progressive neurodegenerative disease with seizures, mild coarsening of the facies, mild skeletal dysplasia and angiokeratoma. Bone marrow transplant may be effective if performed early enough in the course of the disease. Affected children have conjunctival and retinal vascular tortuosity.[25] A bull's eye maculopathy may be seen[26] and central and epithelial "lobulated" corneal opacities.[27]

Sialidosis (neuraminidase deficiency)

Type I: The "cherry-red spot-myoclonus" syndrome. Presenting in late childhood with insidious visual loss, there is a progressive myoclonus, but normal intelligence.[28] A cherry-red spot (Fig. 65.6) fades with age and neuronal loss. Some patients have punctate lens opacities. The diagnosis is made by the finding of a defect in lysosomal neuraminidase with normal beta-galactosidase. Sialyloligosaccharides are excreted in the urine, but mucopolysaccharides are not.

Type II: These patients have coarse features, similar to Hurler disease (Fig. 65.7). They have progressive loss of vision from corneal clouding and bilateral cherry-red spots.[29] They become deaf and mentally retarded, and may have nystagmus. Like type I they excrete sialyloligosaccharides. Histopathological examination has shown lamellated inclusions in retinal ganglion cells and amacrine cells, but not in the optic nerve which showed marked demyelination.[30]

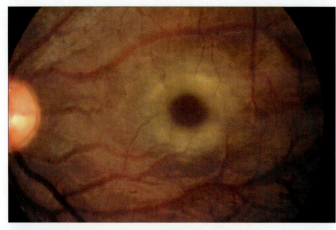

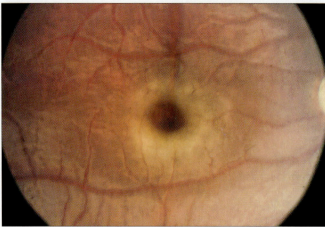

Fig. 65.6 Cherry-red spot in a patient with Sialidosis type I (Mr M.D.Sanders patient).

Galactosialidosis is a disorder which shares many features of sialidosis. There is deficiency of neuraminidase and also of β-galactosidase, due to a defect in cathepsin A.

Sialic acid storage diseases

These result from a block in lysosomal efflux of sialic acid. They range in severity from infantile sialic acid storage disease (ISSD), a severe neurodegenerative disorder with Hurler-like physical features and death in infancy, to Salla disease with slowly progressive mental retardation, ataxia and a near normal life span. In ISSD, children have loss of vision from corneal clouding and cherry-red spots. In Salla disease eye findings are strabismus and nystagmus.

Mucopolysaccharidoses (MPS)

These disorders affect bones, joints, brain, liver, spleen, upper airways and eyes. They can be grouped according to the underlying enzyme deficiency (Table 65.2). The degree of facial dysmorphism, neurodegeneration and extent of eye involvement varies.

An albeit incomplete *aide mémoire* to diagnosis for the ophthalmologist can be based on the facial features, the bone and eye changes:

1. Hurler-like phenotype (Fig. 65.8) with cloudy cornea (Fig. 65.9), retinal degeneration and optic atrophy.
   (a) MPS IH: Hurler syndrome.
   (b) MPS VI: Maroteaux–Lamy syndrome (normal intelligence).
   (c) MPS VII: Sly disease (eye findings not reported).
2. Mild facial changes and cloudy cornea. This can be subdivided into:
   (a) MPS IS: Scheie disease (was MPS V); hand deformity, aortic incompetence, retinal degeneration, normal intelligence.
   (b) MPS IV: Morquio disease: severe skeletal changes and dwarfing, normal intelligence and no retinal degeneration.
3. Mental retardation, facial changes without cloudy cornea.
   (a) MPS II Hunter: occasional mild corneal changes, severe skeletal changes, retinal degeneration, mental retardation.
   (b) MPS III Sanfilippo: severe mental retardation, mild facial changes, moderate skeletal changes, and retinal degeneration present.

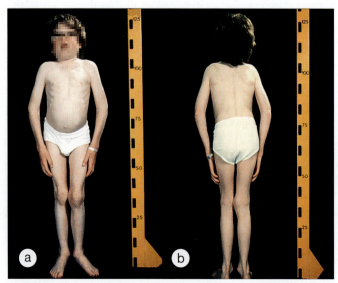

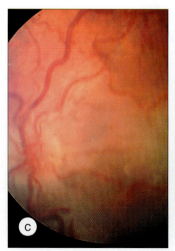

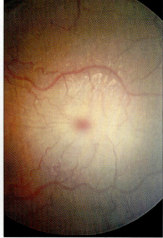

Fig. 65.7 (a & b) Patient with Sialidosis type 2. He has kyphoscoliosis and joint changes. (c) Same Patient as 65.7a & b, showing a cherry-red spot. The picture is hazy because of corneal clouding.

Table 65.2 MPS disorders and underlying enzyme deficiencies

Type	Eponym	Stored material	Enzyme deficiency
MPS IH	Hurler	DS, HS	Iduronidase
MPS IS	Scheie	DS, HS	Iduronidase
MPS IH/S	Hurler–Scheie	DS, HS	Iduronidase
MPS II	Hunter (X-LR)	DS, HS	Iduronidase sulphate sulphatase
MPS IIIA	Sanfillipo	HS	Heparan *N*-sulphatase
MPS IIIB		HS	*N*-acetylglucosaminidase
MPS IIIC		HS	Acetyl-CO-A-glucosaminidase-acetyltransferase
MPS IIID		HS	*N*-acetylglucosamine-6-sulphatase
MPS IVA	Morquio		Galactosamine-6-sulphatase
MPS IVB			β-galactosidase
MPS VI	Maroteaux–Lamy	DS	*N*-acetylgalactosamine-4-sulphatase
MPS VII	Sly	HS, CS, DS	β-glucuronidase

Table 65.3 Corneal opacities in metabolic and other disease

(See Chapter 29)
Whorl-like corneal opacities (differential diagnosis)

1. Well-defined whorls:
(a) Fabry disease
(b) Mucolipidosis IV
(c) Drug deposition—indomethacin, chloroquine, quinacrine, hydroxychloroquine, amiodarone, phenothiazines, especially chlorpromazine, and mepacrine

2. Corneal opacities resembling whorls:
(a) Tangier disease
(b) Melkersson syndrome/amyloidosis V
(c) Tyrosinemia
(d) Corneal edema

3. Other whorl-like opacities:
(a) Fleischer vortex dystrophy
(b) Cornea verticillata
(c) Whorl-like corneal dystrophy

The pediatric ophthalmologist is rarely involved with Hurler or Sanfilippo, because the mental retardation and short lives of the patients often preclude treatment for their corneas. Nevertheless, they are not infrequently asked to see patients with Maroteaux–Lamy, Morquio and Scheie disease whose pathological and ocular clinical features have many similarities, although they are not identical.

Ocular findings and management
Corneal clouding (Table 65.3)
The corneas take on a "ground glass" appearance that, in some instances is better seen with illumination from the side, than on slit-lamp examination. All layers of the corneas are symmetrically infiltrated, both within cells and in the extracellular space, with acid mucopolysaccharide; clouding is due to changes in the corneal stroma, including abnormal spacing and arrangement of collagen fibrils.[31] Although not clinically affected, the conjunctiva (which is readily biopsied) also shows intracellular inclusions which are mucopolysaccharide-containing lysosomes.

The main treatment for the cloudy cornea is corneal transplantation when retinal degeneration, optic atrophy, severe mental retardation or a markedly shortened lifespan are not present. Careful assessment of the patient's needs, together with neurophysiological studies and magnetic resonance imaging (MRI) to establish the viability of the retina and postretinal pathways, are mandatory before embarking on surgery. The visual improvement is rarely long lived but sometimes gives an extended period of vision to children who would otherwise be

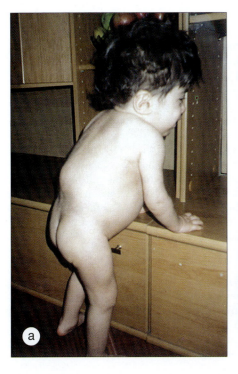
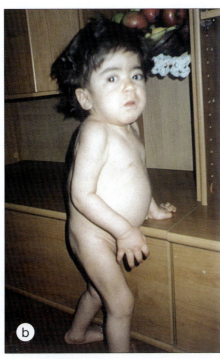

Fig. 65.8 Patient with MPS1 showing the facial features (a) and kyphosis (b). (Patient of Dr Stephanie Grunëwald)

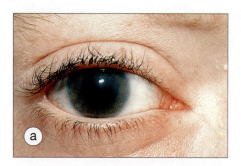

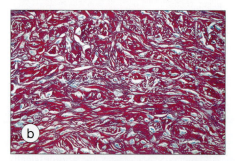

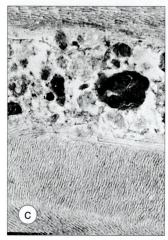
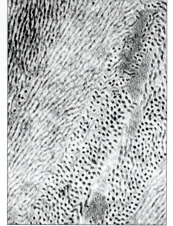

Fig. 65.9 (a) opalescent cornea in MPS1S. The acuity was 6/12. (b) Colloidal iron staining of a corneal graft host button showing the infiltration with acid mucopolysaccharide. (c) Electron microscopy study showing intracellular and extracellular amorphous acid mucopolysaccharide.

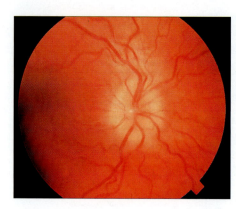

Fig. 65.10 Optic disc swelling in a patient with MPS VI Maroteaux-Lamy syndrome. The picture is hazy due to corneal clouding.

No treatment is available and detection of the retinal degeneration is mandatory before corneal grafting is undertaken. Although the post-BMT ERG stabilizes in the first year, longer follow-up shows progressive retinal decline.[33]

Optic disc swelling and atrophy

Histopathologically, the ganglion cells, retinal nerve fiber layer and optic nerve itself are affected: the optic nerve axons might be compressed or nutritionally compromised by glial cell infiltration. Swelling occurs in most patients (Fig. 65.10) and leads to optic atrophy,[34] which can also be caused by glaucoma. Neurophysiological studies help to delineate optic nerve and cortical visual defect.

Glaucoma

Glaucoma probably occurs in all of the mucopolysaccharidoses and some other metabolic diseases with cloudy corneas. Histopathological studies in MPS IH, -IS and -IV of trabeculectomy specimens show MPS-laden cells in the aqueous draining channels.[35,36] The cloudiness alone often makes the corneas appear large, so glaucoma is a diagnosis easily missed. The incidence is not high enough to warrant routine examinations under anesthetic unless there is clinical suspicion of raised intraocular pressure.

General management

Mucopolysaccharides are widespread throughout connective tissues, resulting in a range of other systemic effects. These include recurrent ENT infections, obstructive sleep apnea, deposits on the cardiac valves and infiltration of the cardiac muscle, inguinal and umbilical hernias, spinal cord compression and pain and stiffness from skeletal dysplasia. Ideally, management is multidisciplinary,[37] coordinated by a pediatrician with input from cardiology, anesthesia, orthopedics, ENT, neurosurgery, physiotherapy, audiology, speech therapy and ophthalmology.

Anesthesia should be undertaken with care in the MPS disorders, particularly in types I, II, IV and VI as these children are difficult to intubate, due to MPS deposition around the airway[38] and vulnerable cervical spinal cords.

Treatment

Symptomatic care is offered in types II, III and IV.

Bone marrow transplant in children with Hurler syndrome reverses many features of the disease: the face remodels, liver and spleen return to normal and ENT problems are improved.[39] Orthopedic complications are the main residual problem due to insufficient bone penetration by the donor enzyme.

blind. Corneal grafts may remain clear for months, rejection is unusual, and the graft reopacifies by involvement with the original process. The host cornea may partially clear in the post-transplant period.[32] They can be regrafted provided that retinal degeneration or optic atrophy has not supervened. After successful bone marrow transplantation, the clearing of the corneas is only partial, but re-accumulation does not occur in further grafts.

Retinal degeneration

This is seen in most forms, not in Morquio disease. Its insidious onset is usually overshadowed by the corneal opacities. Some children with MPS IS or MPS VI may note night-blindness or dimness in addition to the blurring of the corneal disease. Histopathologically, most tissues of the eye are affected, especially the retinal pigment epithelium cells which may be filled with mucopolysaccharide but generally intact. The outer retina is also affected. A macular edema-like change and pseudopapilledema have been described in a patient with MPS IS who had a retinal degeneration.

Enzyme replacement therapy is now available for type I, and is currently being researched for types II and VI.[40] Aimed primarily at the Hurler/Scheie and Scheie ends of the clinical spectrum, it improves lung function and mobility.

Mucolipidoses

The mucolipidosis II and III are due to the same biochemical defect: abnormal transport of lysosomal enzymes into the cell.

ML II or "I cell" disease presents earlier than Hurler, but shares many features with neurological degeneration and death in early childhood. There is retinal degeneration, and corneal clouding (Fig. 65.11).

ML III is milder, with a slowly progressive clinical course and survival to adulthood. There is early joint stiffening with slight facial coarsening and kyphoscoliosis. Eye signs include corneal clouding, hypermetropic astigmatism, optic disc edema and a diffuse retinal haze storage material in ganglion cells. The ERG is normal.

Mucolipidosis IV is seen mainly in the Ashkenazi Jews. Two mutations account for the vast majority of these patients. The biochemical defect is unknown. ML IV is important and has prominent ocular features. Affected children present with early corneal clouding, hypotonia and progressive retardation without skeletal change. Most do not progress beyond a developmental age of 15 months and live until their teens, or occasionally up to their thirties. Mild cases have been described, with the corneal changes being the most prominent problem.[41]

ML IV patients have cloudy corneas,[42] mainly epithelial (Fig. 65.12) and sometimes whorl-like.[41] Rapid regrowth of epithelium makes grafts short lived. Conjunctival transplantation may improve corneal clarity.[43] Sometimes corneal surface irregularities are associated with episodic pain.[44] Retinal degeneration may make treatment unrewarding.

Diagnosis is made by the finding of multiple concentrically lamellated bodies in the cornea and conjunctiva on ultrastructural studies[45] or in informative groups by mutation testing.

Fabry disease (α-galactosidase deficiency)

Fabry disease is caused by a deficiency of the lysosomal enzyme α-galactosidase A (α-Gal A) due to a wide variety of gene

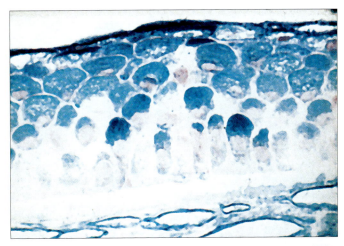

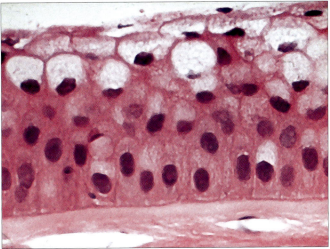

Fig. 65.12 Light microcoscopy showing the enlarged epithelial cells that contain acid mucosubstances staining with colloidal iron (top).

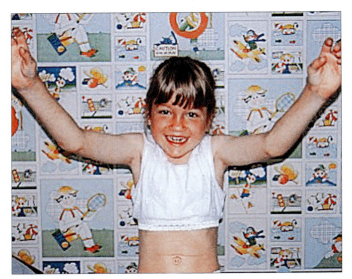

Fig. 65.11 Mucolipidosis 111 showing the facial features and the joint stiffening which prevents her from fully lifting her arms. (Patient of Dr J.E. Wraith, Manchester Children's Hospital).

mutations. This X-linked metabolic defect causes a chronic progressive painful small-fiber neuropathy (Fig. 65.13a), renal dysfunction, heart disease and stroke. Dark red angiectases occurring on the lower abdomen, buttocks and scrotum (bathing-trunk area) are characteristic skin lesions known as *angiokeratoma corporis diffusum*. It presents in males in late childhood or adolescence with pain in the extremities (acroparesthesia) provoked by exertion or change in temperature. The main life-limiting complications are progressive renal disease and hypertrophic cardiomyopathy.

Female heterozygotes may show clinical expression of the disease with acroparesthesia and angiokeratoma. Fabry disease is amenable to enzyme replacement therapy.[46]

In the eye, Fabry disease affects the cornea, lens, fundus, conjunctiva and lids. Slit-lamp examination of the cornea shows one or more lines radiating from a point near the center of the cornea with a whorl-like appearance ("cornea verticillata", Fig. 65.13b). The opacity is made up of myriads of white to yellow-brown dots in the epithelial or subepithelial layers. In young patients the corneal opacities may appear as a diffuse haze.[47] They occur in virtually all hemizygotes and heterozygotes.

Lens opacities, which are probably unique to Fabry disease, occur in two ways: a granular white subcapsular cataract, wedge-shaped with the base at the lens equator, especially inferiorly, and opacities seen in retroillumination that are lines of spots,

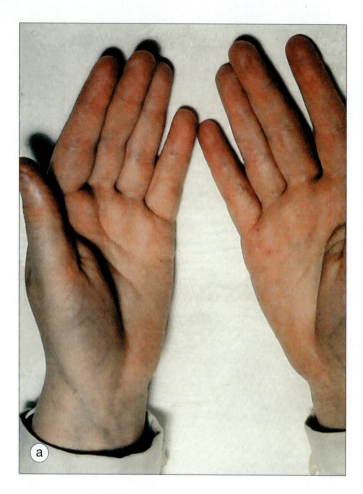

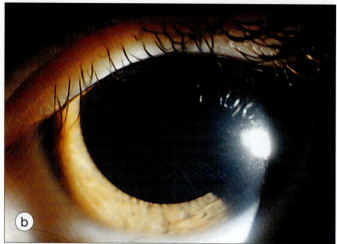

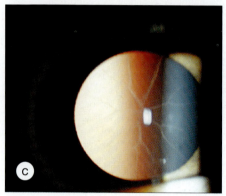

Fig. 65.13 (a) Fabry disease. Hypothenar atrophy from peripheral neuropathy. (b) Fabry disease. Cornea Verticillata can barely be distinguished adjacent to the pupil at 5 o'clock. (c) Fabry disease: characteristic spoke-like posterior cortical sutural cataract on retro-illumination.

radiating from the posterior pole of the lens, along the sutures (Fig. 65.13c).

In the second decade, retinal vascular tortuosity occurs, which especially affects the veins. The vessels become beaded, have sheathing and may develop arteriovenous anastomoses and thromboses. Affected males are more severely affected than the hemizygotes. Retinal vascular occlusion may be the initial symptom, optic disc edema may occur and myelinated nerve fibers.[48]

Neuro-ophthalmological problems include nystagmus, third nerve palsy and strabismus. Optic atrophy, internuclear ophthalmoplegia, seizures and strokes have all been described, but are rare. Visual defects are unusual. Conjunctival vessel tortuosity, lid edema and, rarely, facial angiokeratoma are seen.

Farber disease

This autosomal recessive disease is characterized by the onset in infancy of multiple subcutaneous nodules, lymphadenopathy, a hoarse cry and variable involvement of lung, heart and liver. The course is variable with death between 1 and 18 years. Severely affected children may have eye changes including a cherry-red spot that consists of a faint grey ring around the fovea, nodular corneal opacity and a pingueculum-like conjunctival lesion. The retinal ganglion cells in one child with cherry-red spots were grossly distended with inclusions but most ocular tissues had some involvement. There is no treatment.

Neuronal ceroid lipofuscinosis

The neuronal ceroid lipofuscinoses are the most common pediatric neurodegenerative disease. They are characterized by the accumulation of autofluorescent material in the brain and many other tissues. However, characterization of this abnormal storage product has not yet led to the identification of the underlying biochemical problem. The responsible genes are known to encode either lysosomal enzymes or lysosomal transport proteins: this has led to a firmer classification of the subtypes of the neuronal ceroid lipofuscinosis (Table 65.4). The genetic defects are called CLN genes and genes have been assigned to six of the eight forms of NCL. The common eponym Batten disease strictly applies to the juvenile onset form but in some texts this eponym is applied to all the NCLs.

Infantile neuronal ceroid lipofuscinosis (CLN 1)
Haltia–Santavuori disease

First described in Finnish children where the disease is prevalent, other cases have been reported in several racial groups. Early progress is normal but a slowing of motor skills development is seen around 12–18 months. After this the child becomes floppy and develops limb ataxia and microcephaly. Vision deteriorates around 12 months and by 24 months they are blind, with low amplitude, later absent ERG. Myoclonic jerks start around 16–24 months and repetitive stereotypic hand movements ("knitting"). There is gradual deterioration with hypotonia and

Table 65.4 Classification of neuronal ceroid lipofuscinosis

	Eponym	Also called	Gene product	Storage product
CLN1	Haltia–Santavuori	Infantile	Palmitoyl-protein thioesterase	Granular osmophiliac (GROD)
CLN2	Jansky–Bielschwsky	Late infantile	Peptinase	Curvilinear
CLN3	Batten	Juvenile	Battenin	Fingerprint
CLN4	Kufs	Adult	Unknown	Fingerprint/GROD
CLN5,6,7		Variant infantile	Unknown	
CLN8		Progressive myoclonic epilepsy	Unknown	

opisthotonus, flexion contractures by age 5 and death around 6–7 years.

The retinas show narrow blood vessels, some pigment epithelial changes around the macula and later optic atrophy and clumped retinal pigmentation. Cherry-red spots are not seen. Neurons contain granular osmophilic deposits (GROD or "Finnish snowballs") which can be seen in rectal neurons or leukocytes. The underlying enzyme deficiency is of palmitoyl-protein thioesterase-1 (PPT) and the diagnosis is usually now made with leukocyte enzyme measurement.

Late onset and variable forms of NCL with GROD (CLN1)

About 5–10% of all cases of NCL that present after the age of two years show GROD that are characteristic of the infantile form. It is now recognized that these are due to a milder deficiency of the same enzyme (PPT).

Classical late infantile (CLN2)
Jansky–Bielschowsky disease

These children present between 2 to 4 years of age with mental deterioration, ataxia, myoclonic jerks and epilepsy, with death by 7 years. Blindness occurs early from retinal degeneration most marked at the macula, but later the whole retina is affected and appears thinned with clumped pigment, narrow arterioles and optic atrophy. The ERG is extinguished early but there is an extraordinarily enlarged VER amplitude, many times the normal. The EEG shows large spikes at low rates of photic stimulation.[49]

Juvenile neuronal ceroid lipofuscinosis (CLN3)
Batten disease

Batten disease[50] is the most common neurodegenerative disease seen by pediatric ophthalmologists, and it represents a small but important cause of child blindness in the UK. Perhaps 25% of the children each year registered as blind with acquired retinal or macular disease have Batten disease.[51]

Children with juvenile Batten disease present with visual failure between 4 and 10 years, with a peak incidence at 6 years.[51] The earliest change is a bull's eye maculopathy (Fig. 65.14a) but the whole retina is affected early as shown by the ERG changes, which are present early in the disease.[49,52] Attenuation of the b-wave of the ERG, with initial preservation of the EOG, and later involvement of all elements of the ERG suggests that the retina between the receptors and ganglion cells is primarily affected.[53] Later there is a widespread retinal degeneration with pigment clumping (Fig. 65.14b) and sparse bone spicule pigmentation in the periphery, the disc becomes atrophic and the arterioles thinned (Fig. 65.14c). The whole retina becomes avascular.[54] The children are usually functionally blind within 3 years.

Mental retardation develops slowly and is often noticed at school. These children are not, in contrast to the infantile form, microcephalic. Behavioral disturbances may also be present. Although mental deterioration and behavioral disturbances occur early, often predating the visual deterioration, they are often quite subtle and it is the onset of fits between 7 and 16 years of age that often leads to the diagnosis. The flash VER may show reduced early components initially, but becomes extinguished and the EEG shows runs of large amplitude and slow wave and spike complexes.[49,55] Computed tomographic (CT) scanning shows diffuse supra- and infratentorial brain atrophy.[56,57]

Eccentric viewing (Fig. 65.15) is a characteristic finding at presentation, with the patient tending to overlook the "target";[58] this may be due to a relative preservation of the upper retina. Affected children tend to rub or poke their eye and this may account for the keratoconus and cataracts seen in some patients. Fluorescein angiography may show leakage in rapidly degenerating retinas, but generally only shows evidence of retinal pigment epithelial degeneration.

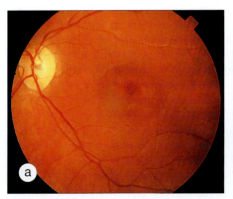 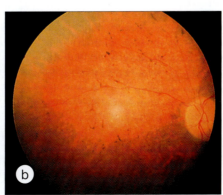 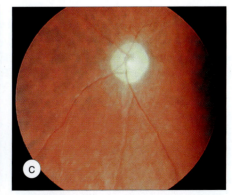

Fig. 65.14 (a) Optic atrophy, arteriolar thinning and bull's eye maculopathy in juvenile Batten disease. (b) Juvenile Batten disease: bone-spicule pigmentation, optic atrophy and arteriolar narrowing. (c) Late retinal changes in juvenile Batten disease including depigmentation, optic atrophy and extreme arteriolar narrowing.

The disease follows a slow downward path with dementia in the teens and death sometimes well into the second or third decade.

Diagnosis is suspected by finding vacuolated lymphocytes in the peripheral blood smears (Fig. 65.16) and is confirmed by the finding of characteristic "fingerprint" inclusions (Fig. 65.17) in neurons on electron microscopy of rectal, skin, conjunctival biopsies and lymphocytes.[59-61] There is no treatment, though prenatal diagnosis is possible. Bone marrow transplantation is not effective.[62] The gene is at 16p12.1[63,64] and it encodes a 438 amino acid protein battenin. The function of this protein is unknown but it is probably a lysosomal membrane protein. There is a common mutation, a 1.02 kb deletion, affecting 85% of affected cases worldwide.[2] There are three mouse models for JCL. The earlier two showed remarkably little retinal pathology but the most recent "knock-in" mouse also has the common deletion and it shows loss of cone-associated markers. It develops the JCL phenotype earlier than the previous mouse models, even showing prenatal pathology. It is hoped that these models can be used to understand the pathophysiology more clearly and then lead onto further attempts at treatment.

Kufs disease

Kufs disease is an adult onset form of Batten's disease with no ophthalmological abnormalities.

Cystinosis

See Chapter 53.

MITOCHONDRIAL DISORDERS:

Mitochondria provide energy in a form that can easily be used (adenosine triphosphate). This is accomplished by the "respiratory

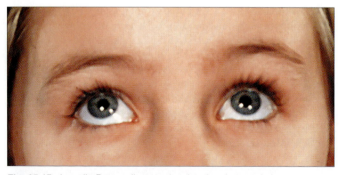

Fig. 65.15 Juvenile Batten disease showing the characteristic 'overlooking' eccentric viewing seen in many cases soon after the onset of the visual loss. Note she is trying to look directly at the camera.

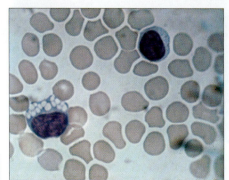

Fig. 65.16 Juvenile Batten disease: lymphocyte inclusions.

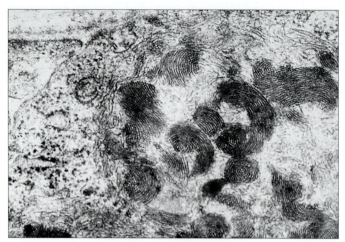

Fig. 65.17 Juvenile Batten disease: 'fingerprint' inclusions in rectal neurons.

chain", a series of five multiprotein complexes located in the inner of the two mitochondrial membranes. Most mitochondrial genes are in the nucleus, but some are on a circular DNA molecule within the mitochondrion itself (mtDNA). MtDNA is, almost exclusively, maternally inherited. Many copies of mtDNA are present in each cell. A mtDNA mutation may be homoplasmic (affects all copies) or heteroplasmic (affects a proportion), the amount varying between different tissues and different pedigree members; the phenotypic severity depends on the level of heteroplasmy. The pathogenesis is poorly understood: energy depletion and generation of free radicals are potential mechanisms.

The eye is frequently affected, along with muscle and brain but multisystem disease is common, particularly in early childhood. Ophthalmological complications of respiratory chain disease include cataracts, various patterns of retinopathy, optic atrophy, subacute visual loss due to optic neuropathy, cortical visual loss, ptosis and ophthalmoplegia. A number of clinical syndromes are recognized, some are associated with particular genetic abnormalities. The syndromes may be incomplete, present in atypical ways or overlap with other syndromes. Moreover, most affected children do not conform to any of the classical syndromes.

If the clinical picture suggests a syndrome associated with particular mtDNA mutations, one can proceed straight to genetic tests. Many mtDNA point mutations can be detected in blood but MtDNA deletions in Kearns–Sayre syndrome can only be detected in muscle. If the clinical features do not suggest a particular mtDNA mutation, the first test will generally be measurement of blood or CSF lactate. Raised concentrations are a useful pointer but normal values do not exclude mitochondrial disorders. Assays of the respiratory chain complexes are usually needed; this should be done by a specialist laboratory with muscle biopsy. Unfortunately, normal results do not completely exclude mitochondrial disease because partial or tissue-specific defects can occur.

Leber hereditary optic neuropathy (LHON)

This is considered in detail in Chapter 60.

Pearson and Kearns–Sayre syndromes

These syndromes are associated with mtDNA "rearrangements" (large deletions or duplications). They are always heteroplasmic;

the concentration of the rearranged mtDNA in different tissues determines the age and manner of presentation: not all conform to the described syndromes.

Pearson et al. reported four infants with sideroblastic anemia, pancytopenia, pancreatic exocrine insufficiency and liver disease.[65] Renal tubular dysfunction, diabetes mellitus and intestinal villus atrophy may also be seen. In patients who survive long enough, the hematological problems generally improve but features of Kearns–Sayre syndrome emerge.

Kearns–Sayre syndrome is a progressive external ophthalmoplegia (PEO) and pigmentary retinopathy with onset before 20 years of age with at least one of: heart block, cerebellar syndrome or CSF protein above 1 g/l. Other features include hearing loss, dementia, cardiomyopathy and endocrine disorders. The most mildly affected patients with mtDNA rearrangements present as adults with isolated ophthalmoplegia and ptosis.

The ophthalmoplegia associated with mtDNA rearrangements appears to result from muscle abnormalities; ptosis is common, as is exotropia, often without diplopia presumably because of the gradual onset. Most patients with Kearns–Sayre syndrome develop a "salt and pepper" fundus. Visual acuity tends not to be severely impaired, unless there is optic atrophy. Other patients have generalized loss of the retinal pigment epithelium.[66]

Pearson syndrome and Kearns–Sayre syndrome are almost always sporadic and, if an unaffected mother has an affected child, the recurrence risk is low. Pearson syndrome has been reported in children of women with Kearns–Sayre syndrome.

In a patient with Pearson or Kearns–Sayre syndrome, all the mtDNA deletions are of the same size and have the same breakpoints. PEO patients occasionally have multiple different mtDNA deletions which result from defects in nuclear genes that are involved in mtDNA replication and inheritance is autosomal dominant or recessive.[67] They usually present as adults with PEO and exercise intolerance. PEO can also be caused by heteroplasmic mtDNA point mutations, most commonly the 3243A→G mutation associated with MELAS syndrome.

MELAS syndrome

MELAS syndrome is characterized by Mitochondrial myopathy, Encephalopathy, Lactic Acidosis and Stroke-like episodes. The strokes start between 5 and 15 years of age, causing visual field defects or cortical blindness and hemiplegia[68]; sometimes the symptoms resolve rapidly. Headaches and vomiting may precede the stroke-like episodes and maternal relatives may have a history of severe migraine. Eighty per cent of patients with MELAS syndrome carry the 3243A→G mtDNA mutation. The severity of problems associated with this mutation depends on the degree of heteroplasmy. Patients with lower levels of mutant mtDNA may present with diabetes and deafness, cardiomyopathy or myopathy. Other manifestations include progressive external ophthalmoplegia, "salt and pepper" pigmentary retinopathy and macular pattern dystrophy.

NARP syndrome

This is characterized by Neurogenic weakness, Ataxia and Retinitis Pigmentosa. It is described in Chapter 53.

Leigh syndrome

This is a neurodegenerative syndrome associated with various biochemical defects. There is symmetrical damage primarily in the brainstem but the spinal cord, corpus striatum, cerebellum, cerebral white matter and optic pathways (Fig. 65.18a) may be involved.[69] The diagnosis is now usually made during life on the basis of the clinical history and MRI (Fig. 65.18b,c). Most cases present in early childhood with non-specific features: feeding problems, failure to thrive and hypotonia. Eye movement disorders, swallowing or breathing difficulties, dystonia or spasticity appear later. The commonest course is chronic and unremitting. Other patients follow a stepwise course with episodes of deterioration and partial recovery separated by periods of stability. CSF lactate concentrations are usually raised. Most but not all have a defect in the respiratory chain or the pyruvate dehydrogenase complex. SURF1 gene mutations are commonest; this gene is concerned with the assembly of respiratory chain complex IV and it is autosomal recessive. Most cases of pyruvate dehydrogenase deficiency are new mutations in an X-linked gene. A few patients with Leigh syndrome have mtDNA mutations and show maternal inheritance. Symptomatic treatment is generally all that can be offered but a few patients have biotinidase deficiency and respond to biotin.

Eye movement disorders are common: nystagmus, strabismus, ophthalmoplegia and ptosis are caused by brainstem involvement. Optic atrophy is common.[70] Pigmentary retinopathy is less common in Leigh syndrome, but may be seen with 8993 "'NARP'" mtDNA mutations.

Alpers syndrome/progressive neuronal degeneration of childhood

Alpers syndrome is an ill-defined childhood neurodegenerative disorder, with progressive cerebral atrophy, particularly of the cortex. Progressive neuronal degeneration of childhood refers to a subgroup who have an explosive onset of seizures in early childhood. Stroke-like episodes are common, typically involving the occipital cortex and leading to cortical visual defects (with or without hemiplegia). Terminally, patients often develop liver failure.[71] The etiology is uncertain but mitochondrial abnormalities have been demonstrated in some patients.

Sengers syndrome

These patients have congenital cataracts, cardiomyopathy and mitochondrial myopathy. The patients, despite prompt management, develop poor vision.[72] The cardiomyopathy is hypertrophic and of variable severity: it may cause death anywhere between the neonatal period and adulthood. Patients have limited exercise capacity. Muscle electron microscopy shows abnormal mitochondria but no defect of the respiratory chain has been demonstrated. It may show autosomal recessive inheritance but it may be genetically heterogeneous. Early onset cataracts may also be seen in other mitochondrial disease, including Kearns–Sayre and MELAS syndromes.

Friedreich ataxia

Typically, this condition presents between 5 and 16 years of age with ataxia or clumsiness, followed by dysarthria. Examination reveals an intention tremor, absent reflexes in the legs, extensor plantar responses and loss of proprioception in the feet. Patients lose the ability to walk at around 25 years. Non-neurological features include pes cavus and cardiomyopathy, which is a common cause of death. Diabetes mellitus and hearing loss are rarer. Some develop fixation instability, nystagmus or optic atrophy

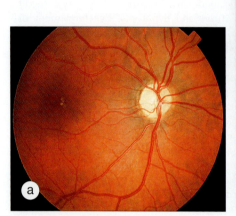
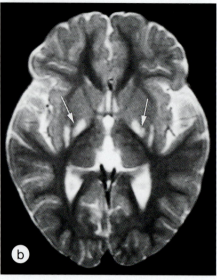
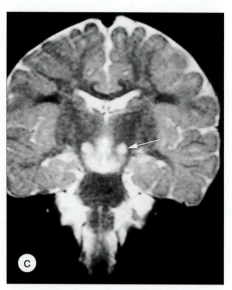

Fig. 65.18 (a) Leigh disease. Optic atrophy is common in later stages. (b) Leigh disease. Abnormal signal in the globus pallidus (arrowed). (c) Leigh disease. Abnormal signal in the upper midbrain (arrowed).

with variable visual impairment,[73] but problems are less common in childhood. It is autosomal recessive and is caused by expansion of a trinucleotide repeat in the frataxin gene. Frataxin is a protein involved in mitochondrial iron handling and respiratory chain defects have been found in cardiac muscle from patients with Friedreich ataxia. Only symptomatic treatment is available.

Autosomal dominant optic atrophy

This is described in Chapter 60.

Propionic acidemia

This is caused by propionyl-CoA carboxylase deficiency. Patients present as neonates or later in childhood with vomitting, drowsiness, acidosis and hyperammonemia. The boys especially may have a progressive, variable optic neuropathy which may be independent of metabolic control.[74]

PEROXISOMAL DISEASES

Peroxisomes contain more than 50 enzymes for the synthesis of plasmalogens, bile acids and isoprenoids and the oxidation of very long chain and branched chain fatty acids (e.g. phytanic acid). Proteins are imported into the peroxisome, dependent on "'PEX genes'", defects of which cause peroxisomal biogenesis disorders, in which several (or all) peroxisomal pathways are impaired. Other peroxisomal disorders are caused by defects of a single enzyme.

Peroxisomal biogenesis disorders

These disorders generally cause congenital malformations, neuro-developmental problems and biochemical abnormalities. There is a wide range of severity but 80% fall within the Zellweger spectrum and the remainder have rhizomelic chondrodysplasia punctata (RCDP).

Patients with severe **Zellweger syndrome** are dysmorphic with a large anterior fontanelle, high forehead, shallow supraorbital ridges and epicanthic folds. They have hypotonia, seizures and feeding difficulties. Ocular abnormalities and impaired hearing are common, as are renal cysts and liver involvement. Most patients die within a few months.

"Neonatal adrenoleukodystrophy" refers to a slightly milder phenotype; some patients survive to mid/late childhood, although they become deaf, blind and profoundly retarded. Most have a leukodystrophy but overt adrenal insufficiency is rare.

Infantile Refsum disease is characterized by mental retardation, deafness, pigmentary retinopathy, anosmia and mild dysmorphism.

In reality, however, the Zellweger spectrum is a continuum, with considerable overlap between the reported phenotypes. At the mildest end of the spectrum, some patients only have deafness and retinitis pigmentosa, which may be misdiagnosed as Usher syndrome: these patients may be mosaics.[75]

Zellweger spectrum patients often have nystagmus and strabismus, associated with poor vision. Anterior segment abnormalities occur at the severe end of the spectrum, such as abnormal insertion of the iris.[76] Commoner findings include corneal clouding, congenital cataracts and glaucoma. Brushfield spots may be present and, with hypotonia, a flattened face and single palmar creases may suggest Down syndrome. Retinal dystrophy is very common (Fig. 65.19). Retinal hypopigmentation is the main fundus abnormality in severely affected patients. Pigment clumping is more prominent towards the mild end of the spectrum. Mildly affected patients lose peripheral vision initially, but ultimately most become completely blind (see Chapter 53).

In **Rhizomelic chondrodysplasia punctata** (RCDP), there is severe shortening of the humeri and femora, vertebral clefts and stippled epiphyses. Most have facial dysmorphism and severe neurological abnormalities: few survive beyond 2 years. Cataracts are found in 75%: they are usually congenital, (Fig. 65.20) but may appear at a few months of age in mildly affected patients.

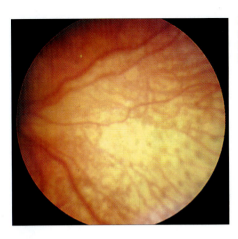

Fig. 65.19 Zellweger syndrome. Retinal Dystrophy with mottled RPE.

Peroxisomal biogenesis disorders may be diagnosed from the concentrations of very long chain fatty acids (VLCFA) and phytanic acid in plasma and plasmalogens in erythrocytes. In the Zellweger spectrum, plasma VLCFA and phytanic acid concentrations are raised and erythrocyte plasmalogen levels are low. In RCDP, phytanic acid concentrations are raised and plasmalogen concentrations are low with normal VLCFA levels. Single peroxisomal enzymes defects can cause phenotypes indistinguishable from the Zellweger spectrum or RCDP. Abnormalities of the initial tests must, therefore, be pursued with further investigations, such as enzymology in cultured fibroblasts.

All the peroxisomal biogenesis disorders are inherited as autosomal recessive traits. To deduce the genetic defect, fibroblasts are fused with cells known to have a particular defect and "complementation" is assessed. Defects in at least 11 PEX genes can lead to the Zellweger spectrum. The phenotype correlates poorly with the gene: some PEX1 mutations cause typical Zellweger syndrome whilst others are associated with neonatal adrenoleukodystrophy or infantile Refsum disease. The RCDP phenotype is usually caused by PEX7 mutations (but it can also result from isolated deficiency of DHAPAT or alkyl-DHAP synthase). Prenatal diagnosis is possible for all peroxisomal biogenesis disorders, using genetic or biochemical tests on a chorionic villus biopsy.

Treatment is largely symptomatic, but docosahexanoic acid (DHA) supplements may improve the retinal and neurological

outcomes.[77] Liver dysfunction may improve with bile acid treatment.

Refsum disease

See Chapter 53.

X-linked adrenoleukodystrophy

In this disorder, VLCFAs accumulate in blood and tissues due to a defect in a peroxisomal membrane protein. The incidence is between 1:20 000 and 1:50 000 males. The clinical phenotype varies markedly, even within a family, the commonest forms being childhood cerebral (35%) and adrenomyeloneuropathy (40%). The childhood cerebral form presents at 4–8 years with behavioral, cognitive and neurological problems, usually leading to a vegetative state within 3 years. Strabismus, visual field defects and decreased visual acuity are early symptoms in a third of patients with this cerebral form. Later these patients become blind due to optic atrophy and cortical visual loss[78] (Fig. 65.21).

Adrenomyeloneuropathy presents with paraparesis in young adults. Most male patients eventually develop adrenal insufficiency, regardless of the neurological phenotype. Heterozygous females may develop mild neurological abnormalities, but only as adults.

Lorenzo's oil combined with a low-fat diet can normalize plasma VLCFA concentrations in patients with X-linked adrenoleukodystrophy, but it is not clear whether this reduces neurological problems. It does not improve the outcome once neurological involvement has started. If undertaken at the first sign of cerebral involvement, bone marrow transplantation may prevent disease progression.[79]

Primary hyperoxaluria type 1

See Chapters 53 and 57.

CONGENITAL DEFECTS OF GLYCOSYLATION

Most extracellular, cell surface proteins and some intracellular proteins are glycoproteins. Oligosaccharides are attached to the amino acid asparagine (N-glycans) or to serine or threonine (O-glycans).

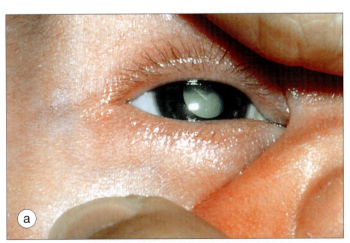
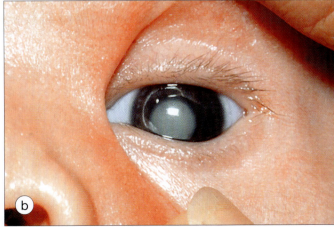

Fig. 65.20 Rhizomelic chondrodysplasia punctata. Bilateral total congenital cataract.

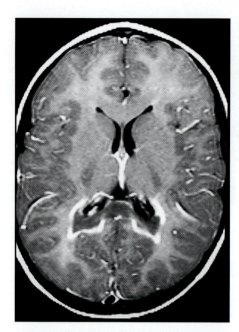

Fig. 65.21
Adrenoleucodystrophy. MRI scan showing characteristically predominant early involvement of the occipital lobes and visual pathway with high signal from the periventricular white matter.

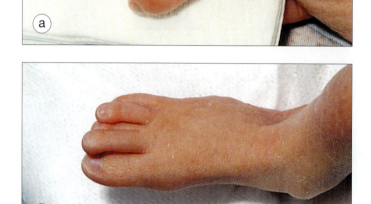

Fig. 65.22 (a) Carbohydrate-Deficient Glycoprotein syndrome1a (CDG1a) showing long fingers. (b)CDG1a showing long toes.

Defects of N-glycan synthesis: the carbohydrate deficient glycoprotein syndromes

N-glycan formation starts in the cytoplasm with the synthesis of precursors, such as GDP-mannose. Oligosaccharides are assembled in the endoplasmic reticulum (ER) and subsequently transferred to the protein. The protein-bound oligosaccharides are then processed in the ER and the Golgi apparatus. Assembly defects are classified as carbohydrate deficient glycoprotein syndromes (CDG) Ia–Ih, whilst processing defects are classified as CDG IIa–IId.[80] Most patients can be detected by transferrin isoelectric focusing, which reveals underglycosylated transferrin molecules. Specific enzyme assays can then be undertaken on fibroblasts.

CDG 1a is the commonest congenital defect of glycosylation, caused by phosphomannomutase-2 deficiency, which interferes with the synthesis of GDP-mannose. Most present as neonates with hypotonia, esotropia and dysmorphism. They may have large dystrophic ears, long fingers and toes (Fig. 65.22), inverted nipples and fat pads over the buttocks. Twenty per cent die in infancy from sepsis, pericardial effusions, nephrotic syndrome or liver failure. Those surviving, or presenting later, show delayed development and ataxia, rarely walking without support. However, they generally have a cheerful personality and regression is rare. Microcephaly and feeding problems are common and 50% of patients have stroke-like episodes.

Esotropia is common, with deficient abduction and nystagmus on attempted lateral gaze.[81] Neonates may also have abnormal vertical or horizontal eye movements. Delayed visual maturation is common.[81] Later, they develop myopia and retinal dystrophy (see Chapter 53).

Ophthalmological complications are less prominent in other N-glycosylation defects. CDG Ic presents with neurological problems similar to those seen in CDG Ia, but with less dysmorphism and retardation. Strabismus is common but retinitis pigmentosa is rare. The reported patient with CDG Id had optic atrophy and iris colobomata, severe retardation and seizures.

Walker–Warburg syndrome and muscle–eye–brain disease

See Chapter 49.

Both conditions result from defects of O-glycan synthesis. Muscle–eye–brain disease is caused by O-mannose–β1,2-N-acetylglucosaminyl-transferase deficiency. Approximately 20% Walker–Warburg patients have O-mannosyltransferase 1 deficiency.[82]

INBORN ERRORS OF CARBOHYDRATE METABOLISM

Galactosemia and galactokinase deficiency

See Chapter 47.

INBORN ERRORS OF AMINO ACID METABOLISM

Classical homocystinuria

See Chapter 46.

Molybdenum cofactor deficiency and isolated sulphite oxidase deficiency

The clinical features are very similar for these two autosomal recessive disorders. Most present in the newborn period with intractable seizures; subsequently, patients develop microcephaly, severe psychomotor retardation and spastic tetraplegia, with early death. A few patients run a milder course with prolonged survival. Ectopia lentis in the first 2 years occurs in over 50%. There may be spherophakia, nystagmus, cortical blindness, enophthalmos and colobomas.

Sulphite, formed during the breakdown of cysteine, is normally oxidized to sulphate. Some features of sulphite oxidase deficiency, such as lens dislocation, are probably mediated by sulphite attacking disulphide bonds, in the same way as homocysteine.[83] Molybdenum cofactor is essential for the function of sulphite oxidase and is also required by xanthine dehydrogenase: patients with deficiency can develop xanthine urolithiasis. Both conditions can be diagnosed by dipsticks that detect urinary sulphite or by demonstrating S-sulphocysteine on urine amino acid analysis. Molybdenum cofactor deficiency is distinguished by xanthinuria and low plasma urate concentrations. There is no effective treatment for the severe form of either condition but mildly affected patients may profit from a diet low in sulphur-containing amino acids.

Maple syrup urine disease

In this autosomal recessive disorder, deficiency of branched-chain α-ketoacid dehydrogenase leads to high concentrations of the amino acids leucine, isoleucine and valine. Leucine is particularly toxic to the brain. Leucine concentrations can be lowered acutely by hemofiltration and subsequently they can be controlled by dietary management.

Most patients present with neonatal encephalopathy. Initial features are lethargy and poor feeding at 4–7 days of age. Later, abnormal posturing, seizures and coma occur. Ophthalmoplegia[84] may be a prominent feature of the encephalopathy, with ptosis and various gaze pareses.[85] Bursts of eye and lid flutter may be seen once treatment is started. If treatment is delayed patients have mental retardation and spasticity. A few patients present later in childhood with recurrent encephalopathy or developmental delay. In older children, ataxia is an early feature of encephalopathy and may be accompanied by nystagmus.

Cbl C (cobalamin C) disease

See Chapter 53.

Gyrate atrophy of the choroid and retina

See Chapter 53.

Tyrosinemia type 2

See Chapter 29.

This autosomal recessive disorder is characterized by corneal ulcers (in 75%), painful hyperkeratotic lesions on the palms and soles (in 80%) and various neurological problems (in 60%). They present in the first year with photophobia, eye pain and conjunctival injection. The corneas have bilateral, central, dendritic corneal erosions. They resemble herpes simplex keratitis[86] but stain poorly, if at all, with fluorescein. Neovascularization may be prominent. Without treatment, corneal scarring may lead to visual impairment and glaucoma.

Tyrosinemia type 2 is caused by deficiency of tyrosine aminotransferase, which catalyses the first step in tyrosine breakdown. Definitive diagnosis requires liver enzymology or mutation analysis, but the diagnosis is likely if plasma tyrosine concentrations exceed 1200 mcmol/l. The eye and skin lesions are probably caused by intracellular precipitation of tyrosine crystals. Tyrosine concentrations can be lowered by dietary restriction of phenylalanine and tyrosine. The eye and skin lesions resolve within a few months when tyrosine concentrations are brought below 800 mcmol/l, but stricter control may be necessary to prevent neurological problems.

Tyrosinemia types 1 and 3 do not have eye complications.

Oculocutaneous albinism

See Chapter 45.

Aromatic L-amino acid decarboxylase deficiency

Eye movement abnormalities are prominent in this rare autosomal recessive disorder, in which the synthesis of catecholamines and serotonin neurotransmitters is impaired. Patients present within a few months of birth with hypotonia, an extrapyramidal movement disorder, irritability and autonomic disturbances, including ptosis, miosis, paroxysmal sweating and temperature instability. Oculogyric crises and convergence spasms are common.[87] Some patients have shown marked clinical improvement when treated with dopamine agonists (such as bromocryptine and pergolide) and a monoamine oxidase inhibitor (tranylcypromine).

Canavan disease

Patients with Canavan disease usually present aged 2–4 months with poor eye contact, hypotonia and seizures. Macrocephaly is apparent by 6 months and leukodystrophy is seen on cerebral imaging. Hypotonia progresses to spasticity with pseudobulbar palsy and opisthotonic posturing. Patients often have cortical visual loss; optic atrophy and nystagmus are common. Most patients die by 3 years of age. It is an autosomal recessive disorder, prevalent in Ashkenazi Jews,[88] caused by aspartoacylase deficiency, which leads to the accumulation of N-acetyl-aspartic acid (NAA); diagnosis is confirmed by demonstrating NAA in the urine. It is normally only present in the brain, where its function is unknown. There is no effective treatment.

DISORDERS OF FATTY ACID AND FATTY ALCOHOL METABOLISM

Long-chain 3-hydroxyacyl-CoA dehydrogenase (LCHADD) deficiency

See Chapter 53.

Sjögren-Larsson syndrome

See Chapters 53–57.

DISORDERS OF STEROL METABOLISM

Early onset cataracts are seen in several disorders of sterol metabolism, including defects of cholesterol synthesis and of bile acid synthesis. The lens membrane has a very high cholesterol content but the pathogenesis of the cataracts is unclear.

Smith–Lemli–Opitz syndrome is caused by deficiency of 7-dehydrocholesterol reductase, which catalyses the final step in cholesterol synthesis. Its incidence in the UK has been estimated at 1:60 000.[89] The clinical severity ranges from mild mental retardation to intrauterine or neonatal death due to malformations. Most patients present in infancy with poor feeding and dysmorphism (microcephaly, ptosis, anteverted nares, cleft palate and cryptorchidism). Malformations of the heart, kidney, gut and brain are common and virtually all patients have mental retardation. One fifth of patients have cataracts (usually congenital). Rarer ophthalmological abnormalities include strabismus, glaucoma, optic atrophy and microphthalmia. Treatment with cholesterol appears to improve weight gain and growth in these patients and *may* improve development and behavior, but the prognosis depends on the severity of internal malformations.

Mevalonic aciduria is caused by deficiency of mevalonate kinase, which catalyses an early step in cholesterol synthesis. Patients with severe deficiency present in infancy with failure to thrive, hypotonia and dysmorphism (dolichocephaly, down-slanting eyes and low set ears). Approximately one-third of patients have cataracts; uveitis and pigmentary retinopathy have also been reported.[90] Many patients die in the first few years and most of the survivors have severe psychomotor retardation. There is no effective treatment. All patients have recurrent febrile crises with vomiting, diarrhea and rashes. Partial deficiency of mevalonate kinase causes similar recurrent fevers with elevated concentrations of IgD, but without the other features of mevalonic aciduria.

Conradi–Hünermann syndrome is caused by deficiency of 3β-hydroxysteroid $\Delta^8\Delta^7$-isomerase. This enzyme lies on an alternative pathway for cholesterol synthesis and deficiency leads to increased levels of (8(9)-cholestenol) and 8-dehydrocholesterol. Inheritance is X-linked dominant: most males die *in utero* and the severity in females is variable. Most patients have ichthyosis or erythroderma from birth, which improves with age, leaving swirls of abnormal pigmentation. Two-thirds of patients develop cataracts during childhood (Fig. 65.23); these are segmental and often unilateral.[91] Orthopedic problems are the most severe complication: X-rays show chondrodysplasia punctata, and asymmetric growth can lead to deformity. They have normal intelligence.

Cataracts are an early feature in **cerebrotendinous xanthomatosis** and may be present as early as 5 years of age.[92] Mental retardation and diarrhea may be present by the age of 10 years. Over the next 20–30 years, most patients develop neurological problems (such as spasticity) and tendon xanthomas. Death is either due to the neurological illness or premature atherosclerosis. Cerebro-

tendinous xanthomatosis is caused by deficiency of sterol 27-hydroxylase, an enzyme involved in the formation of bile acids from cholesterol. Problems result from the accumulation of cholestanol and cholesterol. Treatment with the bile acid, chenodeoxycholic acid, inhibits the synthesis of these sterols and leads to clinical benefit, including improved intelligence. HMG-CoA reductase inhibitors may also be beneficial.

Steroid sulphatase deficiency

Ichthyosis is the main problem in this X-linked disorder. Affected males show skin changes by the age of 4 months. Characteristic corneal opacities are visible on slit-light examination in approximately 25% of affected males and also in heterozygous females.[93] The deposits are located in Descemet's membrane or the stroma anterior to this and they have no effect on visual acuity.

LIPOPROTEIN DISORDERS

Abetalipoproteinemia

See Chapter 53.

Lecithin:cholesterol acyltransferase (LCAT) deficiency and "fish eye" disease

Patients with complete deficiency of LCAT generally present as adults with proteinuria and progress to renal failure. They also have anemia and corneal opacities. Patients with partial LCAT deficiency do not suffer renal failure or anemia and corneal opacification is the only problem: these patients are said to have "fish eye" disease. Corneal opacities are usually detectable in childhood in both complete and partial LCAT deficiency, but they are of variable severity. Grossly, the cornea has a dull grey cloudy appearance and slit-lamp examination reveals small dots in all layers of the cornea except the epithelium.[94]

LCAT converts cholesterol to cholesterol esters by transferring a fatty acid from a phospholipid (lecithin). This is important for the transport of cholesterol to the liver from other tissues ("reverse cholesterol transport"). The diagnosis is suggested by a high plasma ratio of free cholesterol to cholesterol esters (>0.7) and confirmed by low activity of LCAT in plasma. A low fat diet improves the biochemical abnormalities and may slow progression of the disease, although this is not yet proven. Sometimes, visual impairment may be enough to warrant corneal transplantation.

Corneal opacities may also be seen in other rare defects of "reverse cholesterol transport". The main features of **Tangier disease** are enlarged orange tonsils, hepatosplenomegaly and relapsing neuropathy. Corneal opacities occur in one-third of patients, but not during childhood. Corneal clouding has been reported in a few children with **Apo A-I deficiency**. Other features of this condition are premature atherosclerosis and sometimes xanthomas.

COPPER TRANSPORT DISORDERS

Wilson disease usually presents either with liver disease at 5–20 years of age or with neurological problems, typically between 20–40 years, but sometimes during childhood. Hepatic manifestations include chronic active hepatitis, cirrhosis and

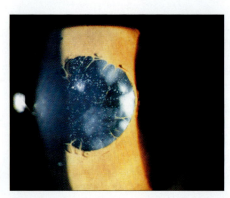

Fig. 65.23 Cataract in a girl with Conradi syndrome.

fulminant hepatic failure. Common neurological features are dystonia, dysarthria, dysphagia, tremor and Parkinsonism and psychiatric problems. Rarer problems include hemolysis, arthritis and Fanconi syndrome. Deposition of copper in peripheral Descemet's membrane leads to golden brown pigmentation: the Kayser–Fleischer ring (Fig. 65.24). Slit- lamp examination reveals these in 95% patients with neurological presentations but they are seldom present in asymptomatic patients and often absent in children presenting with liver disease.[95] Moreover, Kayser–Fleischer rings may occur with chronic cholestasis from other causes.

Wilson disease, an autosomal recessive disorder, is caused by deficiency of an ATPase that transports copper into the Golgi apparatus of hepatocytes.[96] From here, copper is normally excreted into the bile or incorporated into ceruloplasmin and secreted into plasma. In Wilson disease, impaired biliary copper excretion leads to its accumulation at toxic levels in hepatocytes and elsewhere. Plasma ceruloplasmin concentrations may be low. Plasma concentrations of non-ceruloplasmin-bound copper are raised. The diagnosis is confirmed by showing raised 24-hour urine copper excretion or a raised hepatic copper concentration. Treatment aims to remove excess copper from tissues (or to prevent its accumulation in presymptomatic patients). Penicillamine has been used to chelate copper for many years but side-effects are common. Alternative drugs include trientine, zinc and tetrathiomolybdate.

Menkes disease is an X-linked disorder. Affected boys usually present by 2–3 months of age with hypothermia, poor weight gain, seizures and hypotonia. Patients have "pudgy" cheeks, occipital bossing and sparse, brittle, white hair that becomes more obviously abnormal with time. Skeletal and connective tissue abnormalities are common, including osteoporosis and bladder diverticulae. Progressive visual loss is common, due to degeneration of retinal ganglion cells, neuronal loss and optic atrophy. In one series, 40% of patients had very poor visual acuity and more than half had strabismus and myopia.[97] Most patients with Menkes disease have blue irides and iris stromal hypoplasia is common. Patients deteriorate rapidly, with developmental regression, spasticity and lethargy, and most die by 3 years of age. Milder variants are seen in 5–10% of patients. In occipital-horn syndrome, for example, there are skeletal and connective tissue abnormalities but few neurological symptoms.

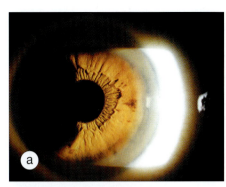

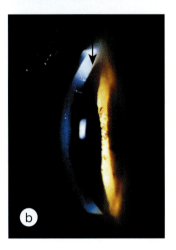

Fig. 65.24 (a) Kayser-Fleischer ring in a child with the neurological presentation of Wilson disease. A brownish haze can be seen in the peripheral cornea. (b) The K-F ring can be seen in the posterior cornea on slit-lamp examination (arrow).

Like Wilson disease, Menkes disease is caused by deficiency of a copper transporting ATPase in the Golgi apparatus. In Menkes disease, however, the ATPase transports copper across the placenta, the intestine and the blood–brain barrier. Symptoms are caused by deficiency of copper and consequently of enzymes that require copper (such as cytochrome oxidase). Serum copper and ceruloplasmin concentrations are low, but low levels can be seen in normal infants during the first few months. The diagnosis should, therefore, be confirmed by copper uptake studies in fibroblasts. Treatment with parenteral copper-histidine may help patients with mild variants and, with early intervention, possibly even those with classic Menkes disease.

REFERENCES

1. Fernandes J, Saudubray JM, van den Berghe G (eds). Inborn Metabolic Diseases. 3rd edn. Heidelberg: Springer-Verlag; 2000.
2. Scriver CR, Beaudet AL, Sly WS, et al. The Metabolic and Molecular Bases of Inherited Disease. 7th edn. New York: McGraw-Hill; 2001.
3. Mehta AB, Lewis S, Laverey C. Treatment of lysosomal storage disorders. BMJ 2003; 327: 463–4.
4. Yeager AM. Allogenic hematopoietic cell transplantation for inborn metabolic diseases. Ann Hematol 2002; 81: S16–9.
5. Butters TD, Mellor HR, Narita K, et al. Small-molecule therapeutics for the treatment of glycolipid lysosomal storage disorders. Phil Trans R Soc Lond B Biol Sci 2003; 358: 927–45.
6. Winchester B, Vellodi A, Young E. The molecular basis of lysosomal storage diseases and their treatment. Biochem Soc Trans 2000; 28: 150–4.
7. Nakai H, Byers MG, Shows TB. Mapping HEXA to 15q 23q24. Cytogenet Cell Genet 1987; 46: 667.
8. Fox MF, Du Toit DL, Warnich L, et al. Regional localization of alpha galactosidase (CLS) to Xpter-q22, hexosaminidase B (HEXB) to 5q31-qter, and arylsulfatase B (ARSB) to 5pter-q13. Cytogenet Cell Genet 1984; 38: 45–9.

9. Godel V, Blumenthal M, Goldman B, et al. Visual functions in Tay-Sachs disease patients following enzyme replacement therapy. Metab Ophthalmol 1978; 2: 27–32.
10. Honda Y, Sudo M. Electroretinogram and visually evoked cortical potential in Tay-Sachs disease; a report of two cases. J Pediatr Ophthalmol 1976; 13: 226–9.
11. Krivit W, Shapiro E, Kennedy W, et al. Treatment of late infantile metachromatic leucodystrophy by bone marrow transplantation. N Engl J Med 1990; 322: 28–32.
12. Krivit W, Shapiro EG, Peters C, et al. Hematopoietic stem-cell transplantation in globoid-cell leukodystrophy. N Engl J Med 1998; 338: 1119–26.
13. Walton DS, Robb RM, Crocker AC. Ocular manifestations of group A Niemann-Pick disease. Am J Ophthalmol 1978; 85: 174–80.
14. Filling-Katz MR, Fink JK, Gorin MB, et al. Metab Pediatr Syst Ophthalmol 1992; 15: 16–20.
15. Vellodi A, Hobbs JR, O'Donnell NM, et al. Treatment of Niemann-Pick disease type B by allogenic bone marrow transplantation. BMJ 1987; 295: 1375–6.
16. Vanier MJ, Pentchev P, Rodriguez-Lafrasse C, et al. Niemann-Pick disease type C: an update. J Inherit Metab Dis 1991; 14: 580–95.

17. Butler JD, Comly ME, Kruth H, et al. Niemann-Pick variant disorders: comparison of errors of cellular cholesterol homeostasis in group D and C fibroblasts. Proc Natl Acad Sci USA 1987; 84: 556–60.

18. Imrie J, Wraith JE. Isolated splenomegaly as the presenting feature of Niemann-Pick disease type C. Arch Dis Child 2001; 84: 427–9.

19. Neville BC, Lake BD, Stevens R, et al. A neurovisceral storage disease with vertical supranuclear ophthalmoplegia and its relationship to Niemann-Pick disease–a report of nine patients. Brain 1973; 96: 97–120.

20. Rottach KG, von Maydell RD, Das VE, et al. Evidence for independent feedback control of horizontal and vertical saccades from Niemann-Pick type C disease. Vision Res 1997; 37: 3627–38.

21. Palmer M, Green WR, Maumenee IH, et al. Niemann-Pick disease – type C. Ocular histopathologic and electron microscopic studies. Arch Ophthalmol 1985; 103: 817–22.

22. Harris CM, Taylor DS, Vellodi A. Ocular motor abnormalities in Gaucher disease. Neuropediatrics 1999; 30: 289–93.

23. Murphree AL, Beaudet AL, Palmer EA, et al. Cataract in mannosidosis. Birth Defects Orig Artic Ser 1976; 12: 319–25.

24. Dietmann JL, Filipi de la Palavesa MM, Trauchant C, et al. MR findings in mannosidosis. Neuroradiology 1990; 32: 485–7.

25. Libert J, Toussaint D. Tortuosities of retinal and conjunctival vessels in lysosomal storage disorders. Birth Defects Orig Artic Ser 1982; 18: 347–58.

26. Snodgrass M. Ocular findings in fucosidosis. Br J Ophthalmol 1976; 60: 508–13.

27. Snyder RO, Carlow TJ, Ledman J, et al. Ocular findings in fucosidosis. Birth Defects 1976; 12: 241–6.

28. Thomas PK, Abrams JD, Swallow D, et al. Sialidosis type I: cherry-red spot myoclonus syndrome with sialidase deficiency and altered electrophoretic mobilities of some enzymes known to be glycoproteins. J Neurol Neurosurg Psychiatry 1979; 42: 873–80.

29. Goldberg MF, Cotlier E, Fichenscher LG, et al. Macular cherry-red spot, corneal clouding and beta galactosidase deficiency. Arch Int Med 1971; 138: 387–9.

30. Usui T, Shirakashi M, Takagi M, et al. Macular edema-like change and pseudopapilloedema in a case of Scheie syndrome. J Clin Neuro-ophthalmol 1991; 11: 183–5.

31. Alroy J, Haskins M, Birk DE. Altered corneal stromal matrix organization is associated with mucopolysaccharidosis I, III and VI. Exp Eye Res 1999; 68: 523–30.

32. Orgül S, Daiker B, Kain H-L. Simultane Hornhaut transplantation bei mucopolysaccharidose. Klin Mbl Augenheilkd 1991; 198: 430–2.

33. Gullingsrud EO, Krivit W, Summers CG. Ocular abnormalities in the mucopolysaccharidoses after bone marrow transplantation. Longer follow-up. Ophthalmology 1998; 105: 1099–105.

34. Collins M, Traboulsi E, Maumenee I. Optic nerve head swelling and optic atrophy in the systemic mucopolysaccharidoses. Ophthalmology 1990; 97: 1445–50.

35. Cahane M, Treister G, Abraham F, et al. Glaucoma in siblings with Morquio syndrome. Br J Ophthalmol 1990; 74: 382–4.

36. Iwamoto M, Nawa Y, Maumenee IH, et al. Ocular histopathology and ultrastructure of Morquio syndrome (systemic mucopolysaccharidosis IV). Graefe's Arch Clin Exp Ophthalmol 1990; 228: 342–9.

37. Wraith JE. The mucopolysaccharidoses: a clinical review and guide to management. Arch Dis Child 1995; 72: 263–7.

38. Walker RW, Darowski M, Morris P, et al. Anaesthesia and mucopolysaccharidoses. A review of airway problems in children. Anaesthesia 1994; 49: 1078–84.

39. Vellodi A, Young EP, Cooper A, et al. Bone marrow transplantation for mucopolysaccharidosis type I: experience of two British centers. Arch Dis Child 1997; 76: 92–9.

40. Wraith JE. Enzyme replacement therapy in mucopolysaccharidosis type I: progress and emerging difficulties. J Inherit Metab Dis 2001; 24: 245–50.

41. Casteels I, Taylor DS, Lake BD, et al. Mucolipidosis IV: presentation of a mild variant. Ophthalmol Paediatr Genet 1992; 13: 205–10.

42. Smith JA, Chan CC, Goldin E, et al. Noninvasive diagnosis and ophthalmic features of mucolipidosis type IV. Ophthalmology 2002; 109: 588–94.

43. Dangel ME, Bremer DL, Rogers GL. Treatment of corneal opacification in mucolipidosis IV with conjunctival transplantation. Am J Ophthalmol 1985; 99: 137–42.

44. Newman NJ, Starck T, Kenyon K, et al. Corneal surface irregularities and episodic pain in a patient with mucolipidosis IV. Arch Ophthalmol 1990; 108: 251–4.

45. Lake BD, Milla PJ, Taylor DS, et al. A mild variant of ML4. Birth Defects Orig Article Serv 1982; 18: 391–404.

46. Desnick RJ, Brady R, Barranger J, et al. Fabry disease, an under-recognised multisystemic disorder: expert recommendations for diagnosis, management, and enzyme replacement therapy. Ann Intern Med 2003; 138: 338–46.

47. Sher NA, Letson RD, Desnick RJ. The ocular manifestations in Fabry's disease. Arch Ophthalmol 1979; 97: 671–6.

48. Sher NA, Reiff W, Letson RD, et al. Central retinal artery occlusion complicating Fabry's disease. Arch Ophthalmol 1978; 96: 815–7.

49. Pampliglione G, Harden A. So-called neuronal ceroid lipofuscinosis. Neurophysiological studies in 60 children. J Neurol Neurosurg Psychiatry 1977; 40: 323–30.

50. Cooper JD. Progress towards understanding the neurobiology of Batten disease or neuronal ceroid lipofuscinosis. Curr Opin Neurol 2003; 16: 121–8.

51. Spalton DJ, Taylor DS, Sanders MD. Juvenile Batten's disease: an ophthalmological assessment of 26 patients. Br J Ophthalmol 1980; 64: 726–32.

52. Hussain AA, Marshall J. Nosological significance of retinopathies in neurodegenerative disorders with emphasis on Batten disease. J Inherit Metab Dis 1993; 16: 267–71.

53. Pinckers A, Bolmers D. Neuronal ceroid lipofuscinosis. Ann Ocul 1974; 207: 523–9.

54. De Venecia G, Shapiro M. Neuronal ceroid lipofuscinosis – a retinal trypsin digest study. Ophthalmology 1984; 91: 1406–10.

55. Westmoreland BF, Groover RV, Sharbrough FW. Electrographic findings in three types of cerebromacular degeneration. Mayo Clin Proc 1979; 54: 12–21.

56. Raininko R, Santavuori P, Heiskala H, et al. CT findings in neuronal ceroid-lipofuscinosis. Neuropediatrics 1990; 21: 95–101.

57. Valavanis A, Friede RL, Schubiger O, et al. Computed tomography in neuronal ceroid lipofuscinosis. Neuroradiology 1980; 19: 35–8.

58. Good W, Crain LS, Quint RD, et al. Overlooking: a sign of bilateral central scotomata in children. Dev Med Child Neurol 1992; 34: 69–73.

59. Lake BD. The differential diagnosis of the various forms of Batten's disease by rectal biopsy. Birth Defects Orig Artic Serv 1976; 12: 455–64.

60. Brod RD, Packer AJ, Van Dyk JL. Diagnosis of neuronal ceroid lipofuscinosis by ultrastructural examination of peripheral blood lymphocytes. Arch Ophthalmol 1987; 105: 1388–93.

61. Bensaoula T, Shibuya H, Katz ML, et al. Histopathologic and immunocytochemical analysis of the retinal and ocular tissues in Batten disease. Ophthalmology 2000; 107: 1746–53.

62. Deeg HJ, Shulman HM, Albrechtsen D, et al. Batten's disease: failure of allogenic bone marrow transplantation to arrest disease progression in a canine model. Clin Genet 1990; 37: 264–70.

63. Gardiner M, Sandford A, Deadman M, et al. Batten disease (Spielemeyer-Vogt disease, juvenile onset neuronal ceroid-lipofuscinosis) gene (CLN3) maps to human chromosome 16. Genomics 1990; 8: 387–90.

64. Mitchison HM, Williams RE, McKay TR, et al. Redefined genetic mapping of juvenile onset neuronal ceroid lipofuscinosis on chromosome 16. J Inherit Metab Dis 1993; 16: 339–41.

65. Pearson H, Lobel J, Kocoshis S, et al. A new syndrome of refractory sideroblastic anaemia with vacuolization of marrow precursors and exocrine pancreatic dysfunction. J Pediatr 1979; 95: 976–84.

66. Petty RK, Harding AE, Morgan-Hughes JA. The clinical features of mitochondrial myopathy. Brain 1986; 109: 915–38.

67. Spelbrink JN, Li F-Y, Tiranti V, et al. Human mitochondrial DNA deletions associated with mutations in the gene encoding Twinkle, a phage T7 gene 4-like protein localized in mitochondria. Nat Genet 2001; 28: 223–31.

68. Ciafaloni E, Ricci E, Shanske S, et al. MELAS: clinical features, biochemistry, and molecular genetics. Ann Neurol 1992; 31: 391–8.

69. Cavanagh JB, Harding BN. Pathogenic factors underlying the lesions in Leigh disease. Brain 1994; 117: 1357–76.

70. Rahman S, Blok RB, Dahl H-HM, et al. Leigh syndrome: clinical features and biochemical and DNA abnormalities. Ann Neurol 1996; 39: 343–51.

71. Harding BN. Progressive neuronal degeneration of childhood with liver disease (Alpers-Huttenlocher syndrome); a personal review. J Child Neurol 1990; 5: 273–87.

72. Cruysberg JR, Sengers R, Pinckers A, et al. Features of a syndrome with congenital cataracts and hypertrophic cardiomyopathy. Am J Ophthalmol 1986; 102: 740–9.

73. Harding AE. Friedrich's ataxia: a clinical and genetic study of 90 families with an analysis of early diagnostic criteria and intrafamilial clustering of clinical features. Brain 1981; 104: 589–620.

74. Ianchulev T, Kolin T, Moseley K, et al. Optic nerve atrophy in propionic acidaemia. Ophthalmology 2003; 110: 1850–4.

75. Raas-Rothschild A, Wanders RJ, Mooijer PA, et al. A PEX6-defective peroxisomal biogenesis disorder with severe phenotype in an infant, versus mild phenotype resembling Usher syndrome in the affected parents. Am J Hum Genet 2002; 70: 1062–8.

76. Cohen SM, Green WR, de la Cruz C, et al. Ocular histopathologic studies of neonatal and childhood adrenoleucodystrophy. Am J Ophthalmol 1983; 95: 82–96.

77. Martinez M, Vazquez E. MRI evidence that docosahexaenoic acid ethyl ester improves myelination in generalized peroxisomal disorders. Neurology 1998; 51: 26–32.

78. Moser HW, Naidu S, Kumar AJ, et al. The adrenoleukodystrophies. Crit Rev Neurobiol 1987; 3: 29–88.

79. Shapiro EK, Lockman L, Jambaque I, et al. Long-term beneficial effect of bone marrow transplantation for childhood onset cerebral X-linked adrenleukodystrophy. Lancet 2000; 356: 713.

80. Jaeken J. Komrower Lecture. Congenital disorders of glycosylation (CDG): it's all in it! J Inherit Metab Dis 2003; 26: 99–118.

81. Jensen H, Kjaergaard S, Klie F, et al. Ophthalmic manifestations of congenital disorder of glycosylation type 1a. Ophthalmic Genet 2003; 24: 81–8.

82. Beltran-Valero de Bernabe D, Currier S, Steinbrecher A, et al. Mutations in the O-mannosyltransferase gene POMT1 give rise to the severe neuronal migration disorder Walker-Warburg syndrome. Am J Hum Genet 2002; 71: 1033–43.

83. Irreverre F, Mudd SH, Heizer WD, et al. Sulphite oxidase deficiency: studies on a patient with mental retardation, dislocated ocular lenses, and abnormal excretion of S-sulfo-L-cysteine, sulfite and thiosulfate. Biochem Med 1967; 1: 187.

84. Gupta B, Waggoner D. Ophthalmoplegia in maple syrup urine disease. J AAPOS 2003; 7: 300–2.

85. Zee DS, Freeman JM, Holtzmann NA. Ophthalmoplegia in maple syrup urine disease. J Pediatr 1974; 84: 113–5.

86. al-Hemidan AI, al-Hazzaa SA. Richner-Hanhart syndrome (tyrosinemia type II). Case report and literature review. Ophthalmic Genet 1995; 16: 21–6.

87. Hyland K, Surtees RA, Rodeck C, et al. Aromatic L-amino acid decarboxylase deficiency: clinical features, diagnosis, and treatment of a new inborn error of neurotransmitter amine synthesis. Neurology 1992; 42: 1980–8.

88. Ungar M, Goodman RM. Spongy degeneration of the brain in Israel: a retrospective study. Clin Genet 1983; 23: 23–9.

89. Ryan AK, Bartlett K, Clayton P, et al. Smith-Lemli-Opitz syndrome: a variable clinical and biochemical phenotype. J Med Genet 1998; 35: 558–65.

90. Hoffmann GF, Charpentier C, Mayatepek E, et al. Clinical and biochemical phenotype in 11 patients with mevalonic aciduria. Pediatrics 1993; 91: 915–21.

91. Happle R. X-linked dominant chrondrodysplasia punctata. Review of literature and report of a case. Hum Genet 1979; 53: 65–73.

92. Cruysberg JR, Wevers RA, van Engelen BG, et al. Ocular and systemic manifestations of cerebrotendinous xanthomatosis. Am J Ophthalmol 1995; 120: 597–604.

93. Costagliola C, Fabbrocini G, Illiano GM, et al. Ocular findings in X-linked ichthyosis: a survey on 38 cases. Ophthalmologica 1991; 202: 152–5.

94. Bron AJ, Lloyd JK, Fosbrooke AS, et al. Primary L.C.A.T. – deficiency disease. Lancet 1975; 1: 928–9.

95. Steindl P, Ferenci P, Dienes HP, et al. Wilson's disease in patients presenting with liver disease: a diagnostic challenge. Gastroenterology 1997; 113: 212–8.

96. Bull PC, Thomas GR, Rommens JM, et al. The Wilson disease gene is a putative copper transporting P-type ATPase similar to the Menkes gene. Nat Genet 1993; 5: 327–37.

97. Gasch AT, Caruso RC, Kaler SG, et al. Menkes' syndrome. Ophthalmic findings. Ophthalmology 2002; 109: 1477–83.

Developmental Dyslexia (Specific Reading Difficulty)

CHAPTER **66**

Frank J Martin

INTRODUCTION

"Reading difficulty" is a generic term for specific reading difficulty, developmental dyslexia, and dyslexia. The terms are frequently interchanged in the literature but "developmental dyslexia" best describes the condition. It can be defined as "a difficulty in reading in children and adults at the level that would be expected with their home background, educational opportunities, motivation, and intelligence." It is a complex problem with no simple solution, and frequently a problem for which the eyes or the visual system is blamed. This misunderstanding has led to myths as to the etiology of the condition and to controversial therapies (Table 66.1).

HISTORICAL BACKGROUND

A general practitioner, Pringle Morgan, first studied developmental dyslexia in 1896 in England. He reported of a case of "congenital word blindness," describing an intelligent fourteen-year-old boy who was severely disabled in reading despite years of individual and classroom instruction. He could read all the letters of the alphabet as well as a few simple common words but could not blend letter sounds and had no appreciation of spelling patterns. He could solve written problems in algebra, and had normal eyes and no visual problem or visual field defect. Morgan concluded that the boy was word blind but not letter blind. On the basis of evidence that pure word blindness after a stroke in adults was produced by a lesion in the angular gyrus, he inferred that the boy's disability was evidently congenital and due, probably, to a similar anatomical defect.

Following the publication of Morgan's paper, the Glasgow ophthalmologist James Hinshelwood postulated that developmental dyslexia was a specific form of aphasia, dismissing the possibility that congenital word blindness was due to any form of visual impairment: he made normal vision a diagnostic criterion.

In 1925 Samuel Orton reported that developmental dyslexia was due to a problem in the visual system. He suggested that an apparent dysfunction in visual perception and visual memory, characterized by perception of letters and words in reverse, causes developmental dyslexia (thus explaining mirror writing). He suggested that the disorder was caused by maturation lag, the consequence of failure of one or other hemisphere of the brain to dominate the development of language.

Between 1930 and 1970 many studies often using unsuitable subjects took place in an attempt to unravel the role of visual and visual motor factors. Many of the findings could not be replicated. Then the focus changed, as the anatomic and physiological basis of the disorder was studied. Research showed that children with developmental dyslexia have a disorder related to the language system, in particular a deficiency in the processing of the distinctive linguistic units called phonemes that make up all spoken and written words.

Linguistic models of reading and developmental dyslexia now provide an explanation as to why some very intelligent people have trouble learning to read and performing other language-related tasks.

EPIDEMIOLOGY[1]

Developmental dyslexia affects 5 to 10% of school populations, although in some unselected population-based studies up to 17.5% of children have been affected. It was believed that developmental dyslexia affected males more than females but recent data indicate similar numbers of affected boys and girls. Boys are probably more easily recognized, as they frequently become disruptive in the classroom due to their frustration in coping with their reading difficulty. Longitudinal studies have shown that dyslexia is a persistent, chronic condition. Over time, readers tend to maintain their relative positions along the spectrum of reading ability (Fig. 66.1). Treatment helps improve the reading ability of children with development dyslexia but can never bring them up to the standard of a normal reader.[2]

PRESENTATION

The child with developmental dyslexia is likely at some stage to present to an ophthalmologist in the belief that a problem in the visual system is the underlying basis of the child's reading difficulty. Such children, despite being above normal intelligence, may have had difficulties with writing letters and recognizing words since beginning school. They may show poor concentration in the classroom and, particularly if they are boys, tend to be disruptive. Their writing may be untidy, their spelling poor, and they may have fallen significantly behind in reading by the time they are seven or eight.

Intervention such as stress-relieving glasses and vision training exercises may have been tried, to no avail. Speech pathologists and

Table 66.1 Key points relating to developmental dyslexia

Due to a linguistic defect and not to a visual problem
Not related to intelligence
Boys and girls have equal prevalence
Early diagnosis followed by appropriate remedial intervention is the only scientifically proven therapy
Persists into adulthood but most children are able to be taught to read accurately even though they tend to read more slowly and not automatically
Therapies not based on a linguistic process remain controversial

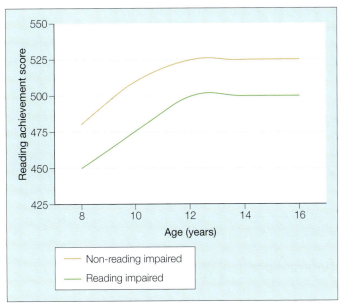

Fig. 66.1 The gap in reading ability between children with developmental dyslexia and nonimpaired readers persists with age. Trajectory of reading skills over time in nonimpaired readers and readers with developmental dyslexia shows reading to improve with age. The gap between the two groups persists. (From Overcoming Dyslexia by Sally Shaywitz MD. Copyright © by Sally Shaywitz MD. Adapted with permission of Alfred A. Knopf, a division of Random House, Inc.)

occupational therapist may also have been consulted. In some instances, if the child continues to be disruptive, they may have been diagnosed as having attention deficit disorder. Despite taking medication, their reading skills may not improve. Their now-desperate parents may search the Internet and find expensive "quick fix solutions" to their child's problem such as tinted lenses or vision training.

The reading difficulties usually continue. In some instances, it will take an ophthalmological opinion to exclude an ocular problem and suspect developmental dyslexia. Referral to an educational psychologist for diagnosis and institution of appropriate remedial intervention is the preferred course.

MYTHS AND REALITY

In order to be able to guide children with developmental dyslexia in the right direction it is important for the ophthalmologist to have a sound understanding of the process of reading.

The ophthalmologist must also be able to dispel the myths that reading difficulties result from:

Defects in visual perception and visual memory;

Visual and ocular defects; and

Eye movement disorders.

The ophthalmologist needs to communicate to parents and to other health and education professionals that the defect lies within the brain and its processing of visual stimuli.

READING

Reading is the process of extracting meaning from print. This involves both visual/perceptual and linguistic processes. There is now a strong consensus that the central difficulty in developmental dyslexia reflects a deficiency within a specific component of the language system, the phonological module, which is engaged in processing the sounds of speech.

Phonological deficit hypothesis[1]

According to the phonological deficit hypothesis, people with developmental dyslexia have difficulty developing an awareness that words, both written and spoken, can be broken down into smaller units of sound and that the letters constituting the printed word represent the sounds heard in the spoken word.

The phoneme is the smallest meaningful segment of language. Different combinations of forty-four phonemes produce every word in the English language; e.g., the word "cat" is broken down into "kuh," "aah," and "tuh." The phonological module automatically assembles phonemes into words.

The language system can be conceptualized as a hierarchical series of components. At the higher levels are neural systems engaged in processing, e.g., semantics (vocabulary or word meaning), syntax (grammatical structure), and discourse (connected sentences). At the lower level is the phonological module that processes the distinctive sound elements that constitute language. To speak a word such as "cat" the speaker retrieves the word's phonemic constituents from the lexicon, and assembles the phonemes. Conversely to read the word "cat" the reader must first segment the word into its underlying phonological elements.

Phonetic reading involves the decoding of the sounds and letters. An inexperienced reader will have to sound out most words and consequently will read rather slowly. Experienced readers quickly recognize most of them as individual units. In other words, during reading, phonetic and whole word reading are engaged in a race. If the word is familiar, the whole reading method will win. If the word is unfamiliar, the whole word method will fail and the phonetic method will take over. Readers spend more time fixating on unusual and longer words.

Psycholinguistic aspects

Children with developmental dyslexia have an impaired ability to segment the written word into its underlying phonological components.[3] Thereby, the access to higher audio-linguistic processes is blocked. As a result, the reader experiences difficulty first in decoding the word and then in identifying it. The phonological deficit is independent of other nonphonologic abilities. In particular, the higher order cognitive and linguistic functions involving comprehension such as general intelligence and reasoning, vocabulary, and syntax are generally intact. This pattern, the deficit of phonologic analysis, contrasted with intact higher order cognitive abilities offers an explanation for the paradox that otherwise intelligent people experience great difficulty in reading.

Reversal of letters is very common in children learning to read and may represent a transitional stage in the reading process. In tests of decoding from left to right and from right to left, normal readers and dyslexics have shown the same performance.

Decoding is a fundamental function of reading and can be made through two separate routes, either phonologically or orthographically.[4] The former is used when reading unknown but regularly spelt words and the latter for irregularly spelt words such as abbreviations. The proficient reader has access to both mechanisms, which probably are used together. Dyslexics may have problems that are larger with one route than the other. It is possible that individuals with orthographic dyslexia have greater problems with visual perception than those with phonological dyslexia.

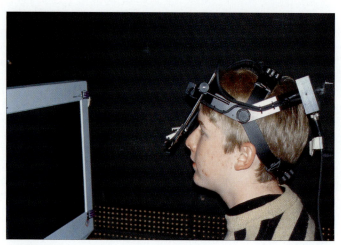

Fig. 66.2 The eye tracker. This device consists of a video camera that tracks the gaze of a person reading by monitoring the position of their pupil.

Eye movements and reading

Eye movements and reading have been studied using an eye tracker (Fig. 66.2), which consists of a video camera that tracks the gaze of a reading person by monitoring the position of their pupil.

When we read we do not move our eyes in a smooth swooping motion across the line of text. Rather, we make a series of short movements called saccades. In saccades, our eyes jump about 6 to 8 character spaces. These last about 20 to 40 ms and virtually no visual information is extracted from the text while the eyes are actually moving. Instead, the saccade brings a new region of the text into central vision for detailed processing. Saccades are separated by short periods of time in which the eyes remain relatively still in what are called fixations. It is during the time that eyes are fixated that new information is acquired for processing. Each fixation lasts approximately 200 to 250 ms. About 10 to 20% of saccades are made from right to left, that is, we move our eyes backward or make regressions in the text, look again at information that has previously been read.

Pavlidis[5] thought that eye movement disorders were the basis of developmental dyslexia, but his work could not be reproduced.[6,7]

Children with developmental dyslexia have shorter forward saccades, longer fixation pauses, and an increased number of regressions, representing their inability to understand the text. The eye movements in developmental dyslexia are similar to that of children beginning to learn to read. It is therefore likely that the difficulties children with developmental dyslexia have in maintaining the proper direction of reading eye movement is a symptom of the reading disorder rather than the cause of the disorder.[4]

NEUROBIOLOGIC EVIDENCE[8]

There is considerable neurobiologic evidence including studies relating to inheritability that developmental dyslexia is not due to visual or ocular defects. A review of this evidence strongly supports the view that developmental dyslexia is due to brain dysfunction.

A range of neurobiologic investigations using postmortem brain specimens, brain morphometry, functional brain magnetic resonance imaging, and electrophysiology suggests that there are differences in the temporoparieto–occipital brain regions between

people with developmental dyslexia and those who are not reading impaired. Some studies suggest differences in the striate or extrastriate cortex, findings that coincide with those in a large body of literature describing anatomical lesions and posterior brain lesions in acquired alexia most prominently in the angular gyrus.

Inheritability

Developmental dyslexia is familial and inheritable.[9] Family history was one of the most important risk factors, with from 23 to 65% of children with a dyslexic parent having the disorder. About 40% of siblings and 27 to 49% of parents of affected children are affected themselves. This allows for early identification of affected siblings. Linkage studies have implicated loci on chromosomes 5 and 15[10] and more recently chromosomes 1 and 2[11] in individuals with reading difficulties.

Neuroanatomical changes

Two different anomalies have been shown in the language-related areas of the brain.[12] The first was the absence of the normal asymmetry between left and right hemispheres: normally, the left planum temporale is the larger but in the dyslexic this asymmetry may be absent or reversed.

The second brain anomaly is the occurrence of a relatively large number of ectopies in the dyslexic,[13] which originate from misdirected migration of neurones during embryonal brain development.

However, differences in the anatomical definitions used and lack of control of other variables such as brain weight, sex, or handedness make it difficult to draw any firm conclusions.[14]

Differences on functional neuroimaging[15]

Several studies have shown differences in spatial and temporal brain activation between normal and dyslexic readers when reading various test materials. This has been best shown with functional magnetic resonance imaging (fMRI) of the brain, which allows for the examination of the brain during the performance of a cognitive task. During the cognitive task there is activation of neural systems in specific brain regions. The neural activity is reflected by changes in brain metabolic activity. Functional MRI maps the brain's response to the specific cognitive task.

A number of neuroimaging studies suggest that fluent word identification reading is related to the functional integrity of two consolidated left hemisphere posterior systems: a dorsal (temporoparietal) circuit and a ventral (occipitotemporal) circuit. This posterior system is functionally disrupted in developmental dyslexia. Reading disabled readers, compared to nonimpaired readers, demonstrate heightened reliance on the left inferior frontal gyrus and right hemisphere portion regions, presumably in compensation for the left hemisphere posterior difficulties (Fig. 66.3). It has been proposed that for normally developing readers the dorsal circuit predominates at first, and is associated with analytical processing necessary for learning to integrate orthographic features with phonological and lexical-semantic features of printed words. The ventral circuit constitutes a fast, late-developing, word identification system that underlines fluent word recognition in skilled readers. The anterior sites are critical in articulation of words and help the child with developmental dyslexia to develop an awareness of sound structures.

Dyslexia-specific brain activation profile has been shown to become normal following successful remedial training.[16] Before

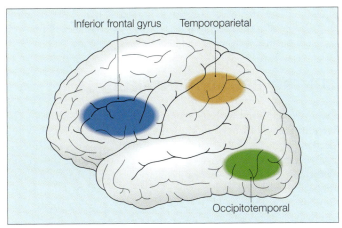

Fig. 66.3 Neural systems used for reading. The three important systems used for reading are in the left hemisphere: (i) Anterior system in the left inferior frontal region; (ii) dorsal temporoparietal system involving the angular gyrus, supramarginal gyrus, and posterior portions of the superior temporal gyrus; (iii) ventral occipitotemporal system involving portions of the middle temporal gyrus and middle occipital gyrus. (Adapted with permission from Shaywitz and Shaywitz.[8])

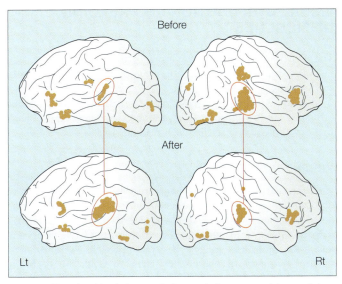

Fig. 66.5 Functional brain images before and after successful remedial treatment. After intervention there is a dramatic increase in the activation of the left temporoparietal region (predominately the posterior portion of the superior temporal gyrus). The profile is similar to that observed in children without reading problems. (Adapted from Simos et al.[16] and reprinted with permission.)

intervention, children with dyslexia showed distinctly aberrant activation profiles featuring little or no activation of the posterior portion of the superior temporoparietal gyrus and increased activation of the corresponding right hemisphere area. After intervention that produced significant improvement in reading skills, activation in the left superior temporoparietal gyrus increased by several orders of magnitude in every participant (Fig. 66.4 and Fig. 66.5).

Electrophysiological changes

Electrophysiological correlates have been examined with brain electrical activity mapping (BEAM) during tests of language and

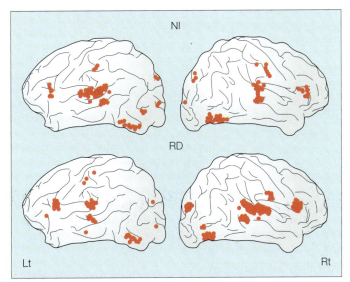

Fig. 66.4 Functional brain imaging. The difference in brain imaging of a normal reader (NI) compared to a reader with developmental dyslexia (RD) is shown. There is a difference in activity in the inferior frontal gyrus, the posterior portion of the superior temporoparietal gyrus, and the corresponding right hemisphere (Adapted from Simos et al.[16] and reprinted with permission.)

nonlanguage functions.[17] Larger differences between dyslexics and normals were seen in the language areas of the parietal and temporal lobes, but they were also found in the frontal regions, which are active in the planning and sequential transformation of different behavioral tasks including reading.

Defects of the magnocellular (or transient) system[18]

The magnocellular deficit theory of developmental dyslexia was originally known as a transient system deficit theory. The visual system is divided into two largely parallel streams: the magnocellular and parvocellular systems. The parvocellular system mediates color vision and the perception of fine spatial details. The magnocellular system responds to rapid changes in visual stimulation such as gross cause by moving stimuli. The magnocellular deficit theory of developmental dyslexia postulated that the magnocellular system suppresses the parvocellular system at the time of each saccade. This suppression, it was thought, caused the activity in the parvocellular system to terminate so as to prevent activity elicited during one fixation from lingering into that from the next fixation. Without this suppression the parvocellular activity from different fixations would be confused. In children with developmental dyslexia it was thought that this suppressive effect was diminished or absent and that the developmental dyslexia was the result of a failure to keep separate neural activity elicited during different fixations. Most of the evidence sighted in support of the magnocellular theory was from contrast sensitivity studies.

The evidence in support of the magnocellular theory is equivocal. In the case of spatial contrast sensitivity there clearly are results consistent with the magnocellular deficit theory. These studies are outnumbered by studies that have found no loss of sensitivity and studies that have found contrast sensitivity reductions inconsistent with a magnocellular deficit. The evidence from studies from contrast sensitivity is highly conflicting with regard to the magnocellular system deficit theory of developmental dyslexia.

VISUAL DYSFUNCTION AND READING DIFFICULTIES[19,20]

There may be many different levels of dysfunction with vision ranging from a problem with the eyes to that with binocularity and/or within the visual cortex.

To consider whether visual dysfunction is related to reading difficulties, it is important to review the specific visual problems that could possibly interfere with reading.

Visual impairment

Children with even severe visual impairment resulting from defects such as bilateral aphakia following cataract surgery, optic nerve hypoplasia, or retinal dystrophy are all able to learn to read using assistance from spectacle correction for refractive errors and low-vision appliances. In general, ocular disease does not seem to affect the ability of children to learn to read. Furthermore, children who are blind are able to learn to read using Braille.

Abnormal eye movements

Children with very abnormal eye movements such as those with congenital motor nystagmus, Duane's syndrome, and Möbius syndrome all have the ability to learn to read fluently. Developmental dyslexia is no more frequent in these children than in the general population.

Refractive errors

Refractive errors have been blamed for developmental dyslexia. The refraction in childhood is usually hyperopic with an average of about 2 diopters in the first five years and gradually decreasing into adolescence. There is no evidence to show that children with high myopia, hyperopia, or astigmatism have any greater difficulty in learning to read than other children.

Binocular vision/accommodation-convergence

Several studies have investigated the connection between reading ability and the binocular and accommodative status of unselected children. True orthophoria occurs very rarely and most people demonstrate a small degree of heterophoria. There is a link between developmental dyslexia and convergence insufficiency and accommodative dysfunction and may be correlated with exophoria at near, low fusional reserve and poor stereopsis. Rather than developmental dyslexia being the result of these problems, it is more likely that these defects interfere with the child's ability to concentrate on print for a prolonged period of time. Following treatment the child with developmental dyslexia is more responsive to appropriate remedial educational therapy.

Studies related to visuospatial dysfunction in dyslexia have implicated more subtle abnormalities of binocular coordination as a contributing factor to the reading problem. Many children with developmental dyslexia describe that the text seems to be moving around, letters jumping and changing places, but there is no unequivocal evidence of beneficial effect of monocular reading and orthoptic exercises on reading ability in developmental dyslexia and little evidence to indicate that strabismus interferes with reading ability.

The most likely scenario is that visual problems coexist with developmental dyslexia. No relationship between visual function and academic performance related to reading ability has been shown.[21] The treatment of visual problems may lead to some improvement in the reading ability of the child with developmental dyslexia but it is extremely unlikely to lead to a cure.

CONTROVERSIAL THERAPIES[22]

Parents of children with developmental dyslexia are often on the lookout for any form of therapy that will "cure" or "correct" the problem quickly. A treatment approach can be considered controversial if the approach is proposed to the public before any research is available or preliminary research has not been replicated; the proposed approach goes beyond what research data support; or the approach is used in isolation when a multimodal approach is needed.

Vision training

Optometric vision training is based on the premise that reading is primarily a visual task. Optometric vision training is proposed to change specific visual function, such as convergence, accommodation, ocular motility, and the range and quality of binocular function. The optometric literature stresses that optometrists do not treat learning difficulties directly, rather, learning disabled children who clinically manifest some type of visual dysfunction. Vision training was popularized by AM Skeffington, regarded as the father of behavioral or developmental optometry, and involves eye muscle exercises, ocular pursuit, and tracking exercises. Training glasses incorporating low plus (+1.00 D) lenses with or without bifocals or prisms are frequently used in conjunction with vision training, as is patterning (Doman and Delacato).

The underlying concept of the Doman and Delacato program is that failure to pass properly through a certain sequence of developmental stages in mobility, language, and competence in the manual, visual, auditory, and tactile areas reflects poor "neurological organization" and may indicate "brain damage." Proposed treatments involve repetitive activities using specific muscle patterns in the order the child should have learnt if development had been normal, e.g., rolling over, sitting, crawling, standing, and walking.

Children with developmental dyslexia frequently are referred to individuals offering vision training combined with neurological organizational training. It is expensive and time consuming, and it is difficult to envisage how patterning is likely to help a child with developmental dyslexia.

Low plus lenses and large print for children who are hyperopic may be of some apparent benefit in that print is slightly enlarged and clearer, but remember that 2 diopters of hyperopia is normal in children up to the age of five years.

Evidence does not support the claim that vision training improves reading.[23] Although ophthalmologists and behavioral optometrists disagree on the value of vision training, there is agreement that if a child has developmental dyslexia it is critical to rule out the presence of any refractive errors, problems with convergence and accommodation, and strabismus and to treat these appropriately.

Applied kinesiology

This is based on the work of Dr Carl A Ferreri, who was under the impression that the displacement of the sphenoid and temporal bones interfered with the so-called "cloacal reflex" and led to "ocular lock." He reported that children with developmental dyslexia respond positively to one to three chiropractic treatments, although he did concede that many children who showed improvement were also receiving remedial intervention.

Parents and professionals should be aware that this form of chiropractic treatment for developmental dyslexia is not based on any known research. Some of the views are based on anatomic and functional concepts not held by the majority of anatomists and that there is no supporting independent research.

Vestibular dysfunction

The claim that there is a cause or relationship between vestibular disorders and poor academic performance involving reading and written language in children with learning disabilities was made by Frank and Levinson. They recommended that such children require specialized therapy before they can benefit from academic input and proposed antimotion sickness medication to correct the vestibular dysfunction as part of the treatment of developmental dyslexia. No evidence supports either. In more recent publications they have suggested there is also a need for special education.

Syntonics

Color vision therapy, known as syntonics, has been used to treat several conditions including myopia, strabismus, amblyopia, headache, visual fatigue, reading problems, and general binocular dysfunction. The published data do not provide convincing support for the claims of therapeutic success for reading disability with the use of syntonics.[24]

Irlen tinted lenses–scotopic sensitivity syndrome

This syndrome was described by Helen Irlen in 1983, who claimed instantaneous improvement in reading performance, comprehension, and distance judgment in children using tinted glasses. In its original form the sufferers from scotopic sensitivity syndrome were diagnosed by a set of questions constituting the Irlen differential perceptional schedule test and treated with colored lenses specific to each individual. No scientific evidence supports the syndrome's existence.

Although scotopic sensitivity syndrome may not exist, colored filters or overlays as a treatment of developmental dyslexia has persisted. Some good studies support it but there is poor test–retest consistency of color selected, and subjects frequently do not persist with the use of the lenses. There is no evidence to suggest that these tints are in any way harmful.[25]

Megavitamins and omega oils

In 1971 it was proposed that learning difficulties could be treated successfully with megavitamins. More recently, similar claims have been made about omega oils. No research supports these claims.

Trace elements

In the 1960s it was proposed that learning disabilities were the results of deficiencies in trace elements. No research data support these claims.

Psycho stimulants

Methylphenidate (Ritalin) and dexamphetamine (Dexedrine) have been reported as helping children with developmental dyslexia. These medications improve symptoms of attention deficit syndrome and make the child more compliant in the classroom. The improvement in concentration improves the ability to respond to instruction and teaching.

NONCONTROVERSIAL THERAPY

Early diagnosis of developmental dyslexia based on a comprehensive evaluation by a skilled educational psychologist will allow the child with developmental dyslexia to gain the maximum benefit from remedial intervention. The diagnosis of developmental dyslexia is reached through an extensive evaluation that involves not only assessment of reading ability, but also assessment of intelligence. Prior to embarking on a remedial program, there is also a need to exclude any sensory deficit involving vision and hearing and to correct these with appropriate glasses, eye exercises, or hearing aids if indicated.

The only form of therapy for developmental dyslexia that has been consistently shown to have results is remediation. To learn to read, all children must discover that spoken words can be broken down into units of sound, phonemes. Children with developmental dyslexia do not easily acquire the basic phonologic skills that serve as a prerequisite to reading. In children with developmental dyslexia phoneme awareness is taught with systemic and highly structured training exercises, such as identifying rhyming and non-rhyming word pairs, blending isolated sounds to form a word, or conversely, segmenting a spoken word into individual sounds (Fig. 66.6). The remedial teacher also guides the child to practice reading stories to allow them to apply their newly acquired decoding skills to reading words in context and to experience reading for meaning. There are a number of different protocols used in remedial teaching that differ in method, format, intensity, and duration.

THE ROLE OF THE OPHTHALMOLOGIST IN THE MANAGEMENT OF DEVELOPMENTAL DYSLEXIA

Developmental dyslexia is a complex problem with no simple solution. The ophthalmologist is part of a multidisciplinary team

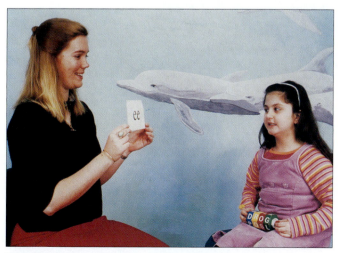

Fig. 66.6 Remedial intervention based on phonetics is most beneficial when performed on a one-to-one basis. Repetition is essential. The child and family need to be prepared for treatment to be ongoing for a considerable period of time.

in the assessment of the child with developmental dyslexia (Table 66.2). Ophthalmologists must have a sound understanding of the process of reading and the role of the eyes and the brain in reading in order to be able to explain to parents in simple terms the mythical and controversial remedial procedures that exist. The ophthalmologist often acts as the advocate for the child and his or her family (Fig. 66.7).

The child with developmental dyslexia usually presents as an intelligent individual with a loss of self-esteem stemming from the inability to read. The thought of having to read aloud in class in front of his or her peers is daunting and often the child is reluctant to attend school. The frustration leads the child to becoming disruptive in the classroom. The child's parents are anxious and unable to understand why their apparently intelligent child is having difficulties with reading.

The consultation is generally time consuming, the majority of the time being taken with explanation of the role of the eyes in developmental dyslexia and discussion of controversial and noncontroversial therapies. A full history of the child's developmental dyslexia and reading problems needs to be documented as well as any intervention that has already occurred. Specific questioning regarding family history of reading difficulties is of paramount importance. The general health of the child, especially relating to low birth weight or neurological deficit, needs to be documented.

A full eye examination is essential. The ophthalmologist should not only check how well the child sees in the distance and at near

Table 66.2 Multidisciplinary approach in management

Ophthalmologist corrects any ocular problem that could interfere with reading
Educational psychologist confirms the diagnosis and assesses the child's reading ability
Pediatrician/general practitioner manages any physical problem
Remedial teacher provides the therapy

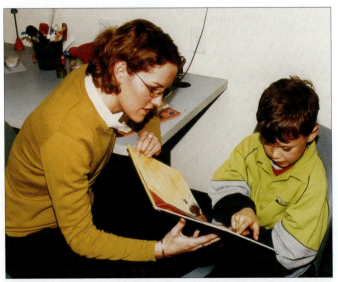

Fig. 66.7 The role of the ophthalmologist. The ophthalmologist performs a full eye examination and corrects any abnormality of ocular function. The ophthalmologist is also the advocate for the child and family and helps guide them in the right direction to ensure the child receives appropriate remedial intervention.

Table 66.3 Ophthalmological examination

Visual acuity at distance and near
Assess child's ability to read age appropriate print
Orthoptic assessment looking for phoria, tropia, problems with convergence and accommodation
Cycloplegic refraction
Ophthalmoscopy

but also how well the child is able to read age-appropriate material to try and gauge the severity of the reading disability. A full orthoptic assessment looking for phorias, tropias, and any weakness of convergence and accommodation is also of importance. The child should then have a cycloplegic refraction followed by a fundus examination (Table 66.3).

The eye examination in most children will be normal. If problems are detected relating to ocular muscle imbalance, weakness of convergence or accommodation, or a significant refractive error, these need to be corrected.

A simple commonsense explanation to the child's parents as to the role of the eyes in reading, and the myth and reality of the etiology and management, must be clearly communicated. Explain that children and adults, even with severe visual problems, are able to read print and that even an individual with vision loss can read using Braille. Discuss examples of severe abnormal eye movements such as congenital nystagmus, Duane's syndrome, and Möbius syndrome that have been shown not to be a barrier to reading. Stress that there is significant evidence to show that developmental dyslexia is due to brain dysfunction and explain how functional magnetic resonance imaging has shown changes after successful remedial treatment.

If the child has not had a comprehensive assessment by an educational psychologist, recommend one. The need for appropriate educational remediation needs to be stressed. Children with developmental dyslexia respond differently to remediation and one form of treatment may not be appropriate for every child. Explain that many of the remedial treatments are based on the phonological deficit hypothesis. Remediation is best on a one-to-one basis. Even with an outstanding remedial teacher, improvement will not occur overnight. Developmental dyslexia cannot be cured but the child can be taught to read and manage adequately and cope, even at the level of tertiary education.

During the consultation it is important to acknowledge that the child has a problem. Do not question the motives and forms of intervention that have been used by other therapists. Most forms of noneducational therapy are harmless and at the very worst may simply delay appropriate intervention. Assuming that the eye examination is normal and the child is already wearing low plus lenses or bifocals or even tinted lenses, explain to the parents that, in your opinion, the child does not require the glasses but if he or she feels more comfortable in them when reading, they can be used for close work.

At the conclusion of the consultation ensure that there is adequate communication with the child's general practitioner. Communication should also occur with the school counselor, educational psychologist, and the remedial teacher if one is already involved. Continue to stress that developmental dyslexia is almost never due to a visual problem and the need for a multidisciplinary approach with the most important aspect being appropriate on-going remedial intervention.

The child and his or her family should leave your office with clear direction and be optimistic that something can be done to overcome the child's reading difficulty. With the use of compensatory mechanisms, the child will cope with the requirements for academic progress.

Brilliant and accomplished individuals who are thought to have had developmental dyslexia abound, including William Butler Yeats, Albert Einstein, and George Patton, all of who have made a significant contribution to society.

REFERENCES

1. Shaywitz SE. Dyslexia. N Engl J Med 1998; 338: 307–12.
2. Shaywitz SE, Fletcher JM, Holahan JM, et al. Persistence of dyslexia: the Connecticut Longitudinal Study at adolescence. Pediatrics 1999; 104: 1351–9.
3. Report of the National Reading Panel. Teaching children to read: an evidence-based assessment of the scientific research literature on reading and its implications for reading instruction. Bethesda, MD: National Institute of Child Health and Human Development, National Institutes of Health; 2000
4. Vellutino FR. Dylexia. Sci Am 1987; 256: 34–41.
5. Pavlidis GT. Do eye movements hold the key to dyslexia? Neuropsychologia 1981; 19: 57–64.
6. Brown B, Haegerstrom-Portnoy G, Adams AJ, et al: Predictive eye movements do not discriminate between dyslexic and control children. Neuropsychologia 1983; 21: 121–8.
7. Stanley G, Smith GA, Howell EA. Eye movements and sequential tracking in dyslexic and control children. Br J Psychol 1983; 74: 181–7.
8. Shaywitz SE, Shaywitz BA. The science of reading and dyslexia. J AAPOS 2003; 7: 158–66.
9. Pennington BF, Gilser JW. How is dyslexia transmitted? In: Rosen GD, Sherman GF, editors. Developmental Dyslexia: Neural, Cognitive and Genetic Mechanisms. Baltimore: York Press; 1996: 41–61.
10. Cardon CR, Smith SD, Fuller DW, et al. Quantitative trait locus for reading disability on chromosone 6. Science 1994; 266: 276–9.
11. Fagerheim T, Raeymaekers P, Tonnessen FE, et al. A new gene (DYX3) for dyslexia is located on chromosome 2. J Med Genet 1999; 36: 664–9.
12. Galaburda AM, Sherman GF, Rosen GD, et al. Development dyslexia: four consecutive patients with cortical anomalies. Ann Neurol 1985; 18: 222–33.
13. Sherman GF, Rosen GD, Galaburda AM. Neuroanatomical findings in developmental dyslexia. In: von Euler C, Lundberg I, Lennerstrand G, editors. Brain and reading. London: Macmillan Press; 1989: 3–15.
14. Beaton AA. The relation of planum temporale asymmetry and morphology of the corpus callosum to handedness, gender, and dyslexia: a review of the evidence. Brain Lang 1997; 60: 255–322.
15. Pugh KR, Mencl WE, Jenner AR, et al. Functional neuroimaging studies of reading and reading disability (developmental dyslexia). Ment Retard Dev Disabil Res Rev 2000; 6: 207–13.
16. Simos PG, Fletcher JM, Bergman E, et al. Dyslexia-specific brain activation profile becomes normal following successful remedial training. Neurology 2002; 58: 1203–13.
17. Duffy FH, McAnulty GB. Brain electrical activity mapping (BEAM): the search for a physiological signature of dyslexia. In: Duffy FH, Geschwind N, editors. Dyslexia: a Neuroscientific Approach to Clinical Evaluation. Boston: Little, Brown; 1985: 105–22.
18. Skottun BC. The magnocellular deficit theory of dyslexia: the evidence from contrast sensitivity. Vision Res 2000; 40: 111–27.
19. Evans BJ, Drasdo N. Review of ophthalmic factors in dyslexia. Ophthalmic Physiol Opt 1990; 10: 123–32.
20. Lennerstrand G, Ygge J. Dyslexia; ophthalmological aspects 1991. Acta Ophthalmol 1992; 70: 3–13.
21. Helveston EM, Weber JC, Miller K, et al. Visual function and academic performance. Am J Ophthalmol 1985; 99: 346–55.
22. Silver LB. Controversial therapies. J Child Neurol 1995; 10s: 96–100.
23. Metzger RL, Werner DB. Use of visual training for reading disabilities: a review. Pediatrics 1984; 73: 824–9.
24. Stanley G. Glare scotopic sensitivity and colour therapy. In: Stein JF, editor. Vision and visual dyslexia. London: Macmillan; 1991: 171–80. (vol 13.)
25. Evans BJ, Drasdo N. Tinted lenses and related therapies for learning disabilities–a review. Ophthalmic Physiol Opt 1991; 11: 206–17.

CHAPTER
67 Pupil Anomalies and Reactions

Creig S Hoyt

Although an understanding of the anatomy (Fig. 67.1), physiology, and pathophysiology of the pupillary pathways is of paramount importance to the pediatric ophthalmologist, they are dealt with so excellently in other books (most notably in Walsh & Hoyt's *Clinical Neuroophthalmology*[1]) that only aspects relevant to children will be discussed here.

DEVELOPMENT

The pupillary light response is absent in infants of 29 gestational weeks or less, but is usually present by 31 or 32 weeks.[2,3] At birth the pupil is small: it enlarges in the first months of life and is probably at its largest at the end of the first decade, before gradually becoming small again in old age. The pupil reactions of term or premature infants are often of small amplitude and because of their small resting size they may be difficult to elicit clinically. The failure of the pupil grating response in infants under one month of age is further evidence of the immaturity of the pupil responses in infancy.[4] Cocaine and hydroxyamphetamine are less potent in infants than in the older children, suggesting that the miosis of the newborn is due to decreased sympathetic tone.[5] In very premature babies the pupil may not have fully formed; during the seventh month the vascular pupillary membrane atrophies and the pupil appears. Until after 32 weeks of gestation mydriasis should not be taken as necessarily indicating a central nervous system lesion and an unresponsive pupil does not necessarily indicate an afferent defect.[3]

Dynamic retinoscopy indicates that the infants from 6 days to 1 month of age exhibit no evidence of accommodation but that normal function is achieved by 3–4 months.[6] The effect of this lack of accommodation is defocusing of the higher spatial frequencies, the detection of which requires a greater discrimination than the younger infant is capable of. However, photorefraction studies have demonstrated an ability to accommodate of over 1 diopter in the neonate, and this increases rapidly in the first month and to a lesser extent in the first few years of life, with high amplitudes from 4 years onward until presbyopia sets in.[7]

THE NEAR SYNKINESIS

When someone looks from a far to a near point, the eyes converge, the pupils constrict, and the eyes focus (accommodate); these three components are separate in origin but linked together as a common response except in some disease states or by pharmacological manipulation when one or more elements may be selectively impaired. Disturbances in the relationship between the amount of accommodation and convergence are important aspects of most childhood squints, and the manipulation of that ratio may be important in management.

In small children the testing of the near pupil response is much more difficult than the pupil response to light. The most important factor in testing is to provide a suitable fixation target, for example, a small internally lit toy for an infant, a mobile toy with sufficient detail to need focusing for a small child, and letters or numbers for the literate.

CONGENITAL AND STRUCTURAL ABNORMALITIES

Congenital, structural, and developmental anomalies in the pupil include the following.

- Aniridia;
- Micropupil (congenital idiopathic microcoria);
- Polycoria and corectopia;
- Coloboma;
- Peninsula pupil: an inherited partial iris sphincter atrophy with dilated oval pupils;
- Persistent pupillary membrane;
- Congenital mydriasis and miosis;
- Irregular pupils; and
- Abnormalities of iris color.

ABNORMALITIES OF PUPIL REACTIVITY

Afferent pupil defects

Amaurotic pupils

A totally blind eye resulting from eye or optic nerve disease usually has no pupil reaction to a light shone on it.[8] If the blindness is unilateral the affected eye has no pupil reaction at all when a light is shone on it but when the light is shifted to the unaffected eye both pupils rapidly constrict, and this is the so-called amaurotic pupil reaction. If both eyes are blind from anterior visual pathway or retinal disease, both pupils are usually dilated if the lesion is recent although they may be nearly normal in size in long-standing blindness.[9] The pupils react to near stimuli in the recently blind child. For instance the recently blind child may be asked to try to imagine looking at his own hand held up in front of him; in long-standing blindness the child usually cannot do this. Sometimes a totally blind person may be found to have preserved pupil reactions, despite careful technique and a cooperative patient who is genuinely blind and not attempting to look near.[10,11] Perhaps there are a few surviving pupillomotor fibers in these cases, or they have a combination of anterior blindness and cortical disease.

Relative afferent pupil defect

When one optic nerve afferent pathway is more affected than the other there may be a difference in the pupil reactions based on the

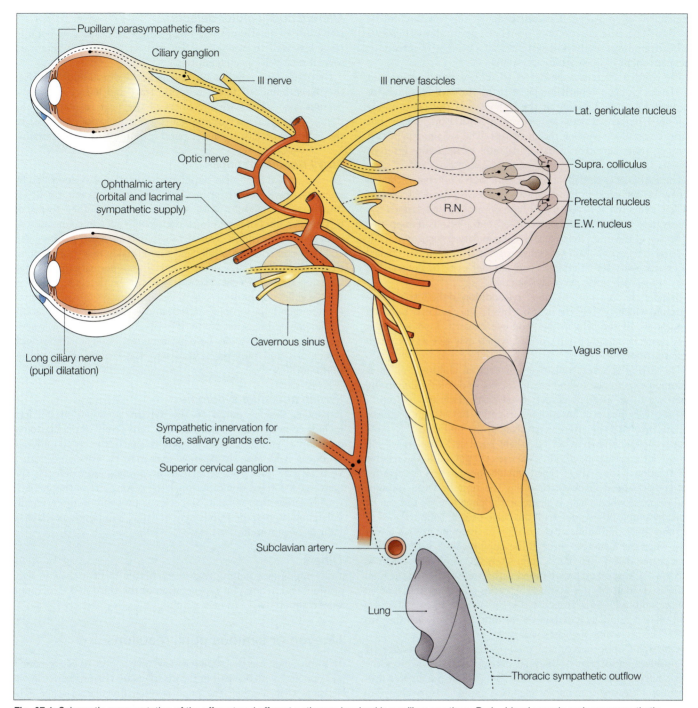

Fig. 67.1 Schematic representation of the efferent and afferent pathways involved in pupillary reactions. Red = blood vessels and parasympathetic. Blue = afferent visual pathways. Green = sympathetic pathway.

relative conduction of the pupillomotor fibers from the two eyes.[12] It is very useful in the preverbal child but requires meticulous technique, the basis of which is to always subject the two eyes to the same stimulus, both in intensity and in direction. It only distinguishes one eye as being more affected than the other and is not an absolute assessment or measurement of pupil function.

The details of the setup and performance of the test are important.[13] In a dimly lit room the observer uses a bright light (hence the alternative name "the swinging flashlight test") that is shone on each eye individually while the child, if possible, has his fixation maintained at one position, preferably in the distance. Any difference in reaction is noted. Then the light is shone on the

expected "better" eye for about 3 s and then rapidly moved to the suspected "worse" eye.[14] If the second eye is really worse both pupils will dilate by a direct and consensual reaction driven by the pupil afferent system from the worse eye. Similarly if the light is moved from the worse to the better eye the pupils will constrict. In either direction of movement there may be a momentary constriction when the pupil is first stimulated.

Although the clinical test is not a measurement it can be graded, usually I–IV, with IV being an amaurotic pupil. Measurement using graded filters or pupillography is usually too difficult in a child.[15] However, in the older child the magnification provided by the slit lamp may be useful in detecting a minimal defect.[16] If there is also a unilateral efferent defect or ocular defect the test can still be performed because the reactions from one eye are always bilateral and the pupil whose efferent system is intact can be observed for the assessment of both afferent systems.

The relative afferent pupil defect (RAPD) is usually attributed to Marcus Gunn, an ophthalmologist at the National Hospitals for Nervous Diseases, London, at the beginning of this century. He described sequential papillary assessment with a bright light but not the so-called swinging flashlight test. The swinging light test is much more sensitive in detecting mild to moderate afferent defects.[8]

The RAPD is essentially a test of optic nerve function although it may be abnormal in patients with extensive retinal disease. As Miller points out it *never* occurs with corneal disease, cataract, a moderately sized vitreous hemorrhage, central serous retinopathy, or drusen of the disc.[1] Relative afferent papillary defects may occur in amblyopic eyes.[17] Recent studies suggest that significant axonal loss is necessary for an afferent papillary defect to be detected in association with optic nerve dysfunction.[18]

In older children a useful subjective addition to the test is to ask the child which eye sees the light brightest. The child may be asked a question, "if the light in the good eye is worth 1 pound/dollar how much is the other one worth?", which may give a very rough quantification.

The RAPD is a very sensitive test even in children, and it is common experience to find normal acuity and color vision in the presence of an afferent defect, most particularly in children in the recovery phase of an optic neuropathy, but also in posterior lesions involving the afferent pathway in the midbrain.[19]

A technique known as the edge-light pupil cycle time may help to give information about individual eyes as opposed to the relative information of the RAPD.[20] The technique needs a very cooperative patient because it involves measuring the time between stimulus and response when a light is shone on the pupil margin; this can be done by simple observation with the beam of a slit lamp reduced to 0.5 mm thick and shone at the margin of the pupil in such a way that when the light goes through the pupil it causes it to constrict to a degree that it then blocks completely the admission of light to the eye. At least 10 cycles are timed with a stopwatch, and the total time is divided by the number of cycles to obtain the time in milliseconds. A normal response is less than 954 ms in either eye, and there is normally less than 70 ms difference between the two eyes. The cycle time increases with age.[21]

Chiasmal, optic nerve, and tract lesions do not produce by themselves anisocoria. A chiasmal defect, unless it involves the optic nerve, does not have a RAPD. Because of the greater proportion of crossing than uncrossing fibers in the chiasm a complete (but not a partial) optic tract lesion may be associated with a contralateral RAPD.[22] This is not easy to detect clinically. A small relative afferent papillary defect may be seen in the smaller pupil when more than 2 mm of anisocoria is present.[23]

Light–near dissociation

When the pupil reacts better to a near than to a light stimulus or vice versa there is said to be light–near dissociation; a relatively poor, rather than an absent, light reaction is much more common. It must be remembered that a bright light is necessary to test the pupil's light reaction; otherwise, the powerful near reflex will always appear better than the light reaction. With the expectation of errors in testing techniques or poor patient cooperation there is no pathological situation where the pupillary light reflex is normal while the near response is defective.

Afferent pupillomotor defects

Any cause of an afferent pupil light reflex will cause the pupil to react less well to near light than to near targets but there are several relatively specific entities.

Damage to the pupillomotor fibers in the dorsal midbrain after they have branched from the optic tract and before they have become associated with the fibers of the near response in the Edinger-Westphal nucleus may cause a relatively poor response to the light with relatively intact pupil response to a near stimulus.

Argyll Robertson pupils

The archetypal light–near pupillary dissociation was described by Douglas Argyll Robertson in 1869. This type of abnormality is usually seen in adults with tabes dorsalis or other forms of tertiary syphilis but is said to be occasionally seen in young persons with congenital syphilis. Typically the pupils are small and irregular, and they constrict more fully and more briskly to a near stimulus than to light. They may dilate less well than normal pupils. If the slit lamp is used, a light response may just be detected. Vision is normal unless there is associated visual pathways disease. The iris is often seen to be atrophic on slit-lamp examination. There is still considerable discussion as to the site of the lesion. Magnetic resonance imaging studies have localized the lesion in patients with sarcoidosis and multiple sclerosis to the region of the dorsal midbrain.[24]

Sylvian aqueduct syndrome

Expanding lesions dorsal to the sylvian aqueduct in children include pinealomas, ependymomas, "trilateral" retinoblastoma, granulomas, and cystic lesions. Compression of the dorsal midbrain produces light–near dissociation that may be associated with a vertical gaze palsy, lid retraction, accommodation defects, and convergence–retraction nystagmus: the resting size of the pupils is usually larger than normal. Sometimes, probably in more rapidly enlarging tumors, the pupils may be large, and poorly reactive to light or near stimuli.[25]

Others

Adie pupils (see below) may react better to near than to light stimuli, and in aberrant regeneration of the third nerve the pupil may respond better to near stimuli.

Uneven or sinuous pupil reactions

In some conditions the pupil reactions may appear to be segmental, or "sinuous," with one part of the iris sphincter reacting better in one segment than another; the pupil is often irregular in shape. The phenomenon may sometimes be seen with the naked eye but it is better seen with magnification by loupe or by slit-lamp examination.

Adie syndrome (tonic pupil syndrome)

This condition may occur in children especially in association with chicken pox infection.[26] It is more frequently found in young adults, especially women.[27] It is usually unilateral but may be bilateral, sometimes with an asynchronous onset.[28]

Children rarely have symptoms related to the onset but they may fail a school near-vision test, or complain of blurred near or distant (if they are hyperopic) vision or photophobia. The potential for the development of anisometropic amblyopia must be considered in the hyperopic child with Adie syndrome. It is the parents noticing an anisocoria that most often brings it to the attention of the doctor.

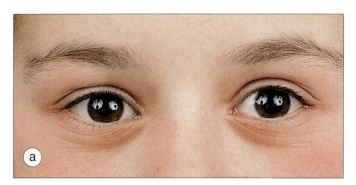 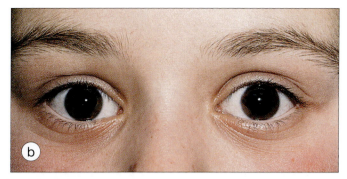

Fig. 67.2 Left Adie pupil (a) in light and (b) in dark. The pupil size difference is less in the dark.

The acutely affected pupil is usually a little larger than its (uninvolved) fellow (Fig. 67.2), but if viewed in darkness, it may be smaller as the normal pupil is free to dilate widely. It always has a segmental paralysis of the iris sphincter that may be extensive with virtually all of the pupil being paralyzed and only reacting sluggishly and in a sinuous fashion (the "tonic" pupil).[29] There is also a defect in accommodation, which is often marked at first but which gradually improves over 2 or more years.[27] Corneal sensation may be reduced when tested with an aesthesiometer or even with a wisp of cotton wool.[30] This is probably due to damage to the trigeminal fibers that also pass through the ciliary ganglion.

Patients with Adie syndrome may be hyporeflexic or areflexic in their extremities. Adie syndrome may be diagnosed by finding an internal ophthalmoplegia, unilateral or asymmetrical with sinuous pupil reactions in a healthy person with normal corrected vision. Denervation hypersensitivity of the pupil may be demonstrated by finding pupillary constriction 20 minutes after instillation of pilocarpine 0.0625%.[31] Stronger concentrations of pilocarpine should not be used since normal innervated pupils may constrict in response to their application.[31] Pharmacological hypersensitivity (Fig. 67.3) may occur with postciliary ganglionic as well as preciliary ganglionic lesions.[32,33]

Deep tendon reflex abnormalities with an intact vibration sense suggest more widespread neural involvement, and this is supported by findings of dorsal root nerve loss.[34]

In time, Adie pupils become smaller and the accommodation paresis becomes less but the other features remain.

Loewenfeld and Thompson have proposed that the site of the lesion of the tonic pupil is in the ciliary ganglion and that many of its features can be explained by aberrant regeneration.[35] The cause is unknown but it may be due to a neurotropic virus. Most patients do not require treatment but they may be helped with their photophobia and occasionally with symptoms due to accommodation paresis by dilute pilocarpine (0.1% three times daily). Young children with Adie or other tonic pupils should have the unaffected or better eye occluded for a short period each day to avoid amblyopia. Spectacle correction of significant hyperopia in the affected eye may be necessary to prevent anisometropic amblyopia.

Iris abnormalities

Damage to the iris by trauma, irradiation, uveitis, ischemia, involvement by leukemia (Fig. 67.4) or hemorrhage, or involvement with a tumor such as lymphoma, leukemia, juvenile xanthogranuloma, leiomyoma, or neurofibroma may all give rise to sinuous pupil reactions.

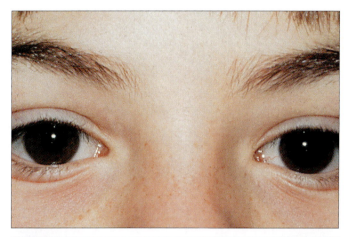

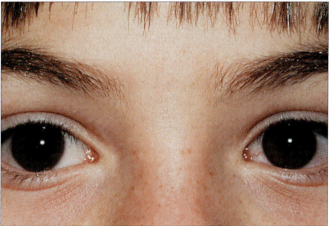

Fig. 67.3 Left Adie pupil (top) before and (bottom) after instillation of 0.1% pilocarpine. The right pupil is unchanged while the left constricts due to denervation hypersensitivity.

Benign episodic unilateral mydriasis ("springing pupil")

The syndrome of idiopathic episodic mydriasis probably is a heterogeneous group of conditions that result in parasympathetic insufficiency of the iris sphincter or sympathetic hyperactivity of the iris dilator.[36] In either case, it results in anisocoria that usually lasts for several hours and then resolves spontaneously. Other signs of oculomotor or sympathetic nerve dysfunction are con-

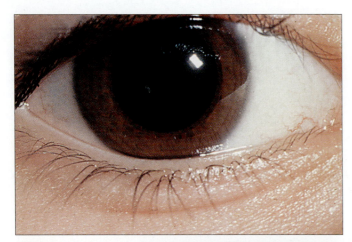

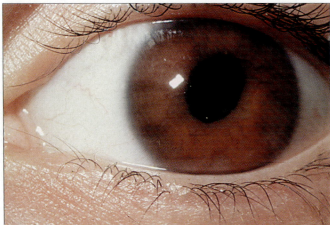

Fig. 67.4 (top) Normal right eye and (bottom) left iris abnormality with sluggish reactions and small pupil due to leukemic infiltration.

spicuous by their absence. The pupil changes are frequently accompanied by headache or orbital pain.[36] Although it occurs primarily in women in the third to fourth decades of life, it has been reported in young children.[37]

Midbrain corectopia

Damage to some midbrain pupillary fibers may give rise to unequal upward and inward distortion of the pupil and an unequal, sinuous pupil reaction to light and near stimuli. The patients described have often but not always been comatose.[38]

Third nerve palsy

In complete third nerve palsy the pupil is unreactive (Fig. 67.5), but in partial or recovering third nerve palsy the ipsilateral pupil reactions may be sluggish and react in an uneven fashion.

Sometimes the pupil shape may be irregular and the reactions sinuous:

1. Acute partial lesions of the third nerve are presumably due to selective loss of function in some but not all third nerve fibers.[39]
2. In oculomotor palsy with cyclic spasm segmental involvement is seen. As patients with oculomotor palsy with cyclic spasms age the spasms of lid and extraocular muscle function may cease but spasms of the pupil may continue.

3. Sinuous iris movements due to sector contractions of the iris sphincter and abnormal spontaneous pupillary contractions occur in aberrant regeneration (Fig. 67.6) following third nerve palsy.[39] The pupil may be small in long-standing lesions (Fig. 67.7).

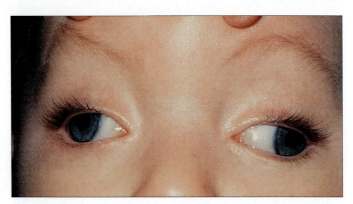

Fig. 67.5 Bilateral congenital third nerve palsy with fixed and unreactive pupils; the pupil made very slow bilateral size changes.

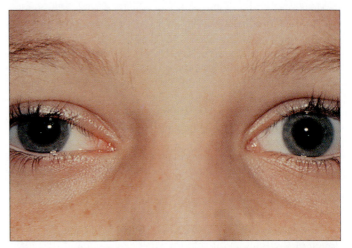

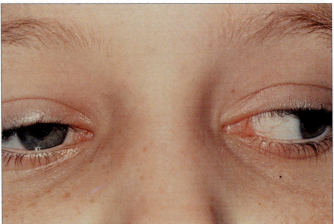

Fig. 67.6 Aberrant regeneration following partial recovery from right traumatic third nerve palsy: the right pupil constricts on attempted adduction.

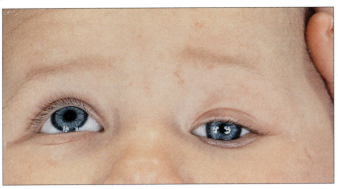

Fig. 67.7 Left congenital third nerve palsy. In long-standing cases the pupil may be small.

Riley-Day syndrome

In the Riley-Day syndrome (familial dysautonomia) there is a hypersensitivity to dilute parasympathomimetic agents (i.e., pilocarpine 0.1%). Although it has been suggested that these children may have a tonic pupil, Korczyn et al. found no evidence of this on pupillography of 10 patients.[40]

Iris sphincter or dilator muscle spasms

Spasm of the iris dilator gives rise to "tadpole-shaped" pupils, which usually occurs in young adults who are otherwise healthy.[41] The pupils are peaked in one direction for a few minutes and it may occur on several separate occasions. This may represent a subset of patients who carry the diagnosis of springing pupil.

Other causes of tonic pupils

Although Adie syndrome is the classic tonic pupil, other causes of ciliary ganglion damage give rise to a similar syndrome, confined to the affected eye, unlike Adie syndrome that may be bilateral and have systemic abnormalities. Congenital or acquired tonic pupils have been described in infants with orbital tumors.[42] Traumatic, infectious, or inflammatory diseases and a wide variety of exanthemas have been described as causing a tonic pupil, and they may also occur as part of a variety of widespread neuropathies including syphilis, diabetes, Guillain-Barré syndrome, Miller-Fisher syndrome, pandysautonomia, hereditary sensory neuropathy, Charcot-Marie-Tooth disease, and Trilene poisoning. Autonomic neuropathy and chronic relapsing polyneuropathy due to paraneoplastic disease have been reported to cause tonic pupils.[43]

Paradoxical pupils

In some people with retinal disease a curious phenomenon may occur in which the pupil size in the light is larger than that in the dark despite the other responses being normal.[44] The parents may occasionally remark on this themselves but it is usually a sign that must be elicited. When clearly present it is extremely helpful as it virtually only occurs in retinal diseases.

A good way to record paradoxical pupils is to take a Polaroid or digital photograph of the child in a fully lit room and in a nearly fully darkened room. The photographs may clearly show the difference and can be kept as a record. Simple observation, however, is perfectly adequate. It is important to leave the child for at least a minute in the dark; the pupils can be observed there by using a flashlight for a moment, or with an infrared viewing device or video. Most typically the response is found in patients with cone dysfunction syndromes, achromatopsia, or congenital stationary night-blindness but it also has been described in Leber's amaurosis, dominant optic atrophy, optic neuritis and other retinal disease, and even amblyopia.[45] Nevertheless, in the young child with nystagmus the presence of the paradoxical pupil suggests an electroretinogram (ERG) should be obtained.

The mechanism has not been adequately explained but it is interesting that dark-rearing chicks to maturity causes them to have paradoxically constricted pupils in the dark.[46]

HORNER SYNDROME

Sympathetic denervation in childhood is not uncommon and may be congenital or acquired.[47]

Clinical characteristics

Miosis

The pupils are unequal with the difference greatest in the dark due to the defect being in a failure of the dilator pupillae muscle (Fig. 67.8). The difference depends on the completeness of the lesion and the alertness of the child. A drowsy child is more likely to have a small resting pupillary tone and the inequality will be less obvious. There is also a lag in the dilatation of the affected side.[48] This lag results in a greater anisocoria at 5 s than at 15 s after

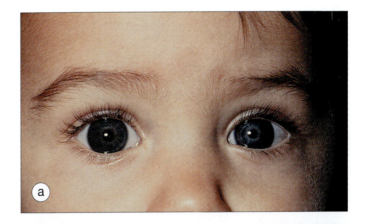

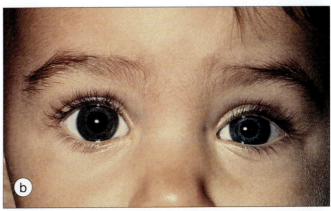

Fig. 67.8 (a) Left Horner syndrome with mild ptosis. Photograph taken in the light. (b) Same patient 5 s after lights turned out showing dilation lag.

the lights are turned out. It is best measured by photographs. Pupil reactions to light and near and accommodation are unaffected.

Ptosis

A 1- to 2-mm ptosis of the upper lid is present but it may be so slight and so variable that it escapes notice. The lower lid may also be affected, giving rise to a more obvious narrowing in the palpebral fissure.[49] This narrowing may give rise to the false appearance of enophthalmos.

Ipsilateral anhidrosis

Lesions before the superior cervical ganglion, where the sweat and piloerector fibers split off to go with the external carotid artery, will damage these fibers and cause an ipsilateral flushed face and conjunctiva and nasal stuffiness in acute lesions. In longer standing lesions there is a defect of sweating with a dry, warm side to the face when the other is cool and sweaty. In chronic lesions the affected side may be pale due to denervation hypersensitivity to circulating catecholamines.

Heterochromia

In congenital Horner syndrome the iris fails to become fully pigmented, giving rise to heterochromia with the light iris on the affected side. This is most marked in heavily pigmented irides. Occasionally heterochromia has been recorded as happening very gradually following injury or surgery to the carotid in childhood.[47] However, progressive heterochromia has been reported following acquired Horner syndrome even in adults.[50] Heterochromia is not invariably present in congenital Horner syndrome especially in light-colored irides or if insufficient time has elapsed.[51] Histopathologically, in one case, the iris pigment epithelium was normal, there were no iris sympathetic fibers, and the stromal melanocytes were reduced in number, but contained normal melanosomes.[52] The anterior border cells were depleted.

Pharmacological responses

Cocaine 10% blocks reuptake of noradrenaline (norepinephrine) by the sympathetic nerve endings. In postganglionic lesions the nerve is dead and contains no noradrenaline (norepinephrine), and since cocaine has no direct effect, the pupil fails to dilate while it dilates in normals and in a preganglionic Horner syndrome, although in the latter situation it does not usually dilate at all well. It is highly effective as one way of distinguishing between normals (even with physiological anisocoria) and anisocoria due to Horner syndrome.[53]

Hydroxyamphetamine 1% releases noradrenaline (norepinephrine) from presynaptic nerve terminal stores; it should be instilled into the conjunctival sac of both eyes at least 24 hr after the use of cocaine. Where the postganglionic neurone is intact noradrenaline (norepinephrine) is present and the pupil is dilated, but if the postganglionic neurone is "dead" it contains no norepinephrine (noradrenaline) and does not dilate. Hydroxyamphetamine takes about 40 min to work.

Adrenaline (epinephrine) 0.1% (1:1000) does not normally dilate the pupil but in postganglionic Horner syndrome there is denervation hypersensitivity and the pupil dilates. Adrenaline (epinephrine) 0.1% has the advantage of being more readily available and it is not a proscribed drug.

A recent report suggests that 0.5% apraclonidine may be useful in establishing a diagnosis of Horner syndrome.[54] Apraclonidine 0.5% causes a reversal of the anisocoria under both dark and light conditions. It is readily available and inexpensive.

Pharmacological testing is frequently not necessary to establish the diagnosis but because ipsilateral ptosis and miosis coexist quite frequently due to the frequency of physiological anisocoria with lid and other abnormalities, it may be diagnostic in some instances.[55] In children, the main problem is measuring the inequality and changes in light and dark; this may be helped by photographs.

Other characteristics

There have been various reports of ipsilateral accommodative increase or decrease but the difference does not seem to be reliably present or easy to measure in children. The ipsilateral central cornea may be thicker on the affected side.[56]

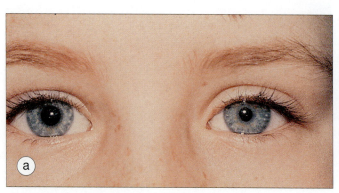
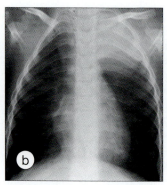
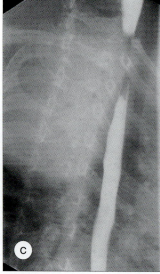

Fig. 67.9 (a) Left Horner syndrome. This child presented with the complaint of a sudden onset ptosis and small pupil. (b) Chest X-ray showing left apical mass. (c) Barium swallow showing constriction of the esophagus. The cause was a large benign ganglioneuroma.

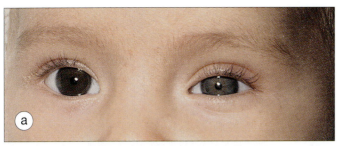
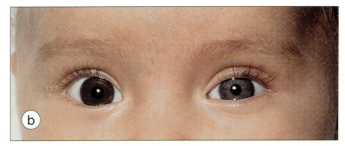

Fig. 67.10 Congenital Horner syndrome showing upper and lower lid ptosis and a difference in iris color with the lighter eye being the affected left eye. (a) In bright light and (b) in the dark.

Congenital Horner syndrome

Weinstein et al. divided congenital Horner syndrome into three causal types:[57]

1. Those who suffered obstetric trauma to the internal carotid artery and its sympathetic nerve plexus. These children were usually delivered by forceps, and they had a postganglionic Horner syndrome on drug testing; i.e., they did not dilate with 1% hydroxyamphetamine. They had no facial anhidrosis.

2. Those who suffered surgical or obstetric trauma to the preganglionic sympathetic pathway (the pupil dilates with 1% hydroxyamphetamine). This group includes patients with brachial plexus injury, known traditionally as Klumpke's palsy. Cardiothoracic surgery is a common cause in most children's hospitals.

3. Those without a history of birth trauma but with a Horner syndrome with evidence of a lesion at, or peripheral to, the superior cervical ganglion. These patients also had anhidrosis (absence of sweating on the ipsilateral face) presumably due to a lesion after the separation of the sweat fibers that pass from the superior cervical ganglion to the external carotid artery. Congenital or early onset Horner syndrome with a preganglionic lesion and anhidrosis have been reported in patients with neuroblastoma.[47,51]

Congenital Horner syndrome may also be found with hemifacial atrophy,[58] cervical vertebral anomalies,[59] congenital tumors,[51] arachnoidal cysts and holoprosencephaly,[47] and congenital varicella syndrome.[60] Despite the above list of causes, it must be said that despite extensive investigation no abnormality has been found in most children with congenital Horner syndrome.[51]

Postnatally acquired Horner syndrome

Some authors have emphasized the seriousness of the causes of acquired Horner syndrome in childhood. It may occur in the following:

1. As a "central" lesion due to brain stem trauma, brain stem tumors and vascular malformations, infarcts and hemorrhages, and syringomyelia.[61] It must be emphasized that other neurologic dysfunction is usually evident in these patients. Bilateral "pinpoint" pupils are found particularly in comatose patients with pontine hemorrhages.

2. As a "preganglionic" lesion, i.e., of the second neurone between the spinal cord and the superior cervical ganglion, due to neck trauma, neuroblastoma, and other tumors.[47,51]

3. As a "postganglionic" lesion, i.e., of the final neurone after the superior cervical ganglion, due to cavernous sinus lesions (tumors, aneurysms, or inflammatory disease), neuroblastoma, and trauma.[51]

Management

Congenital

Since birth trauma or early cardiothoracic surgery are the most frequent causes, further investigations are not usually necessary.[47,51] However, the occurrence of tumors in those children with congenital Horner syndrome of no obvious cause may warrant investigation with a chest X-ray, head and neck tomography, and a 24-hr catecholamine assay.[51]

Treatment with weak adrenergic substances is rarely necessary.[62]

Acquired

Where there is no obvious cause, such as trauma or surgery, a child with acquired Horner syndrome should be investigated by or in conjunction with a neurologist, and the further investigations should include a chest X-ray, computed tomography (CT) or magnetic resonance imaging (MRI) scan, and 24-hr catecholamine assay.[47]

PUPIL CHANGES FROM HIGH SYMPATHETIC "TONE"

Cases have been described in which an intermittent dilated pupil, with or without widening of the palpebral fissure, occurs associated with a cervicomedullary syrinx,[63] post spinal cord injury,[64] lung tumors,[65] or seizures or migraine.[66] In seizures and migraine there may well be a lowering of parasympathetic tone at the same time,[66] but sympathetic-induced spasm is suggested by pallor and sweating.[67]

PUPIL CHANGES FROM DAMAGE TO THE PARASYMPATHETIC SYSTEM

Internal ophthalmoplegia (paralysis of the sphincter pupillae and accommodation) is occasionally seen without external ophthalmoplegia from nuclear lesions. It is bilateral and often associated with other oculomotor palsies.[68]

Damage to the third nerve in the interpeduncular fossa, where the pupillomotor fibers are confined to the superomedial aspect of the nerve, may occur from aneurysm or tumor when it is usually associated with external ophthalmoplegia, but meningitic lesions can cause an isolated internal ophthalmoplegia.

In uncal herniation the comatose patient develops a dilated pupil on the side of the herniation, together with an asymmetrically sluggish reaction to light. The pupil signs may be the only abnormality other than coma for a period of some hours. Flexion of the neck, by stretching the brain stem, may worsen the dilation or even cause both pupils to dilate but this is not a recommended

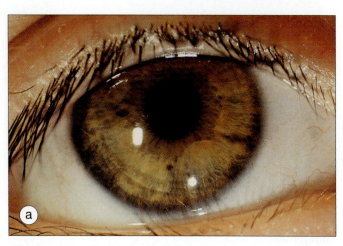
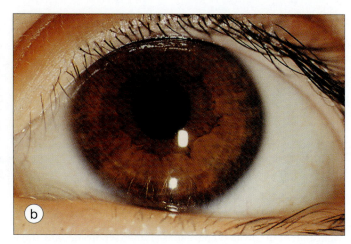

Fig. 67.11 Right congenital Horner syndrome in a teenager. (a) The right iris was noticed to develop a lighter color at the age of 2 although the ptosis and pupil size were noticed at a few weeks of age. (b) The normal left eye.

procedure! Later ipsilateral external ophthalmoplegia and hemiplegia develop, followed by contralateral ophthalmoplegia and then more profound brain stem signs. The syndrome is caused by the uncus of the temporal lobe herniating under the tentorial edge to compress the posterior cerebral artery, third nerve, and the midbrain with the opposite tentorial edge cutting into the cerebral peduncle. Midbrain compression occludes the Sylvian aqueduct, worsening the already-raised supratentorial pressure.

PHARMACOLOGICAL AGENTS

Numerous pharmacological agents affect pupil size and reactivity. Systemic agents usually affect the pupils symmetrically while topical agents are often only instilled into one eye and may be asymmetrical.

Pupil-dilating agents

Parasympatholytic agents
Atropine 0.5–1%, homatropine 2%, cyclopentolate 0.5–1%, and tropicamide 1% are all commonly used agents to dilate the pupil and cause cycloplegia. Homatropine and atropine have a prolonged action and are not often indicated diagnostically or therapeutically unless their long action is desirable as in the case of penalization therapy for amblyopia.[69] Hyoscine 0.5% has an action similar to that of atropine but is less long lived. They may cause respiratory failure in children with congenital central hypoventilation.

Sympathomimetics
Adrenaline (epinephrine) 0.1–1% or phenylephrine 2.5–10% may be used to dilate the pupil in association with a parasympatholytic. They have no action on accommodation but are not sufficient by themselves to produce good dilation. They must be used with great care, and at lowest dilution, if at all, in premature babies, those with cardiac or vascular disease, or those with hypertension.

Pupil-constricting agents

Cholinergic drugs
Pilocarpine 1–4% is commonly used to constrict the pupil. It is now used with decreasing frequency in the treatment of glaucoma. It has little effect on infantile glaucoma.

Anticholinesterases
Phospholine iodide (echothiophate) 0.03–0.125% and eserine 0.5% are infrequently used for treatment of glaucoma. Phospholine iodide is used to cause peripheral accommodation and "unlink" the association between accommodative convergence and accommodation in some cases of high AC:A ratio strabismus.

Sympatholytic agents
Guanethidine 5% (Ismelin) can be used to counter lid retraction in hyperthyroidism. Thymoxamine 1% may also cause pupil construction.

Systemic agents

Atropine, scopolamine, and benztropine can cause pupil dilatation and paralysis of accommodation in sufficient quantities. The seeds of jimson weed, the berries of deadly nightshade, and henbane have all been known to cause a serious or fatal poisoning. The symptoms have been described as "hot as a hare, blind as a bat, dry as a bone, red as a beet, mad as a hen." When proof of atropine poisoning is needed in the absence of facilities for assay it is said that a few drops of the child's urine put into one eye of a cat may suggest the diagnosis. Mydriasis from topical atropine or atropine-like drugs is not counteracted by pilocarpine 1% but in systemic poisoning it may be.

Antihistamines and some antidepressants produce a mydriasis.

Heroin, morphine and other opiates, marijuana, and some other psychotropic drugs cause bilateral pupil constriction.

ABNORMALITIES OF THE NEAR REFLEX

Congenital absence

Children may be born with a defect in the near reflex. They have absent accommodation and poor convergence, and the pupil fails to constrict to a near stimulus, but it constricts to light.[70]

Familial cases of accommodation defect occur.[71] The cause is unknown but it may be peripheral in origin in the ciliary body or lens.

Acquired defects

Psychogenic
Children in the second decade may present with symptoms of difficulty with reading due to nonorganic causes. They can usually

be cajoled into a normal near response or tricked by prisms and minus lenses; the synoptophore is particularly useful here. In older persons, malingering may be suspected especially when compensation for injury is a possibility.

Sylvian aqueduct (Parinaud) syndrome

Premature presbyopia is one of the signs of tumors encroaching on the dorsal midbrain together with the more classic signs of convergence, i.e., retraction nystagmus, vertical gaze defects, eyelid retraction, convergence defect, and pupil light–near dissociation.

Systemic disease

Botulism, diphtheria, diabetes, and head and neck trauma may all give rise to accommodation defects either isolated or associated with eye movement and vergence defects. Wilson disease has been shown to be associated with a defect in the near response in some cases.

Pharmacological agents

See above.

Eye disease

Defective accommodation occurs in children with severe iridocyclitis, dislocated lenses, large colobomas, buphthalmos, very high myopia, and direct eye trauma including retinal detachment surgery.

Other neurological causes

Adie tonic pupil syndrome and third nerve paralysis may cause defective accommodation. Sinus disease, presumably by affecting the short ciliary nerves, may cause cycloplegia and accommodation defect.[72]

Accommodation in schoolchildren

One expects a school-aged child to have a high amplitude of accommodation irrespective of refractive error. Low amplitudes of accommodation have been reported in children who specialize in music as opposed to sport.[73] It has been suggested that there is a causal relationship between a defective near response and some cases of dyslexia.[74]

It is important, however, to distinguish clearly between reading difficulties due to a defective near response, which can be improved by exercises, and dyslexia, which is a specific defect in the perceptual process involved with reading and writing and which cannot be remedied by simple exercises.[75]

SPASM OF THE NEAR REFLEX

Spasm of the near reflex consists of episodes of a combination of:
1. Accommodation-induced pseudo-myopia;
2. Convergence of the eyes; and
3. Miosis.

The symptoms are usually of blurred, double vision, and ocular pain or headache. These cases are rarely due to organic disease and a truly causal relationship with organic pathology is often not easy to establish, although closed head trauma is recognized as a cause in an increasing number of cases.[76,77] Upper brain stem pathology is often suspected but rarely found. In a recent study of two cases related to closed head trauma MR studies revealed no abnormalities in the midbrain but both patients had lesions in the left temporal lobe.[78]

In most cases it is not possible to demonstrate any organic disease and the phenomenon is assumed to be psychogenic. The episodes have a sudden onset and can last many hours and may be very variable. There is blurred vision and photophobia. The eyes are crossed and may mimic a bilateral sixth nerve paresis but the essential finding is of the pupils constricting increasingly as the deviation increases. Pupils that become constricted on attempted lateral gaze are also a clue to the functional nature of the complaint. It is unusual in childhood but may occur. Occasionally symptoms may be recurrent over several years.

The treatment is to reassure the patient and parents, and sometimes they are helped by miotics but more usually by a combination of cycloplegia with bifocal glasses. Unless there are any neurological signs no investigations are required and the prognosis is good.

ANISOCORIA

Anisocoria (unequal pupils) occurs when there is a local abnormality in the iris, or its musculature, or when there is an asymmetrical abnormality in the efferent pathways that drive pupil constriction or dilatation. Afferent (visual) defects never cause anisocoria, even if they are highly asymmetrical, unless they are associated with an efferent defect. Apart from the size abnormality there is usually a change in reactivity that is usually the clue to the diagnosis.

Physiological anisocoria

This is also known as simple anisocoria or occasionally as central anisocoria. Lam et al. determined pupil size in 128 normal individuals: 41% showed anisocoria of 0.4 mm or greater; while 80% showed 0.2 mm or greater.[79] The difference is rarely more than 1 mm between the two sides and may vary from time to time. The size difference is usually apparent in light and dark and the pupil reactions are normal. Direct clinical measurements are often difficult in children and may be avoided by making measurements from photographs.

Anisocoria during reflex responses to unilateral light stimulation, with the direct light reaction exceeding the consensual, can be shown by pupillometry in a significant number of normals.[80] This "contraction anisocoria" was repeatable and the difference was about 6%.

Diagnosis

The diagnosis of anisocoria can be difficult. It is frequently found that the patient and the doctor mistake which is the abnormal pupil, especially in Horner syndrome in which there are no associated visual or ocular motor symptoms.

The abnormality is usually sorted out in three simple stages:
1. The reactions to light and accommodation are determined. If they are abnormal, whether unilateral or bilateral, the diagnosis is of an efferent, parasympathetic, or local cause.
2. Slit-lamp examination will show sinuous pupil reactions and iris anomalies, uveitis, and so on.
3. The size difference in light and dark will help to diagnose sympathetic and parasympathetic lesions. In Horner syndrome the anisocoria is greater in the dark because the dilator pupillae fails to function. In a parasympathetic lesion the difference is greatest in the light because of the failure of the sphincter pupillae.

In nearly all situations the pupil abnormality can be diagnosed by looking at the pupil and by looking for accompanying clinical grounds. It is usually difficult even with the aid of drug testing, especially in small wriggling children who never seem to want to be still at the time you want to measure. The flow chart in Chapter P21 summarizes a clinical approach and has some notes on drug testing for completeness. It is not meant to be absolutely complete or totally foolproof but acts as a guide to diagnosis and is not helpful when both pupils are abnormal.

REFERENCES

1. Miller NR. Newman N. Walsh and Hoyt's Clinical neuro-ophthalmology, 5th ed. Baltimore: Lippincott, Williams & Wilkins; 1997. (vol. 2.)
2. Robinson RJ. Assessment of gestational age by neurological examination. Arch Dis Child 1966; 41: 437–41.
3. Isenberg S, Molarte A, Vazquez M. The fixed and dilated pupils of premature neonates. Am J Ophthalmol 1990; 110: 168–72.
4. Cocker KD, Moseley MJ, Bissenden JG, et al. Visual acuity and papillary responses to special structure in infants. Invest Ophthalmol Vis Sci 1994; 35: 2620–5.
5. Korczyn AD, Laor N, Nemet P. Autonomic pupillary activity in infants. Metab Ophthalmol 1978; 2: 391–4.
6. Haynes H, White BL, Held R. Visual accommodation in human infants. Science 1965; 148: 528–30.
7. Braddick O, Atkinson J, French J, et al. A photorefractive study of infant accommodation. Vision Res 1979; 19: 1319–30.
8. Corbett JJ. The bedside and office neuro-ophthalmology examination. Semin Neurol 2003; 23: 63–76.
9. Girkin CA. Evaluation of the papillary light response as an objective measure of visual function. Ophthalmol Clin North Am 2003; 16: 143–53.
10. Taylor D. Congenital tumors of the anterior visual system with dysplasia of the optic discs. Br J Ophthalmol 1982; 66: 455–63.
11. Lhermitte F, Guillaumat L, Lyon-Caen O. Monocular blindness with preserved direct and consensual pupillary reflex in multiple sclerosis. Arch Neurol 1984; 41: 993–4.
12. Enyedi LB, Dev S, Kox TA. A comparison of the Marcus Gunn and alternating light tests for afferent pupillary defects. Ophthalmology 1998; 105: 871–3.
13. Thompson HS, Corbett J. Asymmetry of pupillomotor input. Eye 1991; 5: 36–40.
14. Thompson HS, Corbett JJ, Cox TA. How to measure the relative afferent pupillary defect. Surv Ophthalmol 1981; 26: 39–42.
15. Bell R, Waggoner P, Boyd W, et al. Clinical grading of relative afferent pupillary defects. Arch Ophthalmol 1993; 111: 938–42.
16. Glazer-Hockstein C, Brookner AJ. The detection of a relative afferent pupillary defect. Am J Ophthalmol 2002; 134: 142–3.
17. Donahue SP, Moore P, Kardon RH. Automated pupil perimetry in amblyopia: generalized depression in the involved eye. Ophthalmology 2003; 104: 2161–7.
18. Kerrison JB, Buchanan K, Rosenberg ML, et al. Quantification of optic nerve axon loss associated with a relative afferent papillary defect in the monkey. Arch Ophthalmol 2001; 119: 1333–41.
19. Forman S, Behrens M, Odel J, et al. Relative afferent pupillary defect with normal visual function. Arch Ophthalmol 1990; 108: 1073–5.
20. Miller SD, Thompson HS. Pupil cycle time. Am J Ophthalmol 1978; 83: 635–42.
21. Manor RS, Yassur Y, Siegal R, et al. The pupil cycle time test: age variations in normal subjects. Br J Ophthalmol 1981; 65: 750–3.
22. Newman SA, Miller NR. The optic tract syndrome: neuro-ophthalmic considerations. Arch Ophthalmol 1983; 101: 1241–50.
23. Lam BL, Thompson HS. An anisocoria produces a small relative afferent pupil defect in the eye with the smaller pupil. J Neuro-ophthalmol 1999; 19: 153–9.
24. Dasco CC, Bortz DL. Significance of the Argyll Robertson pupils in clinical medicine. Am J Med 1989; 86: 199–202.
25. Lee AG. Sylvian aqueduct syndrome. J Neurosurg 1999; 91: 169–70.
26. Hagel T, Kolling GH, Dithmar S. Atypical tonic pupil as complication of chickenpox infection. Ophthalmologe 2003; 100: 330–3.
27. Thompson HS. Adie's syndrome: some new observations. Trans Am Ophthalmol Soc 1977; 75: 587–626.
28. Dulton G, Paul R. Adie syndrome in a child: a case report. J Pediatr Ophthalmol Strabismus 1992; 29: 126.
29. Thompson HS. Segmental palsy of the iris sphincter in Adie's syndrome. Arch Ophthalmol 1978; 96: 1615–20.
30. Purcell JJ, Krachmer JH, Thompson HS. Corneal sensation in Adie's syndrome. Am J Ophthalmol 1977; 84: 496–500.
31. Bourgon P, Pilley SF, Thompson SH. Cholinergic supersensitivity of the iris sphincter of Aide's tonic pupil. Am J Ophthamol 1978; 85: 373–7.
32. Loewenfeld IE, Thompson HS. Mechanism of tonic pupil. Ann Neurol 1981; 10: 275–6.
33. Ponsford JR, Bannister R, Paul EA. Methacholine pupillary responses in third nerve palsy and Adie's syndrome. Brain 1982; 105: 583–7.
34. Selhorst JB, Madge G, Ghatak N. The neuropathology of the Holmes-Adie syndrome. Ann Neurol 1984; 16: 138–9.
35. Loewenfeld IE, Thompson HS. The tonic pupil: a re-evaluation. Am J Ophthalmol 1967; 63: 46–87.
36. Jacobson DM. Benign episodic unilateral mydriasis. Clinical characteristics. Ophthalmology 1995; 102: 1625–7.
37. Balaguer-Santamaria JA, Escofet-Soteras C. Episodic benign unilateral mydriasis. Clinical case in a girl. Rev Neurol 2000; 31: 743–5.
38. Selhorst JB, Hoyt WF, Feinsod M, et al. Midbrain corectopia. Arch Neurol 1976; 33: 193–5.
39. Fisher CM. Oval pupils. Arch Neurol 1980; 37: 502–3.
40. Korczyn AD, Rubenstein AE, Yahr MD, et al. The pupil in familial dysautonomia. Neurology 1981; 31: 628–9.
41. Balaggan KS, Hugkulstone CE, Bremmer FD. Episodic segmental iris dilator muscle spasm: the tadpole pupil. Arch Ophthalmol 2003; 121: 744–5.
42. Goldstein SM, Liu GT, Edmond JC, et al. Orbital neuro-glial hamartoma associated with congenital tonic pupil. J AAPOS 2002; 6: 54–5.
43. Van Lieshout JJ, Wieling W, Van Montfrans GA, et al. Acute dysautonomia associated with Hodgkin's disease. J Neurol Neurosurg Psychiatr 1986; 49: 830–2.
44. Barricks ME, Flynn JT, Kushner BJ. Paradoxical pupillary responses in congenital stationary night blindness. Arch Ophthalmol 1977; 95: 1800.
45. Frank JW, Kushner BJ, France TD. Paradoxical pupillary phenomena. A review of patients with pupillary constriction to darkness. Arch Ophthalmol 1998; 106: 1564–6.
46. Yinon U, Urinowsky E, Barishak Y-TR. Paradoxical pupillary constriction in dark reared chicks. Vision Res 1981; 21: 1319–22.
47. Jeffery AR, Ellis FJ, Repka MX, et al. Pediatric Horner syndrome. J AAPOS 1998; 2: 159–67.
48. Thompson HS. Diagnosing Horner's syndrome. Trans Am Ophthalmol Soc 1977; 83: 840–2.
49. Nielson PJ. Upside down ptosis in Horner's syndrome. Acta Ophthalmol 1983; 61: 952–8.
50. Makley LB, Abbott K. Neurogenic heterochromia: A report of an interesting case. Am J Ophthalmol 1965; 59: 297–9.
51. George ND, Gonzalez G, Hoyt CS. Does Horner's syndrome in infancy require investigation. Br J Ophthalmol 1998; 82: 51–4.
52. McCartney A, Riordan-Eva P, Howes R, et al. Horner's syndrome: an electron microscopic study of human iris. Br J Ophthalmol 1992; 76: 746–9.
53. Kardon RH, Dennison CE, Brown CK, et al. Cortical enucleation of the cocaine test in the diagnosis of Horner syndrome. Arch Ophthalmol 1990; 108: 384–7.
54. Brown SM, Aouchiche R, Freeman KA. The utility of 0.5% apraclonidine in the diagnosis of Horner syndrome. Arch Ophthalmol 2003; 121: 1201–3.
55. Thompson BM, Corbett JJ, Kline LB, et al. Pseudo-Horner's syndrome. Arch Neurol 1982; 39: 108–11.
56. Nielson PJ. The corneal thickness and Horner's syndrome. Acta Ophthalmol 1983; 61: 467–73.
57. Weinstein J, Zweifel TJ, Thompson HS. Congenital Horner's syndrome. Arch Ophthalmol 1980; 98: 1074–8.
58. Mobius PJ. Zur Pathologie des Halssympathicus. Klin Wochenschr 1884; 15–18.

59. Robinson GC, Dikrainian DA, Roseborough GF. Congenital Horner's syndrome and heterochromia iridium: their association with congenital foregut and vertebral anomalies. Pediatrics 1965; 35: 103–7.

60. Borzyskowski M, Harris R, Jones R. The congenital varicella syndrome. Eur J Pediatr 1981; 137: 335–8.

61. Guy J, Day AL, Mickle JP, et al. Contralateral trochlear nerve paresis and ipsilateral Horner's syndrome. Am J Ophthalmol 1989; 107: 73–7.

62. Parsa CF, George ND, Hoyt CS. Pharmacological reversal optosis in a patient with acquired Horner's syndrome and heterochromia. Br J Ophthalmol 1998; 82: 1095.

63. Lowenstein O, Levine AS. Periodic sympathetic spasm and relaxation and role of sympathetic system in pupillary innervation. Arch Ophthalmol 1944; 31: 74–94.

64. Kline LB, McCluer SM. Oculosympathetic spasm with cervical spinal cord injury. Arch Neurol 1984; 41: 61–4.

65. Gadoth N, Margalith D, Bechar M. Unilateral pupillary dilatation during focal seizures. J Neurol 1981; 225: 227–30.

66. Drummond PD. Cervical sympathetic deficit in unilateral migraine headache. Headache 1991; 31: 669–72.

67. Jammes JL. Fixed dilated pupils in petit mal attacks. Neuro-ophthalmol 1980; 1: 155–9.

68. Daroff RB. Ocular motor manifestations of brainstem and cerebellar dysfunction. In: Smith JL, editor. Neuroophthalmology. St Louis: Mosby; 1971: 104–18. (Vol. 5.)

69. Repka MX. Eye drops and patches both in fact work for amblyopia. BMJ 2002; 324: 1397.

70. Chrousos GA, O'Neill JF, Cogan DG. Absence of the near reflex in a healthy adolescent. J Pediatr Ophthalmol Strabismus 1985; 22: 76–7.

71. Hibbert FG, Goldstein V, Osborne SM. Defective accommodation in members of one family. Tr Ophthalmol Soc UK 1975; 95: 455–61.

72. Hein PA. Unilateral paralysis of accommodation. Am J Ophthalmol 1961; 52: 711–12.

73. Mantyjarvi MI. Accommodation in school children with music or sports activities. Pediatr J Ophthalmol Strabismus 1988; 25: 3–7.

74. Hammerberg E, Norm MS. Defective dissociation of accommodation and convergence in dyslexic children. Br Orthopic J 1974: 31: 96–8.

75. Shaywitz SE, Shaywitz BA. The science of reading and dyslexia. J AAPOS 2003; 7: 158–66.

76. Goldstein JH, Schneekloth BB. Spasm of the near reflex: A spectrum of anomalies. Surv Ophthalmol 1996; 40: 269–78.

77. Chan RV, Trobe JD. Spasms of accommodation associated with closed head trauma. J Neuroophthalmol 2002; 22: 15–7.

78. Montiero ML, Curi AL, Pereira A, et al. Persistent accommodative spasm after head trauma. Br J Ophthalmol 2003; 87: 243–4.

79. Lam BL, Thompson HS, Corbett JJ. The prevalence of simple anisocoria. Am J Ophthalmol 1987; 104: 69–73.

80. Smith SA, Ellis CJK, Smith SE. Inequality of the direct and consensual light reflexes in normal subjects. Br J Ophthalmol 1979; 63: 523–7.

CHAPTER
68 Leukemia

David Taylor and David Webb

INTRODUCTION

Combination chemotherapy for acute leukemia in children is highly effective. Five-year survival rates of over 80% are usual for acute lymphoblastic leukemia (ALL) and up to 60% for acute myeloid leukaemia[1] (AML). The majority of treatment failures are due to recurrent leukemia, and treatment-related deaths have become less common with improved supportive care.

Acute lymphoblastic leukemia is the most common cancer in childhood, accounting for more than 30% of cases, with 400–500 new children diagnosed annually in the United Kingdom. Therapy extending over 2 or 3 years is associated with low treatment-related mortality (4%). Several clinical and biological criteria, including age (infants under 1 and children over 10 years suffer high relapse rates), high presenting white blood cell count, slow response to initial therapy, and several chromosomal changes within the leukemic cells, adversely affect prognosis. These adverse factors are used to divide children into subgroups, and treatment strategies adjust for these effects by increasing therapy for those children with higher risk of relapse. This approach has successfully closed the gap in treatment success rates originally identified between the subgroups of patients.

Almost all children are treated with chemotherapy initially, and bone marrow transplantation is reserved for around 10% of children with initial very poor prognosis, or following relapse. Acute myeloid leukemia is relatively rare, accounting for 5% of children's cancers, with only 60–70 new cases in children in the UK each year. Treatment is very intensive over 5 or 6 months with long inpatient stays. Chemotherapy is increasingly effective, and whereas bone marrow transplantation was considered for all children in the early 1990s, fewer are now selected unless chemotherapy has failed. Outcome of therapy is strongly related to chromosomal changes in the leukemic cells and response to initial treatment, and these factors are used to divide children into subgroups in a manner similar to that for acute lymphoblastic disease.

Common sites of disease at presentation are bone marrow, blood, lymph nodes, liver, and spleen. Eye involvement in leukemia is particularly interesting because it is the only site where the leukemic involvement of nerves and blood vessels can be directly observed, because the eye may act as a "sanctuary" for leukemic cells against chemotherapy, and because in the occasional patient the eye complications may be the major residual disability.[2] Serious eye involvement is unusual,[3] although the ophthalmic manifestations of leukemia in childhood may be dramatic, and are more a feature of relapse than of initial presentation. Nonetheless, ocular involvement when it occurs is important and demands prompt diagnosis and treatment.

ORBIT

The incidence in published series has varied with referral patterns, but leukemia is probably a small, but significant cause of proptosis in children. Orbital disease is more likely to be found in uncontrolled disease, and in a postmortem study[4] of patients of all ages orbital involvement was found in 7.3% of patients dying with acute leukemia.

Orbital presentation may occur without eye involvement and it may be the only manifestation, especially in AML.[5] Myeloid leukemia may present as an isolated solid tumor mass (granulocytic sarcoma) at a variety of sites, including the orbit (Figs. 68.1, 68.2). A greenish tinge to the tissue mass led to the term chloroma: this appearance may be due to myeloperoxidase, or from altered blood products.

Orbital involvement in leukemia may be due to bone or soft tissue infiltration, tumor formation, or hemorrhage; the lacrimal gland,[6] or lacrimal drainage apparatus[7] may be primarily involved, with an initially more benign diagnosis. Children with orbital involvement present with proptosis,[8] chemosis, and, rarely, muscle involvement; these may occur early in the course of the disease.[9] It may be difficult to differentiate between primary leukemic infiltration and complications such as hemorrhage or opportunistic infection and a biopsy may be necessary.[10] Exposure keratitis may occur.[11] It is important that any biopsy is representative and from the center of the abnormal area, not from the periphery where secondary inflammatory changes may occur.

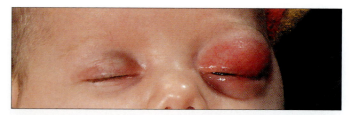

Fig. 68.1 Myeloid leukemia presenting as proptosis and orbital mass.

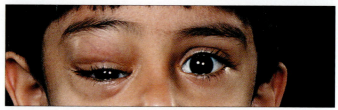

Fig. 68.2 "Chloroma" due to myeloid leukemia.

Review of the blood count and blood film, and thorough clinical assessment prior to biopsy, together with a bone marrow examination at the time of biopsy, are important steps. Close liaison with a pediatric oncologist is essential.

LIDS

The lids are usually only involved as a part of orbital infiltration, but can be due to direct leukemic infiltration.[4,12]

CONJUNCTIVA

The conjunctiva may be involved by hemorrhage (Fig. 68.3), infiltration[13] (Fig. 68.4), or hyperviscosity, when the vessels are tortuous or comma-shaped. Conjunctival mass formation is rare, but can be the presenting sign in acute leukemia.[4]

CORNEA AND SCLERA

Being avascular, the cornea is not often involved in the leukemias, but it may be involved in herpes simplex or zoster in the immune-compromised child, or by other inflammatory disease. Conjunc-

tival staining with fluorescein may be exacerbated by bone marrow transplantation and total body irradiation,[14] due to dry eye and decreased epithelial viability.

Corneal ulcers may be the presenting sign in acute leukemia.[15;16] They may respond to topical antibiotics and steroids. Perilimbal infiltrates have been described in a young adult with acute monocytic leukemia.[17] Scleral involvement has mainly been an autopsy finding.[4]

LENS

Cataracts occur frequently in patients who have had total body irradiation, related not only to the total dose, but also to the rate and fractionation of administration.[14,18] The use of steroids to treat graft-versus-host disease may cause or exacerbate cataracts.[18]

The treatment of cataracts, when visually significant, is usually by lens aspiration with lens implantation: the prognosis is good unless the cataracts are associated with other eye disease, e.g., retinal infections.

ANTERIOR CHAMBER, IRIS, AND INTRAOCULAR PRESSURE

Most reported cases have been of relapse in ALL (Fig. 68.5), but rarely children may present with a leukemic hyphema or hypopyon.[19] The anterior segment is an uncommon site of extramedullary relapse of ALL, accounting for up to 2% of all relapses;[4,20,21] it is very rare in AML.[19,22,23]

The relative infrequency of concurrent central nervous system relapse suggests that seeding from the central nervous system is not important.[22] The infiltration is most likely to be blood-borne and the relatively frequent occurrence of isolated anterior segment relapse supports the concept of the eye as a sanctuary site.[24] Because of the blood–eye barrier, chemotherapeutic agents do not penetrate the eye as well as many other sites, allowing leukemic cells to survive there, therefore causing signs and symptoms after chemotherapy has been stopped.

Symptoms include redness, watering, and photophobia (Fig. 68.6), and the parents may notice changes in the shape or reactions of the pupil or in the color and appearance of the iris (Fig. 68.7). Pain and visual loss may occasionally occur.

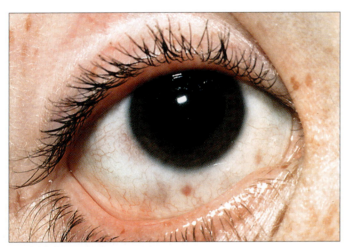

Fig. 68.3 Conjunctival hemorrhages and infiltration in acute lymphoblastic leukemia.

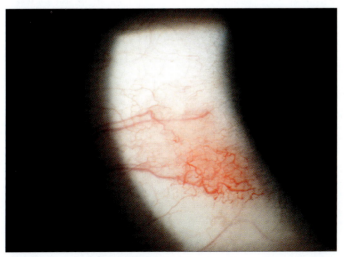

Fig. 68.4 Conjunctival infiltration with leukemic cells.

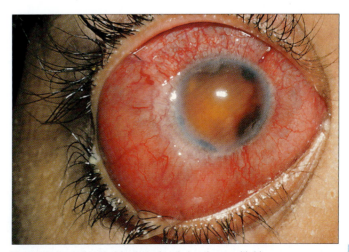

Fig. 68.5 Acute lymphoblastic leukemia in relapse with iris, subconjunctival and scleral invasion, and glaucoma.

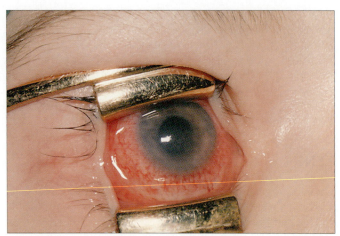

Fig. 68.6 ALL with eye relapse presenting as an acute red and painful eye due to glaucoma.

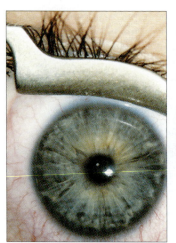 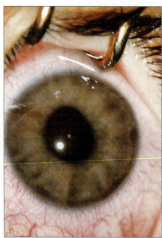

Fig. 68.8 Iris relapse with heterochromia, infiltrated left iris, and sluggish pupil reactions.

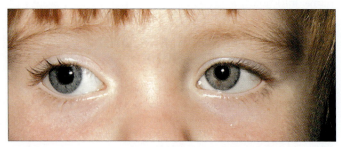

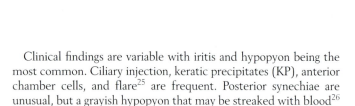

Fig. 68.7 Heterochromia iridis due to iris relapse in the left eye.

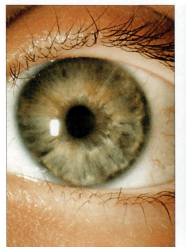 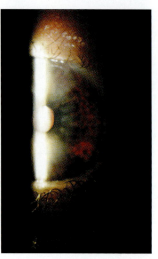

Fig. 68.9 Same patient as that in Fig. 68.8. After treatment with 2500 cGy there is iris transilluminance. The right eye had become affected.

Clinical findings are variable with iritis and hypopyon being the most common. Ciliary injection, keratic precipitates (KP), anterior chamber cells, and flare[25] are frequent. Posterior synechiae are unusual, but a grayish hypopyon that may be streaked with blood[26] is common.

Other causes of hyphema include juvenile xanthogranuloma, retinoblastoma, retrolental fibroplasia, persistent hyperplastic primary vitreous, iridoschisis, unsuspected trauma, iris vascular malformations, rubeosis iridis, and other blood dyscrasias.

Secondary glaucoma is common and is associated with corneal edema, pain, and redness.[19]

The iris may be thickened either diffusely (Fig. 68.8) or in the form of one or more nodules or a mass of variable size; the iris may also be thinned with loss of pigment (Fig. 68.9). The iris color may be changed, usually by a brownish discoloration, and the thickening of the iris obliterates the iris crypts and may give a rather featureless iris. Rubeosis may occur. It is often the failure of standard treatment for uveitis that draws the ophthalmologist's attention to the underlying leukemia. Unless the diagnosis is obvious,[27] it should not be assumed that any uveitis is leukemic: histological confirmation must be obtained. The diagnosis is best established by a combination of an anterior chamber paracentesis and iridectomy[22]: a paracentesis alone may not be sufficient to give an accurate diagnosis. Pathological studies show leukemic infiltration of the iris and trabecular meshwork,[4,28] and the hypopyon consists of leukemic cells, necrotic tissue, and proteinaceous exudate. Leukemic cells may be difficult to find. Patients with glaucoma have histological evidence of leukemic obstruction of the outflow channels and episcleral vessels.

Because children with an apparently localized relapse generally have submicroscopic disease in the bone marrow, retreatment[29] requires full systemic therapy plus local ocular radiotherapy (at least 2000 cGy) and topical steroid treatment. With this approach, long-term survival and likely cure has been achieved in a substantial proportion of patients.[21]

CHOROID

The choroid may be the part of the eye most frequently involved in all types of leukemia,[4,30,31] but it only rarely becomes clinically apparent. The clinical manifestations are the result of serous retinal detachment[32] or retinal detachment[9] associated with a subretinal mass (Fig. 68.10). Retinal infarction occurs with ophthalmic artery occlusion, and chronic or focal ischemia results in retinal pigment epithelial defects and clumping. Fluorescein angiography demonstrates myriads of diffuse leakage points at the level of the retinal pigment epithelium.[33] Similar fluorescein patterns are seen in serous detachments with melanoma, metastatic tumor, Vogt-Koyanagi-Harada disease, and posterior scleritis. Leukemic choroidopathy can be detected by ultrasound.

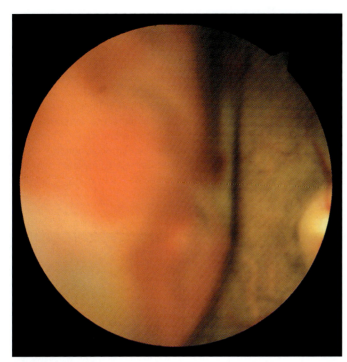

Fig. 68.10 Choroidal mass in ALL.

RETINA AND VITREOUS

The retina, because of its ready visibility, is the part of the eye most frequently found to be involved clinically, and funduscopy is part of the routine follow-up examination of leukemic patients.

Hyperviscosity changes

Hyperviscosity of the blood occurs in many cases of chronic leukemia, but is only clinically significant with very high blood cell counts, as in monocytic AML.

Vascular tortuosity and dilatation with irregularity or "beading" of the veins, sheathing, and hemorrhages are the earliest manifestations.

Fluorescein angiography and trypsin digests[4] show capillary saccular and fusiform microaneurysms, and neovascularization occurs in chronic myeloid leukemia (Fig. 68.11). The latter seems to be more closely related to the longevity of the disease and the increased amounts of blood cells, giving rise to a prolonged hyperviscosity, reduced flow with capillary closure, microaneurysm formation, and neovascularization.[34]

Retinal hemorrhages

Hemorrhages occur as a result of a combination of hyperviscosity, coagulation, infiltration, damage to retinal vessel walls, and vessel occlusion.[35]

Hemorrhages occur throughout the retina and may involve the vitreous. They may be massive and involve the whole eye (Fig. 68.12).

Nerve fiber layer hemorrhages are seen as bright red hemorrhages with at least one margin being "flame-shaped." Deeper hemorrhages are not quite so red and usually more rounded. Subhyaloid hemorrhages have sharply defined margins and can form a fluid level (Fig. 68.13) in which there may be a layer of white cells (Fig. 68.14).

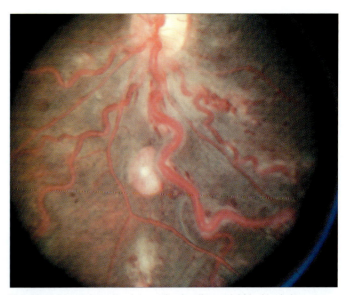

Fig. 68.11 Hyperviscosity changes in chronic myeloid leukemia in a 20-year-old (Dr S Day's patient).

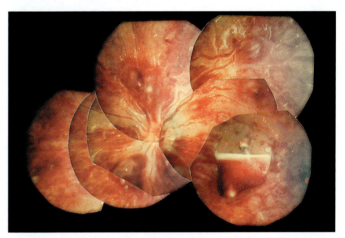

Fig. 68.12 Widespread retinal infiltrates and hemorrhages in all layers of the retina in acute lymphoblastic leukemia.

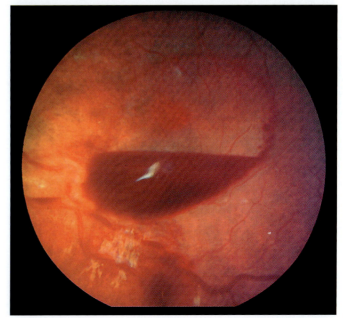

Fig. 68.13 Subhyaloid hemorrhages with fluid levels in acute lymphoblastic leukemia with anemia, and thrombocytopenia.

Some hemorrhages are white centered; this should not be confused with the pinpoint white light reflex from the apex of a hemorrhage, or with hemorrhage around a leukemic deposit. The white area consists of platelet and fibrin deposits that occlude the vessel, or septic emboli. The hemorrhage occurs because of infarction and weakening of the vessel wall, which can also be damaged by leukemic deposits, giving the picture of mixed hemorrhage and infiltration (Fig. 68.15).

Retinal infiltrates and white patches

White areas in the retinas of leukemic children may be caused by the following:

1. Vessel sheathing.[36]
2. Retinal infiltrates: these are leukemic deposits (Fig. 68.16), which, before the era of modern chemotherapy, were commonly seen, often with hemorrhage; they can usually be distinguished from infections by clinical and hematological examination.[37]
3. Cotton-wool spots: these are retinal nerve fiber layer infarcts (Fig. 68.17) and occur frequently in acute leukemia[4] and transiently after bone marrow transplantation. They presumably occur because of retinal vascular occlusion in patients who have recently received bone marrow transplants, whether or not they have been treated with ciclosporin. They can

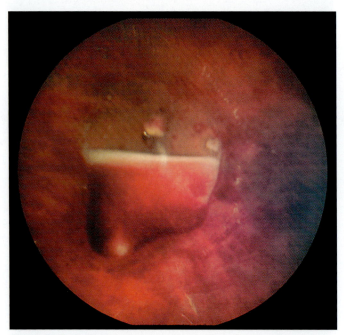

Fig. 68.14 Subhyaloid hemorrhage with a gross leukemic cell content.

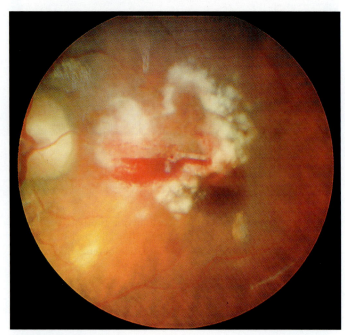

Fig. 68.16 Retinal infiltrates in acute lymphoblastic leukemia.

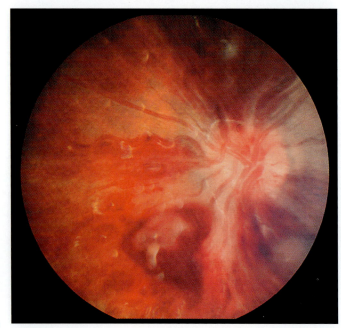

Fig. 68.15 Retinal hemorrhages and infiltrates in acute lymphoblastic leukemia.

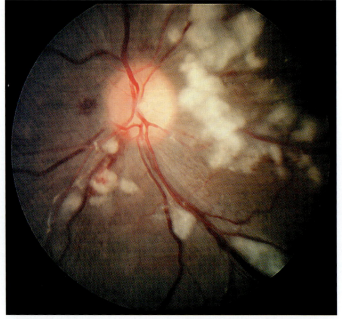

Fig. 68.17 Transient multiple cotton-wool spots after bone marrow transplant.

recover spontaneously and have been shown to be associated with retinal vascular endotheliopathy.[38]

4. Hard exudates: these small yellowish lesions are seen in relation to vessels that are chronically leaking noncellular blood elements and are most frequently seen in chronic leukemias with hyperviscosity.
5. Opportunistic infections with cytomegalovirus or fungus[39] in the immunosuppressed.
6. Retinal infarction in the acute stage: this gives rise to large areas of cloudy swelling of the retinal nerve fibers and ganglion cell layer.

Retinal infarction

Occlusion of larger retinal arterioles or of the ophthalmic artery (Fig. 68.18) occasionally occurs as a preterminal event.[2]

Vitreous cells

Vitreous involvement with leukemic or blood cells is usually but not always[40,41] secondary to retinal or choroidal infiltration[32] or hemorrhage.[4] Occasionally vitreous aspiration may be needed to confirm the diagnosis,[42] especially if the patient is apparently in remission and there is a possibility of an opportunistic infection. Vitreous organization (Fig. 68.19) is an unusual but serious sequel to widespread retinal or optic nerve infiltration.

Other retinal manifestations

Serous retinopathy[33] and retinal pigment clumping occur as manifestations of choroidal involvement.

OPTIC NERVE

Optic nerve involvement in postmortem cases occurs in nearly one-fifth of acute or chronic leukemias,[4] although in clinical series

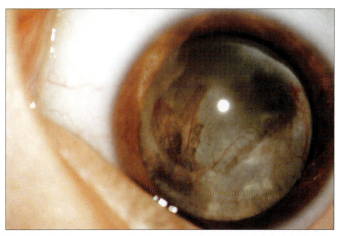

Fig. 68.19 Vitreous organization in acute lymphoblastic leukemia following leukemic retinopathy and choroidopathy.

it is more frequently seen in ALL.[43,44] Optic nerve involvement, which used to presage death, is now less frequently seen presumably due to aggressive chemotherapy.[34]

Leukemic optic neuropathy may cause only minimal visual symptoms despite even massive involvement, but often marked loss of central vision is observed, especially with infiltration behind the lamina cribrosa.[34] With prelaminar infiltration (Fig. 68.20) there is ophthalmoscopically visible fluffy white infiltration with hemorrhage, but on occasion, especially if the infiltration is bilateral, the differentiation from papilledema may be difficult and infectious disease must be remembered.[39]

The response to irradiation at 2000 cGy may be dramatic;[44] whatever the treatment, optic atrophy is a frequent sequel.[45]

An optic neuropathy may also be caused by vincristine treatment[46] or by radiotherapy.

OTHER NEURO-OPHTHALMIC INVOLVEMENT

Central nervous system involvement with leukemia manifests as meningeal irritation, with headaches and vomiting, or cranial nerve involvement. Vessel occlusion gives rise to various defects from transient deafness to an hypoxic encephalopathy,[47] but is usually a feature of leukemia with a very high white blood cell count and hyperviscosity. Communicating hydrocephalus,[48] chiasmal infiltration,[49] and sixth nerve palsies[50] have also been described.

In addition to the disease, many of the drugs and radiotherapy used may have central nervous system side-effects, both short and long term, including fits. Rarely children may develop a leukoencephalopathy due to methotrexate and cranial radiation.

With refinements in therapy, neurological complications of leukemia and its treatment are less common than previously. Better supportive care has reduced the incidence of hemorrhage, and refinements in therapy have reduced leukoencephalopathy. Infection by measles, varicella, or mumps occurred more frequently in older series, but has been reduced by vaccination programs and immunoglobulin prophylaxis in children with proven contacts. Bacterial infections of the CNS are rare.

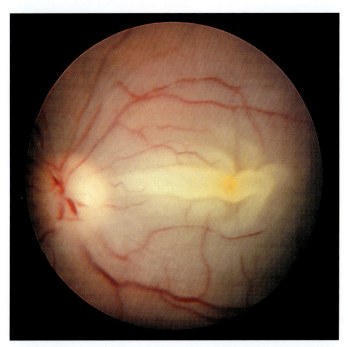

Fig. 68.18 Ophthalmic artery occlusion as a preterminal event.

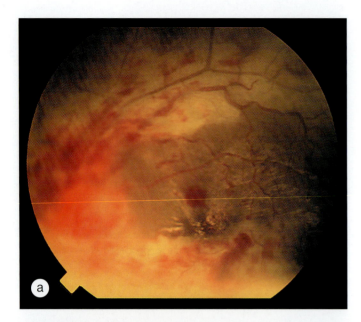

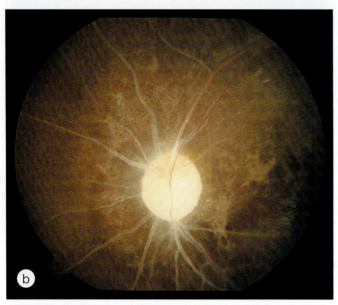

Fig. 68.20 (a) Gross optic nerve head and retinal involvement in acute lymphoblastic leukemia. (b) Profound optic atrophy and vascular attenuation following treatment with radiotherapy (same patient).

COMPLICATIONS OF TREATMENT

Drugs

Vincristine and other vinca alkaloids may cause corneal hypo-esthesia, ptosis, third, sixth and seventh nerve palsies, and optic neuropathy, which may be reversible if the treatment is stopped early. The neuropathy is dose-related and is most frequently seen initially as a peripheral neuropathy with abnormal deep tendon reflexes. Seizures also occur.

L-Asparaginase may occasionally and idiosyncratically be associated with a severe encephalopathy, which may be fatal.

Cytarabine may cause blurred vision from conjunctivitis, corneal epithelial opacities, and microcysts.

Methotrexate is a significant cause of neurological problems including arachnoiditis from intrathecal administration, seizures,

skin rashes, depression, and leukoencephalopathy with ataxia and dementia.

Steroids may cause posterior subcapsular cataracts often not of great visual significance[51] and which have a good prognosis with conventional surgery (Fig, 68.21).

Rapid withdrawal of steroid therapy may cause idiopathic intra-cranial hypertension (pseudotumor cerebri) (Fig. 68.22).

Immune suppression

Anti-leukemia chemotherapy, steroids, and radiotherapy all contribute to immune suppression, which allows infection by opportunistic bacteria, viruses (Fig. 68.23), fungi, or protozoa, some of which do not usually cause significant infection in humans. These complications are related to the intensity of immune suppression and so are most likely following bone marrow transplantation. As broad-spectrum antibiotics have become used aggressively for unexplained fever in neutropenic children, uncontrolled bacterial infections have become less frequent but viruses and fungi have assumed an increasing prominence.

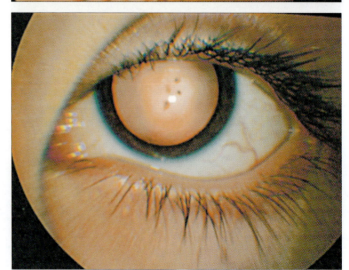

Fig. 68.21 Posterior subcapsular cataracts in a patient after bone marrow transplant. The acuity was 0.0 logMAR.

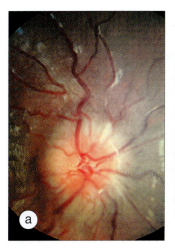
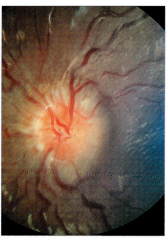

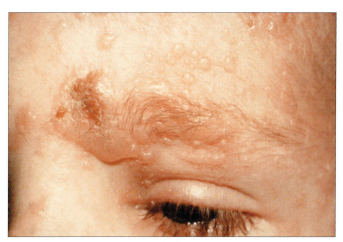

Fig. 68.23 Confluent varicella in a patient with acute lymphoblastic leukemia in relapse.

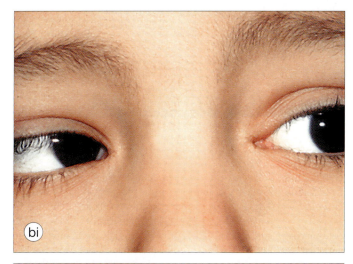

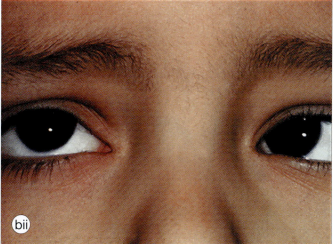

Fig. 68.22 (a) Papilledema and (b) right VI nerve paresis from idiopathic intracranial hypertension in a patient on withdrawal of steroids in ALL.

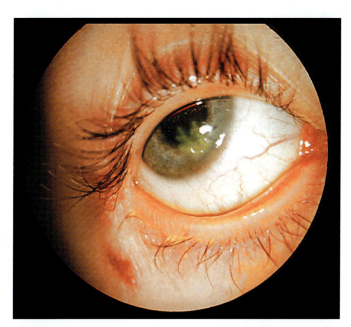

Fig. 68.24 Herpes simplex keratitis in a patient with acute lymphoblastic leukemia on chemotherapy.

Yeast[39] and fungal infections are important complications of neutropenia and, if possible, biopsy is necessary to establish the diagnosis and to plan appropriate treatment. Other infections include mucormycosis, toxoplasmosis, cytomegalovirus,[53] and aspergillosis.[54]

The risk for these infections is related to the severity of immune suppression and therefore highest in children who undergo bone marrow transplantation.

Stem cell transplantation

Bone marrow transplants (BMT) are sometimes necessary in the treatment of childhood leukemia, but as chemotherapy has become increasingly effective, the number of transplants has fallen. Few children now receive BMT as a first-choice therapy, but BMT is often considered in relapsed disease.[55]

In recent years the early hemopoietic progenitor cells required for BMT have increasingly been obtained from blood or cord

Herpes simplex and zoster affect the cornea (Fig.68.24), conjunctiva, and lids. Herpes simplex and cytomegalovirus, which have an affinity for neural tissue, may cause a severe necrotizing retinochoroiditis (Fig. 68.25) that may be difficult to differentiate from leukemic infiltrates, a distinction that can be helped by chorioretinal biopsym[52] but can usually be made by culture of urine or saliva.

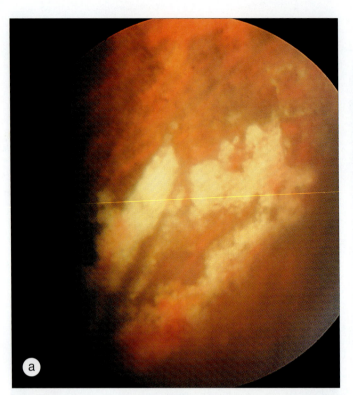
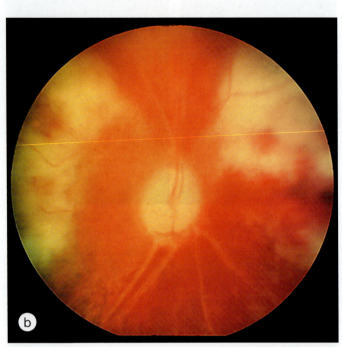

Fig. 68.25 (a, b) Cytomegalovirus retinitis in acute lymphoblastic leukemia in relapse.

blood collections, and the term stem cell transplant (SCT) has supplanted BMT. There are two main types of SCT:

1. Allogeneic, when related or unrelated donor stem cells matched by HLA typing are infused; and
2. Autologous, when the patient's own stored stem cells are used.

Prior to the SCT, children receive chemotherapy alone or combined with total body irradiation (TBI) as both anti-leukemia and immune suppressive therapy, to avoid graft rejection. As the marrow regenerates with new stem cells, all blood cell lineages are donor derived. Ocular changes were found in 50% of children treated with BMT for hematological disorders.[56] The most frequent findings were dry eye (12%), cataracts (23%), and posterior segment complications (13%). These changes did not seriously compromise vision. Another study[57] identified ocular abnormalities in 82% of 29 children, usually in the anterior segment. Tear abnormalities were the most usual finding.

The incidence of eye complications depends on a variety of factors, primarily conditioning regimen, especially the use of TBI, the degree of immune suppression with risk of opportunistic infections, and the occurrence of graft-versus-host disease (GvHD). In one series,[58] cataracts were found in 95% of children given TBI, compared with 23% of children conditioned with chemotherapy alone. Low dose rates and fractionated rather than single-dose radiotherapy appear to be associated with a lower incidence of cataracts.[59] However, it is possible that these differences reflect alterations in the latent period before diagnosis, rather than a true reduction in eventual prevalence.

Because of failure to recognize the transplant recipient as "self," the transplanted T-lymphocytes may attack the recipient and cause graft-versus-host disease. Acute GvHD is characterized by the occurrence–within 4 months of the transplant–of any combination of fever, rash, diarrhea, and liver dysfunction. If the disorder either occurs or persists after this period, it is termed chronic GvHD (cGvHD). Ocular manifestations are common in cGvHD[60–62] and include dry eye, cicatricial lagophthalmos, sterile conjunctivitis, and uveitis. The eye problems are frequently severe and test the ophthalmologist's management of the dry eye. At autopsy the whole eye is affected including the lacrimal gland.[63] About 10% of patients undergoing BMT develop conjunctival involvement with GvHD.[64] Pseudomembranous conjunctivitis was the most frequent manifestation of conjunctival GvHD and carried a poor prognosis for life.

Opportunistic infections are a major risk of BMT, especially in mismatched transplants where depletion of T-lymphocytes from the marrow graft in order to minimize GvHD results in delayed immune reconstitution.

An interesting occurrence is the transient appearance of multiple white cotton-wool spots in BMT recipients.[65] Coskuncan et al. found retinal complications in 12.8% of 397 patients with BMT including retinal or vitreous hemorrhage, cotton-wool spots, optic disc edema, retinitis, lymphoma, and serous retinal detachments.[66]

THE OPHTHALMOLOGIST'S ROLE

Since ocular complications are rare there is probably no need for routine ophthalmological surveillance in these children as long as children at risk of eye complications are identified and examined, and the ophthalmologist usually only becomes involved by the referring oncologist or pediatrician, from whom most ophthalmologists can learn a lot about communication and patient management!

REFERENCES

1. Brenner H, Kaatsch P, Burkhardt-Hammer T, et al. Long-term survival of children with leukemia achieved by the end of the second millennium. Cancer 2001; 92: 1977–83.
2. Taylor DSI, Day SH. In: Smith JL, editor. Neurophthalmology Focus. New York: Massan; 1982: 281–90.
3. Hoover DL, Smith LEH, Turner SJ, et al. Ophthalmic evaluation of survivors of acute lymphoblastic leukemia. Ophthalmology 1988; 95: 151–5.
4. Kincaid MC, Green WR. Ocular and orbital involvement in leukemia. Surv Ophthalmol 1983; 27: 211–32.
5. Zimmerman LE, Font RL. Ophthalmologic manifestations of granulocytic sarcoma (myeloid sarcoma or chloroma). Am J Ophthalmol 1975; 80: 975–90.
6. Johnston DL. Relapse of childhood acute lymphoblastic leukemia in the lacrimal gland. Med Pediatr Oncol 2003; 40: 337–8.
7. Wirostko WJ, Garcia GH, Cory S, et al. Acute dacryocystitis as a presenting sign of pediatric leukemia. Am J Ophthalmol 1999; 127: 734–6.
8. Önder F, Kutluck S, Cosar CB, et al. Bilateral orbital involvement as a presenting sign in a child with acute lymphoblastic leukemia. J Pediatr Ophthalmol Strabismus 2000; 37: 235–7.
9. MacManaway JW, Neely JE. Choroidal and orbital leukemic infiltrate mimicking advanced retinoblastoma. J Pediatr Ophthalmol Strabismus 1994; 31: 394–6.
10. Rubinfeld RS, Gootenberg JE, Chavis RM, et al. Early onset acute orbital involvement in childhood acute lymphoblastic leukemia. Ophthalmology 1988; 95: 116–20.
11. Olson JL, May MJ, Stork L, et al. Acute megakaryoblastic leukemia in Down syndrome: orbital infiltration. Am J Ophthalmol 2000; 130: 128–30.
12. Tabata Y, Yoshihara T, Shirakami S, et al. Eyelid leukemia as a relapse sign of B-cell type acute lymphoblastic leukemia. Med Pediatr Oncol 2001; 36: 505–6.
13. Campagnoli MF, Parodi E, Linari A, et al. Conjunctival mass: an unusual presentation of acute lymphoblastic leukemia relapse in childhood. J Pediatr 2003; 142: 211.
14. Bray LC, Carey PJ, Proctor SJ, et al. Ocular complications of bone marrow transplantation. Br J Ophthalmol 1991; 75: 611–4.
15. Bhadresa GN. Changes in the anterior segment as a presenting feature in leukaemia. Br J Ophthalmol 1971; 55: 133–5.
16. Wood WJ, Nicholson DH. Corneal ring ulcer as the presenting manifestation of acute monocytic leukemia. Am J Ophthalmol 1973; 76: 69–72.
17. Font RL, Mackay B, Tang R. Acute monocytic leukemia recurring as bilateral perilimbal infiltrates: immunohistochemical and ultrastructural confirmation. Ophthalmology 1985; 92: 1681–5.
18. Livesey SJ, Holmes JA, Whittaker JA. Ocular complications of bone marrow transplantation. Eye 1989; 3: 271–6.
19. Tabbara KF, Beckstead JH. Acute promonocytic leukemia with ocular involvement. Arch Ophthalmol 1980; 98: 1055–9.
20. Bunin N, Rivera G, Goode F, et al. Ocular relapse in the anterior chamber in childhood acute lymphoblastic leukemia. J Clin Oncol 1987; 5: 299–303.
21. Somervaille TC, Hann IM, Harrison G, et al. Intraocular relapse of childhood acute lymphoblastic leukaemia. Br J Haematol 2003; 121: 280–8.
22. Novakovic P, Kellie S, Taylor D. Childhood leukaemia: relapse in the anterior segment of the eye. Br J Ophthalmol 1989; 73: 354–9.
23. Perry HD, Mallen FJ. Iris involvement in granulocytic sarcoma. Am J Ophthalmol 1979; 87: 530–2.
24. Ninane J, Taylor D, Day S. The eye as a sanctuary in acute lymphoblastic leukaemia. Lancet 1980; i: 452–3.
25. Zakka KA, Yee RD, Shorr N. Leukemic iris infiltration. Am J Ophthalmol 1980; 89: 204–9.
26. Hinzpeter EN, Knobel H, Freund J. Spontaneous haemophthalmos in leukaemia. Ophthalmologica 1978; 177: 224–8.
27. MacLean H, Clarke MP, Strong NP, et al. Primary ocular relapse in acute lymphoblastic leukemia. Eye 1996; 10: 719–22.
28. Jankovic M, Masera G, Uderzo C. Recurrences of isolated leukemic hypopyon in a child with acute lymphoblastic leukemia. Cancer 1986; 57: 380–4.
29. Patel SV, Herman DC, Anderson PM, et al. Iris and anterior chamber involvement in acute lymphoblastic leukemia. J Pediatr Hematol Oncol 2003; 25: 653–6.
30. Allen RA, Straatsma BR. Ocular involvement in leukemia and allied disorders. Arch Ophthalmol 1961; 66: 490–509.
31. Leonardy NJ, Rupani M, Dent G, et al. Analysis of 135 autopsy eyes for ocular involvement in leukemia. Am J Ophthalmol 1990; 109: 436–45.
32. Birinci H, Albayrak D, Oge I, et al. Ocular involvement in childhood acute lymphoblastic leukemia. J Pediatr Ophthalmol Strabismus 2001; 38: 242–4.
33. Kincaid MC, Green WR, Kelley JS. Acute ocular leukemia. Am J Ophthalmol 1979; 87: 698–702.
34. Rosenthal AR. Ocular manifestations of leukemia: a review. Ophthalmology 1983; 90: 899–905.
35. Kaur B, Taylor D. Fundus hemorrhages in infancy. Surv Ophthalmol 1991; 37: 1–19.
36. Kim TS, Duker JS, Hedges TR. Retinal angiopathy resembling unilateral frosted branch angiitis in a patient with relapsing acute lymphoblastic leukemia. Am J Ophthalmol 1994; 117: 806–8.
37. Gordon KB, Rugo HS, Duncan JL, et al. Ocular manifestations of leukemia: leukemic infiltration versus infectious process. Ophthalmology 2001; 108: 2293–300.
38. Webster AR, Anderson JR, Richards EM, et al. Ischaemic retinopathy occurring in patients receiving bone-marrow allografts and campath-IG: a clinicopathological study. Br J Ophthalmol 1995; 79: 687–91.
39. Song A, Dubovy SR, Berrocal AM, et al. Endogenous fungal retinitis in a patient with acute lymphocytic leukemia manifesting as uveitis and optic nerve lesion. Arch Ophthalmol 2002; 120: 1754–6.
40. Zhioua R, Boussen I, Malek I, et al. [Acute lymphoblastic leukemia and vitreous infiltration. A case study]. J Fr Ophtalmol 2001; 24: 180–2.
41. Reese AB, Guy L. Exophthalmos in leukemia. Am J Ophthalmol 1933; 16: 476–8.
42. Swartz M, Schumann OB. Comma-shaped venular segments of conjunctiva in chronic granulocytic leukemia. Am J Ophthalmol 1980; 90: 326–30.
43. Brown GC, Shields JA, Augsburger JJ, et al. Leukemic optic neuropathy. Int Ophthalmol 1981; 3: 111–6.
44. Rosenthal AR, Egbert PR, Wilbur JR, et al. Leukemic involvement of the optic nerve. J Paediatr Ophthalmol 1975; 12: 84–93.
45. Nikaido H, Mishima H, Ono H, et al. Leukemic involvement of the optic nerve. Am J Ophthalmol 1988; 105: 294–9.
46. Sanderson PA, Kuwabara T, Cogan DG. Optic neuropathy presumably caused by vincristine therapy. Am J Ophthalmol 1976; 81: 146–50.
47. Lilleyman J. Neurological complications of acute childhood leukaemia. J Roy Soc Med 1993; 86: 252–3.
48. De Reuck J, De Coster W, Vander Eecken H. Communicating hydrocephalus in treated leukaemic patients. Eur Neurol 1979; 18: 8–14.
49. Zimmerman LE, Thoreson HT. Sudden loss of vision in acute leukemia. Surv Ophthalmol 1964; 9: 467–73.
50. Abbassidum K. Headaches, vomiting and diplopia in a 16-year-old child. Clin Pediatr 1979; 18: 191–2.
51. Elliott AJ, Oakhill A, Goodman S. Cataracts in childhood leukaemia. Br J Ophthalmol 1985; 69: 459–61.
52. Taylor D, Day S, Tiedemann K, et al. Chorioretinal biopsy in a patient with leukaemia. Br J Ophthalmol 1981; 65: 489–93.
53. Baumal CR, Levin AV, Read SE. Cytomegalovirus retinitis in immunosuppressed children. Am J Ophthalmol 1999; 127: 550–8.
54. Maalouf T, Schmitt C, Crance J, et al. [Endogenous aspergillus endophthalmitis: a case report]. J Fr Ophtalmol 2000; 23: 170–3.
55. Chessells JM. Bone marrow transplantation for leukaemia. Arch Dis Child 1988; 63: 879–82.
56. Suh DW, Ruttum MS, Stuckenschneider BJ, et al. Ocular findings after bone marrow transplantation in a pediatric population. Ophthalmology 1999; 106: 1564–70.
57. Ng JS, Lam DS, Lö CK, et al. Ocular complications of pediatric bone marrow transplantation. Ophthalmology 1999; 106: 160–4.
58. Holmström G, Borgstrom B, Calissendorff B. Cataract in children after bone marrow transplantation. Acta Ophthalmol Scand 2002; 80: 211–5.
59. Leiper AD. Non-endocrine late complications of bone marrow transplant in childhood: part II. Br J Haematol 2002; 118: 23–43.

60. Arocker-Mettinger E, Skorpik F, Grabner G, et al. Manifestations of graft-versus-host disease following allogenic bone marrow transplantation. Eur J Ophthalmol 1991; 1: 28–32.

61. Franklin RM, Kenneth KR, Tutschka PJ. Ocular manifestations of graft-vs-host disease. Ophthalmology 1983; 90: 4–13.

62. Jack MK, Jack GM, Sale GE, et al. Ocular manifestations of graft-v-host disease. Arch Ophthalmol 1983; 101: 1080–4.

63. Jabs DA, Hirst LW, Green WR, et al. The eye in bone marrow transplantation II. Histopathology. Arch Ophthalmol 1983; 101: 585–90.

64. Jabs DA, Wingard J, Green WR, et al. The eye in bone marrow transplantation III. Conjunctival graft-vs-host disease. Arch Ophthalmol 1989; 107: 1343–9.

65. Gratwahl A, Gloor D, Hann H, et al. Retinal cotton-wool patches in bone-marrow transplant recipients. N Engl J Med 1983; 308: 110–1.

66. Coskuncan NM, Jabs DA, Dunn JP, et al. The eye in bone marrow transplantation VI. Retinal complications. Arch Ophthalmol 1994; 112: 372–9.

CHAPTER
69 Phakomatoses

John R Grigg and Robyn V Jamieson

INTRODUCTION

Definition

The phakomatoses are a group of systemic disorders with neurologic, ophthalmic, and cutaneous manifestations. Van der Hoeve first used the term when describing similarities between neurofibromatosis and tuberous sclerosis. No precise definition exists for including a condition. A common feature is the development of multiorgan hamartomas. A hamartoma is a tumor mass arising as an anomaly of tissue formation. It is composed of tissue elements normally present in the involved organ or site. The most important of these conditions are neurofibromatosis, tuberous sclerosis, Sturge-Weber syndrome, and von Hippel-Lindau syndrome. Other conditions sometimes included are Klippel-Trénaunay-Weber syndrome, Wyburn-Mason syndrome, diffuse congenital hemangiomatosis, linear nevus sebaceous syndrome, Osler-Weber-Rendu syndrome, and blue rubber bleb nevus syndrome.

NEUROFIBROMATOSIS

See Chapter 33.

TUBEROUS SCLEROSIS

Tuberous sclerosis complex (TSC) or tuberous sclerosis syndrome (TSS) is a multisystem disease characterized by hamartomatous growths in the brain, skin, kidneys, eyes, and heart but it may affect almost any organ. Malignant tumors are rare and occur predominantly in the kidney.[1] The disease has a prevalence of 4.9/100,000.[2]

Genetic insights

TSC is autosomal dominant with a high spontaneous mutation rate, so that in approximately two-thirds of cases there is no family history. Mutations in the genes *TSC1* and *TSC2* account for the majority of cases. *TSC1* at 9q34 contains 21 exons and encodes the protein hamartin. *TSC2* located at 16p13 contains 41 exons and encodes tuberin. Mutations are more frequently found in *TSC2* than in *TSC1*. Although there is overlap in the spectrum of clinical features of the *TSC1* and *TSC2* mutation patients, sporadic patients with *TSC1* mutations generally have milder disease than those with *TSC2* mutations. *TSC1* patients in general have a lower frequency of seizures, fewer cortical tubers, and less severe kidney and retinal involvement.[3]

Tuberin and hamartin interact directly. The tumor suppressor TSC1–TSC2 complex is integral in pathways regulating cell

growth by interactions with the insulin- and growth factor-stimulated protein kinases, protein kinase B (PKB)/Akt and p70 S6 ribosomal kinase.[4]

Diagnostic criteria

The clinical features are classified into major and minor features (Table 69.1a). Two major features or one major plus two minor features constitute a definitive diagnosis of TSC. One major plus one minor feature indicates a probable diagnosis of TSC. One major or two or more minor features suggest possible TSC.[5]

Neurological features

Epileptic seizures are the most frequent neurological manifestation. The onset of seizures is usually before 2 years of age. Infantile spasms are the predominant form of seizures, occurring in approximately 65% of cases. Partial seizures may precede, coexist with, or evolve into infantile spasms. The seizures may increase in frequency and severity with age. Moderate to severe learning disabilities occur in 38 to 80% of cases. Multiple behavioral problems including sleep disorders, hyperactivity, attention deficit disorder, and autism may also occur.

The CNS lesions include tubers in the cerebral cortex, subependymal nodules (Fig. 69.1a) and subependymal giant cell astrocytomas in the ventricular system (Fig. 69.1b). Tubers are

Table 69.1a Diagnostic criteria for tuberous sclerosis complex[a]

Major features	Minor features
1 Facial angiofibromas or forehead plaque	1. Multiple randomly distributed pits in dental enamel
2. Nontraumatic ungual or periungual fibroma	2. Hamartomatous rectal polyps
3. Hypomelanotic macules (more than 3)	3. Bone cysts
4. Shagreen patch (connective tissue nevus)	4. Cerebral white matter migration lines
5. Multiple retinal nodular hamartomas	5. Gingival fibromas
6. Cortical tuber	6. Nonrenal hamartomas
7. Subependymal nodule	7. Retinal achromatic patch
8. Subependymal giant cell astrocytoma	8. "Confetti" skin lesions (very small white macules)
9. Cardiac rhabdomyosarcoma, single or multiple	9. Multiple renal cysts
10. Lymphangiomyomatosis and or renal angiomyolipoma	

[a]From Hyman and Whittemore.[5] Reprinted with permission.

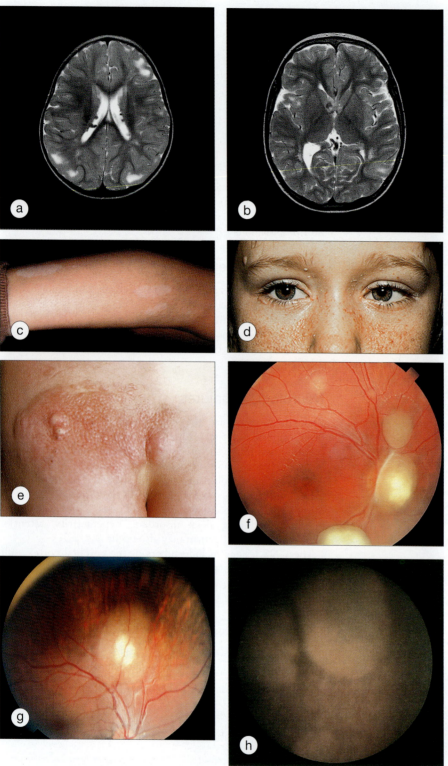

Fig. 69.1 Tuberous sclerosis: clinical features. (a) Cortical tubers show as hyperintense signals and the calcified subependymal nodules as hypointense signals projecting into lateral ventricles. T2 axial MRI scan. (b) Subependymal giant cell astrocytoma partly obstructing the foramen of Monro resulting in mild dilatation of the right lateral ventricle. T2 axial MRI scan. (c) Hypomelanotic macules (ash leaf spots). (d) Facial angiofibromas (formerly adenoma sebaceum) are typically distributed in a butterfly pattern. (e) Shagreen patch on the lower back. (f) Both translucent hamartomas and larger calcified hamartomas are shown in this case. The flat translucent lesions in this case are superior to the fovea within and above the superior vascular arcade. (g) A combined lesion with a flat hamartoma and a central nodular area. (h) A chorioretinal hypopigmented punched-out lesion. These are typically found in the midperiphery.

regions of cortical dysplasia arising from aberrant neuronal migration, cellular differentiation, and excessive cell proliferation. Tubers are static lesions related to the neurological manifestations of TSC, including a topographic relationship with EEG abnormalities. There is also an association of more severe mental retardation with a larger number of cortical tubers.[6]

MRI scanning is better than CT in demonstrating noncalcified subependymal nodules and tubers, although in asymptomatic patients, CT may be preferable because of lower cost and increased specificity. Positron emission tomography (PET) may reveal hypometabolic regions not predicted by MRI.

Dermatological manifestations

The most common of the cutaneous manifestations are hypomelanotic macules (ash leaf spots), which are present in 97% of children (Fig. 69.1c). They are asymmetrically distributed and are usually observed from birth, aided by a Woods ultraviolet light.

Facial angiofibromas (formerly known as adenoma sebaceum) are found in up to 75% of patients and become evident between 5 and 14 years of age (Fig. 69.1d). They are typically distributed in a "butterfly" pattern. Forehead fibrous plaques occur in 25% of cases and may precede facial angiofibromas. They are slightly elevated yellowish-brown or flesh-colored plaques that grow slowly rising several millimeters above the skin surface.

Shagreen patches are found in approximately 50% of cases (Fig. 69.1e). These lesions are flattened yellowish-red or pink with an orange skin texture located on dorsal surfaces particularly the lumbar region. Periungual fibromas also occur, with the toenails a common site. These fibromas arise from the nailbed beneath the nail plate or from the skin of the nail groove.[7]

Visceral features

Cardiac rhabdomyomas may be present in just less than half of TSC children, and may be single or multiple.[7] Echocardiography identifies the tumors that may be present from the neonatal period. They usually do not produce any hemodynamic disturbance and generally regress in childhood.

Renal lesions are a frequent finding in TSC patients by 18 years of age, and include benign angiomyolipomas, malignant angiomyolipomas, cysts, and renal cell carcinoma. Benign angiomyolipomas are the most common, occurring in 70–80% of older children and adults with TSC. Bleeding is a complication with lesions greater than 4 cm in diameter.

Other visceral involvement includes liver angiomyolipomas and lymphangiomyomatosis of the lung,[7] which predominantly affects females.[5]

Ocular features

Retinal hamartomas are one of the major diagnostic criteria for TSC. There are three basic morphological types:
(i) A relatively flat, smooth, noncalcified, gray translucent lesion (Fig. 69.1f);
(ii) An elevated, multinodular, calcified, opaque lesion resembling mulberries (Fig. 69.1f); and
(iii) A lesion that has features of both (Fig. 69.1g).
Retinal hamartomas occur in approximately 50% of TSC patients, are bilateral in approximately a third of cases, and are of multiple morphological types in a third of cases. The flat smooth translucent type is the commonest, occurring in 70% of patients with hamartomas. They may be difficult to see, manifesting as an abnormal light reflex, frequently superficial to retinal vessels located in the posterior pole and approximately 0.25 to 2 disc diameters in size.[1]

The multinodular "mulberry" lesion occurs in approximately 50% of patients with hamartomas. These are located in the posterior pole and are usually within 2 disc diameters of the optic disc. The size ranges from 0.25 to 4 disc diameters. The combined lesions with a flat hamartoma and a central nodular area are less common. Retinal hamartomas are not calcified in infancy but become so later in life. In general the lesions remain static. Rarely vitreous hemorrhage may be a complication presumably due to abnormal vessels involved with the hamartomas.

Other retinal findings include chorioretinal hypopigmented punched-out lesions, which occur in up to 40% of patients.[1] They are less than one disc diameter in size and are distributed in the midperipheral fundus (Fig. 69.1h). Papilledema and optic atrophy may be present as a manifestation of raised intracranial pressure complicating an intracranial lesion.

Nonretinal findings include angiofibromas of the eyelid, nonparalytic strabismus, and pseudo-colobomas of the lens and iris. Sector iris depigmentation has also been reported.[1] Myopia may be slightly more common in this group of patients than age-matched normals.[1]

Ocular management and monitoring of antiepileptic agents

The management of TSC requires a multidisciplinary approach (Table 69.1b). The ophthalmologist plays an important role in screening, assessment of visual development, and progression of lesions, and in the monitoring of ocular complications of antiepileptic medications.

Vigabatrin (GABA agonist) is an effective agent in the management of infantile spasms. A complication of vigabatrin therapy is the development of a specific visual field defect, resulting in bilateral and concentric constriction within a 30° radius from fixation. The defect commences with nasal loss extending in an annulus over the horizontal midline, with relative sparing of the temporal field. Forty to 50% of patients treated with vigabatrin are affected in time.

For monitoring of vigabatrin therapy, children with a cognitive age of ≥ 9 should undergo visual field examination with a Goldmann perimeter (11e or 12e isopter and 14e or V4e isopter) or a Humphrey field analyzer (age-related, three-zone suprathreshold strategy and the 120 degree field) before vigabatrin is prescribed and, ideally, every six months, particularly if they continue to take the drug. For children aged < 9, a full-field electroretinogram ERG looking for altered cone function and/or a multifocal (ERG) looking for a negative b wave are useful for monitoring therapy.[8]

Topiramate is an antiepileptic agent effective in partial seizures. A complication is a supraciliary effusion resulting in anterior displacement of the lens and iris, with induced myopia (up to 8 diopters) and angle closure glaucoma. Symptoms occur within 1 month of initiating therapy.[9] Cessation of topiramate results in clinical improvement. Medical and/or surgical management may be required to control the glaucoma until the drug is eliminated (2–14 days).

Table 69.1b Diagnostic and surveillance screening in tuberous sclerosis complex[a,b]

	"Asymptomatic" parent, child or first-degree relative at time of diagnosis of affected	Suspected case or initial diagnostic evaluation	Child		Adult	
			Known case and no symptoms in referable organ	*Known case and symptoms or findings previously documented*	*Known case and no symptoms in referable organ*	*Known case and symptoms or findings previously documented*
Fundus examination	+	+	–	+	–	+
Brain MRI	+[c]	+	+[d]	+	+[e]	+[f]
Brain EEG	–	–[g]	–	+[f]	–	+[f]
Cardiac ECG and ECHO	–[h]	+	–	+[i]	–	+[f]
Renal MRI, CT, or Ultrasound	+[j]	+	+[k]	+[i]	+d	+[i]
Dermatologic screening	+	+	–	+[f]	–	+[f]
Neurodevelopmental testing	–	+[l]	+[m]	+[f]	–	+[f]
Pulmonary CT	–	–	–	+[f]	+[n]	+[f]

[a] From Hyman and Whittemore.[5] Reprinted with permission.
[b] +, screening recommended; –, screening not recommended; MRI, magnetic resonance imaging; EEG, electroencephalogram; ECG, electrocardiogram; ECHO, echocardiogram; and CT, computed tomography.
[c] With negative physical examination results, CT is generally recommended.
[d] Every 1 to 3 years.
[e] Probably less frequently in children.
[f] As clinically indicated.
[g] Unless seizures are suspected, this is generally not useful for diagnosis.
[h] Unless needed for diagnosis.
[i] Every 6 months to 1 year until involution or size stabilizes.
[j] Ultrasound is generally recommended because of cost, although imaging expertise may vary.
[k] Every 3 years until adolescence.
[l] Generally for children only.
[m] Recommended for children at the time of beginning first grade.
[n] For women at age 18 years.

VON HIPPEL-LINDAU DISEASE

Von Hippel-Lindau (VHL) disease is a rare familial cancer syndrome causing susceptibility to benign vascular tumors of the eye and CNS (angioma or hemangioblastoma), renal-cell carcinoma (RCC), and pheochromocytoma. Cutaneous features are infrequent. VHL affects approximately 1 in 35,000 individuals and is transmitted in an autosomal dominant pattern. The majority of cases are familial, with 4–15% being sporadic due to new mutations.[10] Symptoms typically develop from the second to fourth decade.

Genetic insights

The von Hippel-Lindau disease is caused by a germ-line mutation of the *VHL* tumor-suppressor gene located at 3p25, and conforms to the Knudson 2 hit model. The VHL protein regulates the hypoxia-inducible factor (HIF) protein in an oxygen-dependent manner, which is integral in the process of mammalian cell detection and response to changes in oxygen levels. HIF target genes include growth factors such as vascular endothelial growth factor (VEGF), platelet-derived growth-factor-β chain (PDGF-β), and transforming growth-factor-α (TGF-α). In normoxic conditions, the VHL protein targets HIF for destruction by the proteosome. In VHL disease, where there is loss of VHL activity, HIF is not degraded in the usual manner and there is overproduction of its growth-factor target genes, which contribute to tumor formation.[11]

Some genotype–phenotype correlations have been described with pheochromocytoma particularly associated with missense mutations. VHL has been classified into type 1, VHL without pheochromocytoma, where the mutation causes loss of the VHL gene product, and type 2, VHL with pheochromocytoma, where the mutation is a missense mutation. In type 2 there are three clinical groupings:

- 2A: low risk of renal-cell carcinoma;
- 2B: high risk of renal-cell carcinoma; and
- 2C: pheochromocytoma only.

Diagnostic criteria and screening

Diagnostic criteria have been developed for von Hippel-Lindau disease (Table 69.2a). Clinical variability is common in VHL, so that if a patient is discovered with one manifestation of the condition, they and other family members should be carefully examined and investigated for other features of this disorder (Table 69.2b).

CNS involvement

CNS hemangioblastomas occur in approximately 70% of patients with VHL. These occur particularly in the cerebellum (Fig. 69.2a) and present with typical cerebellar signs or raised intracranial pressure. These tumors may also involve the medulla or spinal cord.

Visceral features

Pheochromocytoma occurs in approximately 18% of VHL patients, with it occurring as a principal manifestation in some

Table 69.2a Diagnostic criteria for Von Hippel-Lindau[a]

Family history[b]	Required feature
Positive	Any one of the following: 　Retinal capillary hemangioma 　CNS hemangioma 　Visceral lesion[c]
Negative	Any one of the following: 　Two or more retinal capillary hemangiomas 　Two or more CNS hemangiomas 　Single retinal or CNS hemangioma with a visceral lesion[c]

[a] Modified from Singh et al.[10] Reprinted with permission.
[b] Family history of retinal or CNS hemangioma or visceral lesion.
[c] Visceral lesions include renal cysts, renal carcinoma, pheochromocytoma, pancreatic cysts, islet cell tumors, epididymal cystadenoma, endolymphatic sac tumor, and adnexal papillary cystadenoma of probable mesonephric origin.

Table 69.2b Protocols for patients with or at risk for von Hippel-Lindau[a]

Test	NIH[12]	Cambridge[13]
Urinary catecholamine	Every year (age 2+)	Every year (age 5+)
Ophthalmoscopy	Every year (age 1+)	Every year (age 5+)
Fluorescein angiography	Not routine	Every year (age 10+)
Enhanced MRI of brain and spine	Every 2 years (age 11–60) Every 3–5 years (age 61+)	Every 3 years (age 15–50) Every 5 years (age 51+)
Abdominal Ultrasound	Every year (age 11–20+)	Every year (age 15+)
CT	Every 1–2 years (age 21+)	Every 3 years (age 15+)

[a] Modified from Singh et al.[10] Reprinted with permission.

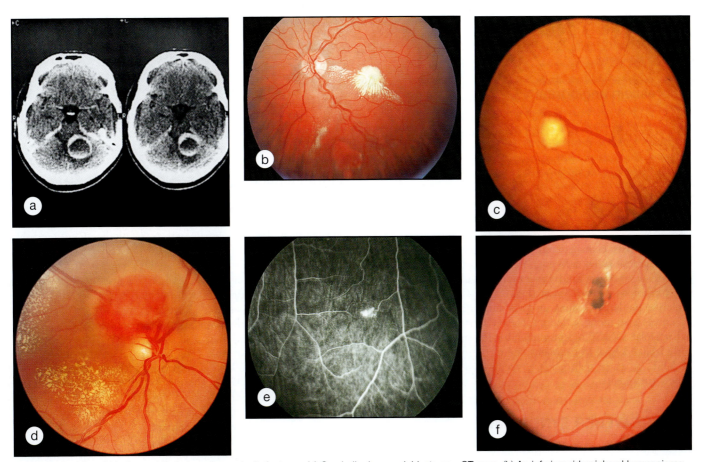

Fig. 69.2 Von Hippel-Lindau: ophthalmic and neurologic features. (a) Cerebellar hemangioblastoma—CT scan. (b) An inferior midperipheral hemangioma with dilated arteriole and venule and exudate consistent with stage III (patient of Professor Frank Billson). (c) Hemangioblastoma with large feeding and draining vessel. (d) A juxtapapillary hemangioma with deep and superficial exudate. (e) Small peripheral angioma fluorescein angiogram (patient of Professor Tony Moore). (f) A lesion shortly after treatment (patient of Professor Tony Moore).

families and not at all in others. Renal-cell carcinoma develops in 24–45% of cases and benign renal cysts also occur. Other systemic involvement includes endolymphatic sac tumors, pancreatic cystic disease, and pancreatic islet cell tumors.

Ophthalmic features

The typical ocular lesions of VHL are retinal capillary hemangiomas and the frequency of occurrence varies from 50 to 85% of cases. These manifest usually by age 30 years and the prevalence is stable thereafter, indicating that the risk of development of retinal capillary hemangiomas may not be lifelong and adults with a normal retina may be at a low risk for developing them.[14] The retinal angioma number may predict the course of VHL later in life, with a greater number associated with renal-cell carcinoma and cerebellar hemangioblastomas.

Retinal capillary hemangiomas can be classified by their location in the retina (peripheral or juxtapapillary), morphology (endophytic, exophytic, or sessile), and effect on the retina (exudative or tractional). The majority of retinal capillary hemangiomas are in the peripheral retina (Fig. 69.2b). Prominent retinal vessels emerging from the optic disk suggest a peripherally located hemangioma. Even small hemangiomas (1.5 mm in diameter) have dilated feeding vessels (Fig. 69.2c). Juxtapapillary hemangiomas (Fig. 69.2d) are less common and tend to be deep retinal tumors associated with exudation.

Five stages of evolution have been described[15]:

Stage I, preclassical: Small capillary clusters, initially the size of a diabetic microaneurysm, difficult to see ophthalmoscopically but revealed on fluorescein angiography. No feeder vessels are seen.

Stage II, classical: Typical retinal angiomas, small red nodules with prominence of the draining vein only.

Stage III, exudation: From leaking vessels of tumors usually larger than 1 disc diameter. Both feeding artery and draining vein are present.

Stage IV, retinal detachment: Exudative or tractional.

Stage V, end stage: Retinal detachment, uveitis, glaucoma, and phthisis.

Fluorescein angiography

Fluorescein angiography reveals a fine vascular pattern in the early stages and helps to confirm the diagnosis (Fig. 69.2e). This is particularly helpful for juxtapapillary retinal capillary hemangiomas and for differentiating the feeder arteriole from the draining vein, which is important when laser therapy is considered.

Treatment

Retinal capillary hemangiomas may be observed if they are small peripheral lesions (< 500 μm), non-vision threatening, with no exudate or subretinal fluid. Laser photocoagulation is most effective for lesions up to 1.5 mm (Fig. 69.2f). Cryotherapy is most effective for larger lesions up to 4 mm in size. Plaque radiotherapy is used for larger lesions. Newer antiangiogenesis therapy, in particular a VEGF receptor inhibitor, has shown potential in an early trial.[16] Visual loss remains one of the major complications of VHL, so early ophthalmic screening is essential to enable timely treatments.

STURGE-WEBER SYNDROME

Sturge-Weber syndrome (SWS) is a neuro-oculocutaneous syndrome characterized by leptomeningeal angiomatosis, usually in the occipital or temporal regions, ipsilateral facial capillary hemangioma (port-wine stain), and glaucoma.

Pathogenesis and genetic insights

SWS is thought to be a disorder of neural crest migration and differentiation, with the affected precursors giving rise to vascular and other tissue malformations in the meninges, the eye, and the dermis.[17] SWS is not usually familial and generally affects both sexes equally. Somatic mosaicism has been suggested as the pathogenesis of lesions in SWS. In two out of four patients examined, chromosomal abnormalities were found in affected tissues while the peripheral blood karyotype was normal.[18]

Cutaneous features

The port-wine stain is a benign, congenital lesion that results from ectasia of cutaneous venules (Fig. 69.3a), which is often unilateral but there may also be bilateral involvement. During infancy, the superficial vascular plexus progressively dilates, without any of the endothelial proliferation that occurs in true hemangiomas. The lesion darkens with age and progresses from a flat to a raised nodular lesion. Dye laser is effective in arresting the progressive skin changes particularly from smooth to lumpy. Multiple treatments may need to be performed (Fig. 69.3b).

Neurological features

Central nervous system involvement manifests usually as ipsilateral leptomeningeal hemangiomas (Figs. 69.3c and 69.3d) (although they may be contralateral or bilateral). This may involve any of the lobes of the cerebral cortex, although the occipital and temporal are more usually affected. Venous drainage is poor so metabolic activity in the underlying cortex becomes increasingly dysfunctional, and the cerebral tissue becomes atrophic and may calcify. Neurological features may include epilepsy, progressive mental retardation, contralateral hemiparesis, hemiplegia, and hemianopsia. Some of these symptoms may be related to the severity of underlying cortical glucose hypometabolism.

Ophthalmic features and management issues

Glaucoma is the principle ocular complication. There is a bimodal presentation with an early onset group (< 2 years) having a developmental angle anomaly with trabeculodysgenesis, and this may lead to buphthalmos (Fig. 69.3d). Glaucoma in the later onset group (> 4 years) is related to conjunctival/episcleral hemangiomas and raised episcleral venous pressure. Virtually all individuals with episcleral involvement (Fig. 69.3e) will develop raised intraocular pressure.[19] Glaucoma may worsen in the early onset group as episcleral venous pressure increases.

Choroidal hemangiomas also occur in SWS and commonly involve the posterior pole (Fig. 69.3f) but may extend to the whole fundus (Fig. 69.3g). Comparison with the other eye assists in diagnosis (Fig. 69.3h). There is loss of the normal choroidal vascular pattern with a diffuse smooth red fundus. Growth occurs slowly, leading to degenerative changes in the overlying retina with serous retinal detachment.

Glaucoma management is a challenge in SWS. Goniotomy is the procedure of choice in the early onset group. Medications are the usual initial management option for the late onset group. The prostaglandin analogues may not be as effective in this group due to the already raised episcleral venous pressure.

Filtration surgery when required mandates alterations in technique to minimize hypotony. For trabeculectomies this entails preplaced scleral flap sutures, viscoelastic or an anterior chamber maintainer during the procedure, and possibly posterior sclerostomies. For tube implant surgery being performed on patients with large choroidal hemangiomas (greatest risk for effusion/hemorrhage) a two-stage procedure should be considered. Intraoperative choroidal effusion presentation may be rapid, requiring immediate wound closure and possible drainage via sclerostomies.

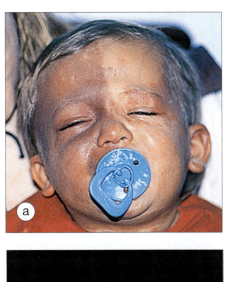

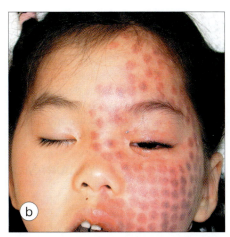

Fig. 69.3 Sturge-Weber syndrome: clinical features. (a) Port-wine stain. Note the deep red-purple coloration typical in the infant. (b) Dye laser therapy. Repeated application to fill in untreated areas. Eyelid spared on this occasion due to recent trabeculectomy.
(c) Leptomeningeal enhancement demonstrating the angiomatosis. Associated cerebral atrophy. Post gadolinium T1 axial MRI scan.
(d) Left temporal lobe leptomeningeal angiomatosis, cortical atrophy with calvarial skull bone thickening and left buphthalmos. T2 axial MRI image. (e) Episcleral hemangioma. Trabeculectomy filtration bleb present in supranasal quadrant. (f) Circumscribed posterior pole angioma. (g) Choroidal hemangioma. Diffuse posterior pole involvement ("tomato ketchup fundus"). (h) Normal left eye same patient.

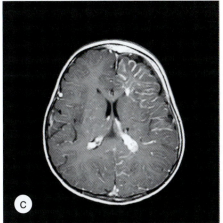

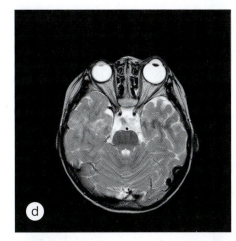

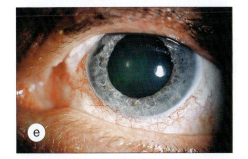

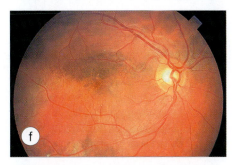

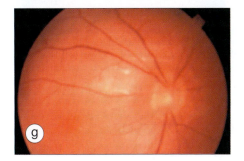

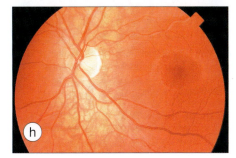

OTHER CONDITIONS SOMETIMES GROUPED WITH THE PHAKOMATOSES

Klippel-Trénaunay-Weber syndrome

Klippel-Trénaunay syndrome (KTS) is defined as a combination of the following:

1. Capillary malformations (usually port-wine stains), which need not extend over the entire affected limb and may be found at sites other than the hypertrophied limb (Fig. 69.4a);
2. Soft tissue or bony hypertrophy (or both) (Fig. 69.4b); and
3. Varicose veins or venous malformations of unusual distribution observed in infancy or childhood (Fig. 69.4c).

KTS can be diagnosed on the basis of any two of these three features. The vascular disorder in KTS is a combined capillary, venous, and lymphatic malformation with no evidence of substantial arteriovenous shunting.[20]

Ophthalmic features include orbital varix, retinal varicosities, angioma of the choroids, heterochromia iridium, and ipsilateral optic nerve enlargement. Glaucoma, when present, has many features in common with the Sturge-Weber syndrome and may also lead to buphthalmos (Fig. 69.4a).

Wyburn-Mason syndrome

See Chapter 55.

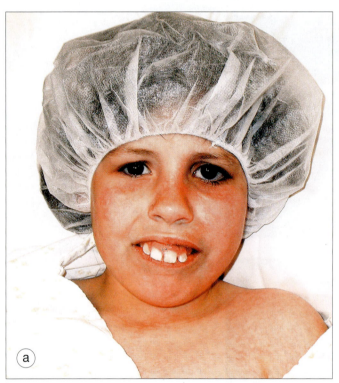
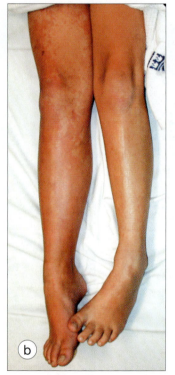
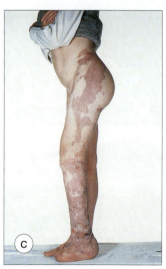

Fig. 69.4 Klippel-Trénaunay-Weber syndrome: clinical features. (a) Facial hemihypertrophy, port-wine stain, and buphthalmos. (b) Leg length inequality due to bone hypertrophy (same patient as that in a). (c) Venous malformations of lower limb.

REFERENCES

1. Rowley SA, O'Callaghan FJ, Osborne JP. Ophthalmic manifestations of tuberous sclerosis: a population based study. Br J Ophthalmol 2001; 85: 420–3.
2. Gomez M. Tuberous Sclerosis Complex. 3rd ed. New York: Oxford University Press; 1999.
3. Dabora SL, Jozwiak S, Franz DN, et al. Mutational analysis in a cohort of 224 tuberous sclerosis patients indicates increased severity of TSC2, compared with TSC1, disease in multiple organs. Am J Hum Genet 2001; 68: 64–80.
4. McManus E, Alessi D. TSC1-TSC2: a complex tale of PKB-mediated S6K regulation. Nature Cell Biology 2002; 4: E214–6.
5. Hyman MH, Whittemore VH. National Institutes of Health consensus conference: tuberous sclerosis complex. Arch Neurol 2000; 57: 662–5.
6. Crino PV, Henske EP. New developments in neurobiology of tuberous sclerosis complex. Neurology 1999; 53: 1384–90.
7. Jozwiak S, Schwartz RA, Janniger CK, et al. Usefulness of diagnostic criteria of tuberous sclerosis complex in pediatric patients. J Child Neurol 2000; 15 :652–9.
8. Vigabatrin Paediatric Advisory Group. Guideline for prescribing vigabatrin in children has been revised. BMJ 2000; 320: 1404.
9. Sankar PS, Pasquale LR, Grosskreutz CL. Uveal effusion and secondary angle-closure glaucoma associated with topiramate use. Arch Ophthalmol 2001; 119: 1210–1.
10. Singh ADC, Shields CL, Shields JA. Von Hippel-Lindau disease. Surv Ophthalmol 2001; 46: 117–42.
11. Kaelin WG. Molecular basis of the VHL hereditary cancer syndrome. Nat Rev Cancer 2002; 2: 673–82.
12. Choyke PL, Glenn GM, Walter MM, et al. Von Hippel-Lindau disease: genetic, clinical, and imaging features. Radiology 1995; 194: 629–42.
13. Maher ER, Yates JR, Harries R, et al. Clinical features and natural history of von Hippel-Lindau disease. Q J Med 1990; 77: 1151–63.
14. Webster AR, Richards FM, MacRonald FE, et al. An analysis of phenotypic variation in the familial cancer syndrome von Hippel-Lindau disease: evidence for modifier effects. Am J Hum Genet 1998; 63: 1025–35.
15. Hardwig P, Robertson DM. Von Hippel-Lindau disease: a familial, often lethal, multisystem phakomatosis. Ophthalmology 1984; 91: 263–70.

16. Aiello LP, George DJ, Cahill MT, et al. Rapid and durable recovery of visual function in a patient with von Hippel-Lindau syndrome after systemic therapy with vascular endothelial growth factor receptor inhibitor su5416. Ophthalmology 2002; 109: 1745–51.

17. Couly GF, Le Douarin NM. Mapping of the early neural primordium in quail-chick chimeras. II. The prosencephalic neural plate and neural folds: implications for the genesis of cephalic human congenital abnormalities. Dev Biol 1987; 120: 198–214.

18. Huq AH, Chugani DC, Hukku B, et al. Evidence of somatic mosaicism in Sturge-Weber syndrome. Neurology 2002;59:780-2.

19. Sullivan TJ, Clarke MP, Morin JD. The ocular manifestations of the Sturge-Weber syndrome. J Pediatr Ophthalmol Strabismus 1992; 29: 349–56.

20. Jacob AG, Driscoll DJ, Shaughnessy WJ, et al. Klippel-Trénaunay syndrome: spectrum and management. Mayo Clin Proc 1998; 73: 28–36.

CHAPTER 70 Accidental Trauma in Children

William V Good

INTRODUCTION

Accidental eye trauma in children is a leading public health concern in all regions of the world. Pediatric eye trauma must be considered contextually. In some cases, a decision must be made as to whether trauma is accidental or nonaccidental. The type of trauma may be helpful in making this discrimination, but the context in which the trauma occurred is an important variable in this decision. Relatively minor trauma can have a significant impact on function when it occurs in special context. For example, corneal abrasions in the setting of malnutrition, or head trauma in a child with co-existent central nervous system pathology may cause substantial morbidity, when they otherwise would not.

A careful history in cases of eye trauma in children is important and yet potentially misleading. Children may try to please adults thereby providing incorrect answers, and may try to deflect blame for an injury by offering misleading statements. Thus any history provided by child or parent must fit the physical findings. The examiner should always consider that something unreported could have occurred.

EPIDEMIOLOGY

The number of serious eye injuries in children has been estimated at 11.8 per 100 000 per year.[1] At least 35% of serious eye injuries occur in children, and the majority of these eye injuries occur in children under the age of 12.[2,3] These epidemiological data hold constant in many countries, including Israel,[3] Ireland,[4] Malawi[5] and Brazil.[6] Eye trauma is the most common cause of unilateral blindness in children.[7,8] Despite the significance and scope of eye trauma in children, the amount of research and effort at prevention and treatment has been less than in other areas of ophthalmic research activity.

Aside from the obvious ramifications of vision loss, significant problems also arise as a consequence of cosmetic problems associated with the disfigurement that often accompanies a serious eye injury. It is difficult to place an objective value or significance on this factor, but studies on the psychosocial consequences of strabismus would suggest that these could be very severe.[9]

Several factors can place a child at particular risk for a serious accidental eye injury.[3,6,10] The first risk factor is youth: children aged between 0 and 5 years of age are probably at greater risk for serious eye injury than children between the ages of 5 and 18. Second, boys are affected far more frequently than girls, particularly in the age group older than 6 years. Third, a lack of parental supervision is a definite and obvious risk factor for serious eye injury. Younger children are more often injured by a fall or being struck with a sharp projectile. Eye injuries in older children are more likely to be related to a sporting event (e.g. ice hockey or baseball).

The prognosis for recovery of vision after accidental eye trauma is also affected by psychosocial factors. Baxter showed that noncompliance with optical correction and patching was an important factor after childhood perforating anterior eye injury.[12] These authors emphasized the importance of parental education. In some cases, the use of social services, home nurses and other ancillary personnel may be helpful in improving the visual prognosis. Amblyopia may limit recovery of vision in children under 7 years of age, even in serious eye injuries that would carry a good prognosis in older individuals.

SELF-INFLICTED INJURY

Self-inflicted injury occurs predominantly in young adults with psychiatric disease. Burning, chemicals or cutting[13] are frequent methods and autoenucleation is also practised by schizophrenics.[14] There is usually evidence of secondary gain from the injury.[15]

Keratoconjunctivitis artefacta, caused by thermal, chemical or mechanical injury, is suggested by sharply demarcated lesions in the inferior and nasal areas of the bulbar conjunctiva and cornea and the skin below the eye (Fig. 70.1) in a patient who shows little concern and has other evidence of psychopathy.[16]

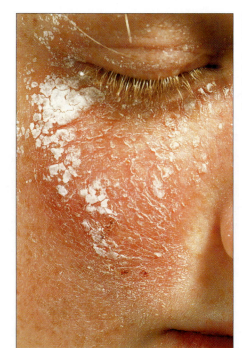

Fig. 70.1 Self-inflicted injury in a teenager. This patient had recurrent attacks of conjunctivitis artefacta and a desquamating skin lesion adjacent to that eye.

In all children with suspected self-induced injury the possibility of underlying metabolic or psychiatric diseases must be entertained. It is also important to look into the possibility of the self-inflicted injury being the manifestation of stress caused by sexual or other abuse. In children, severe self-mutilation occurs in the Smith–Magenis syndrome,[17,18] the Lesch–Nyhan syndrome, Joubert syndrome, and possibly in the Gilles de la Tourette syndrome.

OPHTHALMIC TRAUMA CAUSED BY AMNIOCENTESIS AND BIRTH INJURY

A spectrum of eye injuries can occur in association with amniocentesis. Normally, amniocentesis is performed in the second trimester, with very little risk of fetal loss.[19,20] However, ocular injuries have been the subject of a variety of reports, and clinicians should be aware of the nature of these injuries.

Nonpigmented epithelial iris cysts have been reported after amniocentesis.[21] Presumably, these cysts occur as a result of penetrating injury with the amniocentesis needle. The cysts are located anteriorly and have an adherence to the posterior corneal surface. Peripheral anterior synechiae occur. Congenital aphakia with retinal scar has also been described following in utero perforation of the globe.[22]

Naylor reported five cases of presumed ophthalmic amniocentesis injury.[23] One child had a hemianopia and gaze palsy. Two of the cases had presumed needle perforation of the eye resulting in a peaked pupil in one case and chorioretinal scar in the other. In the remaining two of the five cases one showed a small leucoma, and one a limbal corneal scar.

There have been additional reported cases of injury due to amniocentesis including leucocoria [24], third nerve palsy[25] (Fig. 70.2) and even congenital blindness.[76] Clearly, abnormalities of the anterior segment of the eye or of the retina [27] which could have been caused by trauma should be evaluated in the context of whether a baby or young child was exposed to amniocentesis *in utero*. Real-time ultrasound monitoring of the amniocentesis needle may help avoid this injury.[28]

Ocular adnexal injuries occur rarely after episiotomy. Upper eyelid laceration[29] and lower eyelid laceration[30] have been reported. The instrumentation occasionally used in childbirth may also cause other external trauma, including bruising and subconjunctival hemorrhage.[31] The possibility of ruptured globe as caused by childbirth is discussed below.

Orbital injury due to forceps resulting in inferior rectus fibrosis has been described.[32] Forceps should be suspected as the cause of a congenital corneal abnormality in which vertical ruptures in Descemet's membrane (Fig. 70.3) occur with a contralesional occipital depression caused by the other arm of the forceps.[33]

EYELID AND LACRIMAL SYSTEM TRAUMA

Many eyelid injuries result in superficial lacerations which can be closed with fine silk or nylon suture. Clinicians must be aware of two particular types of injuries which require special attention. The first of these is eyelid margin laceration, and the second is injury to the lacrimal drainage system.

In eyelid margin laceration, attention must be directed towards careful reapproximation of the margins of the eyelid. The usual etiology is sharp or blunt trauma to the lid margin, although other unusual etiologies are known, for example, dog bite or rat bite injuries.[34]

Injuries to the canalicular system will occur if the medial eyelid margin is injured, either of the upper or lower lid. Such injuries usually require intubation with silastic tubing material passed through both ends of the canaliculus and into the nose. With deeper injuries, it is important to close deep edges of the wound with fine grade absorbable suture and close the more superficial edges of the wound with fine suture. Once again, if the eyelid margin is cut, failure to reapproximate the margin precisely may result in the formation of a cosmetically undesirable notch.

Dog bite injuries may affect the eyelid margin and the lacrimal system.[35] In addition, either an inferior oblique palsy or restrictive type of ocular motor problem may occur. Management consists of closure of the laceration, as described above, and strabismus management as required.

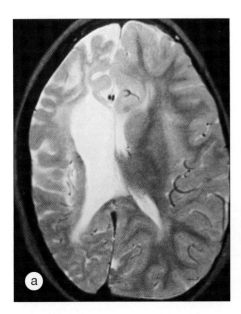
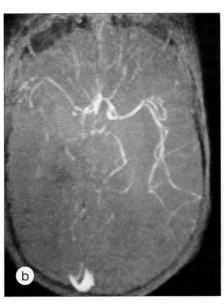

Fig. 70.2 Amniocentesis injury. (a) MRI scan showing right cerebral hemiatrophy. (b) MRI angiography showing occlusion of the right middle cerebral artery.

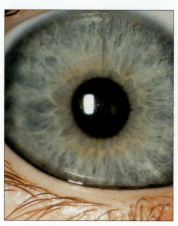
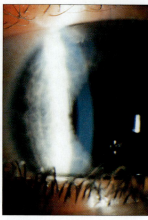

Fig. 70.3 Forceps injury to cornea. The vertically orientated rupture in Descemet's membrane can just be seen to one side of the pupil.

ANTERIOR SEGMENT TRAUMA

Subconjunctival hemorrhage

Subconjunctival hemorrhages can occur spontaneously or as a result of trauma. Despite their dramatic appearance, subconjunctival hemorrhages are of virtually no significance except in a situation where enough swelling occurs near the limbus so as to interfere with normal corneal protection by the eyelids and tear film. In this case a delle may occur. A delle is an excavation of the cornea with or without epithelial defect which occurs adjacent to a mass or bump near the corneal scleral limbus. It is probably caused by localized drying.

Subconjunctival hemorrhages associated with trauma indicate the need for a thorough search for a more serious eye injury (Fig. 70.4). The hemorrhage may mask a penetrating injury, so the examiner should look carefully for other signs of penetrating injury (e.g. uvea in a laceration, distorted pupil, lower intraocular pressure).

Corneal abrasion

Corneal abrasions occur when the corneal epithelium is traumatically removed from its underlying basement membrane. Abrasions can occur in the context of blunt or sharp trauma, and

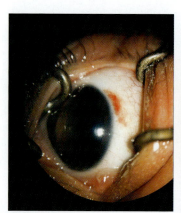
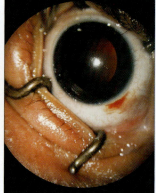

Fig. 70.4 Subconjunctival hemorrhage. In this instance associated with shaking, there were severe intraocular injuries.

are noteworthy for the significant pain that they cause. In some cases, though, persistent abrasions will become asymptomatic, indicating that follow-up may be useful, even when the child has no redness or discomfort.[36] Abrasions are diagnosed with a fluorescein test. Fluorescein instilled into an eye with a corneal abrasion will transiently stain the underlying basement membrane and will fluoresce when exposed to a blue light.

The differential diagnosis for corneal abrasion includes viral illness (e.g. herpes simplex keratitis) and corneal basement membrane disease. Herpes infection is usually suggested by a dendritic appearance, while basement membrane disease occurs in older children and adults and is recurrent, with no history of trauma.

Management of corneal abrasions involves prophylaxis against infection, since the epithelial lining of the cornea is a protective barrier against organisms. Most authorities recommend placing an antibiotic ointment into the eye (broad spectrum, accompanied by cycloplegia in order to reduce pain from iridospasm), and with patching over closed lids. The question of patching and its effectiveness is debated.[37] However, most patients will find the patching to be more comfortable than leaving the eyelids open.

Corneal foreign body

A small foreign body may stick on the cornea if it succeeds in penetrating the corneal epithelium. Patients will complain of pain and foreign body sensation on the eye. There may be a history of injury to the eye, but many patients will not recall anything in particular happening to them.

The foreign body should be removed, usually with irrigation, a rotating "burr", or simply and carefully with a sharp needle brought towards the eye tangentially and used to flick the foreign body away from the surface of the eye.

The eye should be examined carefully for the possibility of a penetrating eye injury and then managed as a corneal abrasion, once the foreign body is gone.

Eye wall injuries

Etiology

Eye wall lacerations can be categorized according to two dichotomies: simple laceration versus rupture; and anterior laceration versus posterior.

In simple lacerations, the eye is cut with a sharp object. Virtually any object imaginable has been responsible at one time or another for an eye wall laceration (Figs 70.5–70.8). Very young children usually suffer injury when they fall on a sharp object, such as a pencil, nail or toothpick. Older children, though, may suffer eye wall lacerations from glass (particularly when they wear spectacles), and projectiles. BB or air guns are notorious for causing ocular penetrating injuries and eye wall lacerations.[38] Bottle rockets and knives are other common causes. Unusual causes include the peck of a chicken, which carries the risk of endophthalmitis caused by unusual bacterial species from the bird's beak. Amniocentesis is also a potential cause of eye wall laceration or other type of injury (see above).[27]

Predisposition ("brittle corneas")

Certain eyes may be more likely to rupture with relatively minor trauma. In Ehlers–Danlos syndrome, defective collagen cross-linkage[39] leads to scleral and corneal weakness (Fig. 70.9). Patients with Ehlers–Danlos show blue sclera (due to scleral thinning), hyperextensible skin, and hypermobile joints. Spontaneous corneal rupture can occur.[40,41]

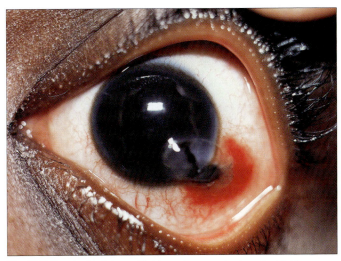

Fig. 70.5 Penetrating injury with iris prolapse and subconjunctival hemorrhage. (Dr William Good's patient.)

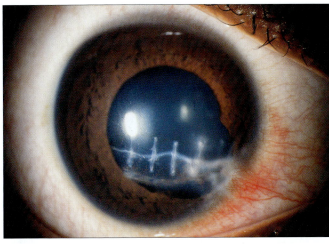

Fig. 70.7 After removal of the corneal sutures a scar persists. Failure to remove suture promptly may cause blood vessel migration and corneal opacification. Note the vessels at the corneoscleral limbus. (Photograph by courtesy of Dr William Good.)

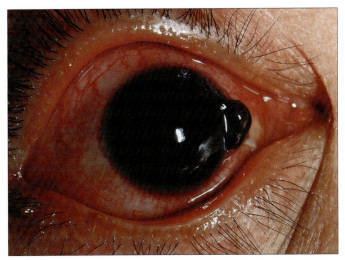

Fig. 70.6 Limbal penetrating injury with iris prolapse. (Photograph by courtesy of Dr William Good.)

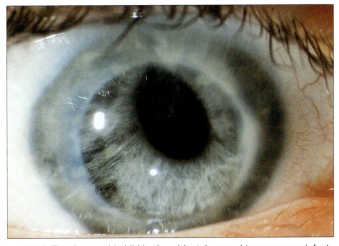

Fig. 70.8 This 5-year-old child had accidental corneal trauma as an infant. Prompt corneal grafting and amblyopia treatment resulted in an acuity of 6/12.

In the brittle cornea, blue sclera and joint hyperextensibility syndrome,[42,43] spontaneous rupture of the globe may occur; patients may have red hair and develop keratoglobus, and, unlike Ehlers–Danlos syndrome, they have normal levels of lysyl hydroxylase.

Osteogenesis imperfecta consists of blue sclera, deafness and bone fractures.[44,45] Children with this syndrome may also be more prone to corneal rupture in the setting of minor trauma.

Rupture

When a globe is ruptured, it is pushed or squeezed so hard that the eye wall breaks under pressure. The results usually are devastating, with partial or complete expulsion of intraocular contents. Expulsion is facilitated due to the increase in intraocular pressure followed by sudden decompression through a hole in the wall of the eye. Events that can cause ruptured globes include encounters with large, usually blunt, objects. A fistfight can result in a ruptured globe, as can injury from the force of a small projectile, such as a handball, squash ball, racquetball or baseball. For example, in North America, hockey puck injuries

were most often responsible for ruptured globes among children prior to the advent of protective eye-wear.[46] In the USA, baseball injuries are now most likely to result in serious eye injuries in older children.

Globe rupture is more common in boys than girls, reflecting the nature of the causal events. When the intraocular contents are affected the prognosis is poor.[47,48]

A ruptured globe has even been reported following parturition, and it is assumed that an increase in intraocular pressure could have been caused by force on the globe by a pelvic bone or some other obstacle.[49] Eyes are more likely to be ruptured or lacerated in areas where the sclera or cornea are thinnest. The areas under the insertions of the rectus and superior oblique muscles and also the corneoscleral limbus are thin and more likely to give way under pressure.

Anterior versus posterior laceration

A second important dichotomy in the diagnosis of globe lacerations is anterior versus posterior positioning. There is no doubt that anterior locations of injuries carry a better prognosis,

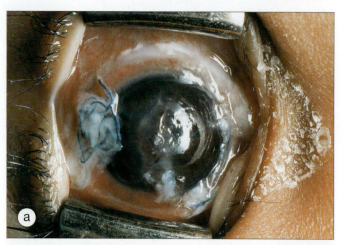
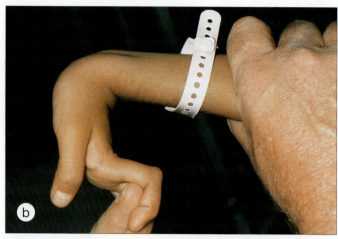

Fig. 70.9 Ehlers–Danlos syndrome. (a) Spontaneous rupture of the cornea. This is an autosomal recessive disease. One of this child's siblings, also affected, had a bilateral corneal rupture at the same time during fisticuffs. (b). Hyperflexible joints.

so long as the inciting agent does not also cut the retina. Injuries anterior to the pars plana (located approximately 5 mm posterior to the corneal scleral limbus) will not cut the retina, and therefore carry a better prognosis.[12,50] If a cataract occurs in conjunction with an anterior laceration, the prognosis for recovery of vision is not as good.[50] Posterior injuries cut the retina and often result in a complicated retinal detachment. Although these retinal detachments may be amenable to treatment, they carry a far worse prognosis than if the laceration were anterior.

One last set of definitions should be mentioned. Penetrating eye injuries are those in which the causative agent enters the eye but does not pass all the way through. Perforating eye injuries are those that pass through two walls of the eye. The same definition holds true when referring to different parts of the eye. For example, a penetrating corneal injury is one that penetrates the cornea but does not pass all the way through it. A perforating injury passes all the way through the cornea into the anterior chamber or further into the eye.

Diagnosis
The diagnosis of penetrating eye injury is obvious when a laceration is apparent. Clues to occult penetration include subconjunctival hemorrhage, distorted pupil, wrinkled lens capsule, and lowered intraocular pressure, particularly compared to pressure in the fellow, uninjured eye. The child's or family's history may or may not corroborate the physical findings.

Management
Prevention
The best form of management for eyeball lacerations is prevention.[51] Education to prevent injuries includes the following.

1. The encouragement of the wearing of suitable safety glasses or goggles by players who participate in games involving a small ball.
2. The encouragement of parents and teachers to supervise play and sport when sharp objects (fencing, archery, etc.) are used and teaching young people to respect the use of handguns, even "low power" or BB or airguns.
3. The use of safety glasses in monocular children is controversial. Although it seems logical to encourage their use, and although compliance may be good[52] there are many children

who will not wear them and it seems to some that their enforcement may be inappropriate except at times of particular risk.
4. A knowledge of when the injuries occur helps[53]: most occur in the home and therefore parental education must be a priority.

Treatment
Once the eye laceration or globe rupture is diagnosed, a protective shield should be placed over the eye. Emergency surgery is indicated, but the patient's overall health status should not be ignored. The eye laceration may accompany head trauma or other head injury. We have had the experience of caring for adolescent patients with multiple gunshot wounds, some of which were nearly ignored due to the focus of attention being placed on the eye injury itself.

Imaging
The role of imaging of the eye in order to determine an intraocular foreign body is an important one. In many cases, a CT scan of the orbits (Figs 70.10, 70.11) will help to identify the location of expected or unexpected intraocular foreign bodies, and ultrasonography also can be very helpful.

Anesthesia
The anesthetic induction of the patient is debated. Some would advocate avoiding a depolarizing agent for fear that the contraction of extraocular muscles (which initially occurs) could press on the eye and express intraocular contents. However, there has been no study that actually documents this, and there is a report[54] which showed no difference in prognosis whether or not a depolarizing agent is used.

Surgery
The main goal of surgery is closure of the eye wall laceration. With anterior lacerations, prompt closure and re-evaluation of the patient's vision and ocular status in the ensuing several days is advisable. We do not administer intraocular antibiotics prophylactically unless there are signs of an infection; but this issue is controversial and some would recommend the use of an intraocular regimen that covers against a broad range of infectious organisms. The prompt closure of an eye wall laceration would

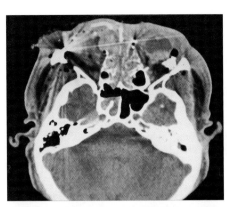

Fig. 70.10 CT scan showing disrupted right globe following a gunshot wound. The left eye was also injured from the concussive effect. Note the vitreous hemorrhage. (Photograph by courtesy of Dr William Good.)

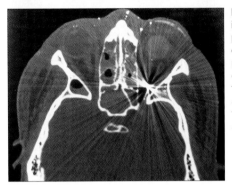

Fig. 70.11 Shotgun injury. CT scanning is particularly helpful in delineating the presence and location of ocular and orbital foreign bodies: this adolescent was shot in the face with a shotgun.

seem to be adequate to greatly reduce the incidence of traumatic endophthalmitis. A concurrent traumatic cataract should be removed at the same time as closure of the laceration in young children. Delay in traumatic cataract extraction runs the risk of inducing amblyopia. In older children (>7 years of age), a second operation could be performed and could include intraocular lens implant, so long as the posterior capsule remains intact.

Posterior lacerations almost always cut through the retina. Even so, the initial goal of surgery is wound closure. Most authorities do not use cryosurgery or scleral buckling at initial surgery. The trauma alone is enough to cause a retinal scar around a break, and cryosurgery releases intraocular factors which may increase the likelihood of posterior vitreoretinopathy (PVR). A posterior vitreous detachment occurs 7–10 days after trauma; after this detachment has taken place, the retinal surgery can be undertaken.

Management continues even after successful closure and repair of the wound. Children under the age of 7 years are at risk for amblyopia.[55] Prompt refractive management in the form of a contact lens over a corneal laceration (or spectacles if appropriate), and patching should be started as soon as possible.[56] Additionally, corneal sutures in children attract blood vessels and scarring much more quickly than in adults. Sutures may need to be removed in a matter of weeks in young children. Failure to remove sutures may result in a completely vascularized cornea, which impedes vision.

Prognosis

Prognosis in eye wall lacerations and ruptures in children is debated.[57,58] Without doubt, anterior lacerations carry a better prognosis than posterior lacerations. But in young children, with the risk of amblyopia, the prognosis may not be so good, even with anterior lacerations. When anterior lacerations are combined with cataract, the prognosis worsens.[12] The prognosis also is highly dependent upon success in the management of amblyopia or the potential for amblyopia.

Traumatic cataracts

Traumatic cataracts can occur either as a result of a sharp penetrating injury to the lens capsule and/or lens, or a blunt concussive force.[59] Traumatic cataracts may occur immediately after the injury, or may occur days to even years after a concussive blow. Cataracts may be partial or complete; trauma may produce a posterior subcapsular cataract which then progresses to a total cataract.

The diagnosis of traumatic cataracts is based on an abnormality in the red reflex. The cataract problem can be confirmed by examining the lens under magnification, either with loupes or a slit lamp. In some cases, a Vossius ring may occur, i.e. a ring of pigment forms on the anterior lens capsule as a result of the posterior (pigmented) aspect of the iris striking the capsule. Examination should establish that there are no other ocular injuries. An effort should be made to search for a rupture in the lens capsule as well, since this usually indicates that the lens opacity will not clear spontaneously, and the lens will need to be removed.

In partial cataracts, an additional important aspect to the examination is an effort at measuring visual function in the involved eye. In older children, of course, this can be done with Snellen acuity. In younger children, an estimate must be made based upon experience with lens clarity and visual functioning under monocular and binocular conditions. Attempts can be made to measure acuity with forced choice preferential looking techniques, but these may be misleading and probably should not be used as the sole determinant to undertaking surgery.[60,61]

If there is doubt as to the value of removing a lens with a cataract, then it should be observed. This is true if the cataract occurs as a result of blunt or penetrating trauma. So long as the child is beyond the age when amblyopia can develop, the initial repair of a corneal or scleral laceration can be followed at a later date with removal of the lens. This "wait-and-see" strategy has no deleterious effects on the child other than the necessity for a second general anesthetic.

Surgical management consists of removal of the lens with or without preservation of the posterior capsule. If a lens is removed at the same time that an eye wall laceration is closed, it may be safer to avoid simultaneous lens implant but simultaneous corneal repair, lens aspiration, and posterior chamber lens implantation has its advocates.[62] One reason for caution is that the implant could conceivably foster survival of bacterial organisms which penetrated the eye as a result of the trauma. Another concerns the choice of power to correct aphakia. In young children, eye growth leads to instability of the refractive power of the eye, making implant power selection problematic.[63] Decisions regarding subsequent implants depend on surgeon preference and the presence or absence of corneal refractive problems. If a child has a significant amount of astigmatism and will require contact lens rehabilitation anyway, then any increased risk of a lens implant can be avoided, since the implant would not avert the need for contact lenses. Contact lenses can be successful in post-traumatic aphakia.[64,65] Amblyopia must also be managed carefully in order to maximize visual potential. Combined keratoplasty and lens implantation may have a role in some cases.[66]

A special type of cataract can occur as the result of electrical injury.[67] A characteristic opacity in the posterior aspect of the lens forms as the result of the transmission of electricity to the eye (Fig. 70.12) itself. If this type of cataract becomes visually

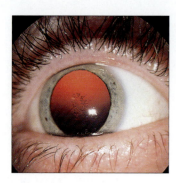

Fig. 70.12 Electric shock. After an electric shock this young man slowly developed a monocular cataract. (Photograph by courtesy of Dr William Good.)

significant it can be cared for in the same fashion as cataracts from other causes.

Hyphema

A hyphema is a collection of blood in the anterior chamber of the eye. In the setting of trauma, hyphema occurs as a result of avulsion of blood vessels, usually at the base of the iris. Bleeding occurs and then ceases after clot formation or an increase in intraocular pressure. A hyphema may be small enough that it can be identified only with a slit-lamp examination, or it can be so extensive as to fill the entire anterior chamber with blood, the so-called "8-ball hyphema". In most instances, a superiorly located meniscus develops due to the effects of gravity (Fig. 70.13).

Knowledge of the various other etiologies of hyphema is important, particularly since children may not reveal that they fell or were hit by a friend or some other object. Herpes zoster iritis can occasionally cause a hyphemia. Spontaneous hyphemas also occur with juvenile xanthogranulomatosis. Most of these cases occur in very young children (<1 year of age), and may or may not be associated with cutaneous lesions. Hyphemas may also occur rarely in association with tumors of the eye, particularly retinoblastoma, but also with iris vascular abnormalities or rubeosis.

The management of hyphemas is debated.[68] The natural history of the hyphema is such that the clot usually retracts between the third and fifth post-traumatic day, at which point the hyphema may recur. There is a general agreement that very small "trickle" hyphemas are less likely to rebleed than larger

ones. However, rebleeding cannot be predicted solely on the basis of the size of the hyphema if it is visible without magnification. For this reason, most advocate some sort of rest regimen for the child. Whether a child should be hospitalized in order to facilitate resting will certainly depend at least on the child's activity level, the family's ability to supervise the child, and perhaps also on the size of the hyphema. Other efforts at enforcing rest include using light sedation. Antiemetics may prevent vomiting (and transient increases in intraocular pressure and eye movement), and should be considered. A quick, substantial rise in intraocular pressure (a complication of hyphema) can cause nausea and vomiting.

The use of eye drops is also of unproven benefit. Many would choose to use a long-acting cycloplegic agent in order to put the iris and pupil "at rest". Short-acting cycloplegics probably are not worthwhile because movement of the iris could potentially lead to disruption of clot and further bleeding. Topical steroids may be useful if an inflammatory component (iritis) occurs.

Systemic steroids have been advocated by Rynne and Romano.[69] The use of epsilon aminocaproic acid has been advocated by some, but its value in children has not been proven conclusively.[70,71] Epsilon aminocaproic acid blocks fibrinolysis. Presumably, it can retard or inhibit the dissolution of the clot, and thereby reduce the risk of rebleeding.

Complications of hyphema are increased intraocular pressure and glaucoma. How much pressure and for how long pressure can be tolerated safely is very individually determined and has not been worked out for children. High pressure runs the risk of causing corneal blood staining and optic nerve damage. To prevent these complications, many would treat pressure and attempt to maintain it below 30 mmHg. Persistent elevation of intraocular pressure may be an indication for surgical evacuation of the hyphema. In many cases, elevated pressure can be managed with eye drops such as beta-blockers (acetylcholine agents are probably ill-advised because they constrict the pupil and may have an effect on the fragile blood vessels). Systemic pressure-lowering agents such as acetazolamide may also be useful.

When a child has sickle cell anemia, the management of glaucoma caused by hyphema is more problematic. The only agent available to the physician is a topical beta-blocker, since other agents may either exacerbate the hyphema (e.g. pilocarpine) or lead to sickle cell crisis. Children with sickle cell with a hyphema may be candidates for early surgical intervention. Surgical intervention consists of a clot evacuation through a corneal scleral incision. In children who do not have sickle cell, but in whom glaucoma remains a refractory problem, such surgical evacuation may also be advisable.

Blood staining occurs when erythrocytes cross the corneal endothelial membrane and stain the cornea. This occurs when the intraocular pressure is elevated, and also in situations where the corneal endothelium is damaged. Corneal blood staining is reversible, but takes several years. Corneal blood staining is particularly problematic in children due to the potential for development of amblyopia.

Months and years later, if the angle of the eye has been traumatized and "recessed", the child may develop a type of open angle glaucoma referred to as "angle recession glaucoma". For that reason, any patient who has had a hyphema probably should have yearly ophthalmology examinations, with intraocular pressure measurements determined. The risk of angle recession glaucoma may be as high as 10% following hyphema, at least in adult patients.[72,73]

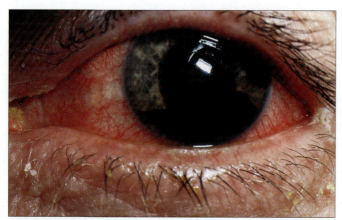

Fig. 70.13 A long-standing hyphema shown by the dark color of the blood in this young man. (Photograph by courtesy of Dr William Good.)

POSTERIOR SEGMENT TRAUMA

Commotio retinae

Commotio retinae, also known as Berlin's edema, can occur after blunt trauma to the front part of the eye. The edema, which occurs in the outer retinal areas, has a funduscopic appearance that is white or grey-white. The macula may be involved, in which case central vision will be at least temporarily diminished.[74,75] But Berlin's edema can also involve extramacular areas and may actually not be noticed by the patient.

In most cases, the edema resolves, but there are some cases where pigment migration in the macula might result in loss of central vision. Also, a full-thickness macular hole can follow the formation of this type of edema.[76] The differential diagnosis consists of retinal infarction, cotton-wool spot and shallow retinal detachment. No particular treatment is available for commotio retinae.

Purtscher retinopathy

Severe trauma to the torso or the head itself can cause a type of retinopathy called Purtscher's retinopathy. Purtscher disease can also be caused by a fat or air embolism.[77,78]

Purtscher retinopathy has the appearance of massive whitening around the optic nerve head associated with hemorrhage. The whitening may represent ischemic areas or exudate. There is no specific treatment for this problem, which may resolve leaving anything from mild to profound vision loss.

Whiplash injury

A macular hole sometimes occurs as a consequence of a severe whiplash injury.[79] Presumably, the head thrusting induces a vitreoretinal interface shearing force which tugs at the fovea and creates a partial or full-thickness hole. The hole resembles solar maculopathy, but this latter problem has an altogether different etiology.

Choroidal rupture

Another potential complication of blunt injury to the front part of the eye is choroidal rupture; it is often associated with widespread damage and vitreous hemorrhage (Fig. 70.14). The choroid may be broken (ruptured) at the level of the inner choroid and retinal pigment epithelium, and often in the most

visually sensitive area of the retina, the macula.[76] The mechanism is mechanical disruption and refraction of tissue. Sometimes the rupture is associated with a serous or hemorrhagic retinal detachment which obscures the nature of the injury. Once the detachment resolves, the patient may be left with diminished vision if there has been scarring or retinal pigment epithelial migration into the area of the macula. Later, choroidal rupture can predispose to a choroidal neovascularization process, which can lead to exudate and hemorrhage under the macula, also diminishing vision. Patients with choroidal rupture should be apprised of this potential consequence, and should monitor their vision on a regular basis, since laser treatment to the choroidal neovascularization may, in some cases, help eliminate the problem.

Retinal hemorrhages

Retinal hemorrhages can be caused by direct head or ocular trauma, or by indirect trauma, as with a shaking injury in non-accidental trauma. Hemorrhages occur in normal infants in the perinatal period (Fig. 70.15) in a large percentage of cases, and may also be caused by trauma. Evidence for the traumatic nature of retinal hemorrhages is found in the fact that occipital presentation at birth, the use of obstetrical procedures, labour induction, and prolonged labour are all associated with an increased incidence in retinal hemorrhages. Retinal hemorrhages are uncommon in children born by cesarean section.

A diagnosis of retinal hemorrhages is made by fundoscopic examination. In older children, retinal hemorrhage may be suspected by complaints of altered or decreased vision. In younger children, hemorrhage will be diagnosed in an incidental examination, or when an examination is performed due to suspected nonaccidental trauma.

Hemorrhages may occur in any of several layers in the retina or vitreous.[80] Subretinal pigment epithelial hemorrhages appear dark with an amorphous boundary. Intraretinal hemorrhages are red in appearance, usually small and round. Superficial retinal hemorrhages have a splinter appearance because they often occur in the nerve fibre layer. Subhyaloid hemorrhages have a characteristic appearance where blood forms a meniscus in a large cystic filled cavity. Finally, vitreous hemorrhages may also occur in the setting of trauma, and may be localized or diffuse depending on their severity.

Any of these hemorrhages may occur with trauma, but pre-retinal hemorrhages are particularly common in children with

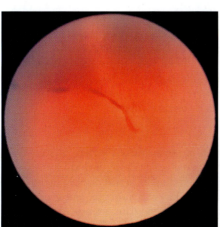

Fig. 70.14 Choroidal rupture. There is a marked vitreous hemorrhage largely obscuring a view of the fundus where a pale organizing clot can barely be made out.

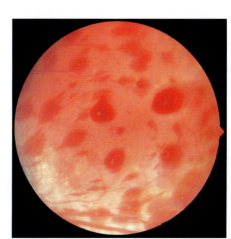

Fig. 70.15 Neonatal retinal hemorrhages in a normal child. (Photograph by courtesy of Dr Andrew Q. McCormick, Vancouver.)

subdural or subarachnoid hemorrhages.[81] Since central nervous system hemorrhage is frequently caused by trauma in children, a traumatic etiology for pre-retinal hemorrhages should be suspected.

Other, nontraumatic causes of retinal hemorrhages include Coats disease[82]; persistent hyperplastic primary vitreous[83]; retinal dysplastic syndrome, including Norrie disease and incontinentia pigmenta[80]; blood dyscrasias[84]; hyperviscosity syndromes; infections of the retina, including cytomegalovirus, rickettsia[85]; endocarditis; protein C deficiency,[86] and retinal tumors such as retinoblastoma. Vitreous hemorrhage may occur in the setting of pars planitis in children.[87] In all of these cases the etiology is usually obvious, but should be searched for prior to diagnosing a traumatic etiology of retinal hemorrhages for reasons discussed under nonaccidental trauma.

There seldom is any particular management for retinal hemorrhages, but the exception would be the baby or young child with a prolonged vitreous hemorrhage. Kaur and Taylor[80] have commented on the fact that vitreous hemorrhages in children may take longer to absorb because the vitreous gel is more solid in this age group. Prolonged obscuration of vision due to vitreous hemorrhage could cause deprivation amblyopia, and is a reason for early vitrectomy,[88] particularly in the first 3–6 months of life. We have encountered children with prolonged vitreous hemorrhage in the setting of profound perinatal hypoxic ischemia and vigorous resuscitation efforts.[89] The children we saw required vitrectomy due to slow absorption of a vitreous hemorrhage.

Traumatic retinal detachment

Blunt trauma to the eye can cause a retinal detachment even if the globe is not cut or ruptured.[90,91] Typically, the detachment occurs as the result of an avulsion of the vitreous base, often in the superonasal quadrant of the eye. Presumably this location is most vulnerable because a blunt blow to the eye arises from 180° away, in the inferotemporal segment. There have been cases where a blunt object strikes the eye and causes a small or large retinal tear which, days, weeks or even months later leads to a delayed retinal detachment. This is known to occur in boxing injuries, for example.

The clinician should be aware of the vulnerability of the vitreous base and should, to the extent possible, inspect this peripheral area of the retina in order to exclude this possible post-traumatic problem. Retinal detachments should be managed promptly, usually with a scleral buckling procedure.

Self-abuse in severely mentally retarded children can also cause retinal detachments by etiologies mentioned above.[92,93] In atopy, constant rubbing to relieve itching increases the risk of retinal detachment.[94,95]

ORBIT TRAUMA

Orbital bone fractures

General

Fractures of the bony orbit are mainly the province of the neurosurgeons and craniofacial team but the high frequency with which the eye is involved (p. 760) demands the involvement of an ophthalmologist in most cases.

Blow-out fractures

The term "blow-out fractures" was probably first used by Smith and Regan.[96] Blow-out fracture refers to the caving in of one of

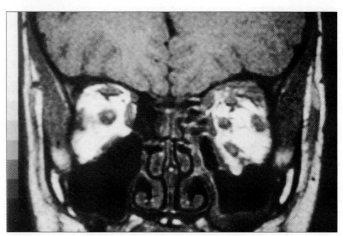

Fig. 70.16 Blow-out fracture showing entrapment of the tissues associated with the inferior rectus in the left orbit.

the orbital bones that surround the eye. In most cases the floor of the orbit is fractured (Fig. 70.16), but the medial wall of the orbit can also be damaged. Blow-out fractures of the superior orbital wall are uncommon and the term "blow-in" fracture is preferable in such cases because most such fractures involve a caving in of the bones in this area into the orbit.[97] Blow-out fractures are unusual in young children, before the sinuses have formed.

Etiology

Blow-out fractures can occur by one or both of two mechanisms. In the first situation, the eye may be compressed into the orbit, thereby increasing the pressure on the orbital contents. This expansion of tissue in the orbit may cause a dramatic increase of pressure on orbital bones. Since the orbital floor appears to be the weakest, it is the most likely to be fractured.[98,99] This first theory is termed the "hydraulic theory". A second mechanism of blow-out fracture involves direct transmission of the force of a blow to the orbital rim to the bones of the floor or medial wall of the orbit. Experimental injuries to the orbital rim have demonstrated that a posterior orbital floor blow-out fracture can be induced in this fashion.[100,101]

Enophthalmos

Generally speaking, there are three types of problems that can result from a blow-out fracture. Enophthalmos can occur as a result of shifting of intraorbital contents into fractures of the floor or medial wall of the orbit. Enophthalmos may not be apparent in the first few days after trauma due to edema and swelling in the injured area. Enophthalmos becomes apparent by 5–7 days after injury and should be evaluated at that point. Its management, if cosmetically significant, requires repair of the fracture and replacement of orbital contents in order to reconstitute the orbit to its original volume.

Strabismus

A second problem is that of strabismus. A variety of strabismus problems can occur after blow-out fracture, including entrapped extraocular muscle, paralysed muscle, actual displacement of the globe in a vertical direction, Brown syndrome, and even cranial nerve injury if the force of the blow damages any of the cranial nerves which innervate the extraocular muscles.

A trapped inferior rectus muscle is the most common cause of strabismus associated with blow-out fracture (Fig. 70.16). The muscle becomes incarcerated in the inferior floor fracture and tethers the eye in a hypotropic position. Almost paradoxically, a posterior floor fracture may tether the eye and cause a hypertropia.[102] Most patients experience vertical diplopia, worsening in upgaze. Patients may be able to use their eyes together (fuse) in downgaze. The results of forced duction testing indicate that traction in the upward direction is more difficult in the involved eye than in the uninvolved eye. Treatment usually consists of freeing of an entrapped extraocular muscle, or recession of the inferior rectus muscle of the involved eye.

In some cases, the inferior rectus muscle may be traumatically paralysed or rendered inefficient. In this case, a hypertropia may exist on the involved side, and the problem worsens in downgaze due to inefficiency of the paralysed inferior rectus muscle. Treatment may consist of recession of the contralateral inferior rectus muscle to alleviate the primary gaze problem, and possibly the use of a posterior fixation suture in the contralateral muscle in order to "match" the downgaze defect in the involved eye.

Occasional cases involve entrapment or tethering of the medial rectus muscle. These cases may emulate a Duane syndrome because abduction is insufficient and enophthalmos may occur on abduction. Forced duction testing plus radiological evaluation should secure the diagnosis. Treatment consists of freeing the medial rectus muscle and recessing it if the eye is esotropic in primary gaze.

Brown syndrome (limited elevation of the eye in adduction) occurs when damage to the superior oblique trochlea or the superior oblique tendon has occurred. Interestingly, Brown syndrome associated with blow-out fracture or orbital trauma can occur with trauma in any location of the orbit. Therefore, Brown syndrome is not diagnostic of superior orbital damage. Treatment may consist of injection of steroid into the area of the superior oblique tendon, or superior oblique weakening procedures, often accompanied by an inferior oblique weakening procedure in order to alleviate the defect caused by iatrogenic superior oblique palsy.

Large orbital floor fractures may allow periorbital pressure to be transmitted to the orbit, for instance on jaw movement.[103]

The third treatment issue with regard to blow-out fractures is whether large fractures should be repaired where there is no functional or cosmetic deficit. Although there is debate, most authorities would not render treatment if there is no functional or cosmetic deficit.

Traumatic optic neuropathy

Etiology
Traumatic optic neuropathy occurs when head or facial trauma causes direct or indirect injury to the optic nerve. The result is unilateral or bilateral loss of vision, and the vision loss may be partial or complete. Perhaps 5% of all head trauma cases result in damage to the visual axis. Even facial fractures have a high degree of association with optic nerve injury.[104] In a very large series of patients, Turner demonstrated that 1% of cases of facial fractures result in an optic nerve injury.[105] Frontal bone trauma is most likely to result in optic nerve injury. Even subtle and apparently insignificant frontal head trauma will occasionally involve an optic nerve lesion. The reports of incidence of traumatic optic neuropathy above involve large numbers of adult patients. The exact incidence and risk of optic neuropathy in children is unknown. There is no doubt, however, that children also are susceptible to traumatic optic neuropathy, and that some cases occur in the setting of apparently minor trauma to the area around the eye(s).

There are several possible mechanisms for traumatic optic neuropathy. The first is optic nerve avulsion where the optic nerve is severed or partially severed near its junction with the globe. The usual source of optic nerve avulsion is severe trauma, although mild cases of trauma also have been reported to cause optic nerve avulsion.[106-108] If the fundus can be visualized ophthalmoscopically through clear media, a hole appears in the previous location of the optic nerve head. Sometimes the avulsion can be visualized with a CT scan.[109] The ultrasonic B scan can also be helpful in demonstrating an avulsed optic nerve and will show a kind of split in the optic nerve head.[110]

One special circumstance bears mentioning. Patients with severe psychiatric disturbances may attempt to enucleate their own eye and in the process sever the optic nerve at some point in its approach to the globe. If the severance is posterior near the chiasm, a unilateral blindness may be accompanied by a temporal hemianopia in the fellow eye due to chiasmal damage.[111] Patients who attempt to remove their own eye often experience temporary relief of their psychiatric symptoms if successful; a resurgence of symptoms may lead them to attempt to enucleate their other eye. Such patients should be guarded very closely and their psychotic symptoms should be managed aggressively.

A second mechanism of vision loss is traumatic anterior ischemic optic neuropathy. The presumed etiology is closure of one or more posterior ciliary arteries.[112] Thrombosis or transient vasospasm caused by the trauma could play a role in the etiology.

In some cases an optic sheath hemorrhage results from trauma and causes an optic neuropathy.[113] In these cases, orbital CT scan or ultrasonography will usually demonstrate enlargement of the optic nerve sheath.[114] Elucidation of this problem is important because optic nerve sheath fenestration may be helpful in restoring vision or preventing further visual loss.[113,115]

The most common etiology of traumatic optic neuropathy is arguably also the most elusive. A posterior traumatic optic neuropathy must be inferred from other aspects of the physical examination, because there are no initial ophthalmoscopic findings.

There are many possible mechanisms for posterior traumatic neuropathy. These include an actual laceration caused by bone fracture, ischemia, contusion and even hemorrhage.[116] Injuries to the posterior optic nerve can also cause cerebrospinal fluid rhinorrhea and even disturbances of cerebral or cortical function.[117]

Diagnosis and treatment
The examiner often must rely on signs of unilateral afferent visual dysfunction (afferent pupil defect, diminished color vision, decreased visual acuity). Unfortunately, many patients who experience such trauma are also neurologically damaged and may not be able to co-operate with a physical examination. The pupillary examination then becomes paramount in establishing the diagnosis.

Treatment of traumatic optic neuropathy can take one of at least three approaches. Although there is increasing evidence that intervention may be useful, in some cases withholding treatment is most sensible, particularly where avulsion is suspected, or where a patient is otherwise so severely injured that surgical or medical intervention is dangerous.

High-dose steroids using methylprednisolone at a dose of 30 mg/kg as an intravenous bolus has been shown to be better than placebo in healing acute spinal cord trauma.[118] These exceptionally high doses of methylprednisolone may also be efficacious in the treatment of traumatic optic neuropathy.[119] In the case of traumatic optic neuropathy, doses are 1 mg/kg per day for 72 hours followed by a rapid taper.

A second option involves surgical intervention. Indications include optic sheath hemorrhage, orbital hemorrhage (focal, diffuse or subperiosteal) and an optic canal fracture causing compression of the optic nerve. The role of optic canal decompression or optic nerve defenestration in "generic" cases of traumatic optic neuropathy is unclear and studies are under way to determine whether surgical intervention is effective in these situations.[119] Transethmoidal decompression may be effective, particularly in younger patients.[120]

Traumatic retrobulbar hemorrhage

Trauma to the eye or orbit will occasionally cause hemorrhage behind the eye. Hemorrhage may be the result of blunt trauma, in which case shearing forces on retrobulbar veins or arteries are suspected. Sharp objects can also penetrate behind the eye without actually injuring the globe itself, and may lacerate blood vessels.

The affected person will have pain with signs of a rapidly increasing mass behind the globe. These signs include proptosis, an increase in intraocular pressure, chemosis and diminished ocular motility.

Trauma is not the only cause of these retro-orbital signs. The clinician should keep in mind that slowly progressive signs may indicate Graves disease, and that conditions such as orbital cellulitis and traumatic carotid-cavernous fistula can also present in the above-mentioned fashion. Cellulitis may be diagnosed when other signs of infection are present (redness, heat in the area, considerable pain). CT scan usually demonstrates a sinusitis extending into the retro-orbital space, and the patient may have fever and leucocytosis. Carotid-cavernous fistula is suspected when there is pulsating exophthalmos and vessels which appear arterialized in the conjunctiva and retina.

Traumatic retrobulbar hemorrhage occasionally is an ophthalmic emergency. When the intraocular pressure is elevated and affecting optic nerve function (as demonstrated by decreased visual acuity, decreased color vision or by an afferent pupil defect) the pressure must be lowered immediately. If there is no visual dysfunction, the pressure can be lowered urgently with medications that may have a more delayed onset of action.

Intraocular pressure can be lowered rapidly (within 1 hour) with carbonic anhydrase inhibitors (acetazolamide) and hyperosmotic agents. A lateral canthotomy can relieve retrobulbar pressure almost immediately. The lateral canthus is excised aggressively to allow orbital contents to shift anteriorly.

Although aqueous paracentesis occasionally is recommended as another method for lowering intraocular pressure, it probably has only a short-term benefit and exposes the patient to the risk of cataract or intraocular infection.

CENTRAL NERVOUS SYSTEM TRAUMA

Prolonged cortical visual impairment following trauma

Many possible mechanisms can account for prolonged cortical visual impairment after head trauma. Trauma that would cause a seizure could then lead to impaired vision on a cortical basis. In addition, a cerebral contusion could result in generalized cerebral edema and this could cause both transient or prolonged cortical visual impairment.[121] Increased cerebral edema could cause the compression of the posterior cerebral arteries which in turn could lead to vascular insufficiency to the visual cortex.[122] One last possible mechanism invokes the watershed zones between the three major cerebral arteries (anterior, middle and posterior). These zones are most vulnerable to severe hypoxia and/or ischemia, and damage there may result in cortical visual impairment. Central nervous system hypoxic ischemia could be a sequel to either generalized trauma with blood loss or even central nervous system vasospasm resulting from more localized trauma. The occipital region is quite susceptible to hypoxia.[123] Thus, the occipital region of the brain may be selectively involved in events that result in hypoxia and ischemia.

Cortical visual impairment following cardiac surgery

Cortical blindness or visual impairment is a well-recognized complication of cardiac surgery. The cause is not known, although embolism by air or fat has been suspected. The prognosis is usually good.

Post-traumatic transient cortical visual impairment

Cortical visual impairment can be defined as complete, or nearly complete, loss of vision with normal pupillary reflexes, and a normal fundus examination.[89] Cortical visual impairment in children may differ in its manifestations from cortical blindness in adults.[89] Children show fluctuating vision, a preference for observing color (versus black and white), light gazing and, occasionally, photophobia.

A relatively minor blow to the head can cause transient cortical blindness. The type of injury that can cause transient cortical blindness is usually a blow to the parieto-occipital region. Alpha rhythm may be suppressed for transient periods after a head trauma.

The clinical picture accompanying transient visual loss is diffuse, and usually nearly complete, visual field loss, with visual acuity loss, along with signs and symptoms of migraine. For example, many children will show headache, irritability, nausea and even vomiting.[124] In fact, the similarities between transient cortical visual impairment and migraine in children have been commented upon by many authorities.[125]

Traumatic cranial neuropathy

Nonfatal head injuries result in cranial neuropathy as much as 13% of the time.[126] The sixth cranial nerve is most commonly traumatized, with the third cranial nerve next in incidence, followed by the fourth cranial nerve.[127] Most cases of traumatic cranial neuropathy occur between the ages of 16 and 25 years, but a wide age range can be involved, including even very young children.[128]

Diagnosis

In sixth nerve palsy, difficulty or inability to abduct the involved eye is noted. The patient demonstrates a large angle esotropia (usually greater than 30 prism diopters) in primary gaze. Bilateral sixth nerve palsies can occur, and should be searched for.

Complete third nerve palsies cause dilated pupil, complete ptosis and inability to abduct, depress or elevate the eye. The resulting eye position is one of exotropia and slight hypotropia. Partial third nerve palsies may occur, and affect the individual oculomotor nerve.

Traumatic fourth nerve palsies may be unilateral or bilateral. Unilateral cases typically show a hypertropia in primary gaze with inferior oblique overaction. Patients may demonstrate excyclotorsion of the eye, and cyclotorsional double vision up to 8°. Bilateral fourth nerve palsies occur in as many as 30% of cases.[129] Bilaterality is suggested by the following physical findings:

(i) a "V" pattern esotropia greater than 25 prism diopters;
(ii) alternating hyperdeviation (right hypertropia on right head tilt, and left hypertropia on left head tilt)[130]; and
(iii) an excyclotorsion which exceeds 15°.[131]

Management

Recovery of cranial nerve function occurs in about 40% of cases when all cases are pooled.[127] The prognosis for recovery of a traumatic fourth nerve palsy is a little better (47%), with sixth nerve palsy at 38.6% or third nerve palsy at 36.2%.[127]

Neuroimaging is often indicated when a cranial neuropathy is present. MRI is probably more sensitive in detecting subtle intraparenchymal lesions or hemorrhages. The CT scan could be more helpful in discerning skull fractures, which could contribute to the development of the cranial neuropathy.

Management of double vision includes monocular patching and the use of prisms. Most authorities would choose to wait 6 months before considering surgical management. The use of botulism neurotoxin may alleviate symptoms of double vision, at least in primary gaze, in the most acute traumatic period of sixth nerve palsy.

Disorders of accommodation following head trauma

A surprising number of patients will complain of trouble focusing their eyes following head trauma.[128] In Kowal's study of referrals to an ocular motility service in Melbourne, Australia, the most common abnormality was paresis of accommodation with no other ocular signs or symptoms. Half of the patients who had trouble accommodating improved within a year. After a year, the prognosis for recovery dropped considerably, and many patients required prolonged reading add treatment. Kowal also noted the occurrence of convergence insufficiency in some of his patients.

Carotid-cavernous fistula

Carotid-cavernous fistulas are rare in children but may occur following severe trauma (Fig. 70.17).

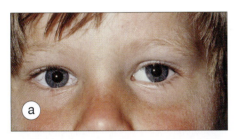
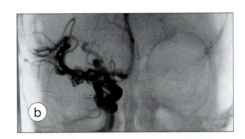
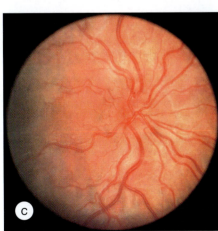
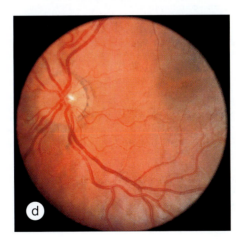

Fig. 70.17 Severe trauma. (a) This 5.5-year-old boy developed right proptosis and a squeaky bruit a week after a severe road traffic accident. (b) Carotid angiogram showing the shunt which was later closed with a balloon catheter. Dilated episcleral veins can be seen on the right. Retinal venous congestion and tortuosity with optic disc edema on the right (c, d).

REFERENCES

1. Morris R, Witherspoon CD, Kuhn F, et al. Epidemiology of Pediatric Injuries from the Injury Registry of Alabama (ERA). Presented at the First International Symposium of Ophthalmology. Bordeaux, France, 9–11 September, 1993.
2. LaRoche GR, McIntyre L, Schertzer RN. Epidemiology of severe eye injuries in childhood. Ophthalmology 1988; 95: 1603–7.
3. Rapoport I, Romen M, Kinek M, et al. Eye injuries in children in Israel: a national collaborative study. Arch Ophthalmol 1990; 108: 376–9.
4. Canavan VM, O'Flaherty MJ, Archer DB, et al. A 10-year survey of eye injuries in Northern Ireland, 1967–76. Br J Ophthalmol 1980; 64: 618–25.
5. Ilsar M, Chirambo M, Belkin M. Ocular injuries in Malawi. Br J Ophthalmol 1982; 66: 145–8.
6. Moreira CA, Debert-Ribeiro M, Belfort R. Epidemiological study of eye injuries in Brazilian children. Arch Ophthalmol 1988; 106: 781–4.

7. Vision Problems in the United States. National Society for the Prevention of Blindness. New York: National Society for the Prevention of Blindness; 1980.

8. Alfaro DV, Chaudhry NA, Walonker AF, et al. Penetrating eye injuries in young children. Retina 1994; 14: 201–5.

9. Satterfield D, Keltner JL, Morrison TL. Psychosocial aspects of strabismus study. Arch Ophthalmol 1993; 111: 1100–4.

10. Scharf J, Zonis S. Perforating injuries of the eye in childhood. J Pediatr Ophthalmol 1975; 13: 326–8.

11. Niiranen M, Raivio I. Eye injuries in children. Br J Ophthalmol 1981; 65: 436–8.

12. Baxter RJ, Hodgkins PR, Calder I, et al. Visual outcome of childhood anterior perforating eye injuries: prognostic indicators. Eye 1994; 8: 349–52.

13. Yang SK, Brown GC, Magargal LE. Self-inflicted ocular mutilation. Am J Ophthalmol 1981; 91: 658–63.

14. Trevor Roper P. The psychopathic eye. Br J Hosp Med 1980;Feb 23: 137–43.

15. Taylor S, Hyler S. Update on factitious disorders. Int J Psych Med 1993; 23: 81–94.

16. Jay J, Grant S, Murray S. Keratoconjunctivitis artefacta. Br J Ophthalmol 1982; 66: 781–5.

17. Finucane BM, Jaeger ER, Kurtz MB, et al. Eye abnormalities in the Smith-Magenis contiguous gene deletion syndrome. Am J Med Genet 1993a; 45: 443–6.

18. Finucane BM, Kurtz MB, Babu VR, et al. Mosaicism for deletion 17p11.2 in a boy with the Smith-Magenis syndrome. Am J Med Genet 1993b; 45: 447–9.

19. Milunsky A. Risk of amniocentesis for prenatal diagnosis (editorial). N Engl J Med 1975; 293: 932–3.

20. Finnegan JA, Quarrington BJ, Hughes HE, et al. Infant outcome following mid-trimester amniocentesis: development and physical status at age six months. Br J Obstet Gynaecol 1985; 92: 1015–23.

21. Rummelt B, Rummelt C, Gottfried O, et al. Congenital non-pigmented epithelial iris cyst after amniocentesis. Ophthalmology 1993; 100: 776–81.

22. Gobert A,Vereecken G, Meire F, et al. J.Ocular perforation in utero. Bull Soc Belge Ophthalmol 1995; 259: 77–80

23. Naylor G, Roper JP, Willshaw HE. Ophthalmic complications of amniocentesis. Eye 1990; 4: 845–9.

24. Admoni MM, Ben-Ezra D. Ocular trauma following amniocentesis as the cause of leukocoria. J Pediatr Ophthalmol Strabismus 1988; 25: 196–7.

25. Patel CK, Taylor DS, Russell-Eggitt IM, et al. Congenital third nerve palsy associated with mid-trimester amniocentesis. Br J Ophthalmol 1993; 77: 530–3.

26. Merin S, Beyth Y. Uniocular congenital blindness as a complication of midtrimester amniocentesis. Am J Ophthalmol 1980; 89: 299–301.

27. Isenberg SJ, Heckenlively JR. Traumatized eye with retinal damage from amniocentesis. J Pediatr Ophthalmol Strabismus 1985; 22: 65–7.

28. Hershey D. Ocular injury from amniocentesis. Ophthalmology 1993; 100: 1601–2.

29. Sachs D, Levin PS, Dooley K. Marginal eyelid laceration at birth. Am J Ophthalmol 1986; 102: 539.

30. Dorfman MS, Benson WH. Marginal eyelid laceration after episiotomy. Am J Ophthalmol 1993; 116: 778.

31. Jain IS, Singh YP, Gupta SL, et al. Ocular hazards during birth. J Pediatr Ophthalmol Strabismus 1980; 17: 14.

32. Hamed LM, Fang EN. Inferior rectus muscle contracture resulting from perinatal orbital trauma. J Pediatr Ophthalmol Strabismus 1992; 29: 387–9.

33. McDonald M, Burgess S. Contralateral occipital depression related to obstetric forceps injury to the eye. Am J Ophthalmol 1992; 114: 318–21.

34. Myers C, Christmann L. Rat bite-an unusual cause of direct trauma to the globe. J Pediatr Ophthalmol Strabismus 1991; 28: 356–8.

35. Jameson NA, Good WV, Hoyt CS. Fat adherence simulating inferior oblique palsy after blepharoplasty. Arch Ophthalmol 1992; 110: 1369.

36. Rittichier KK, Roback MG, Bassett KE. Arch Pediatr Adolesc Med 2002; 154: 370–4.

37. Michael JG, Hug D, Dowd MD. Management of corneal abrasion in children: a randomized clinical trial. Ann Emerg Med. 2002; 40: 67–72.

38. Schein OD, Enger C, Tielsch JM. The context and consequences of ocular injuries from air guns. Am J Ophthalmol 1994; 117: 501–6.

39. Pinnel SR, Krane SM, Kenzora JE, et al. A heritable disorder of connective tissue: hydroxylysine-deficient collagen disease. N Engl J Med 1972; 286: 1013–20.

40. Biglan AW, Brown SI, Johnson BL. Keratoglobus and blue sclera. Am J Ophthalmol 1977; 83: 225–33.

41. Cameron JA. Corneal abnormalities of the Ehlers-Danlos syndrome type VI. Cornea 1993; 12: 54–9.

42. Ticho U, Ivry M, Merin S. Brittle cornea, blue sclera, and red hair syndrome (the brittle cornea syndrome). Br J Med 1980; 64: 175–7.

43. Zlotogera J, Ben-Ezra D, Cohen J, et al. Syndrome of the brittle cornea, blue sclera and joint hyperextensibility. Am J Med Genet 1990; 36: 269–72.

44. Ruedemann AD Jr. Osteogenesis imperfecta congenita and blue sclerotics. Arch Ophthalmol 1953; 49: 6–16.

45. Chan CC, Green WR, de la Cruz ZC, et al. Ocular findings in osteogenesis imperfecta congenita. Arch Ophthalmol 1982; 100: 1459–63.

46. Pashby T. Eye injuries in Canadian amateur hockey. Can J Ophthalmol 1985; 20: 2–4.

47. Cascairo M, Mazow M, Prager T. Pediatric ocular trauma: a retrospective survey. J Pediatr Ophthalmol Strabismus 1994; 31: 312–17.

48. Rudd J, Jaeger E, Freitag S, et al. Traumatically ruptured globes in children. J Pediatr Ophthalmol Strabismus 1994; 31: 307–11.

49. Bachynski BN, Andreu R, Flynn JR. Spontaneous corneal perforation and extrusion of intraocular contents in premature infants. J Pediatr Ophthalmol Strabismus 1986; 23: 25–8.

50. Eagling EM. Perforating injuries of the eye. Br J Ophthalmol 1976; 60: 732–6.

51. Vinger PF. Ocular sports injuries. Principles of protection. Int Ophthalmol Clin 1981; 21: 149–61.

52. Drack A, Kutschke P, Stair S, et al. Compliance with safety glasses wear in monocular children. J Pediatr Ophthalmol Strabismus 1993; 30: 249–52.

53. Luff A, Hodgkins P, Baxter R, et al. Aetiology of perforating eye injury. Arch Dis Child 1993; 68: 682–3.

54. Wang ML, Seiff SR, Drasner K. A comparison of visual outcome in open-globe repair: succinylcholine with D-tubocurarine versus non-depolarizing agents. Ophthalmic Surg 1992; 23: 746–51.

55. Vaegan, Taylor D. Critical period for deprivation amblyopia in children. Trans Ophthalmol Soc UK 1979; 99: 432–9.

56. Epstein RJ, Fernandez A, Gammon JA. The correction of aphakia in infants with hydrogel extended wear contact lenses. Ophthalmology 1988; 95: 1102–6.

57. Sternberg P, De Juan E, Michels, RG, et al. Multivariate analysis of prognostic factors in penetrating ocular injuries. Am J Ophthalmol 1984a; 98: 467–72.

58. Sternberg P, De Juan E, Michels, RG, et al. Penetrating ocular injuries in young patients. Initial injuries and visual results. Retina 1984b; 4: 5–8.

59. Angra SK, Vajpayee RV, Titayal JS, et al. Types of posterior capsule breaks and their surgical management. Ophthalmic Surg 1991; 22: 388–91.

60. Hoyt CS. Cryotherapy for retinopathy of prematurity : 3.5 year outcome for both structure and function. Arch Ophthalmol 1993; 111: 319–20.

61. Kushner BJ. Grating acuity tests should not be used for social service purposes in preliterate children (editorial). Arch Ophthalmol 1994; 112: 1030–1.

62. Anwar M, Bleik J, von Noorden G, et al. Posterior chamber lens implantation for primary repair of corneal lacerations and traumatic cataracts in children. J Pediatr Ophthalmol·Strabismus 1994; 31: 157–61.

63. Crouch ER,Crouch ER, Jr. Pressman SH. Prospective analysis of pediatric pseudophakia: myopic shift and postoperative outcomes. J AAPOS 6: 277–82.

64. Riise R, Kolstad A, Brum S, et al. The use of contact lenses in children with unilateral traumatic aphakia. Acta Ophthalmol 1977; 55: 386–94.

65. Jain IS, Mohan K, Gupta A. Unilateral traumatic aphakia in children: role of corneal contact lenses. J Pediatr Ophthalmol Strabismus 1985; 22: 137–9.

66. Vajpayee RB, Angra SK, Honavour SG. Combined keratoplasty, cataract extraction, and intraocular lens implantation after corneolenticular laceration in children. Am J Ophthalmol 1994; 117: 507–11.

67. Shapiro MB. Lightning cataracts. Wis Med J 1984;83:23–4.

68. Little B, Aylward G. The medical management of traumatic hyphaema: a survey of opinion among ophthalmologists in the UK. J Roy Soc Med 1993; 86: 458–9.

69. Rynne MD, Romano PE. Systemic corticosteroids and the treatment of traumatic hyphema. J Pediatr Ophthalmol Strabismus 1980; 17: 141–3.

70. Palmer DJ, Goldberg MF, Frenkel, M, et al. A comparison of two dose regimens of epsilon-amino caproic acid in the prevention and management of secondary traumatic hyphemas. Ophthalmology 1986; 93: 102–8.

71. Kraft SP, Christianson, MD, Crawford JS, et al. Traumatic hyphema in children: treatment with epsilon-amino caproic acid. Ophthalmology 1987; 94: 1232–7.

72. Wolff SM, Zimmerman L. Chronic secondary glaucoma associated with retro displacement of iris root and deepening of the anterior chamber and angle secondary to contusion. Am J Ophthalmol 1962; 54: 547–63.

73. Blanton FM. Anterior chamber angle recession and secondary glaucoma, a study of the after-effects of traumatic hyphemas. Arch Ophthalmol 1964; 72: 39–42.

74. Blight R, Hart JC. Structural changes in the outer retinal layers following blunt, mechanical, non-perforating trauma to the globe: an experimental study. Br J Ophthalmol 1977; 61: 573.

75. Sipperly JO, Quigley HA, Gass JD. Traumatic retinopathy in primates: the explanation of comotio retinae. Arch Ophthalmol 1978; 96: 2267–70.

76. Gass JD. Berlin's edema. In: Stereoscopic Atlas of Macular Diseases: Diagnosis and Treatment. 3rd edn. St Louis: CV Mosby; 1987: 552.

77. Urbanek J. Über fettemoblie des Auges. Albrecht Graefe's Arch Ophthalmol 1934; 131: 147.

78. Burton TC. Unilateral Purtscher's retinopathy. Ophthalmology 1980; 87: 1096–1105.

79. Grey RH. Foveo-macular retinitis, solar retinopathy, and trauma. Br J Ophthalmol 1978; 62: 543.

80. Kaur B, Taylor D. Fundus hemorrhages in infancy. Surv Ophthalmol 1992; 37: 1–17.

81. Hollenhorst RW, Stein HA. Ocular signs and prognosis in subdural and subarachnoid bleeding in young children. Arch Ophthalmol 1958; 60: 187–92.

82. Quinn G. Vitreous and retina. In: Isenberg SJ, ed. The Eye in Infancy. Chicago: Yearbook Medical Publishers; 1989: 350–1.

83. Karr DJ, Scott WE. Visual acuity results following treatment of persistent hyperplastic primary vitreous. Arch Ophthalmol 1986; 104: 662–7.

84. Baum JD, Bulpitt CJ. Retinal and conjunctival hemorrhage in the newborn. Arch Dis Child 1970; 45: 344–9.

85. Giraud P. Alternations vasculaires retineinnes d'origine riskettsienne. Bull Soc Fr Ophtalmol 1959; 72: 621–31.

86. Pulido JS, Lingua RW, Cristol S, et al. Protein C deficiency associated with vitreous hemorrhage in a neonate. Am J Ophthalmol 1987; 104: 546–7.

87. Lauer AK, Smith JR, Robertson JE, et al. Vitreous hemorrhage is a common complication of pediatric pars planitis. Ophthalmology 2002; 109: 95–8.

88. Ferrone P, de Juan E. Vitreous hemorrhage in infants. Arch Ophthalmol 1994; 112: 1185–9.

89. Good WV, Jan JE, DeSa L, et al. Cortical visual impairment in children. Surv Ophthalmol 1994; 38: 351–64.

90. Cox MS, Schepens CL, Freeman HM. Retinal detachment due to ocular contusion. Arch Ophthalmol 1966; 76: 678–85.

91. Weidenthal DT, Schepens CL. Peripheral fundus changes associated with ocular contusion. Am J Ophthalmol 1966; 62: 465–77.

92. Robertson M, Doran M, Trimble M, et al. The treatment of Gilles de la Tourette syndrome by limbic leucotomy. J Neurol Neurosurg Psych 1990; 53: 691–4.

93. Jan JE, Good WF, Freeman RD, et al. Eye-poking. Dev Med Child Neurol 1994; 36: 321–5.

94. Balyeat RM. Complete retinal detachment (both eyes): with special reference to allergy as a possible primary etiologic factor. Am J Ophthalmol 1937; 20: 580–2.

95. Oka C, Ideta H, Nagasaki H, et al. Retinal detachment with atopic dermatitis similar to traumatic retinal detachment. Ophthalmology 1994; 101: 1050–4.

96. Smith B, Regan WF Jr. Blow-out fracture of the orbit; mechanism and correction of internal orbital fracture. Am J Ophthalmol 1957; 44: 733–9.

97. McLachlan DL, Flanagan JC, Shannon GM. Complications of orbital roof fractures. Ophthalmology 1982;89:1274–8.

98. Pfeiffer RL. Traumatic enophthalmos. Arch Ophthalmol 1943; 30: 718–26.

99. Converse JM, Smith B. Blow-out fracture of the floor of the orbit. Trans Am Acad Ophthalmol Otolaryngol 1960; 64: 676–88.

100. Fujino T. Experimental "blow-out" fracture of the orbit. Plast Reconstr Surg 1974; 56: 81–2.

101. Kersten RC. Blow-out fracture of the orbital floor with entrapment caused by isolated trauma to the orbital rim. Am J Ophthalmol 1987; 103: 215–20.

102. Seiff SR, Good WV. Hypertropia and the posterior blowout fracture: mechanism and management. Ophthalmology 1996; 103: 152–6.

103. Brodsky MC, James C. Ocular protrusion with contralateral jaw movement. Arch Ophthalmol 1993; 111: 1028–9.

104. Gjerris F. Traumatic lesions of the visual pathways. In: Vinken PJ, Bruyn CW, eds. Handbook of Clinical Neurology, Vol. 24. Amsterdam: North Holland; 1976: 27–57.

105. Turner JW. Indirect injury of the optic nerves. Brain 1943; 66: 140–5.

106. Hillman JS, Myska V, Nissim S. Complete avulsion of the optic nerve. A clinical, angiographic, and electrodiagnostic study. Br J Ophthalmol 1975; 59: 503–9.

107. Chow AY, Goldberg MF, Frenkel M. Evulsion of the optic nerve in association with basketball injuries. Ann Ophthalmol 1984; 16: 35–47.

108. Heine J. Optic nerve evulsion. Klin Monatsbl Augeheilkd 1990; 196: 484–5.

109. Christ T, Pillunat L, Wagner P. Computerized tomography in partial avulsion of the optic nerve. Klin Monatsbl Augenheilkd 1985; 187: 531–3.

110. Talwar D, Kumar A, Verma L, et al. Ultrasonography in optic nerve head avulsion. Acta Ophthalmol 1991; 69: 121–3.

111. Krauss HR, Yee RD, Foos RY. Autoenucleation. Surv Ophthalmol 1984; 29: 179–87.

112. Hayreh SS. Anterior Ischemic Optic Neuropathy. Berlin: Springer-Verlag; 1975: 12–23.

113. Guy J, Sherwood M, Day AL. Surgical treatment of progressive visual loss in traumatic optic neuropathy. J Neurosurg 1989; 70: 799–801.

114. Byrne SF, Glaser JS. Orbital tissue differentiation with standardized echography. Ophthalmology 1983; 90: 1071–90.

115. Mauriello JA, DeLuca J, Krieger A, et al. Management of traumatic optic neuropathy-a study of 23 patients. Br J Ophthalmol 1992; 76: 349–52.

116. Kline LB, Morawetz RB, Swaid SN. Indirect injury of the optic nerve. Neurosurgery 1984; 14: 756–64.

117. McDaniel KD, McDaniel LD. Anton's syndrome in a patient with post-traumatic optic neuropathy and bifrontal contusions. Arch Neurol 1991; 48: 101–5.

118. Brachen MB, Shepard MJ, Collins WF, et al. A randomized, controlled trial of methylprednisolone or naloxone in the treatment of acute spinal-cord injury. Results of the Second National Acute Spinal Cord Injury Study. N Engl J Med 1990; 322: 1405–11.

119. Seiff SR. High dose corticosteroids for treatment of vision loss due to indirect injury to the optic nerve. Ophthalmic Surg 1990; 21: 389–95.

120. Levin L, Joseph M, Rizzo J, et al. Optic canal decompression in indirect optic nerve trauma. Ophthalmology 1994; 101: 566–9.

121. Browder EJ, Kaplan HA, Baldwin M, et al. Cerebral concussion and its sequelae. NY State J Med 1961; 61: 1864–1903.

122. Hoyt WF. Vascular lesions of the visual cortex with brain herniation through the tentorial incisura. Arch Ophthalmol 1960; 64: 44–57.

123. Hass DC, Pineda GS, Lourie H. Juvenile head trauma syndromes and their relationship to migraine. Arch Neurol 1975; 32: 727–30.

124. Mitchel EM, Troost BT. Palinopsia: cerebral localization with computed tomography. Neurology 1980; 30: 887–9.

125. Kaye EM, Herskowitz J. Transient post-traumatic cortical blindness: brief versus prolonged syndromes in childhood. J Child Neurol 1986; 1: 206–10.

126. Baker RS, Epstein AD. Ocular motor abnormalities from head trauma. Surv Ophthalmol 1991; 35: 245–67.

127. Rush JA, Younge BR. Paralysis of cranial nerves III, IV, and VI. Cause and prognosis in 1000 cases. Arch Ophthalmol 1981; 99: 76–9.

128. Kowal L. Ophthalmic manifestations of head injury. Aust NZ J Ophthalmol 1992; 20: 35–40.

129. Snydor CF, Seaber BA, Buckley EG. Traumatic superior oblique palsies. Ophthalmology 1982; 89: 134–8.

130. Jampolsky A. Management of vertical strabismus. In: Crawford JS, Flynn JT, Haik BG et al., eds. Pediatric Ophthalmology and Strabismus. Transactions of the New Orleans Academy of Ophthalmology. New York: Raven Press; 1986: 141–71.

131. Ellis FD, Helveston EM. Superior oblique palsy: diagnosis and classification. In: Strabismus Surgery. Boston: Little, Brown; 1976: 127–35.

CHAPTER
71

Child Abuse, Nonaccidental Injury, and the Eye

David Taylor

CHILD ABUSE

Child abuse is a general term used to cover the various forms of damage inflicted on children including neglect, sexual abuse, emotional abuse, induced illness, and physical injury (see Table 71.1).[1] A child may have been subject to more than one kind of abuse. Nonaccidental injury (NAI) is strictly a term that encompasses other forms of injury including some sports, criminal injury, or surgery!

For more complete referencing see Taylor.[1]

In 1946, John Caffey, a New York radiologist published six cases in which there were unaccountable long bone fractures in infants whose principal problem was chronic subdural hematoma, later coining the term "whiplash shaken infant syndrome."[2] Other terms such as battered baby and shaken baby syndrome are sometimes used.

Epidemiology

Rare before the 1960s, a series of papers led to the realization that it is a phenomenon of substantial proportions in many societies today.

In the USA, 300,000 children may be physically abused, 140,000 are sexually abused, and 700,000 are neglected or maltreated each year: this leads to about 1100 annual deaths.[3]

Accident and other referral centers report that nonaccidental injuries are a major, or the most important, cause of serious head injuries, especially in infants.

Indirect evidence comes from studies in the UK of the incidence of subdural hemorrhages, where the incidence has been found to be 12.8 per 100,000 children per year, or 21 per 100,000 infants under 1 year per year.[4]

There is little doubt that child abuse is underdiagnosed,[5] with consequences not only for the undiagnosed children, but in lessening the actions taken to protect children and their siblings from further assault.

Child abuse is under-reported in higher socioeconomic groups who are subject to emotional abuse[6] (see Table 71.2), and burns are probably underdiagnosed.

History taking in suspected child abuse

The taking of a detailed history and recording it is of paramount importance in suspected cases of child abuse (Table 71.3), not only in the clinical management but also in any subsequent legal proceedings. Take the history yourself and write what is said, i.e., "went a bit blue" and not "complained of apnea." Unnecessary history taking at a late stage by the ophthalmologist may damage the future relationship with the family if the child survives. Keep a professional detachment from the issues and stick to the eye examination and management itself and document this well, including photography if possible.

Ophthalmic examination in a patient with suspected child abuse

The eye examination of a patient with suspected child abuse should include the following:

1. Age-appropriate vision assessment;
2. Pupil responses, especially for a relative afferent defect;
3. External eye inspection, including lids, ears, and face;
4. Refraction;
5. Slit-lamp (portable?) examination if possible, looking for iridodonesis, pupil sphincter rupture, cataract, and subtle hyphema;
6. Fundus examination with the pupil dilated, after discussion with the pediatrician, in particular neuro-observations including indirect ophthalmoscopy;
7. Documentation of clinical (including normal) findings with annotated drawings;
8. Fundus photography and external photography, including normal features, correctly timed and dated (wide-angle fundus cameras can enhance documentation);
9. A nonocular examination, which is essential unless the pediatrician or a named doctor has become involved;

Table 71.1 Classification of child abuse

Physical abuse
  Indirect trauma and shaking
  Direct trauma
  Smothering
  Poisoning
Induced illness: Münchausen syndrome by proxy
Sexual abuse
Neglect
Emotional Abuse

Table 71.2 The psychosocial background

Family history of abuse frequent
Parents often abused themselves
All social classes but:
  —Less frequently diagnosed in higher socioeconomic groups[6]
  —More in the socially deprived and stressed
Fathers or mothers male partners[7]
Psychiatric and sociopathic abnormalities frequent in abusers

Table 71.3 Situations that may suggest child abuse in the history and examination

Child and family characteristics
Premature, handicapped, crying colicky babies.
Children of abused parents.
Younger infants are more frequently abused than older ones.
Parents are drug or alcohol abusers.
Other children in the family have been abused.
Family frequently attends (sometimes multiple) A&E departments.
A current family crisis.
Isolated families without help sources.
Families on "at-risk" registers.

Presentation situations
The account or age of injuries inconsistent with appearance.
Injuries of different ages.
Multiple fractures in different stages of healing.
Lack of parental concern.
Delay in seeking medical advice.
Previous seizures, "funny turns," "blue attacks," etc.
Injury occurring at night (when the child would normally be asleep).

Injury types
Head injuries in infants or nonmobile children.
Subdural or subarachnoid hemorrhages.
Human bite marks, black eyes, or fingertip bruising.
Cigarette burns, especially if multiple.
Scalds, especially in the absence of splash marks.
Retinal hemorrhages.
Unusual fractures, e.g., acromion, metaphyseal, and rib fractures.
Bruising in inaccessible sites or unusual cuts or marks.

Behavioral and other signs
"Frozen watchfulness."
Aggressive, highly active playing or acting out.
Unusual closeness or distance between parents.
Hostility or overfriendliness by parents or child to hospital staff.
Male sex of the child and the perpetrator.

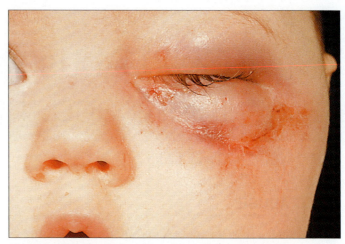

Fig. 71.1 Although mostly accidental in an A&E setting, periocular bruising should always lead to suspicion of a nonaccidental injury, especially in predisposed children and if the circumstances, the age of the child, or the nature of the injury are unusual.

10. Collaboration with the pediatrician especially to exclude a bleeding diathesis; and
11. Follow-up arrangements for those with eye involvement who survive, as visual sequelae are common and often severe.

Ocular signs of child abuse

Direct injuries
Direct injuries are those in which there is a direct blow to the eye or periocular tissues.

Periocular bruising
Lid and subconjunctival bruising is common in Accident and Emergency (A&E): "black eyes" should suggest an examination of the eye for ocular trauma and retinal hemorrhages, which may suggest NAI (Fig. 71.1). If they are bilateral, one must remember a basal fracture.

Lid lacerations, orbital hemorrhage, and inflammation
Punches or slaps may result in periorbital or orbital hemorrhage; lid laceration is less common, implying the use of an instrument.

Unexplained lens dislocation or cataract
In nonaccidentally dislocated lenses and cataracts, the cause may be due to trauma to the lens itself or secondary to intraocular damage.

Conjunctival and corneal injuries
Inflicted corneal injuries are rare, but recurrent kerato-

conjunctivitis,[8,9] though rare, may be more frequent than is currently recognized.

Intraocular hemorrhages and retinal detachment
Retinal detachment and vitreous hemorrhage may be due to direct or indirect trauma. Vitreous base avulsion suggests a contusion injury because vitreoretinal adhesion at the vitreous base is strong in the child and avulsion probably requires more distortive forces than those with shaking injuries alone.[10]

Pupil abnormalities
Abnormalities of the pupil reactions may be due to intracranial problems, but some, predominantly unilateral, cases are due to direct injury to the iris; these are usually accompanied by other intraocular injuries and hemorrhage.

Indirect injuries
Subconjunctival hemorrhages
These are fairly common in the normal neonate, and may be seen in assaulted infants and children when the central venous pressure has been raised.

Hemorrhages in and around the eye
The detection of retinal hemorrhages is a vital part of the work-up of the infant suspected of suffering child abuse: they are an important cause of long-term morbidity and may be important in medicolegal proceedings.[11,12]

Scoring systems
See Jayawant et al.[4]

Age of abused children with retinal hemorrhages
Retinal hemorrhages are more frequent in NAI below 1 year of age, and less frequent and less severe in older children.

Location and type of retinal hemorrhages
Clinically, hemorrhages are seen most easily and frequently at the posterior pole (Fig. 71.2).

Histopathologically, they are more common in the peripheral retina than at the macula or around the optic disc, and least

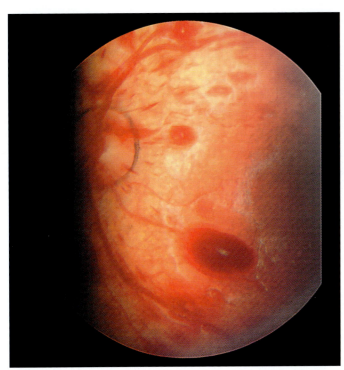

Fig. 71.2 Clinically, hemorrhages in NAI are seen mostly at the posterior pole of the eye. Pathologically, they are widespread. They typically affect more than one retinal layer, subhyaloid are most frequently and easily seen, and they may involve the vitreous. None are pathognomonic of NAI.

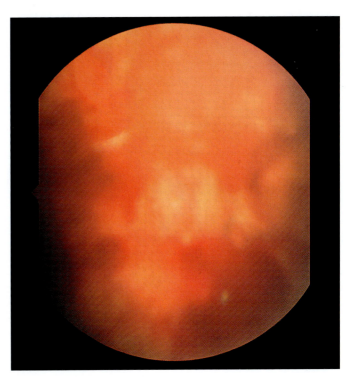

Fig. 71.3 Massive retinal hemorrhages and vitreous hemorrhage. The optic disc can just be seen in the center of the picture.

common at the equator.[13] Typically all layers of the retina are involved,[13] but hemorrhages confined to one layer are also found. They may have white centers that consist of fibrin.[14]

Purtscher's retinopathy, in which there are retinal exudates as well as hemorrhages, is also found in child abuse, since it occurs mostly after chest compression. Air emboli may play a role, and in NAI it is likely that there is a combined effect.

Accidental and nonaccidental trauma

A number of studies have established that retinal hemorrhages are rare after accidental trauma in infants and young children but may be seen after very severe accidental head injury[15,16] causing skull fractures and diffuse or focal intracranial damage.[17-19]

Only a small minority of children attending hospital actually have signs of eye or brain damage.[20,21] In one study of a large number of falls in infancy, 97% involved injury to the head but less than 1% resulted in fractures or concussion. If damage is rare, the chances of a minor injury causing retinal bleeding, which is associated with severe neurological damage, is very unlikely.[12]

When children receive fatal injuries after reportedly short falls, they are more likely to be nonaccidental[22]: although this has been challenged,[23] it has not been done so conclusively. It is vital always to exclude the possibility that an injury has been accidental even in apparently "obvious" circumstances.

Tangential acceleration is associated with much more brain deformation and shear than an equivalent linear acceleration, hence the propensity for retinal hemorrhage to occur with shaking injury in infants.[19]

Although it is much more likely that massive retinal hemorrhages (Fig. 71.3) are caused by a nonaccidental injury, it cannot be said that less extensive hemorrhages (Fig. 71.4) are less likely to be associated with nonaccidental injury.

The biomechanics of retinal hemorrhages

Direct evidence that angular acceleration without impact can produce retinal haemorrhages[24] includes the finding of retinal hemorrhages in adults after emergency aircraft ejection without impact and in experiments in which subjects experienced brief deceleration above 40G. Retinal hemorrhages are also described after road traffic accidents in which there has been no direct trauma to the eye,[25] and they have been described in "bungee-jumpers." Supportive evidence comes from retinal hemorrhages seen after confessed shaking injuries.[19,25]

Much of the indirect evidence linking brain and eye injury is based on the correlation between the severity of ocular injury and the severity of the intracerebral injury. This enables information gathered on the forces required for cerebral injury to be extrapolated to eye injury.[13,26,27] Subdural hematomas and other cerebral hemorrhages and tears were produced by whiplash injury without impact in monkeys. The acceleration threshold for cerebral injury calculated from animal experiments was easily exceeded by shake and impact in life-sized and head weight-equivalent infant models.[28] This threshold could not be reached by violent shaking alone but this may have reflected deficiencies in the model construction.[25] Not all infants with retinal hemorrhages associated with abuse have signs of impact injury.[13,25]

No absolute value can be given for the angular acceleration forces and jerk required to produce retinal bleeding or other injury unlikely to be inflicted accidentally by well-meaning carers, but there is good evidence that they must be considerable.[29] Retinal hemorrhages are not reported in quite severe household falls, even when associated with skull fractures, but occur after very severe motor accidents.[19,25,30]

Geddes et al.[31,32] showed that, in about one-third of infants with inflicted brain injury, there is evidence of axonal damage at the craniocervical junction, which might give rise to damage to the respiratory centers, producing the hypoxic neuronal damage

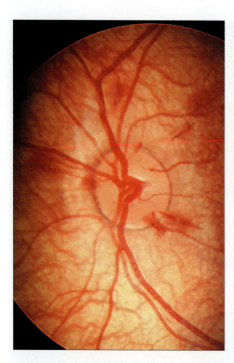
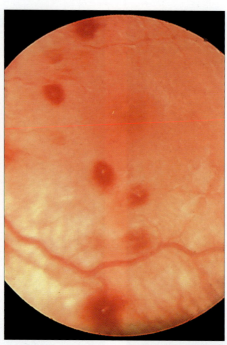

Fig. 71.4 Mild retinal hemorrhages in two NAI cases.

seen in these children rather than the diffuse axonal damage seen in traumatic injury. Their cases all had severe head injury but they suggested that it might not be necessary to shake an infant violently to produce a craniocervical injury. Other high cervical injuries, even when severe enough to induce apnea and hypoxia, from other causes do not give rise to the clinical picture of the shaken baby syndrome.[12]

Retinal hemorrhages are associated with types of cerebral injury that require severe concussive forces. Subdural hemorrhages (which are commonly associated with retinal hemorrhages in NAI) are formed when there is surface vascular damage during short duration angular acceleration loading at high rates of acceleration, as in deceleration-impact injuries in falls. Diffuse axonal injury, mostly seen with motor accidents, is usually seen with coronal plane angular acceleration of longer duration and at a lower rate.[33]

By making comparisons with intracerebral lesions, the finding of retinal hemorrhages with additional features, such as vitreous hemorrhage (Fig. 71.5), perimacular folds (Figs. 71.6, 71.7), subretinal hemorrhages, and choroidal hemorrhage indicates a greater severity of applied force.[13,27] None are pathognomonic.

Blunt head trauma

Blunt head trauma, in addition to angular acceleration, may be necessary to produce the most serious eye problems in child abuse, as the deceleration produced in impact injuries is greater than that produced when the head is flexed or extended to its limits without impact.[19,28] Elner et al.[34] found sometimes occult evidence of head injury at autopsy of all of 10 cases of suspected child abuse. However, evidence of associated head injury is not always present in severe cerebral injury with coexisting eye injuries.[13,35] Gilliland and Folberg[25] found that, of 80 infants dying of NAI, over half had impact injuries without evidence of shaking, over a third had evidence of combined shaking and impact, and the remaining minority had exclusively shaking-induced injuries.

Hypoxia and ischemia

Hypoxia and ischemia, sometimes ongoing, play a significant role in determining the severity of cerebral injuries, whether it is due

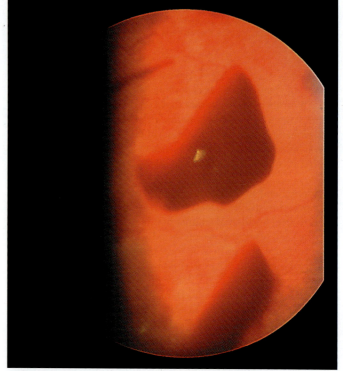

Fig. 71.5 Retinal, preretinal, and vitreous hemorrhages.

to the nature of the trauma itself[36] or to nonspecific trauma-induced apnea[37]: it is likely that similar mechanisms apply to the severity of eye damage.

Increasing retinal hemorrhages

Retinal hemorrhages most rapidly increase in extent and severity while the trauma and its immediate effects are in progress. Many of the intracranial events associated with retinal hemorrhages progress gradually: subdural hemorrhages may progressively

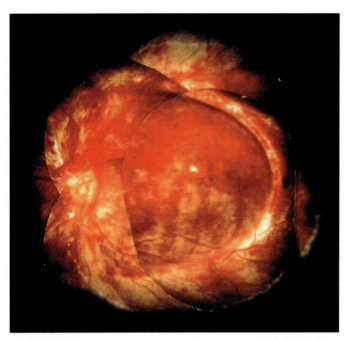

Fig. 71.6 Extensive retinal hemorrhage with a perimacular fold. The optic disc is on the left and the fold extends to surround the macular. There was a severe brain injury.

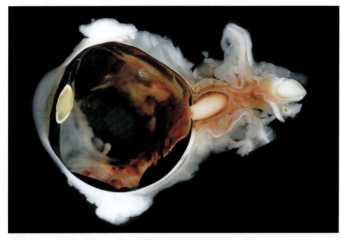

Fig. 71.7 Calotte of the eye shown in Fig. 71.6 showing massive retinal hemorrhage. It was not possible to demonstrate the perimacular fold. (Photograph courtesy of Professor Phil Luthert, London.)

enlarge and further retinal hemorrhages may occur. Therefore, the finding of increasingly extensive intraocular hemorrhages could reflect observer error, further trauma, further hemorrhages as a result of continuation of the effects of the original trauma, or a spread of the hemorrhage from one layer or area of the retina to another.

Birth-related hemorrhages

Retinal hemorrhages are common at birth, occurring in between 2.6 and 59% of newborn infants.[38] The incidence is increased in prolonged labor, assisted delivery, and toxemia, in the children of older primiparae, and possibly with parenteral vitamin E and dinoprostone induction of labor. The incidence appears to be decreased after cesarean section and breech delivery.

The finding of retinal hemorrhages in a large proportion of normal neonates[38] has caused a dilemma in cases of suspected child abuse: are the hemorrhages due to abuse or natural causes?

Table 71.4 Unilateral retinal hemorrhages
Unilateral or highly asymmetrical retinal hemorrhages are not uncommon in child abuse but may also occur in disease and in accidental trauma.[1] The mechanisms may be: 1. Anatomical differences in the optic nerve; 2. Asymmetry in the injury; 3. Shear forces are greater the more peripheral to the center of rotation: one eye receives more accelerative; and 4. Additional local injury.

There are four usual morphological types of neonatal hemorrhages: superficial retinal (splinter- or flame-shaped), intraretinal (dot/blot/domed), preretinal/subhyaloid, and subretinal. Birth-related hemorrhages are thought to occur during labor[38] by leakage from retinal venules and capillaries, and they are similar in appearance to hemorrhages occurring after central retinal vein occlusion or raised intracranial pressure (Fig. 71.8). It is suggested[38] that hypercapnia and hypoxia cause vessel dilatation and compression during labor, leading to raised intracranial pressure and impaired venous return, leading to vessel rupture and hemorrhage. There seems to be no association between neonatal retinal hemorrhages and platelet count, plasma fibrinogen level, or the thrombotest result.[39]

Hemorrhages present after birth disappear rapidly, with very few exceptions; this has been summarized in table form by von Barsewisch.[38] The finest nerve fiber layer (NFL) hemorrhages can disappear in 24 hr, while even extensive NFL hemorrhages are usually gone within a few days. Half of hemorrhages disappear within 48 hr,[40] and Sezen[41] found that 2.6% persisted at 72–120 hr after birth. In one case, the hemorrhage persisted for 6 weeks. Larger subhyaloid and intraretinal hemorrhages seem to persist for the longest time.[39] Most neonatal retinal hemorrhages have no visual sequelae, although occasional cases of long-term visual impairment are reported.

Many of the studies mentioned in more detail in Jayawant et al.[4] were not truly longitudinal and further studies would be helpful.

Both birth related and other retinal hemorrhages in infants can be unilateral (Table 71.4).

The intracranial associations of retinal hemorrhages

There is a close correlation between the severity of retinal hemorrhages and intracranial injuries,[13] although it is sometimes difficult to diagnose intracranial injury on the initial CT scan. It is usual for NAI patients with subdural hemorrhages and other intracranial injuries (Figs. 71.9–71.11) to have retinal hemorrhages, but the association is not invariable;[13] between 11[42] and 39%[43] of abused children do not have retinal hemorrhages. Most subdural hemorrhages in children are associated with child abuse, and they have eye abnormalities.[4]

The differential diagnosis of retinal hemorrhages in childhood

There are numerous conditions that give rise to retinal hemorrhages in infants and children. Mostly, they all have their own special features:

1. Leukemia: 10% of children with acute lymphatic leukemia have intraretinal hemorrhages and 3% have white-centered hemorrhages.
2. Hemorrhagic disease of the newborn.
3. Retinopathy of prematurity.
4. Sickle cell retinopathy.
5. Neonatal arterial hypertension.

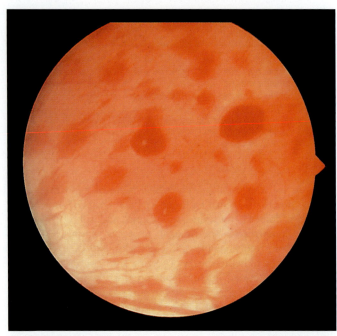

Fig. 71.8 Neonatal retinal hemorrhages. (Photograph by courtesy of Dr Andrew Q McCormick, Vancouver.)

6. ECMO treatment.
7. Metabolic disease: galactosemia, glutaric aciduria type 1.[44]
8. Other bleeding disorders: Henoch-Schönlein purpura, Von Willebrand disease, protein C deficiency, and Hermansky-Pudlak syndrome.[45] However, intracranial hemorrhage is infrequent after accidental head trauma in children with a congenital coagulopathy.[46]

Evidence of a bleeding disorder is not uncommon in child abuse,[47] sometimes due to consumption of coagulation factors in the formation of intracranial hemorrhages.

9. Scurvy.
10. Maternal ingestion of cocaine.
11. Meningitis.
12. Intracranial vascular malformation.
13. Optic disc drusen, in tuberous sclerosis[48] and X-linked retinoschisis.[49]
14. Chronic, severe papilledema associated with diagnosable intracranial pathology may cause peripapillary hemorrhages, and acute, severely raised intracranial pressure may cause widespread hemorrhage.
15. Multiple retinal hemorrhages following intraocular surgery in infants.[50]
16. Severe hypertension.
17. Congenital retinal macrovessels.

Seizures and retinal hemorrhages

In adults with seizures, retinal hemorrhages were not noted in any of 560 visits to an emergency department that resulted in 7

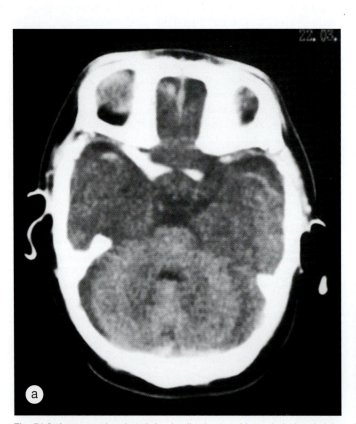

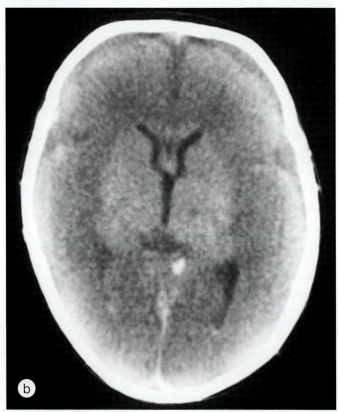

Fig. 71.9 Acute on chronic subdural collections and hypoxic-ischemic injury. Axial CT scans at the level of the (a) cerebellum and (b) third ventricle of a 4-month-old child with generalized seizures. There is widespread low-density change through the cerebral cortex and white matter, and preservation of the cerebellum and central gray structures. In addition, there are bilateral chronic subdural collections (low attenuation) overlying the cerebral hemispheres with evidence of recent hemorrhage (high attenuation) within them anteriorly over the temporal lobes and posteriorly within the interhemispheric fissure. The acute on chronic subdural collections are likely to have been caused by shaking on more than one occasion, and the hypoxic-ischemic injury was most likely caused by suffocation. (Images courtesy of Dr Dawn Saunders, Great Ormond Street Hospital, London.)

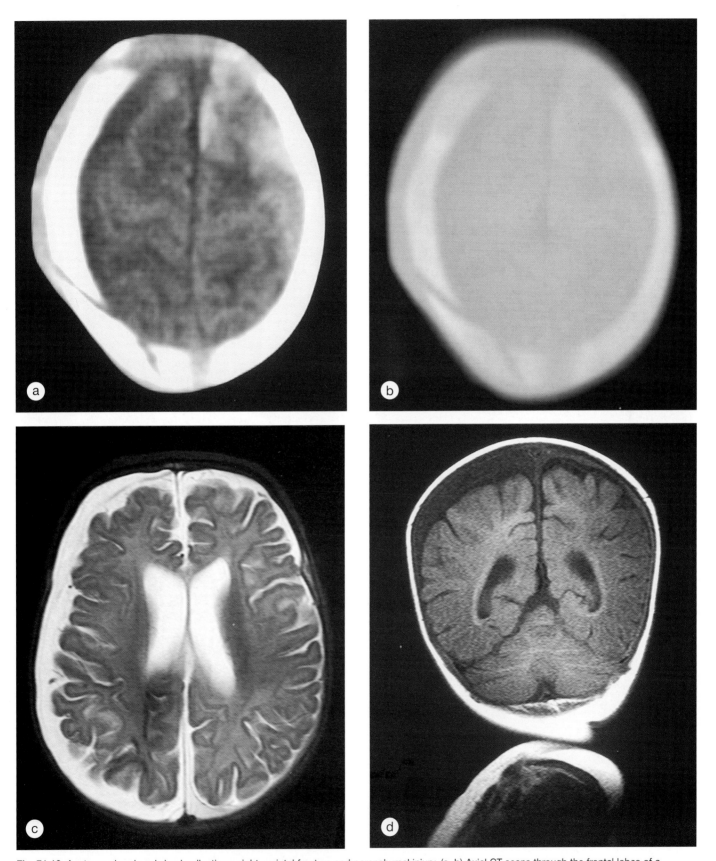

Fig. 71.10 Acute on chronic subdural collections, right parietal fracture and parenchymal injury. (a, b) Axial CT scans through the frontal lobes of a 2-month-old child who presented jittery and generally unwell. A linear fracture through the right parietal bone and overlying soft tissue swelling is seen on both the soft tissue and bone windows. Bilateral subdural collections are seen. The right-sided collection is low density, which implies it occurred more than 7–10 days ago, and the left high-density subdural collection most likely occurred within the preceding 3 days. The acute subdural is seen on the background of a left-side chronic subdural (see MRI). (c, d) T_2-weighted axial and T_1-weighted coronal images reveal bilateral chronic subdural collections, larger and older on the right. Bilateral cortical edema of the parietal lobes, worse on the right, is compatible with recent parenchymal injury. (Images courtesy of Dr Dawn Saunders, Great Ormond Street Hospital, London.)

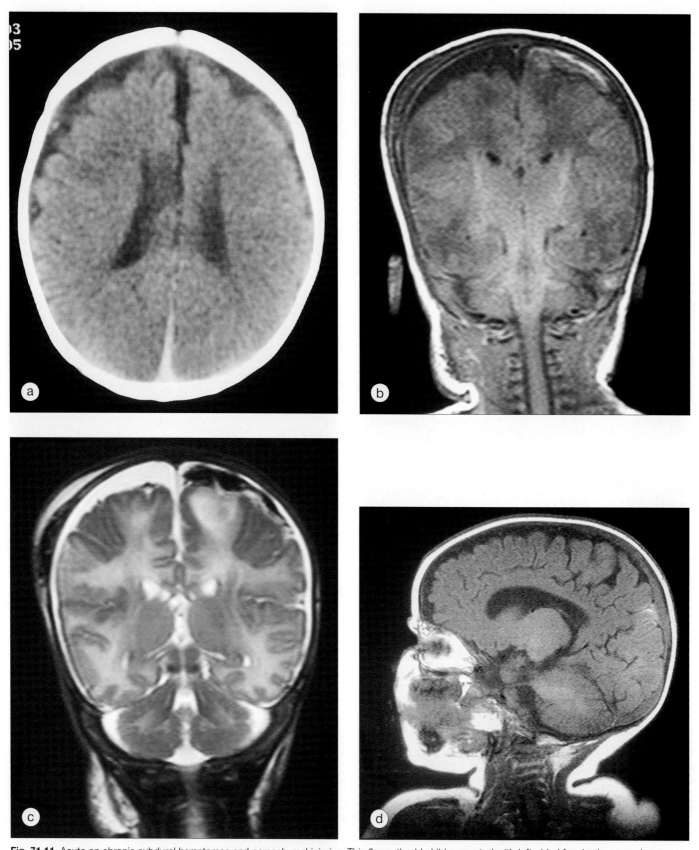

Fig. 71.11 Acute on chronic subdural hematomas and parenchymal injuries. This 3-month-old child presented with left-sided focal seizures and was found to have retinal hemorrrhages, (a) Axial CT scan reveals an acute subdural collection in the posterior interhemispheric fissure and bilateral chronic anterior subdural collections. A focal area of low density is visible in the right side of the corpus callosum. Coronal (b) T_1- and (c) T_2-weighted images through the bodies of the lateral ventricles show evidence of more recent hemorrhage (high signal on T_1-weighted and low signal on the T_2-weighted images) within the chronic subdural collection over the left frontal lobe. Additional cortical edema is seen in the underlying left frontal lobe. (d) The posterior acute subdural hemorrhage can be seen on the sagittal T_1-weighted image to both involve the posterior interhemispheric fissure and lie beneath the tentorium cerebelli. Soft tissue swelling can be seen at the vertex. (Images courtesy of Dr Dawn Saunders, Great Ormond Street Hospital, London.)

deaths and 553 injuries.[51] A case of extensive retinal hemorrhages was described in a 32-year-old man after status epilepticus 3 months after surgery for Arnold-Chiari malformation.[52]

A study in which 33 children were examined ophthalmoscopically within 48 hr of hospital admission for an episode of seizures revealed no retinal hemorrhages despite some having vomited or having had cardiopulmonary resuscitation;[53] later, the authors reported a premature infant who had seizures from 10 days and had unilateral retinal hemorrhages at 23 days. Another study[54] suggested that the upper limit of 95% confidence interval of retinal hemorrhages, following convulsions in children under 14 years old, is less than 5/100. Therefore, convulsions in young children very rarely cause retinal haemorrhages.[11]

Cardiopulmonary resuscitation (CPR), Valsalva's maneuver, and retinal hemorrhages

CPR, even by trained personnel, causes a marked rise in intracranial pressure. Violent chest compression in child abuse may be a cause of retinal hemorrhages, and attempted CPR by untrained individuals has been advanced as an innocent (although NAI was not convincingly excluded) cause of retinal hemorrhages in a single case report.[55]

There have been other reports of retinal hemorrhages occurring after CPR without other explanation for the hemorrhages.[56,57] One neonate with meconium aspiration who had CPR during the first day of life before being put onto ECMO suffered seizures, and vitreous hemorrhages were noted on the 11th day.[58] No case with retinal hemorrhages was found in an autopsy study of 169 cases, 131 of which had had prolonged resuscitation.[59]

Kanter,[60] a pediatrician, found retinal hemorrhages on non-mydriatic ophthalmoscopy in only one of 45 children who had not had prior trauma, and were successfully or unsuccessfully resuscitated: that child had severe arterial hypertension and seizures. This study may have methodological weaknesses.[61]

Experimental evidence from studies on piglets showed no retinal hemorrhages despite high, monitored, intracranial and intrathoracic pressures,[62] although there are a number of differences between pig and human retinas.

CPR alone is unlikely to cause retinal hemorrhages, even if carried out by unskilled individuals.[11]

Valsalva's maneuver may be associated with retinal hemorrhage in adults, but with the possible anecdotal exception of pertussis, no cases have been described in children.[11]

The clearing of retinal hemorrhages

With retinal hemorrhages, the color changes that occur in skin bruising are different, the changes are so gradual, and the retinal background contrast is so variable that accurate dating of retinal hemorrhages to within days, based on their ophthalmoscopic appearance, is not accurate. The color of a retinal hemorrhage is influenced at least as much by its size as by its age. Brown-yellow ochre membranes are consistent with injuries of at least one month old, and the presence of bright red fresh hemorrhage together with ochre membranes strongly suggests hemorrhages of different ages.[11]

Mild retinal hemorrhages in NAI probably clear rapidly; "flame-shaped" birth-related hemorrhages may resolve within 24 hr; and moderately severe retinal hemorrhages clear within a few weeks.[63] Severe, widespread, retinal and vitreous hemorrhages (Fig. 71.12) may take many months to clear, and usually are associated with substantial residual damage. If sub- and intra-retinal hemorrhages are found in the absence of flame-shaped hemorrhages this may suggest that the injury occurred at least

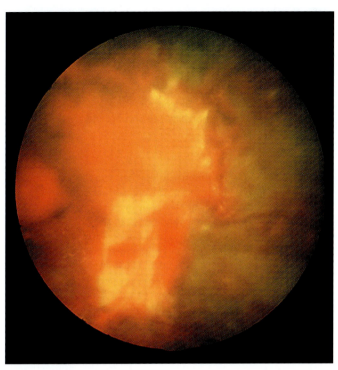

Fig. 71.12 Widespread retinal and vitreous hemorrhages in various stages of organization.

24 hr previously because of different clearing rates, but there are no studies to corroborate this. Dating and timing can be very difficult on morphological grounds alone.[64]

Pathological studies suggest that the finding of hemosiderin in a hemorrhage suggests that it is more than about three days old:[65] in current forensic practice it is generally agreed that hemosiderin begins to appear around 48 hr after injury in bruises in skin and subcutaneous tissue. If there are some hemorrhages with and some without hemosiderin this suggests that the hemorrhages are of different ages,[34,66] but it is possible that there are minor differences in the biochemical ageing of hemorrhages at different sites or even within a single organ. There is no detailed research giving the time of appearance of hemosiderin in retinal tissues.

The persistence of hemosiderin following birth-related hemorrhage at any site is also poorly documented; current opinion favors the disappearance of hemosiderin from soft tissues within 6-8 weeks after birth. Xanthochromic staining of the relatively avascular dura may persist for much longer. If hemosiderin is found in the relatively vascular eye tissues in infants of more than 2–3 months old it is likely that this is from a hemorrhage occurring after birth.

Intrascleral hemorrhages

Hemorrhages in the sclera around the optic disc have been noted histopathologically[14,34,64] associated with trauma,[15] particularly child abuse. A proposed mechanism is that acceleration and deceleration motions tears the intrascleral ciliary vessels that form the circle of Zinn and Haller;[14] the bilaterality seen in many cases suggests that the mechanism is head motion rather than eye or localized trauma.

Optic nerve sheath hemorrhages

Hemorrhages in and around the optic nerve sheath are common in fatally or otherwise seriously injured children.[13,15] When found together with retinal hemorrhages they are very suggestive of child abuse,[64] but cannot be considered pathognomonic.

When at the optic nerve–scleral junction, the pathogenesis may be similar to that of intrascleral haemorrhage,[14] the hemorrhage occurring in the sclera and the adjacent optic nerve sheath. Elsewhere in the optic nerve, a sudden rise in intracranial pressure and cycles of acceleration and deceleration are the most likely causes, giving rise to hemorrhages in and around the optic nerve subarachnoid space.

Perimacular retinal folds

There are no fundus abnormalities that can be described as pathognomonic of child abuse. Severe retinal hemorrhage and perimacular folds are frequently seen in NAI,[34,64,67–69] but they cannot be said to be pathognomonic,[70] as they occur in severe accidental injury and Terson syndrome.[71] However, they are much more likely to be seen in child abuse, and it is likely that the forces generated are sufficient to cause hemorrhages in both the brain and the eye.[12,72] The presence of perimacular folds may suggest that there have been cycles of acceleration and deceleration,[68,69] perhaps also with impact.[34] Perimacular folds may be unilateral.[64]

Defects of pupil reactions

With very severe intraocular or intrasheath hemorrhages, amaurotic pupils may be found; if there is an interocular difference in the extent of the damage, a relative afferent defect may be found.

Third nerve and other cranial nerve palsies are due to intracranial events. The observation of pupil reactions is a vital part of the monitoring of many of children admitted to hospital with head injuries. It may be so important that the pediatrician or intensivist in charge of the case may not wish pupil dilating drops to be instilled: this precludes a full examination of the fundus, but direct ophthalmoscopy or the use of a small pupil indirect ophthalmoscope can help. Short-acting mydriatics, such as tropicamide 0.5–1%, may be useful.

Retinal detachment

Retinal detachments are seen after indirect injuries in child abuse[73] and because they suggest greater trauma,[13] not necessarily direct, has taken place, they are often associated with severe intracranial injuries.[13]

Retinal pigmentation

Peripheral retinal pigmentation or chorioretinal lesions have been noted, presumably due to the various effects of trauma,[73] the frequency of peripheral subhyaloid hemorrhages in less severe trauma[13] may account for the peripheral location.

Ocular sequelae

Because follow-up is frequently erratic in NAI, an accurate prognosis is impossible. It is certain, however, that those with eye signs at the time of admission have a high incidence of residual eye defects[74] and a poor visual prognosis[75] due to both eye and brain damage (Fig. 71.13), especially if the eye problem is severe.[76]

The need for ventilation may be a more important predictor of visual outcome than the acuity at presentation whilst nonreactive pupils and midline shift of brain structures correlate highly with mortality.[77]

Hemorrhagic retinal cysts and retinoschisis[34,64,78,79] are probably much more frequent in child abuse than in accidental trauma. Optic disc neovascularization has been described following severe retinoschisis in a severely shaken infant.[80]

Systemic signs of child abuse

Cerebral trauma and subdural hemorrhage

As in the eye, timing of injury is difficult; the CT changes are not really time-specific. For the ophthalmologist, children with non-accidentally inflicted head injuries may present in a number of ways, including cranial nerve palsies, headaches in older infants and children, or suspected poor vision.

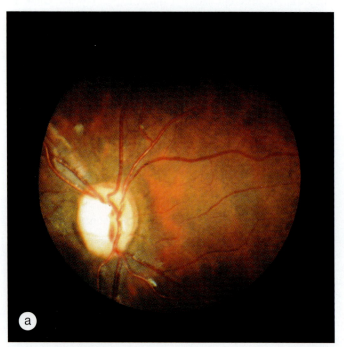
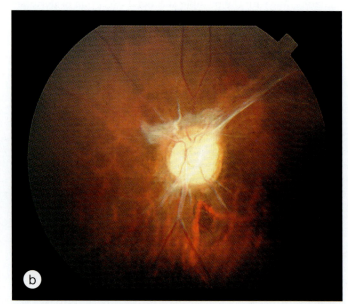

Fig. 71.13 Optic atrophy associated with severe brain damage. (a) Right eye. (b). Left eye with peripapillary retinal and vitreous scarring.

Bruising, burns, and skin marks

It is important to know the prevalence (12%) and distribution of bruises in normal children. They are on the front of the body, mostly single or only a few, on the face, head, and shins, in mobile children.

Tenderness, which must be recorded in the notes, may be present especially if there are underlying fractures.

Bruises cannot reliably be dated even by an experienced clinician on a "balance of probabilities basis," but bruises with some yellowing are likely to be more than 18 hr old. They may change in color at different rates in different sites or if they are of different volume even if of the same age.

It is of concern if the bruising is around the head, especially behind the ear, subscapular bruises, and if there are finger marks at shaking sites or nail gouges. Careful photography can identify a particular bite (note that bites can be self-inflicted). If the child has died, consider calling in the police forensic photographer if there is not a photographer with appropriate experience available.

Burned children tend to be younger; if the burns involve the buttocks or perineum they are more likely to be nonaccidental.

Cigarette burns can be accidental, unless multiple (Fig. 71.14) or linear, especially if they are of different stages of healing or associated with other burns or scalds.

Fractures

Radiographs are important even if the child has died. This is the province of the pediatrician, radiologist, or pathologist not the ophthalmologist. Some fractures, such as rib and metaphyseal fractures, may not be apparent from clinical examination alone.[81]

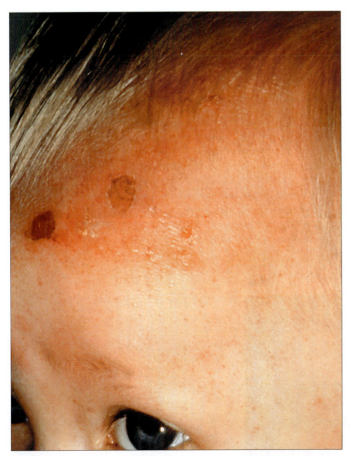

Fig. 71.14 Two supposed cigarette burns are unlikely to have been caused accidentally.

Ribs

Most rib fractures in infants are caused by nonaccidental injury; they are rarely the result of compression from CPR. Similar forces to adjacent ribs leads to a line of fractures or "string of pearls." Anterolateral thoracic compression during shaking is the probable mechanism of the injury of multiple posterior rib fractures near to the costotransverse articulation, caused by the abuser shaking in an anteroposterior direction with the palms laterally and thumbs on the chest.

Scapula

Scapular fractures are rare except in massive direct trauma or child abuse, particularly acromion avulsion by dragging by the arm. Any unusual fracture is considered suggestive of child abuse.

Limbs

Avulsion of a metaphysis, chipped edges of a metaphysis, or epiphysis with isolated small fragments are all suspicious of child abuse. Periosteal new bone formation suggests that the injury is 7–10 days old, which may be significant if there are fractures of different stages of healing. Spiral diaphyseal fractures of long bones are highly suspicious (but not pathognomonic) of NAI if found in children too young to be very mobile.

The doctor's attitude

While being compassionate for the child and the family in the situation that they find themselves in, the doctors involved must be dispassionate in that they need to remember who is the patient and what are the consequences of any management decisions made (Table 71.5). Above all they need to be nonjudgmental.

Giving evidence in court[1]

The consequences of the verdict, whether of guilty or not guilty, to the accused, to the child, to the family, and to friends are so colossal that the medical evidence must be rigorously accurate. An incorrect guilty verdict can have as severe consequences as a correct one.

The evidence given needs to be based on:
1. Factual accuracy;
2. Impartiality and freedom from advocacy; and
3. Clarity.

Prevention

There is a need to draw parents' and other carers' attention to the fact that the effects of shaking may be more severe than expected: this is usually done at prenatal classes or shortly after the birth of the child. Sadly, these campaigns, while useful,

Table 71.5 Investigation of suspected child abuse

Pediatric assessment and management[4]:
    Full multidisciplinary social assessment
    Ophthalmoscopy by an ophthalmologist
    Clinical and eye photographs
    Skeletal survey, and a bone scan or a repeat survey at 10 days
    Coagulation screen
    CT or MRI

usually most effectively reach those less likely to cause injury. Education of personnel involved with childcare is also important.

Conclusion

It is evident that the role of the ophthalmologist in child abuse is an important one, and some of the ophthalmologist's duty to the patient and to the court is based on rather shaky foundations and further studies and evidence-based research is needed.[11]

SELF-INFLICTED INJURY

Dermatitis and keratoconjunctivitis

Self-inflicted injury to the surface of the eye and the skin around the eye is rare in childhood; it may be a warning of much more serious problems such as physical or sexual abuse. In adults there are often a number of associated complex psychological and emotional problems; sometimes these may be of a more serious underlying psychopathology. When dermatitis or kerato-conjunctivitis artefacta affects adults with a long history of psychiatric illness, recovery only occurs with a change in the patient's circumstances. Some adult patients are malingerers, classically trying to escape military service.

Benign neurotic excoriations are diagnosed if the patient admits to the self-destructive nature of their problem. In factitious disease the patients deny the cause of their injury and are deceptive, and their motivation is to play the sick role; they are much more difficult to treat, requiring skilled psychiatric intervention.

The diagnosis is suggested by the combination of sharply delineated lesions in the inferior and nasal quadrants of the cornea and bulbar conjunctiva, an unconcerned attitude ("belle indifférence"), and other psychological features. The dermatitis is very variable in its character. Keratoconjunctivitis was described in an 11-year-old girl who induced it with chalk grains.[82]

It is important to rule out congenital anesthesia, which mostly occurs in young children. In children, self-inflicted injuries mostly occur in mentally retarded children, especially those with Lesch-Nyhan and Smith-Magennis syndromes.

Trichotillomania

Trichotillomania (Fig. 71.15), in which the affected person pulls out hair, sometimes the eyelashes and eyebrows, has a prevalence of between 1 and 5%.

Boys, although affected about half as frequently as girls, have an earlier age at onset, 8 years,[83] but they are less likely to pull

their eyebrows and eyelashes. Trichotillomanics frequently conceal their habit, the hair pulling can become ritualized, with close inspection of the pulled hair, and the hair may be swallowed.

The lids and brows have healthy skin with multiple broken hair shafts. It is not usually a serious condition; the hair loss is reversible when the pulling stops but it may become a severe chronic illness. Some patients are depressed, or have an obsessive–compulsive disorder. Stress is implicated as a precipitating factor in many cases.

Most cases respond to reassurance and explanation, some require behavior therapy, and drug treatment may sometimes help.

Loss of eyelashes occurs with skin diseases such as alopecia, ichthyosis, and ectodermal dysplasia, following radiation or chemotherapy, and after lid infections or endocrine disease.[84] See Chapter 26.

Ocular self-mutilation: direct eye trauma

Ocular self-mutilation typically occurs in young men with a history of severe psychiatric illness, especially schizophrenia, serious criminality, or drug abuse.

In childhood, self-inflicted injuries occur in the severely mentally retarded; the injury may be by laceration,[85] but is more frequently a result of severe direct blows[86] or head-banging.[87] Self-inflicted injuries occur more frequently in certain syndromes, mostly associated with severe mental retardation; the London Dysmorphology Database[88] lists 15 syndromes, of which Lesch-Nyhan and Smith Magennis are the most important to ophthalmologists.

Autoenucleation

This occurs mostly in hallucinating young adult schizophrenics of either sex and is rare in children.[1]

Induced illness: Münchausen syndrome by proxy

Münchausen syndrome was a term used to describe adults who presented with false illness stories; it was adapted[89] using the term "Münchausen syndrome" by proxy to apply to children who were presented with a false illness story by someone else (a proxy).

The illness needs to meet the following criteria:
A. There is intentional production or feigning of physical or psychological signs or symptoms in another person who is under the individual's care.

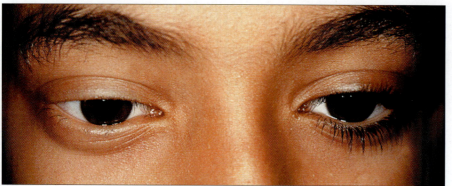

Fig. 71.15 Loss of lashes due to trichotillomania.

B. The motivation of the perpetrator's behavior is to assume the sick role by proxy.

C. External incentives for the behavior (such as economic gain) are absent.

D. The behavior is not accounted for by another mental disorder.

This thus excludes a number of other forms of child abuse, overanxious parents, doctor shopping, and others. It may be seen as a form of attention-seeking behavior.

Ocular involvement in Münchausen syndrome by proxy is rare; orbital cellulitis has been caused by the probable injection of alum by the victim's grandmother who also suffered from Münchausen syndrome,[90] and pupil dilatation was a feature in the child of a potential trainee emergency room technician.[91] The dividing line between Münchausen by proxy and child abuse can be quite fine.

Fabricated illnesss

This is where a carer fabricates an illness in a healthy child for much the same motivation as in induced illness.

REFERENCES

1. Taylor DS. Unnatural injuries. Eye 2000; 14: 123–50.
2. Caffey J. The whiplash shaken infant syndrome: manual shaking by the extremities with whiplash-induced intracranial and intraocular bleedings, linked with residual permanent brain damage and mental retardation. Pediatrics 1974; 54: 396–403.
3. Sedlak A. Study of National Incidence and Prevalence of Child Abuse. 1st ed. Bethesda, MD: Westat; 1987.
4. Jayawant S, Rawlinson A, Gibbon F, et al. Subdural haemorrhages in infants: population based study. BMJ 1998; 317: 1558–61.
5. Lloyd B. Subdural haemorrhages in infants. Almost all are due to abuse but abuse is often not recognized. (Editorial.) BMJ 1998; 317: 1538–9.
6. Hampton RL, Newberger EH. Child abuse incidence and reporting by hospitals: significance of severity, class and race. Am J Public Health 1985; 75: 56–60.
7. Lazoritz S, Baldwin S, Kini N. The whiplash shaken infant syndrome: has Caffey's syndrome changed or have we changed his syndrome? Child Abuse Negl 1997; 21: 1009–14.
8. Ong T, Hodgkins P, Taylor D. Keratitis in child abuse. J Pediatr Ophthalmol Strabismus 2004; in press.
9. Taylor D, Bentovim A. Recurrent nonaccidentally inflicted chemical eye injuries to siblings. J Pediatr Ophthalmol Strabismus 1976; 13: 238–42.
10. Gonzales CA, Scott IU, Chaudry NA, et al. Bilateral rhegmatogenous retinal detachments with unilateral vitreous base avulsion as the presenting signs of child abuse. Am J Ophthalmol 1999; 127: 475–7.
11. The Ophthalmology Child Abuse Working Party. Child abuse and the eye. Eye 1999; 13:3–10.
12. The Ophthalmology Child Abuse Working Party. Update from the Ophthalmology Child Abuse Working Party-Royal College of Ophthalmologists. Eye 2003; 17: 1–5.
13. Green MA, Lieberman G, Milroy CM, et al. Ocular and cerebral trauma in non-accidental injury in infancy: underlying mechanisms and implications for paediatric practice. Br J Ophthalmol 1996; 80: 282–7.
14. Lin KC, Glasgow BJ. Bilateral periopticointrascleral hemorrhages associated with traumatic child abuse. Am J Ophthalmol 1999; 127: 473–5.
15. Gilliland MG, Luckenbach MW, Chenier TC. Systemic and ocular findings in 169 prospectively studied child deaths: retinal hemorrhages usually means child abuse. Forensic Sci 1994; 68: 117–32.
16. Johnson DL, Braun D, Friendly D. Accidental head trauma and retinal hemorrhage. Neurosurgery 1993; 33: 231–5.
17. Betz P, Puschel K, Miltner E, et al. Morphometrical analysis of retinal hemorrhages in the shaken baby syndrome. Forensic Sci Int 1996; 78: 71–80.
18. Buys YM, Levin AV, Enzenauer RW, et al. Retinal findings after head trauma in infants and young children. Ophthalmology 1992; 99: 1718–23.
19. Duhaime AC, Alario AJ, Lewander WJ, et al. Head injury in very young children: mechanisms, injury types and ophthalmologic findings in 100 hospitalised patients younger than two years of age. Pediatrics 1992; 90: 179–85.
20. Maddocks GB, Sibert JR, Brown BM. A four week study of accidents to children in South Glamorgan. Public Health 1978; 92: 171–6.
21. Rivara FP, Kamitsuka MD, Quan L. Injuries to children younger than 1 year of age. Pediatrics 1988; 81: 93–7.

22. Chadwick DL, Chin S, Salerno C, et al. Deaths from falls in children; how far is it fatal? J Trauma 1991; 31: 1353.
23. Plunkett J. Fatal pediatric head injuries caused by short–distance falls. [Comment.] Am J Forensic Med Pathol 2001; 22: 1–12.
24. Caffey J. On the theory and practice of shaking infants. Its potential residual effects of permanent brain damage in mental retardation. Am J Dis Child 1972; 124: 161–9.
25. Gilliland MG, Folberg R. Shaken babies—some have no impact injuries. J Forensic Sci 1996; 41: 114–6.
26. Budenz DL, Farber MG, Mirchandani HG, et al. Ocular and optic nerve hemorrhages in abused infants with intracranial injuries. Ophthalmology 1994; 101: 559–65.
27. Wilkinson WS, Han DP, Rappley MD, et al. Retinal hemorrhage predicts neurologic injury in the shaken baby syndrome. Arch Ophthalmol. 1989; 107: 1472–4.
28. Duhaime AC, Gennarelli TA, Thibault LE, et al. The shaken baby syndrome; a clinical, pathological and biomechanical study. J Neurosurg 1987; 66: 409–15.
29. Duhaime AC, Christian C. In: Choux M, Rocco C, Hockley A, Walker M, editors. Paediatric Neurosurgery. London: Churchill Livingstone; 1999: 373–9.
30. Reiber GD. Fatal falls in childhood. How far must children fall to sustain fatal head injury? Report of cases and review of the literature. Am J Forensic Med Pathol 1993; 14: 201–7.
31. Geddes JF, Vowles GH, Hackshaw AK, et al. Neuropathology of inflicted head injury in children. II. Microscopic brain injury in infants. [Comment.] Brain 2001; 124: 1299–306.
32. Geddes JF, Hackshaw AK, Vowles GH, et al. Neuropathology of inflicted head injury in children. I. Patterns of brain damage. [Comment.] Brain 2001; 124: 1290–8.
33. Gennarelli TA. Head injury in man and experimental animals: clinical aspects. Acta Neurochir Suppl 1983; 32: 1–13.
34. Elner SG, Elner VM, Arnall M, et al. Ocular and associated systemic findings in suspected child abuse. Arch Ophthalmol 1990; 108: 1094–101.
35. Hadley MN, Sonntag V, Rekate HL, et al. The infant whiplash-shake injury syndrome: a clinical and pathological study. Neurosurgery 1989; 24: 536–40.
36. Shaver EG, Duhaime AC., Curtis M, et al. Experimental acute subdural haematoma in piglets. Pediatr Neurosurg 1996; 25: 123–9.
37. Johnson DL, Boal D, Baule R. Role of apnea in nonaccidental head injury. Pediatr Neurosurg 1995; 23: 305–10.
38. Von Barsewisch B. Perinatal retinal haemorrhages: Morphology, aetiology and significance. Berlin: Springer-Verlag; 1979: 1–184.
39. Baum JD, Bulpitt CJ. Retinal and conjunctival haemorrhage in the newborn. Arch Dis Child 1970; 45: 344–9.
40. Giles CL. Retinal haemorrhages in the newborn. Am J Ophthalmol 1960; 49: 1005–10.
41. Sezen F. Retinal haemorrhages in newborn infants. Br J Ophthalmol 1970; 55: 248–53.
42. Billmire ME, Myers PA. Serious head injury in infants: accident or abuse? Pediatrics 1985; 75: 340–2.
43. Riffenburgh RS, Sathyavagiswaran L. The eyes of child abuse victims; autopsy findings. J Forensic Sci 1991; 36: 741–7.
44. Morris AA, Hoffmann GF, Naughten ER, et al. Glutaric aciduria and suspected child abuse. Arch Dis Child 1999; 80: 404–5.
45. Russell-Eggitt IM, Thompson DA, Khair K, et al. Hermansky-Pudlak syndrome presenting with subdural haematoma and retinal haemorrhages in infancy. J R Soc Med 2000; 93: 591–2.
46. Dietrich AM, James CD, King DR. Head trauma in children with congenital coagulation disorders. J Pediatr Surg 1994; 29: 28–32.

47. Hymel KP, Abshire TC, Luckey DW, et al. Coagulopathy in pediatric abusive head trauma. Pediatrics 1997; 99: 371–5.

48. Atkinson A, Sanders MD, Wong V. Vitreous haemorrhage in tuberous sclerosis. Br J Ophthalmol 1973; 57: 773–9.

49. George ND, Yates JR, Bradshaw K, et al. Infantile presentation of X-linked retinoschisis. Br J Ophthalmol 1995; 79: 653–7.

50. Christiansen SP, Munoz M, Capo H. Retinal haemorrhage following lensectomy and vitrectomy in children. J Pediatr Ophthalmol Strabismus 1993; 30: 24–7.

51. Kirby S, Sadler RM. Injury and death as a result of seizures. Epilepsia 1995; 36: 25–8.

52. Feyi-Waboso AC, Beck L. Minerva column. BMJ 1997; 314: 688.

53. Sandramouli S, Robinson R, Tsaloumas M, et al. Retinal haemorrhages and convulsions. Arch Dis Child 1997; 76: 449–51.

54. Tyagi AK, Scotcher S, Kozeis N, et al. Can convulsions alone cause retinal haemorrhages in infants? Br J Ophthalmol 1998; 82: 659–60.

55. Bacon CJ, Sayer GC, Howe J. Extensive retinal haemorrhages in infancy—an innocent cause. BMJ 1978; 1: 281.

56. Goetting MG, Sowa B. Retinal haemorrhage after cardiopulmonary resuscitation in children: An etiologic reevaluation. Pediatrics 1990; 85: 585–8.

57. Weedn VW, Mansour AM, Nichols MM. Retinal hemorrhage in an infant after cardiopulmonary resuscitation. Am J Forensic Pathol 1990; 11: 79–82.

58. Carney MD, Wortham E, al-Mateen KB. Vitreous hemorrhage and extracorporeal membrane oxygenation. Am J Ophthalmol 1993; 115: 391–3.

59. Gilliland MG, Luckenbach MW. Are retinal hemaorrhages found after resuscitation attempts? Am J Forensic Med Pathol 1993; 14: 187–92.

60. Kanter RK. Retinal hemorrhages after cardiopulmonary resuscitation or child abuse. J Pediatr 1986; 108: 430–2.

61. Levin A. Comment on: retinal haemorrhages after cardiopulmonary resuscitation or child abuse. Pediatr Emerg Care 1986; 2: 269–70.

62. Fackler JC, Berkovitz ID, Green WR. Retinal haemorrhages in newborn piglets following cardiopulmonary resuscitation. Am J Dis Child 1992; 146: 1294–6.

63. Giangiacomo J, Barkett KJ. Ophthalmoscopic findings in occult child abuse. J Pediatr Ophthalmol Strabismus 1985; 22: 234–7.

64. Rohrbach JM, Benz D, Friedrichs W, et al. Okuläre Pathologie der Kindesmibhandlung. Klin.Monatsbl.Augenheilkd 1997; 210: 133–8.

65. Gilliland MG, Luckenbach MW, Massicotte SJ, et al. The medicolegal implications of detecting hemosiderin in the eyes of children who are suspected of being abused. Arch Ophthalmol (letter) 1991; 109: 321–2.

66. Elner SG, Elner VM, Albert DM, et al. The medicolegal implications of detecting hemosiderin in the eyes of children who are suspected of being abused (reply to letter from Gilliland et al.). Arch Ophthalmol 1991; 109: 322.

67. Gaynon MW, Koh K, Marmor MF, et al. Retinal folds in the shaken baby syndrome. Am J Ophthalmol 1988; 106: 423–5.

68. Massicotte SJ, Folberg R, Torczynski E, et al. Vitreoretinal traction and perimacular retinal folds in the eyes of deliberately traumatized children. Ophthalmology 1991; 98: 1124–7.

69. Munger CE, Peiffer RL, Bouldin TW, et al. Ocular and associated neuropathologic observations in suspected whiplash baby syndrome. A retrospective study of 12 cases. Am J Forensic Med Pathol 1993; 14: 193–200.

70. Tongue AC. The ophthalmologist(s) role in diagnosing child abuse. Ophthalmology 1991; 98: 1009–11.

71. Keithahn MA, Bennett SR, Cameron D, et al. Retinal folds in Terson syndrome. Ophthalmology 1993; 100: 1187–90.

72. Schloff S, Mullaney PB, Armstrong DC, et al. Retinal findings in children with intracranial hemorrhage. Ophthalmology 2002; 109: 1472–6.

73. Aron JJ, Marx P, Blanck MF, et al. Signes oculaires observés dans le syndrome de Silverman. Annal Ocul (Paris) 1970; 203: 533–46.

74. Hollenhorst RW, Stein HA. Ocular signs and prognosis in subdural and subarachnoid bleeding in young children. Arch Ophthalmol 1958; 60: 187–92.

75. Roussey M, Betremieux P, Journel H, et al. L'ophtalmologiste et les enfants victimes de sévices. J Fr Ophtalmol 1987; 10: 201–5.

76. Matthews GP, Das A. Dense vitreous hemorrhages predict poor visual and neurological prognosis in infants with shaken baby syndrome. J Pediatr Ophthalmol Strabismus 1996; 33: 260–5.

77. McCabe CF, Donahue SP. Prognostic indicators for vision and mortality in shaken baby syndrome. Arch Ophthalmol 2000; 118: 373–7.

78. Greenwald MJ, Weiss A, Oesterle CS, et al. Traumatic retinoschisis in battered babies. Ophthalmology 1986; 93: 618–25.

79. Morris R, Kuhn F, Witherspoon CD. Hemorrhagic macular cysts (letter). Ophthalmology 1994; 101: 1.

80. Brown SM, Shami M. Optic disc neovascularisation following severe retinoschisis due to shaken baby syndrome (letter). Arch Ophthalmol 1999; 117: 838–9.

81. Hall CM, Shaw DG. Non-accidental injury. Current Imaging 1991; 3: 88–93.

82. Cruciani F, Santino G, Trudu R, et al. Ocular Münchausen syndrome characterised by self-introduction of chalk concretions into the conjunctival fornix. Eye 1999; 13: 598–9.

83. Graber J, Arndt WB. Trichotillomania. Compr Psychiatry 1993; 34: 340–6.

84. Mawn LA, Jordan DR. Trichotillomania. Ophthalmology 1997; 104: 2175–8.

85. Noel LP, Clarke WN. Self-inflicted ocular injuries in children. Am J Ophthalmol 1982; 94: 630–3.

86. Ashkenazi I, Shahar E, Brand N, et al. Self-inflicted ocular mutilation in the pediatric age group. Acta Paediatr 1992; 81: 649–51.

87. Spalter HF, Bemporad JR, Sours JA. Cataracts following chronic headbanging. Arch Ophthalmol 1970; 83: 182–6.

88. Winter R, Baraitser M. London dysmorphology database. Oxford Medical Databases. Oxford: Oxford University Press; 1989.

89. Meadow R. Münchausen syndrome by proxy: the hinterland of child abuse. Lancet 1977; 2: 343–5.

90. Feenstra J, Merth IT, Treffers PD. Een geval van het syndroom van Münchausen bij proxy. Tijdschr Kindergeneeskd 1988; 56: 148–53.

91. Wood PR, Fowlkes J, Holden P, et al. Fever of unknown origin for six years: Münchausen syndrome by proxy. J Fam Pract 1989; s28: 391–5.

Blinding Eye Diseases of Childhood in Developing Countries

CHAPTER 72

Clare E Gilbert and Haroon R Awan

INTRODUCTION

The prevalence, magnitude and causes of blindness in children vary widely, being largely determined by levels of socioeconomic development and health care provision. The prevalence of blindness in children is higher in developing countries for the following reasons:

(a) There are conditions in poor communities which are not found in affluent societies (e.g. vitamin A deficiency; cerebral malaria).

(b) Cultural practices may lead to a higher incidence (e.g. use of harmful traditional eye medicines; high rates of consanguinity).

(c) Potentially blinding diseases are not adequately controlled (e.g. measles; rubella; ophthalmia neonatorum).

(d) Services for sight restoration or preservation are not always available, accessible or affordable (e.g. for cataract, glaucoma and retinopathy of prematurity).

Globally, 350 000 children are blind from corneal scarring, and a larger number are visually impaired in one or both eyes.[1] The most important cause of corneal scarring in poor communities is vitamin A deficiency, although particularly in Africa there is close interaction between vitamin A deficiency and measles infection. The use of harmful traditional eye medicines is also more common in sub-Saharan Africa than in other regions, but ophthalmia neonatorum is encountered everywhere in the developing world. Malaria, particularly cerebral malaria, occurs principally in sub-Saharan Africa.

VITAMIN A DEFICIENCY (VAD)

Definition of VAD

Vitamin A deficiency is a systemic condition with multiple adverse effects (including increased mortality), and individuals are at risk even if they do not have symptoms or clinical signs of overt deficiency.[2,3]

VAD: state of inadequate vitamin A nutrition

Vitamin A deficiency usually begins when liver stores are below 20 µg/g, but serum levels can often still be maintained despite this. By convention, serum retinol levels <20 µg/dL (0.70 µmol/L) are deficient.

Vitamin A deficiency disorders (VADD): physiological disturbances secondary to VAD

These may be subclinical (e.g. impaired iron metabolism, disturbed cellular differentiation, reduced immune response), or clinical (e.g. increased morbidity due to infections, increased mortality, growth retardation, anemia and xerophthalmia).

VADD begins long before the development of xerophthalmia, and the clinical manifestations, particularly mortality, increase with increasing deficiency.

Xerophthalmia: clinically evident ocular manifestations of VAD

This term encompasses all the eye signs of the deficiency state (see Table 72.1) many of which are consequences of squamous metaplasia, with loss of goblet cells leading to xerosis and keratinization. Corneal ulceration is a result of coagulative necrosis, and is often associated with secondary infection. The retinal findings are unusual, and are only seen in adults.

It should be noted that this is not a chronological classification: a young child who has VADD but no eye signs can be precipitated into acute deficiency by infection or diarrhea, and develop keratomalacia leading to blindness within a few days. (Figs 72.1 and 72.2)

Sources of vitamin A

The best sources of vitamin A are animal sources, which contain pre-formed retinol (e.g. eggs, milk (including breast milk), butter, liver and oily fish). Plants contain the provitamin A precursors, β-carotene and other carotenoids[4]: these are half as active as β-carotene. The best sources of β-carotene are dark-green, orange and yellow fruits and vegetables (e.g. spinach, carrots, mangos, red palm oil, and sweet potatoes), but the bioavailability is influenced by a range of variables.[4] Cereals and

Table 72.1 Xerophthalmia classification (from WHO)		
	Ocular signs	**Peak age group affected**
XN	Night-blindness	Children 2–6 years; pregnant and lactating women
X1	Conjunctival xerosis	Children 3–6 years
X1A	Bitot's spots[a]	Children 3–6 years
X2B	Corneal xerosis	Children 3–6 years
X3	Corneal ulcer/keratomalacia <$\frac{1}{3}$ of cornea	Children aged 1–4 years
X3A	Corneal ulcer/keratomalacia ≥$\frac{1}{3}$ cornea[b]	Children aged 1–4 years
XSB	Corneal scar	Children aged >3 years
XF	Xerophthalmic fundus	Adults
[a] Fig. 72.1 [b] Fig. 72.2		

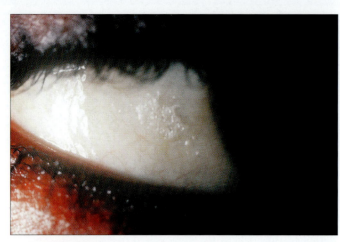

Fig. 72.1 Bitot's spots.

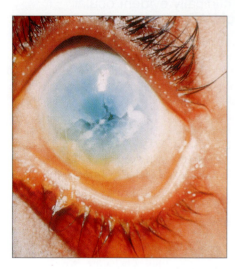

Fig. 72.2
Keratomalacia.

international unit; 1 international unit equals 0.3 μg of retinol; 1 μg of β-carotene equals 0.167 μg of retinol.

Daily requirements

Daily requirements are age and gender dependent: young children need a relatively high intake on account of growth, and pregnant and lactating women also have relatively high requirements (Table 72.2). This in part explains why young children and women of childbearing age are most at risk of vitamin A deficiency.

Metabolism and physiology[4]

Retinol is a requirement of many physiological processes:

- *Vision.* In rod and cone outer segments retinal compounds play a vital role in phototransduction.
- *Gene expression and cell differentiation.* Vitamin A maintains tissue differentiation, particularly of epithelial tissues. Activation of retinoic acid receptors in the nuclear membrane, in the presence of various hormones, affects a number of genes. Vitamin A is required during embryonic development for normal tissue differentiation.
- *Growth.* Vitamin A deficient children have reduced growth.
- *Immune function.* Cell mediated immunity is more adversely affected than humoral immunity.
- *Antioxidant properties.* Vitamin A is one of a group of agents which act to reduce oxidative stress by mopping up free radicals. Antioxidant deficiency has been implicated in cardiovascular disease, cancers, cataract and macular degeneration.
- *Hemopoiesis.* Iron deficiency anemia frequently accompanies vitamin A deficiency.

Risk factors for vitamin A deficiency

Vitamin A deficiency is a condition of poverty, with multiple predisposing conditions and risk factors.

Distal risk factors[5]

These include geographical and ecological factors leading to poverty (e.g. overgrazing, poor soil and climate leading to low production of vitamin A rich foods); political instability and inequitable political and trade systems at the international and national level; poor infrastructure (e.g. poor road networks for transporting food); inadequate primary health care (e.g. poor water supplies and sanitation which lead to diarrhea, low measles immunization coverage); low status of women (lack of female

other staples are poor sources of provitamin A precursors. As the bioavailability of retinol from vegetable sources containing β-carotene and carotenoids is relatively low, larger amounts of these foods need to be consumed to meet daily requirements. As retinol is fat-soluble the diet also needs to contain oil or fat. Biological equivalents for diets with different proportions of retinol and β-carotene, are as follows: 1 USP U equals 1

Table 72.2 Foods that provide the daily requirement				
Age group	Carrots	Sweet potatoes	DGLV	Mango
Children:				
0–5 months	Breast milk	Breast milk	Breast milk	Breast milk
6–11 months	1½ tablespoon	1 tablespoon	⅓ cup	½
1–2 years	1½ tablespoon	1 tablespoon	½ cup	½
2–6 years	2 tablesppon	1½ tablespoon	½ cup	⅔
Females:				
Nonpregnant	¼ cup	2½ tablespoon	1 cup	1
Pregnant	¼ cup	2½ tablespoon	1 cup	1
Lactating	¼ cup	¼ cup	1½ cup	⅔
DGLV: dark green leafy vegetables.				

education); overcrowding and cultural practices (e.g. with holding colostrum; feeding taboos and practices) and inadequate health care services.

Proximal risk factors

These relate to household level factors: lack of a clean water supply, inadequate sanitation, lack of land ownership, uneducated mothers, large family sizes, and feeding practices (such as women and young children eating last).

Individual risk factors

Factors at the individual level include being breast fed by a mother who is herself vitamin A deficient, inadequate intake of foods rich in vitamin A, and infections. Diarrhea (in Asian countries) and measles (in Africa countries) can precipitate a child who is borderline deficient into blinding xerophthalmia.

Mortality from vitamin A deficiency disorders, and infectious morbidity

Many trials have been undertaken in several developing countries in which children aged 6–72 months were randomized to receive either supplements of vitamin A, or placebo. Meta-analyses of these studies show that vitamin A supplementation can reduce all cause child mortality by 23%[6] (34% reduction in the six Asian trials[7]). Morbidity data are fewer, and more difficult to interpret.[3] There is a *vicious cycle* whereby infections lead to vitamin A deficiency (through increased demand, malabsorption, and increased loss in the urine), which itself leads to an increased risk of infection (through loss of the barrier function afforded by intact epithelia and reduced immune responses).

Magnitude and distribution of vitamin A deficiency

Recent estimates suggest that 140 million preschool age children and >7 million women suffer from VADD every year, with 1.2–3 million children and women having signs of xerophthalmia.[5] Individuals living in countries in Asia, Africa and the Western Pacific are most at risk. Within these countries communities living in poor rural areas and in periurban and urban slums are at highest risk. Vitamin A deficiency clusters even within communities, affecting the most marginalized sectors (e.g. migrant laborers; families without a male head of household; low caste).

Recently use of under five mortality rates (U5MRs) has been suggested as a marker to identify countries likely to have vitamin A deficiency: countries with U5MRs >50/1000 live births are likely to have a problem of clinical significance, and countries

with U5MRs in the range 20–50/1000 are likely to have focal areas of VAD, which needs to be confirmed.[8] Vitamin A deficiency is unlikely in countries with U5MRs of <20/1000 live births. Recent data suggest that there are 100 countries with U5MRs of >50/1000 live births. Use of rates of night-blindness during pregnancy is another means of identifying populations with vitamin A deficiency, with a minimum prevalence of 5% considered an indicator of VAD in the wider population.[8]

Control of vitamin A deficiency

Realistic interventions currently concentrate on dietary diversification, supplementation, and food fortification.

Dietary diversification

This is effective[9] but where vitamin A deficiency is prevalent children are unlikely to be able to increase their consumption of vitamin A, particularly where the main sources are vegetables and fruits.[2] Women can consume a large enough quantity of fruit and vegetables, if available, and this is important as breast milk is the best source for infants. Health education combined with home gardening to produce low cost vitamin A rich foods is a strategy employed in Bangladesh, where rice is the main source of calories and where VADD is prevalent. Other approaches include food supplementation of preschool children, as in India.[9]

Periodic supplementation

Supplementing children aged six months to five years with two high-dose vitamin A capsules a year is a safe, cost-effective, efficient strategy for controlling vitamin A deficiency. Dosing takes account of studies involving infants and women of childbearing age (Table 72.3). In the majority of developing countries supplementation is undertaken at the same time as immunization (e.g. with measles immunization at 9 months; during national immunization days), which is an efficient use of resources.[10]

Food fortification

Increasing the vitamin A content of foods frequently consumed by populations with VAD is a strategy adopted in some countries (e.g. fortification of monosodium glutamate in Indonesia and The Philippines).[11] However, the food needs to be consumed by the target population at regular intervals (i.e. women and young children), but in small doses; the fortification process should not change the color, taste, shelf-life, and cost of the product; and the food needs to be manufactured by a small number of companies. There are considerable political, trade and regulatory barriers to overcome.[2]

Table 72.3 Schedule for routine high-dose vitamin A supplementation in populations with vitamin A deficiency		
Population	Amount of vitamin A to be administered	Time of administration
Infants aged 0–5 months	150 000 IU as three doses of 50 000 IU, with at least a 1 month interval between doses	At each DTP immunization contact (6, 10, and 14 weeks after birth) (otherwise at other opportunities)
Infants aged 6–11 months	100 000 IU as a single dose every 4–6 months	At any opportunity (e.g. with measles immunization)
Children aged 12–27 months	200 000 IU as a single dose every 4–6 months	At any opportunity
Postpartum women	400 000 IU as two doses of 200 000 IU at least 1 day apart; and/or 10 000 daily or 25 000 IU weekly*	As soon after delivery as possible but not more than 6 weeks after delivery* and/or during the first 6 months after delivery

*As high-dose vitamin A is teratogenic, vitamin A should not be given during pregnancy, or when a pregnancy is possible.
IU, international units.

Increasing the availability of vitamin A rich foods by genetically modifying crops is another approach. Recent studies have shown proof of concept with the development of "golden rice" which contains a gene from daffodils (a yellow flower). However, there are barriers to overcome in terms of acceptability and cost, before this becomes a viable strategy.

Treatment of xerophthalmia

All children with xerophthalmia should be treated, using the same age-dependant doses as above, but the child should be given three doses: the first on day 1, the second on day 2, and the third on day 10.

Treatment of high-risk groups

All children with malnutrition, diarrhea or measles who live in communities where vitamin A deficiency is prevalent should be treated with high dose vitamin A, on the assumption that they are deficient, or that the condition will lead to acute deficiency and keratomalacia. If the child is too sick to take an oral supplement there is an injectable form. Lactating women should also be supplemented soon after delivery, to improve the retinol content of their breast milk.

International targets and impact of programs

The 1990 World Summit for Children set the goal of virtual elimination of vitamin A deficiency and its consequences, including blindness, by the year 2000. The number of developing countries providing at least one high dose vitamin A supplement to 70% or more of under-fives has risen from only 11 nations in 1996, to 43 in 1999. A million child deaths may have been prevented as a result of vitamin A supplementation. The prevalence and magnitude of vitamin A deficiency is declining in many countries, largely as a result of supplementation. The challenge remains in bringing about the political, economic changes which promote development and reduce poverty to reduce the incidence of vitamin A deficiency, and to develop sustainable and cost effective programs for control that are not dependent on long-term supplementation.

MEASLES

Measles infection

In developing countries measles is a severe and feared disease with a mortality of up to 7% compared with <0.1% in industrialized countries with mortality being higher in infants over 4 months and in older children. It accounts for an estimated 875 000 child deaths per year (10% of all deaths in childhood, and 50% of all vaccine preventable deaths).[12] As well as causing a rash, measles virus infection of the gastrointestinal tract can lead to malabsorption, and infection of the respiratory epithelium causes pneumonia.

The severity of measles in developing countries is due to:

- Overcrowding which increases the infecting dose of virus.
- Pre-existing malnutrition and vitamin A deficiency.
- Inadequate health services to manage life-threatening complications (i.e. pneumonia and diarrhea).

Longitudinal studies have shown that malnutrition and vitamin A deficiency are frequent consequences of measles infection in previously reasonably well-nourished children. The concept that a high infecting dose leads to greater severity of measles infection has been confirmed in other studies, and in relation to other infections.[13]

Corneal ulceration and blindness following measles

In Africa, population-based studies have shown that corneal ulceration follows measles infection in 0.75–3.3% of cases. Blindness from corneal scarring followed measles infection in up to 81% of children in blind school studies, and in 36% of cases in hospital-based studies.[14]

Several inter-related pathogenic mechanisms are implicated in corneal scarring following measles infection, including acute VAD leading to corneal ulceration and keratomalacia; secondary bacterial infection; exposure keratitis; secondary herpes simplex virus (HSV) keratitis (Fig. 72.3); measles keratitis and the use of harmful traditional eye medicines.[14]

All infections increase the metabolic rate, increasing utilization of vitamin A. At the same time the intake of vitamin A may be low, due to anorexia, feeding taboos and customs, and painful herpetic oral ulceration. Infection of the gastrointestinal tract can lead to malabsorption and protein losing enteropathy (with loss of carrier proteins), and infection of the urinary tract can lead to loss of retinol in the urine. Retinol is in great demand during repair and differentiation of all the epithelial tissues damaged by measles. All these factors can precipitate a borderline deficient child into acute deficiency and keratomalacia.

Infection of the corneal epithelium usually gives a self-limiting (albeit symptomatic) keratitis, but occasionally more extensive corneal erosions can occur. This loss of barrier function predisposes towards secondary bacterial infection and suppurative keratitis. Measles infection depresses cell mediated and humoral immunity, which may explain the secondary herpetic infection, which can become ameboid, or involve the corneal stroma. Severe measles can lead to dehydration and prostration–the child may develop exposure keratitis and secondary infection.

Measles immunization

Measles is highly contagious: in nonimmune populations 14 out of 15 individuals would, on average, be infected by one infected individual, who would in turn each pass the infection on to 14 out of 15 further individuals. To be effective, measles immunization needs to be given at an age when maternal antibodies are low in the target population, but before the peak age for epidemics. In developing countries this means at around 9 months of age. Due to the high infectivity coverage needs to be high, and the Expanded Programme of Immunization (EPI) recommends a target coverage of 80%, but even then measles cases are still likely. In 1999 the global coverage was 80% but 13 African and three countries in the Eastern Mediterranean had coverage of <50%.[12]

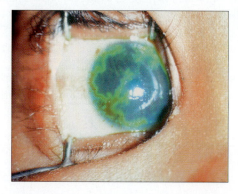

Fig. 72.3 Herpes simplex keratitis.

Control of blindness due to measles infection

The mainstay of control lies in effective immunization programs. Children with measles should all be given high-dose vitamin A, irrespective of whether they have eye signs, to reduce mortality and prevent blindness.[15] In children with corneal ulcers, the underlying cause should be ascertained and treated.

OPHTHALMIA NEONATORUM

See Chapters 19 and Appendix (Red Eye in Infancy).

There are several thousand new cases annually, principally in developing countries.[16] Rates are higher in some areas due to higher rates of sexually transmitted diseases (STDs), high levels of home deliveries and inadequate and poorly distributed health care facilities.

Approaches to the control of ophthalmia neonatorum include control of STDs, and prophylaxis. One percent silver nitrate solution, 1% tetracycline ointment, 0.5% erythromycin, or 2.5% povidone iodine[17] instilled at birth, after cleaning the eyelids, are all effective against gonococcus. The control of gonococcal ophthalmia neonatorum is a challenge in developing countries but programs such as those being implemented by SEARCH in rural India, in which village level community workers provide preventive and therapeutic interventions for neonates, provides a replicable model.[18]

HARMFUL TRADITIONAL EYE MEDICINES

The World Health Organization has defined traditional healing as "the sum total of all the knowledge and practices, used in diagnosis, prevention and elimination of physical, mental or social imbalance and relying exclusively on practical experience and observation handed down from generation to generation, whether verbally or in writing. Traditional medicine might also be considered as solid amalgamation of dynamic medicine know-how and ancestral experience. Traditional African medicine might also be considered to be the sum total of practices, measures, ingredients and procedures of all kinds, whether material or not, which from time immemorial has enabled the African to guard against disease, to alleviate his suffering and to cure himself".

In animist societies diseases are believed to have several origins, and remedies are based on these understandings. They may be supernatural (caused by angering ancestors, by spirits, or be due to breaking of customs or taboos); they may arise as a result of conflict, tension, jealousy or immoral behavior; they may be the result of the "evil eye" or witchcraft, or they may be passed down within the family (usually attributed to the mother). Other conditions are due to lack of respect towards parents or elders, or attributed to weakness or eating unclean food.

The use of harmful traditional remedies, administered on the advice of traditional healers, is an important cause of corneal blindness in children, particularly in sub-Saharan Africa.[19,20] However, traditional practices are widespread: some are harmful, many are benign (e.g. ritual bathing, dances), and some may be beneficial (e.g. direct application of breast milk into the eye, steam baths and inhalations).

Traditional remedies can lead to eye damage and blindness through several mechanisms:

1. Adnexal injuries (e.g. from thermal, acid or alkaline burns) can lead to exposure keratitis and secondary infection (Fig. 72.4).
2. Exposure keratitis can occur if parents hold open the eyes of their child, a practice believed to prevent blindness in children with measles in parts of West Africa.
3. Mechanical damage and burns from objects and material inserted into the eye (e.g. twigs and leaves, ground up cowrie shells, and acidic or alkaline liquids or toxic sap from plants).
4. Fungal infection, particularly if plant material is inserted
5. Bacterial infection (e.g. instillation of urine from someone infected with gonorrhea; use of breast milk expressed into a contaminated container) (Fig. 72.5).
6. Harmless traditional remedies can lead to blindness indirectly, as a consequence of delay in seeking more appropriate treatment.

The practice of traditional healing varies enormously from locality to locality and the tradition and remedies are often passed down within the family. Some healers develop specific areas of expertise, in the area of mental health, for example. Even in settings where eye care services are available, members of the community will often consult the traditional healer first, or want to discuss decisions having already seen an eye-care worker, as they are respected members of the community who share local

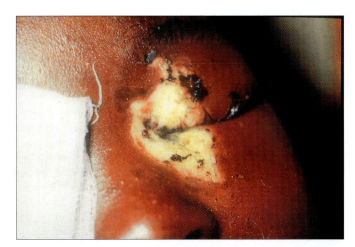

Fig. 72.4 Full-thickness lid burn.

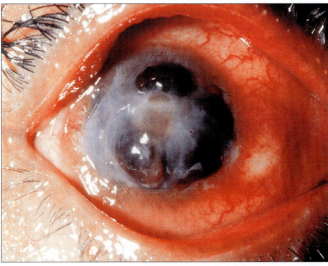

Fig. 72.5 Gonococcal keratitis.

beliefs about the causation of disease. Traditional healers can become important primary eye care workers.[21]

MANAGEMENT OF CORNEAL ULCERS AND SCARRING IN CHILDREN

Correct diagnosis is essential. A history of measles should be sought, and use of traditional medicines enquired after. In countries where vitamin A deficiency is common all children with corneal ulcers should be treated with high-dose vitamin A (see above). If there are facilities for laboratory investigation corneal scrapes should be taken, with Gram staining and culture. In many instances treatment will be empirical: a broad-spectrum antibiotic, with an antifungal agent.

Surgery is not indicated for children with unilateral scarring as these eyes are likely to be amblyopic, and surgical management should be limited to children with bilateral, blinding scarring. If there is a rim of clear peripheral cornea with good light projection an optical iridectomy can restore sufficient sight for independent mobility. Penetrating keratoplasty has a very limited role–in most developing countries corneas are not available for grafting, children present late and the results are poor.[22]

MALARIA

Malaria due to *Plasmodium falciparum* is the most severe form of malaria, leading to severe anemia, hemoglobinuria from massive intravascular hemolysis (black water fever), cerebral malaria and its sequelae, and death. Approximately 10% of children with neurological sequelae of cerebral malaria are cortically blind which represents approximately 1–2000 new cases annually.[23,24]

Children with cerebral malaria can develop fundus findings: papilledema, retinal hemorrhages and Roth spots, cotton-wool spots and extensive areas of retinal whitening (due to intracellular edema), as well as changes in the color and caliber of retinal arterioles and veins (Fig. 72.6). Retinal hemorrhages are of prognostic significance.[25] Retinal changes have been attributed to sequestration of red blood corpuscles, which are often de-hemaglutinized as the corpuscles are full of late stage parasites.

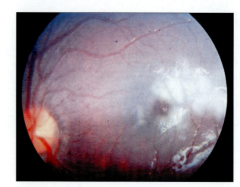

Fig. 72.6 Malaria. Retinal nerve fiber layer whitening.

Management of severe malaria

Management rests on rehydration, and treatment with an effective anti-malarial drug (e.g. quinine or an artemisinin drug). Adjuvant treatment with steroids, mannitol, prophylactic anticonvulsants, and antitumor necrosis factor have shown to have no effect on mortality.[26]

VISION 2020: THE RIGHT TO SIGHT

The International Agency for the Prevention of Blindness (IAPB) together with the World Health Organization, have delineated priorities for the elimination of avoidable blindness by the year 2020. This initiative is called VISION 2020: The Right to Sight.[27] The control of blindness in children is among the priorities, with emphasis on prevention at the community level, and service delivery at secondary and tertiary levels of eye-care delivery. Overall approximately 40% of all blind children are blind from avoidable causes,[1] with up to 70% of children being blind from preventable causes in the poorest communities.[28] Many of these children are blind from corneal scarring, where the role of professionals is to train cadres who work at the primary level, and to be advocates for improvements in primary health care (e.g. measles immunization) and other interventions (e.g. vitamin A supplementation) which have been shown to be highly cost effective at saving lives as well as preserving sight.

REFERENCES

1. World Health Organization. Preventing Blindness in Children: Report of WHO/IAPB scientific meeting (Unpublished document. Geneva: WHO/PBL/00.77; 2000).
2. Sommer A, Davidson FR. Assessment and control of vitamin A deficiency: the Annecy Accords. J Nutr 2002; 132: 2845S–50S.
3. Sommer A, West PW. Vitamin A Deficiency. Health, Survival and Vision. New York: Oxford University Press; 1996.
4. McLaren DS, Frigg M. Sight and Life Manual on Vitamin A Deficiency Disorders (VADD). 2nd edn. Switzerland: Task Force Sight and Life; 2001.
5. World Health Organization. Global Prevalence of Vitamin A Deficiency. Geneva: WHO/NUT/95.3; 1995.
6. Glasziou PP, Mackerras DE. Vitamin A supplementation in infectious diseases: a meta-analysis. BMJ 1993; 306: 366–70.
7. Bellagio Meeting on Vitamin A deficiency and Childhood Mortality. Proceedings of Public Health Significance of Vitamin A Deficiency and its Control. New York: Helen Keller International; 1993.
8. Ramakrishnan U, Danton Hill I. Assessment and control of vitamin A deficiency disorders. J Nutr 2002; 132: 947S–53S.
9. Allen L, Gillespie S. What works? A Review of Efficacy and

Effectiveness of Nutrition Interventions. United Nations Administrative Committee on Coordination Sub-Committee on Nutrition (ACC/SCN). Asian Development Bank; 2001.
10. World Health Organization, Integration of Vitamin A Supplementation with Immunization: Policy and Programme Implications. Geneva: WHO/EPI/GEN/98.07; 1998.
11. West KP Jr, McLaren D. The epidemiology of vitamin A deficiency disorders (VADD). In: Johnson G, Minassian D, Weale R et al. eds. Chapter 15. Epidemiology of Eye Disease. 2nd edn. London: Edward Arnold; 2002.
12. World Health Organization. Vaccines and Biological Annual Report 2000. Geneva: WHO/V&B/01.01; 2001.
13. Aaby P. Malnutrition and overcrowding/intensive exposure in severe measles infection: review of community studies. Rev Infect Dis 1988; 10: 478–91.
14. Foster A, Sommer A. Corneal ulceration, measles, and childhood blindness in Tanzania. Br J Ophthalmol 1987; 71: 331–43.
15. D'Souza RM, D'Souza R. Vitamin A for treating measles in children. Cochrane Database Syst Rev 2002; CD001479.
16. Moseley J. Ophthalmia Neonatorum. In: Wormald R, Smeeth L, Henshaw K, eds. Chapter 11. Evidence Based Ophthalmology. London: BMJ Books; 2004.

17. Isenberg SJ, Apt L, Wood M. A controlled trial of povidone-iodine as prophylaxis against ophthalmia neonatorum. N Engl J Med 1995; 332: 562–6.

18. Bang AT, Bang RA., Baitule SB, et al. Effect of home-based neonatal care and management of sepsis on neonatal mortality: field trial in rural India. Lancet 1999; 354: 955–61.

19. Mselle J. Visual impact of using traditional medicine on the injured eye in Africa. Acta Trop 1998; 70: 185–92.

20. Courtright P, Lewallen S, Kanjaloti S, et al. Traditional eye medicine use among patients with corneal disease in rural Malawi. Br J Ophthalmol 1994; 78: 810–2.

21. Courtright P, Chirambo M, Lewallen S, et al. Collaboration with African traditional healers for the prevention of blindness. Singapore: World Scientific; 2000.

22. Vajpayee RB, Vanathi M, Tandon R, et al. Keratoplasty for keratomalacia in preschool children. Br J Ophthalmol 2003; 87: 538–42.

23. Murphy SC, Breman JG. Gaps in the childhood malaria burden in Africa: cerebral malaria, neurological sequelae, anemia, respiratory distress, hypoglycemia, and complications of pregnancy. Am J Trop Med Hyg 2001; 64S: 57–67.

24. Brewster DR, Kwiatkowski D, White NJ. Neurological sequelae of cerebral malaria in children. Lancet 1990; 336: 1039–43.

25. Lewallen S, Harding SP, Ajewole J, et al. A review of the spectrum of clinical ocular fundus findings in P. falciparum malaria in African children with a proposed classification and grading system. Trans R Soc Trop Med Hyg 1999; 93: 619–22.

26. World Health Organization. Management of Severe Malaria. A Practical Handbook. 2nd edn. Geneva; 2000. ISBN 92 4 154523 2.

27. World Health Organization. Global Initiative for the Elimination of Avoidable Blindness. Geneva: WHO/PBL/97.61; 1997.

28. Kello AB, Gilbert CE. Causes of severe visual impairment and blindness in children in schools for the blind in Ethiopia. Br J Ophthalmol 2003; 87: 526–30.

Supranuclear Eye Movement Disorders, Acquired and Neurological Nystagmus

CHAPTER 73

Richard W Hertle

INTRODUCTION

Abnormal eye movements in the infant or young child can be congenital or acquired, associated with abnormal early visual development or a sign of underlying neurologic or neuromuscular disease or orbital disease. Abnormal eye movements in an apparently well child should never be labeled as congenital or benign without careful investigation including medical history, clinical examination, neuroimaging, laboratory testing, and electrophysiological investigation of the visual sensory system. Ocular motility analysis can indicate the type of eye movement disturbance and whether this is associated with an underlying ocular or neurological condition.

ANATOMY AND PHYSIOLOGY (Table 73.1)

Neural integrator

The neural integrator (NI) is an engineering term applied to an ocular motor "function" carried out by groups of cells in the cerebellum (flocculus and paraflocculus) and the prepositus hypoglossus and medial vestibular nucleus.[1] The NI is needed for all conjugate eye movements. To move the eyes at a constant speed or hold them in an eccentric gaze position, two neural signals must overcome the elastic tendency of the eyes to go back to their "resting" position. These signals are the desired speed (phasic component) and a tonic component that counterbalances the elastic restoring forces. A changing tonic component can be precisely generated by a premotor neural signal that mathematically computes the "integration" of the velocity signal, thus the term NI.[2] The role of the NI in generation of saccades and maintenance of eccentric gaze positions occurs after inhibitory burst neurons (IBN) are inhibited and excitatory burst neurons (EBN) fire rapidly, yielding an intense phasic signal that is transmitted to the appropriate yoked pair of extraocular muscles via the appropriate cranial nerves. The "burst" signal is also transmitted to the NI, which "integrates" that burst signal (counts the number of discharge spikes) and generates a neural signal (again transmitted via the cranial nerves) appropriate to hold the eye steady at the new position (tonic discharge).

The NI is not perfect and the "tonic" signal slowly decays or "leaks" over time. This decay is normally not seen in lighted conditions because visual feedback, with the use of the smooth-pursuit/fixation system, aids in holding the eye steady.[3] At birth the NI is leaky but by about 1 month of age it functions well.[4]

Saccadic system

A saccade is a rapid eye movement, which may occur volitionally (*voluntary saccade*), reflexively, or as part of the fast phases of nystagmus, which serves to purposefully redirect the fovea to a specific target.

Voluntary saccades may be:
1. *Predictive* (in anticipation of a target appearing in a specific location);
2. *command-generated* (i.e., look right);
3. *memory-guided*; and
4. *antisaccades*.[5]

Involuntary saccades include:
1. *the fast phase of nystagmus*, a saccade that resets the eyes after the slow-phase deviation of the vestibular or optokinetic response;
2. *spontaneous saccades*, which are thought to provide the function of repetitive scanning of our environment; and
3. *reflexive saccades*, which occur in response to new visual, auditory, olfactory, or tactile cues and which can be suppressed (see antisaccades).

Table 73.1 Types of eye movements

Type of eye movement	Function	Stimulus	Clinical tests
Vestibular	Maintain steady fixation during head rotation	Head rotation	Fixate on object while moving head; calorics
Saccades	Rapid refixation to eccentric stimuli	Eccentric retinal image	Voluntary movement between two objects; fast phases of OKN or of vestibular nystagmus
Smooth pursuit	Keep moving object on fovea	Retinal image slip	Voluntarily follow a moving target; OKN slow phases
Vergence	Disconjugate, slow movement to maintain binocular vision	Binasal or bitemporal disparity; retinal blur Motion	Fusional amplitudes; near point of convergence

OKN = optokinetic nystagmus

The pathway of saccades originates in the visual cortex and projects through the anterior limb of the internal capsule and then through the diencephalon. It then divides into dorsal and ventral pathways, the dorsal limb going to the superior colliculi and the ventral limb (which contains the ocular motor pathways for horizontal and vertical eye movements) to the pons and midbrain. The superior colliculus acts as an important relay for some of these projections.[6]

In the brainstem, the rostral interstitial nucleus of the medial longitudinal fasciculus (riMLF) and pontine paramedian reticular formation (PPRF) provide the saccadic velocity commands, by generating the "pulse of innervation" immediately before the eye movement, to cranial nerves III, IV, and VI. Horizontal saccades are generated by EBNs in the PPRF, which are found just ventral and lateral to the MLF in the pons, and by IBN in the nucleus paragigantocellularis dorsalis, caudal to the abducens nucleus in the dorsomedial portion of the rostral medulla (Fig. 73.1). Vertical and torsional components of saccades are generated by EBN and IBN in the riMLF, located in the midbrain[6] (Fig. 73.2).

Following a saccade a "step of innervation" occurs during which a higher level of tonic innervation to ocular motor neurons keeps the eye in its new position against orbital elastic forces that would restore the eye to an anatomically "neutral" position in the orbit. For horizontal saccades, the step of innervation comes from the NI, most importantly from the nucleus prepositus-medial vestibular nucleus complex. The eye is held steady at the end of vertical and torsional saccades by the step of innervation provided from the interstitial nucleus of Cajal in the midbrain.[6,7]

In addition to EBNs, omnipause neurons (OPNs), located in the nucleus raphe interpositus in the midline of the pons between the rootlets of the abducens nerves, are essential for normal saccadic activity. Continuous discharge from OPNs inhibits EBNs, and this discharge only ceases immediately prior to and during saccades.[6,7]

Other burst neurons termed long-lead burst neurons (LLBN) discharge 40 ms prior to saccades, whereas EBNs discharge 12 ms prior to saccades. Some LLBN lie in the midbrain, receiving projections from the superior colliculus and projecting to the

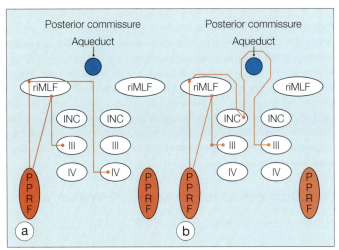

Fig. 73.2 This shows schematics of brainstem pathways coordinating downward (a) and upward (b) saccades. In (a) the PPRF activates neurons in the riMLF that send fibers caudally to synapse upon the inferior rectus subnucleus of the ipsilateral third nerve and the contralateral superior oblique nucleus. Not shown in this diagram, fibers from the contralateral PPRF carry corresponding signals simultaneously. In (b) the PPRF activates neurons in the riMLF that send fibers through the posterior commissure to the superior rectus subnucleus of the contralateral third nerve and fibers to the inferior oblique subnucleus of the ipsilateral third nerve. Not shown in this diagram, fibers from the contralateral PPRF carry corresponding signals simultaneously. riMLF = rostral interstitial nucleus of the medial longitudinal fasiculus, INC = interstitial nucleus of Cajal, III = third cranial nerve nucleus, IV = fourth cranial nerve nucleus, PPRF = paramedian pontine reticular formation.

pontine EBN, medullary IBN, and OPNs. Other LLBN lie in the nucleus reticularis tegmenti pontis, projecting mainly to the cerebellum but also to the PPRF. It appears that LLBN receiving input from the superior colliculus may play a crucial role in transforming spatially coded to temporally coded commands, whereas other LLBN may synchronize the onset and end of saccades.[6,7]

The *saccadic system* is not fully developed until about 1 year of age; infants make multiple hypometric saccades to reach the target.[8] If the head is held still, this hypometria can be seen clinically in infants less than 3 months of age, especially for large saccades. There is a progression toward "normometria" during the first 7 months of life.[9] In healthy adults and children older than 1 year, saccades are typically hypometric, reaching about 90% to 100% of the target distance, followed by secondary saccades–normometria.[10] In optokinetic nystagmus (OKN) and vertical nystagmus, quick phases occur less frequently in children than in adults.[11]

Smooth-pursuit system

The function of smooth pursuit (SP) is to hold fixation on a moving target, and both eye and head movements are required. This requires a prediction to overcome the time delays of the visuomotor system and the ability to suppress the vestibulo-ocular reflex (VOR).[12] VOR suppression is required because, when the head moves, there is a reflexive VOR that moves the eyes equally in the opposite direction. Smooth pursuit and VOR suppression are probably the same ocular motor functions.

The frontal and extrastriate visual cortexes transmit information about the motion of both the target and the eyes to the dorsolateral pontine nuclei (DLPN), thence to the

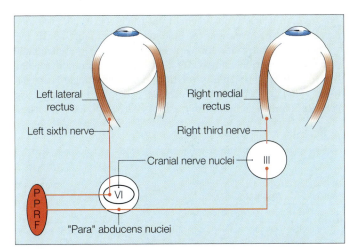

Fig. 73.1 Schematic of brainstem pathways coordinating horizontal saccades. The PPRF, after receiving input from the ipsilateral cortical centers and superior colliculus, stimulates two sets of neurons in the abducens nucleus: those that send axons to innervate the ipsilateral lateral rectus and those whose axons join the MLF and subsequently activate the medial rectus subnuclei of the contralateral third nerve. PPRF = paramedian pontine reticular formation, VI = sixth cranial nerve nuclei, III = third cranial nerve nuclei.

paraflocculus, flocculus, and dorsal vermis, and then via the vestibular and fastigial nuclei to the ocular motor nerve nuclei III, IV, and VI. Unilateral lesions in the cortex and cerebellum affect ipsilateral SP. Brainstem lesions are less well defined clinically.[1]

Smooth pursuit is present in the first week of life but is immature in the young infant. Horizontal gaze probably develops before vertical gaze.[13,14] Smooth-pursuit gain increases with age, and at 5 months the SP is more apparent. It is not known at what point in time pursuit matures to the adult form. It does not appear to happen before 6 months of age, and may not be until late adolescence.[15]

Vestibulo-ocular response (VOR) system

The vestibular apparatus drives reflex eye movements to keep images steady on the retinas as we move our heads. The eyes move in the opposite direction to the head so that they remain in a steady position in space. The three-neuron arc–vestibular ganglion, vestibular nuclei, and ocular motor nuclei–are the principle connections. The direct neuronal pathways include both excitatory and inhibitory contributions. Each semicircular canal influences a pair of extraocular muscles that move the eyes in the plane of that canal (Table 73.2). The anatomy of the vestibular nuclei has been well characterized;[16] they receive projections from the 14,000 to 18,000 axons of the vestibular nerve.[16]

There are four major vestibular nuclei:
1. The medial vestibular nucleus (MVN);
2. The lateral vestibular nucleus (LVN);
3. The inferior or descending vestibular nucleus (DVN); and
4. The superior vestibular nucleus (SVN).

There are also accessory subgroups, including the interstitial nucleus (IN), with its cells distributed among the vestibular rootlets as they enter the brain stem, and the y-group, near the superior cerebellar peduncle. The MVN has the greatest volume and is the longest vestibular nucleus. Its rostral portion is a major receiving area for afferents from the semicircular canals, and its cells project to the III, IV, and VI cranial nuclei, mediating vestibulo-ocular reflexes. Its caudal portion is reciprocally connected to the cervical region of the spinal cord, mediating vestibulocollic reflexes. The caudal MVN is also reciprocally connected to the cerebellum. The rostroventral portion of the LVN receives afferents from the cristae of the semicircular canals and the macula of the utricle. Like the rostral MVN, it participates in vestibulo-ocular reflexes, in part through the ascending tract of Deiters (ATD) to the oculomotor nucleus. The LVN also has projections to the spinal cord, mainly via the ipsilateral lateral vestibulospinal tract but also through the contralateral medial vestibulospinal tract. In its most rostral aspect the DVN also projects to the ocular motor nuclei.

The primary vestibular afferents enter the medulla at the level of the lateral vestibular nucleus. Almost all bifurcate, giving a descending branch to terminate in the MVN and DVN and an ascending branch to the SVN, with a final destination in the cerebellum, especially the anterior vermis and the nodulus and uvula. All canals and otoliths project to the borders of ventromedial LVN, medial MVN, and dorsomedial DVN. All canals also converge on a small patch in the ventromedial SVN. Utricular afferents project to the rostral MVN and saccular afferents project to the y-group. For both the horizontal and vertical VOR, many neurons in the vestibular nuclei that receive inputs from primary vestibular afferents encode head velocity, eye position, and varying amounts of smooth pursuit and saccadic signals. Vestibular nuclei neurons do not project just to motor neurons; they also send collaterals to the nucleus prepositus hypoglossi, the nucleus of Roller, and the cell groups of the paramedian tracts.[16]

When testing the VOR in the infant it is not unusual to find a slightly high VOR gain, which gradually decreases during preschool years, and a short VOR time constant.[17] In the premature infant and in some healthy full-term infants, rotation induces a tonic deviation or "locking up." The eyes deviate in the direction opposite to rotation when the doll's head maneuver or the Barany chair rotation test is used. They deviate in the same direction as the rotation when the infant is rotated at arms' length. A "corrective" fast phase develops at approximately 45 weeks postconceptual age.[8] This lockup up may be prolonged in the infant with delayed visual maturation. Usually there is no more than a couple of beats of postrotational nystagmus when the child stops spinning; if there are more than a few beats of nystagmus, a severe visual deficit, or abnormality of the smooth-pursuit pathway, should be suspected.[18] This test can be influenced by behavioral state and wakefulness.

Vergence system

Vergence is the ability to change the angle between the two visual axes to permit near (convergence), far (divergence), and torsional (cyclovergence) foveation, for binocular vision (Table 73.3).

The neural substrate for vergence lies in the mesencephalic reticular formation, dorsolateral to the oculomotor nucleus where neurons discharge in relation to vergence angle (vergence tonic cells), velocity (vergence burst cells), or both angle and velocity (vergence burst-tonic cells). Although most of these

Table 73.2 Effect of stimulating a single semicircular canal

Canal	Head movement	Eye movement in		Agonist		Antagonist	
		R gaze	*L gaze*	*R*	*L*	*R*	*L*
R Post	R and up	L Tors	Down	SO	IR	IO	SR
R Ant	R and down	Up	L Tors	SR	IO	IR	SO
R Lat	R	L	L	MR	LR	LR	MR
L Post	L and up	Down	R Tors	IR	SO	SR	IO
L Ant	L and down	L Tors	Up	IO	SR	SO	IR
L Lat	L	R	R	LR	MR	MR	LR

Based on Leigh and Zee.[92]
R = right, L = left, Post = posterior, Ant = anterior, Lat = lateral (horizontal canal), Tors = torsional (cyclotorsion with upper poles of eyes moving to subject's right/left), SO = superior oblique, IO = inferior oblique, IR= inferior rectus, SR= superior rectus, MR = medial rectus, LR = lateral rectus.

Table 73.3 Vergence stimuli

1. Retinal image disparity ("fusional" vergence);
2. Motion ("fusional" and "radial flow" vergences);
3. Accommodative blur ("accommodative" vergence); and
4. A "sense" of near (proximal vergence).
A lack of visual stimulation (awake, in the dark) leads to "tonic" vergence: slightly convergent.
Vergence movements are intimately linked to accommodation and pupillary changes.

---

neurons also discharge with accommodation, some remain predominantly related to vergence.[3,19] Like versional movements, a velocity-to-position integration of vergence signals is necessary: the nucleus reticularis tegmenti pontis (NRTP) is important in this integration. The cells in NRTP that mediate the near response are separate from cells that mediate the far response. Lesions of NRTP cause inability to hold a steady vergence angle. NRTP has reciprocal connection with the cerebellum (nucleus interpositus) and receives descending projections from several cortical and subcortical structures.[3,19]

The eyes of neonates, particularly if premature, often appear divergent, and there is little voluntary convergence until 2–3 months. By 3 to 6 months of age, 75% of premature and 97% of full-term infants have no deviation.[13] Fusion is not completely established until 6 months.[14,20] Accommodation-driven vergence can be detected at 2 months of age and disparity-driven vergence at about 4 months, which is when stereopsis and fusion develop.[14,20]

Optokinetic system

The optokinetic system is responsible for conjugate slow following of the eyes to movement of large areas of the visual field. Optokinetic nystagmus (OKN) is a reflex conjugate physiologic nystagmus in which a slow-phase pursuit response to movement of the visual surround (optokinesis) is followed by a corrective saccade or quick phase. OKN is elicited naturally during head and eye movements, or unnaturally by looking out of the window of a moving vehicle. Together with the vestibular system, the optokinetic system holds images steadily on the retina during sustained motion of the head or world or both.

The neural substrate for optokinesis includes the nucleus of the optic tract and accessory optic pathways. Optokinesis can be elicited by either full-field (natural head or eye movements) or small field (foveal) motion (a moving drum or tape). Both smooth-pursuit and optokinetic systems contribute to the stabilization of images of stationary objects during head rotations.

Optokinetic nystagmus is a physiological nystagmus where the slow-phase response is reset by quick phases (saccades). The direction of the OKN is usually referred to by its quick phases, but the optokinetic response itself is the slow phase; the quick phase (saccade) is compensatory or "corrective."

In primates, OKN has two components, each of which has a separate but parallel neural pathway[16]:

A. *Delayed* (indirect, slow) *OKN* (OKNd) has a slow buildup (tens of seconds) and gives rise to optokinetic after-nystagmus (OKAN), which is a gradual decay of the nystagmus after the lights have been extinguished. OKNd is closely related to VOR and is driven by visual motion signals in the visual cortex via the nucleus of the optic tract in the pretectum and the vestibular nuclei.[21,22]

B. *Early* (direct, fast) *OKN* (OKNe) has a rapid buildup (< 1 s) and does not give rise to OKAN; it ceases promptly in the dark. The OKNe pathway is similar to the smooth-pursuit pathway, which is mediated by a corticopontocerebellar route, and it is doubtful that the pretectum has a direct role in OKNe/smooth pursuit, although it may be involved in its adaptive control.

Many authors have not distinguished between OKNe and OKNd, giving a false impression of absent smooth pursuit in the presence of OKN, whereas OKNd was actually being measured.[21,23]

Finally, the cerebellum plays an important role in eye movements. Together with several brainstem structures, including the nucleus prepositus and the medial vestibular nucleus, it appears to convert velocity signals to position signals for all conjugate eye movements through mathematical integration.

CLINICAL ASSESSMENT

General patient investigations

The workup of supranuclear eye movement disorders and nystagmus is directed toward identifying associated ophthalmic and neurologic features with which, if found, the etiology is usually apparent by history, examination, or neuroimaging (Table 73.4).

General examination

The history and physical examination determines whether the nystagmus has been present from early or acquired later. A family history of neonatal eye disease, the pregnancy, labor, delivery, and growth and development since birth should be sought. Neonatal forms are generally benign, while acquired forms require further investigation. Since anxiety can affect nystagmus, the eye movements should be observed at a comfortable distance, in a non-threatening manner, while talking to the child or the parent. The most important features of nystagmus can usually be ascertained while "playing" with the child. Head turns or tilts while the child is viewing distant or near objects should be noted. An adequate fundus examination is a necessary part of the evaluation of eye movement disorders and involuntary ocular oscillations in infants and children.

Vision testing

Subjective accuracy of vision testing depends on the patient's age and their neurologic status. The "binocular acuity" should be

---

Table 73.4 Features of nystagmus suspicious (but not pathognomonic) of underlying neurological abnormality in childhood

Onset
Any acquired nystagmus except LN/MLN
Nystagmus features
Vertical
Circular
Elliptical
Dissociation between the two eyes
Other symptoms and signs
Oscillopsia
Hearing loss
Loss or reversal of developmental milestones
Ataxia or weakness

tested first. The patient must be allowed to assume any anomalous head posture (AHP). During the examination of visual acuity in nystagmus patients with an AHP the direction of the posture must be observed over a 5- to 7-min period. Up to 17% patients with infantile nystagmus and some forms of acquired nystagmus have a periodicity to the direction of their fast phase[24] with a changing head posture.

Binocular acuity is the "person's" acuity and monocular acuity is the "eye's" acuity; they are often very different in patients with nystagmus. In a nonverbal child or adult, various tests can be used to help determine both binocular and monocular acuity. These include fixation behavior, the 10-prism-diopter base-down test, Teller acuity cards, and matching of single, surrounded, HOTV optotypes or Lea symbols. Simple testing of binocular function is always attempted as the results are important if convergence is to be stimulated or fusion is to be aided by refractive therapy, e.g., Worth 4-dot and near stereopsis.

Refraction

In older children a subjective refraction is the foundation for any type of refractive therapy. All refractionists develop their own idiosyncrasies that assist them with rapid and accurate refraction. Try to ignore the oscillation and start with the distance retinoscopy in a phoropter in those patients without an AHP or trial frame (in those with a significant AHP). The next step is to do *binocular* refraction: this is the most important step in these patients because some patients have significant changes in their nystagmus under monocular conditions. The best way to do this is to fog the eye not being refracted with enough extra plus to decrease the vision 1-3 lines.

It is important in infants and young children to perform an objective refraction procedure; a cycloplegic refraction provides additional and important data for treatment decisions. In those patients in whom there is a different refraction under cycloplegia, record *both* subjective and objective refraction for decision making regarding spectacle prescription.

Ocular motility evaluation

Clinical evaluation of the ocular oscillation includes fast-phase direction, movement intensity, conjugacy, gaze effects, convergence effects, and effect of monocular cover. The amplitude, frequency, and direction of the nystagmus in all directions of gaze can be documented with a simple diagram (Fig. 73.3). The clinician can also observe the nystagmus while moving the patient's head. Associated motility systems (e.g., strabismus,

pursuit, saccades, and vestibulo-ocular reflex) can be clinically evaluated and recorded. This is most commonly accomplished with prism cover and/or alternate cover measurements in all gaze positions and at near. In older children fusional and accommodative amplitudes can be measured using prisms and a gradient technique respectively. Changes in the nystagmus with convergence or monocular viewing should be noted. If the nystagmus increases beneath closed eyelids, vestibular or brainstem pathology should be suspected since visual fixation may suppress nystagmus from lesions in these regions. Conjugacy of eye movements should be observed. Conjugacy of nystagmus can be checked by holding a pair of 40-diopter prisms placed base out in front of the nose to bring the images of the eyes closer together so the nystagmus can be compared.

Ocular motility recordings

Eye movement recordings provide a basis for eye movement abnormality classification, etiology, and treatment[25-27] and have impacted on eye movement systems research (Figs. 73.4 and 73.5).

There are three commonly used methods:

Electrooculography: This is useful for gross separation of fast and slow phases, but is limited by nonlinearity, drift, and noise.

Infrared reflectance oculography: This solves the problems of electroculography and can be used in infants and children, but is limited by difficulty in calibration.

Scleral contact lens/magnetic search coils: This is the most sensitive technique and is minimally invasive, but its use in children between 6 months and about 10 years is unpredictable (Figs. 73.4 and 73.5).

Practical applications of eye movement recording technology in clinical medicine include diagnosis/differentiation of eye movement disorders and utility as an "outcome measure" in clinical research.[28,29] Eye movement recordings display the data during continuous periods of time. Position and velocity traces are clearly marked with up being rightward or upward eye movements and down being leftward or downward eye movements. The basic types of nystagmus patterns observed after eye movement recordings are shown in Fig. 73.6.

Specific system evaluation

Neural integrator

To test the neural integrator clinically, observe primary position fixation, fixation in eccentric gaze, saccades, pursuit, and OKN and also test for rebound nystagmus and VOR cancellation. To examine for rebound nystagmus, first ask the patient to fixate on a target from the primary position, then to refixate on an eccentric target for 30 s, and then return to the primary position target. A patient with rebound nystagmus shows transient nystagmus with the slow phases toward the previous gaze position. To evaluate a child's VOR cancellation, it is easiest to place your hand on top of the patient's head to control both the head and a fixation target that will extend in front of the child's visual axis. You may use a Prince rule or a tongue depressor with a target or picture attached. Ask the child to fixate on the target as you passively rotate both the head and the target side-to-side. If the child is unable to cancel the VOR, you will observe nystagmus instead of the steady fixation expected in normal subjects.

"Gaze-evoked" nystagmus is a sign of a leaky neural integrator and occurs with attempts to maintain eccentric gaze. These "beats" of nystagmus toward the eccentric position persist as long

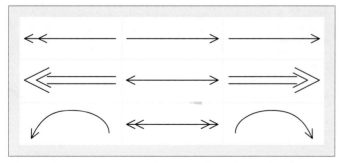

Fig. 73.3 Diagram of nystagmus in nine positions of gaze. Arrowheads indicate direction of jerk fast phase if on one end, pendular nystagmus if on both ends, and increasing frequency with more arrowheads. Additional lines indicate increased nystagmus amplitude. The curved lines indicate torsional nystagmus.

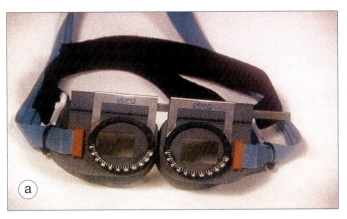

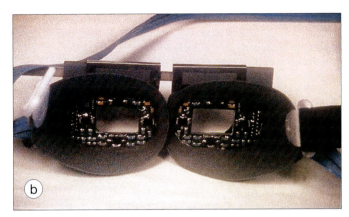

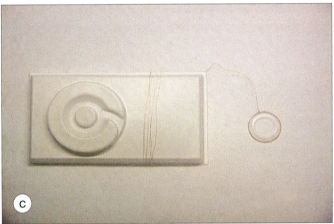

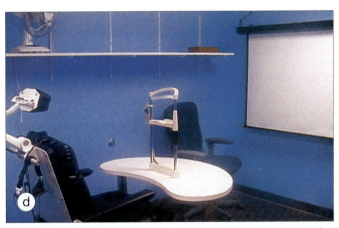

Fig. 73.4 Ocular motility recording equipment. Ocular motor laboratory showing infrared reflectance goggles ((a) front, (b) back), silicone contact lens (c), and flexible exam chair, chin rest, and stimulus screen (d).

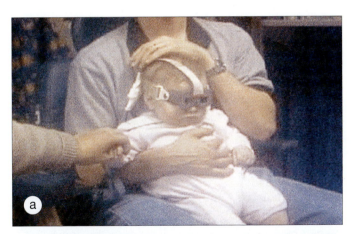

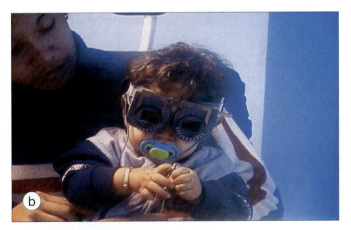

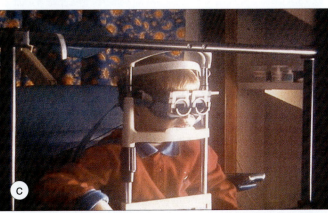

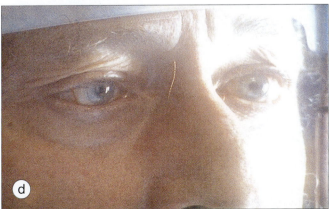

Fig. 73.5 Ocular motility recording techniques. Infrared reflectance performed on an infant (a), toddler (b), and a young child (c) and scleral search coil recordings performed on an adult (d).

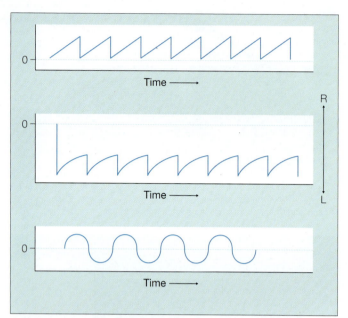

Fig. 73.6 Ocular oscillations. Artist representation of major types of nystagmus waveforms. Continuous periods of time are depicted in each tracing. Rightward eye movements are up and leftward eye movements are down.

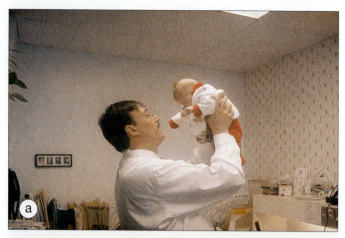

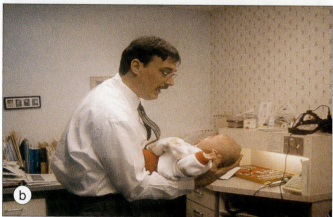

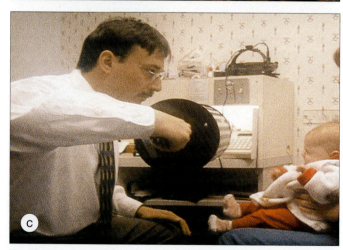

Fig. 73.7 Clinical evaluation of infant eye movements. The child is rotated in the examiner's arms in the vertical (a) and horizontal (b) planes to test the vestibulo-ocular, optokinetic, and saccadic systems. (c) An optokinetic drum is rotated close the child in the vertical direction to assess visual fixation and saccadic and optokinetic functions.

as the child attempts to view a peripherally placed target. This is different to physiologic end-point nystagmus where only a few beats of nystagmus, gradually decreasing in amplitude, are present while viewing eccentrically placed targets.

Saccades (Table 73.5)

If an abnormality of saccadic eye movements is suspected, the quick phases of vestibular and optokinetic nystagmus can be easily evaluated in infants and young children. To produce and observe vestibular nystagmus, hold the infant at arm's length, maintain eye contact, and spin first in one direction and then in the other (Figs. 73.7a and 73.7b). An OKN response can be elicited in the usual manner by passing a repetitive stimulus, such as stripes or an OKN drum, in front of the baby first in one direction and then in another (Fig. 73.7c). In addition, reflex saccades will be induced in many young patients when toys or other interesting stimuli are introduced into the visual field. Older children are asked to fixate alternately upon two targets so that the examiner can closely observe the saccades for promptness of initiation, speed, and accuracy (Fig. 73.8). It is best to

present the targets at large angles, as abnormalities are better visualized in larger-amplitude saccades. The addition of sound helps elicit the saccade. However, do not confuse a saccade toward sound as a visually guided saccade in a child with poor vision; it should first be established that the child could see. In children with strabismus it is necessary to test saccades monocularly. The OKN drum/tape or the VOR response can also be used to assess saccadic function. It is sometimes easier to observe the eyelashes moving vertically while testing vertical saccades using a vertically rotating OKN drum (Fig. 73.7c).

Table 73.5 Types of saccades

A. Voluntary saccades:
a) **Predictive**, in anticipation of a target appearing in a specific location;
b) **Command-generated**, in response to a command such as "look to the right"; and
c) **Memory-guided**; or antisaccades, in which a reflexive saccade to an abruptly appearing peripheral target is suppressed and a voluntary saccade is generated in the equidistant but opposite direction.
B. Involuntary saccades:
a) **Fast phases of nystagmus;**
b) **Spontaneous saccades**, providing repetitive scanning of the environment; and
c) **Reflex saccades**, involuntary in response to new visual, auditory, olfactory, or tactile cues: suppressible by antisaccades.

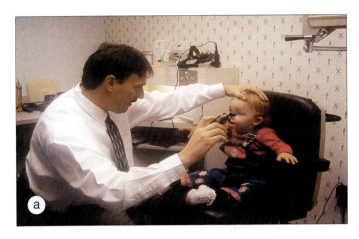

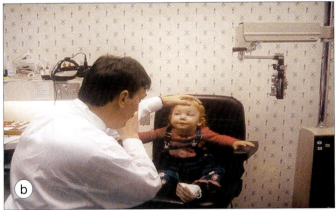

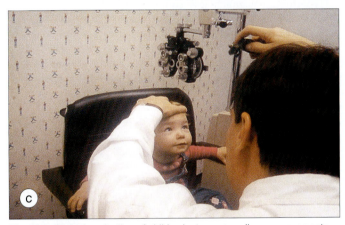

Fig. 73.8 Clinical evaluation of child voluntary saccadic eye movements. The child is seated while the head is held steady and targets are placed in the peripheral visual field horizontally (a, b) and vertically (c).

Smooth pursuit and vestibulo-ocular response systems

Smooth pursuit is tested by having the child follow a slow-moving easily seen target (i.e., a brightly colored toy or mirror), both horizontally and vertically. The child's head should initially be kept still. If the child is uncooperative or is thought to have hysterical blindness, a mirror should be slowly rotated before his/her eyes, or an OKN drum or tape can be used. When examining the pursuit system, one should always include an assessment of VOR suppression, which is an essential component of the smooth pursuit task during motion. In the older child, VOR suppression can be examined by asking the child to hold his/her finger about 14–16 in. in front of their face. The child is

then asked to slowly rotate his/her head with their finger from left to right while maintaining fixation on their finger. If the VOR response is suppressed there is no movement of the eyes relative to the head. Failure of VOR suppression results in a jerk nystagmus beating in the direct of the rotation. In an infant or young child you can test VOR suppression by holding the child in outstretched arms and spinning in both clockwise and counter-clockwise directions, while encouraging the child to fix on your face.

Vergence system

Vergence is usually tested by objective tests such as cover/uncover testing, alternate cover testing, prisms in front of the eye, and manual tests of near point of accommodation and vergence. Subjective aspects of vergence are tested by measuring the child's ability to perceive stereopsis. Many of these tests are dependent on the child's ability to cooperate but alternate cover testing can be performed as soon as the child is able to fix on near object.

Optokinetic system

Both slow and fast phases of OKN can be elicited by using OKN drum, tape, or full-field OKN stimuli (Fig. 73.7c). OKN responses are observed with both eyes open in the full-term infant on the first day of life.[30] In healthy neonates, a monocular OKN response can be obtained when the stimulus is moved in the temporal-to-nasal direction, but not in the nasal-to-temporal direction (physiologic/developmental, monocular OKN asymmetry). After 3 months, this monocular OKN asymmetry declines for moderate stimulus speeds, but persists beyond 6 months of age at high stimulus speeds.

DISORDERS OF SUPRANUCLEAR EYE MOVEMENTS

Neural integrator

Neural integrator dysfunction

Neural integrator dysfunction manifests clinically as gaze-evoked nystagmus and is often associated with low pursuit gain (gaze-holding deficiency nystagmus, eccentric gaze nystagmus) and rebound nystagmus. Quick phases are away from the central position (Fig. 73.6). Neurologic signs and symptoms include vertigo, nausea, dizziness, and oscillopsia. Gaze-evoked nystagmus is induced by moving the eye into lateral or vertical gaze, with sustained attempts to look eccentrically (Fig. 73.9). After the eyes are then returned to the central position, a short-lived nystagmus with quick phases opposite to the direction of the prior eccentric gaze occurs (rebound nystagmus). Abnormal suppression of the VOR and low-gain OKN responses are also associated clinical findings and, again, probably reflect cerebellar disease[31,32] (Fig. 73.9).

Most types of pathological nystagmus increase their intensity as the eyes move in the direction of the fast phase (Alexander's law); this is believed due to a physiologically adapted "leaky" NI responding to the pathological vestibular imbalance that is part of the nystagmus.[31,32]

Most frequently, gaze-holding deficiency nystagmus is seen in conjunction with use of anticonvulsants and sedatives, cerebellar and brainstem disease, or other drug intoxication. MRI/CT scan of brain reflects underlying disease and ocular motility recording show slow phases that have decelerating velocity characteristics.[31,32] Acquired eye movement abnormalities suggesting defective

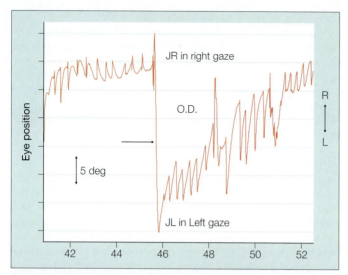

Fig. 73.9 Ocular motility recording of gaze-evoked nystagmus. This is a typical 10 s position trace of ocular motor recordings from a patient with gaze-evoked nystagmus. Right gaze shows jerk right with linear/decreasing velocity slow phases while left gaze shows jerk left with linear and decreasing velocity slow phases. The horizontal arrow points out where the patient's gaze shifted from right 15° to left 15°. O.D. = right eye, R = rightward eye movements and right gaze, L = leftward eye movements and left gaze, Deg = degree, JR = Jerk Right Nystagmus, JL = Jerk Left Nystagmus.

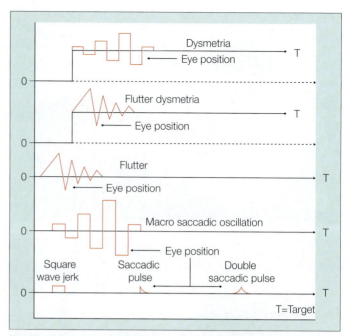

Fig. 73.10 Saccadic intrusions. Artist representation of major types of saccadic instabilities and their ocular motor characteristics. Continuous periods of time are depicted in each tracing. Rightward eye movements are up and leftward eye movements are down. 0 = Primary position fixation, T = target.

neural integration, whether isolated or associated with other neurologic deficits, alert the examiner to investigate for a serious central nervous system abnormality. Structural anomalies affecting the brainstem and cerebellum, e.g., the Arnold-Chiari malformation, as well as metabolic, vascular, and neuro-degenerative disorders may also produce abnormalities of the neural integrator.

Disorders of saccades

Saccadic accuracy
Normal and abnormal saccades are often dysmetric (inaccurate). Saccadic inaccuracy can be a result of gain dysmetria or pulse-step dysmetria. In saccadic dysmetria, the saccade misses the target and corrective saccades are needed for foveation (Fig. 73.10). If the saccades fall short of the target, they are known as hypometric; if they overshoot the target, they are hypermetric. In both cases, one or more secondary saccades are needed to eventually fixate the target. Hypometria is often seen in cerebellar disease, including autosomal dominant spinocerebellar ataxia type 3, and ocular motor apraxia. It is far more common than hypermetria.[33,34] Consistent marked hypometria below 90% that persists beyond 7 months of age suggests neurologic disease.

In homonymous hemianopia, saccades into the blind field are often multiple hypometric, "staircase," or "searching." In basal ganglia disease, voluntary saccades may be hypometric with more or less normal reflexive saccades. During the resolving stages of isolated (type 1) delayed visual maturation (DVM) in infants, saccades may be hypometric for age, but if the hypometria is prolonged, a neurologic explanation should be sought. Hypometric saccades can be secondary to changes in visual magnification; for example, the removal of aphakic spectacles may lead to a temporary hypometria until adaptation takes place.[35]

Hypermetria is much less common and appears flutter-like (but should not be mistaken for ocular flutter). With the exclusion of centripetal saccades, hypermetria is abnormal at any age, and when conjugate, it is almost always associated with cerebellar disease, including spinocerebellar ataxia type 1 (SCA1).[36] If hypermetria is severe, the corrective saccade may be as large as the primary saccade, thus causing the eyes to oscillate back and forth with saccades. This phenomenon has been termed macrosaccadic oscillations. After recovery of opsoclonus, there may be persistent hypermetric saccades (Fig. 73.10).[37,38]

Saccadic velocity
Slow saccades may not be obvious clinically, especially in children. They may result from an abnormality involving the paramedian pontine reticular formation and have been thought to be pathognomonic of burst cell dysfunction. Slow saccades may be seen in mitochondrial disorders, progressive external ophthalmoplegia, myasthenia gravis, basal ganglia disease, Duane syndrome, and families with spinocerebellar ataxia type 2.[34,39,40] Slow horizontal and sometimes vertical saccades may occur in patients with Gaucher type 3 disease.[41] The muscular dystrophies have variable eye movement involvement, and slow saccades have been observed in both Becker and non-Fukuyama-type congenital muscular dystrophy. When saccades are very slow they may be mistaken for a smooth-pursuit response, but a moving target is essential for smooth pursuit.

Saccadic latency
The time between the onset of a stimulus and the beginning of a saccade, and for healthy infants, is up to about 1 s (about 200 ms in adults).[39,42] In childhood, prolonged saccade latencies usually occur in association with saccade initiation failure.

Saccade initiation failure (SIF)/ocular motor apraxia (OMA)

The term saccade initiation failure or ocular motor apraxia is used to specify impaired voluntary saccades and variable deficit of fast-phase saccades during vestibular or optokinetic nystagmus.[41] Congenital ocular motor apraxia is characterized by defective horizontal saccades, but it does not represent a true apraxia since reflex saccades may also be impaired.[43] The incidence of this condition depends on the underlying etiology.

Patients with congenital saccade initiation failure show abnormal initiation and decreased amplitude of voluntary saccades; saccadic velocities in these patients are normal and fast phases of nystagmus of large amplitude can occasionally be generated. This suggests that the brainstem burst neurons that generate saccades are intact.[41,44,45] Acquired SIF may be due to conditions as listed in Table 73.6. Some of these patients with the acquired type, such as those with Gaucher's disease (types 1 and some type 3 patients), have abnormal saccadic velocities.[41] Although the exact cause or localization of the defect in congenital SIF has not been determined, there is strong evidence that most can be localized subtentorially, particularly to the cerebellar vermis.[41,45]

The clinical presentation varies with the age and motor development of the child. Affected infants and children with poor head control are commonly thought to be blind since the expected refixations are not observed. In such an infant demonstration of vertical saccades, vertical pursuit, OKN response in any direction, and normal acuity on visual-evoked response testing suggests the diagnosis of SIF. Another clinical sign in young infants is an intermittent tonic deviation of the eyes in the direction of slow-phase vestibular or optokinetic nystagmus; in these infants fast-phase saccades may be impaired.

By 4 to 8 months of age, the child develops a striking "head-thrusting" behavior in order to refixate. First, the eyelids blink ("synkinetic blink") and the head begin to rotate toward the object of interest (Figs. 73.11 and 73.12). Next, the head

Table 73.6 Congenital and acquired saccade initiation failure

Classification by cause	Specific etiologies
Idiopathic Perinatal problems	Cerebral palsy; hypoxia; hydrocephalus; seizures
Congenital malformations	Agenesis of corpus callosum; fourth ventricle dilation, and vermis hypoplasia; Joubert syndrome; macrocerebellum; dysgenesis of cerebellar vermis and midbrain; Dandy-Walker malformation; immature development of putamen; heterotropia of gray matter; porencephalic cyst; hamartoma near foramen of Munro; macrocephaly; microcephaly; posterior fossa cysts; chondrodystrophic dwarfism and hydrocephalus; encephalocele; occipital meningocele; COACH syndrome (cerebellar vermis hypoplasia, oligophrenia, congenital ataxia, coloboma, hepatic fibrocirrhosis)
Neurodegenerative conditions with infantile onset of SIF	Infantile Gaucher's disease (types 2 and 3); Gaucher's disease type 2; Pelizaeus-Merbacher disease; Krabbe's leukodystrophy; propionic academia; GM1 gangliosidosis; infantile Refsum's disease; 4-hydroxybutyric aciduria
Neurodegenerative conditions with later onset of SIF	Ataxia telangiectasia; spinocerebellar degenerations; juvenile Gaucher's disease (type 3); Huntington's disease; Hallervorden-Spatz disease; Wilson's disease
Acquired disease	Postimmunization encephalopathy; herpes encephalitis; posterior fossa tumors
Other associations	Alagille syndrome; Bardet-Biedl syndrome; carotid fibromuscular hypoplasia; Cockayne syndrome; Cornelia de Lange syndrome; juvenile nephronophthisis; Lowes syndrome; neurofibromatosis type ; orofacial digital syndrome; X-linked muscle atrophy with congenital contractures

Adapted from Cassidy et al.[8]

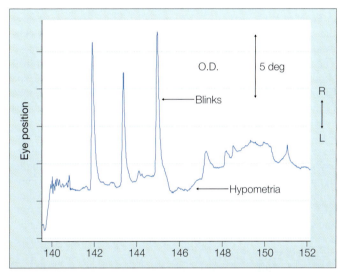

Fig. 73.11 Ocular motility recording of saccadic initiation failure. This is a 12 s position trace of ocular motor recordings from a patient with saccadic initiation failure. "Synkinetic" blinks are followed by hypometric saccades. O.D. = right eye, R = rightward eye movements and right gaze, L = leftward eye movements and left gaze, Deg = degree.

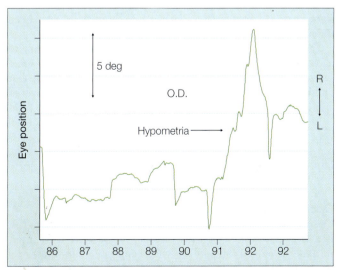

Fig. 73.12 Ocular motility recording of saccadic initiation failure. This is an 7 s position trace of ocular motor recordings from a patient with saccadic initiation failure. Multiple hypometric ("staircase") saccades are illustrated. O.D. = right eye, R = rightward eye movements and right gaze, L = leftward eye movements and left gaze, Deg = degree.

continues to rotate past the intended target allowing the tonically deviated eyes, which are now in an extreme contraversive position, to come into alignment with the target. Finally, as the eyes maintain fixation, the head rotates slowly back so that the eyes are in primary position. This apparent use of the VOR to refixate continues for several years, but with increasing age, patients demonstrate less prominent head thrusting and may even be able to generate some saccades though they are abnormal. The blink-saccade synkinesis adaptation may persist.

In some infants, generalized hypotonia may be associated. This hypotonia seems to be more pronounced in boys and improves with increasing age. These babies later demonstrate the motor delay, incoordination, and clumsiness that has been noted in the literature.[46]

The parents of children are asked about any associated developmental abnormality. An examination is performed to rule out any strabismus or amblyopia, as strabismus has been reported in many of these patients.[47] Vision, ERG, and VEP are normal in the congenital SIF patients. Any coexistent abnormal vision, nystagmus, or abnormal ERG or VEP suggests associated disease. The appropriate subspecialist further investigates neurologic abnormalities or dysmorphic features. A brain MRI is necessary for suspected neurologic disorders, to look for midline malformations, particularly around the fourth ventricle and cerebellar vermis.

Significant structural abnormalities of the central nervous system (CNS), such as lipoma or brainstem tumor, may be associated. Joubert syndrome is associated with cerebellar hypoplasia and agenesis of the corpus callosum. A neuro-radiologic correlation has been made in children with SIF, where 61% of 62 children had abnormal scans, primarily the brainstem and cerebellar vermis, also the cerebral cortex and basal ganglia[47] and at the mesencephalic–diencephalic junction: infarcts due to perinatal hypoxia (Table 73.6).

Gaucher's disease, ataxia telangiectasia and its variants, and Niemann-Pick variants may also present with the inability to generate saccades as well as blinking and head thrusting prior to refixation. Unlike SIF, these disorders generally involve vertical as well as horizontal saccades and eventually manifest systemic signs.

Occasional familial occurrence, increased frequency in males, and occurrence in monozygotic twins suggest a genetic process in some cases.[46] Association with nephronophthisis has been described in two patients with 2q13 deletions.

The prognosis of the congenital type is good. Many adapt to allow gaze shifts with less head thrusting and can generate some saccades, albeit abnormal. There is no treatment for SIF, but children who have this condition should be investigated appropriately and recognized as having learning and living difficulties, and they should receive extra help and other educational benefits at school. Whether the condition improves with age is not known; any apparent improvement may be a result of the improvement of the adaptive strategies these children use to enable rapid shifts of gaze.

Opsoclonus/ocular flutter

Opsoclonus, also referred to as "saccadomania" or dancing eyes, is a rare, but striking saccade disorder, characterized by intermittent involuntary bursts of wild conjugate multidirectional back-to-back saccades.[38] When the eye movement is purely horizontal, it is known as ocular flutter (Fig. 73.13). During resolution, opsoclonus may revert to ocular flutter, and finally saccadic dysmetria, before eventually reverting to normal eye movements. Opsoclonus is often triggered by attempted fixation,

smooth pursuit, convergence, upgaze, eyelid closure, or OKN or vestibular nystagmus. The frequency is high, usually ranging between 5 and 13 Hz, and the amplitude can be tens of degrees, although it may be so small that the oscillations cannot be seen without a slit lamp, ophthalmoscope, or eye movement recordings (Figs. 73.14 and 73.15). Opsoclonus usually persists during sleep, although it may be diminished or even absent.[38] Acquired opsoclonus is often associated with limb myoclonus. In such cases, it is described as opsoclonus–myoclonus, dancing eye-dancing feet syndrome, myoclonic encephalopathy of infants, or infantile polymyoclonia.[38] The opsoclonus–myoclonus syndrome is more common in children.[38]

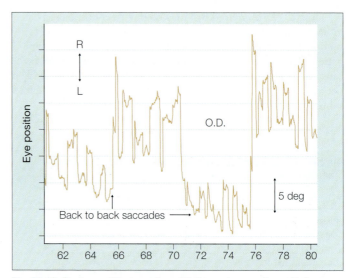

Fig. 73.13 Ocular motility recording of flutter and saccadic oscillations. This is a typical 18 s position trace of ocular motor recordings from a patient with ocular flutter. Back-to-back saccades with (macrosaccadic oscillations) and without (flutter) an intersaccadic interval, both interrupting fixation and occurring on refixation are demonstrated (arrows). O.D. = right eye, R = rightward eye movements and right gaze, L = leftward eye movements and left gaze, Deg = degree.

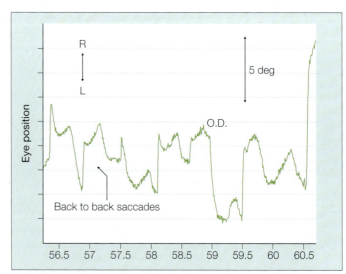

Fig. 73.14 Ocular motility recording of opsoclonus. This is a typical 4 s position trace of ocular motor recordings from a patient with opsoclonus. High-frequency back-to-back saccades without (flutter) an intersaccadic interval are demonstrated (arrows). O.D. = right eye, R = rightward eye movements and right gaze, L = leftward eye movements and left gaze, Deg = degree.

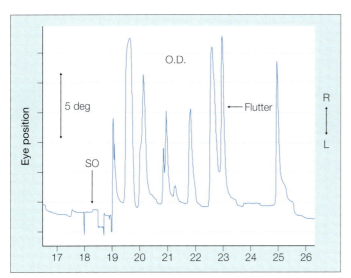

Fig. 73.15 Ocular motility recording of opsoclonus + saccadic intrusions. This is a 9 s position trace of ocular motor recordings from a patient with opsoclonus and saccadic oscillations. Small-amplitude back-to-back saccades with an intersaccadic interval (SO) are followed by large-amplitude back-to-back saccades without an intersaccadic interval (flutter). SO = saccadic oscillation, O.D. = right eye, R = rightward eye movements and right gaze, L = leftward eye movements and left gaze, Deg = degree.

Onset may be acute or subacute and is often accompanied by ataxia, vomiting, and irritability. It may be a manifestation of occult malignancies, in particular, neural crest tumors (neuroblastoma, ganglioneuroblastoma, ganglioneuroma), hepatoblastoma, infection (Coxsackie B, HIV, mumps, parainfluenza virus, psittacosis, salmonella, syphilis, St. Louis encephalitis, rickettsia, enterovirus, Epstein-Barr virus infection), toxic (amitriptyline, cocaine, diazepam, lithium, and phenytoin), or metabolic disorders (biotin-responsive multiple carboxylase deficiency, hyperosmolar nonketotic coma).[8]

In children with neural crest tumors or brain stem encephalitis, opsoclonus is commonly accompanied by diffuse or focal myoclonus. Although opsoclonus–myoclonus is rarely a presenting feature of neuroblastoma, it is seen in about 50% of children with an occult neuroblastoma, and the presence of opsoclonus confers a favorable survival rate.[48] Paraneoplastic opsoclonus is associated with a single copy of the *N-myc* oncogene, and those children with amplification of this oncogene who do not develop opsoclonus and carry a worse prognosis.[49] It is hypothesized that in paraneoplastic opsoclonus, the tumor and some CNS structures share an epitope, and that this common epitope triggers an immune response against the tumor and the CNS, resulting in the neurologic symptoms.[49]

Although extremely rare, congenital opsoclonus has been reported, and it usually resolves spontaneously by 6 months. It is not always benign, and it may be associated with intrauterine anoxia, intracranial hemorrhage, microcephaly, epilepsy, truncal ataxia, mental retardation, and congenitally poor vision.

Opsoclonus may be mistaken for nystagmus and vice versa. Formal eye movement recordings will differentiate the two, demonstrating that opsoclonus is a burst of back-to-back saccades with no intersaccadic interval, without the slow phases of nystagmus (Figs. 73.13–73.15). However, on rare occasions there may be a constant high-frequency acquired pendular nystagmus. Once opsoclonus has been confirmed, children should be screened for urinary vanillylmandelic acid (VMA) and homovanillic acid

(HVA) and have an oncologic workup. This may include chest and abdominal computerized tomography and/or MRI. Elevated levels of urinary VMA and HVA are diagnostic; however, normal levels occur in 26% of children with paraneoplastic opsoclonus.[49] Blood and cerebrospinal fluid (CSF) samples should also be taken and sent for virology and bacteriology. Cerebrospinal fluid pleocytosis has been reported in children with paraneoplastic opsoclonus and there are occasional oligoclonal bands. There have been occasional reports of autoantibodies, including anti-Hu and antibodies against neurofilaments, in the sera of children with paraneoplastic opsoclonus.

Acquired opsoclonus is probably immune-mediated. The evidence for this is its association with:

1. Autoantibodies;
2. Infectious and neoplastic disease;
3. A good oncologic prognosis;
4. The presence of lymphocytic infiltration in tumors in patients with paraneoplastic opsoclonus and a good outcome; and
5. A good response to steroid treatment.[50]

Its neural substrate remains a mystery, and there may be no single site involved in the causation of opsoclonus.

Opsoclonus–myoclonus, especially when it occurs with brainstem encephalitis, may be a benign self-limiting condition.[51] Although children with paraneoplastic opsoclonus tend to have a better oncologic prognosis, the neurologic outcome is unpredictable. Children who have become cancer free may have significant neurologic sequelae. Adrenocorticotrophic hormone (ACTH) or systemic steroid treatment has a dramatic short-term effect on symptoms in 50 to 90% of children with opsoclonus.[50] However, not all children have such a good response, and the opsoclonus and ataxia may become steroid-dependent, reemerging when treatment is tapered or during intercurrent illnesses. Other drugs used to treat opsoclonus–myoclonus include intravenous IgG, azathioprine, propranolol, and divalproex sodium. A combination of systemic steroids and high-dose immunoglobulin can be used for the treatment of opsoclonus–myoclonus in patients who do not respond to first-line therapy with steroids.

Regardless of the short-term response, these children often have long-term developmental problems, including speech, motor, and cognitive disabilities.[51] Abnormal eye movements may persist. Parents, teachers, and carers should be informed of such problems. Occupational therapists, psychologists, and social services should be involved at an early stage.

Antisaccades

An antisaccade requires the subject to suppress a reflexive saccade to an abruptly appearing peripheral target, and generate a voluntary saccade in the equidistant but opposite direction. The ability to suppress reflexive responses in favor of voluntary motor actions is necessary in everyday life, and both of these abilities can be assessed with use of the antisaccade task. The correct execution of an antisaccade requires at least two functioning subprocesses: an intact fixation system and the ability to generate a voluntary saccade in the opposite direction. Infants as young as 4 months have a fixation system adequate to allow inhibition of reflex saccades, but the ability to generate a voluntary antisaccade develops much later, usually over 10 years old, with a steep decrease in the mean error rate from 10 to 15 years, then a more gradual decrease toward 20 years.[52] The antisaccade task requires higher-level control of saccadic eye movements, and in adults, failure of antisaccades has been reported in patients with frontal lobe lesions and basal ganglia disorders, in particular progressive supranuclear palsy. Failure of antisaccades has been reported in both adults and children with obsessive-compulsive disorder; this is thought to be a result of abnormal basal ganglia-frontal interaction. Difficulty in making antisaccades has also been described in people with schizophrenia, children with attention deficit hyperactivity disorder (ADHD), autosomal dominant cerebellar ataxia type 2, male dyslexics, and Tourette syndrome.[53,54]

There are neuroimaging, clinical, and electrophysiologic studies that implicate very many parts of the brain in the generation of antisaccades. Lesions affecting any of these areas may lead to an inability to suppress reflexive saccades, which is necessary to make a successful antisaccade.[55]

Saccadic intrusions and oscillations (SIs, SOs)

There are saccadic eye movements that may intrude on steady primary position fixation or interrupt refixation and, hence, mimic nystagmus (Figs. 73.10, 73.15, and 73.16). Only eye movement recordings can definitively distinguish SIs and SOs from nystagmus.

Square wave jerks may be exaggeration of the normal microsaccadic movements associated with fixation. They consist of a conjugate displacement of the eyes up to 5° from fixation, followed by a refixational saccade after a normal intersaccadic interval of 200 ms. They are seen in normal healthy subjects of any age. However, if they are more frequent (more than nine square wave jerks per minute in a young person should be considered abnormal), they are referred to as square wave oscillations, and are seen in cerebellar disease, progressive supranuclear palsy, and multiple sclerosis.[56] Square wave jerks and oscillations are rarely seen in childhood (Fig. 73.16).

Macro-square wave jerks are also rare in childhood. They consist of conjugate displacement of the eyes away from fixation by more than 5°, and, after a shorter than normal latency of 80 ms, there is a refixation saccade. They occur in bursts and may be mistaken for flutter. The amplitude is variable, and they are present in the dark. They occur in diseases that disrupt cerebellar outflow, i.e., multiple sclerosis or olivopontocerebellar degenerations, including Huntington's disease.[56]

Macrosaccadic oscillations represent a severe form of saccadic hypermetria. They are characterized by conjugate oscillations of the eyes around fixation, with a normal intersaccadic interval of 200 ms. The oscillations increase and then decrease in amplitude during each episode. They are a result of lesions affecting the midline cerebellum and underlying nuclei. They are not present in darkness.

Disorders of smooth pursuit

Smooth-pursuit asymmetry–initiation failure

Monocular smooth-pursuit asymmetries may persist in patients with early-onset, but not with late-onset, strabismus. Impaired smooth pursuit to the side of the lesion has been most frequently reported in patients with lesions restricted to the posterior cortical areas and underlying white matter, but it also occurs with frontal lobe lesions and in hemidecortication. Ipsilateral pursuit deficit may also be seen in unilateral lesions of the lower portions of the pursuit pathway, including the thalamus, midbrain tegmentum, dorsolateral pontine nucleus, and cerebellum. Nuclear vestibular lesions may affect either ipsilateral or contralateral smooth pursuit.[57]

Abnormal smooth pursuit gain

Low pursuit gain, which may be seen clinically as saccadic or jerky pursuits, occurs in the elderly and in patients with basal ganglia disease, and cerebellar disease, large cerebral lesions, or posterior cortical lesions. Low pursuit gain has been described in spinocerebellar ataxia both types 1 and 3. If gaze-holding deficiency nystagmus is associated with saccadic pursuit, the lesion is most likely to be cerebellar, whereas saccadic pursuit in the absence of gaze-holding deficiency nystagmus is more likely to indicate a cerebral lesion. Excessively high pursuit gain can be seen as an adaptive change in extraocular muscle restrictive or paretic disease. There have also been reports of patients with hemidecortication having high-gain smooth pursuit away from the side of the lesion.[34,58,59]

Abnormal visual fixation

Steady fixation may be disrupted by slow drifts, nystagmus, or involuntary saccades. The frequency of square-wave jerks increases in certain neurological conditions, i.e., progressive supranuclear palsy, Friedreich's ataxia, and focal cerebral lesions. Detection of nystagmus during attempted steady fixation is abnormal. If the slow-phase velocity or intensity of nystagmus is similar both during fixation and when fixation is prevented (e.g., by *Frenzel goggles* or in darkness), then a disorder of the fixation system is inferred.

Disorders of the visual system lead to instability of gaze, the extreme example being blindness. Monocular loss of vision may lead to unstable gaze in the affected eye, which is predominantly due to slow, low-frequency vertical drifts. Binocular loss of vision causes loss of gaze stability and a continuous horizontal and vertical nystagmus.[60] This nystagmus characteristically changes direction over the course of seconds and minutes, a feature also encountered following experimental cerebellectomy. Thus, the nystagmus that follows bilateral visual loss reflects a gaze-holding mechanism that has never been calibrated by visual inputs. Acquired lesions of the cerebellum without specific involvement of the visual pathways may disrupt fixation with saccadic intrusions and with slow drifts, especially in the vertical plane, that lead to nystagmus. The pathogenesis of pendular oscillations occurring in association with visual loss is unknown.[61]

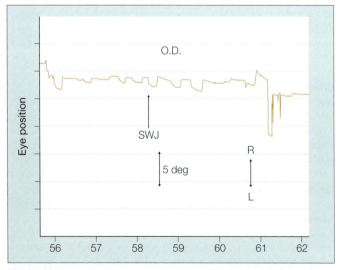

Fig. 73.16 Ocular motility recording of saccadic intrusions. This is a 6 s position trace of ocular motor recordings from a patient with saccadic intrusions (SI). Small- to moderate-amplitude back-to-back saccades with an intersaccadic interval (SWJ) are present throughout the recording at about 1 Hz. SWJ = square wave jerks, O.D. = right eye, R = rightward eye movements and right gaze, L = leftward eye movements and left gaze, Deg = degree.

Disorders of vergence

Strabismus

This is discussed in Chapters 73 to 90.

Spasm of the near reflex (convergence spasm)

Spasm of the near reflex, also referred to as convergence spasm, is characterized by intermittent spasm of convergence, of miosis, and of accommodation. Symptoms include headache, photophobia, eye strain, blurred vision, and diplopia. Patients may appear to have bilateral sixth nerve palsies, but careful observation will reveal miosis and high myopia (8–10 D) on dry retinoscopy, accompanying the failure of abduction.[62] This key clinical clue will prevent misdiagnosis and misdirected testing. Most commonly, spasm of the near reflex is psychogenic, and treatment may include simple reassurance, psychiatric counseling, or cycloplegia with bifocals.

Spasm of the near reflex associated with organic disease has been reported with encephalitis, tabes, labyrinthine fistulas, pituitary adenoma, Arnold-Chiari malformation, posterior fossa lesions, trauma, myasthenia gravis, anticonvulsant toxicities, midbrain lesions, metabolic problems, and cyclic oculomotor palsy. Disturbances that are clearly functional do not exclude coexisting organic disease!

The pathophysiology of organic convergence spasm is not clear, although it has been suggested that it may reflect instability of the vergence integrator. Clinical examination of patients with convergence spasm includes eye movement assessment, as it is important to distinguish between this condition and bilateral sixth nerve palsy. When one eye is occluded, there is often full range of movement and less pupillary constriction of the fixing eye. There may be abducting nystagmus on attempted lateral gaze and the doll's head maneuver may elicit a full range of eye movements.

Divergence insufficiency/paralysis

Divergence insufficiency is characterized by an esotropia for distance and orthophoria for near and normal convergence; the esotropia may be constant or intermittent. The fusional divergence may be reduced or completely absent. Divergence paralysis is characterized by complete loss of divergence amplitude. It appears as a constant esotropia for distance, with normal convergence, and it usually indicates an underlying neurologic problem, such as a tumor or head trauma resulting in elevated intracranial pressure, or the onset of Miller Fisher syndrome. Bilateral sixth nerve paresis should be excluded in these cases.

Convergence insufficiency/paralysis

Convergence insufficiency is characterized by reduced fusional convergence at near and a variable exophoria (occasionally intermittent exotropia) at near. It usually appears in adolescence and gives rise to vague symptoms of eye strain, headache, diplopia, and blurring associated with close work.

On examination, a poorly controlled exophoria on near fixation is found with the cover test. There may also be a phoric or intermittently tropic exodeviation for distance, and if the exodeviation for near is greater by 15 prism diopters or more than that for distance, the patient is demonstrating a convergence insufficiency pattern. Eye movements and reading acuity are normal, and there should be no neurologic abnormalities.

Convergence insufficiency usually has no underlying cause, but it can be associated with stress, fatigue, and anxiety, and it may follow infection or trauma.[63] Underlying intracranial lesions are rare. The child and parents should be reassured that there is no disease, and orthoptic near-point exercises can be tried. If orthoptic exercises fail, prisms may be required.

Complete convergence paralysis is highly suggestive of an intracranial lesion, such as encephalitis, demyelination, neurosyphilis, or a condition resulting from trauma or toxins. The patient is usually completely unable to converge.

Disorders of the vestibulo-ocular response system

Abnormal VOR gain

Vestibulo-ocular reflex gain is the peak slow-phase velocity divided by rotation speed and is higher in infants than in adults. Abnormalities of VOR gain in the small child are not easily detected clinically but require eye movement recordings. If VOR gain is abnormal, a child's visual acuity will deteriorate by several lines while moving the head compared to the acuity taken with the head stationary. Abnormally high gain has been described in lesions of the cerebellar flocculus and the inferior olive. Mildly high gains have also been reported in familial vestibulocerebellar disorders.[64] Abnormally low gain in the young child may indicate vestibular nerve involvement in cases of meningitis or in the CHARGE syndrome. Asymmetrical gain is a more reliable indicator of acquired vestibular disease, but it must be assessed in the context of other ocular motor and possibly auditory abnormalities to distinguish between peripheral, brainstem, cerebellar, and cortical causes.

Abnormal VOR time constant

The time constant is measured as the time taken for the eye velocity of per-rotational or postrotational nystagmus measured in the dark to fall to 37% of its initial value. As a rule of thumb, the nystagmus will persist for a total time of about three times the time constant. Measurements on animals have shown that the time constant of the decay of per-rotatory or postrotatory nystagmus as measured at the vestibular ganglion is about 5 or 6 s. However, the nystagmus takes much longer to decay, with a time constant of approximately 12 s in humans. This augmentation of the cupula time constant is known as the velocity storage mechanism (VSM). It is also under adaptive control by the nodulus and uvula in the cerebellar vermis, and experimental lesions result in a prolonged VSM time constant.[65] Abnormally short time VSM constants can be caused by disease of the end organ, the vestibular nerve, or central disease.[65] Very short time constants have been reported in Chiari type I malformation, olivopontocerebellar degeneration, demyelinating disease, congenital and acquired blindness, and bilateral vestibulopathy secondary to ototoxic drugs. Abnormally long time VSM constant is rarely seen.

Absent VOR quick phases

Absent quick phases are seen in children with SIF. Most of these children will show a similar failure during OKN, but occasionally only vestibular nystagmus demonstrates the failure. This may indicate a very subtle form of saccade failure, and as an isolated phenomenon, it is probably of little clinical significance. Absent quick phases may also be seen in neonates up to 2 to 3 weeks, or in older infants with DVM.[18]

Absent VOR

The VOR appears clinically absent or very erratic in children with infantile nystagmus, whether elicited by calorics, constant rotation, or sinusoidal oscillation.[66] The VOR may be absent in children with the CHARGE association and in children with Usher syndrome type 1.

Disorders of the optokinetic system

Absence of OKN

No OKN can be elicited in a completely blind child, as it is a visually induced reflex. However, the absence of OKN alone must not be used as an indicator of visual acuity as the sighted infant who may appear visually unresponsive may have absence of OKN for another reason. The response to a full-field OKN stimulus is difficult to suppress, so the very presence of OKN demonstrates some vision. Infantile nystagmus is often associated with a clinical failure or "reversal" of OKN.[66] During testing, the nystagmus may persist unabated, persist but with a changing waveform or direction, or become completely quiescent. This is due to an OKN-induced shift in the null position in the direction opposite the smooth-pursuit stimulus. Bilateral lesions of the optokinetic pathway in the cortex, cerebellum, or brainstem may completely obliterate all OKN and smooth pursuit. Infants with cortical dysplasia may have absent OKN, they may be cortically blind, or they can have a normal VEP and no OKN. If the optokinetic response is assessed with a hand-held device in the clinic, quick-phase failure in children with SIF can be mistaken for absent OKN if the eyes are not driven to the limit of gaze. If there is any doubt, the child should have full-field OKN assessment, which will readily demonstrate the typical "locking up" of SIF.

Binocular asymmetry of OKN

Any unilateral lesion in the optokinetic pathway, as it passes through the brainstem, cerebellum, or parietal lobe, can result in asymmetric abnormalities of binocular OKN and smooth pursuit. With brainstem and cerebellar lesions, there may be accompanying localizing neurologic signs, whereas isolated binocular OKN asymmetry is suggestive of a parietal lesion and has been reported in children as young as 4 to 5 months.

Monocular asymmetry of OKN

With early disturbances of binocular vision caused by strabismus, anisometropia, or unilateral congenital cataract, the normal early monocular OKN asymmetry, persists in both eyes;[67] after 1 to 2 years, the monocular asymmetry persists.[67] The persistence of monocular OKN asymmetry and poor binocular vision together with the fact that OKN becomes symmetric in normal infants around the time that binocular function is detectable has led to the hypothesis linking binocularity and OKN asymmetry but they may be separate processes.[19,67] Although OKN asymmetry appears to be a clinical sign of an insult to early binocular motor development it is not a constant feature of early-onset strabismus. Existing monocular OKN asymmetry may appear with both eyes viewing, if vision in one eye is very poor or is suppressed. OKN testing with both eyes open will appear to be binocular OKN asymmetry. Even when there is neurologic impairment in a child, the possibility of a manifest monocular OKN asymmetry must be considered.

Miscellaneous disorders

Induced convergence retraction (dorsal midbrain syndrome)

Lesions of the posterior commissure in the dorsal rostral midbrain may result from many disease processes and can affect a variety of supranuclear mechanisms, including those that control vertical gaze, eyelids, vergence, fixation, and pupils. Other terms such as pretectal syndrome, Koerber Salus-Elschnig syndrome, Sylvian aqueduct syndrome, posterior commissural syndrome, and collicular plate syndrome all refer to this condition.

It may be more common than expected, forming 2.3% of one neurologist's practice.[68] The pretectum is the critical structure in this disorder, and isolated interruption of the posterior commissure in humans produces the entire syndrome of upward gaze palsy, pupillary light–near dissociation, lid retraction, induced convergence retraction, skew deviation, and upbeat nystagmus.[69]

Among the many underlying causes of this condition are hydrocephalus, stroke, and pinealomas. Table 73.7 lists other reported etiologies and systemic associations.

The constellation of deficits is:
1. Vertical gaze palsy;
2. Light–near dissociation of the pupils;
3. Eyelid retraction (Collier's sign);
4. Disturbance of vergence;
5. Fixation instability; and
6. Skew deviation.

Limitation of upward saccades is the most reliable sign of the convergence retraction. Upward pursuit, Bell's phenomenon, and the fast phases of vestibular and optokinetic nystagmus may also be affected either at presentation or with progression of the underlying process. It is rare for up-gaze to be unaffected. Pathologic lid retraction and lid lag are also common (Collier's sign).

When the patient attempts upward saccades a striking phenomenon, convergence and globe retraction, frequently occurs. This is not true nystagmus, despite the common description of this clinical finding as convergence–retraction nystagmus, because there is no true slow phase. This is best elicited with down-moving OKN targets since each fast phase is replaced by a convergence–retraction movement. Cocontraction of the extraocular muscles has been documented during this convergence–retraction jerk.

Unlike the pathways from upward saccades, the pathways for downward saccades do not appear to pass through the posterior commissure (Fig. 73.2). Perhaps because of this, disturbances of down-gaze are not as predictable or uniform. Usually down-going

Table 73.7 Causes of Childhood dorsal Midbrain syndrome

Classification by cause	Specific etiologies
Tumor	Pineal germinoma, teratoma and glioma; pineoblastoma; others
Hydrocephalus	Aqueductal stenosis with secondary dilation of third ventricle and aqueduct, or with secondary suprapineal recess compressing posterior commissure, commonly caused by cysticercosis in endemic areas
Metabolic disease	Gaucher; Tay-Sach; Niemann-Pick; kernicterus; Wilson's disease; others
Midbrain/thalamic damage	Hemorrhage; infarction
Drugs	Barbiturates; carbamazepine; neuroleptics
Miscellaneous	Benign transient vertical eye disturbance in infancy; trauma; neurosurgery; hypoxia; encephalitis; tuberculoma; aneurysm; multiple sclerosis

saccades and pursuit are present, but they may be slow. Sometimes, especially in infants and children, there is a tonic downward deviation of the eyes that has been designated the "setting sun" sign, and downbeating nystagmus may also be observed. The setting sun sign may also be seen in children with hydrocephalus.

Convergence spasm may occur during horizontal saccades and produce a "pseudoabducens palsy" since the abducting eye moves more slowly than the adducting eye. This phenomenon can cause reading difficulties early in the course of dorsal midbrain syndrome since it provides an obstacle to refixation toward the beginning of a new line of text. Indeed, older children may present with numerous pairs of corrective spectacles that have been prescribed due to their "vague" complaints about reading and other near work. In other patients complaining of difficulties with near vision, convergence may be paralyzed. "Tectal" pupils are usually large and react more poorly to light than to near, and anisocoria is not uncommon.

All children with convergence retraction deserve thorough, prompt neurologic and neuroradiologic evaluation, since timely intervention may be decisive. The natural history of this disorder is dependent on the underlying etiology.

The underlying medical cause requires investigation and primary treatment. Once the condition is stable for a period of time, 3 to 12 months, extraocular muscle surgery has been performed with some success. In addition to treatment the coexistent diplopia from skew deviation or horizontal strabismus may be surgically corrected, the anomalous head posture from defective vertical gaze may also be treated by inferior rectus recession or vertical transposition of horizontal recti during simultaneous horizontal strabismus correction.

The medical prognosis is dependent upon the underlying etiology. In the above-mentioned review of 206 patients, only 20 patients died: 11 from tumors, 7 after strokes, and 1 with transtentorial herniation with tuberculous abscess. The good prognosis in this series may have been skewed by the preponderance of patients with cysticercal hydrocephalus.[68] The prognosis of strabismus surgery in alleviating anomalous head posture and diplopia can result in improvement of the deviation.

Transient vertical gaze disturbances in infancy

Vertical gaze abnormalities may be benign and transient in infants. Infants with episodic conjugate up-gaze that became less frequent over time have been described. During these episodes, normal horizontal and vertical vestibulo-ocular responses could be observed.[70]

Tonic down-gaze has been observed in 5 of 242 consecutively examined healthy newborn infants as well as in other infants. Again, the eyes can easily be driven above the primary position with the vestibulo-ocular reflex. Also, the eyes show normal upward movements during sleep. In contrast, infants with hydrocephalus who manifest the setting sun sign do not elevate the eyes during sleep or with an oculocephalic maneuver.

Premature infants with intraventricular hemorrhage may also develop tonic down-gaze, usually in association with a large-angle esotropia. These infants do not elevate the eyes with vestibular stimulation. Up-gaze often returns during the first two years of life, but the esotropia does not resolve when up-gaze returns.

Internuclear ophthalmoplegia

In the absence of peripheral lesions such as myasthenia gravis, failure of adduction combined with nystagmus of the contra-lateral abducting eye is termed internuclear ophthalmoplegia (INO) and localizes the lesion to the medial longitudinal fasciculus (MLF) unequivocally.[71]

The abducens nucleus consists of two populations of neurons that coordinate horizontal eye movements (Fig. 73.1). Fibers from one group form the sixth nerve itself and innervate the ipsilateral lateral rectus muscle; fibers from the second group join the contralateral MLF and project to the subnucleus of the third nerve, which supplies the contralateral medial rectus muscle. In this way, the neurons of the sixth nerve nucleus yoke the lateral rectus with the contralateral medial rectus.

Clearly, lesions of the abducens nucleus will cause ipsilateral conjugate gaze palsy. Lesions of the MLF between the midpons and oculomotor nucleus will, in turn, disconnect the ipsilateral medial rectus subnucleus from the contralateral sixth nerve nucleus and cause diminished adduction of the ipsilateral eye on attempted versions. The signs of INO may be accompanied by an ipsilateral hypertropia or skew deviation.

A subtle adduction deficit is best appreciated when repetitive saccades are attempted; the adducting eye will demonstrate a slow, gliding, hypometric movement in conjunction with overshoot of the abducting eye. Usually, the ipsilateral eye can be adducted with convergence, but convergence will also be impaired if the MLF lesion is rostral enough to involve the medial rectus subnucleus.

Like dorsal midbrain syndrome, INO is an anatomic rather than etiologic diagnosis. A host of structural, metabolic, immuno-logic, inflammatory, degenerative, and other processes can interfere with the function of the MLF and nearby structures. In young adults, multiple sclerosis is by far the most common cause of INO.[71] Multiple sclerosis also underlies most cases of bilateral INO. Although patients with bilateral INO generally remain orthotropic in primary position, they sometimes exhibit an exotropia in the wall-eyed bilateral internuclear ophthalmoplegia (WEBINO) syndrome. Additional causes of INO include Arnold-Chiari malformation, hydrocephalus, meningoencephalitis, brainstem or fourth ventricular tumors, head trauma, metabolic disorders, drug intoxications, paraneoplastic effect, carcinomatous meningitis, and others. Peripheral processes, particularly myasthenia gravis and Miller Fisher syndrome, may closely mimic INO and should be considered in any patient with INO-like eye movements.[72]

Variable diplopia and/or ptosis most often prompt an ophthalmologic evaluation. Patients with these symptoms are evaluated for signs and symptoms of generalized myasthenia such as facial weakness, dysphonia, arm or leg weakness, chewing weakness, and respiratory difficulties. In "ocular myasthenia," however, the findings are restricted to the levator and extraocular muscles. Since there is no stereotypical myasthenic eye movement, this diagnosis should be considered in any child with an unexplained, acquired ocular motility disturbance and clinically normal pupils–particularly when the deviation is variable– whether or not ptosis is present. Any pattern of abnormal motility is suspect including an apparent gaze palsy, internuclear ophthalmoplegia, isolated cranial nerve palsy, one and one-half syndrome, incomitant strabismus, accommodative and vergence insufficiency, and gaze-evoked nystagmus. Prolonged OKN may demonstrate slowing of the quick phases; large saccades may be hypometric; small saccades may be hypermetric; and characteristic "quiver movements, " which consist of an initial small saccadic movement followed by a rapid drift backward, may be seen.[71,72]

ACQUIRED AND NEUROLOGICAL NYSTAGMUS

Eye care practitioners may be among the first to evaluate infants and children with involuntary ocular movements, producing anxiety in the medical care provider as well as the family. The eye care professional choosing to specialize in infants and children may, in fact, see more patients with nystagmus than any other specialist. This is due to the frequent association of nystagmus with strabismus.[29] It may be that nystagmus gets "less press" (e.g., literature, teaching, research, education) because there is less we understand or can do about it than strabismus or other childhood eye diseases.

Historical perspective

Nystagmus comes from the Greek word "nystagmos," to nod, drowsiness and from "nystazein" to doze, probably akin to Lithuanian "snusti," also to doze. It is a rhythmic, involuntary oscillation of one or both eyes. Using the information obtained from a complete history, physical examination, and radiographic and oculographic evaluations over 40 types of nystagmus can be distinguished. Some forms of nystagmus are physiologic, whereas others are pathologic. Although the nystagmus is typically described by its more easily observable fast (jerk) phase, the salient clinical and pathologic feature is the presence of a slow phase in one or both directions. Thus, clinical descriptions of nystagmus are usually based on the direction of the fast phase and are termed horizontal, vertical, or rotary, or any combination of these. The nystagmus may be conjugate or dysconjugate. The nystagmus may be predominantly pendular or jerky, the former referring to equal velocity to-and-fro movement of the eyes, and the latter referring to the eyes moving faster in one direction and slower in the other. Involuntary ocular oscillations containing only fast phases are "saccadic oscillations and intrusions" and *not* nystagmus. It is well documented that these differences may be difficult, if not impossible, to differentiate clinically. Recent advances in eye movement recording technology have increased its application in infants and children who have clinical disturbances of the ocular motor system[66] (Figs. 73.6 and 73.10).

Incidence

In 1991 Stang retrospectively reviewed the records of Group Health Inc. (White Bear Lake, MN) and in their pediatric population of 70,000 found a prevalence of clinical "nystagmus" of 1 in 2,850.[73] Other estimates of its incidence range from 1 in 350 to 1 in 6,550.[74,75] It is difficult if not impossible to give accurate prevalence/incidence on all types of nystagmus combined, but it is known that up to 50% of the infantile strabismic population will have some associated nystagmus. This could increase the prevalence of nystagmus up to 0.5% of the population.

Etiology

All the theoretical neuronal mechanisms of nystagmus are constantly evolving and are beyond the scope of this chapter. Particularly controversial is the role of cortical motion processing in the development of some forms of infantile nystagmus. However, major supranuclear inputs to the oculomotor system are reasonably well accepted for their role in stabilization of eye movements. These include the pursuit system, vestibular system and the neural integrator.

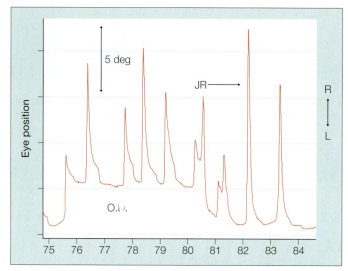

Fig. 73.17 Ocular motility recording of acquired jerk nystagmus. This is a typical 9 s position trace of ocular motor recordings from a patient with acquired jerk nystagmus. The jerk right nystagmus has decreasing velocity slow phases. O.D. = right eye, R = rightward eye movements and right gaze, L = leftward eye movements and left gaze, Deg = degree.

As mentioned above, the pursuit system, previously thought to have only a dynamic function, provides a major input for fixation stability (e.g., pursuit at "0 velocity" is stable fixation). The vestibular system maintains a constant resting firing rate that tends to drive the eyes contralaterally. This tendency is counterbalanced by the vestibular system on the opposite side unless the balance is changed by head rotation. The counter-balance is lost with unilateral vestibular damage, and the eyes tend to drift toward the affected side. A corrective saccade is then made toward the unaffected side. The slow phase of the nystagmus toward the affected side is of constant velocity as recorded by ocular motility recordings. This is a distinguishing feature of vestibular nystagmus. Most forms of acquired nystagmus are due to disease of the vestibular system (centrally or peripherally). Ocular motility recordings show various combinations of; uniplanar or multiplanar, simple pendular, linear, or decelerating velocity slow phases[76] (Fig. 73.17).

Neurological and acquired nystagmus types

Spasmus nutans (SN)

Spasmus nutans is an ocular oscillation beginning in infancy and consisting of the association of high-frequency, small-amplitude, dysconjugate oscillations, a head nodding oscillation, and a head tilt (Fig. 73.18). This usually becomes less noticeable as the infant becomes a toddler. Unlike other forms of infantile or acquired nystagmus, the head nodding may result in improvement of vision and decrease in the nystagmus. The reason for this is unclear. The characteristic feature of spasmus nutans is the very fine, rapid pendular nature of the nystagmus. The eyes appear to have a shimmering movement. It may be horizontal, vertical, or torsional. It is usually asymmetric to the point that it may appear unilateral. Pure unilateral forms are not uncommon. It may appear to switch eyes with changes in direction of gaze, and frequently appears worse in the abducting eye. Tremendous asymmetry is associated with amblyopia of the more involved eye.[29,77,78]

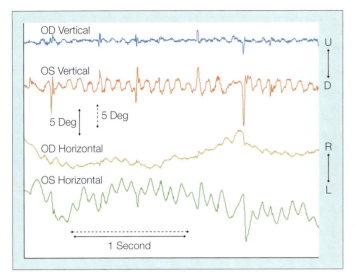

Fig. 73.18 Ocular motility recordings of spasmus nutans. OU open high-frequency (12-14 Hz), asymmetric, dysconjugate, multiplanar, (torsional) pendular nystagmus typical of spasmus nutans. Continuous periods of time are depicted in each tracing. Rightward eye movements are up and leftward eye movements are down. OD = right eye, OS = left eye.

Spasmus nutans may be a completely benign condition with onset in infancy and resolution within 2 years. However, tumors of the diencephalon can cause a condition indistinguishable from spasmus nutans. Consequently, neuroimaging or careful monitoring for visual, neurological, or endocrinological decline is essential. An intracranial tumor should be strongly suspected in any child who develops spasmus nutans after 3 years of age.

Drugs/toxins

Many drugs (some in therapeutic dosages) or toxins can cause nystagmus. The most common of these include anticonvulsants (i.e., phenobarbital, phenytoin, and carbamazepine), sedatives, hypnotics, and alcohol. Aspirin and quinine drugs causing nystagmus include chloroquine, quinidine, and quinine. Loop diuretics causing nystagmus include bumetanide, ethacrynic acid, furosemide, and torsemide. Aminoglycoside antibiotics causing nystagmus include amikacin, dihydrostreptomycin, gentamicin, neomycin, netilmicin, ribostamycin, streptomycin, and tobramycin. Antineoplastic drugs causing nystagmus include carboplatin and cisplatin. Environmental chemicals/toxins causing nystagmus include butyl nitrite, carbon disulfide, carbon monoxide, hexane, lead, manganese, mercury, styrene, tin, toluene, trichloroethylene, and xylene.[79,80]

Intracranial disease

Developmental, traumatic, and inflammatory brain diseases commonly cause acquired nystagmus. Consequently, nystagmus associated with other systemic historical and physical findings nearly always requires further neurological and radiological evaluation. (See "'Localizing' forms of nystagmus" below for further discussion.)

Voluntary flutter

Voluntary flutter ("nystagmus") (present in 7 to 15% of the population) is a misnomer referring to a series of volitional, rapid alternating saccades with little to no intersaccadic interval[25] (Figs. 73.10 and 73.13). They are usually horizontal, but may be vertical or torsional, and can only be sustained for a few seconds. Voluntary

nystagmus is a popular "party trick," and is often seen in patients with functional visual complaints. It is frequently associated with convergence of the eyes or facial grimacing. Voluntary nystagmus warrants no laboratory or radiographic investigation.

"Localizing" forms of nystagmus due to neurological disease (Table 73.8)

(A)periodic alternating nystagmus

(A)periodic alternating nystagmus may resemble infantile nystagmus or be "acquired." The key clinical component is that the null point shifts position in a cyclic pattern. This results in changes in the amplitude and direction of the nystagmus every few minutes. Adequate observation of the patient for several minutes should exclude this diagnosis. However, it should be considered any time a patient's head turn is different from one examination to the next. This is more common in patients with oculocutaneous albinism.[24,81,82]

Table 73.8 Neurological nystagmus types
Seesaw nystagmus Rostral midbrain lesions Parasellar lesions (e.g., pituitary tumors) Visual loss secondary to retinitis pigmentosa
Downbeat nystagmus Lesions of the vestibulocerebellum and underlying medulla (e.g., Arnold-Chiari malformation, microvascular disease with vertebrobasilar insufficiency, multiple sclerosis, Wernicke encephalopathy, encephalitis, lithium intoxication) Heat stroke Approximately 50% have no identifiable cause.
Upbeat nystagmus Medullary lesions, including perihypoglossal nuclei, the adjacent medial vestibular nucleus, and the nucleus intercalatus (structures important in gaze holding) Lesions of the anterior vermis of the cerebellum Benign paroxysmal positional vertigo
Periodic alternating nystagmus Arnold-Chiari malformation Demyelinating disease Spinocerebellar degeneration Lesions of the vestibular nuclei Head trauma Encephalitis Syphilis Posterior fossa tumors Binocular visual deprivation (e.g., ocular media opacities)
Pendular nystagmus Demyelinating disease Monocular or binocular visual deprivation Oculopalatal myoclonus Internuclear ophthalmoplegia Brainstem or cerebellar dysfunction
Spasmus nutans Usually occurs in otherwise healthy children May be caused by chiasmal, suprachiasmal, or third ventricle gliomas
Torsional Lateral medullary syndrome (Wallenberg syndrome)
Abducting nystagmus of internuclear ophthalmoplegia Demyelinating disease Brain stem stroke
Gaze-evoked Drugs: anticonvulsants (e.g., phenobarbital, phenytoin, carbamazepine) at therapeutic dosages Alcohol

Periodic alternating nystagmus is usually congenital and benign. However, it may be associated with vestibulocerebellar lesions, neurodegenerative conditions such as Friedreich's ataxia, or even visual loss. Neuroimaging is warranted in all cases unless the nystagmus has been stable for a prolonged period of time. Periodic alternating nystagmus may respond to treatment with low doses of baclofen in acquired forms of periodic alternating nystagmus.[83]

Gaze-evoked nystagmus

Gaze-evoked nystagmus is a jerk nystagmus that occurs in the direction of eccentric gaze. In contradistinction to infantile nystagmus most forms of gaze-evoked nystagmus can be stabilized by visual fixation and are accentuated by darkness or image blur (Fig. 73.9). Gaze-evoked nystagmus is called *gaze-paretic nystagmus* if it occurs in the direction of limited eye movement, as may be associated with a cranial nerve palsy or myasthenia gravis. Gaze-paretic nystagmus may appear dissociated if the limitation of eye movement is asymmetric between the two eyes.

One form of gaze-evoked nystagmus that is completely benign is endpoint nystagmus. This occurs in extreme positions of lateral or upward gaze. It can be distinguished from pathologic forms of gaze-evoked nystagmus by its low amplitude, symmetry on right and left gaze, poor sustainability, and absence of associated neurologic abnormalities.

Disease in the posterior fossa or drugs, particularly anticonvulsants and sedatives, are the most common causes of pathologic gaze-evoked nystagmus.[84] Such etiologies can usually be elicited by a careful medical history and review of systems. Disease of the cerebellum or vestibular system usually results in asymmetry of gaze-evoked nystagmus between directions of gaze. For example, tumors of the cerebellopontine angle may result in high-amplitude, low-frequency nystagmus (caused by cerebellar damage) when looking to the side of the lesion, and low-amplitude, high-frequency nystagmus (caused by vestibular imbalance) when looking to the contralateral side, a condition known as *Brun's nystagmus*. Associated neurologic abnormalities such as ataxia, hearing loss, tremor, or hemiparesis should always be sought.

Vestibular nystagmus

Certain characteristics of vestibular nystagmus can localize the etiology to the peripheral or central neuronal pathways of the vestibular systems. Central vestibular nystagmus is frequently uniplanar in contrast to peripheral vestibular nystagmus, which is usually torsional or multiplanar (Fig. 73.19). Visual fixation easily inhibits peripheral vestibular nystagmus, but not central vestibular nystagmus. Vertigo and tinnitus are common in peripheral vestibular nystagmus, and uncommon in central vestibular nystagmus.

Acquired pendular nystagmus

Acquired pendular nystagmus may be due to tumors, infarction, inflammation, or degeneration of the brainstem or cerebellum. The nystagmus may be horizontal, vertical, or both. A single lesion in the brain will result in horizontal and vertical components that oscillate at the same frequency of 2 to 7 cycles per second. If the horizontal and vertical components are in phase, the nystagmus will appear oblique. If they are out of phase, it will appear circular or elliptical. Circular or elliptical nystagmus that is constantly changing character is due to horizontal and vertical components oscillating on different frequencies. This implies more than one lesion in the brain.

Certain forms of acquired nystagmus have features so distinct that neuro-anatomic localization of the lesion can be determined by clinical examination alone (Fig. 73.20).

Seesaw nystagmus

Seesaw nystagmus is a pendular, upward incyclotorsion of one eye with a simultaneous downward excyclotorsion of the other eye. The pendular-waveform seesaw nystagmus is commonly due to a midline mesodiencephalic, bilaterally compressing mass[85,86] (Fig. 73.20). Seesaw nystagmus can also be associated with

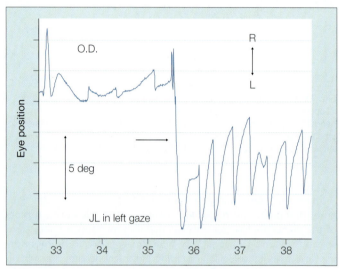

Fig. 73.19 Ocular motility recording of vestibular nystagmus. This is a typical 5 s position trace of ocular motor recordings from a patient with vestibular nystagmus. Primary position and right gaze shows less to no oscillation while in 15° of left gaze there is jerk left with linear and decreasing velocity slow phases. O.D. = right eye, R = rightward eye movements and right gaze, L = leftward eye movements and left gaze, Deg = degree, JL = jerk left nystagmus.

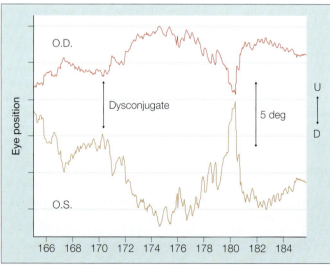

Fig. 73.20 Ocular motility recording of seesaw + pendular nystagmus. This is a 18 s vertical position trace of ocular motor recordings from a patient with seesaw and pendular nystagmus. On a background of a continuous, 2–4 Hz, pendular, small-amplitude, conjugate, ocular oscillation there is a slower, vertically, out-of-phase dysconjugate oscillation representing the seesaw component. O.D. = right eye, O.S. = left eye, U = upward eye movements and up gaze, D = downward eye movements and down gaze, Deg = degree, JL = jerk left nystagmus.

raumatic or congenital chiasmal abnormalities,[85,86] and is mostly due to a unilateral lesion in the mesodiencephalic junction. A current theory assumes a unilateral lesion of the interstitial nucleus of Cajal sparing the rostral interstitial nucleus of the medial longitudinal fascicle. Another concept suggests a lesion of the vertical vestibulo-ocular-reflex. Lesions of the diencephalon usually cause it. Congenital seesaw nystagmus is a rare form of neonatal nystagmus with upward excyclotorsion of one eye and concomitant downward incyclotorsion of the other eye.

Downbeat nystagmus

Downbeat nystagmus is usually produced by lesions in the cerebellum that also damage pathways that control horizontal tracking and visual–vestibulo-ocular interactions.[83,87,88] The most frequent causes are infarction, cerebellar and spinocerebellar degeneration syndromes, and MS and developmental anomalies affecting the pons and cerebellum.[83,87,88] It is also commonly due to drugs (particularly lithium or sedatives) or lesions at the cervicomedullary junction.[83,87,88] In children, it is usually due to Arnold-Chiari malformation or syringomyelia. Without a drug history, downbeat nystagmus should be evaluated in all patients with a sagittal MRI scan of the brainstem and cervical spinal cord. All patients have jerk-down nystagmus in some position of gaze and a few patients have jerk-down nystagmus only with convergence, in the dark, or with positioning of the head and body. Horizontal gaze increases the nystagmus. The nystagmus slow components usually have constant-velocity or increasing-velocity waveforms. Associated patterns of abnormal horizontal eye movements are characteristic of damage to the midline structures of the cerebellum (impaired pursuit, impaired OKN, and inability to suppress VOR).

Upbeat nystagmus

Upbeat nystagmus with its fast upward movement usually increases on extreme up gaze and generally follows Alexander's law.[89] The oscillations may be enhanced by a head tilt, and with convergence the nystagmus can increase or change to downbeat nystagmus. Upbeat nystagmus is probably caused by midbrain dysfunction or cerebellar disease. It is very similar to downbeat nystagmus but is generally less common. Drug-induced upbeat nystagmus could be an exaggerated form of end-point nystagmus. However, the condition is not commonly caused by drugs.[90]

Treatment and prognosis

There are a number of signs and symptoms due to nystagmus that are amenable to treatment. The first and most obvious is *decreased vision* ("central visual acuity," "gaze-angle" acuity, near acuity). Correction of significant refractive errors in children with nystagmus is the single most powerful therapeutic intervention for improving vision and visual function in these patients. Refractive etiologies of decreased "vision" include either one or a combination of conditions, e.g., myopia, hyperopia, astigmatism, and anisometropia. These refractive conditions can contribute significantly to already impaired vision in patients with other "organic" etiologies of decreased vision, e.g., amblyopia, optic nerve and/or retinal disease, oscillopsia, and the oscillation itself. The second is *anomalous head posturing (AHP)*. The etiology of the AHP includes a "gaze-null" due to INS or acquired nystagmus (e.g., chin-down in downbeat nystagmus), an "*adduction* null" due to infantile nystagmus or latent/manifest latent nystagmus (manifest strabismus with the preferred eye fixing in *adduction*), convergence damping ("nystagmus blockage"), and a periodically changing head posture due to (a)periodic alternating nystagmus. The third is *oscillopsia*, which is usually due to either acquired nystagmus or a change in the sensory/motor status of the patient with infantile nystagmus (e.g., "decompensated" strabismus, a change in the gaze null angle, or decreasing acuity).[91] Other less common associated signs and symptoms include hypoaccommodation and photophobia (i.e., congenital cone dystrophy and albinism).

The prognosis of all these ocular oscillations depends on the type of underlying ocular and systemic disease. In general, infantile forms improve with time unless they are associated with a degenerative ocular or systemic disease. Acquired forms are more visually disturbing and follow the course of the underlying neurologic disease.

REFERENCES

1. Cannon SC, Robinson DA, Shamma S. A proposed neural network for the integrator of the oculomotor system. Biol Cybern 1983; 49: 127–36.
2. Robinson DA. The effect of cerebellectomy on the cat's bestibulo-ocular integrator. Brain Res 1974; 71: 195–207.
3. Büttner-Ennever JA, Horn AK, Graf W, et al. Modern concepts of brainstem anatomy: from extraocular motoneurons to proprioceptive pathways. Ann NY Acad Sci 2002; 956: 75–84.
4. Arnold DB, Robinson DA. A learning network model of the neural integrator of the oculomotor system. Biol Cybern 1991; 64: 447–54.
5. Henn V, Büttner-Ennever JA, Hepp K. The primate oculomotor system. I. Motoneurons. A synthesis of anatomical, physiological, and clinical data. Hum Neurobiol 1982; 1: 77–85.
6. Quaia C, Lefevre P, Optican LM. Model of the control of saccades by superior colliculus and cerebellum. J Neurophysiol 1999; 82: 999–1018.
7. Pierrot-Deseilligny C, Rivaud S, Gaynard B, et al. Cortical control of saccades. Ann Neurol 1995; 37: 557–67.
8. Cassidy L, Taylor D, Harris C. Abnormal supranuclear eye movements in the child: a practical guide to examination and interpretation. Surv Ophthalmol 2000; 44: 479–506.
9. Harris CM, Walker J, Shawkat F. Eye movements in a familial vestibulocerebellar disorder. Neuropediatrics 1993; 24: 117–22.
10. Harris PL, Cassel TZ, Bamborough P. Tracking by young infants. Br J Psychol 1974; 65: 345–9.
11. Hainline L, Turkel J, Abramov I. Characteristics of saccades in human infants. Vision Res 1984; 24: 1771–80.
12. Baloh RW, Yee RD, Honrubia V, et al. A comparison of the dynamics of horizontal and vertical smooth pursuit in normal human subjects. Aviat Space Environ Med 1988; 59: 121–4.
13. Nixon RB, Helveston EM, Miller K, et al. Incidence of strabismus in neonates. Am J Ophthalmol 1985; 100: 798–801.
14. Aslin RN, Dumais ST. Binocular vision in infants: a review and a theoretical framework. Adv Child Dev Behav 1980; 15: 53–94.
15. Jacobs M, Harris CM, Shawkat F, et al. Smooth pursuit development in infants. Aust NZ J Ophthalmol 1997; 25: 199–206.
16. Cohen B, Reisine H, Yokota JI, et al. The nucleus of the optic tract. Its function in gaze stabilization and control of visual-vestibular interaction. Ann NY Acad Sci 1992; 656: 277–96.
17. Finocchio DV, Preston KL, Fuchs AF. Infant eye movements: quantification of the vestibulo-ocular reflex and visual-vestibular interactions. Vision Res 1991; 31: 1717–30.
18. Hoyt CS, Jastrzebski G, Marg E. Delayed visual maturation in infancy. Br J Ophthalmol 1983; 67: 127–30.
19. Büttner-Ennever JA, Horn AK. Anatomical substrates of oculomotor control. Curr Opin Neurobiol 1997;7:872–9.
20. Fox R, Aslin RN, Shea SL, et al. Stereopsis in human infants. Science 1980; 207: 323–4.
21. Harris LR, Smith ST. Interactions between first- and second-order motion revealed by optokinetic nystagmus. Exp Brain Res 2000; 130: 67–72.

22. Büttner-Ennever JA, Cohen B, Horn AK. Pretectal projections to the oculomotor complex of the monkey and their role in eye movements. J Comp Neurol 1996; 366: 348–59.

23. Harris LR, Smith ST. Motion defined exclusively by second-order characteristics does not evoke optokinetic nystagmus. Vis Neurosci 1992; 9: 565–70.

24. Shallo-Hoffmann J, Riordan-Eva P. Recognizing periodic alternating nystagmus. Strabismus 2001; 9: 203–15.

25. Yee RD, Spiegel PH, Yamada T. Voluntary saccadic oscillations, resembling ocular flutter and opsoclonus. J Neuroophthalmol 1994; 14: 95–101.

26. Bronstein AM, Morris J, Du Boulay G, et al. Abnormalities of horizontal gaze. Clinical, oculographic and magnetic resonance imaging findings. I. Abducens palsy. J Neurol Neurosurg Psychiatry 1990; 53: 194–9.

27. Dell'Osso LF, Daroff P. Congenital nystagmus waveforms and foveation strategy. Doc Ophthalmol 1975; 39: 155–82.

28. Hertle RW, Dell'Osso LF. Clinical and ocular motor analysis of congenital nystagmus in infancy. J AAPOS 1999; 3: 70–9.

29. Hertle RW, Zhu X. Oculographic and clinical characterization of thirty-seven children with anomalous head postures, nystagmus, and strabismus: the basis of a clinical algorithm. J AAPOS 2000; 4: 25–32.

30. Shawkat FS, Harris CM, Taylor DS, et al. The optokinetic response differences between congenital profound and nonprofound unilateral visual deprivation. Ophthalmology 1995; 102: 1615–22.

31. Zee DS, Leigh RJ, Mathieu-Millaire F. Cerebellar control of ocular gaze stability. Ann Neurol 1980; 7: 37–40.

32. Büttner U, Büttner-Ennever JA. Present concepts of oculomotor organization. Rev Oculomot Res 1988; 2: 3–32.

33. Optican LM, Robinson DA. Cerebellar-dependent adaptive control of primate saccadic system. J Neurophysiol 1980; 44: 1058–76.

34. Zee DS, Yee RD, Cogan DG, et al. Ocular motor abnormalities in hereditary cerebellar ataxia. Brain 1976; 99: 207–34.

35. Cannon SC, Leigh RJ, Zee DS. The effect of the rotational magnification of corrective spectacles on the quantitative evaluation of the VOR. Acta Otolaryngol 1985; 100: 81–8.

36. Rivaud-Pechoux S, Durr A, Gaymard B, et al. Eye movement abnormalities correlate with genotype in autosomal dominant cerebellar ataxia type I. Ann Neurol 1998; 43: 297–302.

37. Bronstein AM, Rudge P, Gresty MA, et al. Abnormalities of horizontal gaze. Clinical, oculographic and magnetic resonance imaging findings. II. Gaze palsy and internuclear ophthalmoplegia. J Neurol Neurosurg Psychiatry 1990; 53: 200–7.

38. Shawkat FS, Harris CM, Wilson J, et al. Eye movements in children with opsoclonus-polymyoclonus. Neuropediatrics 1993; 24: 218–23.

39. Baloh RW, Furman J, Yee RD. Eye movements in patients with absent voluntary horizontal gaze. Ann Neurol 1985; 17: 283–6.

40. Collewijn H, Erkelens CJ, Steinman RM. Binocular co-ordination of human horizontal saccadic eye movements. J Physiol 1988; 404: 157–82.

41. Harris CM, Shawkat F, Russell-Eggitt IM, et al. Intermittent horizontal saccade failure ("ocular motor apraxia") in children. Br J Ophthalmol 1996; 80: 151–8.

42. Pierrot-Deseilligny C, Rosa A, Masmoud K. Saccade deficits after a unilateral lesion affecting the superior colliculus. J Neurol Neurosurg Psychiatry 1991; 54: 1106–9.

43. Cogan DG. Congenital ocular motor apraxia. Can J Ophthalmol 1966; 1: 253–60.

44. Orrison WW, Robertson RM, Jr. Congenital ocular motor apraxia. A possible disconnection syndrome. Arch Neurol 1979; 36: 29–31.

45. Zee DS, Yee RD, Singer HS. Congenital ocular motor apraxia. Brain 1977; 100: 581–99.

46. Gurer YK, Kukner S, Kunak B, et al. Congenital ocular motor apraxia in two siblings. Pediatr Neurol 1995; 13: 261–2.

47. Fielder AR, Gresty MA, Dodd KL, et al. Congenital ocular motor apraxia. Trans Ophthalmol Soc UK 1986; 105: 589–98.

48. Cooper R, Khakoo Y, Matthay KK. Opsoclonus-myoclonus-ataxia syndrome in neuroblastoma: histopathologic features-a report from the Children's Cancer Group. Med Pediatr Oncol 2001; 36: 623–9.

49. Blatt J. Opsoclonus-myoclonus and antineuronal antibodies in neuroblastoma. Pediatr Hematol Oncol 1996; 13: iii–v.

50 Moretti R, Torre P, Antonello RN, et al. Opsoclonus-myoclonus syndrome: gabapentin as a new therapeutic proposal. Eur J Neurol 2000; 7: 455–6.

51. Hammer MS, Larsen MB, Stack CV. Outcome of children with opsoclonus-myoclonus regardless of etiology. Pediatr Neurol 1995; 13: 21–4.

52. Everling S, Fischer B. The antisaccade: a review of basic research and clinical studies. Neuropsychologia 1998;36:885–99.

53. Narita AS, Shawkat FS, Lask B, et al. Eye movement abnormalities in a case of Tourette syndrome. Dev Med Child Neurol 1997; 39: 270–3.

54. McDowell JE, Clementz B. Behavioral and brain imaging studies of saccadic performance in schizophrenia. Biol Psychol 2001; 57:5–22.

55. Sandbach J, Currie B. Central ocular motor disorders. Curr Opin Ophthalmol 1994; 5: 45–51.

56. Dell'Osso LF, Troost BT, Daroff BT. Macro square wave jerks. Neurology 1975; 25: 975–9.

57. Pierrot-Deseilligny C. Saccade and smooth-pursuit impairment after cerebral hemispheric lesions. Eur Neurol 1994; 34: 121–34.

58. Vahedi K, Rivaud S, Amarenco P, et al. Horizontal eye movement disorders after posterior vermis infarctions. J Neurol Neurosurg Psychiatry 1995; 58: 91–4.

59. Rivaud S, Muri RM, Gaymard B, et al. Eye movement disorders after frontal eye field lesions in humans. Exp Brain Res 1994; 102: 110–20.

60. Huo R, Burden SK, Hoyt CS, et al. Chronic cortical visual impairment in children: aetiology, prognosis, and associated neurological deficits. Br J Ophthalmol 1999; 83: 670–5.

61. Good WV, Jan JE, Hoyt CS, et al. Monocular vision loss can cause bilateral nystagmus in young children. Dev Med Child Neurol 1997; 39: 421–4.

62. Meienberg O, Ryffel E. Supranuclear eye movement disorders in Fisher's syndrome of ophthalmoplegia, ataxia, and areflexia. Report of a case and literature review. Arch Neurol 1983; 40: 402–5.

63. van Leeuwen AF, Westen MJ, van der Steen J, et al. Gaze-shift dynamics in subjects with and without symptoms of convergence insufficiency: influence of monocular preference and the effect of training. Vision Res 1999; 39: 3095–107.

64. Yakushin SB, Reisine H, Büttner-Ennever J, et al. Functions of the nucleus of the optic tract (NOT). I. Adaptation of the gain of the horizontal vestibulo–ocular reflex. Exp Brain Res 2000; 131: 416–32.

65. Cohen H, Cohen B, Raphan T, et al. Habituation and adaptation of the vestibuloocular reflex: a model of differential control by the vestibulocerebellum. Exp Brain Res 1992; 90: 526–38.

66. Abadi RV, Bjerre A. Motor and sensory characteristics of infantile nystagmus. Br J Ophthalmol 2002; 86: 1152–60.

67. Aiello A, Wright KW, Borchert M. Independence of optokinetic nystagmus asymmetry and binocularity in infantile esotropia. Arch Ophthalmol 1994; 112: 580–3.

68. Baloh RW, Furman JM, Yee RD. Dorsal midbrain syndrome: clinical and oculographic findings. Neurology 1985; 35: 54–60.

69. Pierrot-Deseilligny CH, Chain F, Gray F, et al. Parinaud's syndrome: electro-oculographic and anatomical analyses of six vascular cases with deductions about vertical gaze organization in the premotor structures. Brain 1982; 105: 667–96.

70. Bhidayasiri R, Plant GT, Leigh RJ. A hypothetical scheme for the brainstem control of vertical gaze. Neurology 2000; 54: 985–93.

71. Crane TB, Yee RD, Baloh RW, et al. Analysis of characteristic eye movement abnormalities in internuclear ophthalmoplegia. Arch Ophthalmol 1983; 101: 206–10.

72. Zasorin NL, Yee RD, Baloh RW. Eye-movement abnormalities in ophthalmoplegia, ataxia, and areflexia (Fisher's syndrome). Arch Ophthalmol 1985; 103: 55–8.

73. Stang HJ. Developmental disabilities associated with congenital nystagmus. J Dev Behav Pediatr 1991; 12: 322–3.

74. DeCarlo DK, Nowakowski R. Causes of visual impairment among students at the Alabama School for the Blind. J Am Optom Assoc 1999; 70: 647–52.

75. Blohme J, Tornqvist K. Visually impaired Swedish children. The 1980 cohort study–a 19-year ophthalmological follow-up. Acta Ophthalmol Scand 2000; 78: 553–9.

76. Stahl JS, Averbuch-Heller L, Leigh RJ. Acquired nystagmus. Arch Ophthalmol 2000; 118: 544–9.

77. Gresty M, Leech J, Sanders M, et al. A study of head and eye movement in spasmus nutans. Br J Ophthalmol 1976 ;60: 652–4.

78. Farmer J, Hoyt CS. Monocular nystagmus in infancy and early childhood. Am J Ophthalmol 1984; 98: 504–9.

79. Leigh RJ, Ramat S. Neuropharmacologic aspects of the ocular motor

system and the treatment of abnormal eye movements. Curr Opin Neurol 1999; 12: 21–7.

80. Jaanus SD. Ocular side effects of selected systemic drugs. Optom Clin 1992; 2: 73–96.

81. Abadi RV, Pascal E. Periodic alternating nystagmus in humans with albinism. Invest Ophthalmol Vis Sci 1994; 35: 4080–6.

82. Leigh RJ, Robinson DA, Zee DS. A hypothetical explanation for periodic alternating nystagmus: instability in the optokinetic-vestibular system. Ann NY Acad Sci 1981; 374: 619–35.

83. Leigh RJ, Das VE, Seidman SH. A neurobiological approach to acquired nystagmus. Ann NY Acad Sci 2002; 956: 380–90.

84. Cogan DG, Chu FC, Reingold DB. Ocular signs of cerebellar disease. Arch Ophthalmol 1982; 100: 755–60.

85. Apkarian P, Bour LJ, Barth PG, et al. Non-decussating retinal-fugal fibre syndrome. An inborn achiasmatic malformation associated with visuotopic misrouting, visual evoked potential ipsilateral asymmetry and nystagmus. Brain 1995; 118: 1195–216.

86. Dell'Osso LF, Williams RW, Jacobs JB, et al. The congenital and see-saw nystagmus in the prototypical achiasma of canines: comparison to the human achiasmatic prototype. Vision Res 1998; 38: 1629–41.

87. Yee RD. Downbeat nystagmus: characteristics and localization of lesions. Trans Am Ophthalmol Soc 1989; 87: 984–1032.

88. Baloh RW, Spooner JW. Downbeat nystagmus: a type of central vestibular nystagmus. Neurology 1981; 31: 304–10.

89. Daroff RB, Troost BT. Upbeat nystagmus. JAMA 1973;225:312.

90. Baloh RW, Yee RD. Spontaneous vertical nystagmus. Rev Neurol (Paris) 1989; 145: 527–32.

91. Hertle RW, Fitzgibbon EJ, Avallone JM, et al. Onset of oscillopsia after visual maturation in patients with congenital nystagmus. Ophthalmology 2001; 108: 2301–7; discussion 2307–8.

92. Leigh R, Zee D. The Neurology of Eye Movements. 3rd ed. New York: Oxford University Press; 1999: 24–9.

CHAPTER 74

Infantile Nystagmus Syndrome (Congenital Nystagmus)

Siobhan Garbutt and R John Leigh

INTRODUCTION AND DEFINITIONS

Nystagmus may be defined as repetitive, to-and-fro, involuntary eye movements initiated by slow drifts of the eyes away from the desired direction of gaze.[1] Most forms of nystagmus consist of an alternation of a slow drift and a corrective quick phase (jerk nystagmus). Thus, each slow phase moves the eyes away from the preferred direction of gaze and a corrective quick phase (a saccade) brings the eyes back towards the visual target. Less commonly, the slow drifts are pendular (to-and-fro), sometimes like a sine-wave oscillation (pendular nystagmus). The main, basic nystagmus waveforms are schematized in Fig. 74.1. Although nystagmus is often described by the direction of its quick phases (e.g., right-beating or "jerk-right"), it is the slow phase that reflects the underlying disorder. Nystagmus should be differentiated from saccadic intrusions and oscillations, in which rapid movements (saccades) take the eye away from the target.

In health, three mechanisms contribute to gaze stability and clear vision:

1. The visual fixation mechanism;
2. The vestibulo-ocular reflex, which compensates for head perturbations, especially during locomotion; and
3. The eccentric gaze-holding mechanism, or neural integrator, which generates tonic contraction of the extraocular muscles to oppose the elastic pull of the orbital tissues.

Disturbance of any of these three mechanisms can lead to drifts of the eyes away from the target, and consequent nystagmus. Although acquired forms of nystagmus can often be attributed to dysfunction of one of these gaze-holding mechanisms, the pathophysiology of infantile nystagmus poses much greater problems. It is important to recognize that nystagmus may be physiological, especially during self-rotation, when vestibular and optokinetic nystagmus act to sustain clear vision of the environment.

There is no widely accepted classification of nystagmus in infancy. For example, it has been suggested that nystagmus with an onset before 6 months be divided into three categories:

A. Congenital idiopathic nystagmus (CIN), in which no visual or neurological impairment can be found;
B. Sensory defect nystagmus (SDN), in which there is a visual sensory abnormality (Table 74.1); and
C. Neurological nystagmus (NN), which is associated with a neurological disorder.[2]

More recently, the Classification of Eye Movement Abnormalities and Strabismus (CEMAS) Working Group (http://www.nei.nih.gov/news/statements/cemas.pdf) has proposed that the term *infantile nystagmus syndrome* (INS) be used to encompass what has previously been called congenital nystagmus, including "motor" or "sensory" varieties. The main criteria for defining INS are infantile onset and accelerating slow-phase waveforms (see Fig. 74.2). A potential problem posed by

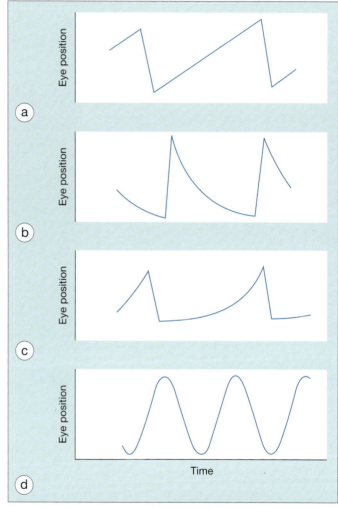

Fig. 74.1 Four common slow-phase waveforms of nystagmus. (a) Constant-velocity drift of the eyes. The added quick phases give a "saw-tooth" appearance. (b) Drift of the eyes back from an eccentric orbital position toward the midline with a decreasing-velocity waveform. (c) Drift of the eyes away from the primary position with a positive exponential time course (increasing velocity), typical of INS. (d) Pendular nystagmus, which approximates a sine wave. Adapted from Leigh and Zee.[1]

the CEMAS classification for some ophthalmologists is that measurement of eye movements, which is necessary to characterize the waveforms,[3,4] may not be available. Nonetheless, reliable measurements of eye movements in children with nystagmus are usually helpful, often diagnostic, and, hopefully, should become the clinical standard. How much visual defects and motor factors contribute to infantile forms of nystagmus has yet to be

Table 74.1 Visual system disorders commonly associated with INS

Ocular and oculocutaneous albinism
Cataracts
Corneal opacities
Optic nerve hypoplasia
Congenital retinal dystrophies
 Leber's congenital amaurosis
 Peroxisomal disorders
 Joubert syndrome
 Cone dystrophy
 Congenital stationary night-blindness
Severe colobomata
Aniridia
Retinopathy of prematurity

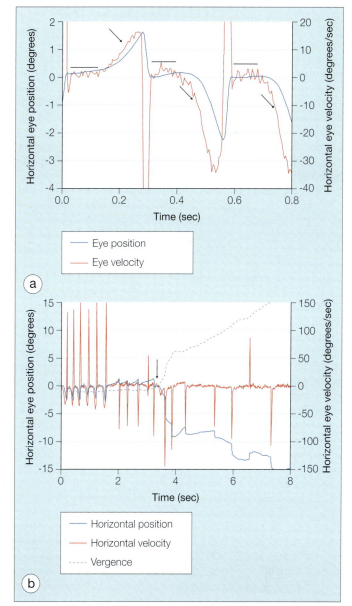

Fig. 74.2 Example of INS. Right eye record. Rightward movements are indicated by upward deflections. (a) One rightward followed by two leftward slow phases all show increasing-velocity waveforms (arrows). Foveation periods, when the eye is pointed at the target (about zero eye position) and eye velocity is less than 5° per second, are demarcated by horizontal bars. (b) Effects of convergence on nystagmus. After the vertical arrow, the subject started to slowly converge (upward deflections) as she viewed an approaching target aligned on her midline; nystagmus was almost completely suppressed.

elucidated. Thus, until the pathogenesis of infantile nystagmus is better understood, it would seem best to use a diagnostic classification that incorporates the broad clinical and laboratory evidence, avoids diagnostic labels based on uncertain pathogenesis, and accepts that overlaps between certain syndromes sometimes occur. Thus, INS is the term that we will use.

Two other forms of nystagmus in children, which have characteristics that differ from INS, include latent nystagmus, which CEMAS has called *fusional maldevelopment nystagmus syndrome* (FMNS), and the *spasmus nutans syndrome* (SNS). These are mentioned briefly in this chapter from the viewpoint of differential diagnosis; and are discussed further in Chapters 73 and 75.

We will first review clinical techniques useful in evaluating the child with nystagmus, and then describe clinical features that are typical. With this background, we discuss the characteristic waveforms of INS, and summarize current ideas on pathogenesis, based on current knowledge of the neurobiology of eye movements. We then discuss the differential diagnosis of nystagmus in infancy and finally summarize current methods for managing these ocular oscillations and their visual consequences.

HISTORY-TAKING AND EXAMINATION IN CHILDREN WITH INS

History

First ask the parents when they first noticed their child's abnormal eye movements, and how these have changed as the child has grown. Determine whether the child's vision has been affected, and document any history of amblyopia, strabismus, and refractive or surgical treatments. Enquire about associated head turns or tilts and head tremors, and look for head turns on early photographs; their presence suggests INS. It is also important to establish whether there is an associated neurological disorder, such as cerebral palsy, developmental delay, or hereditary metabolic disease. Ask whether there is any family history of nystagmus or visual defect, which aids diagnosis, especially if the pattern of inheritance can be established. The genetics of INS are summarized in the section "Genetic factors". Check the child's current medications for agents with effects on the brain (e.g., anticonvulsants).

If the child is old enough, ask whether the nystagmus interferes with vision, and whether associated visual symptoms are worse when viewing far or near objects, during specific directions of gaze (e.g., downgaze), or when the child is in motion (which implies a vestibular disorder). Also ask whether the child has

complained about dizziness or oscillopsia (illusory motion of the visual world). In general, oscillopsia is more common with acquired nystagmus, but up to a third of individuals with INS experience it at some time.[5]

Examination

Before starting an evaluation of nystagmus, note any abnormality of head posture, examine the visual system (acuity and, if the child is old enough, visual fields, color vision, and stereopsis), optic nerves, lids, and pupils, and look for signs of ocular albinism, such as ocular transillumination. Congenital forms of nystagmus are often associated with disorders of the visual system. A full cycloplegic refraction is required as many patients with INS have substantial with-the-rule astigmatism.[6] Vision testing with and without optical correction is an important prelude to management decisions.

Before examining for nystagmus, try to determine whether there is a full range of the movements of each eye, and note any strabismus. Then observe the stability of gaze as the child attempts to fix upon a stationary target at a viewing distance greater than 2 m. With the patient's eyes close to central position, determine whether there is any nystagmus. For each eye, note the directions in which the nystagmus occurs: horizontal, vertical, torsional (rotational around the line of sight), or mixed.

Compare the nystagmus in each eye, and note whether the direction or size of movement differs, or whether there is any asynchrony. If the size of the oscillations differs in each eye, it is referred to as dissociated nystagmus. If the direction of the oscillations in each eye differs, it is called disconjugate or disjunctive nystagmus. Cover each eye in turn to check for reversal of the direction (a "latent component"). Some nystagmus is intermittent and requires sustained observation over several minutes. Low-amplitude nystagmus may only be detected during ophthalmoscopy; note that the direction of horizontal or vertical nystagmus is inverted when viewed through the ophthalmoscope. Attempt to repeat each of these observations as the eyes are brought into right, left, up, and down gaze, and during sustained convergence. If possible, attempt to observe the child fixating a target in the central position for 4 to 5 min to test for periodic alternating nystagmus (see next section), which is important to recognize when surgery for an abnormal head posture is being considered. Arousal and attention may be maintained during this period with the aid of storytelling.[7]

A description of the direction of rotation of the nystagmus in each gaze angle will often indicate the coordinate system to which the nystagmus conforms. Thus, nystagmus that still appears horizontal on upward gaze indicates that the eye is rotating around an eye-fixed axis, characteristic of INS. On the other hand if nystagmus appears horizontal in the straight-ahead position of gaze but torsional on looking far up, the eye is rotating around a rostral-caudal axis relative to the head, characteristic of vestibular nystagmus.

Always examine the effect on nystagmus of removing fixation; nystagmus due to peripheral vestibular imbalance may only be apparent in these circumstances. The best way is to observe the nystagmus behind Frenzel goggles (high-positive lenses with small lights), which prevent fixation of objects and also provide the examiner with a magnified, illuminated view of the patient's eyes. If not available, another technique consists of transiently covering the fixating eye during ophthalmoscopy in an otherwise dark room, and noting the effects on retinal motion in the eye being viewed.

Evaluation of nystagmus is incomplete without a systematic examination of each functional class of eye movements– vestibular, saccades, smooth-pursuit, and vergence; selective defects may indicate the nature of the underlying disorder. It is also important to note the effects of each type of eye movement (such as convergence) on the nystagmus.

It is possible to induce nystagmus in normal subjects with optokinetic or vestibular stimuli. In natural circumstances, visual (optokinetic) and vestibular nystagmus acts to hold images steadily on the retina during self-rotation. In clinical practice, it is convenient to induce nystagmus with an optokinetic drum or tape, which presents a moving pattern of stripes. This stimulus

mainly tests smooth-pursuit tracking (slow phases) and automatic saccades (quick phases). Determine whether the direction of ongoing nystagmus changes so that the quick phases are in the same direction as the optokinetic stripe motion ("OKN reversal"). Nystagmus can also be induced with vestibular stimuli. A simple method is to rotate, by hand, the patient in an office chair for 45 s, and then stop the chair so that induced nystagmus can be viewed. In young children, the child may be held at arms length facing the examiner who turns several rotations clockwise and counterclockwise either standing or sitting in a revolvable chair.

CLINICAL FEATURES OF INS

INS may be present at birth but usually is noted by the age of six months.[5] The common clinical characteristics and eye-movement waveforms of INS begin in infancy, and are associated with abnormal vision (40%), anomalous head postures (37%), strabismus (26%), albinism (28%), and ocular abnormalities (10%). Between 7 and 30% have a positive family history of nystagmus, autosomal dominant being the most common pattern of inheritance.[5,8,9]

Although variable in form, certain clinical features commonly characterize INS (see Table 74.2). It is almost always conjugate and mainly horizontal, even on up or down gaze. A torsional component to the nystagmus may be common,[10] but is usually too small to identify clinically.

Less commonly, INS is mainly seesaw. Seesaw nystagmus is a form of pendular nystagmus in which one half-cycle consists of elevation and intorsion of one eye and synchronous depression and extorsion of the other eye, with the vertical and torsional movements reversing during the next half-cycle (Fig. 74.3). Recent evidence, reviewed under "Pathogenesis of INS," suggests that such patients may have underlying disease of the retina, visual pathways, or cerebellum.[1,11]

INS that is conjugately vertical is rare, and may represent neurological disorders such as familial episodic ataxia.[1]

INS is often accentuated by the attempt to fixate an object, and by attention or anxiety. These psychological factors are important, for example, during testing of vision for driving, when nystagmus is maximized. Convergence often suppresses INS, although occasional patients only develop their nystagmus when they view a near target. Eyelid closure, drowsiness, and a dark environment tend to damp INS.

Often, nystagmus decreases when the eyes are moved into a particular position in the orbit, the null zone, which corresponds to the range of eye positions within which slow-phase eye velocity is minimized. The direction, waveform, and intensity of nystagmus commonly change with different gaze angles. Thus, nystagmus may have a more pendular waveform close to central gaze, but jerk nystagmus on looking laterally.

Table 74.2 Summary of clinical features of INS

Present since infancy
Usually conjugate, horizontal; smaller torsional, or vertical components
Pendular or increasing-velocity waveforms punctuated by foveation periods, during which eyes are transiently still and aimed at the object of interest
Suppresses on convergence or with eyelid closure
Accentuated by visual attention or arousal
Often minimal when the eyes are near one particular orbital position (null zone)
Accompanied by head shaking or head turn

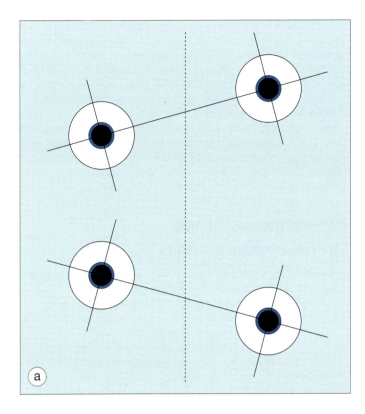

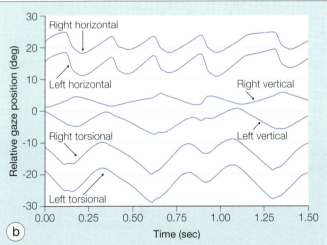

Fig. 74.3 Seesaw nystagmus. (a) Schematic of the oscillation showing that during one half-cycle the left eye rises and intorts, and the right falls and extorts (top); during the next half-cycle, the opposite movements occur (bottom). (b) Example of seesaw nystagmus. The horizontal component has a conjugate "pseudocycloid" waveform typical for INS. There is a disconjugate vertical component and a large conjugate torsional component. Note that as either eye goes up, it intorts, and as it goes down, it extorts. The single position traces are offset for convenience of display; upward deflections indicate rightward (horizontal), upward (vertical), or clockwise (torsional) eye rotations, with respect to the patient. Adapted from Leigh and Zee.[1]

and is sometimes referred to as "congenital nystagmus with a latent component."

Abnormal head postures occur commonly with INS,[5] and are generally used to bring the eye in the orbit close to the null point or zone, at which nystagmus is minimal (Chapters 89 and P24). Thus, a null zone 20° to the right can be best utilized by turning the head 20° to the left. The commonest head posture is a face turn to one side, but chin elevation or depression or a tilt of the head may also be seen. The presence of an abnormal head posture in photographs taken throughout childhood is often valuable evidence in diagnosing INS.

Some patients with INS (and latent nystagmus) purposely induce an esotropia (nystagmus blockage syndrome) in order to suppress the nystagmus (Chapter 80); such an esotropia requires a head turn to direct the viewing eye at the object of regard.

Patients with INS also may show head oscillations, but these can be voluntarily suppressed. Head movements are unlikely to represent an adaptive strategy to improve vision, since the vestibulo-ocular reflex compensates for each head movement. It seems more likely that the head tremor and ocular oscillations are both generated by a similar neural mechanism.[14]

QUANTITATIVE ASPECTS OF INS: WAVEFORMS

The most distinctive feature of INS is its waveforms and, in cases where there is doubt about the diagnosis, measurement of eye movements usually will settle the issue.[1,3,4] Accurate calibration is not essential for recognition of these waveforms, although the noise-free traces obtained by infrared methods are superior to electro-oculography. Babies and children (except around the age of 2 years) can often be coaxed into allowing a record of their eye movements that, although brief, will help make the diagnosis.

The commonest waveforms are jerk with increasing-velocity slow phases (see Fig. 74.1c) and pendular (Fig. 74.1d), both of

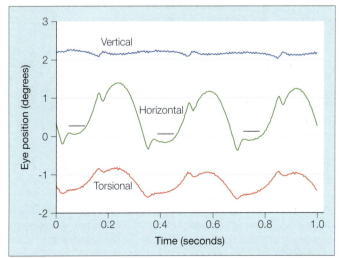

Fig. 74.4 Pendular INS. Pendular type of INS, with superimposed quick phases, showing the large horizontal (green) component, smaller torsional (red) component, and almost absent vertical (blue) component. Note that vertical and torsional channels have been offset to aid clarity of display. Foveation periods follow quick phases and are shown as periods when eye position change is minimal. Upward deflections indicate rightward (horizontal), upward (vertical), or clockwise (torsional) eye rotations, with respect to the patient.

In some patients, jerk nystagmus reverses direction over the course of seconds or minutes; however, this congenital form of periodic alternating nystagmus usually has irregular timing of reversals ("aperiodic alternating nystagmus");[7,12,13] it is common in albinos.[5] In some patients, the direction of the nystagmus is influenced by which eye is viewing, the nystagmus beating away from the covered eye. This is similar to what happens in FMNS, which may be present in some patients. Increasing-velocity slow phases are almost unique to INS but are not always present. Identification of accelerating slow phases does not distinguish between visual and motor factors being the cause, but it does rule out neurological nystagmus. (Acquired nystagmus with accelerating slow phases has been reported with cerebellar lesions, and in such cases the nystagmus is usually in the vertical plane.[1])

Another "signature" of INS is foveation periods (Figs. 74.2 and 74.4): during each cycle–usually after a quick phase–there is a brief period when the eye is still and is pointed at the object of regard. With jerk waveforms, the quick phases (saccades) may "brake" the oscillation, or bring the eye to the target. With pendular waveforms, the oscillation is "flattened" by a foveation period when the eye is closest to the target (Fig. 74.2). Foveation periods are one reason most patients with INS do not complain of oscillopsia, despite otherwise nearly continuous movement of their eyes, and why many patients have good visual acuity. It appears that the visual system can ignore the blur when there is rapid motion of images on the retina, and focus on relatively stable vision during the foveation periods. Whether this is achieved by the visual system's ability to suppress excessive motion of images, or by the brain's monitoring of an efferent copy of neural signals that cause the nystagmus, or both, is not settled. Estimates of the potential visual acuity of INS patients, based on foveation period characteristics, have been developed and applied to clinical treatment trials.[11,15] Patients with albinism (who often lack a well-developed fovea) behave in a similar way and use a specific retinal locus, corresponding to the area of retina that gives maximum vision, during the periods when eye velocity is least.[16] Foveation periods are not an invariable finding in INS waveforms, however. Patients who show absent or poorly developed foveation periods often have visual system disorders. We have only rarely recorded foveation periods in patients whose nystagmus was definitely due to acquired neurological disease.

Even in individuals with INS that have foveation periods, vision may not be perfectly normal. Thus, visual stereoacuity may be reduced,[17] and motion detection thresholds elevated, compared with controls.[18] The association of strabismus with INS depends on the presence or absence of an associated visual disorder, such as bilateral optic nerve hypoplasia, albinism, and congenital retinal dystrophies; it is lowest in children with idiopathic INS.[19]

Another factor that determines the waveform of INS is the child's age. In the first few months of life, it may be large amplitude, with a "triangular" waveform.[20] Later, the nystagmus may become pendular, and finally jerk as the patient reaches about a year of age. These waveforms are so characteristic of INS that reliable records of eye position and velocity will often secure the diagnosis.

PROPERTIES OF EYE MOVEMENTS IN PATIENTS WITH INS

A common finding in INS is so-called inversion of optokinetic nystagmus. Thus, with a hand-held optokinetic drum or tape, quick phases are directed in the same direction as the drum rotates, which is opposite to the normal optokinetic response. In fact, this phenomenon is more likely due to shifts in the position of the null zone of the nystagmus induced by optokinetic stimulation. Precise measurements have shown that smooth pursuit and optokinetic eye movements are preserved in at least some individuals.[21] Furthermore, the vestibular responses during natural head movements have generally been found to be normal in patients with INS as judged by retinal image stability during the foveation period.[22] However, in

those patients with associated visual disorders such as albinism, vestibular responses to lower frequencies of head rotations and optokinetic responses may be impaired. Also, it should be pointed out that the vertical optokinetic response is normal in patients with purely horizontal INS, and in the rare cases of vertical or torsional INS the horizontal optokinetic response is normal.[23]

Occasional patients exhibit their INS only during attempted smooth tracking,[24] and others can voluntarily release or inhibit their INS,[25] suggesting that the fixation mechanism plays some role in their oscillations. INS associated with congenital gaze-holding failure (i.e., leaky neural integrator for eye movements) has been reported in one kindred.[26]

PATHOGENESIS OF INS
The role of visual disorders

Disorders of the visual pathways are often associated with nystagmus (Table 74.3). For example, individuals with complete blindness invariably show nystagmus. At least two mechanisms contribute:

1. Inability to use visual information to generate eye movements to correct for drifts of the eyes (fixation); and
2. Loss of an error signal to drive adaptive properties of eye movements, and tune eye movements to address visual demands.

Thus, retinal disorders causing blindness, such as Leber's congenital amaurosis, cause continuous jerk nystagmus with components in all three planes, which changes in direction over the course of seconds or minutes (Fig. 74.5). Moreover, nystagmus has been reported in association with a variety of hereditary retinal disorders (Table 74.1). However, only some of these patients show the increasing-velocity waveforms (Fig. 74.1c) so characteristic of INS. The same criticism can be leveled at primate models of nystagmus induced by a range of occlusion paradigms;[27] these animals' ocular oscillations have more in common with latent nystagmus.

Optic nerve disease is commonly associated with pendular forms of nystagmus in children. Unilateral optic nerve tumors largely cause nystagmus in the abnormal eye ("monocular nystagmus"), which is low frequency, bidirectional, and prominently vertical[1] (Fig. 74.6).

Pituitary tumors and other parasellar lesions are associated with seesaw nystagmus. Congenital seesaw nystagmus has been reported in a mutant strain of dogs that lack an optic chiasm, and

Table 74.3 Nystagmus associated with disease of the visual pathways

1) Lesions of the eye or optic nerve
a) Bilateral visual loss causes continuous jerk nystagmus, with horizontal, vertical, and torsional components, and a drifting "null" position
b) Unilateral visual loss causes slow vertical oscillations and low-amplitude horizontal nystagmus mainly in the blind eye; in children, especially, pendular nystagmus of the blind eye

2) Lesions at the optic chiasm
Seesaw and other forms of nystagmus with bitemporal visual field loss

3) Lesions affecting posterior cortical areas
If there is any nystagmus at all, it will be a low-amplitude horizontal nystagmus beating toward the side of the lesion

4) Lesions affecting cortical-pontine-cerebellar or olivocerebellar projection
They may be responsible for some forms of acquired pendular nystagmus

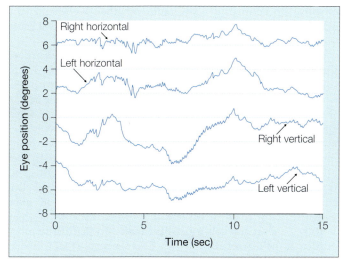

Fig. 74.5 Nystagmus in a patient bilaterally blind since birth due to Leber's congenital amaurosis. In the horizontal plane, there is a wandering null point and changes in direction of the quick phases. Slow-phase waveforms are variably linear, decreasing velocity, or increasing velocity. Upward deflections indicate rightward or upward gaze movements.

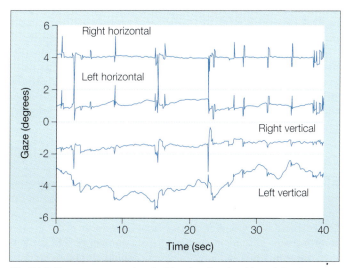

Fig. 74.6 Nystagmus associated with uniocular visual loss, following childhood trauma. During binocular viewing, steady gaze of the left eye is disrupted by slow disconjugate drifts that are more prominent vertically. Upward deflections indicate rightward or upward gaze movements.

in patients in whom imaging and visual-evoked studies suggested a similar developmental defect.[28] It seems possible that visual inputs–especially crossed inputs–are important for optimizing vertical-torsional eye movements. Under natural conditions, seesaw eye movements occur when subjects view a target located off the midsagittal plane during ear-to-shoulder head roll. Visual inputs are presumably necessary to keep this response calibrated and, if compromised, might lead to seesaw oscillations.[1]

Horizontal nystagmus occurs in patients with a unilateral disease of the cerebral hemispheres, especially when the lesion is large and posterior.[1] Such patients show a constant-velocity drift of the eyes toward the intact hemisphere (i.e., quick phases directed toward the side of the lesion). Such patients usually also show asymmetry of horizontal optokinetic nystagmus; the response is reduced when the stripes move toward the side of the lesion. As discussed elsewhere (Chapter 75), latent nystagmus has been

attributed to an abnormality of such cortical motion-vision processing.

In sum, disease affecting various parts of the visual pathways can lead to nystagmus in infants and children. However, in most cases, the clinical features and waveforms are different from "idiopathic INS," lacking increasing-velocity waveforms. Nonetheless, these other conditions are important, since early diagnosis–for example, of optic nerve glioma causing monocular nystagmus in infancy–allows prompt institution of management. Because of the many diagnostic possibilities, a complete ophthalmologic evaluation and an electroretinogram are necessary in children with nystagmus associated with decreased visual acuity or visual dysfunction. Neuroimaging is also sometimes indicated.

The pathogenesis of INS in individuals without associated visual defects is uncertain. It has been variously suggested that disturbances of the smooth-pursuit system, visual fixation, or the gaze-holding mechanism (neural integrator) are responsible, but no compelling case has been put forward to support these hypotheses.[1] Indeed, some properties of the waveforms of INS suggest that these oscillations do not emanate from any of the normal ocular motor systems.[29]

Genetic factors

INS, either with or without associated visual system abnormalities, may be familial. For example, one form of ocular albinism is X-linked.[30] Several modes of inheritance of INS have been reported. INS is most commonly autosomal dominant,[5] and a gene for this form of inheritance has been described on chromosome 6p12.[31] In addition, the genetic substrate for X-linked INS has been clarified.[32] Despite these advances in defining genotypes, the waveforms or other characteristics of the nystagmus may differ considerably between affected family members.

DIFFERENTIATING OTHER CHILDHOOD OCULAR OSCILLATIONS FROM INS

The ophthalmologist needs to keep in mind three main differential diagnoses apart from INS when evaluating the child with nystagmus: fusional maldevelopment nystagmus syndrome (FMNS or latent nystagmus), the spasmus nutans syndrome, and nystagmus due to neurologic disease. Each of these entities is discussed in more detail in other chapters, and here we summarize some of the features that aid diagnosis.

The essential feature of FMNS is that it is affected by monocular occlusion. Classic latent nystagmus appears when one eye is covered: quick phases of both eyes beat away from the covered eye. However, in most patients, nystagmus (which may be of low amplitude) is present when both eyes are uncovered ("manifest latent nystagmus"); in such areas, only one eye is fixating and vision from the other eye (which may be deviated, e.g., esotropic) is suppressed. Usually, the nystagmus reverses direction upon covering of either eye; in some patients, nystagmus is present when one particular eye is covered but is absent when the other is occluded. FMNS is usually associated with strabismus, typically esotropia. Amblyopia is frequent, whereas binocular vision with normal stereopsis is rare. In addition to strabismus, upward deviation of the covered eye (called dissociated vertical deviation or alternating sursumduction) and a torsional component to the nystagmus are frequent.

Some patients with INS also show a change in the direction of their nystagmus when one eye is patched, and strabismus and amblyopia may also coexist. How can a reliable diagnosis be made in such patients? Measurement of eye movements will often settle the issue. The slow phase of FMNS shows a linear or decaying velocity waveform (Figs 74.1a and b), in contrast to the increasing velocity waveform of INS. FMNS usually follows Alexander's law, the nystagmus being greatest on looking in the direction of the quick phases, away from the covered eye. Occasionally, congenital and FMNS coexist and the waveforms may show features of both disorders.

Spasmus nutans syndrome is characterized by the triad of nystagmus, head nodding, and anomalous head positions, such as torticollis (Chapter 89 and P24). Onset is usually in the first year of life. Neurological abnormalities are absent, although strabismus or amblyopia may coexist. Differentiation from spasmus nutans is important, because it resolves, whereas INS generally does not. Unlike INS and FMNS, ocular oscillations in spasmus nutans are intermittent, high frequency, and often with a vertical component and dissociated characteristics. Thus, if the child will cooperate, eye movement records are useful in making the distinction, along with brain imaging and also electrophysiological testing.[33-36]

Consideration should be given to abnormalities of the optic nerve, chiasm, retina, or more posterior visual pathways in children with nystagmus. A careful ophthalmologic evaluation should be performed in all such children; if there is any doubt about the diagnosis, imaging studies should be performed. Not every infant with nystagmus will go on to have life-long INS; those individuals who show regression usually do so within one year.[37]

The prognosis for visual acuity is uncertain, especially in infants and young children with INS. Good early prognostic signs include the use of adaptive behaviors (anomalous head position and head shake/nod), good visual interest, fixation and following, and absence of any other disease. Because their vision, as measured clinically, increases over many years, predictions about final vision and the ability to pass driving tests needs to be guarded.

MANAGEMENT

Surgery

Three surgical procedures on extraocular muscles have been used as treatment for selected patients with INS. The oldest is the Anderson-Kestenbaum operation, which is an approach for the patient with an established null zone in eccentric gaze that causes physical or social discomfort. The aim of this procedure is to move the attachments of the extraocular muscles to shift the null zone to primary gaze. In practice, the Anderson-Kestenbaum procedure not only shifts and broadens the null zone, but also decreases nystagmus outside of the null zone. However, the long-term results of this surgery are variable, as many patients readopt the abnormal head posture after surgery.

The second procedure aims to diverge the eyes. It may be helpful in patients with INS that suppress during fixation of near targets (Fig. 74.2), and who have stereopsis. In some patients, the Anderson-Kestenbaum and divergence procedures can be combined.[38]

A third surgical procedure for INS consists of large recession of the horizontal rectus muscles. Improvement of visual acuity as well as an improvement in abnormal head posture are reported,[39,40] but further studies are required to establish the role of this procedure and determine whether weakening the extraocular muscles will induce adaptive changes that will cause the nystagmus to increase again.

Based on long experience, Dell'Osso noted than any procedure that detached and reattached the extraocular muscles tended to suppress INS. He suggested that simply dissecting the perimuscular fascia and then reattaching them at the same site on the globe might prove effective especially in cases when abnormal head postures are inconsistent and convergence does not dampen the nystagmus. Results of this procedure on a canine model for INS supported this hypothesis.[41] Reported lack of effect in monkeys concerns latent nystagmus, not nystagmus typical of INS.[42,43] Preliminary results of a large, controlled clinical trial suggest that the operation is effective in some patients.[11] How could such a procedure work? Recent studies by Büttner-Ennever and colleagues have indicated that the terminal portion of the extraocular muscles, near their site of attachment, contains multiply innervated muscle fibers.[44] Using Rabies toxin as an anatomic tracer, it has been shown that a separate group of ocular motor neurons (distinct from the classic oculomotor, trochlear, and abducens nuclei, and surrounding each of them) innervates these multiply innervated fibers. Finally, it is known that ocular proprioceptors (palisade organs) lie at the insertion site of the extraocular muscles. Thus, procedures such as those proposed by Dell'Osso may work by disrupting a proprioceptive feedback pathway that normally sets the tone of the extraocular muscles.

There is also some evidence that the tendino-scleral junction may contain neurovascular abnormalities in an INS patient's eye.[45] This proposal is being actively researched and adds to the "orbital revolution" set in motion by the discovery of pulleys for the extraocular muscles.[46] It is possible that new, more selective procedures for treatment of INS will be developed.

Optical methods

All patients need formal refraction, and any refractive correction that would normally be prescribed should be tried. Glasses can improve ocular stability dramatically and even small errors should be corrected.[47] Contact lenses may produce even greater improvement in some individuals.[48] As a number of INS patients are strabismic, this and any amblyopia should also be treated.

Teachers should be informed of the condition, and the child should be seated at an appropriate place in the classroom. (If a face turn is present the child should sit at the same side of the classroom to the direction of the turn: if the face is turned to the left, the child needs to be able to use that posture to maximize vision by turning the head in class. That is, by sitting to the left of the board as the child sees it, to the right as the teacher sees the child.)

Teachers, and indeed parents, also need to be warned that holding items close, an abnormal head posture, or head shaking may help the child see better, and the child should not be discouraged from using such adaptive strategies.

Patients with INS commonly show a reduction of their oscillations with convergence (Fig. 74.2), and experience improvement of visual acuity when they wear base-out prisms. Most patients require about 7-diopter base-out prisms; depending on the age of the individual, a spheric correction may also be needed. Often base-out prisms can improve vision enough to impact on everyday activities. Theoretically, prisms can also be used if an eccentric null zone is present to shift the visual scene to a more central position and improve the head turn. The base of the prism should be in the opposite direction to the null zone and in the same direction for both eyes. However, prisms are only really useful for small head turns, as large power plastic or glass prisms are too thick, heavy, and unwieldy, and Fresnel membrane prisms distort acuity.

Sensory feedback

Following up on the finding that wearing contact lenses may suppress INS,[49] it was documented that electrical stimulation or vibration over the forehead may suppress the oscillations in some patients.[50] These effects may be exerted via the trigeminal system, which receives extraocular proprioception. Acupuncture administered to the neck muscles may suppress INS in some patients, by a similar mechanism.[51] Success has also been reported using auditory feedback coupled to the intensity of the nystagmus.[52,53]

As patients with INS do not usually have oscillopsia they lack any information about the eye oscillation. Thus, these methods may work by providing feedback about the eye oscillation. However, the role of any of these treatments outside the laboratory has yet to be demonstrated, and controlled trials are needed to evaluate these and other measures reported to improve INS.

Drug treatments

Variable success in adults with INS has been reported with baclofen[54] and gabapentin (personal observations). Stimulant drugs such as Dexedrine[55] and diethylpropionate[56] have been found to "paradoxically" improve individual patients with INS.

Botulinum toxin therapy can sometimes be useful in reducing oscillopsia in acquired nystagmus,[1] and it has been suggested that it could be used in INS. However, its effects are transient, and therefore it is only really useful for determining whether surgery is of value.

ACKNOWLEDGMENTS

This research has been supported by the Iris Fund and Help a Child to See (Dr Garbutt), and the Office of Research and Development, Medical Research Service, Department of Veterans Affairs; NIH Grant EY06717; and the Evenor Armington Fund (Dr Leigh). We are grateful to Dr. Louis F. Dell'Osso for helpful discussions.

REFERENCES

1. Leigh R, Zee D. The Neurology of Eye Movements. 3rd ed. New York: Oxford University Press; 1999.
2. Casteels I, Harris C, Shawkat F, et al. Nystagmus in infancy. Br J Ophthalmol 1992; 76: 434–7.
3. Dell'Osso LF, Daroff RB. Congenital nystagmus waveforms and foveation strategy. Doc Opthalmol 1975; 39: 155–82.
4. Abadi RV, Dickinson CM. Waveform characteristics in congenital nystagmus. Doc Opthalmol 1986; 64: 153–67.
5. Abadi RV, Bjerre A. Motor and sensory characteristics of infantile nystagmus. Br J Ophthalmol 2002; 86:1152–60.
6. Dickinson C, Abadi RV. Corneal topography of humans with congenital nystagmus. Ophthalmic Physiol Opt 1984; 4: 3–13.
7. Shallo-Hoffmann J, Faldon M, Tusa RJ. The incidence and waveform characteristics of periodic alternating nystagmus in congenital nystagmus. Invest Ophthalmol Vis Sci 1999; 40: 2546–53.
8. Hertle RW, Dell'Osso LF. Clinical and ocular motor analysis of congenital nystagmus in infancy. J AAPOS 1999; 3: 70–9.
9. Hertle RW, Zhu X. Oculographic and clinical characterization of thirty-seven children with anomalous head postures, nystagmus, and strabismus: the basis of a clinical algorithm. J AAPOS 2000; 4: 25–32.
10. Averbuch-Heller L, Rottach KG, Zivotofsky AZ, et al. Torsional eye movements in patients with skew deviation and spasmodic torticollis: responses to static and dynamic head roll. Neurology 1997; 48: 506–14.
11. Dell'Osso LF. Development of new treatments for congenital nystagmus. Ann NY Acad Sci 2002; 956: 361–79.
12. Shallo-Hoffmann J, Riordan-Eva P. Recognizing periodic alternating nystagmus. Strabismus 2001; 9: 203–15.
13. Gradstein L, Reinecke RD, Wizov SS, et al. Congenital periodic alternating nystagmus. Diagnosis and management. Ophthalmology 1997; 104: 918–28.
14. Dell'Osso LF, Daroff RB. Abnormal head positions and head motion associated with nystagmus. In: Keller EL, Zee DS, editors. Adaptive Processes in Visual and Oculomotor Systems. Oxford: Pergamon; 1986: 473–8.
15. Dell'Osso LF, Jacobs JB. An expanded nystagmus acuity function: intra– and intersubject prediction of best-corrected visual acuity. Doc Ophthalmol 2002; 104: 249–76.
16. Abadi RV, Pascal E. The recognition and management of albinism. Ophthal Physiol Opt 1989; 9: 3–15.
17. Ukwade MT, Bedell HF. Stereothresholds in persons with congenital nystagmus and in normal observers during comparable retinal image motion. Vision Res 1999; 39: 2963–73.
18. Abadi RV, Whittle J, Worfolk R. Oscillopsia and tolerance to retinal image movement in congenital nystagmus. Invest Ophthalmol Vis Sci 1999; 40: 339–45.
19. Brodsky MC, Fray KJ. The prevalence of strabismus in congenital nystagmus: the influence of anterior visual pathway disease. J AAPOS 1997; 1: 16–9.
20. Reinecke RD, Guo S, Goldstein HP. Waveform evolution in infantile nystagmus: an electro-oculo-graphic study of 35 cases. Binoc Vision 1988; 31: 191–202.
21. Dell'Osso LF, van der Steen J, Steinman RM, et al. Foveation dynamics in congenital nystagmus. II: Smooth pursuit. Doc Ophthlmol 1992; 79: 25–49.
22. Dell'Osso LF, van der Steen J, Steinman RM, et al. Foveation dynamics in congenital nystagmus. III: Vestibulo-ocular reflex. Doc Ophthlmol 1992; 79: 51–70.
23. Abadi RV, Dickinson CM. The influence of preexisting oscillations on the binocular optokinetic response. Ann Neurol 1985; 17: 578–86.
24. Kelly BJ, Rosenberg ML, Zee DS, et al. Unilateral pursuit-induced congenital nystagmus. Neurology 1989; 39: 414–6.
25. Tusa RJ, Zee DS, Hain TC, et al. Voluntary control of congenital nystagmus. Clinical Vision Sci 1992; 7: 195–210.
26. Dell'Osso LF, Weisman BM, Leigh RJ, et al. Hereditary congenital nystagmus and gaze-holding failure: The role of the neural integrator. Neurology 1993; 43: 1741–9.
27. Tusa RJ, Mustari MJ, Das VE, et al. Animal models for visual deprivation-induced strabismus and nystagmus. Ann NY Acad Sci 2002; 956: 346–60.
28. Apkarian P, Bour LJ, Barth PG, et al. Non-decussating retinal-fugal fibre syndrome—an inborn achiasmatic malformation associated with visuotopic misrouting, visual evoked potential ipsilateral asymmetry and nystagmus. Brain 1995; 118: 1195–216.
29. Clement RA, Whittle JP, Muldoon MR, et al. Characterisation of congenital nystagmus waveforms in terms of periodic orbits. Vision Res 2002; 42: 2123–30.
30. Faugere V, Tuffery-Giraud S, Hamel C, et al. Identification of three novel OA1 gene mutations identified in three families misdiagnosed with congenital nystagmus and carrier status determination by real-time quantitative PCR assay. BMC Genet 2003; 4:1.
31. Kerrison JB, Koenekoop RK, et al. Clinical features of autosomal dominant congenital nystagmus linked to chromosome 6p12. Am J Ophthalmol 1998; 125: 64–70.
32. Kerrison JB, Giorda R, Lenart TD, et al. Clinical and genetic analysis of a family with X-linked congenital nystagmus (NYS1). Ophthalmic Genet 2001; 22: 241–8.
33. Gottlob I, Wizov SS, Reinecke RD. Spasmus nutans: a long-term follow-up. Invest Ophthalmol Vis Sci 1995; 36: 2768–71.

34. Gresty MA, Ell JJ. Spasmus nutans or congenital nystagmus? Classification according to objective criteria. Br J Ophthalmol 1981; 65: 510–1.

35. Shaw FS, Kriss A, Russel-Eggitt IM, et al. Diagnosing children presenting with asymmetric pendular nystagmus. Dev Med Child Neurol 2001; 43: 622–7.

36. Shawkat FS, Kriss A, Thompson D, et al. Vertical or asymmetric nystagmus need not imply neurological disease. Br J Ophthalmol 2000; 84: 175–80.

37. Good WV, Hou C, Carden SM. Transient, idiopathic nystagmus in infants. Dev Med Child Neurol 2003; 45: 304–7.

38. Graf M. Kestenbaum and artificial divergence surgery for abnormal head turn secondary to nystagmus. Specific and nonspecific effects of artificial divergence. Strabismus 2002; 10: 69–74.

39. Alio JL, Chipont E, Mulet E, et al. Visual performance after congenital nystagmus surgery using extended hang back recession of the four horizontal rectus muscles. Eur J Ophthalmol 2003; 13: 415–23.

40. Kose S, Egrilmez D, Uretmen O, et al. Retroequatorial recession of horizontal recti with loop suture in the treatment of congenital nystagmus. Strabismus 2003; 11: 119–28.

41. Dell'Osso LF, Hertle RW, Williams RW, et al. A new surgery for congenital nystagmus: effects of tenotomy on an achiasmic canine and the role of extraocular proprioception. J AAPOS 1999; 3: 166–82.

42. Wong AM, Tychsen L. Effects of extraocular muscle tenotomy on congenital nystagmus in macaque monkeys. J AAPOS 2002; 6: 100–7.

43. Dell'Osso LF, Hertle RW. Effects of extraocular muscle tenotomy on congenital nystagmus in macaque monkeys. J AAPOS 2002; 6: 334–6.

44. Büttner-Ennever JA, Horn AK, Graf W, et al. Modern concepts of brainstem anatomy: from extraocular motoneurons to proprioceptive pathways. Ann NY Acad Sci 2002; 956: 75–84.

45. Hertle RW, Chan CC, Galita DA, et al. Neuroanatomy of the extraocular muscle tendon enthesis in macaque, normal human, and patients with congenital nystagmus. J AAPOS 2002; 6: 319–27.

46. Demer JL. Pivotal role of orbital connective tissues in binocular alignment and strabismus. Invest Ophthalmol Vis Sci 2004; 45: 729–738.

47. Lee J. Surgical management of nystagmus. J R Soc Med 2002; 95: 238–41.

48. Biousse V, Tusa RJ, Russell B, et al. The use of contact lenses to treat visually symptomatic congenital nystagmus. J Neurol Neurosurg Psychiatry 2004; 75: 314–6.

49. Dell'Osso LF, Traccis S, Erzurum SI. Contact lenses and congenital nystagmus. Clinical Vis Science 1988; 3: 229–32.

50. Sheth NV, Dell'Osso LF, Leigh RJ, et al. The effects of afferent stimulation on congenital nystagmus foveation periods. Vision Res 1995; 35: 2371–82.

51. Blekher T, Yamada T, Yee RD, et al. Effects of acupuncture on foveation charactersitics in congenital nystagmus. Br J Ophthalmol 1998; 82: 115–20.

52. Abadi RV, Carden D, Simpson J. A new treatment for congenital nystagmus. Br J Ophthalmol 1980; 64: 2–6.

53. Sharma P, Tandon R, Kumar S, et al. Reduction of congenital nystagmus amplitude with auditory biofeedback. J AAPOS 2000; 4: 287–90.

54. Yee RD, Baloh RW, Honrubia V, et al. Effect of baclofen on congenital nystagmus. Oxford: Pergamon Press; 1982.

55. Hertle RW, Maybodi M, Bauer RM, et al. Clinical and oculographic response to Dexedrine in a patient with rod-cone dystrophy, exotropia, and congenital aperiodic alternating nystagmus. Binocul Vis Strabismus Q 2001; 16: 259–64.

56. Hertle RW, Maybodi M, Mellow SD, et al. Clinical and oculographic response to Tenuate Dospan (diethylpropionate) in a patient with congenital nystagmus. Am J Ophthalmol 2002; 133: 159–60.

Latent Nystagmus and Dissociated Vertical Divergence

Michael C Brodsky

INTRODUCTION

In evolution, primitive responses to external stimuli are suppressed by newer reflexes. When newer systems fail, phylogenetically retained primitive reflexes may reappear.[1] The emergence of latent nystagmus (LN) and dissociated vertical divergence (DVD) in children with congenital esotropia is this type of atavistic response[2,3]: they reflect our evolution from a lateral-eyed being in which the eyes served as both visual and sensory balance organs that establish central vestibular tone.[2-4]

When congenital strabismus prevents normal binocularity, our eyes revert to this ancestral function; unequal visual input triggers visuo-vestibular reflexes, which alter extraocular muscle and postural muscle tonus in the horizontal plane to generate latent nystagmus, and in the roll plane to generate dissociated vertical divergence (DVD).[2-4]

LATENT NYSTAGMUS (LN)

First described by Faucon in 1872,[5] latent nystagmus develops when congenital esotropia precludes binocular vision early in infancy[6-12]: a conjugate horizontal jerk nystagmus is induced by covering, blurring, or reducing image brightness in one eye.[6,9,12] Fixation with the right eye generates a right-beating nystagmus, whereas fixation with the left eye produces a left-beating

nystagmus[6-12] (Fig. 75.1). In children with alternating fixation, the nystagmus spontaneously reverses direction when fixation is switched from one eye to the other,[9-13] even after surgical realignment. The intensity of LN is maximal in abduction and minimal in adduction, causing a head turn to place the fixing eye in adduction. The intensity decreases when visual attention declines and increases during attempted fixation.[11-18] Some patients can reverse the direction of their latent nystagmus by looking at an imagined target and mentally switching fixation from one eye to the other.[14,18]

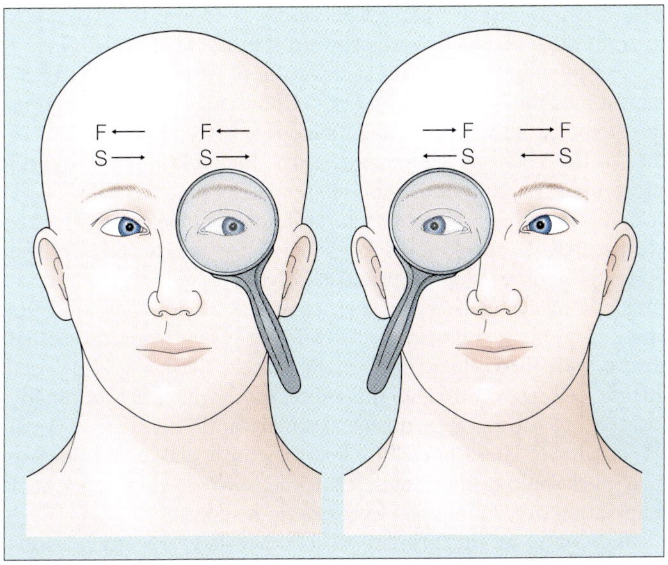

In children with LN, amblyopia or the recurrence of strabismus can make a latent nystagmus become manifest.[19] The magnitude of the *manifest latent nystagmus* (MLN) is proportional to the degree of the interocular visual disparity.[5] Most patients with clinical latent nystagmus have a small spontaneous manifest jerk nystagmus that can be measured with both eyes open using eye movement recording;[11] this can be reversed by treatment of amblyopia or strabismus.[19] LN also occurs in children with unilateral reduced vision from congenital disorders[20,21]: the child often maintains a head turn to position the fixing eye in adduction.[20,21]

Various theories to explain latent nystagmus,[22] including a primitive tonus imbalance,[5] an egocentric disorder,[12] a disorder of the subcortical optokinetic system,[23] subcortical maldevelopment of retinal slip control,[13] abnormal cortical motion processing,[24,25] a cortical pursuit asymmetry,[26] a disorder of proprioception,[27] and an evolutionary preponderance of the nasal half of the retina,[3,28] have been advanced. These disparate theories can be reconciled by considering the evolutionary function of the eyes as balance organs.

Nasotemporal asymmetry and latent nystagmus

In patients with nasotemporal asymmetry, the monocular optokinetic responses to nasally moving targets are brisk, whereas those to temporally moving targets are poor (Fig. 75.2). LN is associated with *nasotemporal asymmetry* of the horizontal optokinetic response during monocular viewing.[24,25] However, not all patients with nasotemporal asymmetry have LN.[29] This nasalward movement bias under monocular viewing conditions corresponds both in direction and in waveform to the nasalward slow-phase drift of the fixating eye in latent nystagmus.[23,29] Roelofs[30] first observed horizontal optokinetic asymmetry in patients with latent nystagmus in 1928, and latent nystagmus may be the consequence of the horizontal optokinetic asymmetry,[31] which persists throughout life in humans with congenital strabismus,[13,23,24,32-34] even after surgical realignment.[36] Nasotemporal asymmetry is seen in rabbits, kittens, monkey infants, and human infants within the first six months of life;[34] its retention in human infants shows ontogeny recapitulating phylogeny.[35,36]

Fig. 75.1 Latent nystagmus. S = slow phase direction; F = fast phase direction.

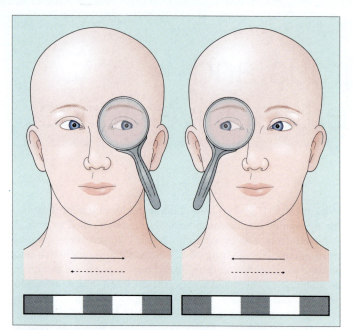

Fig. 75.2 Nasotemporal asymmetry. Unbroken line indicates normal nasally directed slow phase of optokinetic nystagmus. Broken line indicates direction of impaired temporally slow phase of optokinetic nystagmus.

Normally, large parts of the visual field move together during self motion.[37] Optic flow occurs during translation (signaled by the otoliths and linear optic flow) and rotation (signaled by the semicircular canals and rotational optic flow).[37] The low sensitivity to nasal-to-temporal optic flow in afoveate, lateral-eyed animals may prevent the moving animal from responding to the image motion of stationary contours during forward motion while permitting full compensation for rotational input during turning movements[37–39]: this assures that during forward movements, temporalward eye movements do not destabilize images of objects directly ahead of the animal.[37–39] During body turning, the optokinetic responses of both eyes are controlled by whichever eye is stimulated by temporal-to-nasal movement of the visual world.[38] LN recapitulates this monocularly driven horizontal optokinetic movement.

Is latent nystagmus a vestibular nystagmus?

Vestibular eye movements are reflex contraversive rotations of the eyes that occur during involuntary head movements, stabilizing the position of the eyes in space and maintaining visual orientation.[5,6,40,41] Walls states that "vestibularly-controlled reflex eye movements are historically the oldest of all, with all other kinds of eye-muscle controls and operations accreted to them above the primitive fish level of evolution."[42] During head movements, input to the semicircular canals provides the afferent stimulus for the vestibulo-ocular reflex.[5,6,41,43] When the head is rotated in a particular plane, a semicircular canal (whose geometry conforms closely with the orientation of the extraocular muscles[44]) detects angular acceleration and sends excitatory innervation to the corresponding extraocular muscles. Damage to a horizontal semicircular canal pathway produces a nystagmus in the plane of the injured canal.[41,43] Within the brainstem and cerebellum, peripheral vestibular input is summated to innervate the extraocular muscle subnuclei and

maintain the position of the eyes in space. Each horizontal semicircular canal provides excitatory input to the ipsilateral medial rectus muscle and the contralateral lateral rectus muscle.[5,6,41,43]

Visual stabilization mechanisms act in concert with labyrinthine reflexes.[41] Normally, optokinetic responses are elicited mainly by head movements, which also stimulate the vestibular system.[37] Because vestibular neurons receive such prominent visual and vestibular inputs, disrupting either input reduces their tonic activation, disturbing the responses to the other sensory modality.[37] Thus labyrinthectomy eliminates OKN in rabbits,[45,46] whereas blocking optic nerve activity with tetrodotoxin reduces the gain of the vestibulo-ocular reflex.[37,47]

Each sensory modality "has played such a major role in the evolution of the other that it is impossible to understand the operation of either one in isolation."[39] Neuroanatomic, clinical, evolutionary, and experimental evidence suggests that latent nystagmus is a vestibular nystagmus brought about by unequal visual input from the two eyes rather than the two ears (i.e., a visuo-vestibular nystagmus).

That latent nystagmus arises when the two eyes revert to their primitive function as balance organs is evidenced as follows.

Neuroanatomy of latent nystagmus

Primate studies show that latent nystagmus arises as a result of incomplete development of visual input from occipitoparietal cortex to subcortical vestibular pathways.[48,49] In monkeys with LN, there is a loss of binocularity in the nucleus of the optic tract (NOT), the subcortical structure that feeds into the vestibular system, with the majority of cells driven by the contralateral eye. The area that normally provides binocular input to the NOT is area MT/MST in occipitotemporal cortex. When strabismus is surgically induced in infant monkeys during the first two weeks of life, they develop latent nystagmus and area MT/MST loses binocularity. If either eye is covered during infancy, MT/MST and NOT develop normal binocularity but the striate cortex still shows loss of binocularity and these monkeys do not develop latent nystagmus.[49]

Neuroanatomic experiments have confirmed that the NOT is the generator of latent nystagmus.[13,23,48–51] LN occurs in monkeys following artificial induction of esotropia within the first 2 weeks of life.[51] Unilateral electrical stimulation of the NOT in binocularly deprived monkeys induces a conjugate nystagmus with the slow phases directed toward the side of stimulation.[50,51] LN can be abolished by direct injection of Muscimol, a GABAa agonist into the NOT in monkeys.[50] Conversely, latent nystagmus can be increased when the spontaneous activity of the nucleus of the optic tract is enhanced with bicuculline, a GABAa antagonist.[50,51] Simultaneous bilateral blockage of the NOT virtually abolishes LN for the duration of the blockade.[50,51]

Subcortical optokinetic responses are mediated by the pretectal nucleus of the optic tract (NOT).[13,23,31–35] The monocular pathways subserving nasotemporal asymmetry and its neutralization by binocularly driven pathways from the visual cortex were first elucidated in the cat.[32,33] The cat NOT is a diffuse cell aggregation in the pretectum, which are optimally located to integrate direct retinal and diffuse cortical projections.[32] These nuclei are spontaneously active and operate in a push–pull fashion such that the sum of their opponent innervation determines the optokinetic response.[23,32]

Many units in the primate NOT have large receptive fields appropriate for encoding full-field visual motion to support optokinetic eye movements.[50,51] Stimulation of the left and right

NOT results in optokinetic nystagmus to the left and right, respectively.[23] Output from the NOT is maximal for horizontal movements but zero for vertical movements (Fig. 75.3).[32]

Crossed connections from each eye to the contralateral NOT transmit horizontal visual motion information to the vestibular nucleus before impinging on the ocular motor nuclei.[38,52] Pretectal neurons in the left NOT receive only crossed input from the right eye and respond only to leftward motion, whereas those in the right NOT receive only crossed input from the left eye and respond only to rightward motion.[13,23,34] In early infancy, this subcortical system predominates in humans, so that temporally directed monocular optokinetic responses are poor compared to nasally directed optokinetic responses.[34] By 6 months, cortical binocular pathways, which respond to temporally directed-motion, provide a route whereby the NOT with its specialized directional responses can be accessed from either eye.[35,36]

In animals with well-developed foveae and frontal, stereoscopic vision, the visual inputs feeding directly to the pretectum are supplemented by inputs routed through the visual cortex that selectively respond to moving images with no positional disparity in the two eyes.[53] This coupling between optokinetic nystagmus and stereopsis allows frontal-eyed animals to stabilize some moving images while disregarding induced image motion of the visual world at other distances.[38,53] In congenital strabismus, binocularly driven cortico-pretectal pathways never become established, allowing the primitive monocular nasotemporal asymmetry to predominate.

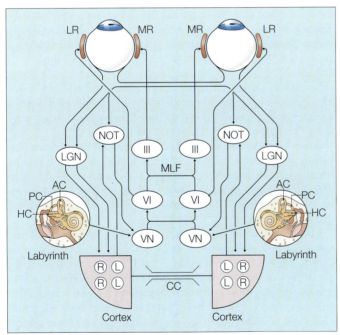

Fig. 75.3 *Proposed* pathways subserving latent nystagmus. Direct crossed pathways to the nucleus of the optic tract provide nasalward subcortical optokinetic responses even when binocular cortical connections are absent (R and L represent monocular cortical cells corresponding to the right and left eyes). Note that the nucleus of the optic tract (NOT) relays horizontal visuo-vestibular information to the vestibular nucleus, where it is integrated with horizontal vestibular input from the labyrinths to establish horizontal extraocular muscle tonus (LGN, lateral geniculate nucleus; CC, corpus callosum; VN, vestibular nucleus; V1, abducens nucleus; III, oculomotor nucleus; LR, lateral rectus muscle; MR, medial rectus muscle). (With permission from the American Medical Association, 2004).

Clinical signs of vestibular origin

Bilateral positioning of the eyes and ears promotes survival by cross-linking input from different sense organs to impart balance. Each eye and its ipsilateral semicircular canals share the same directional bias to movement, so the right horizontal semicircular canal is activated by head rotation to the right (which induces a rotation of the visual world to the left) and inhibited by head rotation to the left (which induces a rotation of the visual world to the right).[6,41,43,54,55] The monaural and monocular directional biases summate, so that activation of the right horizontal semicircular canal during rightward head rotation is reinforced by the physiological activation of the right eye by the induced nasal rotation of the visual world. The close geometrical relationship between the semicircular canals and the extraocular muscles facilitates the integration of head motion and visual movement and their orderly summation to produce transformation to an appropriate ocular motor response.[44,56]

Latent nystagmus usually conforms to Alexander's Law (the intensity of a peripheral vestibular nystagmus increases when the eyes are moved in the direction of the fast phase and decreases when the eyes are moved in the direction of the slow phase).[7,23,57–59] Latent nystagmus damps when the fixating eye is turned toward the nose (also the direction of the slow phase) and increases in intensity when the fixating eye is turned toward the ipsilateral ear (in the direction of the fast phase).[12,13,58,59] A similar damping of horizontal nystagmus is seen in peripheral horizontal vestibular nystagmus after disease or injury to one horizontal semicircular canal. Alexander's law does not apply to congenital nystagmus, which reverses direction in different positions of gaze. The contraversive head turn in latent nystagmus (i.e., a head turn opposite in direction to the deviation of the fixating eye) also characterizes vestibular eye movements.[7]

Additional evidence for the duality of optic and vestibular innervation can be elicited by occluding one eye in the patient with latent nystagmus, spinning the patient, suddenly stopping the spin, then immediately observing the effect of the postrotational nystagmus upon the latent nystagmus when either eye is occluded. A horizontal nystagmus induced by body spinning nullifies or accentuates latent nystagmus, depending on the direction of spin relative to the fixating eye (Fig. 75.4). For example, spinning the patient to the right excites the right horizontal canal and inhibits the left horizontal semicircular canal to induce a nystagmus with a slow phase to the left and a fast phase to the right. If the spin is suddenly stopped (after approximately 10 rotations), a shift in endolymph deflects the cupula in the opposite direction, causing transient excitation of the left horizontal semicircular canal and transient inhibition of the right horizontal semicircular canal and inducing a left-beating nystagmus (termed postrotatory nystagmus). If the left eye is occluded to induce latent nystagmus prior to this maneuver, the latent nystagmus will diminish or disappear immediately following cessation of the spin. If the occluder is quickly moved to cover the right eye, the intensity of the latent nystagmus with the left eye viewing will be correspondingly increased relative to that observed with the left eye fixating before the spin. Thus, the clinician can observe how visual input is summated with vestibular input to establish central vestibular tone in the horizontal plane.

The more visual input is dominated by one eye in latent nystagmus, the higher the velocity of the slow phases in the direction toward the opposite eye.[18] After prolonged occlusion for amblyopia in patients with latent nystagmus, the slow-phase velocity of the nystagmus in the amblyopic eye decreased to the

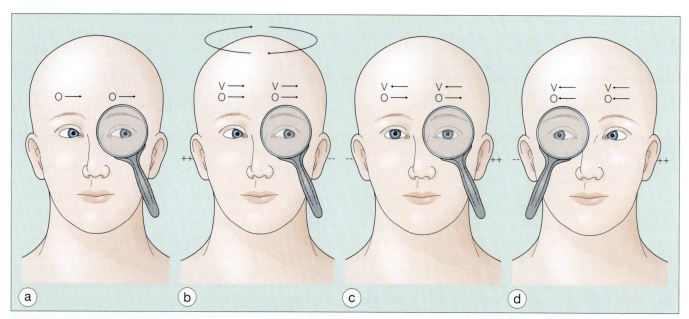

Fig. 75.4 Visual and vestibular interaction in latent nystagmus. Latent nystagmus decreases with spinning toward the fixating eye and increases with spinning toward the occluded eye. O represents direction of ocular (visuo-vestibular) tonus. V represents direction of horizontal vestibular tonus. Both O and V correspond to the slow phase of the induced nystagmus. (a) Occlusion of the left eye increases visuo-vestibular tonus to the left. (b) The patient with latent nystagmus is spun to the right to stimulate the right horizontal semicircular canal, which increases leftward horizontal vestibular tonus causes a slow conjugate drift of both eyes to the left. At this point, the latent nystagmus would be enhanced by vestibular input (if the examiner could observe it). (c) When the spinning is suddenly stopped, the opposite vestibular stimulus is exerted (termed postrotational nystagmus), causing the left semicircular canal to drive the eyes to the right. This rightward vestibular tonus imbalance nullifies the leftward visual tonus imbalance induced by monocular fixation with the right eye, thereby reducing the intensity of the latent nystagmus. (d) When the occluder is quickly switched to the left eye, the visual tonus imbalance is now augmented by an ipsidirectional visual tonus imbalance, increasing the intensity of the latent nystagmus. (With permission from the American Medical Association, 2004).

same extent that the slow-phase speed of the nystagmus in the preferred eye increased.[59] The sum of the two slow-phase velocities remained the same in straight-ahead gaze, demonstrating that visual input to the two eyes (just like rotational input to the two horizontal canals) maintains a push–pull relationship.[23,59] This observation lends further support to a vestibular underpinning for latent nystagmus. The clinical similarities between latent nystagmus and peripheral vestibular nystagmus are summarized in Table 75.1.

Evolutionary underpinnings of latent nystagmus

The evolutionary progenitors of all visuo-vestibular movements use binocular input to establish physical orientation in space.[60]

Table 75.1 Peripheral vestibular nystagmus versus latent nystagmus

Peripheral vestibular nystagmus	Latent nystagmus
Induced by unequal bilateral labyrinthine input	Induced by unequal binocular visual input
Stimulation of right horizontal semicircular canal evokes a conjugate right-beating nystagmus	Stimulation of right eye evokes a conjugate right-beating nystagmus
Nystagmus intensity proportional to degree of horizontal canal imbalance	Nystagmus intensity proportional to degree of binocular visual imbalance
Damps during gaze away from the normal canal	Damps during gaze away from the side of the fixing eye
Conforms to Alexander's law	Conforms to Alexander's law
Modulated by subcortical visual pathways	Modulated by subcortical and cortical neural pathways

These primitive reflexes rely on a dissociated form of binocular vision between the two laterally placed eyes, which has been superseded by normal cortical binocular vision in humans.[2] In congenital esotropia, however, these primitive subcortical reflexes are not erased by binocular cortical input. Eye movement recordings have demonstrated that dissociated vertical divergence incorporates a vertical latent nystagmus, suggesting a shared common origin for these movements.[61]

Given that visual and labyrinthine input are pooled together within the central vestibular system of lower animals,[62–64] a visual counterpart to peripheral vestibular nystagmus would seem necessary on evolutionary grounds. Many authors have referred to latent nystagmus as a tonus imbalance of the horizontal extraocular muscles.[6,12,16,65]

Latent nystagmus corresponds to a vision-induced tonus imbalance that reestablishes binocular equilibrium rather than orients an eye toward incoming light.[66] Ohm recognized the physiologic coaptation of visual and vestibular innervation and its role in the generation of latent nystagmus[67–69]: he stated, "The impulses that originate from both eyes keep both vestibular nuclei in equilibrium. The equilibrium becomes unbalanced when one eye is being occluded. Then, a nystagmus beating towards the side of the open eye appears."[69] LN cannot be attributed to luminance per se, since shining a bright light in the right eye worked like occlusion of the right eye and caused a left-beating nystagmus, and a sharper image on the retina of one eye than that on the other appears to be the decisive stimulus for inducing LN.[9]

Predominance of a primitive visuo-vestibular imbalance provides an evolutionary basis for a shift in egocenter that may explain latent nystagmus[12]: the egocenter is localized to the median body plane under normal binocular conditions but shifts to the side of the fixating eye under monocular conditions. Dell'Osso et al. hypothesized that humans with latent nystagmus retain an abnormal egocenter in the median plane even under monocular conditions, causing the fixating eye to drift toward midline.[12] In the lateral-eyed animal, fixation with the right eye instantaneously shifts the egocenter to the left of the object of regard, necessitating a body turn to frontalize the object and a contraversive eye rotation to maintain fixation.[12]

According to Dichgans and Brandt, "the results of visual and vestibular stimulation on egocentric localization indicate the close similarity in the perceptual consequences of stimulation of the two organs. The assumption of a unitary central representation of egocentric space, based on visual and vestibular (as well as acoustic and somatosensory) afferents, is perceptually obvious."[40]

It remains to be determined whether a higher order egocentric shift could cause the visuo-vestibular imbalance that generates the linear slow phase of latent nystagmus.

Experimental evidence that latent nystagmus is vestibular in origin

Optokinetic responses are fundamentally intertwined with vestibular responses, and a major site of this commingling is the vestibular complex.[37] Single-cell recordings from the medial vestibular nucleus in monkeys showed that single neurons can be activated by either body rotation or optokinetic stimulation.[54,55] Units excited by head acceleration to the left were also exited by motion of optokinetic stripes to the right. Most cells responded to both the whole field visual motion and the vestibular indications of head rotation, and the responses of vestibular neurons followed approximately the same time course as the delayed component of optokinetic nystagmus.[54,55] This underlying vestibular response to both visual motion and body rotational stimuli may explain the overlapping nystagmus response that characterizes latent, optokinetic, and peripheral vestibular nystagmus.[6,16,23,58,68] This overlap suggests that all three movements subserve a similar physiologic function (i.e., detection of rotation of the body and visual environment).

LN, optokinetic nystagmus (OKN), and the vestibulo-ocular reflex (VOR) also show velocity storage, a phenomenon in which constant vestibular input or visual flow in the same direction is stored for up to 20 s in the brain stem, even when the stimulus is terminated (Table 75.2).[21,50] The presence of velocity storage serves to enhance the slow-tracking eye movements to vestibular stimulation and optic flow response at low frequencies of rotation.[6,71] Although LN has been attributed by some investigators to a pursuit deficit or a manifestation of anomalous cortical motion processing,[24,25] the absence of velocity storage mechanism in the pursuit system implicates the vestibular system as the generator of LN.

Summary

Latent nystagmus is a unique form of vestibular nystagmus evoked by unbalanced visual input from the two eyes rather than unequal rotational input from the two labyrinths. The neurophysiologic substrate for latent nystagmus is operative in lateral-eyed animals and in human infants with undeveloped binocular cortico-pretectal pathways. When congenital esotropia disrupts the establishment of these binocular visual connections, visual input from the fixating eye to the contralateral nucleus of the optic tract evokes a visuo-vestibular counter-rotation of the eyes that corresponds to a turning or twisting movement of the body toward the object of regard. In this setting, unbalanced binocular visual input can induce a motion bias in the vestibular nucleus to generate the visual counterpart of horizontal labyrinthine nystagmus, namely *latent nystagmus*. As the eyes rotate frontally during evolution, this visuo-vestibular function is sacrificed, but the central nervous system retains these latent subcortical visual pathways. Latent nystagmus is nature's proclamation that our two eyes can revert to their ancestral function as balance organs.

DISSOCIATED VERTICAL DIVERGENCE (DVD)

DVD is characterized by a slow ascent of one eye followed, after a variable interval, by a slow descent of the higher eye back to the neutral position[74-76] (Fig. 75.5). The deviating eye frequently extorts during its ascent, then intorts as it descends to resume fixation.[75,76] DVD manifests when binocular visual input is mechanically, optically, or sensorially preempted (Fig. 75.6).[74-76] During the period of vertical misalignment, visual input from the hyperdeviated eye is usually suppressed by the brain so that affected individuals do not experience diplopia.[74-76] Since the intermittent hyperdeviation of one eye is unassociated

Table 75.2 Experimental evidence that latent nystagmus is vestibular in origin		
Nucleus of the optic tract (NOT) in monkeys	**Latent nystagmus in monkeys**	**Latent nystagmus in humans**
Electrical stimulation of NOT on one side causes conjugate nystagmus in both eyes whose slow phases are directed to the same side as the stimulated NOT.[72,73]	Covering one eye causes conjugate nystagmus in both eyes whose slow phases are directed to the same side as the activated NOT (contralateral to the viewing eye).[50,51]	Same
The velocity of the slow phases of nystagmus from electrical stimulation of NOT slowly increases. When stimulation is stopped, the slow phase eye velocity slowly decays. This slow increase and slow decay in eye velocity is due to the charging and discharge of the vestibular velocity storage system.[72,73]	When one eye is covered, the velocity of the slow phases of nystagmus slowly increases. When the eye is uncovered, the slow phase eye velocity slowly decays.[51]	Slow rise and slow decay is usually not seen because the eye velocity in humans is much slower (1–5d/s) than that found in monkeys (20–90d/s). In some humans, LN eye velocity can be 20d/s, and in those cases a slow rise and slow decay are found (personal observation and personal communication, Hain 2003).
NOT projects to the vestibular velocity storage system and NOT is responsible for eliciting optokinetic after nystagmus (OKAN), which is the portion of OKN mediated by the velocity storage system.[72,73]	Chemical suppression of NOT blocks OKAN and suppresses latent nystagmus.[50,51]	Unknown

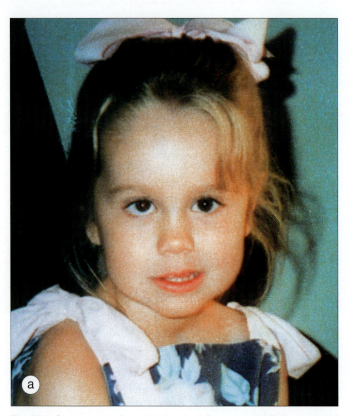
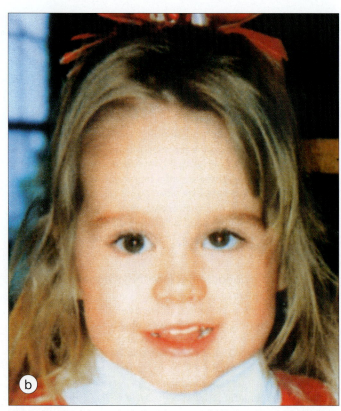

Fig. 75.5 Spontaneous dissociated vertical divergence. (a) Patient seen fixing with left eye, the right eye is deviated upward. (b) Patient has spontaneously switched fixation to right eye: now the left eye is deviated upward.

with a corresponding hypotropia in the nondeviated eye on alternate cover testing, DVD is said to ignore Hering's law and seems to defy explanation according to current concepts of neuroanatomy.[76]

DVD is a postscript to any early disruption of normal binocular interactions.[78] It is seen most commonly in congenital esotropia but also with congenital exotropia and following surgical realignment of the hypotropic eye in congenital "double elevator palsy."[79] According to Helveston, "DVD is a reflex type of event that is programmed to occur if the appropriate mechanisms for nullifying its expression are not functional."[75]

Clinical observations are as follows:

1. "Bilateral" DVD does not exist in that both eyes never drift up simultaneously (Figs. 75.5 and 75.6).[2]
2. An inverse form of DVD, in which an eye drifts downward below horizontal position, has only rarely been observed.[80] Why should DVD manifest only as a hypertropia, and why should it alternate between the two eyes?
3. DVD develops as a delayed phenomenon in children with infantile strabismus. It is usually first noted between 2 and 5 years of age.[76] The amplitude of the hyperdeviation is often asymmetrical, and DVD may be unilateral in amblyopic eyes.[74–76]
4. The vertical amplitude of DVD is variable, making accurate measurement difficult.[74,75]
5. The slow velocity of the upward and downward drift of the deviating eye does not resemble a saccade or pursuit movement but rather a slow divergence in which fixation is constantly maintained by the nondeviating eye.[74,75]
6. A vertical prism placed before one eye induces a corresponding vertical divergence.[74]
7. The amplitude of the vertical deviation is incrementally related to the asymmetry of visual input in the two eyes.[74–76] This effect is clearly shown when filters of increasing density placed before the fixating eye cause the hypertropic eye to descend incrementally, sometimes into a hypotropic position.[74]
8. Eye movement recordings demonstrate that it can be detected in normal nonstrabismic humans.[81]
9. DVD is accompanied by a head tilt in approximately 35% of cases.[82,83]

What is a dorsal light reflex?

In living organisms, light from above and gravity from the earth below have led to the evolution of sensory organs for vision and balance. The bright sky serves as a hemispheric light source that provides a stable visual reference for which way is up. In lower animals, the central vestibular system integrates visual input from the two eyes and graviceptive output from the two labyrinths to modulate postural and extraocular muscle tonus and maintain vertical orientation.[62–64] Although visual input is usually subordinate to vestibular input in establishing postural orientation, some lateral-eyed animals also maintain vertical orientation by equalizing visual input to the two eyes.[66] Many fish and insects exhibit a dorsal light reflex in which illumination from one side evokes a reflex body tilt toward the light.[66,84,85] When a light is shone down from the right side, for example, the right eye receives greater visual input than the left eye (Fig. 75.7). This binocular disparity would only exist in nature if the animal were tilted with its right side toward the sky. This visual imbalance causes the central vestibular system to register a leftward body tilt relative to the body position that would be necessary for the bipeds corresponds to the top of the head. In bipeds such as humans, the back retains its phylogenetic dorsal orientation although it is no longer the upper surface in the upright position. Humans with congenital strabismus who never develop single binocular vision exhibit an atavistic resurgence of the dorsal light reflex in the form of dissociated vertical divergence.[2] When these strabismic humans fixate monocularly, the nonfixating eye exhibits a slow dorsal rotation termed dissociated vertical deviation. In DVD, the dorsal rotation of the visually deprived eye corresponds to the vertical divergence induced by the dorsal light reflex. Although the deviating eye is said to drift "upward" in humans with DVD, the direction of rotation is not necessarily

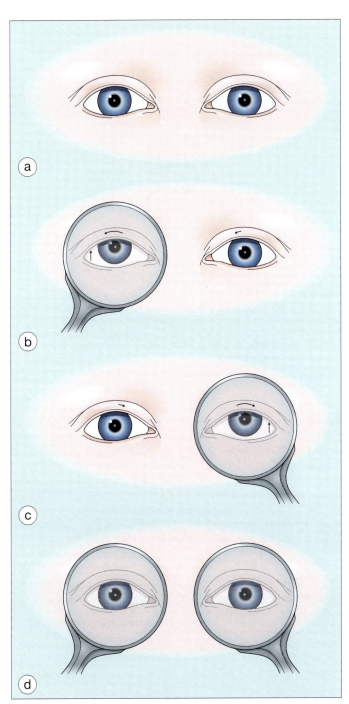

Fig. 75.6 Dissociated vertical divergence induced by monocular occlusion. (a) Absence of hyperdeviation with binocular fixation. (b) Right hyperdeviation and extorsion evoked by occlusion. (c) Left hyperdeviation and extorsion evoked by occlusion. (d) Absence of hyperdeviation during binocular occlusion (as viewed through translucent occluders).

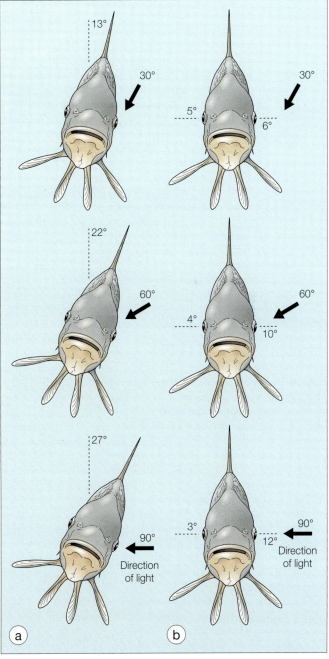

Fig. 75.7 Dorsal light reflex. (a) In the unrestrained fish, the degree of body tilt in the roll plane increases with increasing angles of illumination. (b) In the restrained fish, vertical divergence of the eyes increases with increasing angles of illumination.

two eyes to receive equal binocular visual input, and to reflexively alter postural tonus to correct the tilt[62–64,66] (Fig. 75.7). In a vertically stabilized fish, the same stimulus evokes a vertical divergence of the eyes to reorient the interpupillary axis relative to the new light source, causing the eye with lesser visual input to shift dorsally and the eye with greater visual input to shift ventrally[64] (Fig. 75.7).

The term *dorsal* pertains to the back or upper surface of an animal. The dorsal surface of the head in fish, quadrupeds, and upward in space but always dorsal relative to the head, regardless of whether the patient is positioned in the upright, supine, or head-hanging position.[2,86]

In humans with congenital strabismus, this dorsal rotation can be elicited by reducing visual input to either eye.[2] It can also occur spontaneously when there is a fluctuating degree of sensory suppression in one or both eyes.[2] Eye movement recordings have confirmed that DVD comprises a cyclovertical divergence in which the fixating eye depresses and intorts while the nonfixating eye elevates and extorts.[87,88] Thus, the alternative term *dissociated vertical divergence* provides a more accurate mechanistic description of this movement.[89]

Most animals have a strong drive to maintain verticality in the roll (frontal) plane, which is of paramount importance for balance, navigation, and survival. Primates rely predominantly on graviceptive input to the vestibular system (i.e., gravity receptors within the two utricles) to maintain verticality. However, many lower animals combine graviceptive input with weighted visual information from the two eyes to establish and maintain verticality. (The need for utilizing visual input is evident when one considers that a fish swimming in turbulent waters is subjected to mechanical forces that produce constant fluctuations in vestibular input.[62])

In 1935, Erich von Holst reported that a fish tends to orient its dorsal surface toward the direction of maximal light intensity[62,84] (Fig. 75.7). A fish restrained in an upright position and illuminated from one side will move the eye ipsilateral to the light source downward and the contralateral eye upward[62,84] (Fig. 75.7). These postural and ocular responses to asymmetric illumination are *righting reflexes* that function to reorient the body and eyes with respect to the apparent visual vertical, as judged by the direction of maximal light. Either reflex is only partly compensatory, with its gain determined by the interplay of visual and vestibular drives.[84]

Visual and otolithic signals are yoked in the central vestibular system to establish postural orientation in the roll plane[84,85] (Fig. 75.8). In the restrained, labyrinthectomized fish, labyrinthine input can no longer curb the visually induced postural reflex, and the vertical deviation of each eye in response to a lateral light stimulus is approximately doubled.[84] The enhancement of this visual righting reflex in the absence of vestibular input occurs because it demonstrates the dorsal light reflex is normally held in check by the otolithic input.[64] If the dorsal light reflex in fish resulted from otolithic imbalance, ablation of the otoliths would abolish it rather than increase it. When the right labyrinth is removed and the left eye is blinded, visual and utricular tone summate and the fish will commence permanent rolling to the right[64,85] (Fig. 75.8). When the left labyrinth and left eye are left intact, utricular and visual innervation oppose each other, and normal postural responses are again observed.[64,85] Thus left utricular activation has an effect similar to unilateral illumination of the right eye, and it counteracts the effect of unilateral illumination of the left eye (Fig. 75.8). Visual information pertaining to light asymmetry converges with utricular input pertaining to gravitational asymmetry to modulate postural reflexes at the level of the vestibular nuclei.[63]

The dorsal light reflex bears striking resemblance to DVD[2] (Table 75.3). In fish, the amplitude of the dorsal light response increases with the intensity of illumination. In DVD, the finding of variable vertical amplitudes in the two eyes must also be a function of the degree of visual input asymmetry, as evidenced by the amplitude of the DVD being varied by placing filters of varying density before the fixating eye.[2] This variability is also a prominent feature of the dorsal light reflex. In DVD, the

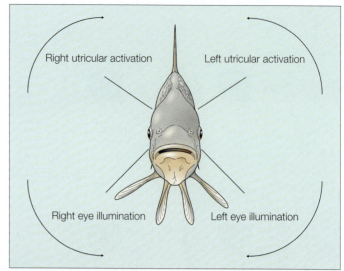

Fig. 75.8 Tilt response to visual and utricular activation in fish: the arrows refer to the rotational movement of the eyes in response to visual or utricular stimulation. For example, a rightward tilt stimulates the right utricle and produces a utricular ocular tilt reaction to the left. Because the eyes are laterally placed, this ocular tilt reaction is associated with a vertical divergence of the eyes with no torsional component. Increased visual input to the right eye produces the opposite reaction.

asymmetry in the hyperdeviation of the two eyes may reflect the momentary visual advantage of one eye, as determined by the degree of amblyopia or by fluctuations in the level of suppression.[80] In the dorsal light reflex and in DVD, the vertical deviation of the eyes occurs slowly and persists for a variable period of time after the inciting stimulus is removed.[64] The rate of each reaction shows a decreasing exponential waveform, suggesting that the driving force is proportional to the deviation from an altered postural equilibrium in each case.[64,87]

Table 75.3 Similarities between dorsal light response in goldfish and dissociated vertical divergence in humans	
Dorsal light response	**Dissociated vertical deviation**
Evoked by asymmetrical light input between the two eyes	Evoked by asymmetrical visual input between the two eyes
Visually deprived eye shifts dorsally	Visually deprived eye shifts dorsally
Tropotactic response[a]	Probably tropotactic
Magnitude of response dependent upon strength of light stimulus	Magnitude of response dependent upon degree of binocular visual disparity
Magnitude of response dependent upon "mood" and external factors	Vertical amplitude variable
Long latency of vertical re-equilibration following prolonged lateral illumination	Slow reversal of hyperdeviation after cessation of monocular occlusion
Decreasing exponential waveform	Decreasing exponential waveform
Body tilts in roll plane toward light (i.e., towards the side of the preferred eye)	Presence and direction of head tilt variable
Right utricular output counteracts right eye illumination	Undetermined
[a] Functions to re-establish binocular equilibrium rather than to directionally orient the eyes toward incoming light.	

That DVD is a dorsal light reflex should not be taken to imply that it is also dependent upon the direction of incoming light. The fact that DVD persists in the supine position[86] suggests that the human dorsal light reflex functions as a binocular-disparity signal that produces a preprogrammed neural output to the extraocular muscles. This neural output retains its innervational characteristics regardless of light direction or body position.

Neuroanatomical studies have shown that direct retinofugal projections to the pretectal accessory optic nuclei and the lateral valvula cerebelli control the dorsal light reflex in goldfish.[90-93] Unilateral lesions of the ipsilateral pretectal nucleus or lateral valvuli cerebelli selectively abolish responses to light stimulation of the contralateral eye.[92] Bilateral lesions completely abolish this visually guided response, whereas lesions of the optic tectum have no such effect. In goldfish, only the caudal portion of the lateral valvuli cerebelli receives visual input from the contra-lateral retina via the ipsilateral pretectal nucleus. The rostral portion receives sensory vestibular (i.e., utricular) input, which is integrated with visual input from the caudal portion to maintain optimal roll orientation. The valvula cerebelli has no analogous structure in the mammalian cerebellum, but it is likely that visuo-vestibular information contributes to postural adjustment through the cerebellum.[90]

Role of fixation in DVD

How would a dorsal light reflex manifest in humans, who have frontally placed eyes with binocular visual fields and stereopsis? The acquisition of binocular vision functions to suppress this reflex since a vertical divergence of the eyes would effectively abolish binocularity and stereopsis. When binocularity is poorly developed, however, this primitive reflex can reemerge if binocular visual input fluctuates.[2] If reduced visual input to one eye is interpreted by the brain as visual tilt, then the dorsal light reflex should act to equilibrate visual input between the two eyes. In the case of DVD, reduced visual input in the left eye activates the left inferior oblique and right superior oblique muscles to produce a cyclovertical divergence movement (Fig. 75.5).[94] Contraction of these muscles produces a clockwise torsional movement of both eyes, together with infraduction of the right eye and supraduction of the left eye. Maintenance of fixation with the right eye would require simultaneous inner-vation to the elevators (superior rectus and inferior oblique muscles) of the right eye to counteract the infraducting action of the superior oblique muscle. By Hering's law, compensatory fixational innervation to the elevators of the fixating eye recruits the same muscles contralaterally, which would augment vestibular innervation to the superior rectus and inferior oblique muscles of the higher eye, and actively drive the vertical component of the deviation (Fig. 75.9). Thus, the observed hyperdeviation in DVD is the composite of two visual righting reflexes: a visuo-vestibular reflex that activates a torsional divergence of the eyes and a compensatory fixational reflex that maintains fixation with the visually advantaged eye and produces an upward (i.e., dorsally directed) movement of the other eye. The pivotal role of the monocular fixation in DVD explains the nonexistence of simultaneous bilateral DVD and dictates that an upward movement of one eye never begins while the other eye is higher (Fig. 75.9). It is only after the higher eye has completed its descent to the mid-position that the other eye may start to ascend.

The interplay between visuo-vestibular and fixational inner-vation explains the perplexing observation that, following

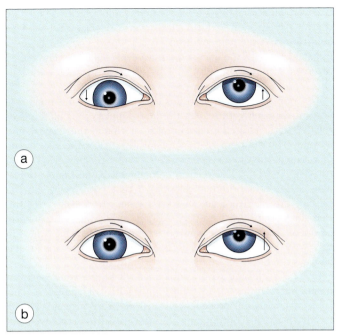

Fig. 75.9 Role of visuo-vestibular innervation (a) and fixational innervation (b) in producing the hyperdeviation of DVD. Compensatory innervation to the elevators of the fixing eye recruits the same muscles contralaterally, which augments vestibular innervation to the superior rectus and inferior oblique muscles of the higher eye.

removal of a cover from an eye of a patient with DVD, the higher eye will sometimes descend below the neutral position before resuming fixation.[74-76] A similar phenomenon is observed when occlusion of the fixating eye induces a downward refixation movement in the hyperdeviated eye, and the covered eye makes a simultaneous downward movement below mid-position before ascending and extorting.[74,76,95,96] In both instances, a fixation shift provides a momentary glimpse into an underlying bias in central vestibular tone.

Perceptual correlates of DVD

In patients with DVD, monocular occlusion evokes a subjective tilt of the visual environment followed by a cyclovertical divergence of the eyes and a perceived rotation of the tilted visual environment back to the vertical.[89] This sequence of perceptual changes suggests that the cycloversion component of the DVD functions to correct a perceived tilt and thereby reestablish vertical orientation under conditions of monocular fixation.

Our perception of true vertical is influenced by graviceptive input to the two labyrinths and visual input to the two eyes. If the subjective vertical is altered by neurologic disease or by abnormal binocular visual input, the patient will perceive a subjective visual tilt.[2] If increased luminance to the right eye of a fish shifts the internal sense of vertical clockwise (as viewed by the animal), a vertical visual stimulus would now appear to be tilted counterclockwise relative to the subjective vertical (Fig. 75.7). The direction of perceived visual tilt in DVD corresponds to the postural responses of lateral-eyed animals that exhibit a dorsal light reflex. The same perceptual shift is reported by strabismic humans with DVD when a binocular visual imbalance is induced by occlusion of one eye (Fig. 75.10).[89] Thus, with occlusion of the left eye, a right eye predominance would shift the subjective vertical clockwise (as seen by the patient), so that true vertical now appears to be rotated counterclockwise relative to the patient's altered subjective vertical (Fig. 75.11). This counterclockwise tilt of the visual world, which is seen monocularly with the uncovered right eye, evokes a cyclovertical divergence movement of the eyes to erase the perceived tilt (Fig. 75.11).

The human dorsal light reflex consists of two movements—a vertical divergence to realign the interpupillary axis of the eyes relative to the altered internal representation of the vertical, and a cycloversion movement that torsionally rotates the eyes in the direction of the tilted visual world to correct the perceived visual tilt (Fig. 75.11).[89] The vertical component of the human dorsal light reflex is a primitive adaptation that corresponds to the purely vertical divergence in fish; it is an *exaptation*, a feature that did not arise as a primary adaptation but was subsequently co-opted to meet the demands of evolution, enhancing fitness in this case by restoring vertical orientation under monocular viewing conditions in the frontal-eyed human.[97]

DVD is associated with a subjective tilt of the visual environment and a reflex cyclovertical divergence of the eyes. This subjective visual tilt precedes the vertical divergence and appears to drive both components of the resulting cyclovertical divergence, suggesting that, as in lower lateral-eyed animals, the human dorsal light reflex serves to restore vertical visual orientation under monocular conditions.[89] In humans with DVD, a subjective sensation of visual tilt under monocular viewing

conditions evokes two compensatory eye movements—a phylogenetically older vertical divergence movement (i.e., a primitive adaptation) to realign the eyes relative to the altered internal representation of vertical, and an exaptive cycloversion movement that torsionally rotates the eyes in the direction of the tilted visual environment to restore vertical visual orientation by neutralizing the perceived visual tilt.[89] The vertical component corresponds to the ancestral dorsal light reflex in fish, whereas the cycloversional component of the human dorsal light reflex appears to be an exaptation that functions to annul subjective visual tilt under monocular conditions when the eyes are frontally placed. This twofold reflex movement corresponds to the ocular motor response that would be necessary to correct a tilted internal representation of the visual vertical. In the human dorsal light reflex, the direction of the cycloversion movement relative

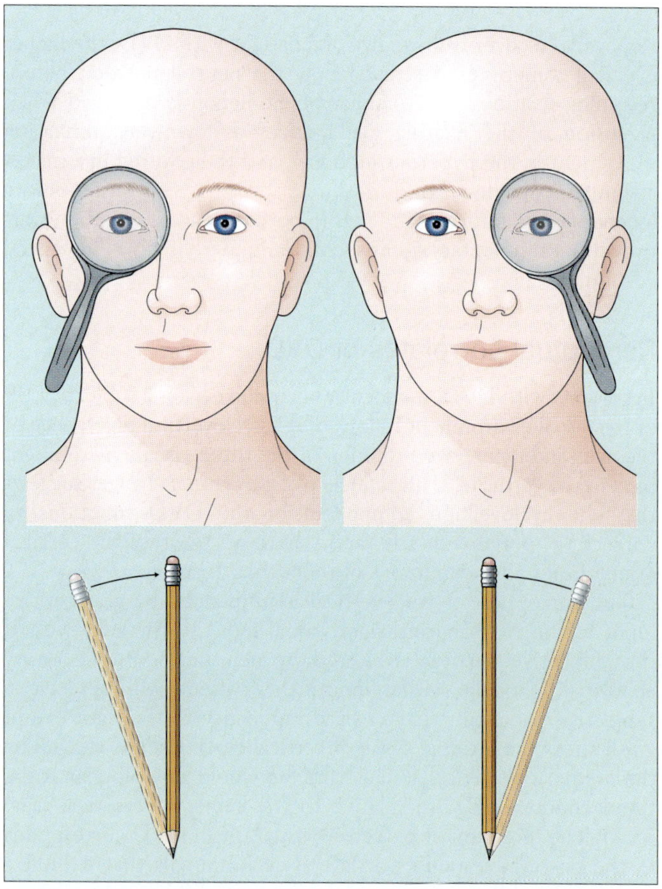

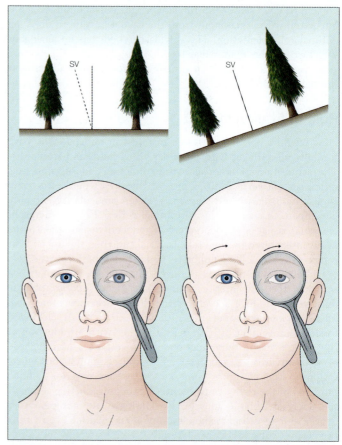

Fig. 75.11 Depiction of perceived visual tilt following monocular occlusion in patients with DVD. SV corresponds to the subjective vertical. A tilt of the subjective visual vertical is determined by the position of vertical objects in the visual world relative to the patient's subjective vertical. (Left) Occlusion of the left eye evokes a monocular tilt in the subjective vertical. Since the visual environment is perceived in relation to the tilted subjective vertical, which the patient perceives as vertical, the monocular visual environment is now perceived as tilted relative to the patient's subjective vertical. (Right) The human dorsal light reflex is a twofold movement consisting of primitive vertical divergence (DVD) that realigns the interpupillary axis with the tilted internal vertical (as in fish), and a phylogenetically newer cycloversional movement that rotates both eyes in the direction of the tilted visual environment. This cycloversional movement (i.e., intorsion of the right eye and extorsion of the left eye) produces a counterrotation in the subject's tilted visual environment to realign it with the tilted subjective vertical (which the subject perceives as vertical); this annuls the subjective visual tilt.

Fig. 75.10 Visual tilt evoked by monocular occlusion in the strabismic human with DVD. Gray image of the pencil denotes perceived visual tilt immediately following occlusion of one eye. Curved arrows denote the perceived rotation of the tilted visual image back to vertical concomitant with the DVD.

to the vertical divergence is opposite to that observed during a head tilt in space, demonstrating that the vertical divergence and the cycloversional component of visual tilt are independently programmed, and that these two extraocular movements can be dissociated by unequal visual input to the two eyes in strabismic humans with DVD.[2,89]

Torticollis as a postural manifestation of DVD

Since DVD is a dorsal light reflex associated with a perceived tilt in the perception of vertical, some patients with DVD maintain a head tilt in the direction of the altered subjective vertical.[98,99] This corresponds to the postural component of the dorsal light reflex in fish. This head tilt is directed away from the side of the hyperdeviating eye and is not compensatory for binocular vision.[98,99] However, other patients maintain a head tilt toward the side of the hyperdeviating eye, which recruits otolithic innervation to neutralize DVD and maintain binocular alignment.[3,4,82,83] For example, DVD with hyperdeviation of the left eye occurs when the right superior oblique and inferior oblique muscles receive simultaneous innervation and a secondary fixational innervation is recruited to maintain monocular fixation with the lower (and visually preferred) right eye.[2,94] A head tilt to the right activates otolithic innervation to the right superior oblique and left inferior oblique muscles and thereby increases the left hyperdeviation, whereas a head tilt to the left would recruit otolithic innervation to neutralize this cyclovertical divergence (Fig. 75.11).[3,4]

This recruitment of otolithic innervation explains why the normal Bielschowsky head tilt response in DVD is characterized by a hyperdeviation of either eye increasing or becoming manifest when the head is tilted to the opposite side.[100] Thus, a head tilt to the side of the hyperdeviating eye can serve as a compensatory means of recruiting otolithic innervation to control the hyperdeviation[100] (Fig. 75.11). A superior rectus contracture can gradually develop in the hyperdeviating eye, which causes a compensatory head tilt toward the side of fixing eye.[101] Various

mechanisms by which DVD is associated with a head tilt are summarized in Fig. 75.12.[100]

DVD induces a situation in which the need for vertical orientation and the need for vertical ocular alignment create conflicting postural drives (Fig. 75.13).[102] On one hand, a head tilt toward the side of the fixing eye, while reestablishing vertical orientation, increases the hyperdeviation of the contralateral eye. A head tilt toward the side of the hyperdeviating eye, while minimizing the DVD-associated hyperdeviation, disrupts vertical orientation. With little binocular vision and an asymmetric DVD, one might expect the drive for vertical orientation to override, resulting in a head tilt toward the side of the fixing eye (i.e., one that is driven by a human dorsal light reflex and non-compensatory for binocular vision). Alternatively, a strong potential for fusion and stereopsis would cause the drive for binocular vision to override, resulting in a head tilt toward the side of the hyperdeviating eye (which is compensatory for binocular vision). The neutral head position adopted by many patients with DVD may therefore represent a compromise position.[102]

Torsional component of DVD

In humans with DVD, the dorsal light reflex acquires a phylogenetically newer cycloversion movement that may annul a perceived tilt of the visual environment by rotating the eyes torsionally in the direction of the tilted visual world.[89] A similar ipsidirectional cycloversion movement can be evoked in humans viewing torsional optokinetic stimuli or a static visual tilt of the visual environment.[103-106] These visual stimuli evoke a reflex cycloversion movement that serves to align the tilted visual environment with the tilted internal representation of vertical.[89]

The variability in the torsional component of DVD[107] can be explained by considering the baseline torsional position of the eyes. When DVD is accompanied by "true" inferior oblique muscle overaction, the dynamic intorsion of the deviated eye is absent as the eye returns to primary position.[76] With DVD and

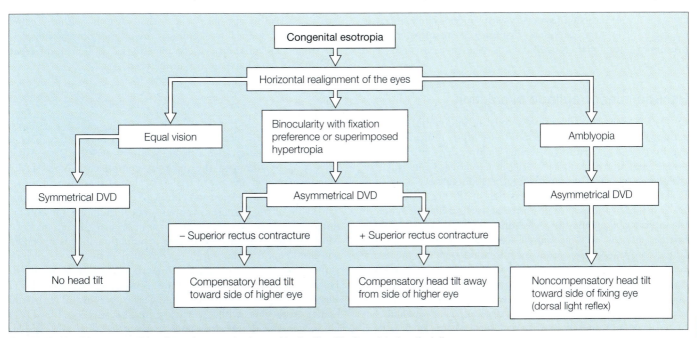

Fig. 75.12 Algorithm summarizing the various mechanisms of torticollis with dissociated vertical divergence.

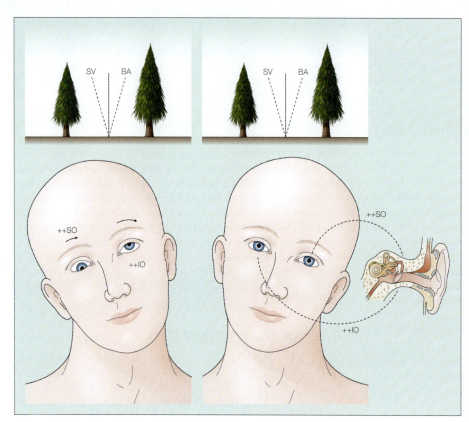

Fig. 75.13 Opposing postural drives for head tilt in DVD. (Left) A dorsal light reflex induces a tilt of the subjective vertical (SV) toward the side of the fixing eye and a vertical divergence of the eyes. A head tilt to align the head with the tilted subjective vertical is necessary to maintain vertical alignment. (Right) A patient can also utilize a compensatory head tilt to recruit otolithic innervation to neutralize the DVD innervation and nullify the vertical divergence and restore binocular alignment (BA).

superior oblique overaction there may be a prominent torsional component that exceeds the vertical component of the deviation.[108] The torsional amplitude of DVD is defined by the disparity between the extorsional position of the hyperdeviated eye during inferior oblique muscle activation and the baseline torsional position of the globe. When the baseline position is one of extorsion (as occurs with inferior oblique overaction) the torsional disparity is minimal and the corresponding torsional movement is small as the extorted eye ascends and descends to an extorted position. When the baseline position of the globes is one of intorsion (as occurs with superior oblique muscle overaction) a large torsional disparity is manifested as a prominent torsional movement as the eye ascends and descends.[108]

Pseudo-inferior oblique overaction

DVD can manifest in adduction, simulating inferior oblique overaction. This is classically attributed to occlusion of the adducting eye by the nose.[76] However, young children have a small nasal bridge[3] and alternate cover testing in lateral gaze confirms that the adducting eye is elevated when the abducting eye is fixing in DVD. The spontaneous hyperdeviation of the adducting eye in DVD begins as the eye rotates into the vertical field of action of the inferior oblique muscle, suggesting that paroxysmal activation of the inferior oblique muscle can excessively elevate the adducted eye.[3] As the eye moves into adduction, the increasing vertical action of the inferior oblique muscle explains how DVD can manifest primarily in adduction without classic inferior oblique muscle overaction (i.e., without hypotropia of the adducting eye, "V" pattern, and extorsion). This spontaneous hyperdeviation represents a different form of true innervational inferior oblique muscle overaction.[3]

Additivity with oblique muscle overaction

In children with early-onset esotropia, DVD often co-exists with primary oblique muscle overaction.[75,76,107,109] Whereas DVD is produced by paroxysmal activation of the oblique muscles (with secondary fixational activation of the vertical rectus muscles), primary oblique muscle overaction generally produces a static cyclovergence of the globes that eventually leads to tight oblique muscles.[60,110] When both conditions are present, their additive effects determine the observed vertical deviation in lateral gaze.[3,79,109] Although some believe that DVD is neither created nor abated by surgical weakening of the inferior oblique muscles, the torsional and vertical components of DVD in different positions of gaze have not been measured.[3]

Treatment

In DVD, as with intermittent exotropia, it is better to have a large latent deviation than a small manifest deviation. The goal of surgery is to eliminate the manifest component. When DVD manifests only in one eye, a trial of occlusion therapy will sometimes reduce suppression and eliminate the manifest component. The value of the numerous touted surgical therapies for DVD is dubious. Recurrence of DVD is common after initial success. Most studies zealously document a reduction in postoperative amplitude in DVD, but rarely document the effect of strabismus surgery on the percentage of time the deviation is manifest. Horizontal strabismus surgery differs fundamentally from DVD surgery in that horizontal muscle surgery preserves full horizontal ocular rotations while vertical muscle surgery for DVD eliminates the dorsal drift only to the extent that it cripples supraduction.

When DVD is cosmetically problematic in one or both eyes, bilateral superior rectus muscle recession has been advocated;[111] unilateral superior rectus recession often induces a postoperative dorsal drift of the contralateral eye and is only indicated when there is amblyopia in that eye. Classic inferior oblique muscle weakening is ineffective, but bilateral anteroplacement of the inferior oblique muscles produces an anti-elevation effect that minimizes the hyperdeviation,[110] but only by crippling supraduction. The same caveat holds true when bilateral superior rectus recession is combined with bilateral inferior oblique muscle weakening to treat severe DVD. Recession of all four oblique muscles may hold promise for eliminating DVD without impairing supraduction.[112]

Summary

DVD is a dorsal light reflex that utilizes unequal visual input to maintain vertical orientation under conditions of monocular fixation. In lower animals, the dorsal light reflex evokes a vertical divergence movement that increases dorsal light input to one eye and decreases it to the other. When human cortical binocular control mechanisms fail to develop properly, a human dorsal light reflex evokes a cyclovertical divergence of the eyes that neutralizes a perceived visual tilt. In the upright individual, the observed ocular drift is necessarily upward because the eye with greater visual input is generally used for fixation and the movement of the visually disadvantaged eye is dorsally directed.[2] The absence of a corresponding hypodeviation on alternate cover testing reflects the instantaneous shift in visual advantage to the uncovered eye that occurs with monocular occlusion.[2] DVD provides testimony to the interplay between visual input and vestibular modulation of extraocular muscle tone, and to the evolutionary role of binocular vision in the suppression of visuo-vestibular reflexes in humans.

REFERENCES

1. Nathan P. The Nervous System. 2nd ed. Oxford: Oxford University Press; 1982: 84–103.
2. Brodsky MC. Dissociated vertical divergence: A righting reflex gone wrong. Arch Ophthalmol 1999; 117: 1216–22.
3. Brodsky MC. DVD remains a moving target! J AAPOS 1999; 3: 325–7.
4. Brodsky MC. Vision-dependent tonus mechanisms of torticollis: An evolutionary perspective. Am Orthop J 1999; 50: 158–62.
5. Faucon A. Nystagmus par insuffissance des Droits externes. J d'Ophtal de Paris 1872; 1: 233.
6. Cogan DG. Neurology of the Ocular Muscles. 2nd ed. Springfield, IL:CC Thomas; 1956: 226–7.
7. Leigh RJ, Zee DS. The Neurology of Eye Movements. 3rd ed. New York: Oxford University Press; 1999: 445–7.
8. Lang J. The congenital strabismus syndrome. Strabismus 2000; 8: 195–9.
9. Kestenbaum A. Clinical Methods of Neuro-ophthalmologic Examination. New York: Grune & Stratton; 1947: 234–5.
10. Shawkat FS, Harris CM, Taylor DS. Spontaneous reversal of nystagmus in the dark. Br J Ophthalmol 2001; 85: 428–31.
11. Dell'Osso LF, Traccis S, Abel LA. Strabismus–a necessary condition for latent and manifest latent nystagmus. Neuro-ophthalmology 1983; 3: 247–57.
12. Dell'Osso LF, Schmidt D, Daroff RB. Latent, manifest latent, and congenital nystagmus. Arch Ophthalmol 1979; 97: 1877–85.
13. Kommerell G. The relationship between infantile strabismus and latent nystagmus. Eye 1996; 10: 274–81.
14. Dell'Osso LF, Abel LA, Daroff RB. Latent/manifest latent nystagmus reversal using an ocular prosthesis. Implications for vision and ocular dominance. Invest Ophthalmol Vis Sci 1987; 28: 1873–6.
15. Ciancia AO. On infantile esotropia with nystagmus in abduction. J Pediatr Ophthalmol Strabismus 1995; 32: 280–8.
16. Gresty MA, Metcalfe T, Timms C, et al. Neurology of latent nystagmus. Brain 1992; 115: 1303–21.
17. Abadi RV, Scallan C. Manifest latent and congenital nystagmus waveforms in the same subject: a need to reconsider the underlying mechanism of nystagmus. Neuro-ophthalmology 1999; 21: 211–21.
18. Kommerell G, Zee DS. Latent nystagmus. Release and suppression at will. Invest Ophthalmol Vis Sci 1993; 34: 1785–92.
19. Zubcov AA, Reinecke RD, Gottlob I, et al. Treatment of manifest latent nystagmus. Am J Ophthalmol 1990; 110: 160–7.
20. Harcourt B. Manifest latent nystagmus affecting patients with uniocular congenital blindness. In: Gregersen E, editor. ESA Proceedings. Copenhagen; 1984: 259–64.
21. Kushner BJ. Infantile uniocular blindness with bilateral nystagmus. A syndrome. Arch Ophthalmol 1995; 113: 1298–300.
22. Sekiya H. Hasegawa S, Mukuno K, et al. Sensitivity of nasal and temporal hemiretinas in latent nystagmus and strabismus evaluated using the light reflex. Br J Ophthalmol 1994; 78: 327–31.
23. Schor CM. Subcortical binocular suppression affects the development of latent and optokinetic nystagmus. Am J Optom Physiol Optics 1983; 60: 481–502.
24. Tychsen L, Lisberger SG. Maldevelopment of visual motion processing in humans who had strabismus with onset in infancy. J Neurosci 1986; 6: 2495–508.
25. Norcia AM, Garcia H, Humphry R, et al. Anomalous motion VEPs in infants and in infantile esotropia. Invest Ophthalmol Vis Sci 1991; 32: 436–9.
26. Kiorpes L, Walton PJ, O'Keefe LP, et al. Effect of early-onset artificial strabismus on pursuit eye movements and on neuronal responses in area MT of macaque monkeys. J Neuroscience 1996; 16: 6537–53.
27. Ishikawa S. Latent nystagmus and its etiology. In: Reinecke RD, editor. Strabismus: Proceedings of the International Strabismological Association, New York; 1978: 203–14.
28. Lang J. A new hypothesis on latent nystagmus and on the congenital squint syndrome. In: van Dalen ATM, Houtman WA, editors. Strabismus Symposium, Amsterdam; 1981. Doc Ophthalmol Proc Ser 1982; 32: 83–8.
29. Shallo-Hoffmann J, Faldon M, Hague S, et al. Motion detection deficits in infantile esotropia without nystagmus. Invest Ophthalmol Vis Sci 1997; 38: 219-26.
30. Roelofs CO. Nystagmus latens. Arch Augenheilk 1928; 98: 401–47.
31. Kommerell G. Beziehungen zwischen Strabismus und Nystagmus. In: Kommerell G, editor. Augenbewegungsstörungen, Neurophysiologie und Klinik. Symposion der Deutschen Ophthalmologischen Gesellschaft, Freiburg; 1977. Munich: Bergmann; 1978: 367–73.
32. Hoffman K-P. Cortical versus subcortical contributions to the optokinetic reflex in the cat. Proceedings of a Wenner-Gren Center and Smith-Kettlewell Eye Research Foundation International Symposium, Stockholm, August 31-September 1981. 1st ed. Oxford; 1981.
33. Hoffman K-P. Neural basis for optokinetic defects in experimental animals with strabismus. Transactions of the 16th meeting of the European Strabismological Association, Giessen, Sept 1987: 35–46.
34. Braddick O. Where is the naso-temporal asymmetry motion processing? Current Biology 1996; 6: 250–3.
35. Atkinson J. Development of optokinetic nystagmus in the human infant and monkey infant: an analogue to development in kittens. In: Freeman RD, editor. Developmental Neurobiology of Vision. New York: Plenum Press; 1979: 277–87. (NATO Advanced Study Institute Series.)
36. Naegele JR, Held R. The postnatal development of monocular optokinetic nystagmus. Vision Res 1982; 22: 341–6.

37. Wallman J. Subcortical optokinetic mechanisms. In: Miles FA, Wallman J, editors. Visual Motion and its Role in the Stabilization of Gaze. Amsterdam: Elsevier; 1993: 321–42.

38. Ohmi M, Howard IP, Eveleigh B. Directional preponderance in human optokinetic nystagmus. Exp Brain Res 1986; 63: 387–94.

39. Miles FA. The sensing of rotational and translational optic flow by the primate optokinetic system. In: Miles FA, Wallman J, editors. Visual Motion and its Role in the Stabilization of Gaze. Amsterdam: Elsevier; 1993: 393–403.

40. Dichgans J, Brandt TH. Visual-vestibular interaction: effects on self-motion perception postural control. In: Held R, Leibowitz HW, Teuber HL, editors. Handbook of Sensory Physiology. Berlin: Springer; 1978: 755–804. (Vol 8.)

41. Markham CH. How does the brain generate horizontal vestibular nystagmus? In: Baloh RW, Halmagyi GM, editors. Basic Vestibular Mechanisms. Oxford: Oxford University Press; 1996: 48–61. (Part 1, Ch 4.)

42. Walls GL. The evolutionary history of eye movements. Vision Res 1962;2:69–80.

43. Cohen BL. Eye movements from semicircular canal nerve stimulation in the cat. Ann Otol Rhinol Laryngology 1964; 73: 153–70.

44. Simpson JI, Graf WG. Eye-muscle geometry and compensatory eye movements in lateral-eyed animals and frontal-eyed animals. Ann NY Acad Sci 1981; 374: 20–30.

45. Baarsma EA, Collewijn H. Changes in compensatory eye movements after unilateral labyrinthectomy in the rabbit. Arch Otorhinolaryngol 1975; 211: 219–30.

46. Barmack NH, Pettorossi VE, Erickson RG. The influence of bilateral labyrinthectomy on horizontal and vertical optokinetic reflexes in the rabbit. Brain Res 1980; 196: 520–24.

47. Collewijn H, Van der Steen J. Visual control of the vestibuloocular reflex in the rabbit: A multi-level interaction. In: Glickstein M, Yeo C, Stein J, editors. Cerebellum and Neuronal Plasticity. New York: Plenum; 1987: 277–91. (NATO ASI Series A.)

48. Mustari JM, Fuchs AF, Tusa RJ, et al. The pretectal nucleus of the optic tract (NOT) subserves latent nystagmus in visually deprived monkeys. Soc Neurosci Abstr 1995; 21: 1916.

49. Tusa RJ, Mustari MJ, Das VE, et al. Animal models for visual deprivation-induced strabismus and nystagmus. Ann NY Acad Sci 2002; 956: 346–60.

50. Mustari MJ, Tusa RJ, Burrows AF, et al. Gaze-stabilizing deficits and latent nystagmus in monkeys with early-onset visual deprivation: Role of the pretectal NOT. J Neurophysiol 2001; 86: 662–75.

51. Tusa RJ, Mustari MJ, Burrows AF, et al. Gaze-stabilizing deficits and latent nystagmus in monkeys with brief, early-onset visual deprivation: eye movement recordings. J Neurophysiol 2001; 86: 651–61.

52. Cazin L, Precht W, Lannou K. Optokinetic responses of vestibular nucleus neurons in the rat. Pflugers Arch Ges Physiol 1980; 38: 31–8.

53. Howard IP, Simpson WA. Human optokinetic nystagmus is linked to the stereoscopic system. Exp Brain Res 1989; 78: 309–14.

54. Waespe W, Henn V. Neuronal activity in the vestibular nuclei of the alert monkey during vestibular and optokinetic stimulation. Exp Brain Res 1977; 27: 523–38.

55. Henn V, Cohen B, Young LR. Visual-vestibular interaction in motion perception and the generation of nystagmus. Neurosci Res Program Bull 1980; 18: 458–651.

56. Ezure K, Graf W. A quantitative analysis of the spatial organization of the vestibuloocular reflexes in lateral-and frontal-eyed animals. I. Orientation of semicircular canals and extraocular muscles. Neuroscience 1984; 12: 85–93.

57. Robinson DA, Zee DS, Hain TC, et al. Alexander's law: Its behavior and origin in the human vestibulo-ocular reflex. Ann Neurol 1984; 16: 714–22.

58. Dell'Osso LF, Jacobs JB. A normal ocular motor system model that simulates the dual mode fast phases of latent/manifest nystagmus. Biol Cybern 2001; 85: 459–71.

59. Simonsz HJ, Kommerell G. Effect of prolonged monocular occlusion on latent nystagmus. Neuro-ophthalmology 1992; 12: 185–92.

60. Brodsky MC, Donahue SP. Primary oblique muscle overaction: The brain throws a wild pitch. Arch Ophthalmol 2001; 119: 1307–14.

61. Irving EL, Goltz HC, Steinbach MJ, et al. Vertical latent nystagmus component and vertical saccadic asymmetry in subjects with dissociated vertical deviation. J AAPOS 1998; 2: 344–50.

62. Pfeiffer W. Equilibrium orientation in fish. Int Rev Gen Exp Zool 1964; 1: 77–111.

63. Meyer DL, Bullock TH. The hypothesis of sense-organ-dependent tonus mechanisms: history of a concept. Ann NY Acad Sci 1977; 290: 3–17.

64. Graf W, Meyer DL. Central mechanisms counteract visually induced tonus asymmetries: a study of ocular responses to unilateral illumination in goldfish. J Comp Physiol 1983; 150: 473–81.

65. Keiner GB. Physiology and pathology of optomotor reflexes. Am J Ophthalmol 1956; 42: 233–49.

66. Duke-Elder S. The effect of light on movement. In: Duke-Elder S, editor. System of Ophthalmology: The Eye in Evolution. London: Henry Klimpton; 1958: 27–81.

67. Ohm J. Der latente Nystagmus bei angeborener einseitiger Blindheit. Von Graefes Arch Ophthalmol vereinigt Arch Augenheilkd 1948; 148: 318.

68. Ohm J. Der latent Nystagmus im Stockdunkeln. Arch Augenheilkd 1928; 99: 417–38.

69. Ohm J. Nystagmus und Schielen bei Sehschwachen und Blinden. Stuttgart: Ferdinand Enke; 1958: 81.

70. Fetter M, Zee DS. Recovery from unilateral labyrinthectomy in Rhesus monkey. J Neurophysiol 1998; 59: 370–93.

71. Cohen B, Henn V, Raphan T, et al. Velocity storage, nystagmus, and visual-vestibular interactions in humans. Ann NY Acad Sci 1981; 421–33.

72. Mustari MJ, Fuchs AF. Discharge patterns of neurons in the pretectal nucleus of the optic tract in the behaving primate. J Neurophysiol 1990; 64: 77–90.

73. Schiff D, Cohen B, Raphan T. Nystagmus induced by stimulation of the nucleus of the optic tract in the monkey. Exp Brain Res 1988; 70: 1–40.

74. Bielschowsky A. Lectures on Motor Anomalies. Hanover, NH: Dartmouth College Publications; 1943: 11–20.

75. Helveston EM. Dissociated vertical deviation. A clinical and laboratory study. Trans Am Ophthalmol Soc 1980; 78: 734–79.

76. von Noorden GK. Binocular vision and ocular motility. Theory and Management of Strabismus. 4th ed. St Louis: Mosby; 1990: 341–5.

77. Spielmann A. Les divergences verticales dissociées: excès de sursumversion lié à la fixation. Ou les divergences verticales dissociées à travers un écran translucide. Ophtalmologie 1987; 1: 457–60.

78. Flynn JT. Strabismus: A Neurodevelopmental Approach. New York: Springer-Verlag; 1991: 71–4.

79. Olson RJ, Scott WE. Dissociative phenomena in congenital monocular elevation deficiency. J AAPOS 1998; 2: 72–8.

80. Guyton JS, Kirkman N. Ocular movement* I. Mechanics, pathogenesis, and surgical treatment of alternating hypertropia (dissociated vertical divergence, double hypertropia) some related phenomena. Am J Ophthalmol 1956; 41: 438–75.

81. van Rijn LJ, ten Tusscher MP, de Jong I, et al. Asymmetrical vertical phorias indicating dissociated vertical deviation in subjects with normal binocular vision. Vision Res 1998; 38: 2973–8.

82. Betchel RT, Kushner BJ, Morton GV. The relationship between dissociated vertical divergence (DVD) and head tilts. J Pediatr Ophthalmol Strabismus 1996; 33: 303–6.

83. Santiago AP, Rosenbaum AL. Dissociated vertical deviation and head tilts. J AAPOS 1998; 2: 5–13.

84. von Holst E. Über den Lichtrückenreflex bei Fische. Pubbl Staz Zool (Napoli) 1935: 15: 143–8.

85. von Holst E. Die Gleichgewichtssinne der Fische. Verh Disch Zool Ges 1935; 37: 109–14.

86. Goltz HC, Irving EL, Hill JA. Dissociated vertical deviation: Head and body orientation affect the amplitude and velocity of the vertical drift. J Pediatr Ophthalmol Strabismus 1996; 33: 307–13.

87. van Rijn LJ, Simonsz HJ, ten Tusscher MP. Dissociated vertical deviation and eye torsion: relation to disparity-induced vertical vergence. Strabismus 1997; 5: 13–20.

88. Inoue M, Kita Y. Eye movements in dissociated vertical deviation. Nippon Ganka Gakkai Zasshi 1993; 97: 1312–9.

89. Brodsky MC. Dissociated vertical divergence: perceptual correlates of the human dorsal light reflex. Arch Ophthalmol 2002; 120: 1174–8.

90. Watanabe S, Takabayashi A, Takagi S, et al. Dorsal light response and changes of its responses under varying acceleration conditions. Adv Space Res 1989; 9: 231–40.

91. Yanagihara D, Watanabe S, Mitarai G. Neuroanatomical substrate for the dorsal light response. I. Differential afferent connections of the lateral lobe of the valvula cerebelli in goldfish (Carassius auratus). Neurosci Res 1993; 16: 25–32.

92. Yanagihara D, Watanabe S, Takagi S, Mitarai G. Neuroanatomical substrate for the dorsal light response. II. Effects of kainic acid-induced lesions of the valvula cerebelli on the goldfish dorsal light response. Neurosci Res 1993; 16: 33–6.

93. Mori S. Localization of extratectally evoked visual response in the corpus and valvula cerebelli in carp, and cerebellar contribution to "dorsal light reaction" behavior. Behav Brain Res 1993; 59: 33–40.

94. Guyton DL, Cheeseman EW, Ellis FJ, et al. Dissociated vertical deviation: an exaggerated normal movement used to damp cyclovertical latent nystagmus. Trans Am Ophthalmol Soc 1998; 96: 389–429.

95. Anderson JR. Latent nystagmus and occlusion hyperphoria. Br J Ophthalmol 1954; 38: 217–31.

96. Caldwell E. The significance of alternating sursumduction. Am Orthop J 1967; 17: 39–43.

97. Gould SJ. Exaptation: a crucial tool for evolutionary psychology. J Social Issues 1991; 47: 43–65.

98. Crone RA. Alternating hyperphoria. Br J Ophthalmol 1954; 38: 591–604.

99. Lang J. Squint dating from birth or with early onset. Transactions of the First International Congress of Orthoptists. London: Henry Klimpton; 1968: 231–7.

100. Jampolsky A. Management of vertical strabismus. In: Pediatric Ophthalmology and Strabismus. Transactions of the New Orleans Academy of Ophthalmology. New York: Raven Press; 1986: 157–64.

101. Jampolsky A. A new look at the head tilt test. In Fuchs AF, Brandt TH, Büttner U, et al., editors. Contemporary Ocular Motor and Vestibular Research: a Tribute to David A Robinson. Stuttgart: Springer-Verlag; 1994: 432–9.

102. Brodsky MC, Jenkins R, Nucci P. Unexplained head tilt following surgical treatment of congenital esotropia: a postural manifestation of dissociated vertical divergence. Br J Ophthalmol 2004; 88: 268–72.

103. Brecher GA. Die optokinetische Auslösung von Augenrollung und rotatorischem Nystagmus. Pflugers Arch 1934; 234: 13–28.

104. Crone RA. Optically-induced eye torsion-II. Optostatic and optokinetic cycloversion. Graefes Arch Klin Exp Ophthalmol 1975; 196: 1–7.

105. Crone RA, Everhard-Hard Y. Optically-induced eye torsion. I. Fusional cyclovergence. Graefes Arch Klin Exp Ophthalmol 1975; 195: 231–9.

106. Goodenough DR, Sigman E, Oltman PK, et al. Eye torsion in response to a tilted visual stimulus. Vis Res 1979; 19: 1177–9.

107. Wilson ME, McClatchey SK. Dissociated horizontal deviation. J Pediatr Ophthalmol Strabismus 1991; 28: 90–5.

108. Brodsky MC. Dissociated torsional deviation. Binoc Vis Q 1999;14:6.

109. Guyton DL, Weingarten PE. Sensory torsion as the cause of primary oblique muscle overaction/underaction and A- and A-pattern strabismus. Binoc Vis Q 1994; 9: 209–36.

110. Santiago AP, Rosenbaum AL. Dissociated vertical deviation. In: Clinical Strabismus Management. Principles and Surgical Techniques. Philadelphia: Saunders; 1999: 237–48.

111. Gamio S. A surgical alternative for dissociated vertical deviation based on new pathologic concepts: weakening all four oblique eye muscles. Outcome and results in 9 cases. Binoc Vis Q 2002; 17: 15–24.

CHAPTER 76 Strabismus: The Scientific Basis

Lawrence Tychsen

One of the goals of clinical science is to understand the mechanisms causing a disease in order to bring about functional cures. The diseases chosen for major study should be those that are: (a) most common and (b) more difficult to cure. Common disorders that are easy to fix do not warrant major attention, and it is difficult to justify placing rare disorders at the top of a list of investigational priorities. By understanding and correcting the paradigmatic disorder in a medical field we should expect to gain derivative insights that could subsequently be applied with major advantage to an entire range of lesser but related disorders.

With regard specifically to the field of strabismus, our efforts should therefore be guided by the answers to a set of simple questions. What is the most common form of strabismus in humans? Can it be prevented or cured currently with a simple single intervention? What are the underlying pathophysiological mechanisms and how do these depart from the mechanisms of normal development? If we understood the major neural mechanisms, would we learn important lessons that would help us treat less common forms of strabismus?

MAJOR SUBTYPE OF DEVELOPMENTAL STRABISMUS

The mean prevalence of developmental strabismus in the Western Hemisphere is ~5%. Graham examined 4748 children in the UK and found manifest strabismus in 5.4%.[1] Lorenz derived a mean prevalence of ~5% from a meta-analysis of data gathered largely from Western European populations.[2] The same prevalence (~5%) for manifest strabismus has been documented in several pediatric surveys conducted in the United States over the past 3 decades.[3-6] Primary, concomitant esodeviations exceed exodeviations in these studies by an average ratio of 10:1.[2,7] Esodeviations (by a ratio 3:1) are predominantly constant, whereas exodeviations (by the inverse ratio) are overwhelmingly intermittent.

Esotropia has a bimodal, age-of-onset distribution. The largest peak (comprising ~40% of all strabismus) occurs at or before age 12-18 months, with a second, smaller "late onset" esotropia peak at age 3–4 years. Children with early-onset esotropia are predominantly emmetropic,[1,7] whereas late-onset esotropia is associated commonly with a substantial hypermetropic refractive error (accommodative esotropia). Thus, the dominant form of developmental strabismus in human is concomitant, constant, nonaccommodative, infantile-onset esotropia. Infantile esotropia may be considered the paradigmatic form of strabismus in all primates, as it is also the most frequent type of natural strabismus observed in monkeys.[8]

RISK FACTORS

If infantile esotropia is the paradigmatic form of strabismus, investigations designed to reveal pathophysiologic mechanisms might begin appropriately by asking which factors contribute to its causation. At highest risk are infants who suffer cerebral maldevelopment from a variety of causes (Table 76.1), especially insults to the parieto-occipital cortex and underlying white matter (geniculostriate projections or optic radiations).[9–12] Periventricular and intraventricular hemorrhage in the neonatal period increases the prevalence of infantile strabismus 50- to 100-fold. Less specific cerebral insults, e.g., from very low birth weight or Down syndrome, increase the risk above that of otherwise healthy infants by factors of 20- to 30-fold.[10,13,14]

The occipital lobes in newborns are especially vulnerable to damage.[12,15–17] Premature infants frequently suffer injury to the optic radiations near the occipital trigone. Balanced binocular input requires equally strong projections from each eye through this region, from lateral geniculate laminae to the dominance columns of the striate cortex. These projections are immature at birth and the quality of signal flow would be critically dependent upon the function of oligodendrocytes, which insulate the visual fibers. Neonatal oligodendrocytes are especially vulnerable to cytotoxic insult.[18] The striate cortex is also susceptible to hypoxic injury because it has the highest neuron-to-glia ratio in the entire cerebrum[19] and the highest regional cerebral glucose consumption.[20]

Genetic factors also play a role. Large-scale studies have documented that ~30% of children born to a strabismic parent will themselves develop strabismus.[2] Twin studies reveal a concordance rate for monozygous twins of 73%.[21] Less than 100%

Table 76.1 Cerebral maldevelopments predisposing to infantile strabismus

Type	Prevalence strabismus	Author(s)
Occipitoparietal hemorrhage and/or leukomalacia	54–57%	Pike et al,[11] Hoyt[12]
Intraventricular hemorrhage with hydrocephalus	100%	Tamura and Hoyt[9]
Very low birth weight infant (<1500 g)	33%[a]	van Hof-van Duin et al[10]
Down syndrome	21–42%	Hiles et al,[13] Shapiro and France[14]
Healthy full-term infants	0.5–1.0%	Archer et al,[23] PEDIG[25]

[a] Additional 17% of infants had persistent asymmetric OKN.

concordance implies that intrauterine or perinatal ("environmental") factors alter the expression of the strabismic genotype. Maumenee and associates analyzed the pedigrees of 173 families containing probands with esotropia onset before age 6 months in the absence of major refractive error.[22] The results suggested a multifactorial or Mendelian codominant inheritance pattern. Co-dominant means that both alleles of a single gene contribute to the phenotype but with different thresholds for expression of each allele.

BINOCULAR DEVELOPMENT AND VISUOMOTOR BEHAVIOR IN NORMAL INFANTS

Classical infantile esotropia is not present at birth. Constant misalignment of the visual axes appears typically after a latency of several months, becoming conspicuous on average between age 2–5 months.[23–25] To understand visuomotor maldevelopment in strabismic infants during this period it is helpful to understand the development of binocular fusion and vergence in normal infants (Table 76.2) during the same 2- to 5-month postnatal interval.

Binocular disparity sensitivity and binocular fusion are absent in infants less than several months of age, as demonstrated by several methods, most notably studies that have used forced preferential looking (FPL) techniques.[26–30] The FPL studies show that stereopsis emerges abruptly in human during the first 3–5 months of postnatal life, achieving adult-like levels of sensitivity (Fig. 76.1A). Sensitivity to crossed (near) disparity appears on average several weeks before that to uncrossed (far) disparity.[27] During this same interval infants begin to display an aversion to stimuli that cause binocular rivalry (i.e., nonfusable stimuli). Visually evoked potentials (VEPs) in normal infants, recorded using dichoptic viewing and dichoptic stimuli, show comparable results.[31–33] Onset of binocular signal summation occurs after, but not before, ~3 months of age.

Fusional vergence eye movements mature during an equivalent period in early infancy (Fig. 76.1B). In the first 2 months of life alignment is unstable and the responses to step or ramp changes in disparity are often markedly inaccurate.[34,35] The inaccuracy cannot be ascribed to errors of accommodation. Accommodative precision during this period consistently exceeds that of fusional (disparity) vergence.[35–37]

Studies of fusional vergence development in normal infants reveal an innate bias for convergence.[34,35] Transient convergence errors of large degree exceed divergence errors by a ratio of 4:1. The fusional vergence response to crossed (convergent) disparity is also intact earlier and substantially more robust than that to divergent disparity. The innate bias favoring fusional convergence in primates persists after full maturation of normal binocular disparity sensitivity. Fusional convergence capacity exceeds the range of divergence capacity by a mean ratio of 2:1.[38,39]

The innate nasalward bias of the vergence pathway has analogs in the visual processing of horizontal motion, for both perception and conjugate eye tracking. In the first months of life, VEPs elicited by oscillating grating stimuli (motion VEPs) show a pronounced nasotemporal asymmetry under conditions of monocular viewing.[40–43] The direction of the asymmetry is inverted when viewing with the right versus left eye. Monocular FPL testing reveals greater sensitivity to nasalward motion.[44] Monocular pursuit and optokinetic tracking show strong biases favoring nasalward target motion when viewing with either eye (Fig. 76.2).[31,45–48] Optokinetic after-nystagmus (slow phase eye movement in the dark after extinction of stimulus motion) is characterized by a consistent nasalward drift of eye position.[49] These nasalward motion biases are most pronounced before onset of sensorial fusion and stereopsis, but systematically diminish thereafter (Fig. 76.1C). If normal maturation of binocularity is impeded by eye misalignment or monocular deprivation, the nasalward biases persist and become more pronounced.[50–53]

Table 76.2 Binocular development and visuomotor behaviors in infant primate

Immature behavior	Chief findings before onset of mature behavior	Investigator(s)
Binocular disparity sensitivity absent before ~3–5 months	• Stereo-blindness • Convergent disparity sensitivity emerges earlier than divergent	Fox et al.,[26] Birch et al.,[27,29] O'Dell and Boothe[107]
Binocular sensorial fusion absent before ~3–5 months	• Equal attraction to rivalrous versus fusible stimuli	Birch et al.,[28,29] Gwiazda et al.[30]
Fusional (binocular) vergence unstable before ~3–5 months	• Binocular alignment errors common despite accommodative capacity	Birch et al.,[28] Horwood,[34] Horwood and Riddell,[35] Aslin,[36] Aslin and Jackson,[37] Hainline and Riddell[108]
Nasalward bias of vergence pronounced before ~3–5 months	• Transient convergence errors 4X divergence errors • Convergent disparity sensitivity present earlier than divergent • Convergence fusion range exceeds divergence by 2:1	Horwood,[34] Horwood and Riddell,[35] Riddell et al.[109]
Nasalward bias of cortically-mediated motion sensitivity before ~6 months	• Motion VEP nasotemporal asymmetry • Stronger preferential sensitivity to nasalward motion	Norcia et al.,[40] Norcia,[41] Brown et al.,[42] Birch et al.,[43] Bosworth and Birch[44]
Nasalward bias of pursuit/OKN before ~6 months	• Nasalward motion evokes stronger OKN/pursuit • Nasotemporal asymmetry resolves after onset binocularity	Wattam-Bell et al.,[31] Atkinson,[45] Naegele and Held,[46] Jacobs et al.,[47] Tychsen,[48] Schor et al.[49]
Nasalward bias of gaze-holding before ~6 months	• Nasalward slow-phase drift of eye position • Persists as latent fixation nystagmus with binocular maldevelopment	Schor et al.,[49] Tychsen et al.,[51] Wong et al.[72]

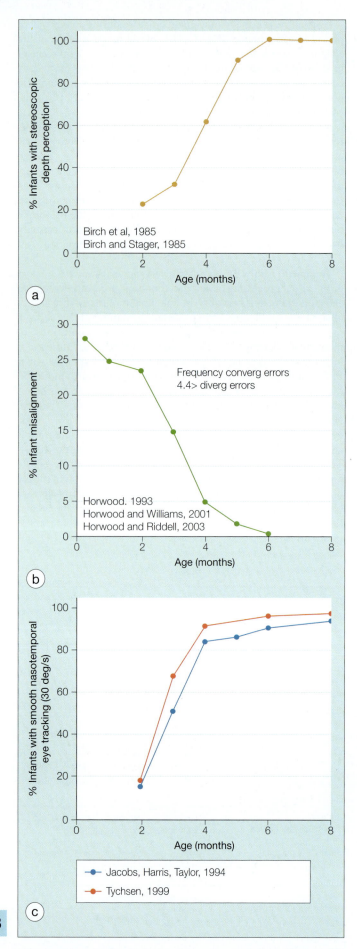

a Birch et al, 1985
Birch and Stager, 1985

b Horwood. 1993
Horwood and Williams, 2001
Horwood and Riddell, 2003

Frequency converg errors
4.4> diverg errors

c Jacobs, Harris, Taylor, 1994
Tychsen, 1999

DEVELOPMENT OF NEURAL PATHWAYS IN NORMAL AND STRABISMIC PRIMATE

Knowledge of visual cortex development (Table 76.3) is important for understanding the neural mechanisms that could cause strabismus, for several reasons. First, the visual cortex is the initial locus in the CNS at which visual signals from the two eyes are combined and a combination of visual signals is necessary to generate the vergence error commands that guide eye alignment. Second, the most common form of strabismus (esotropia) appears coincident with maturation of cortically mediated, binocular, sensorimotor behaviors in normal infants. Third, perinatal insults to the immature visual cortex are linked strongly to subsequent onset of strabismus. Finally, the constellation of sensory and motor deficits in infantile strabismus can be explained by known cortical pathway mechanisms.

Afferents from each eye are segregated in monocular lamina of the LGN and at the input layer (4C) of ocular dominance columns (ODCs) of the striate cortex, or visual area V_1.[54,55] The first stage of binocular processing in the primate CNS is made possible by horizontal connections between ODCs of opposite ocularity, above and below layer 4C (Fig. 76.3).[54,56,57] Physiological recordings in normal neonatal and adult monkeys show monocular responses in layer 4C and binocular responses from the majority of neurons in V_1 layers 4B and 2–6.[54,58,59] The binocular responses in the neonate are cruder and weaker than those recorded in normal adult.[60-62] Binocular disparity sensitive neurons are present in the neonatal cortex, but the spatial tuning is poor, and they are characterized by a high binocular suppression (inhibition) index. The immature neuronal response properties are attributed to unrefined, weak excitatory horizontal binocular connections between ODCs. These axonal connections help define the segregation of ODCs.[62,63] ODC borders are immature (fuzzy) at birth but adult-like (sharply defined) by 3–6 weeks postnatally[64,65] (the equivalent of 3–6 months in human; one week of monkey visual development is comparable to one month of human[66]).

Maturation of binocular connections in V_1 requires correlated (synchronous) activity between right and left eye inputs.[67] Decorrelation of inputs, by natural strabismus,[56,57] or as a consequence of experimental manipulations that produce retinal image noncorrespondence,[67,68] causes loss of binocular horizontal connections (Fig. 76.4). Monocular connections between ODCs of the same ocularity are maintained. The loss is due to excessive pruning of connections, beyond the normal process of axon retraction and refinement that takes place within and between ODCs in the first weeks of life. (Captured in the neuroscience

Fig. 76.1 (*Left*) Postnatal development of stereopsis, eye alignment, and horizontal pursuit eye movement in normal human infants.
(A) Prevalence of stereopsis in a large (*n* = 50 group) of normal infants as a function of postnatal age. Onset of stereopsis occurs between ages 2 and 5 months, approaching 100% prevalence by age 6 months. Tested using polarized goggles and stimuli by the FPL method. Redrawn from data of Birch et al.[29] and Birch and Stager.[1985] (B) Prevalence of large, transient vergence (binocular alignment) errors in a cohort of normal infants, evoked by stimuli located at distances up to 2 m from the eyes in the midsagittal plane. Measured using calibrated video-oculography. Frequency of convergence errors exceeded divergence errors by a ratio 4.4:1. Redrawn from data of Horwood,[34] Horwood and Williams,[2001] and Horwood and Riddell.[35] (C) Prevalence of smooth nasotemporal pursuit eye movements under conditions of monocular viewing in cohorts of normal infants tested at age 2–8 months. Measured using electro-oculography or video-oculography. Redrawn from data of Jacobs et al.[47] and Tychsen.[17]

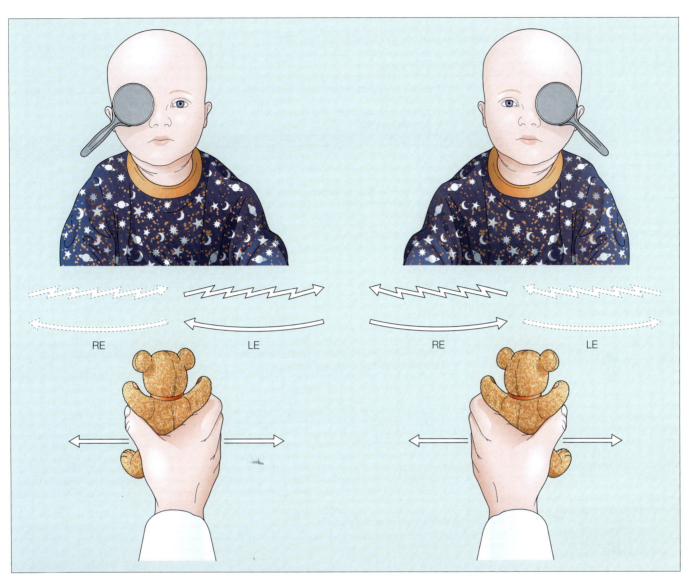

Fig. 76.2 Asymmetry of horizontal smooth pursuit evident during monocular viewing. When a hand-held toy is moved from temporal to nasal before the fixating eye, pursuit is smooth. Pursuit is absent or cogwheel when the target moves nasal to temporal. The movements of the two eyes are conjugate, and the direction of the asymmetry reverses instantaneously with a change of fixating eye, so that the direction of robust pursuit is always for nasally directed targets in the visual field. The asymmetry is seen best by moving the target at a brisk pace. The asymmetry indicates immaturity of binocular connections for pursuit in visual cortex. Dashed lines = conjugate movements of the eye under the cover.

dictum: "Cells that fire together, wire together. Cells that fire apart, depart.") The paucity of binocular connections is accompanied by loss of binocular responsiveness and disparity sensitivity, measured electrophysiologically, in V_1 neurons.[59,69,70] The companion behavioral deficits are stereo-blindness and absence of fusional vergence.[71,72]

Projections, predominantly from V_1 layer 4B, feed forward to regions of extrastriate visual cortex, in particular the middle temporal and middle superior temporal areas (MT/MST).[73] MT and MST mediate pursuit/OKN and a closely related type of tracking movement, ocular following.[74,75] MT/MST neurons are directionally selective and sensitive to binocular disparity, for guiding both conjugate and disconjugate (near-far) tracking.[76-78] With regard to conjugate eye movements, area MST in each cerebral hemisphere encodes ipsiversive eye tracking and gaze holding. Ablations within MST impair ipsiversive pursuit/OKN, and excitation of MST evokes ipsiversive (slow-phase) gaze drift.

Several lines of evidence indicate that the outputs from V_1 to each area MST in the newborn are monocular (Fig. 76.5), with a connectivity bias favoring the contralateral eye (i.e., inputs from the *right* eye make stronger connection–through area V_1 of both hemispheres–to area MST of the *left* hemisphere).[17,79] It is plausible that the innate, contralateral-eye-to-MST connectivity advantage is a carryover from an innate, contralateral-eye-to-V_1 connectivity advantage. (Captured in twin dictums: "First come, first served, " and "Majority rules.") V_1 neurons in each hemisphere, driven by the nasal hemiretinae (contralateral eye), develop earlier and outnumber (by a ratio of ~53:47 in primate) neurons from the temporal hemiretinae (ipsilateral eye). Area MST on the side ipsilateral to the viewing eye can only be accessed through binocular V_1/MT connections.

The innate, monocular, contralateral–MST connectivity bias provides a simple mechanism for the nasalward eye tracking bias, evident before onset of binocularity, in all infant primates (Fig. 76.2). Right eye viewing activates right eye ODCs in each area

Table 76.3 Development of neural pathways in normal and strabismic primate

Neurobiological principle	Physiology/anatomy	Investigator(s)
Striate cortex (area V$_1$) is the first CNS locus for binocular processing	• Right and left eye inputs remain segregated in LGN and input layer (4C) in V$_1$ • Binocular responses recorded from neurons in V$_1$ lamina beyond layer 4C • Neurons in V$_1$ layers 2-6 are sensitive to binocular disparity	Hubel and Wiesel,[54] Hubel,[55] Poggio and Fischer,[58] Wiesel[69]
Binocular structure + function in V$_1$ is immature at birth	• Segregation of RE/LE ODCs immature at birth • Binocular (disparity sensitive) neurons present at birth but tuning poor • Immature binocular neurons have weak excitatory horizontal connections between ODCs and high suppression index	Chino et al.,[60] Chino et al.,[61] Horton and Endo et al.,[63] Horton and Hocking,[64] Hubel et al.,[110] Levay et al.,[111] Horton and Hocking[112]
Maturation of binocular connectivity in V$_1$ requires correlated RE/LE input	• Absence of correlation causes lack of disparity sensitivity and loss of horizontal connections in V$_1$	Tychsen and Burkhalter,[56] Tychsen et al.,[57] Crawford and von Noorden,[59] Lowel and Singer,[67] Trachtenberg and Stryker,[68] Crawford et al.,[70,71] Tychsen et al.[113]
V$_1$ feeds forward to extrastriate visual areas MT/MST which control ipsiversive eye tracking and gaze holding	• Extrastriate areas MT/ MST mediate pursuit/OKN and receive feed forward (binocular)projections from V$_1$ lamina 4B • Lesions of MST impair ipsiversive pursuit/OKN and gaze holding	Ungerleider and Desimone,[73] Dürsteler et al.,[74] Dürsteler and Wurtz,[75] Pasik and Pasik[114,115]
V$_1$ feed forward connections to MT/MST at birth are monocular from ODCs driven by the contralateral eye	• Before maturation of binocularity, a nasalward movement bias is apparent when viewing with either eye (RE viewing evokes leftward pursuit/OKN/gaze drift; LE viewing evokes rightward pursuit/OKN/gaze drift) • Nasalward + temporalward neurons are present in = numbers within V$_1$/MT but nasalward have innate connectivity advantage	Tychsen,[17] Hatta et al.,[62] Kiorpes et al.[79]
MST inputs from the ipsilateral eye require maturation of binocular V$_1$/MT connections MST neurons encode both vergence and pursuit/OKN	• If binocularity matures, monocular viewing evokes equal nasalward/temporalward eye movement + stable gaze • Disparity sensitive neurons in MST also mediate vergence • If binocularity fails to mature, monocular viewing evokes nasalward pursuit/OKN and inappropriate convergence	Tychsen,[17] Wong et al.,[72] Kiorpes et al.[79] Wong et al.,[72] Maunsell and Van Essen,[76] Kawano,[77] Takemura et al.,[78] Yildirim and Tychsen[81]
Convergence motor neurons are more numerous	• Convergence neurons outnumber divergence neurons 3:2 in the midbrain of normal primates	Mays[101,116]

V1. Right eye ODCs connect preferentially to the left area MST (Fig. 76.5A). The left area MST mediates ipsiversive/leftward tracking, which is nasalward tracking with respect to the viewing (right) eye. When binocular connections mature, right eye ODCs gain equal access to neurons within areas MST of the right and left hemispheres (Fig. 76.5B), and the nasalward bias disappears. (Dictum: "Tracking from ear-to-nose will balance as binocularity grows.") If binocular connections are lost, the nasalward bias persists and is exaggerated. The bias is evident clinically as a pathologic nasotemporal asymmetry of pursuit/OKN and a nasalward (slow-phase) drift of gaze-holding (latent nystagmus).[80]

Area MST neurons are sensitive to binocular disparity and appear to mediate, in addition to pursuit/OKN/ocular following, fusional vergence eye movements.[77,78] Eye movement recordings in a primate with infantile esotropia showed inappropriate activation of convergence whenever nasalward monocular OKN was evoked.[81] Neuroanatomic analysis of V$_1$ in this monkey showed a paucity of binocular connections and metabolic evidence of heightened interocular suppression. The conclusion drawn from these observations was that MST neurons promote esotropia (i.e., a bias for nasalward vergence) when binocularity fails to develop in V$_1$. The mechanism is attractive because it:

(a) Parsimoniously explains the nasalward bias of vergence, the nasalward biases of pursuit/OKN (nasotemporal asymmetry), and the nasalward bias of gaze holding (latent nystagmus) that typify infantile strabismus; and

(b) Is localized to one cortical region, known to be vulnerable to perinatal damage.

Outputs from the cortical areas noted above (V$_1$, MT/MST) and related cortical areas descend to brainstem visual relay and premotor neuron pools immediately adjacent to the motor nuclei.[82] Even in the absence of cortical maldevelopments, the vergence system is unbalanced, favoring convergence. In normal primates, midbrain premotor neurons driving convergence outnumber those driving divergence, by a ratio of 3:2.

REPAIR OF CORTICAL VISUOMOTOR CIR CUITS IN INFANTILE STRABISMUS

Is repair of binocular V$_1$ connections possible, restoring normal fusion and stereopsis, while preventing or reversing the constellation of ocular motor maldevelopments? The answer to this question is rooted in a debate between two competing 20th-century schools of treatment philosophy, derived from the eminent British strabismologists, Claude Worth and Bernard Chavasse. Worth postulated in 1903 that esotropic infants suffered "an irreparable defect of the fusion faculty."[83] Their brain was congenitally incapable of achieving substantial binocular vision. Early surgical treatment was therefore unfounded because it was futile. Chavasse on the other hand–attracted by the Pavlovian physiology of the 1920's and 1930's–believed that

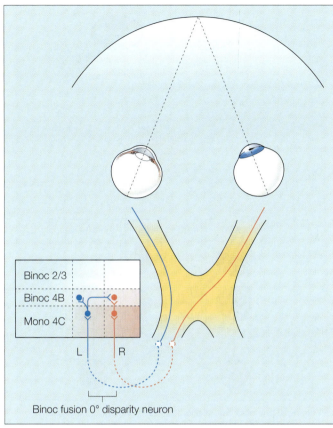

Fig. 76.3 Horizontal axonal connections for binocular vision in area V_1 (striate visual cortex) of normal primate. Monocular retinogeniculate projections from foveae of left (L) and right (R) eye remain segregated at the input layer of ocular dominance columns (ODCs) in V1, lamina 4C. Binocular vision is made possible by horizontal connections between ODCs of opposite ocularity in laminae 4B and 2/3 (as well as 5/6, not shown). Horopter = curved line in front of the eyes.

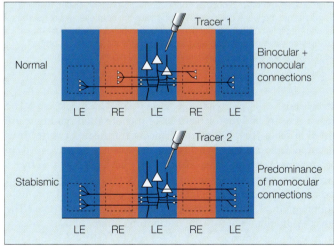

Fig. 76.4 Horizontal connections for binocular vision in V_1 of normal versus strabismic primate, layer 2–4B. V_1 of normal primates is characterized by equal numbers of monocular and binocular connections. In strabismic primates, the connections are predominantly monocular (i.e., a paucity of binocular connections). Neurons interconnecting ODCs have been labeled using a tracer injected into an ODC of V_1. The tracer is taken up by the neuron body and actively transported to reveal the axonal connections. A second tracer, injected into an eye, is transported transsynaptically, from the eye to V_1, to label (reveal) ODCs belonging to the left (LE) versus right (RE) eyes.

the brain machinery for fusion was present in esotropic infants, but the development of "conditioned reflexes" for binocular fusion were impeded by factors such as weakness of the motor limb.[84] He postulated (in his text published in 1939) that if the eyes could be realigned during what he believed to be a period of reflex learning, binocular fusion could be restored.

New knowledge of stereopsis development in the 1980's bolstered the rationale in favor of early surgery, as articulated by disciples of Chavasse in the United States, most notably August Costenbader, Marshall Parks, and a series of Parks' trainees.[85,86] The new knowledge prompted a gradual reexamination of old data and inspired important case studies–in the 1980's and 1990's–on the efficacy of early strabismus surgery.[87–90] These reports showed that if stable, binocular alignment was not achieved until age 24 months, the chances of repairing stereopsis were nil. If stable alignment was achieved by age 6 months, the chances of repairing stereopsis were good, and a substantial percentage of the infants regained robust stereopsis, i.e., random dot stereopsis with thresholds on the order of 60–400 arc sec.

Scrutiny of early alignment data in infantile esotropia has produced more refined and forceful conclusions. Figure 76.6 is replotted data on stereopsis outcomes in over 100 consecutive infantile esotropes.[90] The Y-axis is prevalence of stereopsis after surgical alignment, and the X-axis is age of onset (Fig. 76.6A) or duration of misalignment (Fig. 76.6B) before surgery. The dashed line at 40% represents the average prevalence of stereopsis when all infants operated upon by 2 years of age are grouped together, without regard to age at correction or duration before correction. The noise in the data–relating age at alignment to stereopsis outcome–is related to the fact that onset of strabismus is idiosyncratic, varying considerably from infant to infant, and distributed randomly in the interval 2 to 6 months of age. There is no systematic relationship between age of onset of esotropia and subsequent attainment of stereopsis. However, when the data are reanalyzed with strict attention to duration of misalignment (Fig. 76.6B), a strong correlation between shorter durations of misalignment and restoration of stereopsis is evident. Excellent outcomes are achievable in infants operated upon within 60 days of onset of strabismus ("early surgery").[90] The clinical dictum that follows is that age at surgery should be tailored to age of onset and not chronological age.

Esotropic infants who regain high-grade stereopsis also regain robust fusional vergence.[87,88,90] Clinical observation also suggests that they have a lower prevalence of recurrent esotropia (or exotropia), pursuit/OKN asymmetry, motion VEP asymmetry, latent nystagmus, and dissociated vertical deviation (DVD). However, ocular motor recording is difficult to perform in children and detailed, quantitative information is lacking.

Eye movement studies of strabismic infant monkeys have been particularly helpful. The studies have shown that normal motor and sensory pathway development can be restored when the timeliness of therapy conforms to that of early surgery in human.[72,91] If binocular image correlation is restored in strabismic monkeys within 3 weeks of onset of strabismus (the equivalent of 3 months in human), fusional vergence, pursuit/OKN, and gaze holding return to normal. The repair of ocular motor behavior occurs with repair of stereopsis and restoration of normal motion responses (motion VEPs). If repair in strabismic monkeys is delayed until the equivalent of 12-months-duration in human, esotropia and stereo-blindness persist. Delayed-repair animals exhibit latent nystagmus, pursuit/OKN asymmetry, motion VEP asymmetry, and DVD. The quality of behavioral repair correlates with the quality of neuroanatomic repair in V_1

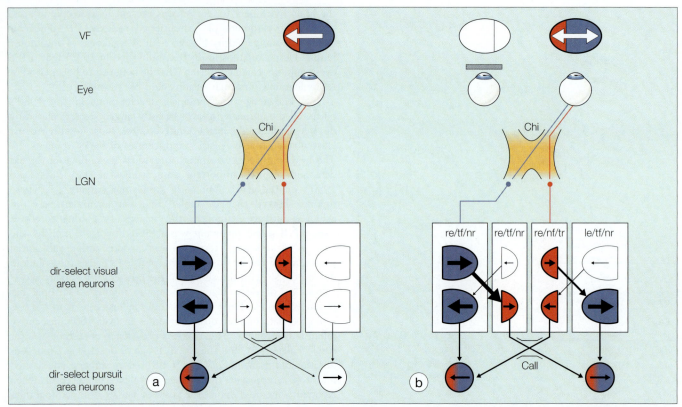

Fig. 76.5 Neural network diagrams showing visual signal flow for pursuit and gaze holding in primates before and after development of binocularity. Paucity of mature binocular connections explains behavioral asymmetries evident as asymmetric pursuit/OKN and latent fixation nystagmus. Note that in all primates, pursuit area neurons in each hemisphere encode ipsilaterally directed pursuit. Signal flow is initiated by a moving stimulus in the monocular visual field, which evokes a response in visual area neurons (i.e., V1/MT). Each eye at birth has access—through innate, monocular connections—to the pursuit area neurons (e.g., MST) of the contralateral hemisphere. Access to pursuit neurons of the ipsilateral hemisphere requires mature, binocular connections. (a) Immature/monocular/asymmetric: Moving from top to bottom, the starting with target motion in monocular visual field of right eye. Retinal ganglion cell fibers from the nasal and temporal hemiretinae (eye) decussate at the optic chiasm (chi), synapse at the lateral geniculate nucleus (LGN), and project to alternating rows of ODCs in V_1 (visual area rectangles). In each V_1, ODCs representing the nasal hemiretinae (temporal visual hemi-field) occupy slightly more cortical territory than those representing the temporal hemiretinae (nasal hemifield), but each ODC contains neurons sensitive to nasally directed versus temporally directed motion (half-circles shaped like the matching hemifield, arrows indicate directional preference). Visual area neurons (including those beyond V1 in area MT) are sensitive to both nasally directed and temporally directed motion, but only those encoding nasally directed motion are wired innately–through monocular connections—to the pursuit area. (b) Mature/binocular/symmetric: Binocular connections are present, linking neurons with similar orientation/directional preferences within ODCs of opposite ocularity (diagonal lines between columns). Viewing with the right eye, visual neurons preferring nasally directed motion project to the left hemisphere pursuit area; visual neurons preferring temporally directed motion project to the right hemisphere pursuit area. Temporally directed visual area neurons gain access to pursuit area neurons only through binocular connections. Call = corpus callosum, through which visual area neurons in each hemisphere project to opposite pursuit area. Bold lines = active neurons and neuronal projections.

(Fig. 76.4). Early repair monkeys have a normal compliment of binocular horizontal excitatory connections between ODCs of opposite ocularity, and delayed repair monkeys a paucity.

MONOFIXATION (MICROESOTROPIA) SYNDROME

As outlined above, recent data on early correction of infantile strabismus suggest that it is a curable disorder. However, early surgery is the exception rather than the rule of current clinical practice in the United States and Europe. The majority of infants who have esotropia are corrected 6 or more months after onset of misalignment. The chances of rescuing bifoveal fusion after this interval are slim. Most infants are aligned to within 8 prism diopters (PD) of orthotropia (microesotropia) and regain a degree of subnormal stereopsis and motor fusion, i.e., monofixation syndrome.

Monofixation syndrome occurs as a primary disorder (prevalence 1%) or, more commonly, as a secondary phenomenon, after (imperfect) treatment of large magnitude strabismus.[92,93] The syndrome also occurs in monkeys.[94] The major sensory and motor features of monofixation syndrome are listed in Table 76.4. Neural mechanisms for the first two features listed in Table 76.4 are not difficult to explain. Receptive fields in V_1–representing the fovea–are tiny and have narrow tolerances. Any defocusing or other decorrelation of one eye's inputs would produce a conflict in neighboring V_1 columns and promote suppression of ODCs corresponding to the weaker eye. The fovea subtends ~5° of the retinotopic map of V_1; thus, a suppression scotoma of = 5° makes sense. Feature 2, subnormal stereopsis, could be explained along similar lines. Stereoscopic thresholds increase exponentially from the fovea to more eccentric positions along the retinotopic map of the visual field. If foveal ODCs are suppressed and parafoveal ODCs are left to mediate stereopsis, stereopsis is degraded but not obliterated. However, it is features 3 and 4 of the monofixation syndrome, the visuomotor signs, that are most intriguing. If binocular development is perturbed so that right and left eye foveal ODCs (receptive fields) do not enjoy perfectly correlated

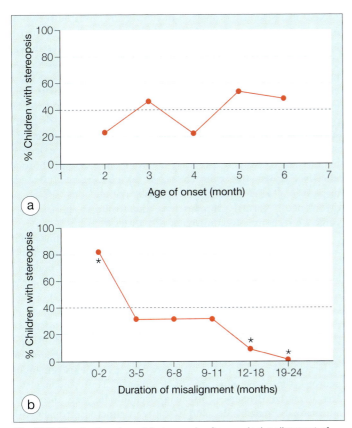

Fig. 76.6 Repair of random-dot stereopsis after surgical realignment of the eyes in children with infantile esotropia. (a) Prevalence of stereopsis as a function of age of onset of strabismus. No systematic relationship is evident. Dashed line = 40% prevalence of some measurable stereopsis for entire study group. (b) High prevalence (~80%) of stereopsis in infants who were aligned within 60 days of onset of strabismus. Probability of stereopsis was negligible in infants who had durations of strabismus exceeding ~12 months. Redrawn from data of Birch et al.[43]

Table 76.4 Monofixation (microstrabismus) syndrome	
Clinical feature	**Possible neural mechanism**
1. Foveal suppression scotoma of 3°–5° in the nonpreferred eye[a] when viewing binocularly	Inhibitory-connection-mediated metabolic suppression of decorrelated activity in V$_1$ foveal ODCs of non-preferred eye
2. Subnormal stereopsis (threshold 60–3000 arc sec)	Broader disparity tuning of parafoveal neurons in V$_1$/MT (foveal neurons suppressed)
3. Stable microesotropia[b] less than ~4-8 PD (~2.5°–5°)	Small angle ≈ average horizontal neuron length in V$_1$, eso by default to convergent disparity coding of major MST population
4. Fusional vergence amplitudes intact for disparities > 2.5°–5° (> 4–8 PD)	V$_1$ excitatory horizontal binocular connections (and V$_1$/MT/MST disparity neurons) intact beyond region of foveal suppression

[a] Subnormal acuity (amblyopia) in the nonpreferred eye in 34% of corrected infantile esotropes and 100% of anisometropes.
[b] Microexotropia in ≤ 10%

Studies of ODCs and neuronal axons in area V$_1$ have revealed a possible mechanism. The overall pattern and width of ODCs in V1 (~400 μm (0.40 mm)) is the same in normal and strabismic monkeys.[65,94] Horizontal axon length was measured for neurons within the V1 region corresponding to visual field eccentricities of 0° to 10° (i.e., the representation of the fovea, parafovea, and macula). The length is similar in both normal and strabismic monkeys, on average ~7 mm.[94,95] In a primate with normal eye alignment, the ODC representing the foveola (or 0° eccentricity) of the left eye is immediately adjacent to the column representing the foveola of the right eye (Fig. 76.7a). The side-by-side arrangement of the "foveolar" columns in normal V$_1$ is well within the range of horizontal axonal connections needed to allow those ODCs to communicate for high-grade binocular fusion.

In a primate with microesotropia and a left eye fixation preference (Fig. 76.8), a neuron within a foveolar (0°) column of the fixating left eye must link up with a nonadjacent column representing the pseudofoveola of the deviated right eye (Fig. 76.7b). Based on retinotopic maps of V$_1$ in macaque monkey, a horizontal axon ~7 mm in length could join ODCs (and receptive fields) that were up to but not further than 2.5° apart, or converting degrees to prism diopters, not more than 4.4 PD. Figure 76.9 is a 2-dimensional map representing V1 from the right cerebral hemisphere (left visual hemi-field) of a microesotropic macaque. The sulci and gyri have been unfolded and the visual field representation superimposed using standard retinotopic landmarks. One horizontal axon, originating within the foveal representation at 0°–1° eccentricity, could link to a receptive field shifted 2.5° or 4.4 PD distant. Two neurons strung

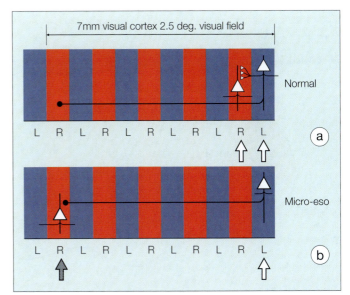

Fig. 76.7 Distance spanned by the average V$_1$ horizontal axon in normal and strabismic primate. (a) Normal: In a primate with normal eye alignment, the ODC representing the foveola (or 0° eccentricity) of the left eye (L) is immediately adjacent to the ODC representing the foveola of the right eye (R). The side-by-side arrangement of the "foveolar" ODCs in this case (white arrowheads) would be well within the range of horizontal connections needed to allow those ODCs to communicate for binocular fusion. (b) Micro-eso: In a primate with microesotropia, a neuron within a foveolar (at 0° eccentricity) ODC of the fixating eye can only span a distance in the visual field corresponding to an angle of strabismus of approximately 4 PD (dark arrowhead = ODC corresponding to pseudofovea position of deviated eye).

activity, why should the fallback position of visual cortex be set so predictably ~2–4° (~4–8 PD) of microesotropia? And if the heterotropia exceeds that range, why is fusional vergence typically absent?

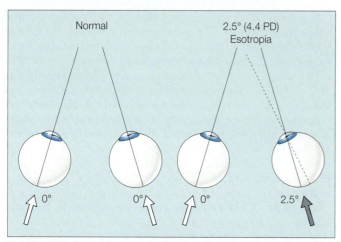

Fig. 76.8 Paradigmatic monofixator/microesotrope exhibits a deviation of the visual axes on cover testing of approximately 4 PD (2.3°), which in this case is shown as a right eye microesotropia. When fusional vergence or prism adaptation is tested in such a patient, the angle of deviation tends to persistently return to that 2.3° angle.

together could join receptive fields 5° or 8.7 PD apart. The conclusion that emerges is that the 4–8 PD "rule" of the monofixation syndrome is explicable as a combination of innate V_1 neuron size and V_1 topography. The visuomotor system of the strabismic primate appears to achieve subnormal, but stable binocular fusion so long as the angle of deviation is confined to a distance corresponding to not more than one to two V_1 neurons.[95]

Neuronal response properties of the vergence-related region of extrastriate visual cortex, MST, may also explain the 2.5° micro-esotropia rule in monofixation syndrome. MST receives down-stream projections from disparity-sensitive cells, both in V_1 and in MT. The majority of binocular neurons in V_1, MT, and MST encode absolute disparity.[78,96] Absolute disparity sensitivity (the location of an image on each retina with respect to the foveola, or 0° eccentricity) guides vergence, as opposed to relative disparity sensitivity (the location of an image in depth with respect to other images), which is necessary for stereopsis. The largest population of vergence-related neurons in MST of normal monkeys drives the eyes to ~2.5° of convergent (crossed) disparity.[78] (The next largest population encodes ~2.5° of divergence.) Normal primates have the strongest short-latency vergence responses to convergent disparities of ~2.5°.[97]

Insults that impair the development of binocular connections in immature V_1 would be expected to impair the (downstream) development of the entire population of binocular MST neurons. The probability of surviving an insult would be greatest for the most populous neurons: those encoding ~2.5° (~4.4 PD) of con-vergence. In the presence of a generally weakened pool of disparity-sensitive neurons, the vergence system may default to the vergence commanded by the surviving population. A 2.5° convergence angle could be kept stable (preventing deterioration to large angle strabismus) by the next most populous remaining neurons, those encoding 2.5° of divergence. These mechanisms are attractive because they can account for the direction, approximate magnitude, and stability of microesotropia, with retention of a capacity for fusional (e.g., prism) vergence responses evoked by disparities > 2.5°.

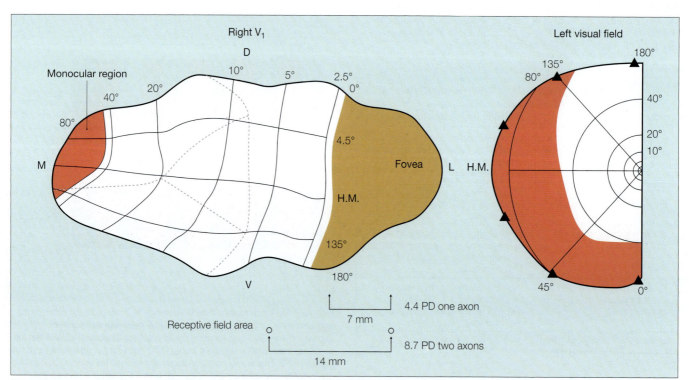

Fig. 76.9 Two-dimensional map representing V_1 from the right cerebral hemisphere (left visual hemi-field) of a microesotropic primate. The sulci and gyri have been unfolded and the visual field representation superimposed using standard retinotopic landmarks. One horizontal axon, originating within the foveal representation at 0°–1° eccentricity, could link to a receptive field shifted 2.5° or 4.4 PD distant. Two neurons strung together could join receptive fields 5° or 8.7 PD apart. The conclusion that emerges is that the 4–8 PD "rule" of monofixation/microesotropia syndrome is explicable as a combination of innate V_1 neuron size and V_1 topography. The visuomotor system of the strabismic primate appears to achieve subnormal, but stable binocular fusion so long as the angle of deviation is confined to a distance corresponding to not more than one to two V_1 neurons.

LESS COMMON FORMS OF CONCOMITANT STRABISMUS

Epidemiologic[1,7] and animal studies[98,99] indicate that the second most common type of strabismus in human and monkey is esotropia linked to accommodation, usually with hypermetropia (accommodative esotropia). Onset of the strabismus occurs at an average age ~3 years, well beyond the early infantile period of rapid maturation of the visuomotor pathways. The majority of children with this disorder regain binocular fusion when the refractive error (and any amblyopia) is corrected, and they do not exhibit the eye-tracking and gaze-holding deficits of infantile esotropia.[51,100] The strong implication is that cortical binocular connections in this disorder are substantially more abundant than those in children with infantile esotropia. A subtle deficit of binocular connections may be inconsequential until the system, normally biased toward convergence, is taxed by the accommodative demands of increasing hyperopia. (Most convergence-related neurons in the midbrain of normal primates encode both vergence and accommodation, with a range of different gains.)[101-103] Whether accommodative esotropia is intermittent or constant would likely depend on a multitude of idiosyncratic variables, e.g., the ratio of convergence to divergence neurons, the average gain of accommodation-linked convergence neurons, the strength of cortical neuron pools encoding corrective, uncrossed (divergent) disparity, the maturity of excitatory horizontal connections between V_1 ODCs mediating fusion, and the strength of inhibitory connections between V_1 ODCs mediating suppression (and loss of fusion). Invasive studies of strabismic nonhuman primates could unravel these competing possibilities.

Exotropia is 10 times less prevalent than esotropia, and the most common form is intermittent.[2,7] Unlike esotropia, exotropia does not have a bimodal distribution of age-of-onset. Onset typically occurs after infancy with slow progression of an exophoria to increasing epochs of exotropia, manifest when viewing distant, nonaccommodative targets. The magnitude of the exotropia tends to increase with age. When the eyes are aligned (exophoria), stereopsis thresholds are normal. Humans with typical, concomitant intermittent exotropia have no evidence of oculomotor nerve dysfunction, midbrain convergence paresis, orbital structural (e.g., pulley) anomaly, or extraocular myopathy.[104] The epidemiologic and clinical observations do not point to a single locus in the CNS that would provide a neural mechanism for the disorder, and laboratory studies of CNS function and structure in naturally exotropic monkeys is lacking (as in human, primary exotropia is much less common than esotropia).

The later onset and progression of the disorder imply that the neural defect promoting exodeviation is present at birth, but controlled (masked or kept subthreshold) by the convergence bias of the infantile visuomotor pathways. As binocularity matures the nasalward bias of these pathways recedes, and the exodrive gradually manifests. A full normal complement of excitatory horizontal connections between ODCs in V_1 would be expected, since stereopsis matured properly during infancy.

Normal V_1/MT/MST binocularity is also connoted by the relative robustness of fusional vergence when accommodation is engaged.

Normal primates have transient exodeviations when executing (superficially conjugate) saccadic eye movements.[105,106] The adducting eye lags the abducting eye, necessitating a pulse of short-latency fusional convergence at the end of a saccade. The saccade-related exodeviation in healthy primates appears to represent a "physiologic internuclear ophthalmoplegia," produced by a normal delay in conducting an adduction signal over inter-neurons, from the abducens nucleus of the pons to the medial rectus subnucleus of the midbrain. It is not known whether this behavior is exaggerated in concomitant exodeviation, which would implicate internuclear, versional gaze pathways. Concomitant exodeviation could also be promoted by other brainstem mechanisms, e.g., an abnormally low ratio of convergence to divergence neurons in the midbrain.

SUMMARY OF STRABISMUS NEUROSCIENCE KNOWLEDGE

- Proper alignment of the eyes requires information sharing (fusion) between monocular visual input channels (ODCs) in the CNS.
- The first locus for fusion in the CNS of primates is the striate cerebral cortex (area V_1).
- Fusion is achieved by excitatory binocular horizontal connections in V_1, which join ODCs of opposite ocularity.
- Fusion behaviors and V_1 binocular connections are immature at birth, maturing during a brief (critical) period in the first months of life.
- Maturation of fusion (and the V_1 binocular connections) requires correlated (synchronized) input from each eye.
- The dominant form of strabismus in primates (esotropia) first appears during the period of normal fusion maturation.
- The strabismus can be produced reliably in normal nonhuman primates by impeding the maturation of fusional connections in V_1.
- The strabismus occurs predominantly in humans who have perinatal insults that could directly or indirectly impair maturation of binocular connections in V_1.
- The strabismus and related maldevelopments of eye movement conform to innate, directional biases present in the neural pathways of normal primates before maturation of binocularity.
- Therapeutic interventions, applied during the brief period of normal binocular maturation, can achieve functional sensory and motor cures.
- If therapy cannot restore bifoveal fusion, subnormal fusion (monofixation) may be achieved within boundaries set by the properties of neurons in V_1 and extrastriate cortex.
- Later-onset forms of strabismus are easier to treat because the fusional connections in V_1 matured before the emergence of minor maldevelopments of vergence.

REFERENCES

1. Graham PA. Epidemiology of strabismus. Br J Ophthalmol 1974; 58: 224–31.
2. Lorenz B. Genetics of isolated and syndromic strabismus: Facts and perspectives. Strabismus 2002; 10: 147–56.
3. U.S. Department of Health, Education, and Welfare. Eye Examination Findings among Children. National Health Survey 1972; 11: 1–47.
4. Simons K, Reinecke RD. Amblyopia Screening and Stereopsis. Transactions of the New Orleans Academy of Ophthalmology. St. Louis: Mosby; 1978: 15–50.
5. Rubenstein R, Lohr K, Brook R, et al. Measurement of Physiological Health for Children, vol 4. Vision Impairments. Rand Health Insurance Experiment Series. Santa Monica: Rand Corporation; 1985.
6. Panel. SAaVP. Vision Research: A National Plan: U.S. Department of Health and Human Services; 1983–1987.
7. Crone F, Velzeboer C. Statistics on strabismus in the Amsterdam youth. Arch Ophthalmol 1956; 55: 455–70.
8. Kiorpes L, Boothe RG, Carlson MR, et al. Frequency of naturally occurring strabismus in monkeys. J Ped Ophthalmol Strabismus 1985; 22: 60–4.
9. Tamura EE, Hoyt CS. Oculomotor consequences of intraventricular hemorrhages in premature infants. Arch Ophthalmol 1987; 105: 533–5.
10. van Hof-van Duin J, Evenhuis-van Leunen A, Mohn G, et al. Effects of very low birth weight (VLBW) on visual development during the first year after term. Early Hum Dev 1989; 20: 255–66.
11. Pike MG, Holmström G, de Vries LS, et al. Patterns of visual impairment associated with lesions of the preterm infant brain. Dev Med Child Neurol 1994; 36: 849–62.
12. Hoyt CS. Visual function in the brain-damaged child. Eye 2003; 17: 371–86.
13. Hiles DA, Hoyme SH, McFarlane F. Down's syndrome and strabismus. Am Orthopt J 1974; 24: 63–8.
14. Shapiro MB, France TD. The ocular features of Down's syndrome. Am J Ophthalmol 1985; 99: 659–63.
15. Bailey P, von Bonin G. The Isocortex of Man. Urbana, IL: Univ Illinois Press; 1951.
16. Volpe JJ. Hypoxic-ischemic encephalopathy: neuropathology and pathogenesis. In: Neurology of the Newborn. Philadelphia: Saunders; 1987: 209–35. (Vol. 22.)
17. Tychsen L. Infantile esotropia: current neurophysiologic concepts. In: Rosenbaum AL, Santiago AP, editors. Clinical Strabismus Management. Philadelphia: Saunders; 1999: 117–38.
18. Noetzel MJ, Brunstrom JE. The vulnerable oligodendrocyte. Inflammatory observations on a cause of cerebral palsy. Neurology 2001; 56: 1254–5.
19. Huttenlocher P, de Courten C, Garey L, et al. Synaptogenesis in human visual cortex: evidence for synapse elimination during normal development. Neurosci Lett 1982; 33: 247–52.
20. Phelps M, Mazziotta J, Kuhl D, et al. Tomographic mapping of human cerebral metabolism: visual stimulation and deprivation. Neurology 1981; 31: 517–29.
21. Paul TO, Hardage LK. The heritability of strabismus. Ophthalmic Genet 1994; 15: 1–18.
22. Maumenee IH, Alston A, Mets MB, et al. Inheritance of congenital esotropia. Tr Am Ophth Soc 1986; 84: 85–93.
23. Archer SM, Sondhi N, Helveston EM. Strabismus in infancy. Ophthalmology 1989; 96: 133–7.
24. Birch E, Stager D, Wright K, et al. Pediatric Eye Disease Investigator Group. The natural history of infantile esotropia during the first six months of life. J AAPOS 1998; 2: 325–8.
25. Pediatric Eye Disease Investigator Group. Spontaneous resolution of early-onset esotropia: experience of the congenital esotropia observational study. Am J Ophthalmol 2002; 133: 109–18.
26. Fox R, Aslin RN, Shea SL, et al. Stereopsis in human infants. Science 1980; 207: 323–4.
27. Birch EE, Gwiazda J, Held R. Stereoacuity development for crossed and uncrossed disparities in human infants. Vision Res 1982; 22: 507–13.
28. Birch EE, Gwiazda J, Held R. The development of vergence does not account for the onset of stereopsis. Perception 1983; 12: 331–6.
29. Birch EE, Shimojo S, Held R. Preferential-looking assessment of fusion and stereopsis in infants aged 1 to 6 months. Invest Ophthalmol Vis Sci 1985; 26: 366–70.
30. Gwiazda J, Bauer J, Held R. Binocular function in human infants: correlation of stereoptic and fusion-rivalry discriminations. J Pediatr Ophthalmol Strabismus 1989; 26: 128–32.
31. Wattam-Bell J, Braddick O, Atkinson J, et al. Measures of infant binocularity in a group at risk for strabismus. Clin Vis Sci 1987; 4: 327–36.
32. Skarf B, Eizenman M, Katz LM, et al. A new VEP system for studying binocular single vision in human infants. J Pediatr Ophthalmol Strabismus 1993; 30: 237–42.
33. Birch EE, Petrig B. FPL and VEP measures of fusion, stereopsis and stereoacuity in normal infants. Vision Res 1996; 36: 1321–7.
34. Horwood AM. Maternal observations of ocular alignment in infants. J Pediatr Ophthalmol Strabismus 1993; 30: 100–5.
35. Horwood AM, Riddell PM. Can misalignments in typical infants be used as a model for infantile esotropia? Invest Ophthalmol Vis Sci 2004; 45: 714–20.
36. Aslin RN. Development of binocular fixation in human infants. In: Eye Movements: Cognition and Visual Perception. Hillsdale, NJ: Erlbaum; 1977: 31–51.
37. Aslin RN, Jackson RW. Accommodative-convergence in young infants: development of a synergistic sensory-motor system. Canad J Psychol/Rev Canad Psychol 1979; 33: 222–31.
38. Mellick A. Convergence. An investigation into the normal standards of age groups. Br J Ophthalmol 1949; 33: 725.
39. Tait EF. Fusional vergence. Am J Ophthalmol 1949; 32: 1223.
40. Norcia AM, Garcia H, Humphry R, et al. Anomalous motion VEPs in infants and in infantile esotropia. Invest Ophthalmol Vis Sci 1991; 32: 436–9.
41. Norcia AM. Abnormal motion processing and binocularity: Infantile esotropia as a model system for effects of early interruptions of binocularity. Eye 1996; 10: 259–65.
42. Brown RJ, Wilson JR, Norcia AM, et al. Development of directional motion symmetry in the monocular visually evoked potential of infant monkeys. Vision Res 1998; 38: 1253–63.
43. Birch EE, Fawcett S, Stager D. Co-development of VEP motion response and binocular vision in normal infants and infantile esotropes. Invest Ophthalmol Vis Sci 2000; 41: 1719–23.
44. Bosworth RG, Birch EE. Nasal-temporal asymmetries in motion sensitivity and motion VEPs in normal infants and patients with infantile esotropia. Am Assoc Pediatr Ophthalmol Strabismus Abst 2003; 38: 61.
45. Atkinson J. Development of optokinetic nystagmus in the human infant and monkey infant: an analogue to development in kittens. In: Freeman RD, editor. Developmental Neurobiology of Vision. New York: Plenum; 1979: 277–87.
46. Naegele JR, Held R. The postnatal development of monocular optokinetic nystagmus in infants. Vision Res 1982; 22: 341–6.
47. Jacobs M, Harris C, Taylor D. The Development of Eye Movements in Infancy, Update on Strabismus and Pediatric Ophthalmology, Vancouver, Canada. Boca Raton, FL: CRC Press; 1994.
48. Tychsen L. Critical periods for development of visual acuity, depth perception and eye tracking. In: Bailey DB Jr, Bruer JT, Symons FJ, editors. Critical Thinking about Critical Periods. National Center for Early Development and Learning, University of North Carolina at Chapel Hill. Baltimore: Brookes; 2001: 67–80.
49. Schor CM, Narayan V, Westall C. Postnatal development of optokinetic after nystagmus in human infants. Vision Res 1983; 23: 1643–7.
50. Schor CM, Levi DM. Disturbances of small-field horizontal and vertical optokinetic nystagmus in amblyopia. Invest Ophthalmol Vis Sci 1980; 19: 668–83.
51. Tychsen L, Hurtig RR, Scott WE. Pursuit is impaired but the vestibulo-ocular reflex is normal in infantile strabismus. Arch Ophthalmol 1985; 103: 536–9.
52. Tychsen L, Lisberger SG. Maldevelopment of visual motion processing in humans who had strabismus with onset in infancy. J Neurosci 1986; 6: 2495–508.
53. Tychsen L, Rastelli A, Steinman S, et al. Biases of motion perception revealed by reversing gratings in humans who had infantile-onset strabismus. Dev Med Child Neurol 1996; 38: 408–22.
54. Hubel DH, Wiesel TN. Ferrier lecture. Functional architecture of macaque monkey visual cortex. Proc R Soc London 1977; 198: 1–59.

55. Hubel DH. Exploration of the primary visual cortex, 1955–78. Nature 1982; 299: 515–24.

56. Tychsen L, Burkhalter A. Neuroanatomic abnormalities of primary visual cortex in macaque monkeys with infantile esotropia: preliminary results. J Pediatr Ophthalmol Strabismus 1995; 32: 323–8.

57. Tychsen L, Wong, AMF, Burkhalter A. Paucity of horizontal connections for binocular vision in V1 of naturally-strabismic macaques: cytochrome-oxidase compartment specificity. J Comp Neurol 2004; in press.

58. Poggio GF, Fischer B. Binocular interaction and depth sensitivity in striate and prestriate cortex of behaving rhesus monkey. J Neurophysiol 1977; 40: 1392–405.

59. Crawford ML, von Noorden GK. The effects of short-term experimental strabismus on the visual system in macaca mulatta. Invest Ophthalmol Vis Sci 1979; 18: 496–505.

60. Chino Y, Smith EL, Hatta S, et al. Suppressive binocular interactions in the primary visual cortex (V1) of infant rhesus monkeys. Washington, DC: Society for Neuroscience; 1996.

61. Chino YM, Smith EL III, Hatta S, et al. Postnatal development of binocular disparity sensitivity in neurons of the primate visual cortex. J Neurosci 1997; 17: 296–307.

62. Hatta S, Kumagami T, Qian J, et al. Nasotemporal directional bias of V1 neurons in young infant monkeys. Invest Ophthalmol Vis Sci 1998; 39: 2259–67.

63. Endo M, Kaas JH, Jain N, et al. Binocular cross-orientation suppression in the primary visual cortex (V1) of infant rhesus monkeys. Invest Ophthalmol Vis Sci 2000; 41: 4022–31.

64. Horton JC, Hocking DR. An adult-like pattern of ocular dominance columns in striate cortex of newborn monkeys prior to visual experience. J Neurosci 1996; 16: 1791–807.

65. Tychsen L, Burkhalter A. Nasotemporal asymmetries in V1: ocular dominance columns of infant, adult, and strabismic macaque monkeys. J Comp Neurol 1997; 388: 32–46.

66. Boothe RG, Dobson V, Teller DY. Postnatal development of vision in human and nonhuman primates. Ann Rev Neurosci 1985; 8:4 95–546.

67. Lowel S, Singer W. Selection of intrinsic horizontal connections in the visual cortex by correlated neuronal activity. Science 1992; 255: 209–12.

68. Trachtenberg JT, Stryker MP. Rapid anatomical plasticity of horizontal connections in the developing visual cortex. J Neurosci 2001; 28: 3476–82.

69. Wiesel TN. Postnatal development of the visual cortex and the influence of environment. Nature 1982; 299: 583–91.

70. Crawford MLJ, Smith EL III, Harwerth RS, et al. Stereoblind monkeys have few binocular neurons. Invest Ophthalmol Vis Sci 1984; 25: 779–81.

71. Crawford ML, Harwerth RS, Smith EL, et al. Loss of stereopsis in monkeys following prismatic binocular dissociation during infancy. Behav Brain Res 1996; 79: 207–18.

72. Wong AM, Foeller P, Bradley D, et al. Early versus delayed repair of infantile strabismus in macaque monkeys: I. Ocular motor effects. J AAPOS 2003; 7: 200–9.

73. Ungerleider LG, Desimone R. Cortical connections of visual area MT in the macaque. J Comp Neurol 1986; 248: 190–222.

74. Dürsteler MR, Wurtz RH, Newsome WT. Directional pursuit deficits following lesions of the foveal representation within the superior temporal sulcus of the macaque monkey. J Neurophysiol 1987; 57: 1262.

75. Dürsteler MR, Wurtz RH. Pursuit and optokinetic deficits following chemical lesions of cortical areas MT and MST. J Neurophysiol 1988; 60: 940–65.

76. Maunsell JH, Van Essen DC. Functional properties of neurons in middle temporal visual area of the macaque monkey. II. Binocular interactions and sensitivity to binocular disparity. J Neurophysiol 1983; 49: 1148–67.

77. Kawano K. Ocular tracking: behavior and neurophysiology. Curr Opin Neurobiol 1999; 9: 467–73.

78. Takemura A, Inoue Y, Kawano K, et al. Single-unit activity in cortical area MST associated with disparity-vergence eye movements: Evidence for population coding. J Neurophysiol 2001; 85: 2245–66.

79. Kiorpes L, Walton PJ, O'Keefe LP, et al. Effects of artificial early-onset strabismus on pursuit eye movements and on neuronal

80. responses in area MT of macaque monkeys. J Neurosci 1996; 16: 6537–53.

80. Tigges M, Tigges J, Fernandes A, et al. Postnatal axial eye elongation in normal and visually deprived rhesus monkeys. Invest. Ophthalmol Vis Sci 1990; 31: 1035–46.

81. Yildirim C, Tychsen L. Disjunctive optokinetic nystagmus in a naturally esotropic macaque monkey: Interactions between nasotemporal asymmetries of versional eye movement and convergence. Ophthalmic Res 2000; 32: 172–80.

82. Leigh RJ, Zee DS. The Neurology of Eye Movements. New York: Oxford University Press; 1999.

83. Worth C. Squint. Its Causes, Pathology, and Treatment. Philadelphia: Blakiston; 1903.

84. Chavasse F. Worth's Squint or the Binocular Reflexes and the Treatment of Strabismus. London: Bailliere Tindall and Cox; 1939.

85. Costenbader FD. Infantile esotropia. Tr Am Ophthal Soc 1961; 59: 397–429.

86. Ing M, Costenbader FD, Parks MM, et al. Early surgery for congenital esotropia. Am J Ophthalmol 1966; 61: 1419–27.

87. Wright KW, Edelman PM, McVey JH, et al. High-grade stereo acuity after early surgery for congenital esotropia. Arch Ophthalmol 1994; 112: 913–9.

88. Ing MR. Surgical alignment prior to six months of age for congenital esotropia. Trans Am Ophthalmol Soc 1995; 93: 135–46.

89. Birch EE, Stager DR, Everett ME. Random dot stereoacuity following surgical correction of infantile esotropia. J Pediatr Ophthalmol Strabismus 1995; 32: 231–5.

90. Birch EE, Fawcett S, Stager DR. Why does early surgical alignment improve stereopsis outcomes in infantile esotropia? J AAPOS 2000; 4: 10–4.

91. Tychsen L, Wong AM, Foeller P, et al. Early versus delayed repair of infantile strabismus in macaque monkeys: II. Effects on motion visual evoked potentials. Invest Ophthalmol Vis Sci 2004; 45: 821–7.

92. Lang J. Evaluation in Small Angle Strabismus or Microtopia, Strabism. Symp. Gieben. Basel: Karger; 1968.

93. Parks MM. The monofixation syndrome. Tr Am Ophth Soc 1969; 67: 609–57.

94. Tychsen L, Scott C. Maldevelopment of convergence eye movements in macaque monkeys with small and large-angle infantile esotropia. Invest Ophthalmol Vis Sci 2003; 44: 3358–68.

95. Wong AM, Lueder GT, Burkhalter A, et al. Anomalous retinal correspondence: neuroanatomic mechanism in strabismic monkeys and clinical findings in strabismic children. J AAPOS 1998; 4: 168–74.

96. Cumming BG, Parker AJ. Binocular neurons in V1 of awake monkeys are selective for absolute, not relative, disparity. J Neurosci 1999; 19: 5602–18.

97. Masson GS, Busettini C, Miles FA. Vergence eye movements in response to binocular disparity without depth perception. Nature 1997; 389: 283–6.

98. Quick MW, Eggers HM, Boothe RG. Natural strabismus in monkeys: convergence errors assessed by cover test and photographic methods. Invest Ophthalmol Vis Sci 1992; 33: 2986–3004.

99. Quick MW, Newbern JD, Boothe RG. Natural strabismus in monkeys: accommodative errors assessed by photorefraction and their relationship to convergence errors. Invest Ophthalmol Vis Sci 1994; 35: 4069–79.

100. Sokol S, Peli E, Moskowitz A, et al. Pursuit eye movements in late-onset esotropia. J Pediatr Ophthalmol Strabismus 1991; 28: 82–6.

101. Mays LE. Neural control of vergence eye movements: convergence and divergence neurons in midbrain. J Neurophysiol 1984; 51: 1091–108.

102. Judge SJ, Cumming BG. Neurons in the monkey midbrain with activity related to vergence eye movement and accommodation. J Neurophysiol 1986; 55: 915–29.

103. Mays LE, Gamlin PDR. Neuronal circuitry controlling the near response. Curr Opin Neurobiol 1995; 5: 763–8.

104. von Noorden GK. Binocular Vision and Ocular Motility: Theory and Management of Strabismus. St. Louis: Mosby; 1996.

105. Collewijn H, Erkelens CJ, Steinman RM. Binocular co-ordination of human horizontal saccadic eye movements. J Physiol 1988; 404: 157–82.

106. Erkelens CJ, Sloot OB. Initial directions and landing positions of binocular saccades. Vision Res 1995; 35: 3297–303.

107. O'Dell C, Boothe RG. The development of stereoacuity in infant rhesus monkeys. Vision Res 1997; 37: 2675–84.

108. Hainline L, Riddell PM. Binocular alignment and vergence in early infancy. Vision Res 1995; 35: 3229–36.

109. Riddell PM, Horwood AM, Houston SM, et al. The response to prism deviations in human infants. Curr Biol 1999; 9: 1050–2.

110. Hubel D, Wiesel T, LeVay S. Plasticity of ocular dominance columns in monkey striate cortex. Philos Trans R Soc London Ser B 1977; 278: 377–409.

111. LeVay S, Wiesel TN, Hubel DH. The development of ocular dominance columns in normal and visually deprived monkeys. J Comp Neurol 1980; 191: 1–51.

112. Horton JC, Hocking DR. Timing of the critical period for plasticity of ocular dominance columns in macaque striate cortex. J Neurosci 1997; 17: 3684–709.

113. Tychsen L, Yildirim C, Anteby I, et al. Macaque monkey as an ocular motor and neuroanatomic model of human infantile strabismus. In: Lennerstrand G, Ygge J, editors. Advances in Strabismus Research: Basic and Clinical Aspects. London: Portland Press; 2000: 103–19. (Wenner-Gren International Series, Vol. 78.)

114. Pasik T, Pasik P. Optokinetic nystagmus: an unlearned response altered by section of chiasma and corpus callosum in monkeys. Nature 1964; 203: 609–11.

115. Pasik P, Pasik T. Ocular movements in split-brain monkeys. Adv Neurol 1977; 18: 125–35.

116. Mays LE. Neurophysiological correlates of vergence eye movements. In: Schor CM, Ciuffreda KJ, editors. Vergence Eye Movements: Basic and Clinical Aspects. Boston: Butterworths; 1983: 649–70.

CHAPTER
77 The Anatomy of Strabismus

Joseph L Demer

An understanding of anatomy is essential to rational diagnosis and treatment of strabismus. Our understanding of the anatomy of the extraocular muscles (EOMs) was significantly clarified by imaging. This chapter reviews the anatomy of the EOMs and associated connective tissues, how anatomical abnormalities may be associated with strabismus, and how the anatomy of the EOMs has been clarified by imaging.

There are six oculorotatory muscles, functioning as antagonist pairs.[1] The medial rectus (MR) and lateral rectus (LR) muscles rotate the eye horizontally, with the MR accomplishing adduction and the LR accomplishing abduction. The superior rectus (SR) and inferior rectus (IR) muscles form a vertical antagonist pair, with the SR supraducting and the IR infraducting the globe. However, the vertical rectus EOMs have additional actions not strictly antagonistic, as detailed later. The superior oblique (SO) and inferior oblique (IO) muscles form an antagonist pair essential for ocular torsion around the line of sight. The SO accomplishes intorsion, while the IO accomplishes extorsion. The oblique EOMs have additional actions also not strictly antagonistic, as detailed later.

STRUCTURES OF THE EXTRAOCULAR MUSCLES

Laminar structure

The oculorotatory EOMs, but not the lid-elevating levator palpebrae superioris (LPS), consist of two distinct layers subserving distinct functions[2] (Fig. 77.1). The global layer (GL), containing a maximum of approximately 10,000-15,000 fibers in the mid-length of the EOM, is located adjacent to the globe in rectus EOMs and in the central core of the oblique EOMs.[3] In the rectus EOMs and the SO, the GL anteriorly becomes contiguous with the terminal tendon and inserts on the sclera.[4] In the IO, the GL inserts directly on the sclera without a tendon. The orbital layer (OL) of each rectus EOM contains 40-60% of all the EOM's fibers. This percentage varies according to the specific EOM, greatest for the MR and least for the SR. The OL does not insert on the eyeball, but instead inserts on connective tissue pulleys. The OL is located on the orbital surface of the rectus EOM, sometimes forming a C-shaped configuration, and constitutes the concentric outer layer of the oblique EOMs. For the GL of rectus EOMs, the maximum number of fibers is in mid-orbit, with the number of fibers diminishing anteriorly and posteriorly.[3]

The OL of each EOM contains two muscle fiber types.[2] About 80% of fibers in the orbital layer of each EOM are fast, twitch-generating, singly innervated fibers (SIFs) resembling mammalian skeletal muscle fibers, while 20% are multiply innervated fibers (MIFs) that either do not conduct action potentials or do so only

in their central portions.[2] Orbital SIFs are relatively small in diameter and contain abundant mitochondria. The metabolism and blood supply of orbital SIFs are tailored to their unique mechanical loading and nearly continuous activity. Orbital SIFs are specialized for intense oxidative metabolism and fatigue resistance.[2] The vascular supply in the OL is higher than that in the GL.[5] Orbital SIFs express unique myosin isoforms, perhaps related to the requirements of fast twitch capability against

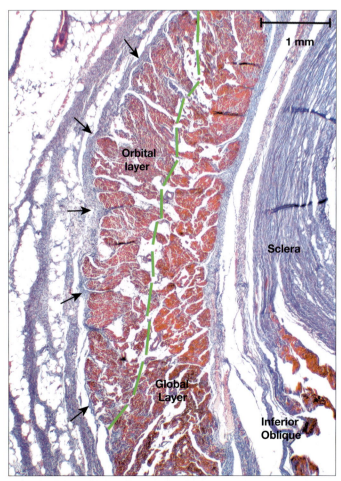

Fig. 77.1 Transverse histological section of 17-month-old human lateral rectus (LR) muscle stained with Masson's trichrome showing the smaller, darker red staining fibers of the orbital layer (OL) to the left of the larger, brighter red staining fibers of the global layer at right. Note insertion of the OL fibers into the dense blue-staining collagen of the LR pulley (arrows). The inferior oblique muscle insertion into the blue-staining collagen of the sclera is seen at lower right.

continuous loading.[6] The relatively sparse and primitive orbital MIFs probably play a proprioceptive role. These MIFs either do not conduct action potentials or do so only in their central portions and not near their origins or insertions.

The GL contains one type of MIF and three designated types of SIFs that really represent a continuum distinguished by their mitochondrial density. The largest and most granular SIF is very similar to the orbital SIF, having almost as many mitochondria, while the other two SIFs have correspondingly fewer mitochondria. Global MIFs are still smaller, contain fewer mitochondria, and correspond to the orbital MIFs. No spindles are present in the GL, but the anterior tendonous termination of the GL of rectus EOMs contains palisade endings. Palisade endings are distributed along the width of each rectus tendon near the insertion, and presumably act as proprioceptive organs.

Extraocular muscles generate force through the interaction of the proteins actin and myosin. Various myosin isoforms are found in EOMs, with the predominant one in orbital SIFs, EOM-specific myosin, occurring only in EOMs.[2] Myosin isoforms vary along the length of individual EOM fibers. Neonatal and embryonic myosin isoforms persist throughout adult life at the anterior and posterior ends of SIFs. This persistence of immature myosins may be related to the capability of EOMs to adjust their total number of sarcomeres. Differences in myosin expression may underlie the susceptibility of the EOMs to disorders such as thyroid ophthalmopathy, as well as their resistance to other disorders such as muscular dystrophy.[7]

Gross structure

The rectus EOMs originate in the orbital apex from the annulus of Zinn, a fibrous ring surrounding the optic nerve. The SO muscle originates from the periorbita of the supranasal orbital wall slightly more anteriorly. The rectus EOMs course anteriorly through loose lobules of orbital fat without mechanical constraint on their paths until they enter their connective tissue pulleys that form sheaths as the EOMs penetrate posterior Tenon's fascia. There is no "muscle cone" of connective tissue forming bridges among the adjacent rectus EOM bellies in the mid- to deep orbit. The SO muscle remains tethered to the periorbita via connective tissues as it courses anteriorly and thins to become continuous with its long, thin tendon. The concentric OL of the SO terminates posterior on a peripherally located sheath. Both the SO sheath and tendon pass through the trochlea, a cartilaginous rigid pulley attached to the supranasal orbital wall. The trochlea typically calcifies in older people. After reflection in the trochlea, the SO tendon passes beneath the SR, thins, and flattens as it spreads out to its broad scleral insertion posterolaterally on the globe. The IO muscle originates much more anteriorly from the periorbita of the inferonasal orbital rim adjacent to the anterior lacrimal crest, and runs laterally to enter its connective tissue pulley immediately inferior to the IR at the point the IO penetrates Tenon's fascia.

The long axes of the bony orbits are angled about 23° laterally from the mid-sagittal plane. The general configuration of the rectus EOMs and the SO is conical. As they continue anteriorly, the rectus EOMs thin to become strap-like bands about 10 mm wide, and ultimately their GLs become continuous with tendons that insert on the globe.

A fundamental, yet recent, insight is that the rectus EOMs do not follow straight-line paths from their origins to their scleral

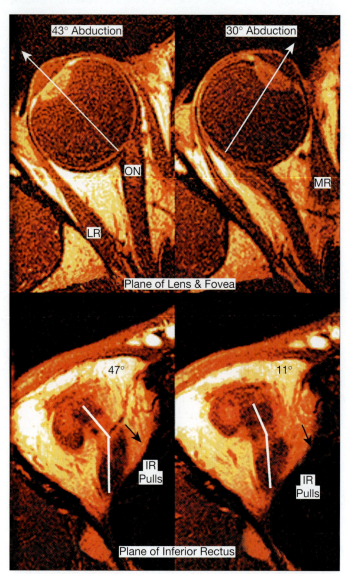

Fig. 77.2 Axial MRI scans (2 mm thickness, T_1 weighted) of a right orbit taken at the level of the lens, fovea, and optic nerve (top row), and simultaneously along the path of the inferior rectus (IR) muscle (bottom row), in abduction (left column) and adduction (right column). Note the bisegmental IR path. For this 73° horizontal gaze shift, there was a corresponding 36° shift in IR muscle path anterior to the inflection at its pulley. This is a direct demonstration of half-angle shift of IR pulling direction with ocular duction.

insertions despite the implications of many textbooks. In eccentric gaze, rectus EOM paths are inflected sharply at discrete points in the anterior orbit (Fig. 77.2). Even in the 19th century it was supposed that inflections in EOM paths might be due to orbital connective tissues acting as pulleys.[8,9] The pulleys cause the anterior paths of the rectus EOMs, and thus their pulling directions, to change in an orderly way as the eye changes position.[10,11] This is shown in the axial magnetic resonance images (MRI) in Fig. 77.2, illustrating that the anterior path of the IR muscle changes by half the change in angle of duction. MRI has shown the same behavior for all the rectus EOMs. In general, the anterior path of a rectus EOM changes in the same qualitative direction as ocular duction, but by quantitatively half as much.[12]

THE PULLEYS

Structural anatomy

The points of rectus EOM inflection in the anterior orbit constitute the functional, mechanical pulleys, whose structure will be described in detail later. Anterior to the pulleys, rectus EOM paths follow the scleral insertions in eccentric gaze. The pulleys thus act as functional, mechanical origins of the rectus EOMs. The line segment between the scleral insertion and the pulley thus defines the pulling direction of each EOM, and profoundly influences EOM action. Pulleys consist of discrete rings of dense collagen encircling the EOM and about 2 mm in length, coaxial with less substantial collagenous sleeves around the EOMs (Fig. 77.3). Anteriorly, these sleeves thin to form slings convex to the orbital wall, and more posteriorly the sleeves thin to form slings convex toward the orbital center. The anterior pulley slings have also been called the "intermuscular septum," a time-honored but relatively vague term that may be supplanted by more specific terminology. Electron microscopy demonstrates the fibrils of pulley collagen in the pulleys to have a crisscrossed configuration suited to high internal rigidity.[13] Elastic fibers in and around pulleys[14] provide reversible extensibility, a spring-like memory. Reversible extensibility, particularly in connective tissue bands that connect the pulleys to bony anchors on the orbital rim, means that the pulleys are suspended under elastic tension that draws them anteriorly. There are bands of smooth muscle in the pulley suspensions, and particularly in a distribution called the inframedial peribulbar muscle between the MR and IR pulleys.[15] The overall structure of the orbital connective tissues is schematized in Fig. 77.4.

The IR pulley is unusual in that it is intimately coupled with the pulley of the IO in a bond that forms part of Lockwood's ligament, the connective tissue "hammock" across the inferior orbit upon which the classical anatomists supposed the globe to be suspended.[15,16] In fact, the pulleys of the IR and IO are formed of a common sheath of collagen stiffened by a heavy elastin deposit at their point of crossing, one that coincides with

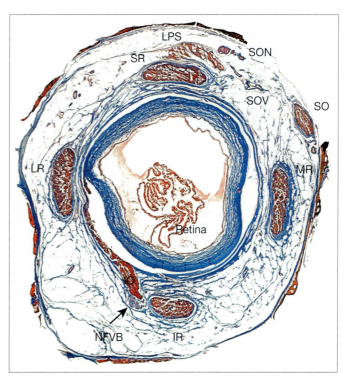

Fig. 77.3 Quasicoronal (perpendicular to orbital axis) histological section of 17-month-old whole human orbit stained with Masson's trichrome showing encirclement of the inferior rectus (IR), lateral rectus (LR), medial rectus (MR), and superior rectus (SR) muscles by the dense, blue-staining collagenous rings of their pulleys. The main part of the inferior oblique (IO) pulley is slightly anterior to this section, but can be seen in part as a dense collagenous mass adjacent the muscle belly and its neurofibrovascular bundle (NFVB). The retina is detached as a postmortem artifact. LPS, levator palpebrae superioris muscle; SO, superior oblique muscle; SON, supraorbital nerve; SOV, superior orbital vein.

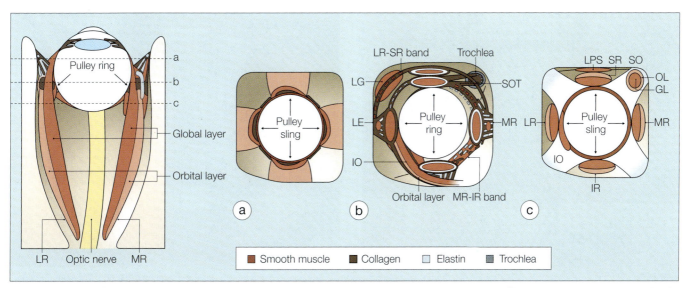

Fig. 77.4 Schematic of orbital connective tissues. Coronal views are depicted at three levels from the axial view. The functional pulleys are at the level depicted at lower right. Tissue composition is color coded as shown at right. GL, global layer; IO, inferior oblique muscle; IR, inferior rectus muscle; LG, lacrimal gland; LE, lateral enthesis, the attachment of the pulley suspension to the orbital wall; LPS, levator palpebrae superioris muscle; LR, lateral rectus muscle; ME, medial enthesis, the attachment of the pulley suspension to the orbital wall; MR, medial rectus muscle; SO, superior oblique muscle; SOT, superior oblique tendon; SR, superior rectus muscle.

Lockwood's ligament. The OL of the IR inserts on its pulley and does not continue anteriorly. The OL of the IO muscle inserts partly on the conjoined IO–IR pulleys, partly on the sheath of the IO muscle temporally and partly on the inferior aspect of the LR pulley. Smooth muscle and elastin are present in the Lockwood's ligament region of posterior Tenon's fascia supporting the combined IR–IO pulley. The inframedial peribulbar muscle has its inferior insertion of the nasal aspect of this conjoint pulley, and is positioned upon contraction to displace the pulley nasally. Inferior oblique contraction in elevation displaces the conjoint IR–IO pulley and the LR pulley inferiorly.[10] The smooth muscle retractors of the lower eyelid ("Muller's inferior tarsal muscle") and connective tissues extending to the inferior tarsus are also anatomically coupled to the conjoint IR–IO pulley, an arrangement that coordinates lower eyelid position with vertical eye position during infraduction.

Although the rigid SO pulley–the trochlea–has been known since antiquity, it is actually unusual in that the trochlea is immobile, and that the SO's OL inserts via the SO sheath on the medial aspect of the SR pulley.[10] The SO pulling direction changes half as much as ocular duction despite an immobile pulley, because of the uniquely broad, thin insertion of the SO tendon as it wraps over the globe.

Most of these anatomical relationships can be demonstrated in gross dissections and in surgical exposures. Following typical conjunctival incision and engagement of a rectus EOM on a surgical hook, the white anterior pulley slings come immediately into view (Fig. 77.5a). These tissues play little role in constraining EOM paths, although they are related to the more posterior pulley rings. The anterior pulley slings can, with the occasional exception of the lateral levator aponeurosis at the superior border of the LR, be posteriorly displaced by blunt dissection, with sharp dissection only occasionally necessary. After this posterior displacement, fine fibrous bands of the OL insertion on the glistening white pulley suspension can be seen (Fig. 77.5a). This insertion site is intimately related to the mechanically effective site of the pulley, the connective tissue

ring, which is slightly posterior but obscured by the overlying white tissue of Tenon's capsule. After transposition of a rectus tendon (for the treatment of, for example, LR palsy), the path of the transposed EOM continues to be toward the original pulley location (Fig. 77.5b). The clinical effect of rectus transposition can be improved by suture fixation from a posterior point on the transposed EOM belly to the sclera adjacent the palsied EOM,[17] which can be shown by MRI to displace the pulley further in the transposed direction.[18]

Functional anatomy

The insertion of each rectus EOM's OL on its pulley translates (linearly moves) that pulley posteriorly during EOM contraction. Direct evidence for this can be seen in the axial, contrast-enhanced MRI scans in Fig. 77.6, which demonstrate the tissues of the MR pulley. The pulley tissues appear to move in precise coordination with the insertion and underlying sclera, although histological examinations show the absence of direct connections between these tissues. Quantitative evidence of the amount of pulley shift during ocular duction is obtained from coronal MRI scans showing changes in the anteroposterior position of the inflections in rectus EOM paths in tertiary gaze positions.[12] These data have confirmed that all four rectus pulleys move anteroposteriorly in coordination with their scleral insertions, by the same anteroposterior amounts.

Being partially coupled to the mobile IR pulley, the IO pulley shifts anteriorly in supraduction, and posteriorly in infraduction This shift is easily seen from the change in the IO muscle's path on MRI in the quasi-sagittal plane parallel to the long axis of the orbit as in Fig. 77.7, which also shows the anteroposterior shift of the IO pulley is much less than that of the limbus and the underlying sclera. Quantitative analysis of MRI scans shows that the IO pulley moves by almost precisely half as much as the IR insertion,[16] an amount necessary to optimal control of the IO's pulling direction.

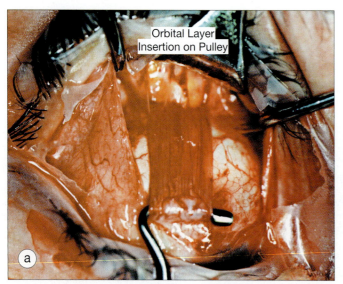

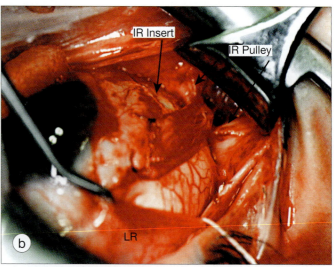

Fig. 77.5 Surgical exposure of right inferior rectus (IR) region, as seen from above the patient, using incision at the conjunctival limbus. The lateral rectus (LR) of this patient was palsied; MRI showed that the deep LR belly was markedly atrophic. (a) Inferior rectus muscle, engaged on hook, courses posteriorly into the glistening white tissue of the IR pulley. Note fine connective tissue bands marking the anterior part of the orbital layer insertion into the pulley. (b) The IR tendon has been disinserted from the sclera, leaving a white line at the original insertion site. The IR tendon has been transposed temporally to adjoin the inferior pole of the insertion of the paralyzed LR muscle. Note the diagonal path of the transposed IR toward the original location of the IR pulley, now more visible as a discrete structure.

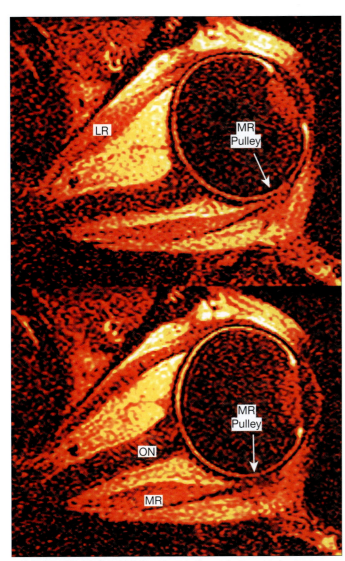

Fig. 77.6 Gadodiamide contrast-enhanced axial MRI scans of a right orbit in central gaze and in abduction. Note that the medial rectus (MR) pulley moves anteriorly in abduction by the same amount as the MR insertion. LR, lateral rectus muscle; ON, optic nerve.

The SR pulley is closely related to the pulley of the LPS muscle, located superior to it. The LPS pulley is a collagenous ring suspended in the superior orbit by Whitnall's ligament and stiffened by a modest amount of elastin and smooth muscle, and it is also closely coupled to the adjacent SR pulley. Not being an oculorotary muscle, the LPS lacks an OL. The LPS has only a GL that passes through its pulley to insert on the anterior border of the collagenous tarsal plate. The LPS pulley inflects the horizontal direction of the muscle belly to the required vertical motion of the upper eyelid. Posterior motion of the LPS pulley during elevation is achieved by that pulley's intimate mechanical coupling to the SR pulley, which is actively translated posteriorly by its insertion from the contracting SR orbital layer. This arrangement tends mechanically to coordinate upper eyelid position with vertical eye position.

The SR pulley also has discrete mechanical couplings to other pulleys.[19] The most prominent such coupling is a dense band extending from the lateral border of the conjoint SR/LPS pulley to the superior border of the LR pulley. This band contains dense collagen and elastin throughout, and divides the orbital lobe of the lacrimal gland.

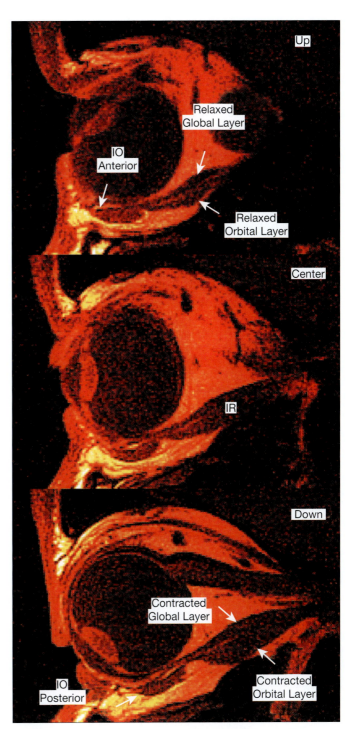

Fig. 77.7 Quasisagittal (parallel to the orbital axis) MRI images (2 mm thickness, T_1 weighted) of orbit in three gaze positions. Note demarcation of the orbital and global layers of the inferior rectus (IR) muscle by a thin, bright, fatty septum. The global layer, in continuity with the scleral insertion, exhibits modest contractile thickening in infraduction. The orbital layer, terminating in the IR pulley (not directly seen), exhibits marked contractile thickening in infraduction. The inferior oblique (IO) muscle shifts posteriorly with infraduction, but only half as far as the lens and other ocular structures. ON, optic nerve.

Although the rectus and IO pulleys are quite mobile along the axes of their respective EOMs, rectus pulleys are located stably and stereotypically in the planes transverse to their long axes. Since the EOMs must pass through their pulleys and the pulleys immediately encircle the EOMs, pulley locations may be inferred from the paths of the EOMs even if the imaging techniques cannot directly show the pulleys. The longitudinal locations of pulleys can be measured by imaging EOM path inflections produced by the pulleys in eccentric gaze positions. In describing pulley location, a coordinate reference system must be clearly understood.

Table 77.1 specifies the coordinates of the rectus pulleys determined by MRI and averaged over 11 normal young adults in a coordinate system originating in the center of the globe, horizontally and torsionally aligned to the interhemispheric fissure of the brain, and vertically aligned to place the MR path in the horizontal plane.[20] (Different numerical results would be obtained using different coordinate systems, markedly so if one were to use a surgically intuitive coordinate system rotationally referenced to globe structures such as the limbus and rectus insertions. Note that the 95% confidence intervals for the horizontal and vertical coordinates of normal rectus pulleys range over less than ± 0.6 mm.[20] This precise placement of rectus pulleys is important since the pulleys serve as the functional mechanical origins of the EOMs, with the rectus pulleys located much closer to globe center than the structural EOM origins in the annulus of Zinn. Aging causes inferior sagging of the horizontal rectus pulley positions, which shift downward by 1–2 mm from young adulthood to the seventh decade.[21] Vertical rectus pulley positions change little.[21]

The globe itself makes translations–linear shifts of its center–during ocular ductions, as determined by high-resolution MRI in normal humans.[21] It translates 0.8 mm inferiorly from 22° infraduction to 22° supraduction, and it also translates slightly nasally in both ab- and adduction (Table 77.2). Although small, these translations do affect the directions of EOM force since the globe center is only 8 mm anterior to the plane of the rectus pulleys.

The pulleys prevent EOM sideslip during globe rotations, but the rectus pulleys do shift transversely under certain physiologic conditions. Changes in rectus pulley positions with gaze have been determined by tracing rectus EOM paths with coronal MRI using a coordinate system relative to the center of the bony orbit.[22] The MR pulley translates 0.6 mm superiorly from 22° infraduction to 22° supraduction. In contrast, due to the insertion upon it of the OL of the IR muscle, the LR pulley translates 1.5 mm inferiorly from infraduction to supraduction. The IR pulley, due to the insertion upon it of the OL of the IO muscle, is drawn 1.1 mm medially by IO contraction in supraduction, but moves 1.3 mm temporally during IO relaxation in infraduction. The SR pulley is relatively stable in the mediolateral direction for

which it is well supported by connective tissue bands and Whitnall's ligament running nasotemporally,[19] but moves inferiorly in supraduction as it is posteriorly displaced by the SR OL, and superiorly in infraduction as the SR OL relaxes. The gaze-related shifts in rectus pulley positions are uniform among normal people (Table 77.3). These shifts are small so they do not produce clinically detectable misdirection of rectus EOM forces. However, recordings made using binocular magnetic search coils confirm a 1°–2° vertical skew misalignment in extreme tertiary gaze positions predicted to result from the differing vertical shifts of the horizontal rectus pulleys in normal people.[10]

Kinematics

Joel M Miller first suggested that orbitally fixed pulleys would make the eye's rotational axis dependent on eye position.[23] Subsequent findings have confirmed that rectus pulleys are fundamental to ocular kinematics, the rotational properties of the eye. Successive rotations of any solid object are not mathematically commutative, so that final eye orientation depends on

Table 77.1 Rectus pulley locations (mm from globe center)

	Lateral	Superior	Anterior
Medial rectus	−14.2 ± 0.2	−0.3 ± 0.3	−3 ± 2
Lateral rectus	10.1 ± 0.1	−0.3 ± 0.2	−9 ± 2
Superior rectus	−1.7 ± 0.3	11.8 ± 0.2	−7 ± 2
Inferior rectus	−4.3 ± 0.2	−12.9 ± 0.1	−6 ± 2

Rectus pulley positions averaged over 11 normal young adults. For lateral and superior positions, error limits represent 95% confidence intervals. For anteroposterior position, the error limits represent the MRI image plane thickness (2 mm). Data from Clark et al.[20]

Table 77.2 Globe translation in orbit (mm)

	Lateral	Superior
Supraduction	−0.1	−0.3
Infraduction	−0.4	0.5
Abduction	−0.2	0.1
Adduction	−0.7	0.0

Data of Clark et al. from 11 normal young adults.[20]

Table 77.3 Positions and duction-related shifts of rectus pulleys (mm from orbital center)

Rectus pulley	Central gaze		Supraduction change		Infraduction change		Abduction change		Adduction change	
	Horizontal	Vertical	Medial	Superior	Medial	Superior	Medial	Superior	Medial	Superior
Medial	12.1 ± 0.4	0.1 ± 0.7	0.1 ± 0.3	0.3 ± 0.4	0.1 ± 0.3	−0.3 ± 0.2	0.4 ± 0.7	0.0 ± 0.2	−0.3 ± 0.4	0.0 ± 0.2
Superior	−1.4 ± 0.3	12.3 ± 0.5	1.0 ± 0.7	−1.6 ± 0.7	0.4 ± 0.6	1.0 ± 0.9	0.2 ± 0.5	0.8 ± 0.4	0.4 ± 0.5	0.1 ± 0.4
Lateral	−11.7 ± 0.3	−0.8 ± 0.4	0.0 ± 0.1	−0.7 ± 0.4	0.0 ± 0.2	0.8 ± 0.7	0.0 ± 0.4	1.0 ± 0.8	−0.5 ± 0.3	−0.5 ± 0.5
Inferior	1.7 ± 0.6	−12.3 ± 0.5	1.1 ± 0.3	−1.0 ± 0.3	−1.3 ± 0.3	1.3 ± 0.3	0.2 ± 0.3	−0.2 ± 0.1	−0.2 ± 0.5	−0.1 ± 0.3

Horizontal and vertical coordinates, relative to orbital center, of rectus EOMs in quasicoronal MRI imaging plane close to the anteroposterior location of the rectus pulleys in central gaze. Data averaged from 10 normal orbits. Errors represent 95% confidence intervals. Data from Clark et al.[22]

the order of rotations.[24] Each combination of horizontal and vertical orientations of an arbitrary sphere could be associated with infinitely many torsional positions,[25] but the eye is constrained (when the head is upright and immobile) by Listing's law: the torsion of the eye in any gaze direction is that which it would have if it had reached that gaze direction by a single rotation from primary eye position about an axis lying in a plane.[26] Listing's law is always satisfied if the ocular rotational axis shifts by exactly half of the shift in ocular duction.[27] For example, if the eye supraducts by 20°, then the vertical axis about which it rotates for subsequent horizontal movement should tip back by 10°. This is called the "half-angle rule." Conformity to the half-angle rule makes the sequence of ocular rotations appear effectively commutative to motor control centers in the brain.[28] This commutativity is the critical feature of the pulley system.

Simple geometric analysis illustrates how appropriate rectus pulley position can implement the half-angle kinematics required by Listing's law. In Fig. 77.8a it is seen from simple small-angle trigonometry that the EOMs pulling direction will tilt posteriorly by half the angle of supraduction if the pulley is located as far posterior to globe center as the insertion is anterior to globe center. This arrangement compels the EOM to exhibit half-angle kinematics consistent with Listing's law. All four rectus EOMs behave identically.[12] Since the rotational axis of each EOM force rotating the globe observes half-angle kinematics, overall ocular rotation conforms to Listing's law.

If primary and secondary gaze positions were the only ones ever required, the rectus pulleys could be rigidly fixed to the orbit in the proper positions. However, tertiary gaze positions such as adducted supraduction require the rectus pulleys actively to shift anteroposteriorly in the orbit along the EOM's length, so that the relationship is maintained in an oculocentric reference (Figs. 77.8c and 77.8d). The *active pulley hypothesis* (APH) states that these shifts are generated by the contractile activity of the OLs of each muscle acting against the elasticity of the pulley suspensions.[1,4,12,29]

Under coordinated control, the rectus pulleys shift anteroposteriorly in the orbit by the same distance as the scleral insertions, while remaining generally stable transversely. Coordinated control could not be the trivial consequence of simple attachment of rectus pulleys to the underlying sclera. Not only does evidence from serially sectioned orbits prove there is no such attachment, but the sclera moves freely relative to pulleys in a direction transverse to the longitudinal EOM axes. Further, anteroposterior rectus pulley movements persist even after enucleation,[30] when the MR path inflection at its pulley continues to shift anteroposteriorly with horizontal gaze of the fellow eye, but the angle of inflection sharpens to as much as 90° at the pulley![30]

Despite coordinated movements, however, ocular rotation by the OL and pulley translation by the GL require different EOM actions and neural commands. The mechanical load on the GL is predominantly the viscosity of the relaxing antagonist EOM, a load proportional to the speed of eye rotation, and slight during sustained eccentric gaze.[31] The mechanical load on the OL, however, is due to the elasticity of the pulley suspension, which is independent of rotational speed, but proportional to the angle of eccentric gaze. Selective electromyography (EMG) in humans shows high, phasic activity in the GL during rapid saccadic eye movements, with only a small sustained change in activity in sustained eccentric gaze.[31] In the OL, EMG shows sustained, high activity in eccentric gaze, but no phasic activity during saccades. Differing mechanical loads on the OL and GL are associated with the corresponding biological specializations of the two layers. The motor nerve arborization for the OL is distinct from that of the GL for all four human rectus EOMs.[32] The ratio of motor axons to EOM fibers is very low in the GL, averaging about one for each human rectus EOM,[32] reflecting the high precision required of ocular rotation. This ratio is higher in the OL, averaging five fibers per axon in horizontal rectus and 2.5 in vertical rectus EOMs.[32] The higher ratio in the OL probably reflects less required precision for pulley control.

The rectus EOMs by themselves seem capable of implementing all the eye movements that conform to Listing's law.[33] However, some important eye movements do not conform to Listing's law. Violations of Listing's law are observed during the vestibulo-ocular reflex (VOR)[34] and during convergence.[35] These violations involve the oblique EOMs.

Considered by itself, the IO muscle also observes half-angle kinematics. For example, as noted above, the IO pulley shifts by half of vertical ocular duction.[16] Although the kinematics are complex, this causes the IO's rotational axis to shift by half of vertical ocular duction, too.[16] Microscopic examination of human and monkey orbits indicates that the IO OL inserts on the IR and LR pulleys.[16] In primary position these two OL insertions constrain the distal IO to lie in the same plane as the IR and LR pulleys, so that IO rotational axis is perpendicular to the primary gaze line, and perpendicular to the rotational axes of the rectus EOMs. In the Listing's coordinate system of the pulleys, this

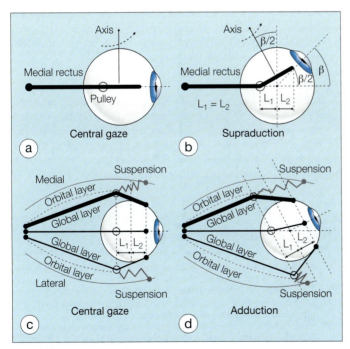

Fig. 77.8 Relationship of pulleys to the rotational axis of horizontal rectus muscles. (a) The medial rectus muscle's rotational axis is perpendicular to the segment between the pulley and the scleral insertion, and is thus vertical in central gaze. (b) In supraduction of angle β, the distance L_1 from the pulley (ring) to globe center is equal to distance L_2 from globe center to the insertion. This causes the medial rectus's rotational axis to tilt posteriorly by approximately angle β/2, the half-angle rule to implement Listing's law. (c) Axial view showing pulleys (depicted as rings) of the horizontal rectus muscles in central gaze. (d) In adduction, the contracting medial rectus orbital layer shifts its pulley posteriorly, while the relaxing lateral rectus orbital layer allows its pulley to move anteriorly.

gives the IO a purely torsional action, capable of nothing other than violating Listing's law. (In other coordinate systems, particularly the coordinate system employed for clinical examination, the IO also exhibits the familiar supraducting and abducting actions.) With oblique gaze shift from supraducted adduction to infraducted abduction, the IO pulley moves anteroposteriorly by half the amount of the coordinated movements of the IR pulley and scleral insertion.[16] Anteroposterior shift of the IO pulley during vertical and horizontal ductions fulfills the kinematic requirements of commutativity, albeit without direct contribution to Listing's law.

The SO, with its immobile pulley at the trochlea, is the exceptional case. The broad, thin SO insertion on the sclera resists sideslip by virtue of its shape. The SO approximates half-angle kinematics because the distance from trochlea to globe center is approximately equal to the distance from globe center to insertion, so that the SO rotational axis shifts by half the horizontal duction.

Stereopsis requires torsional rotations of the eyes to align corresponding retinal meridia.[36] Excyclotorsion occurs in convergence that violates Listing's law.[37] During asymmetrical convergence to a target aligned to one eye, this extorsion occurs in both the aligned and converging eyes, independent of eye position.[35] A form of Herring's law of equal innervation probably exists for the vergence system, such that both eyes receive symmetric version commands for remote targets, and mirror symmetric vergence commands for near targets.[38]

MRI during 22° convergence to a target aligned to one eye can be performed using mirrors.[39] This asymmetrical convergence allows the effect of convergence to be distinguished from the effect of simple adduction. In the orbit aligned to the target, analysis of IR, MR, and SR muscle paths demonstrated a 0.3- to 0.4-mm extorsional shift of the their pulleys in the coronal plane.[39] Although the lacrimal gland prevented determination of LR pulley location, it is likely that all four rectus pulleys shifted extorsionally about 1.9°. This amount is similar to globe extorsion under these conditions.[40] These findings suggest that during convergence, the rectus pulley array rotates in the coronal plane in coordination with ocular torsion, changing the pulling directions of all of the rectus EOMs without altering their fundamental half-angle kinematics that make the sequence of ocular ductions commutative.

Orbital microanatomy suggests the mechanism for rectus pulley shift in convergence. The OL of the IO muscle inserts on the IR pulley and, at least in younger specimens, also on the LR pulley.[16] Contraction of the IO OL would directly produce an extorsional shift of the LR and IR pulleys, and corresponding IO contraction has been directly demonstrated by MRI during convergence.[39] Inferior LR pulley shift could be coupled to lateral SR pulley shift via the dense connective tissue band between them.[19] The OL of the SO muscle inserts on the SO sheath posterior to the trochlea, with both the tendon and sheath reflected at that rigid pulley. Anterior to the trochlea, the SO sheath inserts on the SR pulley's nasal border. Although not directly demonstrated by MRI, relaxation of the SO OL during convergence is consistent with single unit recordings in the monkey trochlear nucleus,[41] and could contribute to extorsional shift of the pulley array. The inframedial peribulbar smooth muscle might also contribute to rectus pulley extorsion in convergence.[15]

The normal ocular counter-rolling response is actually a torsional VOR responsive to changes in the orientation of the head relative to gravity, as sensed by the otolith organs in the inner ear. Since ocular counter-rolling can change ocular torsion without any change in horizontal or vertical eye position, it obviously violates Listing's law. Gravitational stimulation of the otoliths induces counter-rolling of the eyes around the visual axis by 3°–7° in response to sustained 90° head tilt.[42] Imaging by MRI in right as compared with left lateral decubitus positions demonstrates a mean 3.4° difference in conjugate torsional position of the rectus pulley array consistent in direction with the ocular counter-rolling.[43] Intorsion of the pulley array is associated with EOM cross-sectional changes on MRI, indicating SO contraction and IO relaxation.[43] This means that the pulling directions of all of the rectus EOMs change during normal head tilt, very probably due to an interaction with the oblique EOMs. Preliminary MRI evidence suggests that this may not occur to the same extent in the presence of SO palsy.

The full implication of pulleys for the neural control of ocular motility remains controversial. The essence of the argument involves the importance of mechanical versus neural constraints on ocular torsion,[44,45] and whether the central nervous system uses a two-dimensional (2-D, horizontal and vertical) versus a 3-D (horizontal, vertical, and torsional) controller.[46–48] Also controversial is the degree to which neurological lesions might alter ocular torsion independent of pulleys,[49] versus the degree to which pulley behavior itself might be under pathologic neural control.

Pathologic anatomy

The foregoing evidence suggests that the orbital connective tissues play a pivotal role in control of ocular kinematics. It should not be surprising that pathology of the pulleys and their associated connective tissues would be associated with predictable patterns of strabismus. Three forms of pulley pathology appear to cause strabismus (Table 77.4).

Pulley heterotopy

A model of binocular alignment based on static force balances[50] incorporating elastic pulleys[51] is now available as the program *Orbit*, which can model coronal plane heterotopy (malpositioning) of pulleys.[52] Many cases of incomitant cyclovertical strabismus are associated with heterotopy of one or more rectus EOM pulleys >2 standard deviations from normal. Patterns of

---

Table 77.4 Pathologic anatomy of pulleys

1. All six EOMs have pulleys that cause the pulling directions of the EOMs to change by half the angle of ocular duction.
2. This "half-angle" behavior makes ocular rotations mathematically commutative so that binocular alignment during versions does not depend on the sequence of eye rotations.
3. If there were noncommutativity, all of the neural commands to the EOMs would depend on the current eye positions of each of the two eyes and on the history of all of the prior ductions of each eye–an unlikely property of brainstem neurons. Commutative half-angle behavior requires no memory.
4. For visually guided eye movements with the head upright and stationary, half-angle behavior allows conformity of ocular torsion to Listing's law.
5. Non-Listing's law ocular torsion is advantageous in convergence and for the VOR.
6. Rectus pulley reconfiguration coordinated with ocular torsion maintains half-angle behavior even during deviations from Listing's law.
7. Deviations from Listing's law are largely mediated by the oblique EOMs.

incomitance in patients consistently match those predicted by *Orbit* simulation based on measured pulley locations, suggesting that pulley heterotopy *caused* the strabismus.[53–55] Most of these cases had "A" or "V" patterns. In an "A" pattern there is relatively more esotropia in upward than downward gaze, and one or both LR pulleys are located superior to the MR pulleys (Fig. 83.7). The converse is true in the "V" pattern, and the SR may also be significantly temporal to the IR as well. These clinical findings mimic features of what has been heretofore regarded as "oblique" EOM dysfunction,[53] and suggest that clinical nosology be significantly revised to avoid implications of oblique EOM over- or undercontraction.[56] MRI demonstrated no correlation between IO size and contractility, and variations in elevation in adduction in SO palsy.[57] Ocular torsion did not cause the pulley heterotopy because:

1. Typically only one or two pulleys were heterotopic;
2. The amount of ocular torsion was insufficient to account for the amount of pulley heterotopy; and
3. Patients with similar ocular torsion due to SO palsy lack this sort of pulley heterotopy.[54]

Extreme pulley heterotopy is associated with esotropia and hypotropia in axial high myopia, the "heavy eye syndrome."[58,59] Acquired heterotopy may result from aging. The horizontal rectus pulleys of normal older people sag inferiorly and symmetrically,[21] probably a cause of their reduced supraduction.[60] Asymmetric rectus pulley sag would produce incomitant vertical strabismus. Histological examination shows attenuation of connective tissues around the pulleys in the elderly, particularly striking in the attachments of the IO OL to other connective tissues.[19] The OL appears in the oldest specimens to lose its insertion to the temporal IO sleeve and to the LR pulley. These connective tissue changes would compromise EOM kinematics.

Pulley instability

While normal pulleys shift minimally with gaze changes, one or several pulleys may become unstable and shift markedly with gaze to alter EOM action. This shift may occur in one gaze position only. Inferior LR pulley shift in adduction may be acquired, and can mimic the restrictive hypotropia in adduction traditionally attributed to SO tendon sheath pathology (Brown syndrome) or "X" pattern exotropia.[61] This pathology has been termed "gaze-related pulley shift" (GROPS).[62] An exaggeration of the physiologic excyclo-rotation of the rectus pulley array in convergence may produce a marked "Y" or "T" pattern exotropia, one present only in elevated gaze. Pulley instability can be diagnosed only by orbital imaging in multiple gaze positions. The most common instability is downward shift of the LR in supraduction or adduction,[63] the latter producing a restrictive hypotropia clinically identical to Brown syndrome of the SO tendon sheath.[61] Temporal shift of the SR is occasionally associated with inferior shift of the LR.

Pulley hindrance

Abnormally anterior pulley location, or failure of a pulley to move posteriorly during EOM contraction, can result in pulley collision with the scleral insertion and hinder infraduction. As is also the case after fadenoperation,[64] there is restriction to passive forced duction. Hindrance to posterior IR pulley shift due to scarring from inferior orbital[65] or lid[66] surgery creates incomitant, restrictive hypertropia. Release of the adhesions hindering IR pulley motion can ameliorate this form of strabismus, although it is difficult to eliminate the scarring completely.

Pulley surgery

Central to the initial recognition of pulleys was the stability of rectus EOM paths after large surgical transpositions of the scleral insertions. Only slight shifts of pulleys are observed by MRI shows after transposition.[18,67] Posterior suture fixation of the transposed EOMs as described by Foster[17] shifts the pulley farther into the direction of the transposed insertion. This changes the pulling direction to mimic more closely that of the paralyzed EOM, increasing the effectiveness of transposition.[67] It is helpful to aggressively dissect the pulley of the transposed rectus EOM.

Posterior fixation of rectus tendons to the underlying sclera ("fadenoperation," in German) is performed to reduce ocular duction in the field of a particular EOM's contraction.[68] Deep dissection of Tenon's fascia and very posterior scleral placement of the fixation suture were believed essential to success of the operation. The mechanism was believed to be reduction in the EOM's scleral arc of contact and lever arm in rotating the globe.[69] MRI performed before and after posterior fixation surgery shows these concepts to be erroneous.[64] Instead, posterior fixation hinders normal posterior pulley shift during EOM contraction, restricting ocular rotation in that direction only. Based on this, the operation can be modified by placing the suture in a more convenient and safer anterior location.[64] It is counterproductive to dissect the pulley tissues, since their integrity is required for success. Scleral sutures need not be placed posteriorly or even at all: posterior fixation of the MR for esotropia with excessive accommodative convergence is as effective if the sutures simply join the pulley to a more posterior site on the MR muscle belly,[70] increasing the tension of the pulley suspension.

Pulley heterotopy can be treated surgically by large transpositions of the scleral insertions, augmented by posterior fixation to the sclera. Although this conventional sort of strabismus surgery can correct horizontal and vertical incomitances, insertional transposition always has an adverse effect on torsional alignment. A better strategy would be to operate to correct the pulley malpositioning directly. Pulley instability is usually treated by posterior scleral fixation, but might better be treated by surgical reinforcement of the pulley suspensions. Direct pulley surgery is currently in the earliest stages of clinical development and, controversially, might require orbital or craniofacial approaches in some cases.

MUSCLE ABNORMALITIES IN STRABISMUS
Superior oblique

In normals, good quality coronal MRI can resolve the SO muscle belly, trochlea, and reflected tendon to its scleral insertion; axial MRI can separate the tendon and tendon sheath anterior to the trochlea. The intraorbital trochlear nerve also can often be imaged near its entry into the SO. Norms have been published for the size of the SO belly[71]: it is small in SO palsy, as is typically obvious by comparison with the contralateral SO in unilateral pathology. The trochlea and reflected tendon are identifiable and normal in nearly all cases of atrophy of the SO belly, but are occasionally absent when the SO belly is absent.[63] When multipositional MRI is performed in alert patients, SO atrophy is associated with reduced contractile thickening of the SO cross section from supraduction to infraduction. Most cases of SO atrophy or SO absence show clinical features of incomitant hypertropia considered typical of SO palsy. Those cases not typical either are bilateral or involve additional anomalies.[63] Congenital absence of the SO is not uncommon in congenital SO palsy (Fig. 77.9).[72] It should be noted that, prior to imaging, cases of incomitant hypertropia are often clinically diagnosed as being SO palsy, but surprisingly exhibit normal SO size and contractility[73]: these cases probably should not be considered to have SO palsy.[56] Alternative diagnoses might include pulley abnormalities evident from orbital imaging, misinnervation, disorders of rectus muscle stiffness, or mild SO paresis undetectable by MRI. Atrophy of the SO is also readily demonstrable using direct coronal CT.

Inferior oblique

In normals, good quality quasisagittal MRI can resolve the path of the IO from its origin to its insertion.[16] Both quasicoronal and quasisagittal MRI can demonstrate insertion of the motor nerve at the neurofibrovascular bundle is just lateral to the conjoined IO and IR pulleys. MRI following IO surgery can readily verify the expected anatomical changes. Normal IO size and contractile thickening with vertical duction have been measured,[16] but are not correlated with over-elevation in adduction ("inferior oblique overaction") in SO palsy. The clinical diagnosis of "IO palsy," made without orbital imaging, is also seldom associated with MRI evidence of IO atrophy of reduced contractility.[57] Since MRI is so effective in demonstrating the functional anatomy of all of the other EOMs, lack of the expected correlation between orbital imaging and clinically diagnosed IO abnormalities questions the validity of the clinical diagnoses of IO over- and underactions. Since rectus pulley abnormalities can produce the clinical findings historically considered typical of IO dysfunction, abnormalities of pulleys might be considered in these situations.[56]

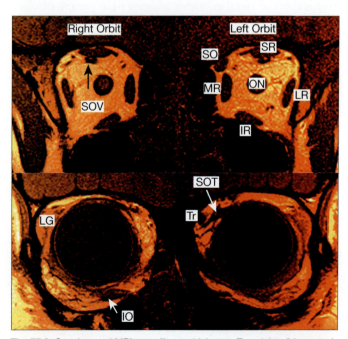

Fig. 77.9 Quasicoronal MRI scan (2 mm thickness, T_1 weighted) in central gaze of both orbits of a 6-year-old girl with congenital right superior oblique (SO) palsy. Posterior images in top row show normal SO belly in the left orbit, but absent SO in the right orbit. Anterior images in bottom row show trochlea (Tr) and reflected superior oblique tendon (SOT) in the left orbit, but absence of these structures in the right orbit. IR, inferior rectus muscle; LG, orbital lobe of lacrimal gland; LR, lateral rectus muscle; MR, medial rectus muscle; ON optic nerve; SOV, superior orbital vein; SR, superior rectus muscle.

Lateral rectus

The normal LR muscle can be imaged by MRI from its origin in the annulus of Zinn, to very near its scleral insertion. The scleral insertion itself can be imaged using high-resolution axial images obtained in adduction, where the relaxed LR tendon pulls sharply away from the sclera. On unenhanced T_1 imaging, the LR pulley is isointense with the LR muscle and surrounding connective tissues of the lateral canthal region and lacrimal gland, so the LR pulley is difficult to resolve. Using bolus intravenous gadodiamide to enhance the highly vascular LR within its less vascular pulley, the pulley itself can be imaged in the coronal plane. Axial images showed an inflection in LR path in adduction, coinciding approximately with the location of the pulley.[74] The normal LR belly typically showed multiple fissures and other internal areas isointense to fat. In the highest resolution images, the abducens nerve can be traced from the orbital apex, to an arborization on and within the global surface of the EOM. Since the motor nerve trunks do not enhance with gadodiamide, this contrast enhancement of the EOM fibers facilitates tracing of intramuscular branches of the abducens nerve. The normal LR shows a striking increase in posterior cross-sectional area from relaxation to contraction.

All patients with chronic abducens paralysis and absent abduction show profound LR atrophy and absent contractile thickening on attempted abduction[63] (Fig. 77.10). LR size is normal in Duane retraction syndrome, despite absent or profoundly limited abduction.[63] An exception of a patient with lifelong history compatible with type I Duane syndrome who developed a large skull base meningioma and exhibited profound LR atrophy compatible with denervation has been reported.[75]

Inferior rectus

The normal IR muscle can be imaged from its origin in the annulus of Zinn, to near its scleral insertion. The normal scleral insertion can be imaged using high-resolution quasisagittal images obtained in central gaze or supraduction. Since the IR pulley is mechanically coupled to the IO pulley, it is difficult to resolve the IR pulley. The normal IR belly normally shows multiple irregular internal areas isointense to fat. In high-resolution coronal images, the motor nerve branch of the inferior division of the oculomotor nerve can be traced from the orbital apex, to an arborization into multiple trunks on the global surface of the EOM, and within the EOM. Coronal images demonstrate a large and obvious contractile increase in normal IR cross section from supraduction to infraduction (Fig. 77.7). In IR palsy, there is atrophy of the IR

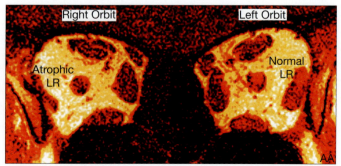

Fig. 77.10 Quasicoronal MRI scan (2 mm thickness, T_1 weighted) in central gaze of both orbits of a 19-year-old adolescent with traumatic right lateral rectus (LR) palsy. Note marked atrophy of right LR muscle.

belly, with absence of the normal contractile thickening in infraduction.

Medial rectus

In coronal images, the normal MR muscle can be imaged from its origin in the annulus of Zinn, to near its scleral insertion. The normal scleral insertion itself can be imaged using high-resolution axial images obtained in abduction. On unenhanced T_1 imaging, the MR pulley is isointense with the MR muscle and surrounding connective tissues of the medial canthal region, so the pulley is difficult to resolve. Using bolus intravenous gadodiamide to enhance the MR muscle within its pulley, the pulley ring itself can be imaged in the coronal plane.[16] The normal MR belly often shows multiple irregular internal areas isointense to fat, particular in older adults. The posterior MR belly normally shows marked contractile thickening from abduction to adduction, obvious on inspection. Chronic MR palsy with limited adduction is associated with atrophy of the MR belly.[63]

Superior rectus

The normal SR muscle can be imaged from its origin in the annulus of Zinn, to near its scleral insertion.[63] The normal scleral insertion can be imaged using high-resolution quasisagittal images obtained in central gaze or supraduction. The LPS muscle can be imaged from its origin on the orbital surface of the SR in the posterior orbit, through an inflection at Whitnall's ligament, and to its insertion on the superior border of the tarsal plate. In the highest resolution images, the motor nerve branch of the superior division of the oculomotor nerve can be traced from the orbital apex, to an arborization into multiple trunks on the global surface of the SR. Coronal images demonstrate an obvious contractile increase in normal SR cross section from infraduction to supraduction. Chronic SR palsy is associated with obvious atrophy of the SR belly, as well as lack of contractile thickening from infra- to supraduction. Atrophy of the SR belly is often but not always associated with LPS atrophy.

MUSCLE ABNORMALITIES IN OCULOMOTOR PALSY

Chronic oculomotor palsy with aberrant innervation is typically not associated with atrophy of EOMs innervated by the oculomotor nerve. Of 9 patients with the clinical diagnosis of chronic partial or complete oculomotor palsy who underwent MRI scanning, only two exhibited atrophy of the EOMs innervated by the oculomotor nerve.[63] This included the MR and IR muscles in both patients, and also the SR in one of them. Neither patient exhibited atrophy of the ipsilesional IO muscle.

TRAUMATIC MYOTOMY OR AVULSION OF EXTRAOCULAR MUSCLES

Imaging is useful to evaluate EOM myotomy or avulsion due either to accidental trauma or complication of surgery. In patients with paralytic strabismus due to such damage,[63] multipositional

MRI can demonstrate residual contractile thickening of the posterior portions of EOMs completely severed from the globe and hence unable to contribute to ocular duction. In some cases, the motor nerve is avulsed, rendering the EOM irreversibly paralyzed: here it may be appropriate to perform inferior transposition of the horizontal rectus EOMs, without futile delay in expectation of spontaneous recovery.

Inadvertent entry into the orbit during endoscopic sinus surgery most commonly results in damage to the MR muscle, also to the SO, and occasionally to the IR, muscles.[63,76] Anterior damage may produce partial or complete tenotomy or anterior myotomy, with the potential for an excellent result from surgical repair of the involved EOM since the bulk of the EOM remains contractile (Fig. 77.11). More posterior damage is permanent and irreversible if the region of the myoneural junction is extirpated. However, incomplete trauma in the region of the myoneural junction can produce profound but reversible EOM paralysis. In such cases, it may be useful to determine the cause of the paralysis by imaging the region of the myoneural junction at high resolution to identify possible intramuscular nerve trauma. With high-resolution techniques and gadodiamide contrast, individual traumatic penetrations of an EOM can be identified and followed in relationship to other evidence of trauma such as edema and hematoma.

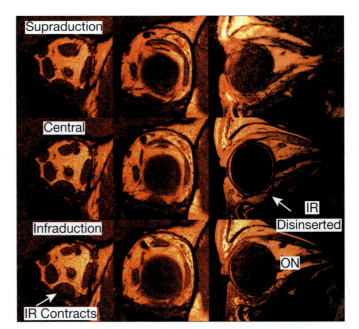

Fig. 77.11 Traumatic avulsion of the left inferior rectus (IR) muscle associated with hypertropia greatest in downward gaze. Quasicoronal (left two columns) and quasisagittal (right column) MRI scans (2 mm thickness, T_1 weighted) of the left orbit during fixation by the normal right eye of targets in supraduction, central gaze, and infraduction. Coronal images show that that the deep belly of the left IR muscle exhibits robust contractile thickening on infraduction, but sagittal images show that the IR tendon is not inserted on the globe. Based on these findings, the IR was recovered by deep orbitotomy and reinserted on the sclera, restoring normal infraduction. Sagittal image in central gaze was performed using intravenous gadodiamide contrast. Compare with normal anatomy in Fig. 77.7.

REFERENCES

1. Demer JL. Extraocular muscles. In: Jaeger EA, Tasman PR, editors. Duane's Clinical Ophthalmology. Philadelphia: Lippincott; 2000: Ch. 1. (vol 1.)

2. Porter JD, Baker RS, Ragusa RJ, et al. Extraocular muscles: Basic and clinical aspects of structure and function. Surv Ophthalmol 1995; 39: 451–84.

3. Oh SY, Poukens V, Demer JL. Quantitative analysis of rectus extraocular muscle layers in monkey and humans. Invest. Ophthalmol Vis. Sci 2001; 42: 10–6.

4. Demer JL, Oh SY, Poukens V. Evidence for active control of rectus extraocular muscle pulleys. Invest Ophthalmol Vis Sci 2000; 41: 1280–90.

5. Oh SY, Poukens V, Cohen MS, et al. Structure-function correlation of laminar vascularity in human rectus extraocular muscles. Invest Ophthalmol Vis Sci 2001; 42: 17–22.

6. Brueckner JK, Ashby LP, Prichard JR, et al. Vestibulo-ocular pathways modulate extraocular muscle myosin expression patterns. Cell Tissue Res 1999; 295: 477–84.

7. Porter JD, Baker RS. Muscles of a different "color": the unusual properties of the extraocular muscles may predispose or protect them in neurogenic and myogenic disease. Neurology 1996; 46: 30–7.

8. Sappey PC. Traite D'Anatomie Descriptive Avec Figures Intercalees Dans Le Texte. Paris: Delahaye et Lecrosnier; 1888.

9. Sappey PC. The motor muscles of the eyeball [translation from the French]. Strabismus 2001; 9: 243–53.

10. Demer JL. Pivotal role of orbital connective tissues in binocular alignment and strabismus. Invest. Ophthalmol Vis Sci 2004; 45: 729–38.

11. Roth A, Muhlendyck H, De Gottrau P. [The function of Tenon's capsule revisited.] J Fr Ophthalmol 2002; 25: 968–76.

12. Kono R, Clark RA, Demer JL. Active pulleys: magnetic resonance imaging of rectus muscle paths in tertiary gazes. Invest. Ophthalmol Vis Sci 2002; 43: 2179–88.

13. Porter JD, Poukens V, Baker RS, et al. Cytoarchitectural organization of the medial rectus muscle pulley in man. Invest Ophthalmol Vis Sci 1995; 36: S960.

14. Demer JL, Poukens V, Miller JM, et al. Innervation of extraocular pulley smooth muscle in monkeys and humans. Invest Ophthalmol Vis Sci 1997; 38: 1774–85.

15. Miller JM, Demer JL, Poukens V, et al. Extraocular connective tissue architecture. J Vis 2003; 3: 240–51.

16. Demer JL, Oh SY, Clark RA, et al. Evidence for a pulley of the inferior oblique muscle. Invest Ophthalmol Vis Sci 2003; 44: 3856–65.

17. Foster RS. Vertical muscle transposition augmented with lateral fixation. J AAPOS 1997;1:20–30.

18. Clark RA, Rosenbaum AL, Demer JL. Magnetic resonance imaging after surgical transposition defines the anteroposterior location of the rectus muscle pulleys. J AAPOS 1999; 3 :9–14.

19. Kono R, Poukens V, Demer JL. Quantitative analysis of the structure of the human extraocular muscle pulley system. Invest Ophthalmol Vis Sci 2002; 43: 2923–32.

20. Clark RA, Miller JM, Demer JL. Three-dimensional location of human rectus pulleys by path inflections in secondary gaze positions. Invest Ophthalmol Vis Sci 2000; 41: 3787–97.

21. Clark RA, Demer JL. Effect of aging on human rectus extraocular muscle paths demonstrated by magnetic resonance imaging. Am J Ophthalmol 2002; 134: 872–8.

22. Clark RA, Miller JM, Demer JL. Location and stability of rectus muscle pulleys inferred from muscle paths. Invest Ophthalmol Vis Sci 1997; 38: 227–40.

23. Miller JM. Functional anatomy of normal human rectus muscles. Vision Res 1989; 29: 223–40.

24. Haslwanter T. Mathematics of three-dimensional eye rotations. Vision Res 1995; 35: 1727–39.

25. van den Berg AV. Kinematics of eye movement control. Proc R Soc Lond 1995; 260: 191–7.

26. Ruete CGT. Ocular physiology. Strabismus 1999;7:43–60.

27. Tweed D, Vilis T. Geometric relations of eye position and velocity vectors during saccades. Vision Res 1990; 30: 111–27.

28. Quaia C, Optican LM. Commutative saccadic generator is sufficient to control a 3-D ocular plant with pulleys. J Neurophysiol 1998; 79: 3197–215.

29. Demer JL. The orbital pulley system: a revolution in concepts of orbital anatomy. Ann NY Acad Sci 2002; 956: 17–32.

30. Detorakis ET, Engstrom RE, Straatsma BR, et al. Functional anatomy of the anophthalmic socket: insights from magnetic resonance imaging. Invest Ophthalmol Vis Sci 2003; 44: 4307–13.

31. Collins CC. The human oculomotor control system. In: Lennerstrand G, Bach-y-Rita P, editors. Basic Mechanisms of Ocular Motility and Their Clinical Implications. New York: Pergamon; 1975: 145–80.

32. Lam H, Poukens V, Oh SY, et al. Laminar analysis of motor unit size in human rectus extraocular muscles (EOMs): evidence for compartmental innervation. In: 2002 Abstracts Viewer/Itinerary Planner. Society for Neuroscience; 2002: 857.7.

33. Porrill J, Warren PA, Dean P. A simple control law generates Listing's positions in a detailed model of the extraocular muscle system. Vision Res 2000; 40: 3743–58.

34. Smith MA, Crawford JD. Neural control of rotational kinematics within realistic vestibuloocular coordinate systems. J Neurophysiol 1998; 80: 2295–315.

35. Steffen H, Walker MF, Zee DS. Rotation of Listing's plane with convergence: independence from eye position. Invest Ophthalmol Vis Sci 2000; 41: 715–21.

36. Schreiber K, Crawford JD, Fetter M, et al. The motor side of depth vision. Nature 2001; 410: 819–22.

37. Bruno P, van den Berg AV. Relative orientation of primary positions of the two eyes. Vision Res 1997; 37: 935–47.

38. van Rijn LJ, van den Berg AV. Binocular eye orientation during fixations: Listing's law extended to include eye vergence. Vision Res 1993; 33: 691–708.

39. Demer JL, Kono R, Wright W. Magnetic resonance imaging of human extraocular muscles in convergence. J Neurophysiol 2003; 89: 2072–85.

40. Allen MJ, Carter JH. The torsional component of the near reflex. Am J Optom 1967; 44: 343–9.

41. Mays LE, Zhang Y, Thorstad MH, et al. Trochlear unit activity during ocular convergence. J Neurophysiol 1991; 65: 1484–91.

42. Bockisch CJ, Haslwanter T. Three-dimensional eye position during static roll and pitch in humans. Vision Res 2001; 41: 2127–37.

43. Demer JL. Magnetic resonance Imaging (MRI) of human extraocular muscles (EOMs) during the static torsional vestibulo-ocular reflex (VOR). ARVO Abstr. 2003; #2736.

44. Misslisch H, Tweed D. Neural and mechanical factors in eye control. J Neurophysiol 2001; 86: 1877–83.

45. Angelaki DE. Three-dimensional ocular kinematics during eccentric rotations: Evidence for functional rather than mechanical constraints. J Neurophysiol 2003; 89: 2685–96.

46. Tweed DB, Haslwanter TP, Happe V, et al. Non-commutativity in the brain. Nature 1999; 399: 261–3.

47. Halswanter T. Mechanics of eye movements: implications of the "orbital revolution." Ann NY Acad Sci 2002; 956: 33–41.

48. Klier EM, Wang H, Crawford D. Three-dimensional eye-head coordination is implemented downstream from the superior colliculus. J Neurophysiol 2003; 89: 2839–53.

49. Wong AMF, Sharpe JA, Tweed D. Adaptive neural mechanism for Listing's law revealed in patients with fourth nerve palsy. Invest Ophthalmol Vis Sci 2002; 43: 1796–1803.

50. Miller JM, Robinson DA. A model of the mechanics of binocular alignment. Comput Biomed Res 1984; 17: 436–70.

51. Miller JM, Pavlovski DS, Shaemeva I. Orbit 1.8 gaze mechanics simulation. San Francisco: Eidactics; 1999.

52. Miller JM, Demer JL. Biomechanical modeling in strabismus surgery. In: Rosenbaum AL, Santiago P, editors. Clinical Strabismus Management: Principles and Techniques. St. Louis: Mosby; 1999: 99–113.

53. Clark RA, Miller JM, Rosenbaum AL, et al. Heterotopic muscle pulleys or oblique muscle dysfunction? J AAPOS 1998; 2: 17–25.

54. Clark RA, Miller JM, Demer JL. Displacement of the medial rectus pulley in superior oblique palsy. Invest Ophthalmol Vis Sci 1998; 39: 207–12.

55. Demer JL, Clark RA, Miller JM. Heterotopy of extraocular muscle pulleys causes incomitant strabismus. In: Lennerstrand G, editor. Advances in Strabismology. Buren (Netherlands): Aeolus Press; 1999: 91–4.

56. Demer JL. Clarity of words and thoughts about strabismus. Am J Ophthalmol 2001; 132: 757–59.

57. Kono R, Demer JL. Magnetic resonance imaging of the functional anatomy of the inferior oblique muscle in superior oblique palsy. Ophthalmology 2003; 110: 1219–29.

58. Krzizok TH, Schroeder BU. Measurement of recti eye muscle paths by magnetic resonance imaging in highly myopic and normal subjects. Invest. Ophthalmol Vis Sci 1999; 40: 2554–60.

59. Demer JL, Miller JM. Orbital imaging in strabismus surgery. In: Rosenbaum AL, Santiago AP, editors. Clinical Strabismus Management: Principles and Techniques. Philadelphia: Saunders; 1999: 84–98.

60. Clark RA, Isenberg SJ. The range of ocular movements decreases with aging. J AAPOS 2001; 5(1): 26–30.

61. Oh SY, Clark RA, Velez F, et al. Incomitant strabismus associated with instability of rectus pulleys. Invest. Ophthalmol Vis Sci 2002; 43: 2169–78.

62. Demer JL, Kono R, Wright W, et al. Gaze-related orbital pulley shift: a novel cause of incomitant strabismus. In: de Faber JT, editor. Progress in Strabismology. Lisse: Swets and Zeitlinger; 2002: 207–10.

63. Demer JL. A 12 year, prospective study of extraocular muscle imaging in complex strabismus. J AAPOS 2003; 6: 337–47.

64. Clark RA, Isenberg SJ, Rosenbaum SJ, et al. Posterior fixation sutures: a revised mechanical explanation for the fadenoperation based on rectus extraocular muscle pulleys. Am J Ophthalmol 1999; 128: 702–14.

65. Goldberg RA, Li TG, Demer JL. Diplopia following porous polyethylene orbital rim onlay implant. Ophthal Plast Reconst Sur 2003; 19: 83–5.

66. Piruzian A, Goldberg RA, Demer JL. Inferior rectus pulley hindrance: Orbital imaging mechanism of restrictive hypertropia following lower lid surgery. J AAPOS 2004; in press.

67. Clark RA, Demer JL. Rectus extraocular muscle pulley displacement after surgical transposition and posterior fixation for treatment of paralytic strabismus. Am J Ophthalmol 2002; 133: 119–28.

68. Cuppers C. The so-called "fadenoperation" (surgical considerations by well-defined changes of the arc of contact). In: Fells P, editor. Transactions of the Second Congress International Strabismological Association. Marseilles: Diffusion Generale de Librairie; 1976: 395–400.

69. Scott AB. The faden operation: mechanical effects. Am Orthoptic J 1977; 27: 44–7.

70. Clark RA, Ariyasu R, Demer JL. Medial rectus pulley posterior fixation is as effective as scleral posterior fixation for acquired esotropia with a high AC/A ratio. Am J Ophthalmol 2004; in press.

71. Demer JL, Miller JM. Magnetic resonance imaging of the functional anatomy of the superior oblique muscle. Invest Ophthalmol Vis Sci 1995; 36: 906–13.

72. Chan TK, Demer JL. Clinical features of congenital absence of the superior oblique muscle as demonstrated by orbital imaging. J AAPOS 1999; 3: 143–50.

73. Demer JL, Miller MJ, Koo EY, et al. True versus masquerading superior oblique palsies: Muscle mechanisms revealed by magnetic resonance imaging. In: Lennerstrand G, editor. Update on Strabismus and Pediatric Ophthalmology. Boca Raton, FL: CRC Press; 1995: 303–6.

74. Demer JL, Miller JM, Poukens V, et al. Evidence for fibromuscular pulleys of the recti extraocular muscles. Invest Ophthalmol Vis Sci 1995; 36: 1125–36.

75. Silverberg M, Demer JL. Duane's syndrome with compressive denervation of the lateral rectus muscle. Am J Ophthalmol 2001; 131: 146–8.

76. Underdahl JP, Demer JL, Goldberg RA, et al. Orbital wall approach with preoperative orbital imaging for identification and retrieval of lost or transected extraocular muscles. J AAPOS 2001; 5: 230–7.

78 Amblyopia Management

Michael X Repka

Amblyopia is the most common cause of visual impairment in children, which often persists into adulthood. The prevalence in childhood is estimated to be 1–4%. It is considered to be the leading cause of monocular vision loss in the 20- to 70-year-old age group.[1] The prevalence of visual loss from amblyopia was 2.9% in one study of adults, indicating the need for improved treatment.[2] Nearly all of the available data on the natural history of amblyopia and success rates of its treatment with either occlusion or penalization are retrospective and uncontrolled. Amblyopia is defined as a "decrease of visual acuity caused by pattern vision deprivation or abnormal binocular interaction for which no causes can be detected by the physical examination of the eye and which in appropriate cases is reversible by therapeutic measures."[3] Amblyopia may be unilateral or less often bilateral.

Most cases are associated with eye misalignment, usually esotropia in infancy or early childhood. Less frequently anisometropia, or a combination of the strabismus and anisometropia, is causally associated with amblyopia. Woodruff and his colleagues performed a population-based study in which they identified 961 amblyopes.[4] They found the cause to be strabismus in 57%, anisometropia in 17%, and a combination of the two in 27%. Shaw et al. reported among 1531 amblyopes that strabismus was the cause in 45%, anisometropia in 17%, a combination of the two in 35%, and deprivation due to cataract or corneal scarring in 3%.[5] The precise percentages vary with the disease definition by the authors.

Visual loss in amblyopia varies from mild to severe. About 25% of cases have visual acuity in the amblyopic eye worse than 6/30 and about 75% 6/30 or better.[4,6–8] Furthermore, the extent of the injury may not be equivalent, but vary by cause. There is evidence that strabismic amblyopia represents a more severe physiological deficit than purely anisometropic amblyopia, and combined strabismic anisometropic amblyopia a more serious deficit still.[9]

METHODS OF DETECTION

Single optotype presentation and picture optotypes are less sensitive and should be used only when a child is unable to perform a test using surrounded or line optotypes. The gold standard for detection is measurement of visual acuity using a crowded or linear letter optotype test. Tests based on the four letters "H," "O," "T," and "V" in a box or with contour surround bars are the basis of several popular test strategies.[10,11] A defined protocol for testing children has been developed in the United States by the Pediatric Eye Disease Investigator Group (PEDIG) for the clinical trials it has conducted.[11] The strategy includes a second chance at threshold determination and a portion designed to get the child back on track with some larger above-threshold stimuli. It has good testability and test-retest reliability, and it has been automated.[12]

For children unable to perform with letter optotypes, clinicians have often used picture optotypes. However, picture optotypes overestimate the visual acuity of amblyopic eyes and are not recommended for screening or diagnosis of amblyopia. Dr. Lea Hyvärinen designed these four picture optotypes to have similar shapes and have contours like the Landolt C, making them more difficult. The objects (apple, circle, house, square) chosen are common in children's experience to improve testability (the proportion of tested patients able to complete a test) among young children and eliminate cultural biases. In one study the surrounded Lea tests systematically overestimated acuity by 1.9 lines compared to the crowded Landolt C in normal eyes.[14] A comparison of the Lea symbols to line optotypes in amblyopic eyes has not been thoroughly studied. Kay's pictures are an alternative.

Fixation preference testing may be used for children unable to perform any optotype-based testing. For strabismic patients the clinician compares the ability to hold fixation with each eye. The child may alternate, be unable to hold fixation after a blink, or be unable to hold fixation. For a patient with no misalignment, the test is performed by placing a 10^Δ prism base down before one eye, having the child fixate a detailed target at distance or near, and assessing the fixation preference. The preference is recorded. If there is a fixation preference for the eye without the prism, switch the prism to the fellow eye and again assess fixation preference. The prism might cause the other eye to be preferred. If the same eye is preferred under each testing condition, then the fellow eye is assumed to have amblyopia. A patient who fixates with the eye without the prism is alternating. Amblyopia therapy may be prescribed for a definite fixation preference as discussed in the sections on treatment. Unfortunately, recent research comparing fixation preference testing to optotype testing has shown it to be very unreliable as a means of diagnosing amblyopia, generally leading to an overdiagnosis of amblyopia. In one study optotype testing confirmed only 17 of 52 patients (33%) diagnosed with amblyopia by fixation preference testing for a disappointing sensitivity of 53%.[15]

Forced choice preferential looking using Teller acuity cards have been used as an alternative method for infants and non-verbal infants[16]: it is time-consuming and requires an experienced tester for reliable results. This test systematically underestimates amblyopia, reducing its clinical utility as a means of screening or detecting a successful treatment endpoint.[17] Visual-evoked potential estimates of visual acuity also underestimate amblyopia but may be useful in documenting changes of acuity during treatment.

METHODS OF TREATMENT

The value of the treatment of amblyopia is widely held. However, there are few data comparing the outcomes of amblyopia treatment to the natural history. Clinicians have noted improvement of acuity when children complied with therapy, but found little improvement when no therapy was completed. Among a case series of amblyopic patients who were not treated, there was no improvement in visual acuity.[18] However, a demonstration of an improvement in acuity of the amblyopic eye without untreated or natural history controls is not sufficient to prove a benefit of therapy. This deficiency led, in the United Kingdom, to a review of screening for and treatment of amblyopia because of a lack of a proven benefit.[19]

A recent retrospective, nonrandomized study suggested that there is value. A group of strabismic patients with amblyopia were treated with spectacles alone ($n = 17$) or spectacles plus occlusion therapy ($n = 69$).[20] Although both treatments led to improvement, the visual acuity improved more in the patients treated with occlusion.

Some of the improvement in acuity reported in uncontrolled studies may represent a combination of age and learning effects with actual treatment benefit, in which a patient performs better because they are older at the time of the outcome exam and they have also performed the test on an earlier occasion. However, the magnitude of the age and learning effects, which has been reported to be about 0.14 logMAR lines over 6 months in a prospective clinical trial, is far less than the improvement typically reported following treatment of amblyopia.[21]

A randomized clinical trial (Amblyopia Treatment Trial, UK) was undertaken to compare an untreated control group of anisometropic amblyopia to a group of children treated with glasses and a third group treated with glasses and occlusion for anisometropic amblyopia. This study found slight improvement with about one line between no treatment and treatment with glasses and occlusion.[22,23] Unfortunately, the cause of the visual loss was not determined. In addition, the control group's acuity at baseline and at final measurement was without correction, whereas the treatment group was measured with best correction.

Refractive correction

The initial intervention is to prescribe any necessary spectacle correction. Indeed, one should not diagnose amblyopia until refractive correction is prescribed, the glasses obtained, and the visual acuity deficit confirmed with the correction being worn. Guidelines for prescribing spectacles for amblyopia vary on clinician's practice and experience and age of the child, but normally should correct any anisometropia above 0.50 D and astigmatism of 1.50 D or more in any patient with amblyopia. Hypermetropia should be fully corrected in younger strabismic patients and corrected with the plus sphere reduced by up to 1.50 D in orthotropic patients. Myopic errors should be fully corrected during office testing with trial frames to confirm the diagnosis, though the prescribed minus sphere may be cut for infants and toddlers.

There is controversy about when to start additional therapy such as occlusion. Some clinicians prefer to prescribe such therapy immediately, some wait a specified time interval, while others wait until improvement with spectacles alone ceases. There are little published data to guide a clinician in this choice. In the United Kingdom, 8 of 12 patients prescribed spectacles for the first time improved 3 or more lines in the amblyopic eye.[24] Additional data are expected from ongoing clinical trials in the United Kingdom and United States.

The author prefers to prescribe any necessary spectacle correction and then wait for at least 6 weeks to reevaluate the acuity. A measure of the visual acuity in trial frames when the glasses are prescribed can be helpful in assessing the change in the vision status at the first follow-up visit. As long as the acuity is improving it is reasonable to continue with just glasses before prescribing additional therapy. The author believes that this graduated approach improves patient compliance with each portion of the therapy.

Occlusion therapy

Occlusion therapy, said to have been originated by Erasmus Darwin, has been the mainstay of treatment despite the lack of data demonstrating its superiority over other modalities. The most common form of this therapy employs an adhesive patch placed over the sound eye so that the amblyopic eye must be used. Opinions vary on the number of hours of patching per day that should be prescribed, ranging from a few hours to all waking hours.[1,3,25-27] Scott and his co-workers have felt that 24 hr per day patching improves compliance.[28]

Only a few reports have evaluated the difference in improvement between full- and part-time occlusion, when the groupings were not established by an assessment of patient compliance. Flynn and co-workers found that the success rates were the same for part- and full-time occlusion based on reported outcomes in 23 studies.[29] Cleary reported in a very small study that full-time occlusion produced a greater improvement in visual acuity and reduction in interocular difference than part-time occlusion, when the acuity outcome was measured at 6 months.[20]

Several authors have shown spectacular improvement in visual acuity using brief daily periods of occlusion (20 min to 1 hr).[30,31] Campbell and co-workers noted that 20 min per day was effective in improving the vision of 83% of children to 6/12. These authors have reported that vision can improve rapidly following brief periods of occlusion, especially when combined with concentration on hard tasks.[32]

The dosages prescribed by clinicians during the past few decades vary greatly and seem to be largely a matter of region or training[33]: more hours are prescribed in German-speaking countries than in the United Kingdom, yet the same outcome is expected.[34]

Recently several clinical trials evaluating varied patching dosages have been organized on the outcome of amblyopia treatment.[21,35] Collectively these are the Amblyopia Treatment Studies, which are prospective multicenter randomized controlled clinical trials, conducted by PEDIG in North America. The studies have included only patients with strabismic and anisometropic forms of amblyopia. The first randomized controlled study compared occlusion to atropine treatment. The dosage of occlusion prescribed was a minimum of 6 hr up to full time, but the investigator chose the actual occlusion dosage. Exploratory analyses of the effect of prescribed occlusion dosage on outcome were reported.[36] Patients with acuity of 6/24 to 6/30 improved faster when a greater number of hours of patching was prescribed, but after 6 months the improvement was not significantly greater than that occurring with a lesser number of hours of patching or with atropine (Fig. 78.1).

The second and third Amblyopia Treatment Studies completed by PEDIG are the only prospective randomized trials designed to compare the efficacy of different occlusion dosages. There are

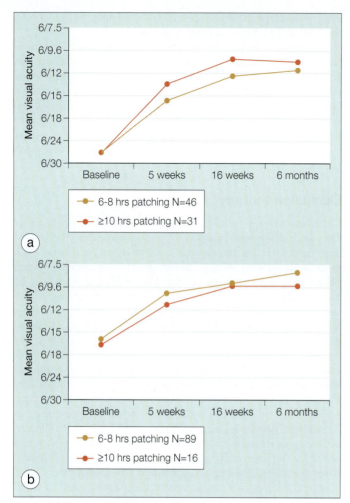

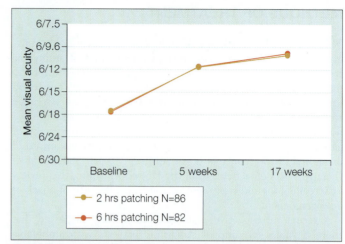

Fig. 78.2 Occlusion dosage of 2 versus 6 hr compared in a randomized controlled trial.[34] No increase in therapy was allowed by the protocol, and patients had an amblyopic eye of 6/12 to 6/24. There was no difference in the rate or magnitude of improvement during the four months of prescribed treatment.

Fig. 78.1 Initial prescribed dosage of patching versus mean visual acuity from a randomized controlled trial.[21] Eighty percent of patients remained on their initial dosage throughout the study. Unsuccessful patients in each subgrouping had patching of 12 or more hours prescribed at the 17-week visit. (a) Patients with amblyopic eye acuity of 6/24 and 6/30. The patients initially treated with 10 or more hours compared to 6 or 8 hr per day had a faster rate of improvement, but by 6 months there was no significant difference in outcome. (b) Patients with amblyopic eye acuity of 6/12 to 6/18. There is no difference in the rate or magnitude of improvement between those initially treated with 10 or more hours and those treated with 6 or 8 hr.

two distinct studies, one for moderate amblyopia 6/12 to 6/24, and one for severe amblyopia 6/30 to 6/120, caused by strabismus, anisometropia, or both. The investigators found that 2 hr of daily patching produces an improvement in visual acuity of magnitude similar to that with 6 hr of daily patching in treating moderate amblyopia in children 3 to less than 7 years of age.[35] Each treatment group improved 2.4 lines over 4 months. Perhaps more interesting was the lack of any benefit in terms of the rate of improvement (Fig. 78.2). The visual acuity gain at 4 months probably does not represent the maximum improvement possible.

A similar study for severe amblyopia found the improvement in the amblyopic eye acuity from baseline to 4 months averaged 4.8 lines in the 6-hr group and 4.7 lines in the full-time group ($p = 0.45$).[37]

Patient dislike of occlusion therapy is well known due to discomfort, poor vision, and social anxiety (see Chapter P29). Reported compliance rates range widely, with rates of both 10 and 90% cited in the literature. Parents have used coercion and clinicians have prescribed punitive measures such as elbow splints to enhance compliance. Lack of parental understanding seems to play a large role. In one study of patching in the United Kingdom, failure to comply with the prescribed regimen at least 80% of the time occurred in 54% of patients.[38] The failure to comply with treatment was directly related to a parental lack of understanding that there is a time limit to effective therapy or a "critical period."

Side-effects from occlusion are relatively uncommon, usually minor skin irritation or the social stigma of a patch.[21] Adhesive sensitivity or allergy to the patches does occur. The clinician should discontinue the patch and treat with an emollient facial crème. In rare instances topical hydrocortisone may be needed.

More serious is occlusion amblyopia, which is a decrease in vision of more than one line in the sound eye. It is more common in younger children, with more intense therapy and longer treatment intervals, especially if the patient is lost to follow-up. In one large prospective study only 1 of 204 occlusion patients was diagnosed with reverse amblyopia in which the majority of patients were treated with 6 or 8 hr per day.[21] Conversely, Pfeiffer and Scott reported in a presentation at the Annual Meeting of AAPOS-2003 a rate of 25% with full-time occlusion. Occlusion amblyopia is usually reversible by stopping the treatment. Rarely, amblyopia therapy needs to be prescribed for the originally amblyopic eye. Another important side-effect is the development of new strabismus. This is infrequent, noted in only 1% of patients during occlusion therapy.[21]

It seems, therefore, that the value of occlusion is well established for anisometropic and strabismic amblyopia. The clinician and the parents should discuss the dosage prescribed for the patient. The number of hours prescribed should be based on many factors including compliance and lifestyle.

An opaque adhesive patch appears to be the best method currently available. Temperature-sensitive patches to help monitor compliance may be available in the future.[39] Spectacle-mounted patches and nonadhesive patches may be less successful because they are easily removed, but there are no published data to confirm this.

Once an occlusion dosage is prescribed the patient must return for visual acuity monitoring. Traditionally these intervals have been 1 week per year of age (i.e., a 3-year-old patient would return in 3 weeks). This approach is necessary when full-time occlusion is prescribed, but may be lengthened with part-time occlusion. An initial follow-up interval of 2 months for 2 to 6 hr per day patching has been sufficient. After the first interval if the amblyopic eye has improved and the sound eye has not been impaired, the treatment interval can be increased, usually 3 months. Therapy should be continued until no improvement occurs between two visits spaced by 3 or more months. If the patient is not cooperative with acuity testing it is best to retest the vision at the same visit or at a subsequent visit to be certain of the lack of improvement.

Most of the treatment of amblyopia is derived from clinical experience with patients who have strabismic, anisometropic, or combined forms of amblyopia. An important group of amblyopic patients have form-deprivation amblyopia, for example, from a treated cataract or media opacity. For these patients, the amblyopia is often severe. Occlusion remains the best choice in the absence of studies demonstrating equivalence of another method. The occlusion dosage should be individualized, as there is no treatment trial available to guide the clinician. For patients with unilateral deprivation amblyopia, occlusion dosages of half waking hours are reasonable to avoid damage to the binocular system or to the sound eye. This dosage can be tapered as the child's vision plateaus to maintain the improvement.

Penalization therapy

Penalization is an alternative to occlusion therapy for amblyopia. Both pharmacological and optical means are used to blur the vision in the better eye for near and/or distance. Use of penalization was first advocated in 1903 by Worth.[3] However, these approaches have not gained widespread use as a primary treatment modality for amblyopia, although a number of authors have noted success in retrospective case series.[40–43] Penalization has mainly been employed as a fall-back treatment, for use with occlusion non-compliance, and for post-occlusion maintenance or titration.[3,44–46]

Pharmacological penalization involves the instillation of a cycloplegic agent into the sound eye: Atropine or, occasionally, short-acting cycloplegic agents have been used. The cycloplegia prevents accommodation, blurring the sound eye at near fixation and forcing the use of the amblyopic eye at near. Some clinicians have augmented the therapeutic effect by reducing or removing any plus sphere from the spectacle correction of the sound eye, effectively blurring the sound eye at all fixation distances.[47] The value of this additional optical blurring has not yet been shown in a randomized comparison to be beneficial. Pharmacological penalization has been recommended for the treatment of moderate amblyopia, but has been effective for patients with amblyopia 6/30 to 6/60.[42] Compliance is good: in one study, 78% of patients had excellent compliance.[21] Penalization may be slower to reach a successful outcome than occlusion, but may be equally effective if adequate time is allowed.

Optical penalization involves the placement of "plus" fogging lenses over the sound eye, blurring that eye at distance, causing the patient to shift fixation at distance to the amblyopic eye. Optical penalization has generally been advocated for mild amblyopia (visual acuity in amblyopic eye 20/60 or better).[40,43] The power of the additional plus before the sound eye may be arbitrarily chosen, usually +2.50 or +3.00 D. It is very convenient for a child wearing bifocals to just extend the power of the bifocal throughout the entire lens. An alternative is to have the patient fixate a distance vectographic target and increase the

plus sphere before the sound eye until the fixation at distance switches to the amblyopic eye.[40]

Compliance is a concern with optical penalization since it is dependent on the child not "peeking" around the glasses: it usually is best reserved for older children and those with milder amblyopia. The clinician should be prepared to continue this treatment for 2 or more years.

Penalization may be effective because the blur produced selectively removes the high-spatial-frequency components of the image to the sound eye, thereby eliminating their suppression of the high-spatial-frequency components perceived by the cortex responsive to the amblyopic eye.[48] This appears to be the critical component of amblyopia therapy, because amblyopia is a deficit of neuronal responses to high spatial frequencies. With penalization, the high spatial frequencies become more dominant in the neurons of the cortex of the amblyopic eye.

Occlusion compared to penalization

One small ($n = 38$) retrospective study reported better visual acuity outcomes in a group of children over 6 years of age treated with atropine penalization than was obtained in a group of younger children who were occluded.[49] Two small ($n = 25$,[50] $n = 36$[51]) prospective studies found no difference in visual acuity outcome between the two methods.

The first Amblyopia Treatment Study was a randomized controlled trial that enrolled 419 patients comparing occlusion to pharmacological penalization.[21] The investigators found both daily patching (6 or more hr) and daily atropine were effective initial treatments for amblyopia throughout the age range of 3 to less than 7 years old and the acuity range of 20/40 to 20/100. Each method produced nearly the same improvement of about 3 logMAR lines over 6 months.

Fogging

An alternative to occlusion or penalization is fogging. This may be done with Bangerter Foils, which reduce the visual acuity in the sound eye. The foils come in a series of graduated densities. The selected filter may reduce the sound eye vision to less than the amblyopic eye. An alternative is to just use the 6/60 (0.1) filter for all patients. An even more readily available and inexpensive alternative is to use an opaque form of adhesive tape placed on the glasses. Each of these is barely visible beyond 0.5 m. This method is ideal for mild visual deficits and long-term maintenance therapy, and in school age children in which compliance with the glasses wear is possible.[52]

Active therapy

Active treatment has long been suggested as an important supplement to occlusion therapy. Duke-Elder emphasized the importance of interesting play activity during occlusion.[53] Physicians have long asked that their patients while patching should not sleep or daydream, but rather be involved in some type of activity, which promotes visual interaction.

The simplest forms have been home-based activities, performed in conjunction with the occlusion, usually involving activities such as tracing, dot-to-dot tasks, coloring, stringing beads, reading, and playing computer/video games. These therapies may be helpful because they:

1. Help overcome compliance problems with occlusion; and
2. May help to improve accommodation and fixation patterns.

François and James showed in a comparison study that 100 patients who were occluded and another 100 who underwent occlusion with active home therapy twice weekly achieved the same visual acuities, but the actively stimulated group reached their zenith 2 months earlier.[54] Campbell and colleagues added intensive close work to 20 min per day of occlusion and found that 83% of children improved to 6/12.[31]

Active therapy has also been shown to be helpful when patching alone did not improve the visual acuity, i.e., 1 hr of video game play for patients previously unsuccessfully treated with occlusion[55]: fifteen of 19 (78%) had an additional 2 lines of improvement, and nearly 50% improved by 3 lines of acuity. Success in older, previously treated children has been reported in small studies[56,57]: these studies have shown improvement in visual acuity, but they were uncontrolled.

The Cambridge Amblyopic Vision Stimulator (CAM) employed more intensive activities.[30] The initial report suggested amazing results. However, subsequent studies included sham visual stimulation arms in which any improvement would be attributed solely to the occlusion. No significant difference in acuity outcomes was found,[58-60] leading to the abandonment of this method. However, with each passing year a new computer-based stimulation program is promoted as the cure. Clinicians need to be vigilant in monitoring the veracity of the outcomes reported!

A reasonable approach to the use of visual stimulation as a part of amblyopia treatment is that a patient should be doing at least some visually challenging activities during the period of occlusion or penalization. Furthermore, the child who is treated only while watching a television program they have seen many times before may not be as likely to improve.

Systemic therapy

Catecholamine neurotransmitters play a role in maintaining plasticity of the visual cortex during development. The administration of oral levodopa–carbidopa (L-dopa) combination therapy does improve the acuity of amblyopic eyes.[61] A standardized dosage regimen is not yet available. When this pharmacological therapy is combined with occlusion therapy the visual acuity improvement was greater than that with occlusion alone.[62] However, each of these studies noted substantial regression after the treatment was stopped, but the outcome acuity was felt to be better when occlusion was combined with L-dopa.[63]

Recently, a randomized trial compared L-dopa alone to L-dopa plus 3 hr per day occlusion and L-dopa plus occlusion for all waking hours in children with amblyopia.[64] An occlusion-only control group was not included. There was no difference in the magnitude of improvement between the three groups. Of the 72 patients, 74% experienced an improvement. The mean improvement was 1.6 lines. Half of the patients who improved maintained their improvement for one year. On the other hand, half of the successful patients experienced a mean 0.8-line regression of acuity after an average of 4 months following treatment. Side-effects of nausea, dizziness, decreased respiration, and decreased body temperature have been reported.[65,66]

Citicoline (Cytidine-5'-diphosphocholine) has been reported to have some success in a study of 50 amblyopic patients.[67] Treatment involved daily intramuscular injections for 10 days. Both the sound and amblyopic eyes improved and were stable for 4 months. This drug has been less widely used because of the requirement for parenteral administration, but few side-effects have been reported.

The high rate of relapse and the lack of compelling evidence of success greater than that found with conventional treatments make it impossible to recommend this approach at this time. However, systemic therapy may play a role in the future treatment of amblyopia.

Combined therapies

It is very common for clinicians to treat amblyopia with more than one approach simultaneously. A common approach is to part-time patch and to prescribe topical atropine, thus allowing the child to be continuously treated. Practically, the child will use the patch when not in school or at other activities where the patch may make them self-conscious. A second alternative is to prescribe topical atropine and reduce the plus sphere in the sound eye to plano (or some other reduction of plus power), thus blurring the sound eye at all fixation distances. Particular care in monitoring these patients for decreasing vision in the sound eye is prudent.

Discontinuation of treatment/maintenance therapy

Most clinicians stop intensive therapy when the patient is no longer showing improvement. However, the duration of treatment before cessation of therapy is unclear. Treatment for a minimum of 3 months with no documented improvement before stopping or reducing therapy is a reasonable approach.

Once therapy is thought to have reached its maximum benefit, this author begins to wean the patient off treatment over months or even a year, preferring to reduce by 50% every 3 months to help prevent a recurrence. However, there are no data to prove that weaning is superior to immediate cessation in retaining the benefit. An alternative would be to carefully follow a child every few months until 7 or 8 years of age without any active treatment besides glasses: this is often more inconvenient because of the increased number of visits needed.

The long-term stability of amblyopia therapy is an important public health goal if the high prevalence of amblyopic adults is to be reduced. The chance of maintaining most of the improvement into adulthood is about 75%.[68-70] These data, however, may represent the best case.

Compliance

Compliance is a key factor in the success of amblyopia therapy: it varies widely, from 30 to more than 90%.[20,71-73] The reasons for the inability to complete the prescribed regimen include visual impairment, skin irritation, and psychosocial reasons. Undoubtedly, poor compliance decreases the effectiveness of treatment. Pilot studies of occlusion therapy with occlusion dose monitors have shown the expected correlation of treatment compliance with outcomes.[74,75]

Compliance with topical pharmacological therapy is much easier, having to put the drop in only once per day: it was reported to be excellent or good in 96% of patients.[21]

Although the children may reject amblyopia therapy, lack of parental understanding about the disease and the time frame of therapy also seem to play a role. In one study of patching from the United Kingdom, failure to comply with the prescribed regimen at least 80% of the time occurred in 54% of patients.[76] The failure to comply was directly related to a parental lack of understanding that there is a time limit to effective therapy or a "critical period." It would appear that compliance can be improved with better education of the parents and some explanatory materials to take home.[38]

Reverse amblyopia

Reverse amblyopia (or occlusion amblyopia) is a form of deprivation amblyopia. It is defined as a reduction of vision in the sound eye of more than one line due to a treatment prescribed for amblyopia in the fellow eye. Reverse amblyopia has been associated with most forms of therapy of amblyopia. It seems to be most commonly associated with full-time occlusion, much less often with part-time occlusion, cycloplegic, and optical methods of treatment. Presumably, the protection afforded the sound eyes with these treatments is a frequent period of use for the sound eye (Table 78.1).

Treatment of adults

It is widely held that amblyopia therapy is more successful in younger patients, especially when less than 7 years of age consistent with the age-specific sensitive periods in development. Several findings question this. No age effect was found in a retrospective study and in two clinical trials for occlusion and pharmacological therapy in patients less than 7 years of age.[4,21,25,35] In addition, successful therapy in older patients has been reported,[71] especially in the setting of the loss of vision in the sound eye from an injury.

An adult who has never been treated should be offered at least one cycle of therapy. Occlusion therapy, dopaminergic drugs, penalization therapy, biofeedback, and repetitive vernier tasks have been associated with improvement in this population. There

Table 78.1 Actions to be taken if reverse (occlusion) amblyopia is suspected

Reverse amblyopia generally recovers quickly, though there are reports of permanent visual impairment or change in fixation.
1. Each patient who develops such a reduction in acuity should be reassessed clinically.
2. Check the refraction with cycloplegia.
3. Retest the vision with the new spectacles.
4. Is there evidence of an optic neuropathy, i.e., an afferent pupil defect, color vision, optic atrophy and nerve fiber layer defect? Other age-appropriate testing may be needed. If there is any doubt consider electrophysiology (Chapter 11) or neuroimaging (Chapter 13).
5. If the acuity reduction is confirmed, either stop the active amblyopia therapy and reexamine the patient in several weeks or continue or reduce therapy with careful monitoring of the sound eye.
6. If the sound eye is worse than the amblyopic eye, stop therapy and reschedule a visit.
7. If the vision in the sound eye is still down on the subsequent visit, consider treating the formerly sound eye.

is no published clinical trial to demonstrate an outcome superior to the natural history. A randomized pilot study of treatment of 10–18 year olds for 2 months with occlusion found that 27% improved two or more lines.[77]

In the absence of a study demonstrating the ideal treatment, it is reasonable to employ every treatment available, often at the same time to maximize the chances of an improvement in acuity. Motivation in this age group is crucial if adequate compliance is to be achieved with the chance of visual acuity improvement.

REFERENCES

1. National Eye Institute Office of Biometry and Epidemiology. Report on the National Eye Institute's Visual Acuity Impairment Survey Pilot Study. Washington, DC: Department of Health and Human Services; 1984: 81–4.
2. Attebo K, Mitchell P, Cumming R, et al. Prevalence and causes of amblyopia in an adult population. Ophthalmology 1998; 105: 154–9.
3. von Noorden GK. Binocular Vision and Ocular Motility: Theory and Management of Strabismus. St Louis: Mosby; 1996.
4. Woodruff G, Hiscox F, Thompson JR, et al. Factors affecting the outcome of children treated for amblyopia. Eye 1994; 8: 627–31.
5. Shaw DE, Fielder AR, Minshull C, et al. Amblyopia–factors influencing age of presentation. Lancet 1988; 2: 207–9.
6. Köhler L, Stigmar G. Vision screening of four-year-old children. Acta Paediatr Scand 1973; 62: 17–27.
7. Winder S, Farquhar A, Nah GKM, et al. The outcome of orthoptic screening in Aberdeen in 1990. Br Orthopt J 1996; 53: 36–8.
8. Bray LC, Clarke MP, Jarvis SN, et al. Preschool vision screening: a prospective comparative evaluation. Eye 1996; 10: 714–6.
9. Simons K. Preschool vision screening: rationale, methodology and outcome. Surv Ophthalmol 1996; 41: 3–30.
10. McGraw PV, Winn B. Glasgow acuity cards: a new test for the measurement of letter acuity in children. Ophthalmic Physiol Opt 1993; 13: 400–4.
11. Holmes JM, Beck RW, Repka MX, et al. The amblyopia treatment study visual acuity testing protocol. Arch Ophthalmol 2001; 119: 1345–53.
12. Moke PS, Turpin AH, Beck RW, et al. Computerized method of visual acuity testing: adaptation of the amblyopia treatment study visual acuity testing protocol. Am J Ophthalmol 2001; 132: 903–9.
13. Hyvarinen L, Nasanen R, Laurinen P. New visual acuity test for pre–school children. Acta Ophthalmologica 1980; 58: 507–11.
14. Becker R, Hubsch S, Graf MH, et al. Examination of young children with Lea symbols. Br J Ophthalmol 2002; 86: 513–6.
15. Atilla H, Oral D, Coskun S, et al. Poor correlation between "fix-follow-maintain" monocular/binocular fixation pattern evaluation and presence of functional amblyopia. Binoc Vis Strabismus Q 2001; 16: 85–90.
16. Teller DY, McDonald MA, Preston K, et al. Assessment of visual acuity in infants and children: the acuity card procedure. Dev Med Child Neurol 1986; 28: 779–89.
17. Rydberg A. Assessment of visual acuity in adult patients with strabismic amblyopia: a comparison between the preferential looking method and different acuity charts. Acta Ophthalmol Scand 1997; 75: 611–7.
18. Simons K, Preslan M. Natural history of amblyopia untreated owing to lack of compliance. Br J Ophthalmol 1999; 83: 582–7.
19. Snowdon SK, Stewart-Brown SL. Preschool vision screening. Health Technol Assess 1997; 1(8): 1–83.
20. Cleary M. Efficacy of occlusion for strabismic amblyopia: can an optimal duration be identified? Br J Ophthalmol 2000; 84: 572–7.
21. Pediatric Eye Disease Investigator Group. A randomized trial of atropine vs patching for treatment of moderate amblyopia in children. Arch Ophthalmol 2002; 120: 268–78.
22. Clarke M, Richardson S, Hrisos S. UK ATT Research Group. The UK amblyopia treatment trial: visual acuity and untreated unilateral straight eyed amblyopia. In: de Faber JT, editor. Transactions of the International Strabismological Association. Sydney, Australia; 2003: 167–86.
23. Clarke MP, Wright CM, Hrisos S, et al. Randomised controlled trial of treatment of unilateral visual impairment detected at preschool vision screening. BMJ 2003; 327: 1251.
24. Moseley M, Fielder AR. Improvement in amblyopic eye function and contralateral eye disease: evidence of residual plasticity. Lancet 2001; 357: 902–3.
25. Hiscox F, Strong N, Thompson JR, et al. Occlusion for amblyopia: a comprehensive survey of outcome. Eye 1992; 6: 300–4.
26. Olson RJ, Scott WE. A practical approach to occlusion therapy for amblyopia. Semin Ophthalmol 1997; 12: 161–5.
27. Rutstein RP. Alternative treatment for amblyopia. Probl Optometry 1991: 351–4.
28. Scott WE, Stratton VB, Fabre J. Full-time occlusion therapy for amblyopia. Am Orthopt J 1980; 30: 125–30.
29. Flynn JT, Schiffman J, Feuer W, et al. The therapy of amblyopia: an analysis of the results of amblyopia therapy utilizing the pooled data of published studies. Trans Am Ophthalmol Soc 1998; 96: 431–53.

30. Banks RV, Campbell FW, Hess RF, et al. A new treatment for amblyopia. Br Orthopt J 1978; 31.

31. Campbell FW, Hess RF, Watson PG, et al. Preliminary results of a physiologically based treatment of amblyopia. Br J Ophthalmol 1978; 62: 748–55.

32. Watson PG, Banks RV, Campbell FW, et al. Clinical assessment of a new treatment for amblyopia. Trans Ophthal Soc UK 1978.

33. Mazow ML, Chuang A, Vital MC, et al. Outcome study in amblyopia: treatment and practice pattern variations. J AAPOS 2000; 4: 1–9.

34. Tan JHY, Thompson JR, Gottlob I. Differences in the management of amblyopia between European countries. Br J Ophthalmol 2003; 87: 291–6.

35. Pediatric Eye Disease Investigator Group. A randomized trial of patching regimens for treatment of moderate amblyopia in children. Arch Ophthalmol 2003; 121: 603–11.

36. Pediatric Eye Disease Investigator Group. A comparison of atropine and patching treatments for moderate amblyopia by patient age, cause of amblyopia, depth of amblyopia, and other factors. Ophthalmology 2003; 110: 1632–7; discussion 1637–8.

37. Pediatric Eye Disease Investigator Group. A randomized trial of prescribed patching regimens for treatment of severe amblyopia in children. Ophthalmology 2003; 110: 2075–87.

38. Newsham D. A randomised controlled trial of written information: the effect on parental non-concordance with occlusion therapy. Br J Ophthalmol 2002; 86: 787–91.

39. Simonsz HJ, Polling JR, Voorn R, et al. Electronic monitoring of treatment compliance in patching for amblyopia. Strabismus 1999; 7: 113–23.

40. Repka MX, Gallin PF, Scholz RT, et al. Determination of optical penalization by vectographic fixation reversal. Ophthalmology 1985; 92: 1584–6.

41. North RV, Kelly ME. Atropine occlusion in the treatment of strabismic amblyopia and its effect upon the non-amblyopic eye. Ophthalmic Physiol Opt 1991; 11: 113–7.

42. Repka MX, Ray JM. The efficacy of optical and pharmacological penalization. Ophthalmology 1993; 100: 769–75.

43. Simons K, Stein L, Sener EC, et al. Full-time atropine, intermittent atropine, and optical penalization and binocular outcome in treatment of strabismic amblyopia. Ophthalmology 1997; 104: 2143–55.

44. Neumann E, Friedman Z, Abel–Peleg B. Prevention of strabismic amblyopia of early onset with special reference to the optimal age for screening. J Pediatr Ophthalmol Strabismus 1987; 24: 106–10.

45. Lithander J, Sjostrand J. Anisometropic and stabismic amblyopia in the age group 2 years and above: a prospective study of the results of treatment. Br J Ophthalmol 1991; 75: 111–6.

46. Ching FC, Park MM, Friendly DS. Practical management of amblyopia. J Pediatr Ophthalmol Strabismus 1986; 23: 12–6.

47. Kaye SB, Chen SI, Price G, et al. Combined optical and atropine penalization for the treatment of strabismic and anisometropic amblyopia. J AAPOS 2002; 6: 289–93.

48. Tychsen L. Discussion. Ophthalmology 1993; 100: 769–75.

49. Ron A, Nawratzki I. Penalization treatment of amblyopia: a follow-up study of two years in older children. J Pediatr Ophthalmol Strabismus 1982; 19: 137–9.

50. Doran RML, Yarde S, Starbuck A. Comparison of treatment methods in strabismic amblyopia, chap. 5. In: Campos EC, editor. Strabismus and Ocular Motility Disorders. London: Macmillan; 1990: 51–9.

51. Foley-Nolan A, McCann A, O'Keefe M. Atropine penalisation versus occlusion as the primary treatment for amblyopia. Br J Ophthalmol 1997; 81: 54–7.

52. France TD, France LW. Optical penalization can improve vision after occlusion treatment. J AAPOS 1999; 3: 341–3.

53. Duke-Elder S, Wybar K. System of ophthalmology. St Louis: Mosby; 1973: 424–32. (Vol. VI.)

54. François J, James M. Comparative study of amblyopic treatment. Am Orthopt J 1955; 5: 61–4.

55. Shippman S. Video games and amblyopia treatment. Am Orthopt J 1985; 32: 2–5.

56. von Noorden GK, Spronger F, Romano P, et al. Home therapy for amblyopia. Am Orthopt J 1970; 20: 46–50.

57. Gould A, Fishkoff D, Galin MA. Active visual stimulation: a method of treatment of amblyopia in the older patient. Am Orthopt J 1970; 20: 39–45.

58. Mitchell DE, Howell ER, Keith CG. The effect of minimal occlusion therapy on binocular visual functions in amblyopia. Invest Ophthalmol Vis Sci 1983; 24: 778–81.

59. Schor C, Gibson J, Hsu M, et al. The use of rotating gratings for the treatment of amblyopia: a clinical trial. Am J Optometry Physiological Optics 1981; 58: 930-8.

60. Lennerstrand G, Samuelsson B. Amblyopia in 4–year-old children treated with grating stimulation and full-time occlusion; a comparative study. Br J Ophthalmol 1983; 67: 181–90.

61. Leguire LE, Narius TM, Rogers GK, et al. Long-term follow-up L-dopa treated amblyopic children. Invest Opthalmol Vis Sci 1996; 37(supp):S941.

62. Leguire LE, Rogers GL, Walson PD, et al. Occlusion and levodopa-carbidopa treatment for childhood amblyopia. J AAPOS 1998; 2: 257–64.

63. Leguire LE, Komaromy KL, Nairus TM, et al. Long-term follow-up of L-dopa treatment in children with amblyopia. J Pediatr Ophthalmol Strabismus 2002; 39: 326–30.

64. Mohan K, Dhankar V, Sharma A. Visual acuities after levodopa adminstration in amblyopia. J Pediatr Ophthalmol Strabismus 2001; 38: 62–7.

65. Leguire LE, Walson PD, Rogers GL, et al. Levodopa/carbidopa treatment for amblyopia in older children. J Pediatr Ophthalmol Strabismus 1995; 32: 143–51.

66. Gottlob I, Wizov SS, Reinecke RD. Visual acuities and scotomas after 3 weeks' levodopa adminstration in adult amblyopia. Graefe's Arch Clin Exp Ophthalmol 1995; 233: 407–13.

67. Campos EC, Bolzani R, Schiavi C, et al. Cytidin-5'-diphosphocholine enhances the effect of part-time occlusion in amblyopia. Documenta Ophthalmologica 1997; 93: 247–63.

68. Scott WE, Dickey CF. Stability of visual acuity in amblyopic patients after visual maturity. Graefe's Arch Clin Exp Ophthalmol 1988; 226: 154, 467–74.

69. Leiba H, Shimshoni M, Oliver M, et al. Long-term follow-up of occlusion therapy in amblyopia. Ophthalmology 2001; 108: 1552–5.

70. Ohlsson J, Baumann M, Sjostrand J, et al. Long term visual outcome in amblyopia treatment. Br J Ophthalmol 2002; 86: 1148–51.

71. Oliver M, Neumann E, Chaimovitch MD, et al. Compliance and results of treatment for amblyopia in children more than 8 years old. Am J Ophthalmol 1986; 102: 340–5.

72. Leach C. Compliance with occlusion therapy for strabismic and anisometropic amblyopia: a pilot study. Binoc Vis Eye Musc Surg Q 1995; 10: 257–66.

73. Parkes LC. An investigation of the impact of occlusion therapy on children with amblyopia, its effect on their families, and compliance with treatment. Br Orthopt J 2001; 58: 30–7.

74. Moseley MJ, Fielder AR, Irwin M, et al. Effectiveness of occlusion therapy in ametropic amblyopia: a pilot study. Br J Ophthalmol 1997; 81: 956–61.

75. Loudon SE, Polling JR, Simonsz HJ. A preliminary report about the relation between visual acuity increase and compliance in patching therapy for amblyopia. Strabismus 2002; 10: 79–82.

76. Newsham D. Parental non–concordance with occlusion therapy. Br J Ophthalmol 2000; 84: 957–62.

77. Pediatric Eye Disease Investigator Group. A prospective, pilot study of treatment of amblyopia in children 10 to <18 years old. Am J Ophthalmol 2004; 137: 581–583

CHAPTER
79

The Clinical Approach to Strabismus

Anthony J Vivian

INTRODUCTION

Although rates of strabismus surgery are declining, the management of strabismus and amblyopia continues to account for a majority of the workload of most pediatric ophthalmologists. Strategies for managing this workload efficiently and effectively are required.

This chapter gives a few ideas about laying out and managing an efficient and effective strabismus practice. It stresses the importance of a friendly, nonthreatening environment (both structural and emotional) and the fundamental principles of accurate documentation and audit to ensure clinically effective management.

THE CLINICAL SETTING

More frequently than not, the structural layout of our clinic space is constrained by immovable walls, doors, and windows often not ideally placed. Occasionally there is an opportunity to start with a blank piece of paper, giving rise to some fundamental questions. How long should an examination room be? Do all the rooms have to be the same size? How can the most be made of a restricted floor area?

Room layout

The dimensions of a typical examination room for assessing children with strabismus have been dictated in the past by the need to measure visual acuity at 6 m (20 ft) using Snellen acuity charts. There is now good evidence that tests based on the logarithmic scale of the minimum angle of resolution (logMAR) are more accurate methods for measuring acuity. Many of these tests can be projected or displayed on computer screens and so testing distances are more flexible.

Other factors determining the length of the examination room are the minimum distance required to prevent accommodation affecting the basic deviation measurement and other distance tests such as distance stereopsis and fusion tests. The maximum amount of accommodation when viewing an accommodative target at 6 m is about an eighth of a diopter, which is clinically insignificant. At 4 m accommodation is not so completely suspended and could theoretically influence the basic deviation measurement (angle of deviation in the primary position for distance with accommodation suspended) in some patients. So, at least some rooms should be 6 m in length to best perform accurate motility testing. However, these rooms do not need to be rectangular and to make the best use of limited floor area the rooms can "interlock" so that there is a wide end for the examiner and patient and a thin end for the fixation and acuity targets (Fig. 79.1).

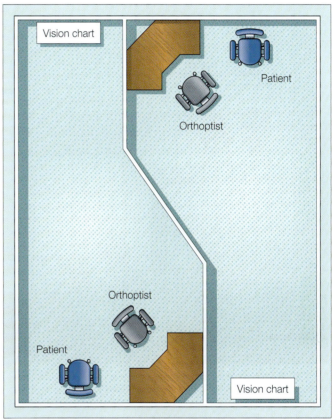

Fig. 79.1 Design for two interlocking 6-m orthoptic rooms making maximum use of available floor space.

Distance fixation and acuity targets

Obtaining accurate results for the basic deviation measurement in children can be challenging. Failure to achieve an accurate measurement for distance is a common cause of surgical error, as many children with strabismus have a disparity between distance and near deviation. Operating on the near angle (which is easier to measure) in these cases may result in an over- or under-correction for distance.

Interesting distance fixation targets are essential items in the management of childhood strabismus. Asking a child to fix on the letters of a Snellen acuity chart will not hold the child's attention for long. A variety of fixation targets are necessary, some requiring greater resolution than others. Cartoon characters and soft toys arranged at 6 m provide more interest for the child. A successful method of maintaining distance fixation in children is using videos on a TV screen at 6 m, which can be controlled from the examination end of the room (Fig. 79.2). A selection of

869

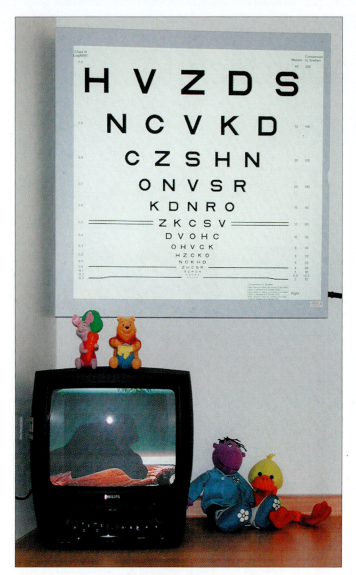

Fig. 79.2 By using a television playing age-appropriate videos, distance fixation is enhanced, allowing better distance measurements.

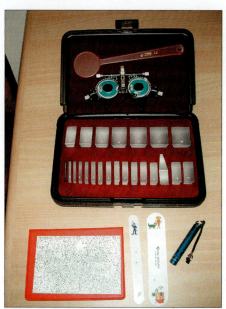

Fig. 79.3 A selection of useful instruments for strabismus assessment.

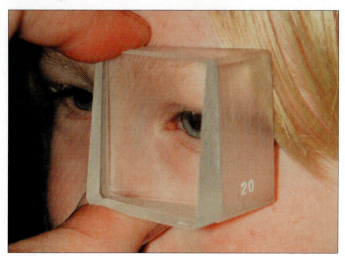

Fig. 79.4 Using single prisms held in one hand, vertical and horizontal deviations can be assessed simultaneously.

videos of interest to different age groups maximizes the chance of prolonged distance fixation to allow prism cover tests to be performed.

Tools of the trade

When assessing children with strabismus, there are a number of items of equipment useful to have on the desk (Fig. 79.3). This list is not exhaustive but serves to emphasize the concept that if the equipment is not at hand, the test will not be done:

1. Occluder for performing cover tests: A transparent (Spielmann) occluder allows visualization of the occluded eye.
2. Single prisms (Berens square prisms are the most accurate) for performing prism cover tests: single prisms have a number of advantages over prism bars. The larger prism area allows better visualization of the fixation targets by the patient, and allows better visualization of the eye by the examiner. Both horizontal and vertical deviations can be corrected simultaneously in front of the same eye (Fig. 79.4).

3. Near acuity target for determining the near angle as accommodative demand is increased (particularly useful in assessing children with convergence excess esotropia).
4. Near stereoacuity tests (Lang, Frisby, TNO, Wirt).
5. Maddox rods or Bagolini lenses to fit in the trial frame for measuring torsion.
6. Fixation light.

INTERACTION WITH THE CHILD AND PARENTS

First meeting

Young children can find their first eye clinic appointment an intimidating experience. They may be too young to understand what is going on and have to wait for a long time to be seen, absorbing the anxiety of their parents. They will need to have dilating drops instilled. It is important to make the first visit a positive experience for both the child and the parents. If the initial visit has not been too traumatic, subsequent visits will yield more information.

The waiting area should be a child-friendly environment. Professional play assistants make a significant difference to the overall mood of the waiting area, relieving some of the stress of the parents, which reflects in the behavior of the child.

Several methods for getting the most information out of the first visit can be employed:

1. Observation: This can be performed while talking to the parents or while the child plays. Look at the visual behavior and look for an abnormal head posture or obvious strabismus.
2. Lang stereotest: This can be made into a game, which can be played first by a parent or sibling. It is a good initial test because it is not intimidating (does not require special glasses to be worn).
3. Distance fixation using videos: Children's videos playing at the far end of the examination room serve as a useful distance fixation target to enable cover testing and diagnosis of amblyopia by determining fixation preference.
4. Cycloplegic drops: Cyclopentolate 1% instilled 30 minutes before refraction is adequate for most children. Best results are obtained if someone other than the examiner, in a separate room, instills them. Topical anesthetic (proxymetacaine 0.5%) used a couple of minutes before reduces the discomfort of the cycloplegic drops considerably and should be considered but it requires two instillations. Atropine 1% can be used if cycloplegia with cyclopentolate cannot be obtained. If the child finds instillation of drops in the clinic very traumatic and as a result examination becomes difficult, atropine ointment can be instilled at home by the parents prior to the clinic appointment.
5. If a fundus view is not achieved, another attempt should be made at a later date. It is occasionally necessary to physically restrain a child for fundus examination if there is suspicion of fundus pathology; otherwise, it can be repeated at another occasion.
6. Examination of the optic nerve should include a magnified view. This can be achieved with a direct ophthalmoscope or by slit-lamp biomicroscopy, which gives a much better view and is not difficult to perform in most children over about 4 years of age. It is particularly important to recheck the fundus and disc appearance in children with amblyopia refractory to treatment to exclude other causes of poor vision such as optic nerve hypoplasia.
7. Hand-held slit lamp: It is possible to look at children on an adult slit lamp, but examining small children is easier with a hand-held slit lamp.

Role of the orthoptist

The orthoptist plays an important role in the strabismus clinic. They have special expertise in the assessment of adults and children with strabismus. However, it is important that the strabismus surgeons are competent at performing a complete examination themselves. Only by examining the patient themselves can they get a feel for the subtleties of strabismus that are not possible to write down.

Strabismus management should involve a multidisciplinary approach. The doctor should be able competently to perform a sensory and motor examination, and increasingly orthoptists are expanding their role to include parts of the examination traditionally the territory of the ophthalmologist such as refraction.

Practical history taking: extracting clinically relevant details

A focussed assessment of symptoms and past history is very useful in the management of child strabismus patients. The history taking does not have to be extensive but should be careful and specific. It is important to find out about:

1. The parent's observations about the strabismus: Whether the eyes turn in or out, which eye is most commonly affected, whether the strabismus is intermittent or constant, and changes in the strabismus when the child is tired or unwell.
2. Other ophthalmic symptoms: Whether there are any associated abnormalities such as closing one eye in bright light, whether double vision is experienced, and whether they have noticed a vertical element to the strabismus or an association with changes in lid height.
3. Past ophthalmic history: Whether there is any history of ophthalmic care (including glasses or patching), trauma, or previous strabismus surgery.
4. Past medical history: Previous history of systemic or neurological disease; the pregnancy, delivery and developmental history; and the drug and allergy history.
5. Family history: Whether there is a family history of glasses wear in childhood, lazy eyes, or strabismus surgery; and whether there is a family history of either ophthalmic or systemic inherited disease.

EXAMINATION

Examination of the strabismus patient should include in all patients:

- A sensory examination (acuity, fixation preference, binocular vision, fusion, accommodation, and convergence);
- Ocular motility testing;
- Ocular examination (slit-lamp examination, media and fundus examination); and
- Refraction (cycloplegic in children).

Further specific examination including a search for dysmorphic or neurological signs may be necessary as a result of other findings.

Sensory examination

Acuity

There are many tests designed to measure visual acuity in preverbal and verbal children, some more successful than others. All of them rely to some degree on experience in both performing and interpreting the tests. A careful measurement of acuity is essential both at the first visit and at subsequent visits for monitoring. Both near and distance acuity should be measured.

In order to maintain reproducible results, acuity measurement techniques and recording in an ophthalmic unit should be standardized with specific acuity tests for children at each level of developmental ability. There is a very large range of different acuity tests, each with its own merits but it is most important to have a hierarchy of tests that give reproducible results at various ages.

Preferential looking techniques

Preferential looking is a behavioral method of assessing visual acuity, which can be performed from a very young age. The principal of these tests is that the child will be more interested in looking at a target with a resolvable pattern on it than looking at a target with no resolvable pattern. The child will therefore make a preferential choice to look at one of a choice of targets, and the resolution of the target can be reduced until the child is unable to make a choice. The point at which the child is unable to make a choice gives an estimate of the visual acuity. For infants and children to the age of about 2 years, grating acuity cards such as Keeler or Teller can be used, and for children between 2 and 3 years of age vanishing optotypes such as Cardiff cards are more appropriate.

Kay pictures

Picture chart acuity tests such as Kay pictures can give some idea about visual acuity although they tend to give an overestimated value. They are certainly useful for comparing the acuity of each eye in children up to the age of about 3 years.

LogMAR-based matching tests

At the age of about $3\frac{1}{2}$ to 4 years most children will be able to perform a logMAR-based matching test, which can be presented on cards[1] or on a screen.[2] These give accurate and reproducible acuity results.

LogMAR

Once the child knows the alphabet, a full logMAR acuity is possible using a logMAR chart (such as a Bailey-Lovie chart). It is important to measure the worse eye first because children have excellent memories.

Fixation preference

Estimating fixation preference is a simple and effective clinical test for detecting amblyopia and can be performed as early as 6 months of age. It is most accurate in patients with strabismus of 10 prism diopters or more. Fixation preference is analyzed by assessing the centrality, steadiness, and maintenance of fixation (CSM method). "Central" fixation requires that the corneal reflex is central in the pupil. "Steady" fixation requires no evidence of nystagmus or oscillatory eye movements. "Maintained" fixation refers to the ability of the nonpreferred eye to maintain fixation after occlusion is removed from the preferred eye. This can be graded to some degree by determining whether the fixation is maintained through a blink or during a smooth pursuit movement, or by observing the time period through which fixation is maintained by the nonpreferred eye when occlusion is removed from the preferred eye.[3]

In orthotropic patients, fixation preference can be assessed by creating a deviation using a 10- or 12-diopter prism either base-up or base-down in front of one eye. The prism is used vertically because vertical fusion is much smaller than horizontal fusion. Fixation should alternate if acuity is equal. If a fixation preference is detected, it can be graded in a similar fashion to strabismic patients.

Binocular single vision, fusion, and stereopsis

Amongst the most confusing and difficult areas of strabismus management to understand are binocular single vision, fusion, and stereopsis. This is partly a result of the terminology and partly reflects our limited understanding of how the eyes work together. The terminology used by physiologists and that used by ophthalmologists are different, which has contributed significantly to our confusion. Although concepts such as "the horopter" and "Panum's fusional area" are useful for the physiologist, they often confound the practical ophthalmologist. The result is that the practical ophthalmologist decides the sensory side of strabismus

is too much to cope with and leaves it to the orthoptist and theorist. This is a pity because if the useful information, which affects management, is separated from the information not useful in making management decisions, it is much easier to use selected sensory evaluations in the overall management plan. In order to achieve this, we must be very clear about our definitions. What follows is a list of definitions, which should help to simplify the sensory assessment of strabismus patients, and an account of how we use this information to our advantage in the management of these patients.

Retinal correspondence

In order to obtain binocular vision, the images from each eye must be superimposed on each other in the occipital cortex. This superimposition is not done as a complete picture but by piecing together many small parts of a picture like a jigsaw. Each piece of the jigsaw requires a contribution from both the right and left retinas. Each retinal area thus has a corresponding mate in the other retina that contributes to the same part of the jigsaw in the cortex. Normal retinal correspondence requires that the foveas of each eye contribute to the same piece of cortical jigsaw. Patients with abnormal retinal correspondence have a situation whereby an area of retina adjacent to the fovea of one eye contributes its image to the same piece of jigsaw as the foveal image from the other eye.

Sensory and motor fusion

The understanding of fusion has been complicated by the use of the word for two separate functions:

- *Motor fusion*: The ability to physically move the eyes so that they are pointing in the same direction, allowing the corresponding areas of the retina in each eye to be pointing at the object of regard.
- *Sensory fusion*: Taking the image from each corresponding retinal area and superimposing them in binocular cells at the level of the occipital cortex.

The two are obviously inextricably linked in that it is not possible to have sensory fusion if the eyes are pointing in different directions, and the brain only knows how much to move the eyes by assessing whether the images arriving at the occipital cortex from the corresponding retinal areas of each eye are similar (the motor fusion mechanism uses sensory fusion as a feedback). When the motor fusion mechanisms have done their job, sensory fusion is possible. If there is no sensory fusion, the motor fusion mechanism has no feedback and may fail, resulting in motor misalignment.

Central (bifoveal) and peripheral fusion

In order to obtain high-quality single images, the foveal images from each eye must be aligned. Only when this is achieved can stereopsis (depth perception) be obtained. This is called central or bifoveal fusion. A cruder form of single image using both eyes is possible without perfect foveal images (for instance, in patients with an amblyopic eye) and without perfect alignment (for instance, in patients with small angle esotropia). This is called peripheral fusion.

Fusion range (fusion amplitudes)

The fusion range refers to the range over which the motor fusion mechanism is able to pull the two eyes together. It is measured by placing progressively more powerful prisms in front of the eyes until the patient experiences diplopia (i.e., the fusional amplitude has been exceeded). The prisms are placed first base in and then base out to measure both the divergence and convergence fusion range. The vertical fusion range is measured using base-up and base-down prisms.

Binocular vision

Binocular vision is another confusing term because it is used in many contexts. Essentially it means seeing with two eyes, but as ophthalmologists we take it to mean more. We assume that using two eyes together and gaining a single image is somehow better than using one eye at a time. Even if one eye is amblyopic and no stereopsis (the perception of depth) is measurable, the combined image from two eyes has a quality superior to that of single eye vision. The term binocular single vision is perhaps preferable as it emphasizes that both eyes are being used and a single image is being obtained. The fact that binocular single vision is even obtainable if the eyes are not aligned (for instance in microtropias) shows that the occipital cortex is lenient in terms of what it will accept from corresponding retinal areas and still perceive single vision. Central (foveal) fusion is not a prerequisite for binocular single vision. Fusion of peripheral retinal areas seems to be enough.

Stereopsis

The most advanced form of vision we possess is stereopsis. This is the perception of depth and the impression of three dimensions. This requires perfect alignment of the eyes and good quality of image from each fovea; foveal fusion is a prerequisite for high levels of stereopsis. A low level of stereopsis is possible in microtropias.

Measuring retinal correspondence binocular vision and fusion

Tests of retinal correspondence

It is not necessary to test retinal correspondence in all patients. The important patients to recognize are those who have a manifest strabismus, but have binocular single vision without suppressing one image. In these patients the fovea of the fixing eye has developed a relationship with an extrafoveal area of the nonfixing eye. If the abnormal retinal correspondence is deep-rooted, operating to straighten the eyes results in a return to the original angle post-operatively.

Bagolini glasses

Bagolini glasses detect abnormal retinal correspondence without dissociating the eyes. They do, however, require a high level of cooperation and understanding and so cannot be used in young children. Because the lenses have striations, a point source of light is seen as a straight line. The lenses in front of each eye are arranged at 90° to each other, so with both eyes open a point source of light (at either 33 cm or 6 m) is perceived as a cross. They give useful information about suppression and they are useful in two other situations:

- The patient with strabismus on corneal reflection, but no movement on cover testing. If the Bagolini glasses result is normal in the presence of an obvious deviation, there must be abnormal retinal correspondence, and if this is well established in a patient who is visually mature, surgery could result in intractable diplopia.
- The patient with microtropia (monofixation syndrome). These patients have ultrasmall deviations (difficult or impossible to detect on cover testing) associated with amblyopia and foveal scotoma. The Bagolini test shows anomalous retinal correspondence with a break in the Bagolini line in the affected eye.

Tests of fusion potential

Strabismus patients with good fusion potential are more likely to maintain alignment after surgery. Testing fusional potential in patients with manifest strabismus is, however, difficult. Fusion potential can be tested using the synoptophore but because this is a dissociative test, results may be difficult to interpret.

Worth four-dot test

Tests such as the Worth four-dot test are of limited value in the management of strabismus. It is a very dissociative test (because red and green glasses are used). All that can be said is that patients able to fuse in such circumstances must have good fusional potential. Patients unable to fuse under the test conditions may still have reasonable fusion if the eyes are not dissociated. This test measures motor fusion rather than sensory fusion.

The test is composed of four lights, two green, one red, and one white. A red glass is worn over one eye (usually the right by convention) and a green glass over the other eye. The test lights are viewed at the appropriate test distance (near or distant, depending on the type of test being used). There are three possible results:

- *Fusion*: If four lights are seen, the patient has fusion capability. At the appropriate test distance the lights fall on the fovea so central fusion is being tested. If the test is negative (shows diplopia or suppression) the patient can be moved closer to the test lights so that the lights fall outside of the fovea, and thus peripheral fusion is tested. If the white light appears green, the left eye is dominant, if it appears red or pink the right eye is dominant.
- *Diplopia*: If five lights are seen the patient has diplopia and no fusion.
- *Suppression*: If only two or three lights are seen, the patient is suppressing one or other of their eyes. If the patient sees two lights and then three, there is alternating suppression.

Testing fusion range (amplitude)

This is best tested using prisms (usually a prism bar) in free space. Prisms are increased in strength until diplopia is reported. If the prisms are placed base-out in front of one eye, the eyes must converge to restore binocularity. The prisms are increased in strength until the patient is no longer able to restore binocularity and reports diplopia. The prisms are then placed base-in in front of one eye and the eyes must diverge to restore binocularity. The vertical fusion ranges can be measured in patients with vertical strabismus.

Motor fusion can be estimated in very young children by putting a 20-diopter base-out prism in front of one eye to see whether the patient is able to overcome the prism. The child fixes on a light, and the prism is placed in front of one eye. If the child has motor fusion potential, a refixation movement will be seen.

Tests of stereopsis

Stereopsis is the most sophisticated form of binocular vision. Patients with measurable stereopsis must have sensory fusion, and so if the stereopsis test is positive, tests of sensory fusion are unnecessary. Stereopsis measurement should be performed before the eyes are dissociated by other tests such as Worth four-dot or cover tests. Patients with obvious manifest deviations are unlikely to have measurable stereopsis (although patients with small angle deviations and good motor fusion may have some stereopsis). The tests are most useful in patients with intermittent deviations or distance/near deviations. Patients who lose stereopsis under either of these conditions need urgent treatment to restore it.

Four commonly used tests of near stereopsis are:

- *Lang stereopsis test*: This test is simple to use, does not involve wearing glasses to dissociate the eyes, and can be used for very young children (even 1 year olds) There are two cards on which stereoscopic images are displayed. Separate random dot images are conveyed to each eye by the cylindrical gratings laminated onto the front of the card. Very young children will point at the images, which can only be seen if some degree of stereopsis is present. Even if the child does not point at the image they may look at each image in turn and it is obvious that they are able to see the images. The disparity of the images ranges from 1200 to 200 sec of arc. This test is very useful in the assessment of the sensory status of children with ocular motility disorders and screening children in the pediatric clinic.
- *Titmus stereo test*: This test uses polarizing glasses to dissociate the two eyes, and can be used from about the age of 2 to 3 years. There are three separate tests (the fly, circles, and animals) that test stereoacuity down to 40 sec of arc.
- *TNO stereo test:* This test uses red and green glasses to dissociate the eyes.
- *Frisby stereo tests*: This test does not require any form of glasses, which is advantageous. It is a nondissociative test.

These tests measure near stereopsis. Some patients have distance stereopsis but no near stereopsis. There are distance stereopsis tests available (Frisby distance stereotest) and are useful in children with convergence excess esotropia with a controlled distance deviation but esotropia for near.

Accommodation and convergence

Accommodation and convergence should be measured routinely when the child is old enough. This can be achieved by using an accommodative near target. The accommodative convergence/accommodation (AC/A) ratio should be measured in those patients with a distance/near disparity. However, measuring the AC/A ratio is difficult in children younger than about 5 or 6 years of age as it requires quite a degree of participation from the child.

Motor examination

Basic deviation

The basic deviation is the angle of strabismus measured with the eyes in the primary position, having ensured full correction of refractive errors. Fixation should be with the preferred eye on a distance target (6 m) in standard room lighting.

Prism cover tests in nine positions of gaze

A full ocular motility examination involves prism cover tests in nine positions of gaze. However, this is not necessary (and not always possible) in all patients. Nine positions of gaze measurements are most important in patients with vertical deviations and require a degree of patient cooperation. In children with horizontal deviations it is important to perform prism cover tests in the primary position, but also in up- and downgaze (to exclude "A" and "V" patterns) and in sidegaze to exclude lateral incomitance (especially in patients with exotropia).

The deviation in nine positions of gaze is determined using prism cover tests. Single prisms are used rather than prism bars. Although errors can be introduced during prism cover testing, being aware of the potential pitfalls and avoiding them can allow

this test to become an accurate measurement method.[4] The patient fixates on a distant target and the head is moved so that the eyes take up the positions of extreme gaze. It is important that the eyes are in extreme gaze positions when performing the prism cover tests to ensure reproducibility. If the nose obscures the vision of one eye, the head can be moved so that vision is just regained. Prisms are held in front of the paretic eye. With single prisms, both the vertical and horizontal elements can be neutralized by holding the appropriate prisms in one hand in front of the paretic eye.

Having performed prism cover tests in nine positions of gaze for distance, the near deviation in the primary position is determined, usually to an accommodative target.

Versions and ductions

Versions are eye movements of each eye tested with both eyes open. The importance of examining the versions is to look at the actions of the six extraocular muscles of each eye for underaction, overaction, or restriction.

Versions are tested using a light as a target with both eyes open, and are scored using a nine-point scoring system. Normal versions score 0, overactions are graded from +1 to +4, and underactions are graded from −1 to − 4. Sclera should be concealed by the canthus in a normal horizontal version. If sclera is just visible, the version is graded -1 and an inability to abduct or adduct the eye more than halfway into the field of action of the muscle is graded −2. Inability to abduct or adduct an eye more than a quarter-way into the field of action of the muscle is graded −3, and if the eye is unable to move at all from the primary position into the field of action of that muscle, the limitation is graded −4. Horizontal rectus overaction is graded according to the amount of cornea covered by the canthus. In extreme overaction half of the cornea is buried, which is graded +4.

Oblique over- and underactions are graded by comparing the height of the inferior limbus of each eye. Overactions are graded from +1, representing a slight overaction, to +4, characterized by abduction of the eye in extreme oblique position (splaying out). Underactions of the obliques are graded from −1 (representing the smallest underaction) to −4 (denoting an inability of the eye to move vertically from the midline in the field of action of the oblique being tested). Examples of the four grades of oblique overaction are shown in Fig. 79.5.

Ductions are the excursion of each eye in the direction of each extraocular muscle with the other eye occluded. If an underaction of one eye is noted on testing the versions, the fellow eye is covered and a comparison between the version and duction is made to differentiate a mechanical from a neurogenic strabismus. A mechanical restriction will show equal limitation in both ductions and versions. If there is a nerve paresis, however, the eye will move more in the direction of limitation with the other eye covered (duction movements will exceed versions).

Head tilts

In patients with a vertical deviation, the primary position deviation with the head tilted to the left and right should be measured using single prisms (Bielschowsky head tilt test).

Torsion measurement

Torsion can be measured using the synoptophore and estimated using Hess charts. Both are dissociative and require special instruments. The synoptophore can measure torsion in various positions of gaze. A simple, clinical method of measuring torsion involves using a trial frame with either Maddox rods or Bagolini

CHAPTER
79

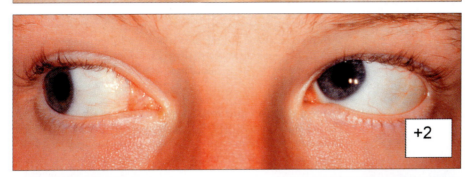

+1

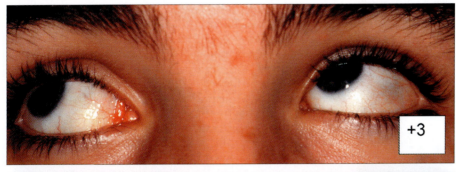

+2

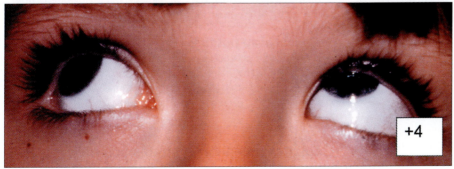

+3

+4

Fig. 79.5 Four grades of inferior oblique overaction.

striated lenses. Torsion should be measured in primary position and downgaze. Both methods can be used in children as young as 5 years of age.

Maddox rods

Two Maddox rods are placed in the trial frame with the cylinders orientated vertically (Fig. 79.6). A patient with torsional diplopia perceives two red lines, one horizontal and one tilted. By turning slightly one Maddox rod and then the other it is possible to get an impression of which side the patient feels is the horizontal side and which is the side with torsion. By turning the Maddox rod in the trial frame until the patient sees both lines as being parallel, the amount of torsion can be determined in degrees from the trial frame (Fig. 79.7). If there is a vertical deviation in addition

to the torsional deviation, which is often the case if torsion is associated with a fourth nerve paresis, the patient sees two lines, one on top of the other and finds it easy to make the lines parallel. If there is no vertical deviation, patients often find it difficult to be sure that the lines are parallel because they merge with each other. In this case, a vertical prism can be put into the trial frame to separate the images, making it easier for the patient to distinguish the lines. Torsional diplopia in downgaze is measured by tilting the patient's head backward and pushing the trial frame down the patient's nose slightly (Fig. 79.8).

Bagolini lenses

Bagolini lenses are used to measure torsion in a trial frame in the same manner as Maddox rods. The patient sees two crosses

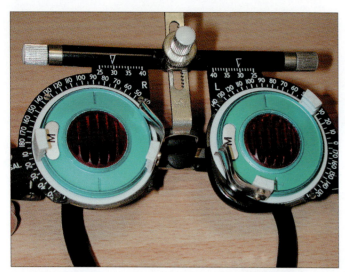

Fig. 79.6 Two Maddox rods aligned vertically in the trial frame are perceived by the diplopic patient as two horizontal lines.

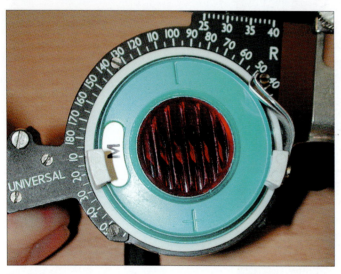

Fig. 79.7 The patient turns one Maddox rod until the lines are parallel and the torsion measurement is read off the trial frame in degrees.

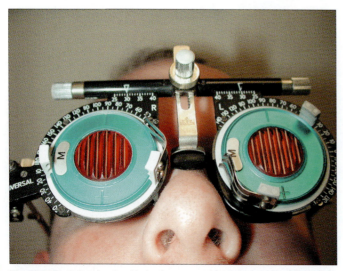

Fig. 79.8 To determine torsion in downgaze, the trial frame is pushed down the nose and the head is tilted back.

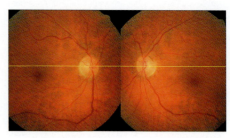

Fig. 79.9 Retinal photography can be used to estimate torsion and gives some idea about whether one eye is contributing more to the torsional diplopia than the other.

because of the striations on the lenses, and superimposes the crosses. Bagolini lenses have the advantage of being nondissociative, allowing cyclovertical fusion.

Indirect ophthalmoscopy
Information about torsion in various positions of gaze can be obtained by looking at the position of the fovea in relation to the disc using an indirect ophthalmoscope or retinal photography (Fig. 79.9).

Forced duction and forced generation tests
Forced duction tests (FDTs) give important information about restrictive strabismus and contribute to decision-making when determining surgical management. In young children, FDTs must be performed under general anesthetic and should be one of the routine procedures at the beginning of each strabismus operation. FDTs can be performed in the clinic setting using topical anesthetic in older, cooperative children.

Forced generation testing (FGT) is an essential part of assessment in patients with nerve paresis (including Duane syndrome). It can only be performed with patient cooperation. This test is important to determine what proportion of the deviation is a result of the nerve paresis itself, and what proportion is the result of restrictive changes in the antagonist muscle. In a patient with lateral rectus paresis, for instance, the eye is held at the temporal limbus with toothed forceps and moved into adduction. The patient is then asked to abduct the eye and the force generated (by the lateral rectus attempting abduction) is estimated by the clinician.

Abnormal head postures
Abnormal head postures (AHP) can be in three dimensions: face turns (to the right or left), chin-up or chin-down, and head tilts (to the right or left). They can be measured simply by using a goniometer borrowed from the orthopedic department (Fig. 79.10).

Ocular examination in strabismus patients
The importance of careful and detailed ocular examination in patients with strabismus or apparent amblyopia cannot be over-emphasized. A number of conditions requiring urgent or prompt treatment present with strabismus or poor vision in one eye that may be diagnosed as amblyopia. Conditions such as raised intracranial pressure (caused by hydrocephalus or intracranial tumor), retinoblastoma, and congenital cataract can be missed if a careful ocular examination is not performed, with sight or life-threatening consequences.

Examination of the lid position and movement may give important information about the underlying strabismus diagnosis. Palpebral aperture changes in Duane syndrome, aberrant innervation in congenital third nerve paresis, and seventh nerve paresis in Möbius syndrome are a few examples where observation of eyelid changes can help in diagnosis.

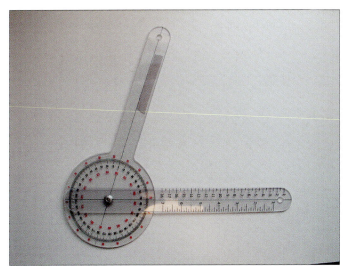

Fig. 79.10 A goniometer, used by orthopedic surgeons to measure joint angles, can be used to measure abnormal head postures.

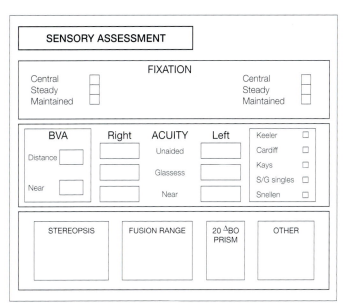

Fig. 79.11 A simple form for recording the findings of the sensory examination.

Suspicions about anterior segment abnormalities are best investigated by slit-lamp examination, using either a regular slit lamp or a portable device. Careful examination of the pupils before dilating drops have been given will exclude an afferent pupil defect. Information about media opacities or leukocoria can be gained at the time of refraction. Indirect ophthalmoscopy is an essential part of the examination of all strabismus patients. Further information about media opacities can be obtained, and a detailed examination of the retina and optic nerve will enable diagnosis of other causes of visual impairment such as optic nerve abnormalities, receptor dystrophies, and macular abnormalities. A more magnified view of fundus changes (with the direct ophthalmoscope or slit-lamp biomicroscopy) should be obtained to exclude conditions such as optic nerve hypoplasia, which can easily be missed with indirect ophthalmoscopy.

Special investigations such as visually evoked potentials or electroretinograms (Chapter 11) may be necessary in unexplained poor vision; neuroimaging (Chapter 13) and orbital imaging may be necessary in a number of conditions.

DOCUMENTATION OF STRABISMUS FINDINGS

Standardization of documentation in strabismus management has contributed significantly to the quality of patient care and to communication both within and between departments. Auditing the outcomes of management is much easier with standardized records, and using a numerical rather than a descriptive documentation system has enabled the development of electronic patient records.

Sensory documentation

Figure 79.11 shows an example of a record for documenting sensory findings. This is not all encompassing and there is still the need for free text documentation in some cases.

Motor documentation

Documentation of motor findings can be standardized by creating a diagrammatic representation of ocular motor findings.[4] On the

same diagrammatic chart, information about prism cover tests, versions and ductions, and abnormal ocular movements can be recorded so that they can be analyzed as if the patient were present. This is a modification of the system first suggested by Jampolsky.[5]

Prism cover tests

The basic template is shown in Fig. 79.12. Prism cover test results in nine positions of gaze are recorded using the notation listed in Table 79.1. Horizontal deviations are recorded above the line and vertical deviations below the line. Although it does take a little time to learn the notation language, once fluent, it is easy to record a lot of information without having to write it all out in longhand. For instance, 25(Δ)E is translated as 25(Δ)esophoria, a

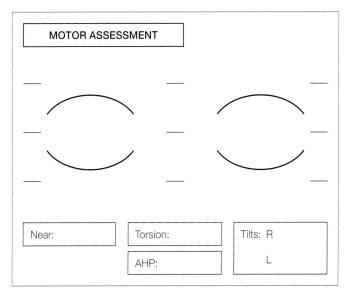

Fig. 79.12 Using this basic template, information including prism cover tests in nine positions of gaze, versions, and abnormalities of ocular movements can be recorded creating a diagrammatic representation of the motility examination findings.

Table 79.1 Notation	
Notation for recording the findings of prism cover tests	
E	Esophoria
X	Exophoria
ET	Esotropia
XT	Exotropia
H	Hyperphoria
HT	Hypertropia
Ho	Hypophoria
HoT	Hypotropia
Notation for intermittent deviations	
E(T)	Intermittent esotropia
E̲(T)	Intermittent esotropia, mainly latent
E(T̲)	Intermittent esotropia, mainly manifest

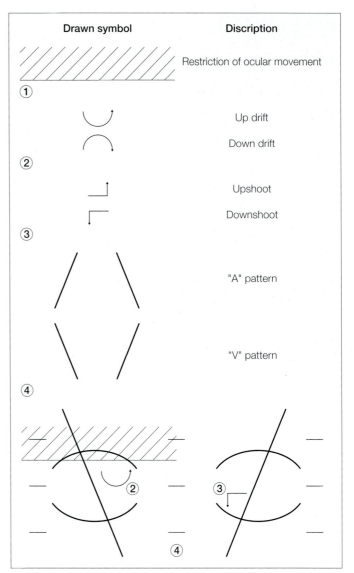

Fig. 79.14 Various characteristics of abnormal ocular movements can be emphasized using a number of symbols. Examples of their use on a basic template are shown.

completely controlled esodeviation, and 25(Δ)ET is translated as 25(Δ)esotropia, a manifest deviation. To give more information without having to resort to free-hand text, the use of brackets and underlining conveys further information. For instance, 25(Δ)E(T) is an intermittent esotropia; 25(Δ)E̲(T) is an intermittent esotropia that is mainly controlled, whereas 25(Δ)E(T̲) is an intermittent esotropia, mainly manifest. Once the language has been learned, recording information is quick and easy, and in a form that is easy to present to others and computerize.

Versions

Six version recordings for each eye are recorded corresponding to the direction of principle action of the six extra-ocular muscles of each eye (Fig. 79.13). As explained in the section "Versions and Ductions," versions are scored using a nine point scoring system where 0 is a normal version, overactions are scored from +1 to +4 and underactions are scored from −1 to −4. The version score for each of the six extraocular muscles of each eye is entered onto the diagram in the appropriate position.

Characteristics of abnormal ocular movements

To further emphasize abnormal ocular movements on the record chart, various symbols can be added (Fig. 79.14). "A" and "V" patterns are emphasized using oblique lines (see Example 1).

Example 1

This eight-year-old boy presented when his parents noticed a strabismus in downgaze. As can be seen from Fig. 79.15 he has a controlled exophoria in the primary position with an esophoria in upgaze. In downgaze, however, he has an exotropia associated with bilateral superior oblique overaction, the right superior

oblique overaction (+4) more than the left (+3). This superior oblique overaction causes an "A" pattern exotropia with left hypotropia in right gaze and right hypotropia in left gaze. The abduction of each eye in downgaze caused by the superior

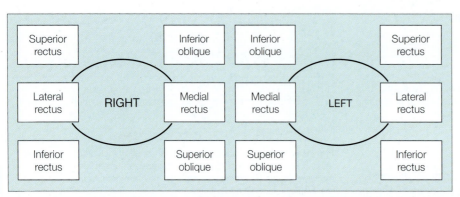

Fig. 79.13 The principle direction of action of the six extraocular muscles of each eye.

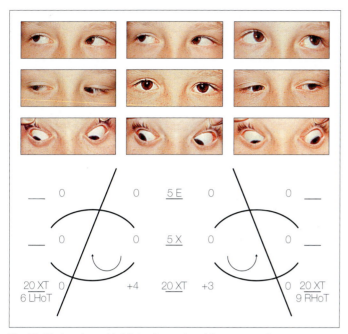

Fig. 79.15 A patient with bilateral superior oblique overaction.

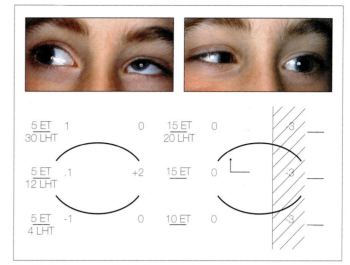

Fig. 79.16 A patient with left Duane syndrome.

oblique overaction is emphasized by the curved arrows, and the "A" pattern by the lines arranged like an "A."

Gradual (up- or downdrift) or sudden movement (up- or downshoot) of an eye on version testing is emphasized using the appropriate arrows. Restriction of eye movement on versions is represented by a hatched line (see Example 2).

Example 2

This 11-year-old boy has bilateral Duane syndrome, more severe in the left eye (Fig. 79.16). He has −3 restriction of left abduction, the left eye only just abducting beyond the midline, which is emphasized using the hatched lines. Abduction of the right eye is only slightly limited (−1). On adduction, the left eye has an upshot, emphasized by the right-angled arrow. This causes a left hypertropia, especially in upgaze. Notice the narrowing of each palpebral aperture in adduction. By convention, horizontal deviations are written above the line in the nine positions, and vertical deviations below the line.

Electronic patient records and audit in strabismus management

Strabismus surgery is well suited to the application of electronic patient records (EPR). Data are easily recorded in an appropriate format (as described earlier) and the power of the EPR can be used to provide a better quality of care.

To allow ease of use and rapid data entry, information must be in a form that is standardized and easily incorporated into drop-down menus. Descriptive terms used in conventional orthoptic reports are not easily adaptable to EPRs, and free-text additions need to be kept to a minimum to prevent data entry from taking too long.

Figures 79.17–79.19 show an example of an EPR developed specifically for strabismus surgery. Figure 79.17 shows the general screen for recording the history, ocular examination, refraction, the final diagnosis, and management plan. Each section has a drop-down menu with a selection of common findings to choose from (although free-text additions can be added).

The screen for entry of sensory and motor findings (Fig. 79.18) is very similar to the paper version and can be filled in very quickly because of the drop-down menus.

The third screen (Fig. 79.19) is for adding surgery details. The top portion of the screen is for audit purposes, showing the strabismus type and the preoperative measurements. This enables easy retrieval of operative data on, for instance, esodeviations to perform an audit of outcomes.

Within each patient's EPR, photographs and videos can be stored. The record automatically creates a diagnostic index.

Computerized clinical records allow much more sophisticated data storage and retrieval. With access to better data it is easier to audit surgical outcomes and adjust personal surgical dosage to optimize outcomes.

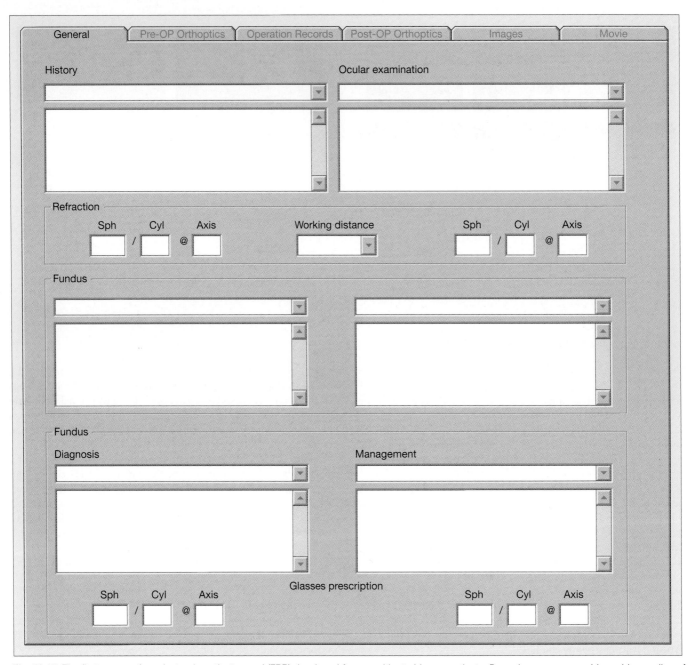

Fig. 79.17 The first screen of an electronic patient record (EPR) developed for use with strabismus patients. Drop-down menus enable rapid recording of information.

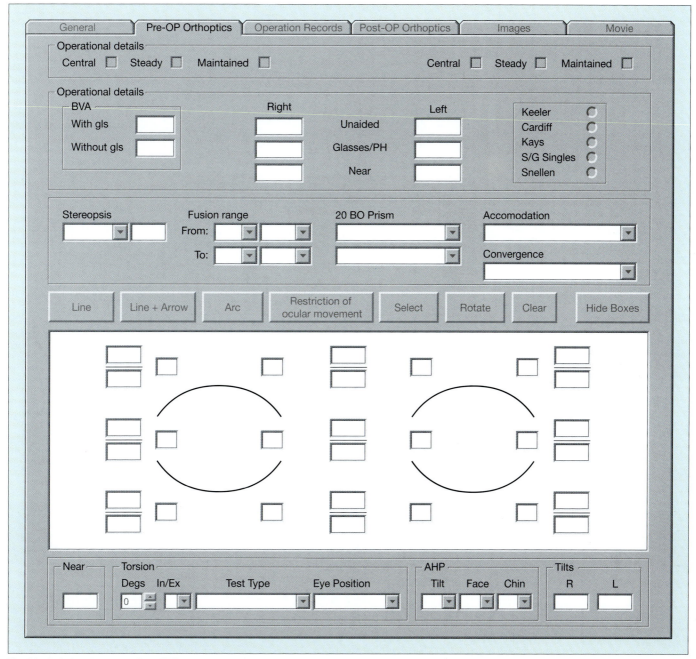

Fig. 79.18 Orthoptic pages of the EPR are designed for recording sensory and motor information from each examination.

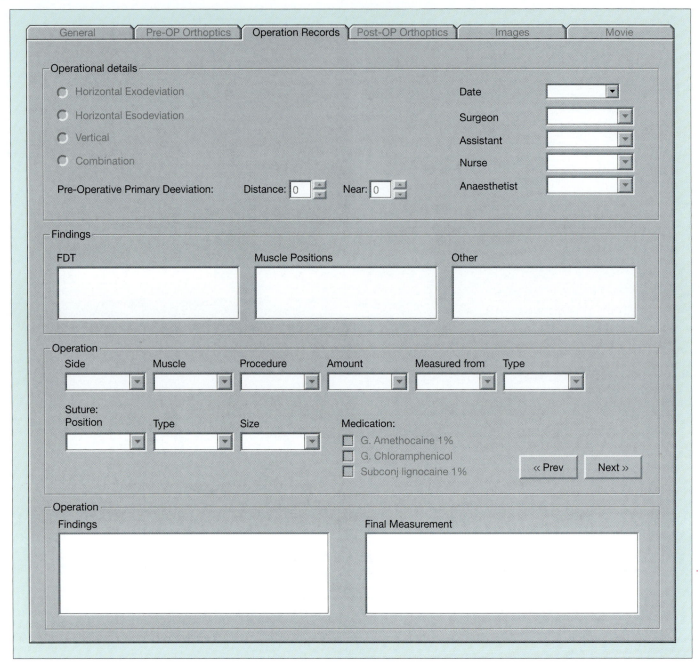

Fig. 79.19 The operation record of the EPR includes data for continuous outcomes audit.

REFERENCES

1. McGraw PV, Winn B, Gray LS, et al. Improving the reliability of visual acuity measures in the young. Ophthalmic Physiol Opt 2000; 20: 173–84.
2. Holmes JM, Beck RW, Repka MX, et al. Pediatric Eye Disease Investigator Group. The amblyopia treatment study visual acuity testing protocol. Arch Ophthalmol 2001; 119: 1345–53.
3. Sener EC, Mocan MC, Gedik S, et al. The reliability of grading the fixation preference test for the assessment of interocular visual acuity differences in patients with strabismus. J AAPOS 2002; 6: 191–4.
4. Thompson JT, Guyton DL. Ophthalmic prisms: measurement errors and how to minimise them. Ophthalmology 1983; 90: 204–10.
5. Vivian AJ, Morris RJ. Diagramatic representation of strabismus. Eye 1993; 7: 565–71.
6. Jampolsky A. A simplified approach to strabismus diagnosis. Symposium on Strabismus: Transactions of the New Orleans Academy of Ophthalmology. St Louis: Mosby; 1971: 34–51.

CHAPTER **80** Concomitant Strabismus: Esotropias

William E Scott and Pamela J Kutschke

PSEUDOESOTROPIA

Pseudoesotropia, the appearance of convergent deviation of the visual axes, accounts for approximately 50% of all suspected esotropia presenting to pediatricians and family practitioners (Fig. 80.1). The apparent crossing is caused by prominent epicanthal folds, which cover the nasal aspect of young children's eyes. They are usually bilateral but may be asymmetric. A flat nasal bridge may also be present.

Pseudoesotropia is the only type of esotropia that a child is able to outgrow. The features that cause the appearance of crossing of the eyes, the epicanthal folds, disappear with growth of the face. Other causes such as a large negative angle kappa or an abnormally small interpupillary distance are less common. The single cover test is the gold standard test to rule out esotropia. If there is no shift on cover test, then the diagnosis of pseudoesotropia may be made.

CONGENITAL (INFANTILE) ESOTROPIA

Congenital esotropia refers to constant esotropia, which is manifest before six months of age (Fig. 80.2). Although this type of esotropia is rarely seen at birth, the term refers to a specific type of esotropia with its associated characteristics. The broader term of infantile esotropia is preferred by some. If the term infantile esotropia is used, one must consider other, rare etiologies of esotropia in the first few months of life, such as nystagmus, high hypermetropia, or certain special forms of strabismus such as congenital fibrosis (see Chapter 85).

Congenital esotropia is usually inherited. In many cases, a careful family history will demonstrate that a family member has had some crossing of the eyes early in life.

As these patients are too young for subjective visual acuity, vision is assessed by fixation pattern—the central, steady, and

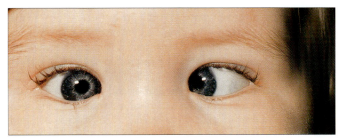

Fig. 80.2 Congenital esotropia. Note the large angle of deviation. The eye movements are full and the child is healthy.

maintained method (see Chapters 9 and 79). The definition of equal vision is fixation that is held or maintained through a blink in both eyes.[1] If fixation is not maintained through a blink, amblyopia is likely to be present.

Many patients with congenital esotropia cross-fixate, or fixate with the eye in an adducted position and never abduct either eye (Fig. 80.3). The diagnosis of congenital sixth nerve palsy may be made erroneously. Abduction can usually be demonstrated by vestibular rotation, the doll's head maneuver, or monocular occlusion. Although cross-fixation is usually a sign that fixation is equal, amblyopia can be present in as many as 50% of cross-fixators.[2] Amblyopia is diagnosed based on the point at which the fixation switch occurs. Fixation change from one eye to the other should occur at the midline of the face. Amblyopia is

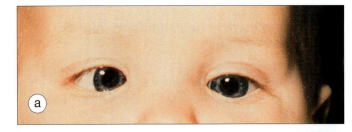

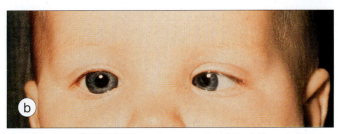

Fig. 80.3 Cross-fixation in congenital esotropia. (a) The left eye is fixing the target and the right eye is deviating inwards. (b) Fixation is reversed spontaneously.

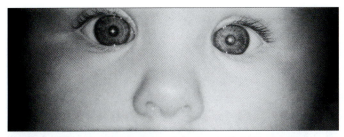

Fig. 80.1 Pseudostrabismus. Although it appears that this child has strabismus, this is a false appearance due to the broad base to the nose. The light reflexes are symmetrical in the pupils, there is no deviation on the cover test, and it is possible to demonstrate normal prism responses.

present if the sound eye continues to fixate beyond midline, into abduction.

The incidence of amblyopia in congenital esotropia is approximately 50%.[3] Occlusion therapy should be undertaken until fixation is maintained through a blink with each eye or until cross-fixation occurs at midline. Amblyopia should be treated early in life as amblyopia probably presents a significant obstacle to binocularity and stability of alignment following surgical correction of congenital esotropia.

Once equal vision has been obtained, the deviation is measured by the prism cover test. The Pediatric Eye Disease Investigator Group found spontaneous resolution of esotropia in 27% of patients studied.[4] It was concluded that early-onset esotropia frequently resolves in patients with intermittent or variable deviations of less than 40$^\Delta$. Prior to contemplating any surgical treatment, two measurements, consistent within 5 prism diopters, done several weeks apart, are necessary to ensure stability of the esotropia.

The deviation is usually large, from 30$^\Delta$ to 100$^\Delta$, with the average angle of 38$^\Delta$, commonly the same at distance and near, and in all positions of gaze. Occasionally a "V" pattern is noted, where the esotropia decreases in upgaze, secondary to inferior oblique overaction. Oblique muscle over- or underaction will be apparent on version testing.

A cycloplegic refraction is necessary to determine refractive error. In children under six months of age, ½% Cyclogyl (cyclopentolate) is used; in children older than the age of six months, 1% Cyclogyl is used. In darkly pigmented children, 2½% Neo-Synephrine (Phenylephrine) is combined with Cyclogyl to improve mydriasis. Neo-Synephrine does not influence accommodation. Two drops, 5 min apart, are administered. The peak effect is 40 minutes after the first drop.

Low degrees of hypermetropia are common in congenital esotropia; less than 3 D of hypermetropic refractive error is considered normal in this young age group. Glasses should be prescribed if the child has greater than 3 D of hypermetropia, to determine the effect on the esotropia. If the deviation is partially corrected by the glasses, the amount of surgical correction necessary may be lessened. The glasses must be worn at the time of corrective surgery because significant, uncorrected hyperopia in the immediate postoperative period may cause the esotropia to recur.

Dissociated vertical deviation and inferior oblique overaction

Dissociated vertical deviation (DVD) is a common associated finding in congenital esotropia–some reporting as high as 48%[5] (Fig. 80.4). Other names for DVD are alternating hyperphoria, double hypertropia, occlusion hyperphoria, alternating sursumduction, and dissociated vertical divergence (see Chapter 83).

DVD is a manifest, spontaneous, upward deviation that does not follow Hering's law of equal innervation. There is no corresponding hypodeviation of the contralateral eye. It may appear early or develop later in the course of the esotropia.[6] The deviation is comitant, i.e., the same in adduction, primary, abduction, and up- and downgaze. It is variable in size, fluctuating from small to large with attention or fatigue. It may be unilateral or bilateral, with the eye drifting up and out upon dissociation. Occasionally, an anomalous head position is present to control the DVD, manifesting as a head tilt to the side of the DVD (see Chapter 89).

DVD must be differentiated from inferior oblique overaction (IOOA), also occurring in congenital esotropia. Like DVD, IOOA is also characterized by an elevation of the eye in adduction. However, IOOA causes a true hyperdeviation, with a corresponding hypodeviation of the contralateral eye, which is greater in the field of action of the inferior oblique (Fig. 80.5). The deviation is constant, reproducible, and not variable. An associated "V" pattern with a larger esotropia in downgaze and a smaller deviation in upgaze is common. No pattern is commonly seen with DVD.

Occasionally in a child with congenital esotropia, both DVD and IOOA can occur simultaneously. If this occurs, then the amount of hypertropia is greater than the amount of hypotropia. The hypertropia, which exceeds the amount of hypotropia, is the DVD. It is important to differentiate these two conditions and determine the amount of inferior oblique overaction versus the amount of dissociated vertical as the treatment of these two conditions is different (see Chapter 89).

Once the determination has been made as to the cause of the elevation in adduction, one needs to measure the degree of inferior oblique overaction and the amount of DVD present. Inferior oblique overaction can be assessed using a five-point scale of 0 (normally acting) to +4 (markedly overacting). If the inferior oblique overaction is greater than +2, significant inferior

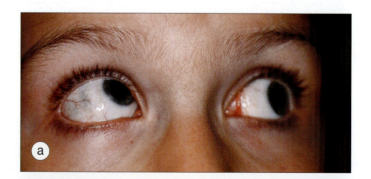

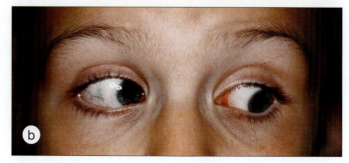

Fig. 80.5 Elevation in adduction caused by inferior oblique overaction. Note (a) true hyperdeviation and (b) corresponding hypodeviation.

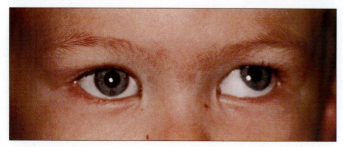

Fig. 80.4 Dissociated vertical deviation. When this child fails to concentrate or "daydreams," the left eye deviates upward and inward, and excyclorotates.

oblique overaction is present, and weakening the inferior oblique should be considered at the time of horizontal deviation correction. For moderate overaction, an inferior oblique recession is adequate, while for marked inferior oblique overaction, an inferior oblique myectomy is recommended.

DVD is measured using the prism cover test. To measure DVD, a base-down prism is placed in front of the eye with DVD until no more downward movement takes place on alternate cover testing. Only the eye with the prism and the DVD should be watched. The contralateral eye has no corresponding hypotropia, so it will look markedly overcorrected on cover testing.

If only DVD is found, the horizontal deviation must be corrected first so that peripheral fusion can be established and the DVD controlled through the fusional mechanism. DVD held latent by peripheral fusion or fixation preference is referred to as an occlusion hyperphoria. This distinction is made as DVD may cause a misalignment requiring surgery. Occlusion hyperphorias do not cause a misalignment and therefore do not need to be treated.

If DVD persists after good horizontal alignment, and there is no associated inferior oblique overaction, a large superior rectus recession is recommended.[7,8] The amount of superior rectus recession is in Table 2 of Chapter 83.

If there is a combination of dissociated vertical deviation and inferior oblique overaction, then it must be determined which is the more significant feature. If the inferior oblique is moderately overacting, a procedure called anteriorization of the inferior oblique is recommended.[9,10]

The inferior oblique is isolated and moved temporal and anterior to the inferior rectus insertion. The anterior portion, or the portion closer to the inferior rectus, can be placed up to 2 mm anterior from the insertion. Care must be taken that the posterior fibers, the part of the inferior oblique most temporal, should not be elevated beyond the inferior rectus insertion. If this is anteriorly displaced further, a limitation of elevation postoperatively could occur. This procedure should be done in both eyes, not monocularly, to avoid overcorrection. This anteriorization of the inferior oblique is performed only for the treatment of the combination of inferior oblique overaction and DVD.

If dissociated vertical deviations are present and manifested bilaterally with alternating fixation, large superior rectus recessions of 10–12 mm are recommended.[11,12]

Dissociated horizontal deviation

Another form of dissociated deviation, dissociated horizontal deviation (DHD), also does not follow Hering's law. Although less frequent than DVD, DHD is seen in patients following surgery for congenital esotropia. DHD manifests as an asymmetric, non-paralytic, dissociated exodeviation, usually in the presence of DVD. The preferred treatment for DHD is a large lateral rectus recession of the eye manifesting the DHD.[13,14]

Latent nystagmus

Latent nystagmus is also frequently associated with congenital esotropia (25–50%).[15] This unique form of nystagmus occurs only upon monocular occlusion and manifests with the beat toward the fixating or uncovered eye. It is reported to worsen when the patient fixates in abduction. Patients often adopt a head turn toward the fixating eye to fixate in adduction. Visual acuity is reduced when the nystagmus is present, and care must be taken to measure visual acuity without reducing the amount

of light entering the visual system. There seems to be an association between the occurrence of DVD and latent nystagmus, although it is not absolute.

Jampolsky et al. recommends full-time alternate occlusion prior to the treatment of congenital esotropia. They feel that occlusion disrupts competitive binocular interaction, which perpetuates motion asymmetry. Preoperative alternate occlusion of infantile esotropes is necessary to produce symmetry of motion processing and to produce a better postoperative result.[16]

Surgical treatment of congenital esotropia

The goal of surgical treatment of congenital esotropia is to align the eyes within 8^Δ of orthotropia so that some degree of peripheral fusion can occur. This is done after the patient has equal visual acuity. Surgery can be performed once amblyopia has been treated, the size of the deviation has stabilized, consistent measurements have been obtained, significant refractive error has been corrected, and the evaluation of inferior oblique overaction versus dissociated vertical deviation has been undertaken. The timing of surgery has been debated. Most feel that early surgery is better although all of the above criteria need to be met.[5] It has been proposed that very early surgery, between 13 and 19 weeks, can produce better sensory results.[17]

The surgical plan for the treatment of congenital esotropia should consist of a selective approach, i.e., changing the amount of surgery done based on the size of the deviation. Table 80.1 shows the surgical amounts in the treatment of congenital esotropia based on cover test measurements.

Once the deviation exceeds 50^Δ, a third muscle, resection of a lateral rectus muscle, is added; once the deviation reaches 70^Δ or greater, a fourth muscle is added, combining bilateral lateral rectus resections with the bilateral medial rectus recessions.

The medial rectus is never left further than 11.5 mm from the limbus. Once a lateral rectus resection is added, the medial rectus is not left further than 11 mm from the limbus. If a resection is done and the medial rectus is placed too far posteriorly, adduction may be limited postoperatively, which could lead to postoperative exotropia. Using this technique, we obtained successful alignment particularly in the larger deviations, in approximately 70% of patients.[18] If two-muscle surgery was used for the larger deviations, it was found that undercorrection occurred approximately 60% of the time.

As can be seen in Table 80.1, medial rectus recessions are measured from the limbus and not from the insertion. The

Table 80.1 Surgical amounts in the treatment of congenital esotropia based on cover test measurements

Preoperative deviation ($^\Delta$)	Bimedial recession	Lateral resection	Bilateral resection
30^Δ	Leave 10 mm from limbus		
35^Δ	Leave 10.5 mm from limbus		
40^Δ	Leave 11 mm from limbus		
45^Δ–50^Δ	Leave 11.5 mm from limbus		
55^Δ	Leave 11 mm from limbus	4–5 mm	
60^Δ	Leave 11 mm from limbus	6 mm	
65^Δ	Leave 11 mm from limbus	7 mm	
70^Δ	Leave 11 mm from limbus		4 mm
75^Δ	Leave 11 mm from limbus		5 mm
80^Δ	Leave 11 mm from limbus		6 mm
90^Δ–100^Δ	Leave 11 mm from limbus		7 mm

Some authorities prefer to use larger bilateral medial rectus recessions and less resection.

medial rectus insertion is classically found 5.5 mm from the limbus. However, variability of the medial rectus insertion has been reported. Helveston et al. measured the distance between the medial rectus insertion and the limbus in 114 eyes and found a range of 3–6 mm, average 4.4 mm.[19] Kushner and Morton measured the distance between the medial rectus insertion and the limbus in 80 eyes with an average of 4.3 mm and a range of 3.5 to 5.5 mm.[20]

Keech et al. measured the medial rectus insertion in 26 eyes of patients ranging in age between 10 and 30 months with preoperative deviations of 25^Δ to 70^Δ.[21] A limbal, conjunctival incision was used. The distance between the surgical limbus and the anterior medial rectus insertion was measured. The average insertion was 5.5 mm from the limbus with a range of 5 to 6 mm. The measurement of the distance between the stump of the disinserted medial rectus muscle and the limbus was then measured. The medial rectus muscle stump moved an average of 1.2 mm toward the limbus (range of 0.5 to 2 mm) upon disinsertion. Once the muscle was disinserted, the muscle stump fixated, the eye placed into abduction, and the caliper placed on the eye once again, the muscle stump moved an additional 0.5 mm closer to the limbus. This is the point at which most eye surgeons measure the amount to be recessed. Because the muscle stump moves forward with disinsertion, yet after grasping it, measurements from the limbus are much more accurate when recessing a muscle.

Helveston et al. reported that recession of the conjunctiva adds to the effective medial rectus recession.[22] The following guidelines are used to determine when to recess the conjunctiva. The eye is grasped with the fixation forceps and abducted. With a small muscle hook, the conjunctiva is palpated. If the conjunctiva is tight, it is recessed to the original muscle insertion at the time of surgery. It is recommended that a limbal incision be used so the conjunctiva can be recessed. If the conjunctiva is loose, recession will not augment the amount of deviation corrected and a fornix or a limbal incision can be used.

Using these guidelines, we find that one procedure can correct approximately 90% of congenital esotropia. At least 50% will develop some degree of peripheral fusion, adding to the stability of alignment. To examine how much stability is added, see the section "Monofixation Syndrome."

A few authors have advocated the use of Botox (botulism toxin), in the treatment of congenital esotropia. They recommend Botox injections of each medial rectus and report a high degree of success.[23] We have not used Botox for the treatment of congenital esotropia, relying more on the conventional surgical approach. There has been no prospective study done comparing conventional surgical techniques to Botox.

SPECIAL FORMS OF EARLY CONCOMITANT ESOTROPIA

Infantile accommodative esotropia

Occasionally a child presents with early-onset esotropia of a moderate angle, and a high degree of hypermetropia is found during cycloplegic examination. These children respond well to their full hypermetropic correction and often alignment is established without surgery, emphasizing the need for all children with early-onset esotropia to undergo a cycloplegic refraction. Once a significant degree, i.e., greater than 3 diopters, of hypermetropia is found, glasses are prescribed to determine their effect on the deviation.

Nystagmus blockage syndrome

This condition was described by Adelstein and Cuppers in 1966.[24] Of 247 patients with congenital esotropia, 12 patients fitted the following criteria: onset of esotropia in early infancy, pseudo-abducens paralysis, head turn toward the side of the fixating eye, absence of nystagmus with the fixating eye in adduction, and the appearance of a manifest nystagmus as the fixating eye moved into primary position and abduction. It was suggested that convergence blocks the nystagmus. The esotropia is caused by sustained convergence and secondary changes in the medial rectus muscles. The differential diagnosis includes cross-fixation and bilateral sixth nerve palsy. The condition was later studied by von Noorden.[25]

In our experience, nystagmus blockage syndrome is a rare cause of early-onset concomitant esotropia. The surgical treatment of nystagmus blockage consists of large medial rectus recession. Some have advocated the use of posterior fixation sutures.[26,27] We feel that posterior fixation sutures have added very little in management of this type of case and are very rarely used in the treatment of congenital esotropia.

Ciancia syndrome

Ciancia syndrome was first described in 1962 as a syndrome of infantile esotropia with abduction nystagmus.[28] The main features were:
1. Esotropia of early onset;
2. Generally large angle of deviation;
3. Bilateral limitation of abduction;
4. Jerk nystagmus with quick phase toward the side of the fixating eye, increasing in abduction and disappearing in adduction;
5. Torticollis with face turned toward the side of the fixing eye;
6. Moderate or absent hyperopia; and
7. Head tilting toward the side of the fixing eye (as was later reported by Lang[29]).

Ciancia syndrome, nystagmus blockage, and large-angle congenital esotropia have very similar characteristics and may be part of a spectrum of the same condition. We have seen conditions of a large-angle esotropia with nystagmus in an attempted abduction similar to that described by Ciancia. The treatment of this condition is the same as that for nystagmus blockage syndrome: large medial rectus recessions to alleviate the tightness and secondary contraction of the medial recti.

ACQUIRED ESOTROPIA

Acquired accommodative esotropia

In 1864, Donders was the first to describe the association of esotropia and uncorrected hypermetropia.[30] In 1897, Duane classified esotropia into three types: convergence excess in which the near deviation exceeded the distance, divergence insufficiency in which the distance deviation exceeded the near, and the basic type in which the distance deviation equaled the near deviation.[31]

Uncorrected hypermetropia, by itself, may not necessarily cause esotropia. Other factors such as the amount of hypermetropia, the AC/A ratio and the strength of the negative relative fusional convergence (fusional divergence) also play a role. An emmetrope will not need to accommodate to see clearly at 6 m. At near, or $\frac{1}{3}$ m, this same person will need to accommodate 3 diopters. Someone with 2 diopters of uncorrected

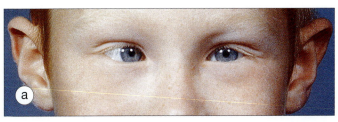 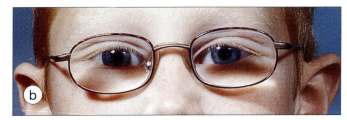

Fig. 80.6 Accommodative esotropia. (a) Large deviation without correction; (b) No deviation with correction.

hypermetropia will need to accommodate 2 diopters at 6 m and 5 diopters at $\frac{1}{3}$ m to see clearly. If the amount of fusional divergence available is not enough to counteract the convergence produced with the accommodation, the eyes will not remain straight and an esotropia will result. However, prescribing the full amount of hypermetropia found on cycloplegic refraction will make the person functionally emmetropic and no excess accommodation will be needed to see the image clearly. Therefore, no esotropia will be produced (Fig. 80.6).

Determining the AC/A ratio

The AC/A ratio can be determined by a number of methods. Although not a true measure of the AC/A ratio, comparing the distance to the near deviation during clinical evaluation is the method most frequently used due to its simplicity. A difference of greater than 10^Δ is considered high.

The heterophoric method uses the distance and near measurements and the interpupillary distance (IPD) to determine the AC/A ratio:

$$AC/A = IPD (cm) + (D_n - D_d)/D,$$

where D = fixation distance at near in diopters, D_n = deviation at near, and D_d = deviation at distance. A normal AC/A by the heterophoric method is $IPD + \frac{1}{2} IPD$.

The most accurate method is the gradient method. The deviation is measured at a constant distance while plus power ophthalmic lenses are used to reduce the amount of accommodation produced:

$$AC/A = (D_l - D_o)/D,$$

where D = power of the lens, D_l = deviation measured with lenses, and D_o = original deviation measured without lenses. A normal AC/A by the gradient method is $3{:}1^\Delta/D$ to $5{:}1^\Delta/D$. The AC/A measured by the gradient method is usually smaller than that measured by the heterophoric method. Because this method uses a constant testing distance, it is not affected by proximal convergence.

The AC/A ratio may be influenced by anticholinesterases, glasses with bifocals or varifocals, surgical correction, orthoptic exercises, or time. Overconvergence secondary to accommodation will lessen as a child matures.

Some patients exhibit a distance–near disparity although their AC/A measurement is normal. This convergence excess at near is not linked to accommodation.

There are several major types of accommodative acquired esotropia.

Fully accommodative esotropia

Fully accommodative esotropia, where uncorrected hypermetropia is the sole cause, accounts for 40% of accommodative esotropia. It is characterized by equal distance and near measurements, an

average age of onset of $3\frac{1}{2}$ years, and an average refractive error of approximately 4.75 D of hypermetropia. Deterioration, where the glasses no longer control the deviation, occurs in approximately 15% of patients.[32]

Esotropia with a high AC/A ratio

In 1958, Parks found approximately 50% of patients with accommodative esotropia had a distance–near disparity where the near deviation exceeded the distance deviation by 10^Δ or more.[33] The average age of onset of these patients was younger than the usual age of onset for accommodative esotropia, at 2.7 years. He felt that a high AC/A ratio was one of the major etiological factors in this form of acquired esotropia. Because greater amounts of accommodation are needed to focus at near, the amount of esotropia at near may be larger than that measured at distance. Fusional divergence is greater at near than distance and may be able to compensate for some of this difference. However, the higher the AC/A ratio, the greater the esotropia will be at near. Parks divided this type of acquired accommodative esotropia into three types based on the severity of the near deviation[33]:

Grade 1 had 10^Δ to 19^Δ greater of near deviation than distance;
Grade 2 had 20^Δ to 29^Δ greater at near; and
Grade 3 had 30^Δ or more at near.

Parks felt that a higher AC/A and lower refractive error increased the deterioration rate. The average deterioration rate of high AC/A accommodative esotropia was approximately 30%. However, a 25% deterioration rate was found in those with grade 1, whereas grade 3 had a higher than 50% deterioration rate. Deterioration was also influenced by an earlier onset of the accommodative esotropia, i.e., the younger the onset of the esotropia, the greater chances of deterioration.[34]

However, an overall deterioration rate in high AC/A esotropia, greater than 5/1, was found to be only 13%.[32] This patient population, however, was different than Parks' original patient population in that only 12 of 93 patients in this study had an AC/A ratio of greater than 9/1. An increase in deterioration rate also occurred with an onset of esotropia before 24 months of age, a delay between the onset of esotropia and the wearing of spectacle correction, and a decreasing or low amount of hyperopia at an early age.

Combined hypermetropic–high AC/A ratio accommodative esotropia

A third type of acquired accommodative esotropia is the combined hypermetropic–high AC/A type. It is characterized by a moderate hypermetropia of approximately 3 diopters, a near esotropia greater than the distance esotropia, and an average age of onset of 3 years. This type of acquired esotropia is felt to be the commonest.

Treatment of accommodative esotropia

Accommodative esotropia is treated by prescribing the proper spectacle correction and equalizing vision with amblyopia treatment. Amblyopia occurs in acquired accommodative esotropia at about the same frequency as it does in congenital esotropia. Approximately 50% of patients will present with either a fixation preference or a difference in subjective visual acuity.

Spectacle correction, based on cycloplegic refraction, can be considered a form of anti-accommodative therapy. By prescribing the full spectacle correction, the patient does not have to accommodate and therefore converge to see clearly. Lesser amounts of the full hyperopic correction can be given only if it renders the eyes in an orthophoric position so that fusion can be reestablished.

Some advocate cutting the amount of hypermetropic correction as the patient matures to try to reduce the hyperopia and stimulate the loss of hyperopia.[35,36] In our experience, hyperopia decreases with age and cutting the full amount of hypermetropic correction may do little to change emmetropization. As the child matures, it is common for the need for hypermetropic correction to decrease. Many grow to be adults who have very little hypermetropia and remain aligned without correction. In others, the hypermetropia remains, and glasses are needed to control the deviation.

Once the distance deviation has been corrected to within a fusional range, i.e., orthophoric to 8^Δ of esodeviation, the patient is evaluated for a distance–near disparity. Some advocate the use of miotics, anticholinesterases such as phospholine iodide or DFP, or pilocarpine to control the difference.[37]

In those patients with more esodeviation at near than at distance, it has been our practice to control the near deviation by the use of bifocals. Before prescribing bifocals, the power should be determined by measurement with different powers of plus lenses at near. Most commonly, it takes a +3.00 lens to control the overconvergence at near and produce fusion. The purpose of the bifocal is not just to reduce the near deviation but to reduce it to a range so that fusion occurs. Children treated with bifocals are monitored until they mature. Bifocals can be gradually reduced as long as fusion is maintained at near. In our experience, most patients are in single-vision lenses before 12 years of age.

For some ophthalmologists, however, experience with bifocals engenders less enthusiasm because it is found difficult to reduce the strength of the near addition and get the children out of bifocals by teenage. This has led some to prefer surgery for the residual deviation once the full hyperopic correction has been worn for at least three months.

Partially accommodative esotropia

Another type of accommodative esotropia is partially accommodative esotropia. Here, the full hypermetropic spectacle correction does not control the entire esodeviation. Any esotropia not controlled by glasses can be treated surgically. Since the treatment of acquired accommodative esotropia is glasses, it is important to use adequate cycloplegia in determining the amount of hypermetropia. Cycloplegic refraction should be performed in the manner discussed previously. However, it is important with accommodative esotropia to be sure that all of the hypermetropia is corrected. The child should be given the full hypermetropic correction and return after wearing it for 6 weeks to 3 months. Repeat cycloplegic refraction will often uncover more hyperopia. Our practice standard is for two cycloplegic refractions that agree within 0.50 diopters to be done within 3 months.[38]

Nonaccommodative acquired esotropia

Nonaccommodative acquired esotropia is a type of acquired esotropia not associated with hypermetropia at all. This usually occurs in older children and young adults. The etiology is unknown. These patients may have had a small-angle esotropia with some degree of peripheral fusion in the past, but over time lost fusion and became more esotropic. The features of these "broken-down monofixators" (see the section "Monofixation Syndrome") are a moderate angle of deviation, usually equal vision, little or no hypermetropia, measurements equal at distance and near, and a normal AC/A. Versions are full and the deviation is comitant, in that the esotropia is the same distance, near and on side gazes. On sensory testing, these patients may show suppression of one eye or anomalous retinal correspondence. This esotropia must be distinguished in young adults from that secondary to neurological disease.

Surgical treatment of acquired esotropia

Surgery is indicated for nonaccommodative acquired, partially accommodative, and deteriorated accommodative esotropia. Once surgery is indicated, it is recommended that the patient undergo prism adaptation prior to surgical treatment.

In the past, patients were operated for the angle of deviation left uncontrolled by the glasses. Undercorrection of these patients was quite common.

Prism adaptation

Preoperative prism adaptation (PA) is used to predict the patient's fusional capability, determine the target angle for surgery, and give an indication of surgical success. The prism adaptation process is fairly simple. Fresnel prisms are worn over the patient's spectacle correction to neutralize the esotropia at distance and near and render the patient orthotropic or slightly exotropic. The prism power is split as equally as possible between the two lenses. This equalizes the effect on visual acuity and thus promotes fusion.

Patients are followed weekly, adjusting the prism until the patient stabilizes at an esotropia of 8^Δ or less. Those exhibiting fusion, either to the original amount of prism or to an increased amount, are classified as *responders*. In responders, surgery is done for the amount of esotropia that has been neutralized when wearing the full amount of prism. Those who do not exhibit fusion, who build to an angle greater than 60^Δ without fusion, or who develop exotropia in their prismatic correction are classified as *nonresponders* (see Fig. 80.7). In nonresponders, the prisms are removed, the deviation returns to the original angle, and surgery is done for the original angle of esotropia.

A randomized clinical trial has compared the overall effectiveness of PA as a preoperative test.[38] Patients were randomly placed into two groups, one for control and one for PA. In the control group, surgery was done for the original angle present at the time of enrollment into the study. Patients that underwent PA were separated into responders and nonresponders. Nonresponders underwent surgery for the original angle. Responders were divided into two groups. One group had the prisms removed and surgery was performed for the original angle of deviation. The second group had surgery for the prism-adapted angle. Two-thirds of patients responded to prisms. Table 80.2 is the surgical table used for this study if bilateral medial rectus recessions were performed. If a recession of the medial rectus combined with a resection of the lateral rectus was performed, the amounts listed in Table 80.3 were used.

Postoperative success was defined as $0-8^\Delta$ by simultaneous prism cover test. At the six-month outcome study, for the prism adaptation group, the results showed a success rate of 83%, and

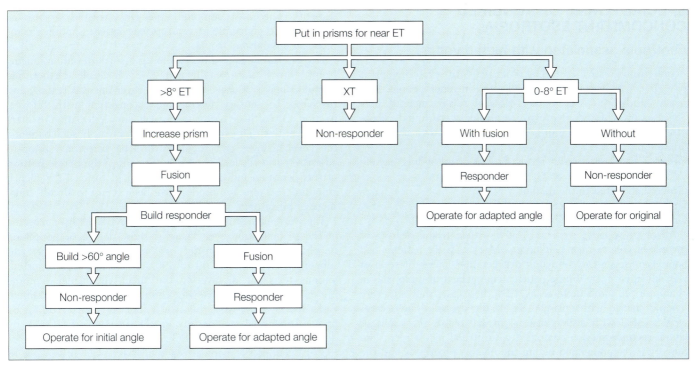

Fig. 80.7 Algorithm for prism adaptation. Adapted from Kutschke PJ. Prisms – are they really helpful? American Orthoptic Journal 1996; 46: 61–4. Reprinted by permission of The University of Wisconsin Press.

Table 80.2 Surgical amounts for bilateral medial rectus recessions used for esodeviations

Target angle (prism diopters)	Medial rectus Amt of recess Both eyes	Lateral rectus Amt of resect One eye
12$^\Delta$–15$^\Delta$	3.0 mm	–
16$^\Delta$–20$^\Delta$	3.5 mm	–
21$^\Delta$–25$^\Delta$	4.0 mm	–
26$^\Delta$–30$^\Delta$	4.5 mm	–
31$^\Delta$–35$^\Delta$	5.0 mm	–
36$^\Delta$–40$^\Delta$	5.5 mm	–
41$^\Delta$–45$^\Delta$	6.0 mm	–
46$^\Delta$–50$^\Delta$	5.0 mm	5.0 mm
51$^\Delta$–55$^\Delta$	5.0 mm	6.0 mm
56$^\Delta$–60$^\Delta$	5.0 mm	7.0 mm

Table 80.3 Surgical amounts for bilateral medial rectus recessions combined with lateral rectus resections used for esodeviations

Target angle (prism diopters)	Medial rectus Amt of recess	Lateral rectus Amt of resect
15$^\Delta$	3.0 mm	4.0 mm
20$^\Delta$	3.5 mm	5.0 mm
25$^\Delta$	4.0 mm	6.0 mm
30$^\Delta$	4.5 mm	7.0 mm
35$^\Delta$–40$^\Delta$	5.0 mm	8.0 mm
> 40$^\Delta$	see Table 80.2	

Some authorities suggest larger bimedial recessions-up to 7 mm, without lateral rectus

The undercorrection rate showed a much greater difference. Of the controls, 25% were undercorrected, defined as greater than 8$^\Delta$ esotropia. Of those that underwent prism adaptation and had surgery for their entry angle, 21% were undercorrected. Only 10% of those that underwent surgery for the full amount of prisms being worn preoperatively were undercorrected. The one-year outcome study showed the disparity in the undercorrection rate in the entry angle group and the prism-adapted surgery group to increase.[40] As a result of this study, we feel that if patients undergo prism adaptation and have surgery for the prism-adapted angle, the predictability of successful surgical outcome is 90%. The rate of undercorrection was low, 10%, without increasing the rate of overcorrection, less than 1%.

PA identifies the group of patients who can receive larger amounts of surgery without fear of overcorrection. Of the prism responders, 45% built their angle of deviation with prism to greater than the original angle. If they had been operated for their original angle of esotropia, they would have been undercorrected. Nonresponders had the lowest rate of postoperative fusion. This study concluded that surgery for the angle of esotropia found following PA produced better postoperative alignment. The recommendation of this study was that PA be done for patients with acquired esotropia to determine the target angle for surgery.

In this original PA trial, if the near deviation exceeded the distance deviation by 10$^\Delta$ or more, bifocals were used at near to control the difference prior to prescribing the prisms. It was thought that if the prisms were mounted to offset the near deviation, the patient would have an exotropia at distance. Subsequently, several studies investigated PA for the near angle of deviation.[41] In one study, when the near deviation was offset preoperatively, 21 of 31 patients fused with prisms without exotropia at distance. Postoperatively, with an average follow-up of over 3 years, 20 of these 21 patients maintained fusion. None required bifocals postoperatively for fusion. A subsequent study with longer follow-up concurred with this result.[42]

in the controls that of 72%. This was statistically significant (p = 0.04). Postoperatively, there were a total of 7 overcorrections, defined as greater than 8$^\Delta$ exotropia. Five of these occurred in controls; the others in patients that underwent prism adaptation.

SPECIAL FORMS OF ACQUIRED CONCOMITANT ESOTROPIA

Esotropia associated with high myopia

Acquired progressive esotropia associated with severe myopia is rare. It occurs without sex predilection in older people. In a recent study,[43] in over 44,000 cases of severe myopia, only 38 cases of acquired progressive esotropia were found. These cases were divided into four groups according to their abduction limitation:

Group 1 had limitation of abduction but could abduct beyond the midline;

Group 2 abducted to the midline;

Group 3 could not abduct to the midline; and

Group 4 was fixed in an extreme adducted position.

All of these cases were associated with extreme degrees of myopia of greater than 12 diopters. Many of these patients had poor vision secondary to myopic degeneration. The earliest onset was 22 years of age. Some patients complained of diplopia. On computerized tomography scans, 12 of these cases showed severe myopic change with enlargement of the eyeball. These cases were treated with either bilateral medial rectus recessions or lateral rectus resection combined with medial rectus recession. Surgery is recommended before the myopia progresses and the limitation of abduction advances to group 4. The groups with better abduction obtained better alignment. Neuroimaging studies suggest that downward displacement of the lateral rectus muscle may be important in the pathogenesis of this syndrome.[44]

Esotropia associated with monocular visual loss

Sensory esotropia is an acquired concomitant esotropia associated with monocular visual loss. Although this may occur at any age, it is usually associated with monocular visual loss early in life. Monocular visual loss later in life is more commonly associated with sensory exotropia. Monocular congenital cataract is a common cause of sensory esotropia. As these children usually cannot achieve equal vision, more than 80% will have a secondary acquired comitant esodeviation. The level of visual acuity ranges anywhere from 20/40 to less than 20/200.

Sensory esotropia does not usually lessen over time. It is not advised, therefore, to ignore this alignment problem. The surgical procedure of choice is a lateral rectus resection combined with medial rectus recession on the nondominant eye (see Table 80.3), leaving a small angle of esotropia without a limitation of adduction. If too much surgery is done and there is a limitation of adduction, a secondary exotropia will likely occur, requiring a second procedure.

Monofixation syndrome

The term monofixation syndrome has become popularized to describe a small, concomitant angle of esotropia. Synonyms used to describe this condition include esophoria with retinal slip, fixational disparity, esophoria with fixational disparity, subnormal binocular vision, small-angle esotropia, and convergence fixation disparity. The most common etiology is treated strabismus, primarily the concomitant esotropia deviations. Another common cause is anisometropia.

Ocular alignment in monofixation is a small deviation ranging from 1^Δ to 8^Δ horizontally and 2^Δ–3^Δ vertically. Orthotropic monofixators, 37%, have no shift on cover/uncover testing, and responses to sensory testing are inconsistent with bifoveal fixation. Often those with a tropia will show a deviation to alternate cover test that exceeds cover/uncover test. In such patients, the cover/uncover test should always be performed prior to alternate cover testing. The ability to control the phoric portion of this deviation indicates some amount of fusional divergence amplitudes. These amplitudes have been found to almost equal those of bifixators.

The constant feature of monofixation is a facultative scotoma in the monofixating eye. There is some degree of peripheral fusion on polarized four-dot or Worth four-dot testing, and subnormal stereopsis of 60 to 300 s of arc has been reported. Various tests for discovering the small, monocular scotoma present under binocular viewing conditions have been described. Parks found it by using the Worth four-dot lights (100%), by finding subnormal stereoacuity on the Titmus test (100%), by doing binocular perimetry (99%), and by using the Bagolini lenses (93%).[45] Jampolsky popularized the 4^Δ base out prism test to detect the presence of a monocular scotoma.[46] Parks found this test to be reliable only 72% of the time.

Amblyopia occurs quite commonly in patients with monofixation syndrome. The incidence varies with the etiology of the monofixation. When monofixation occurs following the treatment of congenital esotropia, the incidence of amblyopia is approximately 34%. When monofixation is secondary to acquired esotropia, the incidence of amblyopia is 67%. Virtually all who have monofixation secondary to anisometropia will have some degree of difference in vision between the two eyes. If strabismus and anisometropia occur together, 88% will have amblyopia.[45]

The treatment for monofixation is the treatment of amblyopia. Surgery or prisms are rarely indicated. It is recommended that monofixators be followed every 6 months to one year, during the years until age 9, looking for the occurrence or reoccurrence of amblyopia.

It is stated that monofixation has great stability and that once it is established, it is as stable as bifixation or bifoveal fusion.[45,47] To investigate this, a study comparing patients having a small angle of esotropia with monofixation syndrome to those without sensory fusion was done.[48] Thirty-eight patients with monofixation syndrome were compared with 42 patients with small-angle esotropia but no monofixation fusion. All patients had surgical treatment for congenital esotropia. The average follow-up for these patients was 17½ years. Comparing the two groups, there was no difference in follow-up time, preoperative esotropia, or alignment immediately postoperatively.

It was found that those who developed monofixation were aligned at an earlier age, 2.6 versus 2.9 years. In the follow-up period, stability of alignment occurred in 74% of monofixators compared with only 45% that did not have monofixation fusion. It was concluded that the fusion is a stabilizing influence regarding motor alignment.

REFERENCES

1. Zipf RF. Binocular fixation pattern. Arch Ophthalmol 1976; 94: 401–5.

2. Dickey CF, Metz HS, Stewart SA, et al. The diagnosis of amblyopia in cross-fixation. J Pediatr Ophthalmol Strabismus 1991; 28: 171–5.

3. Dickey CF, Scott WE. Amblyopia–the prevalence in congenital esotropia versus partially accommodative esotropia–diagnosis and results of treatment. In: Lenk-Schafer M, editor. Orthoptic Horizons: transactions of the VIth International Orthoptic Congress, Harrogate, UK, July 1987. Harrogate: The Congress; 1987: 106–12. (Vol. 106).

4. Pediatric Eye Disease Investigator Group. Spontaneous resolution of early-onset esotropia: experience of the congenital esotropia observational study. Am J Ophthalmol 2002; 133: 109–18.

5. Kraft SP, Scott WE. Surgery for congenital esotropia – an age comparison study. J Pediatr Ophthalmol Strabismus 1984; 21: 57–68.

6. Stewart SA, Scott WE. The age of onset of dissociated vertical deviation (DVD). Am Orthopt J 1991; 41: 85–9.

7. Scott WE, Sutton VJ, Thalacker JA. Superior rectus recessions for dissociated vertical deviation. Ophthalmology 1982; 89: 317–22.

8. Braverman DE, Scott WE. Surgical correction of dissociated vertical deviations. J Pediatr Ophthalmol Strabismus 1977; 14: 337–42.

9. Elliott RL, Nankin SJ. Anterior transposition of the inferior oblique. J Pediatr Ophthalmol Strabismus 1981; 18: 35–8.

10. Burke JP, Scott WE, Kutschke PJ. Anterior transposition of the inferior oblique muscle for dissociated vertical deviation. Ophthalmology 1993; 100: 245–50.

11. Schwartz T, Scott WE. Unilateral superior rectus recession for the treatment of dissociated vertical deviation. J Pediatr Ophthalmol Strabismus 1991; 28: 219–22.

12. Magoon E, Cruciger M, Jampolsky A. Dissociated vertical deviation: An asymmetric condition treated with large bilateral superior rectus recession. J Pediatr Ophthalmol Strabismus 1982; 19: 152–6.

13. Wilson ME, McClatchey SK. Dissociated horizontal deviation. J Pediatr Ophthalmol Strabismus 1991; 28: 90–5.

14. Wheeler DT, Enke ES, Scott WE. Surgical management of dissociated horizontal deviation associated with congenital esotropia. Binoc Vis Strabismus Q 1996; 11: 256–62.

15. von Noorden GK. Binocular Vision and Ocular Motility. St. Louis: Mosby; 1996.

16. Jampolsky AJ, Norcia AM, Hamer RD. Preoperative alternate occlusion decreases motion processing abnormalities in infantile esotropia. J Pediatr Ophthalmol Strabismus 1994; 31: 6–17.

17. Wright KW, Edelman PM, McVey JH, et al. High-grade stereo acuity after early surgery for congenital esotropia. Arch Ophthalmol 1994; 112: 913–9.

18. Scott WE, Reese PD, Hirsch CR, et al. Surgery for large angle congenital esotropia. Arch Ophthalmol 1986; 104: 374–7.

19. Helveston EM, Patterson JH, Ellis FD, et al. En-bloc recession of the medial recti for concomitant esotropia. Symposium on Strabismus: Transactions of the NOAO. St. Louis: Mosby; 1978: 230–43.

20. Kushner BJ, Morton GV. A randomized comparison of surgical procedures for infantile esotropia. Am J Ophthalmol 1984; 98: 50–61.

21. Keech RV, Scott WE, Baker JD. The medial rectus muscle insertion site in infantile esotropia. Am J Ophthalmol 1990; 109: 79–84.

22. Helveston EM, Ellis FD, Patterson JH, et al. Augmented recession of the medial recti. Ophthalmology 1978; 85: 507–11.

23. McNeer KW, Tucker MG, Spencer RF. Botulinum toxin management of essential infantile esotropia in children. Arch Ophthalmol 1997; 115: 1411–18.

24. Adelstein F, Cuppers C. Zum problem der echten und der scheinbaren abducens lahmung (das sogenannte "Blockierung syndrom"). Buch Augenarzt 1966; 46: 271–8.

25. von Noorden GK. The nystagmus compensation (blockage) syndrome. Am J Ophthalmol 1976; 82: 283–90.

26. von Noorden GK, Wong SY. Surgical results in nystagmus blockage syndrome. Ophthalmology 1986; 93: 1028–31.

27. Shuckett EP, Hiles DA, Biglan AW, et al. Posterior fixation suture operation (fadenoperation). Ophthalmic Surg 1981; 12: 578–85.

28. Ciancia AO. Esotropia in the infant—diagnosis and treatment. Arch Chil Oftalmologia 1962; 19: 116–24.

29. Lang J. Der kongenitale oder frühkindliche Strabismus. Ophthalmologica 1967; 154: 201–8.

30. Donders FC. On the Anomalies of Accommodation and Refraction of the Eye. London: New Sydenham Society; 1864.

31. Duane A. A new classification of the motor anomalies of the eye, based upon physiological principles. Ann Ophthal 1897; 6: 84–130.

32. Dickey CF, Scott WE. The deterioration of accommodative esotropia: frequency, characteristics, and predictive factors. J Pediatr Ophthalmol Strabismus 1988; 25: 172–5.

33. Parks MM. Abnormal accommodative convergence in squint. Arch Ophthalmol 1958; 59: 364–80.

34. Ludwig IH, Parks MM, Getson PR, et al. Rate of deterioration in accommodative esotropia correlated to the AC/A relationship. J Pediatr Ophthalmol Strabismus 1988; 25: 8–12.

35. Hutcheson KA, Ellish NJ, Lambert SR. Weaning children with accommodative esotropia out of spectacles: a pilot study. Br J Ophthal 2003; 87: 4–7.

36. Repka MX, Wellish K, Wisnicki HJ, et al. Changes in the refractive error of 94 spectacle-treated patients with acquired accommodative esotropia. Binoc Vision 1989; 4: 15–21.

37. Albert DG, Lederman ME. Abnormal distance-near esotropia. Doc Ophthal 1973; 34: 27–36.

38. Prism Adaptation Study Research Group. Efficacy of prism adaptation in the surgical management of acquired esotropia. Arch Ophthalmol 1990; 108: 1248–56.

39. Kutschke PJ. Prisms–are they really helpful? Am Orthopt J 1996; 46: 61–4.

40. Repka MX, Connett JE, Scott WE, The one-year surgical outcome after prism adaptation for the management of acquired esotropia. Ophthalmology 1996; 103: 922–8.

41. Kutschke PJ, Scott WE, Stewart SA. Prism adaptation for esotropia with a distance-near disparity. J Pediatr Ophthalmol Strabismus 1992; 29: 12–5.

42. Kutschke PJ, Keech RV. Surgical outcome after prism adaptation for esotropia with a distance-near disparity. J AAPOS 2001; 5: 189–92.

43. Hayashi T, Iwashige H, Maruo T. Clinical features and surgery for acquired progressive esotropia associated with severe myopia. Acta Ophthal Scand 1999; 77: 66–71.

44. Krzizoh TH, Kaufmann H, Traupe H. Elucidation of restrictive motility in high myopia by magnetic resonance imaging. Arch Ophthalmol 1997; 115: 1019–22.

45. Parks MM. The monofixation syndrome. Trans Am Ophthalmol Soc 1969; 67: 609–57.

46. Jampolsky A. The prism test for strabismus screening. J Pediatr Ophthalmol Strabismus 1964; 1: 30–4.

47. Vazquez R, Calhoun JH, Harley RD. Development of monofixation syndrome in congenital esotropia. J Pediatr Ophthalmol Strabismus 1981; 18: 42–4.

48. Arthur BW, Smith JT, Scott WE. Long-term stability of alignment in the monofixation syndrome. J Pediatr Ophthalmol Strabismus 1989; 26: 224–1.

CHAPTER

81 Intermittent Exotropia

Alvina Pauline D L Santiago and Arthur L Rosenbaum

INTRODUCTION

Intermittent exotropia is a strabismus condition observed as an outward drifting of either eye interspersed with periods of good alignment or orthotropia. Exodeviations may be caused by an innervational imbalance between fusional convergence and divergence mechanisms. Neuroanatomic substrates, such as the presence of a divergence center, burst cells, or the presence of a divergence nucleus remain controversial. Divergence may be passive, conditioned by the relaxation of accommodation without simultaneous contraction of both lateral rectus muscles. The lateral rectus muscle of the exodeviated eye demonstrates increased innervation electromyographically, whereas the fixing (straight) eye fails to register any change in activity.[1,2] Both static (mechanical and anatomic) and dynamic factors interplay in the development of exodeviations.

Although the literature suggests that exodeviations occur less frequently than esodeviations, and appear to be more common in females, none of the studies published are population-based, and are mostly series from tertiary centers. Many cases of intermittent exotropia (especially those with good control) do not reach the specialists. Exodeviations may be found more frequently in latitudes with higher levels of sunlight.

Maternal smoking during pregnancy, low birth weight, and a genetic predisposition are risk factors for the development of horizontal strabismus.[3,4]

CLINICAL PRESENTATIONS

Natural history

Exodeviation is characterized by visual axes that form divergent angles; in about one third of cases, it appears during the second year of life. It typically begins as a latent deviation–an exophoria. During this phase, patients are bifoveal fixators with normal retinal correspondence. In a mature visual system, or early in the course of the disease, diplopia occurs in the absence of suppression during periods of exodeviation. In young children with visual plasticity, the patient soon develops a temporal hemiretinal suppression of the deviated eye during periods of poor control.

Exophoria may progress to an intermittent exotropia, vacillating between a phoric and a tropic phase. In some cases, the exotropia becomes manifest and constant (Fig. 81.1). In a series of 51 patients aged 5 to 10 years who were observed for an average of 3.5 years, 75% showed progression, 20% remained unchanged, while 16% improved without intervention.[5] The progressive nature of the disease has therapeutic implications. Factors that affect progression may be modified to improve control of the deviation.

Children may close one eye in bright light or direct illumination[6,7] (Fig. 81.2). Bright light disrupts fusion and perhaps causes diplopia and visual confusion despite a lack of its awareness. It may be that monocular eye closure represents photalgia rather than true photophobia–an adaptive response to

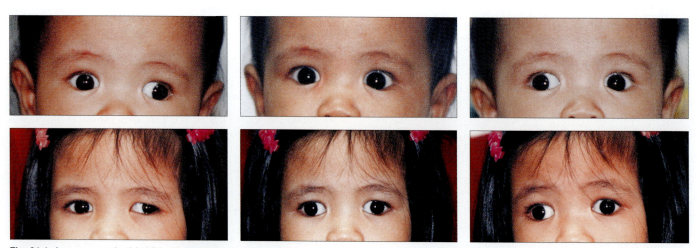

Fig. 81.1 A seven-month-old child with intermittent exotropia that progressed to constant exotropia. (top center) At age seven months note orthotropia in primary gaze; (top left) large angle exotropia with right eye fixing; (top right) large angle exotropia with left eye fixing. Patient was initially managed conservatively with patching and convergence exercises with good control of the deviation after only three months. Patient failed to follow up regularly. (Bottom) At the time of last evaluation at age 2 years, she had a large angle constant exotropia with a left eye preference. Photos also shows deviation with either eye fixing.

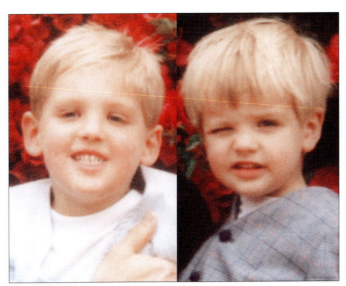

Fig. 81.2 Two brothers standing in Southern California sunshine. Boy on the left has no strabismus. Boy on the right has intermittent exotropia with monocular eye closure, a common sign of intermittent exotropia.

reduce discomfort from high-intensity light in patients already with a subnormal threshold for bright lights. High-intensity lighting also affects the amplitude of fusional convergence in patients with a delicate state of balance between exophoria and intermittent exotropia.

In young children who develop suppression, few symptoms are observed. In older children and adults, asthenopia, blurred vision, headache, diplopia, and visual confusion, as well as reading difficulties especially after prolonged near work, are common complaints. An increase in the reading demand (such as during the first grade, and entry into intermediate or secondary school) and the loss of tonic convergence with advancing age (the onset of presbyopia) bring the patients to the ophthalmologist.

Clinical subtypes

The clinical subtypes elaborate the strength of fusional mechanisms in the different presentations of the intermittent exotrope.[8]
1. *Basic exodeviation*. Distance and near deviation are within 10 PD of each other. Patients have normal accommodative convergence/accommodation (AC/A) ratio.
2. *Convergence insufficiency*. Near deviation exceeds distance deviation by at least 10 PD. Patients may have either a low AC/A ratio or reduced fusional convergence amplitudes. In the early stages of convergence insufficiency, patients complain of asthenopia, visual fatigue, blurred vision, and intermittent diplopia at near. As the process progresses, exophoria deteriorates to a frank intermittent exotropia with near deviation that is larger than the distance deviation. The early stages are most responsive to orthoptic exercises, especially when the deviation is less than 10 PD.
3. *True divergence excess*. The distance deviation exceeds near deviation by at least 10 PD. The AC/A ratio is normal. Measurements at near do not increase with +3.00 D lenses or with prolonged monocular occlusion.
4. *Pseudo-divergence excess*. Initial measurement reveals a distance deviation at least 10 PD more than that at near.
   a. Normal AC/A ratio, tenacious proximal fusion, without pseudo high AC/A. Only monocular occlusion will increase

the size of the deviation at near. Lenses of +3.00 D will not affect near measurements.
   b. High AC/A ratio. Monocular occlusion does not cause an increase in the near exotropic measurement because of absence of tenacious proximal fusion. A high AC/A ratio can be documented with either the gradient method or use of +3.00-D lenses. A small esodeviation may even be measured at distances closer than a third of a meter. The distance deviation may or may not be affected by distance fixation at true infinity (more than 6 m) or by prolonged occlusion.
   c. Normal AC/A ratio, pseudo high AC/A, and tenacious proximal fusion. These patients initially appear to have a high AC/A ratio due to the presence of tenacious proximal fusion, with a smaller deviation measured at near. With prolonged monocular occlusion, the strong fusion at near is disrupted, and the near deviation increases to about equal the distance deviation. When +3.00-D lenses are used to measure the near deviation after monocular occlusion, the deviations at distance and near remain the same.

CLINICAL EVALUATION

Assessing control of the deviation

There are several ways of assessing control of an intermittent exodeviation.

Subjectively, both the parent/guardian and the physician can qualitatively assess whether control is good, fair, or poor. This evaluation depends on frequency, duration, and speed of recovery from a manifest to a latent deviation.

In assessing control of the deviation at home there are four grades of control:
1. *Excellent*–The deviation is manifest less than 10% of waking hours and only at distance, or while daydreaming or fatigued.
2. *Good*–The deviation is manifest less than five times a day and only at distance.
3. *Fair*–The deviation is seen more than five times a day at distance, but near control of the deviation is maintained.
4. *Poor*–The patient breaks into exotropia frequently, both at distance and at near, and only occasionally is orthotropic.[9,10]

In the clinic, the ophthalmologist confirms good control when the patient manifests the deviation only after cover testing. At least motor fusion and realignment spontaneously occur. If a blink or refixation movement is required to regain control of the alignment, the patient has fair control. The patient with poor control spontaneously drifts to an exodeviation despite the absence of fusion disruption.[9,10]

Since loss of control of the distance deviation precedes the loss of control of the near deviation (except for the convergence insufficiency type), an objective measurement of distance stereoacuity may assist in monitoring control of the deviation, or improvement of control of the exodeviation. The Mentor BVAT II BVS measures stereoacuity using both contour circles and random dot stereograms from 240 to 15 sec of arc disparity. Using contour circles, nonstrabismic individuals perform up to 30 sec of arc or better. With random dot E test, controls performed up to 120 sec of arc. Among patients with intermittent exotropia, median performance was only 60 sec of arc or worse on contour circles, and 240 sec of arc for random dot E.[11–13]

Where the Mentor BVAT is unavailable, a red–green filter that splits the Snellen chart into red and green halves may be a useful tool in assessing level of distance control. A red lens is placed in front of the right eye and a green lens in front of the left eye, allowing only the red-filtered letters to be seen by the right eye and the green-filtered letters to be seen by the left. A "Snellen equivalent or letter size" that the patient can fuse at the standard testing distance is demonstrated. The test, however, may be dissociative, and may in itself cause fusion breakdown by mere presentation of the red–green filter, even in patients with good to excellent control of an intermittent exodeviation. Alternate-letter suppression testing may also precede a recordable loss of distance stereoacuity in some cases.[14]

Near stereoacuity fails to correlate well with the early loss of control of an exodeviation, as the exotropia at distance has deteriorated to a significant degree by the time near stereoacuity is affected.

Factors that affect the control of the deviation

Factors that affect the control of the deviation include sensory factors, photalgia, and proximal fusion. Sensory destabilizing factors such as significant refractive errors, amblyopia, and eccentric fixation may disrupt control of a deviation.

Amblyopia is not as frequent in patients with intermittent exotropia as in patients with esotropia. Estimates in retrospective series reach up to 13%.[15] Amblyopia of at least a two-line difference on Snellen linear acuity affects sensory status and deviation control. Understandably, eyes with fairly equal and good vision in both eyes will perform the best on stereoacuity testing. An amblyopic eye limits the level of attainable fusion even in patients without strabismus.[16]

Measuring the deviation

For measurements to be reproducible and repeatable, any significant refractive error must be corrected. This is usually the maximum tolerated plus or the least minus prescription. An accommodative target slightly above threshold must be used as fixation target. A patient with 20/20 vision in both eyes, for example, needs to be presented with a 20/50 line. This permits consistent repeatability of measurements, making the examination more reliable. In preverbal children, videos for children or toys presented as targets should have sufficient detail to control the effects of accommodation.

Distance measurements should be made at a distance of at least 20 ft to eliminate all accommodation. In some cases, distance deviation may have to be measured at true infinity, beyond the confines of the standard visual lane. Breaking fusion by prolonged monocular occlusion for 30 to 60 minutes may be required to eliminate all fusional vergence. In these patients, the patch is removed by the examiner, and fusion, no matter how momentary, is not allowed.

Prism adaptation to measure total preoperative exodeviation, as described for acquired esotropia, has also been used to improve surgical success for patients with intermittent exotropia.[17,18] Preoperative add-on prisms are applied to a patient's spectacle correction, with surgery dictated by the amount of prisms required to neutralize the deviation.

In patients with convergence insufficiency, determining fusional convergence amplitudes and near point of convergence provide useful information for diagnostic and therapeutic purposes. Convergence is a binocular vergence movement that increases the angle formed by the visual axes through simultaneous adduction of both eyes.[19] Convergence amplitudes may be measured using rotary prisms or prism bars for both distance and near. With both eyes open, base-out prisms are gradually added until a *blur point* is reached. Images remain single but with a slight blur. More base-out prisms are added until patient reports diplopia, corresponding to the *break point*. In patients with suppression who do not recognize a second image, the break point is noted when one eye starts to deviate outward under binocular viewing conditions. (Normal convergence amplitudes are 20 PD for distance and 30–35 PD for near.) Finally, base-out prisms are reduced until single vision is reported or motor fusion observed. This *recovery point* is normally 2–4 PD less than the actual break point. In patients where this difference is marked, there is difficulty in regaining fusion that has been disrupted by testing.

In measuring the *near point of convergence*, a fixation object at 30–40 cm is gradually brought closer to the eyes as the patient is instructed to maintain fixation on this object of regard. The near point of convergence is that distance at which one eye starts to lose fixation and drifts out. It should normally be less than 5 cm from the tip of the nose.

Any deficiency in convergence amplitudes (near amplitudes less than 20 PD) or a remote near point of convergence (exceeds 10 cm) constitutes convergence insufficiency. This test is particularly important in patients complaining of asthenopic symptoms related to near work. Reduced convergence amplitudes may precede an exodeviation measured by cover test.

DIFFERENTIAL DIAGNOSIS

Sensory exotropia

A secondary exodeviation or a sensory component can be superimposed on a preexisting intermittent exotropia. Amblyopia or poorer vision in one eye is a common cause. This reiterates the need to address amblyopia and maximize treatment before preoperative surgical treatment planning. Any media opacity, uncorrected refractive error, or organic lesion can predispose to secondary deviations. Correcting the etiology of the sensory deprivation will affect the magnitude and control of the deviation, and should be attempted prior to any surgical decision.

Infantile exotropia

Patients with infantile exotropia present during the first six months of life, typically exhibiting a large angle constant deviation that is not intermittent. They have poor fusion potential. See Chapter 82.

Intermittent exotropia associated with neurologic disease

Variable angles of exotropia are commonly found in the initial stages of delayed visual maturation in patients with global developmental delay, generalized hypotonia, and even cerebral palsy or static encephalopathy. In these patients, the deviation is manifest, not intermittent. Amblyopia, sensory factors, and stability of the deviation need to be addressed before any type of surgical treatment is contemplated.

Craniofacial synostosis/syndromes

Children with craniofacial anomalies are frequently exotropic. Alphabet pattern deviations are common. A "V" pattern mimics inferior oblique overaction while an "A" pattern mimics superior oblique overaction. Dynamic magnetic resonance imaging of the rectus muscles frequently suggest heterotopic rectus muscles[20] (Fig. 81.3). These patients benefit from transposition surgeries correcting the muscle displacements to improve the pattern deviations. Surgical procedure on the oblique muscles is usually unnecessary.

NONSURGICAL MANAGEMENT

Nonsurgical management is indicated in patients with excellent control with normal distance stereoacuity. Young patients at risk of developing monofixational esotropia from persistent surgical overcorrection may also benefit from delay in definitive intervention until the risk for foveal suppression would have passed. Fusional ability is intact and normal if distance stereoacuity compares with normal values. Patients' motor and sensory status should be monitored periodically. In children, the following nonsurgical therapies may prevent or reverse the deterioration of intermittent exotropia by maintaining the potential for equal vision in each eye and preserving binocular vision.[10]

Amblyopia management

Improved vision in an amblyopic eye reduces suppression and allows awareness of a second image (diplopia), which serves as a stimulus to control the deviation. Amblyopia may be associated with anisometropia as a cofactor other than strabismus. Patching remains the mainstay of management although penalization of the better eye with atropine has found increased acceptance and improved patient compliance. However, atropine penalization may adversely affect fusion since normal fusional vergence mechanisms are disrupted because of paralysis of accommodation and convergence. Reports of unilateral patching improving control of an intermittent deviation[21] may be effective because of improvement in mild degrees of amblyopia.[14]

Refractive error

Poor quality of a visual image represents an obstacle to fusion and can facilitate sensory maladaptation such as suppression and amblyopia, contributing to progressive loss of control of an intermittent exotropia. Cylindrical error, myopia, and anisometropia should be corrected.

The hyperopic intermittent exotrope, however, presents a unique dilemma for the strabismus specialist. Children with moderate to severe hyperopia (more than +3.00 D) have been documented to have improved ocular alignment following spectacle correction. Presumably, this occurs because of the influence of improved visual acuity on ocular alignment.[22] Typically, however, many patients have a smaller exodeviation if the hyperopic correction is not worn. Thus, only the minimum plus prescription providing comfort and improved visual acuity should be prescribed. Patients are cautioned that giving of the hyperopic spectacles may lessen a need for accommodation and convergence, allowing for poorer control of the deviation, even augmenting the size of the exotropic deviation. Small amounts of base-in prisms may be added to enhance control of the deviation. Similarly, a presbyopic patient requiring reading glasses may experience deterioration in control of the deviation at near. Only the minimum amount of reading addition should be prescribed.

If control deteriorates and/or surgery is inevitable, the maximum tolerated plus in children above 5 years, and the cycloplegic refraction in younger children, should be worn at least 4 to 6 weeks to obtain consistent and reliable measurements. An attempt is made to push the plus prescription to as close to full cycloplegic refraction as possible at each follow-up visit. The total exodeviation is thus uncovered, dictating the target angle for surgery. This hyperopic correction is maintained after successful alignment surgery.

"Over-minus" lenses

Overcorrection of myopia, or undercorrection of hyperopia, of up to 2.00 to 4.00 D may be used not only as a treatment trial to control the deviation, but also to treat patients with surgical undercorrection who maintain foveal suppression.[23] Prolonged wear may be necessary, sometimes exceeding a year. Improved quality of fusion and a quantitative reduction in the angle of deviation are benefits, although most with improved control of the deviation do not have reduced angles of deviation. A risk of developing esotropia, especially at near, due to excessive accommodative–convergence exists. Patients should be seen no longer than 3 to 4 weeks after the commencement of minus lenses treatment trial. The lenses are discontinued or the power reduced if esotropia develops.

Only younger children with exodeviations less than 15 PD usually benefit from minus lenses. Older children and adults tolerate this poorly, sometimes complaining of asthenopia, headache, and nausea, worse with increased near work. It is helpful when surgery is contraindicated and is most helpful for small undercorrections following surgery. Success may approach 50%, with the control of the deviation lasting up to a year after discontinuation of therapy in 70%.[23]

Prisms and orthoptics

Both base-in and base-out prisms are used in the management of intermittent exotropia. Base-in prisms are used to neutralize small deviations of up to 20 PD to assist control and relieve asthenopia.[24] Patients risk becoming dependent on prisms as they develop a reduced need for convergence effort. In time, patients "eat-up" prisms and gradually develop an increasing exotropic angle–also an argument against prism adaptation in preoperative evaluation of exotropia.

The rationale for base-out prisms, on the other hand, is to stimulate accommodative–convergence. This is reserved for small angle convergence insufficiency type of exotropia. Asthenopia and headache following therapy are common complaints.

Convergence exercises may be used solely or as adjuncts in patients with convergence insufficiency. The objective of the therapy is to increase the range of both fusional convergence and divergence. Among others, they include near-point exercises (e.g., "pencil push-ups"), sliding prisms convergence exercises, and red glass convergence exercises. In near point exercises, the fixation target (we prefer a small toy with sufficient detail to a pencil) is presented at a remote distance (usually an arm's length) where fusion is readily achievable. This is gradually brought toward the nose until the break point is reached. Prism convergence exercises use base-out prism bars with instructions to make images single (fusion). This exploits the patient's awareness of diplopia corresponding to the break point. For patients with suppression, diplopia awareness is taught using a red glass test in front of the dominant eye while viewing a muscle light as a fixation target.

Finally, alternate occlusion therapy to stimulate as well as reduce the hemiretinal suppression scotoma and to improve

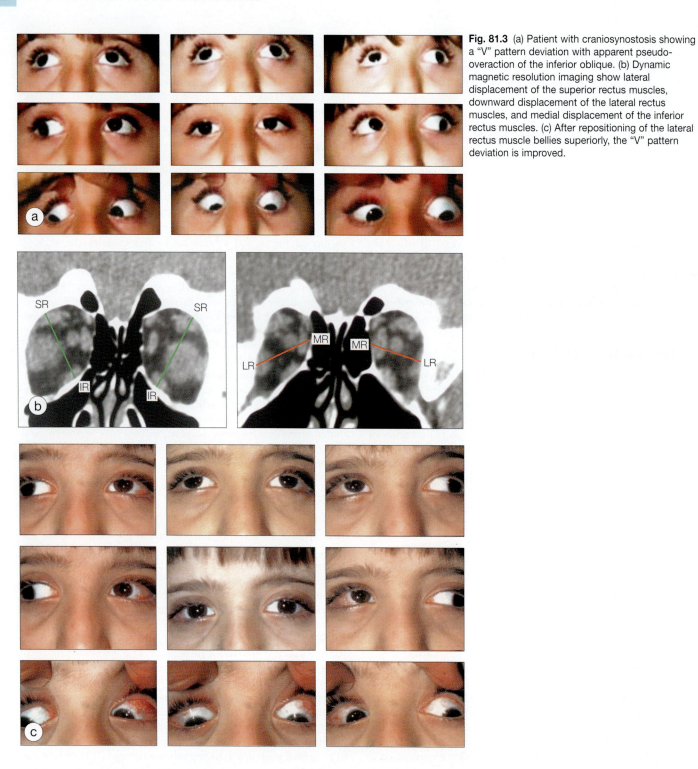

Fig. 81.3 (a) Patient with craniosynostosis showing a "V" pattern deviation with apparent pseudo-overaction of the inferior oblique. (b) Dynamic magnetic resolution imaging show lateral displacement of the superior rectus muscles, downward displacement of the lateral rectus muscles, and medial displacement of the inferior rectus muscles. (c) After repositioning of the lateral rectus muscle bellies superiorly, the "V" pattern deviation is improved.

control may also be tried preoperatively. Although the efficacy of this treatment may be debatable, treatment trial for patients with various reasons for delay of surgical intervention may be indicated.

Chemodenervation

Various reports using botulinum toxin for exodeviation exists[25] but results comparable to surgery were reported only in a few.[26] Satisfactory alignment was achieved in 50% for up to 12 months following the initial injection of botulinum. Chemodenervation remains unlikely to replace surgery but is a reasonable alternative in patients with small angle intermittent exotropia, small postoperative over- or undercorrections, or anesthetic or medical contraindications to surgery. Dose may be titrated based on results, and may start with as little as 1 to 1.5 units for small angle deviations.

SURGICAL MANAGEMENT

Surgical indications

There is no universal agreement nor are there evidence-based guidelines as to the precise indications for intervention, appropriate timing or age at which surgery should be performed, or the most effective surgical procedure.[27] The observation that there is a preclinical exophoric phase, which may deteriorate, and perhaps improve with early treatment alerts the specialist to the need for timely intervention. At any suggestion of worsening (sustained for a few months or more despite nonsurgical treatment), such as deterioration in distance stereoacuity, current data suggest that surgery may be performed. Significantly delaying intervention when deterioration has progressed may reduce the chance of obtaining an optimal outcome.

Serial observations documenting poorer control of the deviation, an increase in the size of the deviation, progressive reduction in stereoacuity especially at distance, a more frequent manifest exotropic than a latent phase, and progressive inability to regain fusion when the deviation has become manifest, with eventual loss of control, are all indications for timely intervention.[9]

Both control at home and in the clinic as described earlier may be used and correlated to assess control of the deviation. An intermittent tropic phase seen more often than phoric or orthotropic phase may be a manifestation of poor control and requires prompt surgical intervention.

Sensory decompensation may be a manifestation of losing control of the deviation before a motor component is observed. In intermittent exotropia, deteriorating or poor control of distance deviation may be the first observation.[9,10] If surgery is performed before the deterioration becomes obligatory, distance stereoacuity improvement also serves as a gauge for successful intervention.[11] Deterioration in near stereoacuity does not come until late in the disease process, especially in patients with good near (proximal) fusion. A patient with consistent subnormal distance stereoacuity despite normal near stereoacuity should be considered a candidate for surgery.

An increase in the size of the exodeviation indicates progression of the exotropia. One should remain cautious in recommending surgery at the earliest suggestion of deterioration as far as size of the deviation is concerned. Various factors should be considered, including a change in refractive error, onset of amblyopia, secondary changes on the lateral rectus muscle, or progressive weakness of convergence among others. At least two consecutive measurements done several weeks apart, with optimal conditions using an accommodative target, may be required before a final decision is made to proceed with surgery.

During the latent or exophoric phase of intermittent exotropia, hardly any sensory adaptation is documented. To resolve the diplopia and visual confusion that ensue during the manifest tropic phase, however, an immature visual system develops a hemiretinal temporal suppression scotoma in the deviated eye. Initially, the suppression may be facultative, later obligatory. In older children and adults, bothersome diplopia or visual confusion is an indication for surgical correction. Both diplopia and visual confusion may occur in the setting of poor vision or amblyopia.

Although many patients with intermittent exotropia are asymptomatic, a significant number, especially those with the convergence insufficiency type of deviation, may have severe asthenopia associated with headache and nausea. The symptoms worsen as the reading demand increases. Asthenopia may also herald deteriorating control. After a failure of orthoptics trial, definitive surgery may be required.

Surgical procedures

Rectus muscle surgery for intermittent exotropia consists of a weakening procedure on the lateral rectus muscle and/or a strengthening procedure on the medial rectus muscle. The lateral rectus muscle is believed to affect the distance deviation more than near, whereas the medial rectus muscle is more effective at near. The choice as to which muscle to perform surgery on is suggested by the clinical pattern of the deviation.

If a patient has true and pseudo- divergence excess type of exotropia, bilateral lateral rectus recession (Table 81.1) is beneficial. Procedures on the medial rectus should be avoided because of its effect at near.

Patients with basic exotropia with equal near and distance deviation are best treated with a recess–resect procedure (Table 81.2). A prospective randomized clinical trial revealed only a 52% success rate in patients with basic exotropia if only lateral rectus recessions are performed. This increases to 82% if a recess–resect procedure was chosen.[28]

A patient with convergence insufficiency may benefit the most from at least one medial rectus resection procedure in combination with a lateral rectus recession. In adults and older children, we prefer an adjustable suture on at least one medial rectus muscle when bilateral medial rectus resection procedure is chosen.[29] Overcorrection at distance is expected up to 6 weeks

Table 81.1 Surgery for exotropia	
Exotropia (PD)	LR recession (mm)
15	4.5
20	5.5
25	6.0
30	7.0
35	8.0
40	9.0
45	9.5
50	10.0

Lateral rectus (LR) recession both eyes for intermittent exotropia. Designed for 5–10 PD of esotropia in the early postoperative period. The numbers in this table should be modified based on clinical findings (such as horizontal incomitance), the surgeon's technique, and results of the surgeon's personal series.

Table 81.2 Surgery for exotropia		
Exotropia (PD)	LR recession (mm)	MR resection (mm)
15	4.0	3.0
20	5.0	4.0
25	6.0	4.5
30	6.5	5.0
35	7.5	5.5

Lateral rectus (LR) recession and medial rectus (MR) resection (recess–resect). The numbers in this table should be modified based on clinical findings (such as horizontal incomitance), the surgeon's technique, and results of the surgeon's personal series.

after surgery. Membrane prisms are added to the distance correction and gradually removed as the distance esotropia resolves. Because of the risk for overcorrection, patient selection and counseling are paramount.

For smaller deviations of up to 16 PD, large unilateral lateral rectus recession of up to 12 mm in the nondominant eye may be effective with only a minimal abduction deficiency.[30]

Medial rectus resection may produce lid fissure narrowing (Fig. 81.4) and overcorrection in the opposite field of gaze of the resected muscle. This small overcorrection in side gaze may be advantageous in eliminating temporal hemiretinal suppression but may predispose to monofixational foveal suppression in the susceptible age group. In left gaze for left-sided driven cars (right gaze for right-sided driven cars), diplopia and visual confusion in this gaze field may cause driving difficulty. The amount of medial rectus resection should be limited to 5.0 mm to avoid introducing horizontal incomitance.

Defining successful intermittent exotropia surgery

Just as there are few consistent guidelines for the timing of surgery, there is disagreement regarding the appropriate criteria for assessing successful or optimal surgical outcome.

If success is measured as good motor fusion and alignment within 10 PD of orthotropia, surgical success rates were estimated at 42–81%,[31–34] improving to 82–90% after a second procedure.[32,34] Yet, motor alignment alone is not a sufficient gauge for success. With a functional goal of achieving sensory fusion or its improvement the results become sobering.

If only some degree of stereopsis at near (Titmus fly stereograms) is required, then success is achieved in 78%.[32] Only 41% of patients achieve bifoveal fixation as measured by stereopsis of 40 sec of arc.[33]

Improved distance stereoacuity is the most stringent criterion of success.[11] In the series that used distance stereoacuity, 75% of patients showed improvement with contour circles, but only 45% with random dot E. From 240 sec of arc preoperatively, 60 sec of arc with contour circles was attained after surgery. Distance stereoacuity levels, however, are not restored to normal values, perhaps reflecting a delay in intervention.

Desired early postoperative alignment

Within the first two weeks, a small angle (5–10 PD) of esotropia is usually desirable.[14] The eyes are brought beyond the temporal hemiretinal suppression scotoma to increase diplopia awareness. This stimulates fusional vergences to stabilize postoperative alignment. Intentional overcorrection has risks in children with an immature visual system. In the immediate postoperative period, base-out prisms to neutralize residual deviation to maintain bifoveal fixation should be used to prevent development of monofixation esotropia with foveal suppression.

In older children and adults who develop intermittent exotropia after the visual system has matured (typically after age 10 years), diplopia and visual confusion occur with little or no suppression. The surgical goal in these cases should be orthotropia even on the first postoperative day. Adjustable sutures optimize postoperative alignment on day one. Base-out prisms are used temporarily to allow patients to function if overcorrection occurs.[14] Nonsurgical management of postoperative overcorrection should be tried for at least a month before reoperating strategies are contemplated because of the high likelihood of spontaneous resolution.[35]

OTHER ASSOCIATIONS

Pattern deviations (see Chapters 84 and 88)

In patients without significant oblique muscle dysfunction, vertical transposition of the horizontal recti is our preference.

In "A" pattern exotropia with superior oblique overaction our preferred procedure is a posterior three-quarters tenectomy of the superior oblique tendon (Fig. 81.5).[36–39]

In "V" pattern deviations with inferior oblique overaction (Fig. 81.6), the patients will benefit from an inferior oblique weakening procedure.

In patients with craniofacial syndromes, dynamic MRI may show that rectus muscles are excyclorotated and that the intermittent exotropia in upgaze is due to the lateral displacement of the superior rectus with downward displacement of the lateral rectus. Repositioning the muscle to its normal anatomic position may improve the pattern deviation[20,40] (see Fig. 81.3).

In patients with long-standing exodeviations, a tight lateral rectus muscle may cause an "X" pattern deviation (Fig. 81.7). Both the inferior oblique and superior oblique muscles appear to

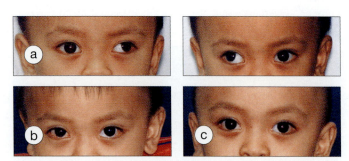

Fig. 81.4 Patient with intermittent exotropia who underwent three muscle surgeries consisting of lateral rectus recession OU and a right medial rectus resection. (b) Preoperative photos showing exotropia. (a) Early postoperative photo showing minimal lid fissure narrowing in the right eye following a recess–resect procedure. (c) Two months postoperative photos show improvement in lid fissure height and symmetry but shows small angle exotropia with dissociated vertical deviation. Amblyopia OD persisted despite occlusion therapy.

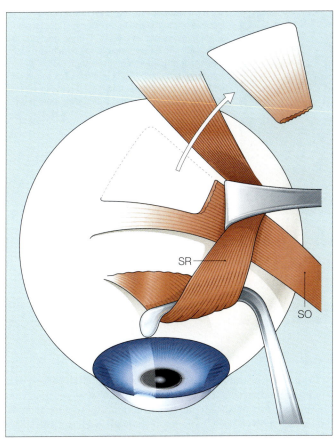

Fig. 81.5 Posterior 3/4 superior oblique tenectomy. A quadrilateral posterior tenectomy is performed on the superior oblique tendon where it fans out, leaving the anterior 1–2 mm of the tendon intact to preserve intorsion. (From Shin et al.[39] Reprinted with permission from Slack, Inc.)

overact. The tight lateral rectus muscles cause a leash effect, creating the pseudo-overaction of the oblique muscles. The apparent oblique muscle dysfunction disappears after lateral rectus weakening.[14] The tight lateral rectus syndrome is uncommon and probably found only in the very large poorly

controlled decompensated intermittent exotropia. It is more commonly associated with long-standing constant exotropia.

Lateral or horizontal incomitance

Patients whose primary position deviation exceeds right and left lateral gazes by 20% or at least 10 PD have significant horizontal incomitance.[41] They may benefit from reducing the intended surgical weakening procedure on the lateral rectus muscle.[42] This modification prevents overcorrection on lateral gazes but risks undercorrection in primary position. Medial rectus resection has also produced satisfactory results.[43]

When the lateral incomitance is due to a tight medial rectus muscle, resection procedures on this muscle worsens the incomitance. Recession of the tight medial rectus with enhanced lateral rectus recession to compensate for the effect of the medial rectus recession is recommended. Adjustable sutures improve results.[42]

Concomitant vertical deviations

Small vertical deviations may occur with intermittent exotropia. Small vertical deviations of less than 10 PD can be corrected by vertical transposition of the horizontal rectus muscles. For example the recessed lateral rectus and the resected medial rectus muscle may be displaced superiorly one-half to a whole tendon width in the hypotropic eye (directions are reversed for a hyperdeviation). This adds an additional upward vector assisting in the control of the vertical deviation. Large vertical deviations should be addressed with the appropriate surgery on the cyclovertical muscle at the time of exotropia surgery.

Dissociated strabismus complex

Just as infantile esotropic patients may have associated dissociated vertical, torsional, and horizontal deviations, patients with intermittent exotropia, especially when it commences in childhood, may also have dissociated strabismus in its various presentations (much less common in exotropia) (see Chapter 75). In determining the true horizontal deviation, neutralization is sometimes confounded by the presence of a dissociated horizontal component. The refixation in dissociated horizontal deviation is slower, and is not accompanied by the same amount

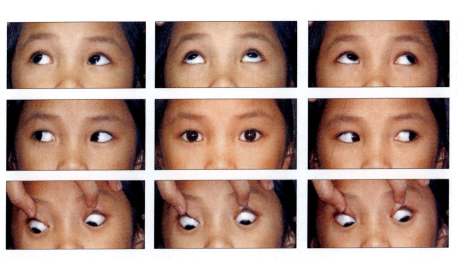

Fig. 81.6 Four-year-old patient with intermittent exotropia with "V" pattern and inferior oblique overaction. Center photograph shows right exotropia that increased in upgaze and reduced in downgaze. Note also the mild overaction of the right inferior oblique in up and left gaze.

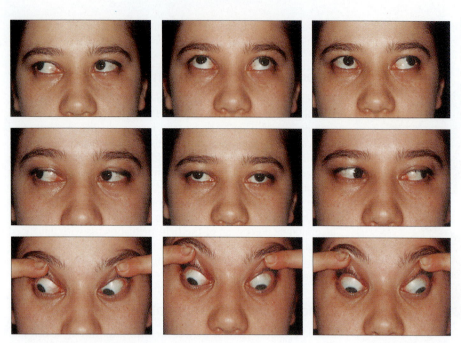

Fig. 81.7 Patient with "X" pattern deviation because of long-standing exotropia. Tight lateral rectus muscles act as a leash. Forced duction testing will show resistance to full adduction. Only weakening procedures on the lateral rectus are necessary to relieve the "X" pattern. No surgery is required on the oblique muscles. (From Fig 12.4 of Santiago et al.[14] Reprinted with permission of WB Saunders (Elsevier Science).

of refixation movement in the other eye. The astute clinician should be alert to this finding to avoid overestimating the amount of exodeviation requiring intervention. Fortunately, dissociated horizontal deviations benefit from lateral rectus weakening procedures as well.

POSTOPERATIVE UNDERCORRECTION

Undercorrection after initial bilateral lateral rectus recession is common, requiring a second surgical intervention in 21–38% of patients.[32,34] The age at the time of initial surgery and the size of the exodeviation at the time of surgery were not contributory factors to this failure. Rather, the following may account for this observation:

1. Increasing constancy of the deviation in viewing distant objects especially beyond 6 m;[44]
2. Small amounts of coexisting vertical misalignment;[33]
3. Failure to identify oblique muscle dysfunction and consequent "A" or "V" pattern exotropia;[14]
4. Failure to reveal the total amount of distance exotropia in preoperative measurements;[8,45] and
5. Uncorrected refractive error, especially significant hyperopia.[14]

The most common clinical presentation of undercorrection is residual deviation at distance. Following lateral rectus recession of both eyes, or a recession on the lateral rectus with a medial rectus resection, orthotropia or a small angle exophoria is observed at near, whereas a small to moderate intermittent exotropia is seen at distance. Although small initially, this residual deviation, without additional therapy, tends to increase with the passage of time.

Base-in prisms to neutralize the distance misalignment are used as a fusion-priming device. Prisms are worn for at least 6 months before a second procedure is contemplated.[46–48] Minus lens therapy may also be used to treat residual deviation of less than 12 PD. Treatment of small undercorrections in this manner may correct 50% of cases in some reports.[23,49]

In the past, waiting 6 months or more after initial surgery was common and acceptable before additional surgery was contemplated for persistent undercorrection. Outcome analysis, however, showed few patients responded well to secondary surgery performed an average of 2 years after the first surgery. Based on these results, additional surgical intervention should be performed earlier, even as early as 8 to 12 weeks after the initial surgery, if residual exotropia at distance remains unresponsive to conservative management.[50]

If maximum or large bilateral lateral rectus recession has been performed, residual distance exotropia with orthotropia at near presents a dilemma. The options include additional recession on an already weakened lateral rectus muscle, between 7.5 to 10.0 mm from the original lateral rectus insertion. Re-recession of the lateral rectus muscle has not been routinely successful. Otherwise, one or both medial rectus muscles may be resected, with no additional surgery on the lateral rectus muscle. This procedure may be used for both early and late undercorrection.

Patients who undergo secondary surgery must be watched for overcorrection. If the initial esotropia from a medial rectus resection does not resolve within 3 weeks, base-out membrane prisms may be prescribed to preserve fusion. Prisms can usually be reduced gradually.

CONSECUTIVE ESODEVIATION

Overcorrection that persists beyond the immediate postoperative period after initial surgery is less common than undercorrection, even when surgery for the largest recorded angle of exodeviation is the target.[32,34] Transient esotropia for near targets is commonly found in the first few postoperative weeks. A small angle esotropia that persists at distance, with only exophoria or orthotropia at near, is usually very stable and best left untreated. Rarely, a large overcorrection following an over-recessed slipped or lost lateral rectus muscle may occur and is most bothersome in the field of gaze of the weakened lateral rectus (Fig. 81.8).

In the early postoperative period, a rather large esotropia may not necessarily mean a poor response to surgery. Long-term stability of alignment after bilateral lateral rectus recession was achieved in patients who demonstrated up to 20 PD of esotropia in the first 10 days after surgery.[51] Esotropia at near that persists beyond 3 weeks is worrisome especially in children susceptible to suppression and deterioration of fusional status. Children can develop monofixational esotropia even if aligned to within 8 PD of orthotropia. Adults, on the other hand, tolerate overcorrection poorly.

Many intermittent exotropic patients may have preoperative distance–near disparity in the deviation. Despite this, most will respond well to surgery, maintaining this disparity after surgery. Infrequently, patients develop a high accommodative accommodation-to-convergence ratio (AC/A) with manifest esotropia at near. Preoperative evaluation to identify patients with high AC/A minimizes postoperative overcorrection.

Older patients will complain of diplopia or visual confusion for either near or distant targets. Monocular eye closure may be observed to avoid diplopia, or patients will tilt the head back or drop the chin down if a pattern deviation is present. Plus lenses (+2.50 to +3.00 D) at near as bifocals will preserve fusion in patients with distance esophoria or exophoria but with esotropia for near targets. Base-out prisms also serve to preserve fusional status and are tapered gradually.

With failure of conservative management, secondary surgical weakening procedures become inevitable. The persistence of a larger angle of esotropia for distance with diplopia can be addressed by advancing the previously recessed lateral rectus muscle, especially if abduction deficit on ductions and versions are apparent. More commonly, if esotropia persists for near, weakening of the medial rectus, through a recession and/or a fadenoperation, may be indicated if esotropia at near persists beyond 3 months.

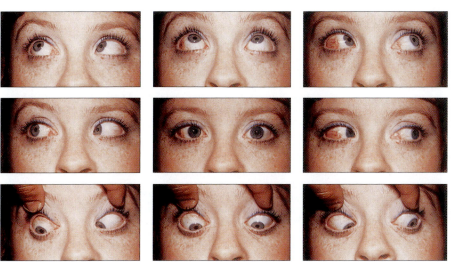

Fig. 81.8 Overcorrection after bilateral rectus recession for intermittent exotropia. Patient developed 25 PD of right esotropia with abduction deficit in right gaze. Differential diagnosis should include slipped or lost lateral rectus muscle. A lost muscle, however, seems less likely because of relatively good right lateral rectus rotation despite the observed deficit. (From Fig. 12.5 of Santiago et al.[14] Reprinted with permission of WB Saunders (Elsevier Science).

REFERENCES

1. Mays LE, Porter JD, Gamlin PD, et al. Neural control of vergence eye movements: neurons encoding vergence velocity. J Neurophysiol 1986; 56: 1007–21.
2. Mays LE. Neural control of vergence eye movements: convergence and divergence neurons in midbrain. J Neurophysiol 1984; 51: 1091–108.
3. Chew E, Remaley NA, Tamboli A, et al. Risk factors for esotropia and exotropia. Arch Ophthalmol 1994; 112: 1349–55.
4. Podgor MJ, Remaley NA, Chew E. Associations between siblings for esotropia and exotropia. Arch Ophthalmol 1996; 114: 739–44.
5. von Noorden GK. The exotropias. In: von Noorden GK, editor. Binocular Vision and Ocular Motility: theory and management of strabismus. 5th ed. St.Louis: Mosby; 1996: 341–59.
6. Wang FM, Chryssanthou G. Monocular eye closure in intermittent exotropia. Arch Ophthalmol 1988; 106: 941–2.
7. Wiggins RE, von Noorden GK. Monocular eye closure in sunlight. J Pediatr Ophthalmol Strabismus 1990; 27: 16–20.
8. Kushner BJ. Richard G. Scobee Memorial Lecture: Exotropic deviations: a functional classification and approach to treatment. Am Orthopt J 1988; 38: 81–93.
9. Rosenbaum AL, Stathacopoulos RA. Subjective and objective criteria in recommending surgery in intermittent exotroia. Am Orthopt J 1992; 42: 46–51.
10. Rosenbaum AL. John Pratt-Johnson Lecture: Evaluation and management of intermittent exotropia. Am Orthopt J 1996; 46: 94–8.
11. O'Neal TD, Rosenbaum AL, Stathacopoulos RA. Distance stereo-

acuity improvement in intermittent exotropic patients following strabismus surgery. J Pediatr Ophthalmol Strabismus 1995; 32: 353–7.
12. Stathacopoulos RA, Rosenbaum AL, Zanoni D, et al. Distance stereoacuity. Assessing control in intermittent exotropia. Ophthalmology 1993; 100: 495–500.
13. Zanoni D, Rosenbaum AL. A new method for evaluating distance stereo acuity. J Pediatr Ophthalmol Strabismus 1991; 28: 255–60.
14. Santiago AP, Ing MR, Kushner BJ, et al. Intermittent exotropia. In: Rosenbaum AL, Santiago AP, editors. Clinical Strabismus Management: principles and surgical techniques. 1st ed. Philadelphia: Saunders; 1999: 163–75.
15. Beneish R, Flanders M. The role of stereopsis and early postoperative alignment in long-term surgical results of intermittent exotropia. Can J Ophthalmol 1994; 29: 119–24.
16. Donzis PB, Rappazzo JA, Burde RM, et al. Effect of binocular variations of Snellen's visual acuity on Titmus stereoacuity. Arch Ophthalmol 1983; 101: 930–2.
17. Dadeya S, Kamlesh, Naniwal S. Usefulness of the preoperative prism adaptation test in patients with intermittent exotropia. J Pediatr Ophthalmol Strabismus 2003; 40: 85–9.
18. Ohtsuki H, Hasebe S, Kono R, et al. Prism adaptation response is useful for predicting surgical outcome in selected types of intermittent exotropia. Am J Ophthalmol 2001; 131: 117–22.
19. von Noorden GK. The near vision complex. In: von Noorden GK, editor. Binocular Vision and Ocular Motility: Theory and Management of Strabismus. 5th ed. St. Louis: Mosby; 1996: 85–100.

20. Demer JL, Clark RA, Kono R, et al. A 12-year, prospective study of extraocular muscle imaging in complex strabismus. J AAPOS 2002; 6: 337–47.

21. Freeman RS, Isenberg SJ. The use of part-time occlusion for early onset unilateral exotropia. J Pediatr Ophthalmol Strabismus 1989; 26: 94–6.

22. Iacobucci IL, Archer SM, Giles CL. Children with exotropia responsive to spectacle correction of hyperopia. Am J Ophthalmol 1993; 116: 79–83.

23. Caltrider N, Jampolsky A. Overcorrecting minus lens therapy for treatment of intermittent exotropia. Ophthalmology 1983; 90: 1160–5.

24. Pratt-Johnson JA, Tillson G. Prismotherapy in intermittent exotropia. A preliminary report. Can J Ophthalmol 1979; 14: 243–5.

25. McNeer KW, Magoon EH, Scott AB. Chemodenervation therapy. In: Rosenbaum AL, Santiago AP, editors. Clinical Strabismus Management: principles and surgical techniques. 1st ed. Philadelphia: Saunders; 1999: 423–32.

26. Buckley EG, Seaber J, Tsironis E. Success of motor alignment in exotropia treated with botulinum toxin versus surgery. Am Orthopt J 1996; 46: 127–32.

27. Richardson S, Gnanaraj L. Interventions for intermittent distance exotropia. Cochrane Database Syst Rev 2003; CD003737.

28. Kushner BJ. Selective surgery for intermittent exotropia based on distance/near differences. Arch Ophthalmol 1998; 116: 324–8.

29. Choi DG, Rosenbaum AL. Medial rectus resection(s) with adjustable suture for intermittent exotropia of the convergence insufficiency type. J AAPOS 2001; 5: 13–7.

30. Feretis D, Mela E, Vasilopoulos G. Excessive single lateral rectus muscle recession in the treatment of intermittent exotropia. J Pediatr Ophthalmol Strabismus 1990; 27: 315–6.

31. Clarke WN, Noel LP. Surgical results in intermittent exotropia. Can J Ophthalmol 1981; 16: 66–9.

32. Hardesty HH, Boynton JR, Keenan JP. Treatment of intermittent exotropia. Arch Ophthalmol 1978; 96: 268–74.

33. Pratt-Johnson JA, Barlow JM, Tillson G. Early surgery in intermittent exotropia. Am J Ophthalmol 1977; 84: 689–94.

34. Richard JM, Parks MM. Intermittent exotropia. Surgical results in different age groups. Ophthalmology 1983; 90: 1172–7.

35. Keech RV, Stewart SA. The surgical overcorrection of intermittent exotropia. J Pediatr Ophthalmol Strabismus 1990; 27: 218–20.

36. Prieto-Diaz J. Posterior tenectomy of the superior oblique. J Pediatr Ophthalmol Strabismus 1979; 16: 321–3.

37. Prieto-Diaz J. Management of superior oblique overaction in A-pattern deviations. Graefes Arch Clin Exp Ophthalmol 1988; 226: 126–31.

38. McCall LC, Rosenbaum AL. Incomitant dissociated vertical deviation and superior oblique overaction. Ophthalmology 1991; 98: 911–7.

39. Shin GS, Elliott RL, Rosenbaum AL. Posterior superior oblique tenectomy at the scleral insertion for collapse of A-pattern strabismus. J Pediatr Ophthalmol Strabismus 1996; 33: 211–8.

40. Oh SY, Clark RA, Velez F, et al. Incomitant strabismus associated with instability of rectus pulleys. Invest Ophthalmol Vis Sci 2002; 43: 2169–78.

41. Knapp P, Moore S. Intermittent exotropia. Am Orthopt J 1960; 10: 118–22.

42. Carlson MR, Jampolsky A. Lateral incomitancy in intermittent exotropia: cause and surgical therapy. Arch Ophthalmol 1979; 97: 1922–5.

43. Diamond GR. Medial rectus resection strategies for laterally incomitant intermittent exotropia. J Pediatr Ophthalmol Strabismus 1987; 24: 242–3.

44. Stoller SH, Simon JW, Lininger LL. Bilateral lateral rectus recession for exotropia: a survival analysis. J Pediatr Ophthalmol Strabismus 1994; 31: 89–92.

45. Kushner BJ. Surgical pearls for the management of exotropia. Am Orthopt J 1992; 42: 65–71.

46. Hardesty HH. Prisms in the management of intermittent exotropia. Am Orthopt J 1972; 22: 22–30.

47. Hardesty HH. Therapeutic uses of prisms in undercorrected intermittent exotropia. Int Ophthalmol Clin 1971; 11: 277–82.

48. Hardesty HH. Treatment of under and overcorrected intermittent exotropia with prism glasses. Am Orthopt J 1969; 19: 110–9.

49. Iacobucci IL, Martoni EJ, Giles CL. Results of overminus lens therapy on postoperative exoceviations. J Pediatr Ophthalmol Strabismus 1986; 23: 287–91.

50. Ing MR, Nishimura J, Okino L. Outcome study of bilateral lateral rectus recession for intermittent exotropia in children. Trans Am Ophthalmol Soc 1997; 95: 433–43.

51. Raab EL, Parks MM. Recession of the lateral recti. Early and late postoperative alignments. Arch Ophthalmol 1969; 82: 203–8.

CHAPTER
82

Special Forms of Comitant Exotropia

Stephen P Kraft

INTRODUCTION

Exodeviations in children can be comitant or noncomitant. The noncomitant exodeviations result from either innervational causes, i.e., third nerve paresis and Duane syndrome, or mechanical etiologies, such as congenital fibrosis of the extraocular muscles.

The most common comitant type in children is intermittent exotropia but there are other comitant exodeviations in infants and children whose management can be challenging. This chapter deals with infantile exotropia, monofixational exotropia, exotropia associated with hemianopic visual field defects, and sensory exotropia.

Although they are considered as comitant deviations, they may develop some incomitance from secondary changes in the lateral rectus muscles, mostly in long-standing cases and especially in sensory exotropia or infantile exotropia with a large deviation or where the exodeviation is due to amblyopia or structural abnormalities in the misaligned eye.

INFANTILE EXOTROPIA

Introduction

Infantile exotropia is an exodeviation that develops within the first 6 months of life and persists.[1–4] It can be primary or secondary to an ocular or systemic problem.

Primary infantile exotropia, unrelated to a systemic or ocular disorder, is rare, roughly 1 per 30,000 births.[5] In primary strabismus in the first 6 months of life, for every case with exotropia there are between 150 and 300 cases with esotropia.[6] Intermittent exotropia can manifest by age 6 months (see Chapter 81).

Infantile exotropia can occur secondary to ocular or systemic disorders: e.g., ptosis, albinism, ocular motor apraxia, optic nerve anomalies, and with diseases that lead to vision loss, including retinoblastoma, retinoschisis, iridolenticular abnormalities, and cataracts.[6–8] Exotropia can be a feature of several congenital strabismus syndromes, including third nerve palsies, Duane syndrome, congenital fibrosis of the extraocular muscles, and strabismus fixus[6,7] (see Chapter 85). It may be associated with systemic disorders, which include cerebral palsy, hydrocephalus, craniofacial syndromes, and various chromosomal anomalies.[1,4,6,8,9]

Ocular or systemic disorders are more common in infantile exotropias than in esotropias. Also, infants with constant exotropia have a much stronger chance than those with intermittent exotropia of having a co-existing problem.[7]

Etiology

Vergence abnormalities

Exodeviations appear in over one-third of healthy neonates, while esodeviations are rare.[10,11] Mostly, they are transient and resolve by 6 months as the vergence system matures.[11] Therefore, primary infantile exotropia is likely caused by arrested development of the convergence system in this sensitive early period.

An abnormal convergence reflex may be a primary or secondary phenomenon. There may be a primary deficit in the convergence system, or it may arise from defective cortical binocular development.[12] Disruption of binocular connections in the immature visual cortex potently disrupts development of vergence reflexes, leading to strabismus and to functional deficits, e.g., loss of fusion, asymmetric monocular smooth pursuit, and asymmetric monocular motion perception.[12] The asymmetries are characterized by better tracking and detection of targets when they are followed from the temporal to the nasal visual field than when they are tracked in the reverse direction.

This directional asymmetry should lead to infantile esotropia, rather than exotropia. Therefore, the severity of a primary or secondary convergence system deficit must override the other abnormal processes such that divergence is the predominant reflex. This is supported by the fact that the identical pursuit asymmetry of infantile esotropia occurs in cases of infantile exotropia (L Tychsen, personal communication, 2001).

Anatomic factors

An asymmetry in the structure of the lateral and medial rectus muscles occurs with the length-tension curve of the lateral rectus showing more stiffness than the medial rectus, or the diameter of the lateral rectus may be congenitally larger than normal, allowing it to "overpower" the medial rectus.[6] Finally, orbital dysmorphism as in craniofacial syndromes can produce a divergent positioning of the eyes.

Genetic factors

Infantile exotropia occurred in three consecutive generations of one family, suggesting autosomal dominant inheritance,[9] and it may be more common in Asians and Africans than in Caucasians.[6]

Clinical features

Infantile exotropia starts by 6 months and requires a diagnosis by 12 months of age.[1,3,6] It can have a wide range of angles, from 20 to 90 prism diopters (PD), mostly more than 35 PD[5,7,9,13] (Fig. 82.1). The angle is usually stable initially, increasing slowly.[6]

Amblyopia occurs in up to 25%, usually caused by strabismus rather than anisometropia.[6] It responds to the usual treatment. There is a normal distribution of refractive errors.[5,6]

If large, an "X" pattern strabismus is common, as in adults with large angle exotropia who have a tight lateral rectus syndrome. The deviation is larger in upgaze and downgaze than in the primary position with mild limitation of adduction in one or both

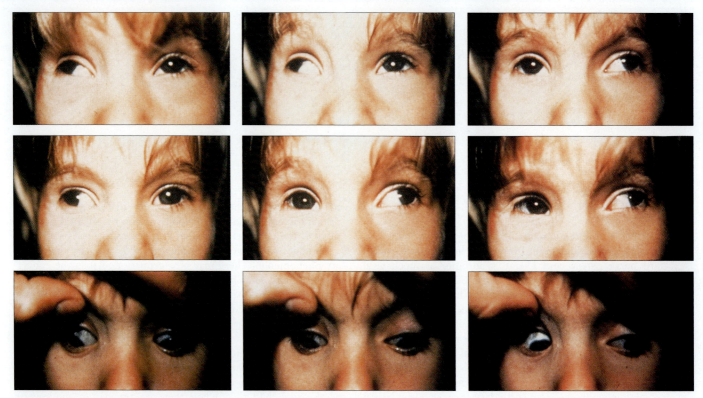

Fig. 82.1 Photos of nine diagnostic gaze positions of a child with infantile exotropia. Note the large angle of exotropia in the primary position (middle photo). There is limited adduction of each eye and an "X" pattern. Each eye shows an upshot and downshoot in the adducted position. (From Kraft,[6] p 177, with permission of WB Saunders.)

eyes, and upshoots and downshoots in adduction (Fig. 82.1). These up- and downshoots have been ascribed to contracture with overactions of the oblique muscles, to sideslip of the lateral rectus around the globe (a "leash effect"), or to the fact the that the globe has more room to elevate and depress when it is not quite fully adducted.[6,14,15] Alternatively, there may be "A" or (more commonly) "V" patterns.[1,4,5,9,13]

Latent nystagmus, dissociated vertical deviations (DVD), and inferior oblique overactions may occur, as with infantile esotropia but less frequently.[1,3,4,13]

Examination

Some pertinent points must be noted in the evaluation of a case of infantile exotropia.

First, the general behavior and physical features of the child may suggest a systemic or orbital association needing referral. Second, an ocular examination rules out anterior and posterior segment disorders, which can be associated with infantile exotropia. A cycloplegic refraction is vital. Third, during the ocular motility examination, the examiner must observe the corneal light reflexes to rule out a positive angle kappa that gives a false appearance of exotropia.[6] The cover test will confirm the presence of a true exodeviation rather than a pseudoexotropia.

Fourth, when the angle is large, the examiner needs to use two prisms oriented base-in and split between the two eyes to get an approximation of the total angle, whether the angle is measured by the Krimsky or prism and alternating cover methods.

Finally, the examiner should search for features of the infantile strabismus complex including dissociated vertical deviations and oblique muscle overactions, and optokinetic testing may detect monocular nasal–temporal motion asymmetries.

Management

Nonsurgical therapy

Infantile exotropia usually requires surgery after any refractive errors and amblyopia have been treated. Although the angle of the deviation is generally stable the strabismus angle may reduce with occlusion.[1]

Botulinum toxin injections have been used for infantile esotropia, but there are no reports on series of cases of the much more rare infantile exotropia. The reported success rates in treating childhood exotropia with botulinum toxin range from 50 to 70%, with bilateral, not unilateral, lateral rectus injections.[16,17] Most had intermittent exotropia: the success rates for exotropia over 35 to 40 PD was much lower, and since most infantile exotropias are larger than this, botulinum toxin may be less successful than surgery for deviations over 35 PD.

Surgery
Timing

Patients with infantile exotropia should be approached in the same manner as those with infantile esotropia: surgery should align the eyes before the age of 24 months to achieve optimal motor and sensory results.[2,3,5,18] Earlier surgery may be beneficial but is controversial. Once the diagnosis of infantile exotropia is confirmed and any refractive error or amblyopia is corrected, the child should be followed for a few weeks to be sure the angle of the strabismus is stable.

Surgical planning

Strabismus surgery techniques are described in Chapter 88, but there are some specific recommendations for surgical treatment of infantile exotropia.

First, the aim is to create a small angle esotropia in the immediate postoperative period, as in most exotropias in older children and adults.[1,5] This principle also applies to children with infantile exotropia and developmental delay or cerebral palsy, as the postoperative drift is usually exotropic despite whether they originally had esotropia or exotropia.[6]

Second, the strategy generally involves weakening (usually recession) one or both lateral rectus muscles, as they are often tight. If the near exotropia is larger than that at distance, then a strengthening (usually a resection) of a medial rectus muscle should be included.[6]

Third, strabismus angles under 40 PD can usually be successfully treated with surgery on two horizontal muscles, either bilateral lateral rectus recessions or a unilateral lateral rectus recession with a medial rectus resection.[1] Treatment of angles over 40 PD may require "supramaximal" amounts of recessions or resections if surgery is planned on two muscles. Alternatively, surgery of more "regular" dosages can be planned on three or four horizontal muscles.[1,3–5,9,13,18]

Finally, surgery for any co-existing dissociated vertical deviations or oblique overactions can be planned for the same sitting or for subsequent surgery, as in infantile esotropia.

Results

The success rates for infantile exotropia surgery are not high. Reoperations are required in up to 50% of patients: undercorrections are more common than overcorrections.[1,3,9,13,18]

Young children who are aligned before age 24 months develop peripheral fusion in up to 50% of cases: some may show gross stereopsis.[1,9,13,18] The best binocular outcomes reported are monofixation syndromes. Realigning patients with infantile exotropia after age 2 can lead to stable long-term results, but sensory fusion is rarely achieved after this age.[5,6]

MONOFIXATIONAL EXOTROPIA

Introduction

The *monofixation syndrome* is characterized by fixation with the fovea of one eye under binocular conditions.[6,19] The sensory features include intact peripheral fusion, preserved gross stereopsis, and frequently, amblyopia of the nonfoveating eye. The motor features include a manifest heterotropia of under 8 PD, a larger heterophoria, and preserved convergence and divergence fusional amplitudes.[19–21] Some cases show no heterotropia on cover test: they are termed *monofixational phorias*. Some show a heterotropia without a heterophoria: these are termed *microtropias*.[21]

In most cases of monofixation syndrome, if there is a small angle heterotropia it is an esotropia, and any associated heterophoria is an esophoria. However, about 20% have an exotropic orientation for the tropia and the phoria.[19,20,22–25] Also, most cases of monofixational exotropia are secondary, either associated with anisometropia or following surgery for exotropia.[23]

Most cases of monofixational exotropia, by virtue of intact vergence amplitudes, retain a stable long-term small exotropia under binocular conditions. In a minority, the fusion control is disrupted and the exophoria becomes predominant: this is termed a *decompensated monofixational exotropia*.[19,20,22] However, most monofixation syndromes underlie cases of intermittent exotropia that reveal their monofixation origin after surgical correction of the exodeviation.[22,23]

Etiology

The monofixation syndrome can be primary or secondary. The secondary form is associated with anisometropia or a macular lesion, or it occurs after surgery for infantile strabismus. Otherwise, it is considered a primary disorder.

Primary monofixation exotropia

Patients with the primary form have a deficit in fovea-to-fovea correspondence: they cannot attain bifoveal fusion.[19] This may be a hereditary error in foveal correspondence that may exceed the capability of Panum's fusional space to compensate for it, leading to suppression of the less dominant fovea.[6] Alternatively, there may be a reversal of the normal dominance of the nasal over the temporal hemifield. As a result, any degree of foveal disparity can lead to a facultative scotoma on the temporal side of the fovea rather than in its usual location on the nasal side.[6,21,26]

A primary monofixational exotropia can decompensate because of an acute illness or chronic fatigue and the "all or none" suppression in exodeviations is less flexible than that in esodeviations.[26,27] If the latent heterophoria begins to manifest, then the strong hemiretinal suppression mechanism may increase the propensity for the exodeviation to decompensate.[6,27]

Secondary monofixational exotropia

The majority of secondary form in children result from surgery for constant or intermittent exotropia.[23] Monofixation after surgery suggests a pre-existing defect in bifoveal fusion.[19,22,23] Anisometropia is a less common cause, but it is a potent obstacle to bifoveal fusion that can lead to suppression of the less dominant fovea.

Finally, a unilateral macular lesion can lead to a progressive manifest exotropia; small lesions can result in a small scotoma with the typical attributes of a monofixation syndrome.[6]

Secondary monofixation exotropia has the same propensity as the primary form for deterioration. There is an abnormal binocular state, and any loss of the "peripheral fusion lock" allows the heterophoria to manifest. If the control deteriorates then the hemiretinal suppression adaptation may take over and increase the likelihood that the exotropia will become constant.[27]

Clinical features

Motor features

Most patients with a monofixation syndrome show a tropia of 2 to 8 PD under binocular conditions. Up to one-third of cases will show no shift on cover test: most commonly in the form secondary to anisometropia.[6,19]

The exophoria uncovered on alternating prism and cover test tends to be larger than that seen in bifoveal patients who have exophoria, although it rarely exceeds 25 PD[20,22] and the fusional amplitudes are often very close to normal.[19]

When exotropia and exophoria co-exist, the simultaneous prism and cover test should be performed initially to measure the static heterotropia. Then the prism and alternating cover test measures the superimposed heterophoria.[6]

Cases of decompensated monofixational exotropia can appear as intermittent exotropia: chronic cases may show a constant exotropia. Children whose monofixation exotropias decompensate may complain of asthenopia, as their deviations stress their range of fusional amplitudes, or give them diplopia if the separation of the perceived images exceeds their suppression scotoma. These symptoms are more common with decompensating monofixation exotropia than for esotropia,[20] but asthenopia in monofixation exotropia is less frequent than in bifoveal patients with exophoria.[20]

Sensory features

Binocular sensory testing in the monofixation state confirms a foveal scotoma in the nondominant eye, with preservation of peripheral fusion. In monofixation exotropia there may be a suppression scotoma extending temporally from the fovea. Depending on the test, the size of targets, the patient's age, and the size of the heterotropia, they can indicate either normal retinal correspondence or anomalous correspondence, even in the same patient.[6,19,24,27] Eccentric fixation may also be demonstrated in the nondominant eye, especially if amblyopia is severe.[24]

Stereopsis is subnormal in this syndrome, although some stereoacuity is often detectable in monofixational exotropia.[22,23] Stereoacuity is higher in the primary than in the secondary form, in both monofixational esotropia and exotropia.[23]

Where the exodeviation has decompensated and manifests almost constantly as an exotropia, sensory testing with the angle offset with prisms may detect subnormal binocular vision, suggesting an underlying monofixation syndrome.[6]

Amblyopia

The incidence of amblyopia in monofixation exotropia ranges from 30 to 65%, slightly less than is reported for monofixational esotropia.[6,19,23–25] It tends to occur most with the anisometropic and least often with the postsurgical form.[19,24] Up to 50% of patients with monofixation and moderate to severe amblyopia may also show eccentric fixation on monocular testing.[24]

Treatment

Once a primary or secondary monofixation syndrome develops, it is difficult to gain bifoveal fixation.[19,21] Aggressive attempts to break down the facultative macular scotoma to achieve this may be contraindicated by the risk of diplopia.[19–21] There are anecdotal cases of successful conversion of monofixation to bifoveal situations with aggressive therapy in children.[21]

In children there are two clear indications for treatment in monofixation exotropia: the reversal of amblyopia and the restoration of alignment in a decompensated exotropia.

Amblyopia

Amblyopia of worse than 6/15 should be treated, even in a monofixation syndrome, including spectacles for refractive errors and anisometropia, and patching or penalization.[21]

In cases of decompensated monofixational exotropia, treatment of the amblyopia can improve control of the exotropia and reduce symptoms such as asthenopia. Success includes improving vision to 6/9 or better and a stable monofixation–a small angle exotropia with peripheral fusion.[6,21]

Alignment

No treatment is indicated for asymptomatic patients with small, infrequently manifest, exodeviations, but those with frequent exotropia who complain of asthenopia or diplopia warrant intervention. The goal is to restore comfortable single vision, usually by achieving a monofixation exotropia result rather than bifoveal fixation.[19,22,27]

Nonsurgical options include part-time occlusion, prisms, and minus lens overcorrection (see Chapter 81). Orthoptic exercises are not usually indicated for decompensated monofixation exotropia as the fusional amplitudes are good and antisuppression therapy is contraindicated, as in decompensated monofixational esotropia, to avoid breaking down suppression.[19]

Botulinum toxin and surgery are used to treat children whose exodeviations have decompensated or are not corrected by amblyopia treatment or nonsurgical interventions. Botulinum toxin has a good success rate for small angles in children[16,17] as the exotropia is rarely more than 20 to 25 PD. Principles of surgical correction exotropia is discussed in Chapter 81. Surgery has about the same rate of success as for the common forms of intermittent exotropia. However, the result is almost always a monofixation syndrome.[6,22]

EXOTROPIA WITH HEMIANOPIC VISUAL FIELD DEFECTS

Introduction

Exotropia occurs with both homonymous and bitemporal hemianopias; binasal hemianopias are very rare. The field loss is usually extensive.

Homonymous hemianopias

Etiology

Exotropia can occur with homonymous hemianopias caused by intracranial disorders that are congenital or acquired before the age of 2.[28,29] The normal binocular visual field is compromised by the bilateral loss of the field on one side. Some children with homonymous hemianopia develop an exotropia in the eye ipsilateral to the field loss, which may be a compensation by which the binocular field can be enlarged[28–30] (Fig. 82.2). Such a theory has been challenged by others who feel that the exodeviation is an epiphenomenon, not adaptive.[31,32]

Clinical features

In contrast to patients who develop homonymous hemianopias later, children with congenital or early-acquired brain lesions adapt well. They are often unaware of their field loss[31–33] and develop eye movement strategies that include saccadic movements into the blind field followed by smooth pursuit into the intact field to fixate a target.[32] They may develop a face turn to the side of the hemianopia in order to better center their remaining hemifield.[6,31,32]

Children who later develop a homonymous hemianopia do not adapt so well: they often bump into objects on the side of the hemianopia and reading is difficult.

Motor features

An exotropia occurring as an adaptation to field loss may be limited to when the cause is congenital or early acquired. The compensatory exotropia can be either in childhood or later.[28–30] They show a constant deviation, which contrasts with the high prevalence of intermittent exodeviations reported with later-acquired hemianopias. The angle in early-onset cases is 40 to 70 PD, often larger for distance fixation than for near.[28–31] It may be associated with a vertical heterotropia or a pattern strabismus.[6,29]

Children with later-acquired hemianopia and exotropia usually have deviations less than 20 PD.[33] They can be an exophoria or an intermittent or constant exotropia. Exotropias in such cases may not be an adaptive phenomenon.[6,28,32,33]

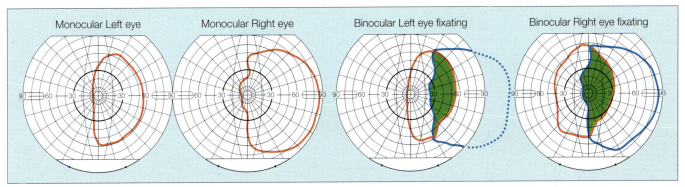

Fig. 82.2 Monocular and binocular visual fields in a patient with congenital complete left homonymous hemianopia and exotropia. The first two plots show the monocular visual fields of the left and right eyes. The third plot shows the binocular field with the left eye fixating, and the fourth plot shows the binocular field with the right eye fixating. The shaded area is the overlap of the monocular fields. Note that the panorama of the binocular field is greater when the right eye is used for fixation than when the left eye takes up fixation. (From Kraft,[6] p 187, with permission of WB Saunders; after Gote et al.,[29] p 131, with permission of Binoculus Publishing.)

Sensory features

Young children adapt better to homonymous defects than do older children; those who develop exotropia have complete and congruous defects.[28–31] The expansion of the visual field to the side of the missing field ranges from 20° to 45°. This strategy is only relevant if the exotropia develops in the eye ipsilateral to the field loss, while the child fixates with the eye on the side of the intact field (Fig. 82.2) and the amount of expansion is proportional to the size of the exotropia.[28–31]

Children with exotropia with congenital or early-onset hemianopia rarely complain of diplopia or asthenopia because they may develop anomalous retinal correspondence (ARC).[28–30] They suppress within the overlapping portions of the monocular fields, and elsewhere they show ARC.[28,29] This can be tested by using the synoptophore, or with sensory tests performed while the angle of exotropia is offset with base-in prisms.[6,28–30]

Patients with later-acquired hemianopias complain of diplopia since they retain normal correspondence, cannot develop ARC,[6,28,33] and cannot develop suppression.

Treatment

Surgery for exotropia with congenital or early-onset homonymous hemianopia is undertaken with caution. First, the realignment of the eyes reduces the panorama of the total binocular visual field. Second, patients who develop ARC in response to the exodeviation may experience paradoxical diplopia if the eye is realigned once the adaptation is complete.[28–30] Patients determined to have surgery should first be tested with a monocular patch to see whether they can adapt to the smaller binocular field and then with a prism to see whether they develop diplopia.

Patients with later-onset hemianopia who develop diplopia or asthenopia because of an exodeviation may be treated initially with prism or a patch, or they may require surgery or botulinum toxin.

Bitemporal visual field defects

Etiology

Bitemporal hemianopia results from lesions of the optic chiasm. In normals, the vergence system tracks targets in depth and responds to stimulation of disparate retinal points. Extensive bitemporal field loss disrupts peripheral fusion and compromises the vergence system, which, in turn, increases the risk that an existing exophoria decompensates.[33,34]

Clinical features

The disruption of the vergence reflex may lead to an exo-deviation, which can cause several sensory phenomena, especially if the field loss in each eye is extensive enough to involve the two maculae.

Motor features

The exodeviation measures a few prism diopters,[6] but it is often variable because of poor fusional vergences and the endpoints of the measurements can be difficult to determine.[33,35] The extraocular movements are usually normal.

Sensory features

Patients with bitemporal hemianopia may have two unusual and often missed symptoms. Firstly, the loss of overlapping visual fields can lead to "hemiretinal slide" as the intact nasal visual fields of the two eyes cannot be synchronized.[33–35] The exotropia in such a situation leads to reduction of the total binocular field and overlap of the partial images seen by the intact nasal fields. Any target would appear elongated, and there would be duplication of features within the target[6,35] (Fig. 82.3). This often leads to reading difficulties.

Secondly, complete bitemporal hemianopia produces "postfixation blindness" from stimulation of nonseeing nasal retina by objects that lie within that area of space beyond the fixation target[6,33] (Fig. 82.4). An exotropia places the area of postfixation blindness further from the eyes and any proximal object including the fixation target may be double, as most patients have normal retinal correspondence (NRC)[6,34,35] (Fig. 82.4). This leads to difficulty with daily chores such as reaching accurately, pouring and picking things up.

Very young children with bitemporal hemianopia and exotropia may not have any symptoms. They may be able to develop suppression as an adaptation to the diplopia.[33,35] Others may adapt to their abnormal binocular vision, in the same way that children can learn strategies to overcome symptoms of bilateral homonymous hemianopia.[6]

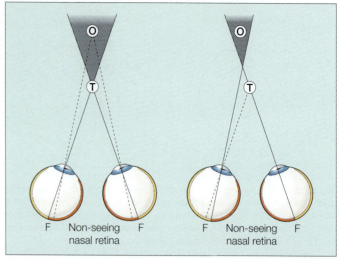

Fig. 82.4 Postfixation blind area in a patient with complete bitemporal hemianopia. (Left) The diagram shows the situation when the eyes are straight. When both foveae (F) fixate on a target (T), the retinal image of any second object (O) located within the shaded area would fall on the nonfunctioning nasal retinas of both eyes and not be seen. (Right) The diagram shows the situation in the presence of a left exotropia with the right eye fixating. The target (T) may be seen as diplopic because the image falls on the fovea of the right eye and on the functioning temporal retina in the left eye. A second object (O) is not visualized as it is located in the postfixation blind area, which is more remote from the patient compared to the orthotropic state. (From Kraft,[6] p 192, with permission of WB Saunders, after Roper-Hall,[33] p 81, with permission of University of Wisconsin Press.)

Treatment

There is no adequate therapy for exotropia with total or almost complete bitemporal hemianopia, whether it appears in young or older children. Prisms can be tried to alleviate diplopia, but they are not always helpful due to the variability of the exodeviation.[35] Patching of one eye will reduce the visual field. Surgery to eliminate diplopia and exotropia can help if the misalignment is reduced to zero. However, the result is rarely stable due to the absence of adequate fusional vergences.[6]

SENSORY EXOTROPIA

The term *sensory exotropia* is applied to a unilateral exodeviation that develops as a result of loss of vision or to chronic poor vision in one eye.[2,6,21] Children under age 5 or 6 years who develop strabismus due to vision loss in one eye have an equal chance of developing esotropia or exotropia. After 6 years exotropia tends to develop.[21]

Etiology

Sensory exotropia occurs in children as a result of a wide range of congenital and acquired ocular disorders. Congenital disorders

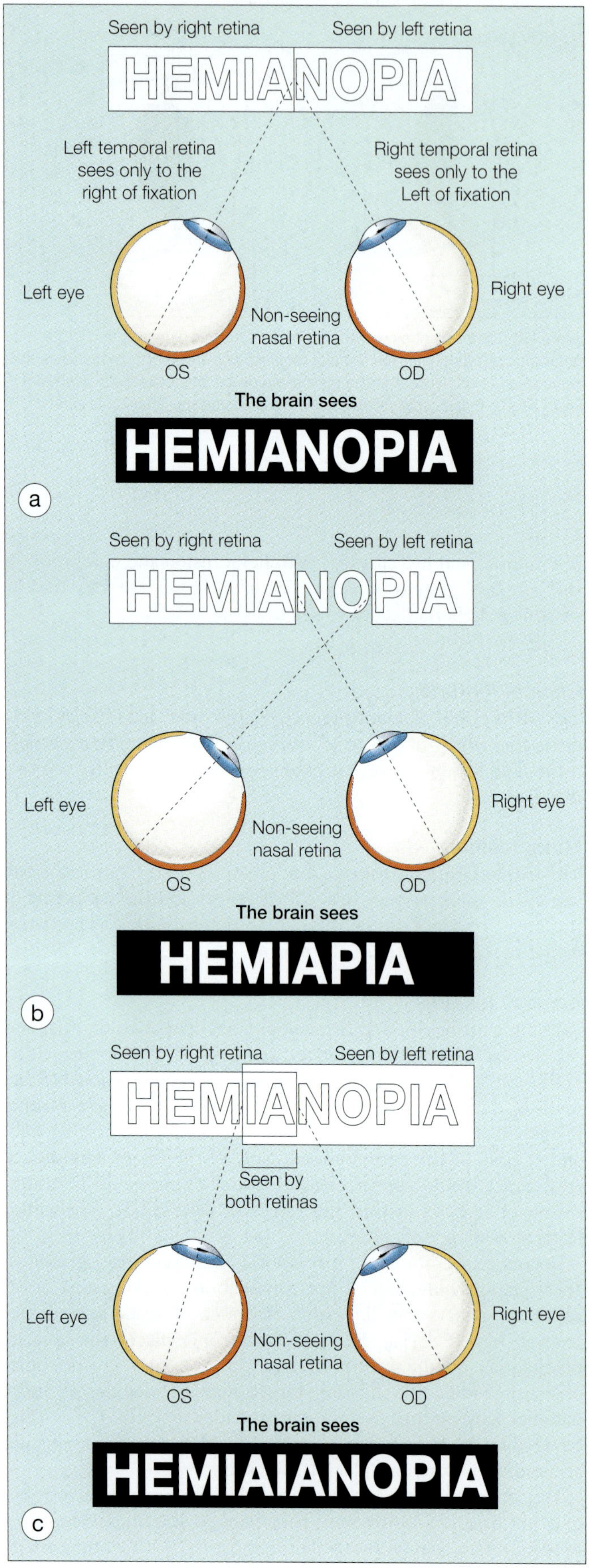

Fig. 82.3 (*Left*) Hemifield sliding and abnormal binocular phenomena in a patient with complete bitemporal hemianopia. (a) Straight eyes: The two separate monocular visual fields juxtapose to form a complete image of the target. (b) Left esotropia: central portions of the target are missing. (c) Left exotropia: central portions of the target are duplicated as a result of redundant reception by the functioning temporal retinas of the both eyes. (From Kraft,[6] p 191, with permission of WB Saunders; after Fritz and Brodsky,[34] p 160, with permission of University of Wisconsin.)

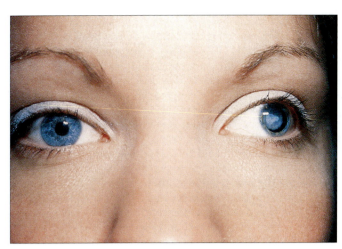

Fig. 82.5 Child with sensory left exotropia due to traumatic cataract. Note the large angle of the deviation. (From Kraft,[6] p 193, with permission of WB Saunders.)

compromise vision development; normal binocular vergence reflexes cannot develop and strabismus is a frequent result. Acquired causes include traumatic and nontraumatic diseases, such as cataracts, that disrupt the fusion reflex[6,21] (Fig. 82.5). One cause that merits specific attention is anisometropic amblyopia. Older children whose vision remains reduced in the eye are at particular risk of developing exotropia.[36-38]

There are several mechanisms for the development of exotropia when vision is lost in one eye: binocular rivalry, decompensation of exophoria, and anatomic factors.

Binocular rivalry

When one eye suffers degradation of its retinal image, it sets up a rivalry between that eye and its fellow eye. The normal visual signals can become inhibitory to the disadvantaged eye: this is even more powerful with partial than with total loss.[36] Also, there is a superiority of the nasal retina over the temporal retina in response to bright and formed stimuli, and this becomes exaggerated when an eye loses vision. These factors lead to disruption of the vergence system, and an active retinomotor divergence reflex takes hold with a progressive exodeviation, especially in older children.[37]

Decompensation of exophoria

A well-controlled exophoria can decompensate from loss of fusion if one eye loses vision. This appears to be a settling of the poorer eye into its elastic rest position, not an active divergence reflex. The divergent position is a result of an imbalance of muscle tone between the lateral rectus and medial rectus muscles.[37]

Mechanical factors

Orbital dysmorphism or muscle anomalies can predispose to an exotropia if one eye suffers a loss of vision. Strabismus in which there is congenital tightness or strictures of the lateral rectus, such as in Duane syndrome, can show progressive exotropia if vision deteriorates in the affected eye.

Clinical features

Motor features

Sensory exotropia is usually over 30 PD.[2,6] If the cause of the vision deficit persists, then the angle can increase progressively. A long-standing large exotropia leads to secondary muscle changes. The lateral rectus contracts and the overlying soft tissues may shorten, creating a tight lateral rectus syndrome (see the Clinical features subsection of Infantile Exotropia): an updrift and downdrift in the adducted position, and possibly an "X" [14] (Fig. 82.1), "A", or less commonly, a "V" pattern.[6,26] The exotropic eye may exhibit a small hypertropia.

Measuring the angle of the exotropia can be tricky when the vision is poor in one eye. The prism and alternating cover test may not be accurate since the poor fixation in the eye does not allow the examiner to see a stable endpoint during the measurement; thus the angle is better measured with the modified prism and light reflex (Krimsky) test: After the angle kappa is noted for the fixating eye, progressive base-in prism power is placed over that eye until the exotropic eye is drawn over sufficiently in the nasal direction to create a matching angle kappa in that eye.[6]

Sensory features

Several adaptations can occur in sensory exotropias. If the vision is very poor, there may be deep suppression and no binocular responses. Children whose vision is not severely reduced and who have exotropia not exceeding 40 PD may develop ARC.[38] Children with anisometropic amblyopia and exotropia may retain NRC.[36] Young children can avoid diplopia by suppressing the displaced image. Older children who develop sensory exotropia may experience diplopia because they cannot develop ARC.

Sensory tests in a patient can vary, ARC or NRC, depending on the depth of suppression and the dissociating ability of the tests,[6,38] influenced by the ambient lighting, the distance of the testing apparatus from the patient, and the size of the exotropia.[6,38]

Management

Treating the underlying cause of the vision loss is paramount: cataracts, corneal opacities, anisometropic amblyopia, ptosis, eyelid hemangioma, retinoblastoma, and retinal detachments are examples of ocular abnormalities that can lead to exotropia but which can be reversed. If the problem is present early in childhood, then the exotropia can be prevented if vision can be restored by vigorous treatment, especially of amblyopia. Irrespective of an early or later onset, if exotropia has already developed, it may still reduce if vision can be recovered.[6]

If exotropia persists despite correction of the underlying disorder, or if the vision loss is chronic and irreversible, it can be treated with either nonsurgical or surgical options.

Nonsurgical therapy

One important aspect of treatment is the prescription of safety lenses for patients with unilateral vision loss. Patients who already wear glasses to correct a refractive error should be sure that their lens and frame designs meet safety specifications.

Patients with diplopia or asthenopia can be helped with prisms if the angle of the exotropia is not over 30 PD. Children who have awareness of the second image but are not helped by base-in prisms may be helped by base-out prisms to further separate the two images. Patients with intractable diplopia may be helped by Bangerter foils to reduce the clarity, and therefore awareness, of the displaced image in the exotropic eye.

Botulinum toxin injections are successful in realigning angles of exotropia under 35 PD.[16,17] However, the angles in sensory exotropia tend to be larger, with a lower long-term success rate. Patients with a large exotropia angle who choose botulinum injections rather than surgery must accept the likelihood that periodic reinjections will be needed indefinitely.[6]

Surgery
Surgical planning

Children with sensory exotropia should undergo preoperative prism testing to see whether they can be realigned without inducing intractable diplopia. If a prism, placed base-in and matching the strabismus angle, is introduced before the misaligned eye and the child does not complain of diplopia, then the surgeon can plan to align the eyes to straight or close to orthotropia. If the child complains of diplopia with exact prism offset, then a reduced amount of prism for determining whether a partial correction is possible can be tried. However, a diplopia response to an offset of the angle does not necessarily mean that the child will experience diplopia postoperatively. In such a case, a prolonged prism trial for determining whether the child can adapt sensorially to a complete correction of the angle can be done.[6]

A complete eye examination is mandatory prior to surgery. The surgeon must be sure that the eye is healthy enough to undergo strabismus surgery. Problems such as phthisis, corneal compromise, and orbit factors may make it risky to perform muscle surgery on the eye. Older children may allow a forced duction test to be done on their eye to detect a contracture of the lateral rectus and any other restrictive phenomena that will help in the planning of surgery.

Most cases of sensory exotropia require surgery on two muscles due to the large angles typically seen in these patients. Weakening of the lateral rectus is almost always a component of the surgery plan, and if the overlying conjunctiva is also tight, it should be recessed as well.[14,39] The medial rectus can be lax and must be strengthened. The surgeon should perform serial forced ductions at surgery as each layer is dealt with, to be sure that any restrictions are released. The addition of inferior oblique and superior oblique weakening to the horizontal rectus surgery can increase the success of surgery for angles over 50 PD.[39]

If the surgical goal is orthotropia, then the immediate postoperative alignment should be a small angle esotropia, as there is typically a drift in the exotropia direction of several prism diopters in the first few weeks after surgery.[6,40] To achieve this result and to improve the chance that the long-term result will be stable, the forced duction at the conclusion of surgery should be slightly limited to abduction and the spring-back balance test should be slightly biased in the esotropic direction.[14] Some authors caution against aligning to orthotropia any older patient with sensory exotropia caused by anisometropia, and they recommend leaving such patients undercorrected.[36]

Results

Patients with preoperative exotropia angles under 40 PD tend to have a 75% chance of achieving a stable small angle heterotropia. Over 45 PD, the results decrease dramatically to 40 to 50% long-term success.[39] Once the eye is realigned, the secondary muscle phenomena such as upshoots and downshoots and "X" patterns often resolve within weeks.[6]

REFERENCES

1. Biglan AW, Davis JS, Cheng KP, et al. Infantile exotropia. J Pediatr Ophthalmol Strabismus 1996; 33: 79–84.
2. Mitchell PR, Parks MM. Concomitant exodeviations. In: Tasman W, Jaeger EA editors. Duane's Clinical Ophthalmology. Philadelphia: Lippincott, Williams, and Wilkins; 2002: 2–4, 14–6. (Vol I, chap 13.)
3. Rubin SE, Nelson LB, Wagner RS, et al. Infantile exotropia in healthy children. Ophthalmic Surg 1988; 19: 792–4.
4. Moore S, Cohen RL. Congenital exotropia. Am Orthoptic J 1985; 35: 68–70.
5. Biedner B, Marcus M, David R, et al. Congenital constant exotropia: Surgical results in six patients. Binocul Vis Eye Muscle Surg Q 1993; 8: 137–40.
6. Kraft SP. Selected exotropia entities and principles of management. In: Rosenbaum AL, Santiago AP, editors. Clinical Strabismus Management. Philadelphia: Saunders; 1999: 176–201.
7. Hunter DG, Ellis FJ: Prevalence of systemic and ocular disease in infantile exotropia: a comparison with infantile esotropia. Ophthalmology 1999; 106: 1951–6.
8. Kushner BJ. Preoperative evaluation of the exotropic patient. In: Long DA, editor. Anterior Segment and Strabismus Surgery. New York: Kugler; 1996: 123–8.
9. Brodsky MC, Fritz KJ. Hereditary congenital exotropia: A report of three cases. Binocul Vis Eye Muscle Surg Q 1993; 8: 133–6.
10. Nixon RB, Helveston EM, Miller K, et al. Incidence of strabismus in neonates. Am J Ophthalmol 1985; 100: 798–801.
11. Archer SM, Sondhi N, Helveston EM. Strabismus in infancy. Ophthalmology 1989; 96: 133–7.
12. Tychsen L. Neural mechanisms in infantile esotropia: What goes wrong? Am Orthoptic J 1996; 46: 18–28.
13. Williams F, Beneish R, Polomeno RC, et al. Congenital exotropia. Am Orthoptic J 1984; 34: 92–4.
14. Jampolsky A. Surgical leashes, reverse leashes in strabismus surgical management. In: Symposium on Strabismus: Transactions of the New Orleans Academy of Ophthalmology. St Louis: Mosby; 1978: 244–68.
15. Capo H, Mallette RA, Guyton DL. Overacting oblique muscles in exotropia: A mechanical explanation. J Pediatr Ophthalmol Strabismus 1988; 25: 281–5.
16. Scott AB, Magoon EH, McNeer KW, et al. Botulinum treatment of childhood strabismus. Ophthalmology 1990; 97: 1434–8.
17. Spencer RF, Tucker MG, Choi RY, et al. Botulinum toxin management of childhood intermittent exotropia. Ophthalmology 1997; 104: 1762–7.
18. Hiles DA, Biglan AW. Early surgery of infantile exotropia. Trans Pa Acad Ophthalmol Otolaryngol 1983; 36: 161–8.
19. Parks MM. Monofixation syndrome. In: Tasman W, Jaeger EA, editors. Duane's Clinical Ophthalmology. Philadelphia: Lippincott, Williams, and Wilkins; 2002: 1–12. (Vol I, chap 14.)
20. Boyd TAS, Budd GE. Monofixation exotropia and asthenopia. In: Moore S, Mein J, Stockbridge L, editors. Orthoptics: Past, Present, Future. Miami: Symposia Specialists; 1976: 173–7.
21. von Noorden GK. Binocular Vision and Ocular Motility. 6th ed. St Louis: Mosby; 2002: 340–5, 370–1.
22. Baker JD, Davies GT. Monofixational intermittent exotropia. Arch Ophthalmol 1979; 97: 93–5.
23. Galloway-Smith K, Kaban T, Cadera W, et al. Monofixation exotropia. Am Orthoptic J 1992; 42: 125–8.
24. Lang J. Lessons learned from microtropia. In: Moore S, Mein J, Stockbridge L, editors. Orthoptics: Past, Present, Future. Miami: Symposia Specialists; 1976: 183–90.
25. Johnson F, Cunha LAP, Harcourt BR. The clinical characteristics of micro-exotropia. Br Orthoptic J 1981; 38: 54–9.
26. Jampolsky A. Management of exodeviations. In: Haik GM, editor. Strabismus: Symposium of the New Orleans Academy of Ophthalmology. St Louis: Mosby; 1962: 140–56.
27. Pratt-Johnson J, Wee HS. Suppression associated with exotropia. Can J Ophthalmol 1969; 4: 136–43.
28. Herzau V, Bleher I, Joos-Kratsch E. Infantile exotropia with homonymous hemianopia: a rare contraindication for strabismus surgery. Graefes Arch Clin Exp Ophthalmol 1988; 226: 148–9.
29. Gote H, Gregersen E, Rindziunski E. Exotropia and panoramic vision compensating for an occult congenital homonymous hemianopia: A case report. Binocul Vis Eye Muscle Surg Q 1993; 8: 129–32.
30. Levy Y, Turetz J, Krakowski D, et al. Development of compensating exotropia with anomalous retinal correspondence after early infancy in congenital homonymous hemianopia. J Pediatr Ophthalmol Strabismus 1995; 32: 236–8.

31. Good WV, Jan JE, DeSa L, et al. Cortical visual impairment in children. Surv Ophthalmol 1994; 38: 351–64.
32. Hoyt CS, Good WV. Ocular motor adaptations to congenital hemianopia. Binocul Vis Eye Muscle Surg Q 1993; 8: 125–6.
33. Roper-Hall G. Effect of visual field defects on binocular single vision. Am Orthoptic J 1976; 26: 74–82.
34. Fritz KJ, Brodsky MC. Elusive neuro-ophthalmic reading impairment. Am Orthoptic J 1992; 42: 159–64.
35. Shainberg MJ, Roper-Hall G, Chung SM. Binocular problems in bitemporal hemianopia. Am Orthoptic J 1995; 45: 132–40.
36. Jampolsky A. Unequal visual inputs and strabismus management: A comparison of human and animal strabismus. In: Symposium on Strabismus: Transactions of the New Orleans Academy of Ophthalmology. St Louis: Mosby; 1978: 358–492.
37. Jampolsky A. Ocular divergence mechanisms. Trans Am Ophthalmol Soc 1970; 68: 730–822.
38. Haldi BA. Annual Richard G Scobee Memorial Lecture. Sensory response in exotropia. Ophthalmology 1979; 86: 2090–100.
39. Velez G. Surgical treatment of exotropia with poor vision. In: Reinecke RD, editor. Strabismus II: Proceedings of the Fourth Meeting of the International Strabismological Association. Orlando: Grune and Stratton; 1984: 263–7.
40. Scott WE, Keech R, Mash AJ. The postoperative results and stability of exodeviations. Arch Ophthalmol 1981; 99: 1814–8.

83 Vertical Strabismus

Burton J Kushner

OVERVIEW AND DEFINITIONS

Vertical strabismus is less common and more challenging than horizontal strabismus. Vertical and horizontal strabismus often occur concurrently; almost half of patients with esotropia will also have a vertical component. When the two do occur together, it is important to determine whether the vertical deviation represents the primary problem, and if it needs specific attention.

When presented with a patient with vertical strabismus, a good approach is to first determine whether the deviation is comitant or incomitant. If the latter, you must next determine if the problem is paretic, restrictive, or a manifestation of primary oblique muscle dysfunction. Finally, it is important to determine early in the workup whether the deviation is dissociated (e.g., does not appear to follow Hering's law with respect to the vertical component).

Conventionally, vertical strabismus was described in terms of the higher eye. Thus even if there was an inferior restriction in the left eye causing a left hypotropia, the convention would call for describing the problem as a right hypertropia. This convention led to confusion and is no longer followed. A preferred convention is to describe the deviation as it is actually manifested, specifically as either a hypertropia of the higher eye or a hypotropia of the contralateral eye, depending upon which eye is habitually used for fixation. If a patient freely alternates, you should default to describing the deviation of the hypertropic eye.

There has also been considerable confusion about the terminology for describing dissociated deviations. They have been variously called dissociated vertical divergence (DVD), alternating sursumduction, alternating hyperphoria, occlusion hyperphoria, and double dissociated hypertropia. Terminology should be appropriately descriptive. It is important that the terms for describing dissociated deviations address three important issues by indicating whether the deviation is:

1. Constant or intermittent;
2. Latent or manifest (e.g., a phoria or a tropia); and
3. Dissociated or not dissociated.

The most common presentation for DVD is for one eye to have a vertical misalignment that is intermittently manifest and for the other eye to have a vertical deviation that is latent (only present in the dissociated state, e.g., under cover). Appropriate terminology for describing such a patient would be intermittent manifest DVD in one eye and latent DVD in the other. An acceptable alternative would be an intermittent dissociated hypertropia in one eye and a dissociated hyperphoria in the other.

PHYSIOLOGY

The cyclovertical muscles each have a triple function that includes a vertical, torsional, and to a lesser degree horizontal action. In order to understand vertical strabismus, one must understand the actions of the cyclovertical muscles during head tilting. Consider the action of the right eye on head tilt to the right. During the active phase of head tilting, a series of intorsional and extorsional movements occur. At first, a slow counter-rolling occurs in the opposite direction of the head tilt (right eye intorts on head tilt to the right), which can be thought of as a rotary doll's head motion. This keeps the visual environment stable on the retina and maximizes vision by decreasing the motion of the peripheral visual field across the retina. However, if this partially compensatory countertorsional (intorsional) movement was allowed to remain, problems with respect to stereopsis and vergence mechanisms would result.[1] Consequently this intorsion is eliminated with a rapid anticompensatory saccadic movement in the direction of the head tilt. This sequence repeats several times during a head tilt. The number, speed, and magnitude of these eye movements are a function of the velocity and size of the head tilt. These dynamic torsional movements can be thought of as a rotary equivalent of optokinetic nystagmus. If the head is kept in the tilted position, there remains a slight partial compensatory intorsion of approximately 5–10% the size of the head tilt. Thus, in the steady-state position with the head tilted, there is increased tonus to the intorters (superior oblique and superior rectus) and partial inhibition of the extorters (inferior oblique and inferior rectus) in the eye on the side to which the head is tilted. This forms the basis for the Bielschowsky head tilt test and the Parks 3-step test for diagnosing superior oblique palsy.[2,3] In the normal situation, after a head tilt is concluded, the vertical actions of the two stimulated muscles (right superior oblique and right superior rectus) cancel one another because one is an elevator and the other a depressor. Consequently there is no shift in vertical alignment. If the right superior oblique is paretic, the right superior rectus is not opposed and the right hypertropia increases.

PATIENT EVALUATION

History

If the patient's initial problem was solely horizontal strabismus and if vertical strabismus developed secondarily, one should suspect either primary oblique muscle dysfunction or DVD, particularly if the patient had infantile esotropia. Diplopia points to an acquired problem that is often paretic or restrictive; if it is present, you should determine whether the image separation is vertical, horizontal, or both.

Specific questions should be asked about the presence of subjective torsional diplopia. If a patient has both a horizontal and vertical component to their diplopia, they often describe the image separation as being "at an angle." This does not necessarily denote torsion. I find it helpful to have the patient look at a vertical line such as the edge of a door or the corner of a room and indicate whether the two lines they see run at an angle with one another. If so, the patient has true subjective torsion. Whether there was significant antecedent trauma or prior eye surgery that may have precipitated the vertical problem should be determined. If the strabismus is acquired, other neurologic symptoms should be specifically inquired about. If reported, checking the appropriate cranial nerve is indicated. A review of the child's growth and developmental milestones is appropriate. Finally, a family history of similar problems should be determined, because certain vertical eye muscle disorders (e.g., chronic progressive external ophthalmoplegia and ocular muscle fibrosis) are familial.

Examination

Before beginning the measurements of the deviation, one should observe whether the child spontaneously assumes a compensatory head posture (tilt, turn, or chin elevation/depression) with visual effort. Often, a compensatory head posture may serve the purpose of placing the eyes in a field of gaze in which the misalignment is smallest, enhancing fusion. Alternatively, some patients may assume an abnormal head posture because it minimizes nystagmus (see Chapter 89). Next, one should observe whether facial asymmetry is present. If a head tilt is longstanding, and particularly if it dates to infancy, there is a shortening of the midface between the horizontal canthus laterally and the corner of the child's mouth on the side to which the head is habitually tilted[4,5] (Fig. 83.1).

The angle of misalignment should be measured in the assumed natural head posture using the prism and alternate cover test, and then in the forced primary position (head erect). One should determine whether the deviation is dissociated. With a non-dissociated deviation, a hypotropia is present in the contralateral eye when the patient fixates with the higher eye. Unless a secondary deviation is present, the hypotropia found in one eye will be of equal magnitude as the hypertropia in the fellow eye. Secondary deviations can occur with paralytic or restrictive strabismus when fixation is with the involved eye. With DVD, the hypotropia of the fellow eye is either smaller or absent when fixation is with the eye with the DVD. For this reason it appears that DVD does not follow Hering's law (see the section "Dissociated deviations").

The alternate prism and cover test should be performed with full optical correction in place at 6 mm. For all patients with vertical strabismus the deviation in the primary position as well as in up- and downgaze and horizontal right and left gaze will need to be determined. However, in order to determine a treatment plan for many patients with vertical strabismus, measurements also must be made in the four oblique fields. The deviation should then be quantified with a head tilted 30° right and 30° left using the alternate prism and cover test. Ductions and versions should be assessed to tell whether there is overelevation or overdepression on side gaze, as well as to help determine whether an "A" or "V" pattern is present. If there is overelevation of the adducting eye on side gaze, it is important to do a cover test in side gaze to tell whether the vertical deviation being viewed is a manifestation of DVD or inferior oblique overaction.

The Parks 3-step test, which is based on the Bielschowsky head tilt test, asks a series of three questions that should determine which of the eight cyclovertical muscles is paretic[2,3]: it works best for unilateral superior oblique palsy. Although this test is

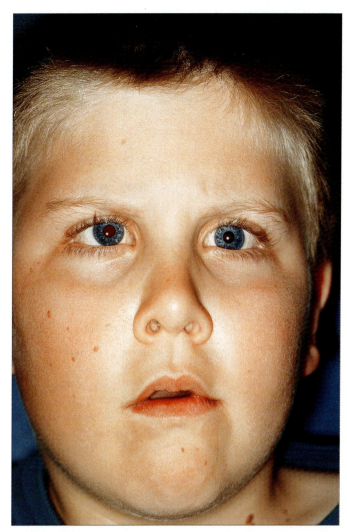

Fig. 83.1 Facial asymmetry. Shortening of the left side of the face in this boy with a long-standing head tilt to the left for control of a right superior oblique palsy.

useful for confirming the diagnosis of a unilateral superior oblique palsy, there are many clinical situations in which it may be misleading.[1,6] Most importantly, the test does not tell *whether* the patient has a palsy of one cyclovertical muscle, but is based on the assumption that he or she does. Table 83.1 lists some of the common situations in which the 3-step test may lead to an incorrect diagnosis (Fig. 83.2).

The presence of torsion should be determined both objectively and subjectively. The latter is accomplished using the double

Table 83.1 Situations in which the Parks 3-step test may be misleading
DVD
Multiple muscle involvement
Bilateral 4th nerve palsy
Multiple other cranial nerve palsy
Superior rectus overaction/contracture
Inferior rectus restriction
Superior rectus palsy
Inferior rectus palsy
Skew deviation
Prior surgery
From Kushner[6] with permission from American Academy of Ophthalmology.

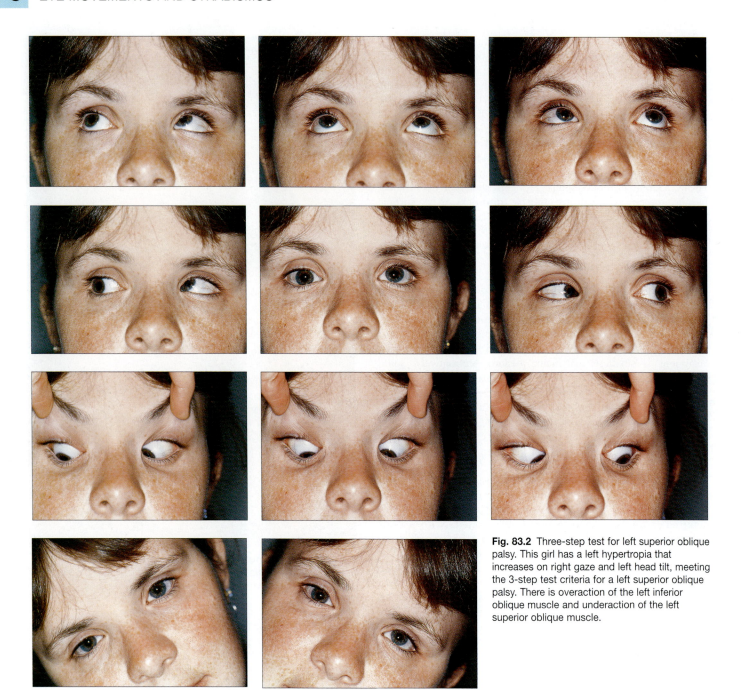

Fig. 83.2 Three-step test for left superior oblique palsy. This girl has a left hypertropia that increases on right gaze and left head tilt, meeting the 3-step test criteria for a left superior oblique palsy. There is overaction of the left inferior oblique muscle and underaction of the left superior oblique muscle.

Maddox rod test. Objective torsion is determined by studying the fundus with the indirect ophthalmoscope.[7] Normally the position of the fovea lies between two imaginary horizontal lines, one at the lower edge of the disk margin and the other through the middle of the disk (Fig. 83.3). One should note whether there is a difference between the objective and subjective determination of torsion. For example, if the fundus depicts objective torsion, but subjectively the patient does not report torsion with the double Maddox rod test, one can assume the deviation is long-standing and sensory adaptations have occurred. If a patient does describe torsion, one should then determine whether the patient can fuse when the horizontal and vertical deviations are offset with prism. This may help in surgical planning. If the patient has comfortable fusion with offsetting prism in place, despite the presence of torsion, it may be possible to ignore the torsion when designing a surgical strategy. If a patient cannot fuse

with the deviation offset with prism, (s)he may have a central disruption of fusion. Testing on the synoptophore (which can offset the torsional misalignment) will determine whether fusion can be expected if the strabismus is successfully treated.

General treatment principles

When determining a treatment plan, an approach that will give the maximum amount of correction in the field of gaze in which the deviation is greatest should be chosen; attention should be paid to the pattern of the deviation. Also, the primary position and downgaze (for reading) are the two most important fields of gaze clinically. Upgaze may be least important, and correction in that field should not be at the expense of alignment in the primary position or downgaze. Also, surgery should be tailored to address any torsional problem if significant, and conversely not

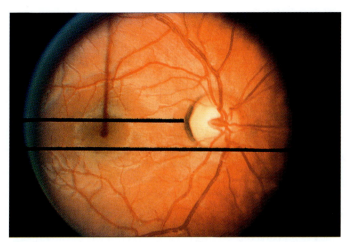

Fig. 83.3 Normal relationship of fovea to disk with respect to torsion. The fovea is normally positioned between two imaginary parallel lines, one level with the lower margin of the disk and the other through the middle of the disk, indicating an absence of objective torsion.

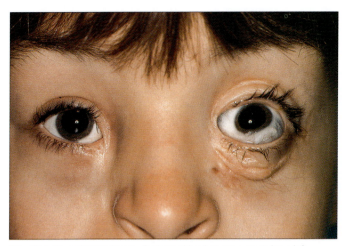

Fig. 83.4 Pseudohypertropia. Patient with what appears to be a left hypertropia. This girl has a type III Tessier maxillofacial cleft and what appears to be a left hypertropia. In fact this is a pseudohypertropia due to distortion of the anterior segment. On cover test there is actually a left hypotropia.

create a torsional problem if it is not already present. Keep in mind that oblique muscle surgery tends to give much more correction in adduction than abduction, but with vertical rectus muscle surgery the difference in correction between abduction and adduction is less dramatic. Also, surgery on the oblique muscles will cause more of a torsional change than on the rectus muscles.

In general, the inferior rectus muscle is the least forgiving muscle and produces the largest effect for a given amount of surgery. Large inferior rectus recessions (5 mm or greater) are apt to cause a lag of that eye in downgaze unless there was a hypotropia that increased in downgaze prior to surgery. Similarly, recessions of the inferior rectus muscle of 5 mm or greater may result in postoperative lower eyelid retraction, which can be minimized with advancement of the capsulopalpebral head at the time of surgery.[8] Large resections of the inferior rectus muscle may cause a narrowing of the palpebral fissure. Large recessions of the inferior rectus muscle using a suspension technique (hang-back, adjustable suture, etc.) appear to have a higher incidence of muscle slippage or nonadherence. This is probably caused by the shorter arc of contact of the inferior rectus muscle, which can cause the muscle to lose apposition with the globe in downgaze after surgery.[9] This complication can be minimized by having the patient avoid downgaze for several weeks after surgery. This may be practical for older patients, the lower half of whose spectacles can be occluded, but it is impractical for younger children.

SPECIFIC CLINICAL ENTITIES

Pseudohypertropia

Some patients may appear to have a hypertropia when in fact they do not. These include cases of orbital dystopia, anterior segment anomalies, or vertical angle kappa (Fig. 83.4). This latter condition may be due to a displaced fovea secondary to retinopathy of prematurity or other causes of retinal dragging.

Comitant deviations

Small comitant hypertropias, not related to prior strabismus surgery, are relatively common. If they are more than several prism diopters, they may cause symptoms of asthenopia or diplopia, and can often be managed with prisms. Large comitant vertical deviations not associated with horizontal strabismus are relatively uncommon. When present, they most likely represent a spread of comitance in a patient that initially had paralytic strabismus. If the deviation is large but comitant, rectus muscle surgery is usually appropriate.

Incomitant deviations

Nonrestrictive nonparetic
Primary oblique dysfunction
Primary overaction of the inferior oblique muscles, and to a lesser degree the superior oblique muscles, is a common accompaniment of primary horizontal strabismus. Usually oblique muscle overaction is not present at birth and typically presents after 1 year of age. Inferior oblique overaction is characterized by an overelevation in adduction and is associated with a "V" pattern; superior oblique overaction is associated with overdepression in adduction and is associated with an "A" pattern (see Chapter 84). Typically objective extorsion is present with inferior oblique overaction and intorsion with superior oblique overaction. Subjective torsion is not present as the patient develops sensory adaptations to this misalignment. Often the antagonist oblique muscle is underacting. Thus in a patient with marked inferior oblique overaction, superior oblique underaction, and a "V" pattern, differentiation between primary oblique dysfunction and bilateral superior oblique palsy may be difficult. The main differential diagnostic factor is found with the head tilt test. With bilateral superior oblique palsy, the Bielschowsky head tilt test should reveal alternating hypertropias (right hypertropia on right head tilt and left hypertropia on left head tilt) for the reasons above. With primary oblique dysfunction, the difference in the vertical deviation with head tilting is minimal.

It is rare for bilateral superior oblique overaction to be secondary to inferior oblique palsy. If superior oblique overaction is bilateral and symmetric, there will be no hypertropia in the primary position, but an "A" pattern is typically present. If the SO overaction is unilateral, there may be a small hypertropia in the primary position.

Paralytic strabismus
Fourth nerve palsy (See Chapter 86)

Fourth nerve palsy is the most common form of paralytic vertical strabismus. The diagnostic criteria include hypertropia of the affected eye that increases on adduction and ipsilateral head tilt (see Fig. 83.2).

Inferior oblique palsy

Inferior oblique palsy is characterized by hypotropia of the affected eye that increases in adduction and on contralateral head tilt. Clinically, the patient shows deficient elevation in adduction and overaction in the field of antagonist superior oblique. It is rare and must be differentiated from Brown syndrome, which has a similar appearance on versions in the inferior oblique field. An important diagnostic criterion is the presence of an "A" pattern, which is typically present with inferior oblique palsy. Brown syndrome more commonly has a "V" pattern as the affected eye cannot move well into adduction in upgaze because of the restriction. With inferior oblique palsy, forced ductions are normal for elevation in adduction; they are abnormal in Brown syndrome. Inferior oblique palsy must also be differentiated from contralateral superior rectus overaction/contracture.[10] This differentiation can be subtle, because forced ductions are often only minimally abnormal in the superior rectus overaction/contracture syndrome. The presence of objective intorsion in the hypotropic eye speaks for inferior oblique palsy. With superior rectus overaction/contracture, there would either be borderline objective intorsion or no objective torsion in the hypertropic eye.

Superior rectus palsy

Superior rectus palsy in children is usually congenital and often associated with ipsilateral ptosis. The differential diagnosis includes ocular muscle fibrosis and other causes of monocular elevation deficiency. The head tilt test is inconsistent with superior rectus palsy.[1,6]

Inferior rectus palsy

Inferior rectus palsy in children is typically congenital but also occurs after trauma. It is the least common form of vertical strabismus in children. There is a hypertropia larger in abduction and associated with a limitation of depression. The 3-step test may be inconsistent in inferior rectus palsy.[1,6]

Dissociated deviations

DVD is a common marker for early-onset strabismus, but it is unusual at birth. Most commonly it appears after about 1 year of age, and may not be evident until after the concurrent infantile esotropia has been surgically corrected. It may present as a subtle deviation, which may be small and only present on cover testing, or it may be associated with a large and frequently manifest vertical deviation that can be as cosmetically disfiguring as was the initial horizontal strabismus. Although DVD is really a bilateral disease, it may appear to be unilateral because often the preferred eye only has a latent deviation. This is particularly the case if amblyopia is present and fixation always occurs with the same eye; however, this presentation can also occur in patients with equal vision.

DVD is characterized by a slow upward drifting of the eye. On close observation, the eye extorts when it elevates: simultaneously, intorsion occurs in the fixing eye. The hallmark of DVD is that when the fixing eye is covered and the patient regains fixation with the deviating eye, the previously fixing eye does not have a commensurate hypotropia. If the DVD is significant bilaterally, the formerly fixing eye will elevate under cover. Thus, it appears that DVD is characterized by an uncoupling of Hering's law. Often DVD appears worse in adduction, when it may simulate inferior oblique overaction. The differentiation includes performing a cover test on side gaze to see whether there is hypotropia of the abducting eye when it is occluded. With DVD, the abducting eye will not show a hypotropia and may, in fact, be hypertropic if the DVD is bilateral (Fig. 83.5). Because of the nature of DVD, and the fact that there is not an equal hypotropia of the contralateral eye, one cannot neutralize this deviation with the alternate prism and cover test.

To accurately measure DVD, one must use the prism under-cover test. This test is carried out by first estimating the size of the DVD. Then a prism equal to the estimated size of the deviation is placed base down in front of the affected eye, while the eye is dissociated behind a cover. The cover should then be rapidly switched to the other eye. If the estimated amount of prism was correct, no movement of the eye being tested should occur. If there is still a downward movement, the test should be repeated with a larger prism; if an upward movement occurs, it

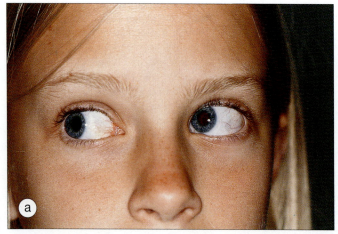
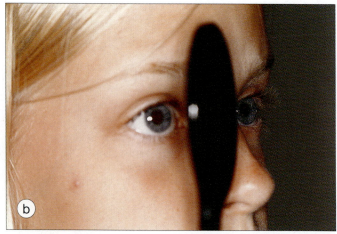

Fig. 83.5 DVD mimicking IO overaction. (a) This girl shows overelevation of the left eye in adduction, which is consistent with left inferior oblique overaction. (b) Under cover, however, a hypertropia is seen in the right eye, confirming that this child in fact has DVD.

should be repeated with a smaller amount of prism. In reality, however, many patients with DVD have a marked redress movement and an accurate endpoint cannot be obtained, even with the prism under-cover test. In that case, the deviation must be estimated by determining whether the upward and downward components of the redress movement were of equal magnitude, or by using a light reflex test.[11]

Approximately one-third of patients with DVD have a spontaneous abnormal head posture.[11] Most patients with DVD show an increase in the size of the DVD on contralateral head tilt (e.g., right DVD increases with left head tilt); however, some show the converse[11] (Fig. 83.6).

The Bielschowsky phenomenon is also characteristic of DVD. As illumination of the fixing eye decreases via the use of a neutral density filter, the size of the DVD in the contralateral eye decreases. Also, DVD is typically associated with latent or manifest latent nystagmus.

Recent theories have shed light on the etiology and pathophysiology of DVD. Considering both the torsional and vertical actions of the muscles, DVD appears to follow Hering's law. The main purpose of DVD may be to damp nystagmus.[12] Consider a patient with DVD in the right eye. According to Guyton, the initial event in DVD is a stimulation of the intorsion of the left eye to damp nystagmus. There is concurrently simulation of the extorters in the right eye (follows Hering's law). Because this torsional change is primarily mediated by the oblique muscles, this results in an infraduction of the fixing left eye and a supraduction of the non-fixing left eye. Then, in order to take up fixation again, the left eye supraducts. There is concurrent stimulation for supraduction in the left eye, according to Hering's law. The added effects of these two vertical movements create the right hypertropia seen as DVD.

Brodsky postulated a similar mechanism for DVD, but he attributed it to being a vestigial remnant of the dorsal light reflex of lower animals.[13]

Surgical management of DVD depends on whether inferior oblique overaction is present, the size of the deviation, and whether it is bilaterally or unilaterally manifest. If it is unilaterally manifest, the possibility that the patient may shift fixation after surgery should be taken into account. If amblyopia is present, a shift in fixation is unlikely.

If inferior oblique overaction is present concurrently with DVD, a common treatment is to anteriorly transpose the inferior oblique muscle to a point level with the inferior rectus insertion.[14] Weakening the inferior oblique without anterior transposition will probably not adequately treat DVD.

If anterior transposition of the inferior oblique is planned, it should be done bilaterally or there will be a resultant hypotropia of the operated eye in upgaze. This procedure should not be performed if the inferior obliques are not overacting, or if there is substantial superior oblique overaction.

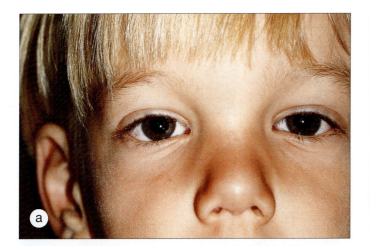
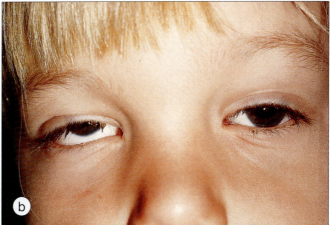
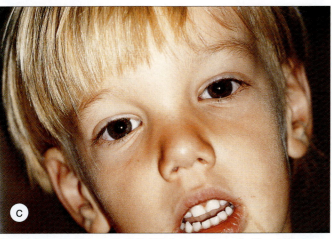
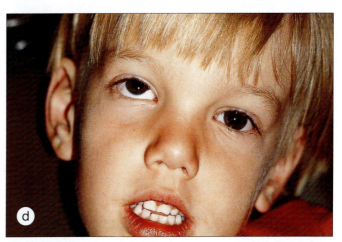

Fig. 83.6 Head tilt test with DVD. This boy has the typical head tilt response for DVD. (a) His DVD is latent and his eyes are often well aligned. (b) A right DVD is intermittently manifest. (c) The deviation is absent on head tilt to the right. (d) The deviation increases on head tilt to the left, which is common for a right DVD.

Table 83.2 Amount of superior rectus recession for DVD

Deviation (pd)	Bilateral superior rectus recession (mm)	Unilateral superior rectus recession (mm)
<10	7	5
10	8	6
15	9	7
20	10	8
25 and up	10	9

If DVD is present and there is no overaction of the inferior obliques, recession of the superior rectus muscles is the treatment of choice. Even if DVD is unilaterally manifest, bilateral surgery is advisable if the dominant eye shows latent DVD under cover and if equal vision is present. If unilateral surgery is performed in this situation, there is a high likelihood the patient will shift fixation postoperatively and then manifest a DVD in the previously preferred eye. For guidelines for the magnitude of superior rectus recession for DVD see Table 83.2. As is depicted in the table, if unilateral surgery is performed (which is desirable if amblyopia is present) the amount of superior rectus recession for a given amount of DVD should be less.

Symmetric inferior rectus resections in the range of 4–7 mm can be used to treat DVD. This procedure is generally reserved for use as a secondary procedure after other treatments have failed. This magnitude of inferior rectus resection will often cause narrowing of the palpebral fissure by raising the height of the lower eyelid.

SPECIAL FORMS OF VERTICAL STRABISMUS
Brown syndrome

Brown syndrome is caused by a mechanical restriction of the superior oblique tendon moving through the trochlea, which results in a restriction of elevation in adduction. On version testing it will mimic an inferior oblique palsy, except that a "V" pattern is present; an "A" pattern would be expected with inferior oblique palsy. Most cases of Brown syndrome are congenital, but it can be acquired due to either trauma or inflammation. If an inflammatory etiology is suspected, a systemic workup for autoimmune disease is appropriate. Inflammatory Brown syndrome may resolve spontaneously. If not it can be treated with steroid injection in the region of the trochlea. Systemic anti-inflammatory medication may play a role; often the results are disappointing with this approach.

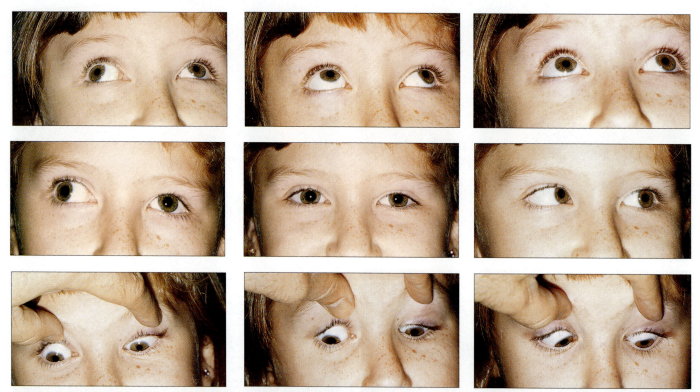

Fig. 83.7 Exotropic Duane syndrome with upshoot. This girl has a left exotropia associated with limited adduction in her left eye secondary to Duane syndrome. There is a marked upshoot of the left eye with adduction and a slight downshoot of the left eye with adduction below the midline. Although this resembles oblique muscle overaction, weakening of the apparent overacting oblique muscle is ineffective but weakening the lateral rectus may be effective (see Chapter 85).

Most cases of congenital Brown syndrome do not resolve spontaneously. Treatment may be indicated if a child needs to assume an unacceptable head posture for fusion. At surgery, forced ductions with attention to elevation in adduction should be performed. They will be positive if Brown syndrome is present and negative if there is an inferior oblique palsy. The surgical treatment of Brown syndrome consists of one of the many procedures to weaken or lengthen the superior oblique tendon. See Chapter 88.

Duane syndrome

Patients with Duane syndrome frequently have an up- or down-shoot of the affected eye on adduction (Fig. 83.7). Although this may appear to be caused by overaction of an oblique muscle, it is in fact caused by co-contraction of the lateral rectus muscle. This causes the lateral rectus to slip above or below the midline on adduction, creating the vertical deviation. Treatment in the form of oblique muscle surgery is usually not helpful. Successful treatment involves releasing the lateral rectus muscle in the form of either recession or Y splitting with recession.

Monocular elevation deficiency

The clinical picture of monocular elevation deficiency can be due to either a congenital fibrosis of the inferior rectus muscle, superior rectus palsy, or a supranuclear problem. (Fig. 83.8) Parents often feel the abnormality is in the unaffected eye, which they see as abnormally elevating on attempted upgaze. The treatment depends on the etiology. If forced ductions are found to be abnormal at surgery, the inferior rectus should be recessed. If forced ductions are normal, superior rectus palsy should be suspected. Depending on the degree to which elevation is limited, surgery should consist of either a vertical recess/resect procedure or a vertical transposition of the horizontal rectus muscles superiorly.

Orbital floor fracture

Orbital floor fracture can occur in children as well as adults. Typically there is diplopia and a hypotropia of the affected eye due to restriction.(Fig. 83.9) Surgical treatment usually involves recessing the affected inferior rectus muscle. In some cases, there may also be concurrent paresis or pseudoparesis of the affected inferior rectus muscle. True paresis can be caused by damage to the nerve to the inferior rectus muscle. Pseudoparesis can be caused by a posterior fracture with entrapment of the inferior rectus muscle, resulting in a loss of mechanical advantage of that muscle for depression.

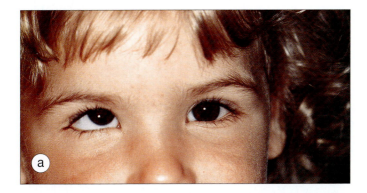
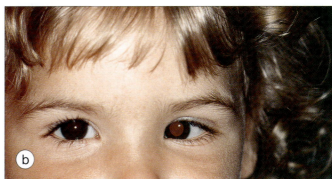
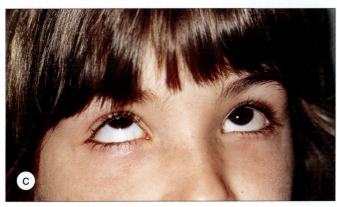
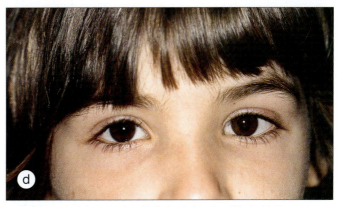

Fig. 83.8 Monocular elevation deficiency secondary to fibrosis. This girl has an esotropia and left hypotropia with limited elevation OS. (a, b) At surgery she was found to have a tight fibrotic left inferior rectus muscle. Several years after bilateral medial rectus recessions and a left inferior rectus recession she is straight in the primary position and shows improved (but still deficient) elevation (c, d).

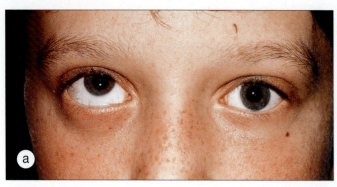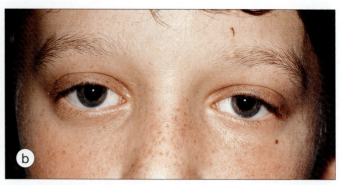

Fig. 83.9 Orbital floor fracture. This boy was struck in the left eye with a baseball and sustained an orbital floor fracture. (a) Limitation of elevation of the left eye is seen secondary to entrapment of the left inferior rectus muscle. (b) With the right eye in the primary position a very small left hypotropia is present.

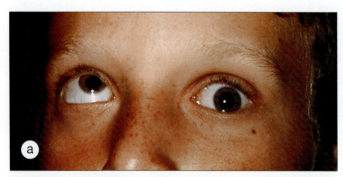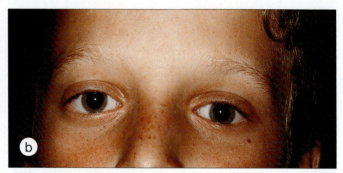

Fig. 83.10 Iatrogenic inferior oblique incorporation in resection. This child has a left hypotropia that developed after undergoing a resection of the left lateral rectus muscle as part of treatment for extropia. (a) In upgaze a large left hypotropia is present. (b) In the primary position the left hypotropia is small.

Iatrogenic

On occasion, the inferior oblique muscle may be inadvertently incorporated in a resection of the lateral rectus muscle and be advanced, often resulting in a postoperative hypotropia of the affected eye (Fig. 83.10).

Heiman Bielschowsky phenomenon

The Heiman Bielschowsky phenomenon is characterized by a peculiar slow vertical floating movement (up and down) of an eye with minimal vision. The mechanism for the phenomenon is not clear.[15]

REFERENCES

1. Kushner BJ. Ocular torsion; rotations around the "WHY" axis. J AAPOS 2004; 8: 1–12.
2. Bielschowsky A. Lectures on motor anomalies: I. The physiology of ocular movements. Am J Ophthalmol 1938; 21: 843–55.
3. Parks M. Isolated cyclovertical palsy. Arch Ophthalmol 1958; 60: 1027–35.
4. Wilson ME, Hoxie J. Facial asymmetry in superior oblique palsy. J Pediatr Ophthalmol Strabismus 1993; 30: 315–8.
5. Rao R, Morton G, Kushner BJ. Ocular torticollis and facial asymmetry. Binoc Vis Strabismus Q 1999; 14: 27–32.

6. Kushner BJ. Errors in the three-step test. Ophthalmology 1989; 96: 127–32.
7. Morton G, Lucchese N, Kushner BJ. The role of fundoscopy and fundus photography in strabismus diagnosis. Ophthalmology 1983; 90: 1186–91.
8. Kushner BJ. A surgical procedure to minimize lower-eyelid retraction with inferior rectus recession. Arch Ophthalmol 1992; 100: 1011–4.
9. Chatzistefanou KI, Kushner BJ, Gentry LR. Magnetic resonance imaging of the arc of contact of extraocular muscles: Implications regarding the incidence of slipped muscles. J AAPOS 2000; 4: 84–93.

10. Jampolsky A. Management of noncomitant ocular deviations. In: Jampolsky A, Scott AB, editors. International Ophthalmology Clinics. Boston: Little Brown; 1964: 675–701.

11. Bechtel RT, Kushner BJ, Morton GV. The relationship between dissociated vertical divergence (DVD) and head tilts. J Pediatr Ophthalmol Strabismus 1996; 33: 303–6.

12. Guyton DL. Dissociated vertical deviation: etiology, mechanisms, and associated phenomena. Costanbader lecture. J AAPOS 2000; 4: 131–44.

13. Brodsky MC. Dissociated vertical divergence: a righting reflex gone wrong. Arch Ophthalmol 1999; 117: 1216–22.

14. Elliott RL, Nankin SJ. Anterior transposition of the inferior oblique. J Pediatr Ophthalmol Strabismus 1981; 1981: 35–8.

15. Smith JL, Flynn JT, Spiro HJ. Monocular vertical oscillations of amblyopia. The Heimann-Bielschowsky phenomenon. J Clin Neuroophthalmol 1982; 2: 85–91.

CHAPTER
84

"A," "V," and Other Alphabet Pattern Strabismus

Burton J Kushner

OVERVIEW AND DEFINITIONS

The terms "A" pattern and "V" pattern describe horizontal strabismus that is vertically incomitant. It is characterized by a substantial increase or decrease in the horizontal deviation in the midline position in upgaze as compared to downgaze. In a patient with a "V" pattern the eyes are more converged in downgaze (more esotropic or less exotropic) than in upgaze (Fig. 84.1). An "A" pattern is characterized by eyes that are more converged (more esotropic or less exotropic) in upgaze as compared to downgaze (Fig. 84.2). By convention, the difference between upgaze and downgaze must be 15 PD (prism diopters) or greater to diagnose a clinically significant "V" pattern, and 10 PD diopters difference to diagnose an "A" pattern. Less commonly there are variations of the "A" and "V" patterns in which the change in the angle of misalignment is not linear from downgaze to upgaze. For example, the deviation may change minimally from downgaze to the primary position and diverge in upgaze resulting in a "Y" pattern (Fig. 84.3). Conversely, the deviation may change little from the upgaze position to the primary position, but diverge in downgaze to form a "λ" (lambda)-pattern (Fig. 84.4). In addition, eyes may diverge in both upgaze and downgaze as compared to the primary position, forming an "X" pattern. A neutralizing pattern is one in which there is orthophoria in the primary position and either divergence in upgaze and convergence in downgaze (neutralizing "V' pattern), or convergence in upgaze and divergence in downgaze (neutralizing "A" pattern).[1]

History

Duane first described a "V" pattern in 1897 in a patient with bilateral superior oblique palsy.[2] Subsequently little attention was given to the importance of measuring the angle of strabismus in upgaze and downgaze in the midline position until Urrets-Zavalia called attention to the relevance of these measurements.[3,4] In 1951, Urist brought attention to the "A" and "V" patterns in the English literature.[5] Initially it was suggested that vertically incomitant horizontal strabismus be referred to as the "V" and "teepee" patterns. However, Dan Albert later suggested the names "A" and "V" pattern, which have stood the test of time.[6]

Occurrence

It is difficult to obtain a prevalence figure for the occurrence of "A" and "V" patterns, because the number would be so heavily influenced by the nature of the series from which it was derived. There are strong ethnic predilections, as well as systemic factors that influence the occurrence of "A" and "V" patterns. Estimates of the percentage of patients with strabismus that have an "A" or "V" pattern range from 12 to 50%.[7-10] However, approximately 25% of patients with strabismus have an associated "A" or "V" pattern.[10,11] Costenbader reported a series of 421 patients that had either an "A" or "V" pattern.

"A" and "V" patterns are relatively frequent in patients who have had congenital strabismus; they are somewhat less frequent in patients with acquired strabismus. In Costenbader's series, 58% had an onset of the strabismus prior to 12 months of age.[10] "A" and "V" patterns occur frequently in patients with paralytic strabismus, due to the common occurrence of dysfunction of the oblique muscles in that patient population. Brown syndrome characteristically has a "V" pattern. This is an important sign that helps differentiate it from inferior oblique palsy. In the latter condition, an "A" pattern is found (Fig. 84.5). Duane syndrome often presents with a "V" or "Y" pattern, and less frequently "A"

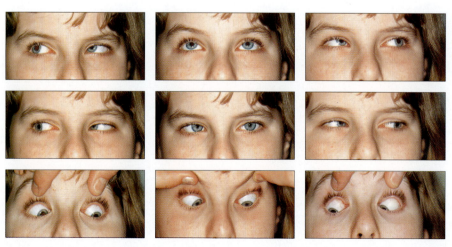

Fig. 84.1 "V" pattern esotropia. This girl has a "V" pattern esotropia with associated inferior oblique muscle overaction and superior oblique muscle underaction.

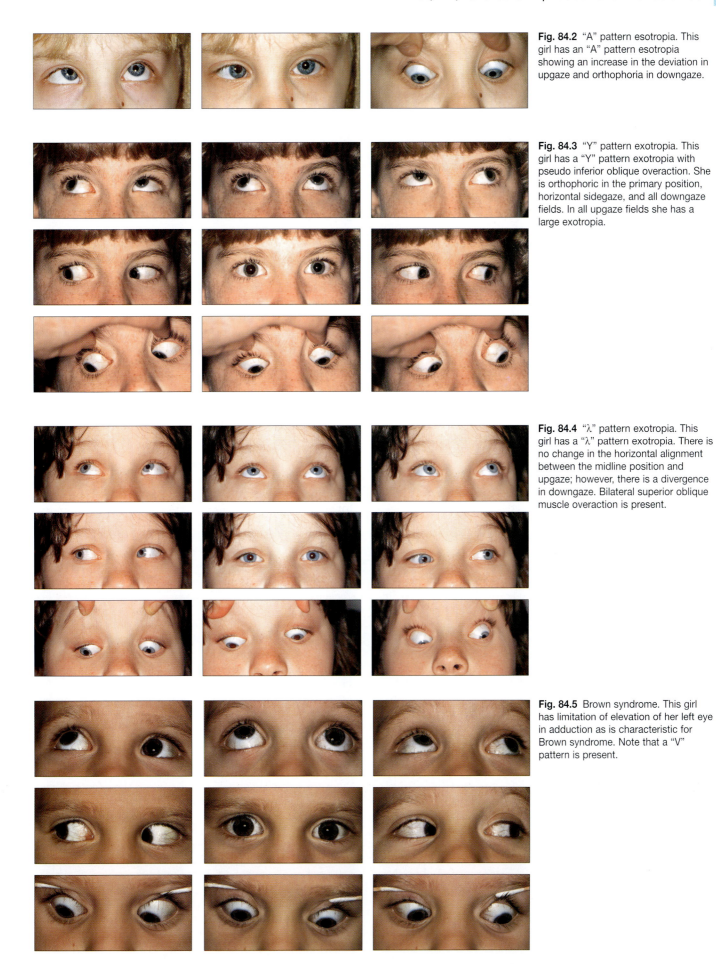

Fig. 84.2 "A" pattern esotropia. This girl has an "A" pattern esotropia showing an increase in the deviation in upgaze and orthophoria in downgaze.

Fig. 84.3 "Y" pattern exotropia. This girl has a "Y" pattern exotropia with pseudo inferior oblique overaction. She is orthophoric in the primary position, horizontal sidegaze, and all downgaze fields. In all upgaze fields she has a large exotropia.

Fig. 84.4 "λ" pattern exotropia. This girl has a "λ" pattern exotropia. There is no change in the horizontal alignment between the midline position and upgaze; however, there is a divergence in downgaze. Bilateral superior oblique muscle overaction is present.

Fig. 84.5 Brown syndrome. This girl has limitation of elevation of her left eye in adduction as is characteristic for Brown syndrome. Note that a "V" pattern is present.

or "λ" pattern (see Chapter 83, Fig. 83.7). There is an association of A-pattern strabismus with concurrent superior oblique muscle overaction in patients with spina bifida and/or hydrocephalus.[12,13] Biglan and Walden reported a 31% incidence of A-patterns in patients with spina bifida who also had strabismus.[13] Although frontal bossing in children with hydrocephalus may provide a mechanical advantage to the vertical vector of the superior oblique muscle in these patients, the exact mechanism is unclear.

ETIOLOGY

There are differing theories as to the etiology of "A" and "V" patterns, in part because different mechanisms may be responsible in different patients.

Oblique muscle dysfunction

The most popular theory, suggested by Knapp in 1959,[8] attributes most cases of "A" and "V" pattern to the role of oblique muscle dysfunction and the contributing effect of the accompanying torsion. Abduction is a tertiary action of the superior and inferior oblique muscles (see Chapter 83). Thus, if the superior oblique muscle is overacting, and the antagonist inferior oblique is underacting, one would expect there to be a relative divergence in downgaze and convergence in upgaze; resulting in an "A" pattern. Conversely if the inferior oblique muscle is overacting and the superior oblique muscle is underacting, one would expect a relative convergence in downgaze and divergence in upgaze, resulting in a "V" pattern. Clinically one frequently finds the oblique muscles are dysfunctional in this manner in patients with "A" or "V" pattern. This clinical observation, combined with the theoretical construct, has lead to the justified popularity of causally implicating the oblique muscles in "A" and "V" patterns.

The torsion that accompanies oblique muscle dysfunction also contributes to the associated "A"-or "V" pattern[14]. If a patient with a "V" pattern has inferior oblique overaction, there is an excyclotropia due to the overaction of the inferior oblique muscles. This results in a rotation of the location of the rectus muscles (counterclockwise in the right eye and clockwise in the left eye). The superior rectus muscles would become partial abductors and the inferior rectus muscles partial adductors (Fig. 84.6). These new force vectors for the vertical rectus muscles cause an exoshift in upgaze and an esoshift in downgaze, thus contributing to the "V" pattern. In addition, the medial rectus muscles have elevating force vectors and lateral rectus muscles depressing force vectors, thus contributing to the elevation seen in adduction found with overacting inferior oblique muscles. Thus the torsion that accompanies the overacting inferior oblique muscles contributes to both the "V" pattern and the vertical deviation on side gaze.

The converse occurs with superior oblique muscle overaction causing an incyclotropia, which enhances the A-pattern for analogous reasons. A lack of fusion may result in a freewheeling torsional drift analogous to the exotropic drift seen in patients with monocular sensory deprivation.[15] This is supported by the finding that torsion is visible in the fundus prior to the observation of elevation in adduction in children with infantile esotropia.[16] However, this finding also suggests that the elevation seen in adduction with inferior oblique muscle overaction is not solely a result of the accompanying excyclotorsion, which can be present in the absence of overelevation in adduction. This suggests that it is subsequent contracture of the inferior oblique muscle (perhaps because the excyclotorsion results in shortening of the muscle) that actually is responsible for the overelevation in adduction. Whether the elevation in adduction seen with inferior oblique muscle overaction is actually caused by the vertical action of the inferior oblique muscle, or is just a manifestation of the torsional changes depicted in Fig. 84.6, is subject to some controversy. Probably both mechanisms are important.

Horizontal muscles

It is mainly of historical interest that Urist felt that overactions or underactions of the horizontal rectus muscles were responsible for "A" and "V" patterns.[5,9] He felt that the medial rectus muscles were more active in downgaze and lateral rectus muscles more in upgaze. Consequently he attributed a "V" pattern esotropia to an overaction of the medial rectus muscles and a "V" pattern exotropia to overaction of the lateral rectus muscles. His surgical recommendations for treating these patterns involved weakening the offending muscles. Although this theory is less compelling than others, it may explain the occurrence of some cases of "A" or "V" pattern where no other cause is apparent. It can also explain the small decrease in "V" pattern observed after bilateral medial rectus recessions in a patient with esotropia.

Vertical rectus muscles

Brown felt that "V" patterns were caused by a weakness of the superior rectus muscles, thus giving rise to the apparent elevation of the contralateral eye on adduction,[17] and inferior rectus muscle weakness was the cause of A-patterns. Where Brown attributed the overelevation or overdepression in adduction to a weakness of the contralateral superior rectus or inferior rectus muscles respectively, most strabismologists today would attribute it to an overaction of the respective yoke oblique muscles. Brown's theory is not consistent with more recent observations regarding objective fundus torsion. The objective fundus extorsion typically seen in a patient with a "V" pattern would be expected if the inferior oblique muscles were overacting; intorsion would be expected if the superior rectus muscles were truly underacting. The converse would be true for an "A" pattern. The common association of objective incyclotropia with "A" patterns suggests it is the superior oblique muscles that are overacting, rather than the inferior rectus muscles underacting. Brown's theory is mainly of historical interest and is not widely accepted.

Sagittalization of the oblique muscles

Gobin presented a theory in which the primary event that causes a "V" pattern is an abnormal sagittalization of the inferior oblique muscles.[18] This means the insertion of the muscle is abnormally posterior, and the course of the muscle is relatively more parallel with the visual axis than normal. This anatomic abnormality serves to decrease the extorsional vector of the inferior oblique muscle, resulting in a shift in balance of opposing torsional forces, resulting in an incyclotropia. Thus, a patient with a "V" pattern would initially have an incyclotropia. Subsequently, for the purpose of eliminating the incyclotropia, there is increased innervation to the excyclorotary muscles (the inferior rectus and inferior oblique muscles in each eye). This eliminates the incyclotropia but also results in the clinical appearance of

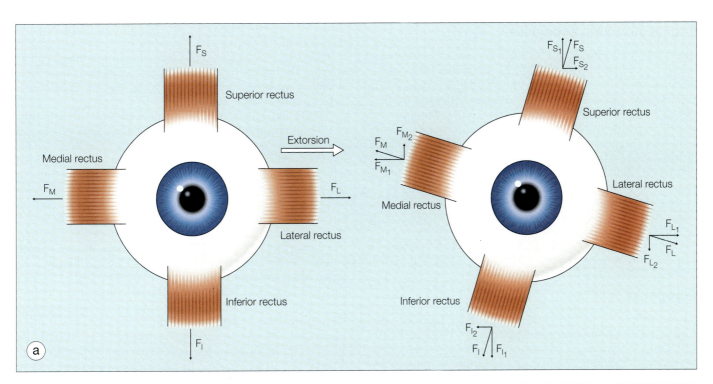

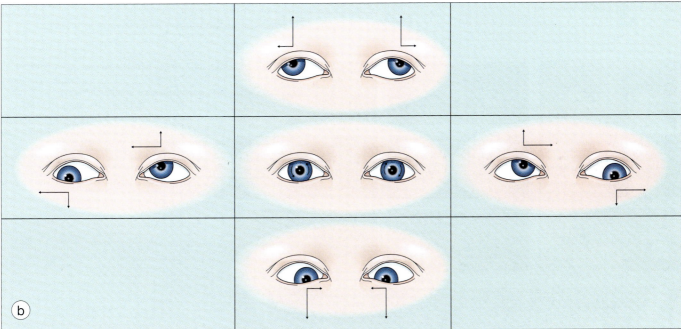

Fig. 84.6 (a) Effect of torsion on individual muscle function. An excyclorotation of the left eye will result in a clockwise rotation of the insertion of the muscles. This will create a vector for elevation of the medial rectus muscle, abduction for the superior rectus, depression for the lateral rectus, and adduction for the inferior rectus. (b) Effect of torsion on motility pattern. If the torsional changes depicted in (a) occurred in both eyes, the new force vectors would cause divergence in upgaze and convergence in downgaze. In addition there would be an elevation of the adducting eye and depression of the abducting eye. Thus, these torsional changes that occurred as a result of extorsion contribute to both the "V" pattern and the elevation seen in adduction.

overacting inferior oblique muscles. In turn, the overacting inferior oblique muscles cause a "V" pattern for the reasons outlined above in the section "Oblique muscle dysfunction."

The inconsistencies in this theory lie in the clinical observations of fundus torsion. According to the sagittalization theory, an incyclotropia should precede the development of a "V" pattern. In reality, an excyclotropia precedes the pattern.[16] Also, if this

theory were valid, the compensatory overinnervation to the inferior oblique muscles should serve the purpose of eliminating torsion. Thus no torsion should be present after the pattern develops. In fact, extorsion is typically present. Finally, it is hard to understand why there would be excessive innervation to the oblique muscles to eliminate torsion, in a patient with a substantial horizontal deviation and hence no fusion.

Orbital structural anomalies

There are strong associations between "A" and "V" patterns and orbital anomalies. There is a frequent occurrence of A-pattern esotropia accompanied by inferior oblique muscle underaction in patients with mongoloid fissures (upslanting palpebral fissures) and an association of "V" pattern exotropia with inferior oblique muscle overaction.[19] In patients with antimongoloid fissures (downslanting palpebral fissures) the opposite occurs. There is an association of "V" pattern esotropia with inferior oblique muscle overaction and "A" pattern exotropia with inferior oblique muscle underaction.

More recently, Clark and co-workers and Demer have attributed some cases of "A" and "V" patterns to orbital pulley heterotopia or pulley laxity[20,21] (Fig. 84.7).

There is also a very high incidence of "A" and "V" patterns in patients with craniofacial syndromes[22,23] (Fig. 84.8).

Iatrogenic

Surgery for an "A" or "V" pattern may result from an overcorrection. An "A"-pattern may develop when there previously had been a "V" pattern; a "V" pattern may develop after surgery to treat an "A" pattern. This may occur after vertical transposition of horizontal rectus muscles or, more frequently, if there is late development of overaction of the antagonist oblique muscle of an oblique muscle that was surgically weakened.

An "A" pattern frequently occurs following large bilateral recessions of the inferior rectus muscles as is commonly done to treat thyroid eye disease. This occurs from loss of the adducting effect of the inferior rectus in downgaze secondary to their being surgically weakened, and by an increase in innervation to the yoke superior oblique muscles.[24]

On occasion, a marked "Y" pattern can occur as a complication of anterior transposition of the inferior oblique muscle.[25] In this operation, for vertical divergence associated with inferior oblique muscle overaction, the inferior oblique muscles are reinserted level with or anterior to the temporal corner of the insertions of the inferior rectus muscles. This changes the vertical force vectors of the inferior oblique muscles from being elevators to being antielevators. If too much antielevation effect is obtained, there is a restriction of elevation in abduction, resulting in overelevation of the contralateral eye in adduction due to fixation duress. This simulates residual contralateral inferior oblique overaction and is associated with a large "Y" pattern (Fig. 84.9). This entity has been labeled the "antielevation syndrome." Interestingly, forced ductions are typically normal for elevation in the antielevation syndrome, because there is not actually a mechanical restriction. The antielevating force, which restricts elevation of the abducting eye, only comes into being when there is innervation for elevation. The antielevation syndrome is more likely to occur if the inferior oblique muscle is advanced to a point anterior to the inferior rectus muscle insertion, and/or if the new insertion of the inferior oblique muscle is spread out so

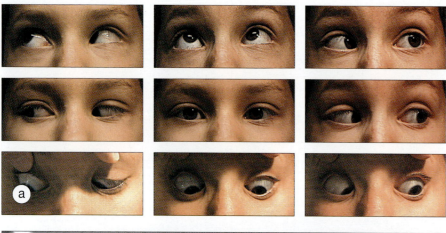

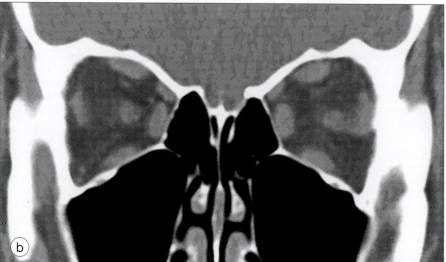

Fig. 84.7 Pulley heterotopia causing A-pattern. (a) This boy has an A-pattern esotropia associated with overdepression in adduction and underelevation in adduction bilaterally. (b) CAT scan shows lateral rectus pulleys superiorly placed relative to medial rectus pulleys. The pattern collapsed with recession and superior transposition of medial rectus muscles bilaterally. (Photographs courtesy of Joseph L Demer, MD, PhD. This work was supported by NIH Grant EY08313.)

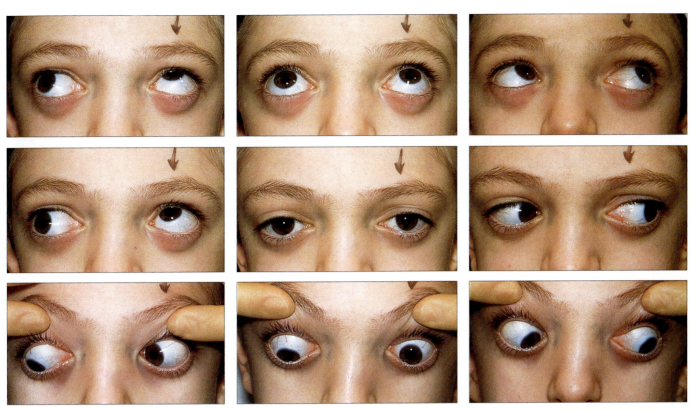

Fig. 84.8 Craniofacial anomaly with associated pattern: Crouzon syndrome. This boy shows the classic "V" pattern seen in Crouzon syndrome. There is overelevation and underdepression of each eye in adduction. (Photo courtesy of Ken K Nischal, FRCOphth.)

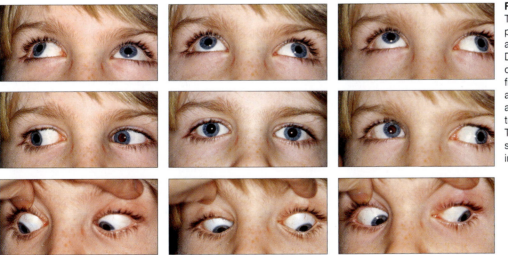

Fig. 84.9 The antielevation syndrome. This boy has a large "V" pattern after previously undergoing inferior oblique anterior transposition bilaterally to treat DVD. What looks like residual inferior oblique overaction is actually a result of fixation duress to the abducting eye on attempted elevation, due to the antielevating property of the transposed inferior oblique muscle. This drives the adducting eye superiorly and mimics contralateral inferior oblique overaction.

that the posterior lateral corner is positioned relatively temporally. When treating a patient with the antielevation syndrome, it is important to know that the restriction of elevation of the abducting eye is what drives the hypertropia of the adducting eye, and surgery should be planned accordingly to relieve that "innervational" restriction.

PRESENTATION

The manner of presentation of a patient with an "A" or "V" pattern depends on the nature of the underlying strabismus and the size of the deviation. If the patient has a substantial horizontal deviation in the primary position, and despite the presence of an "A" or "V" pattern there is no position in which fusion is possible, the pattern may not affect the presentation. If the deviation is small enough that the pattern permits some fusion in either upgaze or downgaze, the patient may assume a chin-down or chin-up head position in order to fuse. A child with a "V" pattern esotropia or an A-pattern exotropia, who assumes a chin-down head posture, may merely be perceived by his or her parents as being shy. The parents frequently will not notice the underlying strabismus. A child with a "V" pattern exotropia or an "A" pattern esotropia may assume a noticeable chin-up head posture. Also, because a child typically must look up to see his or her parents, the strabismus may be more noticeable in these latter two situations. If a pattern occurs mainly in downgaze (A exotropia, V esotropia, or "λ" pattern) the strabismus may be less noticeable, because the eyelids cover the eyes in downgaze. In one series of patients with abnormal head postures due to strabismus, 9% assumed an abnormal head posture because of an "A" or "V" pattern.[26]

Some adults with an "A" or "V" pattern may not become symptomatic until they become presbyopic; their symptoms may not become manifest until they need to get their eyes into downgaze to read through their bifocal segment. Prior to becoming presbyopic, they may have unconsciously held reading material closer than the primary position in order to read.[27] Similarly, some presbyopic patients with strabismus only significant in downgaze may become symptomatic if they switch from a flat-top to a progressive bifocal. This latter type of bifocal has a wide transition zone that requires the eyes to move further into downgaze in order to permit vision through the prescribed add.

EXAMINATION

Motor exam

The diagnosis of an "A" or "V" pattern must be made by measuring the patient with the prism and alternate cover test 25°–30° above and below the midline. Testing should be done at 6 m to eliminate any influence of the near reflex. One can be mislead by simply assessing the size of the deviation seen on versions using a light reflex test, as this will not bring out the latent deviation. Particularly in patients with intermittent exotropia, the deviation may be controlled in the primary position; however, fusion may break down when the eyes are rotated into extreme fields of gaze. The eyes may then diverge in upgaze and/or downgaze, giving the appearance of a "Y","λ", or "X" pattern. When examining young uncooperative children, particular care must be taken to ensure that the comparative measurements obtained in the midline positions are in fact of the full deviation (manifest plus latent deviation). In such patients, it is wise to look carefully for objective torsion in the fundus and for oblique muscle dysfunction to aid in assessing whether an "A" or "V" pattern is truly present.

The testing should be done while full optical correction is in place, and while fixation is maintained on an accommodative target. If not, a pseudo "A" or "V" pattern may be observed.[8] Patients normally tend to accommodate in downgaze but less so in upgaze. If hyperopia is not corrected with spectacles, a patient may appear to have a "V" pattern because accommodation will occur when they look down, thus increasing the esotropia. It is also important to recognize that a "V" pattern may simulate a high AC/A ratio if care is not taken to keep the fixation target in the primary position at near. If the near measurement is inadvertently made with the eyes in slight downgaze, and if a "V" pattern is present, the esotropia may increase due to the downgaze position. It may be incorrectly attributed to a high AC/A ratio.

Special care should be taken to assess any relative overaction or underaction of the oblique muscles. To test versions, the eyes should be taken into extreme fields of gaze even though the criteria to diagnose a clinical "A" or "V" pattern requires that measurements be made in less than extreme rotation. The presence of objective fundus torsion should be noted using the indirect ophthalmoscope through dilated pupils.[28]

Sensory findings

Sensory findings may vary, depending on whether the patient is orthotropic in any field of gaze. Patients with neutralizing patterns, "Y" patterns, or "λ" patterns may be well aligned in the primary position and may have surprisingly good fusion. If a patient is tropic in all fields of gaze, suppression and varying depths of anomalous retinal correspondence (ARC) may be found. Ciancia and Helveston et al. found that in patients with "A" or "V" pattern and ARC, the angle of anomaly varies with the angle of deviation, thus resulting in the ARC being harmonious in all fields of gaze.[29,30] This speaks to the fluidity of ARC.

Surgical treatment

If a pattern needs to be eliminated, the treatment is surgery. However, first, it is necessary to determine whether a pattern needs to be addressed. If a patient has a significant chin-up or chin-down head posture in order to fuse, surgery to address the pattern is appropriate. A continuous change in the size of a deviation with alterations in gaze direction is destabilizing for binocular fusion. Thus if an "A" or "V" pattern is clinically significant, it should probably be addressed in any child undergoing horizontal strabismus surgery, in whom there is any likelihood of gaining some degree of binocularity. This is probably the situation in all children undergoing strabismus surgery, except those with dense amblyopia. One should also pay attention to the location of the pattern. The primary position and downgaze are the two most important fields of gaze. One might ignore the pattern completely in an asymptomatic patient with a "Y" pattern who only manifests in upgaze. This is particularly true if treating the pattern might be at the expense of the good alignment in the primary position and in downgaze. At times, however, the strabismus may be cosmetically unacceptable because of a pattern, in which case surgery to address the pattern is appropriate. Sometimes a "V" pattern may negate the benefit of a bifocal in a patient with an esotropia associated with a high AC/A ratio, because the pattern causes the deviation increases in downgaze. Then surgery to address the pattern is appropriate. For most adults undergoing strabismus surgery, a pattern should be treated if present. Exceptions include patients in whom treating the pattern might adversely affect the outcome in the primary position or downgaze. In adults with dense amblyopia the pattern may be ignored.

Oblique muscle surgery

If it is decided to treat a pattern, and if there is substantial oblique muscle overaction, the offending muscles should be weakened.[8] This addresses all aspects of the problem:
1. It decreases the excessive abducting force in the gaze direction in which the eyes diverge (upgaze for "V" pattern, downgaze for "A" pattern);

2. It decreases the torsion, which contributes to the pattern and may be an obstacle to fusion; and

3. It corrects any cosmetically unacceptable upshoot or downshoot that occurs on adduction.

Oblique muscle surgery should be combined with horizontal surgery, with the latter based on the angle of misalignment in the primary position. No allowance is necessary for the abducting affect of the oblique muscles, which is minimal in the primary position. Weakening the inferior oblique muscles will result in approximately 15–25 PD esotropic shift in upgaze, depending on the degree of overaction of the inferior oblique muscles; the greater is the degree of overaction, the more effect is obtained. It has little or no effect on the horizontal deviation in the primary position. Initially there will also be no horizontal effect in downgaze from weakening the inferior obliques. Later, however, there may be some increased divergence in downgaze because the previously underacting superior obliques will sometimes recover function after the antagonist inferior obliques have been weakened.

The effect one obtains by weakening the superior obliques depends on the technique used. Weakening the superior obliques nasally by any technique has a large effect and can correct up to 40 PD of exotropia in downgaze. Weakening the superior obliques temporally is a less powerful operation, but also less likely to cause complications. The posterior tenectomy as popularized by Prieto-Dias will cause a reduction of approximately 15–20 PD of exotropia in downgaze.[31,32] A slightly more powerful operation is a complete disinsertion of the superior oblique tendon. Still greater effects can be obtained by a tenectomy of the superior oblique tendon near its insertion, or with a graded recession. Weakening the superior oblique muscles has no effect on upgaze. Initially Parks felt that bilateral superior oblique tenectomy resulted in a 15- to 20-PD reduction in exotropia in the primary position, and he recommended that any horizontal surgery be adjusted to take that into account.[33] Subsequently, several studies have found that there is only between 0 and 3 PD of exotropia correction in the primary position after bilateral superior oblique weakening.[34-36] Consequently little or no adjustment should be made in the amount of horizontal surgery performed because of concurrent superior oblique weakening.

When treating a pattern by weakening the obliques, it is important that the surgery is performed symmetrically. Otherwise a vertical deviation may be created in the primary position. A complete weakening procedure of the superior oblique, such as a nasal tenectomy, is a powerful operation. It may lead to disruption of fusion in a patient with bifoveal fusion (such as a patient with intermittent exotropia) and can create postoperative torsional diplopia. Extreme caution should be exercised when weakening the superior oblique of such patients. The posterior tenectomy procedure[31] may be beneficial in addressing the pattern and is safer than doing a complete superior oblique tenectomy. Alternatively, it may be prudent to combine lateral rectus muscle recessions with vertical transposition, and possibly not address the full size of the pattern if it is large. Alternatively, a residual pattern in such a patient could be treated by resecting and raising the medial rectus muscles.

If oblique muscles are not overacting, they should not be weakened when treating an "A" or "V" pattern. Finally, "V" patterns with superior oblique underaction can be treated with superior oblique tucks. Because tucking the superior oblique is a less predictable surgical procedure than others, it is recommended that this operation be limited to surgeons who have experience with that procedure. If possible, a surgeon not experienced at tucking the superior oblique should find a suitable alternative. One should not tuck the superior obliques in a patient with bifoveal fusion unless a preexisting excyclotropia is present. Otherwise they may have postoperative torsional diplopia due to intorsion.

Horizontal rectus transposition

Many patients with "A" and "V" patterns can be treated effectively with transposition of the horizontal rectus muscles combined with the usual recession or resection of the muscles that one would perform based on the primary position deviation. No allowance in the standard surgical formula should be made because of the transposition. This treatment was also initially suggested by Knapp.[8] It is based on the principal that when a horizontal muscle is transposed, its primary action is decreased when the eye rotates into the field of gaze toward which the muscle was moved, and its action increases when the eye moves in the opposite direction (Fig. 84.10a). For example, if a medial rectus muscle is transposed inferiorly, it becomes a weaker adductor when the eye is in downgaze and a greater adductor when the eye is in upgaze. This occurs because the insertion of the transposed muscle has a new relationship to the center of rotation of the globe, as seen in Fig. 84.10a. Thus, for treating a "V" pattern esotropia, one moves the medial rectus muscles down, because that is the direction in which they should have less adducting action. However, when transposing rectus muscles, it is important to note that two additional changes in their function occur simultaneously (see Fig. 84.10b). One effect is the creation of a force vector in the direction in which the muscle is moved. Thus, if the medial rectus muscle is infraplaced, an additional force vector for depression is established. For this reason, it is important to always use this treatment symmetrically; otherwise, an unwanted vertical deviation in the primary position will be induced. The exception might be those circumstances in which one intentionally wishes to treat a preexisting vertical deviation. In such situations the amount of transposition of the rectus muscles may be performed asymmetrically or unilaterally. An additional effect of vertical transposition of a horizontal rectus muscle relates to torsion. When a rectus muscle is transposed, a torsional vector is created in the direction from which the muscle is moved. For example, moving the medial rectus down creates a force vector that results in extorsion. Importantly, this torsional rotation is in the opposite direction of the torsional correction one desires when treating most "A" or "V" patterns. For example, a "V" pattern esotropia is typically associated with inferior oblique overaction and excyclotropia. Moving the medial rectus muscles down treats the "V" pattern but makes the excyclotropia worse. This rarely results in adverse symptoms, probably because most patients with "A" or "V" pattern do not have bifoveal fusion. Similar principles apply when muscles are resected.

Thus, in a "V" pattern esotropia, the medial rectus muscles could be infraplaced, or the lateral rectus muscles supraplaced. Supraplacing a lateral rectus muscle makes it a weaker abductor in upgaze and a stronger abductor in downgaze. This is what one desires when treating a "V" pattern. A simple mnemonic for remembering the direction in which to transpose the horizontal rectus muscles is presented in Fig. 84.11. The medial rectus muscles are always transposed toward the *apex* of the pattern (down for a "V" pattern and up for an A-pattern) and the lateral rectus muscles are always transposed toward the *open space* of the pattern (up for a "V" pattern and down for an "A"-pattern).

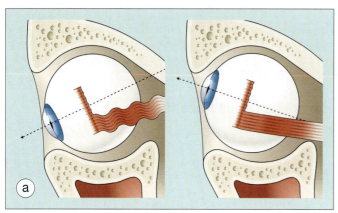

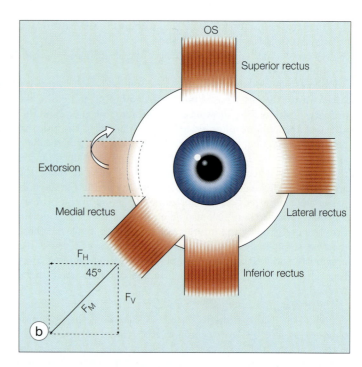

Fig. 84.10 (a) Effect of vertical transposition of rectus muscle on its primary action. If a muscle in infraplaced, there will be more slack in the muscle when the eye is in downgaze (top) than in upgaze. This weakens the primary action of the muscle more in downgaze than in upgaze. (b) Multiple effects of transposition of rectus muscle. If a medial rectus muscle is infraplaced, a new force vector for depression will be created. In addition, a torsional force vector will be created in the direction toward the original insertion. With infraplacement of the medial rectus, a vector for extorsion is created.

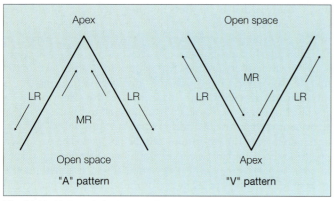

Fig. 84.11 Mnemonic for transposing horizontal rectus muscles. This diagram depicts the directions to move the horizontal rectus muscles for the treatment of an "A" (left) and a "V" pattern (right). The lateral rectus muscles are always moved toward the open space and the medial rectus muscles always move toward the apex of the pattern.

This holds true whether the patient is esotropic or exotropic, or if the muscles in question are being recessed or resected. Transposition of the horizontal rectus muscles is generally effective in treating patients with patterns if there is an absence of significant oblique dysfunction. If significant oblique dysfunction is present, transpositions of the horizontal rectus muscles are less effective in collapsing the pattern than if there is minimal or no oblique muscle dysfunction. Possibly the fact that the transposition worsens the torsion already present if there is oblique muscle overaction, and because torsion contributes to the pattern as indicated earlier, this finding is understandable.

I find that for most cases of "A" or "V" pattern without oblique muscle dysfunction, a symmetric vertical transposition of the appropriate horizontal rectus muscles by one-half tendon width (0.5 mm) is effective in collapsing an average of 15–20 PD of pattern. In most cases in which the pattern is 20 PD or more, there is usually significant oblique muscle dysfunction, and one is usually addressing the pattern with oblique muscle surgery. If for

some reason oblique muscle surgery is not indicated (perhaps it has already been performed but a pattern still persists) transposition of the appropriate horizontal rectus muscles by one-half tendon width (5 mm) or a full tendon width (10 mm) can be effective for treating larger patterns. Also, transpositions of the horizontal rectus muscles can be combined with oblique muscle surgery. For example, a patient with a very large "V" pattern (perhaps 40 PD or more), and inferior oblique overaction plus marked superior oblique underaction, might benefit from receiving bilateral medial rectus muscle recessions with infraplacement combined with bilateral inferior oblique muscle weakening. In this situation weakening the inferior obliques alone would not be expected to address the large increase in esotropia that occurs in downgaze.

The principles of transposition can also be applied when doing unilateral surgery in the form of a recess/resect procedure. One muscle could be raised and the other lowered. Although there are several reports of success with this technique, doing so does not create an equal balance of forces.[37,38] If one raises a weakened (recessed) muscle the same amount as one lowers a tightened (resected) muscle, there should be an increased force in the direction the resected muscle was moved. I have seen vertical deviations created from this surgical approach, although it is often successful. I prefer symmetric surgery if other factors permit.

Horizontal surgery alone

A slight decrease in a "V" pattern may be seen with recession of the medial rectus muscles alone.[5,8] Although this may not be sufficient to treat a clinically significant "V" pattern, it should be taken into account when planning surgery. For example, when treating an A-pattern esotropia, just recessing the medial rectus muscles will aggravate a borderline A-pattern. In this situation, one should address the borderline pattern that otherwise might not have needed treatment. Similarly, although weakening the inferior oblique muscles to treat a "V" pattern will not specifically address downgaze, if the medial rectus muscles are also recessed, one could expect up to 10 PD of collapse of the pattern below primary.

Transposition of vertical rectus muscles

Horizontal transposition of vertical rectus muscle can treat "A" and "V" patterns.[39,40] The theoretical efficacy of this approach is based on a principle different than that of vertical transposition of the horizontal rectus muscles. In the latter, the efficacy of the procedure is based on the principle that the primary (horizontal) force of the rectus muscle is decreased when the eyes rotate in the direction the muscle is moved, as seen in Fig. 84.10a. When the vertical muscles are transposed horizontally to treat patterns, the procedure is based on a different principle, which is depicted in Fig. 84.10b–specifically, that a force vector is created in the direction the muscle is moved. This same principle is the basis for transposition procedures to treat paralytic strabismus. Thus, a "V" pattern esotropia can be treated by temporal transposition of the inferior rectus muscles, a "V" pattern exotropia by nasal transposition of the superior rectus muscles, and an "A" pattern esotropia by temporal transposition of the superior rectus muscles. Typically the transposition performed is 7 mm. For some unexplained reason, this treatment approach has been reported as being unsuccessful for treating A-pattern exotropia.[39,40] A summary of the directions in which to transpose the vertical rectus muscles for treating "A" and "V" patterns is presented in Table 84.1.

Notably, horizontal transposition of the vertical rectus muscles would also create a torsional shift that may exacerbate a pre-existing cyclotropia, as seen in Fig. 84.10b. For example, nasal transposition of the inferior rectus muscles would help collapse an "A" pattern. It would also create an intorsional rotation, and intorsion is often already present preoperatively in patients with "A" patterns. If the patient has bifoveal fusion potential, this may be counterproductive. This is particularly relevant in treating patients with Graves orbitopathy with large bilateral inferior rectus recessions, which often results in a postoperative "A" pattern with intorsion in downgaze. I have seen patients in whom the inferior rectus muscles were transposed nasally in hopes of preventing the occurrence of an "A" pattern, and in whom an unexpectedly large and symptomatic incyclotropia was created. An alternative approach might be to combine large inferior rectus recessions with posterior tenectomies of the superior oblique tendons.[24,31]

Transposition of the vertical rectus muscles is not popular for treating "A" and "V" patterns. If significant oblique dysfunction is present, most surgeons approach the pattern by operating on the oblique muscles. If not, the pattern can be treated with simple transposition of the horizontal rectus muscles, and it is not necessary to additionally operate on the vertical rectus muscles.

Surgery to correct pulley abnormalities

If pulley displacement or pulley heterotopia is a cause of a pattern, surgery can be performed to stabilize or reposition the orbital pulleys.[20,21] Diagnosis of pulley abnormalities requires orbital imaging. This is a relatively new and evolving concept in the management of strabismus (see Chapter 77).

Surgical plan summary

In all cases, do the appropriate horizontal surgery based on the primary position measurement. In cases of weakening the superior oblique muscles, perhaps allow for up to 3 PD of esoshift in the primary position. Table 84.2 summarizes my recommendations for the surgical management of "A" and "V" patterns.

Optical management

Some patients with "A" or "V" pattern may have good alignment in the primary position but have an esotropia or exotropia in downgaze. As stated earlier, such patients may first become symptomatic as they become presbyopic. Some patients of this type can be managed by either using single vision reading glasses, or having a separate bifocal for reading with a segment higher than is typically prescribed.[27]

Special Forms

"X" patterns

"X" pattern strabismus can occur if all the oblique muscles are overacting. This sometimes happens in the presence of long-standing large-angle exotropia, in which case all the oblique muscles are contractured and overacting.[41] In such patients weakening all the oblique muscles may be necessary. Also, some patients with exotropia may have tight lateral rectus muscles, which can result in an "X" pattern. In these patients, weakening the lateral rectus muscles will effectively collapse the pattern.

"Y" patterns

There is a syndrome that strongly resembles marked bilateral inferior oblique overaction, which is associated with a "Y" pattern (see again Fig. 84.3). This has been labeled pseudo inferior

---

Table 84.1 Summary of directions in which to transpose vertical rectus muscle

Strabismus	Transposition
V-esotropia	IR OU temporally
V-exotropia	SR OU nasally
A-esotropia	SR OU temporally
A-exotropia	IR OU nasally
OU = both eyes.	

Table 84.2 Summary of surgical recommendations

Entity	Treatment
If oblique dysfunction is present[a]	
V eso with IO OA	Recess MR or resect LR and weaken IO OU
V exo with IO OA	Recess LR or resect MR and weaken IO OU
A eso with SO OA	Recess MR or resect LR and weaken SO OU[b]
A exo with SO OA	Recess LR or resect MR and weaken SO OU[b]
Without oblique dysfunction[a]	
V eso	Recess MR and infraplace or resect LR and supraplace
V exo	Recess LR and supraplace or resect MR and infraplace
A eso	Recess MR and supraplace or resect LR and infraplace
A exo	Recess LR and infraplace or resect MR and supraplace

eso = esotropia; exo = exotropia; IO = inferior oblique muscles; SO = superior oblique tendons; OA = overaction; MR = medial rectus muscles; LR = lateral rectus muscles; OU = both eyes.
[a] Combine with the usual amount of recession or resection of the horizontal rectus muscles based on the deviation in the primary position.
[b] Avoid a powerful superior oblique weakening procedure in patients with bifoveal fusion.

oblique overaction and is probably a variant of Duane syndrome.[42,43] It is characterized by a marked splaying out that occurs in upgaze with a large exotropic shift. Despite what looks like marked inferior oblique muscle overaction, there is no elevation of either eye on adduction, no superior oblique under-action, and no fundus torsion. It may be associated with orthophoria in the primary position; however, an esotropia or exotropia may be present. It is thought to be due to aberrant innervation to the lateral rectus muscles on attempted upgaze. In this syndrome, weakening the inferior oblique muscle will have no effect on the pattern. Recessing and raising the lateral rectus muscles is an effective treatment.

"λ" patterns

Lambda patterns usually are accompanied by superior oblique overaction and can be treated with appropriate horizontal surgery combined with superior oblique weakening (Fig. 83.4).

REFERENCES

1. Urist MJ. Neutralizing pattern deviations in ocular motility. Br J Ophthal 1970; 54: 191–6.
2. Duane A. Isolated paralysis of the ocular muscles. Arch Ophthalmol 1897; 26: 317–34.
3. Urrets-Zavalia A. Abducción en la elevación. Arch Oftalmol 1948; 23: 124–34.
4. Urrets-Zavalia A. Paralisis bialteral congenita del musculo oblicuo inferior. Arch Oftalmol 1948; 23: 172–82.
5. Urist MJ. Horizontal squint with secondary vertical deviations. Arch Ophthalmol 1951; 46: 245–67.
6. Albert DG. Personal Communication. In Parks MM. Annual review: strabismus. Arch Ophthalmol 1957; 58: 136–60.
7. Harley R, Manley DR. Bilateral superior oblique tenectomy in A-pattern exotropia. Trans Am Ophthalmol Soc 1969 ;67: 324–38.
8. Knapp P. Vertically incomitant horizontal strabismus, the so-called "A" & "V" syndromes. Trans Am Ophthalmol Soc 1959; 57: 666–9.
9. Urist MJ. The etiology of the so-called "A" and "V" syndromes. Am J Ophthalmol 1958; 46: 835–44.
10. Costenbader FD. The "A" and "V" patterns in strabismus. Trans Am Acad Ophthalmol Otolaryngol 1964; 68: 354–86.
11. Knapp P. "A" and "V" patterns. In: Symposium on Strabismus. Transactions of the New Orleans Academy of Ophthalmology. St Louis: Mosby; 1971: 242–54.
12. France TD. Strabismus in hydrocephalus. Am Orthoptic J 1975; 25: 101–5.
13. Biglan AW, Walden PG. Ophthalmologic complications of meningomyolocoele: a longitudinal study. Trans Am Ophthalmol Soc 1990; 88: 389–461.
14. Kushner BJ. The role of ocular torsion on the etiology of "A" and "V" patterns. J Pediatr Ophthalmol Strabismus 1983; 22: 171–9.
15. Guyton D, Weingarten P. Sensory torsion as the cause of primary oblique muscle overaction/underaction and "A" and "V" pattern strabismus. Binoc Vision Eye Muscle Surg Q 1994; 9: 209–36.
16. Eustis H, Nussdorf J. Inferior oblique overaction in infantile esotropia: fundus extorsion as a predictive sign. J Pediatr Ophthalmol Strabismus 1996; 33: 85–8.
17. Brown HW. Vertical deviations. Trans Am Acad Ophthalmol Otolaryngol 1953; 57: 157–62.
18. Gobin MH. Sagittalization of the oblique muscles as a possible cause for the "A,""V," and "X" phenomona. Br J Ophthalmol 1968; 52: 13–8.
19. Urrets-Zavalia A, Solares-Zamora J, Olmos HR. Anthropological studies on the nature of cyclovertical squint. Br J Ophthalmol 1961; 45: 578–96.
20. Clark RA, Demer JL, Rosenbaum AL. Heterotopic rectus muscle pulleys or oblique muscle dysfunction. J AAPOS 1998; 2: 17–25.
21. Demer JL. The orbital pulley system: a revolution in concepts of orbital anatomy. Ann NY Acad Sci 2002; 956: 17–32.
22. Miller M, Folk E. Strabismus associated with craniofacial anomalies. Am Orthoptic J 1975; 25: 27–37.
23. Robb RM, Boger WP. vertical strabismus associated with plagiocephaly. J Pediatr Ophthalmol Strabismus 1983; 20: 58–62.
24. Kushner BJ. Thyroid eye disease–strabismus. In: Dortzbach R, editor. Ophthalmic Plastic Surgery: Prevention and Management of Complications. New York: Raven Press; 1992: 381–94.
25. Kushner BJ. Restriction of elevation in abduction after inferior oblique anteriorization. J AAPOS 1997; 1: 55–62.
26. Kushner B. Ocular causes of abnormal head postures. Ophthalmology 1979; 86: 2115–25.
27. Kushner B. Management of diplopia limited to down gaze. Arch Ophthalmol 1995; 113: 1426–30.
28. Morton GV, Kushner BJ: The use of diagnostic occlusion in strabismus management. Ocular Therapy Surg 1983; 2: 194–200.
29. Ciancia AO. La correspondencia sensorial en los sindromes en A y V. J Pediatr Ophthalmol Strabismus 1965; 2: 15–20.
30. Helveston EM, von Noorden GK, Williams F. Symposium: Sensory adaptations in strabismus: Retinal correspondence in the "A" and "V" pattern. Am Orthoptic J 1970; 20: 22–7.
31. Prieto-Diaz J. Posterior tenectomy of the superior oblique. J Pediatr Ophthalmol Strabismus 1979; 16: 321–3.
32. Shin GS, Elliott RL, Rosenbaum AL. Posterior superior oblique tentectomy at the scleral insertion for collapse of "A"-pattern strabismus. J Pediatr Ophthalmol Strabismus 1996; 23: 211–8.
33. Parks MM. "A"-"V" patterns. In: Ocular Motility and Strabismus. Hagerstown: Harper & Row; 1975: 135.
34. Parks MM. Doyne Memorial Lecture: The superior oblique tendon. Trans Ophthalmol Soc UK 1977; 97: 288–304.
35. Fierson WM, Boger WP, Diorio PC, et al. The effect of bilateral superior oblique tenotomy on horizontal deviation in "A"-pattern strabismus. J Pediatr Ophthalmol Strabismus 1980; 17: 364–71.
36. Diamond GR, Parks MM. The effect of superior oblique weakening procedures on primary position horizontal alignment. J Pediatr Ophthalmol Strabismus 1981; 18: 35–8.
37. Goldstein JH. Monocular values for the "A" and "V" syndromes. Am J Ophthalmol 1967; 64: 265–7.
38. Metz HS, Schwartz L. The treatment of "A" and "Y" patterns by monocular surgery. Arch Ophthalmol 1977; 95: 251–3.
39. Fink WH. The "A" and "V" syndromes. Am Orthoptic J 1959; 9: 105–10.
40. Miller JE. Vertical recti transplantation in the "A" and "V" syndromes. Arch Ophthalmol 1960; 64: 175–9.
41. Jampolsky A. Bilateral anomalies of the oblique muscles. Trans Am Acad Ophthalmol Otolaryngol 1957; 61: 689–700.
42. Scott AB. "V" pattern exotropia: Electromyographic study of an unusual case. Invest Ophthalmol 1973; 65: 232–3.
43. Kushner BJ. Pseudo inferior oblique overaction associated with "Y" and "V" patterns. Ophthalmology 1991; 98: 1500–5.

CHAPTER
85

Strabismus Syndromes: The Congenital Cranial Dysinnervation Disorders (CCDDs)

Neil R Miller

Strabismus syndromes, now known as the congenital cranial dysinnervation disorders (CCDDs), are characterized by abnormal movements of the eyes, eyelids, face, or a combination of these. They include congenital fibrosis of the extraocular muscles (CFEOM), Duane retraction syndrome (DURS), congenital horizontal gaze palsy with scoliosis (HGPS), congenital facial palsy (CFP), Möbius syndrome, and congenital ptosis. The term "congenital cranial dysinnervation disorder" reflects the concept that these disorders result from developmental errors in innervation of the ocular and facial muscles and not from primary dysfunction of the muscles themselves.

The CCDDs encompass congenital, nonprogressive, sporadic, or familial abnormalities of cranial musculature that result from developmental abnormalities of, or the complete absence of, one or more cranial nerves with primary or secondary muscle dysinnervation. Primary dysinnervation in the CCDDs may result from absence of normal muscle innervation because alpha motoneurons of the appropriate cranial nerves either do not develop or are misguided during development. Secondary dysinnervation may occur when a muscle lacking normal innervation becomes aberrantly innervated during development by branches of other nerves. Dysinnervation may be associated with secondary muscle pathology or other orbital and bony structural abnormalities. Disorders involving predominantly vertical ocular motility defects are likely to result from abnormalities in development of oculomotor and trochlear nerves and/or nuclei (e.g., CFEOM variants and congenital ptosis), whereas disorders involving predominately horizontal ocular motility defects are likely to result from abnormalities in the development of the abducens nerve and/or nucleus (Duane syndrome and HGPS). Disorders involving predominantly facial weakness are likely to result from abnormal development of facial nerve and/or nucleus, sometimes with associated ocular motor abnormalities (e.g., congenital facial weakness and Möbius syndrome). In this chapter, only those CCDDs characterized wholly or in part by abnormalities of eye movement will be discussed.

CONGENITAL FIBROSIS OF EXTRAOCULAR MUSCLES (CFEOM)

Johnson[1] was the first to describe two syndromes characterized by defective eye movements that he believed were caused by a primary mechanical process characterized by adherence between two extraocular muscles. In one type, there were adhesions between the sheaths of the lateral rectus and inferior oblique muscles that made it impossible to abduct the eye. The disorder was usually bilateral. Eye second type was characterized by adherence between the sheaths of the superior rectus and superior oblique muscles, preventing elevation of the affected eye.

Following Johnson's descriptions, a variety of authors reported similar cases. Histopathologic findings in some of these cases included replacement of muscle tissue with fibrous tissue and degenerative changes in the muscles. In other patients, however, the muscles were normal or showed minimal pathologic changes, suggesting that fibrosis was a secondary rather than a primary phenomenon. In 1997, extensive neuropathologic analysis of a single case[2] showed absence of the superior division of the oculomotor nerve and its corresponding motoneurons, atrophy and fibrotic replacement of the levator palpebrae superioris and superior rectus, and abnormalities in all of the extraocular muscles, not just those innervated by the superior division of the oculomotor nerve. These findings suggested that CFEOM was caused by an abnormality of development of the innervation of the extraocular muscles and not by a primary abnormality of the muscles themselves.

It was subsequently postulated that the various forms of CFEOM result from primary dysinnervation of oculomotor and/or trochlear-innervated extraocular muscles. The genetic loci for the CFEOM phenotypes are referred to as *FEOM*. To date, three CFEOM phenotypes and four *FEOM* loci have been defined.[3]

CFEOM1 phenotype

This is the most common of the CFEOM phenotypes, and the one pathologically described in detail by Engle et al.[2] It is characterized by congenital bilateral ptosis and a bilateral ocular motility disorder with the globes infraducted in primary position and with restricted upgaze and variably restricted horizontal gaze (Fig. 85.1). These patients commonly have positive forced ductions and misdirected eye movements such as a marked synergistic convergence on attempted upgaze. They are rarely noted to have retraction. Inheritance is autosomal dominant with full penetrance (Fig. 85.2). Neuropathology suggests a primary defect of the superior division of the oculomotor nerve. The main locus for this condition, FEOM1, is on chromosome 12 (12p11.2–q12);[2,3–5] however, a few CFEOM1 families map to the FEOM3 locus on chromosome 16 (16q24.2–q24.3) (see below).[5]

CFEOM2 phenotype

In this rare form of CFEOM, patients have bilateral ptosis and a large-angle exotropia with severely limited horizontal and vertical eye movements. The ptosis is often severe and, combined with the defect in vertical eye movements, is very difficult to treat: the patients often lift their own lid to see better. Inheritance is autosomal recessive, and thus far, this disorder has been identified only in consanguineous families. The main locus for this condition, FEOM2, is the *PHOX2a* gene on chromosome 11 (11q13.2),[6] although other loci apparently exist,[7] and neuro-

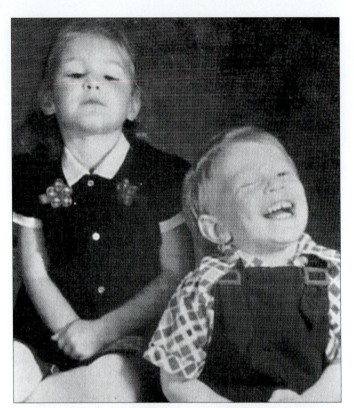

Fig. 85.1 Congenital fibrosis syndrome type I in a brother and sister. Because of the bilateral ptosis and deficient upgaze, both children have adopted a head posture with the chin elevated. (Image courtesy of Dr Stewart M Wolff.)

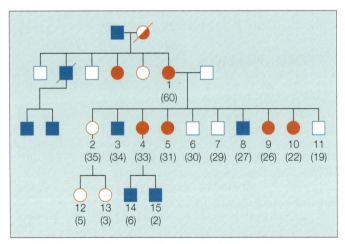

Fig. 85.2 Pedigree of a family with congenital fibrosis syndrome type I showing autosomal dominant transmission. (From Gillies et al.[44].)

pathologic examination of transgenic mice with absence of the *phox2a* gene suggests that the human phenotype results from a primary developmental defect of both the oculomotor and trochlear nuclei.

CFEOM3 phenotype

This is a variable phenotype within some CFEOM1 families in which at least one affected family member does not meet standard CFEOM1 criteria. Examples include unilateral disease, absent or unilateral ptosis, ortho- or hypertropia in primary gaze,

and close to normal elevation of the globe. Affected individuals commonly have positive forced ductions but rarely show misdirected eye movements or retraction. It is proposed that CFEOM3 results from a variable defect in the development of the oculomotor nucleus. Like CFEOM1, inheritance is autosomal dominant; however, in this phenotype there is incomplete penetrance. The main locus is the FEOM3 locus on chromosome 16 (16q24.2–q24.3);[8,9] however, rare CFEOM3 patients map to the FEOM1 locus on chromosome 12 (see above),[5] and one family with a CFEOM3 phenotype has been identified with a chromosomal translocation that is co-inherited in an autosomal-dominant pattern (FEOM4).

Practical management of CFEOM patients

After the diagnosis, helping these patients and their parents to live with their very difficult and unremitting problems is paramount. The outlook must be very guarded, and as the condition is rare, even the most experienced pediatric ophthalmologist can offer little in the way of confidently giving an individual prognosis. The "Everest" phenomenon (doing something because there is a problem there) must be avoided, as many patients are better aided by helping them to live with their problem rather than spending their lives seeking unattainable perfection.

All children with CFEOM should be refracted, and they should be reviewed by an ophthalmologist regularly throughout their visual development and any amblyopia treated.

In all types, the management of the ptosis is difficult because overcorrection is frequent and easily results in exposure keratitis because of the restricted eye movements. Patients with CFEOM2 often adopt the habit of lifting one or other lid to enable them to see better.

The strabismus may be improved by very large recessions and occasionally resections.[3] Muscle transposition surgery is unrewarding. The prognosis is not good, and the parents should be counseled accordingly; any surgery must be done by a very experienced strabismus surgeon.

DUANE RETRACTION SYNDROME (STILLING-TURK-DUANE SYNDROME, DURS)

Duane retraction syndrome is a congenital eye movement disorder characterized by marked limitation or absence of abduction, variable limitation of adduction, and palpebral fissure narrowing and globe retraction on attempted adduction. Vertical ocular movements are often noted on adduction, most frequently in an upward direction. In 1905, Duane described 54 cases, summarized all findings, and offered theories on pathogenesis and treatment.[10] After his original report, several large series of patients were described.

A disorder of horizontal eye movements is common to all patients with DURS. In most cases, the condition is unilateral (Fig. 85.3), but bilateral DURS occurs in 15–20% of affected patients (Fig. 85.4). The syndrome occurs more commonly in females than males, and the left eye is more frequently affected than the right. In most patients, gaze is directed toward the side of the unaffected eye, and in some instances, the face is turned toward the affected side to allow binocular single vision. Visual symptoms are conspicuous by their absence. Vision is almost always normal unless there is associated anisometropia and amblyopia. Thus, in the majority of cases, no treatment is necessary unless the patient has a marked head turn.

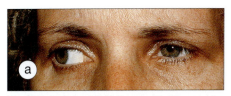
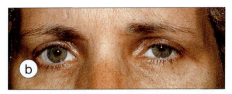
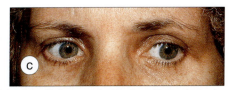

Fig. 85.3 Unilateral (left) Duane retraction syndrome type I in a 42-year-old woman. Note limitation of abduction of left eye and widening of left palpebral fissure on attempted left gaze. On attempted right gaze, there is mild limitation of adduction of the left eye and narrowing of the left palpebral fissure.

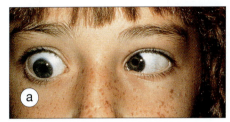
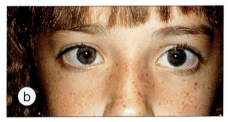
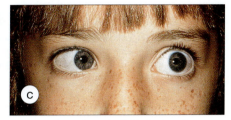

Fig. 85.4 Bilateral Duane retraction syndrome type I in a 4-year-old girl. Note bilateral moderate limitation of abduction, bilateral mild limitation of adduction, and widening of the ipsilateral palpebral fissure on attempted right and left gaze. (Images courtesy of Dr Michael X Repka.)

Early histologic studies demonstrated abnormalities of the lateral or medial rectus muscles and led investigators to the conclusion that DURS was a local, myogenic phenomenon. It was generally believed that the cause of the abduction deficiency was fibrosis of the lateral rectus muscle and that limitation of adduction was caused by a posterior insertion of the medial rectus muscle. Adhesions between the medial rectus muscle and the medial orbital wall were also reported.

In 1957, Breinin used electromyography to examine two patients with unilateral DURS.[11] In one patient, action potentials could be recorded only from a small region of the lateral rectus muscle, and the discharge pattern from the medial rectus muscle was normal. In the second patient, Breinin recorded a discharge pattern from the lateral rectus muscle only when the eye was adducted. Subsequent electromyographic studies suggested that DURS was a neurogenic disorder in which branches of the oculomotor nerve innervated the lateral rectus muscle. These studies also provided evidence that retraction of the globe, once thought to have a mechanical cause, was produced by a co-contraction of horizontal rectus muscles.

Huber et al.[12] distinguished three types of DURS based on electromyographic recordings and speculated on the pathophysiology of each type (Table 85.1). The Duane I type consists of limited or absent abduction with relatively normal adduction (Figs. 85.3 and 85.4); Duane II consists of limited or absent adduction with relatively normal abduction (Figs. 85.5 and 85.6); and Duane III is characterized by limited abduction and adduction. The findings of Huber et al. suggested that in all cases, an anomaly of ocular motor innervation involving the oculomotor and abducens nerves was responsible.

The phenomenon of anomalous oculomotor nerve innervation as the cause of DURS is also consistent with autopsy studies that show the occasional occurrence of anomalous innervation of the extraocular muscles. Until 1980, however, the only pathologic study performed on a patient with DURS was that of Matteuci,[13] who reported the autopsy findings in a well-documented case of unilateral DURS. Gross examination showed no abducens nerve on the affected side. Histologically, the abducens nucleus was hypoplastic, the lateral rectus muscle was fibrotic, and the medial rectus muscle was hypertrophic. The innervation of the lateral

Table 85.1 Types of Duane syndrome and their electromyography findings

	Abduction	Adduction	Retraction	Strabismus	EMG
Type 1	Poor	Good	On adduction	Ortho or small ET	LR discharges on adduction MR normal
Type 2	Decreased	Variable	On adduction	XT	LR discharges on adduction and abduction MR normal
Type 3	Poor	Poor	On adduction	Variable	LR+MR discharge in all positions

After Huber et al.[12]

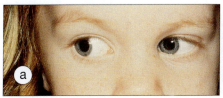
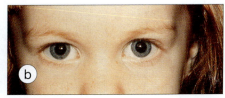
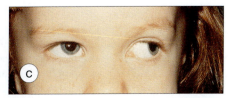

Fig. 85.5 Unilateral (right) Duane retraction syndrome type II in a 3-year-old girl. Note full abduction of right eye on right gaze and moderate limitation of adduction with upshoot of right eye on attempted left gaze.

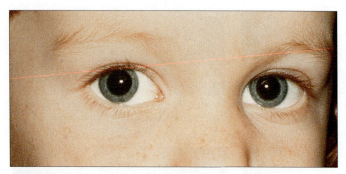

Fig. 85.6 Unilateral (right) Duane retraction syndrome type II. Same patient as that in Fig. 85.5 showing patient's normal head position consists of a face turn to the left to maintain binocularity.

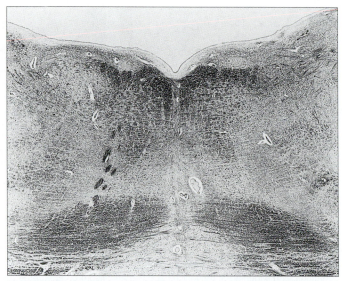

Fig. 85.7 Cross section through pons in a patient with left Duane retraction syndrome type I shows intact right abducens nucleus and fascicle. The left abducens nucleus contains no motoneurons and the left abducens fascicle is absent.

rectus muscle was not discussed, nor were the terminal branches of the oculomotor nerve followed.

In 1980, Hotchkiss et al.[14] reported pathologic findings in a 52-year-old woman with bilateral DURS who died of metastatic carcinoma. The abducens nuclei and nerves were absent bilaterally, and the lateral rectus muscles were partially innervated by branches from the inferior division of the oculomotor nerves. The lateral rectus muscles were fibrotic in areas lacking innervation but appeared relatively normal where innervated. Similar findings were subsequently reported by Hickey and Wagoner[15] in a patient with congenital, bilateral abnormalities of horizontal gaze but in whom the diagnosis of DURS was not apparent prior to death.

Miller et al.[16] reported the complete pathologic findings in a 43-year-old woman with a left-sided DURS (type I). The patient's eye movement disorder was verified clinically and electro-oculographically before her death from metastatic carcinoma. In this patient, the right side of the brainstem, the right cavernous sinus, and the right orbit were normal. The left abducens nucleus contained no cell bodies of abducens motoneurons, but in its rostral portion, there were many small cell bodies believed by the investigators to be internuclear neurons. The left abducens fascicle and nerve were absent (Figs. 85.7–85.9), and the left lateral rectus muscle was innervated by branches from the inferior division of the oculomotor nerve (Figs. 85.10 and 85.11). As in the case reported by Hotchkiss et al.,[14] the affected lateral rectus muscle was fibrotic in those areas not innervated.

The findings of Hotchkiss et al.[14] and of Miller et al.[16] are consistent not only with the results of electromyographic studies, but also with the work of Jay and Hoyt,[17] who found abnormalities of the brainstem auditory-evoked responses in patients with DURS. In those patients with bilateral DURS, the abnormalities were bilateral, whereas in the unilateral cases, the abnormalities were ipsilateral to the affected side. In addition, the presumption by Miller et al.[16] that abducens internuclear neurons were present in the abducens nucleus on the affected side in their patient is consistent with the findings of other investigators that adducting saccades in the normal eye of patients with unilateral DURS (type I) usually have normal velocities.[18]

It thus seems clear that DURS is caused by neurogenic brainstem ocular motor dysfunction. Indeed, 30–50% of patients with DURS have associated congenital neurologic deficits that localize to the brainstem, such as crocodile tears and sensorineural hearing loss or structural defects involving ocular, skeletal, and neural structures.

Most cases of DURS are sporadic, but familial unilateral and bilateral cases occur.[19] Familial DURS usually is transmitted in an autosomal dominant pattern. Affected individuals in such families show substantial clinical diversity.

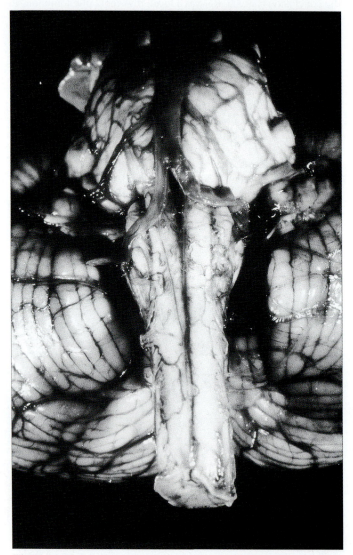

Fig. 85.8 Ventral surface of brainstem in same patient as that in Fig. 85.7 shows abducens nerve on right but no abducens nerve on left.

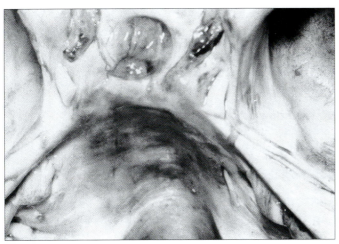

Fig. 85.9 View of clivus in same patient as Figs. 85.7 and 85.8 shows abducens nerve on right but no nerve on left.

DURS1 phenotype

In this phenotype, the syndrome is usually bilateral and, depending on the size of the deletion, may occur in association with other features including mental retardation, branchio-oto-renal syndrome, genital tract anomalies, and other somatic mutations. The gene disrupted by a balanced translocation at the DURS1 locus is *CPAH*, a carboxypeptidase gene.[20] The gene has been reported to reside on chromosome 8 (8q13).[21,22]

DURS2 phenotype

In this phenotype, the syndrome may be unilateral or bilateral. Associated findings can include a variety of vertical deviations such as apparent underaction of the superior oblique and dissociated vertical deviation. Patients have been noted to have decreased abduction with or without decreased adduction. No patients have had adduction defects without abduction defects. Amblyopia is common. No associated somatic abnormalities have been found. Inheritance is autosomal dominant, with the responsible gene being located on chromosome 2 (2q31).[23,24]

DRRS phenotype

This condition, also called the Duane radial ray or the Okihiro syndrome, is characterized by a unilateral or bilateral Duane syndrome plus radial dysplasia. The radial dysplasia can be

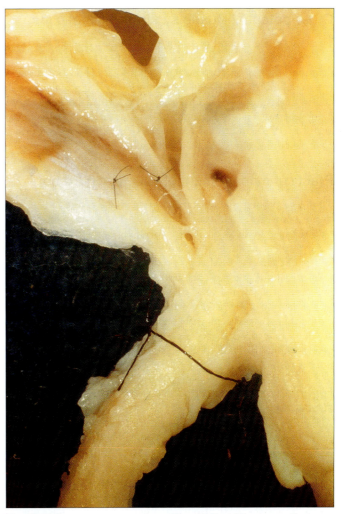

Fig. 85.10 Gross appearance of a portion of left orbit in same patient as that in Figs. 85.7–85.9 shows that the left oculomotor nerve (around which is tied a large black suture) innervates the left lateral rectus muscle (nerve branches tied with small black sutures).

unilateral or bilateral. Thumb hypoplasia is most common, but the defect ranges from hypoplasia of the thenar eminence to phocomelic limbs. The syndrome often includes deafness and somatic malformations. Inheritance is autosomal dominant. Truncating *SALL4* mutations on chromosome 20 (20q13) have been identified in DRRS families.[25,26] *SALL* genes encode putative zinc finger transcription factors.

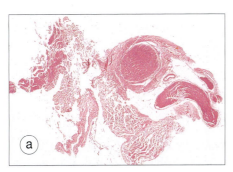
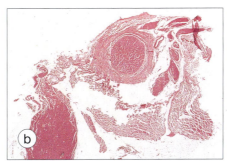
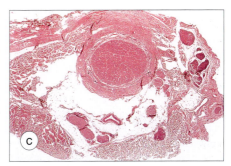

Fig. 85.11 Histopathologic appearance of left orbit in same patient as that in Figs. 85.7–85.10 shows in three successive cross sections (a-c) that the left oculomotor nerve innervates the left lateral rectus muscle.

Other potential Duane syndrome genetic loci

These have been found on chromosome 22 at 22pter→22q11.2 in three isolated cases with supernumerary markers or a deletion[27–29] and on chromosome 4 at 4q27–31 in one subject with a deletion[30] and also in association with Reiger syndrome in another case;[31] however, Ott et al.[32] performed linkage studies in members of a large Hispanic family showing autosomal inheritance for DURS and found no linkage to candidate loci on either of these chromosomes or on chromosome 8.

Practical management of Duane syndrome

The basic problem in Duane syndrome cannot be fixed by any means; however, there are a number of ways in which these children may be helped if their symptoms warrant intervention.

Any associated strabismus, amblyopia, or refractive error must be treated and reviewed appropriately.

The majority of patients with Duane syndrome have few problems other than a head turn and do not require surgery, but reassurance that the head posture is compensatory and, as such, a good thing that is helping the child to use the two eyes together. Teachers may need to be appraised of the situation, and they need to allow the child to sit to the side of the class to which the head is turned.

For an abnormal head posture (AHP) associated with strabismus

AHPs only cause problems if they are large. An AHP will not cause abnormalities of growth of the cervical spine unless the AHP is permanent and large, so indications for treatment are symptoms of neck ache and an AHP that is large and cosmetically significant. If there are complaints of cosmetic problems and teasing when the AHP is small, then the basic problem is probably not the AHP itself but other factors that may not be improved by surgery.

For an AHP with esotropia, ipsilateral medial rectus recession is required; if AHP is large, bilateral medial rectus recession should be carried out, although caution must be exercised to avoid consecutive exodeviations. The amounts of surgery performed are very individual to the surgeon and guidelines are inappropriate. Horizontal transposition of the vertical rectus muscles and posterior fixation sutures have been advocated but results of simple recessions are sufficiently good in nearly all cases to make these procedures unnecessary and may further restrict ductions.

For the rare cases of exotropia, recession of the ipsilateral lateral rectus is required, the amount varying with the angle in the primary position, whether there is marked restriction and retraction.

For marked retraction and narrowing of the palpebral fissure

Eye retraction and the consequent narrowing of the palpebral fissure is a cardinal feature of Duane syndrome; it is caused by co-contraction of the medial and lateral recti. Only very rarely is it severe enough to warrant surgery for this reason alone. Nevertheless, weakening of the medial or lateral rectus for other reasons, such as an anomalous head position, is invariably accompanied by a reduction in the retraction. It is unusual for young children to have sufficient retraction to need surgery but some have an increasing retraction caused by a horizontal rectus, usually the lateral rectus, being "tight," with an abnormal forced duction test. If this becomes cosmetically significant then a large

lateral rectus recession may help: it must be accompanied by a recession of the ipsilateral medial rectus to prevent further strabismus. This an effective procedure but unpredictable, so appropriate preoperative counseling is mandatory and surgical guidelines are inappropriate as the amounts of surgery performed are individual to the surgeon.

Up- and downshoots

"Shoots" are rarely or perhaps never due to a misinnervation: if they were, the up- or downshoot would be present from birth, which it rarely is proven to be. It is usually due to progressive stiffness of the lateral rectus, which on attempted adduction slips under (to give an upshoot) or over (downshoot) the globe. It can be effectively treated by a large recession of the affected lateral rectus, balanced by a medial rectus recession on the same side. The amounts recessed depend on the amount of the shoot, the magnitude of any strabismus, and the presence of marked retraction. Some authorities have suggested the use of posterior fixation sutures on the lateral rectus muscle. A current fashion is to longitudinally split and recess the two split portions of the lateral rectus, thus cradling the eye in between the split portions: a nice idea, effective, but probably no better than a large recession!

HORIZONTAL GAZE PALSY

Congenital paralysis of conjugate horizontal eye movements (Fig. 85.12) may occur as an isolated sporadic finding, or it may be hereditary. Phillips et al.[33] described the autopsy findings in a child with isolated bilateral horizontal gaze palsy. Histologically, abducens nuclei were present but were thought to be hypoplastic. Several nerve fibers extended from the nuclei into the pons for about one-quarter of the normal distance. No abducens nerves could be identified grossly. Brainstem hypoplasia has also been described in familial cases of horizontal gaze palsy associated with scoliosis (see below).

Congenital absence of abduction, either alone or as part of a horizontal gaze palsy, is usually observed in association with other neurologic or systemic anomalies. For example, patients with cerebral palsy seem to have an increased prevalence of congenital abducens paresis. In addition, congenital paralysis of both abduction and horizontal gaze occur in patients with a variety of skeletal abnormalities, including Klippel-Feil syndrome, ear dysplasia, and progressive kyphoscoliosis. In particular, familial cases of kyphoscoliosis in association with congenital horizontal gaze palsy are not uncommon and, as noted above, have been found to be associated with evidence of brainstem hypoplasia. Unilateral agenesis of the abducens nucleus and nerve may occur in the syndrome of oculoauriculovertebral dysplasia and hemifacial microsomia, and the cervico-oculo-acoustic syndrome (Wildevank syndrome) may be associated with a Klippel-Feil anomaly, congenital sensory neural deafness, and bilateral abducens nerve palsy. Other anomalies seen in this syndrome include short stature, microcephaly, mental retardation, and cleft palate.

The only phenotype for which a genetic locus has been identified is the HGPS phenotype, in which there is congenital complete absence of conjugate horizontal gaze and childhood onset progressive scoliosis. Affected individuals have no associated ptosis or somatic abnormalities. Some patients may have nystagmus, esotropia, and/or retraction on adduction.

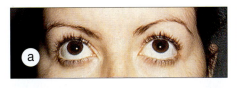
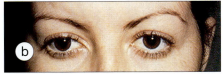
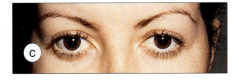
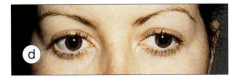
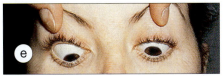

Fig. 85.12 Congenital paralysis of horizontal gaze. Note intact vertical movements. (a) Patient looking up. (b) Patient in primary gaze. (c) Patient attempting to look right. (d) Patient attempting to look left. (e) Patient looking down.

Inheritance is autosomal recessive. The locus is on chromosome 11 (11q23–25).[34]

Congenital horizontal gaze palsy is thought to result from agenesis of the abducens nucleus including both alpha motoneurons and interneurons.

MÖBIUS SYNDROME

Congenital facial weakness can be accompanied by an ocular motility disorder that usually includes abduction weakness. We reserve the eponym "Möbius syndrome" for the combination of facial weakness and either an abduction deficit in one or both eyes or a horizontal gaze paresis. Möbius syndrome is usually a sporadic disorder frequently accompanied by lingual or pharyngeal dysfunction at birth, craniofacial dysmorphisms, and limb malformations. Several cytogenetic abnormalities have been reported in association with Möbius syndrome.

Characteristically, the defect in Möbius syndrome involves the face and horizontal gaze mechanisms bilaterally. Affected patients have a mask-like facies, with the mouth constantly held open (Figs. 85.13 and 85.14). In some infants, this defect prevents adequate nursing and the appearance may interfere with normal bonding and attachment. The eyelids often cannot be completely closed, and in some patients, they cannot be closed at all. There may be excess lacrimation and epiphora. Some patients have only an esotropia (Fig. 85.13) associated with unilateral or bilateral limitation of abduction, and some may even be able to converge. In most cases, however, the eyes are straight but do not move horizontally (Fig. 85.14). Henderson[35] reviewed 61 cases of Möbius syndrome in the literature, commenting that bilateral abducens palsy was present in 43 cases, unilateral abducens palsy in two cases, and horizontal gaze palsy in the rest. In rare cases, vertical eye movements are also abnormal.

Other congenital defects found in patients with Möbius syndrome include deafness, webbed fingers or toes, supernumerary digits, defects of the muscles of the chest, neck, and tongue, and even absence of the hands, feet, fingers, or toes (Fig. 85.15). Abnormalities of lower cranial nerves, with speech and swallowing difficulties, are extremely common. Occurring less frequently are low-set ears, a small mouth opening, micrognathia, epicanthal folds, congenital heart defects, or a combination of these abnormalities. Tachypnea and other respiratory difficulties occur in some patients with Möbius syndrome, whereas others have a combination of anosmia and hypogonadotrophic hypogonadism (Kallmann syndrome). A case of Möbius syndrome associated with a ventricular septal defect has been described, but it is unclear whether these two conditions were related or coincidental. Many patients with Möbius syndrome have some degree of mental retardation, and some degree of autism also is common.

Patients with Möbius syndrome who undergo neuroimaging have the same heterogeneity of findings as their variable clinical presentation would suggest. Some show no abnormalities, where-

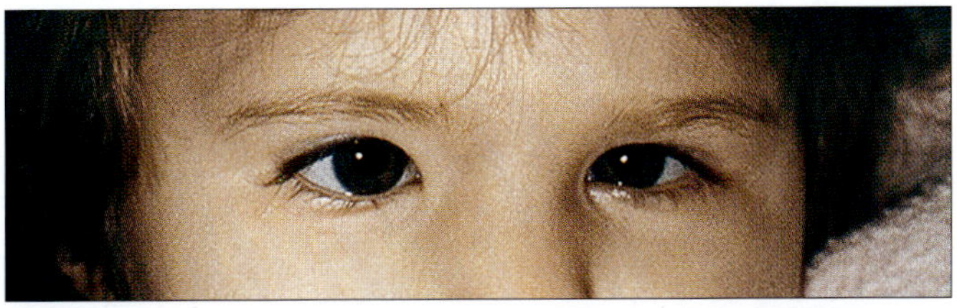

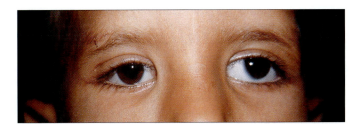

Fig. 85.14 Möbius syndrome in a 6-year-old boy. Note bilateral facial weakness associated with mild bilateral ptosis. The patient's eyes are fairly straight.

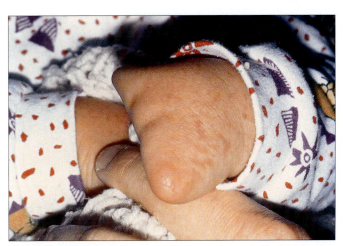

Fig. 85.15 Absent fingers in same patient as that seen in Fig. 85.13. (Image courtesy of Dr Michael X Repka.)

Fig. 85.13 Möbius syndrome in a 3-year-old girl. Note esotropia and bilateral facial weakness. (Image courtesy of Dr Michael X Repka.)

as others show intracranial calcifications, brainstem hypoplasia, or changes consistent with ischemia.

Most cases of Möbius syndrome are sporadic. Although dominant pedigrees occur, the author is aware of only two families with primary skeletal anomalies associated with a Möbius facies and ocular motor dysfunction in more than one member.[36,37] Baraitser[38] concluded that the risk is no greater than 2% for another affected sibling in pedigrees in which the syndrome includes limb abnormalities.

Pathologic findings in patients with Möbius syndrome were separated by Towfighi et al.[39] into four groups according to the neuropathologic findings in the brainstem nuclei. Group I consisted of four cases with hypoplasia or atrophy of cranial nerve nuclei. These cases were associated with an absence of, or decrease in, the number of neurons in the affected cranial nerve nuclei. The remaining neurons in affected nuclei were either small or of normal size. Products of neuron degeneration were absent. Three of these cases had other associated anomalies, including hypoplasia of the inferior olive and other brainstem nuclei, heterotopic immature cells in cranial nerve nuclei, and musculoskeletal or vertebral malformations. Because there were no signs of necrosis or degenerations in these cases, and because of the associated malformations, it was concluded that the CNS lesions were caused by maldevelopment rather than by acquired insults later in life.

Group II consisted of two cases in which, in addition to neuronal loss, there was evidence of active neuronal degeneration in the affected facial nerve nuclei. It was postulated that these neuronal changes were caused by physical injury to the facial nerve, arising from a malformed temporal bone or from application of forceps during delivery. Some of the reported cases of Möbius syndrome associated with peripheral neuropathy or motoneuron disease may belong in this category.

Group III consisted of six cases in which, in addition to a decrease in the number of neurons and reactive changes in the affected cranial nerve nuclei, there was frank necrosis of the tegmentum of the lower pons. The necrotic foci were located in the paramedian pons and generally contained both calcium and iron deposits. These lesions are probably acquired later during fetal life rather than during early embryonic development, and both hypoxia and viral infections are implicated in their etiology. Vulnerability to hypoxia of the brainstem nuclei in the immature brain of humans and experimental animals appears to support the hypoxic theory.

Group IV consisted of three cases in which no lesions were found in the brainstem or cranial nerves. A primary myopathy may have been responsible for these cases.[39]

The diversity of pathologic findings in patients with Möbius syndrome suggests that the syndrome actually is, in fact, a heterogeneous group of congenital disorders caused by developmental defects related to a variety of insults, such as ischemia or toxic effects of prenatal prescribed drugs, such as misoprostol, a synthetic prostaglandin, or one of the benzodiazepines. To date, two phenotypes with responsible genotypes have been identified.

MBS1 phenotype

One patient with unilateral facial weakness, bilateral abduction weakness, tongue hypoplasia, and micrognathia associated with deletion of 13q12.2–13 was reported.[40] In addition, a family with seven members who had facial weakness, ptosis, hearing loss, and finger malformations (flexion contractures) but who lacked abduction weakness was associated with a reciprocal translocation (1:13) (p34;q13).[41]

MBS4 phenotype

A de novo case with the Möbius phenotype and Poland syndrome, cleft palate, dextrocardia, mandibular hypoplasia, and hand deformities associated with a translocation (1:11) (p22;p13) was described.[42] Another de novo case with ptosis, loss of upgaze but normal gaze in other directions, facial weakness, malformed ears, and developmental delay associated with a translocation (1:2) (p22.3;q21.1) was also described.[43]

Practical management of Möbius syndrome

Most patients with Möbius syndrome do not require strabismus surgery because they have bilateral horizontal gaze paresis; however, some children have strabismus characterized by an esotropia. Treatment in such cases includes bilateral medial rectus recessions, medial rectus recession combined with lateral rectus resection, and, in severe cases, muscle transposition. A reasonable cosmetic appearance can be achieved in many cases: one operation to achieve this is aimed at but not often achieved.

If there is an associated corneal anesthesia the cornea is at risk, especially because of the abnormality of blinking, which makes exposure keratitis particularly a problem in infancy. All the usual methods of treating exposure keratitis are used but in infants and young children with a combination of a VII and V nerve palsy, a tarsorrhaphy may be indicated early if the risk of blindness from keratitis outweighs the risk of amblyopia, the management of which is made more difficult by the tarsorrhaphy.

SUMMARY

Based on both neuropathologic and genetic evidence, it is clear that there exists a group of disorders for which absent or anomalous innervation of the extraocular and/or facial muscles is the most likely pathophysiology. These disorders are appropriately referred to as "congenital cranial dysinnervation disorders." As currently conceived, the congenital strabismus syndromes classified as CCDDs would include CFEOM types 1, 2, and 3, congenital ptosis, Duane retraction syndrome, Duane radial ray syndrome, congenital horizontal gaze palsy with scoliosis, and Möbius syndrome. The CCDDs also include developmental disorders of nonocular cranial nerves, such as congenital familial facial weakness. The above list of clinical phenotypes and genetic loci is almost certainly incomplete and will undoubtedly increase with time.

REFERENCES

1. Johnson LV. Adherence syndrome (pseudoparalysis lateral or superior rectus muscles). Arch Ophthalmol 1950; 44: 870–88.

2. Engle EC, Goumnerov BC, McKeown CA, et al., Oculomotor nerve and muscle abnormalities in congenital fibrosis of the extraocular muscles. Ann Neurol 1997; 41: 314–25.

3. Yazdani A, Traboulsi EI. Classification and surgical management of patients with familial and sporadic forms of congenital fibrosis of the extraocular muscles. Ophthalmology 2004; 111: 1035–42.

4. Engle EC, Kunkel LM, Specht LA, et al. Mapping a gene for congenital fibrosis of the extraocular muscles to the centromeric region of chromosome 12. Nat Genetics 1994; 7: 69–73.

5. Engle EC, McIntosh N, Yamada K, et al. CFEOM1, the classical form of congenital fibrosis of the extraocular muscles, is genetically heterogeneous but does not result from mutations in ARIX. BMC Genet 2002; 3: 3.

6. Yazdani A, Chung B, Abbaszadegan MR, et al. A novel PHOX2A/ARIX mutation in an Iranian family with congenital fibrosis of extraocular muscles type 2 (CFEOM2). Am J Ophthalmol 2003; 136: 861–5.

7. Traboulsi IE, Lee BA, Mousawi A, et al. Evidence of genetic heterogeneity in autosomal recessive congenital fibrosis of the extraocular muscles. Am J Ophthalmol 2000; 129: 658–62.

8. Doherty EJ, Macy ME, Wang SM, et al. CFEOM 3: a new extraocular congenital fibrosis syndrome that maps to 16q24.2–q24.3. Invest Ophthalmol Vis Sci 1999; 40: 1687–94.

9. Mackey DA, Chan WM, Chan C, et al. Congenital fibrosis of the vertically acting extraocular muscles maps to the FEOM3 locus. Hum Genet 2002; 110: 510–2.

10. Duane A. Congenital deficiency of abduction, associated with impairment of adduction, retraction movements, contractions of the palpebral fissure and oblique movements of the eye. Arch Ophthalmol 1905; 34: 133–59.

11. Breinin GM. Electromyography: a tool in ocular and neurologic diagnosis. II. Muscle palsy. Arch Ophthalmol 1957; 57: 165–75.

12. Huber A, Esslen E, Kloti R, et al. Zum problem des Duane syndromes. Graefes Arch Klin Exp Ophthalmol 1964; 167: 169–91.

13. Matteuci P. I difetti congenit di abduzione con particolare riguardo alia patogenesi. Rass Ital Ottalmol 1946; 15: 345–80.

14. Hotchkiss MG, Miller NR, Clark AW, et al. Bilateral Duane's retraction syndrome: a clinical-pathologic case report. Arch Ophthalmol 1980; 98: 870–4.

15. Hickey WF, Wagoner MD. Bilateral congenital absence of the abducens nerve. Virchows Arch Pathol Anat Histopathol 1983; 402: 91–8.

16. Miller NR, Kiel SM, Green WR, et al. Unilateral Duane's retraction syndrome (type 1). Arch Ophthalmol 1982; 100: 1468–72.

17. Jay WM, Hoyt CS. Abnormal brain stem auditory-evoked potentials in Stilling-Turk-Duane retraction syndrome. Am J Ophthalmol 1980; 89: 814–8.

18. Gourdeau A, Miller NRM, Zee DS, et al. Central ocular motor abnormalities in Duane's retraction syndrome. Arch Ophthalmol 1981; 99: 1809–10.

19. Chung M, Stout JT, Borchert MS. Clinical diversity of hereditary Duane's retraction syndrome. Ophthalmology 2000; 107: 500–3.

20. Pizzuti A, Calabrese G, Bozzali M, et al. A peptidase gene in chromosome 8q is disrupted by a balanced translocation in a Duane syndrome patient. Invest Ophthalmol Vis Sci 2002; 43: 3609–12.

21. Vincent C, Kalatzis V, Compain S, et al. A proposed new contiguous gene syndrome on 8q consists of Branchio-Oto-Renal (BOR) syndrome, Duane syndrome, a dominant form of hydrocephalus and trapeze aplasia; implications for the mapping of the BOR gene. Hum Mol Genet 1994; 3: 1859–66.

22. Calabrese G, Telvi L, Capodiferro F, et al. Narrowing the Duane syndrome critical region at chromosome 8q13 down to 40kb. Eur J Hum Genet 2000; 8: 319–24.

23. Appukuttan B, Gillanders E, Juo SH, et al. Localization of a gene for Duane retraction syndrome to chromosome 2q31. Am J Hum Genet 1999; 65: 1639–46.

24. Evans JC, Frayling TM, Ellard S, et al. Confirmation of linkage of Duane's syndrome and refinement of the disease locus to an 8.8cM interval on chromosome 2q31. Hum Genet 2000; 106: 636–8.

25. Al-Baradie R, Yamada K, St. Hilaire C, et al. Duane radial ray syndrome (Okihiro syndrome) maps to 20q13 and results from mutations in SALL4, a new member of the SAL family. Am J Hum Genet 2002; 71: 1195–9.

26. Kohlhase J, Heinrich M, Schubert, L, et al. Okihiro syndrome is caused by SALL4 mutations. Hum Mol Genet 2002; 11: 2979–87.

27. Cullen P, Rodgers CS, Callen DF, et al. Association of familial Duane anomaly and urogenital abnormalities with a bisatellited marker derived from chromosome 22. Am J Med Genet 1993; 47: 925–30.

28. Tibiletti MG, Sala E, Colombo D, et al. Chromosome 22 marker in a child with Duane syndrome and urogenital abnormalities. Ann Genet 1996; 39: 168–72.

29. Versteegh FG, von Lindern JS, Kemper J, et al. Duane retraction syndrome, a new feature in 22q11 deletion syndrome? Clin Dysmorphol 2000; 9: 135–7.

30. Chew CK, Foster P, Hurst JA, et al. Duane's retraction syndrome associated with chromosome 4q27–31 segment deletion. Am J Ophthalmol 1995; 119: 807–9.

31. Gregg FM. A case report of both Duane's syndrome and Rieger's anomaly in a single patient. Eur J Ophthalmol 1992; 2: 201–2.

32. Ott S, Borchert M, Chung M, et al. Exclusion of candidate genetic loci for Duane retraction syndrome. Am J Ophthalmol 1999; 127: 358–60.

33. Phillips WJ, Dirion JK, Graves GO. Congenital bilateral palsy of the abducens. Arch Ophthalmol 1932; 10: 355–64.

34. Jen J, Coulin CJ, Bosley TM, et al. Familial horizontal gaze palsy with progressive scoliosis maps to chromosome 11q23–25. Neurology 2002; 59: 432–5.

35. Henderson JL. The congenital facial diplegia syndrome: Clinical features, pathology and aetiology. Brain 1939; 62: 381–403.

36. Hicks AM. Congenital paralysis of lateral rotators of eyes with paralysis of muscles of face. Arch Ophthalmol 1943; 30: 38–43.

37. Wishnick MM, Nelson LB, Huppert L, et al. Möebius syndrome and limb abnormalities with dominant inheritance. Ophthalmic Pediatr Gen 1983; 2: 77–81.

38. Baraitser M. Genetics of Möbius syndrome. J Med Genet 1977; 14: 415–7.

39. Towfighi J, Marks K, Palmer E, et al. Möbius syndrome. Neuropathologic observations. Acta Neuropathol 1979; 48: 11–7.

40. Slee JJ, Smart RD, Viloen DL. Deletion of chromosome 13 in Möbius syndrome. J Med Genet 1991; 28: 413–4.

41. Zitter FA, Wiser WC, Robinson A. Three generation pedigree of a Möbius syndrome variant with chromosome translocation. Arch Neurol 1977; 34: 437–42.

42. Donahue SP, Wenger SL, Steele MW, et al. Broad-spectrum Möbius syndrome associated with a 1;11 chromosome translocation. Ophthalmic Paediatr Genet 1993; 14: 17–21.

43. Nishikawa M, Ichiyama T, Hayashi T, et al. Möbius-like syndrome associated with a 1;2 chromosome translocation. Clin Genet 1997; 51: 122–3.

44. Gillies WE, Harris AJ, Brooks AM, et al. Congenital fibrosis of the vertically acting extraocular muscles. A new group of dominantly inherited ocular fibrosis with radiologic findings. Ophthalmology 1995; 102: 607–12.

Cranial Nerve and Eye Muscle Diseases

John S Elston

INTRODUCTION

An ocular motor palsy (i.e., a third, fourth, or sixth nerve palsy) in a child may be congenital or acquired, isolated or in combination, and may occur with or without additional cranial neuropathy or neurological signs. This chapter is concerned with the presentation, diagnosis, and investigation of such problems, but not with management except in terms of appropriate acute referral.

Epidemiology

Children with third, fourth, and sixth nerve palsies, or combinations of palsies, present to a wide range of different health professionals. Congenital palsies are usually evident in the first weeks or months of life and will initially be assessed by neonatologists and pediatricians. However, some congenital fourth nerve palsies are diagnosed in preschool children on routine examination (screening) by an orthoptist. Acquired palsies may present via primary care physicians to ophthalmologists, pediatricians, pediatric neurologists, or neurosurgeons. The registration and collection of data from these and other sources is variable so it is difficult to obtain representative information on the incidence and prevalence of congenital and acquired ocular motor palsies.

There are two important sources of data. The first is a series of institutional surveys from the 1960's onward originating from tertiary referral centers, which rely on referrals from ophthalmologists, pediatric neurologists, neurosurgeons, and neuro-oncologists as this expertise is usually available on site. There is an over-representation of complicated cases, which have had extensive investigation. In many cases the ophthalmological features will have been discovered as a result of interspecialist referral, and these cases are not representative of those who present primarily to the pediatric ophthalmologist. Moreover, in the earlier studies in the literature the lack of modern imaging and other diagnostic modalities limits the applicability of the findings to contemporary practice.

Harley's review of 121 cases[1] emphasized the frequency of malignancy as an underlying cause: the development of an ocular motor palsy in a child was "an ominous sign." However, in a later study of 160 acquired cases, with a mean age of 9.4 years, trauma was the commonest cause (42.5%) with neoplasm second (16.9%), and in 14.4% the cause was not determined.[2] Fifty percent were sixth nerve palsies, about 25% third, and 10% fourth or multiple. A number of the palsies occurred after surgery or meningitis and a large number of different diagnoses accounted for single cases. In this and in most other more recent surveys boys outnumber girls, probably because of the contribution of trauma.[3,4] The commonest neoplasm listed is brainstem glioma, accounting for 12 of the 33 cases of tumor, and most commonly causing a sixth nerve palsy. However, of the 18 children presenting with sixth nerve palsy due to neoplasm,

15 had other neurological signs and symptoms at presentation, for example, facial palsy, ataxia, dysarthria, or papilledema, making identification of this subgroup easier. Two-thirds of the cases of isolated ocular motor palsy had known metastatic cancer at presentation, leaving only one brainstem glioma presenting with a truly isolated sixth nerve palsy. In a survey of third nerve palsies in children (54 cases) about 25% were congenital and three-quarters of the acquired group were due to trauma. Neoplasm accounted for only 2 cases, and both had additional signs.[3]

The consensus from the recent surveys is that amongst acquired palsies, trauma is the commonest cause and neoplasm next but almost invariably in the context of either known tumor or other predominating symptoms. The tumors responsible are generally primary and infratentorial, and the palsy is often secondary to neurosurgical intervention.

The second source of data on childhood ocular motor palsies is from population-based studies. The important contribution of this sort is from Olmsted County, Minnesota.[5] Over a 15-year period, 36 cases were identified in 35 children. In this semiurban, predominantly white US population, the age- and sex-adjusted annual incidence of pediatric third, fourth, and sixth nerve palsies combined was 7.6 per 100,000. The most commonly affected nerve was the fourth (36%) followed by the sixth (33%), third (22%), and multiple (9%). As much as 94% of the total were unilateral, and overall the commonest cause was congenital, then trauma, then undetermined. Many of the congenital fourth nerve palsies were asymptomatic and found on screening. Of the 3 cases of all palsies due to neoplasm, two had sixth nerve palsies (one bilateral) and one a third but in no case did an intracranial tumor present as an isolated nerve palsy.

Conclusion

The majority of third, fourth, and sixth nerve palsies are referred to the ophthalmologist with an established etiology, or known to be congenital. Occasionally an isolated ocular motor palsy presents and requires full evaluation and investigation. In these cases a detailed history and a full ophthalmological examination are required. Most of these children will then require referral to a pediatric neurologist for investigation, including neuroimaging. The majority are found to have a benign cause.

CRANIAL NERVE PALSIES

Third nerve palsy

Congenital

This is a rare condition and, in the vast majority of cases, unilateral. All bilateral congenital third nerve palsies are associated with additional neurological signs due to anomalous brain development or prenatal brain damage.[6]

Congenital third nerve palsy presents with ptosis, exotropia, and hypotropia of the involved eye. The extent of extraocular muscle and levator involvement varies. The pupil may be normal or either larger or smaller (Fig. 86.1) than the uninvolved side at presentation.

There are two sites of damage. A lesion of the peripheral third nerve may be responsible, in which case the damage occurs in the perinatal period. Alternatively the third nerve fascicles or some or all of the nucleus may be damaged either by:

1. A primary midbrain maldevelopment;
2. Intrauterine injury (vascular, infective, or secondary to a teratogenic agent); or
3. Perinatal damage.

Neurological associations

Approximately 50% of children with a congenital oculomotor palsy have associated neurological or other physical signs.[7] The commonest associations are cerebral palsy, ipsi- or contralateral hemiparesis/plegia, and developmental delay. Neuroimaging may show midbrain hypoplasia or other more widespread developmental brain anomaly. Such abnormalities may be due to a demonstrable lesion (Fig. 86.2), secondary to unknown prenatal

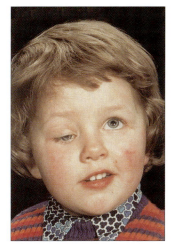
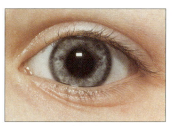
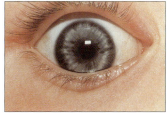

Fig. 86.1 Congenital right third nerve palsy. Congenital third nerve palsy with the smaller pupil on the affected side.

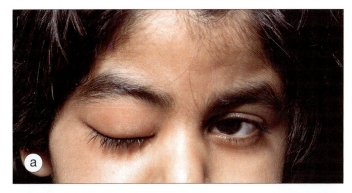

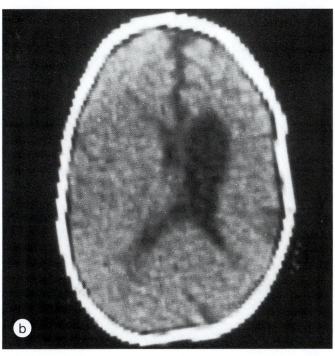

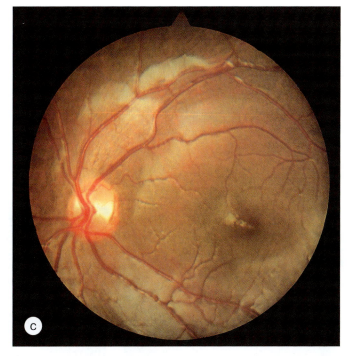

Fig. 86.2 Congenital right third nerve palsy possibly associated with amniocentesis. (a) The right ptosis was present from birth when the child failed to open the eye. (b) There was a right porencephalic cyst. (c) The left optic disc shows band atrophy, reflecting the associated temporal hemianopia in that eye.

insults or as a primary developmental anomaly. Birth hypoxia and trauma may cause third nerve palsy and other deficits.

Natural history

There are four possible outcomes in terms of the extent and pattern of recovery of congenital third nerve palsy:

1. Full (or partial) recovery with a normal innervational pattern. This is usually seen after peripheral trauma from stretching or deformation during delivery.

2. Misdirection-regeneration, probably reflecting more severe axonal damage with retrograde die back (chromatolysis) to the nucleus, and axonal regeneration with misdirection. The pattern of misdirection seen in congenital third nerve palsy usually resembles that seen after acquired third nerve palsy with characteristic features such as elevation of the ptotic lid on attempted adduction (Fig. 86.3) and downgaze and pupil contraction on adduction and upgaze. However, other patterns are also described.

   Peripheral misdirection of regenerating axons is probably responsible for these signs. However, the number and distribution of prenuclear inputs is affected when chromatolysis involves the nucleus, and central synaptic reorganization may be, in part, responsible for the abnormal pattern of third nerve function, explaining the stereotyped pattern of abnormal eye movements.

3. Cyclic oculomotor palsy. The child presents with a complete third nerve palsy, but with superimposed episodic activity in third nerve innervated muscles. The muscles involved are usually the levator, which may elevate to a normal position, or even retract, the superior and medial recti. A dilated pupil may constrict. These "spasms" of third nerve function are usually short-lived, lasting 30 seconds to a minute. The spasms may be induced by contralateral eye movement, or attempted fixation with the paretic eye, and may also occur unpredictably (i.e., spontaneously) and in sleep. It is

presumed that variable prenuclear activation of the motor neurons is responsible for this phenomenon.[8]

Bilateral asynchronous cyclic oculomotor palsy has been observed.

4. There may be no recovery. This applies equally to an isolated palsy, as to one associated with other neurological features.

Amblyopia

Amblyopia of the affected eye is not an invariable feature of congenital third nerve palsy at presentation, but is clearly a highly likely outcome. Anisometropic and astigmatic refractive errors are frequent. In some cases, fixation in the contralateral eye is abnormal, due to either an ocular developmental abnormality or nystagmus, in which case the paretic may be the preferred fixing eye.

Variants and congenital third nerve syndromes

Congenital palsy of an individual third nerve-innervated muscle is occasionally found. The commonest pattern involves the inferior rectus and inferior oblique or superior rectus and inferior oblique (congenital double elevator palsy). Differentiation from primary isolated ocular muscle fibrosis may be difficult, requiring a forced duction test.

Peripheral (orbital) pathology may occasionally present as a partial or complete congenital third nerve palsy. Examples are an anomalous posterior insertion of a medial rectus muscle and a perinatally rupturing dermoid cyst.

Isolated congenital medial rectus palsy with synergistic divergence of the eyes on attempted adduction of the affected eye is a recognized phenomenon. The majority of cases in the literature affect the left eye, and are isolated, i.e., have no associated developmental anomalies or neurology. The palpebral aperture usually narrows on attempted adduction with globe retraction. EMG studies suggest that it is a dysinnervation syndrome, analogous to Duane syndrome with (no) innervation

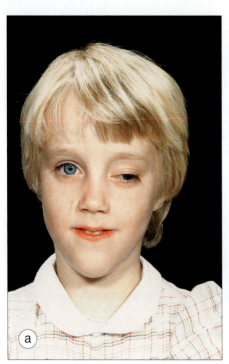 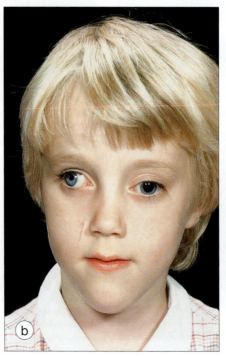 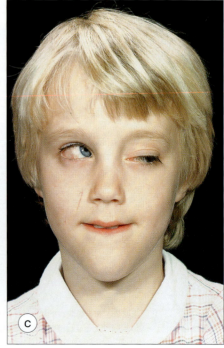

Fig. 86.3 Left third nerve palsy caused by "ophthalmoplegic migraine." (a) In the straight ahead position there is a left ptosis and dilated pupil and the eye is "down and out." (b) Looking right the lid elevates but the relative eye position and the pupil remains the same. (c) On looking left the ptosis increases.

of the medial rectus and aberrant third nerve innervation of the ipsilateral lateral rectus.

The vertical retraction syndrome may also cause confusion; these patients have a congenital abduction deficit with, in addition, globe retraction on up- and downgaze that can be shown on EMG recording to be due to synergistic muscle activity in the lateral rectus and superior rectus or inferior rectus.

There is increasing evidence that congenital fibrosis of the extraocular muscles (CFEOM) is a primary neuropathy, resulting from genetic mutations, causing a primary absence of all or part of the third nerve and other nuclei[9-11] (see Chapter 85).

Management
Awareness of the neurological and developmental deficits that may be associated with congenital third nerve palsy means a pediatric or neurological referral may be indicated.

The parents of a child with a congenital third nerve palsy need a clear explanation of the visual implications of the diagnosis in terms of vision in the affected eye and the lack of binocular development. The extent of recovery of third nerve function will determine what surgical treatment can be offered, and it is important the parents are sympathetically informed about what expectations are reasonable, especially in complete third nerve palsy. The limitations of both eye movement and ptosis surgery on paretic muscles need to be explained.

Amblyopia treatment can be surprisingly successful, even in unrecovered third nerve palsy, if started early enough. Anisometropia and astigmatism are common but accommodation is often relatively well preserved.

The surgical management, which is only undertaken after correction of refractive errors, amblyopia treatment, and allowing sufficient time to pass for maximum spontaneous recovery to take place, depends on the extent of the palsy. Horizontal and vertical rectus muscle recessions and resections (see Chapter 88) are useful in relatively mild cases, with traction sutures and large amounts of surgery in severe cases. Superior oblique transposition may be useful in cases with very limited movement. Ptosis surgery is usually performed, when necessary, after the eye muscle surgery.

Acquired
Introduction
The long-term implications of acquired third nerve palsy in childhood are determined by the age at onset and by the underlying cause. The pattern of recovery is also partly age-dependent, and in infancy cyclic oculomotor palsy may develop. Amblyopia and loss of binocular function are major risks in the visually immature child. The underlying pathology and location of the damage to the nerve will influence the extent of recovery.

Trauma, infection, tumor, and vascular causes, including migraine, are the likely etiologies.[2-4] The damage may involve the third nerve nucleus, the fascicles in the midbrain, or the nerve in the subarachnoid space, wall of the cavernous sinus, superior orbital fissure, or orbit. Topical diagnosis may be aided by the characteristics of the palsy, associated clinical signs, and knowledge of the disease process.

Nuclear third nerve palsies are rare and not well characterized in childhood. Bilateral signs are likely as the superior rectus subnucleus is contralateral to the peripheral nerve, and both levators supplied from a midline subnucleus. However, there is evidence from imaging studies that nuclear third nerve palsies may be partial and unilateral and even involve a single muscle palsy (except the levator). The pupils may be spared. Isolated bilateral ptosis is a recognized presentation.

Nuclear and fascicular third nerve palsy in childhood may be due to an inflammatory brainstem lesion (e.g., acute demyelinating encephalomyelitis, ADEM), infiltration (brainstem glioma), vascular malformation, or vasculitis.

A fascicular third nerve palsy may be complete or partial and can involve those muscles supplied by either the superior or inferior division of the nerve with or without pupil involvement. Monocular elevation ("double elevator") palsy can be due to a midbrain lesion. Topical diagnosis depends on the presence of other signs due to involvement of the adjacent structures, or the demonstration of a causative lesion on imaging.

The syndromes associated with fascicular third nerve palsy are Weber (plus contralateral hemiplegia/paresis) due to involvement of the corticospinal tracts and Benedikt (plus contralateral ataxia/tremor/involuntary movements) due to red nucleus damage. Weber syndrome has been described in hemophilia in childhood.

More commonly, the third nerve is damaged in its course through the subarachnoid space. Major head trauma is the commonest single cause often with additional damage to the brain and elsewhere. Postmortem and imaging studies indicate that the third nerve may be avulsed from the midbrain, and there is also imaging support for this localization in those surviving the trauma.[12] Alternatively, the nerve may be damaged as it enters the dura anteriorly. There may be intraneural hemorrhage. Particularly with structural damage close to the brainstem, secondary nuclear chromatolysis compromises recovery or leads to an abnormal pattern (misdirection-regeneration, see "Natural history").

The occurrence of third nerve (or other ocular motor nerve) palsy, after minor nonconcussive head trauma, should be treated with caution as it may indicate an underlying structural lesion compromising function.

Infection is the next commonest cause and usually a complication of acute bacterial meningitis. The damage is caused by microvascular occlusion and focal demyelination, producing a conduction block. Provided the underlying cause can be successfully treated, the prognosis for recovery is good.[13]

Basal meningitis caused by tuberculosis may involve the third nerve, often bilaterally with damage to the anterior visual pathways; the prognosis is poor.

Neurotropic virus infections, for example varicella and measles, can also rarely be complicated by third nerve palsy. Lyme borreliosis should also be considered. Postsystemic viral infection abducens palsy is well recognized (see "Benign lateral rectus palsy of childhood"), but there is evidence that occasionally a third nerve palsy may also result by the same mechanism.

The subarachnoid third nerve may be involved in infiltrative meningeal malignancies, such as lymphoma, leukemia, or leptomeningeal sarcoma. Raised intracranial pressure damages the third nerve by the mechanism of supratentorial herniation, causing focal ischemia.

Miller-Fisher syndrome
Ophthalmoparesis is a feature of the Miller-Fisher syndrome, a variant of Guillaine-Barré syndrome, associated with the presence of serum anti GQ1b IgG antibodies. The ophthalmoparesis may take the form of progressive, partial, or complete bilateral sixth, third or fourth nerve palsies, with pupil involvement. In partial ophthalmoparesis, oculocephalic maneuvers suggest a supranuclear element. However, the peripheral ocular motor nerves are principally involved and studies have shown that the GQ1b epitope is expressed in the paranodal region of the extramedullary portion of the ocular motor cranial nerves. The third nerve appears to be particularly vulnerable due to the extent of

expression.[14] The effect of the damage is to block impulse generation at nodes of Ranvier, but function slowly recovers either spontaneously or after treatment with plasmapheresis. Prior *Campylobacter jejuni* infection may be demonstrable, and a number of children in the first and second decades with this condition have been reported.[15]

Ophthalmoplegic migraine

A disorder characterized by childhood onset of acute painful unilateral third nerve palsy with pupil involvement spontaneously remitting, but often relapsing, has been designated "ophthalmoplegic migraine." There is an association with other types of migraine and often a family history of migraine. Attacks generally start in the first decade and resolve over weeks; systemic steroids may speed resolution. There is no mass or vascular lesion on brain imaging.

The clinical diagnosis is difficult, and even an initially negative image does not exclude a structural cause for a third nerve palsy in childhood.[16] Characteristic imaging findings have been described in ophthalmoplegic migraine–thickening and gadolinium enhancement of the cisternal segment of the third nerve on MRI at the onset of the palsy, followed by resolution of these signs as the palsy resolves.[17] Whether the cause is migraine or not, the diagnosis should not be made unless the characteristic imaging features are present. Some authors have argued that reversible thickening and enhancement of the third nerve is more likely to have an inflammatory than a vascular etiology and be due to a disease process "similar to Tolosa-Hunt syndrome" (see "Other causes" under "Sixth nerve palsy") or a form of recurrent demyelinating neuropathy.

Other causes

Vascular compression of the subarachnoid third nerve by aneurysm (Fig. 86.4) or arteriovenous malformation in childhood is very rare, but recognized, occurring usually in the second decade.

In all case series of childhood third nerve palsy, a number are unexplained after extensive investigation and designated idiopathic. Some of this group may be due to a third nerve neuroma, which requires thin section gadolinium-enhanced MRI, including coronal views for identification.[17] Characteristically these lesions present in the first decade with a slowly progressive palsy, often initially manifesting as an isolated exotropia. Amblyopia is common. Neuromas have been located in both the subarachnoid and intracavernous portions of the nerve and may associated with neurofibromatosis 2.

In traversing the lateral dural wall of the cavernous sinus the third nerve (and other ocular motor nerves) is vulnerable to involvement in parasellar pathologies, particularly tumors. Both craniopharyngioma and germ cell tumors have been reported to cause third nerve palsy, but always in association with other signs of local anatomical compromise, including involvement of the anterior visual pathways. Third nerve palsy may also occur after neurosurgical intervention for craniopharyngioma.

Isolated third nerve palsy due to tumor in the cavernous sinus has been described with neuroma (see above), lymphoma, rhabdomyosarcoma, and dermoid cyst. The lesion responsible for herpes zoster third nerve palsy may also be in the cavernous sinus. A lesion causing third nerve palsy in the orbit usually also produces an optic neuropathy and other ocular motor dysfunction as well as orbital signs, including proptosis.

Fourth nerve palsy

Congenital

Fourth nerve palsy is the commonest of all congenital ocular motor palsies and nearly half of all isolated fourth nerve palsies are congenital. It is the commonest cause of a congenital vertical strabismus and of ocular torticollis in childhood.

The presentation is often with torticollis–tilting and turning the head to take the eyes out of the field of action of the under-acting muscle and maintain binocularity. The tilt and turn are to the right with a left palsy and vice versa, with the chin held down. Straightening the head produces a manifest vertical strabismus, and head tilt in the opposite direction to the compensatory tilt markedly increases the deviation (positive Bielschowsky head tilt test) (Figs. 86.5 and 86.6). Eye movement testing shows underaction of the superior oblique and overaction of the ipsilateral inferior oblique and contralateral inferior rectus, with secondary underaction of the contralateral superior rectus. Characteristically the primary position vertical deviation with head straight is large, averaging 18 to 20 prism diopters (PD) in most studies. The vertical motor fusion range is also secondarily large, with an ability to control up to 20 PD of height disparity. Stereopsis is usually well developed, but double vision is often not overtly present when the eyes are dissociated. The child is usually aware when the deviation is uncontrolled and does not like this, but does not see double. However, in some children presenting with torticollis, the habitual turn and tilt of the head reduces but does not abolish the vertical deviation and no binocularity is demonstrable. The assumption in these cases is that the compensatory fusional mechanisms have failed, but that the head tilt has persisted or become habitual.

Some children with a congenital superior oblique palsy have, in addition, one or more of the following features: horizontal strabismus (usually esotropia), amblyopia of the hypertropic eye, ipsilateral partial ptosis, and facial asymmetry. Hypodevelopment of the contralateral facial structure is found. The explanation for this latter feature is unclear; it is probably an associated primary hypodevelopment, but could be in some way secondary to the torticollis. Some reports suggest that early surgery for the strabismus may reduce the likelihood of this feature developing.[18]

Decompensated congenital superior oblique palsy

A superior oblique palsy not evident in infancy or early childhood may be detected, or become symptomatic in later childhood, adolescence, or even adult life. The clinical features, including large vertical prism fusion range, are similar to those of congenital palsy, and the suggestion is that the fusional mechanisms have "decompensated." This concept of decompensation appears to be unique to the fourth cranial nerve. Since the fourth nerve supplies a single cyclovertical acting muscle, whose underaction can be compensated for by the head tilting and secondary fusional changes, decompensation is a sustainable concept and also a useful one.

Note that the diagnosis of congenital superior oblique palsy may also be made on routine screening or at an incidental orthoptic or ophthalmological assessment, indicating the parents may be unaware of the presence of the disorder. This lends further support to the concept of later decompensation, and the pre-existing palsy may be suggested by the presence of a compensatory head posture on old photographs. A few reports suggest that the disorder may be familial.

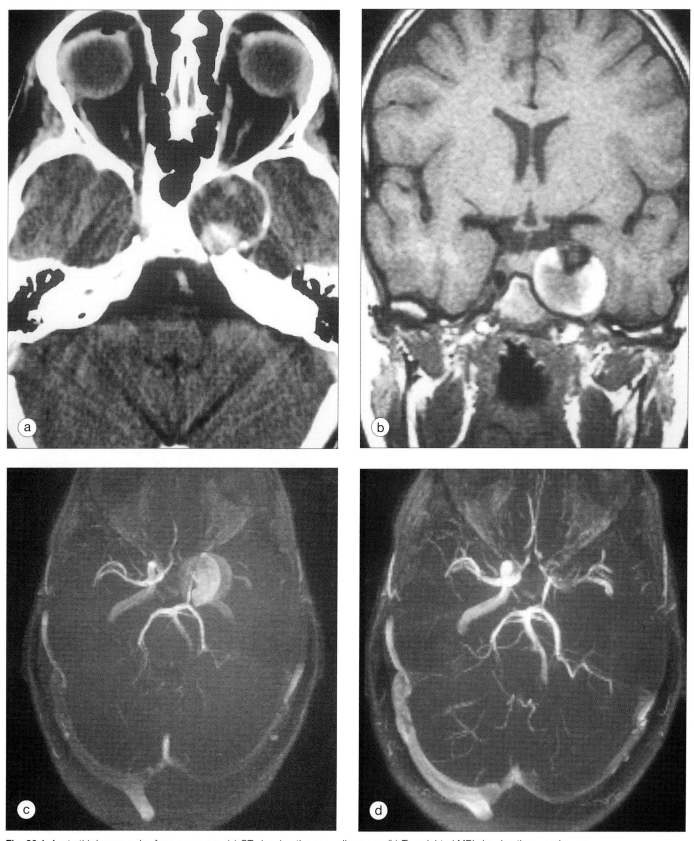

Fig. 86.4 Acute third nerve palsy from aneurysm. (a) CT showing the parasellar mass. (b) T_1-weighted MRI showing the vascular mass. (c) MR angiography demonstrating blood flow in the aneurysm. (d) MRA after balloon occlusion.

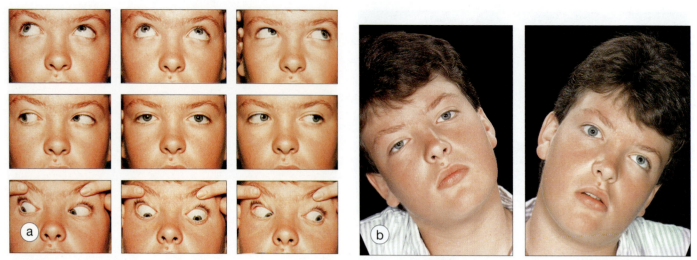

Fig. 86.5 Left congenital superior oblique palsy preoperative. (a) There is underaction of the left superior oblique shown by the defect of depression in adduction and overelevation of the left eye on elevation in adduction. (b) The Bielschowsy head tilt test. The eyes are parallel when the head is tilted to the right (normal) side. When the head is tilted to the left (abnormal) side, the incyclorotation would normally be carried out by both the superior rectus and the superior oblique in combination to maintain the retinal horizon, their vertical actions being opposite, the superior oblique a depressor and the superior rectus an elevator. If the superior oblique action of depression is reduced, the superior rectus is unopposed and elevates the eye.

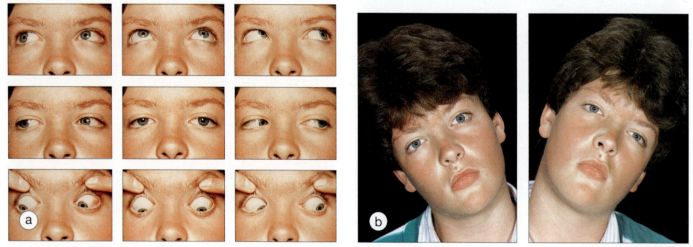

Fig. 86.6 Left congenital superior oblique palsy 3 hours postoperative. (a) The oblique muscle dysfunction is much reduced. (b) The Bielschowsky head tilt test is now normal.

Etiology

Unlike congenital palsies of the other ocular motor nerves, there is no association with prenatal disorders or birth trauma and virtually no associated neurology or developmental abnormality (it has been described in Goldenhar syndrome). The key question is whether the features of congenital superior oblique palsy are due to a neurogenic palsy or a developmental abnormality of the superior oblique tendon or its attachments.

In a study of 36 patients with a congenital superior oblique palsy, as defined above, the tendon was found on the basis of a traction test and direct inspection to be redundant, i.e., slack (the majority), misdirected, inserted into the posterior Tenon's capsule, or absent in about 85% of cases.[19] In traumatic or idiopathic palsies a much smaller proportion had tendon abnormalities.[19–21]

High-resolution MRI studies have demonstrated that the superior oblique muscle volume in these patients is reduced more (65% reduction compared to normal) than it is in acquired palsies (45% reduction).[20] This suggests the muscle is primarily hypo-

plastic, rather than secondarily atrophic. A congenital superior oblique palsy may be simulated by superior oblique muscle dysfunction, secondary to heterotopic muscle pulleys.[22]

Management

In the vast majority of cases there are no developmental or neurological concerns and no indication for pediatric referral or neuroimaging. The diagnosis can be made clinically and the only investigation required, beyond routine ophthalmological examination, including refraction, is orthoptic. Serial measurements are required to establish that the child has normal visual acuities, and sensory and motor binocularity, with the features as described. Cases of "superior oblique palsy plus" should be identified and the amblyopia and the horizontal strabismus treated in the normal way.

The identification of the disorder is not in itself an indication for surgical intervention. A well-compensated congenital fourth nerve palsy can be followed in the orthoptic department, amblyopia treated and refractive errors corrected. Indications for intervention include symptoms due to difficulty controlling the deviation, evidence of deteriorating binocularity, and increasing torticollis, which may cause secondary musculoskeletal problems or, occasionally, cosmesis.

Most superior oblique palsies, especially if the vertical deviation is less than 15 PD, can be adequately treated by weakening the ipsilateral inferior oblique muscle alone. Although this does not necessarily fully treat the underlying problem, any residual deviation is often asymptomatic and any head posture improved. If the deviation is larger or there has been an inadequate response to weakening the ipsilateral inferior oblique, a weakening of the contralateral inferior rectus or an ipsilateral superior oblique tuck may be indicated. If there are symptoms from torsion (most frequent in acquired palsies), a Harada-Ito procedure may be indicated (Chapter 88). If there is any hint of bilaterality, it is usually best to operate on both sides, as "masked" bilaterality is not uncommon.

Acquired

Closed head trauma is responsible for most cases of unilateral and bilateral acquired fourth nerve palsy. A small number of cases are due to miscellaneous causes, such as infection, tumor, and raised intracranial pressure.

The differential diagnosis includes skew deviation, i.e., an imbalance of prenuclear inputs to the vertically acting extra-ocular muscles. In this condition, unlike fourth nerve palsy, there is no subjective or measurable tilt of the involved eye and there are often other associated brainstem signs. Other causes of an acquired vertical strabismus in childhood include myasthenia gravis (which more usually presents with a ptosis) and orbital trauma.

It is not possible to differentiate clinically between a nuclear and a fascicular fourth nerve palsy. They may both be caused by posterior fossa tumors, such as medulloblastoma, ependymoma, astrocytoma, and arteriovenous malformation. The clinical picture is dominated by other symptoms and signs, including those of raised intracranial pressure (including sixth nerve palsy) and cerebellar involvement. In the presence of bilateral sixth nerve palsy, fourth nerve palsy is very difficult to diagnose. In addition there are a number of case reports of fourth nerve palsy in chronic idiopathic intracranial hypertension in children and adults.[23] Distortion of the central infranuclear pathways may be the common factor in these cases, which will resolve if the intracranial hypertension is controlled.

Central (nuclear or fascicular) fourth nerve palsy may be a component of Parinaud dorsal midbrain syndrome, usually due to pineal tumor, or associated with hydrocephalus including that due to aqueduct stenosis.

The vulnerability of the subarachnoid fourth nerve to damage in closed head trauma relates to the dorsal exit of the nerve rootlets after decussation in the superior medullary vellum. Sudden deceleration with neck flexion causes focal damage or avulsion of the nerve rootlets. Slow recovery over months is the rule.

The subarachnoid fourth nerve may also be damaged in acute bacterial meningitis, chronic basal meningitis (e.g., TB), and Lyme borreliosis. Damage in the wall of the cavernous sinus is likely to be accompanied by additional ocular motor signs, and this also applies to orbital pathology, including trauma.

Sixth nerve palsy

Congenital

The finding of an isolated unilateral lateral rectus palsy in an otherwise normal neonate is a rare but well-recognized

phenomenon. The prognosis for full spontaneous recovery is good. In most series, full abduction is demonstrable by 6 weeks and there is no interference with normal binocular development. The assumption is that there has been focal damage to the peripheral nerve, either by stretching or ischemia, but the axons remain intact. This suggestion is strengthened by a study of 6,886 term neonates over a 10-year period. Overall, the incidence was 0.5%, but ranged from nil in those delivered by caesarian section to 3.2% after vacuum extraction. Skull traction and deformation are presumed to cause secondary damage to the sixth nerve.[24]

Congenital sixth nerve palsy may go unrecognized in some cases; examination of the ocular alignment in neonates is difficult and requires patience and practice. It is particularly difficult to demonstrate a full range of eye movement, and may require techniques utilizing the vestibulo-ocular system. Even if an esotropia is detected by the neonatologist its significance may not be appreciated at the time, and as the prognosis is good, there is no long-term adverse outcome.

The differential diagnosis includes infantile esotropia and Duane syndrome. Characteristic signs, such as globe retraction, are difficult to demonstrate in infancy. From informal studies by orthoptists and ophthalmologists it is evident that most cases of infantile esotropia are of postnatal onset, and many of these infants are exotropic (at least intermittently) at birth. Parents of some infantile esotropes date the abnormal alignment from birth, and it is certainly feasible that slow recovery from a congenital sixth nerve palsy could lead to essential infantile esotropia.

Investigation

Given the excellent prognosis and lack of associated neurology, no investigation is required. Orthoptic follow-up to monitor binocular visual development should be arranged.

Acquired

As with other isolated ocular motor cranial neuropathies in childhood the commonest cause of sixth nerve palsy is accidental trauma.[2,4,25] The circumstances can usually be independently corroborated and there are often associated injuries. A wide range of other pathologies may cause sixth nerve palsy, including a potentially life-threatening intracranial tumor or raised intracranial pressure even without the direct effects of a tumor. The history and examination will usually identify such cases at presentation (Fig. 86.7).

A nuclear sixth nerve palsy produces an ipsilateral horizontal gaze palsy, as it involves interneurons passing via the medial longitudinal fasciculus (MLF) to the contralateral medial rectus subnucleus. It may be caused by an infiltrative neoplasm (brainstem glioma), demyelination (e.g., ADEM), AVM, or trauma. Associated neurological findings are common and determined by the extent and location of the lesion. They include:

1. Ipsilateral peripheral facial palsy (Fig. 86.8);
2. Contralateral internuclear ophthalmoplegia (i.e., extension to the ipsilateral MLF)–the 1 1/2 syndrome; and
3. One or more of ipsilateral facial palsy, Horner syndrome, facial analgesia, deafness plus contralateral hemiplegia (Foville and related syndromes–Millard Gubler and Raymond Cesta).

Isolated sixth nerve palsy may be due to a fascicular palsy from a more discrete, usually inflammatory, lesion. If this is adjacent to the sixth nerve nucleus an ipsilateral partial gaze palsy will often be found.

As they ascend in the subarachnoid space the sixth nerves have a close relationship to the clivus. A number of pathologies involving this structure may present with isolated unilateral or bilateral

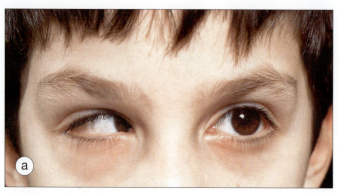

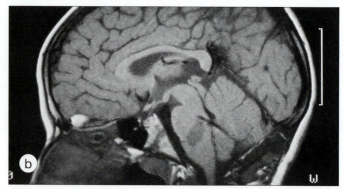

Fig. 86.7 (a) This 10-year-old boy had strabismus surgery as an infant and the strabismus was well controlled for many years, but it deteriorated and it became evident that he had a left sixth nerve paresis. (b) The cause was a brainstem glioma.

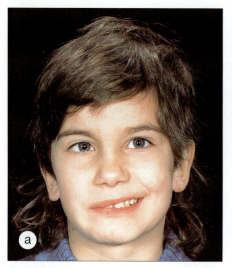

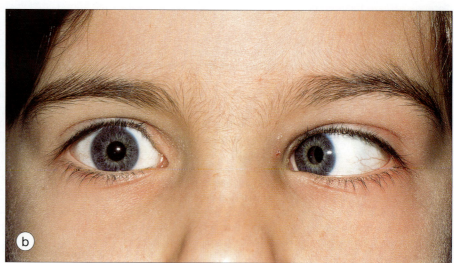

Fig. 86.8 (a) Right traumatic sixth and seventh nerve palsy. The facial paresis shows when she attempts to smile. (b) The right eye fails to abduct.

sixth nerve palsy. These include clivus chordoma, epidural hematoma of the clivus, eosinophilic granuloma of the clivus, Langerhans cell histiocytosis (LCH) of the clivus (or petrous apex), and chondrosarcoma of the skull base.[26] A transverse sphenoidal skull base fracture sustained in major head trauma may damage one or both sixth nerves. Gradenigo syndrome of infected mastoiditis, extending to the petrous apex plus trigeminal pain, reduced hearing, and sixth nerve (± seventh nerve) palsy is now rarely seen.

The subarachnoid sixth nerve may be damaged by stretching due to raised intracranial pressure. The lateral rectus palsy is generally incomplete initially and, if bilateral, often asymmetric. Intracranial hypotension (either post lumbar puncture, trauma, or surgery or rarely spontaneous) usually produces, after a latent period, a complete sixth nerve palsy.

Meningitis of any cause, infective or malignant, can damage the sixth nerve.

Benign lateral rectus palsy of childhood

The diagnosis is by exclusion. A unilateral, usually complete, sudden onset isolated sixth nerve palsy presents in a well child in the first decade. There may have been a prior viral infection or immunization. Neuroimaging and CSF examination are negative, but blood tests may show nonspecific evidence of a recent infection. There is a suggestion of female and left-sided preponderance. The prognosis for full spontaneous recovery is excellent, but not universal. Ipsilateral (and very rarely contra-lateral) recurrences may occur. The condition may continue into adult life.[27]

The etiology is undetermined, and the location of the lesion uncertain. In the visually immature child, the possibility of treating the ipsilateral medial rectus with botulinum toxin, while awaiting recovery to maintain binocularity, should be considered as amblyopia in the affected eye can develop.

Other causes

The sixth nerve may be damaged in the cavernous sinus by a pituitary-based or parasellar tumor, for example, craniopharyngioma or suprasellar germinoma. Almost invariably other neurological symptoms and signs are present, including fifth nerve dysfunction, Horner syndrome, and anterior visual pathway involvement. Other rare pathologies in this location presenting with a sixth nerve palsy in childhood include parameningeal embryonal rhabdomyo-sarcoma, meningioma, and intracavernous carotid aneurysm.[28]

The Tolosa-Hunt syndrome of painful ophthalmoplegia due to presumed granulomatous inflammation (another diagnosis of exclusion) should also be considered. It has been described in the first and second decades, but the diagnosis should be made with caution as, for example, Burkitt lymphoma can also present this way.

The differential diagnosis of sixth nerve palsy in childhood includes (as with all eye movement disorders) ocular myasthenia gravis. Thyroid-associated orbitopathy may also rarely occur in this age group. Medial orbital wall trauma and medial rectus muscle entrapment can simulate a sixth nerve palsy. Spasm of accommodation with pseudoabducens palsy can be differentiated by miosis and varying myopia. It is usually an isolated psychogenic disorder, but may also occur after closed head trauma for reasons that are unclear. Cyclic esotropia may also cause confusion and again has been reported after recovery from traumatic sixth nerve palsy.

Management

Sixth nerve palsies should be left many months to recover spontaneously, during which time botulinum toxin may be used (Chapter 87). Management of refractive errors and amblyopia are essential and diplopia can be helped occasionally in partial palsies by prisms but usually by occlusion. For some part of the day the patch may be worn on the unaffected eye.

For smaller deviations and where there is significant residual muscle function a recession–resection procedure may suffice. If the primary position deviation is larger than 35 PD then a contralateral medial rectus recession may be added. If there is marked incomitance the contralateral medial rectus may be posteriorly fixated ("fadenized," Chapter 88).

With very large deviations and where there is minimal or no residual sixth nerve function an injection of botulinum toxin into the ipsilateral medial rectus plus horizontal transposition of the vertical recti may be indicated (Chapter 88).

Combined ocular motor palsies

A number of the conditions described earlier may present with, or develop, combined third, fourth, and sixth nerve palsies. Examples are brainstem glioma, tubercular meningoencephalitis, and cavernous sinus-based pathologies. The obvious differential diagnosis is ocular myasthenia gravis, in which ptosis is the most common presenting sign. Dynamic abnormalities of eye movement reflect the primary hallmarks of the disease, fatigability, and variability. Other differentials include the Miller-Fisher variant of Guillain-Barré syndrome and botulism.

CHILDHOOD OCULAR NEUROMUSCULAR AND MUSCLE DISEASE

A number of disorders of diverse pathogenesis affect ocular neuromuscular and muscular function in childhood. All are rare. The commonest is myasthenia gravis and this not infrequently presents to the pediatric ophthalmologist. It is very important to make this diagnosis, not only because the condition is treatable but also because there is a risk without, and even with, treatment of severe and occasionally fatal complications. Chronic progressive external ophthalmoplegia is the other condition that may present to the pediatric ophthalmologist. Most of the other disorders discussed in the following will present to other specialists, but the pediatric ophthalmologist may be asked to contribute to diagnosis and help with management. Correct diagnosis is important to ensure appropriate management and referral for any associated systemic features. In some cases genetic counseling is required.

Disorders of the neuromuscular junction

Three disorders are considered in this section. They are the congenital myasthenic syndromes (CMS), comprising about 20% of cases, neonatal myasthenia gravis (5%), and juvenile autoimmune myasthenia gravis (JAMG, 75%).

The congenital myasthenic syndromes

This rare group of disorders can present at any age from birth to early adult life, but usually within the first 2 years with partial bilateral symmetric ptosis and facial and bulbar weakness.[29] The range of eye movement is often limited symmetrically with both up- and downgaze affected. An exotropia is often seen, and probably for this reason amblyopia is uncommon. There is a wide spectrum of severity. There may also be limb weakness. Skeletal muscle bulk is reduced.

Congenital myasthenia may be sporadic or inherited, usually as an autosomal dominant. It is non-autoimmune, and there are no associations with other autoimmune disorders. The diagnosis is confirmed by neuromuscular electrophysiological investigation in the presence of characteristic physical signs. Other aspects of muscle function will also be investigated, including enzymes and sometimes histology on biopsy.

Two groups of disorder are recognized[29,30]:

Presynaptic CMS

These disorders are due to defects in the acetylcholine (Ach) quantal release or resynthesis mechanisms:

1. The Ach quantal release may be inadequate to properly activate the muscle membrane receptors;
2. The neural basal lamina may not properly allow or facilitate the release of normal Ach quanta;
3. Presynaptic resynthesis of Ach, which can be traced to mutations in genes controlling choline acetyltransferase, may be defective; and
4. Released Ach may lack end plate specificity and fail to activate muscle membrane receptors.

This group of disorders tends to slowly improve spontaneously. Anticholinesterase drugs may be helpful in some instances. The ptosis is rarely severe enough to cause problems with visual development, but there is usually an exotropia and reduced range of extraocular movements, so normal binocular functions do not develop.

Postsynaptic CMS

These are a group of disorders of acetylcholine receptor (AchR) number, function, or altered kinetic properties. They prevent normally released presynaptic Ach from activating the muscle. These disorders are secondary to mutations in kinetic or expresser genes in the muscle membrane, or mutations in the *RAPSN* gene, which compromise rapsyn function. Rapsyn is important in the control of AchR numbers and distribution on the postsynaptic membrane.

Postsynaptic CMS may respond to some extent to anticholinesterase drugs. Children with this group of disorders will invariably be under the care of a colleague with pediatric, neurological, or muscle disease expertise. An ophthalmological opinion may be sought in respect of a differential diagnosis (e.g., CPEO; see "CPEO") and aspects of management such as amblyopia and corneal protection.

Neonatal myasthenia gravis

Ten to 20% of the offspring of mothers with autoimmune myasthenia gravis develop transient neonatal MG, since maternal antibodies are able to cross the placenta. The neonates present with generalized weakness, respiratory distress, poor feeding, and bilateral ptosis. The occurrence of the disorder correlates with high AchR levels in the mother in pregnancy and a higher than usual ratio of antiembryonic AchR Abs versus antiadult AchR Abs.[31] The embryonic acetylcholine receptor is antigenically distinct from that of the adult.

Neonatal MG may be severe, and require assisted ventilation. The diagnosis is confirmed by detecting serum AchR Abs in the neonate and by characteristic EMG findings. Treatment is with neostigmine and the condition resolves spontaneously over 4 to 12 weeks dependent on severity. No cases of long-term visual developmental anomalies such as amblyopia and strabismus are described.

Juvenile autoimmune myasthenia gravis (JAMG)

This is defined as autoimmune MG with age of onset of less than 15 years, and it accounts for 10% of all cases. Girls outnumber boys three to one. The mean age at onset varies quite widely in different series between 3 to 4 years and 13.[32,33] Most present with ocular myasthenia in the form of variable, fatigable asymmetric ptosis and strabismus, usually exotropia often with a vertical strabismus as well. Those presenting under the age of 7 are at risk of amblyopia.[33]

On examination eye movements are limited with underaction of the medial and inferior rectus characteristic. As expected variability and fatigability can be demonstrated. Apart from ptosis (Fig. 86.9), the lid signs include upward twitches on vertical saccadic refixation and hops on lateral gaze, as well as orbicularis oculi weakness.

Up to 50% of those presenting with JAMG and ocular signs will go on to generalized MG. There is a risk of developing ventilatory insufficiency and of aspiration and a relatively high risk of myasthenic crisis in this group compared to adults.[32,34] It is therefore very important that ophthalmologists to whom these children present involve a pediatric neurologist at an early stage.

The diagnosis should be suspected with the above clinical signs. A Tensilon test is positive in over 90% of JAMG, and anti Ach RBs are positive in over 60%. Antibody positivity is identical in males and females. Electrophysiological investigation, including repetitive stimulation test (RST) and single-fiber electromyography (SFEMG), is usually positive.[34]

A number of other autoimmune diseases are associated with JAMG. Hyperthyroidism occurs in 8%, juvenile onset diabetes mellitus in 3%, and rheumatoid arthritis subsequently develops in a further 3%.

Differential diagnosis

It is important to recognize that JAMG can mimic any form of pupil-sparing ocular motility disturbance. Meticulous examination looking for the characteristic myasthenic features is required.

Infant botulism can present with facial weakness, bilateral ptosis, and ophthalmoplegia, but with pupillary involvement. It occurs in a much younger age group than that with JAMG with a mean age at presentation of around 3 to 4 months. Constipation, feeding difficulties, and descending symmetric weakness are other features.[35] It is due to intestinal colonization by clostridium botulinum and treated by attempts at intestinal recolonization by normal flora and supportive measures. Bilateral ptosis and ophthalmoplegia may take many weeks to resolve, and normal pupillary responses and accommodation many months. Provided

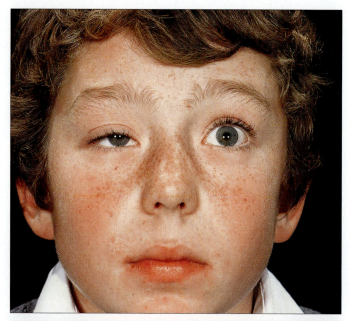

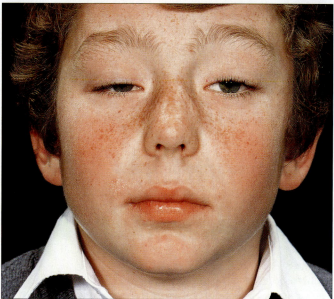

Fig. 86.9 Juvenile autoimmune myasthenia gravis. The bottom picture was taken 10 minutes after the top, during which time the ptosis worsened and the face became weaker.

the child survives without complications, however, there do not seem to be any long-term effects on visual development.

Treatment

Initial treatment in most cases of ocular JAMG is with anticholinesterase drugs, but these are not usually successful in controlling the disorder. There is evidence that the early use of immunosuppression may prevent progression from ocular to generalized MG. This will otherwise occur in over 50% in 2 years. Thymectomy is required in approximately 50% with histology showing thymic lymphoid follicular hyperplasia.[34] In severe cases plasmapheresis and assisted ventilation may be required. Azathioprine is used in those requiring long-term immunosuppression as a steroid-sparing agent. Full spontaneous remission may occur and the majority can be controlled.

Because of the risk of amblyopia, visually immature children should be monitored in the orthoptic department.[33] Corneal exposure may be a problem. In stable ocular myasthenics the possibility of ptosis surgery, either by levator advancement or brow suspension, can be considered. It is important to ensure that corneal sensation is normal and that there is sufficient eye movement to allow protection of the cornea, including Bell's phenomenon, and sufficient orbicularis oculi strength to prevent lagophthalmos. Strabismus surgery may also be considered for a stable, persistent, incomitant or concomitant deviation. Muscle recessions only, on relatively overacting muscles, should be carried out so that the surgery is potentially completely reversible.

Ocular muscle disease

Chronic progressive external ophthalmoplegia (CPEO)

(see also Chapter 53)

This is a heterogenous group of disorders associated with large-scale mitochondrial DNA (mtDNA) deletions or mutations characterized by slow progressive symmetric ophthalmoplegia with ptosis and orbicularis oculi weakness.[36] The muscle weakness is invariable and does not fatigue. On muscle biopsy histology shows ragged red fibers (RRF) on modified Gomori staining.

The clinical spectrum is broad. One of the unexplained features of the phenomenology of mitochondrial mutations is that a specific identifiable mutation (e.g., A3234G) can be associated with either CPEO or another phenotypic manifestation of mitochondrial dysfunction, mitochondrial encephalomyopathy, lactic acidosis, and stroke-like episodes (MELAS).[37] The different phenotypes seemingly being both determined by the same genotype suggests that there are different responses or processes of evolution with time of the same mutation. Rarely the two phenotypes (CPEO and MELAS) may co-exist.

Children with CPEO may present to the pediatric ophthalmologist in the first decade with an exodeviation, with or without a mild bilateral ptosis. Other systemic features, such as growth retardation, may or may not be present at this stage.

CPEO may be classified as:[36]

1. Congenital;
2. Isolated;
3. Oculofacial;
4. Occurring with pigmentary retinopathy (Fig. 86.10);
5. Occurring with pigmentary retinopathy, heart block, cerebellar dysfunction, and raised CSF protein (Kearns-Sayers syndrome, in which the symptoms usually begin in early childhood); or
6. Occurring with other systemic features such as growth retardation or failure to gain weight.

Symptoms in nos. 2 to 6 may become clinically evident in the first or second decade, and present to pediatric ophthalmologists with progressive ptosis and global reduction of eye movement. Definitive diagnosis is by muscle biopsy and genotyping. Systemic features should be sought by referral to a muscle specialist.

The management consists first of all of an explanation of the disorder to the child and parents. The ptosis and ophthalmoparesis are slowly progressive, and surgery for the ptosis in childhood is almost always contraindicated because of the risk of subsequent corneal exposure. Double vision almost never occurs. Upper lid surgery to create a skin crease may improve the appearance.

Muscular dystrophies

Two forms of muscular dystrophy may present to the pediatric ophthalmologist.

Myotonic dystrophy

This characteristically presents in the first decade with muscle weakness and wasting, involving the face, neck, and limbs. It may also rarely present in infancy with poor muscle tone and weakness. The facial appearance is characteristic with ptosis and lower lid retraction. In later life a progressive external ophthalmoplegia becomes evident, but this is rarely symptomatic. The ptosis may occasionally be relatively asymmetric and the diagnosis is occasionally made by the pediatric ophthalmologist in a child referred with ptosis. Myotonia, i.e., slow muscle relaxation is characteristic in skeletal muscles and worse under cold conditions.

The condition has autosomal dominant inheritance with variable penetrance. Systemic features include gonadal atrophy, cataracts, frontal balding, and sometimes cognitive and learning difficulties. Multiple small focal asymptomatic lens opacities are invariably present in myotonic dystrophy and are often polychromatic. The opacities increase in size and coalesce, producing

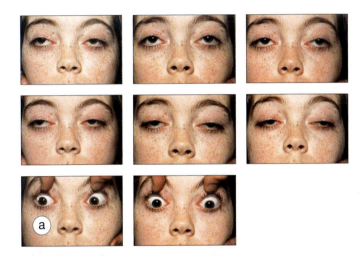

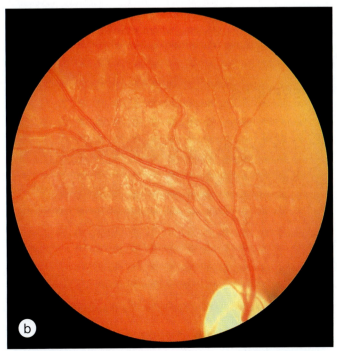

Fig. 86.10 Mitochondrial cytopathy. (a) Bilateral symmetrical ptosis with brow elevation and defective eye movements in all directions. (b) Retinopathy with an abnormal ERG, thinned arterioles, and optic atrophy.

the characteristic "Christmas tree" cataract, or a more diffuse lens opacity.

The condition is due to an unstable trinucleotide repeat (CTG) on the long arm of chromosome 19. This is involved in the encoding of myotin protein kinase, and the number of abnormal repeats determines the severity of the condition.[38]

Management involves confirming the diagnosis and providing the appropriate counseling, including genetic advice. As with other conditions, where there is a combination of ptosis and external ophthalmoplegia, surgical correction of ptosis is generally contraindicated and can lead to major corneal exposure problems.

Oculopharyngeal muscular dystrophy

This is an inherited disorder, usually autosomal dominant, presenting with a slow progressive bilateral ptosis and dysphagia in the fourth to fifth decade. However, it is now recognized that it may occur at a much younger age in the first or second decade with ptosis and exotropia.[39]

The diagnosis is made on muscle electrophysiology and muscle biopsy. A specific genetic defect has been identified with short GCG repeat expansions in the *PABP2* gene.

Congenital myopathy

A number of congenital myopathies classified by the histological features on muscle biopsy, using special histochemical techniques, as well as quantitative EMG, are identified. This group of disorders presents in infancy with delayed motor development and reduced muscle tone and bulk. Ophthalmological involvement is not usually prominent, but both ptosis and ophthalmoparesis are described, for example, in myotubular myopathy.

Neurodegenerative disorders

Ophthalmoplegia and/or ptosis may be a feature of childhood onset neurodegenerative disorders. Examples are:
1. Juvenile spinal muscular atrophy;
2. Infantile progressive spinal muscular atrophy (Werdnig-Hoffman disease type 1);
3. Childhood lactic acidosis, where ptosis is occasionally seen but optic atrophy much more commonly;

4. Abetalipoproteinemia (oculomotor nerve palsies may also occur); and
5. Spinocerebellar degeneration.

Orbital myositis
Graves ophthalmopathy

Childhood onset Graves ophthalmopathy is rare and occurs predominantly in girls. Common features are lid edema, lidlag, and lagophthalmos. Mild proptosis and conjunctival involvement occurs in about 10%. Scanning or ultrasound may show that the extraocular muscles are enlarged, but significant limitation of eye movement is rare and visually threatening complications, e.g., optic neuropathy, have not been reported.[40]

There appears to be a generally good prognosis for spontaneous resolution, usually without recourse to major intervention such as high-dose steroids or orbital decompression.

Isolated extraocular muscle myositis

Isolated extraocular muscle myositis may occur in childhood. It is of acute onset with pain on any eye movement that involves active contraction or passive stretching of the involved muscle. The involved extraocular muscle is swollen and inflamed, often with conjunctival edema and lid swelling and sometimes a small proptosis. Single muscle involvement is usual. Scanning shows diffuse enlargement of the muscle.

Although described in adults in association with a number of systemic inflammatory disorders (e.g., inflammatory bowel disease), extraocular muscle myositis in childhood is usually an isolated disorder without systemic features.

However, it has been described in sarcoidosis in the first and second decades. Bilateral painful external ophthalmoplegia with enlarged muscles on scanning is characteristic. On biopsy sarcoid granulomata are found.[41]

The differential diagnosis of concern is rhabdomyosarcoma. A biopsy must be carried out unless the diagnosis is regarded as secure on clinical grounds, e.g., as a result of spontaneous resolution with nonsteroidal antiinflammatory drugs. A short course of systemic steroids may be required to resolve the condition.

REFERENCES

1. Harley RD. Paralytic strabismus in children. Ophthalmology 1980; 87: 24–43.
2. Kodsi SR, Younge BR. Acquired oculomotor, trochlear and abducent cranial nerve palsies in pediatric patients. Am J Ophthalmol 1992; 114: 568–74.
3. Ing EB, Sullivan TJ, Clarke MP, et al. Oculomotor nerve palsies in children. J Pediatr Ophthalmol Strabismus 1992; 29: 331–6.
4. Afifi AK, Bell WE, Menzes AH. Etiology of lateral rectus palsy in infancy and childhood. J Child Neurol 1992; 7: 295–9.
5. Holmes JM, Mutyala S, Maus TL, et al. Pediatric, third, fourth and sixth nerve palsies: a population-based study. Am J Ophthalmol 1999; 127: 388–92.
6. Flanders M, Watters G, Draper J, et al. Bilateral congenital third cranial nerve palsy. Can J Ophthalmol 1989; 24: 28–30.
7. Tsaloumas MD, Willshaw HE. Congenital oculomotor palsy: associated neurological and ophthalmological findings. Eye 1997; 11: 500–3.
8. Kommerell G, Mehdorn E, Ketelsen UP, et al. Oculomotor palsy with cyclic spasms. Neuro-ophthalmology 1992; 114: 568–74.
9. Brodsky MC, Pollock, SC, Buckley EG. Neural misdirection in congenital ocular fibrosis syndrome: Implications and pathogenesis. J Pediatr Ophthalmol Strabismus 1989; 26: 159–61.
10. Flaherty MP, Grattan-Smith P, Steinberg A, et al. Congenital fibrosis

of the extraocular muscles associated with cortical dysplasia and maldevelopment of the basal ganglia. Ophthalmology 2001; 108: 1313–22.
11. Engle EC. Applications of molecular genetics to the understanding of congenital ocular motility disorders. Ann NY Acad Sci 2002; 956: 55–63.
12. Balcer LJ, Galetta SL, Bagley LJ, et al. Localization of traumatic oculomotor nerve palsy to the midbrain exit site by magnetic resonance imaging. Am J Ophthalmol 1996; 22: 437–9.
13. Amitava AK, Alarm S, Hussain R. Neuro-ophthalmic features in pediatric tubercular meningoencephalitis. J Pediatr Ophthalmol Strabismus 2001; 38: 229–34.
14. Chiba A, Kusunoki S, Obata H, et al. Serum anti-GQ1b IgG antibody is associated with ophthalmoplegia in Miller Fisher Syndrome and Guillain-Barré Syndrome: clinical and immunohistochemical studies. Neurology 1993; 43: 1911–17.
15. Berlit P, Rakicky J. The Miller Fisher Syndrome. Review of the literature. J Clin Neuroophthalmol 1992; 12: 57–63.
16. Norman AA, Farris BK, Siatkowski RM. Neuroma as a cause of oculomotor palsy in infancy and early childhood. J AAPOS 2001; 5: 9–12.
17. Mark AS, Casselman J, Brown D, et al. Ophthalmoplegic migraine: reversible enhancement and thickening of the cisternal segment of the oculomotor nerve in contrast-enhanced MR images. Am J Neuroradial 1998; 19: 1887–91.

18. Goodman CR, Chabner E, Guyton DL. Should early strabismus surgery be performed for ocular torticollis to prevent facial asymmetry? J Pediatr Ophthalmol Strabismus 1995; 32: 162–6.

19. Helveston EM, Krach D, Plager DA, et al. A new classification of superior oblique palsy based on congenital variations in the tendon. Ophthalmology 1992; 99: 1609–15.

20. Sato M, Yagasaki T, Kora T, et al. Comparison of muscle volume between congenital and acquired superior oblique palsies by magnetic resonance imaging. Jpn J Ophthalmol 1998; 42: 466–70.

21. Sato M. Magnetic resonance imaging and tendon anomaly associated with congenital superior oblique palsy. Am J Ophthalmol 1999; 127: 379–87.

22. Demer JL, Miller JM, Koo EY, et al. True versus masquerading superior oblique palsies: muscle mechanisms revealed by MRI. In: Lennerstrand G, editor. Update on Strabismus and Paediatric Ophthalmology. Boca Raton, FL: CRC Press; 1994: 303–6.

23. Speer C, Pearlman, J, Phillips PH, et al. Fourth cranial nerve palsy in pediatric patients with pseudotumour cerebri. Am J Ophthalmol 1999; 127: 236–7.

24. Galbraith RS. Incidence of neonatal VI(th) nerve palsy in relation to mode of delivery. Am J Obstet Gynecol 1994; 170: 158–9.

25. Mutyala S, Holmes JM, Hodge DO, et.al. Spontaneous recovery rate in traumatic sixth-nerve palsy. Am J Ophthalmol 1996; 122: 898–9.

26. Volpe NJ, Liebsch NJ, Muzenrider JE, et al. Neuro-ophthalmic findings in chordoma and chondrosarcoma of the skull base. Am J Ophthalmol 1993; 115: 97–104.

27. Afifi AK, Bell WE, Bale JF, et al. Recurrent lateral rectus palsy in childhood. Pediatr Neurol 1990; 6: 315–8.

28. Mullaney PB, Nabi NU, Thorner P, et al. Ophthalmic involvement as a presenting feature of nonorbit childhood parameningeal embryonal rhabdomyosarcoma. Ophthalmology 2001; 108: 179–82.

29. Shillito P, Vincent A, Newsom-Davis J. Congenital myasthenic syndromes. Neuromuscul Disord 1993; 3: 183–90.

30. Engel AG, Ohno K, Sine SM. Congenital myasthenic syndromes: Progress over the past decade. Muscle Nerve 2003; 27: 4–25.

31. Vernet-der Garabedian B, Lacokova M, Eymard B, et al. Association of neonatal myasthenia gravis with antibodies against the fetal acetylcholine receptor. J Clin Invest 1994; 94: 555–9.

32. Kim JH, Hwang JM, Hwang YS, et al. Childhood ocular myasthenia gravis. Ophthalmology 2003; 110: 1458–62.

33. McCreery KM, Hussein MA, Lee AG, et al. Major review: The clinical spectrum of pediatric myasthenia gravis: blepharoptosis, ophthalmoplegia and strabismus. A review of 14 cases. Binocul Vis Strabismus Q 2002; 17: 181–6.

34. Lindner A, Schalke B, Toyka KV. Outcome in juvenile-onset myasthenia gravis: a retrospective study with long-term follow up of 79 patients. J Neurol 1997; 244: 515–20.

35. Schreiner MS, Field E, Ruddy R. Infant botulism: a review of 12 years' experience at the Children's Hospital of Philadelphia. Pediatrics 1991; 87: 159–65.

36. Lee AG, Brazis PW. Chronic progressive external ophthalmoplegia. Curr Neurol Neurosci Rep 2002; 2: 413–7.

37. Mariotti C, Savarese N, Suomalainen A, et al. Genotype to phenotype correlations in mitochondrial encephalomyopathies associated with the A3243G mutation of mitochondrial DNA. J Neurol 1995; 242: 304–12.

38. Shelbourne P, Johnson K. Myotonic dystrophy: another case of too many repeats? Hum Mutate 1992; 1: 183–9.

39. Lacomis D, Kupsky WJ, Kuban KK, et al. Childhood onset oculopharyngeal muscular dystrophy. Pediatr Neurol 1991; 7: 382–4.

40. Chan W, Wong GW, Fan DS, et al. Ophthalmology in childhood Graves' disease. Br J Ophthalmol 2002; 86: 740–2.

41. Cornblath WT, Elner V, Rolfe M. Extraocular muscle involvement in sarcoidosis. Ophthalmology 1993; 100: 501–5.

CHAPTER **87** # Strabismus: Nonsurgical Management

John P Lee

INTRODUCTION

Most of the management of childhood strabismus is nonsurgical. Surgery is an inappropriate treatment for some specific types of strabismus, such as fully accommodative esotropia. Other conditions, such as sensory deviations in eyes with organic visual defects, merit surgery on cosmetic grounds, and many children do not complain about their appearance until their teenage years. Most strabismus clinics are full of children having their amblyopia treatment monitored and their spectacles checked, in contrast to the handful attending for immediately pre- or post-operative appointments.

Not all parents realize this, and it is not uncommon to have to spend a good deal of time explaining that there are many different types of strabismus, all with their own appropriate therapy, and that "We'd like the operation, please" is not always the best plan of management for their child. All strabismus specialists have had the experience of a patient who disappears immediately after surgical treatment, despite multiple follow-up appointments, because the parents are now satisfied that their child has had the treatment for which they first attended, and see no reason to attend further!

OPTICAL CORRECTION

Spectacles

All children with strabismus or suspected strabismus require a cycloplegic refraction (see Chapter 6). At present, automated refractors lack sufficient reliability, so this must be achieved by retinoscopy. Cycloplegia may be induced by instillation of g. cyclopentolate 1% in children with lightly or moderately pigmented irides, although a repeat instillation may be required. Cyclopentolate, being acidic, stings, and is understandably unpopular with children. Some colleagues have recommended the instillation of a topical anesthetic (oxybuprocaine 0.4%, or proxymetacaine 0.5%) prior to the cyclopentolate. We have found a spray containing cyclopentolate to be effective and acceptable in many children. Children with heavily pigmented irides do not respond well to topical cyclopentolate, and resent the repeated instillation of unpleasant eye drops. These are prescribed atropine 1% ointment to be instilled morning and evening for 3 days prior to the planned day of refraction.

The aim of retinoscopy is to determine the basic refractive state of the eyes without the influence of accommodation. The pupillary dilatation also allows the ophthalmologist to perform ophthalmoscopy to exclude abnormalities of the posterior segments of the eyes.

Once established, the significance of the refraction should be considered in the light of the history and diagnosis. *Anisometropia* is an evident barrier to the development of binocular vision, and

a cause of amblyopia, and should be corrected. Depending on the type of co-existing strabismus, it may be appropriate to correct the full refractive error of both eyes, or simply to prescribe the difference between the eyes. In essential infantile esotropia, moderate *hypermetropia* is common, as it is in most infants, and it is highly unlikely that correction of, say, 2 or 3 diopters of hypermetropia will significantly alter a strabismus angle of 50 prism diopters. However, following surgical alignment, spectacle correction may be of considerable value in improving a small residual esotropia. In acquired esotropia, particularly accommodative esotropia, all degrees of hypermetropia may be significant, and should be corrected with spectacles. When prescribing hypermetropic spectacle corrections, there is no place for the dubious tradition of reducing the spectacle strength by arbitrary amounts to compensate for "ciliary tonus." The aim of correction is to correct fully all hypermetropia, in order to remove all accommodation, and therefore all accommodative convergence.

It has been traditional not to correct moderate hypermetropia in intermittent exotropia, on the argument that the convergence induced by the hypermetropia has a beneficial effect on the control of the exodeviation. This view has recently been challenged by a study suggesting that better binocular outcomes are obtained if hypermetropia is corrected in children with intermittent exotropia.[1]

Myopia is less common in strabismic children, although it may be associated with arrested retinopathy of prematurity and other ocular disorders (see Chapter 6). In the very young child, moderate symmetrical myopia may not require correction until the child starts school. High myopia, which may be associated with esotropia and exotropia, should always be corrected, as binocular vision is unlikely to develop properly if the eyes are constantly presented with blurred retinal images. In intermittent exotropia, where the eyes tend to be straight for near fixation with good binocular function, and divergent with suppression for distance fixation, correction of myopia will allow clear retinal images at all fixation distances and also stimulate some accommodative convergence, which may have a valuable effect on the angle and control of the strabismus. Some authors have deliberately "overminused" patients with intermittent exotropia to obtain this effect,[2] but the author has never seen a case where this strategy has been other than temporarily beneficial.

In all cases, it is important to give children glasses that are acceptable to them, but at the same time light and robust with lenses of plastic rather than of glass. Parents are sometimes keen that their child should have the thinnest possible lenses: they should be apprised of the fact that these expensive lenses carry no advantages from the point of view of vision or strabismus management and little cosmetic advantage from the child's point of view, and if made of glass (for the thinnest lenses) are dangerous.

Tinted glasses

These are mainly used in children with ocular conditions causing photophobia (Chapter P9). Some children with intermittent exotropia close one eye in bright sunshine, probably because of glare rather than diplopia. This is usually of little importance in the UK, with its lack of strong sunshine, but ophthalmologists in areas such as Queensland find tinted glasses for outside wear helpful in this group of strabismic children.

Bifocals

In children with refractive accommodative esotropia (convergence excess esotropia) prescription of the full hypermetropic spectacle correction makes the eyes straight for distance fixation, but residually esotropic for near due to an abnormal relationship between accommodation and accommodative convergence (the AC/A ratio). Prescribing bifocal or varifocal spectacles may compensate this. The aim of the spectacle correction is to ensure that when the child looks down, as when reading, the line of sight will be through the bifocal segment, and this will relax accommodation and control the near esotropia. Some authorities order an add of +3.00 diopters, on the grounds that the average fixation distance at near is in the region of 33 cm. Others have advocated prescribing the minimum near addition which allows control of the near esotropia. The lens form should ensure that the lower bifocal segment is large, so that the child automatically looks through it. The "executive" bifocal is often prescribed.

The recommended strategy is then to gradually reduce ("wean off") the bifocal correction by incremental reductions in the power of the lower segment. Studies of the effects of bifocals[3,4] suggest that this can be achieved in 37 to 60% of cases. Von Noorden[3] has warned of the deleterious effects of extended long-term bifocal wear. Varifocal and progressive lenses have also been suggested as an alternative to bifocals.[5] The advantages are not apparent. They cost more and are more difficult to fit, and younger children may find it difficult adapting to the form of the lower segment of the lens.

Children with unilateral or bilateral aphakia, who cannot accommodate, will also benefit from the use of bifocals.

Contact lenses

Some children with strabismus and gross degrees of anisometropia may benefit from contact lens correction, as this will reduce the aniseikonic effect of spectacle correction and may promote the development of fusion and binocular function. Calcutt[6] reported a series of children with fully accommodative esotropia, but uncooperative with spectacles, where successful management was achieved with contact lens correction. In the author's experience this can be very successful in highly motivated children, usually girls, who are well corrected with glasses, but whose hobbies and pastimes such as ballet, gymnastics, etc. are incompatible with spectacle wear. As the main morbidity of contact lens wear is suppurative keratitis, it is of some importance that the child is old and responsible enough to look after their lenses in an adequately hygienic fashion.

Drugs

Miotics

Miotic drugs are either direct parasympathomimetics, such as pilocarpine, or acetylcholine esterase inhibitors, such as phospholine iodide. The former, which have a short course of action, are not often used in strabismus management, although cases of Adie pupil and third nerve palsy, with unilateral mydriasis may be prescribed pilocarpine to constrict the dilated pupil. As the sphincter is hypersensitive, due to denervation, very weak pilocarpine (0.1%) may be prescribed for the patient to use as required. This is surprisingly popular, and may also improve acuity by improving depth of field.

All miotics constrict the pupil and cause the ciliary body to contract with a change in the refraction in a myopic direction. They were first introduced into strabismus management by Javal[7] (who also advocated bifocals) in the late 19th century. The principle of use is that the child on miotics finds that his or her accommodation is fixed by the effect of the drops, so no active accommodation effort is then made. They are therefore used to control accommodation and thereby accommodative convergence.

Indications have been wider in the past, and these agents are now rarely prescribed. The author has found miotics to be of value in two unusual clinical situations. The first is in the investigation of recalcitrant cases of convergence excess esotropia, where surgery has already been undertaken without success, and the question is whether the child would benefit from further surgical intervention. Sensory testing is often difficult due to the very variable hyperdynamic accommodative convergence. A short course of phospholine iodide 0.06% twice daily will produce good miosis and demonstrate the likely binocular result if surgery was undertaken. Four to six weeks of treatment is normally sufficient for this, and the predictive power is very good. The second indication is persistent consecutive esotropia after surgical overcorrection of intermittent exotropia. Although miotics were often found helpful in reducing the excessive convergence, they have now been superseded in this situation by botulinum toxin injections (see "Botulinum toxin").

Miotics are relatively easy to use, with administration being required once or twice daily. They have several disadvantages; initial instillation usually causes a dull supraorbital headache related to ciliary spasm, although this usually improves over a few days. The child may complain of poor vision, or poor night vision, due to the pupillary constriction. Long-term use may cause iris cysts and lens opacities. As the drops are absorbed through the conjunctival surface and enter the circulation, with phospholine iodide there will be a depletion of plasma cholinesterase. If the child requires medical treatment under general anesthesia, the anesthetist requires being made aware of the therapy and avoiding the use of a depolarizing relaxing agent such as succinylcholine, as prolonged apnea may result. The depletion may last up to six weeks after stopping the drops, and parents should be advised appropriately.

Finally, many manufacturers have stopped making miotic drops. They are expensive, the compounds are basically toxic, and demand is light. It is unlikely that they will remain in the therapeutic armamentarium for childhood strabismus.

Mydriatics and cycloplegics

Pure mydriatics (phenylephrine, adrenaline) are adrenergic agonists, which dilate the pupil by their action on the dilator muscle of the iris, but have little or no effect on ciliary muscle function. Cycloplegics (atropine, cyclopentolate, etc.) are muscarinic parasympathetic blockers, which paralyze the pupillary sphincter muscle as well as the ciliary body.

Mydriatics have little use in the management of strabismus, although they can be combined with cycloplegics to maximize pupillary dilatation for fundus examination, etc. The vasoconstrictive effect of adrenaline makes it valuable as a pre-treatment drop before strabismus surgery or botulinum toxin injection.

Cycloplegic agents are essential in the performance of accurate retinoscopy and refraction in children (see "Spectacles"). Unilateral cycloplegic penalization of the fixing eye can be an effective therapy for amblyopia (see Chapter 78), and may be combined with spectacle penalization and part-time occlusion.

From time to time, one comes across hypermetropic esotropic children who do not tolerate their newly prescribed spectacles and continue to prefer their esotropic uncorrected status. It can be valuable to give their parents a prescription for atropine 1% twice daily (ointment is preferable to drops), which will blur the vision due to uncorrected hypermetropia. The child thereby is given an incentive to wear its glasses. After four or so weeks, the parents are asked to stop the therapy. As atropine is quite slow to wear off, the effect gradually diminishes, and the child is usually then well habituated to its glasses.

Prisms

Prisms have very limited value in the management of childhood strabismus. Where a child has a temporary deviation that might confidently be expected to improve, as in temporary consecutive esotropia after surgery for exotropia, or in a postviral sixth nerve palsy, temporary Fresnel membrane prisms may be attached to glasses to maintain binocularity while the deviation evolves. However, in anything other than the lowest powers, prisms significantly degrade the visual acuity, in addition to attracting dirt, fingerprints, etc.

Prism adaptation

Jampolsky described the prism adaptation test (PAT) for esotropia in 1971.[8] The patient has base-out prisms applied to the glasses to correct the angle of deviation. In cases where the esodeviation increases, "eating up the prisms," the power of the prisms is increased until the angle stabilizes. Subsequent surgery is then based on the maximum prism-adapted angle, and results are claimed to be superior to those based on the manifest angle without prism adaptation. In 1990, the Prism Adaptation Study Research Group[9] reported the results of a prospective randomized controlled clinical trial of prism adaptation in acquired esotropia in which 60% of patients underwent prism adaptation and 40% did not. Of the group that responded to prism adaptation with a stable motor angle and sensory fusion, half had augmented strabismus surgery based on the prism-adapted angle and half had a conventional amount of surgery. The best rates of alignment were obtained in prism responders who underwent augmented surgery (89%), and the lowest were in patients who were not prism adapted (72%). Factors likely to predict prism response were identified in a later analysis[10] as being older age at onset, duration of deviation less than a year, alternating fixation, fusion with the Worth four-dot test when neutralized with prisms for near, and equal visual acuities.

Prisms in nystagmus

In children with congenital nystagmus and a compensatory head posture, when Kestenbaum surgery is being contemplated, it may be helpful to conduct a short trial of prismatic glasses (typically for watching television at home) to allow the parents to confirm that the face turn is abolished. The Fresnel prisms should not be stronger than 15–20 prism diopters, and should be applied with the bases to the side to which the head is habitually turned.

Exercises

In the early years of orthoptics, it was widely believed that children with latent or intermittent deviations could be improved by exercises designed to increase fusional amplitudes, performed with the aid of the synoptophore or major amblyoscope. Indeed, Emile Javal (1839–1907) is credited with having exhorted parents to take their squinting child out of school to allow it to have up to 8 hours a day of stereoscopic exercises.[11] Javal followed up cases over as much as 6 years of treatment and documented them meticulously. He later observed "The first time that I revealed my methods to von Graefe, this colleague, also renowned for his benevolence as well as his professional merits, astonished me by saying that people are not worth the effort. Life's experience has shown me that von Graefe was correct."

Over time, however, enthusiasm for orthoptic exercises has waned, although this has not stopped patients and parents from wondering whether they might be helpful. It is still felt that convergence exercises, with pen convergence and stereogram fixation, are of value in cases of convergence insufficiency. This is, however, a rare entity in children.

Botulinum toxin therapy

In 1979 Alan Scott, an ophthalmologist from San Francisco, published a study of 19 patients treated for strabismus by means of injections into their extraocular muscles of botulinum neurotoxin A, as an alternative to strabismus surgery.[12] Botulinum neurotoxins are taken up by the presynaptic neurone at cholinergic nerve endings supplying striated muscles and exocrine secretory glands. Once internalized, they disrupt the process by which the nerve manufactures vesicles containing acetylcholine. Accordingly, the nerve ending is switched off, and if it supplies a neuromuscular junction, the muscle supplied develops a flaccid paralysis. After a period of time, new endings are established and the paralysis disappears. Scott showed that appropriate doses of botulinum neurotoxin A could be safely and effectively injected into extraocular muscles of adults under local anesthetic, and accuracy maximized by electromyographic monitoring during the injection. The technique was immediately welcomed as an effective and elegant new treatment for strabismus.

The treatment was not initially seen as suitable for children, who, unless they were old enough to be cooperative, had to be admitted to hospital as day cases and undergo treatment under some type of sedation or dissociative anesthesia. However, in 1990 Scott and three colleagues[13] described their experience of treatment of 413 strabismic children with botulinum toxin. In 362 children with follow-up of 6 months or more (average 26 months), 61% were aligned within 10 prism diopters after an average of 1.7 injections. Overall, they found that esotropes responded better than exotropes, and that results were better for smaller angles of strabismus, being especially good for consecutive esotropia. Complications were minor and transient, the commonest being ipsilateral ptosis, which occurred in 31%, and induced vertical deviation in 16%.

Personal experience

We started our botulinum toxin treatment clinic in 1982, and had treated 5860 patients by July 2003, of whom 517 (8.8%) were under the age of 16. There were 290 girls and 227 boys. Figure 87.1 and Table 87.1 show the age distribution of the cases. It can be seen that there is a strong preponderance of older children, with 68% of our cases being 11 or older at first injection. We have found that such children are usually highly motivated and can give informed consent to treatment under local anesthesia. In many ways, they are exactly like our adult patients, many of whom find it entirely acceptable to have maintenance therapy with botulinum toxin, as a superior alternative to incisional surgery.

Figure 87.2 and Table 87.2 show the number of injections given per patient. The total number was 1068 injections, and the vast majority of patients (85%) had 1 or 2 injections and then went on to other therapies, although in some cases the injection was effective in restoring fusion and allowed surgery to be avoided. However, 16 children, 10 girls and 6 boys, received 10 or more injections for strabismus. The age range was from 10 to 15 years, and the average number of previous operations was 1.88. Eight (50%) had consecutive exotropia, 4 (25%) residual esotropia, 2 consecutive esotropia, and 1 each primary esotropia and atypical Duane syndrome. The number of injections given was from 10 to 40 with a mean of 15.

Figure 87.3 shows the diagnoses by category for our strabismic children treated with botulinum toxin. It can be seen that 90% of the total group had concomitant strabismus with 5% paralytic, 4% muscular and restrictive, and 1% miscellaneous indications. Figures 87.4, 87.5, and 87.6 show the subtypes of strabismus treated in each category. Overall the commonest diagnoses were primary esotropia with 118 cases (23%) and consecutive exotropia with 101 cases (19.5%).

We have treated 101 patients as day cases under either ketamine dissociative anesthesia (2 mg per kg intravenously) or with intravenous propofol (2–3 mg per kg) or nitrous oxide inhalation. None of these techniques abolish spontaneous eye movements and all injections were monitored with electro-

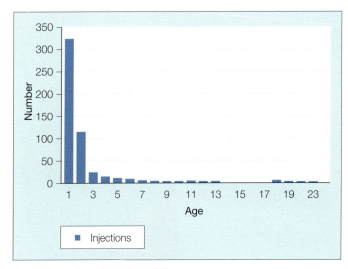

Fig. 87.2 Number of injections–517 cases.

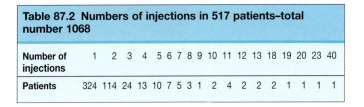

Table 87.2 Numbers of injections in 517 patients–total number 1068																		
Number of injections	1	2	3	4	5	6	7	8	9	10	11	12	13	18	19	20	23	40
Patients	324	114	24	13	10	7	5	3	1	2	4	2	2	2	1	1	1	1

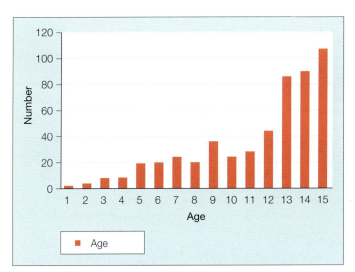

Fig. 87.1 Age at first treatment with botulinum toxin–517 cases.

Table 87.1 Age distribution of 517 children treated with botulinum toxin														
Age	1	2	3	4	5	6	7	8	9	10	11	12	13	14	15
No of patients treated	2	4	8	8	19	20	24	20	36	24	28	44	85	89	106

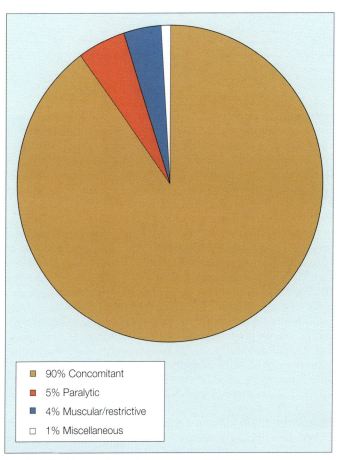

- 90% Concomitant
- 5% Paralytic
- 4% Muscular/restrictive
- 1% Miscellaneous

Fig. 87.3 Strabismus diagnosis by category–517 patients.

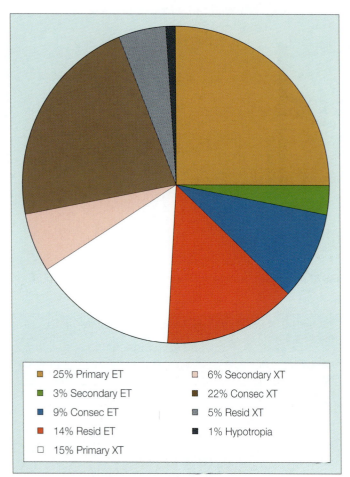

Fig. 87.4 Concomitant strabismus diagnoses–463 patients.

- ■ 25% Primary ET
- ■ 3% Secondary ET
- ■ 9% Consec ET
- ■ 14% Resid ET
- □ 15% Primary XT
- □ 6% Secondary XT
- ■ 22% Consec XT
- ■ 5% Resid XT
- ■ 1% Hypotropia

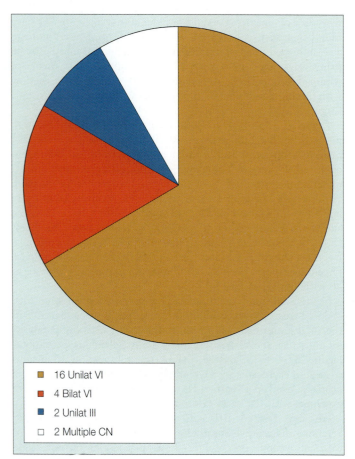

Fig. 87.5 Paralytic strabismus diagnoses–24 patients.

- ■ 16 Unilat VI
- ■ 4 Bilat VI
- ■ 2 Unilat III
- □ 2 Multiple CN

myography to guide needle placement. No problems have been encountered with any of these cases, and the bad reputation of ketamine for causing frightening nightmares has not been encountered in our patients. Nevertheless, our enthusiasm for this approach is less than it was initially. The child requires admission and some type of anesthesia, so the advantages of outpatient clinic management are lost. Also, when children are treated under anesthetic, the rate of ptosis and secondary vertical deviation, which is around 5% in our hands with awake patients, goes up to around 25%. We now tend to reserve the use of botulinum toxin under anesthesia for situations where botulinum toxin is superior to surgery. The main indication is *acquired strabismus (almost always esotropia) in a previously binocular child*. Examples include consecutive esotropia following surgery for intermittent exotropia,[14] sixth nerve palsy beginning to lose a compensatory head posture, acute normisensorial esotropia,[15] and strabismus following temporary uniocular visual deprivation. We have also used botulinum toxin to investigate the sensory status and the possibility of a fusional result from surgery in selected cases of complex strabismus.[16]

Botulinum toxin for other types of childhood strabismus

Other investigators have used botulinum toxin as a primary therapy for essential infantile esotropia. This approach is well described in a large review by McNeer et al.[17] in which they describe the results of several hundred patients reported by investigators in the USA, Spain, France, Argentina, and Italy. Most investigators used bilateral medial rectus injections, and results obtained were judged to be at least as good as those reported after standard strabismus surgery for this condition.

Another approach was described by Tejedor and Rodriguez,[18] who first showed in a randomized controlled trial that botulinum toxin injection was at least as effective as surgery in the retreatment of children with residual esotropia after surgery for acquired esotropia, and then that botulinum toxin was an effective primary therapy for acquired esotropia in children.[19]

Current indications for the use of botulinum toxin in children

Currently when managing children with strabismus with botulinum toxin we are happy to treat older motivated children under local anesthesia in our out patient clinics, reserving the use of day case admission and injection under anesthesia for the specific indications of acquired strabismus in a previously binocular child, and for the investigation of sensory or motor status in complex cases of childhood strabismus.

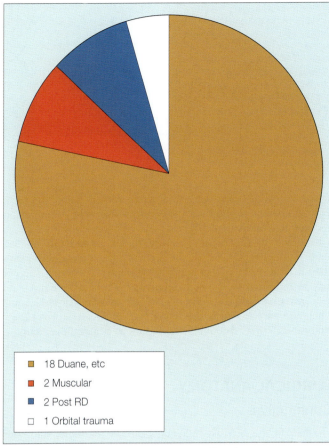

Fig. 87.6 Muscular and restrictive diagnoses–23 patients.

- 18 Duane, etc
- 2 Muscular
- 2 Post RD
- 1 Orbital trauma

REFERENCES

1. Cleary M, Shahid H. In press.
2. Caltrider N, Jampolsky A. Overcorrecting minus lens therapy for treatment of intermittent exotropia. Ophthalmology 1983; 90: 1160–5.
3. von Noorden GK, Morris J, Edelman P. Efficacy of bifocals in the treatment of accommodative esotropia. Am J Ophthalmol 1978; 85: 830–4.
4. Ludwig IH, Parks MM, Getson PR. Long-term results of bifocal therapy for accommodative esotropia. J Pediatr Ophthalmol Strabismus 1989; 26: 264–70.
5. Smith JB. Progressive-addition lenses in the treatment of accommodative esotropia. Am J Ophthalmol 1985; 99: 56–62.
6. Calcutt C. Contact lenses in accommodative esotropia therapy. Brit Orthopt J 1989; 46: 59–65.
7. Javal E. Manuel Théoretique et Practique de Strabisme. Paris: Masson; 1896.
8. Jampolsky A. A simplified approach to strabismus diagnosis. In: Burian HM, editor. Symposium on Strabismus. Transactions of the New Orleans Academy of Ophthalmology. St Louis: Mosby; 1971: 34.
9. Prism Adaptation Study Research Group. Efficacy of prism adaptation in the surgical management of acquired esotropia. Arch Ophthalmol 1990; 108: 1248–56.
10. Repka MX, Wentworth D. Predictors of prism response during prism adaptation. Prism Adaptation Study Research Group. J Pediatr Ophthalmol Strabismus 1991; 28: 202–5.
11. Wybar KC. Anomalies of ocular motility. In: Duke-Elder S, editor. Ocular Motility and Strabismus. London: Henry Kimpton; 1973: 471. (System of ophthalmology, Vol. 6.)
12. Scott AB. Botulinum toxin injections into extraocular muscles as an alternative to strabismus surgery. Ophthalmology 1980; 87: 1044–9.
13. Scott AB, Magoon EH, McNeer KW, et al. Botulinum treatment of childhood strabismus. Ophthalmology 1990; 97: 1434–8.
14. Dawson ELM, Marshman WE, Lee JP. Role of botulinum toxin A in surgically overcorrected exotropia. J AAPOS 1999; 3: 269-71.
15. Timms C, Gregson RM, Lee JP, et al. Sudden onset of concomitant esotropia. In: Kaufmann H, editor. Transactions of the 21st meeting of the European Strabismological Association. 1993.
16. Rayner SA, Hollick EJ, Lee JP. Botulinum toxin in childhood strabismus. Strabismus 1999; 7: 103–11.
17. McNeer KW, Tucker MG, Spencer RF. Management of essential infantile esotropia with botulinum toxin A: review and recommendations. J Pediatr Ophthalmol Strabismus 2000; 37: 63–7.
18. Tejedor J, Rodriguez JM. Retreatment of children after surgery for acquired esotropia: reoperation versus botulinum injection. Br J Ophthalmol 1998; 82: 110-4.
19. Tejedor J, Rodriguez JM. Long-term outcome and predictor variables in the treatment of acquired esotropia with botulinum toxin. Invest Ophthalmol Vis Sci 2001; 42: 2542–6.

CHAPTER 88 Strabismus Surgery

Robert Morris

INTRODUCTION

The management of strabismus involves careful assessment of patients, treatment of amblyopia and refractive errors, and in certain cases surgical correction. Amblyopia should be treated prior to surgery and the different stages in the management of the strabismus should be made clear to parents. Refractive errors should normally be fully corrected and any surgery based on the residual angle in spectacles. Following surgery, children need continued follow-up until at least the age of visual maturity to monitor their vision and refraction, as well as the stability of the strabismus. Adults should be followed for at least six months after surgery to ensure their strabismus is stable. Surgery may be functional, aiming to establish or restore binocular single vision, or indicated to improve ocular alignment in the absence of any potential binocular function.

The assessment of strabismus should include measurement and recording of the deviation, with the appropriate refractive error corrected, at near and distance in primary position and at distance in nine positions of gaze where possible. In patients with vertical strabismus the deviation on head tilting and torsion should also be documented.[1-3] Sensory assessment of strabismus is essential to assess binocular potential or function. All children with strabismus require at least one cycloplegic refraction before surgery. Where appropriate other investigations such as Hess

charts, forced duction tests, and active forced generation tests may be necessary. Only with this information can an informed decision regarding surgery be made.

Parents typically expect surgery to be carried out on the strabismic eye particularly if the eye has poor vision, but in many cases it is advantageous to perform symmetrical surgery. Surgery may be indicated on the nonstrabismic eye when there has been previous surgery on the fixing eye, in cases of paralytic strabismus when the paretic eye is the fixing eye, or in cases of complex strabismus with restriction or limitation of ocular movement.

SURGICAL ANATOMY

Conjunctiva

The conjunctiva is fused to Tenon's capsule anteriorly, and both are fused to the sclera at the limbus. The rectus muscles and anterior ciliary arteries are often visible through the conjunctiva, less so in young patients.

Tenon's capsule and intermuscular septum

Tenon's capsule extends from the limbus fusing posteriorly to the optic nerve. It is a dense white structure (Fig. 88.1), becoming

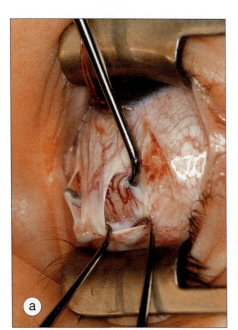
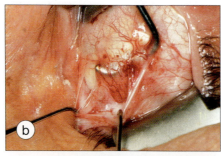
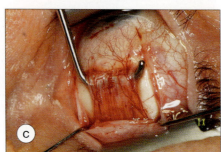

Fig. 88.1 Tenon's capsule overlying the superior rectus: surgeon's view from above. (a) The Tenon's capsule overlying the superior rectus is being held in the lower two strabismus hooks. (b) Intermuscular septum and check ligaments displayed with the two lower tenotomy hooks. (c) Superior rectus after dissection, note anterior ciliary arteries. (Patient of Dr R Morris.)

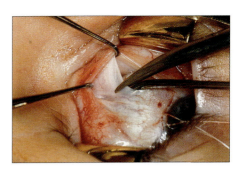

Fig. 88.2
Intermuscular septum and check ligaments over medial rectus. (Patient of Dr R Morris.)

thin in adults. Divided into anterior and posterior parts where the extraocular muscles penetrate it posterior to the equator, it separates the globe and extraocular muscles from the orbital fat. From the under surface of Tenon's, check ligaments extend to the surface of the capsule of the rectus muscles. The intermuscular septum (Fig. 88.2), a thin fascial plane, connects the rectus muscles from the point at which they pierce Tenon's capsule and anteriorly fuses with it and the conjunctiva at the limbus. During strabismus surgery, both Tenon's capsule and the intermuscular septum need to be divided to hook and dissect a rectus muscle. From the outer surface of Tenon's capsule, septae run through the orbital fat to the orbital periosteum.[4] The orbital fat extends anteriorly to within 10 mm of the limbus and can be clearly seen through the conjunctiva in the inferior fornix. Strabismus surgery is carried out within Tenon's capsule, which, if pierced, can lead to orbital fat prolapse and scarring with restriction of eye movements because the fat becomes adherent to the globe and muscles and mobility is restricted by its septal attachment to the orbital periosteum.

The rectus muscles

The rectus muscles originate at the orbital apex, at the annulus of Zinn, are all approximately 40 mm long, and insert onto the sclera anteriorly. There is a variation in the distance between the limbus and insertion (Table 88.1), and the width of the limbus varies, being thinnest medially and widest superiorly.[5]

During strabismus surgery, the insertion may become displaced toward the limbus, making measurements from the insertion inaccurate, and the distance from the limbus to the insertion should be measured before manipulation of the muscle.[6] This displacement may be a combination of shortening of the sclera anterior to the insertion and lamellar tearing of the sclera. V-shaped deformities of the insertion stump, induced by pulling on the insertion stump with toothed forceps, have been also been described.[7] Although careful surgical technique may minimize these artifacts, they are difficult to eliminate.

The medial and lateral rectus muscles act as pure adductors and abductors. The medial has a 6-mm arc of contact with the globe, whereas the lateral is 10 mm.

In primary position, the inferior rectus forms an angle of 23° with the visual axis and function as a depressor, excyclotortor and adductor. In abduction of 23° its only action is depression and in adduction it excyclotorts and adducts the eye. The inferior rectus has a unique relationship with the lower lid and inferior oblique (Fig. 88.3). The capsulopalpebral fascia of the lower lid is analogous to the levator aponeurosis of the upper lid. It arises 5 mm from the insertion of the inferior rectus muscle, splits to surround the inferior oblique, and condenses anteriorly to it, forming Lockwood's ligament. Anterior to Lockwood's ligament, the fascia thickens, being joined by smooth muscle, to form the inferior tarsal muscle, which inserts onto the lower lid tarsus on its anterior, posterior, and basal surfaces. Some of these fibromuscular fibers extend through the preseptal orbicularis muscle, inserting into skin forming the lower lid skin crease. The lower lid is lowered 2 mm by its action and the lashes everted, a movement facilitated by its contact with the globe.

In primary position, the superior rectus forms an angle of 23° with the visual axis and functions as an elevator, incyclotortor, and adductor. In abduction of 23° its only action is elevation, and in adduction it incyclotorts and adducts the eye. Like the inferior rectus muscle there are fascial attachments between the superior rectus and upper lid muscles.

The superior oblique muscle

The superior oblique arises from the orbital apex, and passes through the trochlear as a cord-like tendon and runs posterolaterally at an angle of approximately 54°, before fanning out and passing under the superior rectus, inserting on the supratemporal quadrant of the globe (Fig. 88.4). The anterior end of the insertion lies about 4 mm posterior to lateral insertion of the superior rectus muscle, the posterior end lies approximately 6.5 mm from the optic nerve, and the width of the insertion is about 11mm, but varies considerably. The trochlear acts as its functional origin. The fibers of the posterior two-thirds of the insertion are responsible for the depression action of the muscle in adduction. Intorsion and abduction are maximal in adduction.

The superior oblique tendon is often anomalous.[8] The tendon may be redundant or lax (Fig. 88.5), may be misdirected, may have an anomalous insertion nasal to the superior rectus or into Tenon's and the trochlear, or may be absent.[9] Intraoperative "exaggerated"[10] forced duction testing can demonstrate laxity of the superior oblique tendon. The nasal superior oblique tendon has fascial relationships with the intermuscular septum, which envelops it to form a "capsule." If the nasal intermuscular tendon is removed while performing a nasal tenotomy, the cut tendon ends have no support and will freely separate, and a palsy may result. There is also a frenulum between the undersurface of superior rectus and the superior oblique (Fig. 88.6), which must be divided for effective recession of either muscle.

The inferior oblique muscle

The inferior oblique muscle has a tendon of 1–2 mm. It passes posteriorly, laterally and upward, from its origin adjacent to the lacrimal sac, to its insertion 8–10 mm posterior to the inferior border of the lateral rectus insertion. It runs at an angle of approximately 51° to the vertical plane of the globe. As it passes the inferior temporal quadrant, it overlies a vortex vein. The

Table 88.1 Rectus muscle dimensions

	Distance from limbus to midpoint of insertion	Length of muscle	Width at insertion	Length of tendon
Medial rectus	5.5	40	10.3	3.7
Inferior rectus	6.5	40	9.8	5.5
Lateral rectus	6.9	48	9.2	8.8
Superior rectus	7.7	42	10.8	5.8

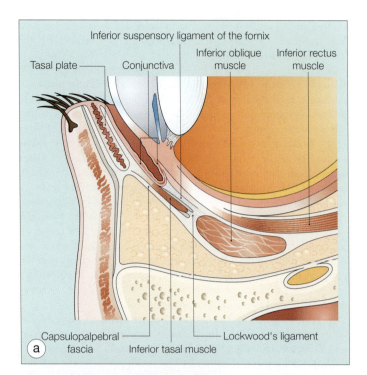

Inferior suspensory ligament of the fornix

Inferior oblique muscle

Inferior rectus muscle

Tasal plate

Conjunctiva

Capsulopalpebral fascia

Inferior tasal muscle

Lockwood's ligament

(a)

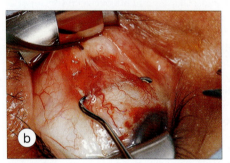

(b)

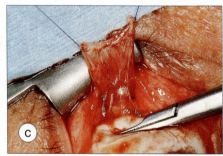

(c)

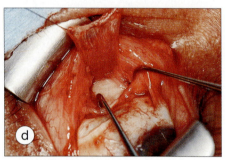

(d)

Fig. 88.3 Relationship of inferior rectus to lower lid: surgeon's view from above. (a) Diagrammatic illustration. (b) Lower lid retractors on surface of inferior rectus muscle being held with forceps. (c) Thickened Tenon's fascia beneath inferior rectus muscle seen as a glistening membrane with ridges between the muscle and the globe. (d) Inferior rectus muscle seen within Tenon's capsule. The original muscle insertion is seen under the left muscle hook. (Patient of Dr R Morris.)

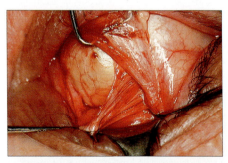

Fig. 88.4 Superior oblique tendon (held in lower hook) inserting beneath the superior rectus: surgeon's view from above. (Patient of Dr R Morris.)

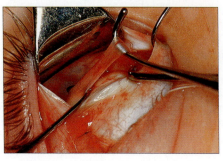

Fig. 88.5 Strabismus hooks beneath superior oblique tendon demonstrating tendon laxity. (Patient of Dr R Morris.)

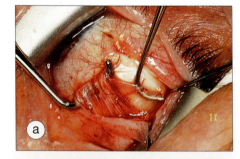

(a)

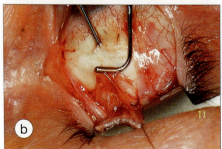

(b)

Fig. 88.6 Relationship between superior oblique and rectus: surgeon's view from above. (a) Chavasse muscle spreading hook (left) beneath superior rectus and Stevens hook beneath the superior oblique showing the fascial attachment between them. It passes obliquely between the crook of the Stevens hook to just by the insertion of the superior rectus. (b) Undersurface of disinserted superior rectus (below, held on sutures) showing fascial attachment between it and the superior oblique tendon. (Patient of Dr R Morris.)

width of the insertion is about 9 mm, and the posterior aspect overlies the macular.[11] The neurovascular bundle enters the muscle as it passes beneath the nasal border of the inferior rectus muscle.

Its primary action elevation is maximal in adduction; its excyclotorsion and abduction actions are maximal in adduction. Inferior oblique overaction is frequent in patients with strabismus, usually congenital esotropia and intermittent exotropia, and superior oblique palsies. Overactions can be graded on a scale of I–IV.[3] Inferior oblique overaction must be distinguished from dissociated vertical deviation (Chapter 75), and the two conditions may co-exist.[12] Inferior oblique underactions are less common and usually secondary to superior oblique overaction; inferior oblique palsies are rare. Inferior oblique underaction can be distinguished from Brown syndrome by a normal forced duction test.

Globe dimensions and strabismus

The anterior portion of the globe of a neonate is proportionately larger than the posterior. The equator of the globe is only a small distance behind the muscle insertion, so a 4-mm recession of the medial rectus may place the muscle behind the equator, thus surgery in infants should be undertaken with caution. During the first 2 years of life there is rapid growth of the eye, mostly post equatorial, the average axial length is 20.3 mm at 6 months and 22.8 mm at 20 months.[13]

Blood supply

The blood supply to the anterior segment is important as some strabismus surgery can lead to anterior segment ischemia. In man there is a collateral blood supply to the anterior segment: an anterior episcleral arterial circle, an incomplete intramuscular arterial circle, and a major arterial circle. The major contribution to this comes from the anterior ciliary arteries; each rectus muscle has two, except the lateral, which has one. The contribution of the two long posterior ciliary arteries is less significant.[14,15]

GENERAL PRINCIPLES OF SURGERY

Anesthetic

In children a general anesthetic is always used. Most children are induced for anesthesia either intravenously or by inhalation and are paralyzed and ventilated. Laryngeal masks and avoidance of premedication enables rapid recovery. Topical local anesthesia and nonsteroidal antiinflammatory agents have all been advocated for the postoperative pain; pain is worse with multiple muscle surgery, reoperations and resections more painful than recessions, and occasionally requires strong analgesia.

Patient preparation

Prior to surgery the patient is positioned so that their head is level and the neck slightly extended (Fig. 88.7). The skin within the surgical field should be cleaned with aqueous povidone iodine and the conjunctival sac irrigated with 5% povidone iodine. The eyebrows should be draped so they are not within the surgical field (Fig. 88.8). A guarded lid speculum keeps the lashes away.

Instruments

A selection of strabismus hooks are invaluable (Fig. 88.9). Long hooks enable rectus muscles to be spread evenly on the hook

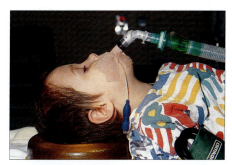

Fig. 88.7 Patient correctly positioned for surgery with neck slightly extended. (Patient of Dr R Morris.)

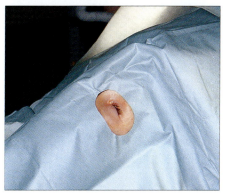

Fig. 88.8 Surgical drape covering brow. (Patient of Dr R Morris.)

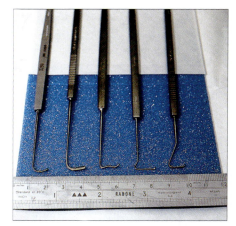

Fig. 88.9 Strabismus hooks. From left to right: a Stevens tenotomy hook, a von Graefe hook, a Chavasse hook, a Helveston hook, and a Green muscle hook.

facilitating dissection and suture placement (Fig. 88.10). Small hooks bunch the muscle on the hook. It is easy to inadvertently split muscles with a hook, but this can be readily identified if a second hook is passed under the muscle from the opposite pole. Stevens tenotomy hooks are useful for retracting conjunctiva and sclera, and essential for oblique muscle surgery. In some cases Desmarres or Fison retractors help exposure. 6-O Vicryl (polyglactin-910) is the most commonly used suture material. It causes minimal tissue reaction, has a high tensile strength, has good knot holding ability, and absorbs in 2–3 months; however, it snags tissues and in rare cases produces an allergic reaction. When reattaching a muscle to the globe, the needle should be placed through the superficial $\frac{1}{3}$ to $\frac{1}{2}$ of the sclera with the tip visible at all times. Spatulate needles, which cut the tissues at the sides and tip, are preferable, and provided the needle is held parallel to the sclera during its intrascleral course the risk of globe perforation is low.[16,17] Usually, a $\frac{3}{8}$-circle needle is preferable, but a $\frac{1}{2}$-circle needle can ease suture placement when access is poor, and it allows a shorter scleral bite of the same depth. A

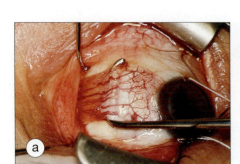
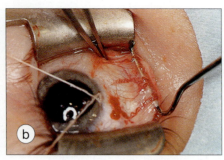

Fig. 88.10 Surgical use of muscle hooks. (a) Chavasse muscle hook under medial rectus. Note even spreading of the muscle tendon on the hook and anterior ciliary arteries. (b) Muscle spread evenly on Helveston hook. (Patient of Dr R Morris.)

reverse cutting needle with a cutting edge on its convex surface has a greater risk of scleral perforation but it does not have to be placed exactly parallel to the scleral surface during its intrascleral course. My preference for conjunctival closure is 8-O virgin silk or 8-O Vicryl.

Strabismus surgery may best be performed with magnification spectacle-mounted loupes or the operating microscope, which has the advantage of good lighting and magnification, but the disadvantages of reducing the field size and depth of focus, and restricting the surgeon's mobility.

Forced duction tests

Forced duction tests (FDTs), the passive movement of a patient's eye to test for mechanical restriction should be conducted before a strabismus operation. They can distinguish mechanical restriction from muscle weakness. Interpretation of the test requires experience but it is still difficult to detect subtle restrictions:

Restriction present: "positive" test;
No restriction: "negative" test.

If positive, the test should be repeated throughout surgery, particularly when the muscle thought to be responsible for the restriction has been disinserted. In adults it can be conducted in the clinic using local anesthesia, but in children it is usually performed under general anesthetic. Succinylcholine may influence FDTs.

The assessment of the rectus and oblique muscles requires different techniques.

To assess the rectus muscles

The globe is held at the limbus with fixation forceps, *pulled forward* to stretch the rectus muscles, and moved in the opposite direction to the muscle's action. To assess restriction of the inferior rectus the eye is held at 6 o'clock and the globe fully elevated. If it can be fully rotated, then no mechanical restriction is present.

To assess the oblique muscles

An "exaggerated" forced duction test[18] aids the diagnosis of congenital superior oblique palsy and Brown syndrome. The eye is held with toothed forceps at 3 and 9 o'clock and *pushed back*, stretching the oblique muscles. The eye is then excyclotorted and elevated in adduction. In Brown syndrome there is restriction to elevation. In congenital superior oblique palsy there may be absence of the normal resistance.[10] The technique assesses the efficacy of superior oblique weakening procedures for Brown syndrome and assesses the tightness of the tendon after a superior oblique tuck. A similar technique can be used to assess the tightness of the inferior oblique.

Active force generation test

Force generation testing, carried out under topical anesthetic, assesses muscle strength by the force generated when the patient looks into the field of action of the muscle in question with the eye held by toothed forceps.

Conjunctival incisions

Limbal incisions

A limbal incision is easy to perform for rectus muscle surgery (Fig. 88.11); it gives good exposure, induces little scarring or adhesions, and can be combined with conjunctival recession. It is good for reoperations or muscle transposition because of the exposure it provides. It may give an unsightly ridge if there is poor reapposition of the conjunctiva. One "relaxing" incision can result in irregular tearing of the conjunctiva and two relaxing incisions should be avoided where the conjunctiva is thin and easily torn.

Cul-de-sac or fornix incisions

The cul-de-sac or fornix incision (Fig. 88.12) is quick, produces minimal scarring, leaves the limbal conjunctiva intact, and a

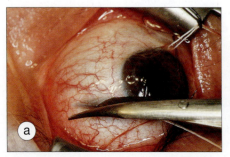
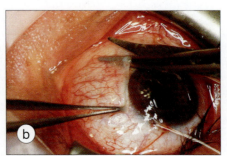
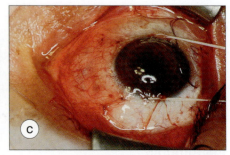

Fig. 88.11 Limbal conjunctival incision: surgeon's view from above. (a) Inferior conjunctival "relaxing" incision. (b) Superior conjunctival relaxing incision parallel to inferior conjunctival incision following completion of peritomy. (c) Accurate apposition of conjunctiva following rectus muscle surgery using four 7–0 Vicryl sutures. (Patient of Dr R Morris.)

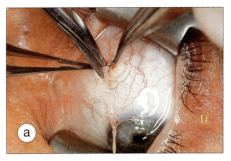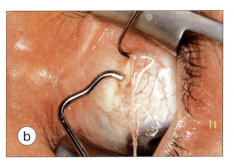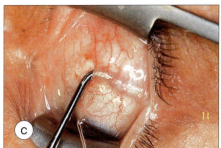

Fig. 88.12 Cul-de-sac conjunctival incision. (a) Incision in Tenon's after a conjunctival incision 8 mm from the limbus. (b) The conjunctiva and Tenon's are held up with a small conjunctival hook (above) while the muscle spreader hook is inserted into the sub-Tenon's space toward the inferior rectus. c) Placement of strabismus hook under the inferior rectus. (Patient of Dr R Morris.)

conjunctival suture may not be needed.[19] As it lies under the lid it is comfortable postoperatively and adjacent rectus muscles can be approached through the same incision. The incision is 8 mm from the limbus (not actually in the fornix, but 1–2 mm limbal to it). The conjunctival incision is pulled over the muscle to expose it. It is more demanding for rectus muscle surgery, particularly for reoperations, and needs a skilled assistant. With thin conjunctiva there is a risk of large conjunctival tears.

The Swan incision
The Swan incision is made over the muscle insertion but is now rarely used. The main disadvantage of this technique is hemorrhage from trauma to the anterior ciliary vessels or muscle when exposing the muscle.[20]

EXTRAOCULAR MUSCLE SURGERY

Principles

Meticulous attention to detail makes surgery easier, outcomes more predictable, and complications fewer. Careful dissection enables good exposure, limits adhesions, and minimizes muscle and vessel trauma and fat prolapse; hemostasis makes surgery easier and reduces postoperative inflammation and adhesions. Any bleeding should be avoided, but, when present, bleeding points identified and cauterized. Saline irrigation can be used to identify bleeding points and prevent charring and shrinkage of conjunctiva, sclera, and muscle.

Rectus muscle surgery

Once a rectus muscle has been exposed, excessive Tenon's should be removed from its surface to allow accurate placement of sutures and reduce snagging on the suture. The anterior ciliary

vessels should then be cauterized before being cut to prevent bleeding. Cauterizing after suture placement risks burning the suture. Whether using a single- or double-ended suture technique, careful suture placement with accurate knots reduces the risk of sutures looping and muscle slippage (Fig. 88.13). A double-ended suture provides support for the center of the muscle and not just the poles and can be used for most muscle recessions, including adjustables, and resections.

Weakening procedures
Recessions
The easiest and most effective technique for weakening a rectus muscle is a recession. Its effect is maximal in the field of action of the muscle, and has a significant effect in primary position. Recessions are faster, easier, more predictable and produce less inflammation and scarring than resections. Suture placement, prior to disinsertion, should be 0.5–1 mm from the insertion with secure lock bites at both poles so that the whole muscle is incorporated into the suture without any Tenon's. This minimizes the amount of induced resection, and the muscle is secure on the suture and can be disinserted safely, reducing the risk of muscle slippage.

The advantage of measuring a recession from the limbus is that it is a fixed anatomical point, whereas the insertion, particularly of the medial rectus, varies;[5] however, the limbus can be up to 1.5 mm wide.[5] If measurements are made from the insertion it should be measured before the muscle is disinserted as it can "creep" toward the limbus after disinsertion.[7]

Most surgeons perform fixed recessions using either single- or double-suture technique (Figs. 88.14a and 88.14b). In fixed recessions the muscle is sutured directly at the desired placement of the recession, and the muscle can be readily supra- or infraplaced. The two sutures should be placed the same distance apart as the poles of the muscle, reducing central sagging, which enhances the recession (Figs. 88.15a and 88.15b). If central

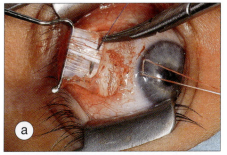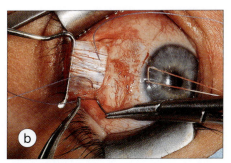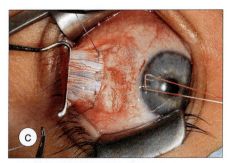

Fig. 88.13 Muscle suture placement: double-armed suture through lateral rectus. (a) Central suture placement. (b) Inferior lock bite. (c) Completed suture placement prior to muscle disinsertion. (Patient of Dr R Morris.)

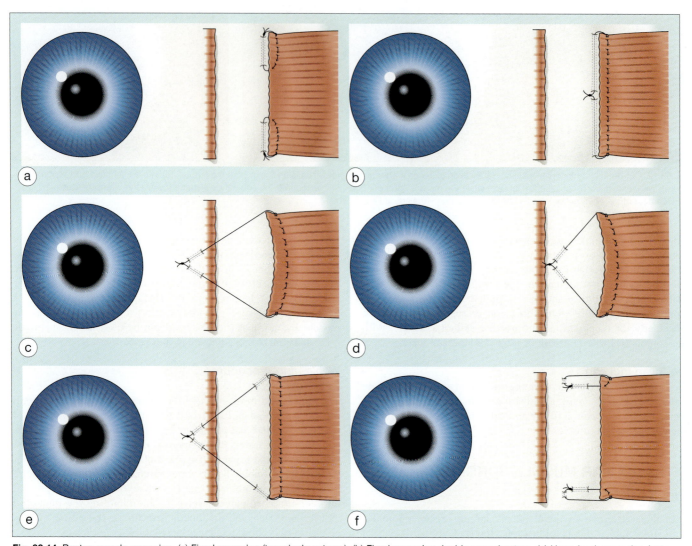

Fig. 88.14 Rectus muscle recession. (a) Fixed recession (two single sutures). (b) Fixed recession double-armed suture. (c) Hang-back recession (note central bowing). (d) Hemi-hang-back recession. (e) Anchored hang-back suture. (f) Gobin's loop recession.

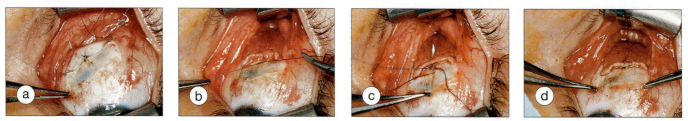

Fig. 88.15 Inferior rectus fixed muscle recession, double-suture technique: surgeon's view from above. (a) Needle placement through two scleral tunnels. (b) Muscle tied in recessed position. (c) Needle placed back through center of muscle. (d) Sutures tied down: note absence of central sag. (Patient of Dr R Morris.)

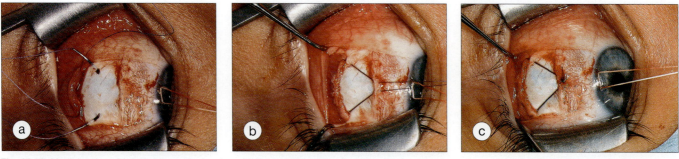

Fig. 88.16 Medial rectus. Anchored hang-back suture. (a) The needles of the double-armed sutures (already attached to the muscle as in Fig. 88.13 and the muscle detached) are passed through the sclera. (b) Sutures passed through muscle insertion. (c) Sutures tied down: note minimal central sag. (Patient of Dr R Morris.)

sagging occurs, the center of the muscle is sutured to the sclera (Figs. 88.15.c and 88.15d). The disadvantages are that the needle passes through the thinnest sclera, increasing the risk of globe perforation, particularly with posterior placement.

Rectus muscles can also be recessed using the "hang-back" or "hemi-hang-back" technique (Fig. 88.14c and 88.14d). The hang-back technique allows the rectus muscle to be suspended, on a single double-armed 6–0 vicryl suture, from its original insertion (Fig. 88.18). It is easier and quicker and may reduce the risk of scleral perforation as the needle is passed through the thick sclera anterior to the insertion of the muscle. The disadvantages are that the muscle width is contracted with central sagging, the muscle might migrate anteriorly, and it is not possible to infra- or supraplace the muscle using this technique. Large recessions of the superior rectus used for dissociated vertical deviation are effectively hang-back recessions. An anchored hang-back suture uses superficial (therefore safer) scleral sutures at the desired point of recession, with deeper scleral bites at or just anterior to the insertion (Figs. 88.14e and 88.16); thus the muscle is placed in the desired position, and it prevents central sag and creeping. Before the knot is tied, the position of the muscle can be checked and the sutures replaced if necessary. The knot is tied anteriorly with less risk of dragging Tenon's into the knot, but it is only covered by thin conjunctiva and can become inflamed.

In the hemi-hang-back technique a single double-armed suture is used and the needles placed posterior to the insertion (Fig. 88.14d). The muscle is then allowed to hang back on the suture. It has been advocated for large recessions where exposure can be difficult but the needle passes through thin sclera. This technique should not be confused with a loop recession where a nonabsorbable suture is placed through each pole of the muscle, which is then sutured to the sclera behind the insertion suspended on a 1.5– to 2.0-mm loop of the suture (Fig. 88.14f).

The amount of recession required to correct a deviation (Tables 88.2 and 88.3) depends on many factors, but correlates most significantly with the preoperative deviation: the axial length and refractive error are not clinically important.[21] A recession of unoperated muscles is more predictable than that of previously operated muscles, which produce a greater effect per millimeter of recession, as does recession of tight muscles associated with mechanical restriction.

Horizontal muscle recessions

The medial rectus can be recessed to 11.5 mm from the limbus without compromising adduction. Curved rulers measure the arc not the chord and are more accurate than calipers for large recessions (Fig. 88.17). Six- to 8-mm medial rectus recessions from the insertion successfully correct large infantile esotropias, but with a frequent consecutive exodeviation,[22] perhaps from the development of medial rectus underaction and the absence of

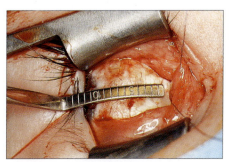

Fig. 88.17 Curved ruler measuring 11 mm from medial limbus. (Patient of Dr R Morris.)

Table 88.2 Esotropia			
Deviation	BMRc	MRc/LRs	BLRs
10–15	3.0	3.0/3.5	5.0
15–20	3.5	3.5/4.5	5.5
20–25	4.0	4.0/5.5	6.0
25–30	4.5	4.5/6.5	6.5
30–35	5.0	5.0/7.0	7.0
35–40	5.5	5.5/7.5	7.5
45–50	6.0	6.0/8.0	8.0
50–60	6.5	6.5/8.0	
60–70	7.0		

BMRc = bilateral medial rectus recessions; MRc/LRs = medial rectus recession and lateral rectus resection; BLRs = bilateral lateral rectus resections.
These guidelines vary depending on the surgeon, the surgical technique, the age of the patient, presence of lateral incomitance, previous strabismus surgery, presence of oblique muscle dysfunction, and the presence of cerebral palsy.

Table 88.3 Exotropia				
Deviation	BLRc	MRs	BMRs	MRs/LRc
15	4.0		4.0	3.0/4.0
20	5.0		5.0	4.0/5.0
25	6.0		6.0	5.0/6.0
30	7.0			6.0/7.0
35	8.0			6.0/8.0
40	7.0	+4.0		7.0/8.0
45	7.0	+5.0		7.5/8.5
50	7.0	+6.0		7.0/9.0
60	7.0		+5.0	8.0/10.0
70	7.0		+7.0	9.0/10.0
80	8.0		+7.0	10.0/10.0

BLRc = bilateral lateral rectus recessions; MRs = medial rectus resection; BMRs = bilateral medial rectus resections; MRs/LRc = medial rectus resection and lateral rectus recession; + = medial rectus surgery in addition to bilateral lateral rectus recession.
These guidelines vary depending on the surgeon, the surgical technique, the age of the patient, presence of lateral incomitance, previous strabismus surgery, presence of oblique muscle dysfunction, and the presence of cerebral palsy.

binocularity.[23,24] Recessions of up to 1.5 mm behind the equator, determined by ultrasonography, do not give underactions, nor do bilateral medial rectus recessions of 11 mm from the limbus usually cause late progressive overcorrection.[25] Three- or four-muscle surgery may be done for large angle congenital esotropia,[26] but large recessions combined with lateral rectus resection may develop limitation of adduction postoperatively.

The lateral rectus has a longer arc of contact with the globe than other rectus muscles, and large recessions, up to 10 or 12 mm, can be performed without limitation of movement, especially with large axial lengths. As the insertion of the lateral rectus is more consistent than the medial rectus, recessions can be measured from the insertion rather than the limbus.

Inferior rectus muscle recession

Indications Inferior rectus recession may be indicated for restricted elevation caused by double elevator palsy, blowout fractures, thyroid orbitopathy, and restrictive ophthalmoplegias. Contralateral inferior rectus weakening may be indicated in inferior rectus paresis, after a blowout fracture or periocular injection and in some superior oblique palsies. If there is a hypertropia in primary position then a recession is indicated, but if there is no significant deviation in primary position and an increasing deviation in downgaze, a posterior fixation suture is preferred.

Principles Forced duction tests should always be performed prior to inferior rectus surgery. In comitant vertical strabismus not associated with restriction, contralateral superior rectus recession is more predictable than ipsilateral inferior rectus recession. One millimeter of inferior rectus recession results in the correction of about 3 prism diopters of vertical deviation in primary position and 5 prism diopters in downgaze.[27] The inferior rectus should not be recessed more than 5 mm, and in patients with a vertical deviation of greater than 15 prisms diopters in primary position, an inferior rectus recession should be combined with contralateral superior rectus recession.

With adjustable sutures, the hypotropia should be slightly undercorrected and the deviation and versions in downgaze should be assessed so that the deviation in primary position is not corrected at the expense of underaction of the inferior rectus in downgaze. Nonabsorbable adjustable sutures or absorbable fixed sutures may be used.

In thyroid orbitopathy, if FDTs indicate restriction of the inferior rectus of the apparently normal eye, then bilateral asymmetrical inferior rectus recessions are indicated. If forced duction tests indicate superior rectus restriction as well, then late slippage might be reduced if both muscles are recessed.

Recession of the inferior rectus may affect the lower lid retractors, giving lid retraction in up to 94% of cases.[28] The degree of retraction seems to be proportional to the amount of inferior rectus recession performed, perhaps by the recession resulting in posterior displacement of the capsulopalpebral head with lowering of the lower lid.

These methods have been advocated for reducing lower lid retraction; none are effective in eliminating it:

1. Dissecting the fascial connections and check ligaments of the inferior rectus as far posteriorly as possible (to the level of the vortex vein);
2. Suturing the lower lid retractors to the inferior rectus;
3. Placing the capsulopalpebral head on an adjustable suture, through the inferior rectus insertion, for adjustment following inferior rectus adjustment;[28,29] and
4. Disinserting the lower lid retractors from the tarsal plate.

Progressive overcorrection following inferior rectus surgery occurs after initially good alignment, especially in patients with thyroid eye disease and those undergoing adjustable sutures. In 10–21% of cases,[30–32] a few weeks after surgery, the eye becomes hypertropic with limited depression and diplopia in downgaze.

This "late slippage" may be due to the following:

1. Thickened Tenon's under the inferior rectus muscle may allow the muscle to slip back after the sutures have absorbed, leading to a pseudotendon anterior to the insertion;
2. The inferior rectus attachment to Lockwood's ligament and the eyelid retractors may be responsible;
3. With adjustable sutures, the newly recessed inferior rectus is held in place centrally as the eye makes horizontal movements, preventing it from moving with the eye and delaying reattachment;
4. Scarring around Lockwood's ligament could pull the inferior rectus muscle anteriorly, slackening the anterior aspect of the muscle and weakening its depressor function;[32]
5. Sideways traction of the inferior oblique may prevent adherence allowing muscle slippage; and
6. After substantial recession the inferior rectus loses apposition to the globe when the muscle is contracting with the eye in

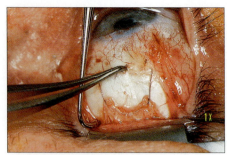

Fig. 88.18 Superior rectus hang-back recession: surgeon's view from above. (Patient of Dr R Morris.)

downgaze.[33] MRI has confirmed that an inferior rectus recession of 6.0 mm and medial rectus recession of 7.5 mm in a normal eye lead to loss of apposition, with lower values found for thyroid patients.[34]

7. In cases of thyroid orbitopathy, ipsilateral contraction of the superior rectus may lead to late overcorrection.

Postoperatively undercorrection of the hypotropia in primary position with associated reversal of the hypotropia in downgaze may be an indication of a tight superior rectus.

"A" pattern exotropia can follow bilateral inferior rectus recessions as not only depression, but also adduction is reduced, particularly in downgaze. Nasal displacement of the inferior recti reduces the effect of the "A" pattern: difficult to achieve with adjustable sutures.

Superior rectus muscle recession

Superior rectus recessions are effective in the management of true vertical deviations and dissociated vertical deviation (DVD). To achieve an effective recession, the fascial attachments between it and the superior oblique must be divided. One-millimeter recession corrects approximately 3 prism diopters of vertical deviation. Recessions of greater than 5 mm are best avoided except in DVD when hang-back recessions of up to 9 mm are indicated (Fig. 88.18). Superior rectus surgery rarely causes significant upper lid retraction.[28]

Because of the complications of inferior rectus recessions, surgery for a comitant vertical deviation of less than 15 prism diopters should be confined to a superior rectus recession. If the deviation increases on upgaze a superior rectus recession is indicated, and if it increases in downgaze an inferior rectus recession is indicated. If the deviation is larger than 15 prism diopters, then surgery should be split equally between the superior rectus and the contralateral inferior rectus.

The faden or posterior fixation operation

The faden operation weakens a muscle by placing two separate nonabsorbable sutures (5–0 Mersilene or 5–0 Dacron) through about 30% of each edge of a muscle behind the equator, usually 12–16 mm from the insertion (as posterior as possible) (Fig. 88.19). A ½-circle needle makes suture placement easier. It weakens the muscle in its field of action with little effect on the deviation in primary position. To be effective, it must produce an underaction of the muscle. It produces its effect by the functional insertion being moved to the point of the faden suture, increasing the arc of contact of the muscle with the globe and reducing the lever arm, thereby weakening the muscle in its field of action.[36] It is most effective on the medial rectus, where it increases the arc of contact from 6 to 12–16 mm, and on the superior and inferior recti, but has little effect on the lateral rectus because it increases the arc of contact very little. It may be combined with a recession of the muscle and enhances the effect of the recession, so that a smaller recession is usually needed.

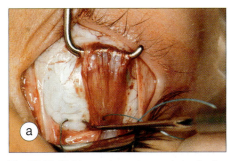 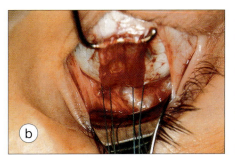 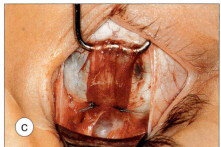

Fig. 88.19 Right superior rectus posterior fixation suture: surgeon's view from above. (a) Scleral placement of suture on a half-curved needle at medial border of superior rectus; it will next be passed through the muscle. The lateral suture is already placed through sclera and muscle. (b) Sutures prior to tying. (c) Completed procedure. (Patient of Dr R Morris.)

The best indication for a faden suture is in incomitant strabismus, when there is little or no deviation in primary position and an incomitant deviation in the field of action of a single underacting muscle. The suture is placed on the contra-lateral overacting yoke muscle. A good example is with inferior rectus underaction after blowout fracture, with no deviation in primary position, but an increasing hyperdeviation on downgaze. The faden suture is placed on the contralateral inferior rectus. Other indications include nystagmus blockage syndrome, convergence excess esotropia, DVD, nystagmus with a face turn, and residual strabismus after recession.

The faden procedure is difficult to perform, but easier when combined with a recession, particularly when a single central suture is used. Good exposure using retractors is essential and extensive dissection is needed before the sutures can be safely placed. The vortex veins are close to the site of suture placement and the insertion of the superior oblique makes placement of the lateral suture in a superior rectus difficult. There is a higher risk of scleral perforation and its effect is relatively unpredictable.

Marginal myotomy

Marginal myotomy of the rectus muscles is an unpredictable and irreversible procedure, which can result in overcorrection. The superior and inferior borders of the muscle are cut 75% of the width of the muscle, about 5 mm apart, so that the all fibers of the muscle are cut (Fig. 88.20). It can be a useful operation if a fully recessed muscle requires further weakening in the presence of a large angle strabismus or if recession is contraindicated because of thin sclera (as in high myopia).

Strengthening procedures
Resections

Resection of a muscle enhances its action, particularly if it is combined with a recession of its direct antagonist muscle.

Resections are more difficult to perform than recessions, with more tissue reaction and redness, particularly if excess conjunctiva is hooded over the cornea. Large resections produce limitation of eye movement in the opposite direction of gaze, by a mechanical leash effect, which is maximal initially, diminishing with time.

Resection requires thorough dissection of the intermuscular septum and check ligaments, ideally 5 mm beyond the extent of the resection so that Tenon's is not advanced as the muscle is repositioned. Care must be taken when resecting a lateral rectus to free the inferior oblique from its lower border to prevent it being included in the resection. Once the muscle has been dissected from its attachments, two hooks are placed under it. There are several suture techniques for rectus muscle resection, the most common being a single double-armed suture, two double-armed sutures, and two single-ended sutures. The aim of resection is to shorten the muscle while maintaining its width without any central sagging. I prefer a single-suture technique (Fig. 88.21), leaving no stump of tissue at the insertion site but removing it and placing the sutures in the sclera just anterior to the insertion which provides a more secure scleral attachment.

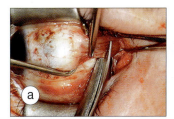 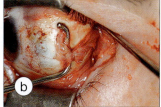

Fig. 88.20 Marginal myotomy. (a) With a strabismus hook under a previously recessed medial rectus, two pairs of scissors are positioned so as to make overlapping myotomy cuts through the muscle. (b) Appearance of muscle postmyotomy: the overlapping cuts allow the muscle to stretch. (Patient of Dr R Morris.)

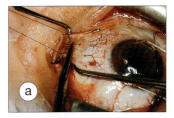 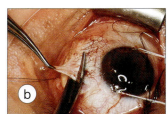 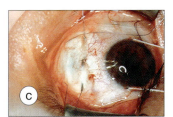 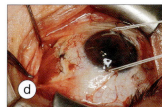

Fig. 88.21 Single-suture, double-armed needle rectus muscle resection. (a) With a suture placed 4 mm from muscle insertion, the muscle is being cut anterior to the suture. (b) Removal of redundant muscle tissue. (c) Scleral placement of sutures anterior to insertion. (d) Final position of muscle following suture tying after a pass through the center of the muscle. Note absence of central sagging of resected muscle. (Patient of Dr R Morris.)

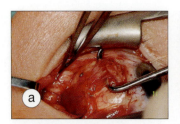
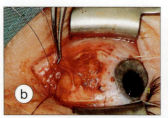
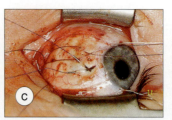
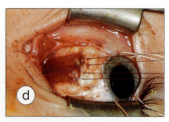

Fig. 88.22 Two-suture, double-armed needle rectus muscle resection.(a) Hook under medial rectus muscle. Note the pseudotendon attached to the muscle, which can be seen on the left. (b) Redundant pseudotendon about to be excised. (c) Sutures placed just anterior to original muscle insertion. (d) Muscle advanced to insertion: the four ends of the two sutures are about to be tied to its corresponding end. This configuration gives minimal central sag. (Patient of Dr R Morris.)

The amount a muscle can be resected for a given deviation varies with the surgical technique. Consistency is essential for predictability. A horizontal muscle can be resected 10 mm or more, but at the expense of limitation of ocular movements in the opposite field, which may lead to incomitant deviations. This may be appropriate in correcting a large deviation in a densely amblyopic eye. Resections greater than 5 mm of the superior and inferior recti should be avoided as they will be associated with lid advancement and narrowing of the palpebral fissure.

Where the resected muscle is tight or a muscle is advanced from a previously recessed position, I use two double-armed sutures: the technique is similar to the single-suture technique but each suture passes through only half the width of the muscle[37] (Fig. 88.22).

Advancement of a slipped or previously recessed muscle enhances the effect of a rectus muscle more per millimeter of advancement than resection, especially if the muscle is advanced 2 mm anterior to the original insertion. The effect varies with the degree of underaction of the muscle, previous surgery, and the findings at surgery. Muscle advancement has the same difficulties as resection, but they are more pronounced, particularly if dissection near the orbital fat is required. For consecutive exotropia a simple advancement of the muscle to the original insertion may suffice, although it is more commonly combined with an adjustable recession of its antagonist.

Tucking and plication procedures

A rectus muscle can also be strengthened using a tuck or plication, which are only indicated if there is a risk of anterior segment ischemia, as it is possible to leave the anterior ciliary vessels intact.

Inferior oblique surgery

Indications

An inferior oblique is usually weakened for primary or secondary overaction especially when associated with "V" pattern strabismus and overaction from superior oblique underaction. Strengthening procedures are rarely performed as they are ineffective. Anterior transposition of the inferior oblique is useful for treating DVD and especially when DVD and inferior oblique overaction co-exist.[38]

In "V" pattern strabismus, inferior oblique surgery is likely, to be most effective when the "V" pattern is greatest between primary and upgaze, as the main inferior oblique abducting effect occurs in upgaze. Bilateral inferior oblique weakening corrects up to 20-prism diopters horizontal deviation in upgaze, having little or no effect on the horizontal deviation in primary position or downgaze.[39]

In symptomatic unilateral superior oblique palsy, inferior oblique surgery is indicated if there is an incomitant hyper-

deviation increasing in the field of action of the inferior oblique and associated with inferior oblique overaction. If the size of the deviation is less than 15 prism diopters then inferior oblique surgery alone suffices, but if greater, then surgery on other muscles should be considered.[40]

Surgical procedures

The inferior oblique is easily approached through an inferolateral fornix incision 8 mm from the limbus. Direct visualization of the muscle is required and good lighting is essential if the posterior fibers of the muscle are to be seen. The assistant places a strabismus hook under the inferior and lateral rectus muscles to expose and protect them from inadvertent dissection. A large strabismus hook retracts conjunctiva, Tenon's, and the orbital fat and a small hook secures the inferior oblique once its posterior border has been identified. Posterior fibers can easily be missed but identified in the "V" formed by the hook holding the anterior fibers, as a strand of muscular tissue running in the original line of the muscle (Fig. 88.25).

Once isolated, a variety of weakening procedures are practiced, the most common being myectomy (Fig. 88.23), disinsertion, and recession[41] (Fig. 88.24). All are effective. Although myectomy (removal of a segment of 5–8 mm of muscle) is effective, myotomy and Z-pasty are less so.

A recession can be graded: a small recession for a small inferior oblique overaction. The muscle is usually placed 2 mm lateral and 3 mm posterior to the lateral border of the inferior rectus, approximately a 10-mm recession. The more medial and anterior the muscle is placed, the greater is the weakening effect.

Anterior transposition of the inferior oblique enhances its weakening effect: It is sutured just anterior and parallel to the inferior rectus insertion, producing a J-shaped deformity of the muscle.[42] The anteriorization can be graded and the muscle placed 1 or 2 mm anterior to the inferior rectus insertion. In this position, anterior to the equator of the globe, the inferior oblique becomes a depressor and there may also be some mechanical restriction to elevation.[43] The more anterior the muscle is placed, particularly the posterior fibers, the greater is this effect, further enhanced by combining it with a myectomy. The mechanism is uncertain but the effective origin of the muscle may be changed to either the anterior end of the neurovascular bundle or Lockwood's ligament, and when the muscle contracts, the globe is pulled downward.[43] It is useful for marked inferior oblique overaction and when inferior oblique overaction and DVD coincide: it is most effective with preoperative deviations of less than 15 prism diopters in primary position.[44] It may also be used when superior rectus surgery has proved ineffective for DVD. It is best performed bilaterally as unilateral surgery may produce a

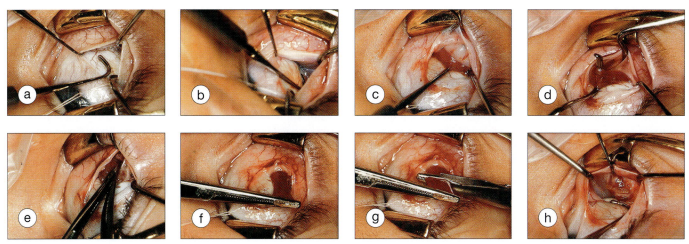

Fig. 88.23 Inferior oblique myectomy: surgeon's view from above. (a) Inferolateral conjunctival fornix incision. (b) Visualization of posterior border of inferior oblique, seen at the tip of the hook. (c) Stevens tenotomy hook under both inferior oblique muscle and orbital fat. (d) Hook under inferior oblique, the orbital fat having been freed, showing the intermuscular septum between inferior oblique and Tenon's capsule. (e) The inferior oblique is held in a straight artery clamp and is being disinserted from the globe. (f) Inferior oblique muscle having been disinserted. (g) A segment of muscle being removed with scissors. (h) Cut border of inferior oblique visible, retracting into Tenon's capsule. (Patient of Dr R Morris.)

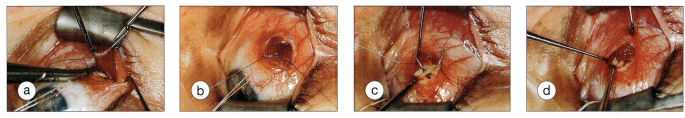

Fig. 88.24 Right inferior oblique recession: surgeon's view from above. (a) Suture being placed at insertion of inferior oblique, the inferior oblique muscle having been disinserted with double-armed Vicryl suture. (b) Double-armed Vicryl suture through inferior oblique muscle. (c) Needles placed lateral and posterior to the lateral border of the inferior rectus (the strabismus hook in the bottom left of the picture is under the insertion of the inferior rectus). (d) Muscle in recessed position. (Patient of Dr R Morris.)

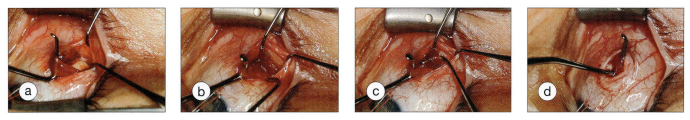

Fig. 88.25 Inadvertently split right inferior oblique muscle: surgeon's view from above. (a) A Green hook placed through apparently intact inferior oblique muscle. (b) The posterior part of the muscle seen in the V formed by the hooked muscle. (c) The Stevens tenotomy hook lifts the split posterior portion of the muscle onto the Green hook to join the two halves together for suturing. (d) No further muscle tissue seen in the V formed by the inferior oblique, which is now complete and held on the Green hook. (Patient of Dr R Morris.)

postoperative hypotropia exacerbated by inadvertent resection of the muscle. In anteriorization, the anterior and posterior borders of the inferior oblique are sutured together in a single scleral bite; rather than spreading out the posterior border laterally, which may restrict elevation. It is also important to dissect the muscle away from its fascial attachments, or the lower lid may appear bulky postoperatively.

Denervation and extirpation may be indicated if other procedures have been ineffective, but should not be used as a primary procedure. The nerve to the inferior oblique is cauterized as it enters the muscle at the lateral border of the inferior rectus, but the muscle function can recover as the nerve regrows. This may be prevented by also removing as much of the inferior oblique as possible.[45]

Specific complications of inferior oblique surgery

1. Persistent inferior oblique overaction can be caused by:
   a. Incomplete division of the posterior fibers (Fig. 88.25); and
   b. DVD, not true inferior oblique overaction, particularly in patients with congenital strabismus.[12]
2. The inferior oblique fat adherence syndrome results in hypotropia and restriction of elevation in adduction following surgery caused by rupture of Tenon's capsule, prolapse of orbital fat, and hemorrhage, leading to scarring.
3. Inadvertent disinsertion of the lateral or inferior rectus muscle.
4. Pupillary dilation.
5. Hemorrhage from the muscle or damage to the inferior temporal vortex vein.

6. The antielevation syndrome[46] follows bilateral anterior transposition of the inferior oblique; patients develop apparent recurrent inferior oblique overaction in the contralateral eye, with a "Y" or "V" pattern and exotropia in upgaze. It may be the result of limitation of elevation in abduction of the operated eye, causing overaction of the contralateral elevators in adduction, especially if the posterior fibers are spread laterally from the inferior rectus insertion: they should be sutured no more than 2 mm lateral to the inferior rectus.[47] If it occurs, bilateral inferior oblique nasal myectomy has been suggested.[48]

Superior oblique surgery

Weakening procedures

The main indications for superior oblique weakening are Brown syndrome and superior oblique overaction with a vertical deviation and an "A" pattern strabismus affecting fusion or causing a significant compensatory head posture. All the procedures described are difficult to quantify, and most are nonselective and produce global weakening of torsion, depression, and abduction.

Superior oblique tenotomies and tenectomies can be performed nasal or temporal to the superior rectus insertion. The closer the tenotomy is to the trochlear, the greater is the weakening effect. Temporal tenotomies have little effect, partly due to the fascial attachment between the superior oblique and the superior rectus, which prevents retraction of the oblique tendon.

Surgically, the nasal portion of the superior oblique tendon can be approached via a nasal (Fig. 88.26) or "a supratemporal fornix incision." The former is easier technically but the latter leaves the nasal intermuscular septum intact, which may reduce postoperative superior oblique palsy, as the cut ends of the tendon are supported by the septum.[49]

Direct visualization of the tendon reduces the complications from blind hooking particularly incomplete tenotomy, and inadvertent transection of the superior rectus.[50] Postoperatively consecutive superior oblique underaction is common. In Brown syndrome, tenotomy leads to consecutive underaction of the superior oblique:[51] Z-tenotomy of the superior oblique may avoid this in 66–85% of cases.[52]

Superior oblique recession is a graded weakening procedure, but it alters function by bunching the tendon fibers anterior to the equator, changing the function from depression and abduction to elevation and adduction. Although recession is more predictable than tenotomy, it may result in undercorrection and has similar complications to tenotomy with no clear advantage over it.

Disinsertion of the tendon produces mild weakening. To be effective, the fascial attachments between it and the superior rectus need to be divided. Disinsertion of the posterior fibers selectively weakens depression.

The use of a superior oblique silicone tendon expander is a method of weakening the muscle.[53] A segment of 240 silicone retinal band is inserted between cut ends of the nasal portion of the tendon (Fig. 88.27). Although globally weakening superior oblique function, the procedure can be quantified using different lengths of silicone band. It is suitable for Brown syndrome and superior oblique overaction, with a low incidence of secondary superior oblique underaction.[54]

Posterior tenectomy with a wedge resection of the posterior and medial fibers, preserving the anterior intorting fibers, may selectively weaken the abduction and depression for mild "A" pattern esotropia yet maintain incyclotorsion.

Preoperative selection minimizes the risks of bilateral superior oblique tenotomies, and fusion was not affected in one series: it should only be carried out for a 45-prism dioptre "A"-pattern with moderate to marked superior oblique overaction and no inferior oblique overaction.[55] In this study up to 12 prism diopters of exodeviation was corrected in primary position and up to 45 prism diopters in downgaze.

Bilateral posterior tenectomies can correct up to 15 prism diopters of "A" pattern and scleral disinsertion up to 25 prism diopters. For larger "A" patterns, superior oblique tenotomy may be combined with horizontal muscle surgery. The magnitude of reduction of the "A" pattern corresponds to its preoperative size: the correction in primary position is greater in patients with exodeviations than in those with esodeviations.

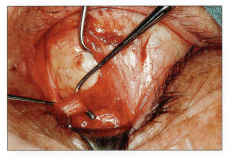

Fig. 88.26 Right superior oblique tenotomy: surgeon's view from above. The superior rectus is held with a Chavasse hook (above). The superior oblique tendon can be identified via nasal approach and is held with two Stevens tenotomy hooks beneath it. The muscle is divided between the hooks for a superior oblique tenotomy. (Patient of Dr R Morris.)

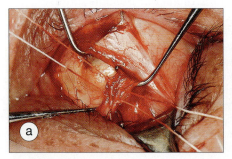
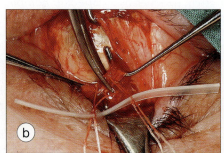
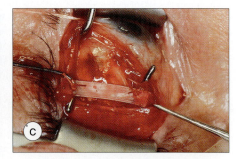

Fig. 88.27 Superior oblique tendon expander: surgeon's view from above. (a) Two nonabsorbable double-armed sutures are passed through superior oblique tendon. (b) A segment of silicone band is inserted and transfixed by each end of the double-armed sutures. The tendon is being divided with scissors. (c) Tendon following division and insertion of the silicone band, which is held by the double-armed sutures. (Patient of Dr R Morris.)

In "de-sagittalization" of the superior oblique, the tendon is disinserted and the anterior tip reattached to the anterior portion of the insertion with a loop of nonabsorbable suture, reducing depression in adduction.[56]

The common complication of superior oblique weakening is secondary underaction: this can usually be treated by ipsilateral inferior oblique weakening; in patients with fusion, superior oblique surgery can induce torsional and/or vertical diplopia. Bilateral superior oblique weakening can cause a postoperative "V" pattern and torsion. Posterior fibers being left intact at surgery may give persistent overaction. Fat adherence can also result if orbital fat is breached at the time of surgery.

The superior oblique can also be weakened by subluxating the tendon out of the trochlear through an anterior orbitotomy, or dislocating the trochlear from the bone by a periosteal approach.[57] The authors report good results, but favor the latter technique as there is less risk of damage to the supratrochlear neurovascular bundle; it can be graded and it is technically easier.

"Strengthening" procedures
Superior oblique tuck
Nonselective "strengthening" of the superior oblique can be achieved by tucking its tendon. Most superior oblique palsies are partial, which suggests a strengthening procedure of the superior oblique tendon is logical.[58] A temporal approach to the tendon avoids disinsertion of the superior rectus.[59] Tuck surgery is helpful for selected patients with both unilateral and bilateral superior oblique pareses. A tuck can be free (Fig. 88.28) or performed using a tendon tucker.[55]

There is no consensus on the role of this procedure; many feel that the complications outweigh the advantages.[60,61] However, a study of 45 patients showed that many cases of superior oblique palsy can be effectively treated with tucks in patients with an incomitant vertical deviation that is greatest in the field of action of the superior oblique, with associated superior oblique underaction, and without inferior oblique overaction.[62]

Quantification superior oblique tucks are difficult. The effect of an isolated tuck ranges from no effect to 11 prism diopters in primary (mean 3.6 prism diopters) and from 0 to 40 prism diopters (mean 14.3 prism diopters) in the field of maximum deviation without any correlation between the size of the tuck and the amount of deviation corrected.[62] Thus, it is not just the size of the tuck that determines the amount of correction obtained; the laxity of the superior oblique tendon and the size of the preoperative deviation are also important. In patients undergoing contralateral inferior rectus recessions in conjunction with a tuck, postoperative adjustment of the inferior rectus on an adjustable suture may improve the accuracy.

Intraoperative adjustment of the tuck by FDTs is essential to prevent a significant postoperative iatrogenic Brown syndrome,[62] although it does not help determine the amount of vertical deviation corrected.[63]

Bilateral superior oblique tucks are indicated for bilateral superior oblique palsies where there is a significant esodeviation on downgaze and alternating hyperdeviations on side gazes; otherwise, bilateral modified Harada Ito procedures are indicated to correct symptomatic torsion.

An alternative to a superior oblique tuck is a resection or advancement of the muscle, but both disinsert the muscle and alter its function.

The Harada Ito procedure
Intortion by the superior oblique can be enhanced by selectively strengthening the anterior muscle fibers. Initially, the anterior fibers were placed anterior and laterally without disinsertion, for excyclotorsion in bilateral superior oblique palsies.[64] Later, the anterior third of the tendon was disinserted and advanced to 8 mm posterior to the superior border of the lateral rectus insertion[65] (Fig. 88.29). This reduces excyclotorsion in patients with bilateral superior oblique palsies in whom torsion is the main problem. It corrects about 11° of excyclotorsion without

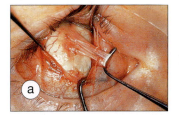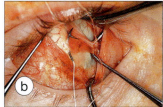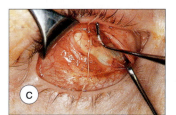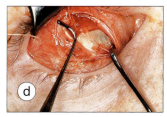

Fig. 88.28 An 8-mm superior oblique free tuck. Right eye, viewed from the front. (a) Superior oblique identified and double-armed nonabsorbable suture placed 8 mm from insertion. The lateral rectus is held to one side by the hook on the left. (b) Needles placed in sclera at insertion of tendon. (c) Muscle tied with Stevens tenotomy hook through redundant loop of muscle. (d) Final position of muscle after tuck. Note Stevens tenotomy hook through redundant loop of muscle. (Patient of Dr R Morris.)

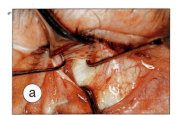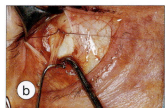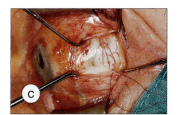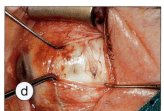

Fig. 88.29 Modified Harada Ito procedure. Left eye, frontal view. (a) After a superior temporal fornix conjunctival and Tenon's incision, the superior rectus is held with a Chavasse hook and the insertion of the superior oblique identified and the tendon held between two Stevens hooks. (b) The anterior third of the tendon is split and a double-armed 6-0 Vicryl suture placed through it at the insertion of the split anterior third. The posterior two-thirds can be seen under the retractor. (c) The anterior third of the tendon is divided from the globe and the double-armed suture placed above the superior border of the lateral rectus 8 mm from insertion. (d) Final position of tendon. (Patient of Dr R Morris.)

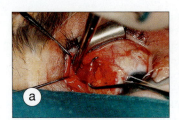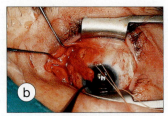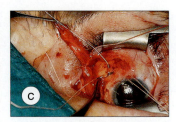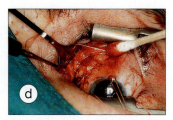

Fig. 88.30 Superior oblique tendon transposition. (a) The tendon is over a Green hook, and an artery forceps is being used to fracture the trochlear. (b) The tendon is disinserted and moved nasally. (c) Suture placed through tendon and sutured above the insertion of the medial rectus. (d) The tendon is sutured to sclera, the redundant tendon tissue having been excised. Note the medial rectus has been resected. (Patient of Dr R Morris.)

inducing a vertical deviation.[66,67] It typically produces an initial postoperative overcorrection that resolves over 2–3 months.

A greater abducting effect in downgaze is achieved if the anterior fibers are placed more posteriorly; this is best for patients with significant esotropia in downgaze.[66] Placing the tendon closer than 8 mm to the lateral rectus insertion may produce an undesirable esotropia. If some posterior fibers are included in the transposition there is a greater depressor effect useful for correcting small hypertropias. It can be combined with other rectus muscle surgery in complex bilateral superior oblique palsies.

Intraoperative adjustment, assessing torsion by examining the fundus with the indirect ophthalmoscope,[68] and an adjustable suture for this procedure,[69] have not gained popularity.

Superior oblique tendon transposition

Transposition of the superior oblique tendon, combined with a large medial rectus resection and lateral rectus recession, is sometimes useful in complete third nerve palsy. The superior oblique tendon is cut at the medial border of the superior rectus, and the tendon is resected and sutured to the globe just above the insertion of the medial rectus (Fig. 88.30). This adducts the globe both mechanically and by exerting some functional rotational action. It can be enhanced by dislocation of the trochlear, allowing the muscle to lie parallel to the medial rectus; postoperatively, traction sutures may hold the eye in adduction, preventing the lateral rectus insertion from creeping forward.[27]

Alternatively, the globe is tethered to the nasal periosteum using an autogenous periosteal flap or superior oblique tendon.[70]

TRANSPOSITION PROCEDURES

Muscle transposition procedures move the muscle out of the normal line of action, changing their function.

Vertical transposition of the horizontal rectus muscles

Vertical transposition of the horizontal rectus muscles may be considered for "A" and "V" patterns[71] if there is no inferior oblique overaction in a "V" pattern and no superior oblique overaction in an "A" pattern.

"V" patterns are significant if there is a difference of 15 prism diopters between upgaze of 25° and downgaze of 25°. A 10-prism diopter difference is significant for "A" patterns. Surgical correction of a pattern may be considered for a chin-up or chin-down head position, or if the pattern is precluding fusion. Surgery on "A" and "V" patterns is rarely indicated for cosmesis.

The horizontal rectus is recessed and transposed in the direction in which the greatest weakening effect is required.[71] In

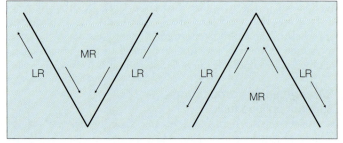

Fig. 88.31 Direction in which medial and lateral recti are moved in "V" and "A" patterns.

"V" pattern esotropia recession and inferior displacement of the medial recti weakens them more in downgaze than in upgaze. Resection and superior displacement of the lateral recti produces less abducting effect in upgaze than in downgaze. Thus:

In "V" patterns, the medial recti are moved inferiorly toward the apex of the "V" (Fig. 88.31) for both resections and recessions. The lateral recti are moved superiorly.

In "A" patterns, the medial recti are moved superiorly toward the apex of the "A" for both resections and recessions. The lateral recti are moved inferiorly (Fig. 88.31).

The effect is inconsistent but depends on how much the muscle is displaced and the size of the preoperative pattern. A half tendon width displacement reduces the pattern by about 10–20 prism diopters, and a full tendon width 25–30 prism diopters. The amount of horizontal surgery performed is based on the deviation in primary position as transposition has little effect on the deviation in this position. Unilateral surgery moving the medial rectus and lateral rectus in opposite directions combined with recession and resection can be performed equally effectively if surgery needs to be confined to one eye.[72,73]

The following are important points to remember:
1. A conjunctival incision is needed with a larger relaxing incision in the direction in which the muscle is to be displaced;
2. The intermuscular septum and check ligaments should be dissected far enough back to allow the muscle to be moved freely; and
3. The displaced muscle, when reattached, should remain concentric with the spiral of Tillaux (Fig. 88.32).

An alternative to vertical transposition in the management of "A" or "V" patterns is to slant the muscle insertion. In "V" pattern esotropia the inferior pole of the medial rectus is recessed more than the upper pole, weakening the muscle more in downgaze. In "A" pattern esotropia the converse applies.

Horizontal muscle transposition can also correct a small comitant vertical deviation associated with a horizontal strabismus.

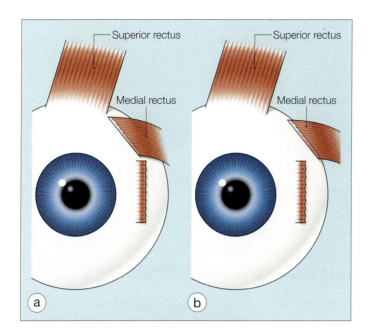

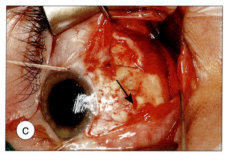

Fig. 88.32 (a, b) Medial recti recessed and supraplaced (anchored hang-back technique). (c) Vertical transposition of the medial rectus for an A-pattern esodeviation. The medial rectus is recessed and supraplaced. The original insertion is arrowed. (Patient of Dr R Morris.)

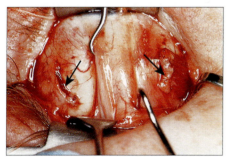

Fig. 88.33 Knapp procedure: surgeon's view of left eye. Vertical transposition of medial and lateral recti parallel to the medial and lateral borders of the superior rectus. The medial rectus has also been resected and the lateral recessed. (Patient of Dr R Morris.)

It can be applied with uniocular surgery, moving the rectus muscle in the opposite direction of the vertical deviation; for example, in the presence of a hypertropia both medial and lateral recti should be lowered. One millimeter of vertical displacement corrects about 1 prism diopter of vertical deviation.[74] The same principle can be used to correct a small horizontal deviation when performing vertical rectus muscle surgery for vertical deviations.

Horizontal muscle transposition is also useful in vertical deviations resulting from underaction or paresis of vertical rectus muscles. Superior vertical transposition of the horizontal recti corrects elevator palsies (Knapp procedure; Fig. 88.33) and inferior transposition corrects depressor palsies (Dunlap

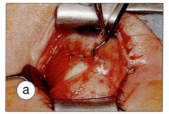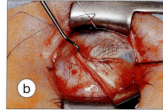

Fig. 88.34 Knapp procedure: surgeon's view of right eye. Vertical transposition of (a) medial and (b) lateral recti on the spiral of Tillaux. The superior rectus is held in a Helveston hook. (Patient of Dr R Morris.)

procedure).[75,76] Knapp transposed both medial and lateral recti alongside the superior rectus, correcting an average of 38 prism diopters of hypotropia. The best indication is a double-elevator palsy with a hypotropia in primary position and a chin-up head posture, without a positive FDT. The horizontal rectus muscles can also be transposed along the spiral of Tillaux (Fig. 88.34). A positive forced duction test indicates inferior rectus restriction, which should be released with an inferior rectus recession prior to a Knapp procedure.

The amount of hypotropia corrected increases over time, does not correlate with the size of the preoperative deviation, and is less predictable after prior inferior rectus surgery.[77]

The same principles apply for inferior rectus weakness: the horizontal recti are transposed inferiorly alongside the inferior rectus or along the spiral of Tillaux, if the FDTs are negative. It is useful in many patients with congenital or acquired inferior rectus weakness, such as after orbital trauma, and in patients with large hypertropias with binocular function.[78,79] If the inferior rectus has residual function then a vertical recess–resect procedure or a graded transposition is indicated to avoid overcorrection.

Both procedures can be combined with a recession/resection of the medial or lateral recti for a co-existent horizontal deviation (Fig. 88.33).

Horizontal transposition of the vertical recti

Because of the risk of anterior segment ischemia associated with earlier techniques that involved disinsertion of part or all of the vertical recti, especially when combined with medial rectus recession, the Jensen procedure was introduced.[80] The rectus muscles are not disinserted, but the superior and inferior recti are split in half and the temporal halves sutured with a non-absorbable suture (5–0 Dacron or 4–0 Mersilene) to the superior and inferior halves of the split lateral rectus. The suture around the muscle is loose to minimize the risk of anterior segment ischemia from constriction of the anterior ciliary arteries; the sutured muscles are fixed to the globe 12–15 mm from the limbus. It is combined with a 5- to 6-mm medial rectus recession, sometimes with preservation of the anterior ciliary arteries or botulinum toxin to the medial rectus. The Jensen procedure is effective, but produces restriction of adduction, although this contributes to stabilizing the surgical outcome and preventing recurrence.[72]

An alternative to the Jensen procedure is full temporal transposition of the superior and inferior recti combined with a medial rectus botulinum toxin injection, which may be done prior to surgery, intraoperatively, or postoperatively.[81,82] These procedures reduce the risk of anterior segment ischemia. The insertion of the vertical recti can be either alongside the lateral rectus, between their original insertion and the lateral rectus, which is easier, or parallel with the upper and lower borders of the lateral rectus, the superior rectus being 3 mm above the superior border and the inferior rectus 1 mm below the inferior border of the lateral rectus (Figs. 88.35 and 88.36). These procedures can be "augmented" by a nonabsorbable suture (5–0 Dacron or 4–0 Mersilene) on both the superior and inferior recti,

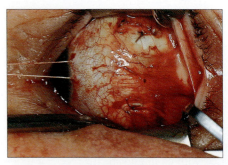

Fig. 88.35 Temporal transposition of superior and inferior recti parallel to the upper and lower borders of the lateral rectus: frontal view, left eye. The superior and inferior recti are sutured above and below the lateral rectus insertion. (Patient of Dr R Morris.)

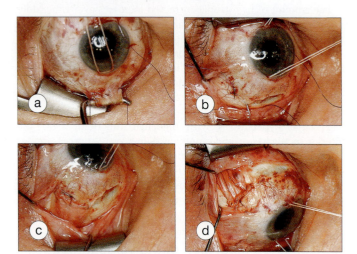

Fig. 88.36 Temporal transposition of the right superior and inferior recti on the spiral of Tillaux. (a) Sutures through the inferior rectus. (b) Position of scleral needle placement after inferior rectus disinsertion. (c) Inferior rectus muscle sutured along the spiral of Tillaux between the insertion of the lateral rectus and the insertion of the inferior rectus. (d) Superior rectus muscle sutured above the lateral rectus. (Patient of Dr R Morris.)

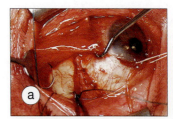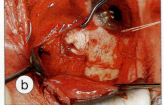

Fig. 88.37 "Augmented" temporal transposition of superior and inferior recti on the spiral of Tillaux: frontal of view right eye. (a) Inferior rectus sutured along the spiral of Tillaux. Note the gap between the lower border of the lateral rectus and superior border of the inferior rectus. A suture is being placed between the superior border of the inferior rectus and the sclera at the lower border of the lateral rectus. (b) Final position of the muscle. Note there is no gap between the lower border of the lateral rectus and superior border of the inferior rectus. (Patient of Dr R Morris.)

through the inferior and superior 25% of the muscle, along the border of the lateral rectus, and secured to the sclera 7–8 mm from the muscle insertion (Fig. 88.37).[83] This can also augment horizontal muscle transpositions.[84]

Vertical deviations can occur with all these techniques, most commonly hyperdeviations that can be overcome by an adjustable suture modification: if there is a hyperdeviation postoperatively the superior rectus muscle is recessed and if there is a consecutive exotropia then both the superior and inferior recti are recessed.

Horizontal transposition procedures can also be effective in carefully selected cases of type 1 Duane syndrome and in lost medial or lateral rectus muscles. The Jensen procedure is contraindicated in Duane syndrome because of the mechanical restriction it produces.

ADJUSTABLE SUTURE TECHNIQUES

Adjustable suture surgery can be carried out under local anesthesia with on-table adjustment, but usually initial surgery is carried out under general anesthesia with postoperative adjustment under topical anesthesia. Most adjustable suture surgery is done on the rectus muscles, but an adjustable Harada Ito procedure has been described.[69]

They are most useful when conventional surgery is unpredictable, particularly in reoperations when scarring, tethering, or contracture is present.[85] They should be considered in any patient having vertical or horizontal rectus muscle surgery for diplopia, to achieve the maximal field of binocular single vision.

Although they require cooperation, they can be performed in children as young as 8 years; girls may be more cooperative than boys. Preoperative assessment indicates the suitability for adjustment: those who can tolerate a cotton bud manipulating the anesthetized conjunctiva, or applanation tonometry, are likely to tolerate the procedure.

The general anesthesia is such that the patient is alert and cooperative with minimal nausea postoperatively: intravenous anesthetic agents can facilitate this. Ideally, the adjustment should be performed within 6 hours; after than 24 hours adjustment may be difficult as the tissues adhere to the globe.

A limbal conjunctival incision is easiest, but it can be difficult to cover the suture knot with conjunctiva after the adjustment, although the conjunctiva can be sutured to cover the knot after adjustment. 6–0 Vicryl has a high tensile strength and little tendency to snag. A colored suture helps identification for adjustment.

There are two main methods for muscle reattachment:
1. *The "bow tie" technique*: The sutures are placed just anterior to the insertion through scleral tunnels emerging 1.5 mm apart (Figs. 88.38 and 88.39). At adjustment, the bow is undone and the muscle advanced or recessed; when in the desired position the knot is tied. Two scleral passes for each suture can be made so that they form a Z[86] (Fig. 88.38b).
2. *The cinch or sliding knot*: A second suture is tied tightly around the two arms of the muscle suture that can be slid up or down the muscle sutures to enable adjustment. It produces a larger knot and more tissue reaction but it is easier to estimate the amount of adjustment.

A scleral fixation suture can be placed through the muscle insertion or adjacent to the limbus to facilitate adjustment. At the end of the initial surgery, the long suture ends of the adjustable can be taped to the lid or tucked into the inferior fornix.

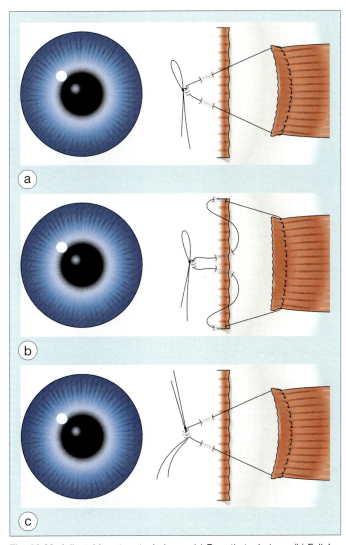

Fig. 88.38 Adjustable suture techniques. (a) Bow-tie technique. (b) Fells' technique. (c) Cinch technique.

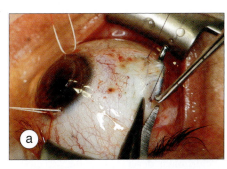

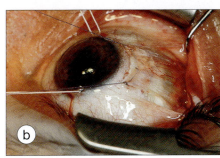

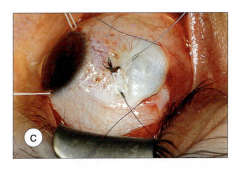

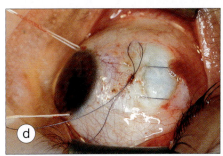

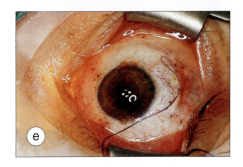

Fig. 88.39 Bow-tie adjustable suture technique using limbal conjunctival approach: left lateral rectus. (a) Double-armed Vicryl suture placed through the muscle, which is then disinserted. (b) The disinserted muscle. (c) Suture needles are placed in "crossed-swords" position anterior to the muscle insertion. (d) A bow-tie knot is placed. (e) The conjunctiva is recessed to the level of the knot to facilitate adjustment of the suture. (Patient of Dr R Morris.)

Most adjustable sutures are put on recessed muscles, and more than one muscle can be placed on an adjustable. The muscle may be deliberately over-recessed as it is easier to advance than recess an adjustment. Resected muscles can be adjustable, but they are more difficult to adjust and there is a risk of muscle slippage.

At adjustment, which can now be performed within a few hours of surgery, the patient needs to be cooperative. The deviation is measured and the movements assessed with their spectacle correction. If they required prisms in their glasses preoperatively they should be adjusted in spectacles that correct the refractive error but have no prisms. Patients with high refractive errors who wear contact lenses can be adjusted in their contact lenses.

The eye is anesthetized with drops and the patient is asked to open their eyes. An assistant helps hold the lids open or a lid speculum can be used and good lighting is essential. Operating loupes should be used. If no adjustment is required the muscle is tied off. If the muscle needs to be recessed, the bow is released and the patient asked to look into the field of action of the muscle while the surgeon moves the eye in the opposite direction. The muscle is retied in a bow and the patient examined again. To advance the muscle the bow is released, the two arms of the suture held in a tying forceps or needle holder and gently pulled while countertraction is applied with a curved forceps at the point at which the sutures leave the sclera. The muscle is retied in a bow and the patient examined again.

Once the desired result has been achieved, the muscle suture is tied off, the ends cut not shorter than 2–3 mm. The knot is covered with conjunctiva. If the cinch technique is used, the knot is moved along the suture instead of the bow being tied and untied. With both techniques, even tension is placed on both ends of the suture so that one pole of the muscle is not advanced more that another and the sutures must not saw through the sclera during adjustment.

At adjustment not only the effect of the adjustment on the deviation in primary position is assessed, but also in other positions of gaze, particularly in the field of action of recessed muscles. A muscle must not be recessed so far that it leads to underaction. With large, especially vertical, deviations it is better to place more than one muscle on an adjustable suture. If more than one muscle is placed on an adjustable suture none should be tied off until the required outcome has been achieved. Postadjustment drift occurs in the first 12 months, horizontal deviations tending to under-correction and vertical deviations to overcorrection.[87]

Adjustable sutures have advantages over conventional surgery and are associated with a reoperation rate lower than that of conventional surgery, with adjustments necessary in about 40%. Nausea induced by the adjustment is the most common; bradycardia, suture breakage, and inability to adjust the suture can occur.

REOPERATIONS

About 25% of patients who have had strabismus surgery require further surgery, the complexity of which depends on the number of previous operations, the type and quality of the previous surgery, which muscles were operated, and the underlying pathology. Reoperations are technically more difficult particularly if there is evidence of restriction, slipped muscles, or scarring.

Prior to a reoperation, FDTs should be performed and the conjunctiva examined. The conjunctiva may be dissected using a microscope to avoid conjunctival scarring. Long oblique rather than parallel conjunctival relaxing incisions should be made to adequately expose muscles, which may have been previously supra- or infraplaced. Hooking a muscle can be difficult and force should not be used, but careful dissection to create a hole in Tenon's to isolate the muscle on a hook should be made. Once isolated, the muscle is freed from adhesions and scar tissue, dissecting only tissues that can be seen. Large "blind" cuts lead to bleeding and the muscle being damaged. Redundant scar tissue and orbital fat may be excised. Sutures are placed in the substance of the muscle, about 2 mm back from the scleral insertion unless a pseudotendon has developed.

Reoperations are unpredictable and most patients benefit from adjustable sutures. Readvancement is more effective than resection, particularly if the antagonist has been recessed. Inferior rectus surgery can lead to severe scar tissue formation between it, Lockwood's ligament, and the lower lid retractors, making reoperations difficult. In reoperations for "slippage" of the inferior rectus a pseudotendon is often found and the muscle is "stiff": advancing this muscle to the insertion may induce a hypotropia with restricted elevation. The muscle is best not fully advanced, and it may be combined with contralateral superior and inferior rectus recessions on adjustable sutures.[88] Careful conjunctival closure after reoperations especially at the plica and caruncle reduces conjunctival scarring. The conjunctiva often needs to be sutured to the sclera so that it stays where intended. Excess and severely scarred conjunctiva can be excised.

COMPLICATIONS

Anesthetic

All general anesthetics carry a small risk but there are some complications of specific interest to the strabismus surgeon. The risks are often stated as being that 1:10,000 anesthetics in a healthy child are complicated by cardiac or respiratory arrest, and that 1:10 of these die or have a permanent disability.

- Traction on any muscle, especially the medial rectus, may induce the oculocardiac reflex (bradycardia): intravenous (IV) atropine can prevent recurrences.
- Postoperative nausea and vomiting is now unusual but it may be more common after strabismus surgery than many other surgical procedures, particularly in children, perhaps related to the use of opiates and related drugs. Droperidol as premedication and IV anesthesia (propofol) may reduce post-operative vomiting. Nowadays most strabismus surgery is done as day cases.
- Patients using phospholine iodide drops are at risk of prolonged apnea if succinylcholine is used during induction; it should be stopped six weeks before surgery.

Hemorrhage

Patients undergoing strabismus surgery should be asked about bleeding disorders and anticoagulant drugs. Bleeding during strabismus surgery relates to surgical technique, the muscle being operated on, and the extent of scarring. Severe bleeding can occur if a muscle or vortex vein is ruptured; this is more likely in reoperations. Delayed hemorrhage is rare, but orbital hemorrhage has been described.

Globe perforation

Scleral perforation occurs during sutures placement in the sclera to reattach muscles. Perforation by stay sutures may lead to shallowing of the anterior chamber or hyphema. Rarely, globe perforation occurs during muscle disinsertion, particularly in reoperations, placement of traction sutures beneath the lateral rectus, and preplacement of muscle sutures.[89] The incidence is around 1%,[17] up to 10.2% in older studies.[90] This decline is the result of the introduction of fine spatulate needles, improved techniques, illumination, and magnification. The incidence is higher for faden sutures as the sutures are being placed through thin posterior sclera.[91]

Scleral perforation can rarely lead to retinal and vitreous hemorrhage, retinal detachment, and endophthalmitis; usually just a localized chorioretinal scar develops (Fig. 88.40a). If scleral perforation is suspected at surgery the retina should be inspected, and antibiotics administered, but the use of cryotherapy is controversial,[90] as retinal detachment is rare and cryotherapy may be detrimental.[92] Late scleral perforation and thinning can occur, including "bleb" formation at the site of limbal traction sutures (Fig. 88.40b) and scleromalacia at the site of muscle disinsertion (Fig. 88.40c).

Conjunctival complications

Most are the result of poor surgical technique.

1. A conjunctival scar is inevitable, but when surgery is meticulous and the conjunctiva well apposed, it is not noticeable. After multiple procedures, vascularization and scarring may be prominent. In reoperations it is often prudent to recess the conjunctiva to reduce scarring and prevent conjunctival restriction. If the plica is drawn toward the limbus, by poor apposition or cicatrization following multiple procedures, unsightly scarring develops (Fig. 88.41c and d). The conjunctiva and plica can be mobilized and recessed, with some improvement. Scarring also develops if the orbital

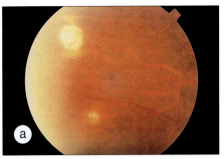 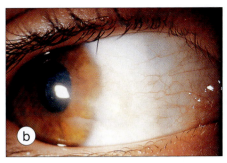 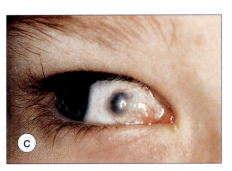

Fig. 88.40 Globe perforation complications. (a) Localized chorioretinal scar following scleral perforation at strabismus surgery. (b) Bleb formation following unrecognized scleral perforation from limbal traction suture 3 years previously. (c) Scleromalacia 4 years after strabismus surgery at site of original muscle insertion. (Patient of Dr R Morris.)

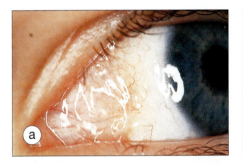 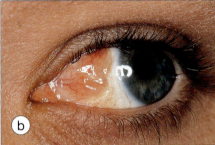 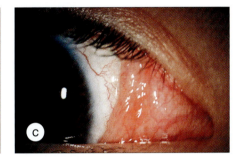

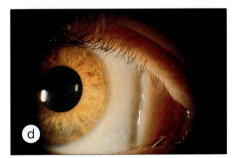 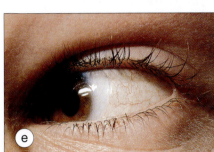

Fig. 88.41 Conjunctival complications. (a, b) Unsightly conjunctival scarring over medial rectus. (c, d) Plica semilunaris drawn toward limbus following medial rectus surgery. (e) Raised conjunctiva at limbus due to early postoperative slippage. (Patient of Dr R Morris.)

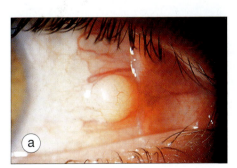 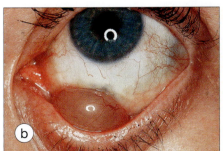 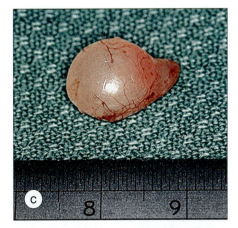

Fig. 88.42 Conjunctival epithelial inclusion cysts. (a) Cyst over medial rectus. (b) Cyst over inferior rectus. (c) Cyst over inferior rectus following excision. (Patient of Dr R Morris.)

fat is penetrated and is advanced subconjunctivally, leaving a pink fleshy appearance. Patients with conjunctival scarring frequently complain of irritable red eyes, especially in dry environments or after swimming.

2. Prolapse of Tenon's through the conjunctival wound, because of incomplete closure, produces a white appearance contrast-

ing with the pinker conjunctiva. It usually shrinks spontaneously, but can be excised if excessive.

3. Conjunctival epithelial inclusion cysts (Fig. 88.42) are uncommon, but may develop years after surgery from small fragments of epithelium within the wound; they may enlarge. If small they can be left, but larger cysts need to be excised intact.

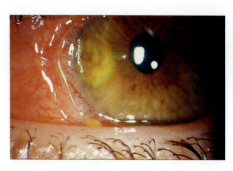

Fig. 88.43 Corneal delle formation following medial rectus readvancement. Staining with fluorescein adjacent to recent strabismus surgery. (Patient of Dr R Morris.)

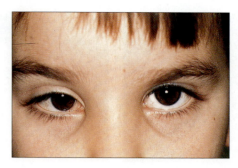

Fig. 88.45 Narrowing of right palpebral fissure following right medial rectus readvancement. (Patient of Dr R Morris.)

4. Dellen, areas of corneal thinning from drying adjacent to the limbus, may follow strabismus surgery, especially resection or advancement of a medial rectus (Fig. 88.43). They are not usually significant but, if symptomatic, treatment is with artificial tears.

Suture and drug-related complications

Allergies to sutures are now uncommon since the advent of synthetic absorbable sutures (Fig. 88.44a). They were common with organic suture materials. They present as a prolonged inflammatory reaction over the site of the sutures, and respond to treatment with topical steroids. Suture granulomas occur in less than 0.5% patients usually over the knot (Fig. 88.44b). In most cases they are small and resolve spontaneously, but can require excision. Superficial conjunctival sutures may cause local irritation (Figs. 88.44c and 88.44d). Nonabsorbable sutures are easily visible through the conjunctiva (Fig. 88.44e).

Allergic reactions to postoperative drops may also occur particularly if they contain neomycin.

Lid changes

In regards to the complication of lower lid retraction, see "Inferior rectus muscle recession." Lower lid advancement is frequent after inferior rectus resection but it is less noticeable than lower lid recession. An upper lid ptosis can occur following large superior rectus resections but upper lid retraction is rarely

seen even with larger recessions of the superior rectus.[28] Narrowing of the palpebral fissure and/or globe retraction may occur after large recession-resections or advancement and resection of a previously recessed or "lost" muscle (Fig. 88.45).

Anterior segment ischemia

Severe anterior segment ischemia following strabismus surgery occurs in 30:400,000 cases, mostly with transpositions.[93] Mild cases are common and not significant. In severe cases the signs include chemosis, corneal edema, uveitis, lens opacities, and hypotony with iris sector perfusion defects occurring in around 20%[14] (Fig. 88.46), particularly with surgery on the vertical rectus muscles. Further surgery on the same muscle does not cause further hypoperfusion because of remodeling of the deep collateral circulation rather than anterior ciliary recanalization. Recovery of the iris circulation occurred in most within 4 weeks and in all by 12 weeks.[94] In children, there is virtually no sector infarction.[15]

The findings in primates are similar, but staged removal of the recti do not suggest remodeling of the circulation.[95] Limbal incisions are said to predispose to more severe ischemia than fornix incisions, by an effect on the anterior episcleral arterial circle, but as this circle lies in the deepest episcleral layers, it is unlikely to be damaged by the reflection of the conjunctiva in a limbal incision.[15]

Two-rectus-muscle surgery rarely causes anterior segment ischemia, unless there is a risk factor such as microvascular disease, sickle cell disease, leukemia, thyroid eye disease, high myopia, and previous scleral buckling or strabismus surgery.

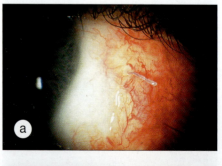
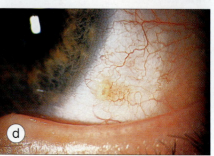
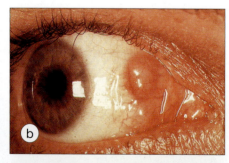
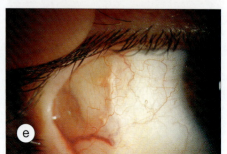
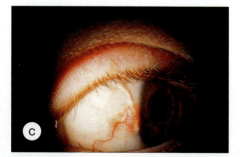

Fig. 88.44 Suture-related complications. (a) Reaction to exposed Vicryl suture. (b) Suture granuloma. (c) Retained stay suture. (d) Delayed absorption of an 8–0 virgin silk conjunctival suture. (e) Muscle suture visible through conjunctiva. (Patient of Dr R Morris.)

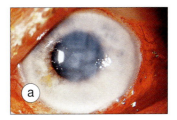 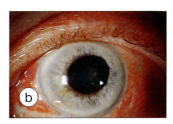 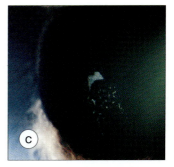 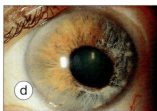

Fig. 88.46 Anterior segment ischemia. (a) Severe ischemia causing corneal edema. (b) Same eye 6 months later; note mid-dilated pupil. (c) Anterior lens opacities following anterior segment ischemia. (d) Iris atrophy following anterior segment ischemia. (Patient of Dr R Morris.)

Horizontal rectus muscle surgery combined with one vertical muscle is safe in children, but surgery of both vertical recti together with a horizontal rectus muscle, especially the medial rectus, may lead to anterior segment ischemia.[15,94] Staged surgery does not produce a cumulative effect and three or even four rectus muscles can be safely detached after a three- to four-month interval, probably because of remodeling of the collateral circulation and an increased contribution from the long posterior ciliary arteries.[15,95] Microvascular dissection may preserve the anterior ciliary arteries in high-risk cases, but its clinical applications and benefits are not yet clear.[96]

Infection

Postoperative infection is rare after strabismus surgery. Preoperative instillation of povidone iodine or topical antibiotics into the conjunctival sac reduces the bacterial load, but their role in reducing infection is not proven. Antibiotics alone or with steroid drops postoperatively are poorly complied with and they are of doubtful benefit. Conjunctivitis is common and usually resolves rapidly with topical antibiotics. Subconjunctival abscesses can occur and respond to surgical drainage and antibiotics (Fig. 88.47).

Orbital cellulitis is rare (1:1000–1:1900 cases) and Gram-positive cocci are the most frequently implicated organisms. Patients present with pain, lid swelling, chemosis, proptosis, limitation of ocular movement, and proptosis, together with systemic signs of infection. They require parenteral antibiotic therapy. Endophthalmitis is rare (1:30,000 cases) and occurs only if the globe has been perforated at surgery.[97] Full-thickness perforation may be followed by early and rapid endophthalmitis, whereas endophthalmitis associated with partial-thickness perforation is more likely to occur after a few days.

Motility and diplopia

The commonest complication in strabismus surgery is over- and undercorrection: about 80% of patients have the desired postoperative outcome, although good initial alignment may change with time. Patients with reduced fusion or amblyopia or those who have had multiple surgical procedures are most likely to have unstable ocular alignment. Limitation of eye movements may occur after inferior oblique surgery, multiple surgery, and excessive resections or recessions.

Surgery on the lateral rectus muscle, if the inferior oblique is included in the insertion, may cause limited elevation in adduction like Brown syndrome, other restrictive motility problems, or vertical strabismus in primary position. It can be prevented by careful dissection but surgery to free the adhesion often fails to correct the vertical deviation.[98]

Postoperatively muscle action may be temporarily reduced by pain, trauma, inflammation, and ischemia. Diplopia is usually transient in children, who suppress the diplopic image. Scott reported a 39% incidence of diplopia in adults 6 weeks postoperatively, but only 1.4% were left with residual diplopia.[99]

Ruptured, slipped, and lost muscles

Rupture of a rectus muscle, usually at its junction of the tendon, can occur during surgery, typically during reoperations when force from a muscle hook is applied to a thin muscle: the muscle may retract into Tenon's. Apart from the medial rectus, which does not have attachments to the obliques, the muscle can usually be identified. The medial rectus can be difficult to identify but it is important not to look for it on the surface of the globe but within Tenon's capsule.

Inferior oblique surgery can lead to disinsertion of the inferior or lateral rectus. Similarly, the superior rectus can be mistaken for the superior oblique, leading to a superior rectus myectomy rather than a superior oblique tenotomy.[50] These complications of oblique muscle surgery can be avoided by visualizing the muscles at surgery and by not blindly sweeping strabismus hooks to engage the muscles.

A "lost" or slipped muscle can develop postoperatively, either immediately or some weeks later.[101,102] It occurs when an operated muscle fails to adhere directly to the sclera, retracting within its capsule, forming a pseudotendon, which is attached to the globe usually where the scleral sutures were placed. It is more common after resections and advancements of previously recessed muscles. It can be avoided by meticulous placement of muscle and scleral sutures, ensuring that sutures are placed through the muscle and not through the capsule. Patients present

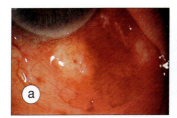 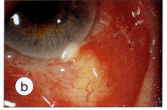

Fig. 88.47 Localized abscess. (a) Localized subconjunctival abscess. (b) Pus released by pressure on abscess. (Patient of Dr R Morris.)

with a deviation and underaction of the muscle (Fig. 88.48). At surgery, FDTs should be performed as the ipsilateral antagonist is often tight and needs to be recessed (ideally on an adjustable suture). The pseudotendon, which is sometimes flimsy, can be stretched by a strabismus hook, and care must be taken as the muscle can often be located by following it posteriorly. A subtle change in color may be seen at the junction of the pseudotendon and muscle, which is usually found at or posterior to the point where Tenon's capsule is penetrated (Fig. 88.48b). Once the muscle has been located by posterior dissection, avoiding hemorrhage and fat prolapse, sutures are placed through the muscle itself, ideally two double-armed sutures (Fig. 88.49). The muscle is advanced and sutured to the sclera. Sometimes it is possible to advance it to its original insertion, but in others it is too tight and should be sutured to a point on the sclera that achieves a small overcorrection. Forced ductions tests out of the

field of action of the muscle are typically positive postoperatively, and versions and ductions reduced: this usually improves with time. It should never be placed on an adjustable suture as it may slip again because of the contracture. The muscle is often narrowed and a horizontal muscle must not be supra- or infraplaced as this induces a vertical deviation.

Refractive changes

There is not usually a change in the spherical power of the eye but horizontal muscle surgery can induce with the rule astigmatism due to corneal rather than lenticular changes.[102,103] Minor changes in astigmatism may occur postoperatively but stabilize by 6–8 weeks, which is the best time for refraction if it is necessary.

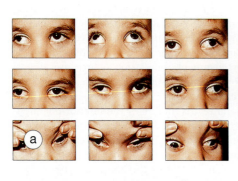
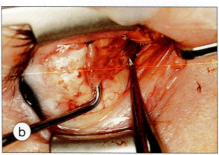

Fig. 88.48 Patient with slipped right medial rectus muscle. (a) Note large exodeviation and underaction of medial rectus. (b) Findings at surgery: Strabismus hook under pseudotendon of medial rectus 11 mm from limbus. Forceps indicating proximal end of medial rectus muscle. Note the change in color between muscle tissue and pseudotendon. (Patient of Dr R Morris.)

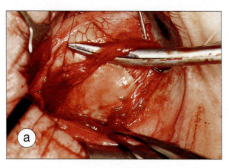
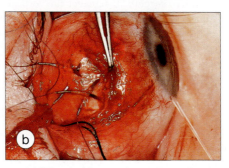
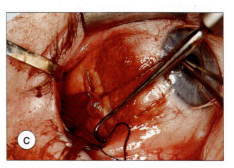

Fig. 88.49 Slipped left medial rectus muscle readvanced. (a) Two double-armed sutures are placed through the muscle. Note the muscle width is contracted and there is a pseudotendon that runs over the curved scissors. (b) Sutures placed behind original insertion as the muscle was tight. (c) The muscle is reattached behind its original insertion. (Patient of Dr R Morris.)

REFERENCES

1. Jampolsky A. In: Symposium on Strabismus. Transactions of the New Orleans Academy of Ophthalmology. St Louis: Mosby, 1971: 34–92.
2. O'Flynn E. Strabismus documentation: an alternative approach. Br Orthop J 1994; 51: 10–4.
3. Vivian AJ, Morris RJ. Diagrammatic representation of strabismus. Eye 1993; 7: 565–71.
4. Koornneef L. New insights in the human orbital connective tissue. Arch Ophthalmol 1977; 95: 1269–73.
5. Apt L, Call NB. An anatomical re-evaluation of rectus muscle insertions. Ophthalmic Surg 1982; 13: 108–12.
6. Keech RV, Scott WE, Baker JD. The medial rectus insertion site in infantile esotropia. Am J Ophthalmol 1990; 109: 79–84.
7. Kushner BJ, Preslan MW, Vrabec M. Artifacts of measurement during strabismus surgery. J Pediatr Ophthalmol Strabismus 1987; 24: 159–64.
8. Helveston EM, Krach P, Plager DA, et al. A new classification for

superior oblique palsy based on congenital variations in the tendon. Ophthalmology 1992; 99: 1609–15.
9. Wallace DK, von Noorden GK. Clinical characteristics and surgical management of congenital absence of the superior oblique tendon. Am J Ophthalmol 1994; 118: 63–9.
10. Plager DA. Traction testing in superior oblique palsy. J Pediatr Ophthalmol Strabismus 1990; 27: 136–40.
11. Fink WH. Surgery of the Vertical Muscles of the Eye. 2nd ed. Springfield, IL: CC Thomas; 1962.
12. Scott WE, Morris RJ. Dissociated vertical deviation and inferior oblique overaction in infantile esotropia. Arch Ophthalmol 1990; 108: 1081.
13. Swan KC, Wilkins JH. Extraocular muscle surgery in early infancy. J Pediatr Ophthalmol Strabismus 1984; 21: 44–9.
14. Lee JP, Olver JM. Anterior segment ischaemia. Eye 1990; 4: 1–6.
15. Olver JM, Lee JP. The effects of strabismus surgery on the anterior segment circulation. Eye 1989; 3: 318–26.
16. Goldstein JH, Prepas SB, Conrad SD. The effect of needle characteristics in strabismus surgery. Arch Ophthalmol 1982; 100: 617–8.

17. Morris RJ, Rosen P, Fells P. Incidence of inadvertent globe perforation during strabismus surgery. Br J Ophthalmol 1990; 74: 490–3.

18. Guyton DL. An exaggerated forced duction test for the oblique muscles. Ophthalmology 1981; 88: 1035–40.

19. Parks MM. Fornix incisions for horizontal rectus muscle surgery. Am J Ophthalmol 1968; 65: 907–15.

20. Swan KC, Talbot T. Recession over Tenon's capsule. Arch Ophthalmol 1954; 51: 32–41.

21. Kushner BJ, Fisher MMJ, Lucchese N, et al. Factors influencing response in strabismus surgery. Arch Ophthalmol 1993; 111: 75–9.

22. Stager DR, Weakley DR, Everett M, et al. Delayed consecutive exotropia following 7–millimetre bilateral medial rectus recession for congenital esotropia. J Pediatr Ophthalmol Strabismus 1994; 31: 147–52.

23. Nelson LB, Calhoun JH, Simon JW, et al. Surgical management of large angle congenital esotropia. Br J Ophthalmol 1987; 71: 380–3.

24. Calhoun JH. Discussion on how far a medial rectus can be safely recessed and delayed consecutive exotropia following 7-millimetre bilateral medial rectus recession for congenital esotropia. J Pediatr Ophthalmol Strabismus 1994; 31: 151–2.

25. Kushner BJ, Fisher MM, Lucchese NJ, et al. How far can a medial rectus safely be recessed? J Pediatr Ophthalmol Strabismus 1994; 31: 138–46.

26. Scott WE, Reese PD, Hirsch CR, et al. Surgery for large angle congenital esotropia. Arch Ophthalmol 1986; 104: 374–7.

27. Pratt-Johnson JA, Tillson G. Management of Strabismus and Amblyopia: a Practical Guide. New York: Thieme Medical; 1995: 175–6.

28. Pacheco EM, Guyton DL, Repka MX. Changes in eyelid position accompanying vertical rectus muscle surgery and prevention of lower lid retraction with adjustable surgery. J Pediatr Ophthalmol Strabismus 1992; 29: 265–72.

29. Kushner BJ. A surgical procedure to minimize lower lid retraction with inferior rectus recession. Arch Ophthalmol 1992; 110: 1011–4.

30. Scotcher SM, O'Flynn EA, Morris RJ. Inferior rectus recession–an effective procedure? Br J Ophthalmol 1997; 81: 1031–6.

31. Sprunger DT, Helveston EM. Progressive overcorrection after inferior rectus recession. J Pediatr Ophthalmol Strabismus 1993; 30: 145–8.

32. Wright KW. Late overcorrection after inferior rectus recession. Ophthalmology 1996; 103: 1503–7.

33. Jampolsky A. In: Symposium on Pediatric Ophthalmology and Strabismus. Transactions of the New Orleans Academy of Ophthalmology. New York: Raven Press; 1986: 154–7.

34. Chatzistefanou KI, Kushner BJ, Gentry LR. Magnetic resonance imaging of the arc of contact of extraocular muscles: implications regarding the incidence of slipped muscles. J AAPOS 2000; 4: 84–93.

35. Scott WE, Sutton VJ, Thalaker JA. Superior rectus recession for dissociated vertical deviation. Ophthalmology 1982; 89: 317–22.

36. Scott AB. The faden operation: mechanical effects. Am Orthop J 1977; 27: 44–7.

37. Parks MM. Atlas of Strabismus Surgery. Philadelphia: Harper & Row; 1983: 116–31.

38. Elliott RL, Nankin SJ. Anterior transposition of the inferior oblique. J Pediatr Ophthalmol Strabismus 1981; 18: 35–8.

39. Stager DR, Parks MM. Inferior oblique weakening procedures: effect on primary position horizontal alignment. Arch Ophthalmol 1973; 90: 15–6.

40. Scott WE, Kraft SP. In: Symposium on Pediatric Ophthalmology and Strabismus: Transactions of the New Orleans Academy of Ophthalmology. New York: Raven Press; 1986: 15–38.

41. Parks MM. Weakening surgical procedures for eliminating overaction of the inferior oblique muscle. Am J Ophthalmol 1972; 73: 107–22.

42. Mims J, Wood RC. Bilateral anterior transposition of the inferior obliques. Arch Ophthalmol 1989; 107: 41–4.

43. Stager DR. Anatomy and surgery of the inferior oblique muscle: recent findings 2. J AAPOS 2001; 5: 203–8.

44. Burke JP, Scott WE, Kutshke PJ. Anterior transposition of the inferior oblique muscle for dissociated vertical deviation. Ophthalmology 1993; 100: 245–50.

45. Gonzalez C. Denervation of the inferior oblique, current status and long-term results. Trans Am Acad Ophthalmol Otolaryngol 1976; 81: 899–906.

46. Kushner BJ. Restriction of elevation in abduction after inferior oblique anteriorization. J AAPOS 1997; 1: 55–62.

47. Stager DR Jr, Beauchamp GR, Wright WW, et al. Anterior and nasal transposition of the inferior oblique muscles 1. J AAPOS 2003; 7: 167–73.

48. Mims JL III, Wood RC. Antielevation syndrome after bilateral anterior transposition of the inferior oblique muscles: incidence and prevention. J AAPOS 1999; 3: 333–6.

49. Parks MM. In: Atlas of Strabismus Surgery. Philadelphia: Harper & Row; 1983: 189–209.

50. Raymond WR, Parks MM. Transection of the superior oblique rectus muscle during intended superior oblique tenotomy: a report of three cases. Ophthalmic Surg 1995; 26: 244–9.

51. Crawford JS, Orton RB, Labow-Daily L. Late results of superior oblique tenotomy in true Brown's syndrome. Am J Ophthalmol 1980; 89: 824–9.

52. Bardorf CM, Baker JD. The efficacy of superior oblique split Z-tendon lengthening for superior oblique overaction. J AAPOS 2003; 7: 96–102.

53. Wright K. Superior oblique silicone expander for Brown syndrome and superior oblique overaction. J Pediatr Ophthalmol Strabismus 1991; 28: 101–7.

54. Manners R, O'Flynn E, Morris RJ. Superior oblique tendon lengthening for acquired superior oblique overactions. Br J Ophthalmol 1994; 78: 280–4.

55. Scott WE, Kraft SP. In: Waltman S, Keates R, Hoyt C, et al., editors. Surgery of the Eye. New York: Churchill Livingstone; 1988: 789–801.

56. Gobin MH. In: Bosch MC, Frosini R, editors. Strabismus Symposium. Florence: 1982.

57. Mombaerts I, Koornneef L, Everhard YS, et al. Superior oblique luxation and trochlear luxation as new concepts in superior oblique muscle weakening surgery. Am J Ophthalmol 1995; 120: 83–91.

58. McGuire W. The surgical correction of paresis of the superior oblique. Trans Am Ophthalmol Soc 1947; 44: 527–49.

59. McLean J. Direct surgery of underacting superior oblique muscles. Trans Am Ophthalmol Soc 1948; 46: 633–51.

60. Helveston EM, Ellis FD. Superior oblique tuck for superior oblique palsy. Aust NZ J Ophthalmol 1983; 11: 215–20.

61. Saunders RA, Tomlinson E. Quantitated superior oblique tendon tuck in the treatment of superior oblique muscle palsy. Am Orthop J 1985; 35: 81–90.

62. Morris RJ, Scott WE, Keech R. Superior oblique tuck surgery in the management of superior oblique palsies. J Pediatr Ophthalmol Strabismus 1992; 29: 337–46.

63. Saunders RA. Treatment of superior oblique palsy with tendon tuck and inferior oblique muscle myectomy. Ophthalmology 1986; 93: 1023–7.

64. Harada M, Ito Y. Surgical correction of cyclotropia. Jpn J Ophthalmol 1964; 8: 88.

65. Fells P. Management of paralytic strabismus. Br J Ophthalmol 1974; 58: 255–65.

66. Mitchell PR, Parks MM. Surgery for bilateral superior oblique palsy. Ophthalmology 1982; 89: 484–8.

67. Price N, Vickers S, Lee J, et al. The diagnosis and surgical management of acquired bilateral superior oblique palsy. Eye 1987; 1: 78–85.

68. Guyton DL. Torsion and elevation under general anaesthesia and during voluntary eye closure. J Pediatr Ophthalmol Strabismus 1984; 21: 78.

69. Metz HL, Lerner H. The adjustable Harada-Ito procedure. Arch Ophthalmol 1981; 99: 624–6.

70. Goldberg RA, Rosenbaum AL, Tong JT. Use of apically based periosteal flaps as globe tethers in severe paretic strabismus. Arch Ophthalmol. 2000; 118: 431–7.

71. Knapp P. Vertically incomitant horizontal strabismus: the so-called "A" and "V" pattern syndromes. Trans Am Ophthalmol Soc 1959; 57: 666–9.

72. Metz HV. Muscle transposition surgery. J Pediatr Ophthalmol Strabismus 1993; 30: 346–53.

73. Scott WE, Drummond GT, Keech RV. Vertical offsets of the horizontal recti in the management of A and V pattern strabismus. Aust NZ J Ophthalmol 1989; 17: 281–8.

74. Metz H. The use of vertical muscle offsets with horizontal strabismus surgery. Ophthalmology 1988; 95: 1094–7.

75. Dunlap EA. Vertical displacement of the horizontal recti 1. Pac Med Surg 1964; 72: 360–2.

76. Knapp P. The surgical treatment of double elevator paralysis. Trans Am Ophthalmol Soc 1969; 67: 304–23.

77. Burke JP, Ruben JB, Scott WE. Vertical transposition of the horizontal recti (Knapp procedure) for the treatment of double elevator palsy. Br J Ophthalmol 1992; 76: 734–7.

78. Burke JP, Keech RV. Effectiveness of inferior rectus transposition of the horizontal rectus muscles for acquired inferior rectus paresis. J Pediatr Ophthalmol Strabismus 1995; 32: 172–7.

79. Maurino V, Kwan AS, Lee JP. Review of the inverse Knapp procedure: indications, effectiveness and results. Eye 2001; 15: 7–11.

80. Jensen CD. Rectus muscle union: a new operation for paralysis of rectus muscles. Trans Pacific Coast Oto-Ophthalmol Soc 1964; 45: 359–84.

81. Fitzsimons R, Lee J, Elston J. Treatment of sixth nerve palsy in adults with combined botulinum toxin chemodenervation and surgery. Ophthalmology 1988; 95: 1535–42.

82. Rosenbaum AR, Kushner BV, Kirschen D. Vertical rectus muscle transposition and botulinum toxin (oculinum) to medial rectus for abducens palsy. Arch Ophthalmol 1991; 109: 1345–6.

83. Foster RS. Vertical muscle transposition augmented with lateral fixation. J AAPOS 1997; 1: 20–30.

84. Paysse EA, Brady McCreery KM, et al. Use of augmented rectus muscle transposition surgery for complex strabismus. Ophthalmology 2002; 109: 1309–14.

85. Morris RJ, Luff A. Adjustable sutures in squint surgery. Br J Ophthalmol 1992; 76: 560–2.

86. Fells P. Adjustable sutures. Eye 1988; 2: 33–5.

87. Rosen P, Morris R, McCarry B, et al. In: Tilson G, editor. Advances in Amblyopia and Strabismus. Transactions of the VIIth International Orthoptic Congress. Germany: Fahner Verlag; 1991: 89–93.

88. Lee J. Corrective measures. Br J Ophthalmol 1997; 81: 1025.

89. Simon JW, Lininger LL, Scheraga JL. Recognised scleral perforation during eye muscle surgery: incidence and sequelae. J Pediatr Ophthalmol Strabismus 1992; 29: 273–5.

90. Gottleib F, Castro J. Perforation of the globe during strabismus surgery. Arch Ophthalmol 1970; 84: 151–7.

91. Lyons CJ, Fells P, Lee JP, et al. Chorioretinal scarring after the Faden operation. Eye 1989; 3: 401–3.

92. Mittelman D., Bakos IM. The role of retinal cryopexy in the management of experimental perforation of the eye during strabismus surgery. J Pediatr Ophthalmol Strabismus 1984; 21: 186–9.

93. France T, Simon J. Anterior segment ischemia syndrome following muscle surgery: the AAPO&S experience. J Pediatr Ophthalmol Strabismus 1986; 23: 87–91.

94. Olver JM, Lee JP. Recovery of the anterior segment circulation after strabismus surgery. Ophthalmology 1992; 99: 305–15.

95. Virdi PS, Hayreh SS. Anterior segment ischaemia after recession of various recti. An experiemental study. Ophthalmology 1987; 94: 1258–71

96. McKeown CA, Lambert HM, Usaf M, et al. Preservation of the anterior vessels during extraocular muscle surgery. Ophthalmology 1989; 96: 499–507.

97. Ing MR. Infection following strabismus surgery. Ophthalmic Surg 1991; 22: 41–3.

98. Moen C, Marsh IB. Inferior oblique syndrome: an under-recognised complication of strabismus surgery. Eye 1998; 12: 970–2.

99. Scott WE, Kutschke P, Lee W. Diplopia in adult strabismus. Am Orthop J 1994; 44: 66–9.

100. MacEwan CJ, Lee JP, Fells P. Aetiology and management of the "detached" rectus muscle. Br J Ophthalmol 1992; 76: 131–6.

101. Plager DG, Parks MM. Repair and recognition of the "lost" rectus muscle. Ophthalmology 1990; 97: 131–6.

102. Bagheri A, Farahi A, Guyton DL. Astigmatism induced by simultaneous recession of both horizontal rectus muscles. J AAPOS 2003; 7: 42–6.

103. Hainsworth DP, Bierly JR, Schmeisser ET, et al. Corneal topographic changes after extraocular muscle surgery. J AAPOS 1999; 3: 80–6.

CHAPTER
89 # Abnormal Head Postures in Children

Stephen P Kraft

GENERAL CONSIDERATIONS

Abnormal head postures (AHPs) are frequent in pediatric ophthalmology. The medical term is *torticollis*, from the Latin prefix "tortus" (twisted), and "collum" (neck).[1,2] This term, used on its own, is applied to muscular or neurologic disorders that cause unnatural positions of the head.[1,3] The eye-related conditions that lead to AHPs are termed *ocular torticollis*.[4,5]

Physiological basis of head postures

Normal head position is maintained by synthesis of input from the labyrinth, the semicircular canals, the proprioceptors in the neck, and the retina. The labyrinth is the sense organ for static and dynamic head movement. The otolithic apparatus within the utricle responds to static head position. It is activated during maneuvers such as head tilting to one shoulder. The semicircular canals respond to dynamic head movements in any of the three dimensions.[1,3,5]

Input from these sources travels to the vestibular nuclei in the brainstem, and from there rostrally to the vestibular cortex and caudally to the cervical cord and neck muscles. There are also direct pathways from the labyrinth to the extraocular muscles in response to changes in the semicircular canals. Cerebellar projections and cervical proprioceptive input are integrated into the system.[2,5] Integration of input from the retinas leads to fine adjustments in head position.[2]

The most important muscles of the neck that maintain the vertical column, which in turn supports the head, are the sternocleidomastoid, thoracic, and semispinalis muscles. Torticollis manifests when the forces in these muscles are unbalanced due to a congenital or acquired problem within the spinal column or the muscles themselves, or as a result of abnormal neural inputs from a variety of sources including the vestibular apparatus.[3] It has also been reported as a rare presenting sign of a psychiatric disorder.[2,3]

Ocular torticollis arises from disturbances in the input from the afferent visual pathway, ocular motor nerves, or the vestibular apparatus. Any of these disorders lead to alterations in the normal balance of inputs to the neck muscles. In ocular torticollis, the abnormal posture is adopted:[2,5–8]

1. To optimize visual acuity;
2. To maintain single binocular vision; or
3. To center a narrowed visual field with respect to the body. When an ocular problem leading to an abnormal posture persists, it can lead secondarily to a musculoskeletal torticollis and even scoliosis,[3-5,8-11] but to do so, it needs to be long-standing and unremitting.

Torticollis is not a diagnosis, but a sign of an underlying disorder[3]: a cause must be sought. The assessment in a child often involves input from pediatricians, orthopedic surgeons, neurologists, and physiotherapists. An ophthalmologist is often asked to rule out ocular causes for torticollis.

GENERAL CATEGORIES OF HEAD POSTURES

By orientation (Fig. 89.1)

Torticollis can involve rotation of the head around any of the three main axes. These include:

1. The vertical axis: the head is rotated to one side or the other away from the primary (straight-ahead) gaze direction;
2. The horizontal axis: the chin is elevated or depressed relative to the primary position;
3. The anteroposterior axis: the head is tilted to one or the other shoulder; and
4. A combination of any of these three orientations.

By onset

Most cases of childhood torticollis are not seen at birth but within a few months. There are cases of true congenital torticollis due to muscular or skeletal anomalies.[1,3] Ocular torticollis almost never presents within the first few weeks of life. Trauma must be ruled out as a cause of any acquired abnormal head posture, whether as a result of damage to the neck or due to disruption of eye muscle balance.[3]

By timing

An AHP can be paroxysmal or persistent. It can be temporary in transient diseases, such as otitis media or benign paroxysmal torticollis of infancy. It can be constant, as with congenital nystagmus with an eccentric null zone or with restrictive strabismus.

The head posture can be consistent in its orientation, as occurs in cases of superior oblique muscle paresis and congenital nystagmus. In some cases it may constantly change, for example in cases of periodic alternating nystagmus.

NONOCULAR CAUSES OF HEAD POSTURES
(Table 89.1)

There are many nonocular causes of torticollis, both congenital and acquired. This discussion will be limited to the most common and serious conditions.

987

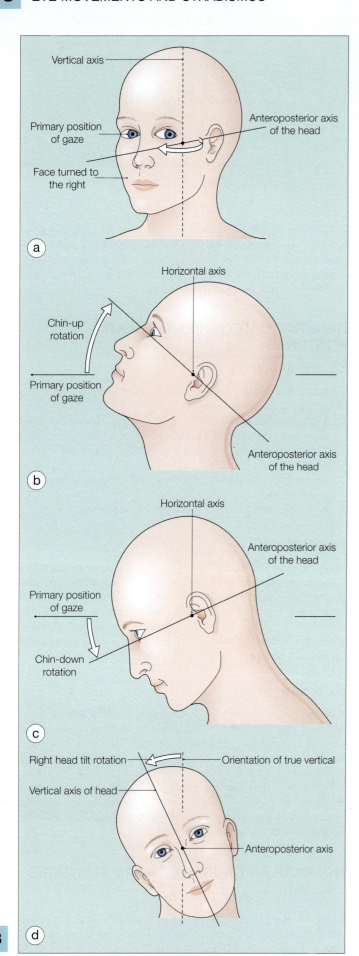

Table 89.1 Nonocular causes of torticollis

I. Congenital
  A. Muscular
    1. Congenital muscular torticollis
    2. Postural torticollis
    3. Absent cervical muscles
  B. Skeletal/Osseous
    1. Atlantoaxial bony deformity
    2. Klippel-Feil syndrome
    3. Sprengel's deformity
    4. Miscellaneous anomalies
II. Acquired
  A. Traumatic
    1 Skeletal/Osseous
      a) Atlantoaxial displacement
      b) Subluxation of C2–C3 joint
      c) Fractures
    2. Ligament
    3. Muscle or soft tissue
  B. Nontraumatic
    1. Skeletal/Osseous
      a) Inflammation
      b) Tumors
      c) Ligamentous laxity
    2. Postural
    3. Neurologic
      a) Syringomyelia
      b) Dystonia
      c) Infections
      d) Posterior fossa pathology
    4. Otolaryngologic
      a) Nasopharyngeal infections
      b) Benign paroxysmal torticollis of infancy
      c) Deafness
      d) Ocular tilt reaction
    5. Miscellaneous
      a) Gastroenterologic
      b) Metabolic
      c) Pharmacologic
      d) Psychogenic/functional

Congenital disorders

Muscular causes
Congenital muscular torticollis

Congenital muscular torticollis (CMT) is the most common type of congenital torticollis: it occurs in 0.4% of newborns. It manifests within 2 to 6 weeks of age, and in many cases there is a painless, discrete "fibroma" on one side of the neck adjacent to the sternocleidomastoid muscle.[1,3,12,13] The infant develops a head tilt to the side of the involved muscle, along with a forward flexion. The mass resolves with time over several months.

As the neck and facial bones enlarge, the fibrotic sternocleidomastoid muscle may fail to elongate properly. As a result, CMT can lead to various deformities including hemifacial hypoplasia, plagiocephaly, and compensatory thoracic scoliosis. The

Fig. 89.1 Orientations of abnormal head postures. (a) Face turn to the right. The anteroposterior axis of the head is rotated from primary gaze direction to the right about the vertical axis. (b) Chin-up posture: The anteroposterior axis of the head is rotated upward from the primary gaze direction about the horizontal axis. (c) Chin-down posture: The anteroposterior axis of the head is rotated downward from the primary gaze direction about the horizontal axis. (d) Head tilt to the right shoulder: The vertical axis of the head is rotated away from the vertical axis about the anteroposterior axis.

changes can usually be arrested by early intervention with passive exercises under the supervision of a physiotherapist.[1,2,12] In a minority of cases surgery is needed.[1,12]

Postural torticollis

The head posture is evident shortly after birth but it is not associated with any mass in the sternocleidomastoid muscle. It may result from an abnormal fetal position. It is usually transient, although some cases require physiotherapy early in childhood to release the muscle stiffness.[1,13]

Skeletal or osseous causes

Abnormalities in the cranial junction or cervical spine, including atlantoaxial rotatory displacement and odontoid hypoplasia, can lead to chronic torticollis.[1,3]

The Klippel-Feil syndrome can lead to torticollis as a result of the associated cervical vertebral anomalies, including congenital vertebral fusion and hemivertebrae, which can lead to reduced neck motion. Sprengel's deformity is seen in 30% of Klippel-Feil cases. It is characterized by an elevated scapula with limited shoulder movement, and it is associated with scoliosis, renal anomalies, and an omovertebral bone.[1,3]

There are several clinical syndromes that place the child at high risk of cervical spine instability as a result of congenital laxity of ligaments or abnormalities of their vertebral bodies. These include Down syndrome, mucopolysaccharidoses, and osteogenesis imperfecta.[1]

Acquired disorders

The acquired causes are divided into traumatic and nontraumatic categories. A traumatic cause must be considered in the evaluation of any case of pediatric torticollis.[1,13,14]

Traumatic causes
Bony trauma

The most common form of trauma affecting the bones of the neck involves rotatory subluxation of the atlantoaxial joint or subluxation of C2 and C3.[1,3,13,14] Fractures of the scapula or clavicle can lead to abnormal head postures.[3] There is usually a great deal of pain and limitation of movement, although there may be little or no neurologic deficit.[3]

Ligament damage

Ligament injuries are much less common than bony injuries. They can be associated with severe neurologic complications, especially if the transverse ligament is ruptured.[13]

Muscle or soft tissue injury

Direct trauma to the neck can lead to hematoma formation in the neck muscles or actual tearing of muscle fibers, especially the sternocleidomastoid or the posterior capitis.[3,13]

Nontraumatic causes
Skeletal or osseous torticollis

Bone erosion in the cranial junction or cervical spine can lead to chronic torticollis. Erosion can arise from inflammation due to osteomyelitis, rheumatoid arthritis, or tuberculosis or from tumors, and it leads to rotatory subluxation or anterior dislocation.[1,3,11]

Atlantoaxial rotatory displacement can arise from excessive transverse ligament laxity following a local infection, especially cervical adenitis or a retropharyngeal abscess.[1,11] It can also arise from intrinsic changes in the ligament as occurs, for example, in

patients who have taken systemic steroids for a long period of time.[3] Most cases resolve spontaneously or once an underlying cause is reversed. A minority require immobilization or cervical traction.[1,3]

Postural torticollis

There is a rare form of torticollis that can be produced by prolonged maintenance of the head in an awkward position that causes undue neck strain. Usually seen in older children, this entity develops over a long period of time and causes gradual but permanent changes in the neck muscles.[3]

Neurologic
Syringomyelia

Acquired torticollis may be the presenting sign of syringomyelia. It can lead to scoliosis and hyperhidrosis. There is also an association with tumors of the spinal cord.[3] Torticollis accompanied by hyperactive tendon reflexes or extensor plantar responses may indicate a cervical cord disturbance; this is an indication for a radiologic study of the cervical spine.[2]

Dystonia

Spasmodic torticollis is a form of dystonia of the facial and cervical muscles that results from neurologic diseases or as an effect of medications that affect the basal ganglia. Loss of interneuron inhibition is a factor.[1,2] Affected patients show sustained muscle contractions with repetitive movements and abnormal head postures.

Spasmodic torticollis in children is usually seen as a reaction to psychiatric medications such as phenothiazine. It may be accompanied by other dystonic reactions such as trismus and oculogyric crises.[2] There are rare cases of idiopathic spasmodic torticollis in children. The childhood form often progresses from a focal dystonia to a more generalized disorder.[1]

Two other conditions that can present in the first two years of life are benign paroxysmal dystonia of infancy and paroxysmal choreoathetosis. Benign paroxysmal dystonia is characterized by episodes of torsion or tilting of the neck or trunk and hypertonic distortions of the upper extremities that can occur up to several times per day. The disease usually subsides spontaneously by age 5 years.[2,3] Paroxysmal choreoathetosis includes abnormal posturing and choreoathetoid movements as well as torticollis and facial grimacing. The episodes can occur up to several times per day.[2]

Infections

Abnormal head postures, usually head tilts, have been reported in association with acute bacterial meningitis, and the mechanism may be involvement of the cranial nerves, especially the fourth cranial nerve.[2] Torticollis can also follow encephalitis, as a result of damage to the basal ganglia.[3] It can also occur after systemic infections including scarlet fever, measles, influenza, poliomyelitis, and diphtheria, as a result of a postinfectious neuritis. Finally, an abnormal head posture can arise as a result of osteomyelitis from a cervical abscess.[3]

Posterior fossa pathology

Torticollis occurs with colloid cysts of the third ventricle and with tumors of the posterior fossa, including ependymomas and hemangioblastomas.[3] Astrocytomas of the cervicomedullary junction can stretch the meninges and lead to head tilts. This can cause neck muscle spasms on attempted passive flexion of the head, especially in young children.[1]

The Arnold-Chiari malformation, in which there is a downward displacement of the cerebellar tonsils in the cervical canal, can lead to a constellation of symptoms and signs including scoliosis, headache, and neck pain with torticollis.[1]

There is a triad of photophobia, epiphora, and torticollis associated with posterior fossa lesions:[15] the postulated mechanism for the torticollis was irritation of the vestibular nuclear complex, herniation of the tonsils, oblique muscle paresis, or a combination of these.[15]

Otolaryngologic

Nasopharyngeal torticollis

Among the most common causes of nontraumatic acute torticollis in children are inflammation and infections of the upper respiratory system, including the pharynx, tonsils, sinuses, mastoids, and the ears.[13] The deep cervical lymph nodes are frequently enlarged and the sternocleidomastoid muscle becomes painful due to spasm[1,3,13]: also termed Grisel syndrome.[13]

The head postures seen with otitis media may be due to disturbance of the labyrinthine apparatus.[3] Retrotonsillar and retropharyngeal abscesses can also lead to torticollis, and a presumed cause is fluid accumulation between the ring of C1 and the odontoid bone.[3,13]

Benign paroxysmal torticollis of infancy

This entity was originally described by Snyder in 1969[16] and consists of recurrent attacks of head tilting often accompanied by vomiting, pallor, and agitation. Its onset is in infancy and it has a female predominance. When the child begins to walk there is an associated ataxia. Older children may also complain of headache or vertigo.[1,2,13,16] It is considered a migraine variant that affects the vestibular system. There is often a strong family history of migraine. The episodes tend to subside over a period of several months or years.[2,13,16]

Deafness

In infants an intermittent unilateral recurring face turn may be the presenting sign of a unilateral hearing deficit.[2,3]

Ocular tilt reaction

This triad of vertical divergence of the eyes, bilateral ocular torsion, and head tilt is a postural reflex originating in the otolithic apparatus. It can be caused by lesions of the vestibular nucleus or its central connections.[2] It will be dealt with in more detail in the section on head tilt postures.

Miscellaneous causes

Gastroenterologic

Hiatus hernia and gastroesophageal reflux can be seen in children, usually those with cerebral palsy. This combination can lead to intermittent neck extensions or head tilts to decrease the amount of reflux, known as Sandifer syndrome.[1,2,5,11,13] Infants with this syndrome rarely present with vomiting.[1,2,13] Treatment with antireflux measures can help. Abnormal neck postures have also been described in infants with pyloric stenosis.[3]

Metabolic disorders

Torticollis may occur in glutaric aciduria, which also causes dystonia and dyskinesia. Children affected with this organic aciduria may also present with severe motor and language deficits and global developmental delays.[1,3]

Pharmacologic

There are a number of drugs that cause torticollis, including the phenothiazines and metoclopramide.[1,3]

Psychiatric and functional disorders

Some head deviations cannot be explained by either nonocular or ocular mechanisms. These may be either functional or psychiatric in nature. The most common form of psychological disorder that leads to torticollis is a conversion reaction[14]: they require close follow-up for signs that would require further investigation.[1]

OCULAR CAUSES OF HEAD POSTURES

General considerations

Children adopt head postures as a result of several ocular conditions. When the patient derives a demonstrable advantage by adopting the head position it is more correctly termed a *compensatory head posture*.[17,18] When a patient is referred to an ophthalmologist, the goal is to determine whether there is an ocular cause for the posture. If an underlying ocular cause is responsible, then treatment can be planned to eliminate or reduce the problem, and restore a normal head posture.

If a primary care physician or specialist is faced with a patient who has an abnormal posture and cannot be sure it is due to a nonocular cause, then an ocular etiology should be considered. Referral for an eye examination should be made early in the assessment protocol:

1. If an ocular cause is left untreated and is prolonged and always present, it can lead to changes in the neck muscles and a musculoskeletal torticollis,[4,5,8] which may persist even if the underlying ocular situation is rectified.
2. A child with incomitant strabismus may adopt a compensatory posture to maintain fusion. If the posture is very pronounced and physically difficult to sustain for long periods, the child may assume a more normal position. If this action creates a heterotropia with loss of fusion in the new preferred position of gaze, then the child is at risk of developing suppression and amblyopia.[2]
3. Some cases of ocular torticollis, especially tilts early in childhood, can lead to changes in the facial bones, resulting in plagiocephaly,. This deformity can be prevented by early detection and treatment.[8-10]
4. The binocular visual acuity of a child with a compensatory posture may not be optimal in the adopted position, especially if nystagmus is the cause. Eye muscle surgery for the head posture may simultaneously improve the binocular acuity.[11,18-20]

Compensatory head postures have four advantages.[5,17] They serve to:

1. Optimize visual acuity;
2. Maintain binocularity;
3. Center the field of binocular vision; and
4. Miscellaneous benefits.

Optimize visual acuity

Children adopt a compensatory posture either to optimize their binocular visual acuity or, if unable to maintain that, to maximize vision in one or the other eye.[2,6,17]

1. Examples in the first category include congenital nystagmus and ptosis. In the case of congenital nystagmus, the vision is best because the nystagmus intensity is least with the AHP.[18,19] The AHPs of spasmus nutans and oculomotor apraxia probably fall into this category.[5,6,18]

2. The second category includes significant refractive errors (especially astigmatism) manifest latent nystagmus in a monocular patient, severe restrictive strabismus, and infantile esotropia with cross fixation. It also includes cases of eccentric fixation associated with macular heterotopia and head tilts adopted in order to reorient the retinal meridians in the presence of cyclotropia.[6,21]

Maintain binocularity

There are many forms of incomitant strabismus with a gaze position featuring zero, or minimal, heterotropia and where fusion is maintained. Usually the posture is adopted to gain the benefit of bifoveal fusion, but it can also achieve anomalous retinal correspondence.[8] The causes can be subdivided into horizontal incomitance (such as sixth nerve paresis, Duane syndrome with esotropia, and oblique muscle paresis) and vertical incomitance (such as monocular elevation deficits and "A" and "V" pattern strabismus).

The causes in each plane can also be grouped under innervational and mechanical causes.[22] Innervational problems include both underaction of muscles (e.g., muscle paresis and myasthenia) and excessive innervation of muscles (e.g., overactions of oblique muscles). Mechanical problems can affect any of the structures within the orbit such as bony abnormalities (e.g., orbit fractures), muscle disorders (e.g., thyroid orbitopathy, Brown syndrome, and congenital fibrosis syndrome), and soft tissue diseases (e.g., pseudotumors and other orbit lesions).

Center the field of binocular vision

Children with congenital severe homonymous hemianopia may turn their faces toward the hemianopic field when they fixate: this strategy may centralize the intact visual field with the body.[2,8,23] Altitudinal field defects may also induce head postures, typically chin up or down.[2] Finally, monocular patients may turn slightly to the blind side to maximize their panorama of vision.[8]

Miscellaneous causes

Children who develop horizontal gaze palsies to one side may adopt a face turn toward the side of the gaze deficit. This strategy may allow the eyes to move in a range that is centered with respect to the body.[2]

Occasionally a patient with diplopia due to an incomitant strabismus will adopt a head posture to maximize the separation of images. This is occasionally seen in acquired unilateral superior oblique paresis whereby the child tilts to the shoulder ipsilateral to the involved eye so that the vertical tropia is maximized.[6,8,17,24]

A head posture may not directly improve vision or binocular functioning. A classic example is the ocular tilt reaction, a reflex of otolithic origin.[2,8] Children may also consciously adopt an abnormal posture for cosmetic reason to hide a physical deformity in the eyes, such as a postsurgical conjunctival scar.[6]

Face turn: Differential diagnosis (Table 89.2)

Nystagmus
Congenital nystagmus
Congenital nystagmus causes face turns for two reasons:
1. Forms with conjugate null zones: The eyes are normally aligned but the nystagmus null zone lies to the same side for both eyes. This is the typical pattern of congenital nystagmus (CN). The child adopts a face turn to the opposite side to fixate in the null zone and optimize binocular visual acuity. For example, if the null zone is located to the right of fixation,

Table 89.2 Ocular causes of a right face turn

I. Nystagmus
  A. Congenital
    1. Conjugate form
    2. Disconjugate form
  B. Acquired
    1. Periodic alternating nystagmus
    2. Spasmus nutans
II. Incomitant strabismus
  A. Horizontal muscle abnormalities
    1. Right eye/left eye
      a) Innervational causes
      b) Mechanical causes
    2. Both eyes: gaze palsy
  B. Vertical muscle abnormalities
    1. Left superior oblique dysfunction
    2. Left inferior oblique dysfunction
  C. Paradoxical face turn
III. Uncorrected refractive errors
IV. Eccentric fixation
V. Right homonymous hemianopia
VI. Miscellaneous etiologies
  A. Oculomotor apraxia
  B. Monocular blindness
  C. Very high myopia with esotropia

the child will adopt a left face turn. Although CN can create any orientation of compensatory posture, at least 80% of patients with a posture have a face turn as the chief component.[17,25] Rarely, there is more than one null zone, sometimes with different locations for distance and near fixation.

2. Forms with disconjugate null zones: this is usually seen with infantile esotropia. The patient presents with a large-angle esotropia with an adduction fixation preference with either eye; they develop nystagmus on attempting to abduct either eye. This is a bilateral manifest latent nystagmus (MLN) or Ciancia syndrome.[18,26] They have a null zone in the adducted position in either eye and adopt a left face turn to fixate with the left eye, and a right face turn to fixate with the right eye.

A similar mechanism accounts for the face turn seen in patients with early-onset disorders of one eye that significantly reduces vision. They are forced to fixate with the better eye. The child may develop a MLN that has an eccentric null zone. The null zone is usually in the adducted position, leading to adoption of an ipsilateral face turn to allow the eye to fixate straight ahead, as steadily as possible.[2,6]

Patients with nystagmus blockage syndrome may converge the eyes as a strategy to dampen the intensity of congenital nystagmus and improve their vision. However, the improved vision is gained at the expense of the alignment of the eyes such that a large esotropia develops. This forces the child to adopt a face turn to fixate with one or the other eye.[5,8]

Acquired nystagmus
Two forms of (usually) acquired nystagmus that can cause face turns are periodic alternating nystagmus (PAN) and spasmus nutans. PAN is a rhythmic shifting of a conjugate null zone from right to left with periods of between 90 s and 10 min. It causes a periodic oscillation of the face turn from right to left and back again. Many cases are benign, but there are reports of posterior fossa pathology.[5]

Spasmus nutans is a triad of a fine rapid frequency nystagmus with head nodding and torticollis. Although the most common head posture is a head tilt, there are cases in which the predominant posture is a face turn.[2,18] It usually resolves by age 2 to 3 years. It is usually benign, but there are cases of chiasmal tumors with a similar picture.[2,5]

Incomitant strabismus

Strabismus incomitant in the horizontal plane can force a child to adopt a face turn to maintain fusion. This allows the child to avoid diplopia and the need to suppress one image. There are two categories of horizontal plane incomitance, one involving the horizontal rectus muscles and the other involving the oblique muscles. For purposes of this discussion the child has a right face turn; the differential diagnosis for a left face turn is the mirror image.

Horizontal rectus muscle abnormalities (Fig. 89.2)

The child may adopt a right face turn to maintain fusion. This implies that there is a horizontal heterotropia whose magnitude is least in the left gaze position. Also implied is the fact that the angle of deviation increases progressively as the eyes move from left gaze into the primary position of gaze and then into the contralateral gaze field. In other cases, fusion may not be a factor, but the preferred eye for fixation may not be able to fixate in the primary position. Therefore, the differential diagnosis of a right face turn includes problems of abduction of the right eye or adduction of the left eye. For each eye, in turn, one must consider both innervational and mechanical disorders.[22]

For the right eye

Innervational causes include such entities as a sixth nerve (lateral rectus) paresis or palsy, Duane syndrome with limited abduction

and esotropia, or a slipped lateral rectus muscle after strabismus surgery.

Mechanical causes include restrictions on the medial side of the orbit, including medial orbital wall fractures, fibrosis syndromes, and thyroid orbitopathy. There can also be a restriction to abduction due to a tumor in the extraconal space on the lateral side of the orbit. Finally, patients with strabismus fixus of each eye are forced to adopt a face turn to maintain the fixating eye in the adducted position.

For the left eye

Innervational causes include a partial third nerve (medial rectus) paresis or palsy, Duane syndrome with exotropia and limited adduction, or a slipped medial rectus muscle after surgery. An internuclear ophthalmoplegia causing limited adduction of the left eye may also force the patient to adopt a right face turn.

Mechanical causes include restrictions from the lateral orbit, including scarring from trauma, fibrosis syndromes, or prior surgery, or tumors on the medial aspect of the orbit, which limit adduction.

For both eyes

A complete gaze palsy to the right side may force the patient to adopt a right face turn to allow easier fixation in the remaining intact field.[2]

Vertical alignment abnormalities (Fig. 89.3)

Strabismus disorders that cause incomitant vertical heterotropias can create face turns. These include oblique muscle anomalies and disorders that create up- or downdrifts in the adducted position of

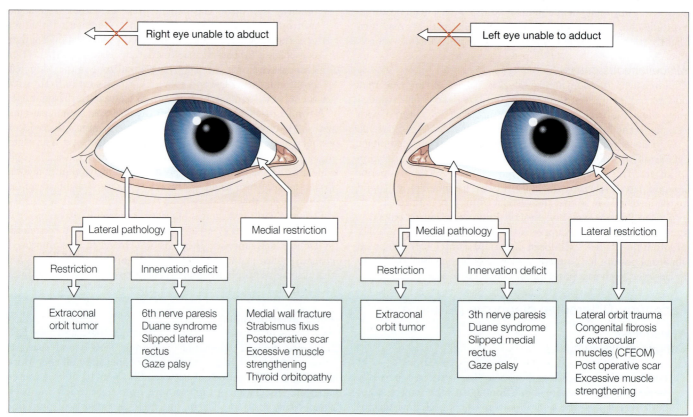

Fig. 89.2 Horizontal strabismus causes of compensatory right face turn. A useful approach is to address the reasons for a deficit of abduction of the right eye or of adduction of the left eye. The causes are classified into innervational and restrictive etiologies, and these are assigned to the lateral or medial sides of the two eyes, as illustrated.

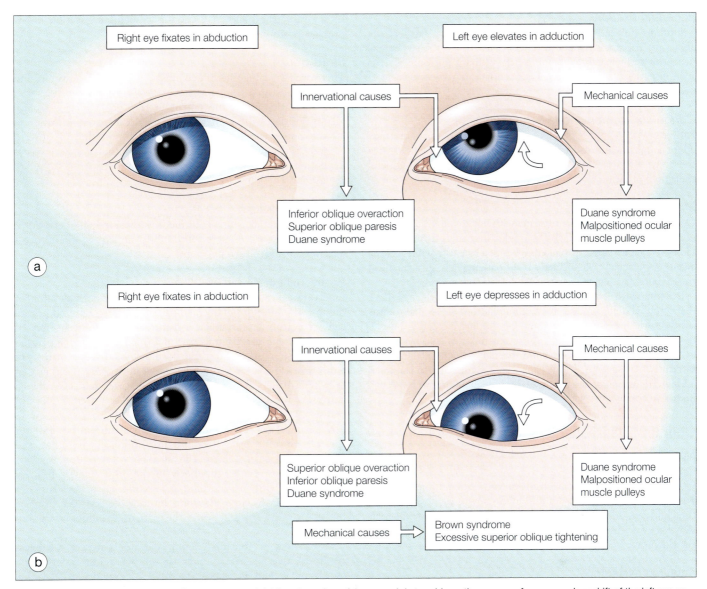

Fig. 89.3 Vertical alignment causes of compensatory right face turn. A useful approach is to address the causes of an up- or downdrift of the left eye on attempted adduction. (a) An updrift of the left eye causes an incomitant left hypertropia that is worse on right gaze. (b) A downdrift of the left eye causes an incomitant left hypotropia that is worse on right gaze. In both situations, the causes are divided into innervational and mechanical etiologies.

one eye. The vertical actions of the inferior and superior oblique muscles are strongest when the eye is in the adducted position and are least effective in the abducted position.

Thus, if an oblique muscle in one eye is overacting or underacting, there is a vertical heterotropia, most marked in the lateral gaze position where the oblique muscle has its strongest vertical action, and least in the opposite gaze field.

Although head tilts are usually the main component of the head posture in oblique muscle disorders, torticollis with mainly a face turn component occurs in a minority.[17] When considering a right face turn, the oblique muscles with abnormal actions would be those of the left eye, including paresis or overaction of either muscle. The child adopts the right face turn to avoid gazing into the right field where the vertical deviation would be most noticeable.

Alternatively, an up- or downdrift of the left eye can result from various mechanical and innervational disorders such as left Brown syndrome, Duane syndrome, or abnormal positioning of the extraocular muscle pulleys in the orbit.

Paradoxical face turn

In rare cases, a patient with diplopia due to an acquired incomitant strabismus will adopt a head posture that brings the eyes into their maximum deviation. For example, a patient with a sixth nerve paresis of the left eye may not have fusion even when a left face turn is adopted. If the diplopia is bothersome in that position due to the proximity of the two images, the patient may chose to adopt a right face turn to spread the diplopic images as much as possible to allow the false image to be ignored.[2,8,17]

Uncorrected refractive errors

The most common uncorrected refractive errors that cause face turns are myopia and against-the-rule astigmatism.[2,5] Correction of the refractive error usually eliminates the face turn. However, if a glasses prescription is too weak, the child may adopt a face turn in order to fixate through the peripheral parts of the lenses: doing so generates added power by taking advantage of astigmatism of oblique incidence.

Eccentric fixation

Children who are forced to fixate with an eye that has lost the ability to foveate may adopt a face turn to position the new eccentric retinal fixation point in the primary position. This is seen in patients with macular heterotopia due to retinopathy of prematurity and in macular dystrophies.[2,6]

Congenital homonymous hemianopia

Patients with a right complete homonymous hemianopia may adopt a right face turn to better center the remaining field with the body. They may also develop an exotropia to further expand their field of vision.[23]

Miscellaneous causes

Oculomotor apraxia usually presents with horizontal head thrusting in order to overcome the lack of saccadic drive to fixate on a target. However, in rare cases the child may adopt a face turn while fixating a stationary target.[6] Monocularly blind patients may turn the head to maximize the panorama of vision in the remaining eye.[8]

Patients with enlarged eyes (e.g., high myopia) may have restricted abduction due to a combination of medial rectus contracture, inferior displacement of the lateral rectus muscle, nasal displacement of the vertical rectus muscles, and herniation of the posterior wall of the globe through defects in the lateral intermuscular septum.[27] This causes a face turn due to the fixed adducted position of the eye. Usually seen in adults, its onset can be in the teenage years.[27]

Chin up: Differential diagnosis (Table 89.3)

Nystagmus

Congenital nystagmus

Congenital nystagmus can lead to any orientation of head posture. If the null zone is located in the downgaze position, then the child may adopt a chin-up posture to maximize the binocular visual acuity.[18] In this case, both eyes have conjugate null zones in the downgaze field.

Acquired nystagmus

Acquired disorders that cause nystagmus exaggerated in the upgaze field may lead to a chin-up posture to maintain optimal visual acuity. One example is the dorsal midbrain syndrome in which there is a limitation of upward movements along with a retraction nystagmus elicited by attempted upgaze movements.

Table 89.3 Ocular causes of a chin-up posture

I. Nystagmus
   A. Congenital
   B. Acquired
II. Strabismus
   A. Elevation deficits
      1. Right eye/left eye
         a) Innervational causes
         b) Mechanical causes
      2. Both eyes
   B. Pattern strabismus
      1. "A" pattern esotropia
      2. "V" pattern exotropia
III. Ptosis
IV. Uncorrected refractive errors
V. Supranuclear gaze disorders
VI. Superior visual field defects

As a result, the child may choose to maintain fixation below primary position.

Strabismus

There are two categories of eye muscle problems that can lead to a chin-up posture.

1. A limitation of eye movements in the vertical plane. A chin-up position will manifest if the child can maintain fusion in the downgaze field. There can be a limitation of upward movement of one or both eyes, and if the process involves both eyes it may be symmetric or asymmetric.
2. "A" and "V" patterns.

Elevation deficits (Fig. 89.4)

The differential diagnosis is formed by considering innervational and mechanical causes for each eye, similar to the process described for face turn positions.

For the right or the left eye

Innervational causes include weakness of one or both elevators of the eye, the inferior oblique and superior rectus. Limited upgaze can occur from an infranuclear disturbance (such as an isolated inferior oblique paresis or as part of a third cranial nerve paresis) or from a supranuclear disorder (see below). Isolated paresis of either muscle can lead to a hypotropia in primary position that may be smaller or absent in the downgaze field. Combined paresis of both muscles is often termed a "double elevator paresis."

Mechanical causes include restrictions arising in the inferior part of the orbit: orbit floor fractures, fibrosis syndromes, and thyroid orbitopathy. There can also be a restriction to elevation due to processes superiorly in the orbit such as primary or secondary Brown syndrome and extraconal masses superior to the globe. A large glaucoma-filtering device can displace the eye downward and force the patient to adopt a chin-up posture.

Most cases of so-called double elevator palsy or weakness are restrictive in nature, due to inferior rectus contracture or fibrosis,[28] and it is best to label it "monocular elevation deficit" until the cause is determined to be innervational or mechanical.

For both eyes

The processes listed for either eye can occur bilaterally. Some entities are particularly prone to affect the two eyes, especially the fibrosis syndromes, thyroid orbitopathy, acquired Brown syndrome, and supranuclear gaze disorders. The involvement can be asymmetric, but a head posture may arise if the vertical and horizontal deviations in downgaze are still small enough to allow fusion.

"A" and "V" patterns

The two entities that are causes of chin-up postures are an "A" pattern esotropia and a "V" pattern exotropia. In both situations the horizontal heterotropia is minimal in the downgaze field, while it increases progressively as the eyes move up to primary position and then into the upgaze field.[5,8]

Ptosis

Ptosis, congenital or acquired, of one or both eyelids can lead to a chin-up posture if the lid margins are at or below the level of the pupil.[5,6,8] This can be a component of hereditary conditions such as the blepharophimosis syndrome.[5]

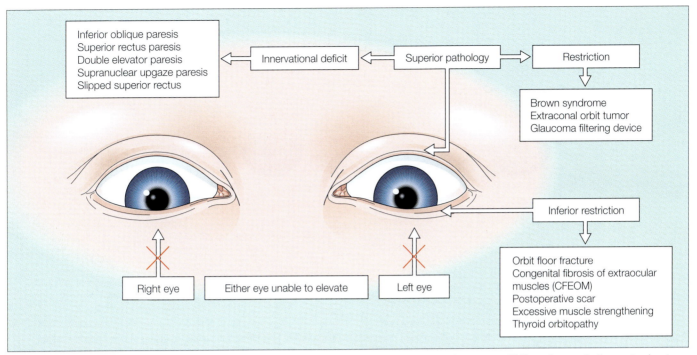

Fig. 89.4 Strabismus causes of a compensatory chin-up head posture. One approach is to address the causes of failure of one or both eyes to elevate. The causes are classified into innervational and restrictive etiologies, and these are assigned to the superior or inferior aspects of the two eyes, as illustrated.

Uncorrected refractive errors

Children with uncorrected or undercorrected refractive errors may adopt a chin-up posture to take advantage of the stenopeic slit effect of the narrowed palpebral apertures. This is most commonly used in the myopia or astigmatism.

Supranuclear gaze disorders

Damage to the vertical gaze centers in the brain stem can lead to paresis of upgaze. The most common causes in children are hydrocephalus and the dorsal midbrain syndrome (Parinaud syndrome).[2] The dorsal midbrain syndrome includes convergence-and-retraction nystagmus, eyelid retraction, and light–near dissociation of the pupils. Most cases of supranuclear gaze deficits are bilateral, but a unilateral monocular elevation deficit can also have a supranuclear etiology.[29]

Visual field defects

Patients who have lost a significant portion of their superior visual fields may adopt a chin-up posture to centralize the range of residual field relative to the body.[2] The most common causes are retina and optic nerve diseases that lead to altitudinal field deficits.

Chin down: Differential diagnosis (Table 89.4)

Nystagmus
Congenital nystagmus

Congenital nystagmus can lead to any head posture. If the null zone is located in the upgaze position then the child may adopt a chin-down posture to maximize the binocular visual acuity. In this case, both eyes have conjugate null zones in the upgaze field.[18]

Acquired nystagmus

Acquired disorders (e.g., lower brainstem trauma or disease) that cause nystagmus whose intensity is greatest in the downgaze field

Table 89.4 Ocular causes of a chin-down posture

I. Nystagmus
   A. Congenital
   B. Acquired
II. Strabismus
   A. Depression deficits
      1. Right eye/left eye
         a) Innervational causes
         b) Mechanical causes
      2. Both eyes
   B. Pattern strabismus
      1. "A" pattern exotropia
      2. "V" pattern esotropia
III. Uncorrected refractive errors
IV. Supranuclear gaze disorders
V. Inferior visual field defects

may induce a chin-down posture for the child to maintain optimal visual acuity.

Strabismus

Eye muscle causes of a chin-down posture include:
1. A limitation of eye movements in the vertical plane: A chin-down position occurs if the child can fuse in the upgaze field. There can be a limitation of downward movement of one or both eyes, and if the process involves both eyes it may be symmetric or asymmetric.
2. "A" and "V" patterns.

Depression deficits (Fig. 89.5)

The differential diagnosis is also formed by considering innervational and mechanical causes for each eye.

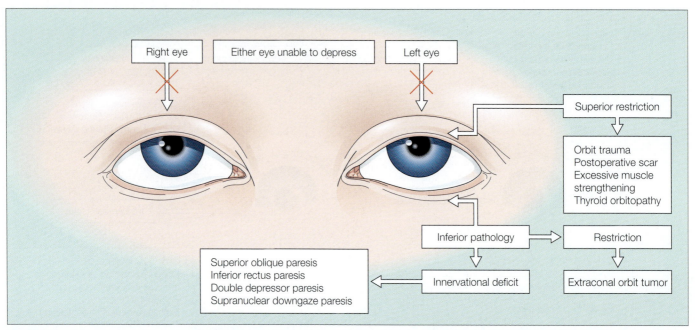

Fig. 89.5 Strabismus causes of a compensatory chin-down head posture. One approach is to address the causes of failure of one or both eyes to depress. The causes are classified into innervational and restrictive etiologies, and these are assigned to the superior or inferior aspects of the two eyes, as illustrated.

For the right or the left eye

Innervational causes include weakness of one or both depressors of the eye, the superior oblique and inferior rectus. This can result from an infranuclear disturbance (third nerve paresis or, rarely, an isolated fourth nerve paresis) or from a supranuclear disorder (see below). Isolated paresis of either muscle can lead to a hypertropia in primary position that may be smaller or absent in upgaze. Combined paresis of both muscles is often termed a "double depressor paresis," usually seen after orbital trauma.

Mechanical causes include restrictions arising in the superior part of the orbit, such as orbit roof fractures, postoperative or posttraumatic scarring, and, in rare cases, thyroid orbitopathy. There can also be a restriction of depression due to mass lesions in the inferior orbit.

For both eyes

Although the processes for either eye can occur bilaterally, some are particularly prone to affect the two eyes, especially bilateral superior oblique paresis after closed head trauma. It can be asymmetric, but a head posture may arise if the vertical and horizontal heterotropias in upgaze are both small enough to allow fusion.

"A" and "V" patterns

The two causes of chin-down postures are an "A" pattern exotropia and a "V" pattern esotropia. In both, the horizontal heterotropia is minimal in the upgaze field, whereas it increases progressively as the eyes move down to primary position and into the downgaze field.[5,8]

Bilateral superior oblique paresis that is fairly symmetric is a common cause of a chin-down posture that compensates for the "V" pattern esotropia and excyclodiplopia.[11,17,24]

Uncorrected refractive errors

Children who have uncorrected or undercorrected refractive errors may adopt a chin-down posture. Children with moderate hyperopia may be more apt to adopt a chin-down posture rather than a chin-up orientation.

Supranuclear gaze disorders

Damage to the vertical gaze centers can lead to paresis of downgaze, especially if it involves the rostral interstitial nucleus of the medial longitudinal fasciculus (riMLF).

Bilateral downgaze paresis may also be a feature of neuropathic Gaucher disease and the DAF variant of Niemann-Pick disease type C.[2]

Visual field defects

Patients who have lost a significant portion of their inferior visual fields, as a result of retina or optic nerve diseases, may adopt a chin-down posture to centralize the range of residual field relative to the body.[2]

Head tilt: Differential diagnosis (Table 89.5)

Nystagmus
Congenital nystagmus

Congenital nystagmus can cause any orientation of head posture. A head tilt can occur as the primary orientation, but there is often an associated face turn.[17,18] The nystagmus intensity

---

Table 89.5 Ocular causes of a right head tilt

I. Nystagmus
   A. Congenital
   B. Acquired
II. Strabismus
   A. Vertical muscle problems
      1. Right eye/left eye
         a) Innervational causes
         b) Mechanical causes
   B. Cyclotropia
   C. Horizontal muscle problems
   D. Paradoxical head tilt
   E. Ocular tilt reaction
III. Refractive errors

decreases when the head is tilted toward one shoulder, whereas it increases as the head is positioned into primary gaze position and then further increases on tilting to the opposite shoulder.

Acquired nystagmus

The most common orientation of the torticollis in spasmus nutans is a head tilt, although a face turn component can accompany the tilt (see above).

Strabismus (Fig. 89.6)

There are several entities that can lead to a head tilt. These include vertical muscle problems, cyclotropia, and horizontal deviations. For the purposes of discussion, the child is assumed to have a right head tilt. The differential diagnosis for a left tilt is the mirror image of that presented.

Vertical muscle problems

The vertical muscle abnormalities that can lead to a head tilt can be divided into innervational and mechanical entities as appropriate for each eye. In each case, the vertical deviation differs on tilting to one shoulder compared to that on tilting to the other shoulder. In most cases the vertical heterotropia is minimal or absent when the compensatory posture is adopted, allowing fusion.

For the right eye

Innervational causes include inferior oblique paresis, inferior rectus paresis, and dissociated vertical deviation (DVD). Inferior oblique paresis creates an incomitant hypotropia, minimized on tilting to the ipsilateral side.[6,30–32] Most cases in children are congenital and benign. Acquired cases are usually caused by facial trauma. The head tilt may be accompanied by a face turn or chin-up position.[31] Inferior rectus paresis can also lead to a head tilt to the ipsilateral shoulder.[32]

Dissociated vertical deviation (DVD) is a frequent finding in the infantile strabismus complex. The spontaneous upward and excyclotropic drift of one eye can be quite large and cosmetically displeasing. It may be associated with a head tilt posture to the side of the eye with the hyperdeviation or to the contralateral side.[9,33,34]

Mechanical causes include a contracture of the inferior rectus muscle. It causes a hypotropia that may be smaller and better controlled on tilt to the ipsilateral shoulder. This can arise, for example, after chronic fixation by the fellow eye affected by a depressor weakness such as a superior oblique paresis.[2] A blowout fracture of one orbit or thyroid orbitopathy can create a head tilt posture by the same mechanism, but an associated cyclodiplopia may also be causative.[6,33] Finally, a unilateral Brown syndrome may cause an ipsilateral head tilt.[6,32]

For the left eye

The most common innervational disorder that leads to a head tilt is a superior oblique paresis.[6,32,33] In a superior oblique paresis a head tilt is usually the dominant posture even if a patient has other components including a face turn or chin-down posture.[5,17,21,24,32] The patient typically has a hypertropia of the paretic eye that increases on gaze to the contralateral side and on ipsilateral head tilt (the Bielschowsky head tilt test). The child compensates by tilting the head to the opposite shoulder to minimize the hyperdeviation and maintain fusion.[24,30,32] In this

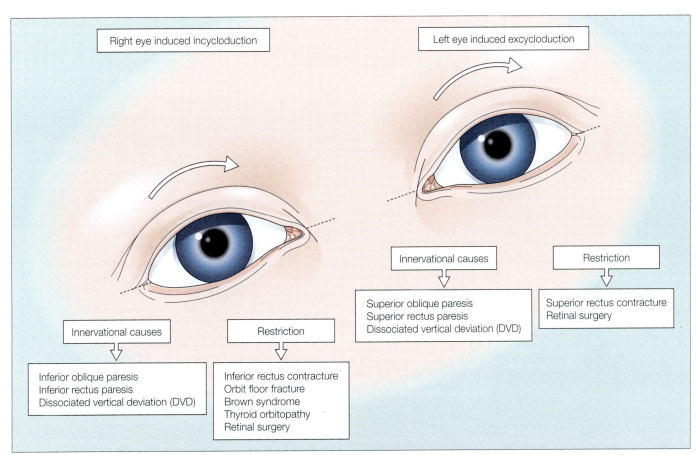

Fig. 89.6 Strabismus causes of a compensatory right head tilt posture. One approach is to address the causes of vertical muscle anomalies or of induced or compensatory cycloduction of one or both eyes. The etiologies are classified into innervational and restrictive etiologies, as illustrated.

case a right head tilt posture would compensate for a left superior oblique paresis.

DVD may show a head tilt to the side contralateral to the eye manifesting the hypertropia.[2,8,33,34] A compensatory head tilt can also arise with the rare isolated paresis of a superior rectus muscle.[6,33] If the left superior rectus were weak, the resulting left hypotropia would be expected to worsen on tilting to the ipsilateral shoulder, and lessen on tilting to the right shoulder. This finding is the outcome of the final step of the three-step test to differentiate a left superior rectus paresis from a right superior oblique paresis.[30] However, there are also cases of superior rectus paresis that lead to compensatory tilts to the ipsilateral side.[32]

A mechanical disorder causing a head tilt is a contracture or fibrosis of a superior rectus muscle. This can be idiopathic or secondary to thyroid orbitopathy or a chronic superior oblique paresis. Contracture of the left superior rectus muscle creates a large hyperdeviation on tilt to the left shoulder, which lessens on tilt to the right shoulder.[35]

Cyclotropia

Cyclotropia of one eye causes a head tilt that may be a sensory compensation for disinclination of the retinal meridians of the fixating eye[5,6,17,21,36]: if a patient fixates with an excyclotropic left eye, it may promote a tilt of the head to the right shoulder.[17,36] It can also occur after retina surgery, either a scleral buckle or macular translocation surgery.[6,24]

Horizontal muscle problems

There are rare cases of horizontal tropias, usually esotropias, that are larger on tilt to one side than the other. Some cases may be due to congenital nystagmus that is worse on head tilt to one side and where convergence is used as a dampening strategy. The patient tends to tilt to the opposite shoulder where the nystagmus intensity is less and little or no convergence dampening is required. However, there are other cases where nystagmus dampening does not seem to be a factor and the esotropia differs on right versus left tilt.[6]

Paradoxical head tilt

Occasionally a patient will adopt a paradoxical head tilt to maximize the separation of images to facilitate suppression or ignoring of one image.[6,8,17,24] This occurs in 2 to 3% of cases of superior oblique paresis presenting with compensatory head posture.[17]

Ocular tilt reaction

This entity is a triad of vertical divergence of the eyes, bilateral ocular torsion, and tilting of the head. It results from a lesion of the central nervous system affecting either the vestibular nucleus or its connections to the contralateral interstitial nucleus of Cajal.[2,8,37] The ocular torsion characteristically is ipsiversive (if the head is tilted to the right shoulder, the right eye is excyclotorted while the left eye is incyclotorted). Also, the ipsilateral eye, in this case the right eye, is hypotropic.[38]

Refractive errors

A high astigmatic refractive error in the fixating eye can induce a head tilt, especially if the cylindrical ametropia is oblique.[5,6,8] The correction of the astigmatic error alleviates the posture.

Bilaterally dislocated lenses may cause a head tilt to place the eyes in a position that optimizes the refractive correction.[39]

DIAGNOSTIC CONSIDERATIONS

The approach to a child with torticollis can be summarized in Fig. 89.7. The main focus is to differentiate ocular from nonocular causes. In the examination of a child with torticollis, the ocular causes must be ruled out before a nonocular basis can be considered.

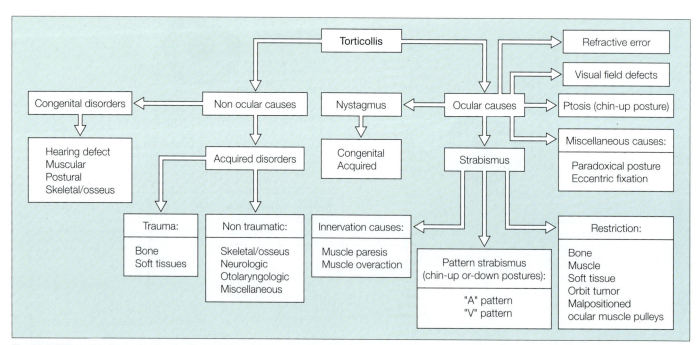

Fig. 89.7 Differential diagnosis of torticollis in children. The causes are divided into nonocular and ocular causes (*ocular torticollis*). The nonocular disorders include congenital and acquired conditions. Nystagmus, strabismus, and refractive errors must be ruled out as possible etiologies for any head posture orientation, whereas other etiologies apply to selected orientations.

There are several clinical tests that are particularly helpful in the assessment (see Chapters 76, 79. and 86). In addition, the treatments for the ocular disorders discussed above are presented in the chapters throughout the book that deal with these entities.

Observation

Physical features

The presence of facial asymmetry or dysmorphism, neck deformities, or anomalies of the trunk or the extremities may suggest either a musculoskeletal cause of the head posture or a chronic ocular muscle palsy. Alternatively, nystagmus or a manifest strabismus can help the examiner focus in on specific ocular conditions.

Prolonged observing of the patient

It is helpful to watch the child for an extended period of time to determine whether the torticollis is consistent. It is important to determine whether it manifests only under certain conditions, such as with fixation on fine visual targets, or with various other vision-related tasks such as reading.

It is mandatory to observe a patient with nystagmus for several minutes. A periodic alternation of a head posture suggests periodic alternating nystagmus, whereas a thrusting of the head with changes in fixation is characteristic of oculomotor apraxia. Finally, the orientation of the posture in all three planes must be noted, especially if it changes slightly or markedly with different tasks.

Review of old photographs or videotapes

Documentation from the early months and years of life can confirm the chronic nature of a head posture especially when the time of onset of the problem is unclear. Serial photographs in a family album, humorously termed a "FAT scan" ("familial axial tomography"), or videos from early years, should be sought whenever possible.

Occlusion of one eye

If a child has ocular torticollis to maintain binocularity, then occluding one eye abolishes or reduces the magnitude of the posture. However, this test can be falsely negative if a chronic problem has led to a "habit" posture in addition to the original compensatory head position.

Eye movements

Conjugate eye movements (versions) are elicited early in the examination. By asking the child to move the eyes into the nine diagnostic positions of gaze the examiner can detect an incomitant strabismus or a nystagmus null zone. An alternative maneuver is to move the head from its abnormal orientation into a position opposite to that adopted as this may expose the presence of a zone of increased nystagmus intensity or a significantly larger heterotropia.

Measuring the head posture

In addition to documenting the orientation of the posture, it is important, where possible, to quantitate the different com-ponents. This can be done using an orthopedic goniometer to measure each component separately. Alternatively, sensitive torticollometers, when placed on the patient's head, accurately measure all three components of the head posture simultaneously.[40] This can allow the examiner to follow a patient serially to observe any change of the posture and to determine the most severe component of a multidirectional orientation.

Visual fields

In cases where strabismus or nystagmus do not seem to be causative factors it is helpful to perform gross or, if possible, formal visual field testing to identify a hemifield or altitudinal field defect.

Refraction

One of the most common causes for vision-driven head postures is an uncorrected or partially corrected refractive error, or an incorrect prescription of glasses or contact lenses. A careful refraction is an essential. If a significant refractive error is found, a trial of spectacles may eliminate the head posture.

Fundus examination

The detection of any anomalies such as retinal traction or fundus pathology can account for some forms of head postures, and the evaluation of the fundus for cyclotropia can help confirm some cases of oblique muscle paresis or overaction. Indirect or direct ophthalmoscopy may also detect low-amplitude nystagmus that may not be seen on direct examination.

Eye movement recordings

In cases where the ocular diagnosis is not clearly evident after a thorough examination, sensitive eye movement recordings may confirm the presence of a nystagmus that is not clinically apparent. The pattern of the nystagmus waveform may also help determine the etiology of the nystagmus and guide further investigation and treatment.

Palpation of the neck muscles

In musculoskeletal torticollis, the neck muscles are tight. Passive straightening of the head is difficult. In congenital muscular torticollis the pseudotumor in the neck can be located. In contrast, it is rare for cases of ocular torticollis to develop the extreme neck muscle contracture seen with congenital or early-onset musculoskeletal anomalies.

Consultations with other specialists

It is important to restate that the evaluation of a child with torticollis may require the involvement of experts in other disciplines, including orthopedic surgeons, otolaryngologists, and neurologists or neurosurgeons. Physiotherapists and occupational therapists may also be part of the treatment team. If serious central nervous system or orbit diseases are suspected in the causation of a child's torticollis, then imaging may be indicated.

REFERENCES

1. Boutros GS, Al-Mateen M. Non-ophthalmological causes of torticollis. Am Orthoptic J 1995; 45: 68–74.
2. Brodsky MC, Baker RS, Hamed LM. Pediatric Neuro-ophthalmology. New York: Springer-Verlag; 1996: 260–2, 350–68.
3. Kiwak KJ. Establishing an etiology for torticollis. Postgrad Med 1984; 75: 126–34.
4. Ruedemann AD Jr. Scoliosis and vertical ocular muscle imbalance. Arch Ophthalmol 1956; 56: 389–414.
5. Rubin SE, Wagner RS. Ocular torticollis. Surv Ophthalmol 1986; 30: 366–76.
6. Kushner BJ. Ocular causes of abnormal head postures. Ophthalmology 1979; 86: 2115–25.
7. Nutt AB. Abnormal head posture. Br Orthoptic J 1963; 20: 18–28.
8. Caldeira JA. Abnormal head posture: an ophthalmological approach. Binocul Vis Strabismus Q 2000; 15: 237–9.
9. Goodman CR, Chabner E, Guyton DL. Should early strabismus surgery be performed for ocular torticollis to prevent facial asymmetry? J Pediatr Ophthalmol Strabismus 1995; 32: 162–6.
10. Greenberg MF, Pollard ZF. Ocular plagiocephaly: ocular torticollis with skull and facial asymmetry. Ophthalmology 2000; 107: 173–9.
11. Fells P, Dulley B. Surgical management of compensatory head posture. Trans Ophthalmol Soc UK 1976; 96: 90–5.
12. Coventry MB, Harris LE. Congenital muscular torticollis in infancy. J Bone Joint Surg 1959; 41: 815–22.
13. Tom LW, Rossiter JL, Sutton LN, et al. Torticollis in children. Otolaryngol Head Neck Surg 1991; 105: 1–5.
14. Webb M. Acute torticollis: identifying and treating the underlying cause. Postgrad Med 1987; 82: 121–8.
15. Marmor MA, Beauchamp GR, Maddox SF. Photophobia, epiphora, and torticollis: a masquerade syndrome. J Pediatr Ophthalmol Strabismus 1990; 27: 202–4.
16. Snyder CH. Paroxysmal torticollis in infancy. A possible form of labyrinthitis. Am J Dis Child 1969; 117: 458–60.
17. Kraft SP, O'Donoghue EP, Roarty JD. Improvement of compensatory head postures after strabismus surgery. Ophthalmology 1992; 99: 1301–8.
18. Hertle RW, Zhu X. Oculographic and clinical characterization of thirty-seven children with anomalous head postures, nystagmus, and strabismus: the basis of a clinical algorithm. J AAPOS 2000; 4: 25–32.
19. Dell'Osso LF, Flynn JF. Congenital nystagmus surgery: a quantitative evaluation of the effects. Arch Ophthalmol 1979; 97: 462–9.
20. Scott WE, Kraft SP. Surgical treatment of compensatory head position in congenital nystagmus. J Pediatr Ophthalmol Strabismus 1984; 21: 85–95.
21. von Noorden GK, Ruttum M. Torticollis in paralysis of the trochlear nerve. Am Orthoptic J 1983; 33: 16–20.
22. Kraft SP. Clues to differential diagnosis in strabismus. Am Orthoptic J 1989; 39: 25–35.
23. Hoyt CS, Good WV. Ocular motor adaptations to congenital hemianopia. Binocul Vis Eye Muscle Surg Q 1993; 8: 125–6.
24. von Noorden GK, Murray E, Wong SY. Superior oblique paralysis. A review of 270 cases. Arch Ophthalmol 1986; 104: 1771–6.
25. Parks MM. Congenital nystagmus surgery. Am Orthoptic J 1973; 23: 35–9.
26. Ciancia A. On infantile esotropia with nystagmus in abduction. J Pediatr Ophthalmol Strabismus 1995; 32: 280–8.
27. Krzizok TH, Kaufmann H, Traupe H. Elucidation of restrictive motility in high myopia by magnetic resonance imaging. Arch Ophthalmol 1997; 115: 1019–27.
28. Metz HS. Double elevator palsy. Arch Ophthalmol 1979; 97: 901–3.
29. Ziffer AJ, Rosenbaum AL, Demer JL, et al. Congenital double elevator palsy: vertical saccadic velocity utilizing the scleral search coil technique. J Pediatr Ophthalmol Strabismus 1992; 29: 142–9.
30. Parks MM. Isolated cyclovertical muscle palsy. Arch Ophthalmol 1958; 60: 1027–35.
31. Pollard ZF. Diagnosis and treatment of inferior oblique palsy. J Pediatr Ophthalmol Strabismus 1993; 30: 15–8.
32. Urist MJ. Head tilt in vertical muscle paresis. Am J Ophthalmol 1970; 69: 440–2.
33. Bechtel RT, Kushner BJ, Morton GV. The relationship between dissociated vertical divergence (DVD) and head tilts. J Pediatr Ophthalmol Strabismus 1996; 33: 303–6.
34. Santiago AP, Rosenbaum AL. Dissociated vertical deviation and head tilts. J AAPOS 1998; 2: 5–11.
35. Jampolsky A. Management of vertical strabismus. In: Caldwell DR, et al., editors. Pediatric Ophthalmology and Strabismus: Transactions of the New Orleans Academy of Ophthalmology. New York: Raven Press; 1986: 141–71.
36. von Noorden GK. Clinical observations in cyclodeviations. Ophthalmology 1979; 86: 1451–61.
37. Hedges TR III, Hoyt WF. Ocular tilt reaction due to an upper brainstem lesion: paroxysmal skew deviation, torsion, and oscillation of the eyes with head tilt. Ann Neurol 1982; 11: 537–40.
38. Donahue SP, Lavin PJM, Hamed LM. Tonic ocular tilt reaction simulating a superior oblique palsy: diagnostic confusion with the three-step test. Arch Ophthalmol 1999; 117: 347–52.
39. Krefman RA, Goldberg MF. Ocular torticollis caused by refractive error. Arch Ophthalmol 1982; 100: 1278–9.
40. Kushner BJ. The usefulness of the cervical range of motion device in the ocular motility examination. Arch Ophthalmol 2000; 118: 946–50.

CHAPTER
90

What Do We Really Know about Strabismus and it's Management?

Arthur Jampolsky

Such an audacious title, which was assigned to me, brings forth several dilemmas. Shall it be approached with some degree of humility, or simply weighted by the degree of selectivity? The editors informed me that this chapter would appear at the end of all of the contributions on strabismus by colleagues and peers. Should it be sort of a "clean-up" chapter deigning from on high that which is selected to be true knowledge, or should it be a muted presentation, polite and restrained, in order not to lose too many friends?

I once believed that "the truth will set you free." However, after more than five decades of practice and research I have learned as a result of my written publications and public remarks that what one may consider to be the truth at any point in time may certainly free you. Free you from colleagues, free you from friends, and free you from other unexpected things.

I considered a more philosophical approach for this chapter: how can one know? What is truth? If one begins with certainties, one will surely end with more doubts. That unfamiliar style might end in a rich morass of conflicting, guarded statements with masked and obfuscated conclusions, not fulfilling the intent of the assignment.

Certainly it would be easier to respond to the assigned title if it were to be written immediately following the early ophthalmology training years. That is the time when one certainly "knows," and really "believes," what has been taught and practiced at the time. The jolt is to discover that in strabismus management there were, and are, many "cults," as the late Gene Folk would have described them. However, one cult may "really know about strabismus," yet may differ considerably from what another cult may "really know," and the followers of each appear to practice a method of thinking that consists of rearranging one's prejudices about new advances, which make traditional beliefs more acceptable to themselves and the cult members. After all, the "blood-letters" of an era long past "really knew or believed" that the noxious toxins of the body would be relieved by that procedure.

I shall, therefore, focus this presentation more on concepts and principles. Our discussion will separate the causes and management of strabismus for infants and for adults. I shall attempt to formulate issues into what we used to know and now really know not to be true. We shall discuss some important principles–well established, well documented–that we really know, and others, unfortunately, that we really know but do not sufficiently use nor apply to the everyday problems of strabismus. Of course it will be highly selective, with a minimum of arm waving as a substitute for evidence, but nevertheless the truth.

WHAT DO WE REALLY KNOW ABOUT THE CAUSES OF STRABISMUS?

The answer to this question is quite different for adult and childhood strabismus: adults usually have already developed a normal sensory and motor binocular system. The usual causes of the adult-acquired strabismus are due to definable diseases, disorders, or injuries. The problem is one of regaining perfection of bifoveal alignment of the eyes wherein a good fusion-lock may occur and good vergences reestablish themselves, even after a dormant period.

Of course, the systemic disease, disorder, or injury needs good management. The strabismus management problems are usually local muscles/orbit in nature and are discussed under the section of balance of muscle forces. We know how to balance the acquired mechanical muscle forces in order to reobtain alignment and fusion, although often with compromised rotations.

An exception to the above is the acquired unilateral sensory exotropia in adults of any age, secondary to an overall (both macula and periphery) blurred image (unilateral acquired cataract, or injury). This intriguing entity deserves further investigation because we do not know very much about its mechanism. I have discussed previously[1] the necessary and sufficient unilateral stimulus, i.e., an overall blur of *both* the macula and periphery of one eye's image relative to its normal fellow eye.

We know the stimulus conditions for this since the acquired exodeviation does not occur with just a unilateral, significant macula lesion, *or* a unilateral peripheral lesion (as in glaucoma) leaving only the macula intact. It must be both macula and peripheral retinal image blur. By descriptive definition, the increasing unilateral exotropia is a vergence, the progression of which may be avoided by instant, total, unilateral visual loss, as by optic nerve severance. So, one does know the exact binocular unequal input stimulus conditions that elicit this not uncommon type of acquired, unilateral exotropia.

Even after a long-standing exodeviation, with restoration of equal inputs (as by extraction of a dense unilateral cataract), good fusion may be restored, with fusion-vergences naturally following in its wake, once fusion either spontaneously or surgically is regained.

What we really need to know, but do not, is why the good fellow eye (in the example just cited), which is always the fixing eye before and after the unilateral blurred image was acquired, under general anesthesia (with muscle relaxants), now usually exhibits more than the usual amount of exodeviation of 5–10 pd. I have previously called attention to this unexpected observation and have mentioned that the arrest and investigation of this exception probably contains some valued secrets of binocular vision.[2]

A second group of adult deviations occurs as a result of decompensated, older, relatively stable strabismus that had an early onset and was previously well compensated by fusion. A good example of this is a well-controlled, intermittent exotropia during childhood, which gradually slips into constant exotropia, equal vision alternating exotropia, which may last for decades as a constant deviation. Even after binocular vision has been dormant for a long time, perfect realignment results in one of the highest rates of bifoveal motor fusion with good amplitudes of vergences, since good fusion was previously present over a long time. The history of such decompensated eso- or exodeviations are easily determined.

We usually know what we need to know about the causes of strabismus in most adult cases.

WHAT DO WE REALLY KNOW ABOUT THE CAUSES OF INFANTILE ESOTROPIA?

One often hears the comment that "*the* cause of infantile esotropia (ET) is unknown." This is unwarranted since there are several clearly identifiable *causes* of infantile ET, sometimes a single cause and sometimes multiple causes; yet each causation factor is identifiable. It is naive to consider that there is *a single cause* of infantile ET; there are many types differing in their individual characteristics, prognosis, and other aspects. Before discussing the different causes of infantile ET, it is well to have an overview and perspective from briefly looking at other diseases.

Let us recognize what is happening to the study of causes and management of glaucoma. Not unexpectedly, there are several different types of glaucoma. Each one may have an identifiable genetic identification. Glaucoma with earlier onset may be particularly severe and have an individual genetic identification. Further, the prognosis and management, even minor details, also have separate genetic identifications. The recent research in glaucoma is most fruitful when conducted in conjunction with the clinical course and responses to management.

With strabismus causes and management, it is to be expected that there may be separate genes identified with the several different causes of ET and the different responses to management, such as the response to hyperopic corrections and whether a given individual has a high or low accommodative–convergence relationship. We shall focus on the usual and ordinary patients with infantile ET, varied enough, and must omit the many congenital syndromes associated with different types of strabismus.

The characteristics of the usual infantile ET are well known. Some of the outstanding ones are onset at two or more months of age (not congenital), associated with some little or a lot of hyperopia, and often dissociated vertical deviations (DVD) and a variable angle of deviation.

Notably absent from this description is the negative bias that there may be some innate defect in the visual system, and/or that full restoration of bifoveal fixation (BFF) is simply unobtainable. One is reminded of a past era when it was held that anomalous retinal correspondence (ARC) was an innate defect that augured poorly for ever obtaining fusion. This has been completely silenced by time.

Similarly, the notion that it is not possible to obtain good BFF or good stereopsis in management is based on the frequent management procedure that, by its nature, never obtains the necessary and sufficient stimulus for obtaining these good results. A result of partial realignment, leaving a residual ET (no matter how small), cannot and will not restore BFF. We now know that one must have good and equal inputs (clear the retinal images of each eye) if one is to have good and equal sensory and motor outputs and BFF.

One should also recall that congenital cataracts were held by most to be accompanied by defective maculae, and therefore good vision could not be obtained. We now "really know" that good vision can indeed be obtained even in unilaterals if, and only if, a clear retinal image is available and used at a very early perinatal age. There must be an "adequate stimulus," as termed by Johannes Mueller (or in its current lexicon: a sufficient and necessary stimulus), present at the right time.

Chavasse,[3] in 1939, made the profound statement that most of the anomalies of binocular vision are arrests, distortions, or exaggerations of normal development. How prophetic! Thus a brief prelude of normal and neonatal development is appropriate at this point. Normal neonates exhibit a modest amount of exodeviation. In normal infants, a binocular fusion-lock first develops for the peripheral retinas. This peripheral sensory binocular fusion-lock becomes more stable as the maculae develop. This is reflected in Panum's areas of single binocular vision, which first develops in the peripheral retinas where they are larger horizontal ellipses, becoming smaller toward the central macular fusion area. This is all reflected in the empirical horizontal longitudinal horopter (Fig. 90.1).

As the macular fusion lock becomes "tighter" and more secure, the extraocular muscles adapt their length appropriate to the eye positions. This is a general muscle adaptation of length that occurs in many instances throughout life.

The motor system early exhibits saccades, which are relatively poorly yoked by the somewhat elastic fusion-lock of first peripheral retinal fusion and later by the more refined and stabilized macular fusion.

On the other hand, congenitally bilateral blind infants exhibit wild, unharnessed saccades, not stabilized by either a fixation or a retinal fusion-lock. It is important here to note the cogent observation by Cogan that congenitally completely blind eyes are relatively aligned. It is interesting to speculate that here there are no abnormal retinal inputs by which misalignment, especially ET, occurs. More particularly, there is not a large degree of esodeviation! Normally, the sensory input systems dominate and control the development of the motor output systems. At this early stage of neonatal development, one factor shapes and determines the destiny of another.

Hering's law itself is an adaptation, since patients with very different interocular distances or protruding or recessed globes end with equal yoked muscle forces in different gazes. This develops even though yoked muscles have quite different mechanical characteristics and cross-sectional areas. For there to be yoked resultant gaze alignments, there must be unequal innervation to unequal mechanical muscles, in order to obtain gaze-balanced alignment of forces in yoke muscles.

First cause

Neural abnormalities, from one or more of the many pre- or perinatal causes of brain damage, is a first cause of infantile ET. The ET may be considered a sign of neural deficits resulting from excessive *general tonus* to the muscles, which cause a differentially greater force in the medial rectus (MR) muscles than in the lateral rectus (LR) muscles, resulting in an eso-deviation. There is no evidence at all to support the old notion of the mysterious, nonretinal, supranuclear convergence balancing or imbalancing a mysterious, nonretinal, supranuclear divergence, with one winning over the other, causing an ET or an exotropia.

There are many pre- and perinatal insults to the nervous system which may result in an increase of innervational tonus to *all* the oculorotary muscles. This may produce an imbalance of agonist/antagonist muscles and result in strabismus. There are

What Do We Really Know about Strabismus and It's Management?

CHAPTER
90

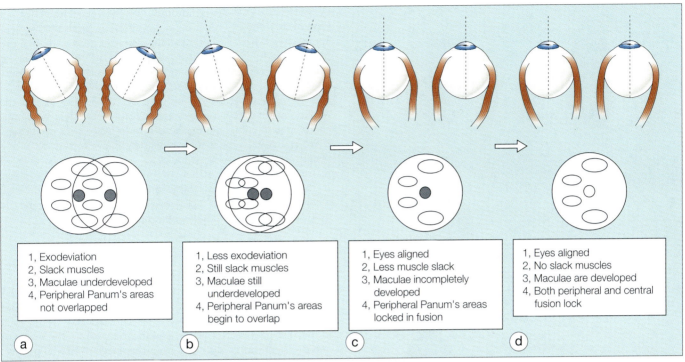

Fig. 90.1 (a) Neonatal exodeviations, slack muscles, maculae undeveloped. (b) Less exodeviation, muscle still slack, still undeveloped maculae, beginning *peripheral* retinal overlap. (c) Eyes aligned, incomplete macula development, peripheral fusion-lock, Panum's areas. (d) Eyes aligned, maculae developed, both peripheral and macula fusion-lock, muscle length adaptations.

imbalances in *each* eye separately and are not indicative of a binocular vergence mechanism.

Maldevelopment of motor subsystems have been indicted as causing ET. It is sometimes difficult to differentiate cause and effect in human and nonhuman primates. The evidence supports the fact that motor subsystem development is, or importantly may become, abnormal in the presence of an early infantile ET. Certainly prenatal central nervous system (CNS) insults may result in abnormal developments of many sorts, and these types of neural deficits are usually identifiable with present-day examination imagery techniques. However, one must take care in applying this neural cause and strabismus effect to those normal infants whose esodeviation begins at 2–4 months of age. In the latter, one must shift one's attention to visual environmental factors (sensory inputs), and it is prudent to take the stance that these infants are born with a potential for a normal sensory and motor binocular system. Nevertheless, neural deficits (overt or soft signs) are an important cause of infantile ET.

Second cause

A second cause of infantile ET is the stimulus of *light* itself on an immature retina. The maturation rates of retinal development amongst infants vary greatly. Each hemiretina of an eye (nasal–temporal) *normally* has a different degree of development at birth, and a different rate of postnatal development. This is physiologically normal and reflects the phylogenetic differences of the nasal hemiretina and temporal hemiretina. Each eye harbors two distinct retinal systems.[4,5] Keiner[6] pointed out what he termed a *monocular* "optomotor reflex," i.e., diffuse light into an eye, which drives an infant's eye into adduction. Every ophthalmologist has experienced (but perhaps not recognized) that observing the fundus of an infant with a direct ophthalmoscope light drives the eye into adduction, presenting only the

nasal retina for observation. Interestingly, a brighter light (light differential) into the fellow eye will drive *it* into adduction wherein the gaze carries the eye to be observed with it so that now the temporal hemiretina is observable.

I here apply the principle of Bender[7] whereby simultaneous stimulation of any bilateral sensory input (right versus left half of retina; right versus left eye; right versus left ear system; right versus left somatic stimuli) results in an exaggeration of any inherent asymmetry. The Bender extinction phenomenon, in short, recognizes that "the better side may inhibit the worse side" of any bilateral sensory system, under simultaneous stimulus conditions, even to the point of extinguishing the percept of the worse side. In this regard, for *an eye* the nasal hemiretina is dominant over the temporal hemiretina, and a light stimulus (simultaneous bilateral stimulation of hemiretinas) results in nasal-retina (temporal field) superiority, an important sensory input (light) cause of infantile ET.

I have extended Keiner's observations, combined with Bender's exaggeration of asymmetries (nasal–temporal asymmetry in an eye) and posit a hypothesis that "very early neonatal visual influences may be responsible for motor misalignment and anomalous motor development. Light stimulus in the premature insufficiently developed eyes (with yet incompletely resolved media diffusers in the vitreous and lens) fulfills the essential overall diffusion stimulus criterion, the chain of *exaggerated* monocular and binocular dominances with altered muscle tonus."[4]

Recall Chavasse's prophetic remark regarding abnormalities that may be *exaggerations* of normal physiology. There is a normal physiologic nasal-hemiretinal dominance. It should not be surprising, therefore, that the superiority and exaggerated dominance of the nasal retina has strabismic consequences (Fig. 90.2).

The hemiretinas in an eye *are* different. After all, there are many adaptations that occur in the nasal retina such as small-angle esotropes (but not exotropes in the temporal retina) and

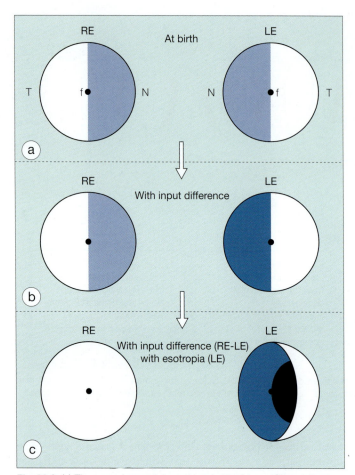

Fig. 90.2 (a) The normal neonatal nasal hemiretina has a different degree of development than does the temporal hemiretina. (b) This nasal–temporal hemiretinal difference is exaggerated with right versus left eye input difference, shown by the increased frequency of the diagrammatic lines on the right. (c) This is further exaggerated with the addition of left ET.

lots of eccentric fixation, while the temporal retina better grows congenital vascular anomalies. The difference is especially exaggerated with diffused light scatter in the eye, which is easily demonstrated in normal adults: with both eyes closed, and the palm covering one closed eyelid, while looking straight ahead, a penlight at a short distance shining onto the uncovered eyelid shows "faulty nasal field projection" (a very old term); i.e., wherever the light is, it appears to come from the temporal field (dominant nasal hemiretina).[4]

Thus, a second cause of infantile esodeviation of an eye is light incident upon an immature retina. Bender's extinction phenomenon exaggerates the inherent normal sensory superiority of the nasal hemiretina under simultaneous nasal–temporal stimulation (light incident to the whole eye), which are important concepts for explaining the cause of light-induced *monocular* adduction.

Clinician and laboratory investigators alike should be alerted to these two phenomena and should ponder the non-real life artifacts from examining a spot of the retina alone versus that same spot when acting with all of the rich retinal interactions that exist under more natural whole-stimulus conditions of both nasal and temporal retinas. I have further called attention to the upper retinas superiority over the inferior retina, which exhibits itself in various forms.[4]

Indeed, some cases of bilateral alternating infantile ET exhibit nystagmus abduction of each eye and exhibit a compensatory head turn with each eye to fix in an adducted position, as the eyes alternate (Ciancia syndrome). This is yet another distinct type of infantile ET, requiring quite different surgical treatment approaches, with a goal of obtaining a straight head with *each* eye fixing separately in the primary area. Vastly different amounts of surgery are required here compared with the usual and ordinary infantile ET. I look upon these cases as "double monocular ET" and the amount of surgery on each eye is based not upon the deviation, but rather upon the degree of abducting nystagmus and degree of compensatory head turn to fixate with each eye.

We know that a monocular adduction of an eye may occur as a result of light per se stimulating a retina with a delayed maturation, especially if there are intraocular scatterers of light. It should be noted that this is a *monocular* esodeviation and, when present in both eyes, one may consider the infantile esotropia as a case of double monocular ET.

Third cause

A third cause of infantile ET is *unequal inputs* (images) to the two eyes. This sensory cause includes *differences* of interocular retinal imagery, with normal retinas. Such interocular input differences occur with uncorrected anisometropia, differences in intraocular light scattering, or anything that makes the image of one eye significantly different from the image of the fellow eye. We "really do know" that unequal retinal images are an abnormal sensory input stimulus condition to the binocular system, which per se may precipitate strabismus.

It has long been observed empirically that a large interocular input difference in infancy results in esodeviation, whereas a large interocular input difference in adults may result in an exodeviation (as in acquired unilateral dense cataract). The following vivid example emphasizes the important difference between equal and unequal inputs. An equal amount of modest congenital nuclear cataract in each eye (*equal inputs*) may result in relatively good vision in each eye, without nystagmus or strabismus. However, the same amount of modest, congenital cataract, when present unilaterally (*unequal inputs*) results in an exaggeration of this modest congenital input difference, so that now the modestly cataractous eye may exhibit profoundly amblyopic vision with strabismus.

To emphasize the important monocular nature (single or double monocular) of some esodeviations, we cite here the example of congenital, severe unilateral microphthalmos (or anophthalmos), which results in the remaining good eye developing a monocular esodeviation, usually with a compensatory head turn to fix. This example may be considered a true monocular infantile esodeviation. Ciancia syndrome may be considered a double monocular esodeviation.

Fourth cause

A fourth cause of infantile ET is uncorrected, or undercorrected, hyperopic refractive errors. Donders' great contribution was to point out that uncorrected, and importantly *undercorrected*, hypermetropia is a major cause of strabismus, because of the accompanying accommodation–convergence relationship (A–C). The problem, and it is a major problem in my view, is that over 100 years later there are many who simply are not listening and are not practicing Donders' significant contribution. Uncorrected, or residual uncorrected hyperopia, abounds and the resultant accommodative action, with its variable effect on the deviation, confuses the uninitiated in both the diagnostic procedures and in the management results.

CHAPTER
90

What Do We Really Know about Strabismus and It's Management?

We really do know that Donders was right. The introductory remarks briefly referred to things that we really do know, but do not implement with sufficient fidelity so as to allow there to be a residual major cause of infantile ET. It is a pervasive problem in both infantile and adult ET. One cannot discuss this topic in terms of causations alone, but rather must include pitfalls in diagnosis and treatment by failing to eliminate the variable of any uncorrected hyperopia.

In infantile ET how much hyperopia is it important to correct and at what age? One not infrequently finds accommodative-ET under 1 year of age with as little as 2 D of uncorrected hyperopia. In my experience, one *can* and *does* observe accommodative-ET at 4 months of age completely corrected with contact lenses. If the examiner sets the threshold for optical corrections at approximately 3 D of hyperopia as found in the initial examination, then one knows that the actual degree of hyperopia is greater than that since all of the accommodation is not fully relaxed even with cycloplegia. To continue the plea to adequately adhere to Donders' principles, consider how many unnecessary surgeries are performed on infants because of lack of a fair and adequate time of *full* optical correction of *all* the hyperopia. Further, examination of the deviation at near, with even a modest amount of uncorrected hyperopia acting, always produces an excessive amount of accommodative–convergence. Examination of the protocol for some studies revealed that "the deviation" was measured at near (without correction if it was not considered to be "significant"). The examiner should not seek to determine the maximum esodeviation at near, but rather the minimum deviation, i.e., the deviation at distance (and it *can* be done at 10–20 ft in infants) with full optical correction in place for a time. It takes time for the tonic A-C to relax. The *basic deviation* is that deviation at the distance without any accommodative–vergence and without any fusion–vergence, to be eliminated by appropriate optical correction and cover test.[8] One cannot begin to think about, or manage, infantile ET without knowing the true *basic deviation*.

The near deviation (especially if measured without glasses) does not represent "the strabismus deviation." One simply must fully correct the accommodative effort, with adequate selection of accommodative targets at the most distant place (10–20 ft) appropriate for the age, with reliable refractive error determination, and full correction fidelity over time.

Appropriate test targets must be attention-getters for infants. There is an array of toys with motion, color, and light that can be sequentially used to maintain such attention. "It's a matter of one toy, one look. Six toys, six looks."[8]

We know that an important cause is any *residual*, uncorrected hypermetropia that may act as a "trigger" to initiate the A–C so that the nasal-suppressed retina is more immediately available to mask the diplopia present in the ET. Even very modest uncorrected hyperopia may act as a trigger during this critical postoperative period of sensory-motor flux, and may be the difference between a stable good result and a recurrence with all of its complications.

What about the hyperopia that allegedly develops after the first surgery for childhood esodeviation? One must ask: how much of this hyperopia may have been present preoperatively though not unmasked with adequate cycloplegic refractions nor adequately treated? There is an interesting phrase in some papers that alerts my curiosity–it is the remark that in management "anti-accommodative efforts were instituted without results." I call this a "fig leaf phrase" that masks uncorrected hyperopia. Holding lenses before the infant's eyes for a few moments time to note any significant change in deviation is a futile gesture. Miotics are a poor substitute for real spectacle correction. A "variable angle" of esodeviation signals uncorrected hyperopia. True, children may indeed have variable deviations, and it is also true that the variability may be markedly diminished or eliminated with adequate correction of even modest hyperopic errors over a sufficient period of time.

One may not expect a significant change in deviation, even with significant hyperopic correction when the degree of esodeviation is very large. The overacting and probably contractured MR muscles control this performance. Postoperatively (MR recessions), this control element is diminished or eliminated, so now the uncorrected hyperopia allows a truly variable esodeviation, which finally may be optically corrected to reaffirm the surgeon's declaration of success.

A cause of near esodeviation is manifest in patients with high hyperopia (over 4 D) and a full and adequate spectacle correction, which make them a simulated emmetrope, but they must exert more accommodation for any given near target than a true emmetrope does. Thus, high-hyperopia patients, who are adequately and fully corrected, have an induced pseudo-high A–C relationship, an optical "cause" of a near deviation. Contact lenses (especially when hyperopia is in the range of 5 D or more) considerably reduce the accommodative demand as well as clarify the peripheral fusion-lock often with considerable benefits to very young children with this type of high hyperopic esodeviation.

What are some of the nuances added to Donders' early causation principles? Both children and adults succumb to the *effort* of accommodation as the controlling cause of the factor of deviations. Even under cycloplegia one may still attempt, with effort, to accommodate and elicit A–C. Early presbyopes exercise greater effort in squeezing out the last increments of accommodation that remain. This increased effort often results in inducing an esophoria, which aggravates the pre-presbyope's problems. So, as it is with the more frequent childhood-related uncorrected hyperopia problems, so it is also with some adult strabismus management problems.

There is less effort of accommodation in downgaze and an increased effort of accommodation in upgaze, which may aggravate occupational symptoms of strabismus for older librarians and pilots viewing the panel of switches above horizontal gaze. The accommodative amplitude of older patients is indeed less when measured for upgazes than that for downgazes.

A cause of intentional self-induced esodeviation is observed in some people (children and adults alike) who learn to manipulate the A-C relationship and may completely fool and baffle the examiner, who may fail to accurately control accommodation on accommodative targets during the examination. I have seen patients "willfully" maintain a continuous A-C and cause an ET, desiring the next of a series of unnecessary operations for an ET caused by psychological/psychiatric reasons. On the other hand, other patients may demonstrate a decreased effort of accommodation for reading (willfully or unconsciously) and may cause convergence insufficiency. It has been my experience that the majority of patients with apparent convergence insufficiency do not (or perhaps will not) accommodate sufficiently to accurately resolve near print. Test conditions *must* control accommodation by demanding resolution of randomly chosen near individual reading letters, *during* the test for near deviations. Simply reading printed paragraphs does not suffice since reading is a skill and may be accomplished with facility even though there is insufficient accommodation and some blurred imagery.

Donders, during his retirement speech, said, "You develop knowledge, *strive persistently* (author's emphasis) to find acceptance, working for the advancement of mankind in the widest sense." It is a noble sentiment from a humanitarian scientist who obviously had to strive for acceptance of his simple, great observation. The persistent strive continues today.

It is my opinion that the major error in current strabismus management is the lack of control of accommodation and its associated convergence as a causation of deviations in infants and adults alike, and as a causation of confusion and errors in diagnosis and treatment.

One hundred and fifty years after Donders, one wonders whether his seed has indeed fallen on such good ground and grown well enough. Inadequate attention to full and proper optical corrections plays an important role in the causation of most cases of childhood strabismus. It is one of the things in strabismus management that we know we know. We also know we can do a lot better by Professor Donders.

Recapitulation of causations of strabismus

The causes and management of adult strabismus pose little problem since the strabismus is a result of acquired disease, disorder, or injury occurring in fully developed, usually normal, sensory and motor systems.

It is heralded from the treetops that little or nothing is known about the causation of infantile ET. However, on the ground it should be recognized that the major causes are known. The majority of causes are postnatal, sensory input factors of several types, acting on immature developing systems and neural deficits.

This is in contradistinction to the known, acquired, localized, mechanical factors in adults. Causation in infants shifts heavily to the nonmechanical and the neural and sensory input causations. Congenital structural mechanical anomalies are statistically a minor causation in infants and children.

THE NORMAL AND ABNORMAL BALANCE OF MUSCLE FORCES

In this discussion the term "muscle force" will mean the combination of neural (innervational) and mechanical contributions to the total resultant muscle force. How does nature successfully balance the resultant (neural and mechanical) muscle forces of agonist/antagonist muscles for binocular alignment and balanced eye rotations? How can we use this knowledge of normality in the *rebalancing* of the resultant muscle forces, to succeed in the goal of reestablishing alignment and balanced rotations?

Collins, the late revered bioengineer at Smith-Kettlewell Eye Research Institute, crystallized the thinking and taught us all about the principle of *balance of muscle forces*. With principles, things can become awfully simple. Without principles, things can become simply awful. We now know that the mechanical characteristics of all "normal" MR muscles do vary, and certainly, we now know that it is a false assumption to hold that the force of any muscle is solely mechanical. Of course, there must be a balance of opposing resultant forces at whatever position an *eye fixates*, else any imbalance would represent an *eye movement*. That might have been obvious to all concerned, but it really was not *known* nor were the ramifications thoroughly examined and the information used in the management of most strabismus cases.

The *normal* alignment in the primary position and the *normal* yoked balanced resultant forces in different gazes come about not

by there being equal and opposite mechanical muscle forces combined with equal and opposite innervational tonus forces. It is important to first get beyond this idealized, but incorrect, notion. Rather, there is abundant evidence that opposing horizontal muscles are mechanically unequal and that opposing vertical muscles are mechanically unequal. Thus, in a normal person, in order for there to be balanced resultant forces of agonist/ antagonist muscles as just described, there must be *unequal* innervation forces (the neural element) to appropriately match the mechanically unequal muscles in order to get resultant force balances. What do we really know about the evidence for these statements?

Horizontal muscle force balances

For normal individuals, under deep surgical anesthesia with intravenous total muscle relaxation, each eye is exodeviated 5–10 pd. This is the mechanical position of rest. In the alert state, when innervational tonus returns to all of the muscles, the resultant neural-mechanical forces of the MRs exceed that of the LRs and the eyes become aligned from the previously (anesthesia) exodeviated position. In short, the MRs lose more force than the LRs when all the innervation to the muscles are eliminated, and the MRs gain more force than the LRs with the innervation restored to both muscles. We have previously discussed the general innervation tonus level.

Further, we have emphasized the importance of future work in what we do *not* know, need to know, and must know, i.e., the sources of normal and abnormal nonretinal-derived innervational tonus to the oculorotatory muscles, in order to more completely understand the causes and management of strabismus. ·

Another excellent example of the mechanical inequality of the horizontal muscles (MRs versus the LRs) is in the condition of *retraction nystagmus*. This is the flip side of the anesthetic loss of innervation to all muscles, since in retraction nystagmus all muscles receive increased bursts (levels) of innervation. As expected, both eyeballs retract from such pulling on all the muscles at the same time, consequent to the burst of innervation to all the oculorotatory muscles, and importantly, during the retraction, the eyes converge (bilateral monocular adduction if you will). Why? Because when the MRs and LRs receive their burst packages of increased innervation, the MR resultant forces are greater than the resultant forces of the LR muscles in such a circumstance. With the cyclic relaxation of this tonic burst to all muscles, the retraction and the esodeviation subside.

Another horizontal muscle example is of the large esodeviation that may be exhibited in the child with cerebral palsy (and other CNS deficits) where there may be 70 pd's of esodeviation in the wakeful stage, which may disappear completely under general anesthesia since it wipes away all of the tonus of the muscles. So, in such cases during their normal awake state, the excessive innervation tonus to all the muscles produces greater resultant forces in the MRs than in the LRs, i.e., an esodeviation. Under anesthesia, when the innervation is wiped away, the esodeviation either considerably diminishes or evaporates because of the reverse situation. It is not unreasonable to suggest that each eye's agonist/antagonist muscle pairs react independently to produce a double monocular esodeviation, if you will.

It is well known that surgically a given length change of an MR produces a deviation change greater than that produced by the same length change in an LR muscle. Such deviation changes are not due solely to the muscle operated upon, but depend also upon the mechanical "pull-over" effect of the antagonist muscle, which in itself differs from the agonist.

In adults, the mechanical half of this equation predominates in the management decisions. On the other hand, for infants, it is the array of neural (innervational) elements to the muscles that predominate in the management decisions. One must recognize these marked differences between the management of adult versus infantile strabismus in order to make predictions and alter treatments accordingly. Models fall far behind in these distinctions if they do not incorporate *both* the neural and mechanical elements that determine the resultant muscle forces.

Vertical rectus and oblique muscle force balances

The vertical rectus muscles are far from being equal and opposite in their surgical effects. For instance, a certain amount of inferior rectus (IR) muscle surgery has considerably more effect on the vertical deviation than an equal amount of superior rectus (SR) muscle surgery, and also insofar as rotations are concerned. Indeed, one may recess the SR muscle as much as 10 mm or more in DVD with very little eventual effect on upward rotations. Also, superior oblique surgery may have a considerable vertical effect in the primary position compared with an equal surgery to the inferior oblique. Also "A"–"V" patterns are affected much more by superior oblique anomalies and surgery than by those of the inferior oblique muscle. We know that agonist–antagonist pairs of oculorotatory muscles are *not* equal and opposite in their mechanical forces.

For example, if one completely detaches the SR from the globe with a patient under just topical drop anesthesia, the fully alert patient cannot elevate the eye beyond horizontal. The inferior oblique muscle in this instance takes the eye from downgaze up to the primary position with saccadic velocity, but alone cannot

elevate the eye beyond the primary position (except perhaps a few degrees in extreme adduction) (Fig. 90.3).

Similarly, in third nerve paralysis, or in traumatic denervation or disinsertion of the IR muscle, the intact superior oblique muscle, acting alone, has an insignificant downward rotatory functional ability.

These cogent, real-life, clinical functional effects relative to muscle actions do not always find their way into oculomotor models.

Continuing the discussion of normal opposing muscle forces, we do know a corollary consideration of importance to both laboratory and clinical people, namely the question of "What are the opposing *horizontal* forces of vertical/oblique muscles?" This is important in predicting the horizontal deviation in up- versus downgaze, as well as in the primary position following acquired weaknesses and overactions of vertical rectus muscles and oblique muscles. It is self-evident that when a normal person moves the eyes up and down (in the primary plane), there is relatively stable horizontal alignment.

Rebalancing of muscle forces (surgery) for stable alignment

The problems in adult strabismics are essentially mechanical. Rebalancing these mechanical elements of abnormal weakness and abnormal strength (contractures) are considerably aided by tests performed during surgery. It is necessary to make certain that the general anesthesia is sufficient, and that muscle relaxants assure that innervational forces are eliminated, leaving mechanical forces to balance. The forced traction test is excellent guidance for diagnosing and correcting limitations of eye movements, and for avoiding producing abnormal and unwanted limitations. The spring-back mechanical balance test and the relative range of the neutral balance zone provide good guidance of when balance is achieved. These tests may be repeated at the beginning, during, and certainly at the end of surgery. A single misplaced conjunctival closure suture may be responsible for recreating an unwanted abnormality.

On the other hand, in infants with infantile ET, there are essentially innervational problems, although muscle mechanical problems also exist. Thus, the above intrasurgical tests guide the surgeon principally in avoiding the production of unwanted limitations or balance of forces. For example, in some "usual" infantile esotropes in whom a resection of the LR may be contemplated, even a 5-mm resection of a virgin LR in an infant may produce a limitation of adduction as demonstrated by forceps-forced duction rotation during surgery. Although unusual, such unusual stiffness muscle characteristics do occur. That's life. It is best to know that at the time of surgery, and a forced duction test for all resected muscles will detect the occasional bad actor and eliminate the overcorrection that, post-operatively, has the appearance of too much recession of the MR. If all resections are first tied with a bow knot, followed by a forced duction test before securing the muscle to the sclera, errors will be avoided. Many surgeons perform a "muscle elongation test" during surgery with similar goals in mind. If the surgeon's forceps reveal a limited globe movement at surgery, the patient will reveal the same limited movement after surgery.

In muscle rebalancing of infantile esotropes, *instability* of position of an eye will occur if the resultant forces of each muscle are not balanced. This is a major consideration if there is muscle slack produced in one or both agonist/antagonist muscles by muscle recession of a large degree. One must consider the rate of

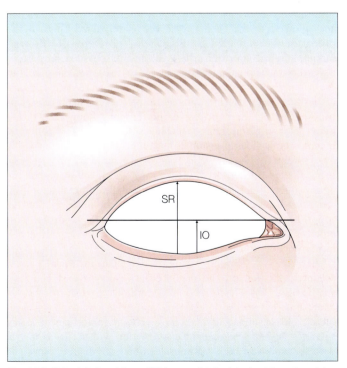

Fig. 90.3 If the inferior oblique (IO) is completely detached from the globe, the superior rectus (SR) can rotate the eye from downgaze to complete upgaze. If the SR is completely detached from the globe, the IO alone (with other muscles still attached) cannot move the eye above horizontal, except for a minor vertical elevation in adduction

muscle length adaptation (taking up the slack) for predicting results. For instance, in an infantile esotrope of large degree, if very large recessions of the MRs are performed, the hope and expectation that stable alignment can be attained often proves false. The recessed, originally stiffer, stronger, now recessed MR is now balanced against the slack produced in the previously stretched out LR when the globe is in the primary position. Since all muscles take up their slack, the stiff, though recessed MR will do so sooner than the slack LR can do, with *instability* of the resultant deviation and not unexpected return of some eso-deviation. This is true for each eye. This is an example of some of the mechanical factors that lead to instability of results. More modest MR recessions have much less of this impending LR slack imbalance develop. In the above-described example of large-degree ET, the addition of a modest resection of one or both LRs mechanically removes the LR slack and the modest resect–recess procedure in one or both eyes more properly balances the resultant opposing forces occurring in the same time frame.

All muscles take up created slack with time, whether it be due to a recessed muscle per se or opposing muscles' slack. Since the sarcomere adaptive adjustments have different rates, one may wish to do less surgery on more muscles, then more surgery on one or two muscles. Strategic considerations vary, of course, with the circumstances.[9] This has been described and discussed many times in the literature as "selective surgery," i.e., select those procedures that best rebalance the mechanical forces and do not leave unattended muscle slack. Intrasurgical tests predict many unwanted results. There is an old dictum stating that a horse-rider should not change horses in the middle of crossing a stream. Whereas that may be good advice for a horse and rider, it is extremely poor advice for a strabismus surgeon. One must be guided by predictive intrasurgical tests.

An alternative surgical method is the "formula approach," usually indicating graded MR recessions for graded deviations. Although we do know that such a formula approach addressing *only* mechanical factors of this neural-mechanical entity may be satisfactory in the majority of instances, we also know that it fails in a large percentage of instances, which should not be surprising. This variable result, and not infrequent, unintended large over-corrections with time, is based upon the false assumption that there are no individual differences in the characteristics of both opposing agonist/antagonist muscles in all infants. The objectives are the preoperative examination stability of deviation, and post-operative stability of deviation to reach the goal of the minimal number of total surgeries.

What do we know about the best times for surgical rebalancing of forces (when indicated) in strabismus, as well as the goals of surgical and nonsurgical realignment?

In *adult* strabismus, these questions are not much of a problem since each acquired disease/disorder entity or type of injury carries its well-established, generally accepted, timing decisions.

The real problem occurs with infantile esotropia. One often hears the clinician's admonition that early surgery to rebalance forces is necessary and is the sole option offered. Others advocate very, very early surgery (under 6 months of age). Some clinician scientists urge these same recommendations based upon elegant laboratory and animal investigations. What do we know about the bases for these positions? What do we know about other nonsurgical options? What are the factors to be considered in making such timing decisions and recommendations?

One of the goals is to fulfill the necessary criteria of rebalanced forces for stable alignment that will *allow* BFF to occur, with a technique that minimizes the total number of surgeries to achieve this, and will have the fewest complications. One cannot expect the development of good stereopsis (40 s Titmus) unless one allows BFF to occur. Any degree of residual esodeviation, after whatever treatment option is selected, means that BFF and perfect stereopsis is impossible. Further, there is a very narrow window of 2 to 6 months of age when stereopsis develops. It is a fact of present life that most infantile esotropes do not begin before 2 months of age and, on average, the referral to the ophthalmologist may not occur until the latter part of the window of opportunity. The stereo boat of exact realignment is simply missed.

Is it possible for an infant esotrope to have the result of normal 40 s of stereopsis? Indeed it is and has been verified by several studies.[10,11] Just as we now know that unilateral dense congenital cataract may result in good acuity with proper surgical timing and vigilant management, so it is with infantile esotropes relative to stereopsis.

WHAT IS THE ROLE OF INTENTIONAL SURGICAL OR NONSURGICAL OVERCORRECTION?

Since one must have perfect realignment in order to develop BFF and perfect stereopsis, it is important to recall the subject of "surgical orthoptics," i.e., intentional surgical overcorrection of an eso- into an exodeviation. Brown (of Brown syndrome fame), a superb observer and surgeon of an era past, always *overcorrected* his infantile esotropes by means of a bilateral LR muscle resection procedure. This, of course, produced 20-30 pd of exodeviation, which because of the strong MRs (unoperated) resulted in the *predictable* partial unwinding of the exodeviation and allowed fusion to occur as the eyes passed through the primary position alignment. Elsewhere,[12] I referred to Brown's unique surgical approach, the goal, and its possible advantages toward establishing better fusion by at least *allowing* BFF to occur. Such intentional surgical overcorrection I termed "surgical orthoptics" since the great advantage of converting an eso into a transient exo is the exposing of the temporal hemiretina rather than the nasal hemiretina to the binocular system. This orthoptic maneuver erases suppression. Surgical orthoptics is "to purposely overcorrect the amount and type of deviation as an orthoptic tool, to alter the sensory-motor status. Specifically, one has the opportunity to enhance the fusion potential, and make the BFF at least possible, by creating postoperative diploplia, minimizing suppression, and altering the anomalous correspondence. Not only can one change the sensory inputs ... but one can affect the motor outflow to the muscles."[13]

Historically, Cüppers[14] mentioned parenthetically that eccentric fixation on the nasal retina (esodeviation) could be ameliorated by overcorrection. Intentional overcorrection of strabismus has special indications, and plays a valuable management role in infant and adults.[12] The natural fear of many surgeons is that a permanent exodeviation will occur, as it may with recessions of both MR muscles of a large degree, especially if there are unhelpful sensory factors, which we have listed as "eso variables," which predict a permanent exodeviation potential. If any one or more of these following factors are present, management caution is appropriate and overcorrection contraindicated: uncorrected hyperopia, high hyperopia even if

CHAPTER

90

What Do We Really Know about Strabismus and It's Management?

fully and adequately corrected, a variable angle of deviation, any significant "A" pattern, unequal inputs (including a little amblyopia), and neural (CNS) deficits. In fact, when one or more of such variable factors are present, one may even expect a modest and small esodeviation to spontaneously convert into an exodeviation *without surgery*. However, for equal-visioned, alternating infantile esotropes without these eso variables, intentional surgical overcorrection of a modest amount (5–10 pd) is a goal.[9]

In adult, long-standing, equal-visioned, alternating exotropes intentional surgical overcorrection is also a goal, in this instance to *reestablish* a long dormant, good fusional stability.

One of the best publications supporting intentional, modest, surgical, overcorrection of infantile esotropia was by Scott and Pressman from the University of Iowa.[15] As expected from this source, good data showed the following: all patients had patching for treatment of amblyopia to equalize the visions, and all patients had a stable angle of deviation manifested by two successive cover test measurements *at the distance* varying not more than 5 pd, and none of the relative contraindications (eso variables) to overcorrection were present. Seventy-six consecutive infantile esotropes were operated upon with "two, three or four horizontal muscle surgeries performed as the primary procedure depending upon the size of the preoperative deviation (selective approach)." All MR recessions (alone or in combination with LR resections) did not exceed 5.5 mm. Those who had an immediate postoperative overcorrection of 4–15 pd had the best results at 6 months postoperatively, compared with those who had immediate postoperative esodeviations. Patients examined between 6 months and 3 years postoperatively showed little tendency for further drift to eso. Those who had more than 4 pd (4–15 pd) had the familiar eso drift through larger postoperative esodeviations. The number of overcorrections at 6 months, in this group, was small and almost equal to the number of significant undercorrections.

Of course, it was well recognized that surgical overcorrection of an amblyopic esodeviation into the exodeviation realm traditionally was to be avoided since the exotropia did not diminish and, if anything, often increased. This observation remains valid today.

So, one must conclude that we *really do know* that a purposeful overcorrection may be indicated in:

1. Adult patients with long-standing, equal vision, alternating exotropias; and
2. Infantile esotropias, equal vision, without the contraindicating factors listed as eso variables.

Intentional overcorrection of infantile ET is routinely achieved by the nonsurgical option of injection of botulinum toxin A (BTA) into both MR muscles.

The marked exodeviation that invariably occurs after this simple bilateral MR procedure makes it a particularly desirable option.[16] Before bilateral MR injections were routinely performed, injection of only one MR considerably reduced the esodeviation without producing an exodeviation, but it is extremely important to note that such patients developed a marked head turn *to fuse* in the position where the incomitancy produced the minimum esodeviation.[17] This is not an incidental point and answers the question of whether fusion is possible in such patients. As one of my most revered mentors, Linksz, would probably say, "This significant occurrence signifies significance."[18]

Bilateral MR injections produce a profound sensory jolt as a result of the intentional significant overcorrection (10–30 pd), which diminishes within weeks. This is precisely comparable to

Brown's intentional surgical overcorrection via bilateral LR resections, discussed earlier. The majority of patients receiving BTA into both MRs are significantly overcorrected, which diminishes within weeks.

As the BTA wears off, the exodeviation diminishes so that at least the eyes are *allowed* to become aligned in the primary position. Pioneers of bilateral MR injections (McNeer, Tucker, Spencer[16,19]) have successfully managed hundreds of infantile esotropes with only BTA injections into both MR muscles. The mean number of injections was two. R. Gomez de Llano[20] in Spain has reported on her successfully managed thousands of such cases. The results of simultaneous bilateral MR injections are comparable to results from very early surgery, without the complications of an occasional lost muscle, operative site scar tissue, repeat hospitalization, and general anesthesia. For very large degrees of esodeviation (stably measured as such over time, for distance–not near–fixations), surgery may be preferable to repeated injections, and surgery may at any time also be utilized if BTA is insufficient.

Currently, the overwhelming majority of *surgical* treatment of infantile esotropia results in undercorrections with residual esodeviations and the expected sensory decrements.

Therefore, early surgery, or very early surgery, is certainly not the only option for rebalancing of forces to realign the eyes in infantile esotropes. BTA is safe and simple, has minimal complications, and incorporates transient exotropia postoperatively. It is interesting and puzzling to note the frequent absence of mention of this available (if one wishes to make it available) and valuable nonsurgical realignment alternative from the concluding recommendations of many publications where there is mention of only one necessary option, i.e., very early surgery as being necessary. Botulinum toxin A may be given very early. (The author and Smith-Kettlewell Eye Research Institute have no financial interest in botulinum A toxin.)

A third alternative option step in the rebalancing/realignment process is that of alternate occlusion (alternate day complete occlusion), or some variation of this schedule. Alternate occlusion allows the practitioner to delay alignment, since alternate occlusion is, in fact, a type of "dark rearing" for the binocular system, and the evidence is clear that, during alternate occlusion, one preserves normal development of binocularity and prevents the occurrence of any bad habits of binocularity from developing.[21] The angle of strabismus often decreases during alternate occlusion since both eyes are not open at the same time and interocular competition is eliminated.

Alternate occlusion may be safely carried out for as long as a year, if one eye is not covered for more than 4-5 days at a time during early infancy. The McNeer/Tucker/Spencer team carried out a brief period of alternate occlusion prior to their BTA injections.

Even if one elects very early surgery, alternate occlusion allows safe delay until all the variable findings of infantile esotropia are known. The surgeon may safely choose a delayed time of surgery, which allows one to determine the quality or inequality of sensory inputs, the refractive errors, the patterns of rotations, and a stabilized angle of deviation–all valuable information, which augurs for a safer visual milieu if surgery is the choice.

To recapitulate the options of timing and goals in the rebalancing/realignment options for the management of infantile esotropia, it may be stated that there certainly is more than the one option of very early surgery. *The options are:*

1. Botulinum toxin A injections into both MR muscles (to be repeated if necessary depending upon the degree of deviation);

2. Alternate occlusion, which allows safe delay in alignment (by any means chosen), until examination findings are fully known, repeatable, and the angle of deviation is stabilized to within 5–10 pd; and

3. Early surgery with its significant rate of reoperations, occasional severe complications, and current absence of the goal of desirable transient exodeviation postoperatively (when not contraindicated by the state of the eso variables).

The ophthalmologist and the alarmed parent, if armed only with the recommendation of the sole option of early surgery, need not leap to that conclusion from either clinical or laboratory investigations (human and nonhuman). (Oh, if only the infant could choose, there would be thousands of fewer operations, and hundreds of fewer complications in the management of infantile esotropia.) The surgeon has an obligation to the infant's parents to always point out and compare the various treatment options.

CONCLUDING COMMENTS

Considering the charge given to me of writing about "What do we really know about strabismus and its management?", it appears appropriate to end the discussion of the issues by asking one final question: "Of all that we know, past and to date, what things best maximize the benefit to today's strabismic patients?" In my mind, there are three answers to this question:

1. The full and adequate correction of hyperopic refractive errors, with time to act, and the care of not leaving residual uncorrected hyperopia. The failure to pay full attention to Donders' 150-year-old teachings is *the* major problem in the management of infantile esotropias. Proper attention to the control of accommodation–convergence by correction of residual uncorrected hyperopia would probably save thousands of operations and thousands of reoperations.

2. Full appreciation of the concept of the balance of muscle forces, and the implementation procedures for rebalancing muscle forces, would greatly simplify the strabismus management task. We need to know much more, about the origins and sources of nonretinal-derived muscle tonus. This would have the potential to open new doors to entirely new treatment avenues.

3. The use of botulinum toxin A (and/or related substances) injected into both MR muscles in infants and children with infantile esotropia would probably save thousands more operations and thousands more reoperations.

REFERENCES

1. Jampolsky A. Ocular divergence mechanisms. Trans Am Ophthalmol Soc 1970; 68: 730–822.
2. Jampolsky A. Treatment of exodeviations. In: Pediatric Ophthalmology and Strabismus: Transactions of the New Orleans Academy of Ophthalmology. New York: Raven Press; 1985: 141–71.
3. Chavasse FB. Squint, or the Binocular Reflexes and the Treatment of Strabismus. 7th ed. London: Baillière, Tindall & Cox; 1939.
4. Jampolsky A. Unequal visual inputs and strabismus management. In: Strabismus Symposium: trans of the New Orleans Academy of Ophthalmology. St. Louis, MO: Mosby; 1978: 358–492.
5. Nawratzki I, Jampolsky A. A regional hemiretinal difference in amblyopia. Am J Ophthalmol 1958; 46: 339–44.
6. Keiner GBJ. New Viewpoints on the Origins of Squint: a Clinical and Statistical Study on Its Nature, Cause, and Therapy. The Hague: Martinus Nijhoff; 1951.
7. Bender MB, Furlow LT. Phenomenon of visual extinction in homonymous fields and psychologic principles involved. Arch Neurol 1945; 53: 29.
8. Jampolsky A. A simplified approach to strabismus diagnosis. In: Symposium on Strabismus: trans of the New Orleans Academy of Ophthalmology. St Louis, MO: Mosby; 1971: 34–92.
9. Jampolsky A. Strategies in strabismus surgery. In: Pediatric Ophthalmology and Strabismus: trans of the New Orleans Academy of Ophthalmology. New York: Raven Press; 1985: 363–98.
10. McNeer KW, Tucker MG, Guerry CH, et al. The incidence of stereopsis following treatment of infantile esotropia with botulinum toxin A. J Pediatr Ophthalmol Strabismus 2002; 2: 1–5.
11. Ing MR, Okino LM. Outcome study of stereopsis in relation to duration of misalignment in congenital esotropia. J AAPOS 2002; 6: 3–9.
12. Jampolsky A. Overcorrections in strabismus. Trans Am Ophthalmol Soc 1965; 8: 75–9.
13. Jampolsky A. Systems of strabismus surgery. In Proc III Congresso del C.L.A.D.E., Mar del Plata, Argentina, 3–6 Nov, 1971: 433–43.
14. Cüppers C. Personal communication; 1982.
15. Scott WE, Pressman SH. Temporary exotropia following surgery for infantile esotropia. In: Orthoptic horizons: trans of the VIth International Orthoptic Congress, Harrogate, Great Britain. Harrogate; 1987: 255–62.
16. McNeer KW, Tucker MG, Spencer, RF. Botulinum toxin management of essential infantile esotropia in children. Arch Ophthalmol 1997; 115: 1411–8.
17. Scott AB. Botulinum toxin injection into extraocular muscles as an alternative to strabismus surgery. J Pediatr Ophthalmol Strabismus 1980; 17: 21–5.
18. Linksz A. Physiology of the Eye, vol 2 Vision. New York: Grune & Stratton; 1952.
19. McNeer KW, Spencer RF, Tucker MG. Observations on bilateral simultaneous botulinum toxin injection in infantile esotropia. J Pediatr Ophthalmol Strabismus 1994; 31: 214–9.
20. Gomez de Llano R, Rodriguez Sanchez JM, Gomez de Llano P, et al. Toxina botulinica tratamiento del estrabismo. Resultado sensorial y motor. Acta Estrabologica 1995; 183–8.
21. Jampolsky A, Norcia AM, Hamer RD. Preoperative alternate occlusion decreases motion processing abnormalities in infantile esotropia. J Pediatr Ophthalmol Strabismus 1994; 31: 6–17.

Clinical Investigation of Bilateral Poor Vision from Birth

CHAPTER **P1**

Ingele Casteels

Normally, full-term babies show visual fixation at birth or shortly afterward. The absence of visual responsiveness in a baby of more than 8 weeks old must be taken seriously and warrants careful investigation. Parents are anxious to understand why the baby seems not to see, and want to know the visual prognosis. The clinician should verify the cause and degree of visual impairment and make a plan of management and counseling for the parents.

The diagnosis of visual unresponsiveness in a baby depends first on a thorough family and clinical history and a complete systematic clinical examination (Fig. P1.1).

HISTORY

The history of the pregnancy and delivery and of postnatal development is important. Maternal infections, trauma, and hypoxia can have significant visual consequences. Visual development in premature babies can be delayed due to the associated retinal or neurological problems. Premature infants with a high-grade intraventricular hemorrhage are at risk of optic atrophy and hydrocephalus. The presence of seizures, developmental delay, and a wide variety of dysmorphic features suggests a brain problem.

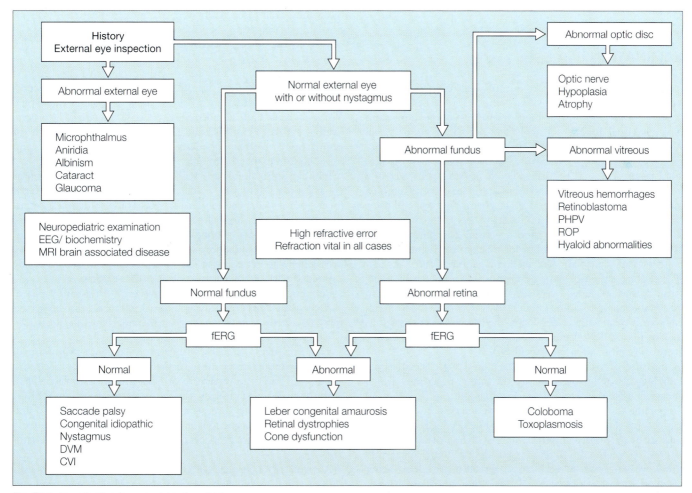

Fig. P1.1 Investigation for poor vision from birth.

A positive family history, or a history of consanguinity, makes certain diseases more likely; for instance, a baby born to first cousin parents with searching eye movements and hypermetropia is very likely to have a congenital retinal dystrophy. The clinician should inquire about other family members; examination of them and the first-degree relatives is also necessary.

Has there been a change in visual behavior since birth? Vision can deteriorate after seizures or with sedation: this visual impairment can be transient.

Specific questions to parents or caregivers on the visual behavior in dark or in light can also give a clue to the diagnosis. Some congenital retinal disorders, especially achromatopsia, cone–rod dystrophy, and Leber congenital amaurosis, may present with photophobia or day-blindness.

Babies with a cerebral visual impairment (CVI) can also show reluctance to look at a light or in contrast will develop light gazing.[1] Lens and corneal opacities, i.e., congenital glaucoma, albinism, and aniridia, can cause photophobia.

Did parents notice wobbling eyes? Nystagmus and searching eye movements can be the presenting symptoms in many babies with poor vision from birth, but usually appears at 2 to 3 months of age. Roving or drifting eye movements are often seen in babies with very poor vision.

Are there any specific hand movements? Blind babies tend to press or poke their eyes. Babies with limited vision due to retinal disorders tend to wave their hands between their eyes and a light source.

EXAMINATION (see Chapters 2 and 9)

In practice, it is often difficult to quantify visual acuity in babies, especially in babies with poor visual contact. Parental estimations of vision can be helpful. It is more relevant to obtain a measure of overall visual function. Establishing normal levels of visual function is, despite research efforts, still primarily one of behavioral observations. By 2 months, a visual following response should be present, and the baby should smile responsively to a parent. At 4 months, a child should reach for an object. Complex stimuli with contrast should be used in a happy and wakeful baby. The presence of neurological problems makes the estimation of vision even more difficult, as there are other possible causes for inattention and a lack of following responses. Techniques to quantify visual acuity[2] are described in Chapter 2.

The presence of optokinetic nystagmus (OKN) in a baby fixing a stripe pattern excludes a very severe current visual problem. In congenital oculomotor apraxia (COMA) the eyes will deviate on being spun around without developing the fast phases of nystagmus ("locking up"); OKN examination in COMA shows the presence of vertical rapid fixation movements.

A measure of vision can also be achieved with the dynamic vestibulo-ocular reflex by evaluating the "after" nystagmus, which is longer in a blind baby due to poor refixation.

Inspecting the pupils and pupillary reactions can be useful. An asymmetrical (i.e., relative) afferent pupil defect suggests anterior visual pathway disease, often compressive or inflammatory. A bilateral symmetrical afferent pupil defect with apparently normal eyes suggests severe bilateral retinal disease, i.e., Leber congenital amaurosis or severe bilateral anterior visual pathway, particularly chiasmal, disease. Paradoxical pupillary responses, with initial constriction in darkness and dilation in brighter illumination, are seen in congenital stationary night-blindness, Leber congenital amaurosis, and cone dystrophies.

Special attention is paid to the eye movements. In addition to the normal immaturity of pursuit and saccadic movements in the newborn, oculomotor apraxia and Duane syndrome may be the cause of poor visual contact. Examination of the external eyes and eye movements will reveal the presence of nystagmus and strabismus. It is difficult to distinguish between nystagmus waveforms clinically. Eye movement recordings have shown some useful clinical information. A high-frequency, low-amplitude pendular nystagmus in otherwise normal eyes is often seen in cone dystrophies.[3] Searching eye movements with very poor vision are seen in Leber congenital amaurosis. Early-onset nystagmus can be divided into three groups: sensory defect nystagmus, in which there is a proven sensory defect; congenital idiopathic nystagmus (sometimes called motor nystagmus), in which no visual or neurological impairment can be found; and neurological nystagmus, which is associated with neurological disease.[4]

In most babies the cause of poor vision from birth is obvious after clinical examination. A structural ocular abnormality (e.g., microphthalmos) may be obvious at a glance. The use of the red reflex to identify media opacities is a useful quick screening technique.

Slit-lamp examination may reveal anterior segment problems: cataracts, colobomas, aniridia, albinism, etc. With the help of an experienced nurse, or a hand-held slit lamp, examination can be performed at any age. It is particularly important in infants with nystagmus, as in cases of albinism, iris transillumination is evident. Slit-lamp examination should be repeated after dilatation of the pupils, with better visualization of lens opacities or lens subluxation.

Bilateral pupillary dilatation with cyclopentolate 0.5% is necessary, with indirect and direct funduscopy and retinoscopy. On funduscopy, attention is paid to the vitreous and the retina. Vitreous haze and hemorrhages, seen in bleeding disorders, uveitis, retinal vasculitis, nonaccidental injury, retinopathy of prematurity, retinal dysplasia, hyaloid abnormalities, and retinoblastoma, may be found.

Indirect ophthalmoscopy will reveal retinal problems such as chorioretinal colobomas, macular toxoplasmosis, retinal detachment, retinal folds, chorioretinal dysplasia, and sometimes, retinal dystrophy. Direct ophthalmoscopy is best for subtle optic disc anomalies such as colobomas and optic disc hypoplasia or dysplasia. An examination under sedation or anesthesia may occasionally be necessary to see the optic nerve in detail, usually combined with another test, such as MRI scanning.

Refraction is vital, as high refractive errors–hypermetropia in particular–can give rise to poor visual contact from birth and refractive errors can give a clue to the underlying diagnosis (see Chapter 6).

When the eyes of a baby with poor visual contact are normal, with or without nystagmus, further investigation is necessary (Table P1.1). As the waveform of nystagmus does not correlate with the underlying etiology, the flash electroretinogram (fERG) may diagnose retinal diseases (see Chapter 11). The fERG and flash VEP have conspicuous immature features during the early months; thus it may be necessary to repeat the fERG at a later age.[5]

A pediatric neurological consultation and further investigations, such as biochemistry and brain MRI, are carried out where indicated. Babies affected with CVI have a normal eye examination and no nystagmus. Delayed visual maturation (DVM) is a term preferably used for a perfectly normal baby with a transient visual deficit (see Chapter 3). It is clear that

Table P1.1 Common causes of poor vision in infants with external normal eyes

Diagnosis	Clinical signs apart from poor vision	Pupils	Slit lamp	Ophthalmoscopy	Refraction	Flash ERG	Flash VEP	Pattern VEP	MRI	Neuropediatric examination/EEG	Visual outcome
DVM	Poor visual contact	Normal	Normal	Normal	Normal	Normal	Normal	Normal	Normal	Normal	Normal
Cerebral visual impairment	Eccentric viewing/light gazing	Normal	Normal	Usually normal	Normal	Normal	Usually abnormal	Usually abnormal	Usually abnormal	Usually abnormal	Usually poor Perceptual defects
Idiopathic nystagmus syndrome	Nystagmus Head tilt	Normal	Normal	Normal	Normal/abnormal	Normal	Normal	Abnormal	Normal	Normal	Good
Leber congenital amaurosis	Roving eyes Photophobia Eye poking	Paradoxical Sluggish or normal	Normal	Usually normal	High hypermetropia	Absent	Abnormal	Absent	Usually normal	Normal	Poor
Retinal dystrophy	Nystagmus Night-blindness	Usually normal	Normal	Usually abnormal	Usually normal	Abnormal	Usually normal	Abnormal	Normal or abnormal	Normal or abnormal	Poor
Achromatopsia/cone dystrophy	Photophobia Day-blindness Color-blindness Nystagmus	Paradoxical or normal	Normal	Normal	Normal or high hypermetropia. Blue cone dystrophy, myopic	Absent cone response	Normal	Abnormal	Not indicated	Normal	Poor, photophobia Stationary
Bilateral optic nerve hypoplasia or atrophy	Poor vision Roving eye movements	Afferent defect	Normal	Abnormal, direct ophthalmoscopy necessary	Normal	Normal	Abnormal	Abnormal	Normal or abnormal	Normal or abnormal + endocrine exam	Variable
Albinism	Nystagmus Photophobia	Normal	Abnormal	Abnormal	Myopia or astigmatism	Normal or enhanced	Crossed asymmetry	Crossed asymmetry	Usually not indicated	Normal	Variable

DVM is a retrospective diagnosis, which can only be made after a long enough follow-up to exclude minor or major neurological problems.[6]

It is sometimes difficult to predict how severe the visual problem will be. In most infants with absent visual contact, there is hope for visual improvement.

However, with a longer follow-up, more neurological problems may emerge.[7,8]

An incorrect or unclear diagnosis of visual impairment in an infant can be devastating to the family. In most infants presenting with poor visual contact, clinical signs are typical, but additional studies may necessary to the correct diagnosis. The use of a clear terminology and classification of poor visual contact and nystagmus is important. A long enough follow-up by the ophthalmologist in collaboration with the pediatrician should be planned.

REFERENCES

1. Jan JE, Groenveld M, Anderson DP. Photophobia and cortical visual impairment. Dev Med Child Neurol 1993; 35: 473–7.
2. Teller DY, McDonald MA, Preston K, et al. Assessment of visual acuity in infants and children: the acuity card procedure: a rapid test of infant acuity. Dev Med Child Neurol 1986; 28: 779–89.
3. Yee RD, Baloh RW, Honrubia V. Eye movement abnormalities in rod monochromacy. Ophthalmology 1981; 88: 1010–8.
4. Casteels I, Harris CM, Shawkat F, et al. Nystagmus in infancy. Br J Ophthalmol 1992; 76: 434–7.
5. Kriss A, Russell-Eggitt IM. Electrophysiological assessment of visual pathway function in infants. Eye 1992; 6: 145–53.
6. Lambert SR, Kriss A, Taylor D. Delayed visual maturation: a longitudinal study: clinical and electrophysiological assessment. Ophthalmology 1989; 96: 524–8.
7. Casteels I, Spileers W, Missotten L. The baby with poor visual contact. Br J Ophthalmol 1998; 82: 1228–9.
8. Weiss AH, Kelly JP, Phillips JO. The infant who is visually unresponsive on a cortical basis. Ophthalmology 2001; 108: 2076–87.

CHAPTER
P2 Red Eye in Infancy

Michael P Clarke

Although other causes of the red eye do occur in infancy, the most common and most important cause of a red eye is neonatal conjunctivitis.

NEONATAL CONJUNCTIVITIS (see Chapter 19)

In 1881, when Credé introduced silver nitrate prophylaxis, gonococcal ophthalmia neonatorum was the principal cause of blindness in infancy and was responsible for a quarter of cases of lost eyesight throughout the world[1]: it remains a significant public health problem in some parts of the world.

Neonatal conjunctivitis is defined as occurring within one month of birth. It presents with a purulent discharge, conjunctival chemosis, and lid swelling. Causative organisms include gonococcus, *Chlamydia*, *Haemophilus*, *Streptococcus pneumoniae*, and *Staphylococcus aureus*.[2]

Neonatal conjunctivitis due to *Neisseria gonorrhoeae*

Symptoms typically begin 24 to 48 hr after birth with purulent conjunctivitis, lid swelling, conjunctival membrane formation, keratitis, corneal ulceration, and perforation.

Topical antibiotic therapy alone is inadequate and is unnecessary if systemic treatment is given.[3] Simultaneous infection with C. *trachomatis* should be considered when a patient does not improve after treatment. Both mother and infant should also be tested for chlamydial infection.

Neonatal conjunctivitis caused by *Chlamydia trachomatis*

Chlamydial conjunctivitis is the most common form of ophthalmia neonatorum in the West. Infants usually present 5–14 days after birth with a purulent discharge and lid swelling. The disease is self-limiting and usually without sequelae, but corneal opacification has been described.

Diagnostic considerations

Sensitive and specific methods used include both tissue culture and nonculture tests (direct fluorescent antibody, enzyme immunoassay, and nucleic acid amplification tests). Specimens must contain conjunctival cells, not exudate alone. Specimens for culture isolation and nonculture tests should be obtained from the everted eyelid using a Dacron-tipped swab or the swab specified by the manufacturer's test kit. Treatment is not only for the neonate, but also for the mother and her sex partner(s). Ocular exudate from infants being evaluated for chlamydial conjunctivitis should also be tested for *N. gonorrhoeae*.

Treatment

Topical antibiotic therapy alone is inadequate for treatment of chlamydial infection and is unnecessary when systemic treatment is administered.

The recommended regime is Erythromycin base or ethyl-succinate 50 mg/kg/day orally divided into four doses daily for 14 days. Tetracycline should not be used in children because of the risk of staining of permanent teeth.

Data on use of other macrolides (e.g., azithromycin and clarithromycin) for the treatment of neonatal chlamydia infection are limited. Twenty to 40% of newborns with chlamydia conjunctivitis develop chlamydial pneumonia by 90 days after birth.

SUBCONJUNCTIVAL HEMORRHAGE

Subconjunctival hemorrhage is very common in perinatal period.[2] In the majority of cases it is caused by elevated venous pressure in the head and neck produced by compression of the fetal thorax and/or abdomen by uterine contractions. A tight umbilical cord around the neck probably represents an additional mechanism.[4] Subconjunctival hemorrhage may also be a feature of child abuse and is found in children with pertussis. See Chapter 27.

VASCULAR MALFORMATIONS AND HEMANGIOMAS

See Chapter 27.

FOREIGN BODIES

Foreign bodies on the cornea or conjunctiva are unusual in infants but may be associated with a (usually localized) redness with watering and pain. Slit-lamp examination may be necessary, and it is important to look under the upper lid.

EPISCLERITIS AND SCLERITIS

Episcleritis and scleritis are rarely diagnosed in infancy but may occur in association with autoimmune vasculitis, dry eye, and graft-versus-host disease.

DRY EYE

Though rare, a number of dry eye conditions can cause redness (see Chapter P8).

UVEITIS

Acute anterior uveitis causing a red eye is very rare in infancy. When it does occur, it is important, as it is usually associated with systemic vasculitis. See Chapter 44.

GLAUCOMA

See Chapter 48. Glaucoma in infancy occasionally has red eye as one of the symptoms, especially in pupil block associated with ROP, PHPV, etc.

MASQUERADE SYNDROMES

Advanced retinoblastoma may present with ocular inflammation and glaucoma. Endophthalmitis may present with a similar picture in the context of ocular trauma or surgery, or a systemic infection such as meningococcal meningitis.

KERATITIS

Neonatal herpes simplex infection usually presents with a systemic meningitic-type illness.[5] HSV neonatal conjunctivitis occurs within the first two weeks of birth. Vesicular eyelid lesions may be present. The conjunctiva is only moderately inflamed, and the discharge is serosanguineous. Microdendrites and geographic ulcers are more commonly seen in the neonatal form than the dendritic ulcer seen more typically in adults and older children. Cataracts and chorioretinitis may develop.

Strategies for prevention of neonatal infection include cesarean delivery and prophylactic acyclovir. Treatment of infected neonates is with systemic acyclovir.

KID (keratitis, ichthyosis, deafness) syndrome (see Chapter 29) is a congenital disorder of ectoderm that affects not only the epidermis but also other ectodermal tissues such as the corneal epithelium and the inner ear. Vascularizing keratitis is present in infancy in some affected individuals, but in others may not arise until later in the course of the disease.[6]

A corneal foreign body should be suspected in infants with a unilateral red eye and corneal staining. Vertical streaks of stain should alert the observer to the presence of a subtarsal foreign body.

REFERENCES

1. Dunn PM. Dr. Carl Credé (1819–1892) and the prevention of ophthalmia neonatorum. Arch Dis Child Fetal Neonatal Ed 2000; 83: 158–9.
2. Bartolomeo SD, Mirta DH, Janer M, et al. Incidence of chlamydia trachomatis and other potential pathogens in neonatal conjunctivitis. Int J Infect Dis 2001; 5: 139–43.
3. Available at http://www.cdc.gov/STD/treatment/4-2002TG.htm#Gonococcal.
4. Katzman G. Pathophysiology of neonatal subconjunctival hemorrhage. Clin Pediatr 1992; 31: 149–52.
5. Enright AM, Prober CG. Neonatal herpes infection: diagnosis, treatment and prevention. Semin Neonatol 2002; 7: 283–91.
6. Caceres-Rios H, Tamayo-Sanchez L, Duran-Mckinster C, et al. Keratitis, ichthyosis and deafness (KID syndrome): review of the literature and proposal of a new terminology. Pediatr Dermatol 1996; 13: 105–13.

CHAPTER
P3 The Sticky Eye in Infancy

David Laws

Any neonate with purulent discharge from the eye should have the diagnosis of ophthalmia neonatorum excluded (Chapter 19). Swabs should be taken for microscopy, culture, and immunofluorescence to exclude *Neisseria* and *Chlamydia* although the former may be clinically suspected by the copious amounts of pus. Both parents should have contact tracing, and the infant should be given systemic therapy to treat other complications such as pneumonitis. Neonatal prophylaxis of ophthalmia neonatorum has been abandoned in the UK and Sweden. Povidone iodine 1.25% is used in some countries,[1] particularly where antenatal care has not been well documented.

Bacteria cause 80% of cases of acute conjunctivitis in infants.[2] Although the majority of cases will clear without treatment, antibiotic therapy causes earlier clinical and microbiological resolution of the disease. Treatment may also prevent more serious complications of conjunctivitis.[3,4] The choice of treatment should be guided by efficacy, cost, and side-effect profile. Most comparative studies of treatment of acute conjunctivitis show little difference between broad-spectrum antibiotics. Chloramphenicol, fluoroquinolones, aminoglycosides, fucidic acid, polymyxin, and sulfacetamide are all used more on national background rather than evidence base.[3]

Viral conjunctivitis makes up the balance of most acute cases with epidemics of adenovirus sweeping through communities in winter months. Primary herpes simplex or chickenpox may also affect the conjunctiva. A small molluscum lesion may be easily missed on the lid margin and result in chronic conjunctivitis. Allergic conjunctivitis is unusual in infancy but should be considered in the presence of other atopic disease.

Chronic or recurrently sticky eyes are more likely to present to the pediatric ophthalmologist in the secondary care setting (Fig. P3.1). The commonest association is with congenital nasolacrimal obstruction with subsequent superinfection or colonization by opportunistic bacteria. The majority of these cases are associated with epiphora (Chapters 31 and P10). Histological studies show that around 60% children have obstruction of the nasolacrimal system at term birth,[5] but clinically 20% have evidence of obstruction in the first year of life.[6] The presence of a lacrimal sac mucocele should be excluded and the child examined for abnormalities of the lacrimal puncta or for supernumerary openings. Initial care of lacrimal obstruction is undertaken by massage to the lacrimal sac and gently cleaning the lids from nasal to temporal using clean cotton wool and water. Persistent epiphora past 1 year of age or intolerable recurrent infection is treated with probing of the nasolacrimal duct.[7] Cases that have persistent watering after one or more probings may undergo silicone rod intubation or other intervention (Chapter 31). The timing of this intervention and whether to intubate both the superior and inferior canaliculi is still debated.

The child should be examined for lid malposition or lashes rubbing the cornea. Epiblepharon is commonly found and usually the soft lashes of small children may be tolerated until the lid fold becomes normal. Persistent corneal staining, however, may be an indication that intervention is required. Multiple rows of lashes (distichiasis, see Chapter 25) or congenital lid anomalies such as lid notch associated with trichiasis may be found. Blepharitis can be associated with recurrent corneal ulceration in children.

Note should be taken of corneal size, clarity, and staining. Epiphora and photophobia raise the possibility of congenital glaucoma, corneal dystrophy, or corneal ulceration. In developing countries malnutrition including vitamin A deficiency may contribute to recurrent infection.

Rarely recurrent conjunctivitis may be associated with systemic disease in children. Lymphadenopathy, a high fever, and conjunctivitis should alert the physician to the possibility of Kawasaki disease, which may have serious complications, e.g., coronary aneurysms. Stevens Johnson syndrome (Chapter 22) may result in a severe cicatrizing conjunctival inflammation. Dry eyes and corneal anesthesia may be associated with familial dysautonomia. Ligneous conjunctivitis also rarely affects infants. All infective disease should be treated with great caution in the immunosuppressed.

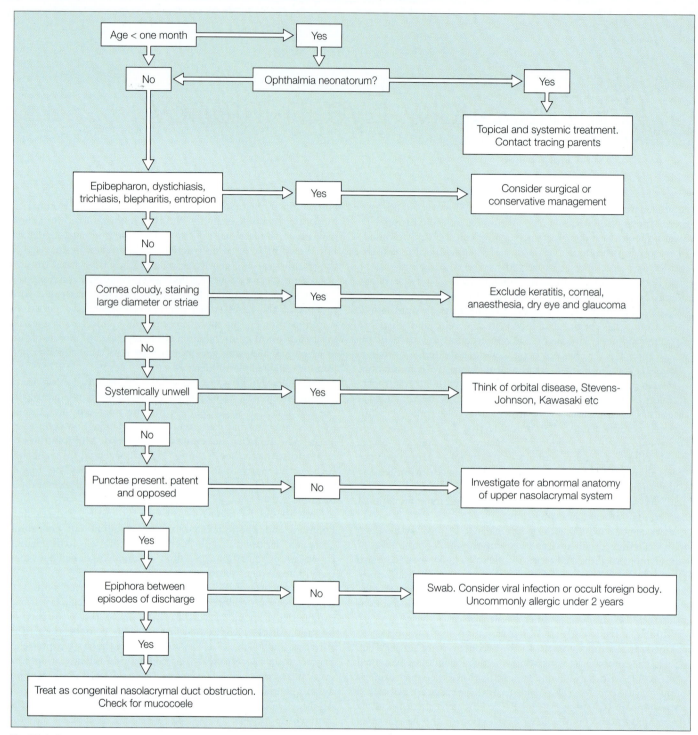

Fig. P3.1 Assessment of recurrent sticky eyes in infancy.

REFERENCES

1. Isenberg SJ, Apt L. Velenton M, et al. A controlled trial of povidone-iodine to treat infectious conjunctivitis in children. Am J Ophthalmol 2002; 134: 681–8.

2. Weiss A, Brinser JH, Nazar-Stewart V. Acute conjunctivitis in childhood. J Pediatr 1993; 122: 10–4.

3. Sheikh A, Hurwitz B. Topical antibiotics for acute bacterial conjunctivitis: a systematic review. Br J Gen Pract 2001; 51: 473–7.

4. Gigliotti F, Hendley JO, Morgan J, et al. Efficacy of topical antibiotic therapy in acute conjunctivitis in children. J Pediatr 1984; 104: 623–6.

5. Busse H, Muller KM, Kroll P. Radiological and histological findings of the lacrimal passages of newborns. Arch Ophthalmol 1980; 98: 528–32.

6. MacEwen CJ, Young JD. Epiphora during the first year of life. Eye 1991; 5: 596–600.

7. Young JD, MacEwen CJ, Ogston SA. Congenital nasolacrimal duct obstruction in the second year of life: a multicentre trial of management. Eye 1996; 10: 485–91.

CHAPTER
P4 The Unusual Appearing Eye

John A Bradbury

Parents find it easier to describe the behaviour of their child than an anatomical abnormality of the eye. For example, parents can usually tell you that their child can't see or has night-blindness rather than describe accurately leucocoria or aniridia. Usually they say that the eye looks "funny" or "unusual". However, a careful history from the parent can often clarify how long the abnormality has been present, whether this has coincided with any deterioration in visual function and if the physical abnormality is static or progressive. Closer questioning may reveal exactly what the abnormality is, but in general this is found by your own careful examination.

If no clue is available from the parent or child's history, the best way to approach the problem is anatomically – looking at each tissue systematically. If an abnormality is found, examining other systems may help in the diagnosis, e.g. umbilical hernia + dental abnormality + corectopia = Reigers syndrome. If the abnormality is not easily explained, examination of parents and siblings is always worthwhile to try and exclude an inherited condition. Also, one must always bear in mind, trauma as a cause of an ocular abnormality.

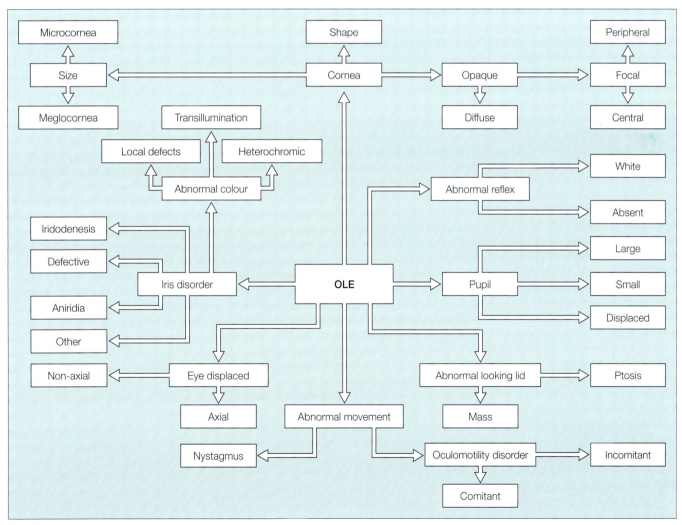

Fig. P4.1 Causes of an odd-looking eye.

CHAPTER
P5 The Lump in the Lid

Gerd Holmström

A lump in the lid is common in children either as an isolated finding or as a manifestation of a systemic disease (Table P5.1). The cause is mostly benign, although malignancies do need to be considered. Some causes are common, while others are extremely rare. The most common causes will be described, while the rare ones are only briefly mentioned.

RHABDOMYOSARCOMA (see Chapter 35)

Rhabdomyosarcoma is a rapidly progressing malignant tumor, which must be considered in the differential diagnosis of a lid lump in children. Although proptosis is the most common feature of ophthalmic rhabdomyosarcoma, manifestation in the lid may also be the presenting finding. The history typically is short, days or weeks, and the tumor often presents before 10 years of age, although infantile presentation may occur.[1,2] The tumor may simulate an inflammatory process or vascular lesions such as capillary hemangioma and lymphangioma.

Table P5.1 Causes of lumps in the lid

Benign
  Nevus
    Acquired melanocytic nevus
    Congenital melanocytic nevus
  Inflammatory
    Chalazion
    Stye/abscess
    Molluscum contagiosum
    Warts
    Sarcoidosis
    Wegener's granulomatosis
    Pseudorheumatoid nodules
  Neural
    Neurofibroma–NF1
    Schwannoma
  Vascular
    Capillary hemangioma
    Nevus flammeus/Sturge-Weber
    Lymphangioma
    Pyogenic granuloma
  Miscellaneous
    Dermoid
    Juvenile xanthogranuloma
    Histiocytosis
    Angiofibroma (in tuberous sclerosis)
    Pilomatrixoma (calcifying epithelioma of Malherbe)
Malign
  Rhabdomyosarcoma
  Lymphoma
  Leukemia
  Metastatic tumor
  Melanoma

If rhabdomyosarcoma is suspected, the child should promptly be investigated with CT or MRI, and a biopsy should be taken for diagnosis and histopathological classification. Molecular diagnostics may sometimes also be helpful in the classification. The child should preferably be taken care of by a team of pediatrician, oncologist, and pediatric ophthalmologist. The prognosis of children with rhabdomyosarcoma is better today than previously. Modern treatment with multiagent chemotherapy, sometimes supported by radiotherapy, has resulted in increased survival rates to more than 90%, although tumors of an alveolar type and presentation of the tumor in infancy show a worse prognosis.[1,2]

DERMOID (see Chapter 40)

Dermoids are commonly seen in children. They are developmental, cystic lesions, usually located at the supratemporal margin of the orbit, less frequently in the medial aspect of the orbit or elsewhere. Histologically they are lined by keratinizing, stratified squamous epithelium and may contain fat, hair follicles, sebaceous glands, and sweat glands. Inflammation occurs if the cyst ruptures.[3] A dermoid usually appears as a smooth mass and is variably movable due to varying attachment to underlying structures. Superficial lesions are most common, although deep dermoids also exist.

Dermoids in the lid usually do not affect visual function, although amblyopia may occasionally occur due to pressure on the eye globe and anisometropia. Treatment may be conservative, i.e., observation only, or surgical. In most cases they are extirpated because of cosmetic disturbance, inflammation, or growth. The dermoids may infiltrate and extend into the orbit. Unless fully movable, a CT scan should therefore be performed prior to surgery. The aim should be to excise the dermoid as a whole cyst and avoid rupture, which may cause chronic inflammation.

CAPILLARY HEMANGIOMA (see Chapters 42 and 26)

Capillary hemangiomas are common and benign tumors, most often affecting the upper lid and the orbit of the child.[4] Superficial hemangiomas have a red, lobulated appearance and are often referred to as "strawberry lesions." Subcutaneous hemangiomas have a more bluish color. The hemangiomas present during the first months of life and grow rapidly during the following months. The final size is variable. In rare cases they are very extended and markedly affect the appearance of the child.[5] After a period of stabilization they slowly regress. Most involution occurs before 7 years and is nearly always complete at the end of the first decade.[4] The capillary hemangiomas are often isolated, but may be associated with ocular and systemic abnormalities.[4,5]

Dealing with hemangiomas of the eye region focuses on prevention of amblyopia, which may occur due to occlusion of the visual axis or distortion of the globe, leading to astigmatism and anisometropia. The child must be followed regularly. Repeated careful refraction with prescription of adequate glasses and occlusion if needed, are important. If the visual axis is threatened, or if a retrobulbar hemangioma threatens the optic nerve, systemic or locally injected steroids usually reduce the hemangioma. Other treatments, such as radiation, interferon, various laser therapies, and chemotherapy, are also described. Surgery, if needed, is usually postponed until the stage of involution.

CHALAZION (see Chapter 26)

Chalazia, though trivial, may cause symptoms. They are lipo-granulomatous inflammation that results from an obstruction of a Meibomian gland duct. They usually present as a localized and painless nodule in the lid or lid margin with a swollen, red lid. Small chalazia usually resolve spontaneously. Warm compresses, lid hygiene, and topical antibiotics can be useful if inflamed. Larger chalazia may need incision and curettage under general anesthesia in young children. Chronic chalazia warrant a suspicion of malignancy, such as rhabdomyosarcoma.

As in all young children with a lump in the lid of any cause, the risk of amblyopia by distortion of the globe or partial occlusion of the visual axis must not be overlooked.

MOLLUSCUM CONTAGIOSUM AND WARTS
(see Chapter 26)

Molluscum contagiosum and warts are common viral infections of the lid in children. Molluscum contagiosum occur anywhere, although the eyelids are frequently affected. The lesions are small (a few millimeters) and often multiple, with an umbilicated center, and if on the lid margin, may be associated with a symptomatic follicular conjunctivitis. They sometimes require treatment with incision, curettage, or diathermy.

STYE/ABSCESS

A stye is a painful abscess of the sebaceous glands of the lid often associated with *Staphylococcus aureus*. The stye may resolve spontaneously, but antibiotic ointment may be helpful and relieve some of the discomfort. Larger abscesses may require systemic antibiotics, incision, and drainage.

OTHER LESS COMMON CAUSES OF LUMPS IN THE LID

Malignancies

Lymphoma, leukemic infiltrates, melanoma, and metastases of other tumors are all rare.

Nevi (see Chapter 26)

Both *acquired and congenital melanocytic nevi* of the lid occur. The acquired nevi usually present between 5 and 10 years of age, they are flat or slightly elevated, and they darken with age. Malignant transformation is rare.

Inflammatory lesions

Sarcoidosis, *Wegener's granulomatosis*, and *pseudorheumatoid nodules* are granulomatous inflammations that may involve the lids.

Neural (see Chapter 33)

A *neurofibroma* of the lid usually occurs with neurofibromatosis, when it often gives the lid a "S-shaped" appearance. Gradual growth of the tumor may cause ptosis, distortion of the globe, and amblyopia. Surgical debulking is therefore often needed but the mass frequently recurs. Ipsilateral glaucoma is frequent.

Schwannomas are tumors arising from the Schwann cells of the peripheral nerve sheath. They may also occur in association with neurofibromatosis.

Other vascular lesions (see Chapter 42)

Lymphangioma presents in infancy and gradually grows during many years. Due to hemorrhage into the tumor, the onset is often sudden. Lymphangiomas are difficult to manage, and unlike capillary hemangiomas, they do not regress spontaneously.

Nevus flammeus may be isolated or associated with the Sturge-Weber syndrome. Congenital or juvenile glaucoma is a common complication, often difficult to handle (see Chapter 48).

Pyogenic granuloma appears as a fleshy red mass and is a proliferative fibrovascular response to a previous trauma such as inflammation or surgery.

Miscellaneous

Juvenile xanthogranuloma is a benign, yellow/orange-colored, granulomatous inflammatory disorder of the skin, which may also affect the eye and the lids. It predominantly occurs in infancy and early childhood. Since the lesions usually regress spontaneously, treatment is often not needed.

Histiocytosis (Langerhan cell histiocytosis, histiocytosis-X) is an uncommon disorder that may affect the lid.

Angiofibromas of the skin and lid often occur in the first decade of life as early manifestations of tuberous sclerosis.

Pilomatrixoma (calcifying epithelioma of Malherbe) is a benign tumor originating from the hair matrix cells. It is usually solitary and appears in the lid or eyebrow as a subcutaneous red to blue, hard mass. The lesion should be surgically excised.

REFERENCES

1. Kodet R, Newton WA, Hamoudi AB, et al. Orbital rhabdomyosarcomas and related tumors in childhood: relationship of morphology to prognosis–an Intergroup Rhabdomyosarcoma Study. Med Pediatr Oncol 1997; 29: 51–60.
2. Shields JA, Shields CL. Rhabdomyosarcoma: review for the ophthalmologist. Surv Ophthalmol 2003; 48: 39–57.
3. Shields JA, Kaden IH, Eagle RC Jr, et al. Orbital dermoid cysts: clinicopathologic correlations, classifications, and management. The 1997 Josephine E. Schueler Lecture. Ophthal Plast Reconstr Surg 1997 Dec; 13(4): 265–76.
4. Garza G, Fay A, Rubin P. Treatment of pediatric vascular lesions of the eyelid and orbit. Int Ophthalmol Clin 2001; 41: 43–55.
5. Holmström G, Taylor D. Capillary haemangiomas in association with morning glory disc anomaly. Acta Ophthalmol 1998; 76: 613–6.

Abnormal Blinking and Eye Closure

CHAPTER **P6**

John S Elston

INTRODUCTION

Eye opening and closure are determined by reciprocal activity in the levator palpebrae and orbicularis oculi. Although the levator subnucleus is an unpaired midline structure, premotor control is partly lateralized, allowing voluntary eye winking (unilateral eye closure) as well as bilateral voluntary and spontaneous (periodic) blinking. Unilateral eye closure is a learnt behavior, which children acquire by mimicry and practice, usually around the age of five or six.

A spontaneous periodic blink lasts about 80 ms. The upper lid movement is due to active muscle contraction when both opening (levator) and closing (orbicularis oculi) the eye. In periodic blinking and gentle eye closure the pretarsal and preseptal portions of the orbicularis oculi are involved, while in forceful eye closure the orbital part is also recruited.[1]

Voluntary blinking and forceful eye closure are controlled by the pyramidal system. Periodic blinking is regulated by the extra pyramidal system. Reflex blinking occurs in response to trigeminal sensory stimulation from the cornea, conjunctiva, or eyelid margin. There is also reflex forceful eye closure to a bright light or loud noise. Reflex blinks also occur in response to threatening movement near to the eyes.[2]

In infancy, blinking or eye closure to a sudden very bright light occurs as a subcortical midbrain reflex, so it occurs in infants with major cortical visual impairment. In some young children sudden bright light may stimulate a reflex sneeze or a startle response as well as blinking.

The fundamental purpose of blinking is the maintenance of the anatomical and optical integrity of the corneal epithelium by periodic reconstitution of the precorneal tear-film. Periodic blink rate depends on a number of environmental conditions. Assessment of the blink rate is difficult and awareness of the individual that the rate is being measured will modify it. Infants and children up to 18 months have a low periodic blink rate (2 to 5 per minute), increasing thereafter to achieve the adult rate (14 to 20 per minute) in the second decade. The period of maturation from early childhood blink rate to that of the adult is usually slow and progressive. The normal adult periodic blink rate is greater than that required for visual purposes.

Many periodic blinks are incomplete but if the pupil is covered, the visual blackout is suppressed by a neural mechanism analogous to that occurring during saccadic eye movement.[3] Periodic blinks are accompanied by a small (1° or 2°) eye movement, usually downward and inward and followed by a refixation saccade. Bell's phenomenon, a large-amplitude upward and outward eye movement, accompanies forceful eye closure.[4] If eye closure is prevented, e.g., with a lid speculum and a maximum attempt to close the eye occurs, globe retraction and Bell's phenomenon occur. Under these conditions supranuclear input to the ocular

motor nuclei is maximal, and a larger range of, for example, upward movement is demonstrable by these means than by, for example, pursuit or voluntary saccadic movement.

Absolute eyelid position changes in response to any change in the vertical eye position in the orbit. The levator and lower lid retractors receive a copy of the input to the vertically acting extra ocular muscles. In extreme downgaze, the lower lid position encroaches beyond the limbus onto the cornea. Modest widening of the palpebral aperture on abduction is normal.

MODIFICATION OF THE PERIODIC BLINK RATE

Excessive blinking

Excessive blinking in children is common and generally benign,[5] although serious causes need to be kept in mind.

The periodic blink rate is relatively constant in an individual under fixed conditions. It is modestly increased by activities such as reading and by anxiety and may be markedly elevated in thyrotoxicosis, schizophrenia, Tourette syndrome, and, to a lesser extent, depression.

Any cause of excessive tear production or poor tear drainage stimulates an increased blink rate, as the tear pump function of the orbicularis oculi is activated. Some children with a large phoria, particularly an exophoria, use blinks to control the ocular deviation, and children with an exodeviation may shut one eye in bright sunlight.

Eye blinks may be used to initiate saccadic eye movements (the blink–saccade synkinesis).[6] The eye blinks are used partly to break fixation, and partly to inhibit pause cells to enable a fast eye movement to be generated. This phenomenon is seen in ocular motor apraxia (saccade initiation failure, SIF), and intermittent forceful blinking, as well as head thrusts, may be a prominent feature. Photophobia with excessive blinking or blepharospasm occurs in photoreceptor dystrophies.

Photophobia, lacrimation, excessive blinking, and blepharospasm are features of ocular surface disorders involving the cornea, conjunctiva, and eyelid margins. The underlying pathologies include corneal abrasion or infection, foreign body, or eyelid or eyelash malposition. This response is reduced by topical anesthesia. Childhood onset corneal dystrophies involving the epithelium, e.g., Reis Buckler, or corneal crystals, e.g., cystinosis, produce similar symptoms.

Inflammatory eye disease (acute anterior uveitis) may present with photophobia and excessive blinking. However, the uveitis of juvenile chronic arthritis (JCA) is usually asymptomatic.

While the periodic blink rate in infancy is characteristically low, many normal infants are quite light sensitive, preferring to shut their eyes to avoid even moderately bright sunlight and reflected light from water, or in motor cars. Parents may need reassurance that this is a normal phenomenon.

Infrequent blinking

Parents may observe that their infants sleep with their eyes open. The palpebral aperture is usually open by 2–3 mm but the eyes are elevated and the cornea protected. This seems to be a variant of normal in infancy and no specific measures are required.

Periodic blinking decreases with alertness, a function of the reticular activating system, and is reduced in hypothyroidism and extra pyramidal disorders. Sometimes the low periodic blink rate of infancy persists into later childhood. In Tourette syndrome (see below), forced staring may be seen.

SPECIFIC DISORDERS OF BLINKING AND EYE CLOSURE

Facial palsy

Lower motor neuron facial palsy, unless accompanied by corneal anesthesia, rarely causes corneal exposure problems in childhood provided the vertical eye movements are intact. Sometimes the eye may have to be taped shut at night. Even in completely unrecovered facial palsy in childhood, facial muscle tone is usually good and the appearance, at rest, reasonably symmetric. In post facial palsy synkinesis (misdirection–regeneration of the facial nerve) there is usually mild persistent weakness of orbicularis oculi and periodic blinks are asymmetric. On attempted forced lid closure synkinetic movements are seen in the mid- and lower face.

Children on ventilators in the ITU are vulnerable to corneal exposure, since lid and orbital edema are common and the eye closure may be incomplete. The high ambient temperature leads to rapid drying. The problem may be overlooked by nursing and medical staff understandably concerned with other very important aspects of the care of an unconscious child, and permanent scarring can rapidly develop unless appropriate protective measures are taken.

Eyelid myokymia

Eyelid myokymia is a repetitive muscle contraction–flickering or twitching–most commonly located in the lower lid laterally. It is common, usually unilateral, and self-limiting and may be seen particularly in children under mild stress, for example, coming up to examinations. If facial myokymia is extensive and persistent a lesion in the dorsal pons should be suspected and an MRI brain scan arranged. Pontine glioma and, more rarely, tuberculoma, may present this way. Bilateral facial myokymia can occur in the Guillain-Barré syndrome or be due to demyelination.

Orbicularis oculi neuromyotonia

This consists of more sustained rippling contractions of the orbicularis oculi, which occurs bilaterally, occasionally spontaneously but more often induced by forceful eyelid closure. Individuals describe a difficulty in opening the eyes after eye closure, and a characteristic symptom is prolonged eye closure after sneezing. It may be a component of more generalized myotonia or occur as an isolated phenomenon. There may or may not be an associated autoimmune disorder and, in some cases, myasthenia gravis. Anti-potassium gated voltage antibodies may be detectable.

Hemifacial spasm

Hemifacial spasm may initially present as eyelid myokymia, but it persists and develops into episodic co-contraction of the facial nerve innervated muscles on one side. Partial eye closure, with synchronous brow elevation, mid-facial movements, and platysma contraction are typical. Bursts of hemifacial spasm occur and may be triggered by talking, eating, or tight eye closure. Sometimes more sustained clonic contraction is seen (Fig. P6.1). In adults it is usually due to microvascular compression of the facial nerve in the root exit zone, and surgical decompression can be curative. Focal botulinum toxin injections substantially relieve the spasm and are the treatment of choice in most cases.

In infancy hemifacial spasm may be the presenting sign of a posterior fossa vascular anomaly[7,8] (Fig. P6.2), an intrinsic pontine lesion[9] (Fig. P6.3), or extra axial compression of the facial nerve by an abnormal blood vessel or tumur.[10] All infantile and childhood cases require neuroimaging. Very rarely hemifacial spasm may be familial, secondary to a familial vascular anomaly, and in such cases start in childhood.[11] Rarely, it may presage accommodative esotropia.[12]

Eye blinking tic

A tic is an abrupt transient purposeless stereotypical coordinated movement, which varies in intensity and is repeated at irregular intervals. Eye winking and eye blinking tics are examples of a simple motor tic and are common in childhood, particularly in boys. There are rapid exaggerated jerky contractions of the orbicularis oculi, bilaterally or unilaterally, which tend to increase with boredom, tiredness, and anxiety. The age of onset is in the second half of the first decade, between the ages of 6 and 10. A tic may start quite abruptly, and the disorder tends to persist for up to about a year.[13]

The evidence suggests that the movements are produced intentionally to suppress an uncontrollable inner urge to perform the tic. The urge is suppressible for variable periods, after which the tic may be performed repeatedly to relieve the urge. Tics reduce with distraction and concentration but are often suppressed during consultation, so the history is usually the most reliable guide to the diagnosis. When the diagnosis is suspected from the referral letter, surreptitious observation of the child in the waiting room may well reveal the characteristic movements, which are not evident in the office.

There may also be a family history of tics. Sometimes the abnormal movements extend to include eyebrow raising, nostril flaring, and grimacing. Simple motor tics, such as eye blinking, usually wax and wane over weeks to months before remitting completely usually within a year. Sometimes other tics develop before or after an eye winking tic, such as head shaking or throat clearing.

A tic is usually idiopathic; there may be a genetic predisposition, and mild focal trauma, such as a foreign body in the eye or the throat, may determine the way in which the tic manifests, i.e., as an eye blinking or throat-clearing tic. Secondary tic disorder may occur after head injury, encephalitis, and neurotropic drug administration. Because of the generally excellent prognosis the parent and child should be strongly reassured and told to expect spontaneous resolution without specific treatment. Parents, teachers and, as far as possible, family members and friends should be encouraged to ignore the tic and the child reassured that the strange compulsion to perform it will resolve. Psychiatric referral is not required. Occasionally, idiopathic simple tics persist to become chronic or lead to Tourette syndrome.[14]

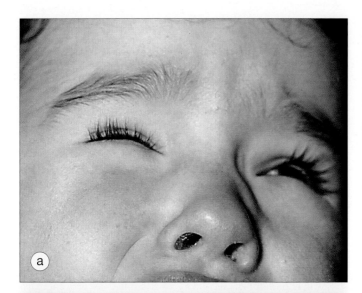

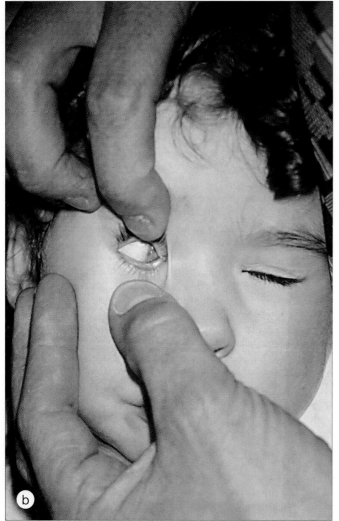

Fig. P6.1. Two-year-old child with intermittent right hemifacial spasm from 1 year of age. The attacks occurred about 20 times a day, were painful, and involved the whole right side of the face (a). There was a Bell's phenomenon during the attacks (b), and no cranial nerve defects in between attacks. Neuroimaging was normal. The attacks resolved spontaneously after 13 months.

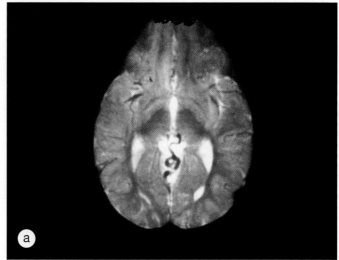

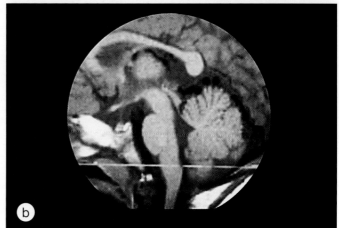

Fig. P6.2. Three-year-old with right hemifacial spasms who had a sigmoid sinus occlusion at the age of 1 year during a high fever. MRI demonstrated an occluded sinus and collateral vessels in the posterior fossa (a, b).

Eye movement tics may occur in isolation or association with other tics. They consist of large-amplitude concomitant and often oblique, saccadic eye movements, and the child may be referred with concern that he or she has opsoclonus or some form of nystagmus. As with other tics they are suppressible and have the characteristic modifying factors. Generally speaking they resolve quickly.[15]

Tourette syndrome

Tourette syndrome may occur in 0.5% of the school population.[16] Eye blinking, eye winking, and facial motor tics may also occur in Tourette syndrome combined with phonic and complex motor tics. The phonic tics include repetitive throat clearing, barks, and clicks as well as complex vocal tics, including echolalia (repetition of someone else's words or phrases), palilalia (repetitions of one's own words or phrases), and coprolalia (shouting of profanities and obscenities). Eye movement tics as well as forced staring and sensory tics, which are brief episodes of subjective sensory disturbance, often in the face or around the eyes, may also be seen. Saccades are dysmetric, and there is a complete failure of anti-saccades (saccades in the opposite direction to the target).[17] Some children exhibit self-injurious behavior, and serious

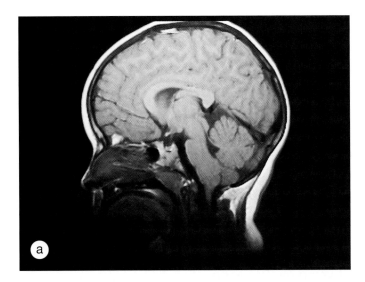

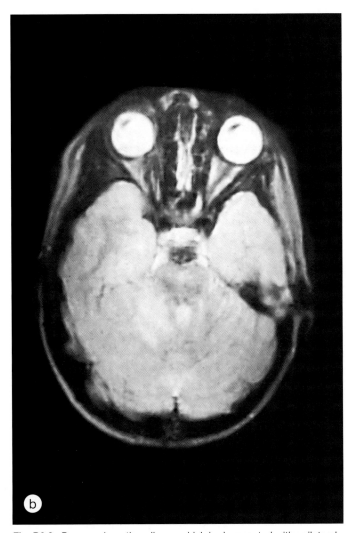

Fig. P6.3. Presumed pontine glioma, which had presented with unilateral facial spasms showing an expanded pons on MRI (a) and an intrinsic pontine lesion (b), which did not change over 15 years.

bilateral eye damage has been reported. Care needs to be taken when examining these children to avoid injury during one of the uncontrollable movements.[18] In florid cases the diagnosis is obvious, but there is a wide spectrum of abnormality.[19]

Tourette syndrome has an autosomal dominant inheritance with variable penetration, and the expression of the gene is, in part, determined by sex, manifesting as Tourette in males and obsessive-compulsive disorder in females. Care has changed substantially;[20] the most common treatment is dopamine receptor antagonists.[21] Intelligence is normal and the prognosis is quite good. Most interference from the tics occurs in adolescence, and nearly half of the adults with Tourette have only mild and suppressible tics.

Idiopathic blepharospasm

Primary or idiopathic blepharospasm is an adult onset focal dystonia, consisting of repeated forceful bilateral eye closure with photophobia and synchronous mid- and lower facial muscle contractions. Childhood or adolescent onset is very unusual,[22] but there is often a prodrome of increased periodic blinking and intermittent blepharospasm, which may begin in the early teens. Some affected adults have had an eye blinking tic in childhood.[23] The onset of a focal dystonia, such as blepharospasm, in the second decade should raise the possibility that the disorder is secondary and not idiopathic: blepharospasm may precede dystonia[24] or Tourette syndrome[25] in children and occurs in Lesch-Nyhan syndrome.[26] It has been described after hypoxic brain damage, and also in metabolic disorders such as Wilson disease. A full neurological assessment to include a metabolic work-up and neuroimaging is therefore indicated if the disorder is diagnosed in childhood.

Reflex blepharospasm, in response to bright light and other stimuli, can occur as a congenital familial characteristic. It consists of prolonged spasms of forceful bilateral eye closure, in response to a stimulus that normally elicits a reflex blink.

MISCELLANEOUS DISORDERS

Myasthenia gravis

Overshooting dynamic upper eyelid movements may be a prominent feature in ocular myasthenia. *Lid hops* are small-amplitude vertical upper lid movements, with a fast upward phase and a slower downward drift that occur with horizontal pursuit eye movements. A series of such upward flicks or hops accompanies large-amplitude horizontal eye movements. *Lid twitches* (Cogan sign) occur on upward vertical movements, both pursuit and particularly saccadic, when the upper lid movement is excessive in relation to the eye movement leading to transient upper lid retraction on upgaze. The lid may settle to a normal or ptotic position.

Lid twitches are explicable on the basis of central adjustment (increase) of the motor input to the vertical eye muscles, to cope with the peripheral deficit of neurotransmission. The "copy" of the increased input to the levator causes an excessive movement, while the viscous drag of the eye and extra ocular muscles prevents this occurring to the globe. For the same reason the initial few degrees of a saccadic eye movement in ocular myasthenia is faster than that in normals. Lid hops are probably due to an analogous mechanism, whereby the vertically acting muscles are involved in side-to-side gaze in keeping the eye position horizontal.

Other signs of ocular myasthenia, i.e., fatigability and variability of both eye and eyelid movement, as well as weakness of forceful eye closure, will usually also be present. This is a useful sign in ocular myasthenia gravis; the upward eye movement (Bell's phenomenon) that accompanies it may be greater than that elicited by voluntary gaze.

Characteristic myasthenic eyelid signs with ophthalmoparesis have been described in a number of cases of low-grade dorsal midbrain tumors. The mechanism is obscure and may involve simultaneous axonal damage and regeneration. The hyperdynamic flickering upper lid movements in these cases of "midbrain myasthenia" are unilateral or highly asymmetric.[27]

Recovered third nerve palsy

Abnormal unilateral upper lid movements accompany misdirection–regeneration of a third nerve palsy on attempted downgaze and adduction, and may have a flicking intermittent quality. This may also be seen in cyclic oculomotor palsy, where the eyelid movement is not sustained.

A number of cases of congenital partial ptosis in the primary position associated with lid elevation on abduction, and an increase in the ptosis on adduction, have been described. In some of these cases what appears to be a Duane-type eye movement disorder is also present.

Brown syndrome

Congenital Brown syndrome may be accompanied by widening of the palpebral aperture on adduction of the affected eye, with upper lid retraction on activation of the ipsilateral superior oblique muscle, i.e., looking down toward the opposite side. This phenomenon is unexplained, but the resemblance to the "pseudo von Graefe" sign of misdirection–regeneration of a third nerve palsy suggests that, at least, some cases of congenital Brown syndrome may be due to a "miswiring" phenomenon.

Marcus Gunn jaw winking phenomenon

This condition is almost invariably unilateral. There is a synkinesis between a pterygoid muscle (lateral or medial) and the levator. There is usually a partial ptosis at rest. The condition presents in infancy with abnormal flicking upper lid retraction, noted on feeding when the pterygoid muscle is activated.

Upper lid retraction

Bilateral upper lid retraction may occasionally be seen in normal neonates. It is usually intermittent and symmetrical, and it resolves spontaneously. In preterm infants intermittent transient conjugate downgaze, with associated relative upper lid retraction, may be seen as a benign phenomenon that resolves spontaneously in the first months of life. So-called "eye popping" consists of a form of startle reflex in normal infants, when ambient illumination is reduced. Both upper lids retract temporarily and the phenomenon may be associated with a backward head movement or jerk.[28]

Dorsal midbrain syndrome

Pathological upper lid retraction is part of the dorsal midbrain syndrome, indicating that the underlying lesion involves the nucleus of the posterior commissure. Lid retraction in these circumstances is due to the pathological process interfering with the normal tonic supranuclear inhibition of the central caudal nucleus of the third nerves.

If the lesion extends to involve the third nerve fascicles on one side, a unilateral, partial, or complete ptosis with contralateral lid retraction may be evident. Other localizing signs will be present.

The commonest cause of the dorsal midbrain syndrome in childhood is hydrocephalus. The combination of bilateral upper lid retraction and a vertical upgaze palsy produces the setting sun sign with the eyes displaced below the horizontal meridian relative to the lower lid position. Other causes of the dorsal midbrain syndrome in this age group include pineal tumors.

Thyroid eye disease

This is unusual but may occur in the pediatric age group. Upper lid retraction is due to either sympathetic overactivity in hyperthyroidism or levator involvement in Graves' ophthalmopathy. Both these processes may occur together. Additional signs of Graves' ophthalmopathy and thyroid dysfunction are usually present.

Eyelid nystagmus

Upper eyelid nystagmus consists of rapid conjugate upward movements of the lids followed by a slow downward drift. It has been described as an unusual component of the dorsal midbrain syndrome, and also rarely in a variety of intrinsic midbrain disorders and less frequently in cerebellar disease. In all cases in the literature there are additional localizing ocular motor, eyelid, and usually other neurological signs. Eliciting eye movements or convergence may trigger the eyelid nystagmus, but it may also occur spontaneously.

Unilateral eyelid retraction

As with bilateral upper lid retraction, unilateral upper lid retraction with either a ptosis or normal position of the contralateral lid may occur as a result of neurogenic, myogenic, or mechanical causes. A contralateral ptosis, either congenital or acquired, may result in ipsilateral upper lid retraction. If the eye with the ptosis is occluded, the upper lid resumes a normal position relative to the globe on the unoccluded side.

A facial palsy may lead to an unopposed ipsilateral levator hyperfunction and an elevated lid.

Local fibrosis in the superior orbit may lead to unilateral upper lid retraction in the primary position, which increases on downgaze. This can occur as a result of local trauma or pathological processes such as focal orbital Langerhan cell histiocytosis. Unilateral proptosis may present as an upper lid retraction.

REFERENCES

1. Carney LG, Hill RM. The nature of normal blinking patterns. Acta Ophthalmol 1982; 60: 427–33.
2. Schmidtke K, Büttner-Ennever JA. Nervous control of eyelid function. A review of clinical, experimental and pathological data. Brain 1992; 115 Pt 1: 227–47.
3. Riggs AL, Volkmann FC, Moore RK. Suppression of the blackout that would otherwise be caused by blinks. Vision Res 1981; 21: 1075–9.
4. Collewijn H, Van Der Steen JP, Stinman RM. Human eye movements associated with blinks and prolonged eye closure. J Neurophysiol 1985; 54: 11–27.
5. Coats DK, Paysse EA, Kim DS. Excessive blinking in childhood: a prospective evaluation of 99 children. Ophthalmology 2001; 108: 1556–61.
6. Zee DS, Chu FC, Leigh RJ, et al. Blink-saccade synkinesis. Neurology 1983; 33: 1233–6.
7. Kobata H, Kondo A, Kinuta Y, et al. Hemifacial spasm in childhood and adolescence. Neurosurgery 1995; 36: 710–4.
8. Milani N, Scaioli V, Giombini S, et al. Hemifacial spasm in a child. Childs Nerv Syst 1991; 7: 466–8.
9. Sandberg DI, Souweidane MM. Hemifacial spasm caused by a pilocytic astrocytoma of the fourth ventricle. Pediatr Neurol 1999; 21: 754–6.
10. Flueler U, Taylor D, Hing S, et al. Hemifacial spasm in infancy. Arch Ophthalmol 1990; 108: 812–5.
11. Carter JB, Patrinely JR, Jankovic J, et al. Familial hemifacial spasm. Arch Ophthalmol 1990; 108: 249–50.
12. Brodsky MC, Thomas AH. Accommodative esotropia: an unrecognized cause of hemifacial spasm in children. Dev Med Child Neurol 2001; 43: 552–4.
13. Lees AJ. In: Tics and Related Disorders. Edinburgh: Churchill Livingstone; 1985: 12–4.
14. Binyon S, Prendergast M. Eye-movement tics in children. Dev Med Child Neurol 1991; 33: 352–5.
15. Shawkat F, Harris CM, Jacobs M, et al. Eye movements tics. Br J Ophthalmol 1992; 76: 697–9.
16. Khalifa N, von Knorring AL. Prevalence of tic disorders and Tourette syndrome in a Swedish school population. DevMedChild Neurol 2003; 45: 315–9.
17. Narita AS, Shawkat FS, Lask B, et al. Eye movement abnormalities in a case of Tourette syndrome. Dev Med Child Neurol 1997; 39: 270–3.
18. Margo CE. Tourette syndrome and iatrogenic eye injury. Am J Ophthalmol 2002; 134: 784–5.
19. Enoch JM, Itzhaki A, Lakshminarayanan V, et al. Gilles de la Tourette syndrome: visual effects. Neuroophthalmology 1988; 8: 251–7.
20. Leckman JF. Tourette syndrome. Lancet 2002; 360: 1577–86.
21. Lavenstein BL. Treatment approaches for children with Tourette syndrome. Curr Neurol Neurosci Rep 2003; 3: 143–8.
22. Khouri AS. Excessive blinking in children. Ophthalmology 2003; 110: 878.
23. Elston JS, Granje FC, Lees AJ. The relationship between eye-winking tics, frequent eye blinking and blepharospasm. Neurol Neurosurg Psychiatry 1989; 52: 477–80.
24. Ohtsu M, Hayashi K, Tanaka T, et al. [A case of idiopathic torsion dystonia showing blepharospasm at the onset]. No To Hattatsu 2002; 34: 254–61.
25. Tatlipinar S, Lener EC, IIlhan B, et al. Ophthalmic manifestations of Gilles de la Tourette syndrome. Eur J Ophthalmol 2001; 11: 223–6.
26. Jinnah HA, Lewis RF, Visser JE, et al. Ocular motor dysfunction in Lesch-Nyhan disease. Pediatr Neurol 2001; 24: 200–4.
27. Ragge NK, Hoyt WF. Midbrain myasthenia: fatigable ptosis, "lid twitch" sign, and ophthalmoparesis from a dorsal midbrain glioma. Neurology 1992; 42: 917–9.
28. Bartley GB. The differential diagnosis and classification of eyelid retraction. Ophthalmology 1996; 103: 168–76.

CHAPTER P7 The Child Who Closes One Eye

John R Ainsworth

There are two broad situations where children present with closure of one eye, acute and long-standing. Acute attendance, such as to a Casualty or A&E department, is common and diagnosis can be challenging in a younger child if the condition is painful. Presentation with a long-standing symptom to a routine clinic is unusual, and though there may be a history of eyelid closure it may not occur during the appointment.

ACUTE LID CLOSURE

In most instances a simple cause can be found. However, the circumstances of the initial eye examination are often less than ideal as care often commences in a general or eye casualty, or general practice. With appropriate skill, time, and equipment an accurate diagnosis is possible without general anesthesia or restraint in the majority of cases. If the child is distressed the examination can be targeted on the basis of history and observation toward a likely cause and exclusion of severe disease (Fig. P7.1).

Useful signs additional to the eye closure will be present and may include the following:

Proptosis, which implies an abnormality behind the globe, such as orbital cellulitis, hematoma, or varix (see Chapters 32, P11).

Eyelid swelling, which may harbor an inflamed chalazion. A classical "lazy S" profile indicates lacrimal gland pathology. Sudden onset of lid and conjunctival edema is most commonly associated with eye rubbing in the presence of allergic conjunctivitis.

Preseptal cellulitis, which in an infant is commonly associated with septicemia and requires systemic antibiotic therapy (see Chapter 20).

Watering, which implies conjunctival or corneal disease.

Photophobia, which occurs in corneal or intraocular disease, including pediatric glaucoma (see Chapter P9).

INTERMITTENT OR LONG-STANDING EYE CLOSURE

Chronic or recurrent *external eye disease* (e.g., Thygeson keratitis) should be excluded (see Chapter 22). However, most cases are likely to be due to less obvious causes.

Tics usually appear between 6 and 12 years of age and are common in boys. In most children the tic will be transient and isolated. On rare occasions there will be an underlying cause such as Tourette syndrome or obsessive-compulsive disorder, of which the tic may be the first feature.[1]

Intermittent exotropia is possibly the commonest association (see Chapter 81), although the child typically presents with the strabismus and the lid is a secondary symptom. It occurs outdoors especially in bright light. The reason for the association is unknown.

Diplopia is an unusual cause of eye closure in children, utilized by the child to eliminate the second image. The diplopia is likely to be of recent onset and often incomitant.

Hemifacial spasm (see Chapter P6) is rare in childhood and is usually associated with underlying disease, particularly fourth ventricle tumors.[2] It has also appeared prior to the development of intermittent esotropia.[3]

Ophthalmoplegic migraine is an atypical migraine that usually commences in childhood. Recurrent oculomotor nerve palsy including ptosis and lasting days or weeks can cause diagnostic uncertainty. MRI may confirm the diagnosis by demonstrating inflammation of the nerve in its interpeduncular course.[4]

Cyclic oculomotor palsy is another rare uniocular disorder that presents in childhood with frequent episodes of eye closure associated with third cranial nerve palsy.[5]

Histrionic ptosis may be unilateral or bilateral. It is much less common than transient tic.

UNILATERAL OR ASYMMETRIC BILATERAL EYE CLOSURE?

Although the child may be reported as closing one eye, examination may suggest a bilateral asymmetric abnormality.

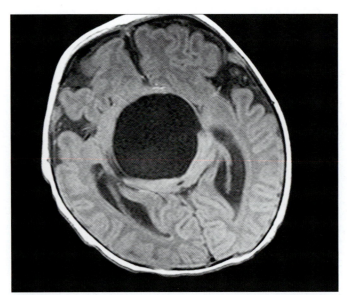

Fig. P7.1 Acquired unilateral eye closure in a 3-day-old infant with poor feeding and drowsiness. MRI revealed midbrain compression from a cystic teratoma. Drainage led to resolution of the ptosis.

Unilateral ptosis may be the presenting symptom of myasthenia or mitochondrial myopathy, but there is usually detectable fatigability or ptosis in the fellow eye, perhaps masked by the increased innervation used to maintain an unobstructed visual axis in the worse eye.

Some conditions commonly regarded as bilateral can occasionally produce uniocular findings, resulting in eye closure.

Blepharochalasis, a focal angioedema that presents as bilateral lid swelling and closure, occurs in a rare unilateral form.[6]

In *Tourette syndrome*, the classical eyelid tic is a bilateral eye blink or stare, but unilateral "eye winks" are also characteristic.

Blepharospasm without obvious external eye cause, whether a unilateral hemifacial spasm, bilateral orbicularis blepharospasm, or intractable orbicularis myokymia, is unusual in childhood. Imaging is indicated if the diagnosis is confirmed clinically (see Chapter P6).

Epilepsy in childhood can produce abnormal unilateral eye movements or bilateral eyelid flutter; unilateral eyelid abnormalities have not been described.

SUMMARY

Specialist referral primarily for a symptom of unilateral eye closure is unusual. If a cause is not apparent and there are no associated ophthalmic or neurological signs the most likely diagnosis is of isolated transient tic.

REFERENCES

1. Chee KY, Sachdev P. The clinical features of Tourette's disorder: an Australian study using a structured interview schedule. Aust NZJ Psychiatry 1994; 28: 313–8.
2. Sandberg DI, Souweidane MM. Hemifacial spasm caused by a pilocytic astrocytoma of the fourth ventricle. Pediatr Neurol 1994; 21: 754–6.
3. Brodsky MC, Thomas AH. Accommodative esotropia: an unrecognized cause of hemifacial spasm in children. Dev Med Child Neurol 2001; 43: 552–4.
4. Carlow TJ. Oculomotor ophthalmoplegic migraine: is it really migraine? J Neuroophthalmol 2002; 22: 215–21.
5. Fells P, Collin JR. Cyclic oculomotor palsy. Trans Ophthalmol Soc UK 1979; 99: 192–6.
6. Huemer GM, Schoeller T, Wechselberger G, et al. Unilateral blepharochalasis. Br J Plast Surg 2003; 56: 293–5.

CHAPTER P8 | Dry Eye and Inappropriate Tearing

Gillian G W Adams

DRY EYE

The eye is protected against damage and infection by the lids and by a lubricating tear film. The surface of an eye dries if the tear film is inadequate to wet it or if the tears evaporate rapidly to allow desiccation.

Abnormalities of lid closure can result in both an increased evaporation of tears and corneal exposure with epithelial drying. The presence of corneal anesthesia exacerbates the effects of drying and exposure and puts the eye at risk of defective epithelial healing, corneal ulceration, and perforation.

The diagnosis of dry eye may be made on the history alone and may simply require a confirmatory examination but it may be the clinical findings that suggest the diagnosis.

Presentation, symptoms, and signs

Children rarely complain of a dry eye, but usually complain of a gritty, itchy, or scratchy eye, a foreign body or burning sensation, or blurred vision and light sensitivity. They may have noticed that their eyes are worse in dry or windy atmospheres where there is increased tear evaporation, or with prolonged reading or use of the computer due to a reduced blink rate.

On examination, the child may have injected, irritable, eyes with photophobia or excessive blinking. The vision is usually normal in cases of mild dry eye but, in more severe forms with significant corneal desiccation, the acuity may be reduced.

Diagnosis

A severe dry eye is easily diagnosed but the milder forms may go unrecognized. A dry eye in childhood is uncommon, and it is underdiagnosed. The diagnosis is based on the history, observation of the ocular signs, and other tests, most commonly Schirmer's test.

Although many cases of dry eye will have a simple explanation such as incomplete eye closure while sleeping in a dry, centrally heated or air-conditioned bedroom, a dry eye in childhood may be the first sign of a rare but serious systemic disorder, and the ophthalmologist, who may be the first physician to examine the child, should be alert to this possibility.

History

A full history should seek relevant information. A dry eye may be associated with a local ophthalmic disorder such as conjunctival scarring, with some systemic diseases including skin, joint, gut, and respiratory problems or with drug medication. Topical beta-blocker or systemic antihistamine can produce ocular dryness. Stevens-Johnson syndrome may occur as an adverse reaction to antibiotics, anticonvulsants, or an infectious agent.[1] Dry eye is a common ocular complication of pediatric bone marrow transplantation.[2] Trachoma is rare in the developed world but not elsewhere.

The parents should be asked if the child produces reflex or emotional tears. It has been said that babies do not produce tears until 6 weeks of age but tears are produced from the first day of life.[3] Congenital alacrima is rare, and even in these cases, the eye surface is often moist despite the absence of reflex or emotional tears.[4] It may occur as a dominant trait due to aplasia or hypoplasia of the lacrimal gland or in association with systemic disturbances including the Riley-Day syndrome, the ectodermal dysplasia syndromes, and the "triple A" syndrome[5] (adrenocorticoid deficiency, achalasia of the cardia, and alacrima). The ocular surface changes in ectodermal dysplasia syndromes may also be due to the primary ectodermal defect.[6]

The parents should be asked whether the child sleeps with their eyes open. This may occur in normal children,[7] in those with craniofacial disorders, proptosis, and lid abnormalities, or after ptosis surgery.

Examination

The following signs will allow the diagnosis to be established:

- Best corrected visual acuity;
- External inspection: face, lid closure and blink rate, external eye, and tear strip;
- Ocular surface examination;
- Staining patterns; and
- Other tests: Schirmer's test, impression cytology, and corneal sensation.

The examination should start with an external inspection of the child, its face, eye, and eyelids and then the ocular surface, if possible using a slit lamp, and other tests as indicated. Some of the tests will only be possible in the older child. In the younger or the less easily examinable child a torch with or without a 20-D lens for magnification can be used. If the child has severe dry eyes it is likely to be photophobic and difficult to examine unless it has corneal anesthesia. Be alert to the possibility of loss of sensation as the combination of dry eye and corneal anesthesia can result in severe keratitis.

External inspection

Look at the whole child, its face, and external eye. If very photophobic the child may not open its eyes. Check for the facies of a syndromic disorder that may be associated with a dry eye such as ectodermal dysplasia or the Marfanoid appearance, thick lips and eyelid neuromas of multiple endocrine neoplasia (MEN) IIb. Inspect whether the lacrimal gland appears swollen as dacryoadenitis can cause an acute keratoconjunctivitis sicca due to lacrimal gland dysfunction.[8]

Assess the blink rate and lid closure. Check for an abnormality that causes ocular surface exposure and drying such as proptosis, a craniofacial syndrome, or a shallow orbit. Look for lid abnormalities such as ectropion, scarring, notches, or colobomas, and for blepharitis and meibomianitis. Meibomianitis and blepharitis may destabilize the tear film and cause surface drying. Assess lid closure, because if inadequate, the tear film cannot maintain corneal wetting and the ocular surface will desiccate. After ptosis surgery a poor Bell's phenomenon or poor upgaze will allow the eye to dry out. If there is evidence of facial weakness or poor lid closure the presence or absence of Bell's phenomenon and corneal sensation should be noted.

Normally, an eye should be "white" with a bright, moist surface. If the eye is mildly injected with a dull surface and little moisture visible in the tear film the child has a dry eye.

Ocular surface examination and staining patterns

If possible this should by undertaken by slit-lamp examination, which is possible in most children from about the age of 3 years, but if not possible a 20-D lens and torch can be substituted. The examination should inspect the conjunctiva, the cornea, the tear film, the tear break-up time, and the surface staining patterns.

In children with significant dry eye the inferior tear strip will be reduced and contain mucus strands and debris.[9] The tear break-up time should be estimated after the instillation of fluorescein drops without anesthetic as fluorescein strips or topical anesthetic will reduce the break-up time. The time is the interval between the end of a blink and the first appearance of dry spots in the fluorescein-stained tear film; less than 10 s is abnormal. Staining of the ocular surface may be assessed with fluorescein or Rose Bengal. Rose Bengal staining of devitalized epithelial cells is a sensitive test of dryness of the cornea and conjunctiva. The dye is instilled as a 1% solution without anesthetic, which can dry the surface, and is uncomfortable so as little solution as possible should be used. The degree of ocular surface dryness can be graded from no staining to staining of the whole cornea and corneal ulceration.

The conjunctiva should be examined for scarring or other abnormality. Severe conjunctival chemosis may cause incomplete lid closure with drying of the eye. The bulbar conjunctiva should be examined and then the lower lid gently pulled down to inspect the tarsal conjunctiva. In the older child it may be possible to evert the upper lid and examine the conjunctiva of the tarsal plate. The conjunctiva may be hyperemic with blisters or pseudomembrane in the early stages of Stevens-Johnson syndrome, followed later by scarring and symblepharon. A mucopurulent conjunctivitis is followed by cicatrization, dry eyes, and corneal scarring in trachoma. The initial signs of hypovitaminosis A occur in the conjunctiva, which is dry and wrinkled with Bitot's spots in the exposed areas followed by keratomalacia as the cornea becomes involved. The presence of dermolipomas and epibulbar dermoids may provide an area for surface drying and suggest a syndrome such as Goldenhar.[10] There may be irregular healing after strabismus surgery, causing conjunctival drying.

The corneal surface should be inspected for dullness, dellen, scarring, ulceration, the presence or absence of corneal nerves, and mucus filaments or plaques. Prominent corneal nerves may be present in patients with MEN IIb.

Other tests
Schirmer's test

The Schirmer's test assesses tear secretion. It can assess basal (unstimulated) secretion if done without anesthetic or reflex (stimulated) secretion if performed after the use of local anesthetic. The test may be difficult to perform in children, and is likely to have to be performed after the instillation of local anesthetic. To perform the test, a filter paper of standard size and width is hung over the lower lid into the conjunctival fornix usually at the junction of the middle and outer one-third without touching the cornea. The child then shuts their eyes gently for 5 min, after which the filter paper is removed and the wetted portion of the paper is measured. An abnormal result is a wetting of 5 mm or less.

Impression cytology

Conjunctival impression cytology, performed by gently rubbing Millipore filter paper against the conjunctival surface, obtains a sheet of cells, which can be stained for epithelial cell morphology and goblet cell density (Fig. P8.1). Epithelial cell cytology is abnormal in damaged eyes and the density of goblet cells, which produce mucus, decreases with an alteration in the normal staining patterns in various diseases including chronic cicatricial change and inflammation (Fig. P8.2). In dry eyes the bulbar ocular surface has been shown to have abnormal epithelium with reduced goblet cell density.[11] This test is only usually possible in the older more cooperative child or in the younger child during an examination under anesthesia.

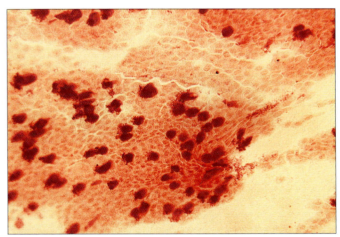

Fig. P8.1 Normal impression cytology showing a confluent sheet of epithelial cells and goblet cells with deep pink-staining intracellular mucus.

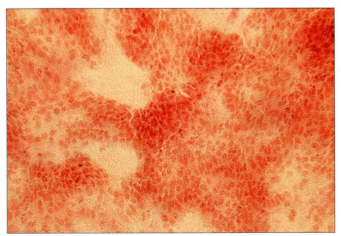

Fig. P8.2 Impression cytology from a child with ectodermal dysplasia showing an almost complete absence of goblet cells.

Corneal sensation

Corneal sensation can be tested using a fine wisp of cotton wool, for example from the tip of a cotton bud, to gently touch the corneal surface. A child with normal sensation will either tell you they can feel it or blink and draw away. Observation of the child's reaction to the instillation of drops will also give an indication of sensation. Corneal sensation is reduced in any severe keratitis and should be unequivocal to be of clinical importance.

Causes of dry eye

Alacrima/tear gland abnormality

- Congenital alacrima;
- Dacryoadenitis; and
- In association with other syndromes (craniosynostosis, Goldenhar syndrome, Duane syndrome, Möbius syndrome, familial glucocorticoid deficiency with achalasia of the cardia ("triple A" syndrome), ectodermal dysplasia syndromes, and multiple endocrine neoplasia type IIb).

External eye abnormalities

- Incomplete lid closure: blink abnormality, post ptosis repair, Down syndrome, proptosis, shallow orbits in craniofacial abnormalities and syndromic conditions;

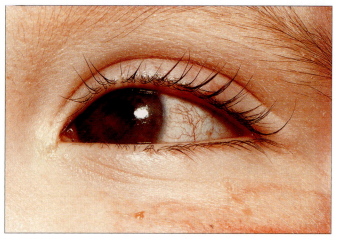

Fig. P8.3 Corneal drying, ulceration, scarring, and vascularization in Riley-Day syndrome. The combination of anesthesia and dryness makes keratitis a significant problem for many of these children.

- Lid defect: notches, scarring, ectropion (see also Chapters 25 and 26);
- Blepharitis, meibomianitis (see also Chapters 22 & 26); and
- Facial palsy.

Ocular surface

- Conjunctival fibrosis: trachoma, vitamin A deficiency, Stevens-Johnson syndrome (see also Chapter 22);
- Conjunctival dermoid, pinguecula, tumors, scarring (see also Chapter 27);
- Corneal dellen;
- Ectodermal dysplasia (see also Chapters 27 and 29); and
- Post chemotherapy, radiotherapy, and bone marrow transplantation (see also Chapter 68).

Associated with reduced corneal sensation/anesthesia

- Riley-Day syndrome;
- Neuroparalytic keratitis; and
- Goldenhar syndrome (see also Chapters 25 and 28).

Riley-Day syndrome

Also called familial dysautonomia, this rare autosomal recessive disorder affects the sympathetic, parasympathetic, and sensory nervous system with neurological, systemic, and ophthalmological manifestations.[12,13] It is mainly but not exclusively found in Ashkenazi Jews (those of European origin) and affects both sexes. Dysfunction of the autonomic nervous system produces labile blood pressure, skin blotching, unstable temperature, and excessive sweating. Sensory disturbance produces insensitivity to pain and reduced taste perception. Other signs are hyporeflexia, motor incoordination, poor swallowing, drooling, anxiety, and emotional lability.

Ophthalmologically the two most significant findings are dry eyes due to absence of tears and either absent or significantly reduced corneal sensation. This combination of deficits produces corneal ulceration (Fig. P8.3). There is evidence of denervation hypersensitivity with pupillary constriction after instillation of dilute (2.5%) methacholine or 0.1% pilocarpine as is seen in Adie syndrome (Fig. P8.4). Other reported findings are exodeviations, myopia, anisocoria, retinal tortuosity, anisometropia, and ptosis.

Nonophthalmic diagnostic features are that an intradermal injection of histamine produces a wheal without the normal

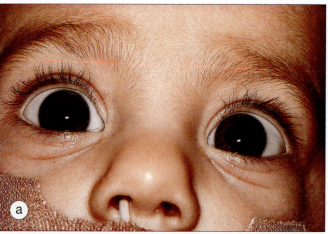
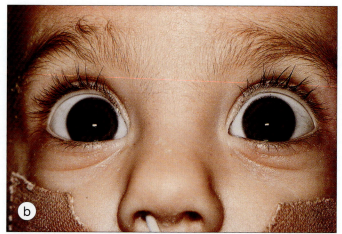

Fig. P8.4 (a) Riley-Day syndrome at the time of instillation of pilocarpine 0.1%. (There is no change in pupil size in normal children.) (b) Same patient, same lighting conditions, 20 min later. The denervation hypersensitivity is indicated by the pupil constriction.

erythematous response and the absence of the fungiform papillae of the tongue.

Neuroparalytic keratitis (NPK)

This may occur unilaterally or bilaterally. There is corneal anesthesia due to damage to the trigeminal nerve. This can be seen with acoustic neuroma or pontine tumors, after trauma or herpes zoster, and has been reported in Goldenhar syndrome and leprosy. If associated with facial palsy or deficient tear production, producing a dry anesthetic eye, there is a high risk of ulceration.

Management

- General advice;
- Avoid drying;
- Lubrication: preservative free medication;
- Acetyl cysteine dropsl;
- Punctal occlusion: temporary, permanent;
- Glasses and moisture-retaining goggles;
- Contact lenses;
- Tarsorrhaphy: temporary, permanent; and
- Salivary gland transplant.

General advice

The aim of treatment is to improve surface wetting and reduce the child's symptoms. If there is an obvious treatable cause of drying such as a lid that cannot close fully after ptosis surgery or where there is a lid defect causing ocular surface desiccation the child should be referred to an oculoplastic specialist. A child with significant ocular exposure due to proptosis from facial deformity or orbital tumor may need to be considered for craniofacial surgery. Drugs contributing to ocular surface drying should be stopped if possible. Vitamin A deficiency should be treated with supplementation. Acute dacryoadenitis is treated with antiviral and anti-inflammatory therapy where indicated.

Whatever the underlying condition, treatment will also be required to prevent further drying. The management becomes more complex if there is also reduced corneal sensation.

Avoid drying

A simple explanation of the problem and advice about the effect of central heating and air conditioning is important. Simple measures for hydrating the atmosphere may be beneficial. Reminding older children to remember to blink when doing computer work and suggesting breaking computer work up into smaller time blocks interspersed with other tasks may be helpful.

In children with significant risk of exposure, for example in intensive care situations or with lack or significant loss of lid closure, protection, in addition to lubrication, should be provided (Fig. P8.5a). The lids may be taped shut but care should be taken to apply tape safely and effectively to provide adequate corneal cover. A protective bubble shield can be taped to the face or a polyacrylamide gel (Geliperm) placed over the eyes[14] (Fig. P8.5b).

Lubrication

The mainstay of treatment is ocular lubrication using topical preparations either drops or ointment. There are many preparations available and different lubricants will help different children. Drops are more useful as ointment will blur the vision, which is unpopular but it may be useful to consider an ointment preparation, preferably preservative free, for use at night. If drops are needed more than four times a day or on a long-term basis it is appropriate to consider the use of preservative-free drops as preservative itself may cause corneal drying and exacerbate the problem. Lubricant drops are now available in a variety of single-dose preparations.

Topical hypotonic hyaluronic acid has also proved helpful and may produce more improvement in symptoms and signs than other artificial tear substitutes.[15]

Acetyl cysteine drops

If the presence of corneal filaments and mucus is significant and contributing to discomfort then topical acetyl cysteine (10 or 20%) may be helpful.

Punctal occlusion: temporary, permanent

The use of drops more than four times a day is difficult unless the child is old enough to instill the treatment for itself. In this situation ointment can be used but this does produce blurring, which may not be acceptable. If considerable lubrication is required then punctal occlusion should be considered. This can be done temporarily with collagen implants or more permanently with lacrimal plugs, which have the advantage that they can be removed if occlusion is over effective with epiphora. They also avoid producing punctal scarring. In small children plugs need to be inserted under general anesthesia but in the older cooperative child this can be performed at the slit lamp. Permanent punctal occlusion using cautery or ligature of the ducts is occasionally required in chronic conditions such as Riley-Day syndrome.

Glasses and moisture-retaining goggles

Glasses with side shields, or for more effect goggles, to reduce tear loss by evaporation and to increase local humidity can be

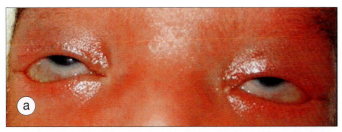
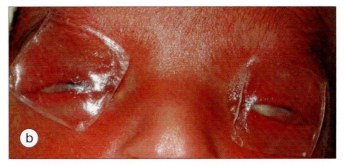

Fig. P8.5 a) Infant with Wolf-Hirschorn syndrome. He had ocular exposure with dryness due to incomplete lid closure. (b) Same patient with the eyes protected with Geliperm and demonstrating a good Bell's phenomenon.

tried. There is likely to be an element of "consumer resistance" from the older child concerned about the appearance of the goggles but if the eyes are sore enough they may be persuaded to wear them.

Contact lenses

These have been advocated but in dry eyes there is a considerable risk of infection, and their use, especially of soft contact lenses, should be approached with caution and close monitoring. The use of lenses must be combined with the frequent instillation of preservative-free lubricant drops. Scleral lenses can be tried as the precorneal reservoir gives better hydration but they are more difficult to fit and insert. Parents should be asked to bring the child back for immediate review if the eyes become sore and cannot be opened or if a discharge is noted (see Chapter P28).

Tarsorrhaphy: temporary, permanent

An anesthetic eye especially if associated with a facial palsy has a significant chance of developing corneal ulceration, which is difficult to treat. In this situation a tarsorrhaphy is often required to produce healing and prevent future damage. The most effective type of tarsorrhaphy for this condition is a central one, which is rarely a popular option with either the child or its parents.

With long-term facial palsy and intact corneal sensation, protection can be provided by a combination of small lateral and medial tarsorrhaphies, which are both more effective and cosmetically better than a large lateral closure. If there is temporary facial weakness, with ocular surface exposure, which is expected to improve, as in a Bell's palsy, then a botulinum toxin protective ptosis should be considered, as it will provide short-acting protection without damage to the lid margins[15] (Fig. P8.6). It is easily achieved by injecting a low dose of botulinum toxin A (BTXA) (usually 2.5–7.5 units, 62.5–187.5 pg of Dysport, i.e., 1–3 times a standard strabismus dose), passing a 25-G, 25-mm needle just beneath the supraorbital margin along the roof of the orbit to its full length prior to injecting the toxin. Complications are reduced by using a small volume and include an induced vertical deviation due to underaction of the ipsilateral superior rectus muscle and preseptal hemorrhage. Full closure may not be achieved in the presence of a facial palsy but the eye will be closed sufficiently to protect the ocular surface. Maximum ptosis will last about two weeks before the lid starts to lift and levator function will have returned to pretreatment level in two to three months. It can be repeated as required. Although it can easily be done in adults and older children without anesthetizing the lid, in the younger, more frightened child the procedure should be undertaken under general anesthesia or sedation.

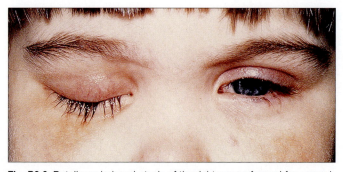

Fig. P8.6 Botulinum induced ptosis of the right eye performed for corneal protection in a 2½-year-old child with Stevens-Johnson syndrome

Temporary lid closure has been attempted with cyanoacrylate glue but in the main is not very effective as it lasts only a short period of time, a few days to about a week, and may be uncomfortable and prevent examination of the ocular surface.

Salivary gland transplant

Submandibular gland autografts have been used in adults for severe dry eyes but, although it improves ocular comfort and wetting, it does not improve vision.[16] It is probably not appropriate for use in very small children but may have a place in the older child with significant problems. Following this procedure the eye is bathed in salivary tears not lacrimal tears, which have a different enzyme and electrolyte composition.[17] Corneal edema occurs in some cases. This is not an option for anything other than severe dry eye.

INAPPROPRIATE TEARING

Presentation, signs, and symptoms

Inappropriate tearing is that occurring out of emotional context or not due to obvious stimulation such as exposure to a noxious smell, e.g., ammonia. The history should ascertain for how long the child's eye has watered, and if of recent onset whether there is a history of any previous eye trauma. Check whether the watering occurs constantly or only with certain activities such as eating.

If the eye is uncomfortable, it may be difficult to examine the child and the instillation of topical anesthetic is useful. If the symptoms improve after local anesthetic then the most likely cause of the tearing is an ocular surface problem. The eye should be examined for possible causes both externally and internally, including foreign bodies, in-growing eyelashes, keratitis or ulceration, and uveitis. Recurrent corneal erosion may follow a minor episode of trauma. A subtarsal foreign body, especially if transparent, is easy to overlook and if the history and corneal-staining pattern suggest this possibility, then the upper lid should be everted and examined. If there is any suggestion of an enlarged eye or cloudy cornea, or any other indicator of glaucoma, the intraocular pressure must be checked. If the child cannot be adequately assessed in clinic, then an examination under anesthetic will be required. A full description of the causes of epiphora is given in Chapter 31.

Causes of inappropriate tearing

- External eye conditions (see also Chapter 22);
- Congenital glaucoma (see also Chapter 48);
- Subtarsal foreign body; and
- Crocodile tears.

Crocodile tears

Profuse lacrimation when eating or drinking is called the gustolacrimal reflex, also known more poetically as crocodile tears from the legend that crocodiles cry hypocritical tears while eating their victims.[18] The condition may be congenital when it can be bilateral or more commonly it is acquired and unilateral. Most are acquired, and follow traumatic or inflammatory conditions of the facial nerve, or the greater superficial petrosal nerve. Acquired causes include post Bell's palsy, zoster infection, following intracranial surgery or head injury, and associated with cerebello pontine angle tumours. Congenital cases are usually associated with abnormalities of lateral rectus function especially

Duane syndrome but have also been reported in the Dandy-Walker and the Treacher-Collins syndromes. This suggests a central pontine location for the causative lesion.

The cause is either an aberrant regeneration phenomenon or due to formation of an artificial synapse with transaxonal transmission and short-circuiting of nerve impulses.[19] This produces hyperlacrimation, which should be distinguished from epiphora due to lower lid laxity and reduced mechanical drainage that may be seen after Bell's palsy.

Treatment

Acquired crocodile tears without a prior history of a facial palsy or intracranial injury or surgery should prompt referral to a pediatric neurologist for further investigation.

Intraorbital injections of alcohol, resection of the lacrimal gland, and anticholinergic drugs have all been tried, mostly without success. The most effective treatment for abolishing hyperlacrimation appears to be intraglandular or periglandular injection of botulinum toxin A.[20] As with all injections of toxin around the eye the side-effects include ptosis and superior rectus underaction; temporary dry eye has also been reported to occur.

REFERENCES

1. Prendiville JS, Hebert AA, Greenwald MJ, et al. Management of Stevens-Johnson syndrome and toxic epidermal necrolysis in children. J Pediatr 1989; 115: 881–7.
2. Suh DW, Ruttum MS, Stuckenschneider BJ, et al. Ocular findings after bone marrow transplantation in a pediatric population. Ophthalmology 1999; 106: 1564–70.
3. Patrick RK. Lacrimal secretion in full-term and premature babies. Trans Ophthalmol Soc UK 1974; 94: 283–90.
4. Sjögren H, Eriksen A. Alacrimia congenital. Br J Ophthalmol 1950; 34: 691–4.
5. Allgrove J, Clayden GS, Grant DB, et al. Familial glucocorticoid deficiency with achalasia of the cardia and deficient tear production. Lancet 1978; 1284–6.
6. Baum JL, Bull MJ. Ocular manifestations of the ectrodactyly, ectodermal dysplasia, cleft lip-palate syndrome. Am J Ophthalmol 1974; 78: 211–6.
7. Katz J, Kaufman HE. Corneal exposure during sleep (nocturnal lagophthalmos). Arch Ophthalmol 1977; 95: 449–53.
8. Merayo-Lloves J, Baltatzis S, Foster CS. Epstein-Barr virus dacryoadenitis resulting in keratoconjunctivitis sicca in a child. Am J Ophthalmol 2001; 132: 922–3.
9. Baum J. Clinical manifestations of dry eye states. Trans Ophthalmol Soc UK 1985; 104: 415–23.
10. Baum JL, Feingold M. Ocular aspects of Goldenhar's syndrome. Am J Ophthalmol 1973; 75: 250–7.
11. Nelson JD, Havener VR, Cameron JD. Cellulose acetate impressions of the ocular surface. Dry eye states. Arch Ophthalmol 1983; 101: 1869–72.
12. Liebman SD. Riley-Day syndrome: long-term ophthalmologic observations. Tr Am Ophthalmol Soc 1968; 66: 95–116.
13. Goldberg MF, Payne JW, Brunt PW. Ophthalmologic studies of familial dysautonomia. Arch Ophthalmol 1968; 80: 732–43.
14. Farrell M, Wray F. Eye care for ventilated patients. Intensive Crit Care Nurs 1993; 9: 137–41.
15. Adams GG, Kirkness CM, Lee JP. Botulinum toxin A induced protective ptosis. Eye 1987; 1: 603–8.
16. Lester M, Orsoni GJ, Gamba G, et al. Improvement of the ocular surface using hypotonic 0.4% hyaluronic acid drops in kerato-conjunctivitis sicca. Eye 2000; 14: 892–8.
17. Geerling G, Sieg P, Bastian GO, et al. Transplantation of the autologous submandibular gland for most severe cases of kerato-conjunctivitis sicca. Ophthalmology 1998; 105: 327–35.
18. Golding-Wood PH. Crocodile tears. Br Med J 1963; 5344: 1518–21.
19. Sadjadpour K. Postfacial palsy phenomena: faulty nerve regeneration or ephaptic transmission? Brain Res 1975; 95: 403–6.
20. Riemann R, Pfennigsdorf S, Riemann E, et al. Successful treatment of crocodile tears by injection of botulinum toxin into the lacrimal gland: a case report. Ophthalmology 1999; 106: 2322–4.

CHAPTER

P9 Photophobia

Abdulaziz H Awad

DEFINITION

Photophobia is light sensitivity that makes the child uncomfortable under normal lighting conditions. Although (in its mild form) it is not uncommon in normal infants and children, it must be taken seriously as it can, rarely, be the presenting symptom of serious disorders like congenital glaucoma or anterior visual pathway tumors. It should, however, be differentiated from epiphora (see Chapter P10).

SIGNS

Children with photophobia may have characteristic facial expression with narrow palpebral fissures and furrowed brow; they may also show:
1. Closure of one or both eyes (with or without squeezing of the lids);
2. Frequent blinking;
3. Epiphora;
4. Ocular pain;
5. Headaches; and
6. Heterotropia.

DIFFERENTIAL DIAGNOSES

There is a lot of variability and overlap in the symptoms but the following may be helpful.

Gauging the *severity of the photophobia* can be important in making a diagnosis:
1. *Severe photophobia*: discomfort under extreme (bright sunlight), normal (standard indoor room illumination), and low (dimmed indoor room illumination) lighting conditions.
   Associated with excessive epiphora
   a. Congenital glaucoma;
   b. Corneal surface disruption, e.g., corneal foreign body, epithelial defect, or corneal burn;
   c. Corneal inflammatory disease (keratitis);
   d. Tyrosinemia type II; and
   e. Cystinosis.
   Associated with less or no epiphora
   f. CNS disorders–including encephalitis, meningitis, migraine, trigeminal neuralgia, and subarachnoid hemorrhage;
   g. Achromatopsia (rod monochromatism);
   h. Oculocutaneous albinism;
   i. Total aniridia; and
   j. Corneal scars.
2. *Moderate photophobia*: discomfort under both extreme (bright sunlight) and normal (standard indoor room illumination) lighting conditions.

a. Iris-hypoplasia (partial aniridia) and colobomas (congenital or surgical/traumatic);
   b. Uveitis (traumatic or associated with corneal inflammatory disorders);
   c. Cataract zonular/lamellar or posterior subcapsular cataract;
   d. Ectopia lentis;
   e. Anterior visual pathway tumors and optic neuritis;
   f. Cortical visual impairment;
   g. Filariasis; and
   h. Drug induced (e.g., pharmacological dilation).
3. *Mild photophobia*: Characterized by discomfort only under extreme (bright sunlight) lighting conditions.
   a. Corneal stromal edema–including conditions such as congenital hereditary endothelial dystrophy (CHED);
   b. Strabismus–most commonly associated with latent or intermittent strabismus (especially with exotropia), but also seen with manifest strabismus;
   c. Posterior fossa tumors; and
   d. Conjunctivitis.

Taking into consideration the *age of the patient* can also be very helpful:
1. Infants
   a. Congenital glaucoma;
   b. Congenital cone dystrophies;
   c. Corneal inflammatory disease, e.g., congenital infections (less common);
   d. Tyrosinemia type II; and
   e. Birth trauma (e.g., forceps delivery).
2. Toddlers
   a. Trauma (corneal abrasions, foreign body); and
   b. Keratitis.
3. Preschool children
   a. Albinism;
   b. Aniridia; and
   c. Monochromatism.
4. School-age children
   a. Nonorganic visual loss;
   b. Latent or intermittent strabismus; and
   c. Migraine.

ETIOLOGY

Conjunctiva

Mild photophobia is an uncommon manifestation of mucopurulent conjunctivitis; however, certain conjunctivitis maybe associated with significant photophobia, either by concomitant keratitis as in epidemic acute follicular conjunctivitis or by disruption of the normal ocular surface and tear function as in membranous or pseudomembranous conjunctivitis, e.g., Stevens-Johnson syndrome (see Chapter 22).

Cornea

Corneal disorders are the most common cause of photophobia. One or more of the following mechanisms may contribute to photophobia (see Chapter 29):

A. Epithelial injury as with corneal abrasions, foreign bodies, corneal burns, or complicated contact lens use. It should be suspected with the history of recent onset of severe photophobia with epiphora associated to a variable extent with conjunctival hyperemia and eyelids edema. Examination is usually facilitated by installation of topical anesthetic eye drops to reduce the pain and enhance patient cooperation. Fluorescein staining readily stains the abraded corneal surface and would help to exclude penetration (Seidel test).

B. Failure of restoration of the normal corneal surface as with xeroderma pigmentosa.[1] See Chapter 27 or Tyrosinemia type II (Richner-Hanhart Syndrome), where photophobia may be the presenting symptom as early as two weeks of age.[2,3]

C. Corneal stromal changes.
   1. Edema as with congenital hereditary endothelial dystrophy (CHED)–see Chapter 30. Photophobia is not marked due to sparing of the corneal epithelium.
   2. Scarring–corneal scars are an important cause of photophobia in children particularly if the visual axis is involved probably due to light scattering.
   3. Deposition of unusual material as with cystinosis, especially with recurrent erosions.[4] See Chapter 29.
   4. Corneal inflammatory diseases (keratitis)–keratitis is a very important cause of photophobia as it is usually associated with corneal surface disruption, and uveitis, which makes the photophobia even more prominent. In children, keratitis can be of variable etiology. See Chapter 22.

Glaucoma

Congenital glaucoma is by far the most common cause of photophobia in infancy; it should always be suspected. See Chapter 48.

Acute pupillary block glaucoma is rare in children: it is secondary to anterior subluxation of the lens, complicating microspherophakia, or vitreous block in aphakic eyes.

Uvea

One or more of the following abnormalities account for photophobia:

a. Aniridia–loss of pupil function (see Chapter 43)–ocular surface disturbance (aniridia keratopathy).

b. Ocular and oculocutaneous albinism[5,6] (see Chapter 45).

c. Uveitis–(see Chapter 44) photophobia is most commonly associated with anterior uveitis (iridocyclitis). It is most frequently reported by children whose uveitis has traumatic etiology as well as by those with endophthalmitis, or is secondary to corneal inflammatory disorders or secondary to neoplastic infiltration of the iris and ciliary body. However, anterior uveitis associated with juvenile rheumatoid arthritis (JRA) is usually silent, and photophobia is an uncommon complaint. These patients are usually picked up through the screening process.

Lens

Partial cataracts, particularly posterior subcapsular and lamellar or zonular cataracts, and ectopia lentis are the most likely lenticular conditions that can lead to photophobia (see Chapters 46 and 47). Light scattering or glare is the most likely mechanism for photophobia in zonular or lamellar cataract and in ectopia lentis, while in posterior subcapsular cataract the significant impairment in vision with incrossing illumination is probably the cause of photophobia.

Retina

Photophobia is particularly common among patients with congenital cone dystrophies. Cone dystrophies can be of variable severity and are often associated with poor vision and nystagmus. The nystagmus is usually of the high-frequency, low-amplitude variety. Many of these children will experience a remarkable increase in visual acuity with decreased ambient illumination.[7] Photophobia is most prominent in achromatopsia (rod monochromatism); however, various cone dystrophies are associated with variable severity of photophobia (see Chapter 54).

Optic nerve

A variable degree of photophobia has been reported in some patients with optic neuritis. The severity of the photophobia maybe significant despite extremely poor vision. The exact mechanism is poorly understood (see Chapter 61).

Central nervous system

Several disease processes affecting the central nervous system could account for photophobia (see Chapters 61–63). It can be severe in children with encephalitis, meningitis, subarachnoid hemorrhage, and trigeminal neuralgia, and in migraine. Photophobia is less pronounced, but still significant, in patients with anterior visual pathway tumors and optic neuritis and in children with cortical visual impairment. When cortical impairment is congenital the photophobia is present from birth, and when it is acquired it follows immediately the brain insult. The intensity of light sensitivity tends to diminish with time.[8]

The pathophysiology of photophobia in central nervous system disorders is unclear; however, it could be related to the trigeminal nerve, which is responsible for much of the sensation in the periorbital region and the meninges.

Strabismus

Mild to moderate photophobia is common in patients with latent and dissociated deviations (see Chapter 81); however, even patients with manifest strabismus may display these behaviors, which most commonly include monocular closure under bright outdoor lighting conditions. Photophobia rather than diplopia-avoidance is the most likely cause of the monocular closure.[9] The mechanism of photophobia in these cases is still unclear.

Less common causes

a. Nonorganic factors – a common attention-seeking behavior among prepubertal children with frequent blinking associated with headache, periorbital pain, diplopia, and photophobia. Although a complete examination may be in order to rule out factors such as a foreign body, corneal abrasion, or mild conjunctivitis, simple compassionate reassurance of the benign nature of this entity is usually all that is required.

b. Fair skin and ocular pigmentation–it has been observed that nonalbino children who simply have a very fair complexion will complain of photophobia. This situation demands that ocular albinism is ruled out. Usually these symptoms would dissipate with age.

EXAMINATION

The direction of the patient examination is dependent upon the suspected etiology by history and appearance of the patient's photophobic symptoms. As is always the case in pediatric ophthalmology, there will be limitations imposed according to the level of cooperation obtained. However, all possible attempts should be made to ensure that the examination is as complete as possible.

Some recommended examination paths would include:

1. Look for signs of buphthalmos when glaucoma is suspected. This should be followed by a careful measurement of the patient's intraocular pressure.
2. Visual acuity assessment with careful attention for nystagmus.
3. Local anesthetic to evaluate patients with suspected corneal abrasions or intraocular foreign bodies followed by fluorescein staining.
4. Transillumination to rule out either oculocutaneous or ocular albinism.
5. An evaluation of extraocular motility, including a very careful cover–uncover test to rule out a latent or dissociated strabismus.
6. Fundus examination may disclose ocular albinism with foveal hypoplasia.
7. Electropsychological studies (electroretinography and visually evoked response) and neuroradiological imaging are desirable in certain cases to confirm the diagnosis or rule out certain disease processes.

8. In very uncooperative children with significant photophobia, sedated exam or examination under general anesthesia should be undertaken for proper evaluation with biomicroscopy, intraocular pressure evaluation, and fundus examination.

MANAGEMENT

Identifying the underlying etiology is the first step toward the appropriate management. Congenital glaucoma is a surgical disease, and surgery should be undertaken as soon as possible to avoid further damage to the cornea that can lead to permanent scarring and visual impairment. Cataract surgery may be undertaken to improve visual performance and relieve photophobia. Corneal surface disorders are treated according to the underlying etiology, e.g., corneal foreign body removal and patching for corneal abrasion and appropriate treatment with antibiotic agent for microbial keratitis.

Iris-colored IOL implants have been reported to help patients with aniridia and cataract who underwent cataract surgery; however, this procedure has not yet gained wide acceptance probably because the majority of these patients have other associated anomalies, e.g., keratopathy, which contributes to the photophobia. On the other hand iris-colored IOL would be a very appropriate choice for patients with traumatized/surgical aniridia.

In addition to the management certain supportive measures help alleviate the specific symptom of photophobia, e.g., use of sunglasses and hats and avoidance of bright outdoor illumination is recommended. These measures are particularly important in patients with albinism, aniridia, and monochromatism; however, very little objective evidence has been provided to support anecdotal reports of improvements in visual performance using tinted lenses or filters.[10]

REFERENCES

1. Goyal JL, Rao VA, Srinivasan R, et al. Oculocutaneous manifestations in xeroderma pigmentosa. Br J Ophthalmol 1994; 78: 295–7.
2. Roussat B, Fournier F, Besson D, et al. À propos de deux cas de tyrosinose de type II (syndrome de Richner-Hanhart). Bull Soc Ophtalmol Fr 1988; 88: 751–7.
3. Burns RP, Gipson IK, Murray MJ. Keratopathy in tyrosinemia. Birth Defects 1976; 12: 169–80.
4. Elder MJ, Astin CL. Recurrent corneal erosion in cystinosis. J Pediatr Ophthalmol Strabismus 1994; 31: 270–1.
5. Traboulsi EI, Green WR, O'Donnell FJ Jr. The eye in albinism. In: Tasman W, Jaeger EA, editors. Duane's Clinical Ophthalmology. Philadelphia: Lippincott-Raven; 1995: Chap 38. (vol. 4.)

6. O'Donnell FJ Jr, Green WR, Fleischman JA, et al. X-linked ocular albinism in blacks: ocular albinism cum pigmento. Arch Ophthalmol 1978; 96: 1189–92.
7. Simunovic MP, Moore AT. The cone dystrophies. Eye 1998; 12: 553–65.
8. Jan JE, Groenveld M, Anderson DP. Photophobia and cortical visual impairment. Dev Med Child Neurol 1993; 35: 473–7.
9. Wiggins RE, von Noorden GK. Monocular eye closure in sunlight. J Pediatr Ophthalmol Strabismus 1990; 27: 16–20.
10. Eperjesi F, Fowler CW, Evans BJ. Do tinted lenses or filters improve visual performance in low vision? A review of the literature. Ophthalmic Physiol Opt 2002; 22: 68–77.

CHAPTER P10 The Watering Eye

Anthony G Quinn

Up to 20% of infants having a watery eye in the first month of life,[1,2] the vast majority have congenital nasolacrimal duct obstruction; the rest may have potentially serious problems. Acquired watering eyes present another range of diagnoses.

Congenital nasolacrimal duct obstruction and its management is discussed elsewhere (Chapter 31).

SIGNS AND SYMPTOMS

History

A child with excessive tearing causes parents and primary care doctors concern. Buildup of mucus in the tear film causes "stickiness," and constant spillage of tears can cause redness and irritation of the lower lid skin. The lids may be stuck together on waking and require frequent cleaning. Parents complain that the appearance "ruins" photographs, and they may feel the child's appearance reflects poorly on them as a parent. The primary care physician may feel compelled to prescribe repeated courses of topical antibiotics, to no lasting effect.

It is important to establish whether the watering had its onset soon after birth or if it is recent. Photophobia must specifically be asked about, as it is a common finding in congenital glaucoma. The typical presentation is a child who avoids opening their eyes in normal daylight, often burying the eyes behind an arm or hand. Photophobia is also a symptom of corneal disease, uveitis, and foreign body in the conjunctival sac. The possibility of trauma needs to be kept in mind, as children cannot always give a detailed history. The child with excessive lacrimation, rather than blocked tear drainage, may have a watery nose on the same side as the watery eye. A history of eye rubbing or poking and concerns about whether the child can see suggests a retinal dystrophy, such as Leber's congenital amaurosis.

EXAMINATION

External inspection

Tearing, red, macerated skin and stickiness may be seen. In naso-lacrimal duct obstruction, the tear film is thickened, brimming the lower lid margin. Normally the tear film is virtually invisible, and with fluorescein staining of the tear film, measures less than 1 mm. With obstruction, it typically measures 2 mm or more. Secondary bacterial conjunctivitis can occur, causing generalized conjunctival redness, whereas perilimbal injection may be more specific for keratitis or uveitis. Generalized corneal haze may be a sign of glaucoma, with secondary corneal epithelial edema. An estimate should be made of horizontal corneal diameters using a ruler held close to the lid. A congenital swelling over the nasolacrimal sac is probably a dacryocystocele.

Slit-lamp examination

This is best done with a portable slit lamp in young children. Look for presence or absence of puncta, puntual ectopia, or epiblepharon with in-turned eyelashes. Inspect the inferior conjunctival fornix looking for a diffuse redness and swelling of the conjunctiva, suggesting chlamydia conjunctivitis. Everting the upper lid is very unlikely to be possible in a young, awake child, but it is possible to retract the upper lid digitally and inspect the tarsal conjunctiva and fornix with the portable slit lamp, looking from below. Corneal abrasions, scars, ulcers, and foreign bodies can be excluded, as can signs of uveitis, e.g., hypopyon, posterior synechiae, or cataract (also check red reflex). Haab's striae and corneal edema should be actively excluded.

Fluorescein testing

This is a very sensitive test for detecting any defect in the corneal epithelium, and fluorescein will diffusely stain the cornea with epithelial edema. The fluorescein dye disappearance test is excellent for confirming nasolacrimal duct obstruction (see Chapter 31). It may also appear in the nose, confirming drainage.

Intraocular pressure (IOP)

It is possible to check this in the majority of awake infants or young children with a "Tono-Pen," or if this is not possible, an "air puff" tonometer[1] (see Chapters 9 and 48). If congenital glaucoma is likely, an examination under anesthesia or sedation may be necessary. Tactile measurement is inaccurate and may mislead.

Cycloplegic refraction, fundus examination

Refraction and fundus examination will highlight unilateral myopia in a child with unilateral glaucoma, posterior synechiae, disc cupping, and any posterior segment pathology such as retinoblastoma, which can present as a red, watery eye with a "pseudo-hypopyon."

CAUSES AND TREATMENT

Nonpatent nasolacrimal drainage system
(see Chapter 31)

Spontaneous resolution will occur in most affected children with about 70% being free of symptoms by 3 months of age and over 90% having resolved by 1 year.[4–9] Spontaneous resolution may also occur later than 12 months,[5,9,10] and those children whose epiphora does not resolve spontaneously after age 2 years are likely to have more complex lacrimal drainage problems. Children with white eyes (no evidence of conjunctivitis) should not be treated with antibiotic drops. Antibiotics should only be given when there is clinical evidence of infection. Many physicians have advocated massage of the lacrimal sac, but its efficacy is not known.[4] Lid cleaning may help prevent secondary infection and skin excoriation.

Treatment

There are a number of treatments (see Chapter 31), the commonest, probing, is safe but even in the best circumstances can have complications; it is sometimes traumatic and may, rarely, cause canalicular stenosis.[10,11]

Foreign body/corneal abrasion

A history of sudden onset of pain, epiphora, conjunctival redness, and a foreign body sensation suggests either a corneal/conjunctival abrasion or a foreign body in the conjunctival sac or cornea. A careful history from the child and/or others present at the time is essential in understanding the likely injury and predicting its severity. Fluorescein stains a corneal or conjunctival abrasion very clearly, and suggests a superior subtarsal foreign body by staining vertical scratches on the cornea, caused by the foreign body being dragged over the corneal surface with blinks. If there is a full-thickness corneal laceration, the Seidel test will sometimes be positive. If a portable slit lamp is not available for the examination, loupes or a +20-diopter lens, with a good light, may be useful.

Corneal abrasions usually settle quickly with antibiotic ointment and no patching is required. Removal of an embedded corneal foreign body in a child may require general anesthesia. Loosely adherent foreign bodies in the conjunctival sac or on the cornea may be removable with a sterile cotton bud.

Keratitis and conjunctivitis (see Chapter 22)

A watery eye is a common symptom in keratitis (Fig. P10.1). There is frequently associated photophobia, conjunctival injection, increased mucus production, and a foreign body sensation. Visual acuity is often reduced in keratitis. Conjunctivitis is not associated with photophobia, unless there is an accompanying keratitis. Conjunctivitis is commonly infective (viral, bacterial), allergic, or traumatic. Allergic conjunctivitis typically presents as itchy, watery eyes, and is usually a bilateral problem. There may be a family history of allergic disease, and a clinical history of exacerbations in spring/summer, or of other allergic diseases such as eczema, hay fever, or asthma. "Shield" ulcers secondary to giant subtarsal conjunctival papillae produce a characteristic loss of corneal epithelium and are easily seen with fluorescein and slit-lamp microscope.

Contact lens-related epiphora

In the older child or the aphakic infant with contact lenses, epiphora may result from numerous causes. Poor fitting, change in

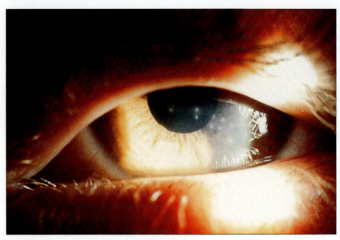

Fig. P10.1 Thygeson keratitis. This eight-year-old child had a variably watering right eye for nine months that did not respond to a variety of treatments.

corneal curvature, buildup of deposits on the contact lens, and chips or tears at the edge of the contact lens can all cause watery eyes from epithelial trauma or drying. The superior tarsal conjunctiva must be assessed for giant papillary conjunctivitis (GPC) in the long-term contact lens wearer.[12] Treatment may include revising contact lens hygiene, replacing lenses, refitting lenses, replacing lenses with a different material or edge design, and treatment of GPC with appropriate pharmacological agents (see Chapter 22). Infectious keratitis or corneal abrasion should be excluded and parents warned to remove the lens and seek ophthalmological advice within a few hours if the child's eye becomes red, sticky, watery, or photophobic.

Congenital glaucoma

Epiphora with photophobia may indicate congenital glaucoma. Buphthalmos, corneal clouding, Haab's striae, increased intraocular pressure (compared to normal for infants), and enlarged optic disc cup are also usually present. Anisometropia and strabismus may occur (see Chapter 48). Prompt treatment, usually surgical, is needed to prevent further optic nerve damage.

Crocodile tears

One peculiar form of tearing occurs only when the patient salivates, most typically when eating or just thinking of a good meal.[13] This can be congenital, and is an example the "congenital cranial dysinnervation disorders" (see Chapter 85).[14] Congenital crocodile tears have been reported in association with Duane syndrome,[15] after trauma or surgery on the ear,[16] or as a sequel to Bell's palsy,[17] in these situations representing aberrant nerve regeneration.

REFERENCES

1. Guerry D, Kendig EL. Congenital impatency of the nasolacrimal duct. Am J Ophthalmol 1948; 31: 773–80.
2. MacEwen CJ, Young JD. Epiphora during the first year of life. Eye 1991; 5: 596–600.
3. Lim JI, Blair NP, Higginbotham EJ, et al. Assessment of intraocular pressure in vitrectomized gas-containing eyes. A clinical and manometric comparison of the Tono-Pen to the pneumotonometer. Arch Ophthalmol 1990; 108: 684–8.
4. Young JD, MacEwan CJ. Managing congenital lacrimal obstruction in general practice. BMJ 1997; 315: 293–6.
5. Price HW. Dacryostenosis. J Pediatr 1947; 30: 302–5.
6. Paul TO. Medical management of congenital nasolacrimal duct obstruction. J Pediatr Ophthalmol Strabismus 1985; 22: 68–70.
7. Petersen RA, Robb RM. The natural course of congenital obstruction of the nasolacrimal duct. J Pediatr Ophthalmol Strabismus 1978; 15: 246–50.
8. Nelson LB, Calhoun JH, Menduke H. Medical management of congenital nasolacrimal duct obstruction. Ophthalmology 1985; 92: 1187–90.
9. Nucci P, Capoferri C, Alfarano R, et al. Conservative management of nasolacrimal duct obstruction. J Pediatr Ophthalmol Strabismus 1989; 26: 39–43.
10. Young JD, MacEwen CJ, Ogston SA. Congenital nasolacrimal duct obstruction in the second year of life, a multicentre trial of management. Eye 1996; 10: 484–91.
11. Lyon DB, Dortzbach RK, Lemke BN, et al. Canalicular stenosis following probing for congenital nasolacrimal duct obstruction. Ophthalmic Surg 1991; 22: 228–32.
12. Allansmith MR, Greiner JV, Henriquez AS, et al. Giant papillary conjunctivitis in contact lens wearers. Am J Ophthalmol 1977; 83: 697–708.
13. Golding-Wood PH. Crocodile tears. Br Med J 1963; i: 1518.
14. Engle EC. The molecular basis of the congenital fibrosis syndromes. Strabismus 2002; 10: 125–8.
15. Ramsay J, Taylor D. Congenital crocodile tears: a clue to the aetiology of Duane's syndrome. Br J Ophthalmol 1980; 64: 518–22.
16. Axelsson A, Laage-Hellman JE. The gusto-lacrimal reflex: the syndrome of crocodile tears. Acta Otolaryngol 1962; 54: 239–42.
17. McGovern FH. Paroxysmal lacrimation during eating following recovery from facial palsy. Am J Ophthalmol 1940; 23: 1388–92.

CHAPTER
P11 Proptosis

Christopher J Lyons and Jack Rootman

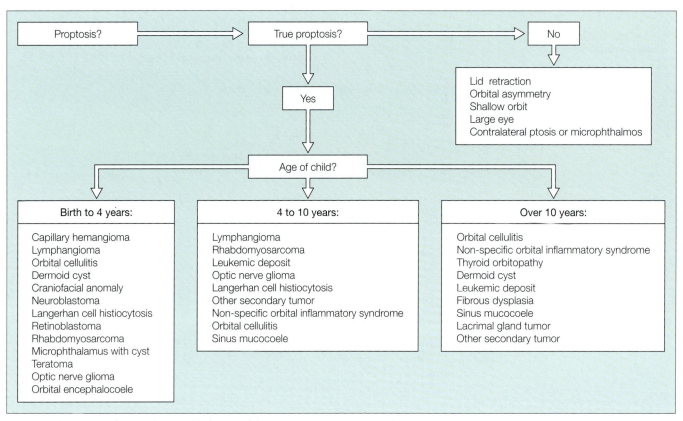

Fig. P11.1 The causes of proptosis vary with the age of the child and there is considerable overlap between both the age groups and the various centres. This figure lists causes in approximate order of frequency. Details of each condition should be sought in the text. In making a clinical diagnosis, the history and progression of the condition as well as the clinical findings are of vital importance. See Chapter 32 for a more detailed and different approach.

CHAPTER
P12 Eye Pain

Peter Hodgkins

Eye pain is a subjective complaint, which does not always match the physical findings. In a young child, it may manifest as eye rubbing, light sensitivity, excessive blinking, and irritability. The older child is able to complain of eye pain when the underlying cause may be anything from a foreign body to an attention-seeking device.

ANATOMY

Two fiber systems, myelinated and unmyelinated, transmit pain. The former transmits sharp transient pain sensations, and the latter dull aching sensations. Pain fibers innervating the eye and periorbital structures arise from the trigeminal or fifth cranial nerve. The first (ophthalmic) division is the most important division for eye pain.[1] It innervates the globe, forehead, lacrimal gland, canaliculi, and lacrimal sac as well as the frontal sinus, upper lid, and side of the nose. Its intracranial source is the Gasserian ganglion, from which it extends through the cavernous sinus. Branching just behind the superior orbital fissure into the lacrimal, frontal, and nasociliary nerves, it enters the superior orbital fissure. An important intracranial branch of the ophthalmic division supplies the meninges. The second major branch (V2), the maxillary nerve, supplies the cheek, lower eyelid, sometimes a small lower segment of the cornea, upper lip, side of the nose, maxillary sinus, roof of the mouth, and temporal region; it too arises from the Gasserian ganglion and courses either within or just lateral to the cavernous sinus. It then passes through the inferior orbital fissure after giving rise to dural branches. Although coursing within the orbit, its terminal branches *do not* include intraorbital structures. The third (V3) division, or mandibular nerve, supplies sensation to other regions of the cheek, within the mouth and the preauricular area. From the Gasserian ganglion, it passes through the foramen ovale to the intratemporal fossa. Although pain is most commonly generated at the site of the insult, referred pain may occur if the sensory pathway is stimulated in other regions: dural stimulation may result in retrobulbar pain.

The cornea has one of the areas of greatest density of pain nerve endings with the greatest concentration in the central cornea. Noncorneal structures that show less sensitivity are in descending order eyelids, caruncle, and conjunctiva.[2] Other ocular structures that can be associated with pain include the uvea, sclera, and optic nerve sheaths (Table P12.1).

Some are left with no pathology to explain their eye pain and one is left with a diagnosis of eye strain, atypical facial pain, or attention seeking. Careful review and working with the parents and child is necessary to achieve a satisfactory outcome.

Table P12.1 Causes of eye pain

1. Obvious eye problems
2. Nonobvious eye problems: refractive; accommodative
3. Quiet eyes but localizing neuro-ophthalmic findings
4. No ocular and neuro-ophthalmic findings
5. Others
   a. Specific short or long-lasting headaches or eye pain syndromes;
   b. Pains referred to the eye from other pathology (secondary eye pain);
   c. **Pain from orbit, superior orbital fissure, cavernous sinus, intracranial infiltrative, neoplastic, or inflammatory disease process.**

From Brazis et al[3]

NONACCIDENTAL INJURY (NAI)

A child's cornea may be scratched by fingernails: this usually occurs rather innocuously since a toddler's eyes are at the height where an adult's hand rests. However, beware nonaccidental injury can also be a cause if it is recurrent or unusual. Before jumping to this conclusion in the recurrent cases, however, examine siblings and parents to see whether it might be an inherited corneal dystrophy (Chapter 30) or whether there might be an anesthetic cornea. In recurrent or inexplicable situations, involvement of a pediatrician is wise. There are also reports of nonaccidental chemical injuries to the eyes, which are probably underreported as they go unrecognized.[4]

CORNEA

Infection is a common cause of eye pain. Corneal scraping and culture and sensitivity should be performed although a trial of broad spectrum treatment with cefuroxime and ofloxacin could be tried where a general anesthetic is not indicated. Keratitis is seen as part of an adenoviral keratoconjunctivitis but may be present with other viral causes. Herpetic keratitis, although uncommon in children, is also seen in an infant born vaginally to a mother with genital herpes or where a relative with an active cold sore has come into contact. The child may develop the typical primary vesicles and swelling but this may have been missed, and the presentation is with a dendritic ulcer or a disciform corneal change. Treatment needs to be instituted to minimize scarring and a watchful eye on the development of acute amblyopia.

Exposure keratopathy can occur in children with especially prominent eyes and shallow orbits, such as occurs with craniofacial abnormalities. Children with Down syndrome may fail to close their eyes sufficiently when sleeping, resulting in chronic keratopathy. Their symptoms may be aggravated by chronic blepharitis.[5] Beware also the child with recurrent corneal ulceration and chronically red eyes yet relative indifference to the changes, where instead of NAI it may be a situation of corneal hypoesthesia that can be seen in the Riley-Day syndrome but can be seen on its own. Tyrosinemia type 2 and biotinidase deficiency may present with keratitis: they are treatable (Chapter 65).

CONJUNCTIVA

Acute conjunctivitis can be uncomfortable, probably as the lid becomes swollen. Beware, however, if this pain is excessive or there is marked photophobia as this implies another pathology. Another common circumstance in which the conjunctiva is apparently responsible for eye discomfort is in the postoperative strabismus patient. The conjunctiva suture often causes a foreign body sensation probably by corneal stimulation.

LACRIMAL GLAND

Pain secondary to dry eyes is an uncommon occurrence in children. Dry eyes may occur as a side-effect of chemotherapy, radiotherapy, or graft-versus-host disease. These children should be given artificial tears prophylactically and especially ointment at nighttime. Absent tear production associated with Riley-Day syndrome, although a cause of dry eyes and recurrent corneal ulceration, is devoid of any eye pain since corneal sensation is absent.

Lacrimal gland swelling is rare in children though it may occur with parotid gland swelling in mumps. Dacryoadenitis occurs rarely in association with a childhood viremia and produces vague discomfort around the eyes. Lacrimal gland infarction associated with sickle cell disease can result in rapid swelling of the gland and mimic acute bacterial cellulites. Childhood inflammatory orbital disease, with signs and symptoms compatible with orbital pseudotumor, is often associated with pain.[6]

LACRIMAL SAC

Acute dacryocystis may occur in infants with a nonpatent nasolacrimal system. The pain is accompanied by redness swelling in the region of the nasolacrimal sac as well as other signs of acute infection and requires systemic antibiotics. Probing should be performed when it has settled down. Differentiation should be made from a dacryocystocele, which should be pain free (Chapter 31).

GLAUCOMA

The eye pain of congenital glaucoma is also associated with photophobia. Both result from corneal abnormalities as the neonate's cornea is stretched by the high pressure. With breaks in Descemet's membrane, stromal edema and epithelial irregularities develop, leading to pain and photophobia. The child whose pressure is brought under control may continue

to have light sensitivity as a consequence of corneal scarring (Chapter 48).

UVEA

Since the iris is supplied with pain fibers, iritis is associated with pain, which may be augmented by ciliary spasm. The symptoms of pain may be difficult to distinguish from photophobia: the combination results in an extremely uncomfortable eye. Childhood iritis may occur in association with infection (measles, chicken pox), often in conjunction with keratitis. The iritis of juvenile rheumatoid arthritis is only occasionally painful. Iritis may occur in conjunction with hyphema, which is usually traumatic. If not associated with trauma, infiltrative processes such as childhood leukemia or juvenile xanthogranuloma must be considered, and in these situations secondary glaucoma may also cause pain. More posterior forms of childhood uveitis include pars planitis and toxocara lesions. These inflammations usually present as visual loss rather than eye pain (Chapter 44).

OPTIC NERVE

The retina and optic nerves do not contain pain fibers but the optic nerve sheath does. Eye pain may occur with childhood optic neuritis. As with adult optic neuritis the pain is most commonly initiated by looking from side to side; this causes the inflamed nerve sheath to stretch, eliciting pain. More chronic distention of the nerve sheath such as occurs with optic nerve sheath glioma in childhood does not cause pain.

LIDS

Acute distension of all or part of the lids results in vague pain. A stye (hordeolum) or an acute chalazion can cause pain out of context to what you see due to the stretching of local lid tissues. Preseptal cellulitis also results in tremendous stretching of the lid tissue, and pain is one of the hallmark symptoms. Lids of children with chronic allergy may itch rather than cause true pain. Their skin becomes scaly with the eczematous reaction.

ORBIT AND CENTRAL NERVOUS SYSTEM

Orbital pain may result from local irritation of pain fibers. Such pain usually implies an acute event, such as rapidly expanding mass or infection.[6] The pain, however, may be referred pain from intracranial irritation of the dura (V2). Cavernous sinus inflammation such as occurs in individuals with Tolosa-Hunt syndrome causes pain within the orbit, but does not often occur in children.[7] Rarely brain stem glioma may present with episodic pain, sometimes with facial spasm.

PAINFUL THIRD NERVE PALSY

Third nerve palsy is often congenital even with pupil involvement or due to road traffic accidents. New onset painful third nerve palsy implies serious pathology and needs full investigation. The diagnosis of ophthalmoplegic migraine is a diagnosis of exclusion and needs to fulfill certain criteria: it is not usually painful.

PAINFUL SIXTH NERVE PALSY

In childhood the sudden onset of a sixth nerve palsy, the sudden worsening of an existing concomitant squint with the appearance of features of incomitance, or the onset of a convergent squint worse in the distance, together with the facial pain, should make one think of petrous apex osteitis secondary to mastoiditis or suppurative otitis media (Gradenigo syndrome). This was common in preantibiotic days but now painful sixth nerve palsy is probably more frequently seen with orbital or retro-orbital disease. It is still crucial in these children, however, to carry out a cycloplegic refraction as the illness may just have broken down an esophoria.

HERPES ZOSTER OPHTHALMICUS

Although relatively unusual in children this does occur, and it may give rise to severe discomfort in the acute phase. Post-herpetic neuralgia, however, seems to be unusual in children. As opposed to adults with herpes zoster ophthalmicus, children with this condition have a significant incidence of systemic disease, including immune deficiency and leukemia. Treatment with antiviral agents and steroids may reduce the incidence of post-herpetic neuralgia and it is essential in the immune suppressed.

TRIGEMINAL NEURALGIA

Trigeminal neuralgia is predominantly a disease of old age but cases have been described in early childhood.[8] It may be secondary to pontine tumors or tumors including vascular anomalies that press on the fifth nerve. It had been associated with multiple sclerosis but, especially in childhood, this is probably not significant. The pain is severe and paroxysmal, lasting seconds but leaving the child shaking and upset for a while afterward. The fact that it is facial pain causing the problem is not obvious in the smaller child who may not be able to communicate his problem so well. Detailed neuroradiology of the course of the fifth nerve is indicated.

HEADACHE

A child may occasionally talk about eye pain when in fact the complaint is a more generalized headache. The interpretation as "eye pain" may be an important localizing symptom for a further discussion of childhood headache (see Chapter P18). History is the key to diagnosis: Where is it? How long has it been there? How often? What type of pain? What are the relieving/exacerbating factors?

Migraine is derived from the word hemicrania. Its incidence is approximately 50/1000 in school-age children. It increases in frequency with age but is rare under 2 years. In the prepubertal period boys outnumber girls by 2:1. At puberty this lessens in boys, resulting in the female excess in adults. The accepted subdivision is as follows:

Classic migraine – aura and hemicranial pain
Common migraine – diffuse headache and unwell
Cluster migraine – repeated pain in orbit with swelling
Complicated migraine – ophthalmoplegic; abdominal convulsive; basilar.

Ophthalmoplegic migraine usually has an onset before 10 years of age with the third nerve affected much more commonly than the sixth (10:1). The pupil and accommodation are frequently involved, and the ophthalmoplegia occurs at the height of the headache, persisting when the headache clears. This may last weeks and the criteria for diagnosis are strict: onset in first decade; history of typical migraine; ophthalmoplegia ipsilateral to the headache, when present; negative investigations.

REFRACTION

When refractive errors are large the presenting symptom is reduced vision. When the error is smaller, however, it can present in a variety of ways. These other symptoms arise as a result of the effort to see clearly. Sustained excessive accommodation may be seen in hypermetropia, or discrepancies in the accommodation–convergence association can give rise to strain in the effort to maintain binocular single vision. Myopia may cause peering and periocular pain. These symptoms tend to be grouped together as eyestrain. These symptoms, however, may be diverse and do not appear in proportion to the causal defect.

Visual symptoms

These are characteristically intermittent, and the symptoms may be most marked in those with good vision who try hard to keep the vision up. There are periods of particular strain, however, when the vision may fall, especially with excessive reading or detailed tasks when there may be sudden confusion, temporary blurring, or the letters running together. The eyes become more tired and the lids heavy with a progressive weariness.

Ocular symptoms

These symptoms are collectively spoken of as asthenopia. The symptoms of eyestrain are due to the increased muscular work involved and the direct muscular fatigue that ensues. After long periods of close work the eyes feel hot, tired, and uncomfortable. If work is continued then quite severe pain may actually develop in the eyes. These eyes lead to a watery red look when it may be associated with chronic blepharitis or recurrent conjunctivitis. These low-grade infections are exacerbated by the rubbing with unclean hands.

Referred symptoms–Headaches are the most common symptom, and it may take almost any form.

Accommodative spasm–The patient presents with diplopia, blurred vision, macropsia, or headaches and eye pain. There will be a variable esotropia, pupil constriction, and pseudomyopia. Refraction is important for the uncorrected hypermetropia; it can also be seen with intermittent exotropia where the patient is using convergence and accommodation to control the exotropia. It can also be functional where no cause can be found.

Convergence insufficiency/paresis–Typical symptoms are frontal headaches and eyestrain associated with close work and blurred vision. Exophorias can also give rise to these symptoms.

FUNCTIONAL EYE PAIN

The child between 5 and 8 years has learned that complaining about pain leads to parental attention. Occasionally this complaint may center on the eyes. The child may really be asking for glasses as further questioning may reveal this motive. Siblings of children with bona fide eye problems may have observed the extra commotion and attention given the sibling and hope for equal treatment by complaining of eye pain. Nevertheless, a diagnosis of a functional disorder is purely one of exclusion in any child, which usually can be made with ease after listening to and observing the child.

DIAGNOSTIC TECHNIQUES

It is important to take a careful history looking for acute events that may explain a foreign body. Have there been contacts with cases of conjunctivitis or mumps? Is there a family history of eye problems and/or a previous history of any eye problems? Examine other family members first to allow the child to see what is going to happen as well as to gain useful information. An orthoptic examination is also helpful to record the vision and look at the eye movement and visual system.

Then conduct a full eye examination. The slit-lamp examination can be performed on children of all ages but in children who cannot cooperate for a slit lamp, a +20-diopter lens or operating loupes may provide adequate magnification. If there is undue difficulty in achieving a good examination one could wait a while before trying again or proceed through to an examination under anesthesia, depending on the situation. A cycloplegic dilation and refraction and fundus examination is also important.

Intraocular pressure measurement when required with the pneumotonometer can often be achieved but examination under sedation may be necessary. It is also important to measure the axial length and have a good look at the optic discs with photos where possible in suspicious cases.

Neuroradiological studies are required whenever orbital swelling persists or when the quality of retro-orbital pain and presence of associated symptoms suggests intracranial pathology. Orbital disease, optic nerve sheath pathology, and lacrimal gland swelling are all usually detectable with these studies. A bone scan is rarely indicated when concern about a lacrimal gland infarct in association with sickle-cell disease is present. Debate as to when a neuroradiological study should be performed in cases of presumed periorbital cellulites often occurs. If the child fails to respond to intravenous antibiotics after 36–38 hr, then computed tomography (CT) or magnetic resonance imaging (MRI) should be performed to exclude the possibility of orbital mass (such as retinoblastoma, rhabdomyosarcoma, or abscess).

TREATMENT

The treatment of eye pain depends upon achieving the correct diagnosis even if this involves a general anesthetic examination. Once the diagnosis is made, treatment can be tailored appropriately. It will be necessary in some cases to perform investigations such as CT or MRI scans or electrodiagnostics. The compounding factor in pediatric ophthalmology is amblyopia, which can appear very quickly. Always beware of this and ensure a refraction is carried out and some patching instituted early when this seems to be happening. Also remember to examine the family and siblings for clues as to the problem. Treatment of conjunctivitis with chloramphenicol did wane with the reported association with the gray baby syndrome, and many use Fucithalmic where indicated.[9] Nevertheless the use of chloramphenicol does seem to be returning. When treating the cause, remember to institute analgesics in age-dependent doses.

REFERENCES

1. Miller N. Anatomy and physiology of the trigeminal nerve. In: Walsh and Hoyt's Clinical Neuro-Ophthalmology. 4th ed. Baltimore: Williams and Wilkins; 1985: 999–1043.
2. Norn M. Conjunctival sensitivity in normal eyes. Acta Ophthalmolol 1973; 51: 58–66.
3. Brazis PW, Lee AG, Stewart M, et al. Clinical review: the differential diagnosis of pain in the quiet eye. Neurologist 2002; 8: 82–100.
4. Ong T, Hodgkins PR, Marsh C, et al. Blinding keratoconjunctivitis and child abuse. J Ped Ophthalmol Strabismus 2004; in press.
5. Shapiro MB, France TD. The ocular features of Down's syndrome. Am J Ophthalmol 1985; 99: 659–63.
6. Mottow LS, Jakobiec FA. Idiopathic inflammatory orbital pseudo-tumour in childhood. I. clinical characteristics. Arch Ophthalmol 1978; 96: 1410–7.
7. Kline L. The Tolosa-Hunt syndrome. Surv Ophthalmol 1982; 27: 79–95.
8. Poser CM. Facial pain: diagnostic dilemma, therapeutic challenge. Geriatrics 1975; 30: 110–5.
9. Haider S, Craft AW. The grey toddler: chloramphenicol toxicity. Arch Dis Child 1974; 49: 913.

CHAPTER
P13 Blurred and Weak Vision

Hanne Jensen

MODE OF PRESENTATION

Children who come to the clinic complaining of blurred or weak vision are older and observant; they have to be old enough to speak, and to be able to understand that what they see is not normal. There will be no complaints if a child has never had normal vision, nor when the change is chronic.

With the younger child, blurred or weak vision is often based on information from parents, teachers, or caretakers, together with the eye examination, or the nurse may detect reduced visual acuity at screening examinations. Older children often detect the blurred or weak vision when they have problems with their schoolwork or in daily living.

The mode of presentation therefore depends on the age of the child, when and how quickly the problem has developed, and how reduced the vision is compared with the child's needs. The reduced visual acuity is often the only, often subtle symptom. Severe symptoms such as headache, seizures, and failure to thrive make it more obvious that the child needs to be examined. The symptoms might vary during the day, and are often most marked when the child is tired.

In the following the signs and symptoms that should lead to the suspicion of blurred or weak vision in the different age groups are presented.

SIGNS AND SYMPTOMS (Table P13.1)

Infants

If eye contact does not develop in the first few weeks of life, the parents are usually concerned and referred. Reduced visual acuity from birth might occur with nystagmus, roving eye movements,

---

Table P13.1 Sign and symptoms of blurred or weak vision

Abnormal eye contact
Nystagmus or roving eye movements
Rubbing the eyes/eye poking
Watery eyes
Abnormal reaction to light: photophobic or light fixating
Abnormal reaction in dark: becoming scared
Difficulties in walking/falling over play toys or tumbling into things
Only interested in things with sounds
Only interested in things nearby/comes close to the TV
Only interested in things at a distance/or does not like close eye contact
Squeezing the eye lids/abnormal head posture
Lack of concentration
Problems with colors
Strabismus
Abnormalities or malformations, leukocoria, red eye, microphthalmia

---

or congenital malformations; in these cases it is not difficult to detect that the child has a problem. The parents might say that the child does not like eye contact, or looks over their heads–a symptom also seen in autistic children. There might be epiphora or photophobia–however, if the child is born in the autumn the reduced light makes it take longer for the parents to be aware of the problem. Rarely, an infant with normal early visual development suddenly loses vision; this may occur in some neurological or neurometabolic diseases: it is accompanied by other symptoms (Chapter 65).

Preschool children

Children aged 1–5 years are normally very curious and love to investigate. The child will try to do the same as it observes, e.g., smile when the parents smile, use toys as others use them, and later use them in its own way. With reduced vision, he will not be able to copy what he sees, and development will seem slow. The child does not complain: it is the parents or the caretakers who bring the child. A very common complaint is that the child sits close to the television–but normal-sighted children do this as well–it is easier for them to fix and follow the pictures on the screen when it occupies the total visual field. This symptom is therefore not very specific.

Parents will register whether the child prefers toys with sound or with colors, small subjects or only the large ones, or only the nearest things. They will react if the child begins to squint, if the eyes become red or watery, or if the child does not want to go out because of photophobia or gets scared in dim light, but one can only expect a preschool child to complain about blurred or weak vision if it is massive or has a sudden onset.

A child often goes through kindergarten with moderate visual reduction without being diagnosed, dealing with life without problems, as most tasks are so undemanding that minor visual deficits are not detected. The children might be thought distractible or immature, and no referral made.

Schoolchildren

Schoolchildren with slightly reduced vision, which has not been detected before the start of school, will often do reasonably well in the beginning. However, the problems become pronounced when demands increase; e.g., the letters are smaller, the tempo is higher, the tasks are more complex, and it becomes difficult for the child to use imagination or skill to compensate for the blurred or weak vision. The child will have a hard time, but not all will complain of visual difficulties and so it is important for the teachers to be aware.

Schoolchildren that suddenly get blurred or weak vision will of course complain; they know what to expect and what they have lost. However, if the visual reduction is monocular, they will complain only if they shut the good eye by chance.

With increasing age; the demands are higher not only at school, but also recreations, computer games, and sport need detailed vision.

Finding a child with weak and blurred vision is therefore a job for all concerned.

DIAGNOSIS

History

In small children, the history is from the parents or other care-takers, but when there is a suspicion of child abuse, reliance should not be placed on the parents' story. Is there a story of trauma? Children who have done something they know their parents will not approve of may not speak about this spontaneously, and it is sometimes necessary to talk with the child without the parents. Has the situation always been as now, or has a change to do with higher demands? Does the child like to play where is it dark, does the child like to walk on its own, or does she always want to hold hands? Has the child suddenly changed her behavior? Aggression or passivity can be symptoms of progressive visual reduction. Specific questions are necessary because people will often not associate visual problems with change in behavior. Any other systemic symptom must be noted.

A distinction between blurred and weak vision can only be made by the older child who can describe the defocused image versus the vision that is just not so good as it ought to be. Blurred vision implies an optical problem. A complaint of decreased acuity after strenuous exercise or after warm baths suggests Uhthoff's sign of demyelinating disease.

Examinations

It is essential to observe the child entering the clinic; are there difficulties, is the child afraid or curious, does the child reach for toys that match its age, and very important, can the child hear? Children who have been attending several different clinics through-out their childhood are often afraid and shy with professionals. This is understandable, and it is important to make the child feel safe and cooperative.

Ocular examination

It is important to begin with easy and fun examinations and proceed as in Chapters 9 and 10.

The media should be examined by the retinoscope before and after the pupils are dilated, and with the slit lamp if necessary. Refraction (see Chapter 6) is a vital and often forgotten part of the examination. The direct ophthalmoscope is used for fundus details, e,g., changes in the retinal nerve fiber layer and in the fovea, whereas indirect ophthalmoscope gives a panoramic view.

The optic nerve is examined by pupillary responses, contrast sensitivity, color vision and visual field, and ophthalmoscopy. Visual-evoked potentials can be used (see Chapter 11).

Color vision and pupillary responses often are normal in retinal diseases with marked reduced visual acuity while they are abnormal even in mild optic nerve disease.

Field testing in small children is difficult–see Chapter 10.

Neurological examination

Neurological examination is necessary in children with reduced vision but normal eyes and many eye symptoms can be part of a

systemic disease. It is important to enquire about other symptoms, including hearing problems, in every child with visual loss. Children with concentration deficits must be examined by a neurologist to exclude seizure disorders, and it is necessary to make sure that no medicine has been given that might influence the vision or the visual field, e.g., vigabatrin.

CAUSES AND TREATMENT (Table P13.2)

Amblyopia

Refractive errors
See Chapter 6.

Accommodative anomalies
Older schoolchildren often have problems when looking at the blackboard but not when reading a book. This may be due to a high accommodative tonus that makes them appear myopic, and it is important to measure the refraction with cycloplegia (Fig. P13.1); otherwise, the diagnosis will be missed and glasses prescribed. Occasionally, a period with cycloplegic eye drops and reading glasses is the only way to help the child to relax accommodation. In low hypermetropia they may accommodate to compensate, but some children cannot (e.g., Down syndrome), and they develop asthenopia: reading glasses may help. Children with convergence insufficiency can get the feeling of blurred vision while reading; they seldom describe the

Table P13.2 Conditions with blurred or weak vision
Amblyopia
Refractive errors (Chapter 6)
Uncorrected hypermetropia
Uncorrected myopia
Uncorrected astigmatism
Accommodative anomalies (Chapter 6)
Reduced accommodation
Reduced convergence
Orbital diseases (Chapter 32)
Tumor
Inflammation
Media opacities
Lid anomalies (Chapters 25 and 26)
Ptosis
Hemangioma
Corneal diseases (Chapters 29 and 30)
Corneal clouding
Keratitis
Keratoconus
Corneal dystrophies
Anterior chamber anomalies (Chapters 28, 43, and 48)
Chronic anterior uveitis
Glaucoma
Persistent pupillary membrane
Lens anomalies (Chapter 46)
Dislocated lens
Cataract
Inherited
Acquired/infection/trauma
Metabolic
Corpus vitreous disorders (Chapter 49)
Vitreoretinal degeneration (Stickler)
Juvenile X-linked retinoschisis
Hemorrhage
Vitreitis due to infections/tumor

Table P13.2 *(Cont'd)* Conditions with blurred or weak vision

Retinal disorders
  Retinopathy of prematurity (Chapter 51)
  Retinoblastoma (Chapter 50)
  Congenital vascular disorders (Chapter 55)
  Retinal dystrophies (Chapter 52)
  Systemic disease (Chapters 53 and 68)
    Diabetes/metabolic/infections
    Leukemic retinopathy

Optic nerve diseases
  Neuritis (Chapter 61)
  Inherited (Chapter 60)
    Leber's neuropathy
    Dominant optic atrophy
  Papilledema (Chapter 59)
  Coloboma (Chapter 59)
  Tumor (Chapters 33 and 34)
    Glioma
    Optic nerve sheath meningioma
CNS diseases
  Tumor (Chapters 62 and 63)
    Meningioma
    Chiasmal glioma
  Hydrocephalus (Chapter 63)
  Infections
    Meningitis sequelae
    Encephalitis sequelae
  Cerebral visual impairment (Chapter 63)
Nonorganic visual disorders (Chapter 64)

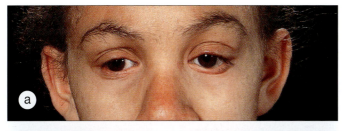
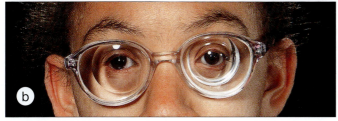

Fig. P13.1 (a) This patient with the diagnosis of hypomelanosis of Ito (which does not often cause defective vision) had acuities of 2/60 in each eye. Despite several examinations (she was difficult to examine), no cause was found. (b) When eventually refracted she was found to be a-25 myope. Corrected, her binocular acuity was 6/12.

problem as double vision. Orthoptic treatment may help these cases, but surgery may be necessary.

Orbital disease

An inflammation or a tumor may present with proptosis, but the presenting symptom might be reduced vision accompanied by restriction of movement and eventually pain and redness. Distortion of the globe tends to result in astigmatism and hyperopia that, left untreated, is an important cause of amblyopia.

Media opacities

Lid anomalies

Ptosis can occlude the visual axis or induce astigmatism, creating blurred vision, often unilateral. Capillary hemangioma can also interfere with the visual axis and create reduced vision or astigmatism.

Corneal diseases

Corneal clouding due to keratitis from any cause may reduce acuity with irritation and watery discharge. Symptoms due to keratoconus usually present during the second decade as slowly progressive visual loss, often with multiple attempts at correction with glasses or contact lenses. Dystrophies presenting within the early years of life can result in recurrent epithelial defects or reduced vision.

Anterior chamber anomalies

Blurred vision due to anterior segment inflammation is usually associated with pain, redness, and photophobia. In uveitis, vision may be reduced without symptoms (see chapter 44).

Lens anomalies

See Chapters 46 and 47.

Dislocation of the lens is an important cause of reduced vision, as a consequence of either the dislocated lens or high myopia. Glaucoma and retinal detachment can arise. Congenital cataract can be seen in any age; in young children the cataract is usually asymptomatic, its presence being detected by the parents or by professionals. In older children, blurred vision or photophobia can occur and be complained of, particularly if the child has a predisposing condition such as diabetes mellitus or steroid treatment to cause him to be more aware of any symptom.

Vitreous disorders

Vitreoretinal degenerations such as Stickler or juvenile X-linked retinoschisis might be diagnosed because of reduced visual acuity at or before school age from myopia or retinal detachment.

Vitreous opacities including hemorrhage, vitreitis, and retinoblastoma seedlings are uncommon causes of blurred vision. When the vitreous is too opacified to allow visualization, other diagnostic tests must be performed, e.g., ultrasound and/or computer tomography (CT) or magnetic resonance (MRI) scanning of the eyes or orbits.

Retinal disorders

ROP (retinopathy of prematurity)

ROP is an important diagnosis as children who have had it might develop myopia and retinal detachment, and any complaint about vision should be taken seriously.

Retinoblastoma

Approximately 5% of children with retinoblastoma have visual difficulties as a presenting feature. Slower growing and unilateral tumors may present at a later age, and retinoblastoma must be excluded in any child presenting with poor vision or strabismus.

Congenital vascular disorders

Von Hippel-Lindau disease and Coats disease can present with blurred vision.

Retinal dystrophies

The visual disturbances with retinal dystrophies are variable. A family history of bilateral visual loss may be present, and there may be systemic findings. Blurred vision is rarely a complaint in retinitis pigmentosa in the early stages; night-blindness and loss of peripheral visual field are more usual. These children often have high ametropias (hypermetropia or myopia).

Systemic disease

It is important to consider a retinal involvement from systemic disease because the ocular findings may lead directly to the systemic diagnosis. Blurred vision may also occur as a consequence of side-effects of treatment.

Diabetes may present early, but retinopathy is uncommon during the first decade of the disease and is reduced by good control of blood sugar. Blurred vision may result from myopia from rapid shifts in blood glucose levels, cataract, or optic atrophy associated with DIDMOAD.

Many neurometabolic disorders, including Batten's disease, mucopolysaccharidoses, and mucolipidoses can create blurred vision on a retinal basis.

Infections (especially cytomegalovirus (CMV) and toxoplasma) can cause retinitis.

In leukemia, vision may be affected by retinal, choroidal, or iris hemorrhage or infiltration.

Optic nerve diseases

When poor acuity or color vision, a central scotoma or constricted fields, poor pupil responses (an afferent defect), and a variably swollen optic disc is found in a child, it indicates an optic neuropathy (see Chapters 60 and 61). Optic atrophy without ocular postinflammatory or hereditary causes suggests a central nervous system abnormality. It is usually bilateral but can initially be unilateral. Congenital optic nerve anomalies (coloboma) can be associated with poor vision and can be discovered late at school testing.

Central nervous system diseases

Blurred or reduced vision can result from involvement of the visual pathways; a lesion proximal to the chiasma more readily results in optic atrophy. Increased intracranial pressure may cause papilledema, usually without visual symptoms, but if it is severe there may be episodic, then permanent loss of vision. A severely atrophic optic nerve cannot appear swollen despite increased intracranial pressure because there is no retinal fiber layer to become swollen. A child with a central nervous system tumor (especially in the posterior fossa) is often ill, vomiting, and complaining of headache. He may also have varying and evanescent double vision from cranial nerve palsy.

The parachiasmal syndrome of visual defect, growth, and other hypothalamic disturbances in children is often caused by optic gliomas or craniopharyngiomas. Various combinations of optic atrophy and papilledema occur, depending on the duration of the process and how fast the intracranial disease has developed.

Hydrocephalus is a cause of visual loss in children; the usual cause of the visual loss is the papilledema with subsequent bilateral optic atrophy.

Cerebral visual impairment represents a particularly frustrating diagnosis, since there are so few ophthalmological findings. It often follows perinatal anoxia, but also occurs with meningitis or encephalitis. The children will have reduced visual acuity, but it will change during the day, depending on the state of the child (see Chapter 63).

Nonorganic visual disorders

These are often seen in teenage girls with problems either in the family or among their friends or related to schoolwork. They can be very difficult to diagnose, and some children have gone through several tests in order to be sure that was no other diagnosis (Chapter 64).

Varying degrees of acuity and visual field loss are often found, often becoming worse with time, but rarely to an extent that the child becomes blind. It is remarkable how well the child behaves despite marked visual loss.

CHAPTER P14

Investigation of Acquired Poor Vision in Childhood

Luis Carlos F de Sa

Poor vision in childhood may result from congenital problems, as indicated by apparent visual inattention within the first weeks of life, or may be acquired, when the child develops normal visual behavior followed by chronic or acute visual loss (such as ceroid lipofuscinosis or optic neuritis) (Fig. P14.1). Consequently, when investigating acquired visual loss, a comprehensive medical history is essential and should include questions about pregnancy, delivery, gestational age, birth weight, perinatal problems, developmental milestones, ocular and medical anomalies, medications, and family history of systemic and/or visual problems (Fig. P14.2). Details about photophobia and eye movement disorders, including strabismus and nystagmus, may help in the diagnosis. It is also important to consider that the apparent acquired visual loss could be congenital, since parents often think their infant's behavior is normal or merely delayed. Irrespective of whether the onset of visual loss is acute or chronic, ophthalmic examination in most cases may reveal abnormalities in the anterior and/or posterior segment, although the site of visual loss may be intracranial (see Chapters 57 to 63).

CLINICAL EXAMINATION

The examination starts with observation of the infant's visual behavior. A child may present with different degrees of visual loss, including visual inattention, and may not respond to visual stimuli such as lights, faces, or toys. The examiner should avoid the use of animated and noisy objects, since children may be attracted to the sound rather than the visual stimulus, but these can be helpful to attain the child's interest. Whenever possible, visual acuity should be measured with age- and neurological status-appropriate methods (Chapter 9).

Evaluation of pupillary responses (grade of reactions, presence of an afferent pupillary defect, or paradoxical reaction) and assessment of alignment and eye movement disorders provide the clinician with important diagnostic clues.

Anterior segment

Cornea

Various diseases may affect the cornea in terms of its size, transparency, and shape. Developmental glaucoma may present with increased corneal diameter in the first three years of life because collagen fibers are softer and more elastic than those of older children and adults. Corneal transparency may be reduced by several conditions including developmental glaucoma (Chapter 48), infectious keratitis (syphilis, rubella, measles, herpes; Chapters 18 and 22), and metabolic diseases (mucolipidoses, mucopolysaccharidoses, and cystinosis; Chapter 29). Corneal shape may be progressively altered in cases of keratoconus

(Chapter 29), which can be present since childhood and may progress at puberty.

Iris

Iris abnormalities are usually not associated with acquired visual problems, although colobomas (Chapter 43) and iris transillumination (albinism; Chapter 45) may be related to congenital visual loss.

Lens

The lens should be carefully evaluated, since developmental cataracts can be secondary to trauma and metabolic/storage diseases, drug-induced, or associated with genetic syndromes that may develop later in childhood (Chapter 46). Ectopia lentis may also be observed and can be related to trauma, genetic/syndromes, and metabolic diseases.

Posterior segment

Vitreous

The vitreous body may show signs of inflammation and/or hemorrhage that may be related with uveitis, trauma, or tumors. Frequently vitreous changes are part of a vitreoretinopathy (Chapters 49, 56, and 58). Past medical history of prematurity and high refractive errors or familial history of retinal detachment, joint pains, or cataracts may suggest a diagnosis of retinopathy of prematurity, Stickler syndrome, familial exudative vitreoretinopathy (FEVR), or congenital stationary night-blindness. Electroretinogram (ERG) can be helpful in certain cases (Chapter 11). Ultrasound and/or magnetic resonance imaging (MRI)/computed tomography (CT) scan are indicated when vitreous opacities impede observation of the retina, or when there is calcification in order to rule out retinoblastoma (Chapter 50).

Retina/Choroid

The retina/choroid should be carefully evaluated because subtle anomalies are not always readily observed. Retinal dystrophy and metabolic/storage diseases (Chapters 49, 53, and 54) commonly start without the pigmentary changes that may develop as the disease progresses (Leber's congenital amaurosis, ceroid lipofuscinosis). When the condition is bilateral and present since birth, nystagmus develops as in cases of Leber's congenital amaurosis. Color vision abnormalities and presence of paradoxical pupil reaction may suggest cone dysfunction. Some retinal dystrophies may require further evaluation with ERG for specific diagnosis. Severely reduced electro-oculogram (EOG) is observed in cases of incipient vitelliform dystrophy (Best's disease; Chapter 54), and it is important for specific diagnosis. Fluorescein angiography, although difficult in small children, is particularly useful for diagnosis of Stargardt's disease ("dark choroid" sign), when visual

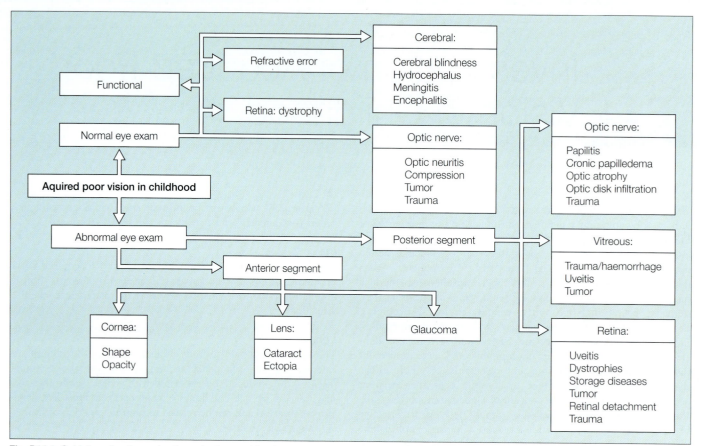

Fig. P14.1 Guidelines for diagnosis of acquired poor vision in childhood.

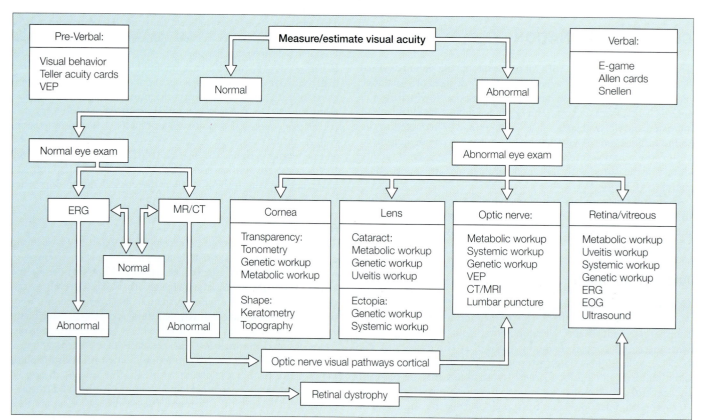

Fig. P14.2 Guidelines for investigation of acquired poor vision in childhood.

loss and macular changes are minimal (Chapter 54). Workup for uveitis (Chapter 44) and retinal detachment (Chapter 56) may be necessary because both conditions develop at any age and are important causes of acquired visual loss.

Optic nerve

The size, color, and contour of the optic disc merit special attention, since anomalies of the optic disc may be related to congenital or acquired visual loss. Evaluation of the presence or absence of optic atrophy is frequently done by examining the color of the optic nerve. It is important to emphasize that the optic discs are often pale in the first weeks compared with older children. Inherited optic atrophy may not manifest in the first year of life. Optic atrophy may also be the result of panretinal degeneration as occurs in retinal dystrophies, and retinal evaluation with ERG may occasionally be necessary.

Optic atrophy may occur secondary to long-standing papilledema or compressive lesions of the anterior visual pathway, and neuroimaging studies may also be indicated.

Intracranial causes

Diseases affecting the intracranial optic nerve, the chiasm, and the posterior visual pathways are important to diagnose because many of them are treatable or their effects may be ameliorated by treatment. Early diagnosis is paramount. (See Chapters 62 and 63).

WORKUP

Normal eye exam

When a child presents with acquired visual loss and there is no ocular explanation for poor vision, it is always important to rule out functional visual loss (Chapter 64) and refractive errors (Chapter 6). Further evaluation with electrophysiological tests and neuroimaging studies are mandatory to rule out organic disease. In some patients, acquired visual loss is part of a multisystem disorder. Full evaluation may require a multidisciplinary approach with pediatrician, neurologist, geneticist, radiologist, and other specialists. Laboratory workup may also include a variety of blood tests and occasionally cerebral spinal fluid (only if imaging has excluded a propensity to coning) studies.

Electrophysiological tests (see Chapter 11)

The ERG is an invaluable tool for diagnosing poor vision in children. The ERG and a normal ocular examination should be performed in every child with poor vision because many retinal disorders are not associated with any visible pigmentary changes early in the course of disease. EOG is rarely indicated for small children since Best's disease, as an example of a condition in which EOG is indicated, rarely manifests in the first decade.

Visual-evoked potential (VEP) can also be helpful not only for measuring objectively visual acuity, but also for providing information about the visual pathway, as in cases of optic neuritis that may show a longer latency. The decision to perform electrophysiological tests before neuroimaging studies should be based on the individual child, depending on age, availability of an electrophysiological test laboratory, and possibility of associated CNS pathology.

Neuroimaging studies (see Chapter 13)

Magnetic resonance imaging and/or CT scan are indicated when clinical examination and electrophysiological tests fail to explain the cause of poor vision. Resolution of MRI is superior to that of CT scan, providing better images of the CNS, and it does not expose the child to radiation. However, MRI acquisition time is longer, it does not visualize the bone as well as CT scan, and it may require anesthesia in small children. Neuroimaging studies are important in cases of compressive lesions of the visual pathways, cortical abnormalities, and the demyelinating process, as these conditions may present with acquired visual loss in childhood.

CHAPTER
P15 The Deaf-Blind Child

Isabelle M Russell-Eggitt

Early diagnosis of sensory impairment is important in young children, especially if the defect is dual, for the child to achieve their maximum potential. An awareness of syndromes and associations will encourage screening for occult defect and clarify diagnosis so that prognosis and genetic counseling can be given. There is a high incidence of visual defects in deaf children and hearing impairment is frequent in children with visual defects. History taking is vital; often there have been family concerns considerably preceding medical diagnosis. Hearing tests performed in infants and young children include simple distraction tests similar to those used to assess field of vision and transient-evoked otoacoustic emission recording.[1]

HIGHER SENSORY PATHWAYS IN SEVERE CONGENITAL DEPRIVATION

Functional MRI imaging supports the hypothesis that perceptual functions may be organized differently in children with early severe damage to one or more sensory inputs. Blind individuals may have faster speech processing. During speech comprehension sighted individuals activate left hemisphere perisylvian language areas. Blind individuals in addition also display activation of extrastriate and striate cortex.[2] Deaf individuals may have enhanced motion processing, particularly in their right visual field, if they use sign language early compared to hearing individuals learning signing from their deaf parents.[3] Auditory deprivation from birth leads to compensatory changes within the visual system that enhance attentional processing of the peripheral visual field.[4]

MANAGEMENT OF THE DEAF-BLIND CHILD

Many children have useful residual sight or hearing or even both. However, a small group has profound dual handicap often also with other disabilities (see Tables P15.1–P15.7). It may be very difficult for a deaf-blind child, especially if both handicaps are profound, to acquire very basic skills such as spatial awareness and self/nonself differentiation. The early relationship between parents, especially the mother, and the infant is important for the child to achieve his or her full potential and not to develop frustrated, inturned, and often self-injurious behavior. There are several excellent books detailing care programs such as *The Deaf/Blind Baby* written by the mother of a multisensorially handicapped girl.[8] Other useful texts are referenced.[9,10] The family unit when first faced with a devastating diagnosis needs more than just information from the ophthalmologist. Support groups such as SENSE in the UK will need to be involved at an early stage (see Useful Addresses).

Table P15.1 Congenital or infantile severe vision and hearing impairment

Congenital infection
Rubella (Chapter 18)
Toxoplasma (Chapter 18)
Cytomegalovirus (Chapter 18)
Premature birth (Chapters 51 and 63)
CHARGE association (Chapter 24)
Genetic disorders
Cockayne syndrome (Chapter 53)
Zellweger syndrome (Chapters 53 and 65)
Infantile Refsum syndrome (Chapter 53)
Osteopetrosis (Chapter 53)
Mitochondrial mutations (Chapter 53)
Norrie syndrome (Chapter 55)
Tay-Sachs disease (Chapter 65)
KIDS (keratitis, ichthyosis, and deafness)
Trisomy 13 (Chapter 24)
X-linked ataxia, posterior column demyelination, deafness, optic atrophy (Chapter 61)
Yemenite deaf-blind hypopigmentation syndrome[5,6]
3-methylglutaconic aciduria, severe or type III (OPA3) (Chapter 65)
Alpers' progressive infantile poliodystrophy
Alpha-*N*-acetylgalactosaminidase deficiency (Chapter 65)
Krabbe (globoid) leukodystrophy
Fetal methylmercury exposure

Table P15.2 Congenital or infantile vision with subsequent hearing impairment

Alström syndrome (Chapter 53)
Norrie syndrome (Chapter 55)
Leber amaurosis–deafness (Chapter 53)
Peroxisome disorders (Chapters 53, 65)
X-linked ocular albinism–deafness (Chapter 45)

Table P15.3 Juvenile vision loss of vision with subsequent hearing loss

Refsum syndrome (Chapter 53)
Peroxisomal disorders (Chapters 53, 65)
Wolfram (DIDMOAD) syndrome (Chapter 60)

EDUCATION

In recent years, more deaf children are educated in mainstream schools than previously. Specialist deaf schools now have a higher proportion of children with dual handicap.[11] A child with a severe early-onset dual handicap is more likely to suffer from multiple-organ abnormality and severe learning difficulties. Education may be as basic as teaching self-feeding skills.[12] There

Table P15.4 Congenital or infantile hearing loss with subsequent vision impairment

Rubella (Chapter 18)
Norrie syndrome (Chapter 55)
Cockayne syndrome (Chapter 53)
Usher syndrome (Chapter 53)
Beighton syndrome (autosomal recessive sensorineural deafness, progressive rod–cone retinal dystrophy and renal failure)[7]
Hallgren syndrome (Chapter 53)
Premature birth (Chapters 51, 63)
CHARGE syndrome (Chapter 59)
Alström syndrome (Chapter 53)
Osteopetrosis (Chapter 53)
Albinism–late-onset deafness (Chapter 45)
Deafness-choroideremia deletion syndrome
Stickler, Kniest, and Marshall syndromes (Chapter 56)

Table P15.5 Acquired hearing and vision loss during childhood

Meningitis
Craniostenosis syndromes (Chapter 39)
Hydrocephalus (Chapter 63)
Trauma (Chapters 70 and 71)
Mitochondrial cytopathy (Chapter 53)
Biotinidase deficiency (Chapter 65)
Cockayne syndrome (Chapter 53)
Mucopolysaccharidoses (Chapter 65)
Friedreich's ataxia (Chapter 60)

Table P15.6 Congenital hearing loss with eye signs

Waardenburg syndrome (Chapter 45)
The Möbius complex (Chapter 85)
Wildervanck syndrome (Chapter 85)
Goldenhar syndrome (Chapters 25 and 28)

Table P15.7 Juvenile hearing loss with eye signs

Alport syndrome (Chapters 46 and 57)
Neurofibromatosis type 2 (Chapter 33)

is a goal of developing a sign system so that the child may communicate and acquire some control over his or her environment.[13] Videotapes illustrating an American "easy to feel, easy to relate to the referent, and easy to make" sign system are available to teachers and families.[14] Many children have some potentially useful residual sight and hearing, and early sensory training may improve outcome.[15]

PSYCHOSOCIAL SUPPORT

Both deaf and blind children may have difficulty in coming to terms with their handicap and difficulty with social and communication skills.[16] A dual-sensory defect can be even more disabling, and in severe early-onset disorders as yet only a partial communication system can be achieved.[17] Any residual vision is very valuable and use should be encouraged.[18]

COCHLEAR IMPLANTATION

Cochlear implantation may lead to the successful development of speech in some severely hearing-impaired children.[19] Congenitally severely hearing-impaired children who will later become blind, such as in Usher syndrome, have a high priority. Hearing must be stimulated early for sound to be understood and not just interpreted as noise. The hearing equivalent of derivational amblyopia requires that implantation is undertaken within the first two years.

REFRACT ALL CHILDREN WITH SEVERE HEARING IMPAIRMENT TO IMPROVE THEIR HEARING!

There is an increased incidence of ocular problems in children with hearing impairment apart from the conditions that lead to severe visual loss.[20] Paramount amongst these are refractive errors.[21] Obtaining the clearest possible vision is especially important to the hearing-impaired child, for lip reading, signing, and reading.

USEFUL ADDRESSES (See also Appendix P32)

SENSE (The UK National Deaf/Blind and Rubella Association), http://www.sense.org.uk

11–13 Clifton Terrace, London N4 3SR, UK
Tel: +44 (0)20 7272 7774; fax: +44 (0)20 7272 6012
- Advice, help, and provide information to deaf-blind people and their families.
- Support to families through a national network and local branches.
- Holiday program for deaf-blind children and adults.
- Education, residential, respite, and day services.
- Communicator-guides and one-to-one intervener support.
- Training and consultancy.

CAF (Contact a Family) UK, http://www.cafamily.org.uk

209–211 City Road, London EC1V 1JN, UK
Tel: +44 (0)20 7608 8700; fax: +44 (0)20 7608 8701
Helpline: 0808 808 3555, or Textphone: 0808 808 3556. Freephone for parents and families.
E-mail: info@cafamily.org.uk
- Expert and comprehensive knowledge about rare disorders and all aspects of disability.
- A wealth of personal experience and contacts.
- An approach driven first and foremost by parents' points of view.

American Association of the Deaf-Blind (AADB), http://www.aadb.org

814 Thayer Avenue, Suite 302, Silver Spring, MD 20910–4500, USA
Tel: +1 (800) 735-2258, +1 (301) 588-6545; fax: +1 (301) 588-8705
E-mail: info@aadb.org
- Consumer advocacy organization for people who have combined hearing and vision impairments.

- Open to all persons who are deaf-blind and individuals directly concerned with their well being.
- Seeks to encourage independent living for individuals who are deaf-blind.
- Provides technical assistance to persons who are deaf-blind, families, educators, and service providers.
- Services: Training of consumers, info and referral, social/recreational.

The Deafblind Association, Australia, http://www.dba.asn.au

616 Riversdale Road, Camberwell, Victoria, Australia 3124
PO Box 1213, Camberwell, Victoria, Australia 3124
Tel: +61 (03) 9882 7055; fax: +61 (03) 9882 9210

The Anne Sullivan Centre for Deaf-Blind

Brewery Road, Stillorgan, Co. Dublin, Republic of Ireland
Tel: +353 (0)1 289 8339; fax: +353 (0)1 289 8408

Toys for Children with Hearing and Vision Impairment

ROMPA Goyt Side Road, Chesterfield S40 2PH, UK
Tel: +44 (0)1246 211777; fax: +44 (0)1246 221802

Playring Limited

53 Westbere Road, West Hampstead, London NW2, UK
Tel: +44 (0)20 7794 9497

REFERENCES

1. Norton SJ, Gorga MP, Widen JE, et al. Identification of neonatal hearing impairment: summary and recommendations. Ear Hear 2000; 21: 529–35.
2. Roder B, Stock O, Bien S, et al. Speech processing activates visual cortex in congenitally blind humans. Eur J Neurosci 2002; 16: 930–6.
3. Bosworth RG, Dobkins KR. Visual field asymmetries for motion processing in deaf and hearing signers. Brain Cogn 2002; 49: 170–81.
4. Proksch J, Bavelier D. Changes in the spatial distribution of visual attention after early deafness. J Cogn Neurosci 2002; 14: 687–701.
5. Bondurand N, Kuhlbrodt K, Pingault V, et al. A molecular analysis of the Yemenite deaf-blind hypopigmentation syndrome: SOX10 dysfunction causes different neurocristopathies. Hum Mol Genet 1999; 8: 1785–9.
6. Hennekam RC, Gorlin RJ. Confirmation of the Yemenite (Warburg) deaf-blind hypopigmentation syndrome. Am J Med Genet 1996; 65: 146–8.
7. Beighton P, Bartmann L, Bingham G, et al. Rod-cone dystrophy, sensorineural deafness, and renal dysfunction: an autosomal recessive syndrome? Am J Med Genet 1993; 47: 832–6.
8. Freeman P. The deaf/blind baby: a programme of care. London: Heinemann; 1985.
9. Wyman R. Multiply Handicapped Children. London: Souvenir Press; 1986.
10. McInnes JM, Treffry JA. Deaf-blind Infants and Children: a developmental guide. Toronto: University of Toronto Press; 1993.
11. Admiraal RJ, Huygen PL. Changes in the aetiology of hearing impair-
ment in deaf-blind pupils and deaf infant pupils at an institute for the deaf. Int J Pediatr Otorhinolaryngol 2000; 55: 133–42.
12. Luiselli JK. Training self-feeding skills in children who are deaf and blind. Behav Modif 1993; 17: 457–73.
13. Ronnberg J, Borg E. A review and evaluation of research on the deaf-blind from perceptual, communicative, social and rehabilitative perspectives. Scand Audiol 2001; 30: 67–77.
14. Watkins S, Clark TC. A coactive sign system for children who are dual-sensory impaired. Am Ann Deaf 1991; 136: 321–4.
15. Michael MG, Paul PV. Early intervention for infants with deaf-blindness. Except Child 1990; 57: 200–10.
16. Abolfotouh MA, Telmesani A. A study of some psycho-social characteristics of blind and deaf male students in Abha City, Asir region, Saudi Arabia. Public Health 1993; 107: 261–9.
17. Downing JE. Communication intervention for individuals with dual sensory and intellectual impairments. Clin Commun Disord 1993; 3: 31–42.
18. Ronnberg J, Samuelsson E, Borg E. Exploring the perceived world of the deaf-blind: on the development of an instrument. Int J Audiol 2002; 41: 136–43.
19. Edwards LC. Candidacy and the Children's Implant Profile: is our selection appropriate? Int J Audiol 2003; 42: 426–31.
20. Siatkowski RM, Flynn JT, Hodges AV, et al. Visual function in children with congenital sensorineural deafness. Trans Am Ophthalmol Soc 1993; 91: 309–18.
21. Guy R, Nicholson J, Pannu SS, et al. A clinical evaluation of ophthalmic assessment in children with sensori-neural deafness. Child Care Health Dev 2003; 29: 377–84.

Optic Atrophy in Infancy and the Child with Optic Atrophy and Neurological Disease

Yoshikazu Hatsukawa

Presentation and diagnosis

Small children with optic atrophy do not have a pathognomonic mode of presentation connected with the optic atrophy itself. Rather, they present with either the general behavioral characteristics of visual loss or the ocular motor consequences thereof. The history is vital and particular attention should be paid to any family history of poor vision, consanguinity of the parents, the progress of the pregnancy and suspicion of the lack of weight gain as well as any immediate perinatal problem. The most important time in a child's life for acquiring non-refractive visual defects is in the perinatal period, particularly if the baby is premature or of low birth weight. The parents of these children should be questioned in detail about their baby's early life: whether the child had to be in the incubator, have added oxygen, be ventilated, or had any difficulty in breathing. Episodes of bradycardia or apnea must be noted; also whether the child had to be resuscitated, or the parents warned by the neonatologist that survival was in jeopardy.

If the onset was in postnatal life the mode of onset and the progression of any visual field defect should be detailed as well as possible, including the child's visual behavior. Many observant parents will make relevant observations about the vision and even about the state of the pupils, presence of nystagmus, strabismus or structural abnormalities of the eye. Their observations should be noted because they will be useful in determining progression, especially in the preverbal child who cannot perform standard subjective visual acuity tests.

An assessment of a child's visual function should be made together with the state of the pupil reactions, which if reacting sluggishly to light or showing a relatively afferent pupillary defect, will suggest anterior visual pathway disease. In older children, an acquired defect of color (usually red/green) vision may help in identifying optic nerve disease, especially if asymmetrical.

A careful examination of the fundus with both direct and indirect ophthalmoscopy is mandatory in order to establish the diagnosis of optic atrophy. The optic disc itself will appear pale with fewer than normal vessels on the surface. The pallor may be diffuse or segmental, and it is most important to pay attention to the presence of the nerve fiber layer atrophy which will show as an enhancement of the normal reflex from the retinal vessels, which normally do not stand up greatly against the internal limiting membrane: in optic atrophy where the nerve fiber layer has atrophied, the vessels stand out. If the optic atrophy is severe the vessels stand out like cords seen in the light reflected in parallax from the internal limiting membrane as it passes over the vessels.

The differential diagnosis on fundoscopy is between optic atrophy and optic disc hypoplasia or other congenital disc anomalies or even glaucoma. Here it is most important that the optic disc be examined by direct ophthalmoscopy. Structural anomalies of the optic disc may also be mistaken if the outline of the disc is not grossly abnormal and similarly glaucoma may be missed if the cup of the disc is not noticed during a hasty examination without adequate magnification. It is most important to pay very close attention to the state of the optic disc in order to be certain that it is either abnormal or entirely normal and that the visual defect may be attributed appropriately to either an optic disc problem or to some other cause, for instance, delayed visual development.

It is not possible to establish a cause in every case[1] and in published series the cause varies enormously between centers; the tertiary referral teaching center will see cases biased by a close association with neurology, neurosurgery or metabolic departments while developmental centers will see mainly cases associated with cerebral palsy.

Causes

Fig P16.1 provides guidelines for diagnosis (see text for details).

Optic atrophy occurs in late prenatal or early postnatal life.[2] Early prenatal onset damage to the anterior visual system results in a hypoplastic or anomalous optic disc. In postnatal life optic atrophy is an indication that the damage is anterior to the lateral geniculate. When the optic atrophy is definitely unilateral, the cause is anterior to the chiasm and when it is definitely bilateral it is either due to bilateral disease or disease involving pathways posterior to the chiasm. It is possible that late prenatal brain damage may, by trans-synaptic degeneration, give rise to optic atrophy without hypoplasia, but there is little clear evidence for this in human studies. Prenatal causes of optic atrophy include the hereditary optic neuropathies and metabolic causes. If there is a history of pre- or perinatal problems they may well be the cause, especially if there is a history of significant perinatal hypoxia.

Conversely, one should be cautious about attributing optic atrophy to a relatively mild perinatal insult and it is rare for optic atrophy caused by perinatal problems to not be associated with other obvious central nervous system damage. Postnatal causes include tumors invading or encroaching on the visual pathways. Clues to this in the diagnosis may be in the history of progression of the visual defect and associated eye movement disorders or the presence of systemic diseases such as neurofibromatosis. There may be a clear history of trauma or meningitis and a careful history should be taken of any drug ingestion.

Hydrocephalus may also result in optic atrophy but it is an entirely unusual presenting symptom of this disorder. The child with repeated shunt failures or infections is particularly prone to develop optic atrophy. Optic atrophy in hydrocephalus may be difficult to assess even in later life as acuity may be preserved much later than other aspects of vision. Babies with lactic

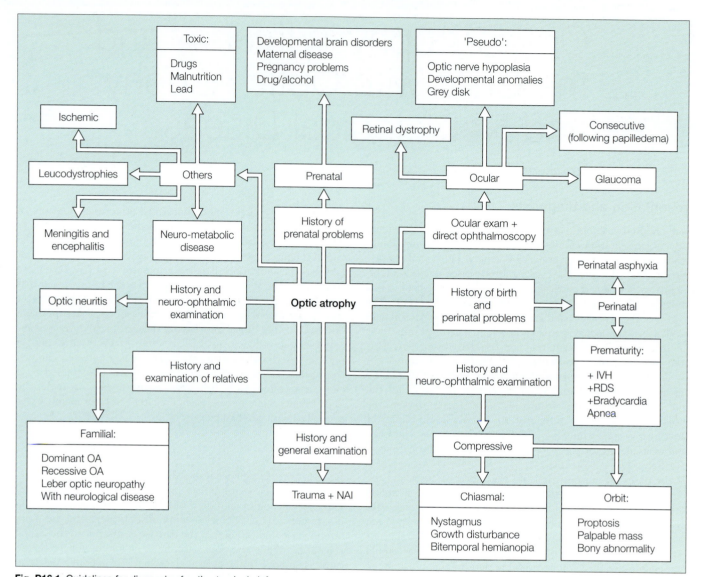

Fig. P16.1 Guidelines for diagnosis of optic atrophy in infancy.

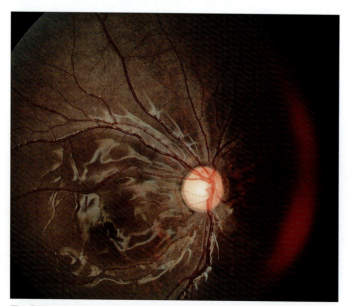

Fig. P16.2 Post-traumatic optic atrophy of the right eye discovered by vision screening at the age of three years. The acuity is 1/60. The child had an episode of head trauma at the age of 7 months.

acidosis (i.e. Leigh disease, mitochondrial cytopathy, pyruvate decarboxylase or cytochrome oxidase deficiency) have a high incidence of optic atrophy, sometimes profound.[3] Other optic neuropathies in many of the hereditary optic neuropathies present later in childhood or the teens.

Investigation

Structure eye disease must be excluded, especially retinal disorders, even if the retina appears normal. An electroretinogram is important in establishing that optic atrophy is not associated with a primary retinal disorder. The integrity of the visual pathways may also be assessed by visually evoked responses. A CT or MRI scan may also be indicated. Systemic investigations are carried out where appropriate.

Prognosis

The prognosis depends on the diagnosis and the natural history of the condition. Much caution should be used in giving a prognosis to parents whose child has recently suffered optic atrophy from an acute cause such as tumor or hydrocephalus, since very dramatic recovery can take place up to 2 or occasionally more

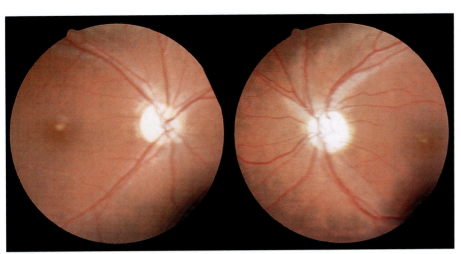

Fig. P16.3 Bilateral optic atrophy in a 10-year-old boy with adrenoleucodystrophy.

years after the onset of the visual loss. As a general rule it is better to be optimistic rather than pessimistic and this should especially be so if there is still some response to a flash stimulus on the visual evoked responses. Every pediatric ophthalmologist has seen examples of remarkable late recovery in vision with optic atrophy or cerebral disorders in infancy.

The uncertainty about prognosis, however, should not inhibit the ophthalmologist from registering the visual handicap with the appropriate authority, although re-assessment should be suggested periodically.

REFERENCES

1. Repka M, Miller NR. Optic atrophy in children. *Am J Ophthalmol* 1988; 191: 181–4.
2. Hoyt CS, Good WV. Do we understand the difference between optic nerve hypoplasia and atrophy? *Eye* 1992; 6: 201–4.
3. Hayasaka S, Yamaguschio K, Misuro K, Miyabayashi S, Narasawa K, Tada K. Ocular findings in childhood lactic acidosis. *Arch Ophthalmol* 1986; 104: 1956–8.

CHAPTER P17 Optic Disc Swelling in Children

David Taylor

PAPILLEDEMA

Papilledema is optic disc swelling associated with raised intracranial pressure. The vision is usually normal, even when the discs are markedly swollen although in later or very severe cases there may be a progressive loss of vision. The swelling comprises congested neurons and dilated blood vessels, and these spread into the surrounding tissues, causing retinal disturbance, radial retinal folds (Paton's lines), and choroidal folds. A hypermetropic refractive error is induced by the raised retina, and enlargement of the blind spot is noted on visual field testing. An enlarged blind spot also occurs in optic nerve infiltration, developmental anomalies, and trauma and as part of a centrocecal scotoma or as an event of presumed retinal origin in an otherwise normal optic disc. If visual loss is progressive, nerve fiber bundle field defects and peripheral constriction occur.

The earliest signs of papilledema include a blurring of the disc margins (Fig. P17.1), an elevated disc, a dilated peripapillary capillary plexus, dilated retinal veins with absent pulsation at the optic disc, and swollen nerve fiber bundles (Figs. P17.2–P17.4).

Splinter hemorrhages, a more markedly elevated disc, nerve fiber infarcts ("cotton-wool spots"), exudates (Fig. P17.5), and macular star formation follow. The retinal and disc capillaries become more engorged and tortuous and hemorrhages more widespread (Fig. P17.6).

Children with a chronic but mildly raised intracranial pressure (as in some cases of craniosynostosis) may have papilledema for

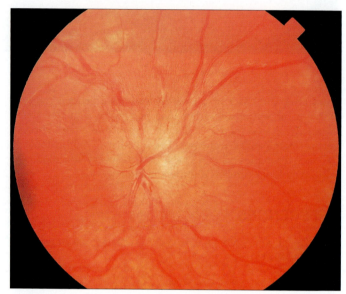

Fig. P17.2 Moderate papilledema with swollen disc and peripapillary nerve fiber layer with dilated capillaries and veins and nerve fiber layer hemorrhages.

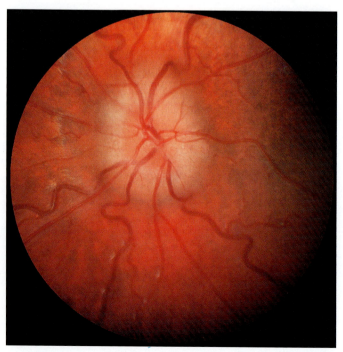

Fig. P17.3 Chronic papilledema in a patient with craniosynostosis; note the elevated optic disc and tortuous dilated veins.

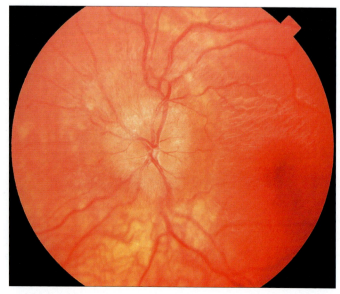

Fig. P17.1 Mild papilledema with mildly swollen disc and peripapillary nerve fiber layer.

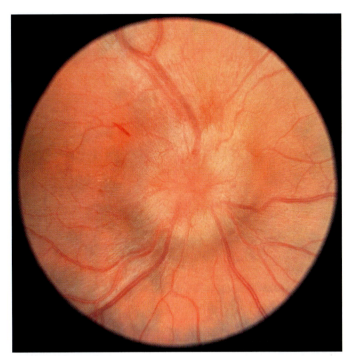

Fig. P17.4 Papilledema secondary to raised intracranial pressure; note the elevated disc, swollen nerve fiber layer, dilated veins, and small hemorrhages radiating around the disc.

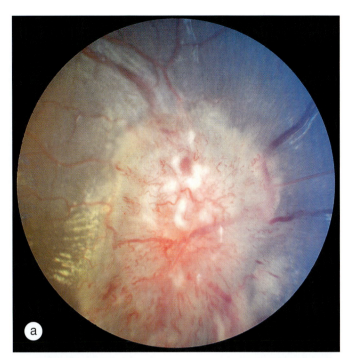

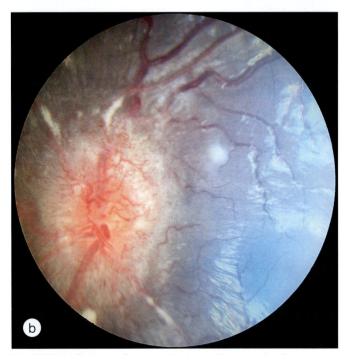

Fig. P17.6 (a) Right eye. Severe papilledema with gross elevation, hemorrhages, exudates, macular star, dilated veins, and cotton-wool spots on the optic disc. (b) Same patient. The left eye is less affected. Asymmetry is frequent in papilledema and may be due to anomalous optic nerve sheaths.

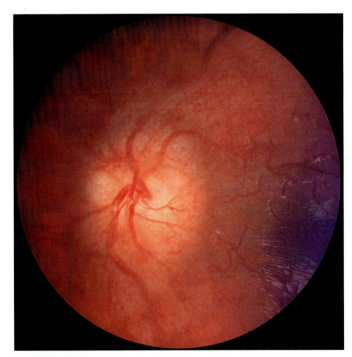

Fig. P17.5 Papilledema in a patient with neurofibromatosis and a chiasmal glioma. The swelling of the optic disc with dilated veins, hemorrhages, a few exudates, and dilated capillaries is most marked in the upper and lower poles. This eye has a temporal hemianopia and the fibers swollen are those subserving the intact nasal field. The horizontal band of relative lack of swelling is in the area of the disc that is atrophic from loss of nerve fibers. The superior poles, although also atrophic, are covered by the fibers from the intact nasal field.

many years without loss of vision, the clinical dilemma being the decision of whether the papilledema is or will be associated with neuronal loss. If the intracranial pressure is very high there is a progressive loss of neurons, accompanied by increasingly frequent visual symptoms. Optic atrophy ensues as the neurons die, the disc becoming flat again after a period of being swollen and pale (Fig. P17.7).

The symptoms are those of headache and episodic visual loss in the form of posture-related obscurations, which consist of

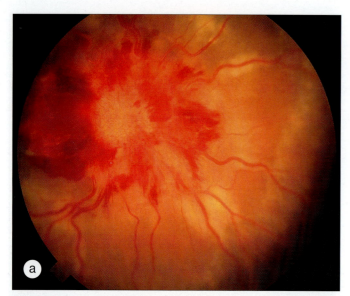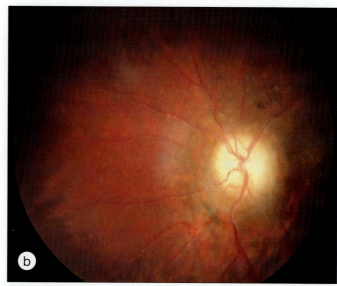

Fig. P17.7 (a) Severe papilledema with widespread hemorrhages. (b) The optic nerve has decompensated and there is marked consecutive optic atrophy. The eye is blind. The 7-year-old child had severe papilledema due to a posterior fossa tumor (same eye).

seconds-long blackouts or grayouts. In many children, for instance, with long-standing shunted hydrocephalus in which the shunt is malfunctioning, there are very few symptoms of progressive visual loss. When there is likely to be visual loss reliance needs to be placed on acuity, color vision, and visual field examinations supplemented by serial pattern visual-evoked potential (VEP) studies, neuroimaging, eye ultrasound (to identify optic disc drusen), and intracranial pressure monitoring, but so often the child is uncooperative and difficult to test that it is inevitable that some patients will be less than optimally managed. For management of papilledema see Chapters 63 and P18.

THE DIFFERENTIAL DIAGNOSIS OF THE SWOLLEN OPTIC DISC IN CHILDHOOD

(See Table P17.1)

Bilateral

1. Papilledema: raised intracranial pressure:
   - Hydrocephalus (Chapter 63); and
   - Idiopathic intracranial hypertension: pseudo-tumor cerebri (Chapter P18).
2. Hypertension: usually has associated retinal vascular signs.

3. Papillitis: optic neuritis and other optic neuropathies (Chapters 60 and 61).
4. Optic disc swelling in diabetes mellitus (mostly bilateral):
   - Idiopathic;
   - Hypertension; and
   - Raised ICP from sinus thrombosis.
5. Bilateral cases of unilateral causes of unilateral disc edema or pseudopapilledema (see below).

Unilateral

1. Pseudopapilledema:
   - Drusen (Chapter 59);
   - Myelinated nerve fibers (Fig. P17.8), (Chapter 59);
   - Hypermetropia, "crowded" disc (Chapter 6);
   - Myopia, "tilted" disc (Chapter 16);
   - Glial anomalies (Fig. P17.9), (Chapter 59); and
   - Idiopathic swelling in Down syndrome.
2. Tumors, Infiltrations, and compression:
   - Solid tumors:
     - Hemangioma (Chapter 55);
     - "Mulberry tumor" of tuberous sclerosis (Fig. P17.10), (Chapter 69);

Table P17.1 Common causes of swollen optic discs in childhood						
	Acuity loss	Field defect	Color vision	Pain?	Biomicroscopy	Optic nerve appearance
Optic neuropathy	Early	Central/centrocecal	↓↓↓	On eye movement	Cells in anterior vitreous	Usually mild swelling. Few hges
Papilledema	Late or very late	Large blind spots	Normal	Headache only	No cells	Mild to marked swelling. Hges+
Pseudopapilledema	None/minimal in Drusen	None/minimal	Normal	None	No cells	No hges. Drusen/other findings.
Optic nerve compression	Early	Variable. Often central	↓↓	Depends on cause	No cells	Swollen. No hges
Optic disc infiltration	Variable but usual	Variable but usual	↓	Not usually	Often abnormal + cells	Variable/swollen/hges and exudates

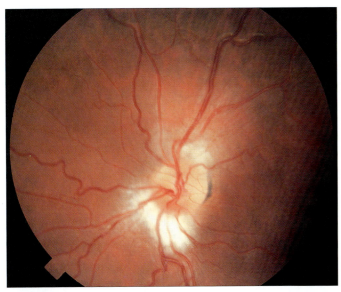

Fig. P17.8 Bilateral peripapillary myelinated nerve fibers and papilledema in a patient with hydrocephalus.

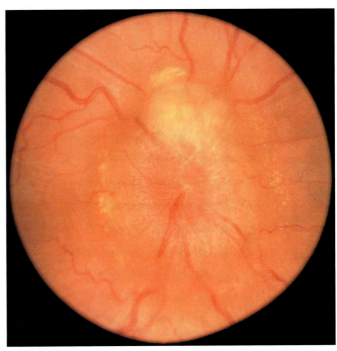

Fig. P17.10 Papilledema in a child with tuberous sclerosis and hydrocephalus. Note that at the superior pole there is a phakoma, which gave rise to a form of pseudopapilledema in addition to the papilledema.

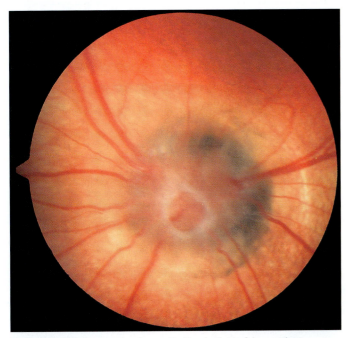

Fig. P17.9 "Glial" anomaly of an optic disc (unilateral) in a patient presenting with headaches suspected of having unilateral papilledema by the referring doctor.

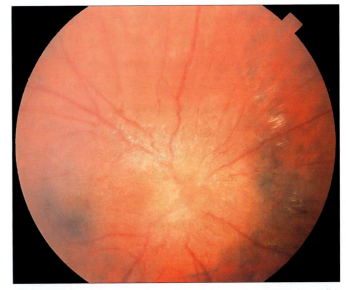

Fig. P17.11 Combined hamartoma of the optic nerve and retina in a child who presented with strabismus and mild documented visual loss aged 7 years.

- ▪ Retinal hamartoma (Fig. P17.11), (Chapter 55); and
- ▪ Retinoblastoma (Chapter 50).
- ▪ Infiltrations, etc.:
  - ▪ Optic nerve glioma with or without disc invasion (Fig. P17.12), (Chapter 34);
  - ▪ Leukemia (Chapter 68);
  - ▪ Juvenile xanthogranuloma (Fig. P17.13), (Chapter 38);
  - ▪ Sarcoidosis (Chapter 44); and
  - ▪ Mucopolysaccharidoses (Chapter 65).
- ▪ Other forms of compression (Chapters 32-42):
  - ▪ Bone disorders (craniometaphyseal dysplasia, osteopetrosis, etc.);

- ▪ Dysthyroid eye disease (unusual in childhood); and
- ▪ Orbital tumors.
3. Uveitis (Chapter 44):
   - ▪ *Toxocara* involving the disc (Fig. P17.14);
   - ▪ Lyme disease;
   - ▪ Other uveitis (Fig. P17.15); and
   - ▪ Swollen disc secondary to hypotony.
4. Ischemic optic neuropathy:
   - ▪ Hypertension; and
   - ▪ Vasculitis.

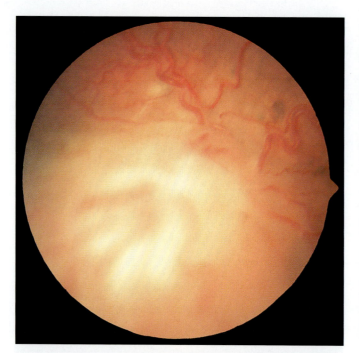

Fig. P17.12 Optic nerve involvement with glioma. There is a large swelling extending anteriorly from the lower part of the optic disc that consists of edema and tumor involvement. Four year old with no signs of neurofibromatosis.

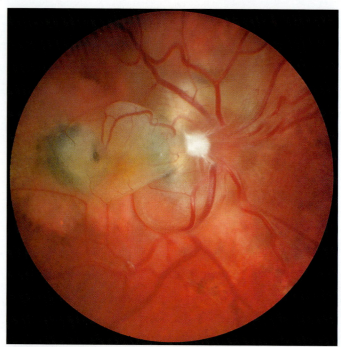

Fig. P17.14 *Toxocara* involving the optic disc. At presentation there was a marked uveitis and swelling of the optic disc obscuring all details.

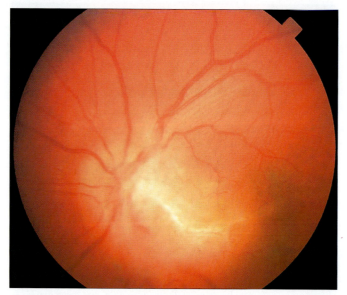

Fig. P17.13 Optic disc swelling, peripapillary retinal edema, and swelling from infiltration by juvenile xanthogranuloma.

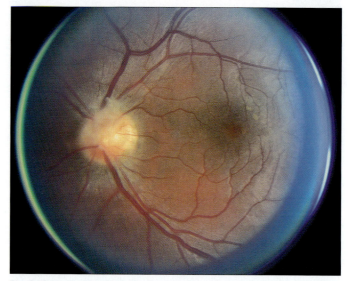

Fig. P17.15 Uveitis with optic disc swelling and opacities in front of the disc.

5. Papillitis/optic neuropathy (Chapters 60 and 61):
   ■ Optic neuritis;
   ■ Leber hereditary neuropathy; and
   ■ Other optic neuropathies.

6. Papilledema.

Papilledema may be asymmetrical, perhaps due to unilateral acquired or congenital lesions in one optic disc, but it is rarely unilateral.

CHAPTER
P18 Headaches

Abdulaziz H Awad

INTRODUCTION

Headaches are common among children and adolescents. The pain is of great concern to both the parent and child but medical attention is usually sought to find the cause of the headache: parents are aware that headaches can be a sign of more serious disease. It is the first responsibility of the doctor to find the cause of the headache and, if possible, provide assurance that the headache is not associated with a serious condition.

It is often possible to differentiate between benign and more sinister headaches with a history and physical examination alone. When this is not possible, appropriate clinical, laboratory, and diagnostic investigations are mandatory and referral to other medical specialists may be appropriate.

The following points in the history or examination warrant careful attention for an organic cause:

1. A headache that begins in the early morning or awakens the child during sleep and especially if it is increasing in frequency or severity.
2. A headache in a very young child and of recent onset. Young children are often unable to adequately express that they are suffering from headache. When they do, it is often severe.
3. Coexistence of headache or migraine with (especially focal) seizures.
4. Recent history of school failure or a change in behavior.
5. A headache that is associated with, or relieved by, significant cough or vomiting.
6. Focal neurologic symptoms or signs developing during a headache (i.e., complicated headache).

The role of the ophthalmologist is primarily to distinguish between ocular and nonocular causes for the patient's symptoms. Pediatric ophthalmologists frequently hear the histories of headaches and acquire expertise in headache diagnosis and management.

NONOCULAR HEADACHE: SOURCES OF PAIN IN THE HEAD AND NECK

Blood vessels are a major source of pain inside the skull. Head pain can be generated by dilation, inflammation, and/or traction-displacement of intracranial and extracranial blood vessels. The brain parenchyma, ependymal lining, and meninges are not pain sensitive. The trigeminal nerve transmits pain from the supratentorial intracranial vessels while the first three cervical nerves are responsible for pain transmission from the infratentorial intracranial vessels. Scalp arteries are also pain sensitive, and produce pain when they are dilated or stretched. The periosteum (especially in the sinuses and near the teeth), the muscles attached to the skull, the cervical roots, and cranial nerves are sensitive to mechanical traction from injury or deformation.

Vascular headache

Migraine

Migraine is a recurrent clinical syndrome characterized by combinations of neurological, gastrointestinal, and autonomic manifestations. Cervico-trigemino-vascular dysfunction may be the primary cause.[1-3] It is often hereditary. Although headache is a prominent feature, it is not always present.

The diagnosis of migraine in children is established by a personal profile, attack profile, family history, and the absence of organic disease. Often, the child with migraine has a history of early-onset migraine equivalents including colic, abdominal pain, cyclic vomiting, night terrors, and paroxysmal torticollis.[4] The migraine sufferer will often be highly reactive to extraneous visual, auditory, gustatory, and thermal stimuli: bright lights, strong smells, and abrupt motion may trigger migraines. Parents must be questioned for a family history of migraine or migraine-like headaches. When doubt exists about the diagnosis clinical and laboratory investigations and neuroimaging may be carried out to rule out organic disease.

Epidemiology and triggering factors

Migraine accounts for 75% of headaches in young children referred for neurological consultation.[5] The prevalence of migraine is 2.5% under the age of 7 years with both sexes equally affected. From age 7 to puberty, the prevalence is 5% and the ratio of affected females to males is 3:2. In postpubescent males, the prevalence remains at 5%; while in postpubescent girls, the prevalence rises to 10%.[6,7] The prevalence data for preschool children are probably higher than what is typically reported, as migraine is underdiagnosed in young children. The higher incidence in postpubescent girls may be related to the menstrual cycle.

Triggering factors for migraine can be somewhat nebulous; however, there are several that are commonly reported: stress, exercise, foodstuff, missed meals, head trauma, and the premenstrual decline in circulating estrogen. Allergies have also been cited (but substantiated) as potential triggering factors.

Migraine without aura (common migraine)

This is the most common form of migraine in children and adolescents. Children with common migraines frequently have physical and emotional changes leading up to an attack, including malaise, irritability, and lethargy. The headache is usually bifrontal or bitemporal, but can be unilateral. Often, children have difficulty localizing the pain and/or describing the quality; however, when it is possible, it is usually described as a pounding pain. While it can be difficult to differentiate migraine from other childhood headaches, there are several clues. Children with migraines feel sick, want to rest, and are often highly sensitive to light and sound.

Severe nausea and vomiting may occur during the attack, and often continue after the headache has subsided.

Migraine with aura (classic migraine)

The hallmark of classic migraine is the visual, autonomic, or somatosensory auras that precede an attack. It occurs more frequently in adults than in children and adolescents. The pain is usually described as throbbing and severe. Visual auras are the most common type of aura, and often consist of one or more of the following features: sparking lights, colored lines, "fortification spectra," blind spots, blurred vision, hemianopia, transient blindness (amaurosis fugax), micropsia, and, rarely, visual hallucinations. About 40% of children with migraines have visual symptoms,[4,8] which vary from child to child, but are usually perceived in only one eye or in one field, and without localization. Somatosensory auras include speech disturbances, focal motor weakness, and focal sensory change. Autonomic auras include distortion of body image, malaise, pallor, and irritability. Generally, the aura associated with classic migraine lasts less than 20 minutes. It is commonly reported that if an aura is lateralized, then the subsequent headache will be contralateral. Of special interest to the ophthalmologist is the *headache-less migraine:* an aura without a headache–though it would be unlikely for a child to present with this.

Complicated migraine

Complicated migraines are migraine attacks associated with transient neurological disturbances. They may be the result of ischemia and edema with secondary intracranial vasoconstriction. The neurological deficit is dependent upon the location of the affected vessels. The neurological symptoms are infrequently permanent. Patients usually recover completely and rarely do symptoms persist. The presence of neurological symptoms can be distressing and a more sinister etiology should be excluded, usually by investigations including EEG, MRI, and MR angiography (MRA).

Ophthalmoplegic migraine

Localized headache in the orbital region associated with partial or complete paralysis of the oculomotor nerve is called ophthalmoplegic migraine. The pain is sometimes severe, lasts several hours, and is accompanied by the typical symptoms of a partial or complete third nerve palsy–a combination of the following: strabismus (usually an exotropia with hypotropia in the affected eye), ptosis, diplopia, and variable pupillary dilation. Sometimes there is no pain at all. Recurrent attacks may lead to permanent dysfunction of the third cranial nerve. Enhanced MRI studies suggest that this disorder may represent an inflammatory process similar to Tolosa-Hunt syndrome occurring in the interpeduncular segment of the oculomotor nerve. Patients with ophthalmoplegic migraine may, therefore, benefit from the use of steroids.[9] These findings have been supported by a more recent study that concludes that ophthalmoplegic migraine is not truly a migraine but is caused by a trigeminovascular migraine epiphenomenon consisting of a thickened and enhancing ipsilateral oculomotor nerve at its exit from the midbrain.[10]

Hemiplegic migraine

Hemiplegic migraine is headache associated with hemiplegia. It may be familial or sporadic. The hemiparesis usually precedes the headache, and patients may have additional cortical deficits including visual field defects and aphasia. Many have a mutation that maps to the *CACNA1A* gene on chromosome 19p13.[11] There is heterogeneity of the symptoms associated with mutations of this gene.[12]

Differential diagnosis includes occlusive cerebral vasculature disease, arteriovenous malformations, cerebral hemorrhage, brain tumor, vasculitis, mitochondrial encephalopathy with acidosis, moya-moya disease, and stroke. Treatment with calcium channel blocking agents has proven to be effective in both the sporadic and familial forms of the disease.[13]

Basilar artery migraine

Basilar artery migraine affects the basilar artery and its branches. It typically presents as an occipital headache preceding, coexisting, or following blurred or tunnel vision and one or more of the following: paresthesias, ataxia, vertigo, dysarthria, obtundation, hemiparesis, quadriparesis, or loss of consciousness. It is most common in adolescent females. The differential diagnosis should include seizures, demyelinating disease, infection, trauma with vertebral artery dissection, and congenital anomalies of the occipital cervical region.[14]

Confusional migraine

Migraine followed by confusion is called confusional migraine. It is mainly a condition of adolescence, and can be mistaken for drug abuse. The duration of confusion is usually less than 24 hr.[15] Other findings may include a positive history of mild head trauma, agitation, past history of headache, and a family history of migraine on the maternal side. MRI and CT scans are usually normal.[16] EEG may reveal slowing over the dominant hemisphere. Management of a child with confusional migraine must take into consideration underlying causes, such as seizures, encephalitis, and substance abuse.

Management of migraine

Many cases of migraine can be managed by explanation, reassurance, and simple measures to avoid the attacks if they are precipitated by specific factors such as foods or exercise. Resting or sleep may be all that some children need. Other nonpharmacological treatment regimens include relaxation therapy, counseling, and biofeedback. Simple analgesia with ibuprofen or paracetamol may be effective.

Recently published evidence-based guidelines advocate migraine-specific drugs, such as serotonin 5-HT (1B/1D) agonists (the triptans) and dihydroergotamine mesylate, for patients with moderate to severe migraine. Additional therapeutic options include other ergotamine derivatives, phenothiazines, nonsteroidal anti-inflammatory agents, and opioids. Preventative medication therapy is indicated for patients experiencing frequent and/or refractory attacks.[1]

Vascular nonmigrainous headache

Other than migraine, vascular headache can be due to the following:

1. Traction displacement of the intracranial vessels as in increased intracranial pressure.
2. Vasodilation of the intracranial or extracranial vessels as in:
   a. Hypertension;
   b. Fever;
   c. Effort headache (exertional headaches);
   d. Post-trauma headaches; and
   e. Secondary to drugs or toxins.
3. Vasculitis.

Cerebral vasculitis is uncommon in children and usually occurs as part of an autoimmune disorder (e.g., systemic lupus erythematosus), hypersensitivity reaction (e.g., serum sickness, Henoch-Schönlein purpura, and cocaine abuse), or secondary to infectious process. Diagnosis would depend on the patient history and on the accompanying clinical signs and symptoms.

Increased intracranial pressure

Headaches and transient visual obscurations are the main presenting symptoms from elevated intracranial pressure. Nausea, vomiting ("sometimes projectile"), persistent visual loss, and diplopia are also reported. Characteristically, however, the headaches are frequently present upon awakening. The older child is often manifestly distressed by the pain and may describe it as "bursting" or "blowing up." Younger children just go "off color" or babies become disgruntled and unhappy.[17] The visual obscurations can be of "gray outs" or "fuzz out," lasting a few seconds. They occur upon bending over or standing up or with Valsalva pressure. Papilledema is the main sign of elevated intracranial pressure; however, in children it may or may not be present.

Intracranial mass lesions are the primary diagnostic considerations. They can elevate intracranial pressure by acting as space-occupying lesions, by producing focal or diffuse cerebral edema or by blocking the flow of cerebrospinal fluid or compressing a venous sinus. Rarely it is due to excessive production of cerebrospinal fluid as in choroid plexus papilloma.

Pseudotumor cerebri in children/idiopathic intracranial hypertension

Idiopathic intracranial hypertension (IIH) is a condition characterized by symptoms and signs of increased intracranial pressure without evidence of a mass lesion or hydrocephalus. The level of consciousness is not affected.[18] As the diagnosis in primary cases is essentially one of exclusion the following criteria have been recommended for the diagnosis of primary IIH:

1. Signs and symptoms of increased intracranial pressure;
2. Absence of localizing findings on neurological examination;
3. Otherwise normal neurodiagnostic studies, except for increased cerebrospinal fluid pressure;
4. Alert and oriented patient; and
5. No other cause for the increased intracranial pressure is present.

Although it is considered to be a disease of obese women of childbearing age, it can occur in children of all ages. Unlike adults, the male–female ratio in prepubescent children is approximately equal. Starting at puberty, however, there is a distinct female predominance. Obesity is less common in children than in adults with primary IIH. Spontaneous remissions are more common in children than in adults.

Infants and young children may present with irritability, somnolence with or without dizziness, or ataxia. In older children apathy or nervousness may be the presenting complaint. Generalized seizures have also been reported. Infants with open fontanelles may still develop papilledema. Lateral rectus paresis, skew deviation, and facial paresis are seen more often in children than in adults.

Children and adults share a similar, significant, risk of visual loss secondary to pseudotumor cerebri; hence the term *idiopathic intracranial hypertension* is now favored over benign intracranial hypertension. Optic atrophy secondary to chronic papilledema is the main cause of visual loss, which can evolve in a period of weeks in severe cases. Hence, there is the need for urgent and aggressive intervention at the earliest sign of decreased vision. Other rare causes of visual loss including central retinal artery occlusion, peripapillary subretinal neovascularization, anterior ischemic optic neuropathy, and macular edema should also be sought.

Secondary IIH can be due to several disease processes. It can be associated with neurological diseases including dural venous thrombosis, arteriovenous malformations, or gliomatosis cerebri. It can be secondary to systemic disease: malnutrition, systemic lupus erythematosus, Addison's disease, or severe anemia. IIH can be secondary to the withdrawal of corticosteroid or the ingestion of tetracycline, vitamin A, nalidixic acid, thyroxine, or danazol.

Treatment is primarily of the underlying cause in secondary IIH. In primary cases treatments include oral steroids (which may be more effective in children), furosemide, and high-dose acetazolamide.[19] Surgical intervention includes optic nerve sheath fenestration and lumboperitoneal shunt.[19] Shunting is effective but it carries the risk of shunt failure, infection that may be life threatening, and tonsillar herniation. Optic nerve sheath fenestration may have the lowest risk, and be the most effective way for restoring or preserving vision in pseudotumor cerebri. It is the surgical treatment of choice in some centers. It relieves the headache in two thirds of the patients. Optic nerve sheath fenestration is indicated when there is evidence of progressive optic neuropathy, i.e., visual acuity or field loss despite medical treatment.[19]

Hypertension

Headaches are rarely caused by hypertension, but they can be the most common symptom of childhood hypertension. Sudden rise in systemic blood pressure (hypertension crisis) causes explosive throbbing headache. Childhood hypertension headache is usually severe (Fig. P18.1), may wake the child, or may be present upon waking. It is made worse by lifting heavy objects. Hypertension retinopathy or papilledema is often present.[20] It is certain that the improved medical care has increased the survival of children with chronic illnesses especially renal or renovascular disorders. Therefore, childhood hypertension is more frequent. It is easily overlooked though it can account for serious neurological disability and blindness.

Early recognition and treatment avoids those complications and improves the survival and well being of the child. Pediatric ophthalmologists should be able to measure blood pressure of their patients.

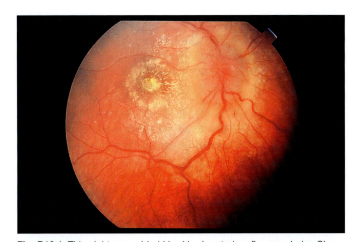

Fig. P18.1 This eight-year-old girl had had ureteric reflux as a baby. She had intermittent headaches for six months, gradually becoming more frequent and worse, before her blood pressure was taken. She made a full recovery but had chronic renal disease. Early diagnosis of hypertension (which is often not suspected in children) is essential to prevent devastating complications. The picture shows gross papilledema and a macular star.

Fever headache

Fever is the most common cause of vascular headache. Vasodilation of the intra- and extracranial vessels, which parallels the rise of body temperature, accounts for the headache. It is bitemporal or diffuse in location and throbbing in quality. The underlying etiology is usually self-evident and does not need further diagnostic studies unless infection of the nervous system or subarachnoid hemorrhage is suspected.

Effort headache (exertional headaches)

As the name indicates these headaches are precipitated by exertion, including coughing, running, and swimming. It may interfere with training as it may occur during or after the activity and may be associated with nausea and vomiting. The pain may be brief and generalized, or sharply localized and may last up to 12 hr. It is believed that the increase in intrathoracic pressure and sudden increase in blood pressure lead to extracranial vasodilatation and headache. In the majority of cases the headaches are benign; however, special attention should be paid to the patient's blood pressure at rest and during exercise. Treatment is usually conservative; however, indometacin may be used before specific activities.

Post-traumatic headache

Several different kinds of headaches of different mechanisms may be associated with head trauma. Vascular headache accounts for a significant percentage of the headache experienced in the first day or two after head injury. It is diffuse, pounding in nature and is made worse by head movement or straining. It usually subsides spontaneously. Meningism, sinus diseases, or direct skull or muscle trauma can also account for post-trauma headache. Behavioral disorders and lack of concentration are also sequelae of head injury.

Drugs and toxins

Many psychotropic drugs, analgesics, and cardiovascular agents have vasodilating properties and consequently can give rise to headache. Cocaine may produce a migraine-like headache in individuals who do not have migraine otherwise.[21] It should be suspected in any child who experiences vascular headache following the administration of, or exposure to, any drug, toxin, or food additive. Treatment is by avoidance of the substance.

Psychogenic (stress/tension) headache

It is estimated to account for 75% of childhood headache affecting all ages and both sexes.[22] The pain is characteristically a dull ache or pressure squeezing around the head. The neck muscles may feel stiff. It is most commonly caused by stress; however, fatigue, exertion, or hunger may produce tension headaches. It is important to remember that children may not be able to communicate their fears and often headaches may be the first symptom of their stress.

The mechanism is probably prolonged contracture of the muscles attached to the skull with the induced relative ischemia. Vascular headaches and tension headaches may be concurrent. Nausea, vomiting, and other symptoms of vascular headaches are not usually present in tension headaches.

Tension headaches should be differentiated from chronic mixed headaches, which may have similar clinical features but persists for weeks, months, and years. Tension headaches on the other hand are often self-diagnosed, limited, and respond to relaxation, rest, and mild analgesia. The most important treatment is explanation and reassurance of the parent and child.

Headache due to intracranial disease

Irritation of the meninges (meningism) may produce a headache and a stiff neck that is worse on flection. It can be due to meningitis or to blood in the cerebrospinal fluid as in subarachnoid hemorrhage. Acute subarachnoid hemorrhage with cerebral aneurysm is usually preceded by "a sentinel" headache, which is immediate, severe, and unique for the patient "like a thunder clap in a clear sky." If diagnosed early, it may lead to satisfactory treatment.[17] Arteriovenous malformation, on the other hand, is well known to produce the triad of hemorrhage, seizures, and recurrent headaches. Children are more likely to present with hemorrhage, whereas adults are more likely to present with headaches.[23] Intracranial tumors particularly posterior fossa tumors usually give rise to headaches by increasing intracranial pressure. Arnold-Chiari malformations may give rise to suboccipital or occipital headaches aggravated by cough or Valsalva maneuver. Other intracranial lesions give rise to headaches by one or more of the above mechanisms.

OCULAR HEADACHE

Ocular disease

Several intraocular disease processes can cause a deep, throbbing pain localized to the orbital region. In children especially, this eye pain may be described as headache. These include the following.

Uveitis (see Chapter 44)
Inflammation of the iris or ciliary body can be very painful and is associated with ciliary injection at first, then an overall red eye.

Angle-closure glaucoma (see Chapter 48)
A sudden upward surge of intraocular pressure can cause intense intraorbital pain.

Other
Other causes of ocular pain include endophthalmitis, scleritis, and corneal disease; however, these conditions have clinical characteristics (e.g., red eye or pain only on blinking) that easily differentiate them from headache.

Orbital disease

Young children can describe pain localized to the orbital region as headache, which can include orbital inflammation of any kind. Some examples would include the following.

Orbital myositis
Orbital myositis is an inflammation of one or more of the extraocular muscles, and is characterized by pain when the eye is moved into the field of the affected muscle (see Chapter 41).

Optic neuritis
Inflammation of the optic nerve, causing retrobulbar pain, is often made worse on extreme movement and is associated in children with profound visual loss (see Chapter 61).

Orbital pseudotumor
See Chapter 41.

Orbital cellulitis/abscess
See Chapter 20.

Latent strabismus

In addition to the minimum convergence, divergence, or vertical fusional amplitudes required to simply control a latent deviation, one must also have a sufficient reserve of fusional amplitudes to comfortably maintain binocular single vision throughout the course of one's normal activities.

If a patient does not have sufficient fusional amplitudes, the patient may experience asthenopic symptoms, including frontal headaches. Characteristically, these start after "using the eyes" and rarely on resting or waking.

Patients with headache stemming from latent strabismus will find relief when one eye is occluded for a significant period of time. Headaches that are the result of accommodative deficiencies will not be improved with monocular occlusion.

Headache sufferers with pain secondary to latent strabismus can benefit from well-selected orthoptic exercises, e.g., convergence exercises, "pencil push-ups," or strabismus surgery. Orthoptics is effective in small- to medium-sized exodeviations and may help with very small-angle eso- and vertical deviations. Strabismus surgery is the choice only for larger deviations.

Convergence and accommodation disorders

Convergence insufficiency

A remote near point of convergence in combination with decreased fusional convergence at near fixation is the hallmark of convergence insufficiency. Frontal headaches are one part of a constellation of symptoms that appear after prolonged near fixation. The associated symptoms include eyestrain, blurred near vision, and crossed diplopia. The patient reports the need to close one eye to read comfortably. They usually present during adolescence or early adulthood due to the visual demands of high school, college, or university.

Long-lasting relief from symptoms can be achieved with convergence exercises, including "pencil push-ups" and stereogram convergence training.[24,25] Surgery is only for those rare cases that persist despite exercises: postoperative symptoms are frequent.[26]

Spasm of the near reflex (convergence or accommodative spasm)

Patients with spasm of the near reflex produce sustained maximal convergence in association with accommodative spasm and miosis. They may have frontal headaches, diplopia, and blurred distance visual acuity. It is usually attributed to psychogenic causes.[27] Nonetheless, posterior fossa abnormalities should be ruled out.[28]

If no organic cause can be determined, instillation of atropine to both eyes over an extended period (months to years) may help and referral to a psychiatrist or psychologist may be appropriate.

Refractive error

High hyperopia

Children with a large amount of uncorrected hyperopia will need a lot of accommodative effort to see clearly. This may cause frontal headaches. However, it is far more likely for a child with high hyperopia to exhibit an esotropia as the presenting sign.

Muscular contraction to produce a pinhole effect

Individuals with uncorrected or poorly corrected refractive error will often squeeze the palpebral fissures ("peer" or "squint") in order to improve visual acuity by a pinhole effect; over an extended period this can produce a periorbital headache.

Misplacement of the optical center of a spectacle correction

Misaligned optical centers produce a prismatic effect and may cause an induced latent strabismus, giving frontal headaches. This is likely to occur in children who have a large refractive error, as the amount of prismatic effect is dependent upon the amount of decentration and the power of the lens (see Section 6 and Chapter 6).

REFERENCES

1. Diamond S, Wenzel R. Practical approaches to migraine management. Headache 2003: 304.
2. Barlow CF. Migraine in infant and toddler. J Child Neurol 1994; 9: 92–4.
3. Elser JM, Woody RC. Migraine headache in the infant and young child. Headache 1990; 30: 366–8.
4. Campbell JK. Manifestations of migraine. Neurol Clin 1990; 8: 841–55.
5. Chu ML, Shinnar S. Headache in children younger than 7 years of age. Arch Neurol 1992; 49: 79–82.
6. Deubner DC. An epidemiologic study of migraine and headache in 10–20 year olds. Headache 1977; 17: 173–80.
7. Sillanpaa M. Changes in prevalence of migraine and other headaches during the first seven school years. Headache 1983; 23: 15–9.
8. Bille B. Migraine in school children. Acta Pediatr Scand 1962; 51: 1–151.
9. O'Hara MA, Anderson RT, Brown D. Magnetic resonance imaging in ophthalmoplegic migraine of children. J AAPOS 2001; 5: 307–10.
10. Carlow TJ. Oculomotor ophthalmoplegic migraine: is it really migraine? J Neuro-ophthalmol 2002; 22: 215–21.
11. Joutel A, Bousser MG, Biousse V, et al. A gene for familial hemiplegic migraine maps to chromosome 19. Nat Genet 1993; 5: 40–5.
12. Ducros A, Denier C, Joutel A, et al. The clinical spectrum of familial hemiplegic migraine associated with mutations in a neuronal calcium channel. N Engl J Med 2001; 345: 17–24.
13. Yu W, Horowitz SH. Treatment of sporadic hemiplegic migraine with calcium-channel blocker verapamil. Neurology 2003; 60: 120–1.
14. Caplan LR. "Top of the basilar" syndrome. Neurology 1980; 30: 72–9.
15. Ehyai A, Fenichel GM. The natural history of acute confusional migraine. Arch Neurol 1978; 35: 368–9.
16. Shaabat A. Confusional migraine in childhood. Pediatr Neurol 1996; 15: 23–5.
17. Taylor D. Headaches. In: Taylor D, editor. Pediatric Ophthalmology. Second edition. Oxford: Blackwell Science; 1997: 1064.
18. Couch R, Camfield PR, Tibbles JA. The changing picture of pseudotumor cerebri in children. Can J Neurol Sci 1985; 12: 48–50.
19. Shin RK, Balce LJ. Idiopathic intracranial hypertension. Curr Treat Options Neurol 2002; 4: 297–305.
20. Trompeter RS, Smith RL, Hoare RD, et al. Neurological complications of arterial hypertension. Arch Dis Child 1982; 57: 913–7.
21. Dhuna A, Pascuel-Leone A, Belgrade M. Cocaine-related vascular headaches. J Neurol Neurosurg Psychiatry 1991; 54: 803–6.
22. Children headaches: An information guide for young sufferers, their parents and school health professionals. Chicago: National Headache Foundation; 2002. Available at http://www.headaches.org/consumer/educationalmodules/childrensheadache/chhome.html
23. Mori K, Murata T, Hashimoto N, et al. Clinical analysis of arteriovenous malformations in children. Childs Brain 1980; 6: 13–25.
24. van Leeuwen AF, Westen MJ, van der Steen J, et al. Gaze-shift dynamics in subjects with and without symptoms of convergence insufficiency: Influence of monocular performance on the effect of training. Vision Res 1999; 39: 3095–107.
25. Alder P. Efficacy of treatment for convergence insufficiency using vision therapy. Ophthalmic Physiol Opt 2002; 22: 565–71.
26. von Noorden GK. Resection of both medial rectus muscles in organic convergence insufficiency. Am J Ophthalmol 1976; 81: 223–6.
27. von Noorden GK. Binocular vision and ocular motility: theory and management of strabismus. Fifth edition. St Louis: Mosby; 1996: 472.
28. Dagi LR, Chrousos GA, Cogan DC. Spasm of the near reflex associated with organic disease. Am J Ophthalmol 1987; 103: 582–5.

CHAPTER
P19 Peculiar Visual Images

David Taylor and Katharine Barr

INTRODUCTION

Children probably have visual experiences that are not "usual" much more frequently than is realized but they have difficulty in describing them, preferring to call their vision blurred or fuzzy or just "funny." Their parents, quite understandably, often do not report the symptoms because they do not understand them. Ophthalmologists rarely ask children whether they have odd visual images because of a mistaken fear of being misunderstood. Nonetheless, they are important symptoms[1] that deserve to be listened to.

DYSMETROPSIA

Dysmetropsia involves changes in the size or shape of an object.

METAMORPHOPSIA

Distortion of central vision–which the child reports as "lines are bent," "objects appear broken up," or in younger children, that things are blurred or that they just cannot see properly–occurs only with organic disease, usually of the anterior visual system. It is accompanied by clinical or neurophysiological evidence of central visual disorders.

MICROPSIA

A sensation that objects are smaller than they should be is a common experience in childhood, and it is usually not based on any organic disease unless associated with other symptoms. Micropsia with metamorphopsia, hallucinations, or visual defects is always organic.

Benign global micropsia

Most children with this condition are between 7 and 15 years, of either sex, and it is an isolated complaint. Often they have been reading in bed in the evening and have noticed a progressive diminution in the size of their book; looking up they see familiar surroundings clearly but greatly diminished in size; if they walk around they have a peculiar sensation that they are in Lilliputian land. There is no distortion of reality other than the size, and no hallucinations. The sensation frightens only the most timid. It lasts a few minutes and usually goes more quickly than it comes. Sometimes the disappearance is instantaneous, whereas the onset is so gradual that it is difficult to say when it began.

This sensation can be reproduced by a pseudoscope (Fig. P19.1), which has a system of mirrors that alters vergence without altering accommodation. There is no adequate explanation of the cause

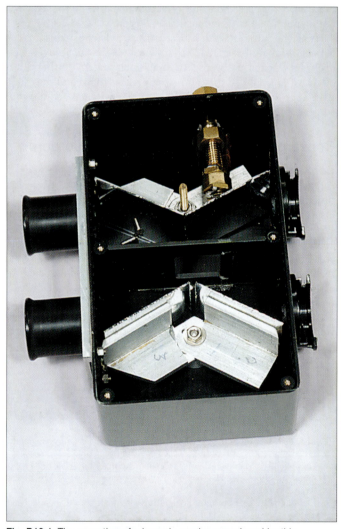

Fig. P19.1 The sensation of micropsia can be reproduced by this instrument, a pseudoscope. The lid has been removed to view the mirror system: the viewer holds the instrument like a pair of binoculars; the eyepieces can be seen on the left. Vergence is varied by the screw at the top of the picture, but accommodation is unchanged by the plane mirrors. When divergence is induced without a change in accommodation or change in image size, an increase in the perceived size of the image is experienced. The reverse occurs when convergence is induced.

but it could be related to a "mismatch" between accommodation and vergence because when divergence is induced by a pseudoscope in the absence of a change in accommodation or change in image size, an increase in the perceived size of the image is experienced. The reverse occurs when convergence is induced.

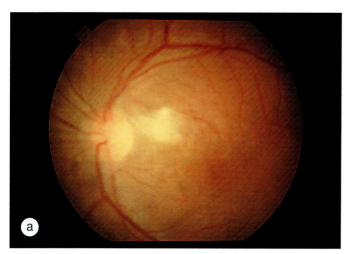 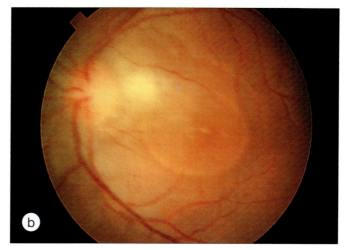

Fig. P19.2 (a) Neuroretinitis with micropsia. This 9-year-old girl complained of dullness of vision in both eyes and smallness of objects with distortion on the left. The white area temporal to the optic disc represents retinal nerve fiber swelling and vascular leakage, extending to the fovea. (b) As the retinal edema increased and extended across the macula, the acuity dropped to 6/36 and the micropsia disappeared.

The symptoms usually disappear in a few months and reassurance is the only treatment.

Micropsia with macular disease

Micropsia also occurs with macular disease, particularly with macular edema or any disease in which the retinal elements are abnormally separated including dystrophies and neuroretinitis (Figs. P19.2a, P19.2b). In retinal micropsia there is usually an uncorrectable acuity defect, only a minimal color defect, and the child notices blurred or distorted central vision especially if the disorder is bilateral.

Refractive micropsia

Micropsia may be noticed at the first wearing of myopic spectacles or contact lenses for hypermetropia, and it may be prolonged if the lenses are too strong.

Cerebral micropsia and the "Alice in Wonderland" syndrome

Cerebral abnormalities have been reported as causing micropsia, including migraine, cortical defects, and a chiasmal tumor,[2] which gave rise to a nasotemporal field size difference, and frontal lobe epilepsy.[3] Lilliputian images occur in a number of infections: in a child with scarlet fever,[4] with Coxsackie B1 virus infection,[5] and with varicella.[6]

Cerebral metamorphopsia is sometimes accompanied by hallucinations, visual field defects, or both. A variety of dysmetropias, erythropsia, and metamorphopsia have been reported in the course of infectious mononucleosis (Epstein-Barr virus infection).[7,8] The bizarre images of the body and external objects have prompted the term "Alice in Wonderland" syndrome. Although generally benign, serious or recurrent neurological complications may ensue.[9] MRI changes, which are transient, show brain swelling,[10] which may be due to reduced brain perfusion.[11,12]

Diagnosis and management of micropsia

Micropsia therefore can be an entirely benign condition or one with more serious implications. The key to diagnosis is the history and clinical examination of the child: in a healthy child with isolated micropsia without hallucinations or distortions of reality, with no field defect, and with a normal eye examination, there is no need for further investigation, and reassurance of the child and parents is all that is needed. Cases with an abnormal history or examination, or with persistent symptoms, warrant investigation including for infective causes and by neuroimaging.

MACROPSIA

Macropsia is much rarer than micropsia. It may occur with retinal diseases where foveal cones are pushed together or with cortical disease. Rarely, it is found as a nonorganic or benign disorder in the same way that micropsia occurs.

ERYTHROPSIA AND "COLORED CLOUDS"

A sensation that everything is red (erythropsia) is sometimes noted by patients, including children, for a few days or weeks after cataract surgery. It does not seem to have any significance and usually does not trouble the child very much.

"Colored clouds" are a sensation reported by some children and adults when lying in a sleepy state in oblique sunlight or bright light. They see whorls of multicolored lights, predominantly red and blue, which swirl in their vision when the lids are closed; it is normal and probably an entoptic phenomenon.

ENTOPTIC PHENOMENA

Entoptic phenomena are visual observations of normal phenomena within the eye made under unusual viewing conditions. Examples include the viewing of retinal vessels by rubbing the eye with a light through closed lids, or seeing spots moving when looking at a bright clear sky or an open field of snow (Scheerer's phenomenon).

PHOSPHENES AND PHOTOPSIAS

Phosphenes are transient tiny spots of light in an otherwise intact field of vision, which usually occurs because of retinal stimulation. There are many examples of phosphenes including the following:

1. The bright lights seen when the eye is rubbed through closed lids.
2. Bright lights may occur as a result of retinal traction in vitreous disease. When associated with seeing spots these are an indication for careful ophthalmoscopy since they are the cardinal symptoms of a retinal tear.
3. "Moore's lightning streaks" are larger blue or white lights that meander in the vision for a second or so especially when the lights are dimmed. Their origin is unknown and they seem to be harmless.
4. Eye movement or "flick" phosphenes are the eye movement-related spots of light caused by retinal traction at the scleral insertions of eye muscles.
5. Transient flashes of light may be seen in retinal embolic disease.

Photopsias are larger, longer-lasting visual phenomena that may also be related to movement:

1. They were described in patients with optic neuropathies,[13] the relationship to movement presumably being due to traction on the optic nerve.
2. Rarely a patient with an optic neuropathy may complain of seeing a bright light or a flash of light when stimulated by sound.[14,15]

Thus some of the transient flashes of light seen by children can be of serious significance and should not necessarily be dismissed as being "invented." Complaints about poor vision under special lighting conditions should never be dismissed. They may be a form of photophobia (see Chapter P9), due to an optic neuropathy causing altered visual perception, or due to retinal disease or to a cerebral defect.

MONOCULAR DIPLOPIA

Monocular diplopia in children requires especially careful questioning to determine its true nature. It is most often due to small axial cataracts or corneal disease, cataracts where one part of the lens has a higher refractive index than another, or occasionally retinal disease or simple refractive errors.[16] Careful questioning may also reveal more than two images, each of varying sharpness.

An interesting example of monocular diplopia occurs when, in a child who has anomalous retinal correspondence associated with squint, the eyes are realigned surgically; he sees two images with the eye that was squinting before surgery. It fades gradually over weeks or months as one or other image predominates, depending on the success of the realignment. With both eyes open there can be binocular triplopia. Diplopia may occur in brain disease[17] when either eye is viewing but is very rare. In many cases no cause can be found, and the underlying problem may be nonorganic (see Chapter 64) or stress-related.

HALLUCINATIONS

Hallucinations are entirely personal subjective phenomena, defined by Esquirol as "false sensory impressions not due to disease of the sense organs." There is no totally satisfactory definition of these images, which the patient thinks are real but which arise within the mind in the absence of sense organ stimulation.

Pseudohallucinations are described as hallucinations where the subject realizes they are not "real" images. Illusions are misinterpretations of actual images.

Social deprivation

Children deprived, intentionally or otherwise, of social contact may develop elaborate visual and auditory images of imaginary friends or animals that can last hours and are usually enjoyed by the child, who is preoccupied by them.[18] They are probably extensions of the normal imaginary companions that many children have.[19]

Sensory deprivation and visual loss

People who have been isolated for prolonged periods, especially under conditions of total sensory deprivation, may develop elaborate visual and other sensory hallucinations that are often quite pleasant.

Hallucinations occur quite frequently in visual loss; this is a common experience in age-related macular degeneration or senile cataract, and the phenomenon is enhanced by the patient's nervousness and exposure to drugs, especially alcohol (and its withdrawal) and premedication drugs.

Patients with sudden cortical visual loss have formed hallucinations that usually, but not always, occur in the area of the defective visual field.[20] These hallucinations are "irritative" phenomena similar to those that occur after encephalitis[21] or with epilepsy. However, they occur in any part of the visual field. Patients with eye disease may develop hallucinations that diminish in their clarity, frequency, and duration as the blindness progresses.[22] When vivid hallucinations occur in patients with preserved intellectual functions and eye disease, they are known as the Charles Bonnet syndrome[23–25] (Fig. P19.3). I have seen a child with adrenoleukodystrophy, cortical blindness, and optic atrophy who had vivid and pleasant hallucinations of animals. White and Jan[26] described a fascinating case of a child who was blind after surgery for optic glioma; the child's mental state was normal, and he was initially frightened by the vivid images of familiar objects.

Visual phenomena with localized brain disease

Hallucinations should not be thought of as arising from disease of any particular part of the brain, but some phenomena are more common with disease of certain areas of the brain.[27] Disease of the posterior visual pathways and particularly the occipital cortex usually gives rise to unformed, crude, repetitive hallucinations. These are usually "irritative," i.e., due to an epileptic form of discharge, as opposed to hallucinating due to the anterior visual pathways disease, which "releases" the brain from vision, which normally suppresses unwanted discharges.[28]

Temporal lobe lesions are said to give rise to formed and detailed visual and olfactory hallucinations. In one case, that of an elderly man with a stroke, the hallucinations were exclusively provoked by watching television.[17]

The evidence for midbrain disorders giving rise to hallucinations is less clear. L'Hermitte[29] and Van Bogaert[30] described cases with pathological confirmation; the latter coined the term peduncular hallucinosis because he believed that involvement of the cerebral peduncles was a vital feature. The name is so euphonic that it has remained. The hallucinations are remarkably vivid,[31–33] like a film in many cases, colored and occasionally accompanied by unformed sound.

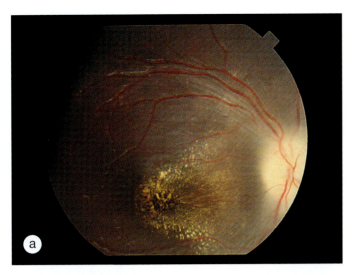

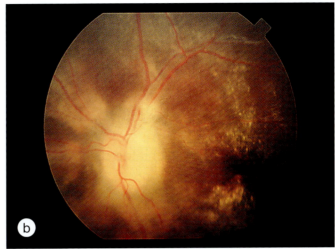

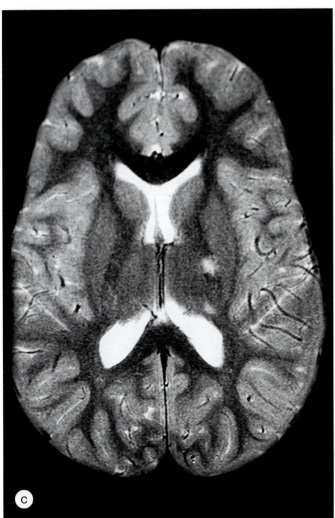

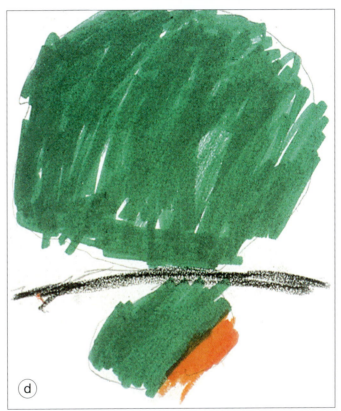

Fig. P19.3 (a, b) Fundi of a boy with neuroretinitis as part of a disseminated encephalopathy with preserved intellect. (c) MRI scan showing foci of white matter inflammation. (d) His vision at this stage, four weeks after the onset, was "counting fingers." He later (when his vision had partially recovered) drew the figures that he had seen.

Hypnagogic and hypnopompic hallucinations

Hallucinations on going to sleep (hypnagogic) or waking (hypnopompic) are quite common in adults. They are often pleasant and have the frustrating quality that when they are concentrated on they disappear. Although said to be common, occurring in perhaps one-fifth of a population of doctors,[34] I have found them so rarely in children that I am reluctant to ask.

Drug-induced hallucination

Barbiturates, Valium, and alcohol withdrawal after chronic intoxication may all be associated with hallucinations. Chronic abuse is very rare in childhood, but must be remembered with the withdrawal of barbiturates in epileptic children.

Atropine, cyclopentolate, and some other cycloplegic drugs are causes of visual hallucinations, which occur as part of an organic psychosis with confusion and signs of intoxication (hot, red-faced, dilated pupils, tachycardia).

Ketamine, widely used for examinations under anesthesia, produces visual and frightening hallucinations especially if the child is wakened roughly.

LSD and mescaline cause hallucinations that may occur long after taking the drug but usually within the first 6 hr, starting shortly after ingestion. Micropsia, macropsia, palinopsia, and remarkably formed visual hallucinations that are not stereotyped also occur.[34]

Psychoneuroses and psychiatric disease

Hallucinations, particularly auditory, occur in about 15% of children with behavioral problems.[18] Powerful auditory and visual hallucinations, often religious or persecutory and frightening, are characteristic of schizophrenia, which may have its onset in later childhood. They are true hallucinations, believed by the patient. In adolescent psychoses, hallucinations occur in 75% of children and are most frequently auditory or auditory and visual.[35]

Children with conduct or emotional disorders who also suffered from hallucinations were older than similar children without hallucinations. They also had lower IQs and were more frequently admitted to hospital for the disorder. The hallucinating children were more likely to be depressed, to have a family history of mood changes, and to have more symptoms suggestive of cognitive perceptual disorder.[36] When followed to adulthood the association with hallucinations did not carry an increased risk for psychoses, depressive illness, organic brain disease, or other psychiatric disorder.[37]

Visual perseveration

Perseveration is the persistence of the perception of an object in the absence of its original external stimulus.

PALINOPSIA

Visual perseveration in time, palinopsia, is when there is a "flashback" of part of a visual scene that was experienced seconds, minutes, or hours previously. Part or whole of the visual field may be affected by the palinopsic image (Fig. P19.4), and there may also be auditory perseveration, palinacousis,[34] and polyopia,[38] or previously seen objects may become incorporated into new images.[38] It occurs in evolving lesions of different types, usually in defective areas of the visual fields. It has been described in schizophrenia. There is almost invariably a visual field defect, and the nondominant parietal lobe is most frequently affected.[39] A similar phenomenon may be seen in patients on or in withdrawal from a number of drugs, such as LSD, maprotiline, mirtazapine, paroxetine, nefazodone, and risperidone.

VISUAL PERSEVERATION IN SPACE– POLYOPIA

In polyopia, the same object is seen a number of times simultaneously in the visual field, usually in a line, one in front of and

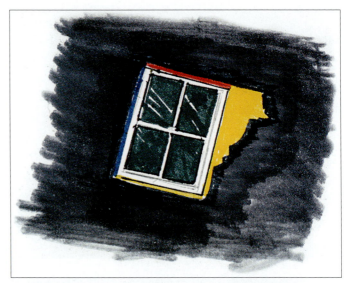

Fig. P19.4 Picture drawn by a right-handed young person with an ultimately fatal metastatic carcinoma in the right parietal lobe. The presenting symptom was the recurrence of an image of the kitchen window that impinged itself involuntarily on the visual environment in different circumstances for several hours after the original stimulus.

overlapping the others. It may occur simultaneously with palinopsia and seems to have similar causes.

OCCIPITAL EPILEPSY

Benign occipital epilepsy of childhood is a condition that may be familial[40] and gives rise to stereotyped unformed visual experiences of multiple brightly colored spots, circles, or balls starting in a temporal hemifield and moving contralaterally[41] or to the center where they may be flashing. They may multiply and increase in size in the course of the seizure and may progress to other nonvisual occipital seizure symptoms and more rarely to extraoccipital manifestations and convulsions. The visual phenomena are completely different to those of migraine. Transient loss of vision occurs from early in the attack, and there is a postictal headache similar to migraine. They occur in brief attacks up to several times a day. Electroencephalography shows interictal epileptiform discharges over the occipital region that are abolished by eye opening.[42] Symptoms may be improved by antiepileptic drugs,[40] carbamazepine in particular[41].

Occipital epilepsy also occurs as a condition with very serious implications; Lortie et al.[43] reported 12 neonates with often generalized seizures who had severe visual and general developmental abnormalities. Other unformed visual hallucinations occur in patients with developmental anomalies of the occipital lobes (Fig. P19.5).

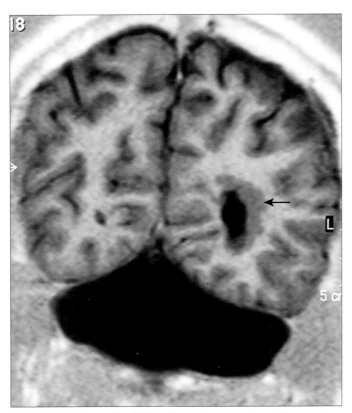

Fig. P19.5 This boy with a Möbius-like syndrome started, at the age of 18, to get unformed hallucinations in the right half of his visual field accompanied by nausea followed by sleepiness, without seizures. The MRI shows an area of dysplastic ectopic gray matter in the left posterior parieto-occipital region (arrow).

REFERENCES

1. Wright JR, Boger WP III. Visual complaints from healthy children. Surv Ophthalmol 1999; 44: 113–21.
2. Bender MB, Savitsky N. Micropsia and teleopsia limited to the temporal fields of vision. Arch Ophthalmol 1943; 29: 904–8.
3. Zwijnenburg PJ, Wennink JM, Laman DM, et al. Alice in Wonderland syndrome: a clinical presentation of frontal lobe epilepsy. Neuropediatrics 2002; 33: 53–5.
4. Savitsky N, Tarachov S. Lilliputian hallucinations during convalescence from scarlet fever in a child. J Nerve Ment Dis 1941; 93: 310–2.
5. Wang SM, Liu CC, Chen YJ, et al. Alice in Wonderland syndrome caused by coxsackievirus B1. Pediatr Infect.Dis J 1996; 15: 470–1.
6. Soriani S, Faggioli R, Scarpa P, et al. "Alice in Wonderland" syndrome and varicella. Pediatr Infect.Dis J 1998; 17: 935–6.
7. Cinbis M., Aysun S. Alice in Wonderland syndrome as an initial manifestation of Epstein-Barr virus infection. Br J Ophthalmol 1992; 76: 316.
8. Copperman SM. "Alice in Wonderland" syndrome as a presenting symptom of infectious mononucleosis in children. Clin Paediatr 1977; 16: 143–6.
9. Hausler M, Ramaekers VT, Doenges M, et al. Neurological complications of acute and persistent Epstein-Barr virus infection in paediatric patients. J Med Virol. 2002; 68: 253–63.
10. Kamei A, Sasaki M, Akasaka M, et al. [Abnormal magnetic resonance imaging in a child with Alice in Wonderland syndrome following Epstein-Barr virus infection]. No To Hattatsu 2002; 34: 348–52.
11. Lahat E, Berkovitch M, Barr J, et al. Abnormal visual evoked potentials in children with "Alice in Wonderland" syndrome due to infectious mononucleosis. J Child Neurol 1999; 14: 732–5.
12. Kuo YT, Chiu NC, Shen EY, et al. Cerebral perfusion in children with Alice in Wonderland syndrome. Pediatr Neurol 1998; 19: 105–8.
13. Davis FA, Bergen D, Schauf C, et al. Movement phosphenes in optic neuritis: a new clinical sign. Neurology 1976; 26: 1100–4.
14. Jacobs L, Karpic A, Bozian D, et al. Auditory-visual synesthesia. Arch Neurol 1987; 38: 211–6.
15. Page NG, Bolger JP, Sanders MD. Auditory evoked phosphenes in optic nerve disease. J Neurol Neurosurg Psychiatr 1982; 45: 7–12.
16. Coffeen O, Guyton DL. Monocular diplopia accompanying ordinary refractive errors. Am J Ophthalmol 1988; 105: 451–9.
17. Safran AB, Kline LB, Glaser JS, et al. Television-induced formed visual hallucinations and cerebral diplopia. Br J Ophthalmol 1981; 65: 707–11.
18. Bender L. In: A Dynamic Psychopathology of Childhood. Springfield, IL: CC Thomas; 1954.
19. Bender L, Vogel BF. Imaginary companions of children. Am J Orthopsychiatr 1941; 11: 56–65.
20. Lance JW. Simple formed hallucinations confined to the area of a specific visual field defect. Brain 1976; 99: 719–34.
21. Mize K. Visual hallucinations following viral encephalitis; a self report. Neuropsychologica 1980; 18: 193–202.
22. White NJ. Complex visual hallucinations in partial blindness due to eye disease. Br J Psychiatr 1980; 136: 284–6.
23. Brown GC, Murphy RP. Visual symptoms associated with the choroidal neovascularisation: photopsias and the Charles Bonnet syndrome. Arch Ophthalmol 1992; 110: 1251–6.
24. Damas-Mora J, Skelton-Robinson M, Jenner FA. The Charles Bonnet syndrome in perspective. Psychol Med 1982; 12: 251–61.
25. Siatkowski RM, Zimmer B, Rosenberg PR. The Charles Bonnet syndrome. Visual perception dysfunction in sensory deprivation. J Clin Neuroophthalmol 1990; 10: 215–8.
26. White CP, Jan JE. Visual hallucinations after acute visual loss in a young child. Dev Med Child Neurol 1992; 34: 259–65.
27. Gittinger WW, Miller NR, Keltner JL, et al. Sugar plum fairies. Visual hallucinations. Surv Ophthalmol 1982; 27: 42–8.
28. Cogan DG. Visual hallucinations as release phenomena. Klin Exp Ophthalmol 1973; 188: 139–50.
29. L'Hermitte J. Syndrome de la calotte du pédoncule cérébral. Les troubles psycho-sensoric dans les lésions du mésocéphale. Rev Neurol 1922; 2: 1359–65.
30. Van Bogaert L. L'hallucinose pédonculaire. Rev Neurol 1927; 47: 608–17.
31. Geller T, Bellur SN. Peduncular hallucinosis. MRI confirmation of mesencephalic infarction during life. Ann Neurol 1987; 21: 602–3.
32. Kölmel HW. Peduncular hallucination. J Neurol 1991; 238: 457–9.
33. Serra Catafu J, Rubio F, Peres Serra J. Peduncular hallucinosis associated with posterior thalamic infarction. J Neurol 1992; 239: 89–90.
34. Lessell S. High disorders of visual function. In: Glaser JS, Smith JL, editors. Neuro-ophthalmology. St Louis: Mosby, 1975: 27–44. (vol 8).
35. Garralda ME, Ainsworth P. In: Coleman J, editor. Working with Troubled Adolescents. London: Academic Press; 1987.
36. Garralda ME. Hallucinations in children with conduct and emotional disorders I. The clinical phenomenon. Psychol Med 1984; 14: 589–96.
37. Garralda ME. Hallucinations in children with conduct and emotional disorders II. The follow-up study. Psychol Med 1984; 14: 597–604.
38. Smith PE, Shah P, Sharpe J, et al. Palinopsia. Lancet 2003; 361: 1098.
39. Bender MB, Feldman M, Sobin AJ. Palinopsia. Brain 1968; 91: 321–38.
40. Nagendran K, Prior PF, Rossiter MA. Benign occipital epilepsy of childhood: a family study. J R Soc Med 1989; 82: 684–5.
41. Panayiotopoulos CP. Elementary visual hallucinations, blindness, and headache in idiopathic occipital epilepsy: differentiation from migraine. J Neurol Neurosurg.Psychiatry 1999; 66: 536–40.
42. Andermann F, Zifkin B. The benign occipital epilepsies of childhood: an overview of the idiopathic syndromes and of the relationship to migraine. Epilepsia 1998; 39: S9–23.
43. Lortie A, Ploulin P, Pinard J-M, et al. Occipital epilepsy in neonates and infants. In: Andermann F, Beaumanoir A, Mira L, et al., editors. Occipital Seizures and Epilepsies in Children. London: John Libbey, 1993: 121–32.

CHAPTER
P20 The Child Who Fails in School

Alison Salt

WHY DO CHILDREN WITH SCHOOL DIFFICULTIES PRESENT TO THE EYE CLINIC?

Many children present to the eye clinic because of failure to progress in school. Parents and teachers quite reasonably ask whether a problem with vision could be interfering with learning. This chapter provides a brief outline of the problems that may present with school failure and suggests appropriate referral routes.

Most children with severe learning difficulty are identified before they start school. However, some, with less severe problems, will become apparent with the increased demands of a formal curriculum. Schools will usually monitor a child's progress and may take several routes in seeking advice when a child is not reaching expected targets; an educational psychologist may be asked to undertake an assessment of a child's abilities, a pediatrician may be asked to exclude a medical diagnosis, and the child may be referred to an eye clinic or an audiologist to exclude a visual or hearing impairment.

POSSIBLE REASONS FOR FAILURE IN SCHOOL

Global learning difficulty

Mild or moderate learning difficulties affecting all areas of development may not present until the child starts school. These problems have been reported to occur in around 3–10% of children. The most common known cause of these difficulties are chromosomal anomalies–Down syndrome and fragile X syndrome being the most common. However, in a majority no cause can be identified. Nevertheless, referral to a pediatrician to consider etiology and intervention is appropriate.

Specific learning difficulty

Some children with general cognitive abilities within the average range have specific problems in a one area of development. However, these problems may also present in combination.

Dyslexia or specific difficulties with reading are described in detail in Chapter 66. These problems frequently lead to referral to the eye clinic so that vision problems as a cause of reading difficulty can be excluded. The diagnosis will be confirmed by a detailed assessment by an educational or neuropsychologist and special educational support will be required.

Developmental coordination disorder (DCD) (or dyspraxia) is a specific problem of motor coordination affecting the coordination of large and fine movements and may lead to difficulty with physical education, writing, and speech clarity. In addition these children may have difficulty with general organization and self-help skills, e.g., dressing. Problems with visual and spatial perception may also be recognized. They may also experience additional emotional and social difficulties. A physiotherapist or an occupational therapist can provide assessment, advice, and treatment for this disorder.

Speech and language disorders usually present prior to starting school, but more subtle difficulties of comprehension may not be recognized without detailed assessment. Assessment and support from a speech and language therapist will be necessary and may include a language program delivered as part of the school curriculum. Difficulties with literacy may follow particular speech and language disorders.

Other developmental disorders

Problems with attention and concentration may lead to underachievement and may present with behavior difficulties. The possibility of attention deficit hyperactivity disorder (ADHD) should be considered in these children. The diagnosis is based on the recognition of early onset and pervasive (occurring in all environments) problems with overactivity and impulsivity and problems with attention and concentration. The diagnosis usually requires collection of information about behavior from parents and teachers using standardized questionnaires. Treatment may include medication with methylphenidate (Ritalin) or similar psychostimulant medications but will also require modification of the environment with reduction in distraction and additional adult support to assist with concentration. Referral to a pediatrician for diagnosis may be appropriate.

Problems with concentration may also indicate a hearing difficulty. Most severe hearing difficulties present early with concern about hearing behavior in the young child, or speech delay. However, conductive hearing loss is very common in childhood, and some of the progressive sensorineural hearing impairments will present after the age of routine screening. Hearing assessment should always be considered if a child appears to have problems of attention or concentration in the classroom.

Children may also present with difficulties with peer relationships and social interaction. When these children also have problems with the use of language for communication and limited or obsessional interests, a diagnosis of autistic spectrum disorder may be considered. If this type of problem is suspected, a referral to a pediatrician will be necessary.

Other problems with peers may be secondary to external factors. School failure or reluctance to attend school may result from emotional and social difficulties in school through difficult relationships with peers, e.g., bullying, or a difficult interaction with the teacher. Difficulties at home may also lead to school failure.

Beware of the child who appears to be losing skills, as this suggests a neurological degenerative condition (see Chapters 53 and 65). Vision loss may also occur under these conditions. Urgent referral to a pediatrician or pediatric neurologist is essential.

ASSESSMENT AND INTERVENTION

Assessment by a pediatrician, psychologist, and other therapists can provide a description of a child's strengths and weaknesses in verbal and nonverbal abilities. A child's learning needs can therefore be identified and appropriate suggestions made for intervention. This may include additional support in the classroom, specific educational interventions, e.g., for reading difficulty, or intervention and advice from other therapists, e.g., a speech and language therapist, occupational therapist, or physiotherapist (Fig. P20.1).

THE ROLE OF THE OPHTHALMOLOGIST

The ophthalmologist will need to exclude significant eye disease, refractive error, or oculomotor dysfunction. Subtle visual problems are a rare cause of educational difficulties but mild refractive errors or problems such as convergence insufficiency may be playing a role.

When there is a significant visual impairment and failure in school it will be important to consider how the child's visual difficulties are being supported.

SCHOOL DIFFICULTY IN A CHILD WITH VISUAL IMPAIRMENT

Children with visual impairment may also present with school failure. These children may have additional learning difficulty or they may be experiencing difficulty because educational material is not being sufficiently adapted either at a distance or near to meet their visual needs (Table P20.1).

Table P20.1 The child with visual impairment failing in school

Ensure visual material is appropriately adapted
Distance material
 Board work
 Sit close to front of class
 Reproduced near
 Prepared in advance

Near
 Appropriate enlargement (font size read at approx. 30 cm)
 Sloping desk
 Good contrast
 CCTV
 Other low-vision aids

Alternatives for written work
 Laptop
 Audiotape
Lighting
 Sufficient
 Not too bright

Social
 Playground assistance
 Use auditory and not visual cues

Exclude other learning difficulties (see Fig. P20.1)

Distance

For those with mild visual impairment simply ensuring that they are sitting at the front of the class with appropriate lighting condition may be all that is required. In those with moderate to severe visual impairment (worse than 6/18), it is likely to be necessary for work copied from the board at the front of the class

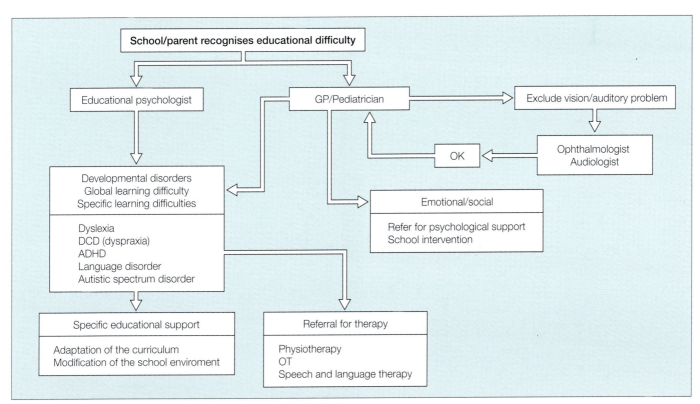

Fig. P20.1 Referral pathways and possible reasons for educational difficulties.

1077

to be reproduced for them close to their desk or to provide ready-prepared material that has been appropriately enlarged.

Children may also experience difficulties in the playground. They may not be able to identify their friends at a distance so that support systems to assist them at playtime need to be put in place. They may also have difficulty identifying facial expression and body language at a distance and therefore do not pick up on social cues.

Near

For near work it will be important to ensure that print is appropriately enlarged. In the early stages of reading it is essential that text is enlarged and that good contrast is ensured. Print size used should be that which is read easily at standard reading distance (approx. 30 cm). Some early reading books have print overlying pictures, thus reducing contrast. This should be avoided.

Low-vision aids and magnifiers are usually only useful for accessing small amounts of text and rarely useful for prolonged spells of reading, especially in younger children. A sloping desk will help children to come closer to text without adversely affecting the child's posture and the lighting of the text. A closed circuit TV (CCTV) can be useful where small amounts of text are too difficult to enlarge or for maps or pictures.

Some children, e.g., those with albinism and cone dystrophies, find bright lighting conditions uncomfortable or will actually have reduced vision under these conditions; therefore lighting conditions in the classroom need to be carefully considered.

The effort involved in reading, for children with visual impairment, should not be underestimated. Children will often tire toward the end of a school day. If possible therefore tasks with high visual demand should be confined to the early part of the school day.

Alternative means for producing written work will also be necessary, e.g., access to a laptop or audiotape.

A specialist advisory teacher for children with visual impairment should be available to give advice to the class teacher and to monitor progress.

CHAPTER P21
Abnormal Pupil Appearance in Infancy

Susan M Carden

Neonates are sometimes referred from the nursery because of suspected pupillary abnormalities and concern about possible associated anomalies or syndromes. Referring neonatologists may have difficulty describing pupillary abnormalities because the palpebral fissures of premature babies are small, making examination difficult. Premature babies in the nursery may be intubated and have edematous eyelids, which further makes examination difficult.

Infants are easier to examine but, again, pediatricians may have difficulty describing the abnormality.

The vagueness of any description by referring doctors (nurses or parents) should not be dismissed nor criticized because it is rarely a finding without foundation. A full eye examination usually reveals the cause. A portable slit lamp can be helpful. Funduscopy should be performed as associated retinal problems are not infrequent.

In children, the pupil is smallest during infancy, which adds to the difficulty for pediatricians in their assessments, particularly in babies with dark irides. An increase in size begins to occur sometime during the first six months.[1] It is not until adolescence that the pupils attain their fullest size (see Chapter 5).

Some patients have an intermittent alteration in pupil size. Alternating anisocoria has been described.[2] It is important to listen carefully to the history given by parents and to encourage them to describe what they think they have seen as these conditions might not be present on the day the child visits for the clinical examination.

Table P21.1 gives guidelines on the causes of abnormal pupils in infancy, the details of which should be sought in the text of Chapters 43 and 67.

Table P21.1 Guidelines on the causes of abnormal pupils in infancy

Abnormal shape
Coloboma (inferonasal)
Atypical coloboma
Polycoria/corectopia
Partial aniridia
Persistent pupillary membrane

Abnormal size
1. Relatively too small
Horner syndrome
Microcornea
Uveitis with posterior synechiae
Drugs (e.g., narcotics)
Severe retinopathy of prematurity (failure of pupils to dilate)

2. Relatively large
Third nerve palsy
Tonic pupil (Adie)
Drugs
Aniridia/partial aniridia
Coloboma
Trauma – sphincter rupture
Surgical mydriasis for a congenital problem

Abnormal position
Corectopia
Polycoria
Coloboma

Abnormal iris color
Congenital heterochromia
Waardenburg syndrome[3]
Hirschsprung associated heterochromia[4]
Postuveitis or severe intraocular congenital defects
Congenital Horner syndrome
Incontinentia pigmenti
Heterochromic cyclitis
Neovascularization/rubeosis
Trauma
Rubella

Other pupil abnormalities observed by parents
Unusual reflection from the pupil (see leukocoria in Chapter 50)
Persistent pupillary membrane

REFERENCES

1. MacLachlan C, Howland HC. Normal values and standard deviations for pupil diameter and interpupillary distance in subjects aged 1 month to 19 years. Ophthalmic Physiol Opt 2002; 22: 175–82.
2. Brodsky MC, Sharp GB, Fritz KJ, et al. Idiopathic alternating anisocoria. Am J Ophthalmol 1992; 114: 509–10.
3. Mullaney PB, Parsons MA, Weatherhead RG, et al. Clinical and morphological features of Waardenburg syndrome type II. Eye 1998; 12: 353–7.
4. Lai JS, Lan DS, Yeung, CK, et al. Bilateral iris sector heterochromia with or without Hirschsprung's disease. Eye 1998; 12: 1024–7.

CHAPTER P22
Clinical Investigations for Anisocoria

Susan M Carden

When anisocoria is found in a child, a simple stage-by-stage routine can be followed as outlined in Fig. P22.1. This is designed as a guide. In most cases, a concern about possible Horner syndrome will be evaluated. Anisocoria caused by congenital oculomotor palsy is rare and virtually always accompanied by some degree of ocular motility disturbance[1-3] (see Chapters 43 and 67).

Pharmacological testing may be helpful, but most cases of anisocoria can be diagnosed clinically by the pupil size variation under different lighting conditions and by neurological accompaniments.[1] In contrast to adult ophthalmologists, pediatric ophthalmologists rarely use pharmacological adjuncts to aid diagnosis.

Slit-lamp examination reveals developmental abnormalities of the pupil and sinuous (uneven) pupillary reactions. Hippus (physiologic pupillary unrest of the entire pupil) is present in normal pupils.

The pupil reactions to a bright light and to a near stimulus are noted.

It may be useful to perform retinoscopy while eliciting a visual response to a near target. A dynamic change in retinoscopy reveals important information about reaction to accommodation of the pupil, and also about visual response per se (accommodation is induced by a sense of a near visual target).

The pupil sizes in the dark and in bright light are recorded and photographed when possible. Physiological anisocoria is common in minor degrees and occurs in as many as 21% of healthy newborn infants;[4] it is usually equal in light and dark and the reactions are normal.

One concern in the evaluation of congenital Horner syndrome is whether the pupil defect is caused by a neuroblastoma. The question arises as to how far such a child should be investigated. Experts are divided, with some arguing in favor of investigations, others preferring repeated testing;[5,6] we believe that the child should be investigated only if there is any question about its congenital onset, if the child is unwell in any way, or if there are signs of involvement of the superior cervical ganglion such as in anhidrosis.

Anisocoria can be thought of as being due to one of four problems:

1. Structural abnormality of the iris (congenital or acquired);
2. Abnormality of the parasympathetic nervous supply to the iris;
3. Abnormality of the sympathetic nervous supply to the iris; and
4. Benign, physiologic.

Figure P22.1 provides a flow diagram as an aid in differentiating which of the above problems is the issue.

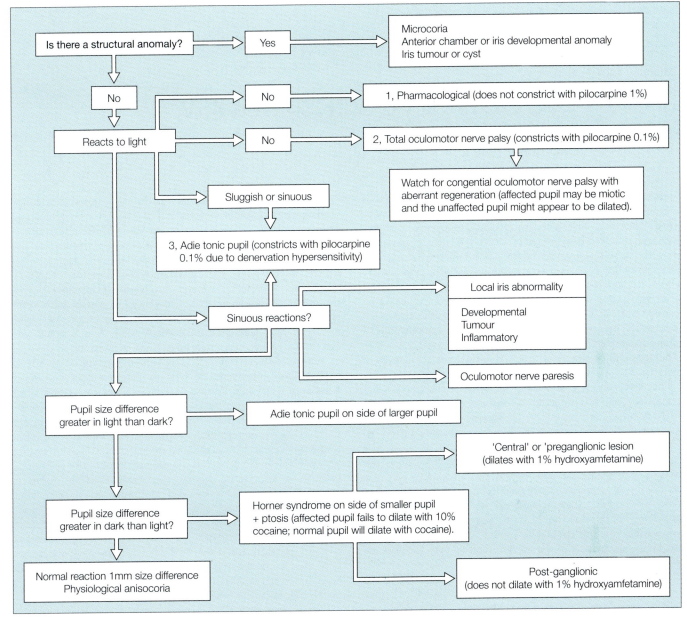

Fig. P22.1 A guide to the routine investigation of anisocoria.

REFERENCES

1. Balkan R, Hoyt CS. Associated neurologic abnormalities in congenital third nerve palsies. Am J Ophthalmol 1984; 97: 315–9.
2. Good WV, Barkovich AJ, Nickel BL, et al. Bilateral congenital oculomotor nerve palsy in a child with brain anomalies. Am J Ophthalmol 1991; 111: 555–8.
3. Sun CC, Kao LY. Unilateral congenital third cranial nerve palsy with central nervous system anomalies: report of two cases. Chang Gung Med J 2000; 23: 776–81.
4. Roarty JD, Keltner JL. Normal pupil size and anisocoria in newborn infants. Arch Ophthalmol 1990; 108: 94–5.
5. Musarella MA, Chan HS, De Boer G, et al. Ocular involvement in neuroblastoma: prognostic implications. Ophthalmology 1984; 91: 936–40.
6. George ND, Gonzalez G, Hoyt CS. Does Horner's syndrome in infancy require investigation? Br J Ophthalmol 1998; 82: 51–4.

CHAPTER
P23 Wobbly Eyes in Infancy

J Raymond Buncic

It sometimes comes as a surprise to young parents to learn that the jiggling or wobbly movement of the eyes of their infant is not normal. They may have failed to recognize the problem themselves, and it is often first spotted by a friend, relative, or physician during the first few months of life. Sometimes what is more noticeable is the associated strabismus, ocular structural abnormalities, e.g., microphthalmos, or poor visual responsiveness. The questions asked by the parents are: what is the problem, can it be repaired, and can/will the child see? Generally, the two main issues are the presence of spontaneous abnormal eye movements and any accompanying impairment of vision.

The *two main categories* of motor abnormalities of the eyes in general are:

1. The less common abnormal *saccadic (rapid movement) disorders*, and often related to fixational changes; and
2. Those which are repetitive oscillations (*nystagmus*), more constant though variable and not as closely related to fixational changes.

The most important of the saccadic disorders clinically is the bursts of spontaneous saccades, multidirectional, often part of a startle response, seen as an early manifestation of the generalized clonic movements that accompany a neuroblastoma: this "opsoclonus" of the eyes should always alert the physician toward investigation for this treatable tumor. On the other hand, opsoclonus may be part of the benign "dancing eyes and dancing feet" syndrome of childhood.

Spontaneous jiggling of the infant's eyes is clinically more commonly due to nystagmus, which can be regarded as either ocular or neurologic in origin. The ocular types, more often seen in infants than the latter, can be due to some form of definable visual impairment (sensory infantile nystagmus) or idiopathic (formerly referred to as a motor congenital nystagmus).

CLINICAL "WAVE FORMS"

In infants, as in older age groups, nystagmus can take many forms in its movement, usually variations of pendular and jerk type of oscillations, as well as in direction and speed. Some movements form a pattern that is helpful in diagnosis, but many times, other clues in the history of examination lead the way in investigation and definition of the problem. Some patterns of nystagmus are highly characteristic and suggestive of a typical ocular problem, while, less commonly, others suggest a topographically localizing neurological problem.

As is usual in children's problems, the history of prenatal/natal difficulties (maternal diabetes, drug ingestion, difficult delivery) and a stormy neonatal and developmental course need to be considered as well as the child's visual responsiveness, ocular symptoms (poor vision, photophobia, head nodding, strabismus), and the family history of any visual impairment and nystagmus.

Most infantile nystagmus disorders shows horizontal oscillations, but sometimes vertical or rotatory or combinations of several planes of movement occur. Visual fixation may appear to be good or vision clinically may be poor. Sometimes, the eye movements are typical of *idiopathic infantile nystagmus*, sometimes called "congenital nystagmus" or "motor congenital nystagmus" (horizontal, variable in intensity, changing with gaze movements, dampening by convergence, increasing with visual effort, and no conversion to vertical nystagmus on vertical gaze, i.e., remaining horizontal on vertical gaze). A null point with compensatory head turn may be present. Nystagmus on the basis of sensory defects (*sensory congenital nystagmus*) may appear similar. It is not always possible to detect milder degrees of associated visual loss. Vertical nystagmus in infants is more often ocular in origin than neurological. *Severe visual impairment* commonly produces more irregular, slow, wandering horizontal movements with intermittent vertical jerking and little response to the usual clinical stimulation strategies and optokinetic testing. Very valuable is the history of the time of onset of the nystagmus, because visual system gliomas may *masquerade* as forms of infantile nystagmus with good vision, even the so-called "congenital nystagmus" and spasmus nutans. In most cases, infantile wobbly eyes are recognized early in life by the parents but sometime the "time of onset" may be unclear. In this regard, a useful practical rule is that in cases with onset not recognized until after approximately 3 months of age, neuroimaging of the head and visual system, preferably with MRI, should be carried out to rule out structural brain abnormalities.

Latent or occlusion nystagmus often accompanies infantile esotropia, with or without congenital nystagmus. This is a binocular horizontal jerk form of oscillation, precipitated by occlusion of one eye, resulting in conjugate nystagmus jerking toward the fixating eye. Sometimes, the same form of nystagmus exists without being initiated by occlusion, usually in the presence of strabismus, either esotropia or exotropia, but is further exaggerated by an additional occlusion maneuver, i.e., a spontaneous binocular deficiency nystagmus syndrome (sometimes called by the oxymoron "manifest" latent nystagmus). Latent nystagmus is a motor sign of strabismic loss of binocular vision and, for isolated cases, usually requires no electrophysiologic or neurological investigation.

Monocular nystagmus in infancy is an unusual form and usually is associated with amblyopia that requires occlusion therapy. Occasionally, it is the harbinger of a brain tumor such as a hypothalamic glioma, and for this reason, an MRI of the head is necessary.

Symptoms related to the visual system (poor vision, head nodding, anomalous head positions, photophobia, strabismus) in the absence of CNS problems point the way to ocular causes of the infant's nystagmus.

In general, the *ocular examination* may reveal the cause of the nystagmus, e.g., bilateral macular toxoplasmosis, bilateral optic

The Evaluation of Abnormal Head Postures

CHAPTER P24

David G Hunter

INTRODUCTION

This chapter describes a practical clinical approach to the patient who presents with an abnormal head posture of unknown etiology.[1-3] The companion chapter (Chapter 89) details the causes, types, and physiologic basis of abnormal head postures.

NOMENCLATURE

The three axes of rotation of any 3-dimensional object are described as "yaw" (rotation about the vertical axis), "pitch" (rotation about the anteroposterior axis), and "roll" (rotation about the left-to-right axis) (Fig. P24.1). An abnormal head posture may be described in terms of these axes–*yaw* corresponds to *head turn* or *face turn*, *pitch* to *head tilt*, and *roll* to *chin-up* or *chin-down*. A head turn is referred to as either a "face turn" or a "head turn." "Torticollis" may refer to any head posture, although some authors reserve this term for head tilt. "Compensatory head posture" refers to a head position adopted specifically to improve vision.

PATIENT HISTORY

Although it is important to inquire about the age of onset of a head posture, this information is available only infrequently, as the patient and family do not routinely recognize an abnormal head posture, except in extreme cases (Figs. P24.2 and P24.3). Often the only family recollection relates to a photographer's frustrated attempts to straighten the child's head for a portrait. Old photographs provide the most reliable historical information about the onset and severity of the problem.

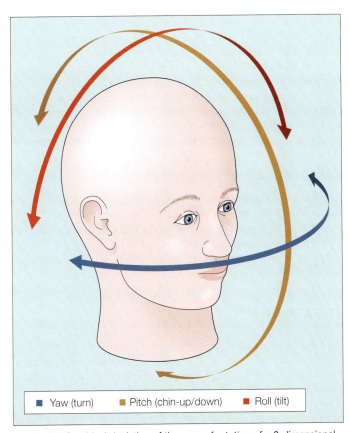

Fig. P24.1 Graphical depiction of the axes of rotation of a 3-dimensional object.

Legend: ■ Yaw (turn)   ■ Pitch (chin-up/down)   ■ Roll (tilt)

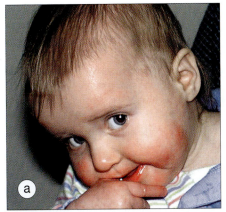

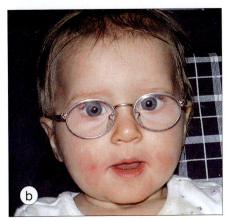

Fig. P24.2 (a) This 6-month-old girl presented with a 3-month history of a head turn and tilt. The magnitude of the head turn was variable, and the patient did not resist forced head repositioning. Motility was full. Cycloplegic refraction was +8.50 +0.50 × 90 OU. Note use of brow for "pinhole" effect on right eye. (b) Three months later the patient returned wearing partial hyperopic correction of +6.50 +0.50 × 90 OU. The head posture had completely resolved.

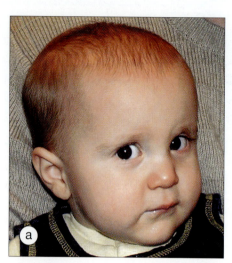

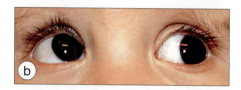

Fig. P24.3 (a) This 11-month-old boy presented with a constant left head turn and a slight chin-down position. He strongly resisted left gaze. (b) On forced gaze left, a right hypertropia was noted. High-resolution imaging revealed no orbital or extraocular muscle abnormality. Strabismus surgery is under consideration.

CHARACTERIZATION OF THE HEAD POSITION

Clinicians typically estimate the angle of head positions in degrees. Orthopedic goniometers and other more complex devices have been used to improve the precision of the estimate. Placing a prism (or yoked prisms) of increasing power in the line of sight until the head appears straight may also be used to measure the head position. Clinical photographs are a convenient and reproducible way to document a head position, but care is required to accurately depict the condition in a photograph. To obtain an accurate photograph, provide a target requiring fine visual resolution to assure that the patient is trying to obtain best acuity as the photograph is taken. Eliminate confounding objects from the background. Have the child sit up straight, off of the parent's lap if possible, to minimize leaning. Obtain similar photographs with each eye covered if head position changes with monocular viewing.

It is informative to force the head in the opposite direction and observe the response. The drive to maintain the head position against resistance may also be characterized. This is best performed while the patient is absorbed watching a movie or reading an eye chart and oblivious to the purpose of the observation. Strong resistance to movement may represent either a strong drive for binocularity with obvious strabismus or a nonocular, musculoskeletal anomaly. Lower resistance followed by a prompt return to the position with high acuity demands is suggestive of a desire to improve vision related to nystagmus or dissociated vertical deviation (DVD). Minimal resistance, with prolonged maintenance of the newly forced head position, suggests habitual head turn or possibly periodic alternating nystagmus with variable head posture, but may also be acuity-based positioning. This evaluation should be repeated with one eye occluded to determine whether the head posture is used to preserve binocular function.

EXAMINATION
Visual acuity/refraction

Uncorrected refractive error may cause a compensatory head posture (Fig. P24.2). The head position allows use of the brow or eyelid margins to achieve a pinhole effect without eyelid squeezing. Subnormal visual acuity in the absence of uncorrected refractive error is a cue to the examiner to vigorously seek other ocular causes of a head posture, such as subtle nystagmus. When the head posture persists after monocular occlusion, measure visual acuity with the head held straight; remeasure acuity after allowing the patient to adopt the preferred head posture, or observe for a change in head position as the patient reads progressively smaller letters.

External examination

Palpate the neck muscles—unusual tightness suggests a nonocular etiology. Ptosis is obvious when severe enough to produce a head posture. Assess for facial asymmetry by imagining two roughly horizontal lines, one connecting the lateral canthi and the second connecting the corners of the mouth. These lines should be parallel; if not, there is facial asymmetry. In congenital superior oblique palsy, the side where the lines diverge (larger orbit) is the side of the paresis.

Ocular motility

When nystagmus causes an abnormal head position, it is frequently obvious to the specialist. More subtle cases can be missed without careful observation. To identify subtle nystagmus as a cause of a head posture, hold the head in the position opposite to the preferred position and assess the stability of the eye. Magnification may help. Assess ductions and versions, and perform prism-and-cover testing in the diagnostic positions of gaze, as any incomitant strabismus may lead to a compensatory head posture. Occasionally a comitant, intermittent exotropia may lead to a head turn as control decompensates. Perform sensory testing with and without the abnormal head posture. Dissimilar target projection tests (Hess screen, Lancaster red-green) map the gaze position in the nine diagnostic gaze positions, revealing the direction with the smallest binocular misalignment.

Other aspects of the examination

Slit-lamp evaluation and indirect ophthalmoscopy may reveal micronystagmus not visible to the unaided eye. Visual field evaluation can reveal a hemifield defect that could rarely cause an abnormal head position. Detection of fundus torsion by indirect ophthalmoscopy may reveal unrecognized malfunction of a cyclovertical muscle.

TREATMENT[4–6]

Although treatment of an underlying condition (e.g., refractive error, ptosis, or strabismus) normally eliminates its symptoms (such as an abnormal head posture), there are exceptions. Head positions may become habitual, though this may be over-diagnosed when the examiner cannot locate a cause. Other causes of persistent abnormal head posture after surgery (including, most commonly, undercorrection of the condition) must be ruled out before concluding that it is habitual. Marked facial asymmetry may create the appearance of a head tilt no matter what the head position. DVD is difficult to treat, and even surgery that eliminates the vertical drift may not alter the head tilt. DVD may also coincide with other conditions causing abnormal head postures, such that treatment of those conditions does not eliminate either the DVD or the head posture. In nystagmus, surgery may reposition the null point but the nystagmus may persist, and the null point may drift.

Correction of an anomalous head posture secondary to nystagmus may present a formidable clinical challenge (see Chapter 74 for details). Head turns may respond to bilateral recess/resect procedures, but the surgical dosage must be selected to avoid inducing heterotropias and adjusted to compensate for preexisting horizontal strabismus. Chin-up or chin-down head postures may respond to symmetric vertical recess/resect procedures, or to weakening matched vertically acting muscles in both eyes (e.g., the superior rectus muscle recession combined with inferior oblique muscle recession and anterior transposition for a chin-down head posture). For head tilts, horizontal transposition of the vertical rectus muscles to induce torsion may be effective.

SUMMARY

An abnormal head posture is more often a diagnostic clue than a presenting complaint. When a patient presents with an anomalous head position, the comprehensive eye examination and sensorimotor evaluation may need to be supplemented by:
1. Assessing resistance to head repositioning;
2. Measuring function in primary position, preferred position, and the position opposite the preferred position; and
3. Determining the response to monocular occlusion.

Nonocular causes should be considered only after no ocular cause can be identified.

REFERENCES

1. Kushner BJ. Ocular causes of abnormal head postures. Ophthalmology 1979; 86: 2115–25.
2. Caldeira JA. Abnormal head posture: An ophthalmological approach. Binoc Vis Strabismus Q 2000; 15: 237–9.
3. Hertle RW, Zhu X. Oculographic and clinical characterization of thirty-seven children with anomalous head postures, nystagmus, and strabismus: the basis of a clinical algorithm. J AAPOS 2000; 4: 25–32.
4. Kraft SP, O'Donoghue EP, Roarty JD. Improvement of compensatory head postures after strabismus surgery. Ophthalmology 1992; 99: 1301–8.
5. Repka, MX. Surgery to correct nystagmus. In: Tasman W, editor. Duane's Clinical Ophthalmology on CD-Rom. CD-ROM. Philadelphia: Lippincott Williams & Wilkins; 2003.
6. Guyton DL. Dissociated vertical deviation: etiology, mechanism, and associated phenomena. Costenbader lecture. J AAPOS 2000; 4: 131–44.

CHAPTER
P25

The Uncooperative or Difficult Parent

Mark G Wood

"Time is the currency of care in medicine," according to the pediatrician Eisenberg.[1] In the era of managed care in the USA and global changes in health care systems, doctors have less and less time to spend with each patient. A thorough exam and the time taken to discuss exam findings and treatment options become, for parents, a major indicator of a physician's competence. Creating enough time for discussion is also the best way to avoid conflict with difficult and uncooperative parents. This chapter will describe why parents are most likely to become angry and the preventative strategies to avoid creating angry parents before they decide to visit another physician.

PREVENTION STRATEGIES TO AVOID ANGRY PARENTS

Waiting too long to see the doctor

Assuming that check-in and evaluation by your team takes 20 minutes, then a half-hour from the time the parent walks through the door should be an acceptable waiting time target (assumes no waiting for referring doctor approval). Unless they are the first patient this is rare. It is best to time your average waiting time and lower expectations by mentioning this in an introductory leaflet for parents. Also, give the average waiting time when patients phone for an appointment. On the first visit, you may wish to tell new patients to expect a longer wait because their child will require two separate exams to complete a refraction and fundus exam after using dilating drops.

In a perfect world, the physician would personally complete an entire eye examination. In some health systems this is not realistic: other than portions of the ocular motility, slit-lamp, fundus exam, and perhaps refraction, the rest of the initial eye exam may be delegated to trusted assistants. Appropriate delegation of portions of the eye exam increases the all-important face-to-face time with parents. There is a compromise between seeing enough patients to allow a practice to thrive and ensuring enough time for face-to-face explanations with parents.

Where the waiting time exceeds an acceptable limit, recognize the value of parents' time by apologizing for the delay. If you anticipate the waiting time will exceed an hour, parents should be given the option of rescheduling within a week as the first patient of the morning or afternoon to be certain they will not be delayed again. Reducing the patient waiting time in a successful practice is a never-ending struggle since the prevention strategy described here creates overwhelming demand for the practitioner's services!

Impersonal care and poor communication skills

A famous study found that the average time before a patient was interrupted by the physician was 18 seconds![2] Nothing is more satisfying to a parent than active listening and honest discussion on the part of the physician.[3] A good way to start is to take a verbatim statement of the chief complaint, e.g., "Last week his eyes crossed as he looked in the mirror up close."

Most parents have already had negative experiences with physicians. They are usually searching for someone to trust and with whom they can form a lasting partnership. Once this occurs, cooperation and compliance follow.

Not only the physician but the office staff as well must demonstrate a caring attitude. The physician's caring and patience can be undone by unprofessional behavior by office staff. Usually, parents will let the doctor know who is uncaring among office staff. Pay attention to, counsel the staff member, and replace them if they do not improve on repeated written warnings.

Preoperative counseling

Preoperative counseling is critical to continued compliance postoperatively. If more than one strabismus surgery is a possibility (virtually true with every strabismus surgery), the best time to talk about this is preoperatively. I always mention the possibility of complete loss of vision as a complication of strabismus surgery. If the parent accepts the complete loss of vision as a possibility, lesser complications including retinal detachment, diplopia, and the need for multiple procedures are likely to be accepted as well.

It is important to lower expectations for success in any surgery but particularly strabismus surgery, laser treatment for retinopathy of prematurity, cataract surgery especially if unilateral, and ptosis surgery. Even the most thorough preoperative discussions may not counteract unrealistic expectations on the part of parents.

The advantages of well-educated parents

Doctors must help people with very different backgrounds and abilities. The more you can take parents into your thinking process, the more likely they will participate and cooperate in the care of their child. Also, parents who are educated about their child's condition make rational choices about their care. Your office should have information brochures of your own creation or from national or subspecialty organizations. You might have a list of reliable Web sites for each diagnosis and the Web site to search for medical literature at the National Institutes of Health (keyword: PubMed).

When an initial diagnosis is suggested, a parent may continue to ask the same questions in another form again and again. You must be willing to repeat the answer several times in clear language and then write down the diagnosis in order to help parents absorb what may be devastating news. Copy pages from a text describing the diagnosis or give parents an information brochure.[3]

If you dictate a letter to a referring physician do this at the time of the exam in front of the parents. Send a copy to the parents. If some facts are not quite correct, the parents will correct you. This permits parents to participate, and they will know exactly what is being said to the primary care physician. When the dictation is completed you should ask again "Do you have any other questions?" If they have no more questions and you have done a complete exam and explained the diagnosis and treatment plan, this constitutes reassurance therapy.[4]

COMMUNICATING BAD NEWS

Occasionally, you will have to tell parents their child is totally blind with no hope of recovery or there is a cancer or a fatal tumor, etc. Be certain you are alone and sitting down behind closed doors, preferably with a senior nurse or counselor. Often there is a flood of emotions between you and parents that should only be shared with parents or their trusted friend. Try to give a reasonable but not hopeless prognosis if possible. For instance, cortical visual impairment and retinitis pigmentosa usually do not cause complete blindness.

After a catastrophic event parents may have unrealistic expectations for recovery, and it is clear at the time of your exam perhaps years after the event that there is no longer any hope for any significant recovery of vision. Extremely bad news should, if possible, be approached over several follow-up visits. If the same guarded prognosis can be repeated over several visits, parents are more likely to accept the reality based on their own evaluations.

If a patient is significantly visually impaired, parents and child will need rehabilitation services from an agency providing aid and special education for the visually handicapped. Your dictation to the referring physician copied to the parents can serve as a letter of introduction to the school but direct communication with the education authorities, in language that is appropriate to education, is best.

As an advocate for both your patients and parents you should plan to see visually handicapped children for at least several successive years, not just for "medical" reasons but to celebrate the child's and parents' successes at their new adaptations. Also, if services are not being rendered appropriately you can advocate for more services with a copy of your letter to the primary care physician.

Of equal importance for the physician is to recognize no matter how handicapped and disadvantaged some patients may appear, there remains dignity in every life. Parents will never forget the dignity you show toward their handicapped child. Kindness and hope should be dispensed generously to every child and every parent even in what appears to be a hopeless situation. This is the essence of what it means to be a caring physician.

COMMUNICATING BAD SURGICAL RESULTS

I see all surgical patients on the first postoperative day. Surgical complications from strabismus surgery in the form of slight over- or undercorrections are not unusual (especially small-angle esotropias after correction of an exotropia). Parents should be told preoperatively that 3 months must pass to "let the dust settle" after surgery. Use of correct wording is important and should not be self-incriminating or suggest the fault might be the child's or parent's. At 10 days postoperatively if you are not happy with a postoperative result you can say something like "The eye deviation is certainly better but not perfect. Let's wait to see if it will improve." The physician can be reassuring that time will usually improve a deviation. For instance, I waited several months as a 30-diopter overcorrection from a 90-diopter four-muscle exotropia surgery finally improved until the patient developed perfect stereopsis!

PARENTS WHO DO NOT FOLLOW ADVICE

Compliance with eye patching or using daily eye drops for treatment of amblyopia can be challenging for even the most intelligent and conscientious parents. Expect compliance in most circumstances to be marginal at best. A lecture from the physician is not needed. Reassurance and repetition in your confidence that patching will eventually work is usually all that is required. More information both written and what you say in encouragement will serve to reinforce your common goal. In fact, on a return visit even 1 or 2 lines of improvement in visual acuity will eventually lead to a successful outcome.

Responses to neglectful parents who will not patch at all vary in different societies from no response through a gentle reminder in the form of a certified letter to a court order.

PERSONAL INCOMPATIBILITY

Whether it is because you brought unwanted bad news or whether for unknown reasons parents decided they did not like you or the outcome was less than desired, you will never be able to satisfy every patient. You should be the first to recognize, however, when a parent is not happy with you or with the news you bring, or simply expresses a lack of confidence in your diagnosis or treatment. You should be the first to offer a second opinion especially if there is some uncertainty in the diagnosis or treatment regimen.

SUMMARY

A thorough exam with enough time to give a detailed explanation of your findings with heartfelt interest and a rationale for your treatment plan constitutes reassurance therapy. This is the best prevention to avoid difficult parents. Recognizing all parents' concerns calmly during a difficult exam will make you be appreciated by the vast majority. Most parents will soon realize they have found a rare commodity: a caring physician who listens. It is rare for parents to leave angry when these techniques are used. Parents have protective instincts and intuition: the secret is to listen to them to help you discover the problem and to be their partner in carrying out a mutually agreed treatment plan. Good cooperation follows naturally from this form of parent–physician interaction.[1]

REFERENCES

1. Eisenberg L. Whatever happened to the faculty on the way to the agora? Arch Intern Med 1999; 159: 2251–6.
2. Barrier P, Li J, Jensen N. Two words to improve physician-patient communication: what else? Mayo Clin Proc 2003; 78: 211–4.
3. Dawn A, Santiago-Turla C, Lee P. Patient expectations regarding eye care. Arch Ophthalmol 2003; 121: 762–8.
4. Sapira J. Reassurance therapy. Ann Intern Med 1972; 77: 603–4.

CHAPTER P26 The Uncooperative or Difficult Child

Mark G Wood

If your patience with screaming and uncontrollable children has a limit, some established techniques can rescue you from the unruly children in your office. Even if you are a pediatric ophthalmologist with infinite patience who loves playing with children, there are many times when techniques can be employed to reduce a long line of patients waiting to see you. This chapter will review how to establish rapport, what specific "tools" you'll need to keep children's interest, and finally how to hold children for a fundus exam when their cooperation is no longer possible.

DEVELOPING RAPPORT

A large part of pleasing parents depends on your ability to develop rapport with children. This chapter is written for those without God-given talents in talking to and sustaining children's cooperation and interest. A child's eye exam requires active patient participation and cooperation. Creating enough rapport for a 3-year-old to be willing to say what picture they see on a distant wall from a total stranger with one eye occluded challenges even the most experienced ophthalmologist.

Developing rapport starts from the moment you meet after introducing yourself to the parents. You turn to the child who is most at ease sitting in Mom's lap (especially if less than age 4) and introduce yourself waving your hand in a greeting making direct eye-to-eye contact. An observational comment about what a child is wearing can often break the ice: "Oh my goodness what a beautiful dress you're wearing!" If less than age 5 the physician is often met with pursed lips and not an utterance of sound. When frightened, sitting alone or shy, their lips become sealed unless you can tease them open. So how can a total stranger (hopefully without a white coat) bring a tight-lipped pouting child to utter a sound and finally do a visual acuity measurement?

It is often best not to approach the child first, but talk to the parents while the child assesses his surroundings and you. Each person's techniques are individual and personal. You might begin with direct eye-to-eye contact with a multitude of facial expressions starting with a "mouth open, eyes wide open" expression of amazement trying to generate a smile or some facial expression followed by an assortment of sounds from tongue snapping or clicking to humming to singing to imitation of cartoon characters. Occasionally "head bonking" forehead to forehead will generate a response, or occasionally the question "Do you need to be tickled?" followed suddenly by tickling of the ribs will generate a smile and later verbal response; a balance needs to be made between what is perceived as too personal for a stranger to do and what the child enjoys.

Asking the child to imitate animal sounds such as a cow or pig also works. Once a few words are uttered, some nonthreatening whispers from the physician will usually open a floodgate of responses. Several single syllable responses are all that is needed before the barrier is broken and verbal cooperation begins. It is a matter of judgment how long one should persist. Failure on the first round does not spell disaster. Wait until the patient has returned after instilling dilating drops before concluding the patient does not want to utter a sound.

The overwhelming characteristic practiced ophthalmologists have above others is tolerance and tremendous amounts of patience. After parents have witnessed all the contortions and effort you have expended to make their child cooperate, they will conclude, as you have, that sometimes it is preferable to wait for a better day.

GATHERING ACCURATE DATA

Part of developing rapport is also having the best "tools." The best of these "tools" can be just as important as an ophthalmoscope or a retinoscope in your exam room. You will need some interesting illuminated targets for near fixation in a darkened room. The lighted finger puppet of the Muppet "Bert" (Fig. P26.1) has magical qualities to attract some of the most frightened infants. Infants cannot resist trying to suck on Bert's nose. Allow the infant to grab onto Bert and as you shake Bert to loosen their grip, cover each eye for prolonged periods to check near fixation.

The best distance fixation targets make lots of movements and varied sounds, the more "bells and whistles" the better. An interesting distance fixation target (Fig. P26.2) becomes

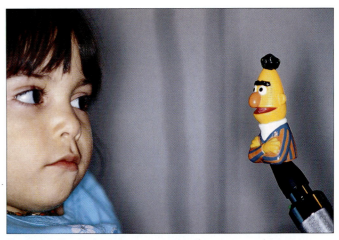

Fig. P26.1 Illuminating a finger puppet at close range can interest even the most frightened children. © 2003 Sesame Workshop. "Sesame Workshop" and its logo are trademarks of Sesame Workshop. All rights reserved.

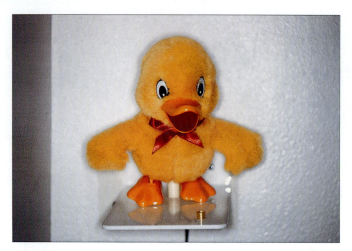

Fig. P26.2 Movement and sounds in a distant fixation target encourage prolonged fixation. (Duck, Distance Fixation Animals. Richmond Products, Boca Raton, FL, USA.)

indispensable in determining the presence or absence of strabismus, amblyopia, and poor distance fixation seen for instance in cortical visual impairment. Children's curiosity will overcome their fear of your occluder or your thumb. If the occluder is held motionless and just out of their reach a child will eventually allow determination of fixation preference and the recognition of small-angle strabismus. Another acceptable distance fixation target includes video recordings in continuous play mode.

Refraction after cycloplegia is one of the cornerstones of the eye examination of children since it is pivotal in curing accommodative esotropia and revealing an anisometropic amblyopia. An interesting near or distant fixation target after cycloplegia may save the day for retinoscopy. Unfortunately, children with larger refractive errors will try the patience of the examiner, the child, and the parent.

Children are cooperative enough by age 3 to use a standing autorefractor after cycloplegia. In a prospective study of 100 children by the author, 96% of the children read the 20/30 line perfectly with the result from the autorefractor alone.[1] In unreliable or uncooperative children the autorefractor results can be used as the basis for a prescription without a subjective refraction. Follow-up confirmation with visual acuity testing and a repeated refraction is required.

If a child is less than age 3 and too uncooperative for a standing autorefractor, the portable extremely short fixation time (0.05 s) autorefractor can be very helpful even in a screaming child, with the head held by the parent (Fig. 26.3). Because of the short fixation time the lids can be pried open and even with very brief fixation multiple measurements can be made. It is the author's experience that using this technique narrows the refractive error to within 1 diopter of accurate retinoscopy. The portable autorefractor result can then be refined with retinoscopy even with brief glimpses of the red reflex. This approximate refraction can later be confirmed in follow-up exams.

For bottle-fed infants, reserving use of the bottle for just those moments when the most cooperation is required (fixing and following, retinoscopy, and fundus exam) can save the day. The mother should withhold feeding until the most cooperation is required. It is not uncommon for hungry bottle-feeding infants to tolerate even the brightest indirect ophthalmoscope.

As a last resort, especially in the instance when no pathology is suspected (no anticipated need to go to the operating theater) or

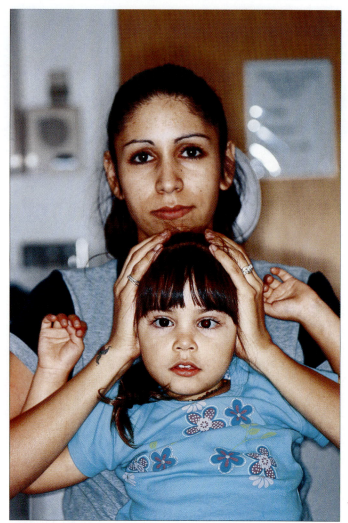

Fig. P26.3 The parent can secure the head and arms at the same time crossing their legs to prevent the patient's legs from moving.

a cursory exam is all that is required, an eyelid speculum can be used with parents' permission. It is best to demonstrate the function of the speculum before using it and explain that using it could avoid a trip to the operating room. Employing the holding technique to be demonstrated below, a great deal of information can be gleaned using either a portable slit lamp or a 30-diopter indirect lens to magnify both the anterior and posterior segments of the eye. This instrumentation can only be employed in infants using a technique described in the next section, namely the "burrito wrap."

EXAM TECHNIQUES

Much of the essential data needed for a thorough eye examination can be obtained while the patient is sitting in the secure environment of a parent's lap, well removed from the physician. Perhaps the best "pearl" in technique is using the Bruckner red reflex test[2]: inspecting the red reflexes at a distance of one-half meter with the ophthalmoscope set at +2.00. This allows the examiner to check pupil symmetry and reactivity, determine symmetrical positions of the tiny white corneal reflexes, and determine whether the red reflexes appear symmetrically bright in each eye as an indication of poor fixation on the light of the

Fortunately, at this point, the fundus exam requires no co-operation in younger infants since the parent can restrain the head and feet well enough to permit indirect ophthalmoscopy (Fig. 26.3). In children less than age 2, to avoid examinations under anesthesia or sedation, the "burrito wrap" (Fig. 26.4) can permit ophthalmoscopy or other parts of an eye exam, including a search for a retained foreign body. Using a sheet both arms are placed tightly and parallel along the torso and one edge of the sheet is wrapped across one arm and tucked snugly underneath the other arm held closely against the torso so that the weight of the infant's body holds the sheet tightly. The other side of the sheet is wrapped in the same manner in the opposite direction so that both arms are doubly wrapped tightly against the torso. An assistant holds the head securely allowing safe placement of an eyelid speculum. In the case of a retained foreign body, double eversion of the upper eyelid with a Desmarres lid retractor can be completed to expose the extreme apex of the superior cul-de-sac. (The author found a 1-cm serrated-edged insect carapace using this technique!)

RECOGNIZING BAD DAYS

With experience, the ophthalmologist will recognize when achieving only a portion of the exam is a qualified success. Both doctor and patient can have bad days. If the patient is known to have combative behaviors or is mentally challenged and making no attempt to cooperate then one has several choices:
1. Sometimes behavior improves with time or after dilating pupils.
2. Try performing the remote exam as described above.
3. Set limited goals and ask parents to try again on a better day.

The physician can also have a bad day especially if exhausted and not feeling well. If you are short on time or patience then it is important to set limited goals for yourself and the patient. Explain the situation to parents, apologize, and complete only a portion of the full exam.

The decision to perform an exam under anesthesia or sedation (which carry the same risks) include the following:
1. Known or suspected glaucoma, retinal detachment, or retinal pathology such as retinoblastoma or retinopathy of prematurity.
2. A combative older or mentally challenged child.

In summary, overwhelming patience and the luxury of having enough time to wait out bad behavior episodes are essential assets. For those without patience or time, these techniques and the "tools" described work surprisingly well even in the youngest patients.

REFERENCES

1. Wood M, Mazow M, Prager T. Accuracy of the Nidek ARK-900 objective refractor in comparison with retinoscopy in children ages 3 to 18 years. Am J Ophthalmol 1998; 126: 100–8.
2. Tongue A, Cibis G. Bruckner test. Ophthalmology 1981; 88: 1041–4.

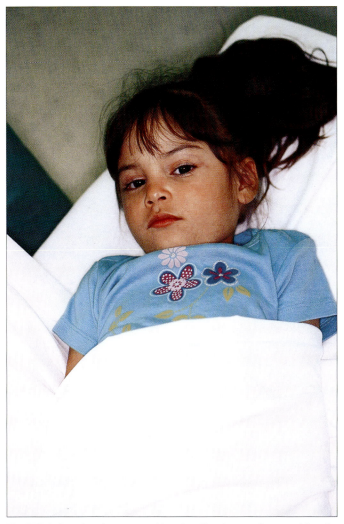

Fig. P26.4 Securing the arms and legs in a "burrito wrap" can avoid a trip to the operating room.

ophthalmoscope. With practice some practitioners can recognize less than 10 prism diopters of horizontal deviation.

The eye exam can be entertainment for most children. It begins with the ride up in the examination chair followed by looking at the ophthalmoscope light for red reflexes or the light of the retinoscope. To test extraocular motility it is time to "follow my friend Bert. He's looking very closely at you." Cover testing at distance requires an interesting fixation target and willingness of the patient to allow covering one eye. Testing stereopsis becomes using "the funny glasses," finding the pictures of the Lang stereoacuity plates, or "touching the colors" of the Worth 4-dot test. The slit-lamp exam is called "riding the motorcycle." Finally, indirect ophthalmoscopy is called "going on a rocket ship ride" as the chair is reclined into a recumbent position.

CHAPTER P27 Hand Defects and the Eye

Luis Carlos F de Sa

The combination of hand and eye defects is frequent and may be observed in a variety of disorders, given that similar phenotypes may result from different etiologies. There may be genetic causes, including specific genes and/or new mutations, but due to incomplete penetrance, sporadic events, and association with environmental factors, it is not always possible to determine the underlying mechanism.

Structural defects may result from three kinds of developmental pathology:

1. *Malformation* is an inadequate tissue formation and rarely allows survival, when it occurs prior to 23 days.
2. *Deformation* occurs in normal tissue, resulting generally from mechanical forces.
3. *Disruption* results from a breakdown of a previously normal tissue. Furthermore, an initial malformation may induce secondary deformation or disruption and vice versa.

It is important to briefly consider the embryology and the timing of eye and hand development to understand why such defects may occur simultaneously. During the third week of gestation, at about 22 days, the optic primordium becomes identifiable in the human embryo, and it is the first morphological evidence of the eyes. Soon after (25 days) as optic cup and embryonic fissure emerge, upper limb buds appear. By 36 days, closure of retinal fissure is almost complete and the retina is now incompletely pigmented. At the same time, the hand plate has formed with condensation of mesenchyme. In the hand plate, a central carpal region is surrounded by a crescentic flange, the digital plate, which originates the five-finger rays. Ten days later (45 days) the fingers are partially separated.

The etiology of most limb defects (Table P27.1) is unknown. Familial associations indicate a genetic basis for some cases; however, environmental agents such as drugs and hyperthermia may be related with the development of limb defects. Developmental abnormalities such as amniotic bands, oligohydramnios, and local vascular disruption are also associated with limb abnormalities.[1] Eye defects and hand/finger anomalies originate usually between the third and the fifth week of gestation.

The various hand and eye defects are grouped in Table P27.2 according to their similarity in overall features or according to one major feature among the patterns of malformation, in the same manner as the classic *Smith's Recognizable Patterns of Malformation*.[2] Many conditions may present occasional hand and eye defects, but only the most important and consistent associations are described.

Table P27.1 Common terms used for limb and fingers malformation

Anomaly	Definition
Arachnodactyly	Long and thin bones of the fingers
Brachydactyly	Abnormal shortness of the fingers
Camptodactyly	Permanent and irreducible flexion of fingers
Clinodactyly	Deviation or deflection of one or more fingers
Ectrodactyly	Absence of any numbers of fingers
Macrodactyly	Abnormal largeness of the fingers
Meromelia	Absence of part of a limb
Micromelia	Abnormal smallness of a limb
Polydactyly	Extra digits or parts of digits
Syndactyly	Fusion of digits
Oligodactyly	Reduced number of digits
Phocomely	Hands/feet without arms/legs

Table P27.2 Disease and related eye/ocular region and hand/finger anomalies

Group/disease	Eye/ocular region anomalies	Hand/finger anomalies
Chromosomal syndromes Down syndrome[3] (Trisomy 21)	Upslanting palpebral fissures, epicanthal folds, Iris Brushfield spots, keratoconus, strabismus, nystagmus, myopia, cataracts	Short metacarpals and phalanges, fifth finger mid-phalanx hypoplasia, single transverse palmar (simian) crease
Trisomy 18	Short/slanted palpebral fissure, ptosis, hypertelorism, iris coloboma, cataract, microphthalmos	Clenched hand, overlapping of fingers, absence of distal crease, hypoplasia of nails, hypoplastic or absent thumb, syndactyly, polydactyly, ectrodactyly, short fifth metacarpals
Trisomy 13 (Patau syndrome)	Microphthalmia, iris coloboma, retinal dysplasia, hypotelorism, hypertelorism, anophthalmos, cyclopia, slanting palpebral fissures, shallow orbital ridges, absent eyebrow	Flexion of fingers, overlapping, camptodactyly, polydactyly, syndactyly, retroflexilble thumb
Triploidy syndrome and diploid triploid mixoploidy syndrome	Hypertelorism, coloboma, microphthalmia, iris heterochromia	Syndactyly, simian crease, clinodactyly, proximally placed thumb
Aniridia-Wilms tumor association (Chapter 28)	Aniridia, cataracts, nystagmus, ptosis, glaucoma	Clinodactyly

Table P27.2 (*Cont'd*) Disease and related eye/ocular region and hand/finger anomalies

Group/disease	Eye/ocular region anomalies	Hand/finger anomalies
Very small stature, not skeletal dysplasia		
Cornelia de Lange syndrome[4]	Bushy eyebrow, synophrys, long, curly eyelashes	Micromelia, phocomelia, oligodactyly, simian crease, proximal implantation of thumbs
Rubinstein Taybi syndrome[5]	Heavy/highly arched eyebrows, long eyelashes, epicanthal folds, strabismus, nasolacrimal duct stenosis, ptosis	Broad thumbs with radial angulation, fingers broad, clinodactyly, persistent fetal fingertip pads
Moderate stature, facial, genital		
Smith-Lemli-Opitz syndrome	Ptosis, epicanthal folds, strabismus	Simian crease, occasional flexed fingers, short fingers, polydactyly
Williams-Beuren syndrome[6]	Epicanthal folds, stellate iris pattern, occasional strabismus, hypotelorism	Hypoplastic nails, occasional clinodactyly
Noonan syndrome	Hypertelorism, downslanting palpebral fissures, prominent corneal nerves, myopia, keratoconus, strabismus, nystagmus	Clinodactyly, brachydactyly, blunt fingertips
Unusual brain and/or neuromuscular findings with associated defects		
Cohen syndrome	Decreased visual acuity, strabismus, constricted visual fields, chorioretinal dystrophy, optic atrophy	Narrow hands, mild shortening of metacarpals, simian crease
Zellweger syndrome	Cataracts, optic nerve hypoplasia, retinal pigmentary changes, glaucoma, nystagmus	Variable contractures, camptodactyly
Facial defects as major feature		
Möbius sequence[7] (Fig. P27.1)	Sixth and seventh nerve palsy, strabismus	Syndactyly, limb reduction defects
Fraser syndrome	Cryptophthalmos, associated with eye defects	Partial cutaneous syndactyly, occasional absent phalanges/thumb
Facial-limb defects as major feature		
Miller syndrome	Eyelids coloboma, ectropion	Absence of fifth digits, syndactyly
Oculodentodigital syndrome	Microphthalmos, microcornea, short palpebral fissures, epicanthal folds, fine porous iris	Syndactyly, camptodactyly, phalangeal hypoplasia
Stickler syndrome[8] (Hereditary arthroophthalmopathy)	Myopia, chorioretinal degeneration, retinal detachment, cataract	Severe arthropathy, occasional arachnodactyly
Ectrodactyly-ectodermal dysplasia-clefting syndrome (EEC syndrome)	Blue iris, photophobia, blepharophimosis, lacrimal system anomalies, blepharitis	Syndactyly, ectrodactyly, nail dysplasia
Craniosynostosis syndromes (Chapter 39)		
Apert syndrome (acrocephalosyndactyly) (Fig. P27.2)	Hypertelorism, strabismus, shallow orbits, down slanting of palpebral fissures	Osseous and/or cutaneous syndactyly, broad distal phalanges of thumb, fingers may be short
Pfeiffer syndrome (Fig. P27.3)	Ocular hypertelorism, shallow orbit, proptosis	Broad distal phalanges, syndactyly
Carpenter syndrome	Cornea opacity, microcornea, optic atrophy	Brachydactyly, syndactyly, polydactyly, clinodactyly, camptodactyly
Other skeletal dysplasia		
Weill-Marchesani syndrome (Chapter 46)	Spherophakia, ectopia lentis, myopia, glaucoma	Brachydactyly, broad metacarpals and phalanges, stiff joints (hands)
Connective disorders		
Marfan syndrome (Fig. P27.4) (Chapter 46)	Lens luxation/subluxation, myopia, retinal detachment, glaucoma	Arachnodactyly
Homocystinuria syndrome (Chapter 46)	Lens subluxation (inferiorly), myopia, cataract, glaucoma, optic atrophy	Arachnodactyly
Ehlers-Danlos syndrome[9]	Blue sclera, myopia, microcornea, glaucoma, ectopia lentis, keratoconus	Hyperextensibility of joints
Osteogenesis imperfecta[10]	Blue sclera (thin and translucent), keratoconus, embryotoxon posterior	Hyperextensibility of joints, fractures, occasional syndactyly
Hamartoses/phakomatosis		
Linear sebaceous nevus sequence	Esotropia, lipodermoid, cloudy cornea, coloboma, optic atrophy, microphthalmia	Polydactyly, syndactyly
Klippel-Trénaunay-Weber syndrome[11]	Glaucoma, cataracts, heterochromia	Asymmetric limb hypertrophy, occasional macrodactyly, syndactyly, polydactyly, or oligodactyly
Environmental agents		
Fetal-alcohol syndrome[12]	Optic nerve hypoplasia, occasional ptosis, microphthalmos	Small distal phalanges, small fifth finger nail
Miscellaneous syndromes associations		
Bardet-Biedl syndrome (Laurence-Moon-Biedl syndrome)	Retinal dystrophy (retinitis pigmentosa) astigmatism, nystagmus, cataracts	Polydactyly, syndactyly, brachydactyly

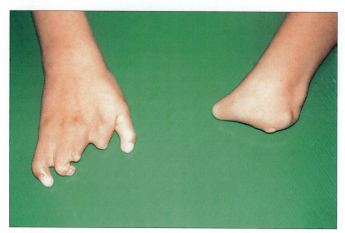

Fig. P27.1 Möbius syndrome. Ectrodactyly and meromelia.

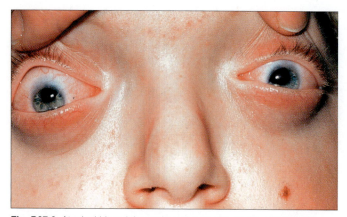

Fig. P27.3 Atypical iris coloboma in a patient with Pfeiffer syndrome.

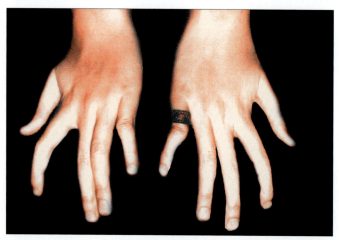

Fig. P27.4 Arachnodactyly frequently found in patients with Marfan syndrome.

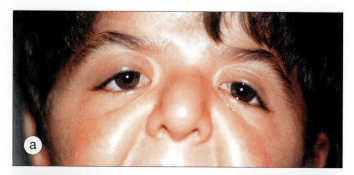

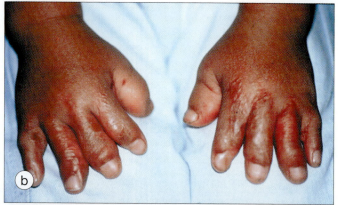

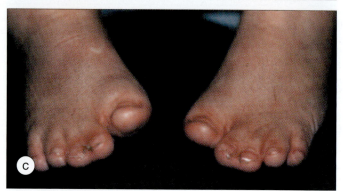

Fig. P27.2 (a) Apert syndrome. (b) Same patient after surgery for syndactyly. (c) Syndactyly of toes.

REFERENCES

1. Larsen WJ. Development of the limbs. In Larsen WJ. editor. Human Embryology. 2nd ed. New York: Churchill Livingstone; 1997: 311–44.

2. Jones KL, editor. Smith's Recognizable Patterns of Human Malformation. 5th ed. Philadelphia: Saunders; 1997.

3. da Cunha RP, Moreira JB. Ocular findings in Down's syndrome. Am J Ophthalmol 1996; 122: 236–44.

4. Allarzon JE, Hennekan RC, Ireland M. DeLange syndrome: subjective and objective comparison of the classical and mild phenotypes. J Med Genet 1997; 34: 645–50.

5. van Genderer MM, Kinds GF, Riemslag FC, et al. Ocular features in Rubenstein-Taybi syndrome: investigation of 24 patients and review of the literature. Br J Ophthalmol 2000; 84: 1177–84.

6. Winter M, Pankau R, Ann M, et al. The spectrum of ocular features in the Williams-Beuren syndrome. Clin Genet 1996; 49: 28–31.

7. Cronemberger MF, de Castro Moreira JB, Brunoni D, et al. Ocular and clinical manifestations of Möbius' syndrome. J Pediatr Ophthalmol Strabismus 2001; 38: 156–62.

8. Stickler GB, Hughes W, Houchin P. Clinical features of hereditary progressive orthro-ophthalmology (Stickler syndrome): a survey. Genet Med 2001; 3: 192–6.

9. Pollack JS, Custer PL, Hart WM, et al. Ocular complications in Ehlers-Danlos syndrome type IV. Arch Ophthalmol 1997; 115: 416–9.

10. Chan CC, Green WR, de la Cruz ZC, et al. Ocualr findings in osteogenesis imperfecta congenita. Arch Ophthalmol 1982; 100: 1658–63.

11. Teekhasaenee C, Ritch R. Glaucoma in phakomatosis pigmentovascularis. Ophthalmology 1997; 104: 150–7.

12. Hug TE, Fitzgerald KM, Cibis GW. Clinical and electroretinographic findings in fetal alcohol syndrome. J AAPOS 2000; 4: 200–4.

13. Spaggiari E, Salati R, Nicolini P, et al. Evolution of ocular clinical and electrophysiological findings in pediatric Bardet-Biedl syndrome. Int Ophthalmol 1999: 23: 61–7.

Contact Lens Management Problems

Lynne Speedwell

Many conditions in infancy and childhood benefit from contact lenses but a contact lens is a foreign body and can induce adverse corneal and conjunctival changes. Extended or overnight wear is best avoided to reduce the risk of infection. Many parents are nervous of dealing with their children's lenses especially in a resistant infant but with time most overcome their fears.[1]

The care regime needs to be simple and effective and strict hygiene stressed from the outset. Solutions that could cause an allergic response should be avoided.

If an eye shows any sign of irritation, the lens must be removed immediately and the eye examined by an ophthalmologist.

CONTACT LENS MATERIALS

Children can wear all types of contact lenses but the optimum lens depends on the eye condition, the age, and the child. General anesthesia is not required for lens fitting with the possible exception of impression scleral lenses (see Scleral Lenses).

Soft lenses

Soft lenses contain water and absorb whatever fluid they are soaking in. Water contents vary from 38% to more than 80%. The amount of oxygen permeating through the material is limited by water content and thickness. Lenses can be made in spherical or toric (astigmatic) form.

Soft lenses are prone to deposition, which is avoided by using disposable lenses. However, lenses required for most of the conditions discussed below are rarely available in disposable lens parameters.

There are numerous contact lens solutions available to clean and disinfect soft lenses. Alternatively, if parents have a steam sterilizer for babies' bottles, lenses can be cleaned with a surfactant cleaner, rinsed, and placed in a case with saline and then into the sterilizer.

Soft lenses are inserted by "posting" the lens underneath the top eyelid and removed by scooping the lens out as for a rigid lens.

Silicone hydrogels

Silicone hydrogels are soft lens materials that hold less water but are more oxygen permeable because they contain silicone.[2] To date they are only available in a limited range of low spherical powers.

Cleaning these lenses is the same as for soft lenses although heat should be avoided.

Rigid lenses

Rigid lenses can be made of polymethyl methacrylate (PMMA), which is now rarely used, or a rigid gas permeable (RGP) material to allow oxygen of varying amounts to permeate through the lens. For conditions requiring high-power lenses or where there is a risk of corneal neovascularization, a high Dk (oxygen permeability) material is used. RGP lenses can be fitted for most conditions and prescriptions but may be less comfortable than soft lenses and are dangerous to insert into a tightly squeezed eye.

Various cleaning and disinfecting solutions are available for RGP lenses.

They are inserted directly onto the cornea and removed by scooping them out. Where necessary, a rubber suction holder can be used to remove the lens.

Silicone rubber

Silicone rubber is a hydrophobic material, which is coated to make it hydrophilic and comfortable to wear. Oxygen permeation through the lens is 100% but the surface degrades with wear and the lenses are difficult, time-consuming, and expensive to fit. Silicone rubber is useful in conditions where the tears or blink rate are poor or other types of lenses are constantly being rubbed out.[3]

Surfactant cleaners with an abrasive action should be avoided but otherwise RGP lens solutions can be used.

Silicone rubber lenses are inserted the same way as soft lenses and removed by scooping them out. Where necessary, a rubber suction holder can be used to remove the lens.

Scleral lenses

Scleral lenses are large lenses, covering the whole eye. They are available in RGP materials or PMMA and can be either pre-formed or fitted by impression technique. A general anesthetic may be necessary if an impression is taken. Scleral lenses are used only rarely for children except in the form of a cosmetic shell although they do have the advantage of being easy to handle.

CONTACT LENSES FOR REFRACTIVE CONDITIONS

High myopia

High myopes benefit from wearing contact lenses, as the visual acuity is better (spectacles minify the retinal image). Lenses should only be fitted if a child is keen; otherwise, the novelty soon wears off. Both soft and RGP lenses can be fitted. It may be easier to start with spherical soft lenses for an astigmatic child, especially if they are nervous, and progress to RGP or toric soft lenses later.

Lenses used to retard myopia

Fitting young myopes with RGP lenses may retard any increase in refractive error. Conventionally fitted rigid lenses appear to slow the progression of myopia,[4,5] but this is controversial (see Chapter 6). *Orthokeratology* (moulding corneal shape to reduce myopia) can be carried out on young myopes and can be temporarily successful if the child is compliant (see Chapter 6).

High hypermetropia and strabismus

Contact lenses are often fitted for cosmetic reasons. Visual acuity is not as good in contact lenses as in spectacles due to the magnifying effect of the convex spectacle lenses.

Unilateral ametropes

Unilateral ametropes demonstrate reduced aniseikonia for both axial and refractive myopia[6] when wearing contact lenses instead of spectacles. However, amblyopia is usually a problem, and a lot of patching is needed. Unilateral high myopia (over -9.00 D) and amblyopia do not usually respond well with patching.[7]

Unfortunately, children do not notice any difference when wearing their lens, as they are rarely binocular so compliance may be difficult.

PATHOLOGICAL CONDITIONS

Aphakia

Aphakia is the most common indication for contact lenses in infancy (Chapter 47).[1,8] Spectacles also have advantages and a combination of devices may be necessary, for example, an intraocular lens together with a contact lens or spectacle lens.

Retinoscopy should be on-axis and with the trial lens held close to the eye (the effective power of a +20.00-D trial lens with a back vertex distance of 16 mm is +29.41 D at the cornea). Because babies tend to be interested only in their immediate environment, they are overcorrected by 2–3 D. The power of the first lens required by the infant aphake is typically +32.00 D. As the child grows the overcorrection is reduced, so that by school age, they are wearing a distance contact lens correction with bifocal spectacles for close work. Astigmatism need not be corrected in infants as it frequently alters or disappears in the first two years.[9]

Bifocal contact lenses are rarely fitted, as they require good subjective feedback for accurate results. However, aspheric RGP lenses can be designed to give reasonable near acuity.

Aphakic spectacles magnify the image, giving better acuity than spectacles but the field of vision is reduced. Therefore if vision is about 6/18 or less in spectacles, they will not manage well with contact lenses for school or work but they may appreciate contact lenses for social occasions. Aphakes who are considering secondary implants should wear contact lenses regularly for three months before surgery to be certain they are comfortable with the anticipated lower acuity.

What lens to fit?
Soft lenses
- Where keratometry (K) readings are not measured, radius is fitted on known average keratometry (K) reading (7.10 mm (47.54 D) for a neonate).[10]
- The total diameter (TD) is 2 mm larger than corneal diameter although it may assist centration to make it larger.

- The lens should center well and move slightly on versions and upgaze.
- Microphthalmic patients who are also aphakic can require powers of up to +50 D. TD can be as little as 10 mm.

RGP lenses

RGP lenses can be used for all ages but are easier to fit in patients under 6 months or over 5 years.
- It can help to instill local anesthetic drops before inserting the lenses.
- Take K readings if possible (this is easier if a hand-held keratometer is available). Fit on flattest K and then check the fit using fluorescein and blue light. If K readings are not obtainable, fit empirically on known average K (7.1 mm (47.54 D) for a neonate) then check the fit and alter accordingly.
- The first trial lens should be an aspheric design with reduced edge clearance, and the TD is larger than normal, 1–1.5 mm smaller than corneal diameter, to lessen the risk of the lenses falling out.

Silicone rubber lenses

Silicone rubber lenses are available in limited parameters only.[3]
- Take K readings and fit on flattest K or 0.1 mm flatter.
- Total diameter is 11.30 mm.
- Check immediately with fluorescein and then after 10 minutes. Allow settling for at least 45 minutes before final assessment.
- If at any time the lens appears steep, remove it at once.
- The lens should show light central touch and moderate edge clearance (Fig. P28.1).

Changes as the child grows

The power decreases from around +32.00 D in infancy (including overcorrection for close focus) to about +22.00 D by age 2 and +16.00 D in an adult. Emmetropization continues in some aphakic children who would otherwise have been myopic. Those given implants in infancy may need to have the power of the IOL changed later.[11] Many children with Down syndrome become myopic and, if aphakic, the prescription may reduce to +5.00 D or less. (A myopic shift may be a sign of glaucoma.)

The corneal diameter increases from 10 mm in a neonate to 11.5–12.5 mm in an adult. The corneal radius increases from

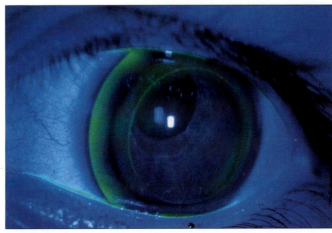

Fig. P28.1 A silicone rubber contact lens. The fit of the lens is assessed with fluorescein, which shows adequate central fit and excessive edge clearance.

7.1 mm (47.54 D) in a neonate to 7.86 mm (42.94 D) for an adult.[10]

Lenses for microphthalmic adults are only slightly flatter and larger than those fitted to an infant but the power decreases.

Unilateral aphakes

Unilateral aphakes are often densely amblyopic and the phakic eye needs to be patched extensively. The results of treatment are variable,[12] but the outcome can be good if treatment starts early,[13] often with graded patching until 7 years or more[14] (see Chapter 47). Unilateral aphakes may complain of photophobia in the aphakic eye and benefit from a tint in the contact lens.

Ectopia lentis

Flat corneas are common in Marfan syndrome: possibly 8.50 mm (39.71 D) or flatter. These eyes do better with soft lenses although if Ks are less flat, RGP lenses can work. Phakic eyes have irregular astigmatism, which is not fully corrected by toric lenses either soft or RGP. Spectacles are required with an astigmatic correction to wear over the lenses.

The dislocating lens itself and an increased axial length cause myopic astigmatism. When one eye is surgically aphakic or the lens has dislocated sufficiently to use the aphakic portion of the pupil (Fig. P28.2), the prescription is highly hypermetropic with gross anisometropia if unilateral. Contact lenses provide binocularity although where the child is averse to contact lens wear, spectacles can be an interim measure. Amblyopia can slowly improve with either form of correction.[15]

Simple ectopia lentis is treated similarly, but the Ks are not as flat. In ectopia lentis et pupillae, an aphakic prescription is usually required from the outset as the lens is dislocated in the direction opposite to the pupil.

Keratoconus

Keratoconus is not common in young children but where it does occur, RGP lenses are the first choice although scleral lenses may be necessary from the outset. It is more common in the second decade, with Asians having a greater risk of developing keratoconus.[16]

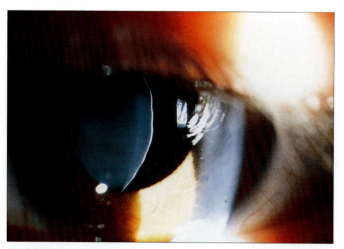

Fig. P28.2 Dislocated lens. The edge of lens is cutting across the pupil. The patient will see better out of the corrected aphakic portion of the pupil than through the myopic lens.

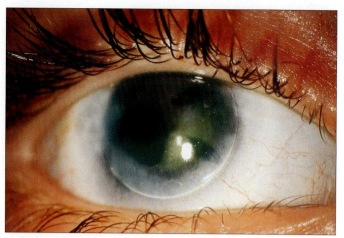

Fig. P28.3 A rigid gas permeable lens on a corneal graft for Peters' anomaly. There is inadequate edge lift although this is not the cause of the neovascularization.

Penetrating keratoplasty (PK)

Contact lenses may be fitted postoperatively to infants who have had a PK. The graft tissue is often larger than the host, which has the effect of making the cornea steep, and the eye can become increasingly myopic as it heals. The lens of choice is an RGP keratoconic lens with a small total diameter. Adequate edge clearance may be difficult to achieve (Fig. P28.3). At aftercare, the cornea may have steepened and care is needed if there is any neovascularization.

When contact lenses are fitted to older children who have had a PK for keratoconus or corneal dystrophy, care is needed to avoid pressure on the graft.

Nanophthalmos

Nanophthalmic eyes are highly hypermetropic (+20.00 D or more). The same type of lens as required for aphakia is used, but no allowance is necessary for accommodation.

COSMETIC CONDITIONS REQUIRING CONTACT LENSES

It is not always practical to fit a perfectly matched tinted lens to a young child as lenses are easily lost and broken. However, fitting a cosmetic lens to a school-age child with an unsightly eye can make an enormous difference to how they see themselves and how others respond to them.

A clear lens can be fitted initially to accurately assess the fit and to teach good lens handling and a tinted lens can be ordered later.

Aniridia

Tinted lenses do not improve acuity in congenital aniridia but older children do appear more comfortable with tinted soft lenses, especially if there are lens opacities. Tinted soft lenses can be fitted but care must be taken due to the corneal stem cell deficiency, as pannus is common. In adults the cornea may become opacified, and RGP lenses will give better acuity and may delay the need for a stem cell graft.

Traumatic aniridia is usually unilateral. Any photophobia is reduced by a cosmetic contact lens and the appearance is better.

Albinism

Infants with oculocutaneous albinism occasionally appear more sensitive to having contact lenses inserted. Lenses do not improve visual acuity, and the dark tints required are cosmetically unacceptable (unless hand-painted lenses, which cannot be slept in and are prohibitively expensive, are used). Wearing dark glasses and a hat or shading the pram is more practical.

Some older children appreciate tinted lenses but the cylindrical correction, common in albinos, may not improve acuity much, so spherical soft lenses are adequate. Where the astigmatic correction is required, RGP lenses work better.

Iris coloboma

Cosmetic iris lenses are of little use to young children with iris coloboma but, if unilateral, they may help older children. Color matching is easier if a tinted segment is incorporated (Figs. P28.4 and P28.5).

Achromatopsia

Patients with achromatopsia are photophobic and require a tint. Soft, tinted-pupil lenses that leave the iris color unaffected can work well but some light still enters the pupil obliquely. A soft, tinted-iris lens or a tinted RGP lens often works better. Outdoors, dark spectacles are required in addition to contact lenses.

The optimum color of the tint varies between individuals (reds, browns, and grays are the most common). Where patients have sunglasses with their "perfect" color, a sample spectacle lens can be sent for the contact lens laboratory to match.

Microphthalmos

Microphthalmos can occur with or without cataracts. When unilateral, a soft lens is fitted with matching iris color and size. A prescription can be incorporated into the lens for a sighted eye; a plano cosmetic lens is prescribed if the eye is amblyopic. Where the eye is severely microphthalmic or phthisical, a cosmetic shell will be required.

Scars and opacities

In infants where the eye is unsightly it is worthwhile fitting even if the lens is not a perfect match (Figs. P28.6 and P28.7).

OCCLUSIVE CONTACT LENSES

These can be used instead of patching for unilateral aphakes or strabismic amblyopes who do not comply with adhesive patches

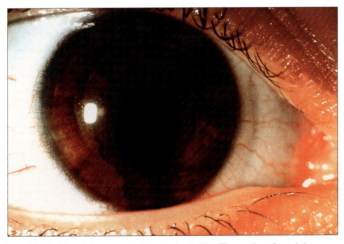

Fig. P28.4 Iris coloboma causing photophobia. The patient found the appearance unsightly.

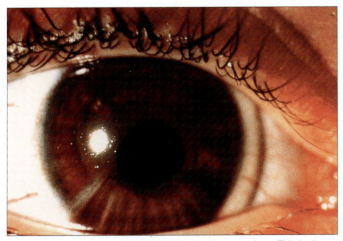

Fig. P28.5 Iris coloboma fitted with a cosmetic contact lens. This is the same eye as that in Fig. P28.4 with a hand-painted iris segment on a soft contact lens fitted to cover the coloboma.

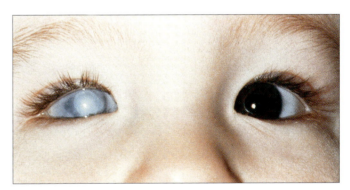

Fig. P28.6 Iris dysgenesis in Peters' anomaly. At the age of 14 months, the appearance was of concern to the parents only. As the child grows older, he will be bothered by the cosmesis.

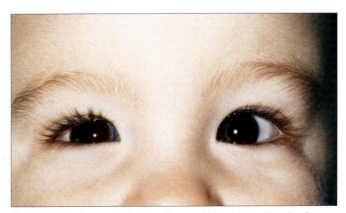

Fig. P28.7 Iris dysgenesis in Peters' anomaly fitted with a tinted soft contact lens. This is the same child as that in Fig. P28.6 with a tinted lens in situ. Although it is not a perfect match, it looks better and the child can continue thus until he is able to wear a hand-painted lens.

(see Chapter 78). They do not often work as children soon learn to rub the lens out.[17] It is important to consider the risks to the phakic or better eye when an occlusive lens is fitted. Many clinicians do not feel that the benefits are worth the potential risks.

Occlusive lenses can also be used in older children who have intractable diplopia, but every alternative option should be attempted first.

THERAPEUTIC LENSES

Therapeutic lenses are used infrequently for conditions similar to those in adults–corneal dystrophies, leaking blebs, or corneal grafts and perforations. They are worn temporarily while the eye heals or until an alternative form of treatment is found.

Lenses used are high-water-content soft for epithelial erosions; silicone hydrogel or silicone rubber lenses for perforations and leaking grafts; and large high-water-content soft lenses for leaking blebs.

PRACTICAL POINTS

- Involve both parents, where possible, in handling the lenses. If only one parent is available, a grandparent or friend may help until the parent is more adept.
- With young infants, where lens insertion and removal are difficult, try while the child is asleep.
- Insist on daily lens removal and cleaning. Warn parents of potential hazards and the importance of good hygiene.

- Vision does not develop better in contact lenses although there is more chance of binocularity developing in cases of anisometropia.
- Do not fit lenses to please the parents except in rare instances (e.g., fitting a cosmetic lens to an unsightly eye). Explain why the child may be better to remain in spectacles.
- Parents who cannot persuade their child to wear glasses may have difficulty following instructions on contact lens care.
- In a slightly older uncooperative child, it is better to make several short appointments, rather than one long one to help the child become familiar with the practitioner and the surroundings.
- If the child wants lenses but is too nervous, give them artificial tears to practice with and encourage them to touch the white of the eye with a clean finger. In most cases, patching can be carried out with spectacle correction as an interim step before fitting a contact lens.
- Many children, having worn lenses since infancy, start to rebel against having them inserted at about eighteen months of age. At that stage they can wear spectacles and return to lenses later. Parents may be reluctant for their child to change from contact lenses to spectacles, but they usually find it worthwhile. Warn them early on that this may happen.
- At the first sign of soreness, irritation, watering or if a child has a cold or infection, the lenses should be removed and left out until the condition has been clear for three days. Remove lenses from both eyes and treat each eye the same.
- Contact lenses should not be worn for swimming because of risk of infection.
- Lenses should be removed or rewetting drops used when flying, as aircraft cabins are very dry.

REFERENCES

1. Ma JJ, Morad Y, Mau E, et al. Contact lenses for the treatment of pediatric cataracts. Ophthalmology 2003; 110: 299–305.
2. Tighe BJ. Silicone hydrogel materials–how do they work. In: Sweeney D, editor. Silicone Hydrogel: the Rebirth of Continuous Wear Contact Lenses. London: Butterworth Heinemann; 2000: 1–21.
3. Cutler SI, Nelson LB, Calhoun JH. Extended wear contact lenses in pediatric aphakia. J Pediatr Ophthal Strabismus 1985; 22: 86–91.
4. Stone J. The possible influence of contact lenses on myopia. Br J Physiol Optics 1979; 31: 89–114.
5. Perrigin J, Perrigin D, Quintero S, et al. Silicone-acrylate contact lenses for myopia control: 3-year results. Optom Vis Sci 1990; 67: 764–9.
6. Winn B, Ackerley RG, Brown CA, et al. Reduced aniseikonia in axial anisometropia with contact lens correction. Ophthalmic Physiol Opt 1988; 8: 341–4.
7. Roberts CJ, Adams GG. Contact lenses in the management of high anisometropic amblyopia. Eye 2002; 16: 577–9.
8. Amaya LG, Speedwell L, Taylor D. Contact lenses for infant aphakia. Br J Ophthalmol 1990; 74: 150–4.
9. Atkinson J, Braddick D, French J. Infant astigmatism: its disappearance with age. Vision Res 1980; 20: 891–3.
10. Asbell PA, Chiang B, Somers ME, et al. Keratometry in children. CLAO 1990; 16: 99–102.
11. Vanathi M, Tandon R, Titiyal JS, et al. Case series of 12 children with progressive axial myopia following unilateral cataract extraction. J AAPOS 2002; 6: 228–32.
12. Taylor D, Wright KW, Amaya L, et al. Should we aggressively treat unilateral congenital cataracts? Br J Ophthalmol 2001; 85: 1120–6.
13. Birch EE, Stager DR. The critical period for surgical treatment of dense congenital unilateral cataract. Investi Ophthalmol Vis Sci 1996; 37: 1532–8.
14. Lloyd IC, Dowler JG, Kriss A, et al. Modulation of amblyopia therapy following early surgery for unilateral congenital cataracts. Br J Ophthalmol 1995; 79: 802–6.
15. Speedwell L, Russell-Eggitt IM. Improvement in visual acuity in children with ectopia lentis. J Pediatr Ophthalmol Strabismus 1995; 32: 94–7.
16. Pearson AR, Soneji B, Sarvananthan N, et al. Does ethnic origin influence the incidence or severity of keratoconus? Eye 2000; 14: 625–8.
17. Eustis HS, Chamberlain D. Treatment for amblyopia: results using occlusive contact lens. J Pediatr Ophthalmol Strabismus 1996; 33: 319–22.

CHAPTER
P29 Difficulties with Patching

Chris Timms

PRACTICAL DIFFICULTIES WITH PATCHING

See also Chapter 78.

Amblyopia is the most common cause of poor vision in children, affecting between 1 and 4% of the population. Most commonly it is associated with strabismus and/or anisometropia but may also be the sequelae of other children's eye conditions, e.g., congenital glaucoma, ptosis, and congenital cataract. Since it was introduced by Erasmus Darwin, the standard treatment has been occlusion of the better eye. With an effective patching regime the visual acuity in the amblyopic eye can be improved to within one line of the vision in the better eye in up to 89% of cases,[1,2] but as most practicing orthoptists and ophthalmologists attest, patching is only successful in treating amblyopia if the parents or carers of the patient apply the patch and keep it on for the required period of time each day. Compliance is a very important factor in the success or failure of occlusion therapy.[3]

Early diagnosis and treatment of amblyopia produce better results: treatment of amblyopia after the age of 8 or 9 years of age is less likely to be successful, although there are some notable cases where late patching has been successful. The earlier treatment is started, the better are the results and the less time the patching is needed. We ask parents to patch difficult toddlers, and patching is difficult and unpleasant for both the child and the parent. It is unpleasant because it is a new sensation for a young child, being made to wear a sticky patch and forced to use an eye with poor vision, but with patience most children get used to the patch quite quickly, particularly once the difference between the amblyopic eye and the better eye is lessened and the vision improves. Any strategy for improving compliance with patching should involve detailed information to the parent or carer about the following:

1. *The need for the patch*: the parents need to know the patch is to improve the vision in the amblyopic eye, not to improve the appearance of the strabismus. Many parents will give up if they cannot see an immediate change in the cosmetic appearance.
2. *The reason patching must be carried out while the child is young*: Poor compliance often results from a misunderstanding of the purpose and urgency of occlusion treatment, which can be helped by an information leaflet given to the parent at the start.[4,5]
3. *Tips for helping them to get the child to wear the patch.*

As much of this information as possible must be conveyed to the child, too.

Regular reviews in the clinic to monitor progress are an encouragement to the patient and his parent. Some orthoptic departments have instigated patch clubs where groups of children who are having difficulty complying with their treatment are invited along with their supervised activities while wearing their patches.

Poor understanding of the purpose of the treatment or memory of what the parent was told in the clinic may lead to ineffective treatment, e.g., the patch being put on the wrong eye or for an inadequate period of time each day. Clear and concise instructions, giving the eye to be covered and daily period of patching, are tailored to each child.

It is helpful if the parent keeps a record of how much patching is achieved each day. Older children can help with this record keeping by making a logbook or star chart: this is to assist the progress of the treatment and not used in a critical way. It is important that the parents know that we understand that patching is difficult, especially at certain times in a child's development. The role of the professional must be supportive and not judgmental; good compliance should be rewarded by the parent with a treat or small gift rather than punishment for not wearing the patch (Fig. P29.1).

There is little evidence on the dose-effect of occlusion but dose-monitored patching[6,7] shows that it is probably the total period of the patching over a period of time that achieves the result rather than the exact time the patch is on each day. The amount of patching given must be reasonable and achievable for the family's circumstances. This may mean a compromise: some parents like the idea of full-time patching for a relatively short period of time, others prefer shorter periods each day, knowing it will take longer to reach the required improvement in visual acuity. It is also vital to explain that, in certain circumstances, too much patching may be harmful. The risk of occlusion amblyopia and intractable diplopia is small but significant in younger children.

Sticky patches worn on the face are probably the ideal method of occlusion, particularly at the beginning of the treatment when the vision in the amblyopic eye is poor. Most bright children will take the opportunity to peep over the glasses if the patch is stuck to the lens. There are several patches that have enough "stick" to keep them in place (Fig. P29.2), but not too sticky to cause trauma to the skin when the patch is removed. For most children, the adhesive used on the patch will not cause any difficulty with the skin of the face other than a possible mild temporary redness when the patch is taken off. This can usually be alleviated with some face cream, but if the patch does cause irritation to the skin it is worth changing the brand of patch, as they do not all use the same adhesive agent. Using a hole punch to remove some of the sticky part of the patch may help. There are also some cloth patches that fit entirely around the spectacle lens (Fig. P29.2) to minimize the chances of peeping over the patch. In the maintenance phase of treatment a frosted lens or patch on the glasses will be enough to ensure that the better eye is disadvantaged.

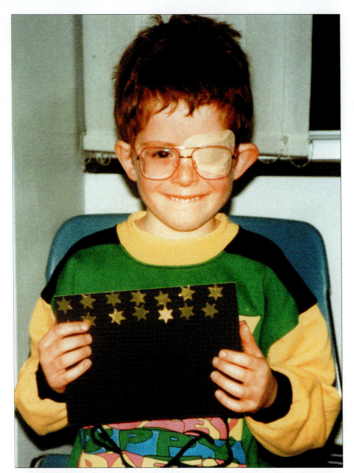

Fig. P29.1 Reward in the form of stars for each successfully completed day of patching makes a child proud of his success.

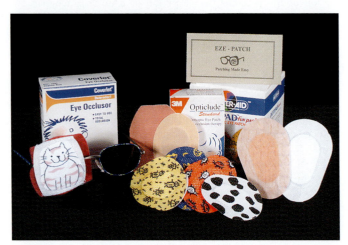

Fig. P29.2 Various adhesive patches can be used, either to cover spectacles (left of display) or to stick on the skin.

Most orthoptists have a list of their favorite ways of ensuring that recalcitrant patients comply with treatment! Of primary importance is to give the parent the confidence to be firm with their child: "This treatment will work if the patch is worn!" Here are few things we have found that help:

- Choosing the right time to patch is important, e.g., not, when the child is tired. For older children patching is much more effective when combined with close work. Often the teachers at school or nursery will undertake some of the patching,

relieving the parents of all the stress of having to enforce the occlusion regime all the time. In this respect grandparents may also be very useful in supervising some of the patching.

- The patch sticks better to grease free skin so clean the skin before the patch is put on.
- If the child pulls the patch off easily, use a stickier patch for a week or so until he gets used to it.
- Sticky tape over the top of the patch means it takes longer to take the patch off, thus giving the parent a few valuable moments to distract the child before he manages to take the patch off.
- Several devices can be used to stop the child being able to manipulate his fingers to take the patch off: In a young child a sock pulled up to the elbows over the hands especially if he then wears a sweater over the top. In general gloves don't work as well as they are too easy to remove. For a slightly older child sticky tape on the tips of the thumb and first two fingers of both hands make it very difficult to take the patch off.
- Splints applied to the elbows will still allow the child to play with his toys but he will be unable to bend his elbows to get to the patch. These are available commercially or can be made by the physiotherapy department in the hospital. Elbow restraints can be improvised by taping a cardboard tube to the upper and forearm or by using swimming arm bands inflated over the elbows (Fig. P29.3).

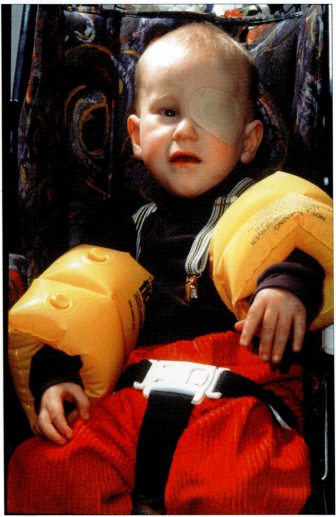

Fig. P29.3 Swimming arm bands used as elbow restraints.

■ These methods may seem rather cruel but in practice they do not need to be worn for very long, as the child soon realizes that the patch is better than the restraints! They also stress to the parents the importance we place on the treatment of amblyopia. If these mechanical restraints fail, as a last resort some clinics admit children to hospital for a few days, where the nursing staff can supervise the patching–not often done in today's environment!

■ If it proves impossible to keep the patch in place it is possible to penalize the better eye with a cycloplegic drop (Chapter 78). The Amblyopia Treatment Study suggests that a daily drop of atropine worked as well as patching.[8]

REFERENCES

1. Lithander J, Sjorstrand J. Anisometropic and strabismic amblyopia in the age goup 2 years and above: a prospective study of the results of treatment. Br J Ophthalmol 1991; 75: 11–6.
2. Hiscox F, Strong N, Thompson JR, et al. Occlusion for amblyopia: a comprehensive survey of outcome. Eye 1992; 6: 300–4.
3. Woodruff G, Hiscox F, Thompson JR, et al. Factors affecting the outcome of children treated for amblyopia. Eye 1994; 8; 627–31.
4. Newsham D. A randomised controlled trial of written information: the effect on parental non-concordance with occlusion therapy. Br J Ophthalmol 2002; 86: 787–91.
5. Newsham D. Paraental non-concordance with occlusion therapy. Br J Ophthalmol 2000; 84: 957–62.
6. Simonsz HJ, Polling JR, Voorm R, et al. Electronic monitoring of treatment compliance in patching for amblyopia. Strabismus 1999; 7: 113–23.
7. Stewart CE, Fielder FR, Stephens DA, et al. Design of the Monitored Occlusion Treatment of Amblyopia Study (MOTAS). Br J Ophthalmol 2002; 86: 915–9.
8. Pediatric Eye Disease Investigator Group. A randomized trial of atropine–the patching for treatment of moderate amblyopia in children. Arch Ophthalmol 2002; 120: 268–78.

Sleep Disorders in Children with Poor Vision

CHAPTER **P30**

James E Jan

Sleep disturbances are common in children and are among the leading concerns about which parents approach physicians. Most are transient and respond to stricter regulation of the sleep environment. Most sleep problems fall into three main categories: sleeplessness or excessive sleepiness (dyssomnias), and episodes of disturbed behavior during sleep (parasomnias). Visually impaired children, with or without neurodevelopmental disabilities, for several reasons, commonly experience often severe and long-standing sleep difficulties.[1] With increasing severity of visual loss, the prevalence of sleep difficulties tends to increase[2] because vision is important for sleep regulation. The enforcement of sleep "hygiene" by parents must be strong and consistent since in the presence of visual loss it is harder to understand environmental cues (*zeitgebers*) required for establishing healthy sleep habits. Excessive parental permissiveness can harm blind children in many ways. Visually impaired children often have additional neurodevelopmental and physical disabilities, and these may lead to various sleep disorders. Although researchers have been concentrating on the sleep difficulties associated with ocular visual disorders, severe, long-standing sleep disturbance is far more common in children with cortical visual impairment, as they tend to be severely disabled.

Chronic sleep disorders can adversely affect the child's development, as sleep plays a major role in the early maturational process. It can lead to delayed development, learning and behavioral difficulties, decreased attention span, difficulties with memory formation and recall, mood changes, impaired social interactions, and ill health, and when the children do not sleep, neither do the caregivers. Chronic sleep deprivation can lead to such an emotional, health, and economic burden on the parents that they are often forced to request alternate care. Thus, sleep disorders must be appropriately diagnosed and treated as early as possible.

CAUSES OF SLEEP DISORDERS RELATED TO VISUAL IMPAIRMENT

Visually impaired children, like the sighted, can be affected by a great variety of sleep disorders. However, they can also have sleep difficulties related to their visual loss because through the retinohypothalamic visual pathway the retina regulates the suprachiasmatic nucleus of the hypothalamus (SCN), called the "sleep clock." This small structure in turn controls the production of the pineal hormone melatonin, which is required for sleep induction and maintenance. Light inhibits melatonin secretion, whereas darkness promotes it. In this process, the rods and cones are not involved, but an unidentified photoreceptor. This explains why some individuals without light perception still have normal sleep–wake cycles.

In total ocular blindness, the SCN is deprived of visual input, and as a result, it often assumes its own endogenous rhythm. Such blind individuals frequently, but not always, develop free-running sleep–wake cycle rhythms and fall asleep sometimes up to 1 hour or even more later every day. Children with enucleated, destroyed, or congenitally absent globes have the highest incidence of free-running sleep–wake cycle rhythms. Since total blindness is uncommon in childhood, this type of sleep disorder is rare. When visually impaired, low-functioning children are unable to understand their environmental *zeitgebers*, which train the SCN and dictate when and how long to sleep, their sleep may resemble an infantile, fragmented pattern.

DIAGNOSIS AND MANAGEMENT

Sleep problems in children with impaired sight and neurodevelopmental disabilities are often preventable if they are exposed to a well-structured and vigorously enforced sleep environment from infancy. Once the sleep difficulties are noted, it is essential to identify the underlying cause, because only then can the management chosen from a wide range of therapies be successful. Early treatment is important because long-standing sleep disorders often continue into adulthood. A detailed sleep history, together with a physical examination, is always necessary. The caregivers then should be asked to document the child's sleep pattern for several days (somnologs). Actigraphs, which record limb movements and thereby identify periods of wakefulness and sleep, can also be very helpful. At times polysomnography, especially for parasomnias, together with specific medical investigations is required (Fig. P30.1).

Hypnotic drugs are rarely justifiable in the treatment of sleep disorders in children, as they offer only temporary benefits and are associated with potentially adverse effects. Behavioral management with promotion of healthy sleep habits is frequently successful in visually impaired children. In contrast, chronic sleep–wake cycle disorders, such as delayed sleep phase onset, day–night reversals, early morning awakenings, sleep fragmentation, and free-running sleep–wake cycles, are more resistant to behavioral treatment. These conditions should be viewed as disorders of the sleep clock. Since this brain structure regulates pineal melatonin metabolism, reduced or inappropriately timed melatonin secretion is generally present. For these individuals, when vigorous enforcement of healthy sleep habits has failed, melatonin administration can be beneficial.

Melatonin is a hormone with chronobiotic properties required for sleep induction and maintenance. It is not a sleeping pill and should not be used as such. In the United States it is available without prescription, but in most other countries it can only be released by special permission. Ideally, it should be prescribed by

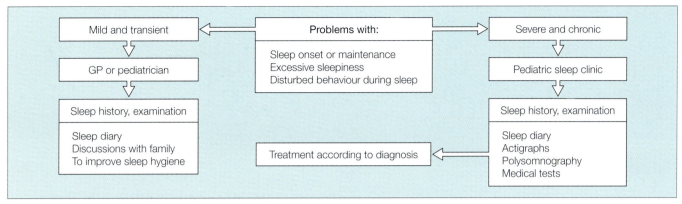

Fig. P30.1 Approach to sleep difficulties.

qualified physicians who can correctly diagnose the cause of the sleep disorder. Sleep is a highly complex biological function, and as a result numerous medical, neurological, and psychiatric disorders can cause a variety of sleep disturbances. Melatonin should not be used indiscriminately for all sleep problems.

Melatonin administration, which is the only effective treatment for free-running sleep–wake cycle disorders, should be started when the sleep phase has shifted to night time.[3] It is useful for multidisabled visually impaired children who are unable to understand the environmental cues for healthy sleep patterns. Delayed sleep phase onset also tends to respond to this treatment. The dose ranges from 0.5 up to 10 mg, given orally at the desired bedtime. Fast-release formulations are the best for sleep induction, whereas the controlled release is more useful for sleep maintenance. The treatment is most effective when the sleep hygiene is strictly enforced simultaneously.[4] It is free from significant adverse effects although very few long-term studies are available.[5]

There is a common misconception that children only rarely have sleep difficulties, which are usually the parents' fault. There needs to be more professional and public awareness that disturbed sleep is neurodevelopmentally damaging and devastating for the families. Sleep disorders should be treated early, and the majority do respond to appropriate management.

REFERENCES

1. Leger D, Prevot E, Philip P, et al. Sleep disorders in children with blindness. Ann Neurol 1999; 46: 648–51.
2. Stores G, Ramchandani P. Sleep disorders in visually impaired children. Dev Med Child Neurol 1999; 41: 348–52.
3. Sack RL, Lewy AJ. Circadian rhythm sleep disorders: lessons from the blind. Sleep Med Rev 2001; 5: 189–206.
4. Jan JE, Hamilton D, Seward N, et al. Clinical trials of controlled-release melatonin in children with sleep-wake cycle disorders. J Pineal Res 2000; 29: 34–9.
5. Palm L, Blennow G, Wetterberg L. Long-term melatonin treatment in blind children and young adults with circadian sleep-wake disturbances. Dev Med Child Neurol 1997; 39: 319–25.

Is My Child's Development Normal?

Alison Salt

Many eye conditions are associated with developmental disorders. The ophthalmologist will need to recognize when to make a referral for a further opinion about a child's development.

Concerns may arise about children both with normal vision and with severe visual impairment. Children with visual impairment may develop more slowly than their sighted peers, and therefore their progress should be judged against developmental norms appropriate to their level of visual impairment.

The first step in considering whether there is a risk of developmental delay is to take a careful history. It is important to remember that parents are the best observers of their child's development and their concerns should always be taken seriously.

Some common risk factors associated with developmental problems, which should be inquired about, are as follows:

1. Pregnancy–infection (especially cytomegalovirus, toxoplasmosis, and rubella), consumption of drugs or alcohol, smoking, hypertension, and exposure to irradiation.
2. Health of the fetus–poor growth, reduced fetal movements, or reduced or excessive amniotic fluid.
3. Delivery–the need for resuscitation and signs of significant encephalopathy in the infant, such as significant drowsiness, poor feeding, and seizures soon after birth may suggest that damage was sustained around the time of birth. If no such signs are present then the birth is unlikely to have a causal relationship to later developmental problems. A difficult delivery in fact accounts for a very small proportion of subsequent neurological and developmental problems, although parents may often worry about difficulties that they experienced.[1]
4. Premature birth (<37 weeks gestation)–gestational age is strongly correlated with the risk of subsequent developmental problems. Whether the child was ventilated and for how long, whether there were complications, e.g., intraventricular hemorrhage, or whether a poor prognosis was given at any stage. When considering whether a premature child is reaching developmental milestones it is generally considered appropriate to take account of gestational age up to the age of 2 years.
5. Serious infection–meningitis or septicemia especially in the early weeks or months of life.
6. Jaundice in the first days of life–prolonged and severe jaundice (> 340 micromol/litre).
7. Conditions of the eye known to be associated with developmental problems.

Next, consider whether a child is reaching expected developmental milestones.

DEVELOPMENTAL MILESTONES IN THE FULLY SIGHTED CHILD

Some key milestones are described in Table P31.1. These are based on observation and normative data from Sheridan,[2,3] and the revised Denver developmental screening test.[4] This table shows the average age or the age at which the majority of children achieve particular milestones.

Parents will usually remember the age their child reached major developmental milestones with reasonable accuracy–independent sitting and walking, the development of first words, and when their child was speaking clearly.[5]

In reviewing current development, consideration should be given to the following areas of development:

- Mobility and coordination of movements (gross motor);
- Eye–hand coordination (fine motor);
- Speech and language;
- Personal/social skills;
- Vision; and
- Hearing.

When should delay in milestones cause concern?

Table P31.2 provides a list of potential developmental warning signs that will help the clinician to recognize when to be concerned about delay in a particular milestone and therefore request further assessment.

Variation in patterns of normal development

Some patterns of normal development are associated with delay in milestones but may not be associated with pathology. A good example of this is the child who does not crawl but moves around on his/her bottom. This is known as bottom shuffling or scooting and is seen in almost 10% of children.[6] This pattern of prewalking mobility is usually benign and is often familial. Children with this pattern of development on average achieve independent walking at around 18 months but this may be as late as 25 months in a minority.[7] However, this pattern may also be seen in children with neurological disorders, e.g., cerebral palsy or muscular dystrophy, and therefore if delay in walking is beyond 18 months or if there are other concerns, a further opinion should be sought.

As there are a number of conditions that affect both vision and hearing, always enquire about hearing concerns. Delay in speech development should always lead to referral for a formal assessment of hearing.

Table P31.1 Key developmental milestones in the fully sighted child

Age	Gross motor	Fine motor	Speech and Language	Personal/social	Vision
4–6 weeks	Pulled to sit—head lags Held sitting curved back	Hands fisted	Vocalizes not crying	Social smile by 6 weeks	Looks at mother's face Follows dangling ball through 90°
3 months	Prone-lifts head and chest Pulled to sit—little head lag Held sitting—lumbar curve only Held standing, sags at knees	Hands open Hands together in midline Holds rattle briefly	Different vowel sounds	Laugh Social response to nearby friendly faces	Follows dangling ball through 180° Horizontal and later vertically Converges on near object
4–5 months	Pulled to sit—no head lag Rolls prone to supine – then supine to prone Bears some weight on legs	Reaches for objects			
6 months	Prone-lifts head and chest on extended arms Supine-lifts head Sits with support—back straight Held standing, legs are straight and takes weight	Takes toys to mouth Passes toy from hand to hand Uses whole hand in palmer grasp Holds two cubes	Vocalizes tunefully single and double syllables	Socially alert and curious Plays peek-a-boo	Visually attentive for near and far Watches small rolling balls at 5+ feet Full conjugate eye movements
9 months	Sits alone for 10–15 minutes Stands holding on Can get to sitting from lying down Stands momentarily (from 10 months)	Uses index finger approach to objects Immature pincer grasp (between thumb and index finger but not using finger tips) Throws toys to the ground deliberately Looks for fallen toy (even when falls out of sight) Removes object from container	Babbles in long repetitive strings of syllables Situational understanding developing	Feeds self with biscuit Distinguishes strangers from familiars and may be wary	
12 months	Walks holding on to furniture Stands alone well Crawls rapidly Walks hands held	Uses a neat mature pincer grasp Casts repeatedly Retrieves toy hidden in view under cup or cloth Puts object into container	Jargons with conversational cadence Indicates wants (e.g., by pointing) Knows and turns to own name Understands simple commands, e.g., give me and wave "bye-bye"	Holds spoon but does not use Drinks from cup with help Cooperates in dressing	Sustained visual interest for near and far
18 months	Walks well (75% by 14 months) Stoops without overbalancing	Builds a tower of three cubes Spontaneous scribble Looks at pictures in books and turns pages Tips object out of container	6 to 20 recognizable words and understands many more Shows body parts on request	Uses a spoon Drinks from cup Copies domestic activities Removes some clothing, e.g., simple shoes/socks	
2 years	Walks up and down stairs two feet per step Runs Jumps on the spot Throws a ball overhand Kicks a ball	Builds tower of 6 cubes Imitates circular scribble (Copies a circle by 2.5 yrs)	Uses 50 or more words Puts two or more words together Much of speech may not be intelligible Asks "what" questions	Uses spoon well Lifts and replaces cup without spilling	Letter matching test possible (BEO) from 2.5 yrs in > 80%
3 years	Stands on one foot momentarily	Builds tower of 9 cubes	Large vocabulary (200+ words) Speech may be unintelligible to strangers	Can undress with fastenings undone	

Table P31.1 (Cont'd) Key developmental milestones in the fully sighted child

Age	Gross motor	Fine motor	Speech and Language	Personal/social	Vision
3.5 years	Hops on one foot	Copies bridge of 3 cubes and copies the drawing of a cross	Uses personal pronouns, regular plurals, and most prepositions Knows some colors Concepts of size and number developing Asks "who" and "why" questions	Dresses self with some help	
4 years	Balances on one foot for 5 seconds Goes up and down stairs adult fashion	Mature tripod grasp of pencil Draws a man 3 parts	Speech mature and intelligible Knows full name	Dresses without supervision and can manage buttons	Completes letter-matching task with each eye
5 years	Can skip on alternate feet	Draws a man 6 parts Copies a square (By 5.5 years a triangle)	Comprehension of abstract meaning and verbal reasoning Asks 'why', 'When' and 'How' questions	Understands the need for rules and cooperates with other children	

All cells equal average based on Sheridan, Egan, and/or achieved by >50% on Denver Developmental Screening Test.

Table P31.2 Developmental warning signs

At any age	Excessive hypotonia (floppiness) or hypertonia (stiffness) Marked asymmetry of posture, movements, or muscle tone Persistent hand fisting Persistent tremor, clonus, jerky movements Tendency to push head back and arch body Parental concern about hearing or vision
0–3 months	Feeding problems—weak suck
4 weeks	Not fixing on mother's face
3 months	Not smiling responsively Not fixing and following Inability to hold toy placed in hand
4 months	Poor head control (head lag when pulled to sit) Not lifting head up supine or chest up in prone Not engaging hands in midline Persistence of infantile reflexes
After 4 months	Grasp reflex
After 5 months	ATNR (asymmetric tonic neck reflex) Moro (startle reflex) Stepping reflex
6 months	Persistent hand regard Not showing interest in surroundings Little interest in sounds or does not turn head to sound
7 months	Not reaching, transferring, or taking toys to mouth
9 months	Not sitting steadily unsupported Lack of social engagement
10 months	Not using tuneful repetitive babble
12 months	Not mobile on the floor No pincer grip Showing hand preference before 12 months No response to sound Has not babbled or has stopped babbling Does not participate in vocal interactive play
18 months	Persistence of casting or mouthing Does not understand or respond when familiar objects are named Showing no interest in communicating his/her needs through pointing or gesture or attempts at words

Table P31.2 (Cont'd) Developmental warning signs

24 months	Unsteady walking, not running Not pushing or pulling toys No constructive or imaginative play Poor social interaction
2.5 years	Not using 50+ words Not joining 2 words together (e.g., "look bus") Does not understand simple commands (e.g., "sit down")
3 years	Unable to throw/kick ball without falling Cannot generally be understood by strangers Does not use 4-word phrases ("I want a big biscuit")
4 years	Poor vocabulary or sentence construction Speech not fully intelligible (except for a few minor articulation difficulties)
4.5 years	Unable to stand on one leg for 3-5 seconds Cannot follow stories or a sequence of commands

The history is key to providing warning signs of developmental problems; tables P31.1 and P31.2 are designed to provide guidance on expected developmental stages and to alert the ophthalmologist to the need for further assessment by a pediatrician.

While a pediatric ophthalmologist is not expected to be as expert in general history taking and examination as a pediatrician, it is essential that he/she understands the rudiments of examining children from a general developmental perspective. It is also important that the ophthalmologist is familiar and confident with the handling of children of all ages. The confidence of parents is greatly enhanced by pediatric ophthalmologist who is confident handling babies and children.

A close collaborative working relationship between the pediatric ophthalmologist and the pediatrician will be essential when there are developmental concerns.

DEVELOPMENT IN CHILDREN WITH VISUAL IMPAIRMENT

Severe visual impairment (SVI) constrains all areas of development and has a wide-ranging and cumulative impact related to the level of vision. Parents play a major role in promoting the development of their infants. However, when their child is diagnosed as visually impaired they need support not only to come to terms with the shock and sadness associated with the knowledge of their child's visual impairment but also to understand how to help their child learn about their world.

The early months are critical in the development of drive to learn. If the child's natural interest and responsiveness is not stimulated early, then it becomes increasingly difficult to promote them. Therefore it is essential that parents receive early support and education about how to help their child. In the UK each Education Authority has an advisory service for visually impaired children, and in most areas a specialist peripatetic teacher will visit the family at home to provide practical advice and support.

The impact of SVI on development means that children will not always follow the same developmental trajectory as their fully sighted peers. Therefore it is important that these children are seen by a pediatrician experienced in assessment of the developmental profiles of children with visual impairment. Norms for the development of "blind" and "partially sighted" children were produced by Reynell and Zinkin in the early 1970s.[8] They represented a landmark in the recognition that developmental scales for sighted infants were inappropriate for visually impaired infants, and continue as the main psychological tool available for assessment of this population. Although these scales remain the best available there is a need for improved developmental scales that fulfill contemporary rehabilitative and educational aspirations and meet scientific requirements of modern developmental tests.

Some of the key developmental milestones for the blind infant are set out in the following and highlight the need for early intervention.

Motor development

Poor vision constrains development of motor skills through a number of complex and interacting mechanisms.[9] These include reduced drive or motivation to move and explore; the child's poor realization of the potential functional capacity of hands for reaching and legs for mobility; reduced opportunity to observe and practice movements; delay in understanding of concepts such as permanence of people and objects and the floor as a concrete base and continuous surface; integration of vestibular and proprioceptive sensory inputs to develop postural reactions to changes in position; and fear of moving beyond a secure base. Blind babies therefore show variable delays in motor development with delay in achieving sitting and becoming mobile. Independent walking may not be achieved in some until 2 years or sometimes later.[10]

Exploration of different textures

At 3 to 6 months both the sighted and blind infant begin to actively explore objects in the hands and mouth. The sighted infant will be motivated by sensory feedback and move on by 6 months to active exploration of shape and texture. The blind

It is important to introduce different shapes and textures early as some children may become alarmed by these different sensations and become "tactile defensive." That is, they refuse to touch new objects and textures and become distressed if these are introduced. This will severely limit their introduction and learning through more complex play and manipulation.

Speech and language/communication

Blind children tend to develop first words later than sighted children. The content of these words tends to emphasize people's names and is related to body movements. Social phrases are initially imitated as a whole and then used in context. Expressive language on average lags behind sighted peers by 2 to 3 months and comprehension may also lag behind expressive language. For example, the first meaningful word is usually associated with understanding of a simple request ("give me the cup") but in the blind child there may by a 9-month lag in comprehension of simple phrases. In other blind children first words may not appear until age 2 years.[11]

Sound localization

Understanding where sounds come from requires the integration of hearing, vision, and recognition that sound implies the presence of an object. This is usually integrated with reach at ear level by 5 months, but not above ear level until 8 to 9 months. Blind babies need to be actively taught this skill and without this teaching delay may be even more marked. Parents need to guide their child's arm toward the sound initially in front of them and then in different directions.[12]

Developmental vulnerability

Recent research has found that 31% (10/32) of children with profound visual impairment (awareness of light or light-reflecting objects only) were at risk of stasis or regression in cognitive development during the second year of life.[13,14] In this group disordered social communication was most prominent. This phenomenon was not specific to any particular visual disorder and was seen in children with a number of different diagnoses. There are likely to be a number of interrelated factors that lead to this vulnerability including underlying associated structural brain anomalies and genetic factors. In addition there are the challenges of development in the second year of life including the development of attention control, shared attention, and independence in the toddler. This highlights the need for intensive support and monitoring of development in these developmentally vulnerable children. The presence of even limited form vision appears protective.

In some visual conditions there is potential for promoting the visual performance, and a carefully designed visual promotion program has been shown to be effective in a randomized control trial.[15] The above emphasizes that even an improvement from light awareness to limited form vision will have significant benefits.

To be born with SVI is a crisis that requires experienced developmental and visual management as soon as possible after the diagnosis and requires close working between the ophthalmological and developmental teams.

REFERENCES

1. Stanley F, Blair E, Alberman E. Cerebral palsies: epidemiology and causal pathways. London: MacKeith Press; 2000. (Clinics in developmental medicine; vol 151).
2. Sheridan M. The developmental progress of infants and young children. London: HMSO; 1975. (Reports on public health and medical subjects; vol 102).
3. Egan DF, Illingworth RS, MacKeith RC. Developmental screening 0–5 years. London: Heinemann Medical Books; 1969. (Clinics in developmental medicine; vol 30).
4. Denver Developmental Screening Test. High Wycombe, Bucks, UK: The Test Agency Ltd.
5. Capute AJ, Shapiro BK, Palmer FB, et al. Normal gross motor development: the influences of race, sex and socioeconomic status. Dev Med Child Neurol 1985; 27: 635–43.
6. Robson P. Shuffling, hitching, scooting or sliding, some observations in 30 otherwise normal children. Dev Med Child Neurol 1970; 12: 608–20.
7. Robson P. Prewalking locomotor movements and their use in predicting standing and walking. Child Care Health Dev 1984; 10: 317–30.
8. Reynell J, Zinkin P. New procedures for developmental assessment of young children with severe visual handicaps. Child Care Health Dev 1979; 1 61–9.
9. Sonksen PM, Levitt S, Kitsinger M. Identification of constraints acting on motor development in young visually disabled children and principles of remediation. Child Care Health Dev 1984; 10: 273–86.
10. Fraiberg S. Insights from the Blind. London: Souvenir Press; 1977.
11. McConachie H, Moore V. Early expressive language of severely visually impaired children. Dev Med Child Neurol 1994; 36: 230–40.
12. Sonksen P, Stiff B. Show Me What My Friends Can See: a developmental guide for parents of babies with severely impaired sight and their professional advisors. London: The Wolfson Centre; 1999.
13. Cass HD, Sonksen PM, McConachie HR. Developmental setback in severe visual impairment. Arch Dis Child 1994; 70: 192–6.
14. Sonksen P, Dale N. Visual impairment in infancy: impact on neurodevelopment and neurobiological processes. Dev Med Child Neurol 2002; 44: 782–91.
15. Sonksen PM, Petrie A, Drew KJ. Promotion of visual development of severely visually impaired babies: evaluation of a developmentally based programme. Dev Med Child Neurol 1991; 33: 320–5.

FURTHER READING

Dale N, Sonksen P. Developmental outcome, including setback, in young children with severe visual impairment. Dev Med Child Neurol 2002; 44: 613–22.

Worldwide Resources for Parents of a Visually Handicapped Child

CHAPTER P32

Angela Tank and David Taylor

We found this section, put at the back of the second edition, proved useful for parents and ophthalmologists who wanted to find out about facilities for visually impaired (VI) children in other countries–for instance, if a family with a VI child was moving abroad. Angela Tank completely revised the list through our personal contacts, by searching Web sites and search-engines, through blind societies' contact lists, etc.

The list cannot be comprehensive but will hopefully serve to help some people to get a start into the complex business of bringing up a VI child.

USEFUL WEB SITES

RNIB: Helping you live with sight loss: http://info.rnib.org.uk/exe/Agencies
http://www.tiresia.org

ALBANIA

Albanian Blind Association

Rruga Nikolla Lena nr 62, Tirana
Tel: +355 42–59611
Fax: +355 42–59635
E-mail: *stafaj@yahoo.com*

ALGERIA

Organisation Nationale des Aveugles Algériens

4 Boulevard Mohamed Khemisti, Algiers
Tel: +213 2264 2716
Fax: +213 271 4415

ANGOLA

Associação Nacional de Apoio aos Deficientes Visuais

National Association of Support for the Blind
Caixa Postal No 14010, S Paulo, Luanda
Tel: +244 2–3 43665
Fax: +244 2–3 43665

ANGUILLA

Anguilla Society of and for the Blind c/o Valley Secondary School,

The Valley, Anguilla, West Indies
Tel: +1 809 497 2416

ANTIGUA

Antigua and Barbuda Society of and for the Blind

All Saints Road, St John's, Antigua, West Indies
Tel: +1 809 462 0663

ARGENTINA

Federación Argentina de Instituciones de Ciegos y Amblíopes

Argentinian Federation for Organizations of the Blind
46 Medrano Street, Piso 6 Dto. A, Buenos Aires 1178, Argentina
Tel: +54 11 4981 5012
Fax: +54 11 4981 5012

Instituto Helen Keller (HKI)

Mtro Marcelo Lopez S/N, Ciudad Universitaria, Cordoba, 5000
Tel: +54 51–334547
Fax: +54 51–692768
E-mail: *ehelen@proedu.edu.ar; ihk@onenet.com.ar*

ARMENIA

Armenian Association of the Blind

18 Isaakian Street, Erevan, 375025
Tel: +374 2–56 05 21
Fax: +374 2–58 22 66
E-mail: *armblind2000@yahoo.com*

ARUBA

Fundashon Arubano di Esnan Visualmente Incapacita (FAVI)

Aruban Foundation of the Visually Handicapped
Campanastraat 5, Aruba
Tel: +297 8–25222 or 25051
Fax: +297 8–20306
Web page: http://www.athaaruba.org

AUSTRALIA

Royal Blind Society of Australia: http://www.rbs.org.au
Royal Victorian Institute for the Blind: http://www.rvib.org.au

Forsight Foundation for the Deafblind

PO Box 240, Carlingford, New South Wales, 2118
Tel: +61 2–9630 5599
Fax: +61 2–9630 6888

Australian DeafBlind Council (ADBC)

PO Box 1213, Camberwell, Victoria, 3124
Tel: +61 03–0427 435 243
Fax: +61 39–486 2092
E-mail: *segrave@connexus.net.au*
Web page: http://home.vicnet.net.au/~dbansw/

Australian and New Zealand Association of Educators of the Visually Handicapped (ANZAEVH)

333 Burwood Highway, Burwood, Victoria, Vic 3125
Tel: +61 3–9808 6422
Fax: +61 3–9808 2914

Association for the Blind of Western Australia

16 Sunbury Road, PO Box 101, Victoria Park, Western Australia, WA 6979
Tel: +61 8–9311 8202
Fax: +61 8–9361 8696
E-mail: *mailbox@abwa.asn.au*
Web page: http://www.abwa.asn.au

AUSTRIA

Odilien Blindeninstitute

Leonhardstraße 130, Graz, A-8010
Tel: +43 316 322 66750
Fax: +43 316 32266749
E-mail: *foerderverein@odilien.at*
Web page: http://www.odilien.at

Federal Institute for the Education of the Blind

Wittelsbachstraße 5, Vienna, A-1020
Tel: +43 1–728 0866
Fax: +43 1–728 0866–275
E-mail: *bbi@bbi.at*
Web page: http://www.bbi.at

AZERBAIJAN

Azerbaidzhan Association of the Blind

40 Chuluflu Street, Baku, 370052, Azerbaidzhan
Tel: +994 12 645294

BAHAMAS

Salvation Army Institute for the Blind

31 Mackey Street, PO Box N-205, Nassau
Tel: +1 242–393 2745
Fax: +1 242–393 2189
E-mail: *salarmy@batelnet.bs*

BAHRAIN

Saudi-Bahraini Institute for the Blind, The

PO Box 33484
Tel: +973 780818
Fax: +973 780786
E-mail : *sbiblind@batelco.com.bh*
Web: http://www.blindinstitute.org

BANGLADESH

Assistance for Blind Children

2/11 Tajmahal Road, Block C, Mohammadpur, Dhaka 1207, Bangladesh
Tel: +880 2 819320
Fax: +880 2 819320

Helen Keller International

PO Box 6066, Gulshan, Dhaka, 1212, Bangladesh
Tel: +880 2 811 6156/4234
Fax: +880 2 811 3310
E-mail: *cd@hkidhaka.org*

BARBADOS

Barbados Association for the Blind and Deaf

The Workshop for the Blind, St Paul's Avenue, Beckles Road, St Michael, Barbados, West Indies
Tel: +1 809 426 3438
Fax: +1 809 429 4854

BELARUS, REPUBLIC OF

Belarussian Association of the Visually Handicapped

7 Amuratorskaya Str, Minsk, 220 004
Tel: +375 172–232 506
Fax: +375 172–238 641
E-mail: *typhlo-bel@mail.ru*

BELGIUM

Belgische Confederatie van Blinden en Slechtzienden

George Henrilaan 278, 1200 Brussel
Tel: 02–7325324
Fax: 02–7356453

Association des Parents d'Aveugles et Malvoyants de Belgique Francophone (APAM bf)

Association of Parents of Blind and Partially Sighted
Rue Sur les Thiers, 322, Herstal, 4040
Tel: +32 0381 21 84
Fax: +33 0381 26 65

VZW Anna Temmerman voor Auditief-Visueel Gehandikapten

Anna Temmerman Association for Deafblind Persons
Snaggaardstraat 9, Bruges, B-8000
Tel: +32 50 34 03 41
Fax: +32 50 33 73 06

BELIZE

Belize Council for the Visually Impaired (BCVI)

1 Gabourel Lane, PO Box 413, Belize City, C A
Tel: +501 22–77776
Fax: +501 22–32907
E-mail: bcvi@btl.net
Web page: http://www.bcvi.org

BENIN

Association of the Blind and Partially Sighted of Benin

BP 540, Cotonou
Tel: +229–33 17 47
Fax: +229–30 13 65 s/c Gbedi Gilbert
E-mail: blind@avu.org

BERMUDA

Bermuda Society for the Blind

Beacon House, Dundonald Street West, Hamilton, Bermuda

BOLIVIA

National Federation of the Blind of Bolivia

C. Colombia 472 (Interior), Casilla Postal 07432, La Paz
Tel: +591 2–32 67 53
Fax: +591 2–358530

Aprecia Santa Cruz Escuela para Niños Ciegos y Deficientes Visuales, Centro de Rehabilitacion (School for Blind and Visually Handicapped Children, Rehabilitation Centre)

Casilla 3538, 3er Anillo, Detras del HoTel:, "Los Tajibos,"
Santa Cruz, Bolivia
Tel: +591 42 0666
Fax: +591 42 9920

BOSNIA HERZEGOVINA

Bosnia and Herzegovina Blind Union

Blind Union Republic of Serpska, Sime Matavulja 6,
Banja Luka
Tel: +387 51–216 469
Fax: +387 51–216 469
E-mail: ssrs@ssrs.org.yu

BOTSWANA

Botswana Association of the Blind and Partially Sighted

PO Box 229, Serowe, Botswana
Tel: +267 430006
Fax: +267 431500

BRAZIL

Conselho Brasileiro para o Bem-Estar dos Ciegos (CBBEC)

Brasilian Council for the Welfare of the Blind
Rua Clarimundo de Melo, 216 Encantado, Rio de Janeiro,
20740–322 RJ
Tel: +55 21–594 0284
Fax: +55 21 275 1405
E-mail: tjonir@quindim.nc-rj.rnp.br

Brasilian Council for the Welfare of the Blind

Rua Rosa, S/N(UNICEP), 29104–730-Vila Velha,
Espirito Santo, Brazil
Tel: +55 27 229 8743
Fax: +55 21 229 5233
Web page: http://www.rionet.com.br/~cbbec

Associaçao Brasileira de Educadores de Deficientes Visuais (ABEDEV)

Brazilian Association for the Education of Visually Impaired
People
Rua Rui Barbosa, 1961 Apt 14, Campo Grande,
79001–431 MS
Tel: +55 67–382 1581 or 6896

BRITISH VIRGIN ISLANDS

British Virgin Islands Friends of the Blind Association

Road Town, Tortola, British Virgin Islands
Tel: +1 809 49 43428

BULGARIA

Central Union of Blind and Partially Sighted People

172 Naicho Zanov Street, Sofia, 1309
Tel: +359 2–22 34 35 or 21 18 61
Fax: +359 2–22 00 18
E-mail: skarlatov@ssb.sofianet.net

Varna School for the Blind

kv Asparuhoro, Varna, 9003, Bulgaria
Tel: +359 52 77 42 70
Fax: +359 52 77 42 70

BURKINA FASO

Association Burkinabé pour la Promotion des Aveugles et Malvoyants (ABPAM)

Association for the Blind and Partially Sighted of Burkina Faso
BP 5588, Ouagadougou 01
Tel: +226–30 33 54
Fax: +226–30 33 54

BURMA

Mission to the Blind of Myanmar

196 Kyundaw Road, San Chaung PO 1111, Yangon (Rangoon)
Tel: +95 1–33326

CAMBODIA

Helen Keller International

House #60, Street 310, Sangkat Boeng Kend Kang, Khann Chamcar Mon, PO Box 168, Phnom Penh, Cambodia
Contact person: Thong Chun Leng, Eye Health Officer
Tel: +855 23 21 0851
Fax: +822 23 21 0852
E-mail: *tleng@bigpond.com.kh*

CAMEROON

Association Nationale des Aveugles du Cameroun (ANAC)

National Association for the Blind of Cameroon
Accueil Notre-Dame de la Paix, BP 190, Dschang
Tel: +237–45 12 51
Fax: +237 45 19 55

CANADA

Canadian Council of the Blind (CCB)

401–396 Cooper Street, Ottawa, Ontario, K2P 2H7
Tel: +1 613-567 0311
Fax: +1 613-567 2728
E-mail: *ccb.national@on.aibn.com*
Web page: http://www.ccbnational.net

Canadian National Institute for the Blind (CNIB), The

320 McLeod Street, Ottawa, Ontario, K2P 1A3
Tel: +1 613–563 0000
Fax: +1 613–232 9070
E-mail: *irc@lib.cnib.ca*
Web page: http://www.cnib.ca

Canadian Deafblind and Rubella Association (CDBRA), The

The W Ross Macdonald School, 350 Brant Avenue, Brantford, Ontario, N3T 3J9
Tel: +1 519–754 0729
Fax: +1 519–754 5400
E-mail: *cdbra.nat@sympatico.ca*
Web page: http://www.cdbra.ca

Association Québécoise des Parents d'Enfants Handicapés Visuels (AQPEHV)

10, boul. Churchill, Bureau 203, Greenfield Park, Quebec, J4V 2L7
Tel: +1 450–465–7225
Fax: +1 450–465–5129
E-mail: *info@aqpehv.qc.ca*
Web page: http://www.aqpehv.qc.ca

CAPE VERDE

Associacão dos Deficientes Visuais de Cabo Verde (ADVCV)

Association of the Visually Impaired of Cape Verde
CP 831, Achodo Santo Antonio, Praia
Tel: +238 61 11 12 or 61 33 15
Fax: +238 61 33 15

CENTRAL AFRICAN REPUBLIC

Association pour la Promotion Sociale des Handicapés Visuels Centrafricains

Association of the Visually Handicapped of Central African Republic
BP 38, Bangui-Lakouanga
Tel: +236–61 89 53
Fax: +236 61 21 89

CHAD (see TCHAD)

CHILE

Unión Nacional de Instituciones Tiflológicas de Chile

Casilla 87–C, Concepción
Tel: +56 41–22 63 92 or 23 40 76
Fax: +56 41–23 80 88
E-mail: *urcae@ctcinternet.cl*

Escuela Hogar para Ciegos Santa Lucia

Hogar School for the Blind
Salesianos 1190, San Miguel, Santiago

CHINA

China Association of the Blind

44 Beichizi Street, Dongcheng District, Beijing 100006, China
Tel: +86 10 65139719
Fax: +86 10 65139722

Hong Kong Society for the Blind, The

248 Nam Cheong Street, Shamshuipo, Kowloon, Hong Kong
Tel: +852 2778–8332
Fax: +852 2788–0040 & 2778–1336
E-mail: *genadmin@hksb.org.hk*
Web page: http://www.hksb.org.hk

COLOMBIA

Instituto Nacional para Ciegos (INCI)

Carrera 13, 34–91, Bogota
Tel: +57 1–232 90 77/78
Fax: +57 1–2232 90 76
Web page: http://www.inci.gov.co

CONGO (DEMOCRATIC REPUBLIC OF)

Association Nationale des Aveugles et Déficients Visuels du Congo (ANADVC)

BP 13205, Brazzaville, Republique du Congo
Tel: +242 664145
Fax: +242 810330

Union Nationale des Aveugles du Congo (UNAC)

BP 23 Kin 8, Congo. Fax: +243 1 262937

COSTA RICA

Instituto de Rehabilitacion para Ciegos Helen Keller (HKI)

Helen Keller Institute of Rehabilitation for the Blind
Apartado 456–1011 y Griega SJ, San José
Tel: +506–263705

CROATIA

Hrvatski Savez Slijepih

Croatian Association of the Blind
Draskoviceva 80, PO Box 736, Zagreb, 10 000
Tel: +385 1–431 039
Fax: +385 1–430 355
Web page: http://www.savez-slijepih.hr

National Association of Deafblind People in Croatia

Vodnikova 8, 10000 Zagreb
Tel/fax: +385 1 / 4875 431, 4875 432
E-mail: *dodir@zg.tel.hr*
Web page: http://www.dodir.hr

CUBA

Asociacion Nacional del Ciego (ANCI)

National Association of the Blind
Apartado 4129, Havana, 4
Tel: +53 7–32 04 49
Fax: +53 7–33 41 34

Escuela Especial para Ciegos y Débiles Visuales "Abel Santamarino"

Special School for Blind and Partially Sighted Children
29-F y 86, Ciudad Escolear Libertad Marianao, Havana
Tel: +53 7–20 0207

CURACAO (see NETHERLANDS ANTILLES)

CYPRUS

Pancyprian Organization of the Blind

PO Box 23511, Nicosia, 1684
Tel: +357 22 81 33 83 or 99 65 74 67
Fax: +357 22 49 5395
E-mail: *pot@logos.cy.net*
Web page: http://www.pot-cyprus.com

St Barnabas School for the Blind

PO Box 3511, Nicosia
Tel: +357 2–422131
Fax: +357 2–420256

Kibris Türk Görmezler Dernegi

Cyprus Turkish Blind Association
Kutlu Adali Street No.12, PO Box 100 Krzrlay, Lefkosa (Nicosia), via Turkey
Tel: +90 392–227 2452/8228 or 228 6376
Fax: +90 392–227 5809

CZECH REPUBLIC

Czech Blind United (SONS)

Krakovska 21, Prague, 110 00
Tel: + 420 2–21 46 22 46
Fax: +420 2–21 46 21 45
E-mail: *sons_zahr@braillnet.cz*
Web page: http://www.braillnet.cz

DENMARK

Dansk Blindesamfund

Danish Association of the Blind
Thoravej 35, Copenhagen NV, DK-2400
Tel: +45 38–14 88 44
Fax: +45 38–14 88 00
E-mail: *info@dkblind.dk*
Web page: http://www.dkblind.dk

Instituttet for Blinde og Svagsynede

Institute for the Blind and Partially Sighted
Rymarksvej 1, Hellerup, DK-2900
Tel: +45 39 45 25 45
Fax: +45 39 45 25 25
E-mail: *ibos@ibos.dk*
Web page: http://www.ibos.dk

Danish Resource Centre on Congenital Deafblindness, The

Langagervej 4, Aalborg Oest, DK-9220
Tel: +45 98 155313
Fax: +45 98 155323
E-mail: *vcdbf@hum.auc.dk*
Web page: http://www.videnscenterdbf.dk/

National Institute for Blind and Partially Sighted Children

Kystvejen 112, Kalundborg, DK-4400
Tel: +45 5957–0100
Fax: +45 5957–0101
E-mail: *refsnaes@inet.uni-c.dk*

DOMINICAN REPUBLIC

Organización Dominicana de Ciegos Inc (ODC)

C/30 de marzo, 57, Apartado Postal 22424, Santa Domingo
Tel: +1 809–682 5558
Fax: +1 809–682 9927

ECUADOR

Federacion National de Ciegos de Ecuador

National Federation for the Blind of Ecuador
Rocafuerte 10–54 y Av 9 de Octubre, Casilla 480, Riobamba
Tel: +593 3–96 58 52
Fax: +593 3–94 05 67

EGYPT

National Committee of the Blind

Demonstration Centre for the Rehabilitation of the Blind,
PO Box 302, Tareht El Gabal Street, Zuetoun, Egypt
Tel: +20 243 40 97

Al Nour Wal Amal School

16 Abu Bakr El-Seddik Street, Heliopolis, Cairo, Egypt
Tel: +20 2 24 37 772

EL SALVADOR

Asociacion de Ciegos Salvadoreños

Association of the Blind of El Salvador
1a Avenida Norte No 920, San Salvador
Tel: +503–222 6065
Fax: +503–222 6065

ESTONIA

Estonian Federation of the Blind (EFB)

Lai Str 9, Tallinn, EE-0001
Tel: +372 64 11 972
Fax: +372 64 11 831

ERITREA

Eritrean National Association of the Blind

Lbne Dngel Street, House No.40, PO Box 615, Asmara, Eritrea
Tel: +291 1 122 435
Fax: +291 1 122 435
E-mail: *ernab@gemel.com.er*

ETHIOPIA

Ethiopian National Association of the Blind (ENAB)

PO Box 30057, Addis Adaba
Tel: +251 1–12 06 98/550542

FIJI

Fiji Society for the Blind

Nanuku Street, PO Box 521, Suva
Tel: +679–382966
Fax: +679–387950

FINLAND

Näkövammaisten Keskusliitto ry./Synskadades Centralförbund rfv (NKL)

Finnish Federation of the Visually Impaired
Mäkelänkatu 50, Helsinki, FIN-00510
Tel: +358 9–3960 4700
Fax: +358 9–3960 4710
E-mail: *ffvi@nkl.fi*
Web page: http://www.nkl.fi

Finnish Deafblind Association, The

Uudenmaankatu 28A, Helsinki, 00120
Tel: +358 9–54 95 35 18
Fax: +358 9–54 95 35 17
E-mail: *heikki.Majava@kuuros.sci.fi*

FRANCE

Association Nationale des Parents d'Enfants Aveugles ou Gravement Déficients Visuels (ANPEA)

National Association of Parents of Blind or Seriously Visually Impaired
12 bis Rue de Picpus, Paris, Ile-de-France, 75012
Tel: +33 043 42 40 40
Fax: +33 043 42 40 66
E-mail: *anpea@wanadoo.fr*
Web page: http://www.anpea.asso.fr

National Federation of Associations of Parents of Visually Impaired Children

28 Place Saint-Georges, Paris, Ile-de-France, 75009
Tel: +33 045 26 73 45
Fax: +33 045 26 05 24
E-mail: *fndv@wanadoo.fr*

Institut des Jeunes Aveugles et Amblyopes l'Arc en Ciel

Rainbow Institute for Young Blind and Partially Sighted
3 Rue Abbé Dassy, Marseille, Bouches du Rhone, 13007
Tel: +33 091 39 68 00

Comité de Liaison et d'Action des Parents d'Enfants et d'Adultes Atteints de Handicaps Associés (CLAPEAHA)

Liaison and Action Committee of Parents for Children and Adults with Associated Handicaps
18 rue Etex, Paris, Ile-de-France, 75018
Tel: +33 142 63 12 02
Fax: +33 146 27 80 92
E-mail: *CLAPEAHA@wanadoo.fr*

Association des Aveugles de la Manche (AAM)

Manche Blind Association
25 Rue de la réauté, Vaudrimesnil, Manche, 50490
Tel: +33 02 33 46 69 75
Fax: 02 3 47 35 19
E-mail: *aam@ifrance.com*

Amicale des handicapés visuels de Bretagne (AAHVB)

Visually Impaired Group of Brittany
BP 243, 5 Rue Mancel, Lorient Cedex, Morbihan, 56102
Tel: +33097 84 45 45
Fax: +33097 64 53 19
E-mail: *Aahvb@wanadoo.fr*

GABON

Union nationale des Aveugles et Malvoyants du Gabon

BP 18 155, Libreville, Gabon
Tel: +241 72 65 02
Fax: +241 76 24 59

Centre d'Education et de Réhabilitation des Aveugles et Malvoyants (CERAM)

Centre for the Education and Rehabilitation of Blind and Partially Sighted People
BP 20311, Libreville
Tel: +241 72 49 94
Fax: +241 77 46 40

GAMBIA

Gambia Organization of the Visually Impaired (GOVI), The

PO Box 2053, Serrekunda
Tel: +220–227001
Fax: +220–224131
E-mail: *AmieJahateh520@hotmail.com*

GERMANY

Deutscher Blindenverband Sehbehinderteuverband eV

German Federation of the Blind and Visually Impaired People
Bismarckallee 30, Bonn, NRW, D-53173
Tel: +49 228–955820
Fax: +49 228–357719
E-mail: *info@dbsv.org*
Web page: http://www.dbsv.org

GEORGIA

School for Visually Impaired Children

6 Gutanskaia str, 380022 Tiblisi, Georgia
Tel: +995 32 771483
Fax: +995 32 983262
E-mail: *info@edvisors.com*

GHANA

Ghana Society for the Blind (GSB)

PO Box 3065, Accra
Tel: +233 21–22 16 14
Fax: +233 21–23 08 31
E-mail: *socblind@ghana.com*

GREECE

Panhellenic Association of the Blind

31, Veranzerou Street, Athens, 104 32
Tel: +30 1–5228333
Fax: +30 1–5222112
E-mail: *pab@otenet.gr*
Web page: http://www.pst.gr

GRENADA

Society of Friends of the Blind, The

PO Box 1235, St George's, Grenada, West Indies
Tel: +473 440 9233
Fax: +473 440 9233

GUATEMALA

Association of the Blind of Guatemala

1 Calle 2–03, Zona 2, Guatemala City, CP 01001
Tel: +502 221 3614
Fax: +502–221 3614
E-mail: *acc@guate.net*

GUINEA

Association Guinéenne pour la Promotion des Aveugles (AGUIPA)

Association for the Blind of Guinea
BP 3494, Conakry
Tel: +224 41 28 90
Fax: +224 41 20 12

GUINEA BISSAU

Associaçao Nacional dos Deficientes (ANDE)

National Association for Disabled People
BP 62, Bissau
Tel: +242–21 18 91 or 21 11 67
Fax: +245–20 11 97

HAITI

École St Vincent pour les Enfants Handicapés, Haiti

St Vincent's School for Handicapped Children
119 Ave Paul VI, PO Box 1319, Port-au–Prince
Tel: +11 509 22–5844
Fax: +11 509 22–0120
E-mail: *fcasseus@yahoo.com*

HONDURAS

Union Nacional de Ciegos de Honduras

Colonia 21 de Octubre, Sector 9, Bloque 1, Tegucigalpa
Tel: +504 38 50 93
Fax: +504 36 24 68

HUNGARY

Magyar VAkok és Gyengénlátok Országos Szövetsége

Hungarian Federation of the Blind and Partially Sighted
Hermina út 47, Budapest, H-1146
Tel: +36 1–384 5028
Fax: +36 1–384 5028
E-mail: *mvgyosz@axelero.hu*

ICELAND

Icelandic Association of the Blind

Hamrahlid 17, Reykjavík, 105
Tel: +354 525–0000
Fax: +354 525 0001
E-mail: *blind@blind.is*
Web page: http://www.blind.is/

INDIA

National Federation of the Blind

2721 Chowk Sangtrashan, 2nd Floor, Hotel Little Star, New Delhi, Delhi, 110 055
Tel: +91 11–355 0277
Fax: +91 11–752 2410 or 685 4133

International Council for Education of People with Visual Impairment–West Asia Region (ICEVI)

Blind People's Association
Vastrapur, Ahmedabad, Gujarat, 380 015
Tel: +9109 630 3346
Fax: +9109 630 0106
E-mail: *srkvcoe@md3.vsnl.net.in*

National Association for the Blind, India

11 Khan Abdul Gaffar Khan Road, Worli Seaface, Mumbai, Maharashtra, 400 025
Tel: +91 22–493 5370 or 493 6930
Fax: +91 22–493 2539
E-mail: *nab@giasm01.vsnl.net.in*

Helen Keller Institute for the Deaf and Deafblind

Municipal Secondary School, South Wing, Gr floor, Nr 'S' Bridge, Mumbai, Maharashtra, 400 011
Tel: +91 22–308 7052
Fax: +91 22–287 2735
E-mail: *hkidbind@bom5.vsnl.net.in*

INDONESIA

Indonesian Association of the Blind

Jl Wartawan IV/14, Buahbatu, Bandung, 40264
Tel: +62 22–305 504
Fax: +62 22–316 584

Helen Keller International (HKI)

Bina Mulia Building, 9th Floor, Jl. HR Rasuna Said, Kav 10, Jakarta

IRAN

Iranian Society of Blind, The

Darros Street, Hassan Tash Street, No.10 code 19436, Tehran, Iran
Fax: +98 21 256 0255

Roudaki Complex for the Blind

State Welfare Organisation
Shahid Fayazbakhsh Ave, PO Box 11365–9187, Tehran
Tel: +98 21 670 7090
Fax: +98 21 311 1294
E-mail: roudaki@neda.net

IRELAND

National Council for the Blind of Ireland (NCBI)

Whitworth Road, Drumcondra, Dublin, 9
Tel: +353 1–830 7033
Fax: +353 1–830 7787
E-mail: info@ncbi.ie
Web page: http://www.ncbi.ie

ISRAEL

Society for the Blind and Prevention of Blindness

Herzlia Street 11, Haifa, 33302
Tel: +972 4–851 5506 or 852 5831
Fax: +972 4–851 5506
E-mail: sbhil@net.vision.net.il

Israel National Association of Parents of Visually Impaired

Variety Center, 17 Diskin St, Jerusalem
Tel: +972 2 5391911
Fax: +972 2 5391913
E-mail: ofek@ofek-liyladenu.org.il
Web page: http://www.ofek-liyladenu.org.il

ITALY

Italian Union of the Blind

Unione Italiana Ciechi
Vis Borgogna 38, Rome, 00187
Tel: +39069 98 83 75
Fax: +39069 98 83 28
E-mail: inter@uiciechi.it
Web page: http://www.uiciechi.it

Fondazione Robert Hollman Centro di Intervento Precoce per Bambini con Deficit Visivo

Robert Hollman Foundation, Early Therapeutic Intervention Centre for Visually Impaired Children
Via Oddone Clerici 6, Cannero Riviera (VB), 28824
Tel: +39023 78 84 85
Fax: +39023 78 81 98
E-mail: info@fondazionehollman.it
Web page: http://www.fondazionehollman.it

IVORY COAST

International Network for the Prevention of Blindness in Africa Inc (INPBA)

06 BP 368, Abidjan, 06
Tel: +225 2345 5480
Fax: +225 3236 49

JAMAICA

Jamaica Society for the Blind

111 1/2 Old Hope Road, Kingston 6, Jamaica
Tel: +1 809 92 73760, +1 927 6758 9
Fax: +1 809 92 76757

JAPAN

Japan Federation of the Blind

1–10–33 Takadanobaba, Shinjuku-ku, Tokyo, 169
Tel: +81 3 3200 0011
Fax: +81 3 3200 7755

Japan Deafblind Association

2-2-3 Nishiwaseda, Shinjuku-ku, Tokyo, 162
Tel: +81 3–5272 1691
Fax: +81 3–5272 1692

JORDAN

Friendship Association for the Blind

PO Box 7063, Amman
Tel: +962 6–656228
Fax: +962 6–641570

Aldhia Society for Visually Handicapped Children

PO Box 129, Khalda-Omsumag, Amman, 11821

KAZHAKSTAN

Kazakhstan Association of the Blind

Kirova Street 21, Astana, PO 473000
Tel: +7 3172–261 568
Fax: +7 3172–216 749

KENYA

Kenya Union of the Blind

PO Box 34510, Nairobi
Tel: +254 2–822915, 823989
Fax: +254 2–822915 (AFUB)

African Union of the Blind

North Airport Road Embakasi, PO Box 72872, Nairobi
Tel: +254 2 823989
Fax: +254 2 823776

KOREA

Korea Welfare Foundation for the Visually Handicapped (KWFVH)

Sangil-Dong 126, Kangdong-gu, Seoul, 134–090
Tel: +82 2–427 9111
Fax: +82 2–427 2687
E-mail: *kswvh@chollian.net*

KUWAIT

Kuwait Society of the Blind (KSB)

PO Box 43244, Hawalle, 32047
Tel: +965 562–2245 or 2300
Fax: +965 562–4700

KYRGYZSTAN

Kyrgyz Association of Deaf and Blind People

Bokonbaev s 191, Bishkek C, 720300
Tel: +7 3312-244222
Fax: +7 3312–244760

LATVIA

Latvijas Neredzigo Biedriba

Latvian Society of the Blind
Pales 14/1, Riga, LV-1024
Tel: +371 7–532 607
Fax: +371 7–532 607
E-mail: *lnbcv@e-apollo.lv*
Web page: http://www.lnbrc.lv

LEBANON

Lebanese School for the Blind

Box 40021, Baabda
Tel: +961 0 920 601

Lebanon Evangelican School for the Blind

Rashid Nakhleh Street, Zarif, PO Box 166, Beirut
Tel: +961 1 327 416
Fax: +961 1 887 134

LESOTHO

Lesotho National League of Visually Impaired Persons

PO Box 0262, Maseru West, 105
Tel: +266 31–7428 or 325885
Fax: +266–311340

LIBERIA

Liberian National Association of the Blind

PO Box 4336, Monrovia
Tel: +231–226507
Fax: +231–227838 or 226356

LIBYA

Association for the Blind

PO Box 583, Jumaheriya, Benghazi
Tel: +218 61–90040 or 90044 or 95831
Fax: +218 61–909 5831

LITHUANIA

Lithuanian Association of the Blind and Visually Handicapped

7/11 Labdariu Str, Vilnius, 2600
Tel: +370 2–62 48 66
Fax: +370 2–22 14 64
E-mail: *audra@lass.aiva.lt*

LUXEMBOURG

Association des Aveugles et Malvoyants du Luxembourg (ASBL)

Association of the Blind of Luxembourg
47 rue de Luxembourg, Berschbach/Mersch, L-7540
Tel: +352–32 90 31 ext 300
Fax: +352–32 91 81
E-mail: *roger.hoffmann@blannenheem.lu*
Web page: http://www.blannenheem.lu

MACEDONIA

Macedonian Republic Union of the Blind

st."29 Noemvri" 46, Skopje, 1000
Tel: +389–2 113 662
Fax: +389 112 292
E-mail: *pajdakov@mail.com*

MADAGASCAR

Association des Aveugles Malgaches (AAM)

Association of the Blind of Madagascar
1 bis, Rue Patric Lemumba Tsaralalana, Antananarivo, 101
Tel: +261 2–223 56
Fax: +261 2–339 02

MALAWI

Malawi Union of the Blind (MAB)

Malawi Council of the Blind, PO Box 5971, Limbe
Tel: +265–645449 or 632 928 (c/o Polio Association)

Malawi Council for the Handicapped (MACOHA)

PO Box 5971, Limbe, Blantyre
Tel: +265 643684
Fax: +265 645449

MALAYSIA

Malaysian Association for the Blind (MAB) (Persatuan Bagi Orang Buta Malaysia)

PO Box 10687, 50722 Kuala Lumpur, Malaysia
Tel: +603 2272 2672/2677/2679
Fax: +603 2272 2676
E-mail: *mablind@po.jaring.my*
Web page: http://www.mab.org.my

Sarawak Society for the Blind

Kuching Division Branch, Ong Tiang Swee Road,
PO Box 515, Kuching, Sarawak, 93710, Malaysia
Tel: +60 82 424046
Fax: +60 82 429597

Sabah Society for the Blind

PO Box 10720, 88807 Kota Kinabalu, Sabah, Malaysia
Tel: +60 88 218130
Fax: +60 88 260753

MALI

Union Malienne des Aveugles

BP 377, Bamako
Tel: +223–22 3267
Fax: +223 23 84 23

Institute National des Jeunes Aveugles (Mali) (National Institute of the Young Blind)

PO Box 377, Bamako, Mali

MALTA

Malta Society of the Blind

54 Carini Street, Saint Venera
Tel: +356 440 145
Fax: +356 440 690

MARTINIQUE

Union des Aveugles de Martinique (Union of the Blind of Martinique)

Centre des Aveugles de Terreville, 97200 Terreville
Schoelche, Martinique
Tel: +596 421972

MAURITANIA

Association Nationale des Aveugles de Mauritanie

Blind Association of Mauritania
Siege Immeuble ex-El Mouna 1er etage U14, BP 1037,
Nouakchott
Tel: +222 292 448 or 290 915
Fax: +222 292 021or 259 224
E-mail: *anam@iiardd.mr*

MAURITIUS

Lizie Dan La Main' Union des Aveugles de l'Ile Maurice

Eyes in the Hand, Union of the Blind of Mauritius
Royal Road, St Jean, Belle Rose, Quatre-Bornes
Tel: +230 465 4801
Fax: +230 464 6019/466 6500

MEXICO

Instituto de Capacitacion del Niño Ciego, AC

Capacitation Institute for Blind Children
Calle 56 No 385 SR, Guadalajara, Jalisco, 44410
Tel: +52 36 35 3192
Fax: +52 36 35 3192

Escuela Nacional para Ciegos "Lic Ignacio Trigueros"

National School for the Blind
Calle Mixcalco No. 6, Centro Histórico, Mexico DF
Tel: +52 5–702 3037
Fax: +52 5–709 3324

Organización de Invidentes Unidos de Monterrey AC

Calle Rayón No. 744 Sur, Monterrey NL, 64000 CP
Tel: +52 83–429884
Fax: +52 83–429884

MOLDOVA

Societatea Orbilor din Moldova

Union of the Blind in Moldova
Directia Centrala, Columna Stret 101, Kishinev, MD-2012
Tel: +373 2–225378/225191
Fax: +373 2–225224

MONGOLIA

Mongolian Association for the Blind

PO Box 511, Ulan Bator 210136, Mongolia
Tel: +976 1 417 50
E-mail: *mnblindassoc@magicnet.mn*; *ectacis@mongol.net*

MOROCCO

Association Nationale des Aveugles au Maroc

National Association for the Blind of Morocco
93 Avenue Mohamed V, Rabat
Tel: +212 7–863762
Fax: +212 7–778135

MOZAMBIQUE

Associaçao de Cegos e Ambliopes de Moçambique (ACAMO)

Association of the Blind and Partially Sighted of Mozambique
c/o Institute for the Partially Sighted, Rua Mouzinho de Albuquerque, Beira
Tel: +258 3–327759 or 323999
Fax: +258 3–328549

MYANMAR (see BURMA)

NAMIBIA

Namibian Association of Visually Disabled People

c/o ELCIN Rehabilitation Centre, Private Bag 2018, Ondagwa, 9000
Tel: +264–6756 4056
Fax: +264–6756 40566

NEPAL

Nepal Association for the Welfare of the Blind (NAWB)

PO No 3255, Tripureshwar, Kathmandu
Tel: +977 1–236 583 or 229 219
Fax: +977 1–226 057
E-mail: *hki@hkipc.mos.com.np*

Helen Keller International (HKI)

PO Box 3752, Min Bhawan, Kathmandu
Tel: +977 1–480 921
Fax: +977 1–480 234
E-mail: *hki@hkipc.wlink.com.np*

NETHERLANDS (see THE NETHERLANDS)

NETHERLANDS ANTILLES

Sociedad Nacional pa Siegunan

National Society for the Blind
Corrieweg 16, POB 2122, Curaçao
Tel: +599 9–379758/642094

NEW ZEALAND

Royal New Zealand Foundation for the Blind

Private Bag 99941, Newmarket, Auckland
Tel: +64 9–309 6333
Fax: +64 9–366 0099
E-mail: *library@rnzfb.org.nz*
Web page: http://www.rnzfb.org.nz

Parents of Vision Impaired (NZ) Inc (PVI)

PO Box 21 141, Flagstaff, Hamilton
Tel: 0800–213 019
Fax: +64 7–855 5520
E-mail: *paul@pvi.org.nz*
Web page: http://www.pvi.org.nz

Deafblind New Zealand (DBNZ)

National Office, Box 24–136, Auckland
Tel: +64 07–828 9554
Fax: +64 07–828 9424
E-mail: *pmclark@paradise.net.nz*
Web page: http://www.deafblind.org.nz

NICARAGUA

Centro de Rehabilitacion para Ciegos

Carlos Fonseca Amador, 1/2 Cuadra al Sur a Mano, Managua

NIGER

Union Nationale des Aveugles du Niger

National Union of the Blind of Niger
BP Box 2393, Niamey Balafon
Tel: +227 753850
Fax: +227 753313

NIGERIA

Nigerian National Advisory Council for the Blind

Plot 255/256 Johnson Street, Off Bode Thomas Street, Surulere, Lagos, Lagos State
Tel: +234 1–03323594

NORWAY

Norges Blindeforbund

Norwegian Association of the Blind and Partially Sighted
PB 5900 Hegdehaugen, Oslo, N-0308
Tel: +47 23–21 50 00
Fax: +47 22–69 35 55
E-mail: info@blindeforbundet.no
Web page: http://www.blindeforbundet.no

OMAN

School for the Blind at Soor El Sharkia

PO Box 30178, Soor
Tel: +968 44–0357

PAKISTAN

Pakistan Association of the Blind (PAB)

356 Usmania Colony, Karachi, Sindh, 406
Tel: +92 51–5558959

Pakistan Foundation Fighting Blindness (PFFB)

PO Box 1652, Islamabad, Punjab, 44000
Tel: +92 51–290261 or 290262/290264
Fax: +92 51–290465
E-mail: hhk@pffb.sdnpk.undp.org

PALESTINE (PALESTINIAN AUTONOMOUS TERRITORY)

Friends of the Blind Association

Street address: Hay Al-Janayen, Al-Bireh, Ramallah, Palestine
Postal address: PO Box 4450, Ramallah, Palestine
Tel: +972 2 240 0398
Fax: +972 2 240 5336
E-mail: fblind@palnet.com
Web page: http://www.fblind.org

Al-Alayiyeh School for the Blind

PO Box 20, Bethlehem

PANAMA

Union Nacional de Ciegos de Panama

via Esteban Ysern Cervera, Las Cumbres, Panama
Tel: +507–268 0526
Fax: +507–268 2979

Escuela de Ciegos Helen Keller (HKI)

Apartado 11349, Panama City, 6
Tel: +507 613441

PAPUA NEW GUINEA

St John Association for the Blind

PO Box 6075, Boroko NCD
Tel: +675 325 1238
Fax: +675 325 4637/1238

PARAGUAY

Asociacion de Ciegos del Paraguay

Association of the Blind of Paraguay
Carrera Saguier 730, Apartado de Correo 2548, Asuncion
Tel: +595 21–60 38 10/60 92 20
Fax: +595 21–44 33 59

PERU

Unión Nacional de Ciegos del Peru

Plaza Bolognesi 479, Barranco, Lima
Tel: +51 14–230 941 or 238 380
Fax: +51 14–300 614

PHILIPPINES

Helen Keller Institute, Philippines

2139 Fidel A Reyes Street, Malate, Manila, Philippines
Tel: +63 2–523 8223
Fax: +63 2–524 1526
E-mail: *73312.702@compuserve.com*

Philippine Blind Union, Inc

71 Appaloosa, St. Rancho Estate IV, East Conception II, Marikina, Metro Manila, Philippines
Tel: +63 2 9415611
Fax: +63 2 9420030
E-mail: *ojtaleon@pacific.net.ph*

POLAND

Polski Zwiazek Niewidomych Zarzad Glowny

Polish Association of the Blind
ul. Konwiktorska 9, Warsaw, 00–216
Tel: +48 22–635 5793
Fax: +48 22–635 5793 or 635 7652
E-mail: *international@pzn.org.pl*
Web page: http://www.pzn.org.pl

PORTUGAL

Associação dos Cegos e Ambliopes de Portugal (ACAPO)

Portuguese National Association of the Blind and Partially Sighted
Rua de S José 86–1°, Lisbon, 1150
Tel: +351 21–342 20 01
Fax: +351 21–342 85 18
E-mail: *dn@acapo.pt*
Web page: http://www.acapo.pt; http://www.acapo-centro.rcts.pt

PUERTO RICO

Blind Rehabilitation Centre (124) VA Medical Center

One Veterans Plaza, San Juan, 00927–5800
Tel: +809 758–7575 x 4020
Fax: +809 766–6021

QATAR

Al Noor Institute

School of Light
PO Box 6618, Doha
Tel: +974 593–8292
Fax: +974 888113

REPUBLIC OF CONGO (see CONGO)

ROMANIA

Asociatia Nevazatorilor din Romania

Romanian Association of the Blind
str Vatra Luminoasa, nr 108 bis, Sector 2, Bucharest, 73302
Tel: +40 1–2506525 or 0519
Fax: +40 1–2500519

Sense International (Romania)

Blv. Timisoara 27, BI D, sc. B, et.5. ap23, Bucharest, Romania
Tel/Fax: 00 401 413 9040
E-mail: *csalomie@senseint.org.ro*

RUSSIA

All Russia Association of the Blind (VOS)

14 Novaya Ploschod, Moscow, Russia, 103 672
Tel: +7 95 923 6160
Fax: +7 95 923 91 49
E-mail: *oms@vos.org.ru*
Web page: http://www.vos.org.ru

Association of the Parents of the Visually Impaired

117–13 pr.Vernadskogo, Moscow 117571, Russia
Contact person: Elena Nasibulova, Director
Tel: +7 95 4335306
Fax: +7 95 1575411

RWANDA

Union Rwandaise des Aveugles (URA)

BP 1527, Kigali
Tel: +250 76097
Fax: +250 77543

SAMOA

Association of the Blind and Visually Impaired

c/o PREB, PO Box 3295, Apia
Tel: +685–24998
Fax: +685–24000

SANTO DOMINGO

Fundacion Dominicana de Ciegos Inc (FUDCI)

c/o Sanchez #40, Bo. 30 de Mayo, Santo Domingo

SAUDI ARABIA

Saudi-Bahraini Institute for the Blind, The

PO Box: 33484
Tel: +973 780818
Fax : +973 780786
E-mail : *sbiblind@batelco.com.bh*

General Secretariat for Special Education

Department of Education of the Visually Handicapped, Riyadh, 11148
Tel: +966 1 488 1623
Fax: +966 1 488 0308

Rehabilitation Society for Disabled Persons, Eastern Province

PO Box 9119, Damman, 31431
Tel: +966 3–842 5340
Fax: +966 3–842 5340

SENEGAL

Amitié des Aveugles du Sénégal

Friends of the Blind of Senegal
Champ des Courses 2, Plle 5624 Pikine Icotaf, Dakar
Tel: +221 34–4419
Fax: +221 22–1117 (Hotel de l'Indépendence)

SEYCHELLES

Seychelles Union of the Blind

PO Box 613, Victoria, Mahe, Seychelles
Tel: +248 321333
Fax: +248 225507

SIERRA LEONE

Sierra Leone Association of the Blind (SLAB)

5 Walpole Street, Freetown, Sierra Leone
Postal address: PM Bag 851, Freetown, Sierra Leone
Tel: +232 22 227657
Fax: +232 22 224439

SINGAPORE

Singapore Association of the Visually Handicapped

47 Toa Payoh Rise, Singapore, 298 104
Tel: +65 6251–4331 ext. 131
Fax: +65 6253–7191
E-mail: *webmaster@savh.org.sg*
Web page: http://www.savh.org.sg

SLOVAK REPUBLIC

Unia Nevidiacich a Slabozrakych Slovenska (UNSS)

Slovak Blind and Partially Sighted Union
Sekulská 1, Bratislava, 842 50, Slovak Republic
Contact person: Branislav Mamojka, President
Tel: +421 7 654 20 796
Fax: +421 7 654 20 842
E-mail: *unss@unss.sk*
Web page: http://www.unss.sk

SLOVENIA

Zveza drustev slepih in slabovidnih Slovenije

Association of the Blind and Partially Sighted of Slovenia
Groharjeva 2, Ljubljana, SI 1000
Tel: +386 61–1700211
Fax: +386 61–1700220
E-mail: *zdss@zveza-slepih.si*
Web page: http://www.zveza-slepih.si

SOLOMON ISLANDS

Siloam Dominican Centre for the Visually Handicapped

Nila, Western Province, Solomon Islands

SOMALIA

Somalia Society of the Blind

PO Box 1566, Mogadishu, Somalia
Tel: +252 13473

SOUTH AFRICA

South African National Council for the Blind (SANCB)

PO Box 11149, Hatfield, Pretoria, Gauteng, 0028
Tel: +2702 346 1171
Fax: +2702 346 1177
E-mail: *admin@sancb.org.za*
Web page: http://www.sancb.co.za

Deafblind South Africa

Suite 80, PO Box 3105, Worcester, Western Cape, 6849
Tel: +27 23–347 7542
Fax: +27 23–347 7581
E-mail: *dbsa@lando.co.za.*
Web page: http://www.deafblind.com/africa.html

SPAIN

Organizacion Nacional de Ciegos Españoles (ONCE)

Spanish National Organization of the Blind
José Ortega y Gasset 18, Madrid, 28006
Tel: +34 1–436 5300
Fax: +34 1–575 6053
E-mail: *efd@once.es* or *ramm@once.es*
Web page: http://www.once.es

SRI LANKA

Sri Lanka Council for the Blind

No. 74A Church Street, Colombo, National, 02
Tel: +941–329 564
Fax: +94 1–329 564

ST KITTS, WEST INDIES

St Kitts and Nevis National Society for the Blind (St Kitts and Nevis Society of and for the Blind)

Basseterre, Parsoris Village, St. Kitts, West Indies
Tel: +869 465 6226 or 6227
Fax: +869 465 8557

ST LUCIA, WEST INDIES

St Lucia Blind Welfare Association

PO Box 788, Castries
Tel: +809 452 4691

ST VINCENT, WEST INDIES

St Vincent Society of the Blind

PO Box 54, Kingstown, St Vincent, West Indies
Tel: +809 456 1111

SUDAN

Sudanese National Association of the Blind (SNAB)

PO Box 271, Khartoum North
Tel: +249 11–613 212
Fax: +249 11–451 949

Al Nour Institute for Blind Children

PO Box 1284, Khartoum North
Tel: +249–13 331858
Fax: +249–13 3331173

SWAZILAND

Ekululameni

Swaziland Association of the Visually Impaired (SWAVI)
c/o Central Bank of Swaziland, PO Box 546, Mbabane
Tel: +268 43221 or 40013
Fax: +268 45417

SWEDEN

Swedish Association of the Visually Impaired (SRF)

Sandborgvagen 52, Enskede, Sweden, 5 122 88
Tel: +46 8 3990 00
Fax: +46 8 3993 22
E-mail: *info@srfriks.org*
Web page: http://www.srfriks.org

SWITZERLAND

Swiss Federation of the Blind and Partially Sighted

Zentralsekretariat, Laupenstraße 4, Berne, 3008
Tel: +41 31–390 8800
Fax: +41 31–390 8850
E-mail: *info@sbv-fsa.ch*
Web page: http://www.sbv-fsa.ch

Schweizerische Stiftung für Taublinde

Swiss Foundation for the Deafblind
Heim Tanne, Furhstraße 15, Langnau am Albis, CH-8135
Tel: +41 1–713 1440
Fax: +41 1–713 1435
E-mail: *tanne@swissonline.ch*

Swiss National Association of and for the Blind

Schützengaße 4, St Gallen, CH-9000
Tel: +41 71–223 3636
Fax: +41 71–222 7318
E-mail: *sekretariat@szb.ch*
Web page: http://www.szb.ch

Stiftung für Blinde und Sehbehinderte Kinder und Jugendliche

Foundation for Blind and Visually Handicapped Children and Youth
Kirchlindachstraße 49, Zollikofen, CH-3052
Tel: +41 31–911 2516
Fax: +41 31–911 3041

SYRIA

Conseil des Aveugles au Moyen Orient

Victoria Circle, Mardam Building, Damascas, Syria
Tel: +963 11 223 0600
Fax: +963 11 333 6131

TAIWAN

Blind Welfare Association (BWA)

Department of Special Education, National Chang Hua University of Education, Chang Hua City
Tel: +886 2–7223 2105 ext 2440

Institute for the Blind of Taiwan

384 Chungcheng Road, Hsinchuang, Taipei, 242
Tel: +886 2–998 5588
Fax: +886 2–996 3306

TAJIKISTAN

Tajikistan Society of the Blind

Karamov Street 205, Dushanbe 734027, Tajikistan
Tel: +7 377 373231

TANZANIA

Zanzibar National Association of the Blind

PO Box 3441, Zanzibar Town, Urban West Region
Tel: +255 54–233 299
Fax: +255 54–31730

Tanzania League of the Blind

Street address: 8 Chui Street, Kariakoo, Dar es Salaam, Tanzania
Postal adress: PO Box 22408, Dar es Salaam, Tanzania
Tel: +255 51183280
Fax: +255 51183281

TCHAD

National Association for the Visually Impaired of Tchad

BP 3068, N'Djamena
Tel: +235–51 54 16
Fax: +235–51 85 93

THAILAND

Foundation for the Blind in Thailand

420 Rajavidhi Road, Rajathevee, Bangkok, 10400
Tel: +66 2–246–0070
Fax: +66 2–248 1369
E-mail: *panna@mozart.inet.co.th*

THE NETHERLANDS

Netherlands Federation of the Blind and Partially Sighted

PO Box 2062, Utrecht, 3500 GB
Tel: +31 30–299 2878
Fax: +31 30–293 2544
E-mail: *federatie@sb-belang.nl*
Web page: http://www.sb-belang.nl

TOGO

Centre des Aveugles de Togoville

Centre for the Blind of Togo
BP 205, Aneho

Association for the Blind of Togo

BP 8242, Lomé
Tel: +228 21 6580
Fax: +228 21 2038

TRINIDAD AND TOBAGO

Trinidad and Tobago Blind Welfare Association for the Blind and Visually Impaired (T&TABVI)

Street address: 116–118 Duke Street, Port of Spain, Trinidad and Tobago
Postal address: PO Box 1179, Port of Spain, Trinidad and Tobago
Contact person: Mrs. Diane Borneo, Executive Officer
Tel: +1 868 624 1613/4675/3809
Fax: +1 868 624 1613

TUNISIA

Union Nationale des Aveugles de Tunisie (UNAT)

21 Boulevard Bab Bénat, Tunis, 1006
Tel: +216 1–565630 or 566747 or 565634
Fax: +216 1–566749

TURKEY

Federation of the Blind of Turkey

GMK Bulvan 32/6, Demirtepe, Ankara
Tel: +90 312–231 8243
Fax: +90 312–229 1662

Türkiye Körler Vakfi Genel Merkezi

Turkish Foundation for the Blind
Fevzi Çakmak Sokak 14/3, Kizilay, Ankara
Tel: +90 312–230 1483
Fax: +90 312 230 7311

TURKMENISTAN

Society of Blind People of Turkmenistan

Kekilova St. 49, 744012 Ashgabat, Turkmenistan
Tel: +993 12 347413
E-mail: *fsc@cpart.org*

UGANDA

Uganda National Association of the Blind (UNAB)

PO Box 6938, Kampala
Tel: +256 41–241659 or 268296
Fax: +256 41–250445 or 268296 (c/o ADD)

UKRAINE

Ukrainian Association of the Blind (YTOC)

3 Pechortsky spusk, Kiev, 252 023
Tel: +380 44 224 1127 or +380 44 225 6257
Fax: +380 44 225 4342.

UNITED ARAB EMIRATES

Emirates Society for the Rehabilitation of the Blind

PO Box 3128, Sharjah, United Arab Emirates
Contact person: Adel Al_Zamar, Vice President
Tel: +971 6 5247 7000
Fax: +971 50 652 1021

Ministry of Labour and Social Affairs

Handicapped Centre, PO Box 261, Abu Dhabi
Tel: +971 2–668524

Sharjah City for Humanitarian Services (SCHS)

PO Box 5796, Sharjah
Tel: +971 6 5671117/5660667
Fax: +971 6 5664461
E-mail: *shjchs@emirates.net.ae*
Web page: http://www.elcnewmedia.com/demo/schs3/

UNITED KINGDOM

Royal National Institute for the Blind

105 Judd Street London WC1H 9NE
Tel: +020 7388 1266
Fax: +020 7388 2034
Helpline: +0845 766 9999
Web page: http://*www.rnib.org.uk*

National Blind Childrens Society

Bradbury House, Market Street, Highbridge, Somerset
TA9 3BW
Telephone: +01278 764 764
Fax: +01278 764 790
E-mail: *enquiries@nbcs.org.uk*
Web page: http://www.nbcs.org.uk

Royal London Society for the Blind

Dorton House, Seal, Nr Sevenoaks, Kent TN15 0ED
Tel: +44 1732 592500
Fax: +44 1732 592506
E-mail: *enquiries@rlsb.org.uk*
Web page: http://www.rlsb.org.uk

UNITED STATES OF AMERICA

American Council of the Blind

1155 15th Street, NW, Suite 720, Washington,
District of Columbia, DC 20005
Tel: +1 202–467 5081
Fax: +1 202–467 5085
E-mail: *wfo@acb.org*
Web page: http://www.acb.org

American Foundation for the Blind

Web page: http://www.afb.org

Blind Babies Foundation

Web page: http://blindbabies.org/links.htm

Foundation for the Junior Blind (Los Angeles)

Web page: http://www.fjb.org

URUGUAY

Union Nacional de Ciegos del Uruguay

National Union of the Blind of Uruguay
21 de Setiembre 2268, Montevideo
Tel: +598 2–411187 or 400485

UZBEKISTAN

Union of the Blind in Uzbek

Bobour Street 22, Tashkent
Tel: +7 371–55 75 90 or 55 65 59
Fax: +7 371–53 53 81

VENEZUELA

Federacion Venezolana de Instituciones de Ciegos (FEVIC)

Federation of Organization for the Blind of Venezuela
Res Jardin Botanico, Edif Buca, Re"A," NW El Plaza, Caracas,
1010-DF
Tel: +58 2–577 8065
Fax: +58 2–577 5966

VIETNAM

Vietnam Blind Association

139 Nguyen Thai Hoc Street, Hanoi, Vietnam
Tel: +84 48 452060
Fax: +84 48 452537

Nguyen Dinh Chieu School for the Blind

184 Nguyen Chi Thanh Street, District 10, Saigon/Ho Chi Minh City
Tel: +848 835 2959 or 839 7470
Fax: +848 822 2136

YEMEN

Yemen Association of Blind Care and Rehabilitation

PO Box 60, Sana'a
Tel: +967 1–262809 or 262800 or 262804
Fax: +967 1–262806

YUGOSLAVIA

Union of the Blind and Partially Sighted of Yugoslavia

Federal Board, Knez Mihailov 42/11, Beograd, 11000
Tel: +381 11–186726/635962
Fax: +381 11–635962
E-mail: *ssyu@eunet.yu*

ZAIRE

Institut pour les Aveugles

BP 14859 KinI, Kinshasa

ZAMBIA

National Federation of the Blind

PO Box 32847, Chilimbulu Road, Lusaka
Tel: +260 1–212260 (264602)
Fax: +260 1–260516

ZIMBABWE

Zimbabwe National League of the Blind

PO Box 641, Bulawayo
Tel: +263 9–76049
Fax: +263 9–61768

Index

INDEX